CLINICALLY ORIENTED ANATOMY

With Illustrations from Grant's Atlas

CLINICALLY ORIENTED ANATOMY

Keith L. Moore, Ph.D., F.I.A.C., F.R.S.M.

Professor and Chairman, Department of Anatomy, University of Toronto, Faculty of Medicine, Toronto, Ontario, Canada
Formerly Professor and Head of Anatomy, University of Manitoba, Faculty of Medicine, Winnipeg, Manitoba, Canada

Illustrated primarily by Dorothy Chubb, Nancy Joy, A.O.C.A., and Nina Kilpatrick, B.Sc., AAM.

SANS TACHE

WILLIAMS & WILKINS
Baltimore/London

Made in the United States of America

Reprinted 1981
Reprinted 1982

Library of Congress Cataloging in Publication Data

Moore, Keith L
Clinically oriented anatomy.

Includes index.
1. Anatomy, Human. I. Title. [DNLM: 1. Anatomy. QS4 M822c]
QM23.2.M67 611 80-13362
ISBN 0-683-06146-1

Composed and printed at the
Waverly Press, Inc.
Mt. Royal and Guilford Aves.
Baltimore, MD 21202, U.S.A.

COVER ILLUSTRATION:

The Anatomy Lesson of Dr. Nicolaes Tulp by Rembrandt van Rijn. From a mezzotint in The Bettman Archive.

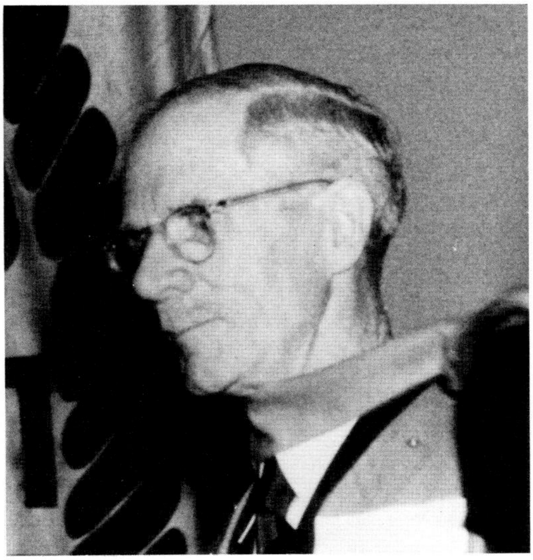

Dedicated to the memory of

Professor J. C. Boileau Grant

M.C., M.B., Ch.B., Hon. D.Sc.(Man.), F.R.C.S.(Edin.)

Late Professor Emeritus of Anatomy in the University of Toronto and Curator of the Anatomy Museum; for many years Visiting Professor of Anatomy in the University of California, Los Angeles; formerly Professor of Anatomy in the University of Manitoba. The photograph above was taken in 1956 when Professor Grant was awarded an honorary degree by the University of Manitoba, where he began his academic career in North America.

Foreword

The author of this book has endeavoured to continue the tradition of clinically oriented teaching of basic medical science established by the late Drs. *J. C. Boileau Grant* and *William Boyd* who came to the University of Toronto from the University of Manitoba many years before Dr. Moore. To write this new textbook *Moore* imagined himself in the position of a student commencing his medical studies and endeavouring to overcome the difficulties with which many students are faced at this time. Students beginning the study of anatomy are presented with a vast new vocabulary of anatomical terms, many of them in Latin and Greek, together with a large amount of factual information.

The desire for students to acquire an adequate knowledge of anatomy can be greatly increased if it is clearly demonstrated to them that what they are learning will be important to them in their subsequent studies and throughout their careers in medicine. Anatomy is the foundation of all branches of medicine and unfortunately the amount of time allotted to this discipline in the average medical course is far too short, with the result that many students are at a loss when they come to examine a patient. Thus, it is most important that anatomy be presented in a concise and stimulating manner and that the clinical importance of anatomy be clearly explained. Dr. Moore is an experienced writer with a remarkable ability to organize material so that it is interesting and flows logically. In this new textbook the achievement of his established aims has been carried out in the following manner.

First, the meaning of the majority of the Latin and Greek terms has been carefully explained so that the student can relate the words to the structures they describe. This leads to "understanding" rather than "memorization."

Second, keeping in mind that a good illustration is worth a thousand words, Dr. Moore was most fortunate in being able to use the majority of the very accurate illustrations from the *Atlas of Anatomy* produced by the late Professor J. C. B. Grant. The chapters in this book and those in the *Atlas* are keyed in the same manner, making cross reference easy. Further anatomical illustration is presented in a large number of radiographs illustrating both normal and abnormal radiographic anatomy. These have been carefully selected and described with the aid of one of us (DLM). The author has also included numerous photographs and line drawings demonstrating the important surface features of the body which will prove valuable in the clinical examination of patients.

Third, in order to stimulate students to learn, a large number of case studies in anatomy have been placed at the end of each chapter, followed by comments on the anatomy involved in each case. *Learning is more than mere teaching.* It includes questioning, correlation, and justification. Hence, the author has attempted to make this book a learning tool by including in each chapter many clinically oriented comments and patient oriented problems. The clinical comments and patients' problems are at a level that is suitable for beginning medical students who may have similar questions and problems or who will be asked similar questions and posed with similar problems by their friends and relatives. We know of no other text in which this type of anatomy teaching has been carried out to this extent.

We have both read and commented upon this text since its early stages and we feel that the clinical comments and patient oriented problems are worded so as to avoid controversy and to present current medical knowledge. Dr. Moore has produced a textbook with a refreshingly new approach to anatomical teaching which we feel sure will be appreciated by students, doctors, and teachers alike. We wish him and the text every success.

J. W. A. Duckworth, M.B., Ch.B., M.D.

Professor Emeritus of Anatomy and former Chairman, University of Toronto and Consultant in Anatomy and Embryology, Department of Pathology, The Hospital for Sick Children, Toronto, Ontario.

D. L. McRae, M.D., F.R.C.P. (C), F.A.C.R.

Professor Emeritus of Radiology, University of Toronto. Formerly Chief of Radiology at the Montreal Neurological Institute and Head of Radiology, Sunnybrook Medical Centre, Toronto, Ontario.

Preface

The invitation to write a book on patient oriented anatomy using illustrations from *Grant's Atlas* was one that could not be refused by this medical writer, who believes that learning anatomy can be *especially* exciting when its relevance to medicine is emphasized. This book is written primarily for students studying anatomy for the first time.

The title **Clinically Oriented Anatomy** was chosen to indicate that *the book highlights those features of anatomy which are of clinical importance.* Every good teacher of anatomy recognizes that nothing stimulates the student more than correlating anatomy with a problem presented by a patient. Because there is often difficulty relating what one sees in the cadaver to what is seen in patients during physical examinations and in the operating room, *emphasis is placed on living anatomy.* For example, the pancreas is described as a soft, grayish-pink gland to emphasize that it is not a hard, almost colorless organ that one sees in the cadaver or colored yellow or red as depicted in some books and atlases.

Surface anatomy is stressed because ignorance of this aspect is a serious handicap when interpreting the results of a physical examination. Furthermore, the performance of tests requiring the insertion of needles requires a good knowledge of structures that lie under the skin. Throughout the book, *students are urged to examine their own bodies* and those of others because a good knowledge of surface anatomy makes it unnecessary to learn by rote. Used properly, *the body is a "living textbook."*

This book is not designed primarily as a guide to clinical anatomy which would be of concern to practicing doctors. It is *patient oriented anatomy* that was written to stimulate the interest of beginning students so that they can appreciate what is involved anatomically in nerve injuries, stab wounds, surgical approaches, etc. Care has been taken not to expect students to make diagnoses, and treatments have not been suggested for conditions discussed in the patient oriented problems. Errors in surgery may result from failure to appreciate variations in the body (*e.g.*, in the anatomy of the biliary system); therefore *common variations of form and structure are illustrated.*

The *many radiographs in this book* give a clinical orientation to bones, joints, and organs, enabling students to begin identifying normal structures and how they can change in form and appearance in diseased states. At the University of Toronto, 1st year students are expected to be able to interpret normal radiographs of the body and to recognize obvious fractures and developmental abnormalities such as cervical ribs. With this in mind, radiographs are used to illustrate some of the clinically oriented comments and patient oriented problems.

This book is not intended to be a core textbook of anatomy; several of this kind are available for students who wish to know the minimum amount required for them to pass their 1st year examinations. *Neither is it overly detailed;* several excellent books already fulfill this need. An attempt has been made to cover areas that are most important for students to know and to arouse in them an interest in revising their knowledge of anatomy as they progress in their medical studies. The regional plan has been used because most anatomy courses are based on regional dissection and *the chapters in this book follow the same order as in Grant's Atlas and Grant's Dissector.*

Boldface type and *italics* have been used to highlight important concepts and essential terminology. Explanatory notes and supplementary information appear in intermediate type so they can be read once and passed over during reviews. *Clinically oriented comments are screened* for special attention and quick referral.

The terminology in this book adheres to the internationally accepted *Nomina Anatomica* (4th ed.) approved by the Tenth International Congress of Anatomists at Tokyo in August, 1975. In accordance with international agreement, the terminology in this book departs from strict Latin in some cases by anglicizing terms or by using direct English translations. *Eponyms commonly used clinically appear in parentheses, e.g.*, **sternal angle** (angle of Louis), to assist students in translating the clinical terminology used in hospitals and patients' charts. In all cases, the official term is printed in **boldface** as in the example just given.

This book is freely illustrated because much of the difficulty encountered by students results from their inability to visualize the form and structure of parts of the body. The selected line drawings and photographs based on Grant's dissections are familiar to students, physicians, and surgeons around the world. These illustrations form the nucleus around which this book was written. In addition there are many new illustrations (photographs of models, drawings, radiographs, and clinical photographs). *Studying anatomy at the dissecting table with a good teacher, where the parts may be seen, felt, and dissected, is the best way to learn anatomy.* A well illustrated book with accompanying observations, clinical comments, and discussions of patient oriented problems is probably the next best way. *The legends to the figures from Grant's Atlas have not been significantly changed*; hence students who use this classical atlas will be afforded a review when they re-examine them in the present book. Almost all specimens illustrated in this book may be seen in the anatomy museum of the University of Toronto and students are encouraged to come and see them. You will observe, as *Professor Grant said in the Preface to his Atlas*, "Little, if any liberty has been taken with the anatomy; that is to say, the illustrations profess a considerable accuracy of detail."

Sir Isaac Newton once said, "*If I have seen further, it is by standing on the shoulders of giants.*" Much of my knowledge of clinically oriented anatomy was taught to me by a "giant in Anatomy," **Professor I. Maclaren Thompson,** former Professor and Head of Anatomy at the University of Manitoba, who conducted weekly *anatomical clinics* in the Winnipeg General Hospital using patients to illustrate the anatomically related problems. I owe much to this fine gentleman, scholar, and teacher. When I became the Professor of Anatomy and a Consultant at the Health Sciences Centre in Winnipeg, I continued his method of teaching clinically oriented anatomy.

Thanks are due my colleagues in the Department of Anatomy, University of Toronto, especially **Dr. W. M. Brown,** Associate Professor of Anatomy, **Dr. J. W. A. Duckworth,** Professor Emeritus of Anatomy, and **Dr. D. L. McRae,** Professor Emeritus of Radiology. Drs. Duckworth and McRae have commented on the book in the Foreword. Several other members of the Department also gave much help: Mrs. E. J. Akesson, Dr. E. G. Bertram, Dr. B. Liebgott, Dr. R. G. MacKenzie, Dr. A. Roberts, Dr. C. G. Smith, Dr. I. M. Taylor, and Dr. J. S. Thompson. All these colleagues, most of whom have many years of teaching and clinical experience, were generous with their time and thoughts. I thank all of them most sincerely.

I owe much to the following *Williams & Wilkins authors* who kindly consented to let me use illustrations from their books: Drs. J. E. Anderson, T. A. Baramki, M. Bartalos, J. V. Basmajian, R. F. Becker, M. B. Carpenter, W. M. Copenhaver, P. V. Dilts, Jr., J. A. Gehweiler, J. W. Greene, Jr., D. E. Kelly, J. Langman, J. W. Roddick, Jr., R. B. Salter, E. K. Sauerland, J. W. Wilson, and R. L. Wood. I am also grateful to Mr. A. E. Meier, Vice President and Editor-in-Chief, Health Sciences, W. B. Saunders Company, for allowing me to use many illustrations from my book *The Developing Human: Clinically Oriented Embryology*. I should also like to thank all other authors and publishers, acknowledged elsewhere, who have given me permission to use illustrations from their books.

The medical illustrators for this book merit special attention. Mrs. **Dorothy Chubb,** a pupil of Max Brödel, and Professor **Nancy Joy**, Chairman of the Department of Art as Applied to Medicine in the University of Toronto, prepared most of the illustrations in this book. Their expert skill is unsurpassed. Most new illustrations were prepared by Mrs. **Nina Kilpatrick**, a recent graduate of the University of Toronto program in Art as Applied to Medicine. I am grateful to her for her work which was carefully and cheerfully done.

The medical photographers also set high standards. The photographs were taken by Messrs. Paul Schwartz, B.A., Mr. John Kozie, B.Sc., Associate Professor of Art as Applied to Medicine and Director of Photographic Services, and Mark Sawyer, B.Sc. Their expertise and friendly help were much appreciated.

My secretaries, especially my wife Marion and Jill Parsons, deserve my most sincere thanks. They have worked hard and cheerfully, often under pressure. *Marion* spent many hours proofreading and discussing the manuscript with me.

Finally I thank the Publishers, Williams & Wilkins—particularly *Sara A. Finnegan,* the Vice President and Editor-in-Chief—for inviting me to write this book and for her enthusiasm, unfailing courtesy, and consideration in endeavoring to fill my many requests.

TORONTO, Canada

Keith L. Moore

Acknowledgments

Throughout the text, liberal use has been made of illustrations from the following Williams & Wilkins publications, which the author and publisher acknowledge with sincere thanks:

Anderson, J. E. *Grant's Atlas of Anatomy*, Ed. 7, 1978.

Bartalos, M., and Baramki, T. A. *Medical Cytogenetics*, 1967.

Basmajian, J. V. *Grant's Method of Anatomy*, Ed. 10, 1980.

Basamajian, J. V. *Primary Anatomy*, Ed. 7, 1976.

Basmajian, J. V. *Surface Anatomy*, 1977.

Becker, R. F., Wilson, J. W., and Gehweiler, J. A. *The Anatomical Basis of Medical Practice*, 1971.

Carpenter, M. B. *Core Text of Neuroanatomy*, Ed. 2, 1978.

Copenhaver, W. M., Kelly, D. E., and Wood, R. L. *Bailey's Textbook of Histology*, Ed. 17, 1978.

Dilts, P. V., Jr., Greene, J. W., Jr., and Roddick, J. W., Jr. *Core Studies in Obstetrics and Gynecology*, Ed. 2, 1977.

Langman, J. *Medical Embryology*, Ed. 3, 1975.

Salter, R. B. *Textbook of Disorders and Injuries of the Musculoskeletal System*, 1970.

Sauerland, E. K. *Grant's Dissector*, Ed. 8, 1978.

Stedman's Medical Dictionary, Ed. 23, 1976.

The author and publisher also gratefully acknowledge the use of illustrations from the following sources:

Campbell, J. Sunnybrook Medical Centre, Toronto (Fig. 2–118).

Connor, T. Women's College Hospital, Toronto (Figs. 6–11 and 6–183).

Cooper, L. Z., Green, F. H., Krugman, S., Giles, J. P., and Mirick, G. S. *Am. J. Dis. Child. 110:* 416, 1965 (Fig. 7–103).

Eastman Kodak. *Fundamentals of Radiology* (Fig. I–18).

General Electric Medical Systems, Ltd. (Fig. I–22).

Ham, A. W., and Cormack, D. H. *Histology*, Ed. 8. J. B. Lippincott Co., 1979 (Fig. 7–102).

Haymaker, W., and Woodhall, B. *Peripheral Nerve Injuries*, Ed. 2. W. B. Saunders Co., Philadelphia, 1953 (Fig. 6–104).

Healey, J. E., Jr. *A Synopsis of Clinical Anatomy*. W. B. Saunders Co., Philadelphia, 1969 (Figs. 3–99, 3–100, 3–111, and 4–156).

Laurenson, R. D. *An Introduction to Clinical Anatomy by Dissection of the Human Body*. W. B. Saunders Co., Philadelphia, 1968 (Figs. 3–78, 3–84, and 3–88 (illustrations by Mrs. D. M. Hutchinson)).

McCredie, J. A. *Basic Surgery*. Macmillan Publishing Co., New York, 1977 (Fig. 2–53).

McRae, D. L. Professor Emeritus of Radiology, University of Toronto (Figs. I–19, I–20, 4–142, and 5–77).

Moore, K. L. *The Developing Human: Clinically Oriented Embryology*, Ed. 2. W. B. Saunders Co., Philadelphia, 1977 (Figs. 1–62, 1–98, 1–99, 1–101, 1–103, 2–18, 2–22, 2–152, 3–103, 3–104, 3–108, 3–110, 5–28, 5–30, 5–61, 5–70, 5–71, 7–10, 7–11, 7–25, 7–139, 7–152, 9–48, 9–67, and 9–89).

Moore, K. L. *Before We Are Born. Basic Embryology and Birth Defects*. W. B. Saunders Co., Philadelphia, 1974 (Fig. 3–106).

Moore, K. L., and Barr, M. L. *Lancet 2:* 57, 1955 (Fig. 3–109).

Norman, D., Korobkin, M., and Newton, T. H. *Computed Tomography.* C. V. Mosby Co., St. Louis, 1977 (Fig. 2–201).

Persaud, T. V. N. Professor of Anatomy and Head of the Department, University of Manitoba, Winnipeg, Canada (Fig. 7–86).

Smith Kline Corporation. *Essentials of the Neurological Examination.* 1978 (Figs. 8–14, 8–16, and 8–24).

Contents

CHAPTER 3

CHAPTER 4

CHAPTER 5

CHAPTER 6

CHAPTER 7

CHAPTER 8

CHAPTER 9

INTRODUCTION

Anatomy is. . .

THE OLDEST BASIC MEDICAL SCIENCE

Anatomy is one of the disciplines taught in the fourth century B.C. by **Hippocrates**, often called the "*Father of Medicine.*" In addition to the **Hippocratic Oath** attributed to him, he wrote several medical books, and in one of them he stated, "*The nature of the body is the beginning of medical science.*"

Another famous Greek physician and scientist, **Aristotle** (384-322 B.C.), made many new observations, especially concerning **developmental anatomy** or **embryology**. He is also credited with being the first person to use the word "*anatome,*" a Greek word meaning "to cut up" or, as we now say, "*to dissect.*" In those days, to perform an "anatomy" was to do a dissection. These two words are no longer synonymous. Dissection is a *technique* used to learn gross anatomy, whereas anatomy is a *discipline* or field of scientific study dealing with all branches of knowledge which are concerned with *the study of bodily structure.*

A STUDY OF STRUCTURE AND FUNCTION

Anatomy is the **basic medical science** dealing with the *structure* and *function* of the human body. In the early days the science of anatomy was mainly concerned with the form and function of parts of the body that could be demonstrated by dissection. This method of study is still widely used because it provides an orderly and consecutive display of the structures of the body. It also helps in obtaining a three-dimensional concept of its parts. *You must learn to make and to trust your own observations.* You will also find that it is impossible to find two bodies that are identical in structure. Even monozygotic (identical) twins are anatomically dissimilar in *some* respects. During dissection you will observe, feel, move, and dissect the parts of the body. Although this method of studying the body, called **macroscopic** or **gross anatomy**, is closely associated with surgery (Fig. I-1), it forms *an essential basis for all branches of medicine and dentistry.*

Although essentially a morphological science, anatomy has never been just that; even in the writings of Hippocrates and Aristotle there were descriptions of the functions of the various parts of the body. Although many of their ideas were correct, some of them later proved to be false. However, *discussion of the function of a part or organ has always been included in anatomy.* An anatomy course that does not discuss the function of the parts of the body would be analogous to a course in auto mechanics in which the parts of the engine were described but the function of them was not. At one time **physiology** was part of the discipline of anatomy, but as many new methods of investigating function were developed, it became a separate discipline. However, the division between the two sciences is not so sharp as the names imply. When the word anatomy is used without qualification, it is gross anatomy that is generally meant, but the discipline includes all the other **anatomical sciences** (histology, cytology, neuroanatomy, and embryology).

Much can be learned from observing the surface of the body. The diagnostic approach begins when the doctor or dentist

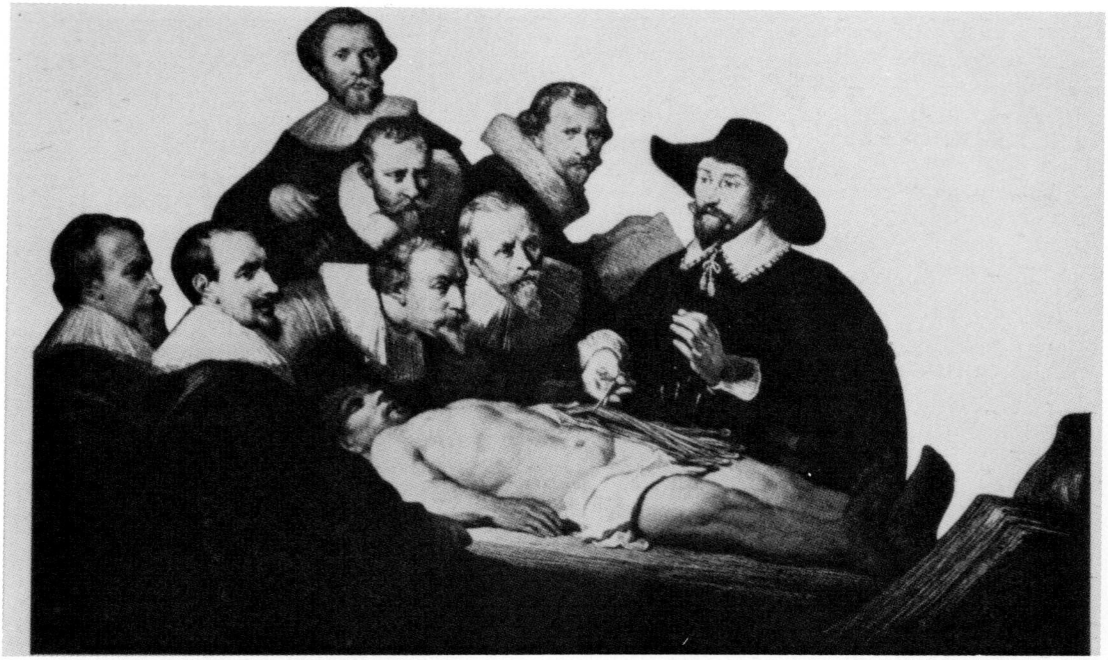

Figure I-1. Rembrandt van Rijn's famous painting, *The Anatomy Lesson*, showing Dr. Nicolaes Tulp teaching **clinically oriented anatomy** to a small group of Amsterdam surgeons in 1632.

first sees a patient; hence, you must practice *the art of observation* as you learn anatomy. For example, you are already aware of the "collar bones" or **clavicles** because they are well known *bony landmarks.* Observe them in the man shown in Figure I-2*A*. **Palpation**, or examining with the hands and the fingers, is another clinical technique you will use in anatomy. Almost everyone has taken his/her own pulse. *Palpation of arterial pulses is part of every routine evaluation* of the living body. Practice palpating with the pads of your fingers. Do not jab with your fingertips and fingernails.

Children study surface and living anatomy. They soon begin to observe and to feel their muscles and are fascinated when they see them move. Before long you will learn how to use various instruments to observe parts of the body (*e.g.*, the eye using an **ophthalmoscope**) or to listen to the functioning parts of the body (*e.g.*, the heart and lungs using a **stethoscope**). You will also learn to use a **reflex hammer** for examining the functional state of nerves and muscles.

Most students soon associate the facts of surface and living anatomy with those of descriptive anatomy. Hence, their own bodies become useful and honest **memory aids** during examinations. The study of the surface features of bones (**bony landmarks**) and of other structures (*e.g.*, ligaments) that are visible or palpable (perceptible to touch) is called living or **surface anatomy**. The fundamental aim of surface anatomy is the visualization (in the "mind's eye") of structures which lie beneath the skin and are hidden by it. For example, in patients with stab or **gunshot wounds** or other penetrating injuries, the doctor must visualize in his mind's eye the structures beneath the wound that might have been injured. Furthermore, *surface anatomy is the basis for the physical examination of the body that forms a part of physical diagnosis.* The thorough study of a patient's body, with emphasis on the area of complaint, is most helpful in making the correct diagnosis of the anatomical basis for the patient's complaint, *e.g.*, chest pain (see Case 1-1 of **Patient Oriented Problems** at the end of Chap. 1).

The best way to learn surface anatomy is by examining living persons. Recording what you see, feel, and hear is an essential part of **clinical diagnosis**. Begin developing your powers of observation by determining how the **anatomical position** of the persons shown in Figure I-2 differs from the way people usually stand. Check your observations with the subsequent description of this important position. Observe the many **surface features** visible in these young adults.

As methods of investigating structure and function became increasingly complex and following the development of the microscope and good staining procedures, another branch of anatomy was formed. *The study of the make-up of the tissues and organs of the body* under the microscope is called **microscopic anatomy** or **histology**. Again, microscopy (light or electron) is a *technique*, whereas histology is a *subdiscipline* of anatomy, a field of scientific study. It deals with the normal structure and function of cells, their growth and differentiation, and their interrelations in the tissues, organs, and systems of the body.

When **x-rays** were discovered in the 19th century, some new observations were made about the structure and function of the skeleton of the body. The bones and joints were readily visualized on **radiographs** (x-

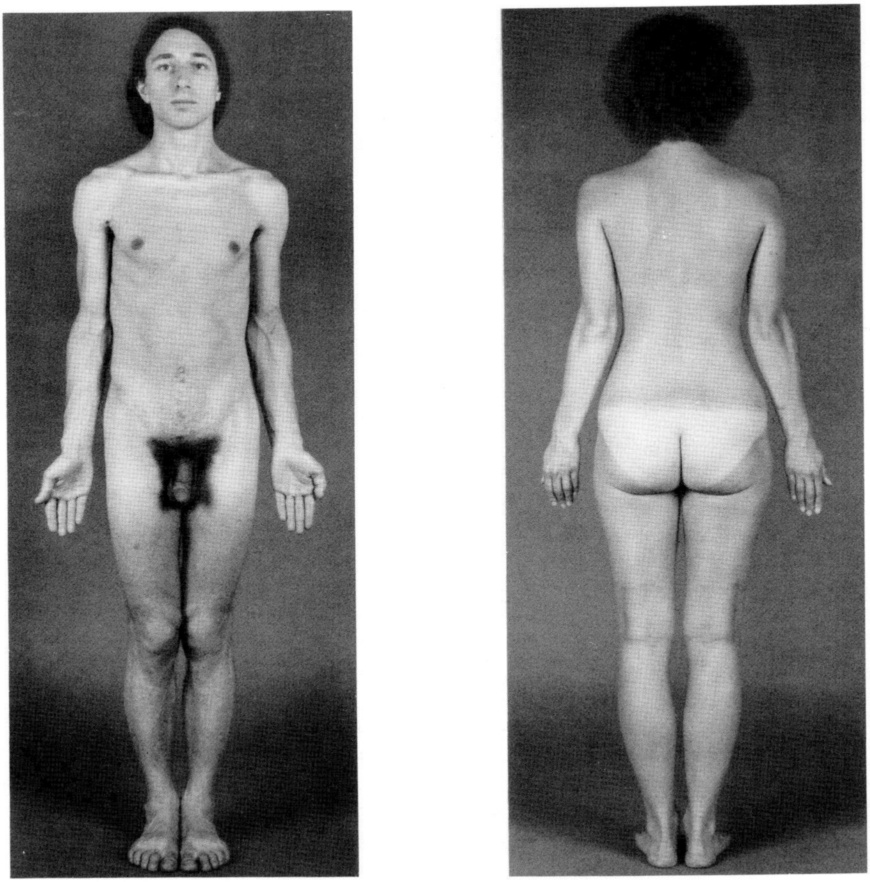

Figure I-2. Photographs of a 27-year-old man and woman *standing in the anatomical position. A*, anterior view of a male. Note particularly the bony landmarks formed by his clavicles (collar bones) and the position of his hands and feet. *B*, posterior view of a female. Note the effect ultraviolet has had on the areas of exposed skin. You can also see the bony landmarks of her scapulae (shoulder blades).

ray films). Later, by introducing radiopaque or radiolucent substances, the form and function of various organs and cavities could be studied (*e.g.*, during swallowing). **Radiographic anatomy** is the study of the structure and function of the body using radiographic techniques. It is an important part of gross anatomy and is the anatomical basis of **radiology**, the branch of medical science dealing with the use of radiant energy in the diagnosis and treatment of disease. The sooner you learn to identify the normal structures of the body on radiographs, the easier it will be for you to recognize and understand the changes visible on radiographs that are caused by disease and injury.

The study of the structure and function of the nervous system is specialized because of the intricacies of neuronal connections. Courses in **neuroanatomy** deal with the gross, microscopic, developmental, and radiographic anatomy of the nervous system, with special emphasis on the *central nervous system*, consisting of the brain and spinal cord.

Just as anatomy and physiology overlap, so do gross anatomy, histology, and neuroanatomy; *e.g.*, the contents of the skull and the vertebral canal are studied in both gross anatomy and neuroanatomy. In addition, the microscopic anatomy of the nervous system forms an important part of courses in histology and physiology. Hence, you must integrate information on the nervous system that is presented in the various disciplines called the **neurosciences**.

The study of growth and development is called **developmental anatomy** or **embryology**. Much can be learned about the structure and function of the adult body by studying the changes that occur during its development from a single cell (the **zygote**) into a multicellular adult person. Growth and development occur throughout life, but developmental processes are most pronounced during *prenatal life* (i.e., before birth), particularly during the **embryonic period** (4 to 8 weeks). The rate of growth and development slows down after birth, but there is active ossification (bone formation) and other important changes during infancy and childhood.

Many developmental changes occur during puberty, the period between 12 and 15 years in girls and 13 and 16 years in boys (*e.g.*, the development of **secondary sexual characteristics** such as breasts in females). Although sometimes given as a separate course, embryology is often integrated with gross anatomy, histology, and neuroanatomy because it explains how structures develop and acquire their adult structure and functions.

Although the anatomy of the body is studied in various ways and is often taught in three or four different courses, you must strive to **learn anatomy as an integrated subject**, keeping in mind that the various subdisciplines arose as new techniques for studying anatomy were developed and more knowledge was obtained. Your professors in the various courses are specialists who will help you learn which facts are of clinical importance and what is **essential knowledge** for you to retain in order to perform adequately as a doctor or a dentist. You will find that *many clinical problems can be understood by using knowledge acquired in anatomy courses*. This explains why this book is called **Clinically Oriented Anatomy**. The many references to the clinical significance of anatomy are inserted in this book as **clinically oriented comments** and **patient oriented problems** to indicate what is *essential knowledge* and to add interest to your anatomical studies.

The body is generally examined regionally, *i.e.*, by regions such as the thorax (Chap. 1), the abdomen (Chap. 2), and the pelvis (Chap. 3). The study of all structures in one area or region, including their relationships to each other, is known as **regional anatomy** or topographical anatomy. During regional anatomy, the body is generally divided into the following regions: (1) the **thorax**, (2) the **abdomen**, (3) the **perineum** and **pelvis**, (4) the **lower limb**, (5) the **back**,(6) the **upper limb**, (7) the **head**, (8) the **cranial nerves**, and (9) the **neck**. The chapters in this book and in Grant's *Atlas* are arranged in this order. For purposes of description, some regions are further subdivided; *e.g.*, the upper limb, which you probably call the arm, is subdivided into (1) the shoulder, (2) the arm, (3) the forearm, and (4) the hand.

Although you are familiar with the common or layman's terms for many of the parts and regions of the body, you should use the internationally adopted nomenclature; *e.g.*, use the word "**axilla**" instead of "armpit" and "**clavicle**" instead of "collar bone." Despite this, you must know what the common terms mean so that you can understand the words your patients use when they describe their complaints to you. In addition, you must be able to explain their problems to them in terms that they can understand.

From the functional standpoint, it is helpful to describe the parts and organs of the body by systems. This is referred to as **systemic (systematic) anatomy**. The systems of the body are:

1. **The integumentary system,** consisting of the skin and its appendages (*e.g.*, hair and nails).
2. **The skeletal system,** composed of the bones and their articulations (joints).
3. **The muscular system,** comprising the muscles that, with few exceptions, move the joints. Sometimes the muscular and skeletal systems are considered together as the musculoskeletal or locomotor system.
4. **The nervous system,** consisting of nerves, the brain, and the spinal cord, including their coverings (**meninges**).
5. **The circulatory (vascular) system,** comprising the heart and blood vessels and including the **lymphatic system** composed of lymph nodes and lymph vessels. The heart and the blood vessels are often referred to as the **cardiovascular system**.
6. **The visceral system,** exclusive of the heart, is usually considered separately as the **alimentary** or **digestive system**, the **respiratory system**, the **urinary system**, and the **genital system**. Because of their close association during development and in the adult, especially in the male, the urinary and genital systems are often described together as the **urogenital system**.
7. **The endocrine system** consists of ductless glands which produce secretions, called **hormones**, that pass into the circulatory system and are carried to all parts of the body.

THE FOUNDATION OF MEDICAL LANGUAGE

Anatomy is the basis of the language of medicine and dentistry. As a beginning student you will learn a **fascinating new language** consisting of at least *7500 words*; however, do not be overwhelmed! You will learn these words gradually and when you can speak the anatomical language fluently, you will feel at ease talking to your clinical colleagues because *the anatomical language constitutes about three-fourths of the words making up the medical language.*

To describe the relationship of one structure to another, the accepted **anatomical nomenclature** should be used. *To be understood you must express yourself clearly, using the official terms in the correct way.* If you are like most people, you have not studied the classics, Latin and Greek; consequently you may not pick up the anatomical language as quickly as those who have studied these old languages. Many anatomical and medical terms are derived from *Greek* because of the studies of **Hippocrates** and **Aristotle**, two famous Greek physicians. Similarly, many terms come from *Latin* mainly because of the influence of **Vesalius** (1514–1564), a great Flemish anatomist who was the Professor of Anatomy at the University of Padua in Italy for many years. His gross anatomy textbook, emphasizing the importance of *human dissection*, was used for over two centuries. Some words also stem from French, Italian, and Arabic. If you have not studied any of these languages, do not feel depressed! You can learn all you need to know by using a good medical dictionary. The study of the derivation of words (**etymology**) can help you remember anatomy and, at the same time, you are likely to find the process enjoyable. The following are good examples. (1) The term **cecum** is from the Latin word *caecus* meaning "blind." Your cecum is a blind pouch or **cul-de-sac** (French words meaning "bottom of a sac") lying below the terminal portion of your **ileum** (from a Latin verb meaning "to roll up or twist"). The jejunum and ileum are the highly coiled or rolled up parts of the small intestines. (2) **Decidua**, used for *the lining of the uterus during pregnancy*, is from Latin and means "a falling or cutting off." This is an appropriate term because this lining layer "falls off" or is shed after the baby is born, just as the leaves of deciduous trees fall off after the summer.

DESCRIPTIVE TERMS

To describe the body and to indicate the position of its parts and organs relative to

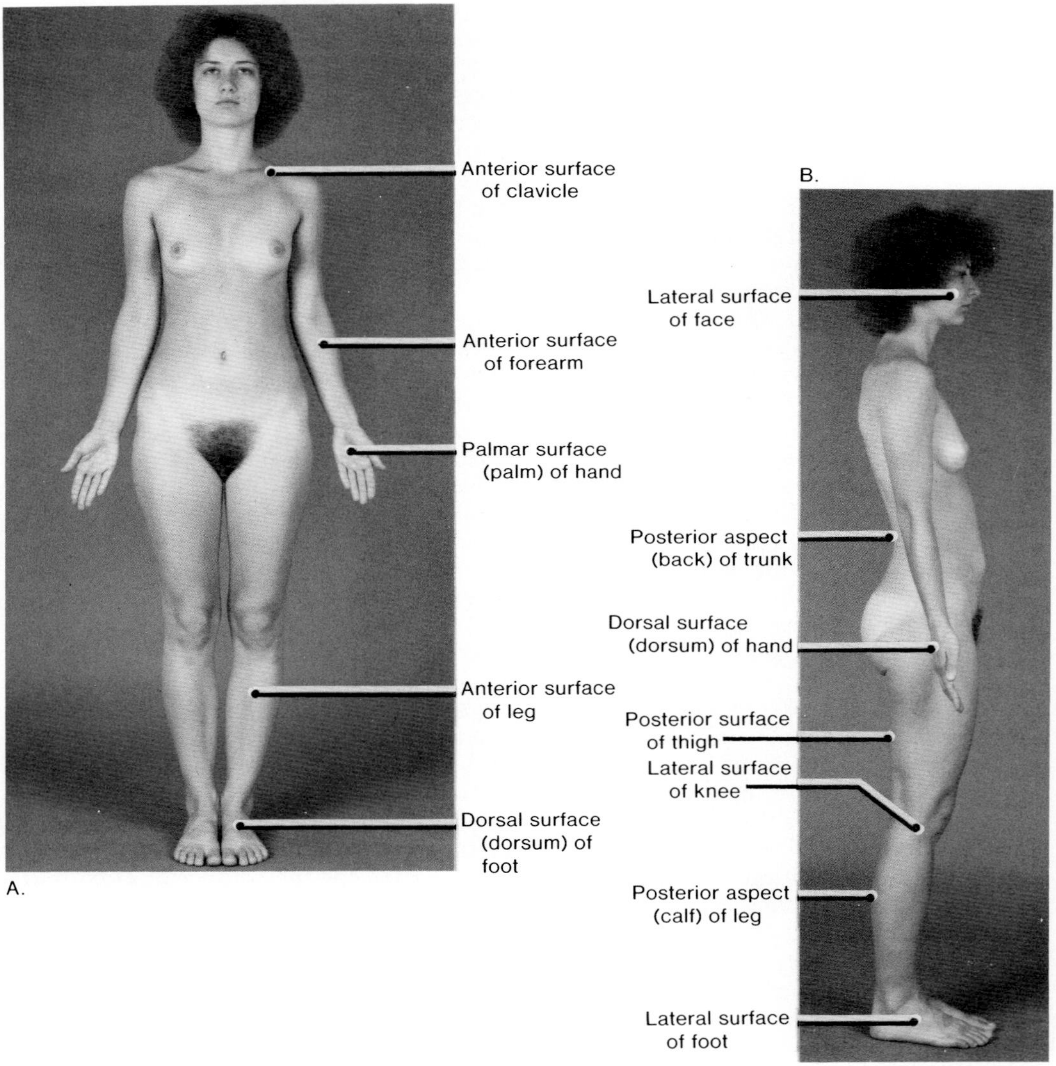

Figure I-3. Photographs of a 27-year-old woman demonstrating *the anatomical position* and some anatomical terms. *A*, anterior view. *B*, lateral view. Note: (1) she is standing erect; (2) her face and eyes are directed forward; (3) her hands are by her sides with the palms directed forward or anteriorly; (4) her heels are together; (5) her toes are pointed anteriorly; and (6) her great toes are touching.

each other, *anatomists around the world have agreed to use several terms of position and direction and various planes of the body.* Because **clinicians** (practicing doctors) also use these terms, it is important for you to take time at the beginning of your medical or dental career to learn them well and to practice using them so that it will be clear what you mean when you describe parts of the body in **patients' histories** or during discussion of patients with your clinical colleagues.

Use of the correct terminology will also be required when you write reports for medical and other journals. Persons who examine your reports or patients weeks, months, or years later should be able to understand clearly the descriptions, *e.g.*, the size of a tumor, the exact site of a fracture, or the kind of abnormality present. Be assured that the time you spend learning descriptive terms now will be well spent.

The Anatomical Position (Figs. I-2 to I-5). *This position of the body is adopted worldwide* for giving anatomical descriptions and must be thoroughly understood. *By using this position, any part of the body can be related to any other part of it.* **All descriptions of the body are based on the assumption that the person is standing erect with the head, eyes, and toes directed forward (anteriorly), the**

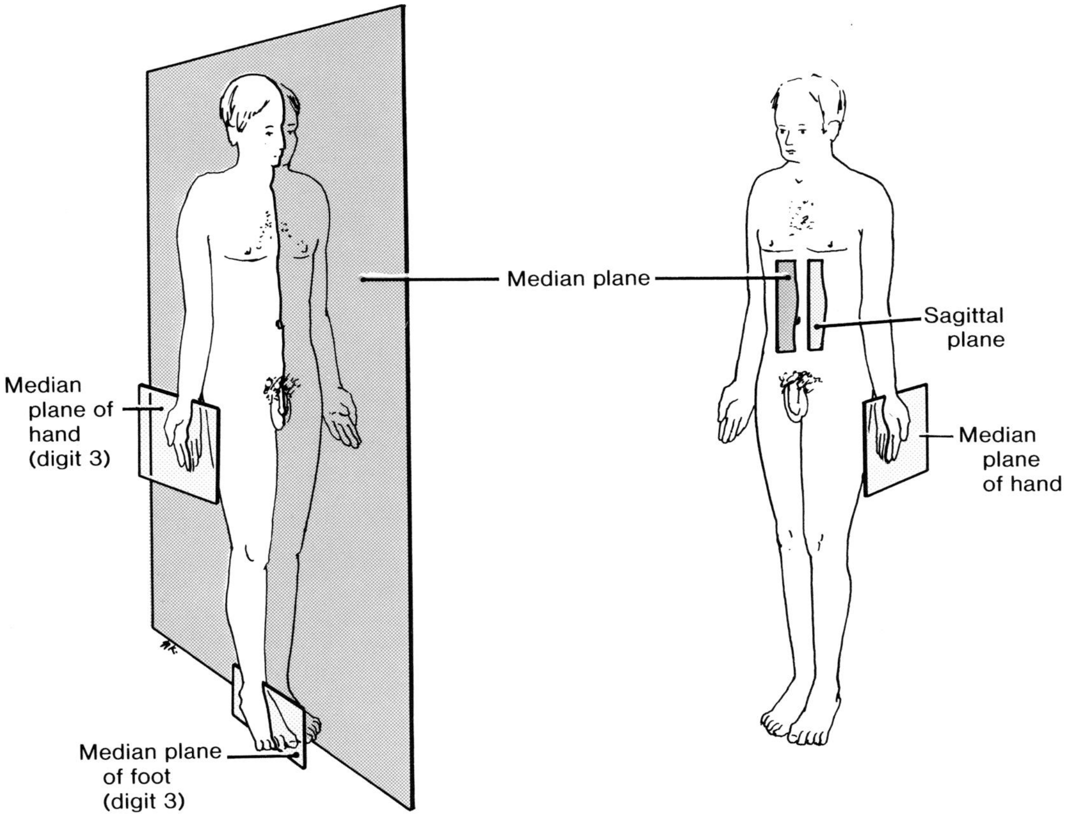

Figure I-4. Drawing illustrating *the median and sagittal planes* of the body, two of the four main anatomical planes. Observe that the median plane is a vertical plane passing through the body from front to back, dividing it into equal and superficially symmetrical right and left halves. Understand that there are many sagittal planes, because a sagittal plane is *any* vertical plane passing through the body parallel to the median plane. The sagittal plane that passes through the median plane is called the midsagittal plane. For another illustration of the median plane of the hand, see Figure I-14.

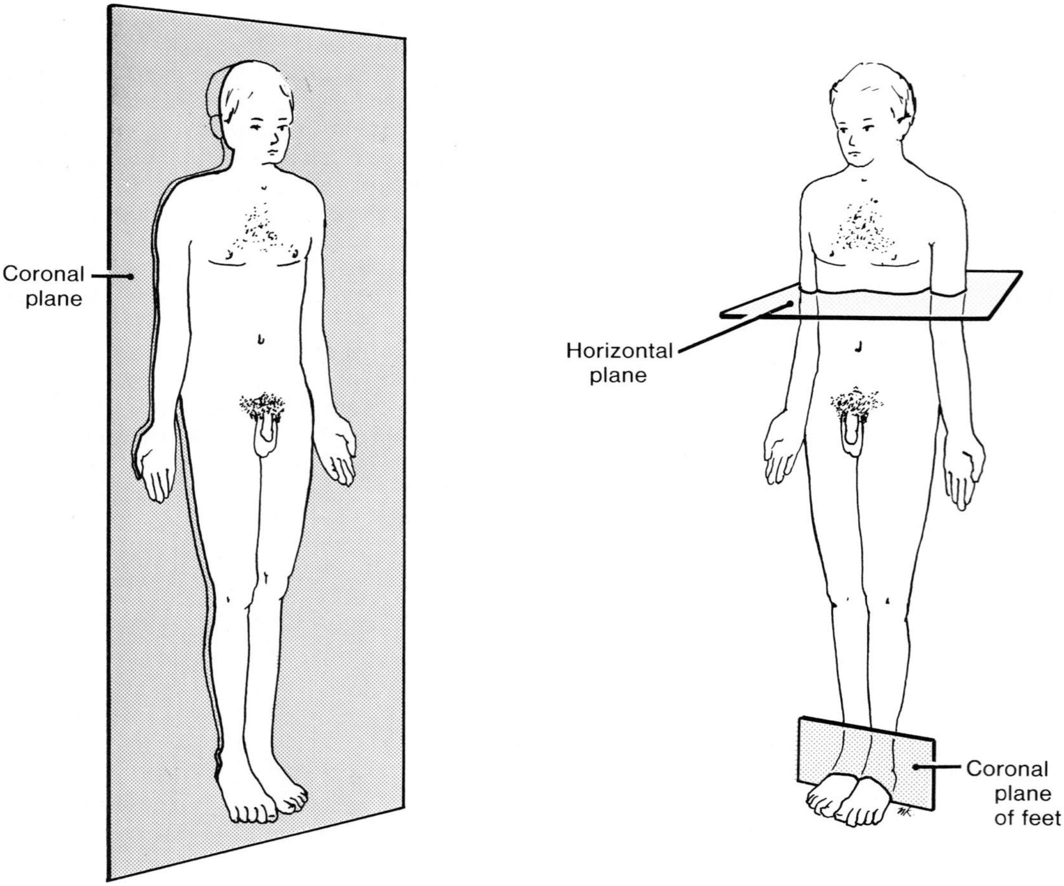

Figure I-5. Drawings illustrating *the coronal and horizontal planes*. Coronal planes are any vertical planes passing through the body at right angles to the median plane. A horizontal plane is any plane passing through the body at right angles to both the median and coronal planes (*i.e.*, parallel to the surface on which the subject is standing). Note that the coronal plane of the feet *shown here* does not pass through the trunk of the body. Coronal planes of the body usually pass through the ankles and the posterior parts of the feet.

heels and toes together, and the upper limbs hanging by the sides with the palms facing forward. You must always visualize this position when describing patients (or cadavers) lying on their backs (the **supine position**), sides, or fronts (the **prone position**). *Regardless of the patient's position, you must always think of the person as standing erect in the anatomical position*; otherwise, confusion as to the meaning of your description will exist and serious consequences could result.

Because the anatomical position is not the natural way of standing and differs from the military position of attention, special effort should be made to learn how the body is positioned. In Figures I-2 and I-3 observe that:

1. *The palms of the hands face anteriorly* (ventrally, forward) because the forearms are supinated; *i.e.*, they have been rotated laterally, away from the median plane of the body (Figs. I-4 and I-17). When you stand casually, your forearms are partly pronated; *i.e*, the palms almost face posteriorly (dorsally, backward). Hence, the anatomical position is not a casual stance.

2. *The great (big) toes touch.* In the usual stance, the heels are together but the toes are directed anterolaterally (toward the front and the sides). Because the anatomical position is such a fundamental concept, you are urged to practice standing in this position.

The Planes of the Body (Figs. I-4 and I-5). Many descriptions are made using *imaginary planes* passing through the body in the anatomical position. There are median, sagittal, coronal, and horizontal planes.

The Median Plane (Fig. I-4). This is the vertical plane passing lengthwise through the midline of the body from front to back and *dividing it into equal right and left halves*, except for such internal organs as the heart and the liver that do not lie in the midline. (See Fig. I-14 for an illustration of the median plane of the hand).

The Sagittal Plane (Fig. I-4). This is *any vertical plane passing through the body parallel to the median plane.* The sagittal plane that passes through the median plane of the body is called the **median sagittal plane** or **midsagittal plane**. It is in the same plane as the **sagittal suture** of the skull (Fig. I-39*A*), which lies between the parietal bones of the skull (Fig. 7-3). The sagittal planes that divide the body into right and left portions but do not pass through the median plane of the body are sometimes referred to as **paramedian** or **parasagittal planes** (G. *para*, beyond, beside). You are certain to hear neurologists, neurosurgeons, and neuroradiologists refer to **parasagittal tumors** (*i.e.*, tumors that are alongside or near the median sagittal plane). It is always helpful to give a point of reference, *e.g.*, a sagittal plane passing through the midpoint of the clavicle.

The Coronal (Frontal) Plane (Fig. I-5). This is *any vertical plane that passes through the body at right angles to the median plane,* dividing it into anterior (front) and posterior (back) portions. It is in the same plane as the **coronal suture** of the skull (Fig. I-39*A*) that unites the frontal bone with the parietal bones (Fig. 7-8). The coronal planes of the body pass through the ankles and the posterior parts of the feet. Hence, the coronal planes of the anterior parts of the feet do not pass through the trunk of the body.

The Horizontal (Transverse) Plane (Fig. I-5). This is *any plane that passes through the body at right angles to both the median and the coronal planes.* The horizontal plane divides the body into superior (upper) and inferior (lower) portions. Again it is always helpful to give a reference point, *e.g.*, a horizontal plane passing through the umbilicus (navel) which usually lies at the level of the intervertebral disc between L3 and L4 vertebrae (Figs. 2-1 and 2-68).

Sections Through the Body. In order to describe and display many internal structures, sections of the body and its parts are cut in various planes.

Longitudinal Sections (Fig. I-6). These sections (L. *longitudo*, length) *run lengthwise in the direction of the long axis of the body or any of its parts* and they are applicable regardless of the position of the body. Longitudinal sections may be cut in the median, sagittal, or coronal planes.

Vertical Sections. These are the same as longitudinal sections except that they denote that the sections are taken through the body when it is in the anatomical position. *Vertical sections pass toward the vertex* (L. whirl or crown) of the skull (Fig. 7-1).

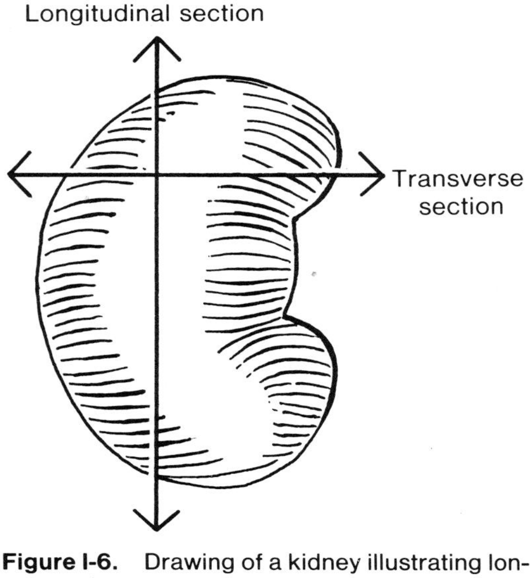

Figure I-6. Drawing of a kidney illustrating longitudinal and transverse sections of it.

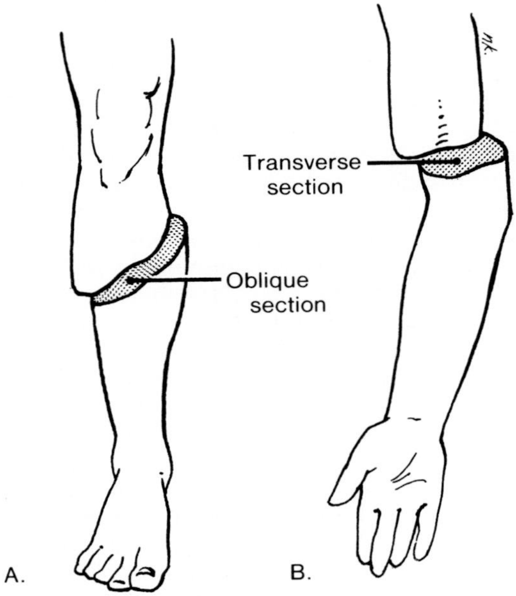

Figure I-7. Diagrams illustrating oblique (*A*) and transverse (*B*) sections of the limbs.

Transverse (Cross) Sections (Figs. I-6 and I-7*B*). These sections of the body or its parts are *cut at right angles to the longitudinal axis of the body or its parts.* Transverse sections of the whole body (*e.g.*, Fig. 2-119) do not necessarily cut vessels or internal organs transversely because they may not be located in the long axis of the body. For example, a transverse section in a horizontal plane through the chest at the level of the heart does not cut the ventricles horizontally because the heart is not centered in the median plane (Figs. I-22, 1-52, and 1-53). To make a transverse section of an organ or a part (*e.g.*, of the upper limb), the section must be cut at right angles to its longitudinal axis.

Oblique Sections (Fig. I-7). These are sections of the body or any of its parts that are not cut in one of the main planes of the body; *i.e.*, they slant or deviate from the perpendicular or the horizontal.

Terms of Relationship (Fig. I-8). Various terms are used to describe the body in the anatomical position. Because anatomy is a descriptive science, many clearly defined and unambiguous terms are used to indicate the positions of structures to each other and to the body as a whole.

Anterior (Ventral, Front). **Nearer the front** surface of the body; *e.g.*, the nipples and the umbilicus (navel or "belly button") are on the anterior surface of the body (Figs. I-2*A* and I-3*A*). Usually the anterior surface of the hand is called the **volar** or **palmar surface** (Fig. I-3*A*) and the inferior surface of the foot is called the **plantar surface** or the **sole** (Fig. I-13*A*). *Ventral is equivalent to anterior* and is commonly used in descriptions of embryos because they cannot be placed in the anatomical position. The term ventral is commonly used in neuroanatomy where it has an advantage because it is equally applicable to man and the four-footed animals that are commonly used in studies of the nervous system.

Posterior (Dorsal, Behind). **Nearer the back** surface of the body; *e.g.*, the buttocks (gluteal region) are on the posterior surface

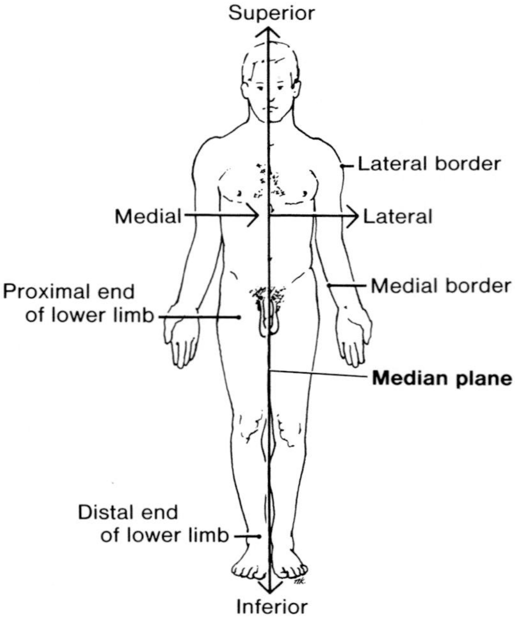

Figure I-8. Diagram of an anterior view of a man standing in the anatomical position. Understand that *medial means toward the median plane* and *lateral means away from the median plane* of the body. The terms median and medial are sometimes confused. Median means "*in* the median plane," whereas medial means "*toward* the median plane."

(Fig. I-2*B*). *Dorsal is interchangeable with posterior* and is commonly used in descriptions of embryos and of the nervous system. When describing the posterior or dorsal surface of the hand, the term **dorsum** is commonly used (Fig. I-3*B*). Similarly, when describing the superior or upper surface of the foot, the term dorsum is used (Figs. I-3*A* and I-13*C*) because this surface faced dorsally in the early embryo. *During the late embryonic period, the upper and lower limbs rotate in different directions*; as a result, following the embryonic period, the dorsal surfaces of the feet come to lie anterosuperiorly.

Superior (Cephalic, Cephalad, Cranial, Above). **Toward the head** or upper part of the body (Fig. I-8); *e.g.*, the heart lies superior to the diaphragm, *i.e.*, higher or closer to the head, cranium, or superior end of the body. *Cranial and cephalic are interchangeable adjectives* that are commonly used in descriptions of embryos and the nervous system; *e.g.*, the spinothalamic fibers run cranially, *i.e.*, from the spinal cord toward the thalamus in the brain. The Greek word for the brain is *enkephalos*. Rostral is often used synonymously with anterior, particularly in descriptions of the brain. It is derived from the Latin word *rostrum*, meaning beak; thus, structures nearer to the nose are rostral to structures that lie posterior to it.

Inferior (Caudal, Caudad, Below). **Toward the feet** or lower part of the body; *e.g.*, the diaphragm is inferior to the heart, *i.e.*, nearer to the feet or inferior end of the body and further from the head. The term **caudal** is derived from the Latin word *cauda*, meaning "tail." It is commonly used in descriptions of embryos where the term is applicable because human embryos have a tail until near the end of the embryonic period. Caudal is also used frequently in neuroanatomy to indicate structures that are **nearer the tail** or inferior end; *e.g.*, corticospinal fibers run caudally from the head, *i.e.*, from the cerebral cortex of the brain to the spinal cord located inferior or caudal to it. Again, the term has an advantage because it is equally applicable to man and to the animals that are frequently used in neuroanatomical studies.

Medial (Figs. I-4 and I-8). **Toward the median plane** of the body, *e.g.*, the external openings of the nose (**anterior nares** or nostrils) are medial to the eyes. The term **mesial** (G. *mesos*, middle) is equivalent to medial and is used interchangeably with it. Because medial, as applied to the limbs, is sometimes misinterpreted, depending upon whether one is thinking of the median plane of the body or the midline of the limb, it is common to describe the limbs in terms of the position of their paired bones. In the upper limb, the **radius** is the lateral bone of the forearm (Fig. I-17) and the **ulna** is the medial one. Thus, the terms "ulnar" and "medial" and "radial" and "lateral" are synonymous and refer to the little finger and the thumb sides of the hand, respectively.

Lateral (Figs. I-4 and I-8). **Away from the median plane** of the body. Understand that the little toe is lateral to the great toe, but the little finger is medial to the thumb.

Intermediate. **Between two structures**, one of which is medial and the other lateral; *e.g.*, the ring finger is intermediate between the little and middle fingers. The little finger is medial and the middle finger is lateral to it.

Terms of Comparison. These terms are used to compare the relative position of two structures to each other.

Proximal (L. *proximus*, next). **Nearest the trunk** or the **point of origin** of a vessel, nerve, limb, or organ; *e.g.*, the thigh is at the proximal end of the lower limb (Fig. I-3). In the limbs the terms proximal and superior are synonymous. When referring to a limb muscle, the proximal attachment is its origin.

Distal (L. *distans*, distant). **Farthest from the trunk** or the **point of origin** of a vessel, nerve, limb, or organ; *e.g.*, the foot is at the distal end of the lower limb. In the limbs the terms distal and inferior are synonymous. **Distad** means **toward the periphery** or in a distal direction. When referring to a limb muscle, the distal attachment is its insertion. In dental anatomy, distal means away from the median plane of the face, following the curve of the dental arch. In addition, **labial** means toward the lip (L. *labium*), whereas lingual (L. *lingua*, tongue) means toward the tongue.

Superficial (L. surface). **Nearer to the skin surface** (Fig. I-9*A*); *e.g.*, the superficial fascia is closer to the skin surface of the body than the deep fascia. Similarly the scalp is superficial to the skull.

Deep (Fig. I-9*A*). **Further from the skin surface**; *e.g.*, in the arm the bone (humerus) is deep to the muscles and the skin.

Interior (Inside, Inner, Internal). **Nearer to the center** of an organ or cavity (Fig. I-9*B*); *e.g.*, the interior of the urinary bladder. The term is also used to describe structures that pass from the front to the back of the body or enclose other structures (*e.g.*, as the ribs enclose the thoracic viscera). Hence, the internal surface of the rib is the surface farthest from the skin. Also, the **internal carotid artery** passes to the *inside of the skull.* In older textbooks you may find inner used incorrectly to mean medial (toward the median plane of the body).

Exterior (Outside, Outer, External). **Farther from the center** of an organ or cavity (Fig. I-9*B*); *e.g.*, the external surface of the urinary bladder is farther from the center of the organ than the internal surface. Similarly, the external surface of a rib is the surface closer to the skin and the **external carotid artery** passes to the *outside of the skull.* In older textbooks you may find outer used incorrectly to mean lateral (away from the median plane of the body).

Ipsilateral (L. *ipse,* same, + *lateralis,* side). **On the same side** of the body; *e.g.*, the right thumb and the right great (big) toe are ipsilateral.

Contralateral (L. *contra,* opposite, + *lateralis,* side). **On the opposite side** of the body; *e.g.*, the right hand and the left hand are contralateral.

Ambiguous Terms. **Do not use the terms on, over, and under** because it may not always be clear what you mean; *e.g.*, when you say a structure passes over another one, do you mean anterior, superior, or superficial to it.

Combined Terms. Often terms are combined to indicate a direction; *e.g.*, **inferomedially** means toward the feet and the median plane. Initially the ulnar artery passes inferomedially in the forearm (Fig. 6-97). There are many other combinations of terms, *e.g.*, **anteroinferior, anteroposterior.** In a posteroanterior (**PA**) radiograph of the chest (Fig. 1-38), a beam of x-rays passes through the thorax of a patient from posterior to anterior; *i.e.*, the x-ray tube is posterior to the patient and the x-ray film is anterior to him/her.

Terms of Movement. As anatomy is primarily concerned with the living body, there are various terms to describe the var-

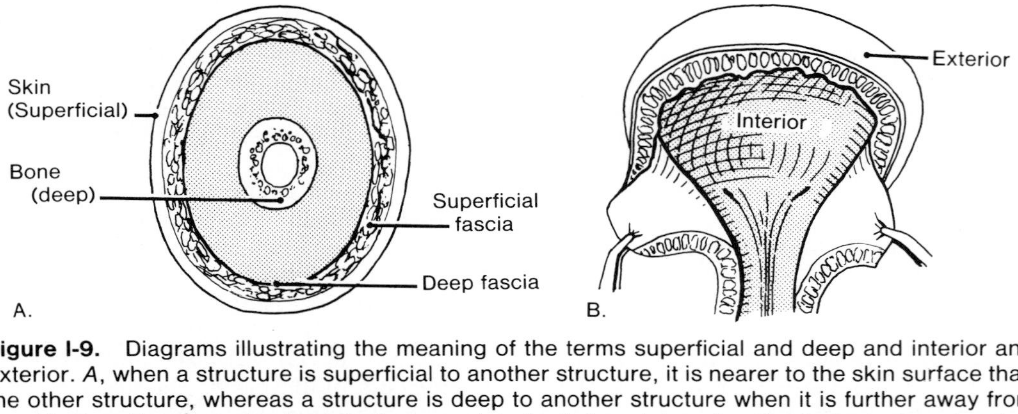

Figure I-9. Diagrams illustrating the meaning of the terms superficial and deep and interior and exterior. *A*, when a structure is superficial to another structure, it is nearer to the skin surface than the other structure, whereas a structure is deep to another structure when it is further away from the skin than the other structure. *B*, the terms interior (internal, inner) and exterior (external, outer) are often used to describe cavities of hollow organs such as the uterus. The skull is also described as having an internal surface and an external surface; *e.g.*, a bullet lying on the internal aspect of the skull would lie between the skull and the brain, whereas a bullet lying on the external aspect would lie in the scalp. The terms inner and outer should not be used when you mean medial (toward the median plane) or lateral (away from the median plane).

ious types of movement of the limbs and other parts of the body. Movements take place at certain joints (articulations) where two or more bones meet one another. (For details, see subsequent discussion of joints.)

Flexion (Figs. I-10 to I-13). This indicates **bending or making a decreasing angle between the bones or parts of the body.** Usually the movement is an anterior bending in the sagittal plane, *e.g.*, flexion of the forearm at the elbow joint (Fig. I-10*B*), but flexion of the leg at the knee joint is a posterior bending of the limb (Fig. I-10*C*). To indicate flexion or bending in the dorsal direction, as in the ankle, the term dorsiflexion is used (Fig. I-13*A*).

Extension (Figs. I-10 to I-13). This is a **straightening of a bent part or joint** and is the movement opposed to that of flexion. It therefore usually occurs in the posterior direction. If the movement is continued beyond that which is necessary to straighten the part, it is referred to as **hyperextension** (*e.g.*, as occurs to the neck in rear end collisions; see Case 5-2 at the end of Chap. 5). Extension of the foot, *e.g.*, when standing on the tiptoes, is referred to as **plantarflexion** (Fig. I-13*B*) to indicate that the ankle is in extension toward the sole or plantar surface of the foot.

Abduction (Figs. I-14*A* and I-15*A*). This term means **moving apart** or **away from the median plane** of the body in the coronal plane, *i.e.*, drawing away laterally, as when moving the upper limb away from the body. The prefix *ab-* is the Latin preposition meaning "*away from.*" In abduction of the fingers or toes, the term means spreading them apart, *e.g.*, fanning or moving the fingers away from the middle finger or median plane of the hand (Fig. I-14*A*) and the toes away from the second toe. **Lateral**

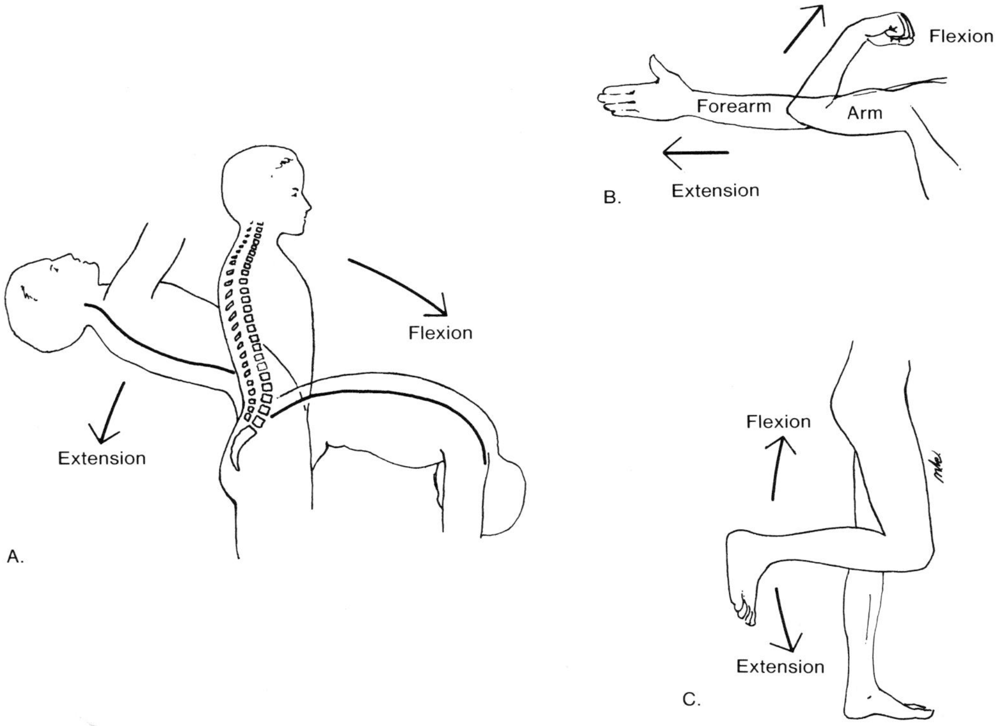

Figure I-10. Drawings illustrating *flexion* and *extension*. *A*, movements of the trunk or neck in a sagittal plane are known as flexion or forward bending and extension or backward bending. *B*, movements of the forearm in a sagittal plane are known as flexion and extension. In flexion the angle between the forearm and the arm is reduced, whereas in extension the angle is increased. *C*, note that flexion of the leg at the knee joint is a posterior bending of the limb.

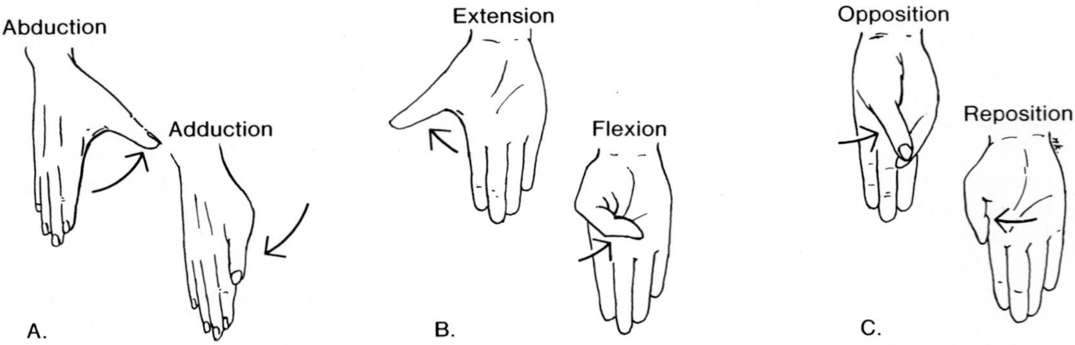

Figure I-11. Drawings illustrating the various types of movement of the thumb.

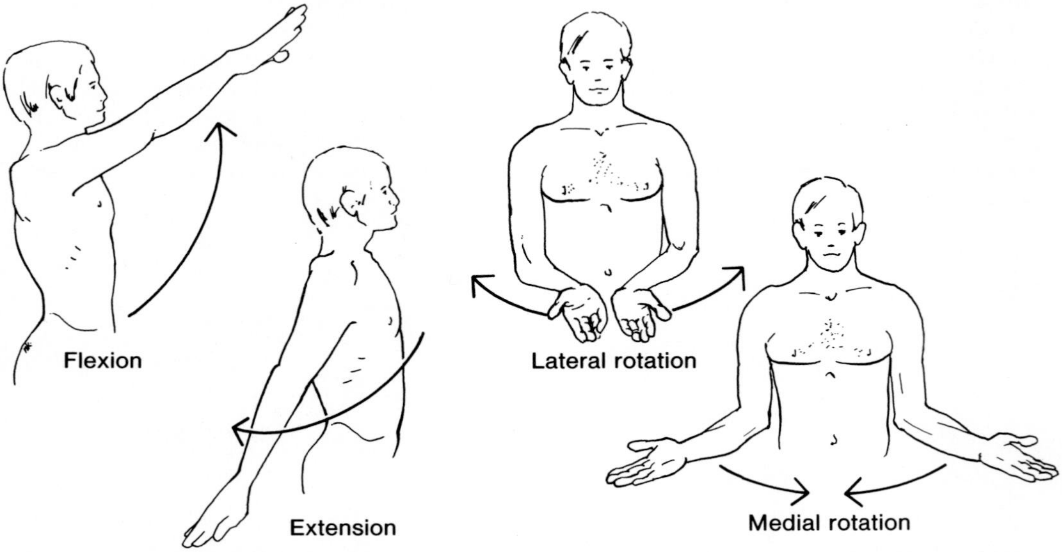

Figure I-12. Drawings illustrating some movements at the shoulder joint. Note that the forearms are flexed to 90° during rotation at this joint.

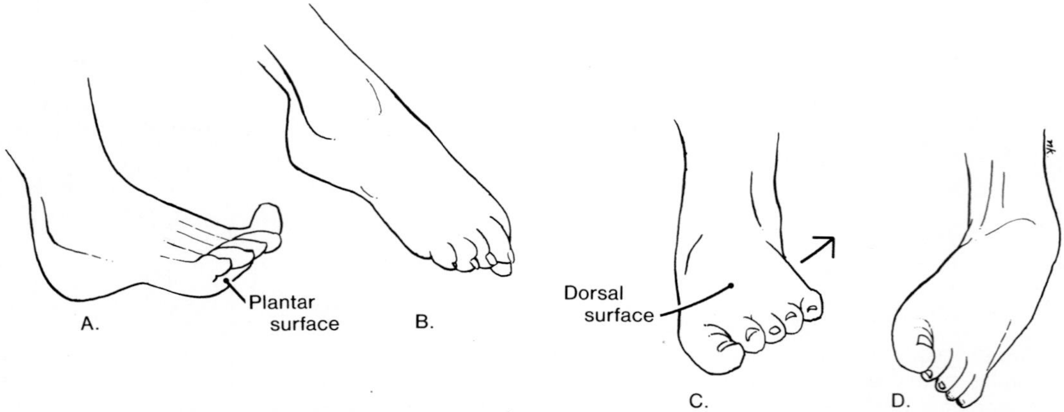

Figure I-13. Drawings illustrating movements of the foot. *A*, dorsiflexion. *B*, plantarflexion. *C*, eversion. *D*, inversion.

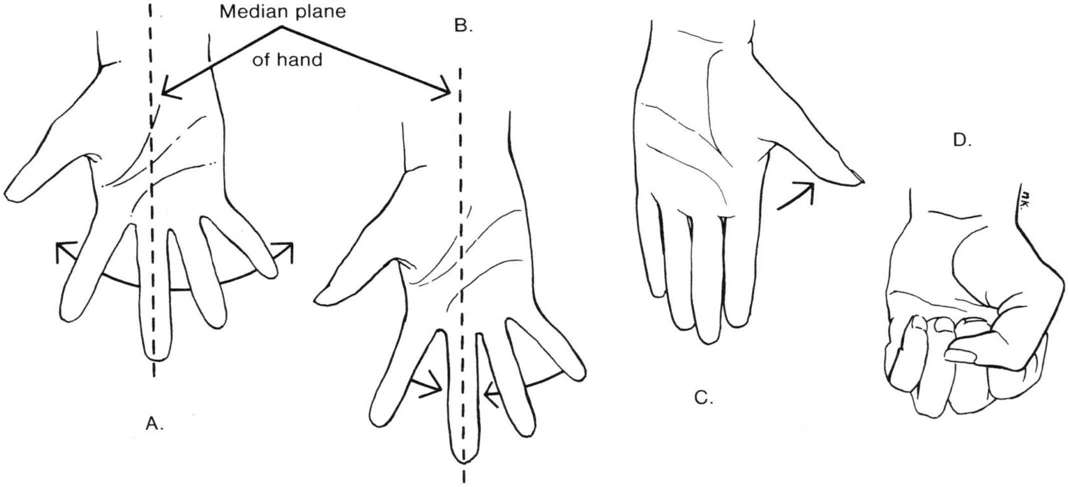

Figure I-14. Drawings illustrating various movements of the fingers and the thumb. *A*, abduction of the fingers. *B*, adduction of the fingers. *C*, extension of the thumb and the fingers. *D*, flexion of the fingers and the thumb. Note that the median plane of the hand passes through the midline of the middle finger. The median plane of the foot passes through the second toe.

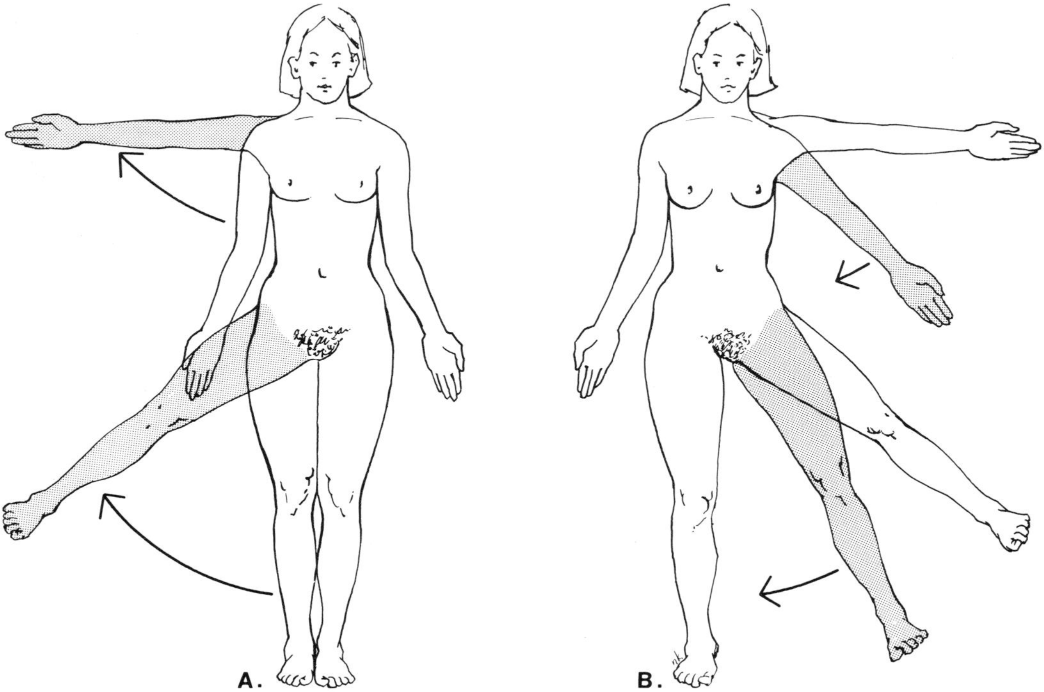

Figure I-15. Drawings illustrating *abduction* of the right limbs in *A* and *adduction* of the left limbs in *B*. Observe that abduction of a limb is the *movement away* from the median plane of the body in the coronal plane, whereas *adduction* of a limb is the *movement toward* the median plane of the body in the coronal plane.

bending (flexion) is movement of the trunk laterally (*i.e.*, away from the median plane of the body) in the coronal plane (Fig. 5-9).

Adduction (Figs. I-11*A*, I-14*B*, and I-15*B*). This is the opposite movement to abduction. It refers to a **moving together** or **toward the median plane** of the body in the coronal plane, *e.g.*, when moving the upper limb toward the body. The prefix *ad-* is a Latin preposition meaning "*to or toward*." In adduction of the fingers or toes, the term means moving them toward the median plane of the hand or foot, *e.g.*, moving the fingers toward the middle finger and the toes toward the second toe.

Opposition (Fig. I-11*C*). This is the movement during which **the thumb pad is brought to a finger pad** and held there. We frequently use this movement to hold a pen, to pinch, or to grasp a cup handle.

Reposition (Fig. I-11*C*). This is the term used to describe the movement of the thumb from the position of opposition back to its anatomical position.

Protraction. This is a **movement forward**, as occurs in moving the jaw forward (*i.e.*, sticking the chin out) or in drawing the shoulders forward.

Retraction. This is a **movement backward** as in moving the jaw backward (*i.e.*, tucking in the chin) or in drawing the shoulders backward, *e.g.*, squaring the shoulders in the military stance.

Elevation. This term means **lifting, raising,** or **moving a part superiorly,** *e.g.*, elevating the shoulders, as occurs when shrugging them or in raising the upper limb above the shoulder.

Depression. This is a **letting down, lowering,** or **moving a part inferiorly**, *e.g.*, depressing or lowering the shoulders, as occurs when standing at ease.

Circumduction (Fig. I-16). This term is derived from the Latin words *circum*, meaning around, and *duco*, meaning to draw. Hence, it means to draw around or to form a circle. *Circumduction is the combination of successive movements of flexion,*

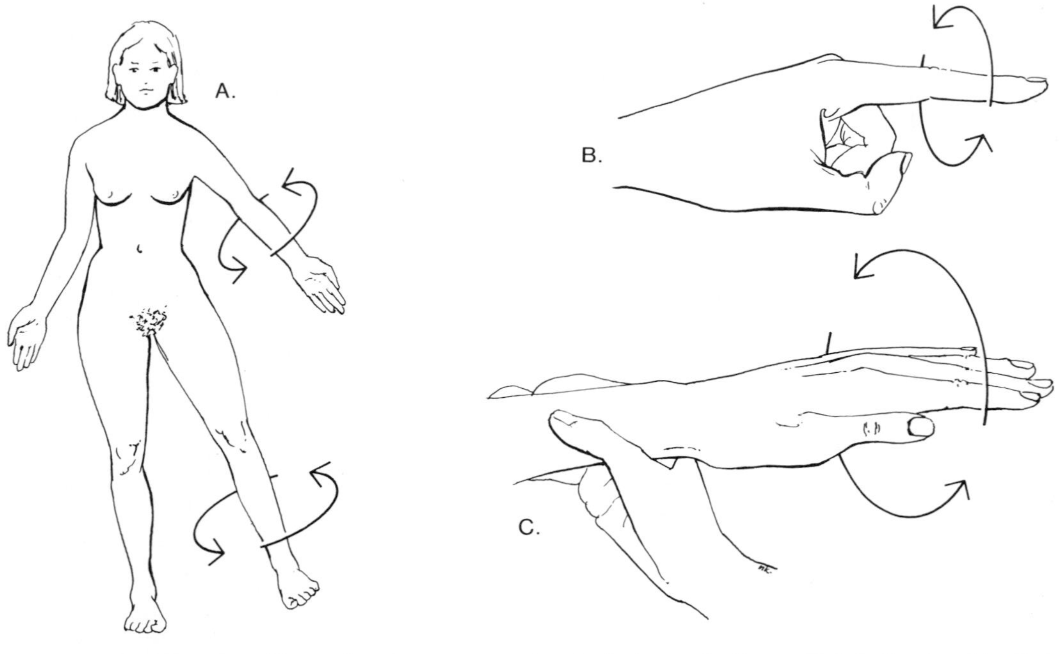

Figure I-16. Drawings illustrating the movement called *circumduction*, which is the combination in sequence of the movements of *flexion*, *extension*, *abduction*, and *adduction*. *A*, circumduction of the left upper and lower limbs at the shoulder and hip joints, respectively. *B*, circumduction of the index finger (digit 2). *C*, circumduction of the hand at the wrist joint. Understand that circumduction does not involve rotation of the joint; *i.e.*, the joint remains stationary as the distal (peripheral) end of the moving part describes a circle.

abduction, extension, and adduction in such a way that the distal end of the part being moved describes or forms a circle. *The sequence of movements resulting in the formation of a cone of movement* can occur at any joint at which the above mentioned four types of movement are possible, *e.g.*, the hip, the wrist, and the metacarpophalangeal joints of the fingers. You may observe this movement by extending your leg and moving it in such a way as to produce an imaginary circle or a cone of movement (Fig. I-16*A*). A person with a paralyzed lower limb swings the stiffly extended limb in a partial arch when walking; this is called the **circumducted gait.** You can observe circumduction of the shoulder by drawing a circle on a blackboard while the upper limb is extended and abducted to the horizontal level. The thumb and index finger can also be circumducted (Fig. I-16*B*), but it is not so easy to circumduct the other fingers.

Rotation (Fig. I-12). This is a turning or revolving of a part of the body or a bone around its long axis, *e.g.*, rotation of the humerus of the arm at the shoulder joint and the femur of the thigh at the hip joint. *Rotation toward the median plane* of the body is **medial rotation,** whereas *rotation away from the median plane* is **lateral rotation.** During these movements, the anterior aspect of the limb moves medially in medial rotation and laterally in lateral rotation.

Eversion of the Foot (Fig. I-13*C*). This movement turns the plantar surface or *sole of the foot away from the median plane* of the body (*i.e.*, the sole faces laterally).

Inversion of the Foot (Fig. I-13*D*). This movement turns the plantar surface or *sole of the foot toward the median plane* of the body (*i.e.*, the sole faces medially).

Supination (Fig. I-17*A*). This is the movement that rotates the radius of the forearm laterally around its long axis, so that *the dorsum (back) of the hand faces posteriorly and the palm faces anteriorly* when the body is in the anatomical position (Figs. I-2 to I-4). When the elbow is flexed 90°, supination moves the forearm so that the palm of the hand is turned upward (*i.e.*, faces superiorly), as when begging. The **supine position** of the body is lying on the back with the head and toes directed anteriorly.

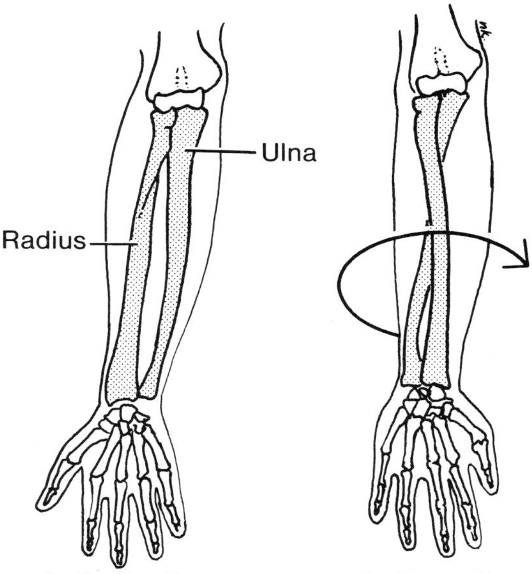

Figure I-17. Drawings illustrating *supination* (*A*) and *pronation* (*B*) of the forearm. Observe that pronation is a medial rotation of the radius from its anatomical position (*A*) so that the dorsum (back) of the hand faces anteriorly. Supination of the pronated forearm returns the hand to its anatomical position shown in *A* and in Figure I-3. Note that the positions of the radius and the ulna change during pronation.

Pronation (Fig. I-17*B*). This is the movement that rotates the radius of the forearm medially around its long axis so that *the palm of the hand faces posteriorly and the dorsum faces anteriorly* when the upper limb hangs by the side in the anatomical position. When the elbow is flexed 90°, pronation moves the forearm so that the palm of the hand faces inferiorly or is turned downward, *e.g.*, when the palm of the hand is placed on a table. During this movement, the radius of the forearm crosses the ulna diagonally, moving the thumb medially (Fig. I-17). The **prone position** of the body is lying face downward with the tips of the toes touching the table or the ground.

General Comments on Terminology. It should be obvious now that *one of the first essentials in learning anatomy is the understanding of anatomical terms.* They are used loosely by some students who have never bothered to learn their exact meaning. These students usually do poorly on examinations. You are urged to learn and use the correct terms so that your colleagues and examiners will understand what you are describing or discussing. *Medical slang, local abbreviations, and imprecise use of words leads to loose thinking and may lead to error.*

As anatomy is a descriptive science, many anatomical terms are in themselves descriptive indicating the shape, size, location, function, or resemblance of a structure to some other structure; *e.g.*, the appendix of the cecum is appropriately referred to as the **vermiform appendix** (L. *vermis*, a worm) because it is shaped like a worm. You will quickly learn that muscles are given descriptive terms to indicate their characteristics, *e.g.*, the **biceps** (L. *bi*, two, + *caput*, head), the **triceps** (L. *tri*, three) and the **quadriceps** (L. *quattuor*, four) because they have two, three, and four heads, respectively. Some muscles are named according to their shape, *e.g.*, the **piriformis** (L. pear-like form), the **rectus** (L. straight) abdominis, and the **quadratus** (L. square) muscles. Other muscles are named by location, *e.g.*, the **temporalis**, a major muscle of the **temporal region** of the skull. In other cases actions are used to describe muscles, *e.g.*, the **levator scapulae**, as you have probably guessed, raises the scapula. Thus, there are good reasons for the names given to the parts of the body and if you learn them and think about them as you dissect you should have less difficulty remembering their names.

Abbreviations. As abbreviations are commonly used in this and other anatomy books, especially for structures in illustrations, they must be explained. They are easy to understand if you know the word(s) being abbreviated; *e.g.*, "**fl. carpi ulnaris**" refers to the flexor carpi ulnaris muscle in the forearm (Fig. 6-90). Frequently on illustrations you will also see abbreviations for arteries and ligaments (*e.g.*, "**post. circumflex humeral a.**" refers to the posterior circumflex humeral artery and "**sup. glenohumeral lig.**" refers to the superior glenohumeral ligament). As "**a.**" is used for an artery, the abbreviation for arteries is "**aa.**" Similarly, "**v.**" is used for a vein and "**vv.**" for veins, "**m.**" for muscle and "**mm.**" for muscles, "**n.**" for nerve and "**nn.**" for nerves. In most cases the abbreviation "m." (muscle) is omitted when it is obviously a muscle (see the muscles of the arm in Fig. 6-71).

When referring to vertebrae and spinal nerves, they are designated both by region and by number, *e.g.*, for the third cervical, it is common to use the abbreviation C3. Later, you will learn that the ulnar nerve supplying structures in the forearm and hand carries nerve fibers from C7 to T1, meaning that it receives them from the 7th and 8th cervical and first thoracic segments of the spinal cord.

As most medical words stem from Greek (**G.**) and Latin (**L.**), the derivation of a word is often given because it helps in understanding its meaning; *e.g.*, **cancer** (L. crab) was so named because it gnaws away at the body like a crab. Similarly, **coccyx** (G. cuckoo) indicates that this bone is shaped like the beak of a cuckoo. If in doubt about the meaning of an abbreviation or word, *check your medical dictionary.*

THE BASIS OF RADIOLOGY[1]

Anatomy is essential for understanding radiology (L. *radius*, ray, + G. *logos*, study). During 1st year medicine and when you begin to practice this art, you will examine *the anatomy of the body in radiographs* (*i.e.*, radiographic anatomy) nearly every day. You will see anatomical structures this way much more frequently than you will see them displayed at operation or autopsy. For this reason, many **radiographs** (x-rays[2], x-ray films, or roentgenographs) have been used in this book. Familiarity with normal radiographs allows you to recognize abnormalities, *e.g.*, tumors or **fractures.**

---

[1] By D. L. McRae, M.D., F.R.C.P. (Canada), F.A.C.R., Professor Emeritus of Radiology, University of Toronto.

[2] You are urged not to use the term "x-rays" when you mean radiographs; x-rays emerge from the x-ray tube producing images on x-ray films called radiographs.

The study of radiographs also improves your understanding of the anatomy of bones, joints, and many internal organs and prepares you for the study of physiology, pathology, and the **clinical sciences.** When faced with an injured patient, *you must be able to visualize in your "mind's eye" the injured part and its surroundings.* When you examine a sick patient, you must be able to visualize the diseased organ and its associated structures. Knowledge of radiological anatomy helps you to do these things.

Each image on normal radiographs should be studied and identified on a skeleton and in your dissection, because learning by doing is the best and most permanent way to learn. The essence of the radiological examination is that a highly penetrating beam of x-rays "transilluminates" the patient, showing tissues of differing densities within the body as images of differing densities on x-ray film (Fig. I-18) or on the screen of a fluoroscopic device of some kind.

Density is the ratio of the mass of a homogenous portion of a material to its volume. Its dimension is mass/volume, *e.g.*, the density of water is 1 g/cm^3. It is analogous to specific gravity, the ratio of the weight of a given volume of a homogenous portion of a material to the weight of an equal volume of water. The specific gravity of water is 1. *A tissue or organ that is relatively dense absorbs (or stops) more x-rays than a less dense tissue.* Consequently, a dense tissue or organ produces a relatively transparent (erroneously called white) area on the x-ray film because relatively fewer x-rays reach the silver salt/gelatin emulsion in the film at that point. Therefore, relatively fewer grains of silver are developed at this area when the film is processed. *A very dense substance is said to be radiopaque, whereas a substance of small density is said to be radiolucent* (Table I-1). The density of fat is approximately 0.9 g/cm^3, whereas water and most soft tissues of the body have a density of 1.00 to 1.04 g/cm^3. Cancellous bone varies in density, but can be considered to be about 1.3 g/cm^3; compact bone has a density of approximately 1.8 g/cm^3.

As the image is a two-dimensional image of a three dimensional object, images of structures at different depths in the body overlap each other. When "filming" a part of the patient, at least two projections or views must be made, usually at right angles to each other in order to obviate the overlap of one object by another and to help your mind reconstruct the three-dimensional part (Figs. I-19 and I-20). **Stereoscopic films** of a part will give you a three-dimensional image also.

Body section radiography can be utilized to give three-dimensional information also. There are two types. **Conventional tomography** (G. *tomos*, a cutting or section), also called *laminography*, is a method of moving an x-ray tube in the opposite direction to a moving x-ray film during the exposure so that images of a predetermined plane in the body remain stationary on the film while images in other planes move on the film and are blurred and become invisible (Fig. I-21). The second type of body section radiography, using **CT (computerized tomographic) scanners,** shows sections of the body resembling anatomical sections (Fig. I-22). In this process a small beam or pencil of x-rays is passed through a plane of the body while *the x-ray tube*

Table I-1
The Basic Principles of X-ray Image Formation

Most Radiolucent ↑		Least Radiodense ↑
	Air	
	Fat	
	Water and Most Tissues*	
	Cancellous Bone	
	Compact Bone	
↓ Least Radiolucent		↓ Most Radiodense

* Includes cytoplasm and uncalcified intercellular substances.

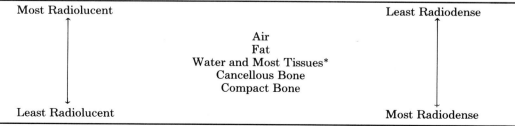

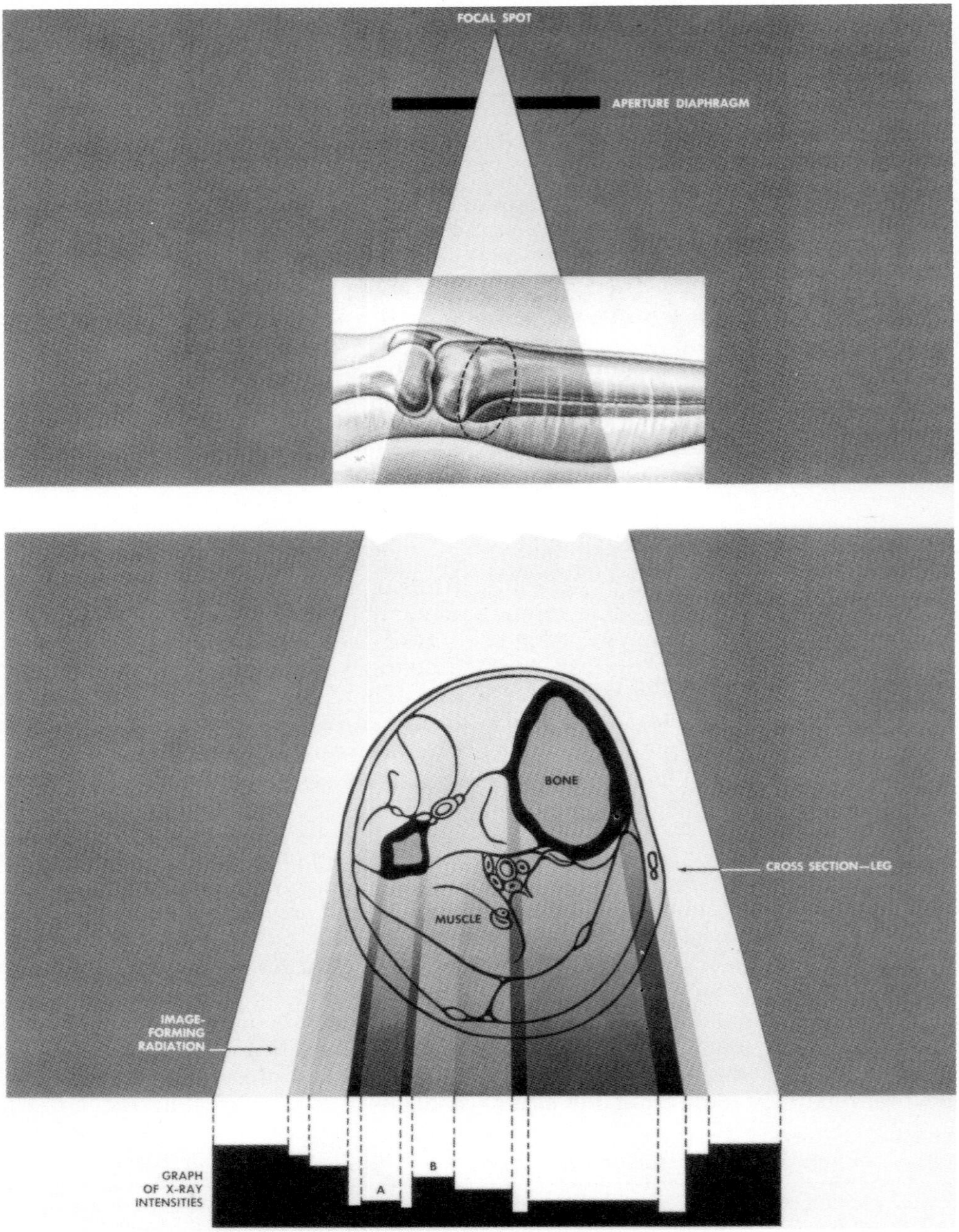

Figure I-18. Diagram illustrating how a beam of x-rays passes through the leg and forms images on an x-ray film. On each side of the leg, the x-rays pass through air only, resulting in maximum x-ray intensity in the film and maximum film blackening as indicated on the graph. The greatest thickness of the most dense tissue (compact bone of the cortex of the tibia, the larger bone) stopped the most x-rays, resulting in minimum x-ray intensity in the film and minimum film blackening under the tibia.

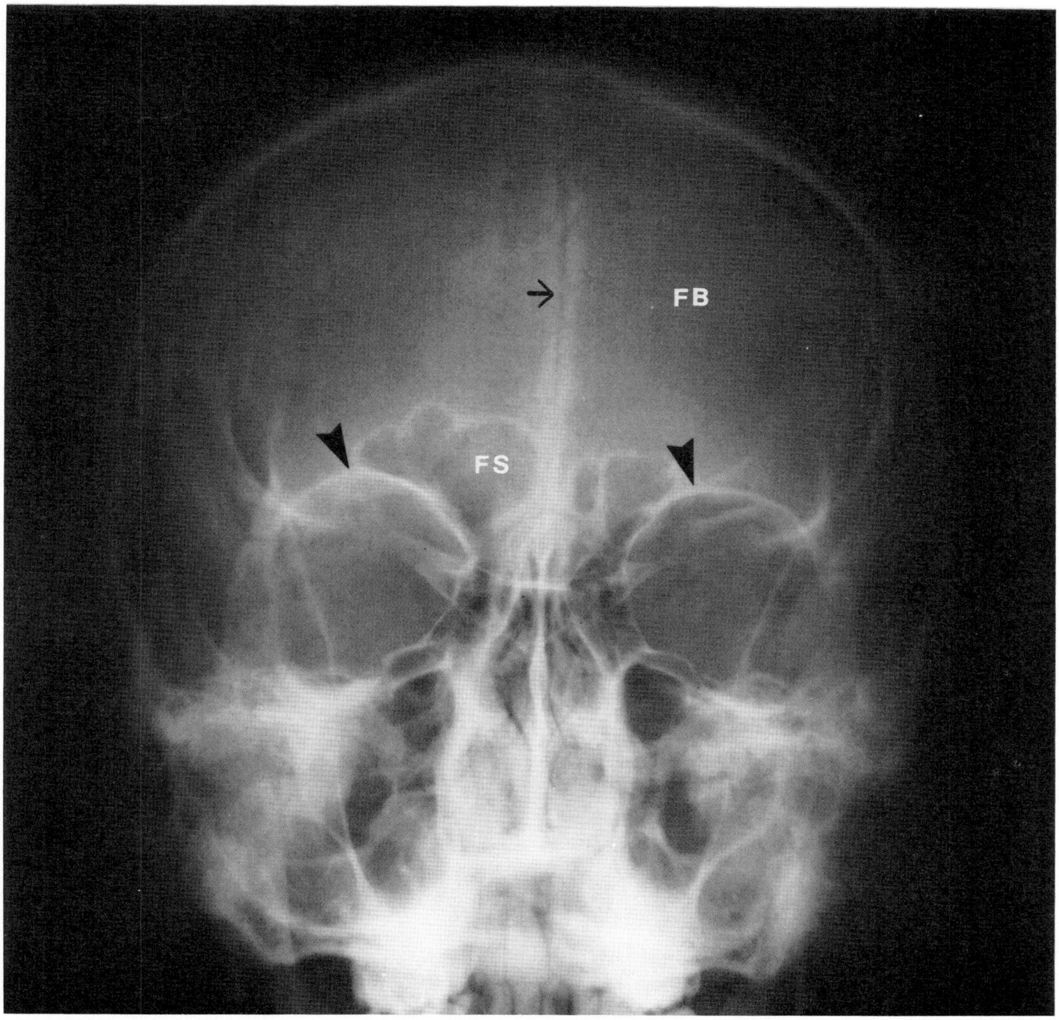

Figure I-19. Frontal projection of the skull. The *arrowhead* points to the roof of the orbit (eye socket). *FS*, frontal sinus; *FB*, frontal bone. The *arrow* indicates a persistent frontal (metopic) suture between the two halves of the frontal bone. Usually union of the halves of this bone begins during the 2nd year and the suture is usually not visible after the 8th year. The remains of this suture are visible in 1 to 2% of adult people (see Fig. 7-1).

moves in an arc or a circle around the body. The amount of radiation absorbed by each different volume element of the chosen plane varies with the amounts of fat, water density tissue, and bone in each element. A multitude of linear energy absorptions is measured and passed to a computer. The computer matches the many linear energy absorptions to each point within the section or plane that is scanned and displays the result on a print-out or on a **CRT** (cathode ray tube).

Nowadays, x-rays for medical diagnosis are produced in a highly evacuated tube containing a hot cathode and a cold anode. The **x-ray tube** and its terminals are enclosed in a *shockproof* and *rayproof* housing which is filled with insulating oil. The terminals of the tube are connected internally to heavily insulated shockproof cables

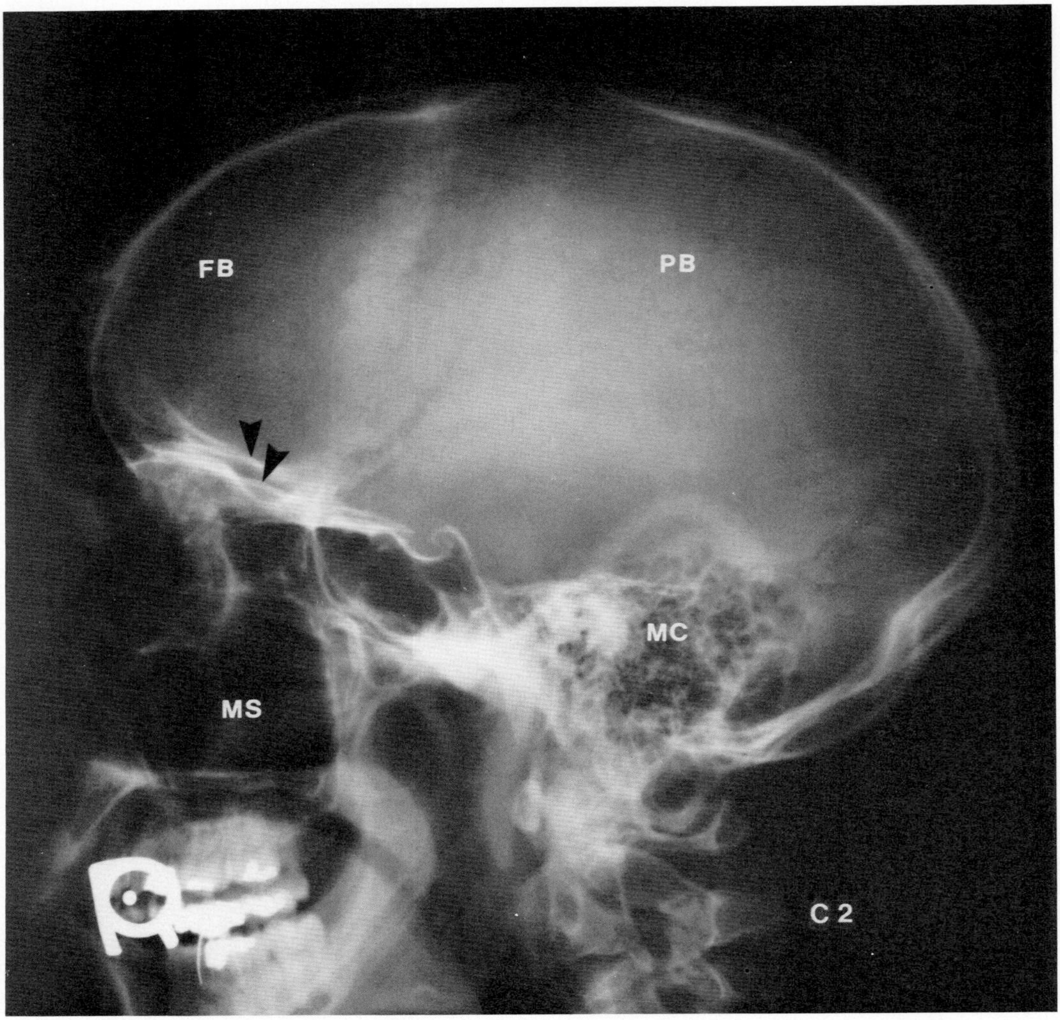

Figure I-20. Lateral projection of the skull with arrows pointing to the roof of each orbit (compare with Fig. I-19). *FB*, frontal bone(s); *PB*, parietal bone(s); *MC*, mastoid air cells; *MS*, maxillary sinus(es). The right and left parietal bones are projected on each other. They can be seen separately if stereo films are made. *C2* is the spinous process of the second cervical vertebra (axis) in the neck. (For other illustrations of the sinuses, see Figs. 7-18 and 7-175).

leading to the **x-ray generator.** The rayproof housing of heavy metal has one small area opposite the anode which is made of radiolucent material, often glass, called the port or **portal.** Through the portal a slightly divergent beam of x-rays emerges. *No x-rays leave the tube housing elsewhere.*

This x-ray beam originates in a heavy metal target, usually tungsten on the anode. The x-rays are produced when electrons from the hot cathode are pulled to the anode by a momentary large potential difference between the anode and the cathode. This potential difference varies from 40 to 150 kv, thus the need for a shockproof housing and cables. As x-rays leave the anode in all directions, a rayproof housing is necessary.

As the **x-ray beam** emerging through the portal is composed of slightly diverging x-rays, structures far from the x-ray film

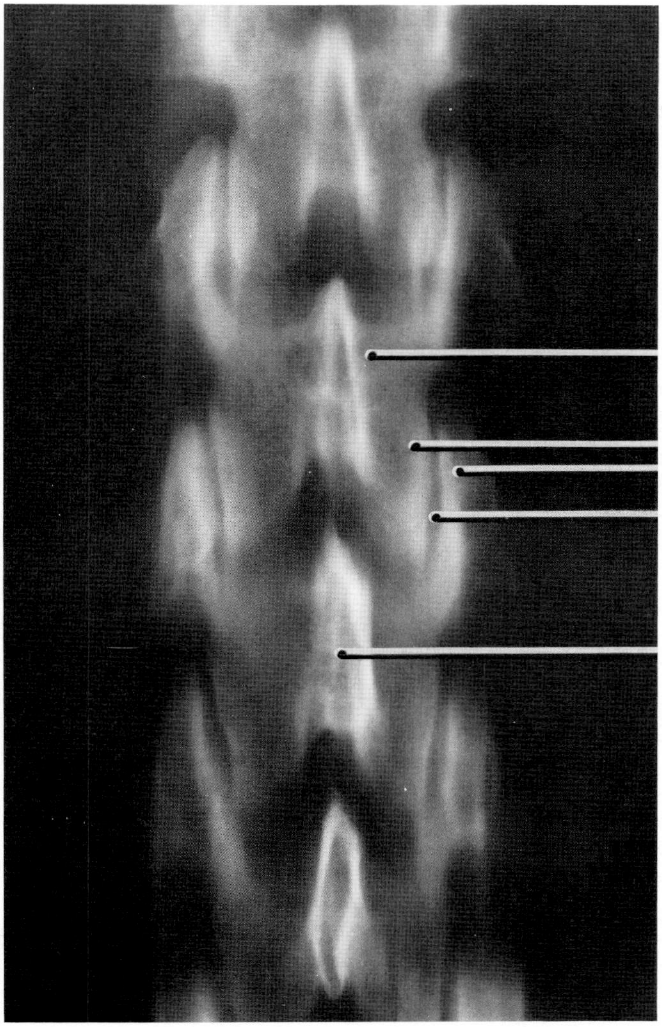

Figure I-21. Tomogram of the arches of the lumbar vertebrae. (For an illustration of the parts of a lumbar vertebra, see Fig. 5-13. For a conventional radiograph of the lumbar region of the vertebral column, see Fig. 5-27*A*.) To make the above tomogram, circular movement of the x-ray tube and x-ray film 180° out of phase with each other was made during the exposure. The images of the vertebral bodies are so blurred that they are invisible. Observe that the image of a vertebral arch has a frog-like appearance. The right and left laminae appear as the trunk of the frog, the superior articular processes resembling arms and the inferior articular processes resembling legs. The clarity of the zygapophyseal joint "spaces" results from the articular cartilages on the opposing articular facets being of soft tissue density. The "spaces" are spaces in the image on the x-ray film, but in the patient they are cartilage filled areas between bones (the articular processes).

will be magnified and may give you an incorrect idea of their size (Fig. I-18). Because some parts of the body are oblique to the x-ray beam when frontal or lateral views are made, their images may be foreshortened, giving you an incorrect idea of their size and shape. The radiologist sometimes makes **oblique projections** (views) of a part of the body to show the image of the part as close as possible to its true shape and size. Oblique projections may also be made to project overlapping images away from the part of greatest interest.

The correct radiological nomenclature

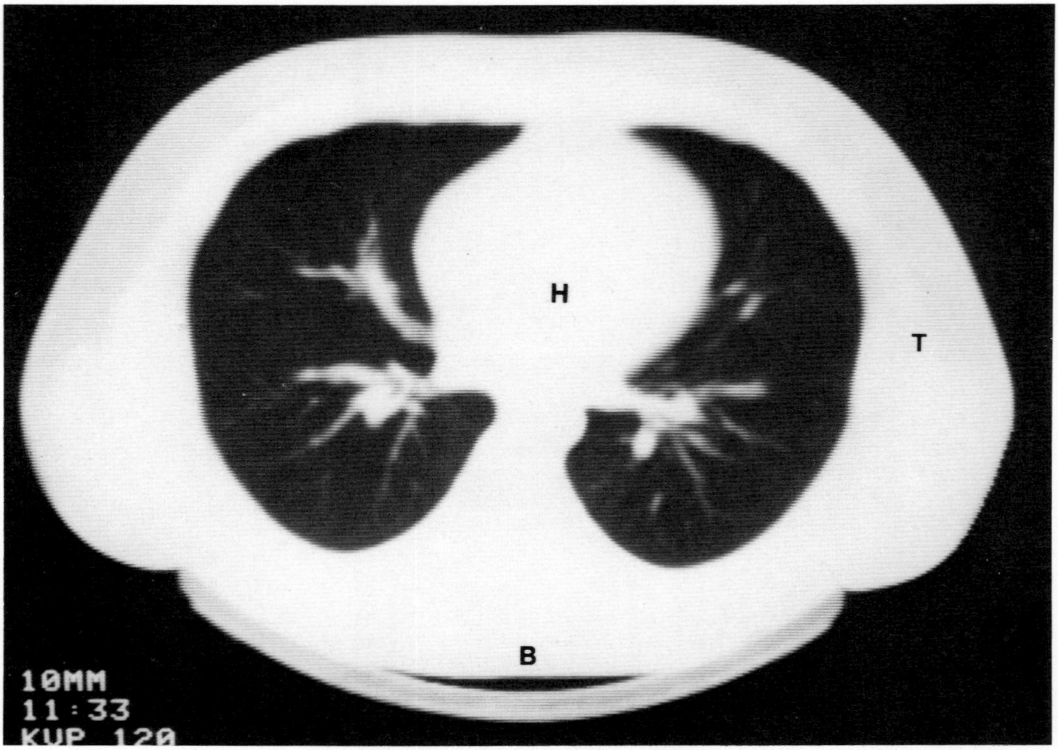

Figure I-22. CT scan of the thorax showing the upper part of the heart (*H*) in the midline anteriorly and bulging to each side. Also observe the arteries (*A*) supplying the lungs. The thoracic wall (*T*) and the back (*B*) appear featureless. In this CT scan, detail within the chest wall is not visualized because the group of linear absorptions chosen for display was for maximum contrast between air-filled lung and soft tissue densities within it, such as pulmonary arteries and tumor nodules.

should be understood. An **AP projection** is one in which the rays traverse the patient from the anterior (**A**) to the posterior (**P**) surfaces of the body. This indicates that the x-ray tube is in front of the patient and that the x-ray film or fluoroscopic screen is behind. The reverse is a **PA projection**; *most frontal chest films are PA projections* (Fig. 1-38). Frontal projection is used for both AP and PA projections. A **left lateral projection** is made with the patient's left side close to the film and a right lateral is made with the right side close to the film. A left anterior oblique (**LAO**) **projection** is made with the patient's left anterior surface against the film, whereas a right posterior oblique (**RPO**) **projection** is made with the patient's right posterior surface against the film. Note that the x-rays pass along the same axis of the patient in both LAO and RPO projections, but that they pass through it in different directions; therefore structures on different sides are magnified to different degrees.

Historical Note. *X-rays were discovered in 1895* by the Professor of Physics at the University of Würzburg, Germany, **Dr. Wilhelm Conrad Röentgen**. He discovered them accidentally while investigating cathode rays (streams of electrons as we now know them) produced in a Crookes tube, a partly evacuated glass bulb containing two electrodes, a cold cathode, and a cold anode. When the cathode and anode are connected to an external source of high voltage, electrons come from the cathode and pass through the thin air in the tube, causing it to glow. They then continue through the walls of the tube to penetrate a few centimeters of air, causing it to become electrically conductive. It had been shown that these cathode rays would also cause darkening of a photographic emulsion, make certain chemicals and minerals fluoresce, and could be deflected by a magnet.

Röentgen had covered his Crookes tube with a jacket of black paper to block out the luminescence produced by the residual air in the tube, darkened the room, and energized the tube. To his surprise, he noticed a screen of barium platinocyanide glowing, even though it was too far away to be reached by cathode rays. He did not ignore his chance observation but gave it some thought. When he realized that a previously unknown radiation of great penetrating power was coming from the tube, he conducted experiments to demonstrate many of the properties and effects of the new kind of "rays" he called **x-rays**.

His first paper, entitled "*On a New Kind of Rays*," published on December 28, 1895, about 6 weeks after his first observation, astounded both the scientific and nonscientific world. An x-ray "picture" of a hand showing images of the bones and joints appeared on the front pages of newspapers all over the world. Many people began to call the new rays "Röentgen rays" in honor of the discoverer, but **Röentgen** modestly refused to use this designation, preferring the term x-ray. Even today you may hear **radiographs** referred to as **roentgenograms.** His discovery stimulated physicists to feverish activity at a time when there seemed little more to discover in nature. For his revolutionary discovery, Dr. Röentgen was awarded the first **Nobel prize** in physics in 1901. Röentgen is only one of many nonmedical persons whose discoveries have led to progress in medicine. **Louis Pasteur** is another.

The discovery of x-rays ushered in a new age in medicine as well as in science in general. For the first time, doctors were able to see the images of bones, joints, some organs, and foreign bodies inside the intact patient. Soon, as contrast materials were developed (materials denser or lighter than body tissues), nearly every organ of the human body could be demonstrated in the living patient. Contrast materials allowed some physiological processes to be followed (*e.g.*, gastric peristalsis after ingesting a barium meal). X-ray examinations thus became dynamic as well as static.

BONES AND JOINTS

The adult **skeleton system** or skeleton (G. dried) consists of over 200 bones which *form the supporting framework of the body.* A few cartilages are also included in the skeletal system (*e.g.*, the **costal cartilages,** connecting the anterior ends of the ribs to the **sternum** or breastbone). The junctions between skeletal components are called **joints** or **articulations;** most of them permit movement.

BONE OR OSSEOUS TISSUE

The study of bones is called **osteology** (G. *osteon*, bone, + *logos*, study). Although the bones studied in the laboratory are lifeless and dry owing to the removal of protein from them, *bones are vital living organs* in your body that will change considerably as you get older. Like other organs, bones have blood vessels, lymph vessels, and nerves, and they may become diseased (*e.g.*, **osteomyelitis** is an inflammation of the bone marrow and the adjacent bone). When broken or fractured, a bone heals. Unused bones **atrophy** (*e.g.*, in a paralyzed limb). Bone may be absorbed, as occurs following the loss or extraction of the teeth when the walls of the sockets disappear (Fig. 7-24). Bones also **hypertrophy** (*i.e.*, become thicker and stronger) when they have increased weight to support.

The bones from different people exhibit considerable anatomical variation. They vary according to age, sex, physical characteristics (**body habitus**), health, diet, race, and with different genetic and endocrinological conditions. *These anatomical variations are useful in identifying skeletal remains*, one aspect of **forensic medicine** (the relation and application of medical facts to legal problems).

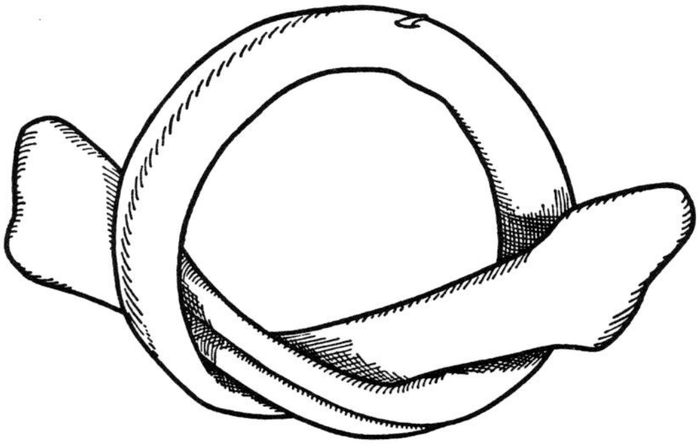

Figure I-23. A decalcified fibula, a long bone of the leg (Fig. 4-65) that has been tied in a knot.

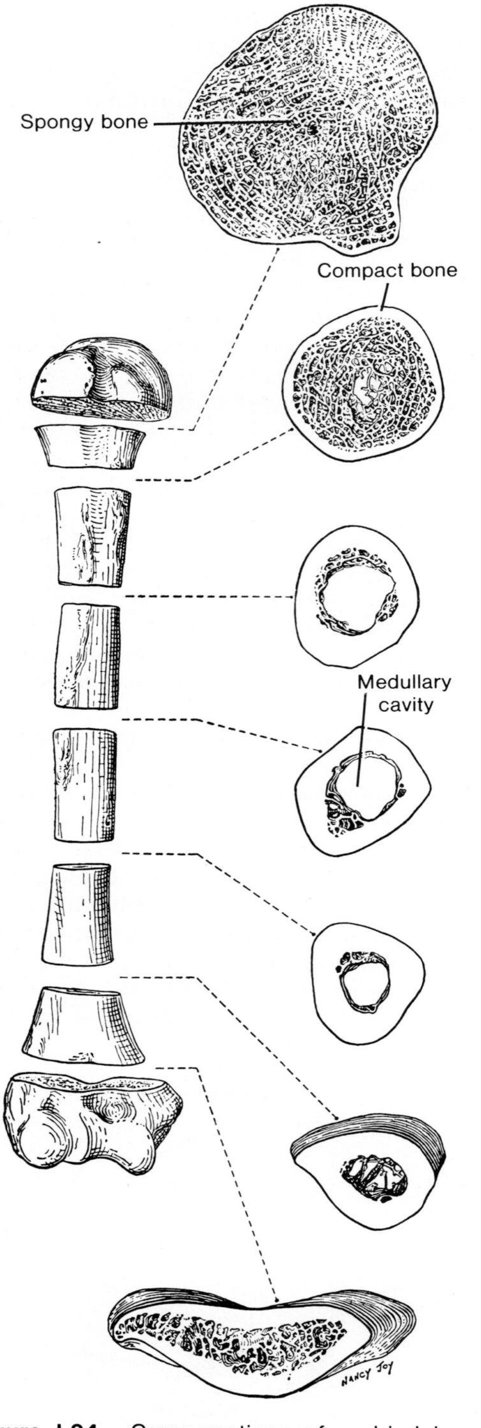

Figure I-24. Cross-sections of a dried long bone (the humerus of the arm, Fig. 6-1). Observe that it consists of an outer shell of compact bone, an inner core of cancellous or spongy bone, and often a medullary (marrow) cavity. These sections demonstrate the variations in thickness of the compact and spongy bone at different levels and at different parts of the same level. The extent of the medullary cavity is also demonstrated.

Living bones are plastic tissues containing organic and inorganic components. They consist essentially of intercellular material impregnated with mineral substances, mainly hydrated calcium phosphate, *i.e.*, $Ca_3(PO_4)_2$. Collagen fibers in the intercellular material give the bones resilience and toughness, whereas the salt crystals in the form of tubes and rods give them hardness and some rigidity. When a bone is decalcified in the laboratory by submerging it in dilute acid for a few days, its salts are removed, but the organic material remains. It retains its shape, but it is so flexible that it can be tied into a knot (Fig. I-23). A bone that is burned also retains its shape, but its fibrous tissue is destroyed. As a result, the bone becomes brittle and inelastic and crumbles easily.

Types of Bone. There are *two main types* of bone, **spongy** (cancellous) and **compact** (dense), but there are no sharp boundaries between the two types of osseous tissue because the differences between them depend upon the relative amount of solid matter and the number and size of the spaces in each of them. *All bones have an outer shell of compact bone around a central mass of cancellous bone,* except where the latter is replaced by a **medullary cavity** (Fig. I-24) or an air space, *e.g.*, the **paranasal air sinuses** (Figs. I-19 and 7-18).

Spongy bone consists of slender, irregular *trabeculae* or bars of compact bone which branch and unite with one another to form intercommunicating spaces that are filled with **bone marrow** (Figs. I-24 and I-30). The trabeculae of the spongy bone are arranged in lines of pressure and tension (Fig. I-25). In radiographs these pressure lines are seen to pass across joints from bone to bone.

Red marrow is active in blood formation (**hematopoiesis**, G. *hemato*, blood, + *poiein*, to form), whereas **yellow marrow**

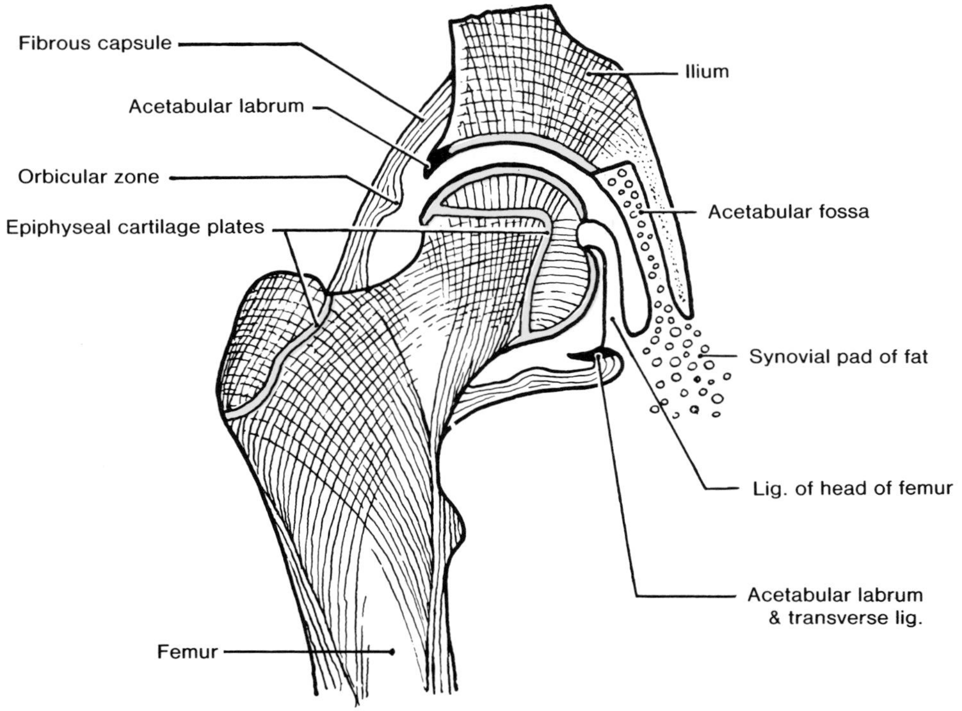

Figure I-25. Drawing of the hip joint in coronal section illustrating the lines of strain and stress. Observe the bony trabeculae of the ilium projected into the head of the femur as lines of pressure and the trabeculae that cross these as lines of tension. Note the epiphyseal cartilage plates of the head and greater trochanter of the femur.

is mainly inert and fatty. In most long bones there is a **medullary cavity** (marrow cavity) in the body or shaft of the bone that contains yellow marrow in adult life.

Compact bone appears solid except for microscopic spaces (Figs. I-24 and I-34). Its crystalline structure gives it hardness and rigidity and makes it opaque to x-rays.

Classification of Bones. Bones may be classified regionally as **axial bones** (skull, vertebrae, ribs, and sternum) or as **appendicular bones** (upper and lower limb bones and those associated with them). Bones are also classified according to their shape.

1. **Long bones** (Figs. I-24 and I-26) are tubular in shape and have a body or shaft and two ends or extremities which are either concave or convex. The length of long bones is greater than their breadth, even though some long bones are quite short (*e.g.*, in the fingers and toes). The ends of long bones articulate with other bones and they are enlarged, smooth, and covered with hyaline cartilage. Usually the **body (shaft)** of a long bone is hollow (**medullary center**) and typically has three borders separating its three surfaces.
2. **Short bones** are cuboidal in shape and are found only in the foot and the wrist, *e.g.*, the carpal or wrist bones (Fig. 6-87). They have six surfaces, four or less of which are articular and two or more for the attachment of tendons and ligaments and for the entry of blood vessels.
3. **Flat bones** consist of two plates of compact bone with spongy bone and marrow between them, *e.g.*, the bones of the skullcap, the sternum, and the scapula (except for the thin part of this bone). The marrow space between the tables (external and internal cortices) of flat bones in the skull (Fig. 7-

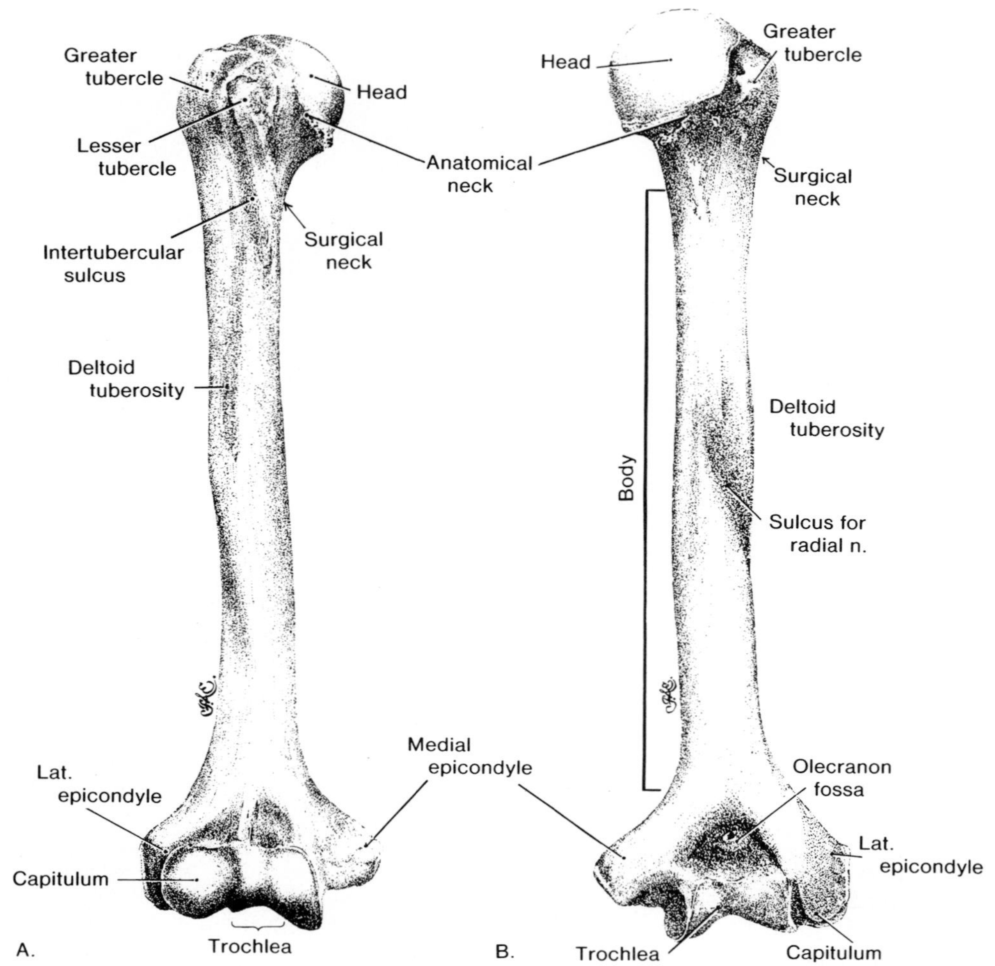

Figure I-26. Drawings of the right humerus showing its features. Note that the articular condyle (G. knuckle) is divided by a ridge into two parts, the capitulum and the trochlea (L. pulley). *A*, anterior view. *B*, posterior view.

43*A*) is known as **diploë** (G. double). *Most flat bones help to form the walls of cavities* (*e.g.*, the cranial cavity); hence, most of them are gently curved rather than flat. In early life a flat bone consists of a thin plate of compact bone but marrow (*e.g.*, the diploë) appears in it during childhood, resulting in compact plates on each side of the spongy medullary or marrow cavity.

4. **Irregular bones** have various shapes (*e.g.*, the facial bones and the vertebrae). The bodies of vertebrae (Fig. 5-12) possess some of the features of long bones.
5. **Pneumatic bones** contain air cells or sinuses (*e.g.*, **mastoid air cells** in the mastoid part of the temporal bone (Figs. I-20 and 7-72) and the **paranasal air sinuses** (Fig. 7-18). Outgrowths (evaginations) of the mucous membrane of the middle ear and of the nasal cavities invade the marrow space, producing the air cells and sinuses, respectively.
6. **Sesamoid bones** are round or oval nodules of bone (Figs. 4-70 and 4-101)

that develop in certain tendons (*e.g.*, the **patella**, or kneecap in the quadriceps femoris tendon, Fig. 4-125, and the **pisiform** in the tendon of the flexor carpi ulnaris muscle, Fig. 6-133). They received their name because of the resemblance of the very small sesamoid bones to **sesame seeds.** *Sesamoid bones are commonly found where tendons cross the ends of long bones* in the limbs (*e.g.*, at the knee, Fig. 4-124, and the wrist, Fig. 6-133). Not only do they *protect the tendon from excessive wear*, but they *change the angle of the tendon* as it passes to its insertion. This results in a greater mechanical advantage at the joint. The articular surface of a sesamoid bone is covered with articular cartilage, whereas the rest of it is buried in the tendon and may be attached to the fibrous capsule of the joint concerned (Figs. 4-101 and 4-125).

7. **Accessory (supernumerary) bones** develop when an additional ossification center appears, giving rise to a bone, or one of the usual centers fails to fuse with the main bone. The separated part of the bone gives the appearance of an extra bone. *Accessory bones are common in the foot* and it is important to know about them so that they will not be mistaken for fractures in radiographs.

Bone Markings (Figs. I-26, 4-1, and 5-12). The surface of bones is not smooth and glossy or even in contour, except over areas covered by cartilage and where tendons, blood vessels, and nerves move in grooves (*e.g.*, the **intertubercular sulcus** in the head of the humerus and the **sulcus for the radial nerve** in its body, Fig. I-26*B*). *Bones display a variety of bumps, depressions, and holes.* Markings appear on dried bones wherever tendons, ligaments, and fascia were attached. The attachment of the fleshy fibers of a muscle make no markings on a bone. Bone markings become prominent during **puberty** (12 to 16 years) and become progressively more marked as adulthood occurs. The surface features of bones are given names to help distinguish them.

Elevations (Fig. I-26). The various kinds of elevation that are visible on bones are listed in order of prominence. Examine each type on the bones of a skeleton.

A linear elevation is referred to as a **line** (*e.g.*, the *superior nuchal line* of the occipital bone, Fig. 7-8) or a **ridge** (*e.g.*, the *medial supracondylar ridge*, Fig. 6-1). Very prominent ridges are called **crests** (*e.g.*, the *iliac crest*, Fig. 4-1).

A rounded elevation (Fig. I-26) is called (1) a **tubercle** (small raised eminence); (2) a **protuberance** (swelling or knob, *e.g.*, *external occipital protuberance*, Fig. 7-3); (3) a **trochanter** (large blunt elevation, *e.g.*, the *greater trochanter* of the femurs Fig. 4-1); (4) a **tuberosity** or **tuber** (large elevation); and (5) a **malleolus** (a hammerhead-like elevation, Fig. 4-65).

A sharp elevation or projecting part is called a **spine** (L. *spina*, a thorn), *e.g*, the *anterior superior iliac spine* (Fig. 4-1), or a **process** (L. to go forward), *e.g.*, the *spinous process (spine) of a vertebra* (Fig. 5-12).

Facets (F. little faces). The term facet is used by gem cutters to describe the small, cut, polished surfaces of a precious stone. In anatomy the term facet is applied to a small, smooth, flat area or surface of a bone, especially where it articulates with another bone (Fig. 4-125). Facets covered with hyaline (articular) cartilage are called **articular facets** (*e.g.*, of vertebra, Fig. 5-21).

A rounded articular area of a bone is called a **head** (*e.g.*, the *head of the humerus*, Fig. I-26) or a **condyle** (G. knuckle), *e.g.*, the *lateral condyle* of the femur (Fig. 4-1). An **epicondyle** (G. *epi*, upon) is a prominent process just above a condyle (Fig. I-26).

Depressions (Fig. I-26). Small hollows in bones are described as pits or **fossae** (L. pits), whereas long narrow depressions are referred to as grooves or **sulci** (L. furrows or ditches). An indentation at the edge of a bone is called a notch or **incisura** (L. a cutting into). When a notch is bridged by a ligament or by bone to form a perforation or hole, it is called a **foramen** (*e.g.*, the *foramen magnum*, Fig. 7-52). A foramen that has length is called a **canal** (*e.g.*, the *facial canal*, Fig. 7-185). A canal has an

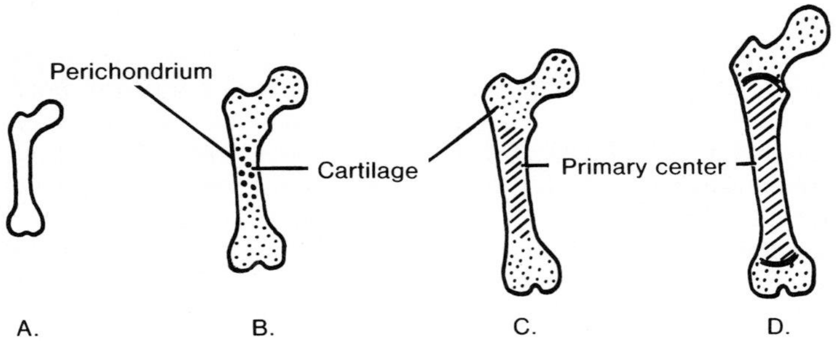

Figure I-27. Drawings illustrating the prenatal development of a long bone during the first 6 months. *A*, the mesenchymal model, 5 weeks. *B*, the cartilage model, 6 weeks. *C* and *D*, the beginning of ossification, 7 to 12 weeks. Ossification begins in long bones by the end of the embryonic period; *i.e.*, primary centers of ossification have appeared. By 12 weeks primary centers have appeared in nearly all limb bones.

orifice (opening, ostium) at each end, but a **meatus** (L. a passage) is a canal that enters a structure but does not pass through it, *e.g.*, the *external acoustic meatus* or ear canal (Figs. 7-7 and 7-180).

Development of Bones (Fig. I-27). *Bones develop from condensations of mesenchyme* (embryonic connective tissue). The mesenchymal model of a bone which forms during the embryonic period may undergo direct ossification (**intramembranous ossification** or membranous bone formation), or it may be replaced by a densely cellular *cartilage model* which later becomes ossified by **intracartilaginous ossification** or endochondral bone formation. *Simply, bone replaces membrane or cartilage.* The process of ossification is similar in each case and the final histological structure of the bone is identical.

Intramembranous ossification occurs rapidly and takes place in bones that are urgently required for protection (*e.g.*, the flat bones of the skullcap). Intracartilaginous ossification, occurring in most of the skeleton, is a much slower process.

Development of Long Bones (Figs. I-27 to I-30). The first indication of ossification in the cartilaginous model of a long bone is visible near the center of the future shaft. This is called the diaphyseal or **primary center of ossification.** Primary centers appear at different times in different developing bones, but *most primary centers appear between the 7th and 12th* weeks of prenatal life. Virtually all of them are present by birth. By this time, ossification from the primary center has almost reached the ends of the cartilage model of the long bone (Fig. I-28). *The part of a bone ossified from a primary center is called the* **diaphysis** (G. *dia*, through, + *physis*, growth).

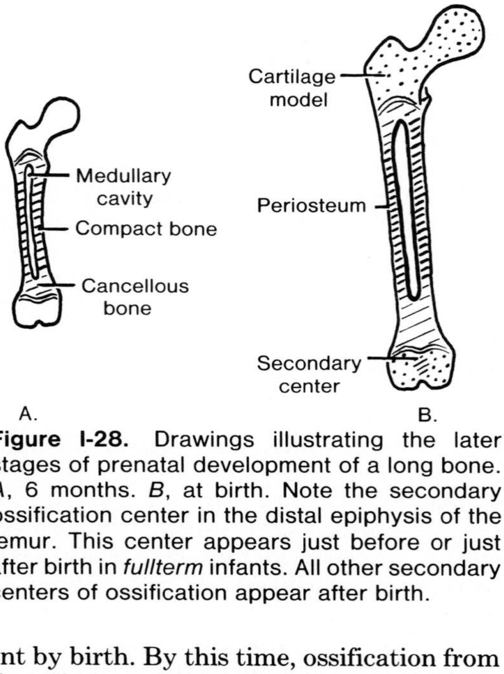

Figure I-28. Drawings illustrating the later stages of prenatal development of a long bone. *A*, 6 months. *B*, at birth. Note the secondary ossification center in the distal epiphysis of the femur. This center appears just before or just after birth in *fullterm* infants. All other secondary centers of ossification appear after birth.

Around birth an additional ossification center may appear in the cartilaginous end of a long bone. This is referred to as the epiphyseal or **secondary center of ossification** (Fig. I-28). *Most secondary centers of ossification appear after birth.* The part of a bone ossified from a secondary center is called the **epiphysis** (G. *epi*, upon,

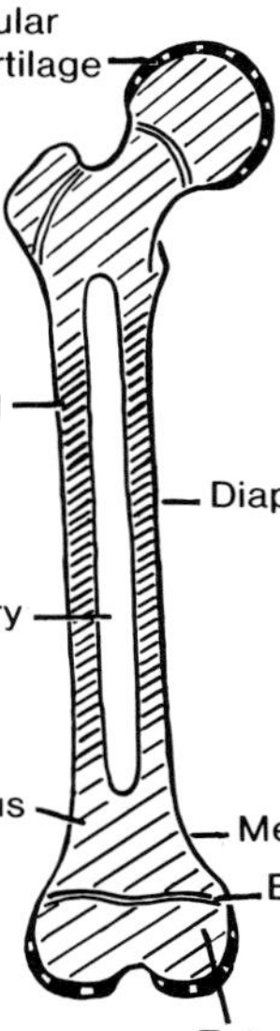

Figure I-29. Drawing illustrating the growth of a long bone (the femur) during childhood. In freely movable joints the ends of the bones are capped with cartilage that is called articular cartilage. It provides smooth slippery surfaces where the bones of the joint meet so that friction is minimized.

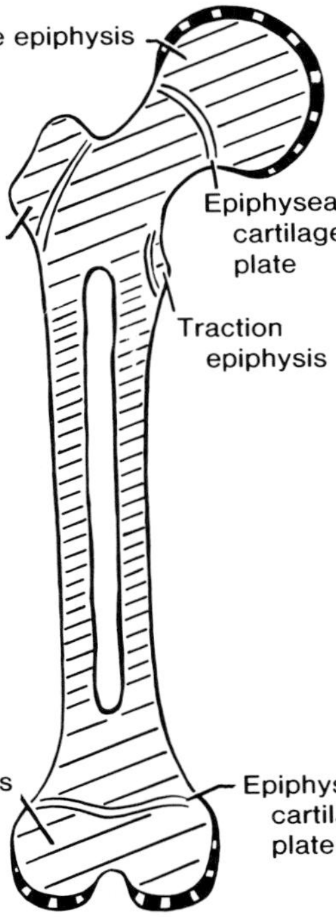

Figure I-30. Drawing of a young long bone (the femur) illustrating the types of epiphysis. The epiphyseal cartilage plate provides for the longitudinal growth of the bone.

+ *physis*, growth). The secondary ossification centers of the bones at the knee (lower femur and upper tibia, Fig. 4-1) are the first to appear. They may be present at birth in a fullterm infant.

The cartilage at the bone ends, **the epiphyses**, undergoes much the same change that occurs in the diaphysis, as you will learn in histology. As a result, the body or shaft of the bone becomes capped at each end by bone that is developing from the secondary centers (Fig. I-29).

The part of the **diaphysis** (body) nearest the **epiphysis** is referred to as the **metaphysis** (G. *meta*, beyond, + *physis*, growth). *The diaphysis grows in length by proliferation of cartilage at the metaphysis.* To enable growth in length to continue until the adult length of a bone is attained, the bone formed from the primary center in the diaphysis does not fuse with that formed from the secondary centers in the epiphysis until the adult size of the bone is reached. During growth a plate of cartilage, known as the growth plate or **epiphyseal cartilage plate**, intervenes between the diaphysis and the epiphysis (Figs. I-28 and I-29).

The **diaphysis** consists of a hollow tube of compact bone surrounding the medullary (marrow) cavity, whereas the epiphyses and metaphyses consist of spongy (cancellous) bone covered by a thin layer of compact bone (Fig. I-24). The compact bone over the articular surfaces of the epiphyses is covered with **hyaline cartilage** (Figs. I-29 and I-30). Hyaline (G. *hyalos*, glass) cartilage is pure cartilage and was given its name because of its pearly white, somewhat translucent, glassy appearance.

During the first two postnatal years, secondary ossification centers appear in many epiphyses that will be exposed to pressure (*e.g.*, at the knee and the hip, Fig. I-30). These centers, often referred to as **pressure epiphyses**, are located at the ends of long bones where they are subjected to pressure from opposing bone at the joint which they form. Some secondary ossification centers ossify parts of bone associated with the attachment of muscles and strong tendons. These centers are often referred to as **traction epiphyses** (*e.g.*, the tubercles of the humerus, Fig. I-26, and the tuberosities of the femur, Figs. I-30 and 4-1). These epiphyses are subjected to traction rather than pressure. As most of them do not enter into the formation of a joint, they do not contribute to the longitudinal growth of the bones concerned.

Atavistic epiphyses may represent parts of bones that were separate in some earlier evolutionary stage. The **coracoid process** of the scapula (Figs. I-31 and 6-1) is formed by a small ossification center that is thought to have given rise to a separate bone in earlier vertebrates.

The epiphyseal cartilage plate is eventually replaced by bone development at each of its two sides, diaphyseal and epiphyseal (Fig. I-32). When this occurs, growth of the bone ceases and the diaphysis has fused with the epiphysis by bony union or **synostosis** (G. *syn*, with, together + *osteon*, bone, + *osis*, condition). The bone formed at the site of the epiphyseal cartilage plate is particularly dense and is still recognizable on the radiographs of young and even middle-aged adults. Knowledge of this prevents their confusion with fracture lines.

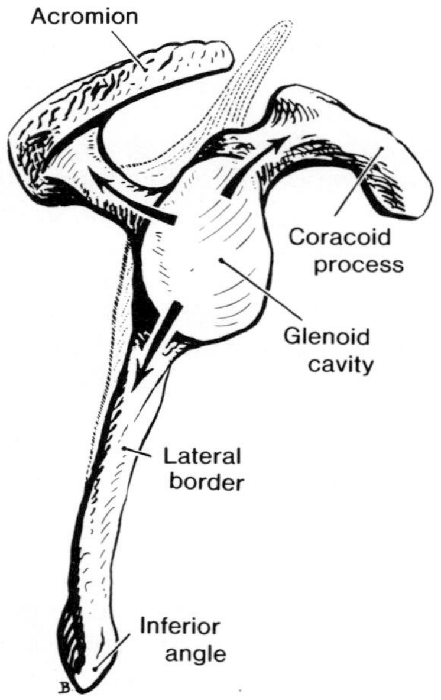

Figure I-31. Drawing of an anterolateral view of the right scapula. The coracoid process, which is ossified by a separate center, is an example of an atavistic epiphysis.

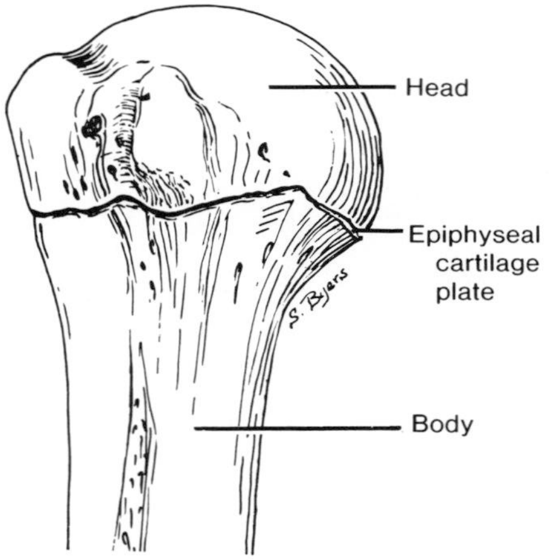

Figure I-32. Drawing of the proximal end of the humerus of a 19-year-old man, just before fusion of the epiphysis with the diaphysis. Observe the thin layer of cartilage (epiphyseal cartilage plate) which is responsible for allowing the body (shaft) of the bone to lengthen until full growth is obtained.

In general, the epiphysis of a long bone whose center of ossification is the last to appear is the first to fuse with the diaphysis. When an epiphysis forms from more than one center (*e.g.*, the proximal end of the humerus), the centers fuse with each other before union of the epiphysis occurs with the diaphysis.

Development of Short Bones. The development of short bones is similar to that of the primary center of long bones and only one, the calcaneus (Fig. 4-71), develops a secondary center of osssification (epiphysis).

Blood Supply of Long Bones (Fig. I-33). Bones are richly supplied with blood vessels that pass into them from the **periosteum**, the fibrous connective tissue membrane investing them, except at the articular surfaces. Near the center of the body of a long bone, a **nutrient artery** passes obliquely through the compact bone.

Some pressure epiphyses are largely covered by hyaline **articular cartilage** (Figs. I-29, I-30, and I-33). They receive their

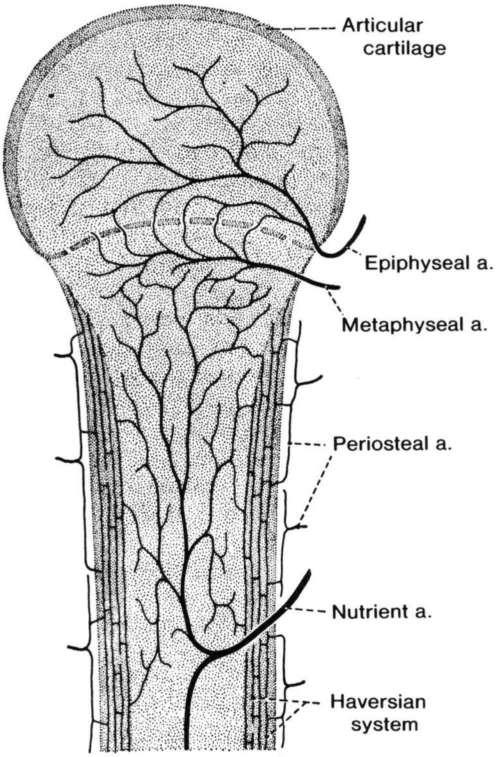

Figure I-33. Schematic drawing of part of a long bone illustrating its blood supply.

blood supply from the region of the epiphyseal cartilage plate. These pressure epiphyses (*e.g.*, the head of the femur) are almost completely covered by articular cartilage (Fig. I-29) and receive their blood supply from vessels that penetrate just outside the edge of the articular cartilage.

Nerve Supply of Bones. The periosteum of bones is rich in sensory nerves, called **periosteal nerves**. Hence, pain from injured bones is usually severe. The nerves that accompany the arteries into the bones are probably **vasomotor** (*i.e.*, ones causing constriction or dilation of the vessels).

CLINICALLY ORIENTED COMMENTS

Loss of blood supply to an epiphysis or to other parts of a bone results in *death of bone tissue*, a condition referred to as **avascular necrosis** (ischemic or aseptic necrosis) of bone. After every fracture adjacent minute areas of bone undergo avascular necrosis. In a few fractures, there may be avascular necrosis of a large fragment of bone if its blood supply has been cut off. A number of clinical disorders of epiphyses in children result from avascular necrosis of unknown etiology (cause). They are referred to as **osteochondroses** and usually involve a pressure epiphysis at the end of a long bone (*e.g.*, the head of the femur).

Architecture of Bones. The structure of a bone varies according to its function. In long bones, designed for rigidity and for providing attachments for muscles and ligaments, compact bone is relatively greatest in amount near the midshaft (Fig. I-24) and where it is liable to buckle, *e.g.*, the concavity of a bend. The compact bone of the shaft or body provides strength architecturally for weight bearing. In addition, as described previously, long bones have elevations (lines, ridges, crests, tubercles, and tuberosities) that serve as buttresses wherever heavy muscles attach (Fig. I-26).

Living bones have some elasticity (flexibility) and great rigidity (hardness). Their elasticity results from their organic matter (fibrous tissue) and their rigidity results from their lamellae and tubes of inorganic calcium phosphate. The salts, representing about 60% of the weight of a bone, are deposited in the matrix of the collagenous connective element of the bone. *Bones are like hardwood in resisting tension and like concrete in resisting compression.*

Inside the outer shell of **compact bone**, particularly at the ends of long bones, is **spongy bone** that has a trellis-like appearance (Figs. I-24 and I-34). Spongy bone is not laid down in a haphazard fashion but is composed of tubes and lamellae (L. plates) which are arranged like struts along lines of pressure and tension (Fig. I-25 and I-34). *The architecture of these bony trabeculae is distinctive for each person,* a fact of value in identifying skeletal remains, which is an important part of forensic medicine.

Functions of Bones. The main functions of bones are to provide:

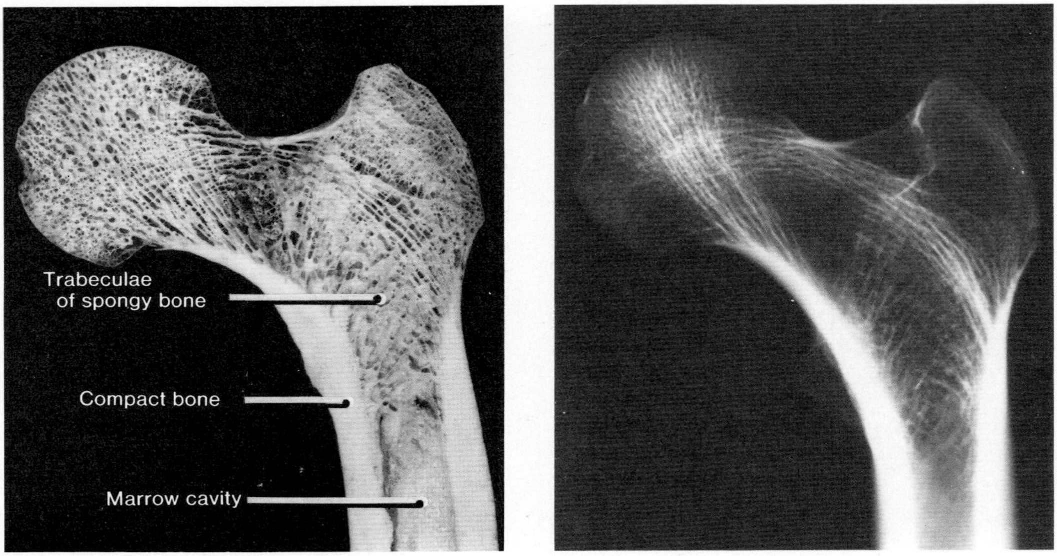

A. B.

Figure I-34. *A*, photograph of a coronal section of the proximal end of the femur showing its bony trabeculae and its lines of pressure and tension. *B*, radiograph of this bone showing the same lines.

1. **Protection** by forming the rigid walls of cavities (*e.g.*, the *cranial cavity* that contains vital structures).
2. **Support** (*i.e.*, the rigid framework) for the body.
3. **A mechanical basis for movement** by providing attachments for muscles and serving as levers for ones that produce the movements permitted by the joints.
4. **Blood cells.** The bone marrow in the ends of long bones, in ribs, in vertebrae, and in the diploë of the flat bones of the skull (Fig. 7-43*A*) are the sites for the development of red blood cells, some lymphocytes, granulocytic white cells, and platelets of the blood.
5. **A store of salts.** The calcium, phosphorous, and magnesium salts in bones provide a mineral reservoir for the body.

CLINICALLY ORIENTED COMMENTS

The relative amount of organic to inorganic matter in bones varies with age. Organic matter is greatest in childhood; hence, the bones of children will bend somewhat. In some metabolic disturbances such as **rickets** and **osteomalacia** there is inadequate calcification of the matrix of bones. As calcium provides the hardness to bones, the uncalcified areas bend, particularly if they are weight-bearing bones, resulting in progressive deformities (Fig. I-35).

Although the diagnosis of rickets is suggested by clinical enlargement at the sites of the **epiphyseal cartilage plates**, the diagnosis is confirmed by the typical radiographic changes that occur in the growing ends of the long bones and ribs in these patients.

Fractures are more common in children than adults owing to the combination of their slender bones and carefree activities. Fortunately many of these breaks are hairline, buckle, or green-stick fractures that are not so serious. In a green-stick fracture, the bone breaks like a willow bough. However, epiphyseal cartilage plate fractures are serious because they may result in premature fusion of the diaphysis and the epiphysis with subsequent shortening of the

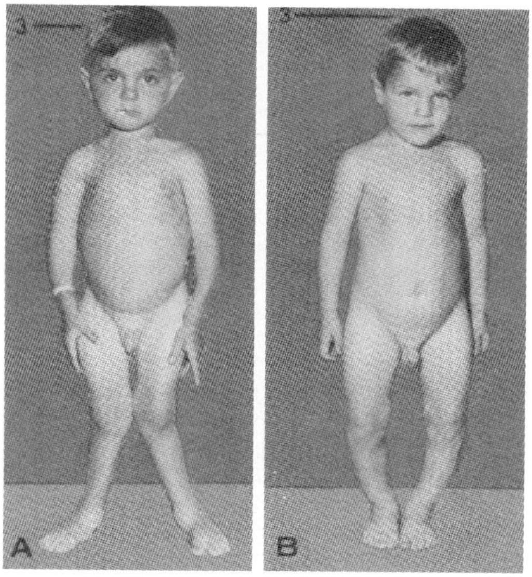

Figure I-35. Photographs of boys with rickets. *A*, genu valgum (knock-knee) in a 5-year-old with vitamin D-refractory rickets. Note the enlargement at the sites of epiphyseal cartilage plates (*e.g.*, ankles and knees). *B*, genu varum (bowleg) in a 4-year-old with a similar condition. Note their short stature (about 3 feet).

bone; *e.g.*, premature fusion of a radial epiphysis results in progressive radial deviation of the hand as the ulna continues to grow. The existence of unfused epiphyses in young people can be helpful in treating them; *e.g.*, placing staples across the epiphyseal cartilage plate at the knee will arrest growth in the lower limb. Understand that it is the normal leg bones that are stapled in order to permit the bones of the short leg to catch up.

Fortunately fractures heal more rapidly in children than in adults. A femoral shaft fracture occurring at birth is united in 3 weeks, whereas union takes up to 20 weeks in persons 20 years and older. During old age both the organic and inorganic components of bone decrease, producing a condition called **osteoporosis** (G. *osteon*, bone, + *poros*, pore). There is a reduction in the quantity of bone (**atrophy of skeletal tissue**) and as a result the bones of old people lose their elasticity and fracture easily. For example, elderly people may catch a foot on a slight projection while walking, feel and hear the neck of their femur (thigh bone) snap, and fall to the ground. *Fractures of the upper femur are especially common in elderly females* because osteoporosis is more severe in them than in elderly males. For a typical case of a fracture of the upper femur, see Case 4-1 at the end of Chapter 4. Doctors and dentists, especially radiologists, pediatricians, orthodontists, and orthopaedic surgeons, must be knowledgeable about bone growth. *The time of appearance of the various epiphyses varies with chronologic age.* As good reference tables are available, it is not useful to memorize the dates of appearance and disappearance of the ossification centers for all bones.

A radiologist determines the bone age of a person by assessing ossifiication centers. Two criteria are used: (1) *the appearance of calcified material in the diaphysis and/or epiphyses*; the time of its appearance is specific for each epiphysis and diaphysis of each bone for each sex; and (2) *the disappearance of the dark line representing the epiphyseal cartilage plate.* This indicates that the epiphysis has fused to the diaphysis and occurs at specific times for each epiphysis. *Fusion occurs 1 to 2 years earlier in females than in males.* Determination of bone age is often used in determining the approximate age of human skeletal remains in medicolegal cases.

Some diseases speed up and others slow down ossification times as compared to the chronological age of the individual. The growing skeleton is sensitive to relatively slight and transient illnesses and to periods of **malnutrition**. Proliferation of cartilage at the metaphysis slows down during starvation and illness, but degeneration of cartilage cells in the columns continues, producing a dense line of provisional calcification which later becomes bone with thicker trabeculae, called **lines of arrested growth** (Fig. I-36).

Without a basic knowledge of bone growth and the appearance of bones on radiographs at various ages, *an epiphyseal cartilage plate could be mistaken for a fracture*, and separation of an epiphysis could be interpreted as normal (Fig. I-37).

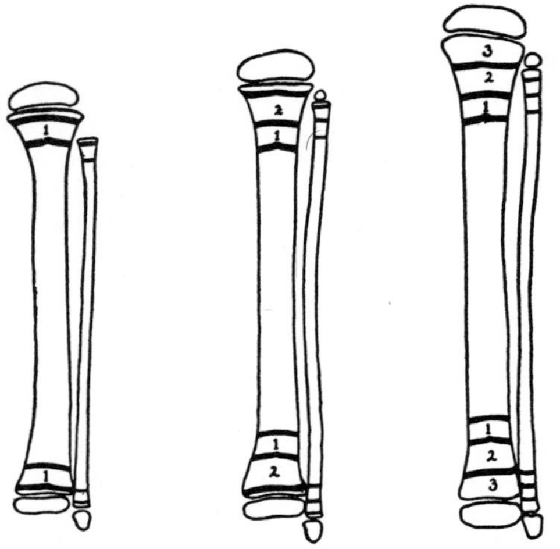

Figure I-36. Outlines of three radiographs of the leg bones of a young girl taken over a period of 2 years. Observe that the three lines of arrested growth, denoting three successive illnesses, remain equidistant.

If you know the age of a patient and the location of the epiphyses, these errors can be avoided, especially if you note that the edges of the diaphysis and epiphysis are smoothly curved in the region of the epiphyseal cartilage. A fracture leaves a sharp, often uneven edge of bone. An injury that causes a fracture in an adult may cause displacement of an epiphysis in a young person (Fig. I-37).

JOINTS OR ARTICULATIONS

The **articular system**, consisting of the articulations or joints where two or more bones are related to one another at their region of contact, is often considered to be a part of the **skeletal system**. The study of joints is called **arthrology** (G. *arthros*, joint, + *logos*, study). Joints with little or no movement are classified according to the type of material holding the bones together. In joints where bones move freely, the only tissue joining the bones is the **fibrous capsule** with its lining of *synovial membrane* (Fig. I-38).

Fibrous Joints. The bones involved in these articulations are *united by fibrous tissue*. The amount of movement permitted at the joint depends on the length of the fibers uniting the bones.

Sutures (Figs. I-38, I-39, and 7-4). The bones are separated yet held together by a thin layer of fibrous tissue. The union is extremely tight and there is little or no movement between the bones. *Sutures occur only in the skull*; hence they are sometimes referred to as "skull type" joints. The edges of the bones may overlap (**squamous type**) or interlock in a jigsaw fashion (**serrate type**).

In the skull of a newborn infant, the growing bones of the skullcap do not make full contact with each other (Fig. I-39). At places where contact does not occur, the sutures are wide areas of fibrous tissue known as **fonticuli** or **fontanelles**. The terms *fonticuli* (L.) and *fontanelles* (F.) mean little springs or fountains. Probably they were given this name because in earlier times openings may have been made in the skull at these points in infants with bulging fontanelles resulting from high intracranial pressure. In these cases, the spurting cerebrospinal fluid (CSF) and blood that would well out probably reminded them of a spring of water. The most prominent of these is the **anterior fonticulus** (**anterior fontanelle**). The separation of the bones at the sutures and fontanelles of the newborn skull allow them to overlap each other during birth, permitting the infant's head to pass through the birth canal (Figs. 3-22 and 3-106). *The anterior fontanelle is not present in* normal children after 18 to 24 months (*i.e.*, it is the same width as the adjacent parts of the sutures). Union of the bones at the **pterion** (Fig. 7-7), located at the site of the anterolateral fontanelle (Fig. I-39B), has taken place by 6 years in about 50% of children.

Complete fusion of the bones across the suture lines (**synostosis**) begins on the inner side of the skullcap during the early 20s and progresses throughout life. Nearly all sutures of the skull are obliterated in very old people.

Syndesmosis (G. *syndesmos*, ligament). In this type of fibrous joint, *the two bones are united by a sheet of fibrous tissue*. The tissue may be a ligament or an interosseous fibrous membrane; *e.g.*, the interosseous

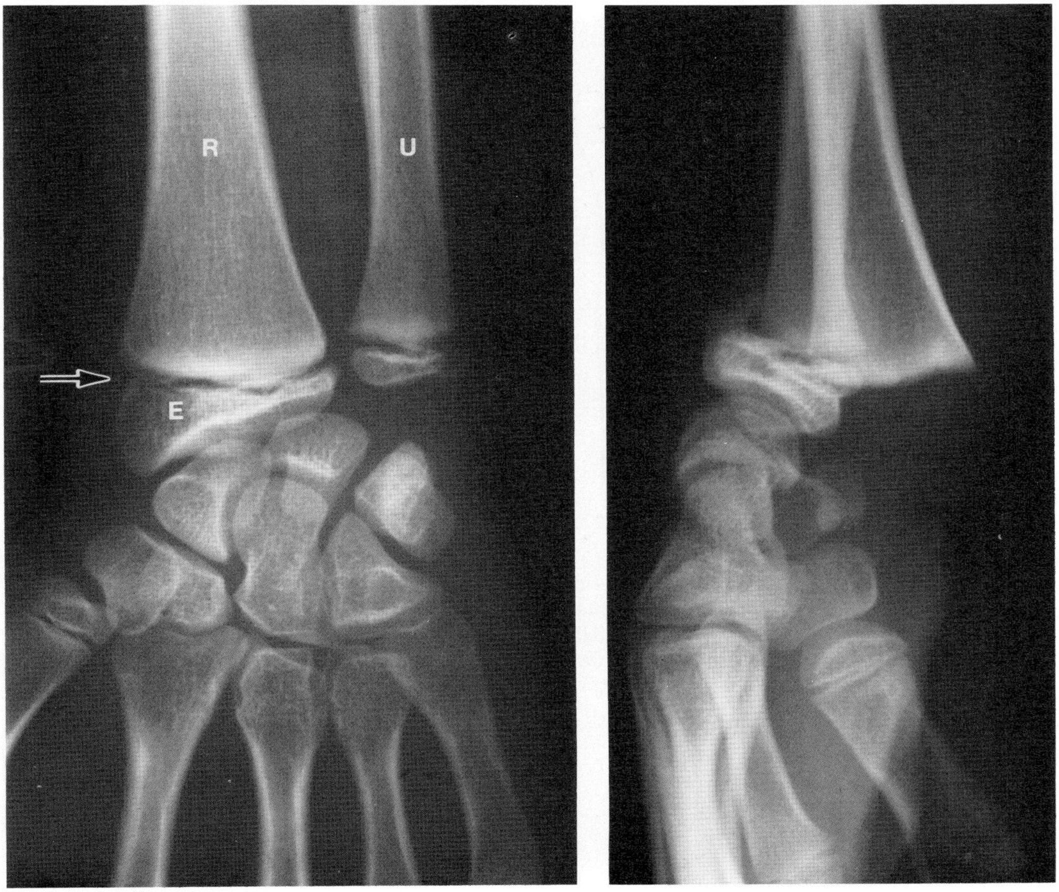

A B

Figure I-37. Radiographs of the wrist. *R*, radius; *U*, ulna; *E*, epiphysis at the distal end of the radius. The *arrow* indicates the site of the epiphyseal cartilage plate. *A*, frontal projection of the left wrist showing the apparently normal position of the epiphyses at the distal ends of the radius and ulna. *B*, lateral projection of the right wrist showing dorsal displacement of the epiphysis at the distal end of the radius. A fragment of the posterior cortex of the shaft of the radius is also broken off. As growth of this bone depends on a normally functioning epiphyseal cartilage plate, treatment involves replacing the epiphysis in its normal position.

border of the radius is attached to the interosseous border of the ulna by an **interosseous membrane** (Figs. I-38 and 6-167). In syndesmoses, slight to considerable movement can be achieved. The degree of movement depends upon the distance between the bones and the degree of flexibility of the uniting fibrous tissue. The interosseous membrane between the radius and ulna of the forearm is broad enough and sufficiently flexible to allow considerable movement, such as occurs during pronation and supination of the forearm (Fig. I-17).

Cartilaginous Joints (Fig. I-40). The bones involved in these articulations are *united by cartilage.*

Primary Cartilaginous Joints (Synchondroses). The bones in these joints are united by **hyaline cartilage**, which permits slight bending during early life. **Synchondroses** usually represent temporary conditions, *e.g.*, during the period of endo-

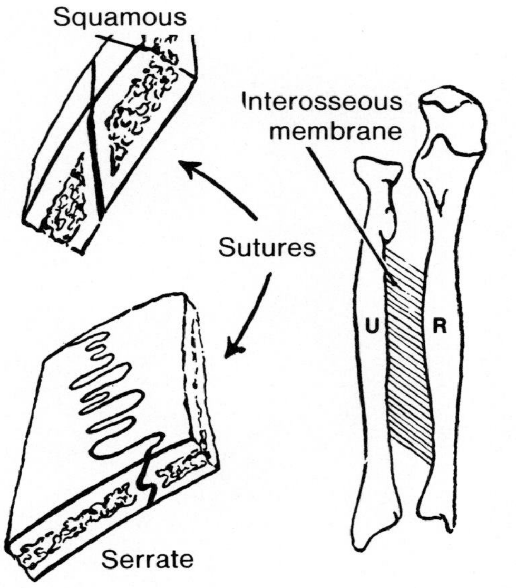

Figure I-38. Drawings illustrating the various types of fibrous joint. The interosseous membrane joining the radius (*R*) and the ulna (*U*) of the forearm is strong but relatively thin (Fig. 6-167). The leg bones are similarly joined (Figs. 4-64 and 4-74).

chondral development of a long bone. As previously described, an **epiphyseal cartilage plate** separates the ends (epiphyses) and the body (diaphysis) of a long bone (Fig. I-40*A*). *This joint permits growth in the length of the bone.* When full growth is achieved, the cartilage is converted into bone and the epiphysis becomes fused with the diaphysis; *i.e.*, a **synchondrosis** is converted into a **synostosis**. Other synchondroses are permanent, *e.g.*, where the costal cartilage of the first rib joins it to the manubrium of the sternum (Fig. I-40*B*).

Secondary Synchondroses (Symphyses). The articular surfaces of the bones in these joints are covered by **hyaline cartilage** and these cartilaginous surfaces are united by fibrous tissue and/or fibrocartilage (Fig. I-40*C*). *Symphyses are strong, slightly movable joints.* The **anterior intervertebral joints** with their **intervertebral discs** are classified as symphyses (Fig. 5-33). They are designed for strength and shock absorption (Fig. 5-8). The bodies of vertebrae are bound together by **longitudinal ligaments** and the *anuli fibrosi* of

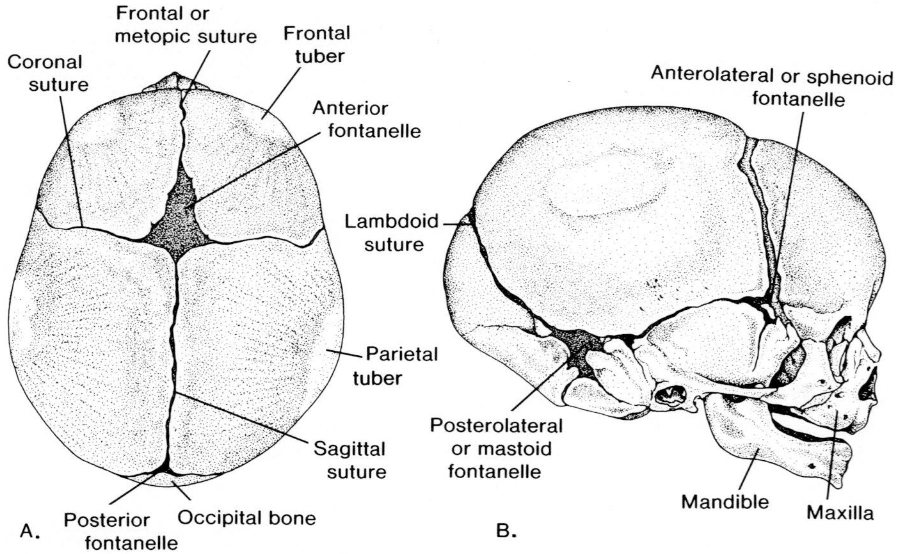

Figure I-39. Drawing of the skull of a newborn infant. *A*, from above. *B*, from the right side. Observe the fonticuli or fontanelles (also see Fig. 7-5). At these sites, called "soft spots" by laymen, the bones are attached to each other by fibrous tissue. The arterial pulsations of the brain may be felt at the anterior fontanelle.

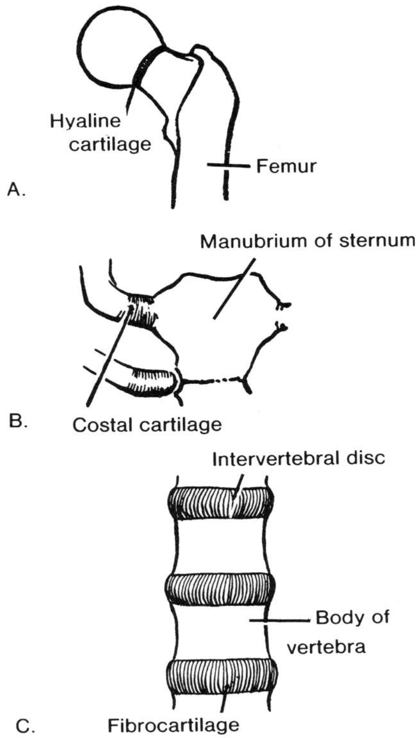

Figure I-40. Drawings illustrating the various types of cartilaginous joint. *A* and *B* are primary synchondroses, whereas *C* illustrates secondary synchondroses.

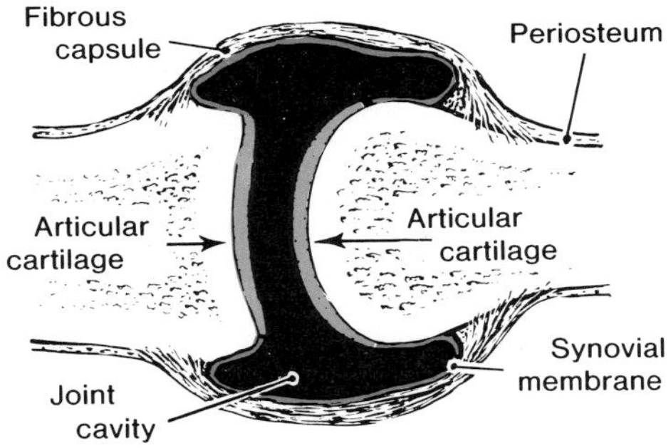

Figure I-41. Drawing illustrating the scheme of a synovial joint and its four distinguishing features. For clarity, the two bones have been pulled apart and the capsule has been inflated. Normally the joint cavity is more potential than real.

the **intervertebral discs** (Fig. 5-33). Cumulatively, these fibrocartilaginous discs give considerable flexibility to the vertebral column (Fig. I-10*A*).

Other examples of symphyses are the **symphysis pubis** between the bodies of pubic bones (Fig. 3-8) and the **manubriosternal joint** between the manubrium and the body of the sternum (Fig. 1-96). The "*symphysis menti*" of the mandible is a misnomer; it is a fibrous joint in infants, not a secondary cartilaginous one (symphysis). The symphysis menti in the adult mandible (Fig. 7-1) is a bony ridge in its median plane which indicates where the two halves of the bone (Fig. 7-5*A*) fused after birth, usually by the end of the 2nd year.

Synovial Joints (Fig. I-41). These joints, *the most* common and most important functionally, normally provide free movement between the bones they join. *The four distinguishing features of a synovial joint are that they have* (1) a **joint cavity**, (2) **articular cartilage**, (3) a **synovial membrane**, and (4) an **articular capsule** (fibrous capsule lined by a synovial membrane). Friction between the bones in a synovial joint is reduced to a minimum because the articular surfaces are covered with a thin layer of hyaline cartilage which is lubricated by **synovial fluid** produced by the *synovial membrane* (Fig. I-41). The synovial fluid was given its name because it is slippery like egg white (G. *syn*, together, with, + L. *ovum*, egg). The articular cartilages have no nerves or blood vessels, but they are nourished by the synovial fluid.

The unique feature of synovial joints is the joint cavity, but it is potential space rather than a real one because it contains only a trace of synovial fluid. The part of the cavity not covered by articular cartilage is lined by **synovial membrane**. It invests the inside of the **fibrous capsule** and any other intra-articular structures not covered by cartilage (*e.g.*, the medial aspect of the surgical neck of the humerus, Fig. I-26).

The articular capsules of synovial joints are usually strengthened by **accessory ligaments** (connective tissue bands) which are either part of their fibrous capsules (**intrinsic ligaments**) or separate from them (**extrinsic ligaments**). These ligaments are designed to limit movements of the joint in undesirable directions. The joint capsule and its associated ligaments are important in maintaining the normal relationship between the bones. For example, trauma to the knee joint results in **torn knee ligaments**, a common injury in contact sports such as football (see Case 4-4 at the end of Chap. 4).

The joint cavity is lined by a **synovial membrane** which (as described previously) invests the inside of the fibrous capsule, except for the surfaces of the articular cartilages. There are nerve fibers in the fibrous capsule and in the synovial membrane but not in the articular cartilages. *Some synovial joints have other features besides the four distinguishing features listed previously.* Three additional features are relatively common. (1) **Articular discs** or cartilages (*e.g.*, the articular disc of the wrist joint, Fig. 6-172), which are usually fibrocartilaginous pads that may help to hold the bones together, as in the example given. In some cases, however, they are attached to only one of the bones (*e.g.*, in the knee, Fig. 4-132). The articular discs have no nerves except at their attached margins. (2) A **labrum** (L. lip), which is a pliable, fibrocartilaginous ring that helps to deepen the articular surface for the bones, *e.g.*, *the labrum of the glenoid cavity* of the scapula (Figs. I-29 and 6-149). (3) A **tendon** may pass within the capsule of the joint; *e.g.*, the tendon of the long head of the biceps brachii muscle runs within the shoulder joint (Fig. 6-151). The intracapsular part of this tendon is covered with synovial membrane.

Types of Synovial Joint. There are various types of synovial joints in the body which are classified according to the type of movement they permit. They are described in ascending order of movement as follows:

1. **Plane joints** (arthroidal or gliding joints) are numerous and are nearly always small. They *permit only gliding or sliding movements*, *e.g.*, the **zygapophyseal joints** between the articular processes of the vertebrae (Figs. I-21 and 5-33); the joints between two carpal (wrist) bones; and the **acromioclavicular joints** (Fig. I-42). The opposed surfaces of the bones in these articulations are flat or almost so. Most plane joints may be moved in only one axis; hence, they are called **uniaxial joints**; but some may be moved in several axes and so are referred to as **multiaxial joints.** *Movement of plane joints is limited by their articular capsules.*
2. **Hinge (ginglymus) joints** permit movement in one axis (*uniaxial joints*) at right angles to the bones involved (*e.g.*, the humeroulnar joint at the elbow and the interphalangeal joints of the fingers). The Greek word *ginglymus* means hinge joint (Fig. I-43). *These articulations permit flexion and extension only.* The articular

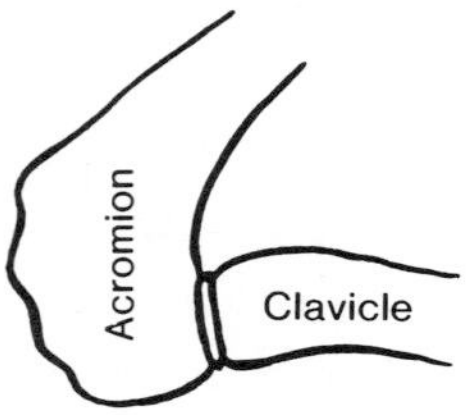

Figure I-42. Diagrammatic illustration of a multiaxial plane joint, the acromioclavicular joint. Here the oval articular surface of the lateral end of the clavicle articulates with the medial border of the acromion of the scapula (see Fig. 6-145 for a better illustration of this articulation).

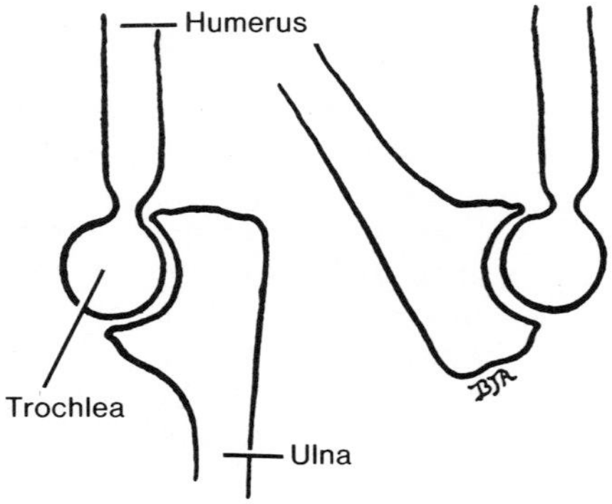

Figure I-43. Diagrammatic illustration of the humeroulnar joint, one of the two articulations at the elbow joint. This is classified as a *hinge joint*. Here the rounded trochlea of the humerus articulates with the trochlear notch of the ulna.

capsule of these joints is thin and lax where the movement occurs, but *the bones are joined by strong collateral ligaments.*

3. **Pivot (trochoidal) joints** are *uniaxial joints* which allow *rotation around a long axis* (*e.g.*, the proximal radioulnar joint permits rotation of the radius about the ulna (Fig. I-17). The word trochoidal is from Greek words meaning *"resembling a wheel,"* *e.g.*, the **dens** (odontoid process) of the axis revolves in a collar formed by the anterior arch of the **atlas** and the transverse ligament (Fig. I-44). In each case, a rounded piece of bone (*e.g.*, the dens) rotates within a sleeve or ring composed of a bone and a strong ligament.
4. **Condyloid joints** (G. knuckle-like) allow movement in two directions (*i.e.*, biaxial joints at right angles to each other. *They permit flexion and extension*, as in a hinge joint, *as well as abduction and adduction.* These joints are sometimes referred to as **ellipsoid joints** because the articulating surfaces are ellipsoidal or oval in shape, *e.g.*, the metacarpophalangeal (knuckle) joints between the heads of the metacarpal bones and the bases of the corresponding proximal phalanges (Fig. I-45).
5. **Saddle joints** are appropriately named because the opposing surfaces of the bones are concave and convex, opposite to each other (Fig. I-46). The carpometacarpal joint of the thumb is a good example of a multiaxial type of saddle joint (Fig. I-46). *It allows movement in several directions.*
6. **Ball and socket joints** are the freest moving of the multiaxial articulations (Fig. I-47). *Universal movements are permitted* (*i.e.*, in an almost infinite number of axes), such as flexion and extension, abduction and adduction, medial and lateral rotation, and circumduction (Figs. I-12 and I-15). *The hip and shoulder joints are good examples of ball and socket joints.*

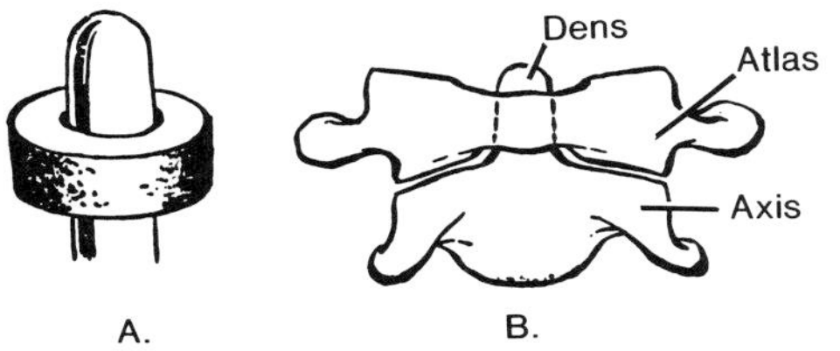

Figure I-44. Diagrammatic illustration of the atlantoaxial joint, a uniaxial and pivot joint of the cervical region of the vertebral column. *A*, schematic drawing illustrating movement around a longitudinal axis. *B*, the finger-like dens of the axis (C2 vertebra) rotates in the collar partly formed by the anterior arch of the atlas (C1 vertebra) and partly by the transverse ligament (see Fig. 5-19).

Nerve Supply of Joints. There is a rich supply of nerves to joints. Nerve endings are located in the articular capsule, both in

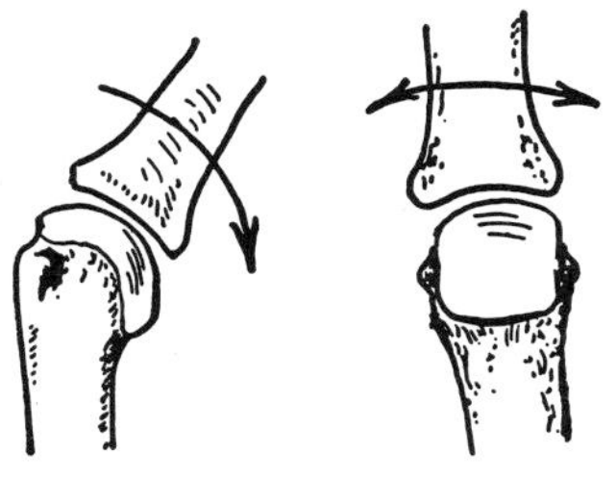

Figure I-45. Diagrammatic illustration of a metacarpophalangeal (knuckle) joint of a finger, a biaxial condyloid articulation. Note that this joint permits movement in two directions.

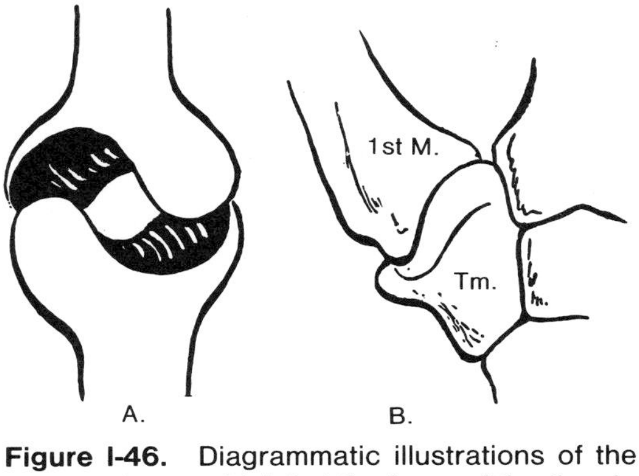

Figure I-46. Diagrammatic illustrations of the carpometacarpal joint at the base of the thumb, a multiaxial saddle joint. *A*, schematic drawing illustrating the saddle-like shape of the articulating bones. *B*, drawing of the first metacarpal (*1st M*) and the trapezium (*Tm*), a carpal bone, articulating in a saddle joint.

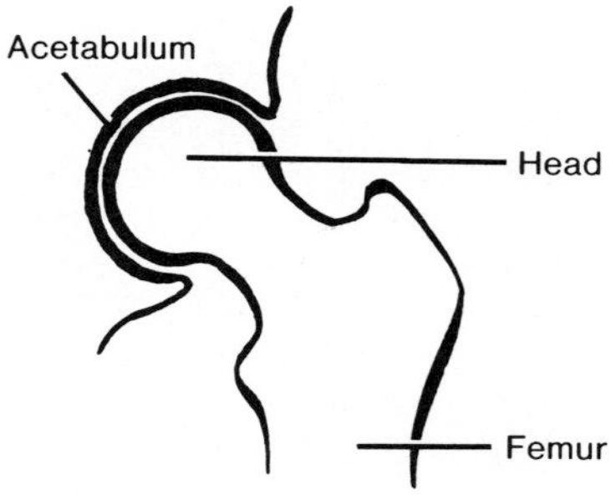

Figure I-47. Diagrammatic illustration of the hip joint, a multiaxial ball and socket articulation. The head of the femur is permitted universal movements in the acetabulum of the pelvis (also see Figs. I-25, 4-1, and 4-109).

the fibrous capsule and in the synovial membrane. The nerves are branches of the ones supplying the overlying skin and the muscles moving the joint. **Hilton's law** states that *the nerves supplying a joint also supply the muscles moving the joint and the skin covering the insertion of these muscles.*

The main type of sensation from joints is proprioception (L. *proprius*, one's own, + *receptor*, receiver), which provides information concerning the movement and position of the parts of the body. Impulses pass from nerve endings in the articular capsule to the spinal cord and the brain and act in reflex mechanisms concerned with the control of the muscles acting on the joints.

Pain fibers are numerous in the capsule and accessory ligaments. Their sensory endings respond to twisting and stretching such as occurs with distention of the joint with fluid owing to injury (see Case 4-4 at the end of Chap. 4).

Blood and Lymphatic Supply of Joints. Numerous articular arteries supply the joints. They arise from the vessels around the joint which often anastomose (join) to form a network (*e.g.*, th *anastomoses around the elbow joint*, Fig. 6-74). Veins accompany these arteries and a lymphatic network is present in the articular capsule. Details of the blood and nerve supply of joints are given with subsequent descriptions of each joint in the region concerned.

CLINICALLY ORIENTED COMMENTS

Beginning early in adult life and progressing slowly thereafter, **aging of articular cartilage** occurs on the ends of the bones involved in joints, particularly those of the hip, knee, vertebral column, and hands. These *irreversible degenerative changes* result in the articular cartilage becoming less effective as a shock absorber and as a lubricated surface. As a result, the articulation becomes vulnerable to the repeated friction that occurs during movements of the joint and to **subclinical trauma**. In some cases these changes do not produce significant symptoms, but in other cases they cause considerable pain.

Degenerative joint disease (also called *osteoarthritis, osteoarthrosis*, and *degenerative arthritis*) is the most common type of **arthritis**. *Degenerative joint disease is most common in weight-bearing joints* such as those of the hip, the knee, and the lumbar region of the vertebral column. Obviously obesity aggravates the condition.

MUSCLES

Muscles enable us to move from place to place (**locomotion**) and to move various parts of our body with respect to other parts. *Contractility is highly developed in muscular tissue* and its component cells are organized into long units called **muscle fibers** (Figs. I-52 and I-59).

Two general categories of muscle are recognized, **striated** and **nonstriated**. Striated muscle exhibits regular microscopic *transverse bands* along the length of the muscle fibers (Fig. I-59), whereas nonstriated or smooth muscle is composed of individual muscle cells without striations. *Striated muscle is commonly subdivided into two types*, **skeletal** and **cardiac**. The contraction of skeletal (voluntary) muscle fibers is under voluntary control, whereas the rhythmical contraction of cardiac muscle is involuntary. The muscle (flesh) of the body walls and of the limbs is composed of **striated skeletal muscle**, whereas the walls of heart are made up of **striated cardiac muscle**.

STRIATED SKELETAL MUSCLE

This type of muscular tissue is what most people refer to as muscle. It is commonly called "skeletal" because most of it is attached by at least one end to some part of the skeleton. *Most skeletal muscles move the skeleton.* It comprises the red or lean meat (flesh) of the animals we eat. About 43% of the weight of our bodies is composed of striated skeletal muscle.

A muscle is composed of a collection of muscle fibers (cells) that are bound together and surrounded by connective tissue. The entire muscle is enclosed by **epimysium** (G. *epi*, upon, + *mys*, muscle), a tough sheath of relatively dense connective tissue (Fig. I-48). **Perimysium** (G. *peri*, around, + *mys*, muscle) is the connective tissue that surrounds each bundle of muscle fibers. **Endomysium** (G. *endon*, within, + *mys*, muscle) lies in between the various muscle fibers and contains the extensive capillaries and many nerve fibers supplying the muscle fibers. Blood vessels, lymphatics, and nerves enter and leave a muscle through the epimysium. They course along the fibrous partitions formed by the perimysium and end as capillaries and nerve terminals on and in the endomysium.

At each end of a skeletal muscle the connective tissue blends with the strong connective tissue that anchors it to the structure on which it pulls (*e.g.*, bone, cartilage, or articular capsule). In some cases the muscle tapers into a long **tendon** of collagenous fibers (*e.g.* the *tendo calcaneus* or tendon of Achilles, Fig. 4-83). In certain regions the muscles are attached by **aponeuroses** (G. *apo*, away, + *neuron*, tendon). These are fibrous membranous expansions of muscle, such as those of the flat muscles of the abdomen (Fig. 2-9). The fleshy part of a muscle is often called its *belly*.

Attachments of Striated Skeletal Muscle. A skeletal muscle has at least two attachments. *Most muscles are attached to bone or cartilage* and their tendons are anchored by means of **Sharpey's fibers** into the bone or cartilage. These fibers are located where the collagen bundles of the

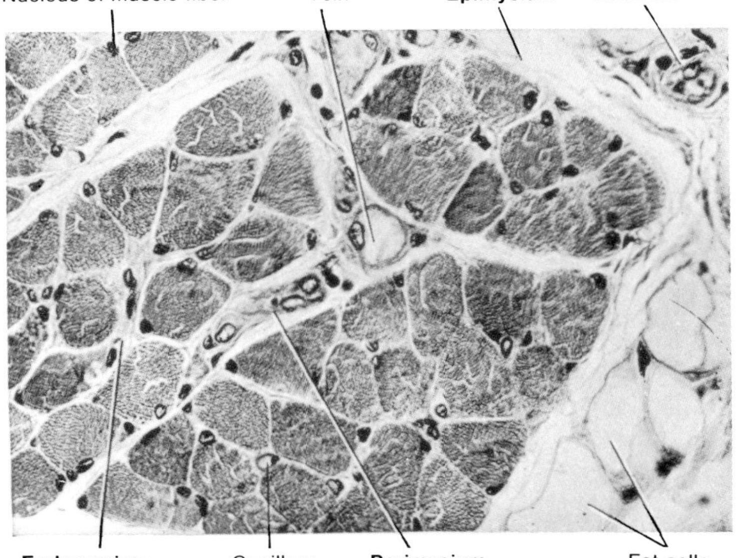

Figure I-48. Photomicrograph of a cross-section of a striated skeletal muscle from the human tongue, showing its connective tissue components and its organization into bundles of muscle fibers. Note that *epimysium* encloses the entire muscle and that *perimysium* surrounds each bundle of muscle fibers. The *endomysium* lies between the individual muscle fibers. Hematoxylin and eosin stain. ×510.

tendon lie buried in bone. Some muscles (*e.g.*, the facial muscles) are inserted into the dermis of the skin, whereas other muscles (*e.g.*, those of the tongue) are attached to the mucous membrane. A few muscles are attached to fascia (*e.g.*, the tensor fasciae latae, Fig. 4-23) and other muscles form circular bands called **sphincters** (*e.g.*, the external anal sphincter, Fig. 3-2).

For purposes of description, most muscles are described as having an **origin** and an **insertion**. *The origin is the attachment that moves the least, whereas the insertion is the attachment that moves the most.* Some people *erroneously* refer to the origin as the fixed end and to the insertion as the moving end. This is wrong because one end of a muscle moves in some activities and the other end in others. Because the freedom of movement of a muscle varies, the terms origin and insertion are interchangeable. *Generally the origin is the more proximal attachment and the insertion the more distal* and the attachment of a muscle closest to the long axis of the body is its origin.

Muscles are usually inserted near the proximal end of a bone (Fig. I-49*B* and *C*), but some are inserted near the middle of its body or shaft (*e.g.*, the deltoid, Fig. 6-55). Skeletal muscles are frequently part of a lever system; hence, the power exerted by a muscle depends in part on its angle of pull. The optimum angle of pull is a right angle and as its angle of pull increases, the power of its pull decreases.

Architecture of Muscles (Figs. I-50 and I-51). Most fibers of some muscles run parallel to the long axis of the muscle, but a few of them run the whole length of a muscle (*i.e.*, they form bundles of overlapping relays). *Muscles with their fibers disposed in parallel can lift a weight through a long distance.*

In some muscles the fibers are oblique to the long axis of the muscle. Because of their resemblance to feathers, they are called **pennate muscles** (L. *pennatus*, feather). They are known as (1) *unipennate muscles* when their fibers have a linear or narrow origin resembling one-half of a feather; (2) *bipennate muscles* when their fibers arise from a broad surface resembling a whole feather; (3) *multipennate muscles* when septa extend into the origin and insertion of the muscles, dividing them into several feather-like portions (e.g., the deltoid, Fig. 6-55); and (4) *circumpennate muscles* when the fibers converge on a tendon extending into their substance.

In other muscles the fibers converge from a wide origin or base to a fibrous apex. This

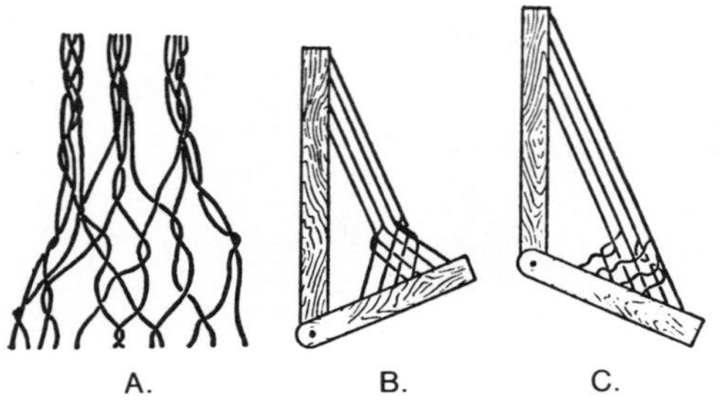

Figure I-49. *A*, diagram of the inferior end of a tendon showing that its component fibers are plaited (braided, intertwined). This structure provides added strength. *B* and *C* illustrate that in different positions of a joint, different fibers take the strain. Tendons are very strong. The fan-shaped way most tendons are inserted into a bone ensures that successive parts of it take the strain as the angle of the joint changes.

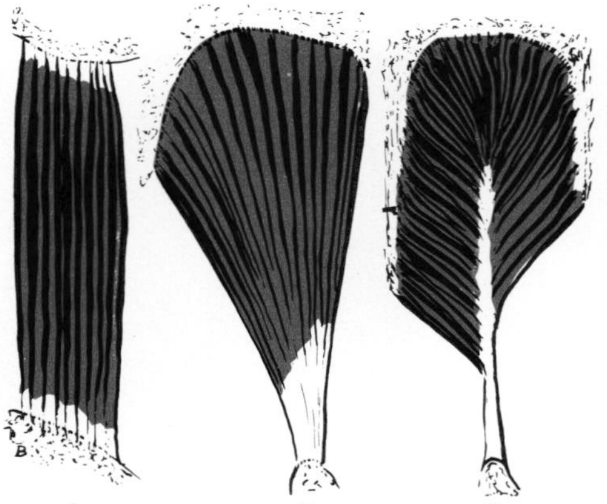

Figure I-50. Drawings illustrating the three types of architecture in muscles. *A*, parallel fibers end to end. *B*, nearly parallel fibers, *i.e.*, fan-shaped. *C*, pennate fibers which converge on a central tendon. Note the two chief components of a striated skeletal muscle, the fleshy belly (*red*) and the fibrous tendon (*white*).

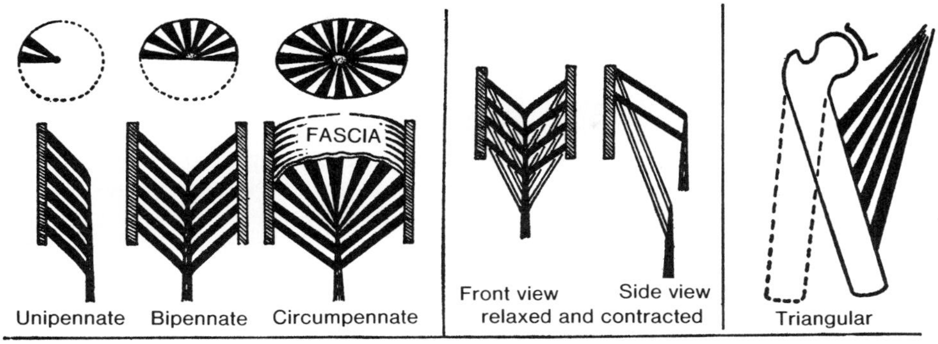

Figure I-51. Diagrams showing the architecture or internal structure of pennate and triangular muscles. Obviously pennate muscles are powerful (*e.g.*, the large deltoid muscle that gives the rounded contour to the shoulder, Fig. 6-55). *Top left*, cross-sections of the pennate muscles.

type of muscle is referred to as a fan-shaped or **triangular muscle**. On contracting, its fleshy muscle fibers shorten by a third to a half of their resting length. Hence they "swell," as illustrated by your biceps brachii muscle when you flex your forearm (Fig. I-10*B*). It forms a bulge as it changes from its relaxed state to its contracted state.

Muscle Action (Fig. I-52). *The structural unit of a muscle is a muscle fiber.* The **functional unit**, consisting of a motor neuron and the muscle fibers it controls, is called a **motor unit**. The number of muscle fibers in a motor unit varies from one to several hundred, but usually there are about 100. This number varies according to the size and the function of the muscle. Large motor units, where one neuron supplies several hundred muscle fibers, are found in the large trunk and thigh muscles, whereas in the small eye and hand muscles (where precision movements are required) the motor units contain only a few muscle fibers.

When a nerve impulse reaches a motor neuron in the spinal cord (Fig. I-52), a nerve impulse may be initiated which will make *all the muscle fibers of the motor unit supplied by that motor neuron contract simultaneously* (Fig. I-59).

Movements result from an increasing number of motor units being put into action while antagonistic muscles are relaxing. During maintenance of a given position or posture, the muscles involved are in a state of *reflex contraction* or **tone**. The maintenance of tone depends upon impulses

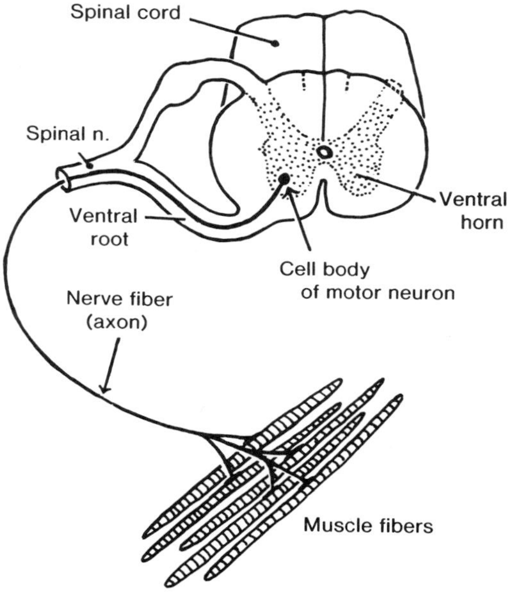

Figure I-52. Diagram illustrating one motor unit consisting of a motor neuron and the muscle fibers innervated by it. The fewer muscle fibers per nerve fiber, the more precise is the movement produced by the muscle. Observe that the motor neuron is in the anterior gray horn of the spinal cord. The gray and white rami communicantes have been omitted for simplicity (see Figs. I-64 and I-65).

reaching the brain and spinal cord (**CNS**) from the sensory endings in the muscles, tendons, and joints. *Tone is abolished by anesthesia*; hence, dislocated joints or fractures are more easily reduced when the patient is given an **anesthetic agent**, a

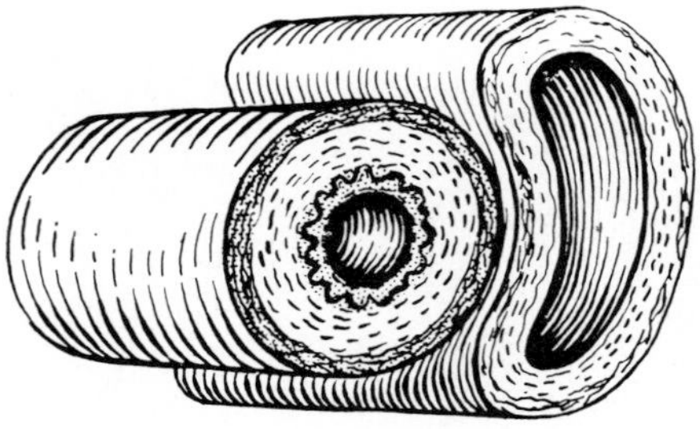

Figure I-53. Schematic section of an artery (*left*) and its accompanying vein (*right*). Note that the wall of the artery is much thicker than the vein. Observe the three layers in its wall.

compound that reversibly depresses neuronal function.

During movements of the body, certain principal muscles are called into action. These muscles, called **prime movers** or agonists (G. *agon*, a contest), contract actively (shorten) and produce the desired movement. *A muscle that opposes the action of a prime mover* is called an **antagonist**. As a prime mover contracts the antagonist(s) progessively relax, thereby producing a smooth coordinated movement. The antagonists are called into action at the end of a violent movement to protect the joint involved. When a prime mover passes over more than one joint, certain muscles prevent movement of the intervening joints. These muscles are called **synergists** (G. *syn*, together, + *ergon*, work); thus, synergists complement the action of the prime mover. Other muscles, called **fixators**, steady the proximal parts of a limb (*e.g.*, the arm) while movements are occurring in distal parts (*e.g.*, the hand). *Understand that the same muscle may act as a prime mover, antagonist, synergist, or fixator under different conditions.*

Muscle action can be tested in various ways. This is usually done when nerve injuries are suspected. There are *two common ways of determining the status of motor function*: (1) the patient performs certain movements against resistance produced by the examiner, and (2) the examiner performs certain movements against resistance produced by the patient. For example, when testing flexion of the forearm at the elbow joint (Fig. I-10*B*), the patient is asked to flex the forearm while the examiner resists the effort. The other way is to ask the patient to keep the forearm flexed while the examiner attempts to extend it. The latter method enables the examiner to gauge the power of the movement (flexion in this case). Try flexing your forearm against resistance and you can see your biceps brachii muscle stand out and you can feel it become firm.

Electrical stimulation of muscles is used by physiotherapists as part of the treatment for restoring the action of muscles. This kind of stimulation is also used for testing muscles. **Electromyography** is a good method of testing the action of muscles. Electrodes are inserted in the muscle and then the patient is asked to perform certain movements. The differences in electrical action potentials of the muscles are amplified and recorded. Using this technique, it is possible to analyze the activity of an individual muscle during different movements.

STRIATED CARDIAC MUSCLE

The heart muscle or **myocardium** surrounds all the chambers of the heart, but it is much thicker around the ventricles than the atria. The fibers of cardiac muscle fit together so tightly that they give the impression under a light microscope that they form a network or syncytium. However, electron microscopy shows that cardiac muscle fibers are composed of individual cells joined end to end at the cell junctions. Although cardiac muscle is striated, *its rhythmic contractions are not under voluntary control.* The heart rate is regulated by a **pacemaker** composed of special cardiac muscle cells which are innervated by the **autonomic nervous system** (see subsequent discussion). The myocardium will contract spontaneously without any nerve supply.

CLINICALLY ORIENTED COMMENTS

Heart muscle responds to increased demands by increasing the size of its fibers. This is called **compensatory hypertrophy**. When heart muscle is damaged, fibrous scar tissue is formed. When this muscle is rendered **necrotic** (*i.e.*, dies), the lesion is called an **infarct**. It is usually called a **myocardial infarct** (**MI**), even though in most cases there is some involvement of the endocardium and/or epicardium, its inner and outer layers, respectively. A person suffering a heart attack (**MI**) usually describes a crushing substernal pain that does not disappear with rest (see Case 1-1 at end of Chap. 1).

NONSTRIATED OR SMOOTH MUSCLE

Nonstriated or smooth muscle forms the muscular layers of the walls of the GI tract and of blood vessels. As its name implies, nonstriated or *smooth muscle cells have no microscopic cross striations*. Smooth muscle is generally arranged in two layers in the walls of the viscera (L. the soft parts, internal organs). In some parts of the GI and respiratory tracts and in arteries, the smooth muscle cells are arranged spirally.

Smooth muscle, like cardiac muscle, is innervated by the autonomic nervous system. Hence it is **involuntary** and can partly contract for long periods (*i.e.*, maintain **tonus**). This is important in regulating the size of the lumen (L. light, window) of tubular structures. In the walls of the GI tract, uterine tubes, ureters, etc., the smooth muscle cells undergo rhythmic contractions. These are called **peristaltic waves** and it is the process known as **peristalsis** which propels the contents along the tubular structures.

CLINICALLY ORIENTED COMMENTS

Like skeletal and cardiac muscle, smooth muscle undergoes **compensatory hypertrophy** in response to increased demands. During pregnancy the smooth muscle cells in the wall of the uterus not only increase in size (**hypertrophy**), but they also increase in number (**hyperplasia**).

BLOOD VESSELS

There are three types of blood vessels: *arteries*, *veins*, and *capillaries*.

ARTERIES

Arteries carry blood away from the heart and distribute it to various parts of the body. There are three main kinds of artery: elastic, muscular, and arterioles, but they are not sharply divided.

Arterioles. *These are the smallest arteries.* They have a relatively narrow lumen and thick muscular walls. The degree of pressure within the arterial system (**arterial pressure**) is mainly regulated by the degree of tonus in the smooth muscle in the arterial walls. If the tonus of this smooth muscle becomes increased above normal, **hypertension** (high blood pressure) results.

Muscular Arteries. These arteries distribute the blood to various parts of the body. The walls of these distributing arteries consist chiefly of circularly disposed smooth muscle fibers which constrict the lumen of the vessel when they contract. They are under the control of the **autonomic nervous system**. Hence, they regulate the flow of blood to different parts of the body as required (*e.g.*, the blood flow to the skeletal muscles in the limbs increases during exercise).

Elastic Arteries. *These are the largest arteries in the body* and their walls consist chiefly of elastin, a yellow elastic fibrous mucoprotein. The maintenance of blood pressure within the arterial system between contractions of the heart results from the elasticity of the largest arteries. This elasticity allows them to expand when the heart contracts and to return to normal caliber between cardiac contractions.

VEINS

The veins return blood to the heart largely because contracting skeletal muscles compress them, "milking" the blood along. The smallest veins are called **venules**. Small veins or tributaries unite to form larger veins which commonly join together, forming **venous plexuses** or networks (*e.g.*, the dorsal venous network of the hand, Fig. 6-82). The two veins that commonly accompany medium-sized arteries, one on each side, are called **venae comitantes** (L. accompanying veins). Generally, systemic veins are more variable

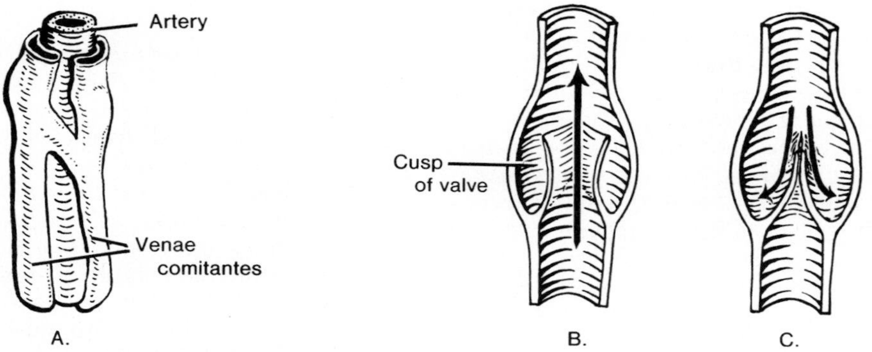

Figure I-54. *A*, drawing of an artery accompanied by two veins (venae comitantes), one on each side. Small and medium-sized arteries are generally accompanied by a pair of veins, whereas larger arteries usually have only one accompanying vein (Fig. I-53). Some arteries, however, have no companion veins. Observe the communication (anastomosis) between the venae comitantes. Blood flows in one direction only through a vein, *i.e.*, toward the heart. *B* shows a bicuspid (two cusps) valve in the open position. *C* shows the valve closed by the back pressure of the blood. The *arrows* indicate the direction of blood flow.

than the arteries and **anastomoses** (communications) occur more often between them.

Many veins contain **valves** (Fig. 6-44), which prevent backflow of blood and encourage the flow of blood toward the heart.

CLINICALLY ORIENTED COMMENTS

Varicose veins have a caliber greater than normal and their cusps do not meet or have been destroyed by inflammation. In these cases the valves are said to be **incompetent** because they are unable to perform their function competently. Varicose veins are common in the posterior and medial parts of the lower limbs (see Case 1-10 at the end of Chap. 1).

CAPILLARIES

Capillaries are generally arranged in communicating networks called **capillary beds** or networks (Fig. I-55). The blood flowing through a capillary bed is brought to it by arterioles and is carried away by venules. The volume of blood flowing through a capillary bed is under the control of the autonomic nervous system (discussed subsequently).

Capillaries are microscopic vessels that connect the arterioles to the venules. In some regions of the body (e.g., in the fingers and the toes), there are direct connections between the arteries and the veins; *i.e.*, there are no capillaries between them. These alternative channels, called **arteriovenous anastomoses** (*AV shunts*), permit blood to pass directly from the arterial to the venous side of the circulation without having to pass through capillaries. **AV shunts** are fairly numerous in the skin, where they are important in conserving the heat of the body.

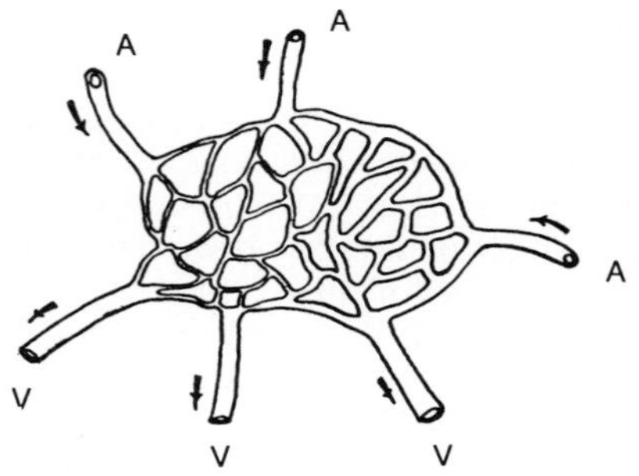

Figure I-55. Drawing of a capillary bed or network. Observe that arterioles (*A*) convey blood into the network and that venules (*V*) drain blood from it.

LYMPHATICS

The vessels in the body that conduct lymph are called *lymphatics*. **The lym-**

phatic system (Fig. I-56) consists of: (1) **plexuses** (networks) of very small lymph vessels called **lymph capillaries** which begin in the intercellular spaces of most tissues in the body; (2) **lymph nodes** (Fig. I-57) composed of small masses of **lymphatic tissue** arranged along the course of the lymph vessels (Fig. I-56) through which

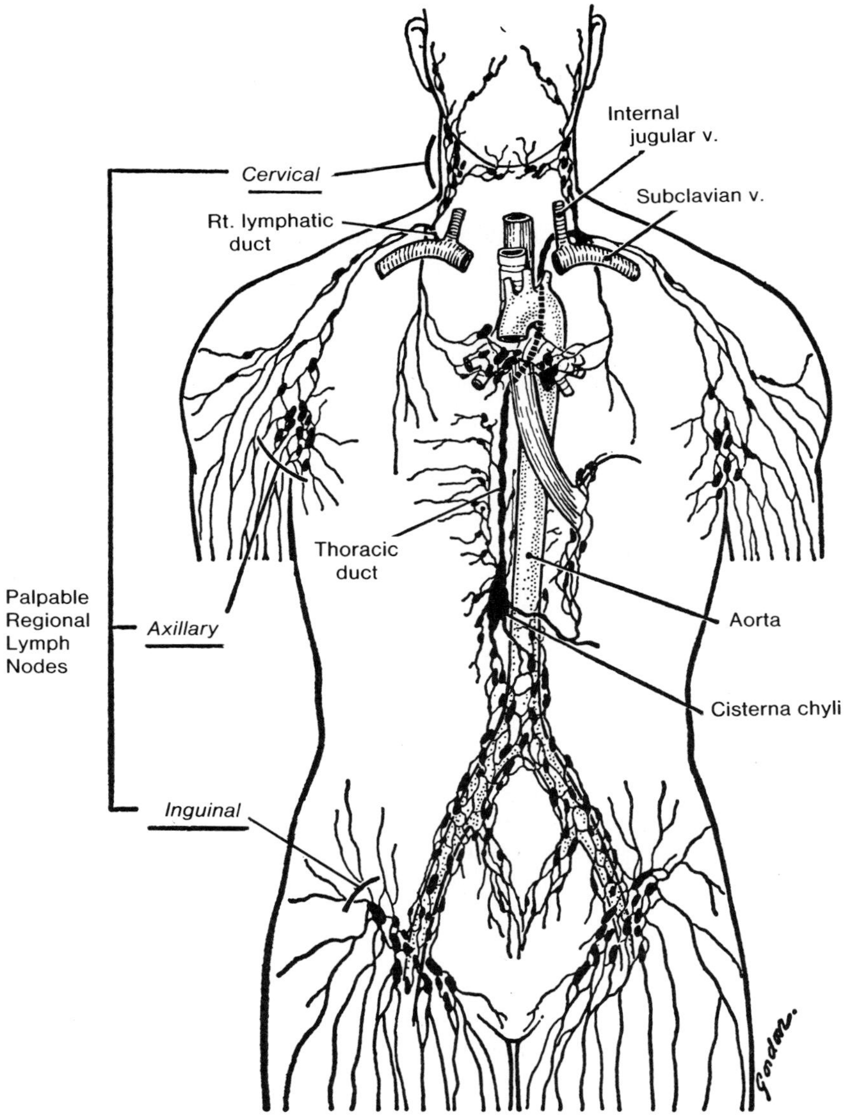

Figure I-56. Drawing illustrating the scheme of the lymphatic system. Note the regional lymph nodes which become palpable when inflamed or invaded by tumor cells. Observe that (1) the lymphatics of the upper limb converge upon *axillary lymph nodes* in the axilla (armpit); (2) those of the head and neck drain into *cervical lymph nodes* grouped especially around the vessels of the neck (L. *cervix*, hence the adjective cervical). Note that the lymph from the entire body drains into the *thoracic duct*, except for the right side of the head and neck, the right upper limb, and the right half of the thoracic cavity; (3) most of the lymphatics of the lower limb converge on the *inguinal lymph nodes* in the groin or upper thigh region. The *cysterna chyli* is a dilated sac at the inferior end of the thoracic duct into which the intestinal and two lumbar lymphatic trunks empty. Note that the thoracic duct and the right lymphatic duct open into the venous system (see the text for details).

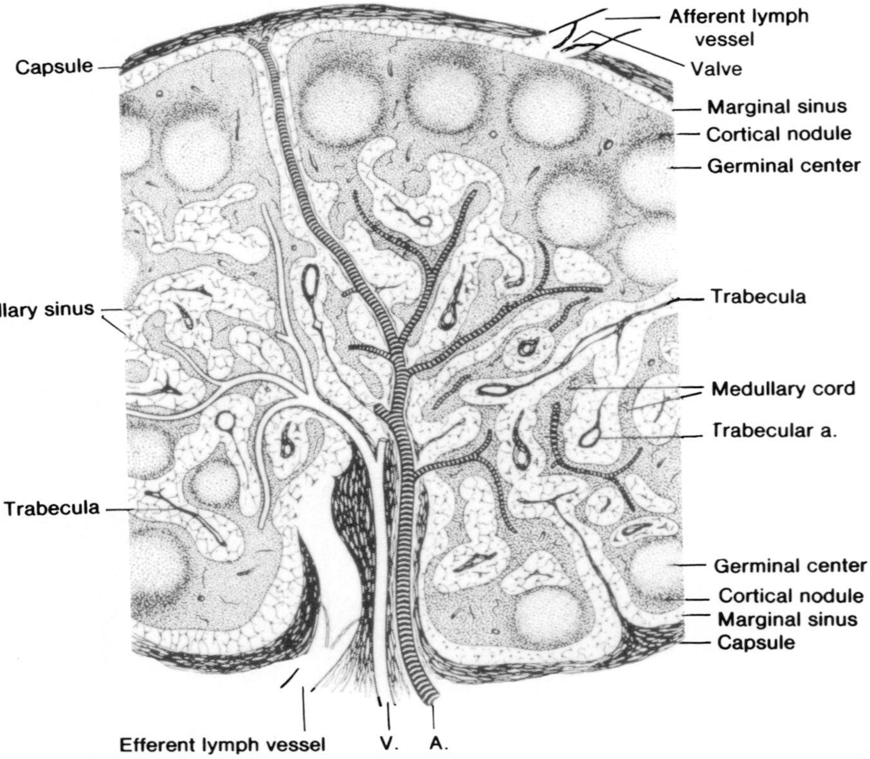

Figure I-57. Diagram of a lymph node. Observe the hilum through which the blood vessels enter and leave the node. The efferent lymph vessel, usually single, also emerges from the node at the hilum. The afferent lymph vessels (usually multiple) bringing lymph to the node enter it at many different parts of the capsule. Both kinds have flap-type valves which prevent lymph from passing backward toward its point of origin.

lymph, the clear fluid in the vessels, passes on its way to the venous system; (3) **aggregations of lymphoid tissue** located in the walls of the alimentary canal (the mouth, pharynx, esophagus, stomach, and intestines) and in the spleen and thymus; and (4) **circulating lymphocytes** which are formed in (a) lymphoid tissue located throughout the body (*e.g.*, in lymph nodes, spleen, thymus, and tonsils) and (b) in myeloid tissue located in the bone marrow. T-lymphocytes are produced in the thymus and B-lymphocytes are formed in myeloid tissue.

LYMPH VESSELS

Most lymph vessels are not visible in dissections, but they can be demonstrated in vivo (L. in the living person), as shown in Figures I-56, 4-38, and 6-47. **Lymph capillaries** begin blindly in most tissues of the body and join to form larger and larger collecting vessels or trunks that pass to nearby or regional lymph nodes. *As a general rule, lymph traverses one or more lymph nodes before it enters the bloodstream.*

The wall of a lymph capillary consists of a single layer of endothelial cells, resembling that of a blood capillary. As the lymph capillaries unite to form larger vessels, thin connective tissue is added to their walls. The largest lymph vessels, called **lymph trunks** and **ducts**, also contain smooth muscle in their walls.

The lymphatics carrying lymph to the lymph nodes are called **afferent lymph vessels** (Fig. I-57), whereas those leaving a lymph node are called **efferent lymph**

vessels. Understand that the efferent lymph vessel of one lymph node becomes an afferent lymph vessel of another lymph node in a chain. After traversing one or more lymph nodes, the lymph enters larger lymph vessels called lymph trunks. These trunks unite to form either (1) the **thoracic duct** (Figs. I-56, 1-48, and 1-84), which enters the junction of the left internal jugular and left subclavian veins, or (2) the **right lymphatic duct** (Figs. I-56 and 1-48), which enters the junction of the right internal jugular and right subclavian veins. *In general, the thoracic duct drains lymph from the entire body, except for* (1) the right side of the head and neck, (2) the right upper limb, and (3) the right upper half of the thoracic cavity.

Superficial Lymph Vessels. These vessels are located *in the skin* (L. *cutis*) and in the subcutaneous tissue (i.e., *beneath the skin*). They also form a network on the deep surface of the epithelium lining cavities. The lymph capillaries run parallel to the superficial vessels of the skin and then join to form slightly larger vessels. The superficial lymph vessels eventually drain into deep lymph vessels.

Deep Lymph Vessels. These vessels run in the *deep fascia* (subcutaneous connective tissue), located between the muscles and the *superficial fascia* (tela subcutanea). The deep vessels also accompany the major blood vessels of the region concerned. These lymph vessels have thick walls containing connective tissue and smooth muscle. They also have valves.

LYMPH NODES

Lymph nodes are round, oval, or bean-shaped structures which are easily palpated when they are swollen. Many lymph nodes are located in the **axilla** (armpit) and the **inguinal region** (groin), but there are numerous lymph nodes distributed along the large vessels of the neck (Fig. I-56) and there are large numbers in the thorax and abdomen.

Lymph nodes consist of aggregations of lymphatic tissue (Fig. I-57) and vary in size from about the size of a pinhead to a fingerbreadth or more in diameter. Generally there is a slight depression on one side of a lymph node, called the **hilum** (hilus), through which the blood vessels enter and leave the node. The afferent lymph vessels bringing lymph to the node enter different parts of the capsule. The efferent lymph vessel (usually single) carrying lymph from the node, emerges from the node at the hilum.

Each node has (1) a thick outer part called the **cortex** (L. bark) and (2) an inner part called the **medulla** (L. marrow). Connective tissue *trabeculae* (L. little beams) pass inward from the capsule at the hilum, providing support and carrying the blood vessels (Fig. I-57). Trabeculae also pass inward from the capsule covering the external surface of the node.

The cortex contains collections of lymphatic cells called **germinal centers** (Fig. I-57), whereas the medulla contains cords of cells. **Reticuloendothelial cells** are located along the trabeculae and have the ability to remove foreign material from the lymph as it passes through the node (*e.g.*, the lymph nodes draining the lungs of persons who smoke and/or inhale dark colored dust have a blackened appearance, as do those receiving lymph from a darkly tattooed area of skin).

LYMPH

Lymph (L. *lympha*, clear water) is usually a clear, transparent, watery fluid. Sometimes it is a faintly yellow and slightly opalescent fluid. Lymph is collected from the intercellular spaces in various tissues of the body. Usually more tissue fluid is produced at the arterial ends of capillaries than is absorbed at their venous ends. This extra fluid is drained away by the lymph capillaries. Lymph contains the same constituents as blood plasma (*e.g.*, protein and many lymphocytes). Lymph coming from the intestine also contains fat, fatty acids, glycerol, amino acids, glucose, and other substances (*e.g.*, medicine given to the patient).

FUNCTIONS OF THE LYMPHATIC SYSTEM

Drainage of Tissue Fluid and Protein. Lymph capillaries are mainly involved in absorbing plasma from the tissue spaces and transporting it back to the venous system. On its way the lymph passes through the lymph nodes where particulate matter (*e.g.*, dust inhaled into the lungs) is largely filtered out by the phagocytic (G. *phagein*, to eat) activity of the scavenger cells, called **macrophages**, in the nodes. In a similar way, bacteria and other microorganisms drained from an infected area are trapped and ingested by the phagocytic cells, thereby preventing them from entering the bloodstream.

Absorption and Transport of Fat. The lymphatics draining the intestine contain considerable amounts of emulsified fat after a fatty meal. This creamy lymph is called **chyle** (G. *chylos*, juice). The turbid, white or pale yellow fluid is taken up by the **lacteals** of the intestine during digestion (Fig. 2-103) and consists of lymph and emulsified fat. After passing through various lymph vessels, it is conveyed by the **thoracic duct** to the left subclavian vein (Fig. I-56), where it becomes mixed with the blood.

Part of the Defense Mechanism of the Body. The lymphatic system provides an *important immune mechanism for the body*. When minute amounts of foreign protein are drained from an infected area by the lymphatic capillaries, **immunologically competent cells** produce a specific antibody to the foreign protein, or lymphocytes are dispatched to the infected area. The antibody is carried to this area via the bloodstream and the tissue fluid. This is referred to as the **humeral mechanism** of the immune reaction. When foreign tissue is transplanted, lymphocytes are active in rejecting the graft.

CLINICALLY ORIENTED COMMENTS

The lymph vessels and lymph nodes draining an infected area often become inflamed. *Inflammation of the lymph vessels* is called **lymphangitis** (G. *angeion*, vessel), whereas *inflammation of a lymph node (s)* is called **lymphadenitis** (G. *adēn*, gland). Lymph nodes used to be called lymph glands, but this term is not used now because they are not designed for secretion. Laymen usually refer to inflamed lymph nodes as *swollen glands*.

Chronic lymphangitis or inflammation of lymph vessels that has persisted for a long time (G. *chronos*, time), together with blockage of many lymph vessels, can be produced by the escaped ova (L. eggs) of a minute parasitic worm called *Microfilaris nocturna*. The resulting condition, called **elephantiasis**, is common in the tropics and is characterized by enormous enlargement of some parts of the body (*e.g.*, the legs and the scrotum in males).

The extensive spread of cancer cells via the lymphatic system can also cause blockage of lymph vessels and **lymphedema** (G. *oidēma*, swelling), an accumulation of a large amount of fluid in the affected region. Similarly, the widespread removal of lymph nodes (e.g., as may occur during a **radical mastectomy**, the surgical removal of a breast) can cause swelling of the limbs owing to poor drainage of lymph from them. For a discussion of breast cancer and its spread to the regional lymph nodes, see Case 6-12 at the end of Chapter 6.

The lymphatic system is involved in the metastasis (spread) of cancer cells. This is referred to as **lymphogenous dissemination of malignant cells**. Cancer can spread by permeating the lymph vessels as solid cell growths from which minute cellular **emboli** (G. *embolus*, a plug, wedge, or stopper) may break free and pass to regional and distant lymph nodes. This shifting of malignant disease from one part of the body to another is called metastasis and the transportation of cancer cells via the lymphatic system is called **lymphogenous metastasis**.

The radiographic study of lymph vessels and lymph nodes, called **lymphography**, is possible after the cannulation of appropriate peripheral lymph vessels and the injection of a radiopaque contrast material.

NERVES

Nerves are strong whitish cords in living persons. They are made up of many **nerve fibers (axons)** arranged in **fasciculi** or fascicles (L. bundles) which are held together by a connective tissue sheath (Fig. I-58). *Nerves carry impulses to and from the central nervous system* (**CNS**), *i.e.*, the **brain** and the **spinal cord**. The peripheral nervous system (**PNS**) sends impulses to and receives impulses from the CNS. These impulses come and go to all parts of the body, external and internal. Together, the CNS and PNS serve conscious perception, voluntary movement, and automatic (autonomic) functions and integrate messages received from the body. The nerves connected with the brain situated in the **cranium** (G. *kranion*, skull) are called **cranial nerves**, whereas those connected with the spinal cord are called **spinal nerves**.

The **brain** lies in the cranial cavity (Fig. 7-76), where it is *surrounded by the meninges* (*G. membranes*) *and the skull.* The spinal cord is in the vertebral canal where it is *surrounded by the meninges, the vertebrae, and their interconnecting ligaments* (Figs. 5-59 and 5-65).

The **cranial nerves** leave the cranium or skull through various **cranial foramina** in it (Figs. 7-51 and 7-54), and the **spinal nerves** leave the vertebral (spinal) column via the **intervertebral foramina** (Fig. 5-59). In the limbs they form plexuses (**brachial plexus**, Fig. 6-25, and **sacral plexus**, Fig. 2-139) which are networks where the nerves intermingle. Hence, the nerves to the limbs contain fibers from several segments of the spinal cord.

The neuron (*nerve cell*) *is the anatomical unit of the nervous system (Fig. I-60)*; *it includes the nerve cell body and all its extensions.* Some neurons are very long, extending from the brain to the inferior end of the spinal cord. The processes extending from the cell body are specialized for different functions. The **dendrites** (G. *dendron*, tree) *receive impulses* and the **axons** *conduct impulses away from the cell body, e.g.*, to the muscles or the skin.

A neuron can be divided into three portions: (1) a **receptive portion** (cell body and dendrites), (2) a **conductile portion** (axon), and (3) an **effector portion** (collateral branch or the end of the axon which produces an effect on other neurons or on a muscle or a gland, Fig. I-59).

A **nerve fiber** consists of an *axon, a myelin sheath* (in some cases), and the *neurolemmal sheath* (of Schwann). Both the neurolemma and the myelin sheath are components of Schwann cells. The components of all but the smallest peripheral

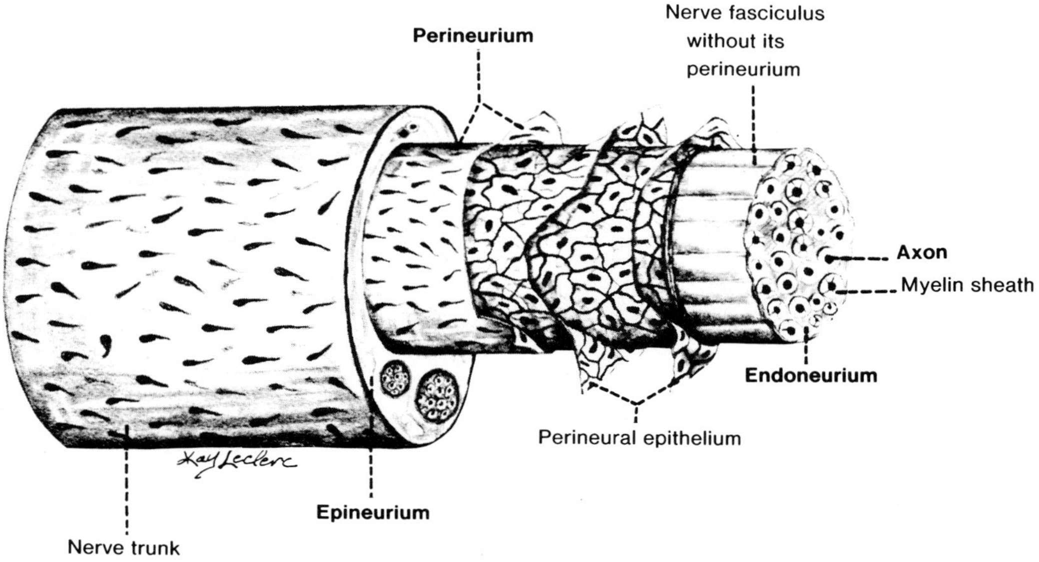

Figure I-58. Drawing illustrating the connective tissue sheaths around a peripheral nerve. Observe that the cells of the perineurium are disposed as an epithelium which forms a barrier against the penetration of certain materials into the nerve fasciculus.

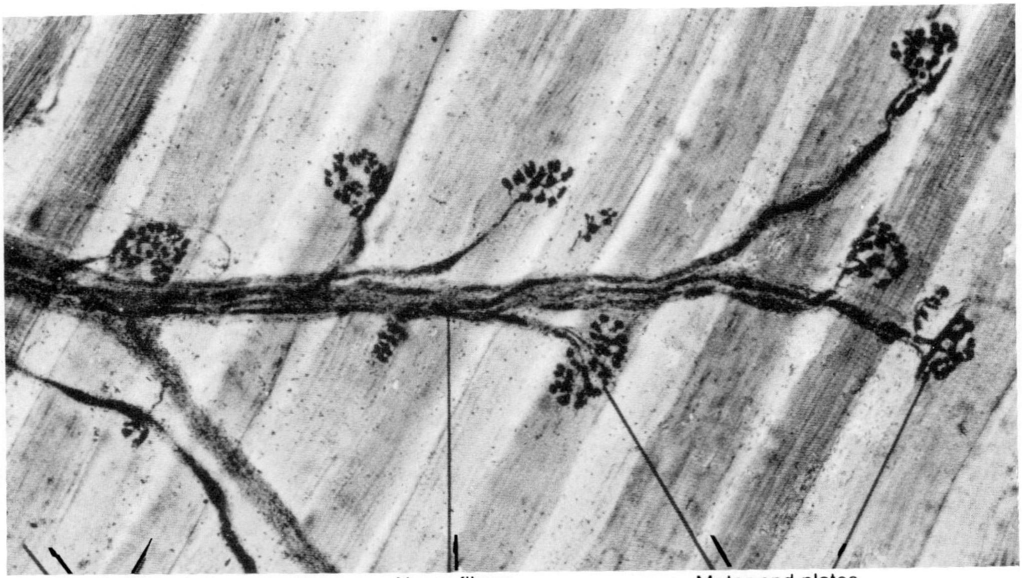

Figure I-59. Photomicrograph of the motor nerve endings in an intercostal muscle, a striated skeletal muscle. Observe the regular alteration of light and dark striations across each muscle fiber. Examine the motor endplates or myoneural junctions, noting that these synapse-like structures have two components, the ending of the motor nerve fiber and the subjacent part of the muscle fibers. A motor unit consists of a motor neuron and the muscle fibers innervated by that neuron (also see Fig. I-52). Gold chloride stain. ×215.

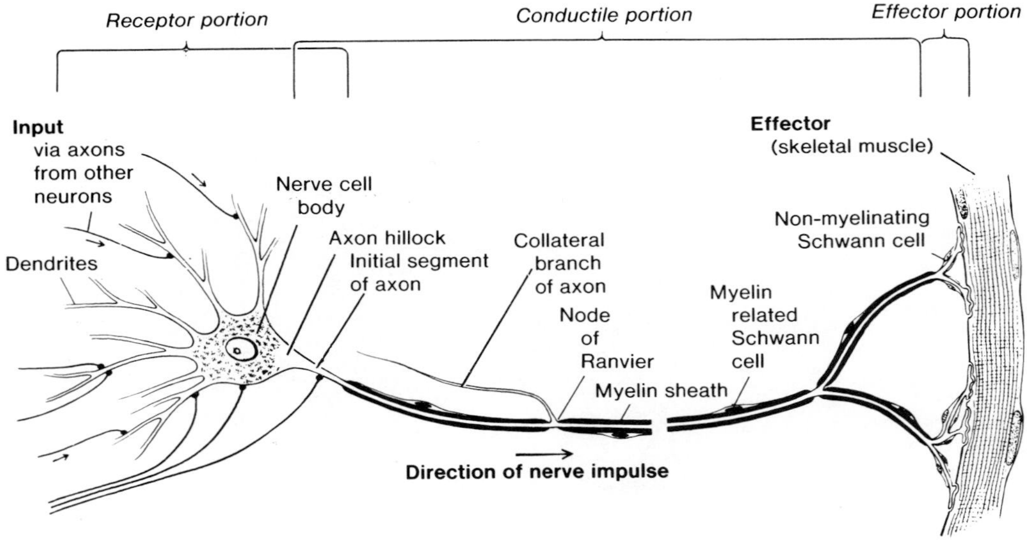

Figure I-60. Diagram illustrating the receptor, conductile, and effector portions of a typical large motor neuron. Observe the effector endings on skeletal muscle (for a better view of them, see Fig. I-59). The presence of the myelin sheath on the axon (the conductile portion of the neuron) increases conduction velocity. Understand that the axon is much longer than is illustrated here. Some are 90 to 150 cm long.

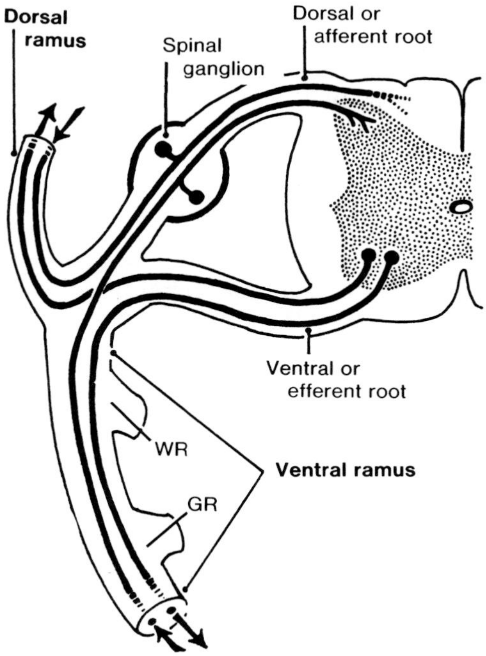

Figure I-61. Diagram illustrating the nerve fibers in the two roots and two primary rami of a typical spinal nerve. *WR* and *GR* indicate the white and gray rami communicantes (only the stumps of them are shown; see Fig. 1-65).

nerves are arranged in nerve **fasciculi** (fascicles, bundles, Fig. I-58). *The delicate nerve fibers are strengthened and protected by connective tissue coverings* (Fig. I-58) as follows. The entire nerve is surrounded by a thick sheath of loose connective tissue, called the **epineurium**, which contains fatty tissue and blood and lymph vessels. A more delicate connective tissue sheath enclosing a fasciculus of nerve fibers, called the **perineurium**, provides an effective barrier to the penetration of substances into or out of the nerve fiber. The individual nerve fibers are surrounded by a delicate covering of connective tissue called the **endoneurium**.

The regions of specialized attachment between neurons or between neurons and effector organs are called **synapses** (G. *synaptō*, to join). They are *the sites of contact between neurons* at which one neuron is excited or inhibited by another neuron.

A typical spinal nerve arises from the spinal cord by two roots. The **ventral root** contains *motor* (*efferent*) *fibers* from a motor neuron in the ventral horn of the spinal cord (Figs. I-52 and I-61). The **dorsal root** *carries sensory* (*afferent*) *fibers* of the spinal or dorsal root ganglion cells. In or

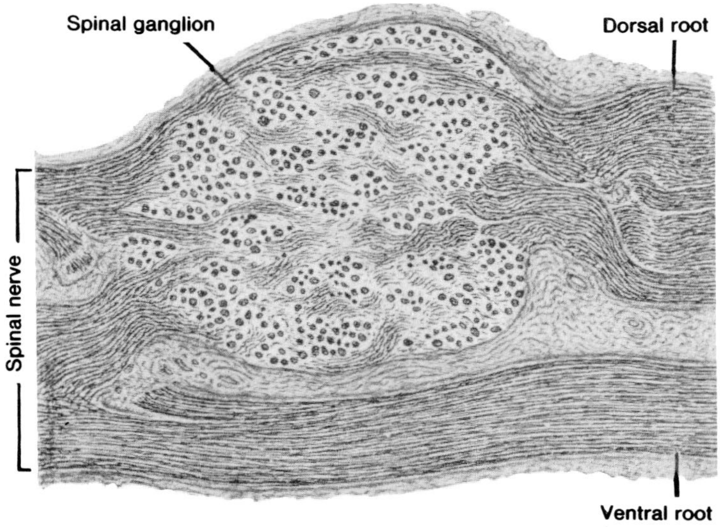

Figure I-62. Drawing of a longitudinal section of a spinal (dorsal root) ganglion of a 2 month-old infant (also see Fig. I-61). Both cranial and spinal ganglia consist of nerve cell bodies of afferent neurons. Each ganglion cell is surrounded by a connective tissue capsule which is continuous with the epineurium and the perineurium of the spinal nerve. Cajal silver stain. ×28.

close to the **intervertebral foramen** (Figs. 5-59 and 5-60), *the dorsal and ventral roots unite to form a spinal nerve.* The sensory **spinal ganglion** (dorsal root ganglion) forms a swelling on the dorsal root (Fig. I-62). It lies in or close to the intervertebral foramen (Figs. 5-59 and 5-60).

As soon as the spinal nerve leaves the intervertebral foramen, it divides into two parts: a **dorsal (posterior) primary ramus** and a **ventral (anterior) primary ramus**. The dorsal rami supply nerve fibers to the **back**, whereas the ventral rami supply nerve fibers to the lateral and anterior regions of the trunk and to the limbs.

The autonomic nervous system (ANS) is a system of nerves and ganglia *concerned with the distribution of impulses to* (1) the **heart**, (2) nonstriated or **smooth muscle**, and (3) **glands** (Fig. I-63). The ANS also receives afferent impulses from these parts of the body. *The autonomic nervous system has two parts*: (1) the **sympathetic system** and (2) the **parasympathetic system**. The sympathetic system has connections with the thoracic and lumbar regions of the spinal cord from T1 to L2 or L3 segments. The parasympathetic system has cranial and sacral parts which are connected (1) with the brain through **cranial nerves III**, **VII**, **IX**, and **X**, and (2) with the spinal cord through **spinal nerves S2** to **S4** (the S2 connection is not always present).

There are neurons in the sympathetic system which correspond to the efferent or

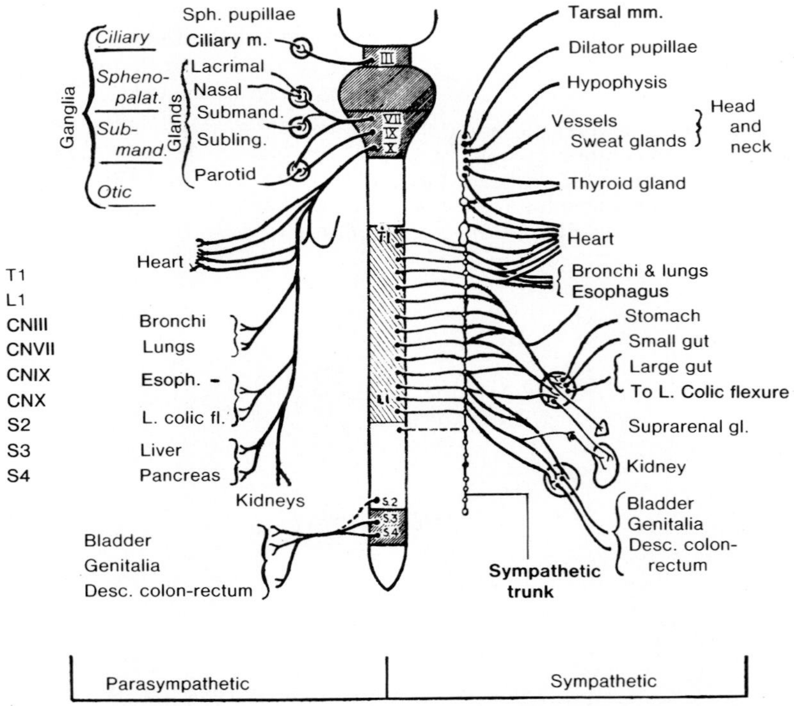

Figure I-63. Diagram illustrating the general plan of the autonomic nervous system (ANS). It is so named because it is concerned with involuntary activity. The ANS is a subdivision of the motor portion of the nervous system. Note that it consists of two parts, *sympathetic* and *parasympathetic*. These parts are anatomically separate and usually functionally reciprocal. The ANS carries nerve impulses to the heart, smooth muscle, and glands. The ganglia of the *sympathetic trunk* form a longitudinal series of swellings, one in front of each spinal nerve (also see Figs. I-64 and 1-25). The nerve fibers of the parasympathetic division of the ANS leave the CNS in cranial nerves III, VII, IX, and X and in sacral nerves 2, 3, and 4.

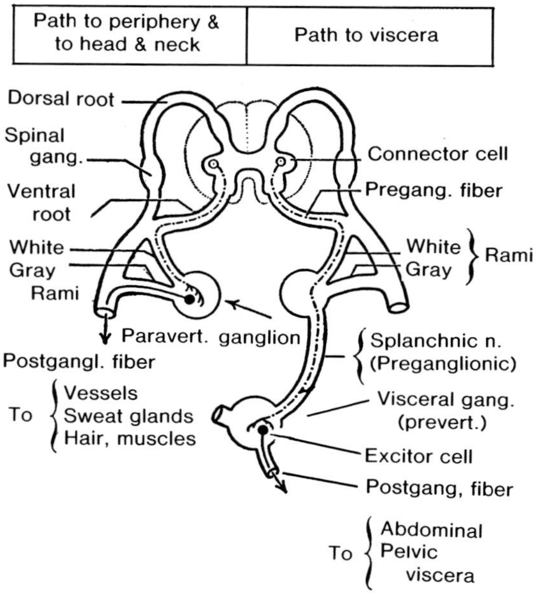

Figure I-64. Diagram illustrating the general plan of a sympathetic ganglion. Note that the fibers of sympathetic nerves leave the spinal cord in the ventral roots (T1 to L2 or L3) and enter a ventral primary ramus to run to a point just lateral to the vertebral column. From this point they pass anteromedially as the white ramus communicans to enter a paravertebral ganglion (ganglion of sympathetic trunk, Fig. I-63).

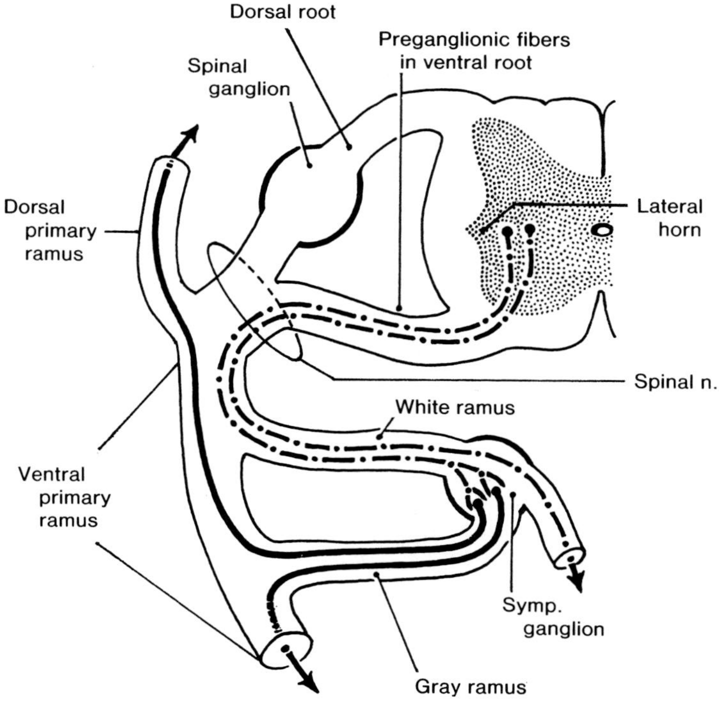

Figure I-65. Diagram illustrating the typical sympathetic contribution to a spinal nerve. Most autonomic ganglia resemble dorsal root or spinal ganglia as far as their connective tissue capsule and structure; however, unlike these ganglia, synapses occur in autonomic ganglia. Note that the neurons in the small lateral horn of gray matter, extending from segment T1 through L2 or L3, are the source of the preganglionic sympathetic fibers. Observe that these fibers reach the sympathetic trunk by way of the ventral root and the white ramus communicans.

motor neurons of the PNS. These efferent neurons are located (1) in **paravertebral ganglia** or ganglia of the **sympathetic trunk** (Figs. I-63, I-64, 1-25, and 2-131); (2) in **prevertebral ganglia** or visceral ganglia (*e.g.*, the **celiac ganglion**, Fig. 2-111); and (3) in the medulla of the **suprarenal gland** (Fig. 2-140).

In Figures I-64 and I-65, observe that the axon of a sympathetic neuron sends a **preganglionic fiber** via the ventral root and the **white ramus communicans** (connecting branch) to a paravertebral ganglion. Here it may synapse with excitor neurons, but some preganglionic fibers ascend or descend in the **sympathetic trunk** to synapse at other levels. Other preganglionic fibers pass through the paravertebral ganglia without synapsing to form **splanchnic nerves** to the viscera (Figs. I-64 and 2-127).

The **postganglionic fibers** or axons of excitor neurons course through the **gray ramus communicans** (Figs. I-64 and I-65) and pass from the sympathetic ganglion into the spinal nerve. They run to blood vessels, sweat glands, sebaceous glands, and the arrector pili muscles (associated with hairs). Other postganglionic fibers pass upward to the cervical sympathetic ganglia and supply structures in the head. Others pass downward to supply the lower limbs. Hence, the sympathetic trunks (Figs. I-63, 1-25, and 1-26) are composed of ascending and descending fibers (preganglionic efferent, postganglionic efferent, and afferent fibers).

It should now be clear that the *dorsal and ventral primary rami of spinal nerves contain* (1) **motor (efferent) fibers** from the ventral horn cells of the spinal cord, (2) **sensory (afferent) fibers** of spinal ganglion cells, and (3) **autonomic fibers**.

SUGGESTIONS FOR ADDITIONAL READING

1. Basmajian, J. V. *Primary Anatomy*, Ed. 7, The Williams & Wilkins Company, Baltimore, 1965.

This book, written as a textbook for elementary courses in anatomy, has been found useful by many medical and dental students as *an introduction to anatomy*. Unlike many anatomy books, including this one, it stresses the systemic approach, which is very helpful to a beginning student. Furthermore, the illustrations are simple and schematic, which quickly convey basic concepts in anatomy.

2. Basmajian, J. V. *Grant's Method of Anatomy*, Ed. 10, The Williams & Wilkins Company, Baltimore, 1980.

Grant's method of teaching anatomy made him a world renowned scholar. In addition to this book, his *Atlas* and *Dissector* are still widely used several years after his death. *His method teaches you to reason anatomically.* His review of the systems of the body would be profitable reading before you begin the detailed study of anatomy. Many illustrations from these sections are incorporated into this book because of their usefulness in helping beginning students to understand that human anatomy is rational and interesting, with direct applications to problems in medicine and surgery.

3. Ham, A. W. and Cormack, D. H. *Histology*, Ed. 8, J. B. Lippincott Company, Philadelphia, 1979.

The descriptions of bones, joints, muscles, lymphatics, and nerves in the present chapter are summaries. For more details, you are urged to read the descriptions in this classical textbook, which explains histology "simply enough for undergaduate students to learn the subject, not merely to memorize bits and pieces of it." You will particularly enjoy reading the well-illustrated description of bone and bones, muscle tissue, and nervous tissue.

4. Smith, C. G. *Basic Neuroanatomy*, Ed. 2. University of Toronto Press, Toronto, 1971.

If you are like most students, you will initially have trouble understanding the nervous system because of the intricacies of neuronal connections and the necessity of being able to visualize structures in three dimensions. This book has been used at the University of Toronto for over 18 years and is popular because of its easy-to-read style and its easy-to-follow illustrations. Students who cannot cope with more detailed texts turn to this book with gratitude.

CHAPTER 1

The Thorax

The thorax (G. chest) is the upper part of the trunk between the neck and the abdomen. The superficial structures covering the thoracic cage (Fig. 1-1), consisting of the pectoral (L. *pectus*, chest) muscles and the breast, are mainly described with the upper limb (see Chap. 6). These muscles act from the upper thorax to move the humerus (arm bone).

Chest pain is a common occurrence, the significance of which varies from negligible to very serious. Most people have had a local sharp and sudden pain in the side ("stitch in the side") or a burning pain behind the sternum (heartburn owing to gastric upset). However, a person with a **heart attack** (**MI,** myocardial infarction) will probably describe a **crushing substernal pain** that does not disappear with rest.

The evaluation of a patient with chest pain is largely concerned with discriminating between serious conditions and the many minor causes of chest pain. To perform a thorough clinical examination, a good knowledge of the anatomy of the thorax is required. Because a patient's life may be "hanging in the balance," there is no opportunity to consult an anatomy book.

The terms **thorax** and **chest** refer to the same region of the body. The pectoral region lies anteriorly on the thoracic or chest wall.

The heart (including the great vessels) and lungs are the most important viscera (L. soft parts) within the thorax. As these organs are constantly moving in living persons, the thorax is obviously one of the most dynamic regions of the body.

THE THORACIC WALL

The thoracic (chest) wall illustrates the correlation between structure and function in that the anatomical structures provide the mechanism for the functions of breathing, protection of the underlying viscera, and the venous return from areas inferior to the thorax.

BONES OF THE THORACIC WALL

The osseocartilaginous **thoracic cage** is formed by (1) the **12 thoracic vertebrae** posteriorly; (2) the **12 pairs of ribs** and their **costal cartilages**; and (3) the **sternum** anteriorly.

The Thoracic Vertebrae (Figs. 1-1 to 1-3, 5-1, 5-4, 5-15, 5-17, 5-21, and 5-22). These vertebrae are described with other parts of the vertebral column in Chapter 5. Their special features related to the thorax are as follows: they have (1) **facets on their bodies** for articulation with the heads of the ribs; (2) **facets on their transverse processes** for the rib tubercles, except for the lower two or three; and (3) **long spinous processes** (spines).

The spinous processes vary in their posterior direction. Those of T5 to T8 are nearly vertical and overlap the vertebrae below like roof shingles or tiles. This arrangement covers the small intervals between the laminae of adjacent vertebrae, preventing sharp objects from penetrating the vertebral canal and injuring the spinal cord when the vertebral column is flexed. The spinous processes of T1, T2, T11, and T12 are horizontal and those of T3, T4, T9, and T10 are directed obliquely downward. *Check the above statements* on an articulated vertebral column.

The Costal Facets (Figs. 1-2, 1-3, and 5-15). Thoracic vertebrae are unique in that they have facets on their bodies and transverse processes for articulation with the ribs (T11 and T12 are exceptions). Two demifacets are located laterally on the bod-

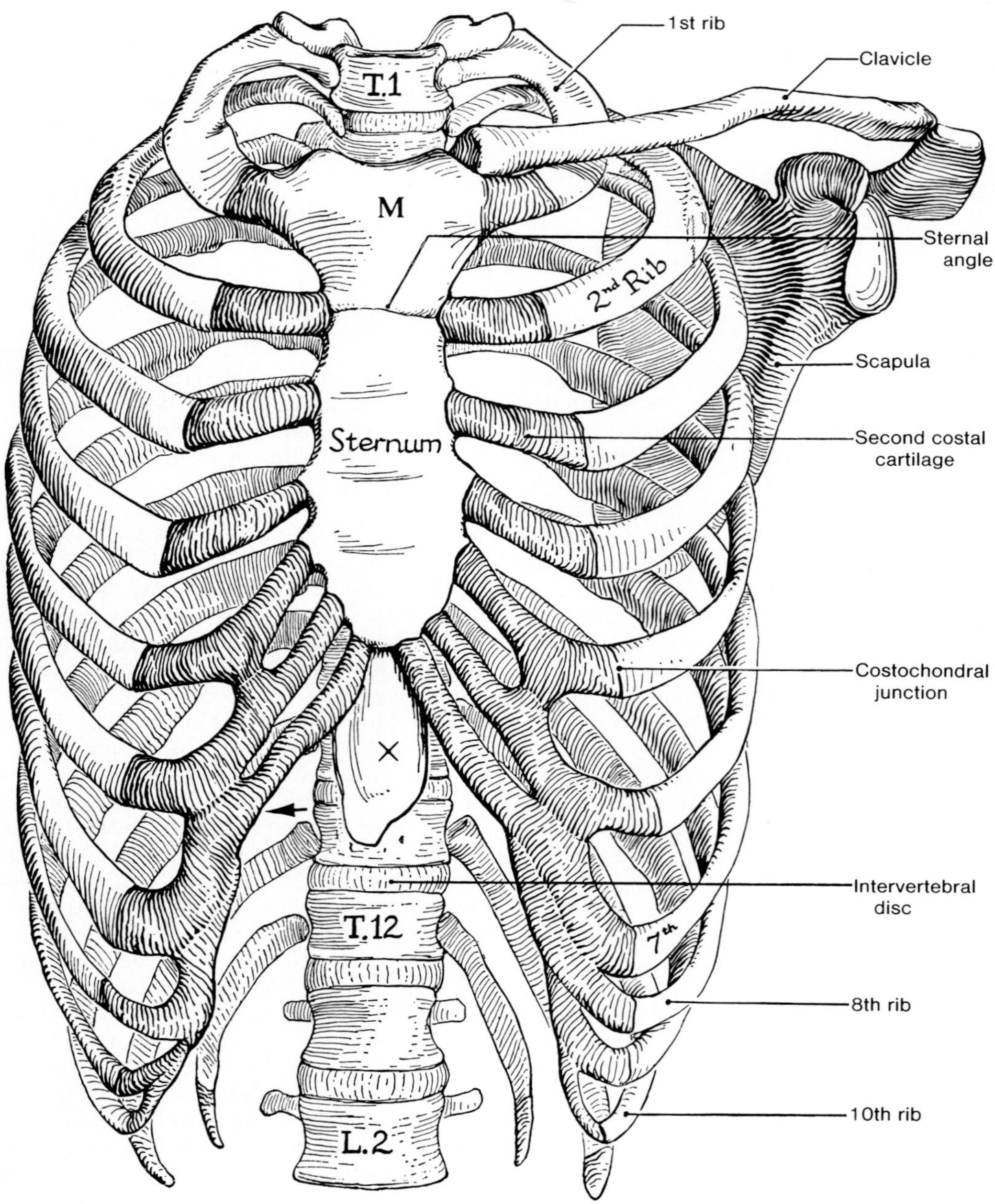

Figure 1-1. Drawing of the anterior aspect of the bony thorax of an adult female. Observe its component parts: 12 thoracic vertebrae (T1 to T12), 12 pairs of ribs and costal cartilages, and the sternum. Note that each rib articulates posteriorly with the vertebral column. Observe that the costal cartilages of the upper seven pairs of ribs articulate directly with the sternum. (The eighth pair may do so also). Note that the 8th, 9th, and 10th costal cartilages articulate with the cartilages next above and that the 11th and 12th cartilages are free or floating anteriorly and have cartilaginous tips. Observe the downward inclination of all ribs. Note that the costal cartilages of the 3rd to 10th ribs incline upward. Observe that the tip of the 12th costal cartilage is at the level of the 2nd lumbar vertebra. Note that the 10th ribs and costal cartilages are the lowest ribs and cartilages visible from the front. Observe that the clavicle lies over the first rib making it difficult to palpate anteriorly in living persons. The second rib is easy to locate because its costal cartilage articulates at the junction of the manubrium (*M*) and the body of the sternum. This sternal angle, opposite the second costal cartilage, is a key landmark in the chest that is used when counting the ribs. Observe the costal margin (*arrow*) formed by the upturned costal cartilages of the 7th to 10th ribs (also see Fig. 1-11). *X* indicates the xiphoid process of the sternum.

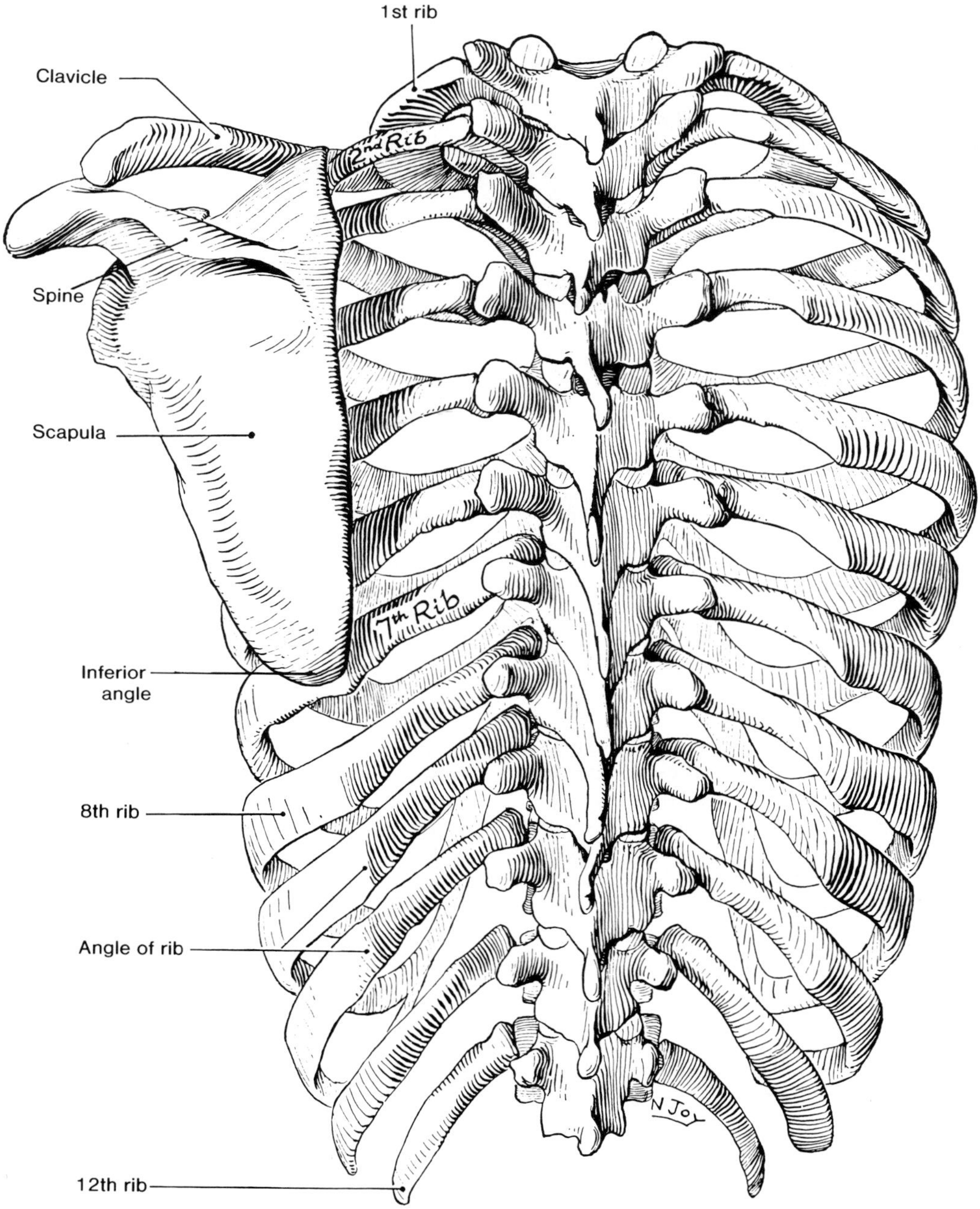

Figure 1-2. Drawing of the posterior aspect of the bony thorax shown in Figure 1-1. Observe the progressive increase in length of the first seven ribs and of the first seven costal cartilages. Although the seventh rib is the longest rib, the eighth and ninth ones are more oblique. Observe that the sternal end of the first costal cartilage is about 4 cm below the level of the head of the first rib. Note that the scapula crosses 50% of the 12 ribs, namely the second to seventh inclusive. Verify that the distance between the spinous processes of the vertebrae and the angles of the ribs diminish from the eighth rib upward. Note that the seventh intercostal space is located just below the tip of the inferior angle of the scapula. Observe that only the left pectoral girdle (clavicle and scapula) is illustrated in Figures 1-1 and 1-2. (For details on the pectoral girdle, see Chap. 6).

ies of T2 to T9. The **superior demifacet** on the superior edge is for articulation with the caudal part of the head of its own rib. The **inferior demifacet** on the inferior edge is for articulation with the cranial part of the head of the rib immediately below.

The costal facets on the other vertebrae vary somewhat. T1 has a single costal facet for the head of the first rib and a small demifacet for the cranial part of the second rib (Fig. 1-3*A*). T10 has only one costal facet, part of which is on the body and part on the pedicle. T11 and T12 (Fig. 1-3*C*) have only a single costal facet on their pedicles.

CLINICALLY ORIENTED COMMENTS

Movements between adjacent vertebrae are relatively small in the thoracic region. The limited movement of this part of the vertebral column serves to protect the thoracic viscera.

The bodies of T5 to T8 vertebrae are related to the descending thoracic aorta (Fig. 1-19) and sometimes it forms an impression on their left sides. If the aorta develops an **aneurysm** (localized dilation) in this region, these vertebrae may be partly eroded by pressure from this vessel. In some cases these bony changes are visible on chest radiographs. The intervertebral discs are apparently unaffected by pressure from a dilated aorta.

Surface Anatomy of the Thoracic Vertebrae (Fig. 5-10). The spinous processes of all the thoracic vertebrae can be palpated in the posterior median line. When the vertebral column is flexed, the first spinous process that is visible is usually C7 (the **vertebra prominens**), but the spinous process of T1 is sometimes just as prominent as that of C7.

A line drawn through the tip of the spinous process of **T3** indicates the base of the *spine of the scapula* when the arm is at the side (Fig. 1-2). Similarly, a line through the middle of the spinous process of **T7** indicates the *inferior angle of the scapula.* Verify these landmarks on a dried skeleton and on a colleague; then ask the person to elevate his/her shoulders. Note that the inferior angle of the scapula rises. The trapezius and levator scapulae muscles perform this action (see Chap. 6). It is important to know about this because you may sometime use the base of the spine of the scapula and the inferior angle of the scapula as a guide to thoracic vertebral levels or to the level of an intercostal space.

The Ribs (Figs. 1-1 to 1-7). These elongated **flat bones** form the largest part of the **thoracic cage**, which houses the lungs, the heart, and most of the great vessels. In addition, the thorax protects the liver and the spleen. The sternum, the costal cartilages, and the vertebrae form the other parts of the thoracic cage.

The ribs are long, thin, curved, slightly twisted arches of bone. **There are usually 12 pairs of ribs,** but the number may be increased by the development of cervical **ribs** (Fig. 6-38) or lumbar ribs (Fig. 5-50), or it may be decreased by **agenesis** (failure of formation) of the 12th pair.

The True Ribs (Fig. 1-1). The **first seven pairs** of ribs are called true ribs or **vertebrosternal ribs** because they *articulate with the sternum through their costal cartilages.* Examine an articulated skeleton and observe that the *true ribs increase in length from above downward.*

The False Ribs (Figs. 1-1 and 1-2). The **8th to 12th pairs** of ribs are called false ribs or **vertebrocostal ribs** because they are *attached to the sternum through the costal cartilage of another rib or not at all.* The 8th, 9th, and 10th ribs join the sternum indirectly through articulation of their costal cartilages with each other and fusion of this combined cartilage with the seventh costal cartilage.

The 11th and 12th ribs are called "**floating ribs**" because they are so short that they do not attach to the sternum (*i.e.*, their anterior ends lie free and end amongst the muscles of the lateral abdominal wall). Understand that *the last two ribs are not really floating*; they articulate with the body of their own numbered vertebra. Examine an articulated skeleton and observe

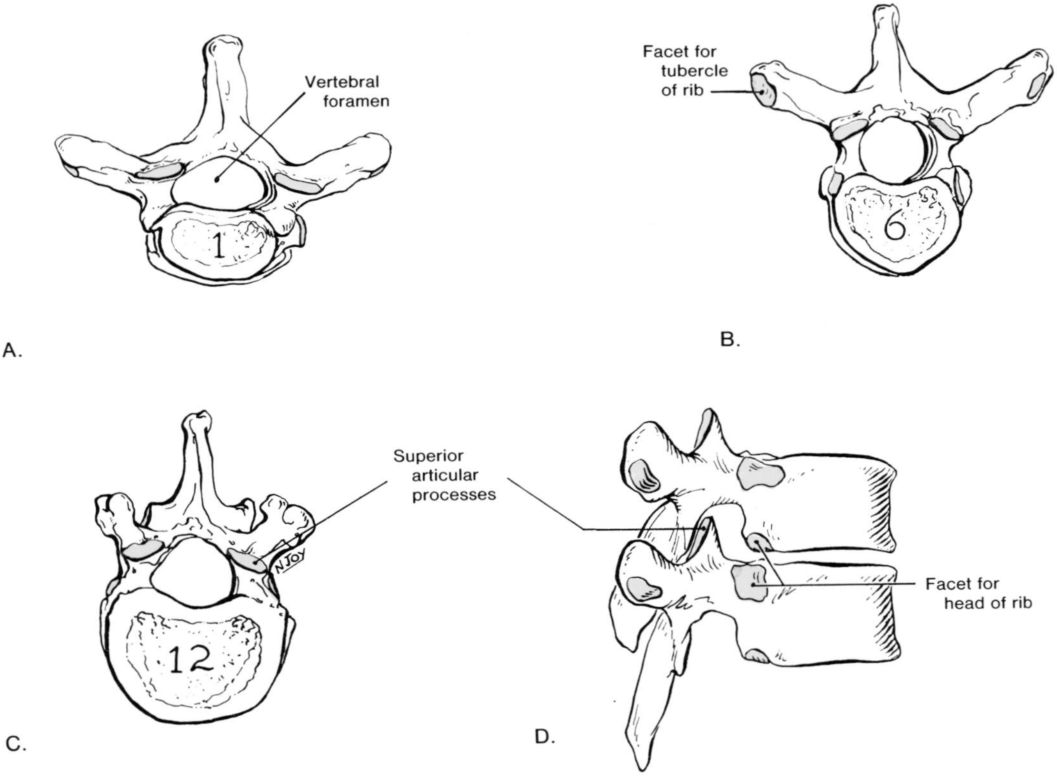

Figure 1-3. *A* to *C*, drawings of thoracic vertebrae from above. *D*, drawing of a lateral view of two typical midthoracic vertebrae. Observe the variation in the size and shape of these vertebrae and the variation in the shape of the vertebral foramen. Thoracic vertebrae differ from other vertebrae in that they have costal facets (*yellow*) on their bodies and transverse processes for articulation with ribs, except for T11 and T12, which have only a single costal facet located laterally on their pedicles. Differentiate between costal facets and those for the articular processes, which are also colored yellow.

that the *false ribs* (*8 to 12*) *decrease in length from above downward.*

Variations in the sternocostal junctions are not uncommon. Although the first seven costal cartilages nearly always join the sternum, sometimes only six cartilages articulate with it (Fig. 1-14). In other people, the eighth costal cartilage (especially on the right) joins the sternum (Fig. 1-20).

The Typical Ribs (Figs. 1-4 and 1-5). **Ribs 3 to 10** are regarded as typical ribs; however, the 10th rib is atypical in that it has only one articular facet on its head. Note that *typical ribs vary slightly in length* and in other characteristics. Each typical rib has a head, a neck, a tubercle, and a body (shaft).

The head of a rib is wedge-shaped and presents **two articular facets** for articulation with the numerically corresponding vertebra and the vertebra superior to it. These facets are separated by the **crest of the head**, which is joined to the **intervertebral disc** (Fig. 1-1) by an intra-articular ligament.

The neck of a rib is the stout, flattened part (about 2.5 cm long) that is *located between the head and the tubercle.* The neck lies anterior to the transverse process of the corresponding vertebra. Its upper border, called the **crest of the neck**, is sharp and its lower border is rounded.

The tubercle of a true rib is on the posterior surface *at the junction of its neck*

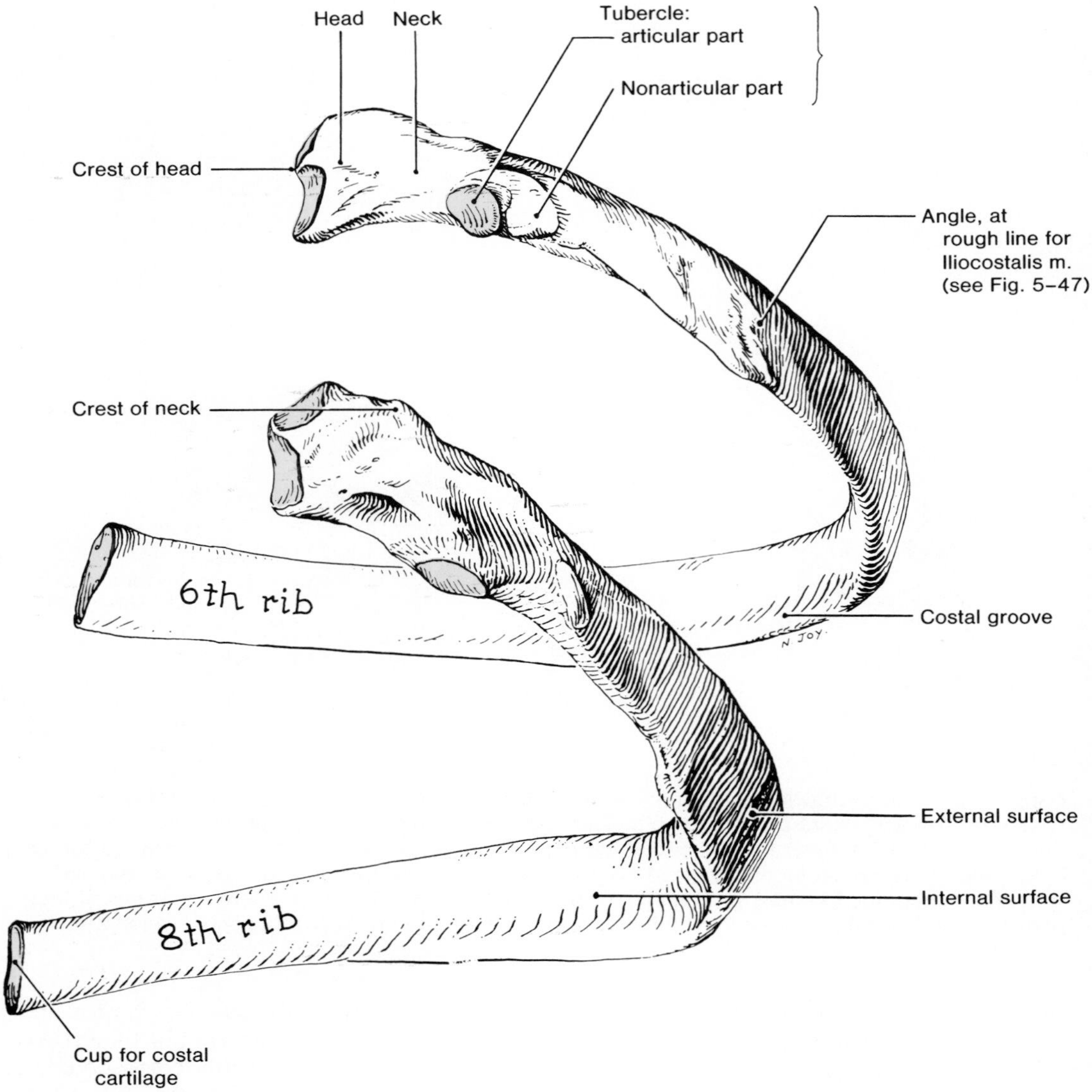

Figure 1-4. Drawings of two typical right ribs viewed from behind (see Fig. 1-2). Ribs 3 to 10 are called "typical" ribs, but the ones shown here are most typical of ribs in general. *They will not lie flat on the table* because they bend relatively sharply at their angles. Observe the wedge-shaped *head*, with a larger lower facet for its own vertebra (sixth or eighth) and a smaller facet for the vertebra above. Note the crest of the head which is joined to the intervertebral disc (Fig. 1-1) by an intra-articular ligament. Examine the posterior surface of the *neck*, which is rough where the costotransverse ligament attaches (Fig. 1-23). Note the sharp *crest of the neck* for the superior costotransverse ligament. Observe the nonarticular part of the tubercle for the lateral costotransverse ligament. Examine the convex, articular part of the tubercle (*yellow*) which is on the posterior aspect of the upper seven ribs. Note that the posterior part of the body (shaft) is round on cross-section and that the anterior part is flattened and, being articular, slightly enlarged. Observe the rough line for the attachment of the iliocostalis muscle, where the rib takes not only a bend but also a twist. Examine the costal groove which lodges the intercostal vein, artery, and nerve (Fig. 1-28). The side to which a detached rib belongs may be determined at a glance by the fact that the front of its neck faces upward and forward. This does not apply to the uppermost two or three ribs.

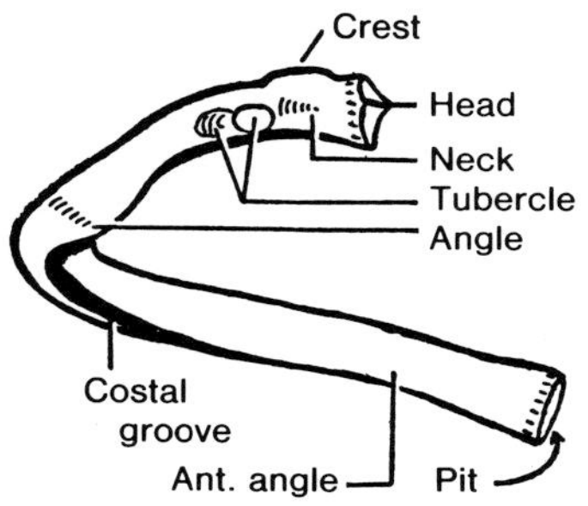

Figure 1-5. Drawing of a typical rib, viewed obliquely from behind. Observe that it has (1) a *posterior* (*vertebral*) *end* that is slightly enlarged to form (2) a *head* that has a crest (see Fig. 1-4); (3) a *neck* that also has a crest; (4) a *body* (shaft) between the neck and the anterior end; (5) a *tubercle* on the posterior end at the junction of the neck and the body; (6) an *angle* where the rib abruptly changes its direction (this main angle must not be confused with the anterior angle where there is a sudden increase in curvature as the anterior end is reached); and (7) the *anterior* (sternal) end which has a rough oval pit or cup where it becomes continuous with its costal cartilage.

and body. It is most prominent on the upper ribs and has a smooth convex facet which *articulates with the corresponding transverse process.* It also has a rough nonarticular part for attachment of the **lateral costotransverse ligament** (Fig. 5-51). The tubercles of the 8th to 10th ribs have *flat facets* for articulation with similar facets on the transverse processes.

The body (shaft) of a rib is thin, flat, long, and curved. Forming the greatest part of a rib, the body has external and internal surfaces, thick rounded superior borders, and thin, sharp, inferior borders. A short distance beyond the tubercle (5 to 6 cm), the body ceases to pass backward and swings rather sharply forward. The point of greatest change in curvature is called the **angle of the rib**; here, the rib is both curved and twisted. The sharp inferior border of a rib projects downward and is located external to the **costal groove** on the internal surface of the body, near its inferior border. This groove and the flange formed by the inferior border are for the accommodation and protection of the intercostal vessels and nerve that accompany the rib (Fig. 1-28). Examine a typical dried rib and note that the costal groove fades out as the anterior (sternal) end is approached (Figs. 1-4 and 1-5). Also observe that this end is cupped for reception of the costal cartilage.

The Atypical Ribs (Fig. 1-6). Certain features of the four atypical ribs warrant description.

The first rib (Figs. 1-1, 1-2, and 1-6) is the broadest and most curved of all the ribs and is the shortest of the true ribs. *The first rib is clinically important* because many structures cross or attach to it. It is flattened from above downward and has a prominent **scalene tubercle** on the inner border of its superior surface for the insertion of the **scalenus anterior muscle** (Figs. 1-20 and 9-33). The subclavian vein crosses the first rib in front of this tubercle and the subclavian artery and the lower trunk of the **brachial plexus** (network of nerves to the upper limb (Fig 1-20)) pass behind it. Examine the grooves formed by the **subclavian vessels** on a dried first rib.

The first rib has a single facet which articulates with the body of the first thoracic vertebra and slightly with the intervertebral disc above. The prominent **tubercle of the first rib** articulates with the transverse process of the first thoracic vertebra.

The second rib (Figs. 1-1, 1-2, and 1-6) has a curvature similar to that of the first rib, but it is thinner, much less curved, and about twice as long. It can easily be distinguished from the first rib by the presence of a broad rough eminence, the **tuberosity for the serratus anterior muscle**. Actually only part of this muscle originates here (see Fig. 6-21).

The 11th and 12th ribs (Figs. 1-1, 1-2, and 1-6) are **short**, especially the 12th pair. They are capped with cartilage and have a single facet on their heads and *no neck or tubercle.* The 11th has a slight angle and a shallow costal groove. The 12th has neither of these features.

CLINICALLY ORIENTED COMMENTS

Despite their ability to bend under stress, the ribs may be fractured by direct violence or indirectly by crushing injuries. On some

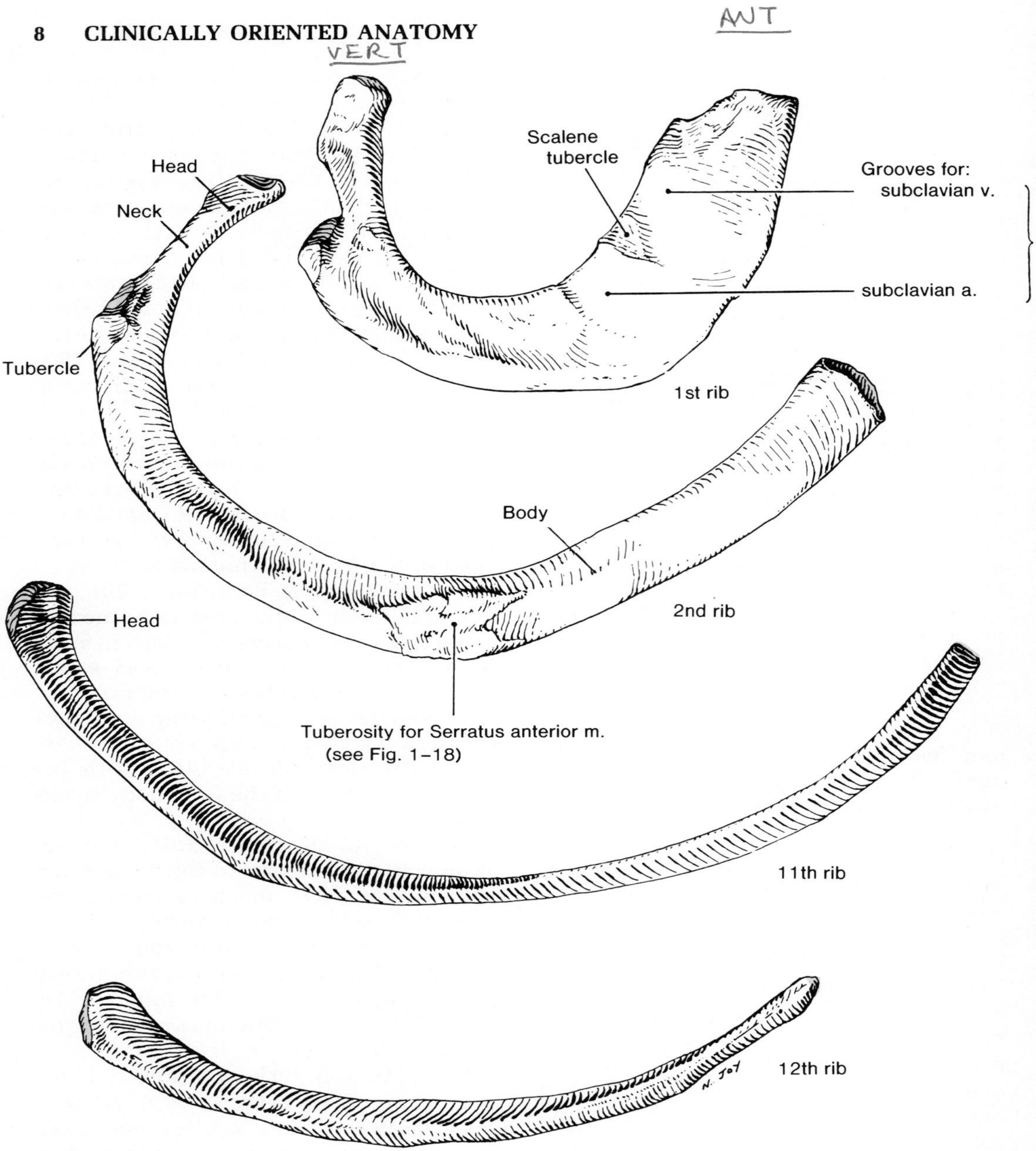

Figure 1-6. Drawings of four atypical ribs, viewed from above. These four ribs have faint angles (*i.e.*, twists); hence, they will *lie flat* on the table. Observe that the first rib is the highest; shortest, broadest, strongest, and most curved of these ribs. Note that its head and neck are directed medially and downward and its head has a single facet. Observe that its tubercle is the most prominent of all, for here the tubercle and the angle coincide. The tubercle for the scalenus anterior muscle on the upper (external) surface of the body separates the groove for the subclavian vein in front from the groove for the subclavian artery (Fig. 1-85) and the lowest trunk of the brachial plexus behind (see the brachial plexus in Fig. 6-25). Note that the second rib is marked by the tuberosity for the serratus anterior muscle. Observe that, for the 11th and 12th ribs, called floating ribs, each has a single facet on the head for articulation with the body of their own number vertebra, no tubercle, and a tapering end. The heads of all the ribs lie on a plane which is anterior to their most posterior parts (Fig. 1-1).

occasions ribs have been fractured by muscular men hugging frail women too vigorously. *The middle ribs are the ones most commonly fractured.* The first two ribs (which are protected by the clavicle) and the last two (which are free and movable) are the least commonly injured. The chest walls of infants and children are very elastic; hence, rib fractures are rare in them.

Crushing injuries tend to break the ribs at their weakest point, *i.e.*, the site of greatest change in curvature, which is just anterior to the costal angle. **Direct injuries** may fracture a rib anywhere and the broken ends may be driven inward and injure the thoracic and/or upper abdominal organs (*e.g.*, lungs and/or spleen). Understandably, patients with fractured ribs experience pain in the region of the fracture when asked to take a deep breath. Similarly, careful palpation along the broken rib often reveals local tenderness, *even when a fracture may not be visible on a radiograph.*

Flail chest (**"stove-in chest"**) occurs when a sizeable segment of the anterior and/or lateral chest wall is freely movable because of multiple rib fractures. This allows the loose segment of the chest wall to move paradoxically (*i.e.*, inward on inspiration and outward on expiration). This impairs ventilation and thereby affects oxygenation of the blood; if severe, death results. Current treatment is to fix the loose segment of chest wall by hooks and/or wires so that it cannot move.

To remove a well defined **collection of pus** in the pleural cavity, called **empyema,** sometimes a partial **rib excision** is performed. The piece of rib is removed in a manner similar to that described for excision of a piece of costal cartilage (Fig. 1-20). When removed from its periosteum, access to the pleural cavity (Fig. 1-15) is gained by making an incision in the bed of the rib (*i.e.*, periosteum and fascia). Following the operation, the rib regenerates from the remaining periosteum. Any cutting operation on the thoracic wall is called a **thoracotomy.** Sometimes a piece of rib is used for **autogenous bone grafting** (*e.g.*, for reconstruction of the mandible following excision of a mandibular tumor).

Cervical ribs are present in about 0.5 to 1% of people and articulate with the seventh cervical vertebra (Fig. 6-38). Commonly they have a head, neck, and tubercle, with varying amounts of body. A cervical rib extends into the posterior triangle of the neck (Fig. 9-15), where its anterior end may lie free or be attached to the first rib or its costal cartilage or even the sternum. Often cervical ribs are incidental observations on routine radiographs and may not be reported unless **neurovascular symptoms** have been reported in the upper limb. For clinically oriented comments on this condition, see chapter 6.

Lumbar ribs are more common than cervical ribs. They consist of a head, neck, tubercle, and short (usually less than 5 cm) pointed body. Lumbar ribs articulate with the first lumbar vertebra or are attached to the tips of its transverse processes (Fig. 5-50). *Lumbar ribs have significance* in that they may confuse the identification of vertebral levels in radiographs. In addition, a lumbar rib may be erroneously interpreted as a fracture of a lumbar transverse process by an inexperienced observer of radiographs.

On rare occasions, the 12th ribs fail to develop; hence, persons may have only 11 pairs. *Otherwise normal people may have 11 to 14 pairs of ribs,* but in some persons with spinal anomalies the number may even be less. Accessory cervical or lumbar ribs represent the costal elements (Fig. 1-7) that have developed (abnormally) into ribs.

In **coarctation of the aorta,** narrowing of the distal part of its arch (Fig. 1-99) results in considerable enlargement of the intercostal arteries and other arteries as a means of providing a **collateral circulation** to lower parts of the body (Fig. 1-103). These enlarged intercostal arteries erode the inferior borders of the corresponding ribs. Radiographic demonstration of this characteristic **notching of the ribs** is very useful in confirming suspected congenital malformation of the aorta (Case 1-9). A significant coarctation occurs about once in every 1000 persons.

Bifid ribs or **forked ribs** (Fig. 1-8) are not uncommon and this possibility must be considered when a rib count seems to indicate that the cartilages of the upper eight

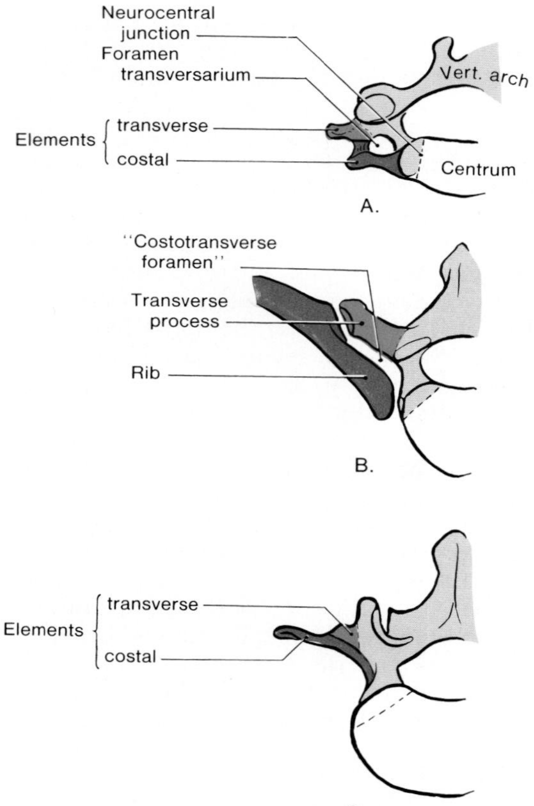

Figure 1-7. Diagrams illustrating the homologous parts of vertebrae. The vertebral (neural) arch lies lateral and posterior to the spinal cord and meninges. The centrum is the ossification center of the central part of the body of a vertebra. (For details about the above two structures see Chap. 5). *Red*, rib or costal element; *blue*, vertebral arch and its processes; *uncolored*, centrum. *A*, in the cervical region the costal element is represented by the anterior part of a transverse process of a cervical vertebra. In about 0.5% of people the costal element of C7 develops into a cervical rib. *B*, in the thoracic region the costal element develops into a rib. *C*, in the lumbar region the costal element usually becomes the anterior part of a transverse process, but often develops into a short lumbar rib (Fig. 5-50).

ribs articulate with the sternum. Usually the condition is unilateral; hence, unilaterality of eight apparent true ribs favors the suspicion of a bifid rib. However, in some cases (Fig. 1-20) eight normal ribs articulate with the sternum.

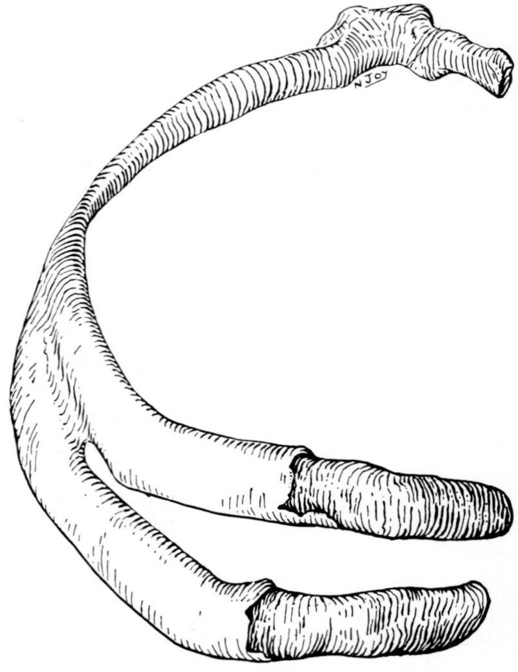

Figure 1-8. Drawing of bifid right third rib. The upper part, which is supernumerary, articulated with the side of the first sternebra (segment) of the body of the sternum (Fig. 1-10*B*); the lower part articulated in the normal situation for the costal cartilage of a third rib, *i.e.*, at the junction of the first and second sternabrae. This rib abnormality is not uncommon and it is usually unilateral.

Fused ribs are uncommon and are often associated with a vertebral abnormality, *e.g.*, a **hemivertebra** (failure of half of a vertebra to form, Fig. 5-7).

The Costal Cartilages (Figs. 1-1 and 1-14). These flattened bars of **hyaline cartilage** extend from the anterior ends of the ribs and contribute significantly to the elasticity and the mobility of the ribs. Actually the costal cartilages are unossified parts of the embryonic cartilaginous ribs. Their perichondrium blends with the periosteum of the ribs associated with them (Fig. 1-20).

The upper seven costal cartilages are connected with the sternum. Those of the 8th to 10th articulate with the lower border of the cartilage just above them. The lowest

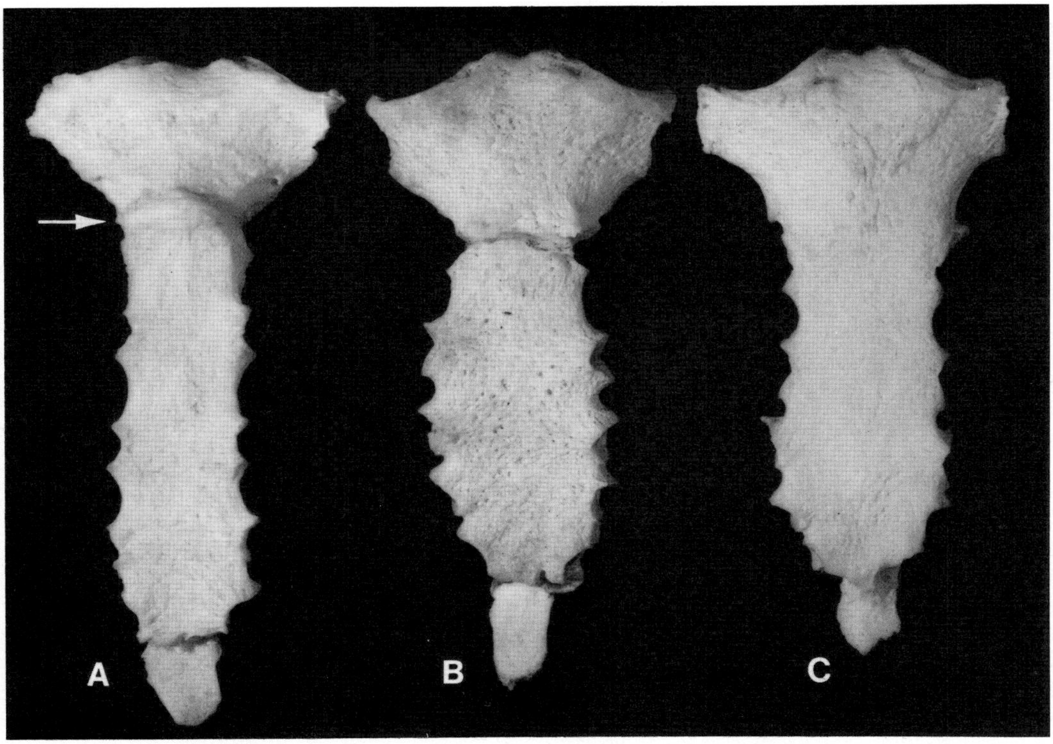

Figure 1-9. Photographs of anterior views of three sterna. *A*, from a male; *B* and *C*, from females. Observe that the bodies of the sterna from the females are shorter and broader than that from the male and less than twice the length of the manubrium. Note that the sternal angle (*arrow*) forms a prominent ridge in *A* and that the manubrium has fused with the body in *C*.

two cartilages have pointed tips which end in the muscular wall of the abdomen. The costal cartilages increase in length from the first to the seventh and then gradually become shorter. They also diminish in breadth from above downward.

The Costal Margin (Figs. 1-11 and 1-13). The 7th to 10th costal cartilages meet on each side and their inferior edges form the costal margin. The diverging costal margins form an **infrasternal (subcostal) angle** below the xiphisternal joint (Fig. 1-53). The apex of the angle is at the above joint.

The medial end of the first costal cartilage joins the **manubrium** with no joint between them; its perichondrium blends with the periosteum of the sternum. The medial ends of the second to seventh costal cartilages are rounded and articulate with the body of the sternum. *These sternocostal articulations are synovial joints.* The costal cartilages of the 8th to 10th ribs do not reach the sternum; they taper to a point and articulate with the cartilage just above. The costal cartilages of the 11th and 12th ribs are mere tips which are pointed and free.

CLINICALLY ORIENTED COMMENTS

The costal cartilages of young people provide resilience to the thoracic cage, preventing many crushing injuries or direct blows from fracturing the ribs and/or the sternum. In older adults the costal cartilages often undergo superficial calcification, losing some of their elasticity and becoming brittle. This calcification makes them radiopaque (*i.e.*, visible on radiographs) which may be confusing to inexperienced observers.

Separation of a rib (separated rib cartilage) refers to a dislocation between the rib and its costal cartilage and not to the breach of continuity in the bone that may be detected in a fractured rib, especially in a thin person. One of the costal cartilages of the lower ribs, usually the 10th, separates from the inferior border of the costal cartilage immediately above. Consequently, the cartilage of this **slipping rib** can move upward and override the one above, causing pain. Slipping ribs are most common in young women, but the reason for this is unclear.

The Sternum (Figs. 1-1 and 1-9 to 1-12). The sternum (breastbone) is an elongated **flat bone,** resembling a short broadsword, that lies in the anterior midline of the thorax. The sternum (G. *sternon,* the chest) *consists of three parts*: the manubrium, the body, and the xiphoid process. The sternum is covered anteriorly only by skin, superficial fascia, and periosteum, except where the pectoralis major muscle and the sternal head of the sternocleidomastoid muscle arise from it (Figs. 6-19 and 6-21).

The Manubrium (Figs. 1-1, 1-9, and 1-10). The manubrium (L. handle), or superior part of the sternum, is wider and thicker than the inferior two parts. Although generally quadrilateral, its narrow inferior end gives it a somewhat triangular shape. Broad and thick above, it slopes downward and forward. The superior surface of the manubrium is indented by a median **jugular notch** (suprasternal notch). On each side of this is an oval articular facet, called the **clavicular notch,** for articulation with the medial end of the clavicle. In Figures 1-1 and 1-11 note that the sternal end of the clavicle projects above the manubrium. Just below each clavicular notch, the costal cartilage of the first rib is fused with the lateral margin of the manubrium. This is a flexible but strong union, known as a **synchondrosis**, where the hyaline cartilage of the costal process unites with the manubrium.

The inferior border of the manubrium is oval and rough where it articulates with the body of the sternum at the **manubriosternal joint,** which is usually a **symphysis.** In this union, fibrocartilage and ligaments join the bones.

The manubrium and the body of the sternum lie in slightly different planes, hence their line of junction at the manubriosternal joint forms an anteriorly projecting obtuse **sternal angle** (of Louis). This very **important bony landmark** is about 5 cm inferior to the jugular notch.

The Body of the Sternum (Figs. 1-1 and 1-9 to 1-12). This is the longest of its three parts. It is longer, thinner, and narrower than the manubrium, but its width varies as a result of the scalloping of its lateral borders by the costal notches. It is broadest at about the level of the fifth sternocostal joints and then gradually tapers inferiorly. The body of the sternum is usually significantly shorter in the female than in the male and is less than twice the length of manubrium. This **sex difference** is useful in identifying the sex of skeletal remains.

The anterior surface of the body is slightly concave from side to side (nearly flat) and is directed slightly forward. It is variably marked by three transverse ridges, representing the lines of fusion of the four **sternebrae.** The centers of ossification for these segments appear before birth (20 to 24 weeks) and begin to fuse at puberty from below upward. *By 25 years all the sternabrae have fused to form the body of the sternum;* in old age no evidence of their former existence is detectable (Fig. 1-9*C*). Frequently there is an opening in the body of the sternum called the **sternal foramen.** This common anomaly resulting from a defect in ossification is of no clinical significance, except that its possible presence should be known so that it will not be misinterpreted as a bullet hole.

The posterior surface of the body is slightly concave and transverse ridges marking the lines of fusion of the sternabrae may be visible, but they are less distinct than those on the anterior surface and disappear in old age.

The Xiphoid Process (Figs. 1-1 and 1-9 to 1-11). This thin broadsword-like pointed process is the *smallest and most variable part of the sternum.* Although it may be

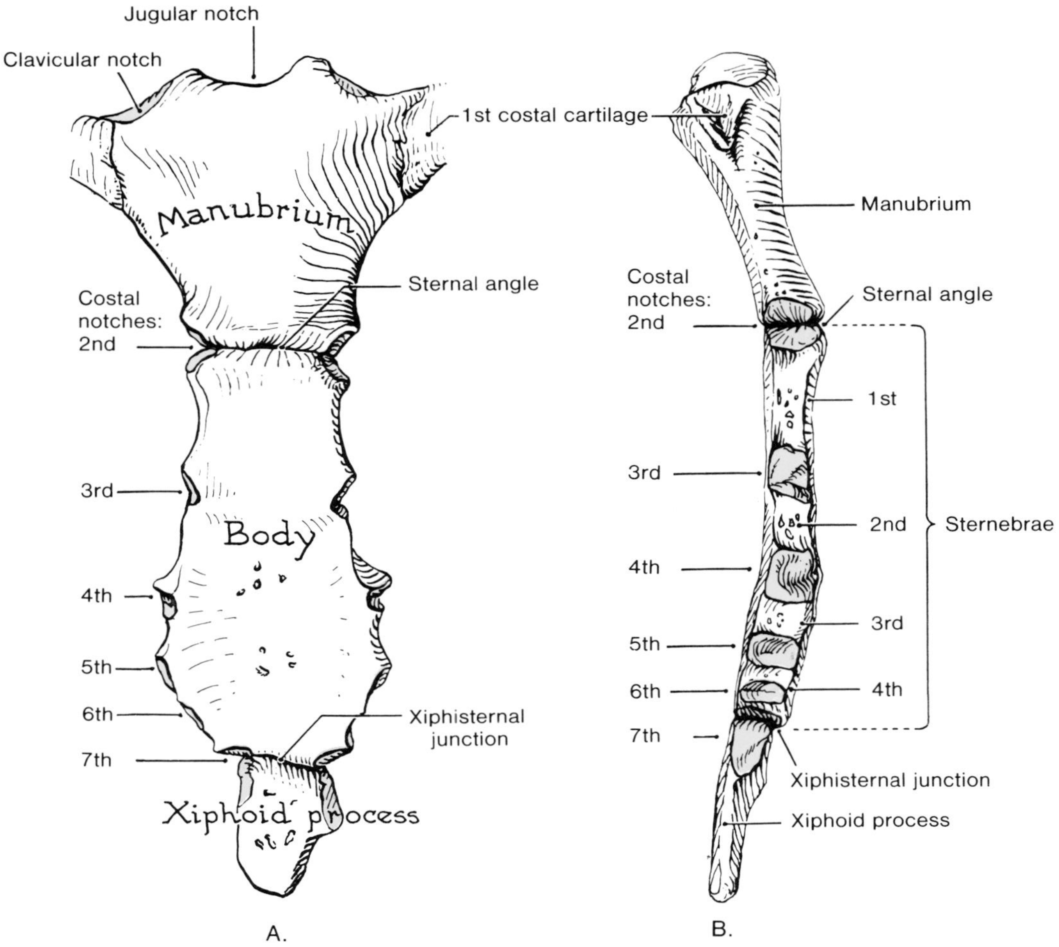

Figure 1-10. Drawings of the adult sternum. Observe its resemblance to a broadsword. *A*, anterior view. *B*, lateral view. Observe that the sternum is a flat elongated bone that somewhat resembles a short broadsword. The manubrium (L. handle) represents the handle and the xiphoid (G. sword-like) its pointed end. Observe the considerable thickness of the upper third of the manubrium between the clavicular notches. On a dried manubrium verify that its anterior surface is smooth and slightly convex, whereas its posterior surface is concave and featureless. Note the thin and tapering tip and sides of the xiphoid process. Examine two landmarks: (1) the sternal angle at the junction of the manubrium and body at the level of the second costal cartilage, and (2) the sharp lower edge of the body at the xiphisternal junction. Observe where the first seven pairs of costal cartilages articulate with the sternum. The other ribs do not articulate with it, except for the eighth which may do so (Fig. 1-20).

pointed (G. *xiphos*, sword + *eidos*, appearance), it is often blunt, bifid, curved, deflected to one side or the other, or directed anteriorly. Although commonly perforated in old persons owing to incomplete ossification, this observation is of no clinical significance.

The xiphoid process is cartilaginous at birth and remains so during infancy and early childhood. It may begin to ossify during the third year, but usually this process does not begin until much later. The xiphoid process usually ossifies and unites with the body of the sternum around the 40th

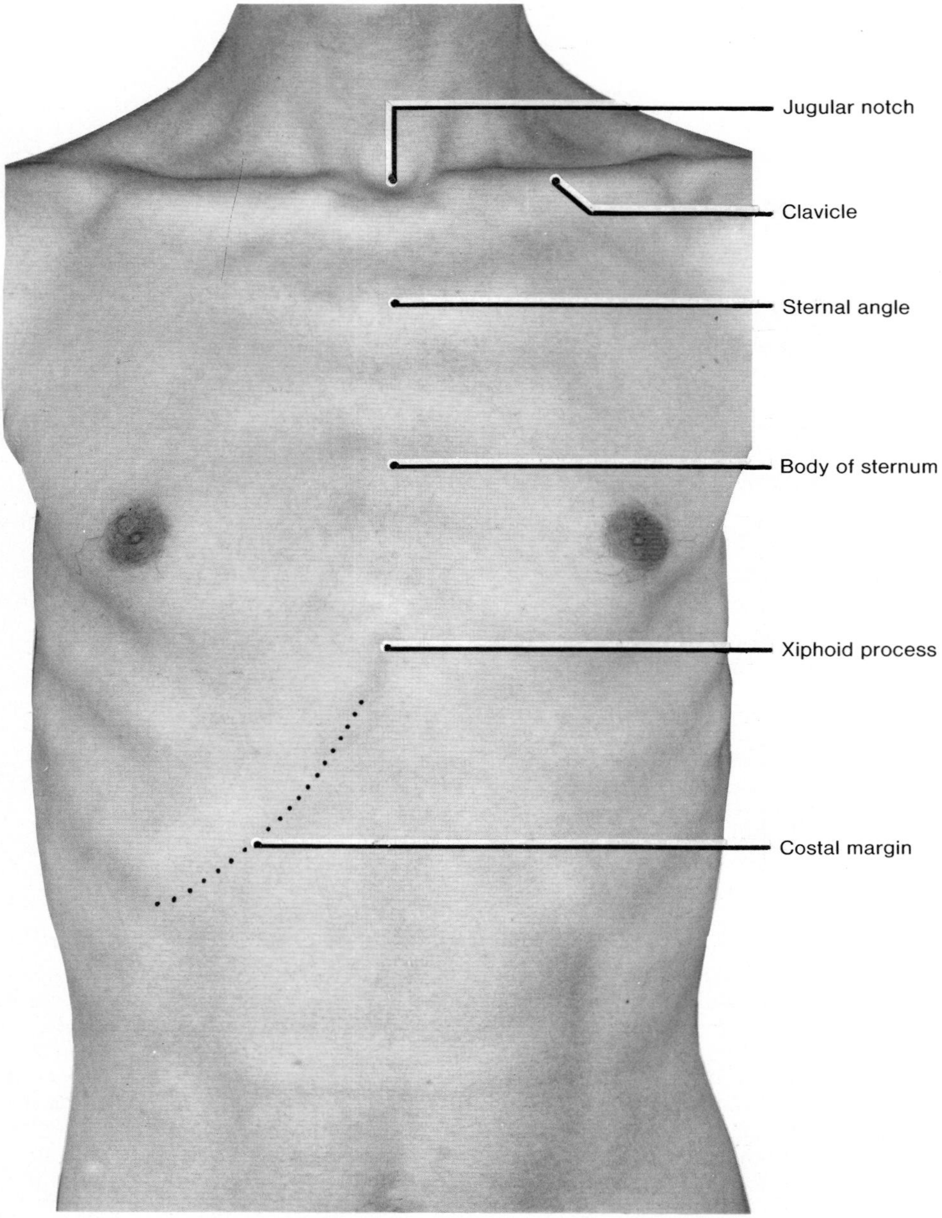

Figure 1-11. Photograph of an anterior view of the thorax of a 27-year-old man showing the surface features of the clavicles, ribs, and sternum. Observe the sternal angle at the junction of the manubrium and the body of the sternum (also see Figs. 1-9 and 1-10). This ridge is usually visible and is almost invariably easily palpable. It is an important bony landmark clinically in connection with the identification of ribs. Visualize the following two lines of orientation: (1) the *midsternal line* lies in the median plane over the sternum, and (2) the *midclavicular line* runs vertically downward from the midpoint of the clavicle and runs about 9 cm from the anterior median line. Study this photograph while examining the anterior aspect of the bony thorax as illustrated in Figure 1-1.

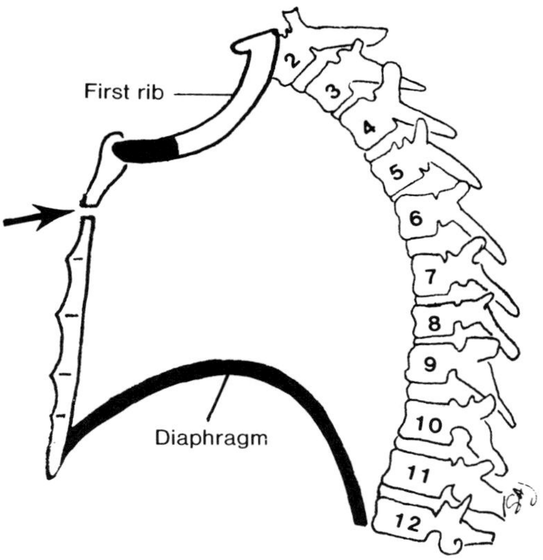

Figure 1-12. Diagrammatic sketch of a median section of the bony thorax, indicating various levels and lengths. The *arrow* indicates the sternal angle where the manubrium meets the body of the sternum. Note the costal cartilage of the first rib (*black tip*) joining with the manubrium. (See Fig. 1-96 for details).

year, but it may remain ununited even in old age (Fig. 1-9*A*).

CLINICALLY ORIENTED COMMENTS

Fracture of the sternum is uncommon, except in automobile accidents when the driver's chest is driven into the steering wheel. The body of the sternum is commonly fractured in the region of the sternal angle and it is often a **comminuted fracture** (broken into pieces). Fortunately the ligamentous coverings confine the fragments in most cases so that a compound fracture does not occur (*i.e.*, a fracture in which there is an open wound). However, in severe accidents, the body of the sternum separates from the manubrium at the manubriosternal joint and is driven posteriorly, rupturing the aorta and/or injuring the heart. This may result in sufficient loss of blood and/or damage to the heart muscle (**myocardium**) so that the patient dies.

Not uncommonly, men in their early forties suddenly detect their ossified xiphoid processes and consult their doctor about the "hard lump in the pit of their stomach." Never having felt it before, because it is mainly cartilaginous until around the 40th year, they fear they have developed a cancer in the stomach.

The sternum is important to the hematologist because it has a readily accessible marrow cavity (Fig. 1-96). During a procedure called **sternal puncture**, a large bore needle is inserted through the cortex of the sternum into the red bone marrow deep to it for aspiration of a sample of it for laboratory evaluation.

Access to the anterior mediastinum (region anterior to heart, Fig. 1-49) to reach the heart and great vessels may be gained by splitting the sternum in the median plane (*i.e.*, lengthwise).

In some people the body of the sternum projects downward and backward rather than downward and forward (Fig. 1-53). This presses the heart posteriorly and widens it, making it appear large on frontal chest radiographs. A lateral chest radiograph reveals the true cause. This condition, usually congenital (present at birth), is called **pectus excavatum** (funnel chest) and is characterized by curving backward of the lower part of the sternum.

In other people, the chest is flattened on each side and the sternum projects anteriorly. This keel-like condition, called **pectus carinatum**, was given this name because the chest looks like the keel of a boat (L. *carina*, keel).

Surface Anatomy of the Ribs, Costal Cartilages, and Sternum (Figs. 1-11 to 1-13). The smooth superior border of the sternum is easily felt because it has a shallow concavity which forms the floor of the **jugular notch** at the root of the neck. As you palpate this notch with your forefinger on yourself and your colleagues, verify that the concavity here is much deepened by the medial (sternal) ends of the clavicles. Their knobby ends project above and behind their articulation with the manubrium because they are too large for the clavicular notches provided for them at the supero-

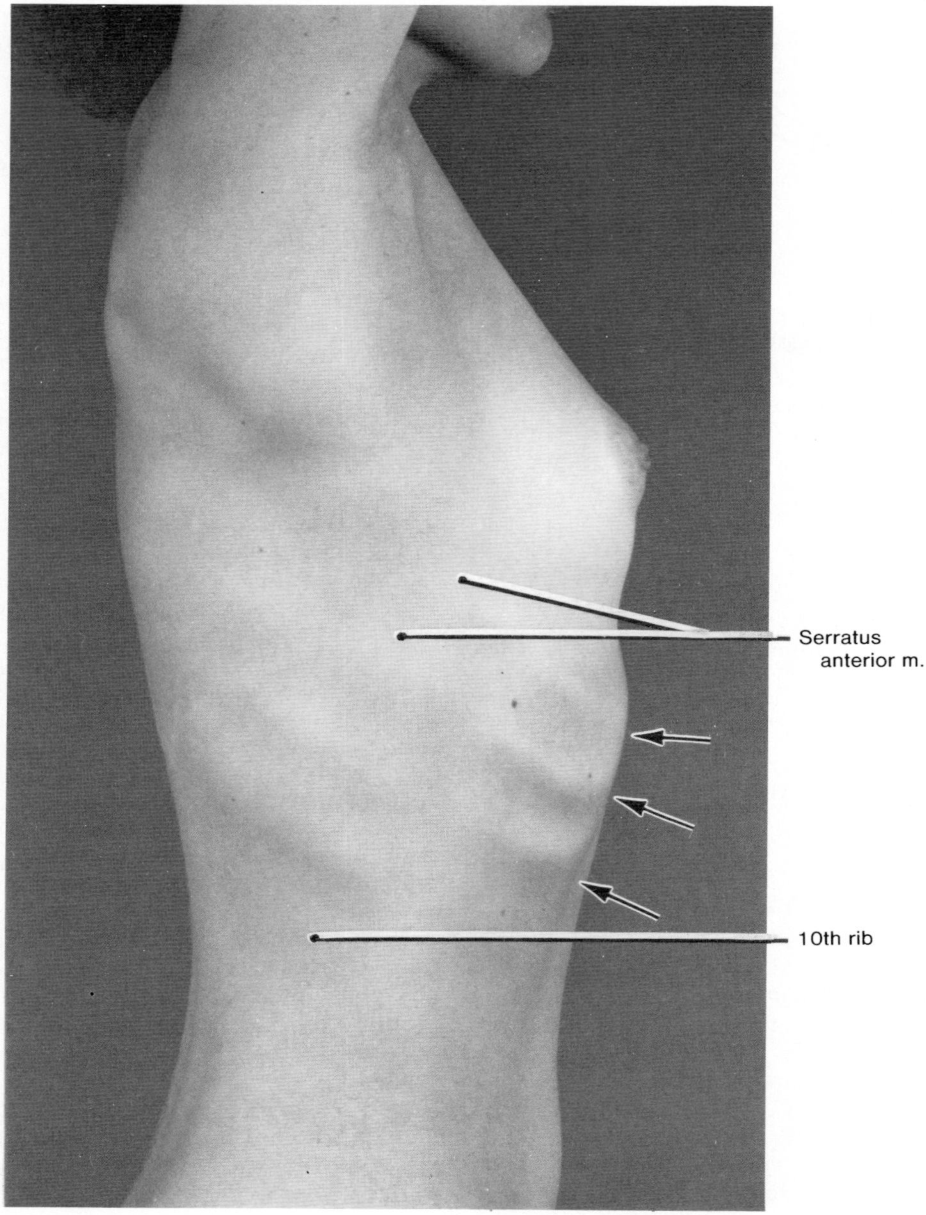

Figure 1-13. Photograph of a lateral view of the thorax of a 27-year-old woman from the right side with her arm abducted over her head. Because she is thin, most of her ribs are visible. In this position the digitations of the serratus anterior muscle are often visible (also see Fig. 1-18), particularly in muscular persons (Fig. 6-53). Most of the region lateral to her sternum is occupied by the breast which lies in the superficial fascia anterior to the pectoralis major muscle and forms most of the contour of her pectoral region. The gross structure of the breast is described in Chapter 6 (see Figs. 6-7 to 6-9). Her right costal margin is indicated by *arrows.* Also see Figs. 1-11 and 1-18.

lateral angles of this bone (Fig. 1-10*A*). Note that the upper border of the jugular notch is at the level of the junction of the second and third thoracic vertebrae (Fig. 1-49).

Slide your forefinger and middle finger slowly down the midline of your manubrium until you feel a horizontal ridge at the junction of the manubrium and the body of the sternum. As fat does not accumulate anterior to the manubrium, this ridge, called the **sternal angle** (Fig. 1-10), is usually visible and is almost invariably easily palpable, *especially on inspiration.* This angle is located about 5 cm inferior to the jugular notch and forms where the manubrium joins the body of the sternum at the manubriosternal joint, a **synchondrosis** (bones united by cartilage).

The sternal angle is situated at the level of the second sternocostal articulation (Fig. 1-1) and is at the level of the junction of the fourth and fifth thoracic vertebrae (Fig. 1-49). When traced laterally, this transverse ridge that indicates *the sternal angle accurately directs the palpating finger to the second costal cartilage, the starting point from which the ribs should be counted.* As the accurate identification of ribs is of considerable importance, you are urged to practice the identification of each rib by this method.

CLINICALLY ORIENTED COMMENTS

Often there is a need to count the ribs (*e.g.*, to determine which rib is diseased or injured). First the sternal angle is found and the palpating finger is passed directly laterally from it on to the second rib; then the ribs are counted downward from this point. *On rare occasions* (Fig. 1-14*B*), the sternal angle occurs at the level of the third costal cartilage. You should suspect this condition if the manubrium seems longer than usual and the sternal angle is 6 to 7 cm below the jugular notch.

As will be discussed later, access to the lung is gained through the intercostal spaces (spaces between ribs). In conventional posterolateral **thoracotomy**, the incision is made along the line of the sixth rib. Obviously, accurate identification of this rib is very important.

The first rib is difficult to feel because it lies deep to the clavicle and is covered by muscles (Figs. 1-1, 1-11, and 9-14). The other ribs may be palpated by placing your fingertips in your axilla and slowly drawing them inferomedially over your thoracic cage.

The ribs can be counted posteriorly by counting upward from the short 12th one, which can be palpated in most people but with difficulty in obese persons. Sometimes the 12th rib is so rudimentary that it does not project beyond the lateral border of the erector spinae muscle (Figs. 5-11 and 5-48), in which case it is not palpable. Count the ribs on the back of a colleague (pick a thin one!). Note that the spine of the scapula lies over the third rib or third intercostal space (Fig. 1-2). The inferior angle of the scapula is at the level of the seventh rib and is a good guide to the seventh intercostal space. Understand that scapular surface markings are not so accurate for identifying the ribs as is the sternal angle.

The costal margins are palpable with ease, extending inferolaterally from the sternum (Figs. 1-1, 1-11, and 1-13). The highest part of the costal margin is usually formed by the seventh costal cartilage and its lowest part, when viewed from the front, is usually formed by the 10th costal cartilage. The degree of prominence of the costal margin varies and should be examined in several persons. It is very obvious in thin persons when they inspire (Fig. 1-18).

The infrasternal angle also varies in size from person to person and increases during inspiration. The depressed area included within this angle is called the **infrasternal fossa** (epigastric fossa, "pit of stomach"). The **xiphisternal joint** is felt as a transverse ridge at the superior end of the infrasternal fossa (Figs. 1-9 to 1-11).

The xiphoid process (lying in the bottom of the infrasternal fossa) can easily be felt extending inferiorly for a varying distance. Observe that the xiphoid process occupies a plane posterior to that of the body

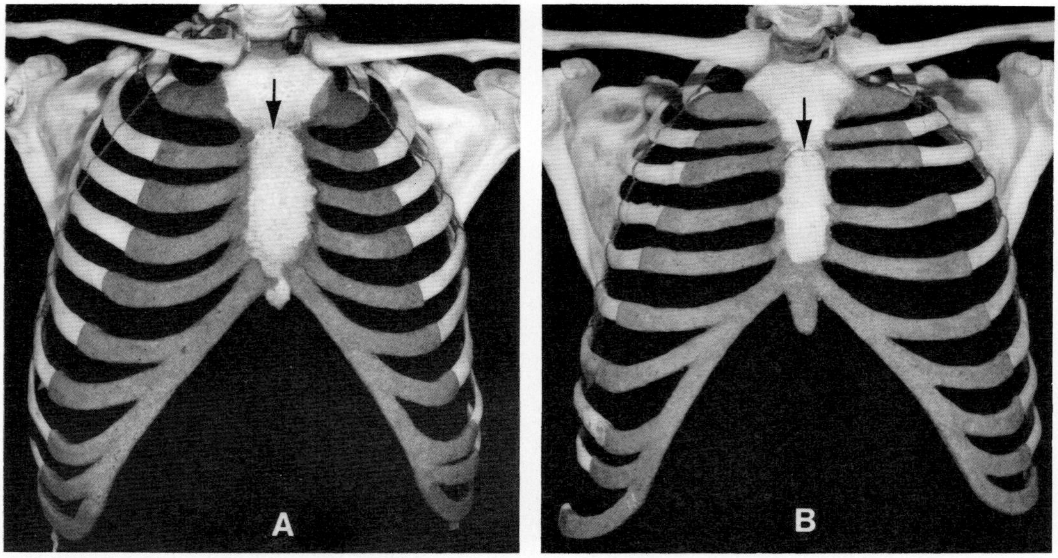

Figure 1-14. Photographs of anterior views of the thoracic cages of two articulated skeletons. In each photograph the *arrow* indicates the *sternal angle* between the manubrium and the body of the sternum. *A*, a typical specimen of a person over 40 years of age. Note that the xiphoid process is small, blunt, ossified and joined to the sternum. Probably the hyaline cartilage surrounding the bony xiphoid was lost during preparation. Observe the jugular notch and that the medial (sternal) ends of the clavicles project above the manubrium. *B*, an atypical specimen. Note that the sternal angle is at the level of the third costal cartilage. Although usual in the gibbon (a small ape), it is *rare* in man. In this unusual specimen the sternal angle does not indicate the level of the second costal cartilages. The anatomical sign of the presence of this unusual variation is the long manubrium (here 6 cm; usually 5 cm). Also observe the pointed cartilaginous xiphoid process. Understand that the xiphoid process is quite variable in size, shape, and thickness. In some people it never completely ossifies or unites with the body of the sternum. It is not uncommon for the xiphoid process to deviate from the midline. Note the short body of the sternum in *B* compared with that in *A*.

of the sternum. If you check an articulated skeleton, you can observe the anatomical basis for this. The xiphoid process is thinner anteroposteriorly than the body and its posterior aspect is at the same level; hence, its anterior aspect is posterior to that of the body of the sternum (Fig. 1-9).

MOVEMENTS OF THE THORACIC WALL

Movements of the thorax are primarily concerned with increasing and decreasing the intrathoracic volume. The resulting changes in pressure result in air being alternately drawn into the lungs (**inspiration**) through the nose, mouth, larynx, and trachea and expelled from the lungs (**expiration**) through the same passages.

To increase the volume of the thorax, *the chest can increase in diameter in three dimensions.* Each of these increases the volume, but most increase occurs when all three dimensions are increased at the same time.

The Vertical Diameter (Fig. 1-15). This dimension of the thorax is increased primarily when the **diaphragm** contracts, lowering it (Fig. 1-58). The upper ribs are raised slightly during very deep breathing, which also increases the vertical diameter. During expiration the vertical diameter is returned to normal by the subatmospheric pressure produced in the pleural cavities by the elastic recoil of the lungs. As a result, the diaphragm moves upward, diminishing the vertical diameter of the thorax (Fig. 1-59). It is also important to understand that

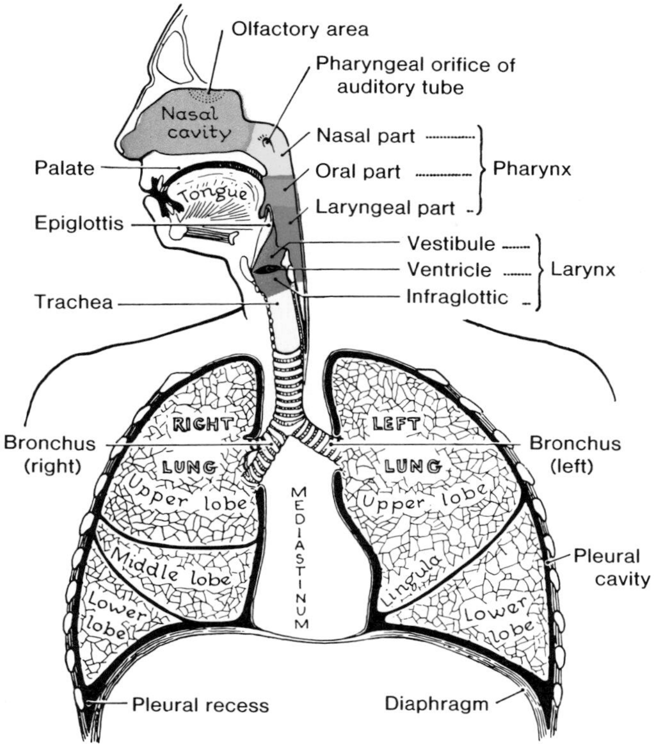

Figure 1-15. Diagram illustrating the respiratory system. Observe the dome-shaped diaphragm which is attached to the sternum, the ribs, and the vertebral column. This partly muscular partition is the main muscle of respiration. During inspiration the diaphragm contracts and lowers its domes (cupolae), whereas during expiration the relaxed diaphragm moves upward. The vertical diameter of the thorax is increased by the descent and flattening of the domes of the diaphragm.

the weight of the abdominal viscera will push the diaphragm upward in the recumbent position.

The Transverse Diameter (Fig. 1-16). This dimension of the thorax is increased by the ribs swinging outward during the so-called "bucket-handle movement," which elevates ribs 2 to 10 approximately and everts their lower borders. This pulls the lateral portions of the ribs away from the midline, thereby increasing the transverse diameter of the thorax.

The Anteroposterior Diameter (Fig. 1-17). This dimension of the thorax is also increased by raising the ribs. Movement at the costovertebral joints through the long axes of the necks of the ribs results in raising and lowering their sternal ends, the "pump-handle movement." The second to sixth ribs are the ones mainly involved in this movement. Because the ribs slope downward, any elevation during inspiration (Fig. 1-58) results in an upward movement of the sternum at the manubriosternal joint and an increase in the anteroposterior diameter of the thorax. This is most noticeable in young people.

During expiration, the elastic recoil of the lungs produces a subatmospheric pressure in the pleural cavities. This and the weight of the thoracic walls cause the lateral and anteroposterior diameters of the thorax to return to normal.

APERTURES OF THE THORAX

The Superior Thoracic Aperture (Thoracic Inlet). The thoracic cavity communicates with the root of the neck via an opening commonly called the inlet of the

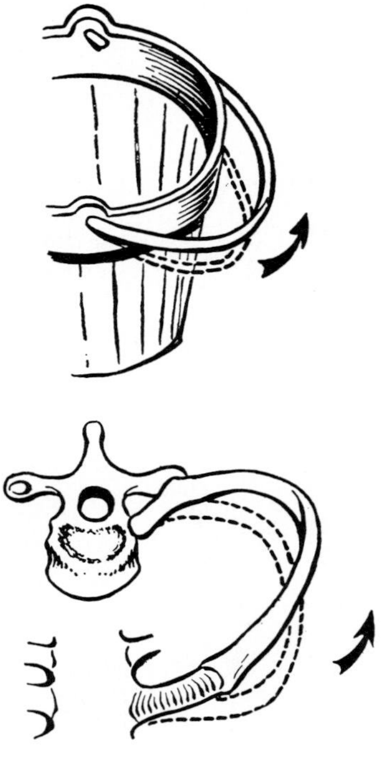

Figure 1-16. Diagrams illustrating the "bucket-handle" inspiratory movement. The lower ribs move laterally when they are elevated, thereby increasing the transverse diameter of the thorax. Movement at the costovertebral joint about a front-to-back axis leads to elevation of the middle of the rib. This movement takes place mainly at the 7th to 10th costotransverse joints.

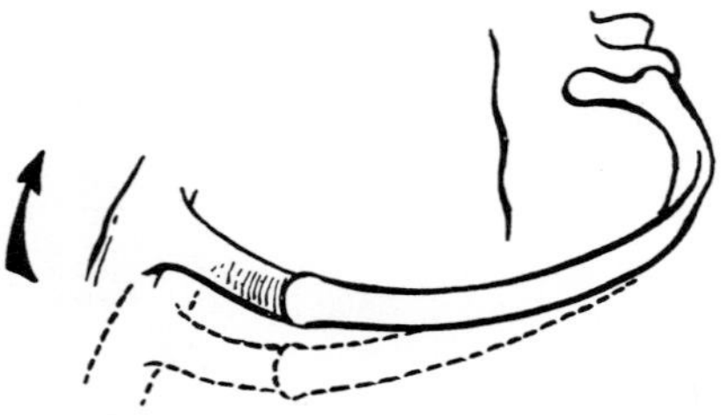

Figure 1-17. Diagram illustrating the "pump-handle" inspiratory movement. When the upper ribs are elevated, the anteroposterior diameter of the thorax is increased. Movement at the costovertebral joint about a side-to-side axis results in raising and lowering of the sternal end of the rib, the so-called pump-handle movement.

thorax. Through this relatively small opening (about 5 cm anteroposteriorly and 11 cm transversely) pass structures joining the thorax to the upper limbs and neck (*e.g.*, trachea, esophagus, vessels, and nerves). To visualize its size oppose the thumb and forefinger of one hand with those of the other to form a kidney-shaped opening.

The superior thoracic aperture is bounded by the body of the **first thoracic vertebra** posteriorly, the medial borders of the **first ribs** and their **costal cartilages** laterally, and the superior end of the **manubrium** anteriorly (Fig. 1-1). The margin of the superior aperture slopes steeply downward and forward; hence, the apex of each lung and its covering of pleura project upward through the lateral parts of the inlet (Fig. 1-30).

The Inferior Thoracic Aperture (Thoracic Outlet). The thoracic cavity communicates with the abdomen via a wide opening commonly called the outlet of the thorax. In the living state it is closed by the diaphragm, which is pierced by the structures passing between the mediastinum (the median partition of the thoracic cavity) and the abdomen. The inferior aperture is uneven and is much larger than the superior aperture. It slopes downward and backward.

The inferior aperture is bounded by the **12th thoracic vertebra** posteriorly, the **12th pair of ribs** and the curved **costal margins** laterally, and the **xiphisternal joint** anteriorly (Fig. 1-1).

CLINICALLY ORIENTED COMMENTS

As the lower trunk of the brachial plexus leaves the neck to enter the axilla, it crosses over the first rib (Fig. 6-25) and often produces a groove in it. The subclavian artery on its way to the upper limb also runs over the first rib, producing a distinct groove (Figs. 1-6 and 1-30). Sometimes these structures are compressed where they pass over the first rib, producing **vascular symptoms** (*e.g.*, pallor, coldness, and cyanosis or bluishness of the hands) and less frequently **nerve pressure symptoms** (numbness and tingling in the fingers). These conditions have been described under several different terms, depending on what was thought to be the cause of the symptoms. Generally the condition is called the **neurovascular compression syndrome**. *The compression generally involves the lower trunk of the brachial plexus* (Fig. 6-24) at or close to the level at which it crosses the first rib. In some cases it is attributed to carrying the shoulder abnormally low so that the nerves are pulled over the first rib.

A condition called *the thoracic inlet syndrome* results from the development of a **lymphosarcoma** (malignant lymphatic tumor). There are multiple enlarged lymph nodes and infiltration of tissues in the supraclavicular fossae and the thoracic inlet. As a result, blood cannot drain from the head, neck, and upper limbs to the heart, so these parts become congested with blood and appear to be swollen.

MUSCLES OF THE THORACIC WALL

Many muscles are attached to the ribs, including some back muscles (Fig. 5-45) and anterolateral muscles of the abdomen (Fig. 1-20).

The Platysma (Figs. 9-8 and 9-9). This paper-thin muscle in the superficial fascia originates in the deep fascia over the pectoralis major and deltoid muscles in the upper chest and extends through the neck to the chin. As it is a muscle of facial expression and tenses the skin of the neck, it is described with the head (Chap. 7) and the neck (Chap. 9).

The Pectoral Muscles. These anteriorly located chest muscles act on the upper limb and connect it to the thoracic skeleton. (For a full description of them, see Chap. 6).

The Pectoralis Major Muscle (Figs. 1-20, 6-19, and 6-21). This large, fan-shaped muscle has an extensive origin from the clavicle, the sternum, and the upper six costal cartilages. It flexes, extends, adducts, and medially rotates the arm, but by fixing the arm it can be used as an accessory muscle of respiration to expand the thoracic cavity. The pectoralis major is active when inspiration is deep and forcible.

The Pectoralis Minor Muscle (Figs. 1-20 and 6-23). This flat, triangular muscle lies immediately deep to the pectoralis major muscle. It arises from the third, fourth, and fifth ribs and inserts on the coracoid process of the scapula. It stabilizes the scapula by drawing it forward and downward and elevates the ribs from which it arises.

The Serratus Anterior Muscle (Figs. 1-18, 1-20, 6-31, 6-52, and 6-53). This major muscle covers much of the lateral aspect of the thorax and the intercostal muscles. It arises by fleshy digitations from the outer surfaces of the upper eight ribs, about midway between their angles and costal cartilages. Its upper fleshy slips of origin are under cover of the pectoralis major and minor muscles, but the lower ones are visible in most males, particularly muscular ones, where they interdigitate with the origins of the external oblique muscle of the abdomen from the middle four ribs (Fig. 1-20). The serratus anterior inserts along the entire costal aspect of the medial border of the scapula. It functions principally in protracting the scapula and in holding it against the thoracic wall. Other actions of this powerful muscle are described in Chapter 6.

Muscles of the Back (Figs. 1-23 and 5-45). The back muscles inserting into the ribs (*e.g.*, the iliocostalis part of the erector spinae muscle) are discussed in Chapter 5. The two muscles concerned with inspiration will be described here.

The Serratus Posterior Muscles (Fig. 5-44). These flat muscles run from the vertebrae to the ribs. Both muscles are innervated by intercostal nerves, the superior ones by the first four and the inferior ones by the last four.

The serratus posterior superior muscle arises from the lower part of the **ligamentum nuchae** (a median ligamentous band at the back of the neck) and the spinous processes of the **seventh cervical** and **first three thoracic vertebrae.** It runs inferolaterally to insert into the upper borders of the second to fourth (or fifth) ribs (Figs. 5-44 and 5-45).

The serratus posterior inferior muscle arises from the spinous processes of the last two thoracic and first two lumbar vertebrae. It runs superolaterally to insert into

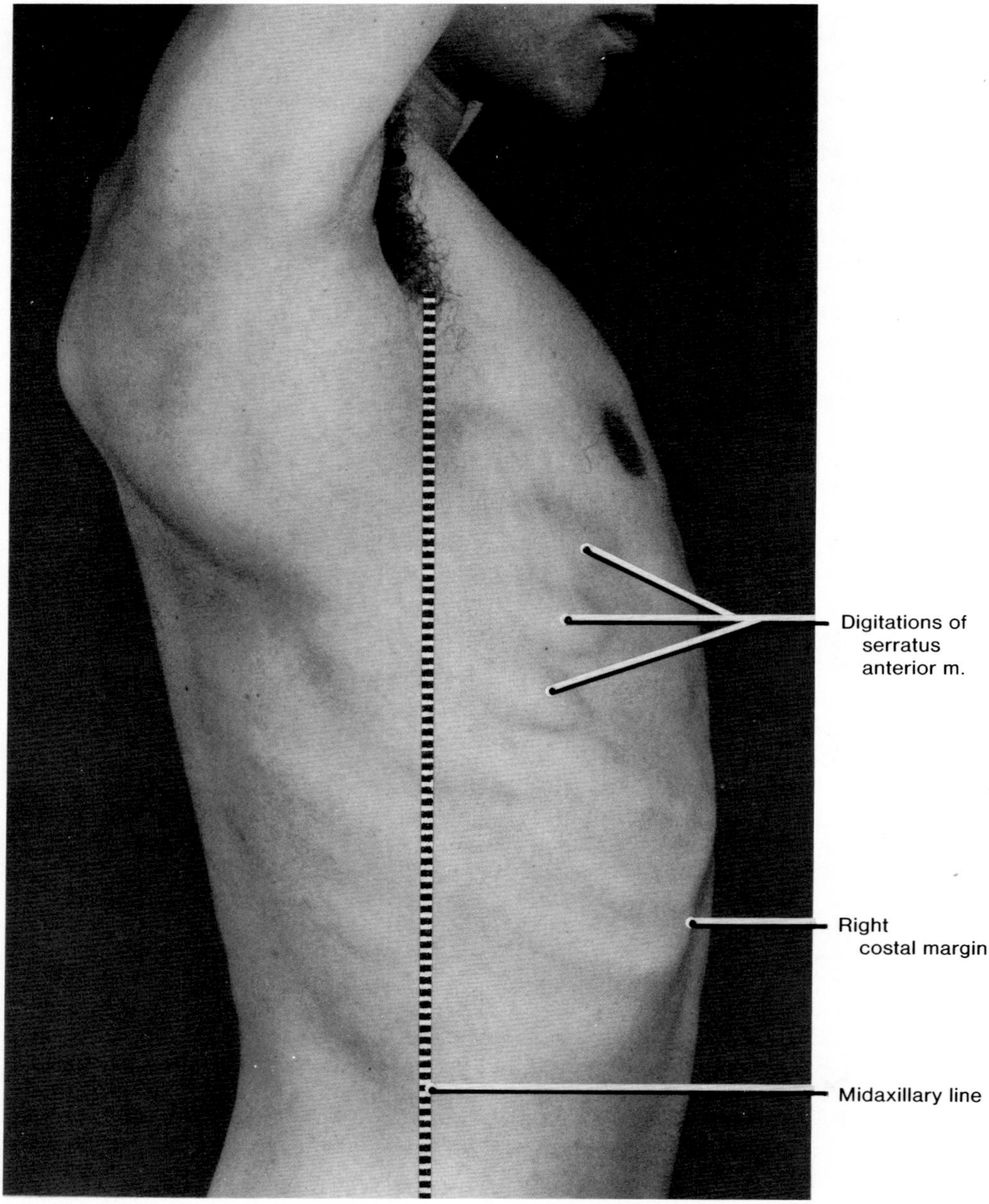

Figure 1-18. Photograph of a lateral view of the thorax of a 27-year-old man from the right side with his arm abducted over his head. Observe the midaxillary line which is an imaginary perpendicular line passing through the center of the axilla (armpit). The upper fleshy slips of the serratus anterior muscle are invisible from the surface because they are covered by the pectoral muscles. Most of the contour of the pectoral region in males is formed by the pectoralis major muscle (Fig. 6-19), whereas in females the breast produces varying contours depending upon its development (Fig. 1-13). The nipple in the male usually lies at the level of the fourth intercostal space (*ie*, between the fourth and fifth ribs). In the female the position of the nipple is not a reliable guide to the intercostal spaces because its position varies according to the size and shape of the breast. Note that the digitations of his serratus anterior muscle are much more prominent than those of the woman shown in Figure 1-13.

the lower borders of the lower three or four ribs near their angles (Figs. 5-44 and 5-45).

Both serratus posterior muscles are inspiratory ones. As you might expect, the serratus posterior superior elevates the upper ribs and the serratus posterior inferior depresses the lower ribs, preventing them from being pulled upward by the action of the diaphragm.

The Intercostal Muscles (Figs. 1-19 to 1-24 and 1-28). There are *three incomplete layers of muscle* in each intercostal space: **external, internal,** and **innermost** intercostal muscles. In a deeper plane there are two muscles (transversus thoracis and subcostals) that extend over more than one intercostal space. The intercostal muscles are supplied by intercostal nerves.

The External Intercostal Muscles (Figs. 1-19, 1-22 to 1-24, and 1-28). Each of the 11 pairs of thin external intercostal muscles runs obliquely downward and forward from the **rib above to the rib below**. These muscles arise from the bodies of the ribs, beginning just lateral to their tubercles and extending anteriorly almost to their costal cartilages. Between the costal cartilages, the external intercostal muscles are replaced by the **external intercostal membranes**. In the lower intercostal spaces, the external intercostal muscles become continuous with the external oblique muscle of the anterior abdominal wall (Fig. 1-20).

The Internal Intercostal Muscles (Figs. 1-19 to 1-23 and 1-28). The fibers of these 11 pairs of muscles run deep to and at right angles to those of the external intercostal muscles. The fibers of the internal intercostal muscles run obliquely from the edge of the **costal groove of one rib** downward

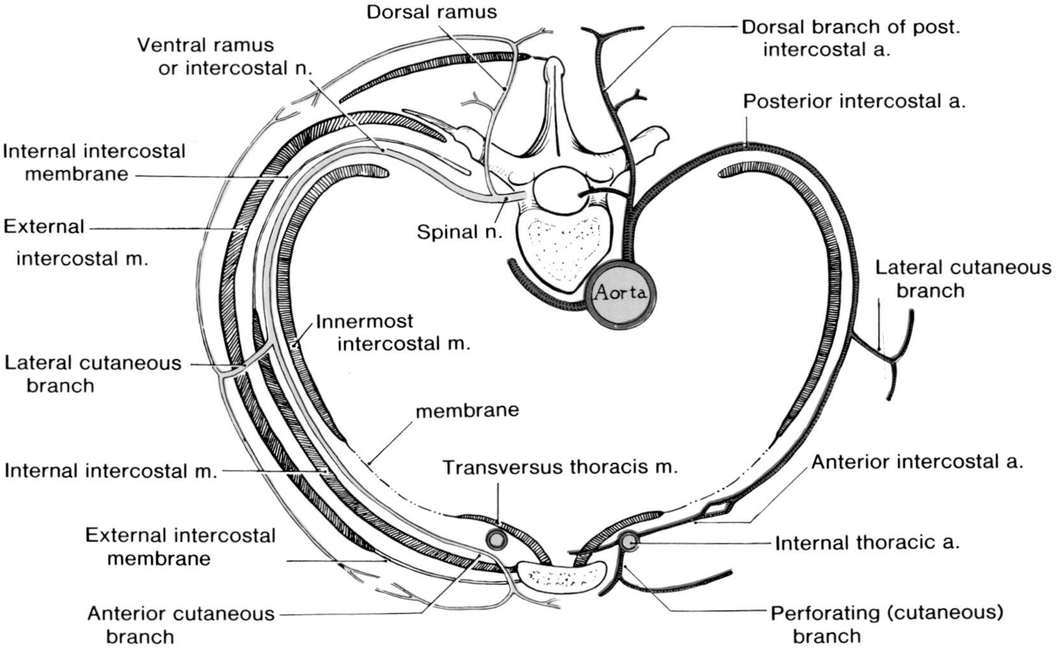

Figure 1-19. Diagram of a horizontal section of the thorax showing the contents of an intercostal space. For purposes of illustration, the nerves are shown on the right (*yellow*) and the arteries on the left (*red*). Observe the three muscular layers: (1) external intercostal muscle and external intercostal membrane; (2) internal intercostal muscle and internal intercostal membrane; and (3) innermost intercostal and transversus thoracis muscles and the membrane connecting them. Examine the intercostal vessels and nerves running in the plane between the middle and innermost layers of muscle. Subsequently, the lower intercostal vessels and nerves occupy the corresponding morphological plane in the abdominal wall. Note that the posterior intercostal arteries are branches of the aorta and that the anterior intercostal arteries are branches of the internal thoracic artery.

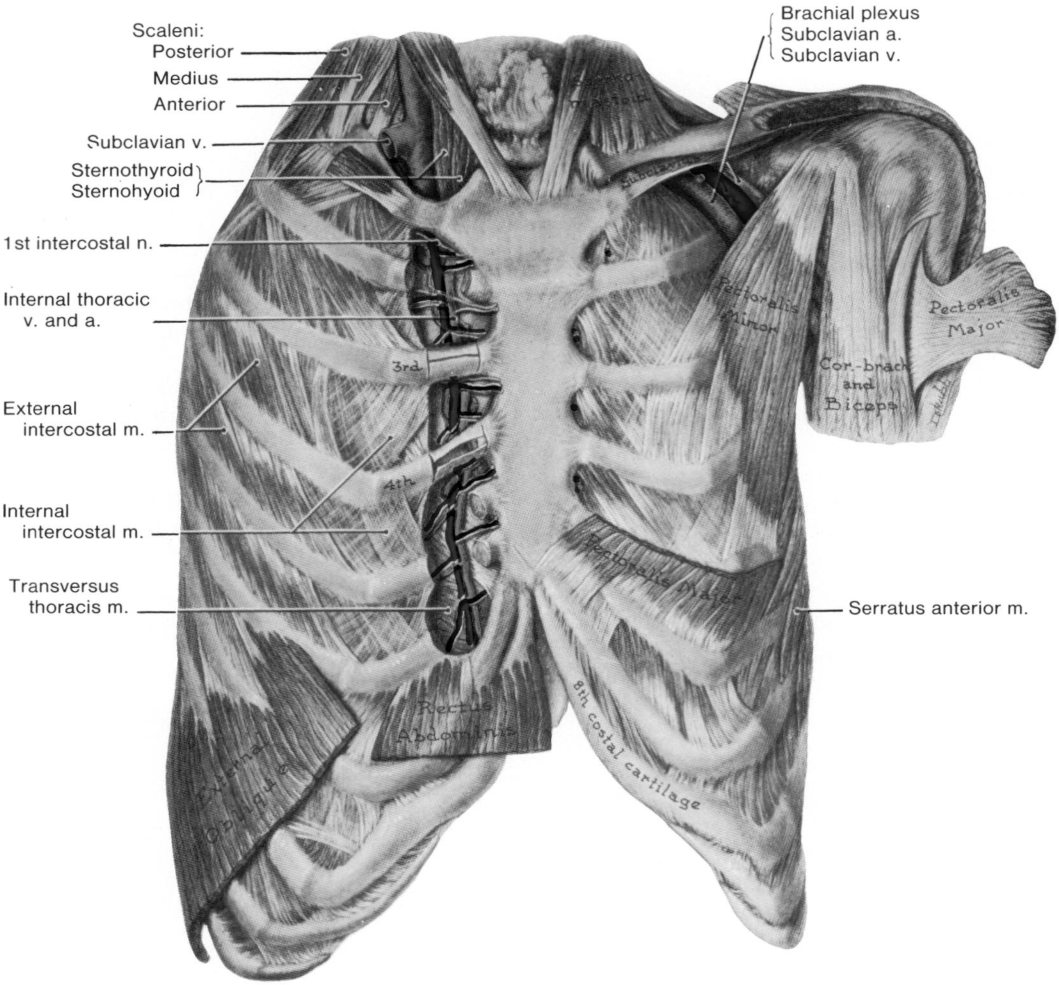

Figure 1-20. Drawing of a dissection of the anterior wall of the thorax. Observe the internal thoracic vessels running downward about a fingerbreadth from the edge of the sternum. Note their intercostal branches. Examine the parasternal lymph nodes (*green*) which receive lymph vessels from the intercostal spaces, the costal pleura, the diaphragm, and the medial part of the breast. It is by this route that a cancer of the breast may spread to the lungs and mediastinum (see Chap. 6). Observe that the subclavian vessels are sandwiched between the first rib and the clavicle (padded by the subclavius muscle). Although the seventh costal cartilage is usually the last one to reach the sternum, it is not uncommon, as in this specimen, for the eighth to do so. The H-shaped cut through the perichondrium of the third and fourth costal cartilages was used to shell out segments of cartilage as an illustration of a surgical approach to the thoracic cavity.

and backward to the **upper margin of the rib below**. The muscles arise from the bodies of the ribs and their costal cartilages as far anteriorly as the sternum and as far posteriorly as the angles of the ribs. Between the ribs posteriorly the internal intercostal muscles are represented by the **internal intercostal membranes**. The lower internal intercostal muscles are continuous with the internal oblique muscle of the anterior abdominal wall (Fig. 1-22).

The Innermost Intercostal Muscles (Figs. 1-19 to 1-23 and 1-28). These muscles (also called intercostales intimi) appear similar to the internal intercostal muscles. *The innermost intercostal muscles are sep-*

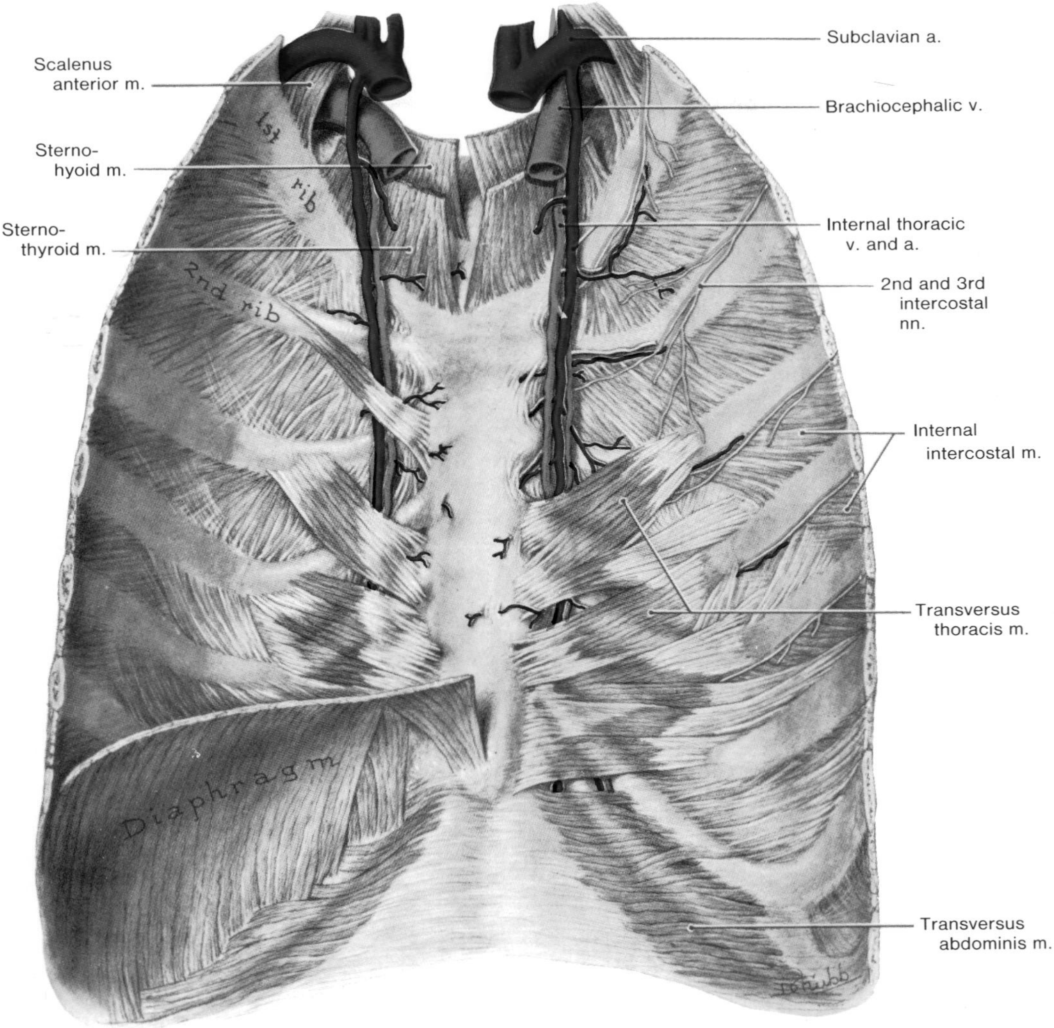

Figure 1-21. Drawing of the anterior thoracic wall from behind. Observe that the internal thoracic artery, arising from the first part of the subclavian artery, is accompanied by two veins (venae comitantes) up to the third or second intercostal space and above this by a single vein (internal thoracic vein), which proceeds to the brachiocephalic vein. Note that the lower portions of the internal thoracic vessels are covered posteriorly by the transversus thoracis muscle. Observe the continuity of the transversus thoracis muscle with the transversus abdominis muscle, the innermost layer of the three flat muscles of the thoracoabdominal wall.

arated from the internal intercostal muscles by the intercostal nerves and vessels. These muscles pass between the internal surfaces of adjacent ribs and cover approximately the middle two-fourths of the intercostal spaces. They are usually best developed in the lower thorax.

The Subcostal Muscles (Fig. 1-24). These thin muscular slips, variable in size and shape, extend from the inside of the angle of one rib to the internal surface of the rib below, crossing one or two intercostal spaces. They run in the same direction as the internal intercostal muscles and lie internal to them. These muscles probably depress the ribs.

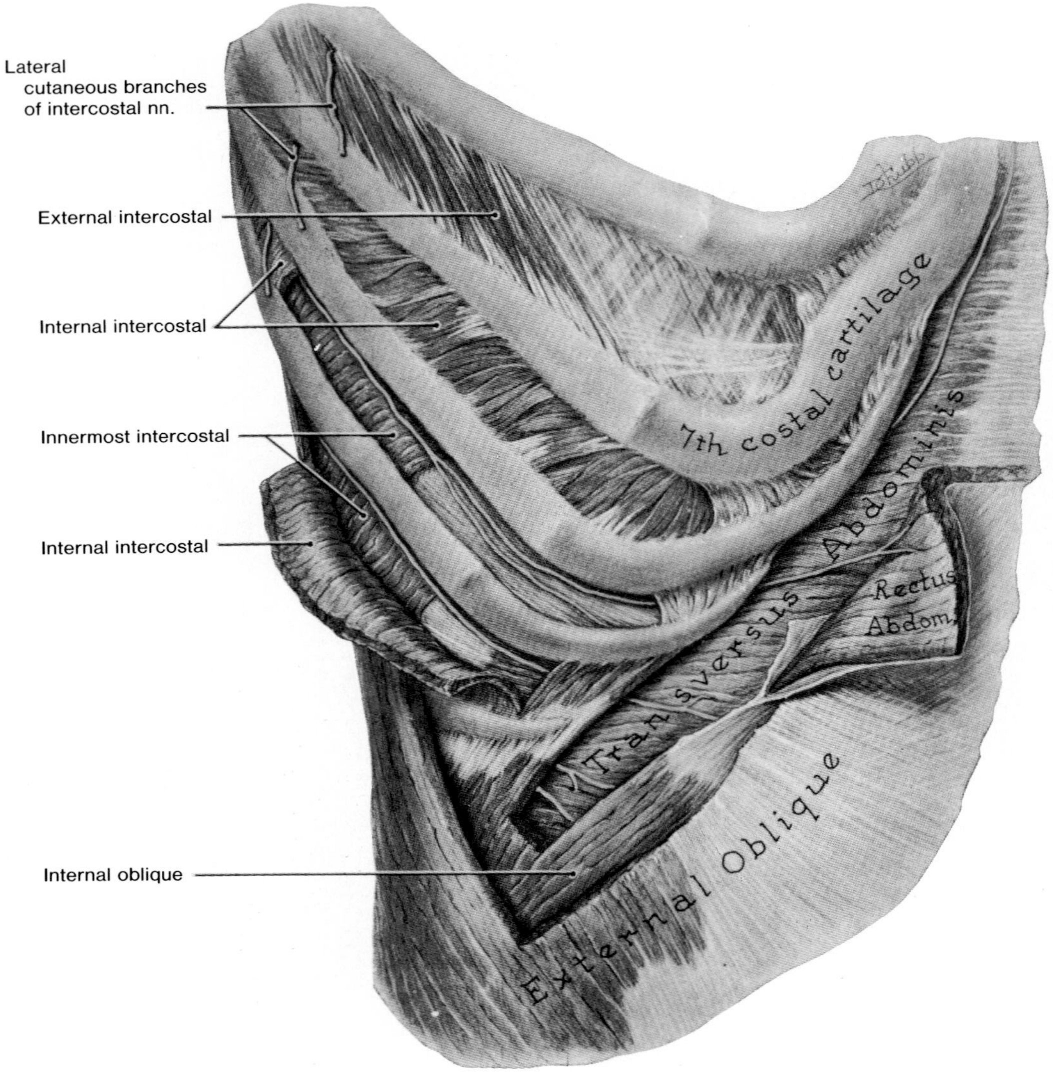

Figure 1-22. Drawing of the anterior ends of the lower intercostal spaces, right side. Observe the common direction of the fibers of the external intercostal and external oblique muscles and the continuity of the internal intercostal muscle with the internal oblique muscle at the anterior ends of the 9th to 11th intercostal spaces. Note the morphological plane in which an intercostal nerve lies deep to an internal intercostal muscle but superficial to an innermost intercostal muscle and either the transversus thoracis or the transversus abdominis, according to the level. Observe the direction in which an intercostal nerve runs: first parallel to the ribs immediately above and below and then parallel to the costal cartilages. Thus, on gaining the abdominal walls, nerves T7 and T8 continue upward, T9 continues nearly horizontally, and T10 continues downward toward the umbilicus.

The Transversus Thoracis Muscle (Figs. 1-19 to 1-21). This thin muscle consists of four or five slips which arise from the xiphoid process and lower part of the sternum and pass superolaterally to the second to sixth costal cartilages. It becomes continuous with the transversus abdominus (Fig. 1-22). The internal thoracic vessels run anterior to this muscle, between it and the costal cartilages and the internal intercostal

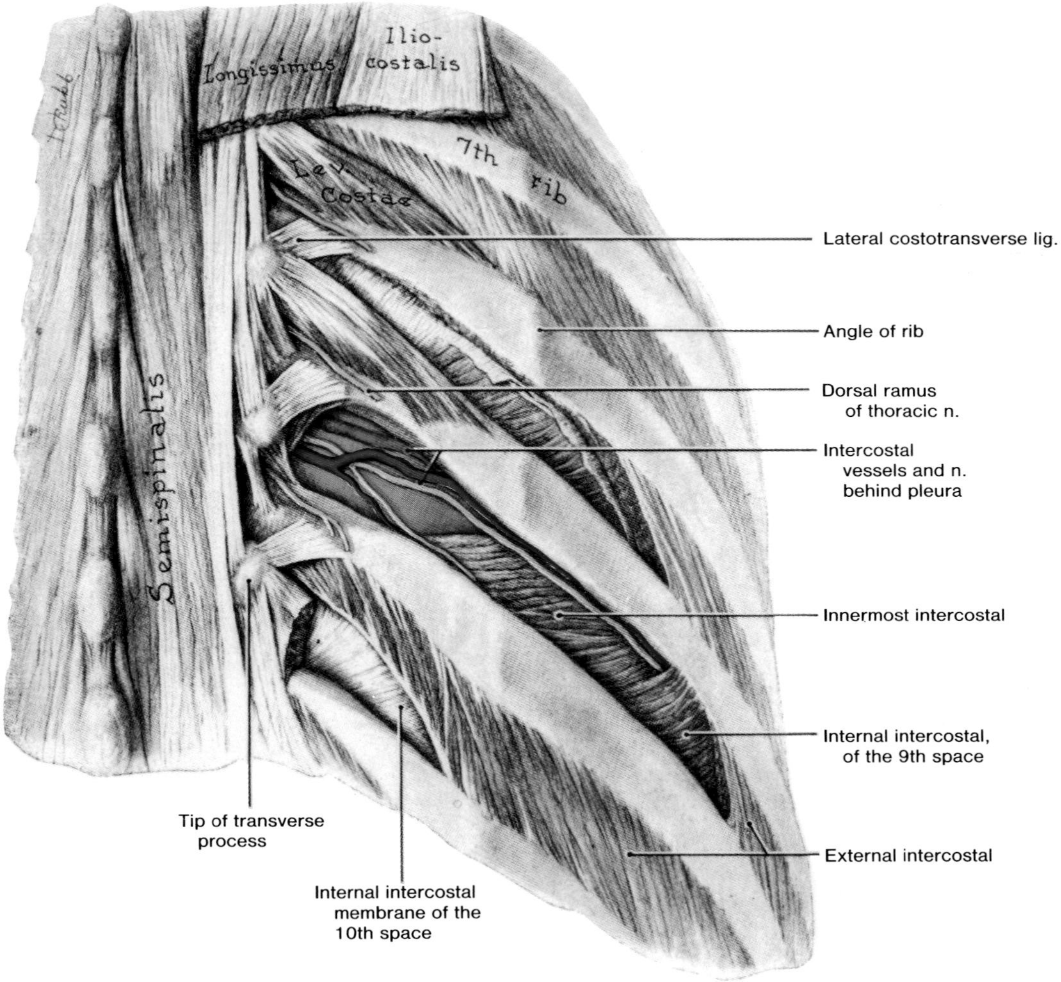

Figure 1-23. Drawing of a dissection of the posterior end of an intercostal space. Medial to the angles of the ribs, the iliocostalis and longissimus muscles have been removed to expose the levatores costarum muscles. In the five intercostal spaces depicted observe that (1) the upper two (sixth and seventh) are intact; (2) from the lowest or 10th space the levator costae muscle and the underlying part of the external intercostal muscle have been removed to reveal the internal intercostal membrane; (3) from the eighth space more of the external intercostal muscle has been removed and the internal intercostal membrane is seen extending laterally as an areolar sheet; and (4) in the ninth space this sheet has been removed in order to show the intercostal vessels and nerve appearing medially between the superior costotransverse ligament and the pleura and disappearing laterally between the internal intercostal and the innermost intercostal muscles.

muscles (Fig. 1-21). This muscle probably depresses the second to sixth ribs.

The Levatores Costarum Muscles (Fig. 1-23). These 12 fan-shaped muscles arise from the transverse processes of C7 and T1 to T11 and pass inferolaterally to insert on the ribs below, close to the tubercle. As their name indicates, they elevate the ribs to which they are attached.

Actions of the Intercostal Muscles. Inspiration and expiration radiographs (Figs. 1-58 and 1-59) show that the intercostal spaces widen on inspiration, but the exact role of the intercostal muscles in this move-

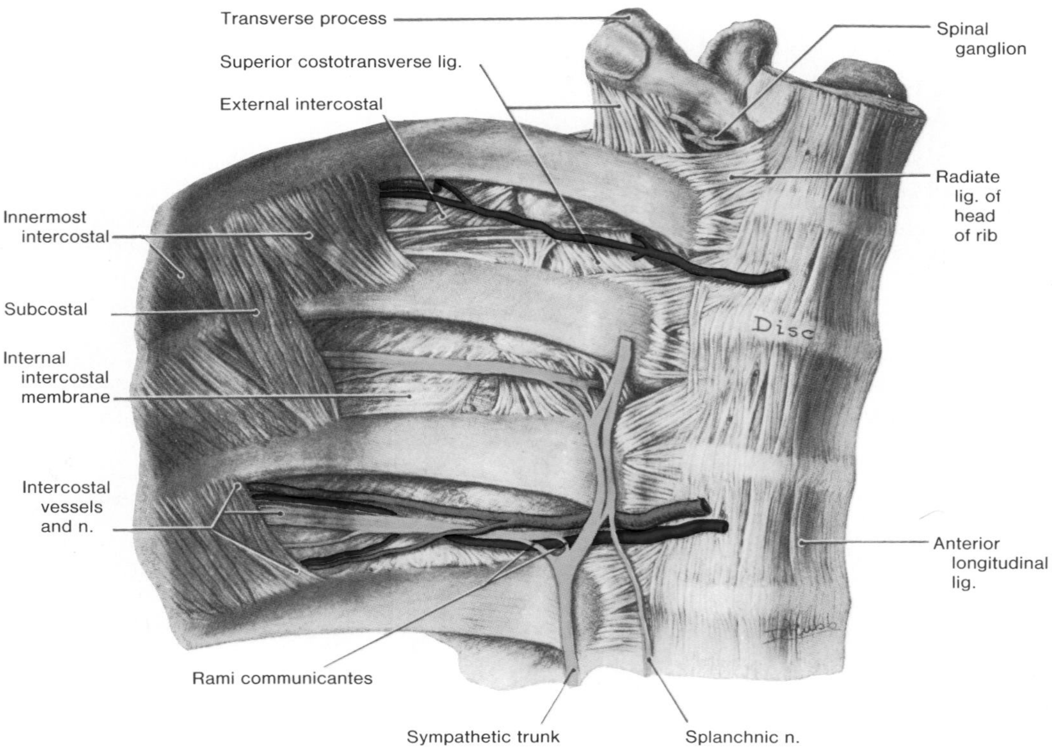

Figure 1-24. Drawing of an anterior view of a dissection of the vertebral end of an intercostal space. Observe the portions of the innermost intercostal muscle that bridge two intercostal spaces, called subcostal muscles. Note the external intercostal muscle in the uppermost space and the internal intercostal membrane in the middle space that is continuous medially with a superior costotransverse ligament. Observe the order of the structures in the lowest space: intercostal vein, artery, and nerve. Note the ventral ramus of a thoracic nerve crossing in front of a superior costotransverse ligament and a dorsal ramus crossing behind it. The rami communicantes are well shown (also see Figs. 1-25 and 1-26).

ment is controversial. It is known that all three layers of intercostal muscles act together in keeping the intercostal spaces rigid, thereby preventing them from bulging out during expiration and from being drawn in during inspiration.

When the first rib is fixed by the scalenus anterior and scalenus medius (neck muscles) during quiet respiration, the intercostal muscles elevate the anterior parts of the other ribs, except for the lower ones which are held in position by the serratus posterior inferior and abdominal muscles (Fig. 1-22). Elevation of the ribs increases the anteroposterior diameter of the thorax (Fig. 1-58).

When the 12th rib is fixed by the abdominal muscles, the other ribs are lowered by the intercostal muscles during expiration, which decreases the anteroposterior diameter of the thorax (Fig. 1-59).

THE INTERCOSTAL NERVES

As soon as they pass through the intervertebral foramina, the thoracic spinal nerves divide into ventral (anterior) and dorsal (posterior) primary divisions or rami (Figs. 1-19 and 5-59).

The dorsal rami pass backward, immediately lateral to the articular processes, to supply the muscles, bones, joints, and skin of the back.

The ventral rami of the first 11 thoracic nerves are called **intercostal nerves** because they enter the spaces between the ribs, called **intercostal spaces**. The 12th intercostal nerve, being below the 12th rib, is not intercostal and so is called the **subcostal nerve**.

Each intercostal nerve is connected to a ganglion of the **sympathetic trunk** by small branches, called rami communicantes (Figs. 1-24 to 1-26). The **white ramus communicans** carries preganglionic sympathetic fibers to the sympathetic trunk and/or the prevertebral ganglion from the intercostal nerve, whereas the **gray ramus communicans** carries postganglionic sympathetic fibers from the sympathetic trunk to the intercostal nerve. These fibers are distributed through all branches of the intercostal nerve to blood vessels, sweat glands, and smooth muscle.

Typical Intercostal Nerves (Figs. 1-19 to 1-26 and 1-28). A typical intercostal nerve (*third to sixth*) enters the intercostal space between the parietal pleura and the internal intercostal membrane. At first it runs more or less in the middle of the intercostal space, across the internal surface of the internal intercostal membrane and muscle (Fig. 1-19). Near the angle of the rib, it passes between the internal intercostal and the innermost intercostal muscles. Here it enters and is sheltered by the **costal groove**, where it lies just below the intercostal artery (Figs. 1-25 and 1-28). It continues forward between the internal and innermost intercostal muscles, giving off muscular branches to the intercostal and other muscles and a lateral cutaneous branch. Anteriorly it appears on the inner surface of the internal intercostal muscle (Fig. 1-20), but external (anterior) to the transversus thoracis muscle and internal thoracic vessels. Near the sternum (about 1 cm) it turns anteriorly and ends as an anterior cutaneous branch.

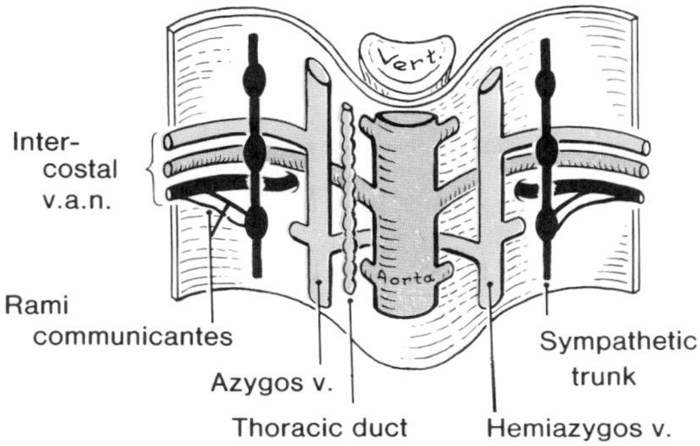

Figure 1-25. Diagram of an intercostal space showing its relationships. *From above downward*: vein, artery, nerve (*VAN*). Order of entry *from medial to lateral*: artery, vein, nerve. The sympathetic trunk is a bilateral series of sympathetic ganglia that lies a little lateral to the vertebral column.

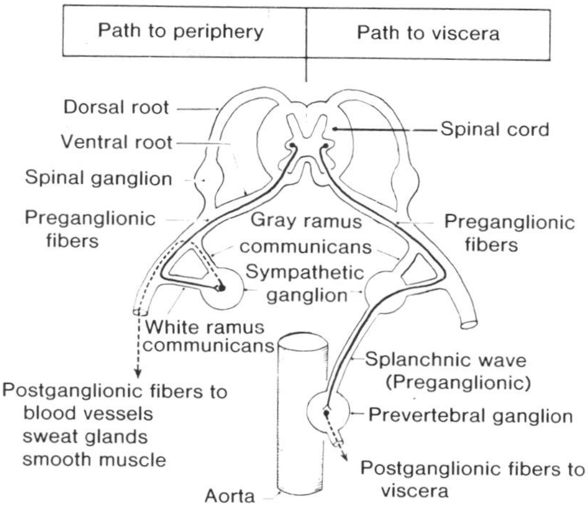

Figure 1-26. Diagram showing the general plan of sympathetic nerve distribution. Observe that each ventral ramus (intercostal nerve) is connected to a sympathetic ganglion of the sympathetic trunk (Fig. 1-25) by two branches (rami communicantes). The white ramus communicans carries preganglionic nerve fibers to the ganglion, whereas the gray ramus communicans carries postganglionic fibers from the ganglion to the nerve for distribution to blood vessels, glands, and smooth muscle.

Branches of a Typical Intercostal Nerve (Figs. 1-19, 1-22, 1-25, and 1-26). The branches mentioned previously are only briefly referred to here.

1. **Rami communicantes** (Figs. 1-24 to 1-26) connect the intercostal nerve to the sympathetic trunk. The nerve sends a white ramus communicans to a ganglion of the sympathetic trunk and receives a gray ramus communicans from a ganglion of the trunk.
2. **A collateral branch** (Figs. 1-22 and 1-24) arises near the angle of a rib and runs along the upper margin of the rib below to supply the intercostal muscles.
3. **A lateral cutaneous branch** (Figs.

1-19 and 1-22) arises beyond the angle of a rib and pierces the internal and external intercostal muscles about halfway around the thorax. The cutaneous branches divide into anterior and posterior branches which supply the skin of the thoracic and abdominal walls.

4. An **anterior cutaneous branch** (Figs. 1-19 and 1-20) supplies the skin and subcutaneous tissue on the front of the chest.
5. **Muscular branches** (Figs. 1-21 and 1-22) supply the subcostal, transversus thoracis, levator costae, and serratus posterior muscles. Note that the intercostal nerves do not supply the muscles connecting the upper limb and the thoracic wall (*i.e.*, the pectoral muscles, Fig. 1-20) or those connecting the upper limb and the vertebral column (*i.e.*, trapezius, latissimus dorsi, rhomboids, and levator scapulae, Fig. 5-45). These muscles are supplied through the accessory nerve (CN XI) and the cervical and brachial plexuses.

Atypical Intercostal Nerves (Figs. 1-21 to 1-23 and 6-25). The preceding description of a typical intercostal nerve applies only to the third to sixth intercostal nerves. In the first part of their course, the first and second intercostal nerves pass on the pleural surfaces of the first and second ribs.

The first intercostal nerve has no anterior cutaneous branch and usually has no lateral cutaneous branch. It divides into a large upper and a small lower part. The upper part joins the **brachial plexus**, supplying the upper limb (Fig. 6-25). The lower part becomes the first intercostal nerve.

The second intercostal nerve may also contribute a small branch to the brachial plexus. Its lateral cutaneous branch is called the **intercostobrachial nerve** because it supplies the floor of the axilla and then communicates with the **medial cutaneous nerve of the arm** to supply the medial side of the upper limb as far as the elbow (Figs. 6-102 and 6-103).

The 7th to 11th intercostal nerves (thoracoabdominal nerves) supply the abdominal as well as the thoracic wall. They pass forward and downward to the anterior ends of the intercostal spaces (Figs. 1-22 and 1-23), where they pass into the abdominal wall deep to the costal cartilages to lie between the internal oblique and transversus abdominus muscles (Fig. 1-22).

The subcostal nerve runs below the 12th rib and passes into the abdominal wall. Its lateral cutaneous branch supplies skin in the gluteal region (buttocks).

Dermatomes (Figs. 1-26 and 1-29). The *area of skin supplied by a dorsal or sensory root of a spinal nerve* is called a dermatome (G. skin slice). The dermatomes were determined by plotting (1) the areas of vasodilation that resulted from stimulation of individual dorsal nerve roots, and (2) the areas of "remaining sensibility" after cutting three roots above and three roots below a given nerve root. The areas plotted represent the average finding for each dorsal root based on pain sensation. Areas determined for temperature sensation have similar limits, but those for touch are more extensive. Note that *there is considerable overlapping of contiguous dermatomes*; *i.e.*, each segmental nerve overlaps the territories of its neighbors. As a result, no anesthesia results unless two or more consecutive dorsal roots have lost their functions. In Figure 1-29, observe that the first two intercostal nerves (T1 and T2), in addition to supplying the thorax, supply the upper limb. Also note that the lower six intercostal nerves (T7 to T12) supply the abdominal wall as well as the thoracic wall. Note that T10 supplies the area of the umbilicus.

CLINICALLY ORIENTED COMMENTS

When the **herpes zoster virus** invades the spinal ganglia of the thoracic spinal nerves, a sharp burning pain is produced in the area of skin supplied by the dorsal roots involved. A few days later, the involved dermatomes become red and a vesicular eruption appears in a segmental distribution (Fig. 1-29).

Local anesthesia of an intercostal space may be produced by injecting an anesthetic agent around the origin of an intercostal nerve, just lateral to the vertebra concerned (Fig. 1-19). This procedure is known as an **intercostal nerve block**. Because there is considerable overlapping of contiguous dermatomes, complete anesthesia results only when two or more consecutive intercostal nerves have been anesthetized.

Pus originating in the region of the vertebral column tends to pass around the thorax along the course of the **neurovascular bundle** (Figs. 1-23 and 1-28) and to point (pass to the surface) where the cutaneous branches of the intercostal nerves pierce the muscles to supply the skin, *e.g.*, in the **midaxillary line** (Figs. 1-18 and 1-19) and just lateral to the sternum (Fig. 1-20).

THE INTERCOSTAL ARTERIES

Three arteries, a large **posterior intercostal artery** and small paired **anterior intercostal arteries**, supply each intercostal space.

The Posterior Intercostal Arteries (Figs. 1-19, 1-23, 1-30, and 1-91). The first two posterior intercostal arteries arise from the **superior intercostal artery**, a branch of the **costocervical trunk** of the subclavian artery. Nine pairs of large posterior intercostal arteries and one pair of subcostal arteries arise from the back of the **thoracic aorta**. Each posterior intercostal artery gives off a *posterior branch* which accompanies the posterior ramus of the spinal nerve and supplies the spinal cord, vertebral column, postvertebral muscles, and skin.

The *anterior branch* of the posterior intercostal artery accompanies the intercostal nerve across the intercostal space. Close to the angle of the rib it enters the **costal groove**, where it lies between the intercostal vein above and the intercostal nerve below (Figs. 1-25 and 1-28). At first the artery runs between the pleura and the internal intercostal membrane (Figs. 1-19 and 1-23). It then runs between the innermost intercostal and the internal intercostal muscles.

Each posterior intercostal artery also gives off a small *collateral branch* that crosses the intercostal space and runs along the upper border of the rib below the space (Fig. 1-23). The terminal branches of the posterior intercostal artery anastomose anteriorly with the anterior intercostal artery.

The Anterior Intercostal Arteries (Figs. 1-19 to 1-21 and 1-30). The paired anterior intercostal arteries supplying the upper six intercostal spaces are derived from the **internal thoracic artery.** Those supplying the seventh to ninth intercostal spaces are derived from its musculophrenic branch. These arteries pass laterally, one near the lower margin of the upper rib and the other near the upper margin of the lower rib. At their origins, the first two arteries lie between the pleura and the internal intercostal muscles, whereas the next four arteries are separated from the pleura by the transversus thoracis muscle (Fig. 1-21). These arteries supply the intercostal muscles and send branches through them to the pectoral muscles, the breast, and the skin.

There are no anterior intercostal arteries in the lower two intercostal spaces. These spaces are supplied by the posterior intercostal arteries and their collateral branches in these spaces.

The Internal Thoracic Artery (Figs. 1-19 to 1-21, 1-30, and 1-93). This artery arises from the inferior surface of the first part of the subclavian artery in the root of the neck, at the medial border of the scalenus anterior muscle. It descends into the thorax posterior to the clavicle and the first costal cartilage. It lies on the pleura behind and is crossed by the **phrenic nerve** (Figs. 1-30 and 1-93). It passes downward in the thorax behind the upper six costal cartilages and the intervening intercostal muscles, about 1 cm from the margin of the sternum. At the level of the third costal cartilage, it continues inferiorly in front of the transverse thoracis muscle to end in the sixth intercostal space by dividing into superior epigastric and musculophrenic arteries. The **superior epigastric artery** supplies the diaphragm and the muscles of the abdominal wall, and the **musculophrenic artery** gives origin to the anterior intercostal arteries which supply the seventh to ninth intercostal spaces.

THE THORACIC CAVITY

DIVISIONS OF THE THORACIC CAVITY

The thoracic cavity is divided into three major divisions: right and left **pleural cavities** and the **mediastinum.** The pleurae and lungs occupy most of the thoracic cavity (Fig. 1-15), with the heart between them and the esophagus and aorta behind the heart. The mediastinum (Fig. 1-49) is a median partition that contains the heart and great vessels and other important structures (*e.g.*, the trachea, esophagus, thymus, and lymph nodes).

The Pleurae and Pleural Cavities (Figs. 1-15 and 1-27). The pleural cavity on each side is almost completely filled by a **lung**. The two pleural cavities occupy the lateral parts of the thoracic cavity (Fig. 1-33).

Each lung is completely covered with a smooth glistening membrane, the **visceral (pulmonary) pleura**, except at the narrow **root of the lung** where each lung is attached to the mediastinum. Here, the visceral pleura is continuous with the parietal pleura, which lines the walls of the pleural cavity (Fig. 1-32).

Understand that *the two pleural cavities are two separate and closed potential spaces.* Normally there is only a capillary layer of serous lubricating fluid in the pleural cavity. This substance lubricates the surfaces and reduces friction between the parietal and visceral layers of pleura so that respiratory movements can occur without interference.

The above arrangement develops as the embryonic lungs grow laterally into the pleural cavities, carrying the medial walls of the cavities before them, which become the visceral layer of pleura covering the lungs. You can visualize how this occurs by pushing your fist into a balloon. Note that the inner and outer walls of the balloon are continuous at your wrist, just as the visceral and parietal layers of pleura are continuous at the root of the lung (Fig. 1-32). If your fist were to swell it would reduce the cavity of the balloon just as the developing lung reduces the pleural cavity and brings the visceral and parietal layers of pleura together (Fig. 1-27). The original site of outgrowth of the embryonic lung is indicated by the root of the lung through which the airways and blood vessels enter and leave the lung.

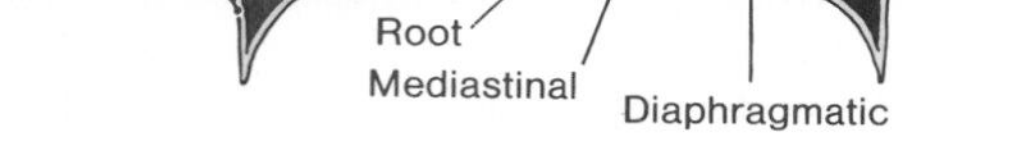

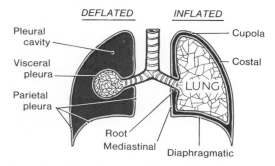

Figure 1-27. Drawing showing the scheme of the pleural cavities and pleurae. In the inflated lung, note that the parietal pleura is applied to the visceral (pulmonary) pleura but separated from it by a narrow interval, the pleural cavity which contains a little fluid.

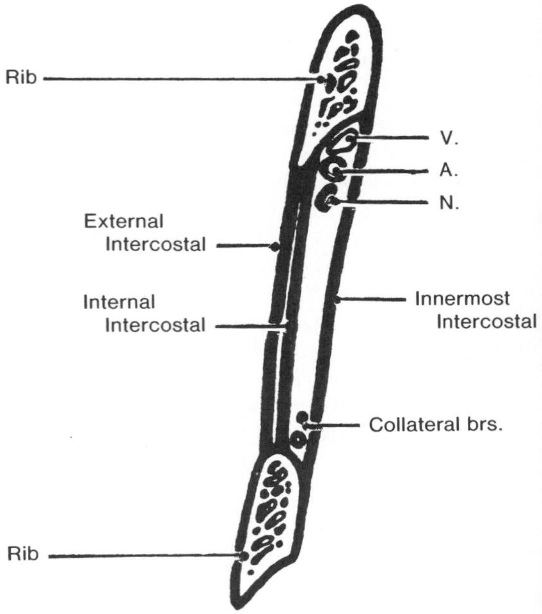

Figure 1-28. Diagrammatic sketch of a coronal section through two ribs illustrating the position of the intercostal nerve and vessels between the intercostal muscles. The key to remembering the relationships of the neurovascular bundle is VAN (*i.e.*, vein, artery, nerve). Observe that a needle passed into the chest (*e.g.*, to enter the pleural cavity) immediately above the rib will avoid the neurovascular bundle.

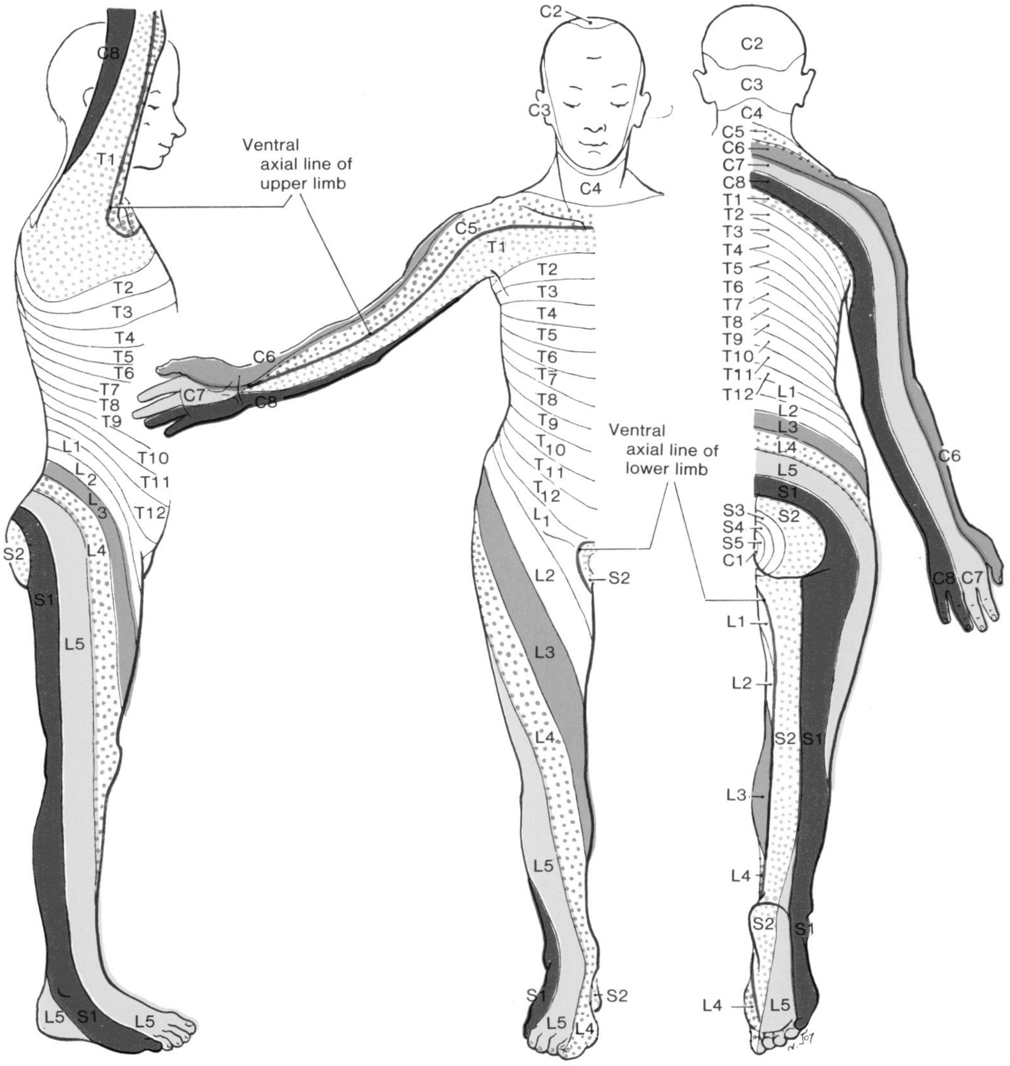

Figure 1-29. Diagram showing the dermatomes of the body, the strip-like areas of skin supplied by one pair of spinal nerves. When the function of even a single dorsal nerve root is interrupted, faint but definite diminution of sensitivity can be demonstrated in the dermatome. The method for detecting and plotting the area of diminished sensitivity is by using a light pin scratch for pain sensation, although it can be found for temperature and tactile sensation also.

The Parietal Pleura (Figs. 1-27, 1-30, and 1-32 to 1-34). The parietal pleura, the outer wall of the pleural sac, covers the different parts of the thoracic wall and the thoracic contents. It is given four names for descriptive purposes, according to the part it covers.

The costal pleura, the strongest part of the parietal pleura, covers the internal surfaces of the sternum, the **costal cartilages**, the ribs, the intercostal muscles, and the sides of the thoracic vertebrae. It is separated from these structures by a thin layer of loose areolar tissue called the **endothoracic fascia**. It provides a natural cleavage plane for surgical separation of the costal pleura from the thoracic wall.

The mediastinal pleura (Figs. 1-32 and

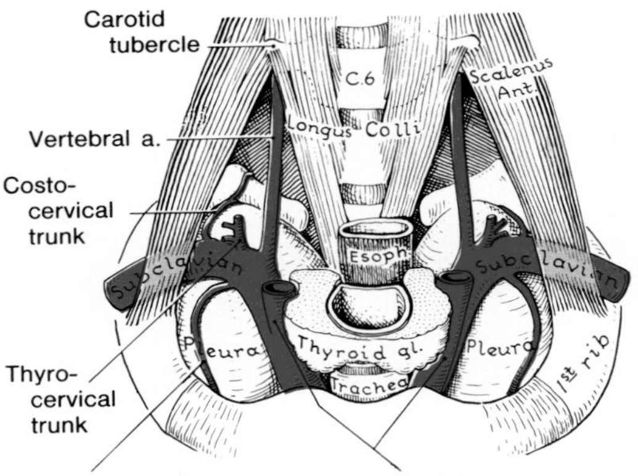

Figure 1-30. Drawing of a dissection showing the subclavian artery and its main branches. The first two posterior intercostal arteries arise from the superior intercostal artery, a branch of the costocervical trunk of the subclavian artery. The paired anterior intercostal arteries supplying the upper six intercostal spaces are derived from the internal thoracic artery and those supplying the seventh to ninth spaces are derived from its musculophrenic branch.

1-83) covers the **mediastinum** and is continuous with the costal pleura anteriorly and posteriorly, with the diaphragmatic pleura inferiorly, and with the dome or **cupola** of the pleura (Figs. 1-27 and 1-40) superiorly. *Above the root of the lung*, the mediastinal pleura is a continuous sheet between the sternum and the vertebral column. *At the root of the lung*, the mediastinal pleura passes laterally, enclosing the structures of the lung root, and becomes continuous with the visceral pleura (Fig. 1-32). *Below the root of the lung*, the mediastinal pleura passes laterally as a double layer from the esophagus to the lung, where it is continuous with the visceral pleura. This double layer, called the **pulmonary ligament** (Figs. 1-36 and 1-37), is continuous above with the mediastinal pleura, enclosing the lung root and ends below in a free border. The parietal layers of mediastinal pleura come into close apposition between the aorta and esophagus, just above the diaphragm (Fig. 1-34).

The diaphragmatic pleura (Figs. 1-27 and 1-34) is thin and covers the superior surface of the diaphragm lateral to the mediastinum (*i.e.*, most of the diaphragm except the central tendon).

The dome or cupola of the pleura (cervical pleura) covers the apex of the lung (Fig. 1-27) and extends through the thoracic inlet into the root of the neck (Fig. 1-40). This dome-shaped roof of the pleural cavity is the continuation of the costal and mediastinal parts of the pleura over the apex of the lung. *It extends upward to but not above the neck of the first rib* (Fig. 1-30). This is at the level of the spinous process of the seventh cervical vertebra, or **vertebra prominens** (Fig. 5-10). Because the first rib slopes downward, the lung and the pleura rise 3.5 cm above the anterior end of the first rib and 1 to 2 cm above the middle third of the clavicle (Figs. 1-30 and 1-40). The cupolae are separated by the trachea and the esophagus and the blood vessels passing to and from the neck (Figs. 1-30 and 1-84).

The cupola is strengthened by a layer of dense fascia, called the **suprapleural membrane**, which is attached to the inner margin of the first rib and the anterior border of the transverse process of C7. This membrane usually contains some muscle fibers (scalenus minimus) which give it added strength.

The lines of pleural reflection are sites

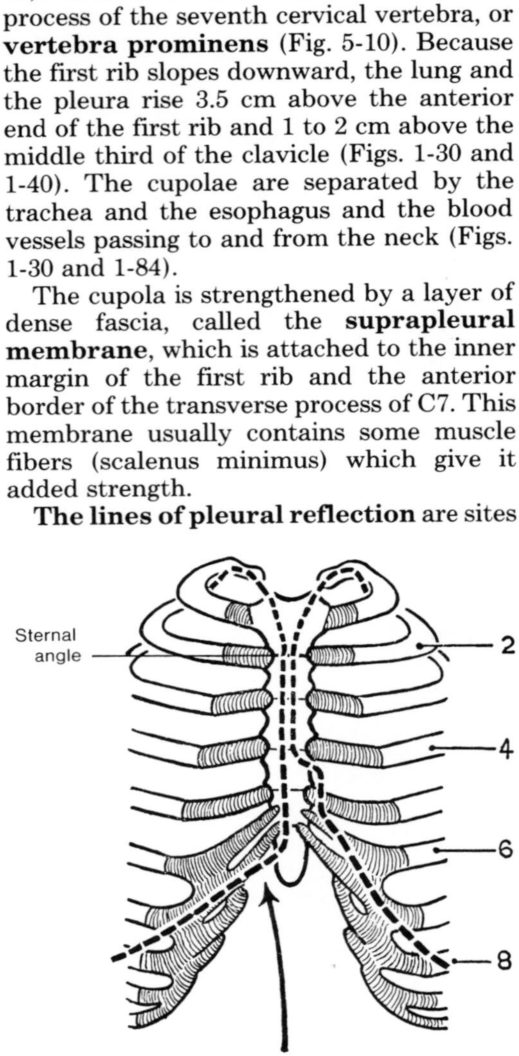

Figure 1-31. Diagram illustrating the sternal and costal lines of pleural reflection. The numbers indicate the even numbered ribs which are related to the lines of pleural reflection. The truncated apex of the infrasternal angle is at the xiphisternal joint.

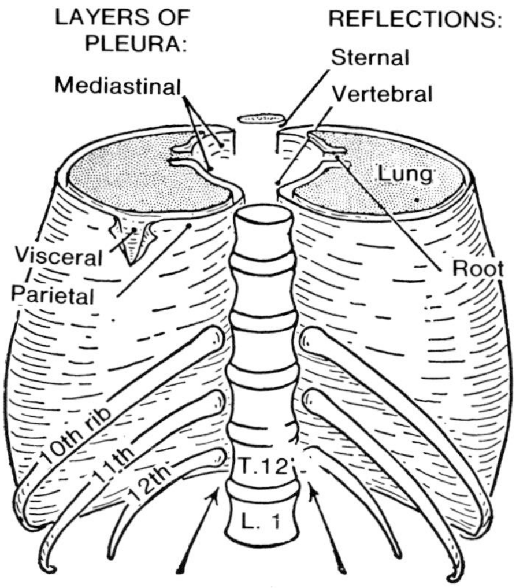

Figure 1-32. Drawing of the thorax from behind illustrating the sternal and vertebral pleural reflections.

at which the costal pleura becomes continuous with the mediastinal pleura anteriorly and posteriorly and with the diaphragmatic pleura inferiorly (Figs. 1-31, 1-32, and 1-39). *The sternal and costal lines of reflection are clinically important.*

The sternal reflection is where the costal pleura is continuous with the mediastinal pleura **behind the sternum**. The right and left sternal reflections are indicated by lines that pass inferomedially from the sternoclavicular joints to the median line at the level of the **sternal angle**, which lies at the level of the *second costal cartilages.* Here the two pleural sacs come in contact (Fig. 1-31) and may slightly overlap each other. **On the right side**, the reflection continues downward in the midline to the back of the xiphoid process. **On the left side**, the reflection passes downward in the midline to the level of the *fourth costal cartilage.* Here it passes to the left margin of the sternum and then continues downward to the *sixth costal cartilage.*

The costal reflection is where the costal pleura is continuous with the diaphragmatic pleura **near the chest margin**. It passes obliquely across the *8th rib* in the **midclavicular line**, the *10th rib* in the **midaxillary line**, and the *12th rib* at its **neck** or lower.

Review the lines of pleural reflection, noting that the costal cartilages or ribs printed in italics give a memory key composed of even numbers from **2** to **12**.

CLINICALLY ORIENTED COMMENTS

The pleurae descend below the costal margin in three regions where an abdominal incision might inadvertently enter a pleural sac: (1) the right xiphisternal angle (Fig. 1-40); (2) the right costovertebral angle; and (3) the left costovertebral angle (Fig. 1-32). In cases where the 12th rib is very short, the pleura lies below the costal margin after crossing the 11th rib and is, therefore, in surgical danger.

The parietal pleura is visible radiographically only in certain regions and in special views. The visceral pleura is usually not visible radiographically, except in certain views that demonstrate the fissures of the lung. However, any disease process that causes thickening of the pleura may make it visible in radiographs.

There are two other pleural reflections that need mention. The costal pleura is continuous with the mediastinal pleura along a vertical line which descends along the sides of the bodies of the thoracic vertebrae, just anterior to the heads of the first to the twelfth ribs. This is called the **vertebral reflection** (Fig. 1-32). The costal pleura is continuous with the diaphragmatic pleura along the line connecting the lower ends of the sternal and vertebral reflections. This **mediastinodiaphragmatic reflection** is deep and does not have the clinical importance of the other reflections.

The Visceral Pleura (Fig. 1-27). The visceral or pulmonary pleura **covers the lung closely and is adherent to all its surfaces.** It also passes into its fissures so that the lobes are also covered with visceral pleura. In these fissures the pleura of one lobe is in contact with the pleura of the adjacent lobe. Elsewhere the opposed surfaces of parietal and visceral pleura slide smoothly against each other during respiration.

The visceral pleura is continuous with the parietal pleura at the **root of the lung** (Figs. 1-15, 1-27, and 1-32), where the bronchi and blood vessels pass from the mediastinum to the lung.

The Pleural Recesses (Figs. 1-15, 1-33, and 1-34). During full inspiration the lungs fill the pleural cavities, but during quiet respiration three parts of them are not occupied by the lungs. At these sites the pleural reflections are so acute that the two portions of the parietal pleura are not only in continuous apposition, but are also in contact with one another at their inner or serous surfaces. No lung tissue with its covering of visceral pleura intervenes between these opposed layers. These three sites of reflection of parietal pleura are known as pleural recesses.

The right and left costodiaphragmatic recesses (Figs. 1-15, 1-33, and 1-34) are the slit-like intervals between the costal and diaphragmatic pleurae on each side. Here these parts of the pleura are separated by only a capillary layer of fluid. These recesses become alternately smaller and larger as the lungs move in and out of them during inspiration and expiration (Figs. 1-58 and 1-59).

The costomediastinal recess (Fig. 1-34) lies along the anterior margin of the pleura. Here the costal and mediastinal parts of the left pleura come into contact at the **cardiac notch** (Fig. 1-35) in the anterior border of the left lung where it overlies the heart. The slit-like costomediastinal recess is to the *left of the sternum* owing to the bulge of the heart to this side and lies at the anterior ends of the fourth and fifth interspaces. During inspiration and expiration, a thin edge of the left lung, called the **lingula** (Figs. 1-35*B* and 1-37), slides in and out of the costomediastinal recess.

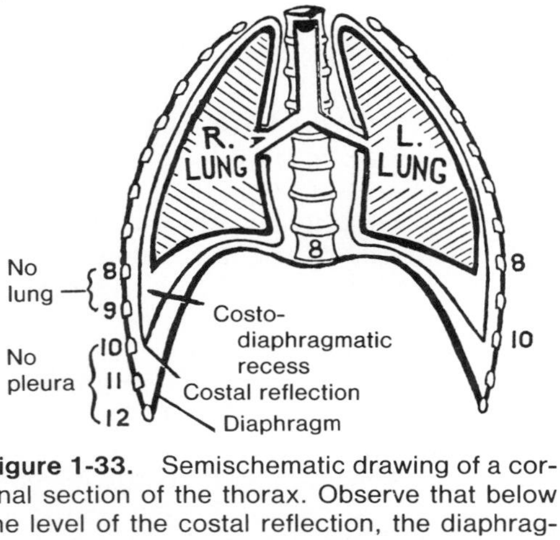

Figure 1-33. Semischematic drawing of a coronal section of the thorax. Observe that below the level of the costal reflection, the diaphragmatic pleura lies in direct contact with the costal pleura because the sides and back of the lower border of the lung do not descend to the level of the costal reflection.

CLINICALLY ORIENTED COMMENTS

The pleural cavity is only a potential space containing a thin film of lubricating fluid separating the opposing surfaces of pleurae. The potential pleural space, filled with a capillary thin film of fluid, facilitates movements of the lung, but its obliteration by disease or surgical removal (**pleurectomy**) does not cause appreciable functional consequences. In other surgical procedures, adherence of the visceral and parietal layers of pleura is purposely induced by covering the opposing pleural surfaces with a slightly irritating powder (**pleural poudrage** or powdering). This operation may be performed to prevent recurring spontaneous **pneumothorax** (presence of air in the pleural cavity) resulting from disease of the lung.

During inspiration and expiration, the normal moist smooth pleurae make no detectable sound during **auscultation**; however, inflammation of the pleurae (**pleuritis** or pleurisy) causes the surfaces to become rough and the resulting friction (**pleural rub** or friction rub) may be heard with a stethoscope. Pleuritis usually leads to the formation of **pleural adhesions** between the parietal and visceral pleurae. You may encounter such adhesions in a cadaver, which must be broken down before the lung can be completely mobilized.

The accumulation of significant amounts of fluid in the pleural cavity (**hydrothorax**) may result from a variety of causes. In advanced cases of pleurisy, serum

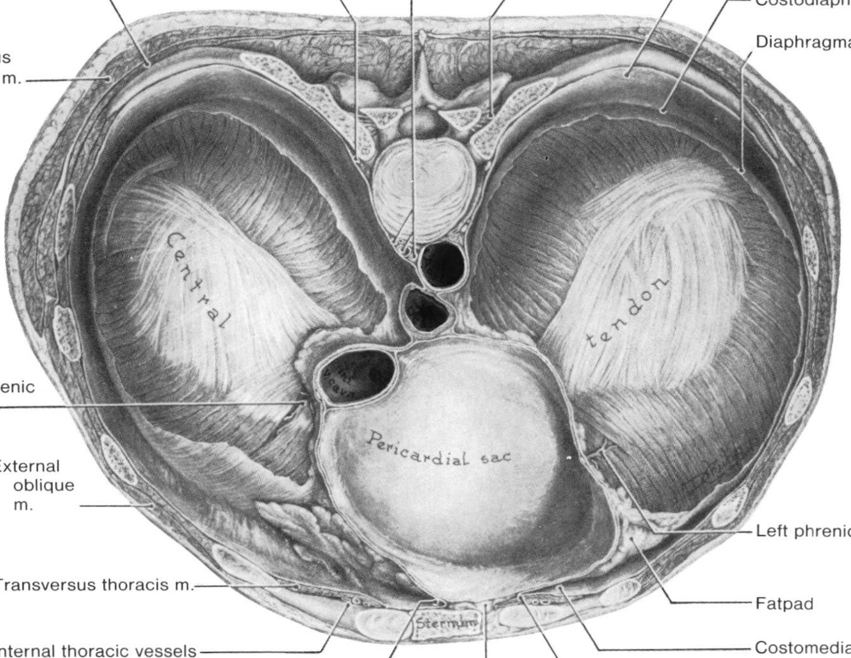

Figure 1-34. Drawing of a superior view of a dissection of the diaphragm and the pericardial sac. Most of the diaphragmatic pleura is removed. Observe the sternal reflexion of the left pleural sac which fails to meet that of the right sac in the median plane, ventral to the pericardium. Note that the right and left pleural sacs almost meet between the esophagus and the aorta to form a mesoesophagus. Examine the costodiaphragmatic recess which is deepest about the midlateral line. Observe that the costal pleura on reaching the vertebral column imperceptibly becomes the mediastinal pleura.

from the inflamed pleurae may exude or effuse from the blood vessels of the pleurae into the pleural cavity, forming a **pleural exudate**. As the fluid accumulates, the subatmospheric pressure is lessened, allowing the lung to retract toward the hilum. After the lung is completely retracted, additional fluid will cause the heart and mediastinum to become displaced toward the opposite side. If the inflamed pleurae become infected, the fluid contains leukocytes and the debris of dead cells (*i.e.*, pus). Pus in a body cavity is called **empyema** and when used without qualification refers to **pyothorax** (pus in the pleural cavity). One of the common causes of noninflammatory fluid accumulation in the pleural cavity is **congestive heart failure** (excessive accumulation of fluid resulting from failure of the heart to function normally), especially left heart failure.

Blood may also appear in the pleural cavity (**hemothorax**). The accumulation of blood may result from a chest wound or may be caused by a tumor. In rare cases, **chyle** (lymph and emulsified fat) may pass into the pleural cavity from a thoracic duct that is ruptured as it passes through the

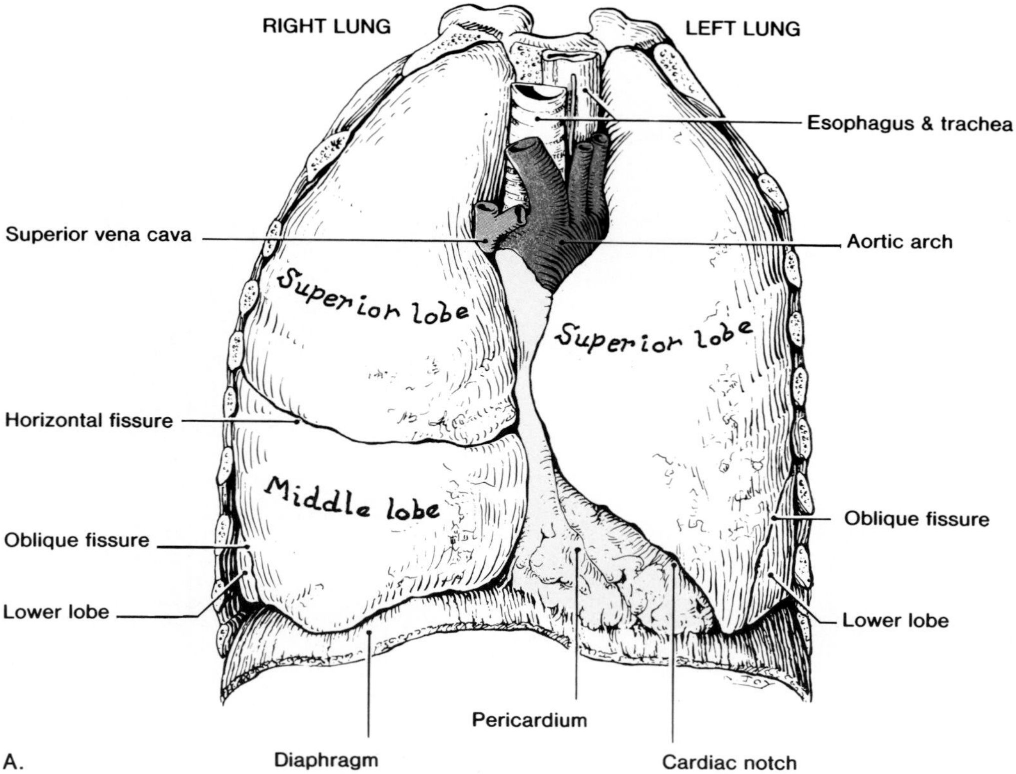
RIGHT LUNG
LEFT LUNG
Esophagus & trachea
Superior vena cava
Aortic arch
Superior lobe
Superior lobe
Horizontal fissure
Middle lobe
Oblique fissure
Oblique fissure
Lower lobe
Lower lobe
Pericardium
Diaphragm
Cardiac notch

A.

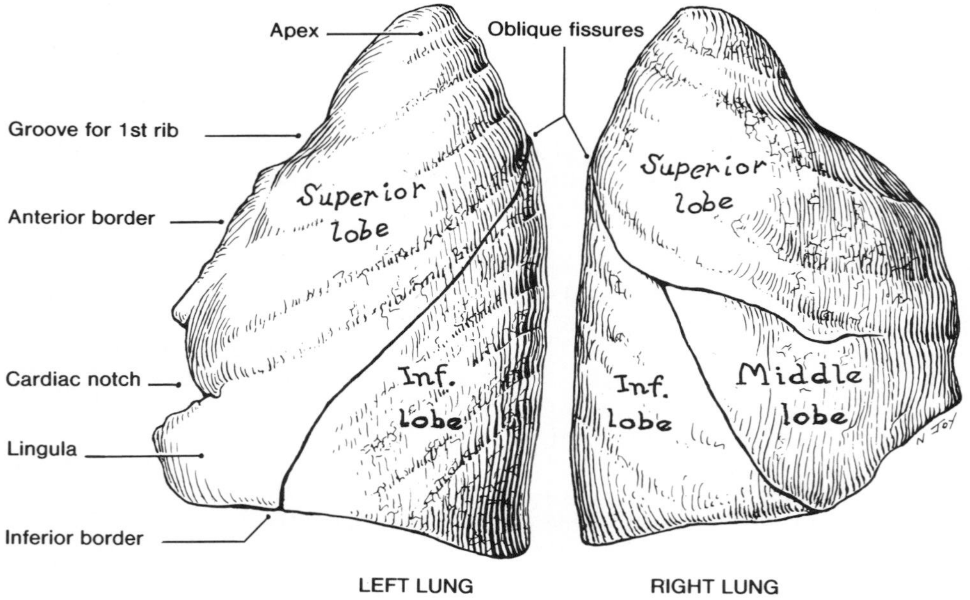
Apex
Oblique fissures
Groove for 1st rib
Anterior border
Superior lobe
Superior lobe
Cardiac notch
Inf. lobe
Inf. lobe
Middle lobe
Lingula
Inferior border
LEFT LUNG
RIGHT LUNG

B.

posterior mediastinum (Figs. 1-90 and 1-92). This condition is called **chylothorax**.

Fluid can be drained from the pleural cavity by inserting a wide-bore needle through an intercostal space (usually posteriorly through the seventh). Aspiration of material (*e.g.*, serous fluid, blood, pus) from the pleural cavity is called a **pleural tap** and is of significant diagnostic value. If the needle is inserted below intercostal space 8 or 9 and pushed too deeply, it is in danger of penetrating the diaphragm. After penetration of the diaphragm, the needle might reach the spleen on the left side or the liver on the right side and injure them.

Entry of air into the thorax (**pneumothorax**) following an external penetrating wound or rupture of a lung results in partial collapse of the lung. *Fractured ribs often produce a pneumothorax,* but the most common type is **spontaneous pneumothorax** that often results from rupture of bullae (blebs) on the surface of the lungs.

As the cupolae of the pleurae and the apices of the lungs extend up into the neck about 2.5 cm above the medial third of the clavicle (Fig. 1-40), they are vulnerable to stab wounds in the root of the neck. These wounds may penetrate the pleural cavity and the lung, producing an **open pneumothorax**. In these cases there is communication between the atmosphere and the pleural cavity; hence, you may hear this condition referred to as a "**blowing** or **sucking**" **pneumothorax**. Most cases of uncomplicated pneumothorax are not dangerous, but if the opening in the visceral pleura has a flap over it, air can enter the pleural cavity on inspiration but cannot leave it during expiration. In such cases, the amount of air in the pleural space increases (**positive pressure pneumothorax**), pushing the mediastinum to the other side, compressing the opposite lung, and killing the patient. Thus, *positive pressure pneumothorax is a medical emergency*!

The pleurae may also be injured by an anesthetist's needle when a **stellate ganglion block** or a nerve block of the brachial plexus (nerves supplying the upper limbs, Fig. 6-24) are being performed. The needle tears the pleura as the lungs move.

Because the pleura crosses the 12th rib (Figs. 1-32 and 1-40), it may be injured during removal of a kidney (**nephrectomy**). When the 12th rib is very short, the 11th rib may be mistaken for it and a posterior incision reaching it would result in opening of the pleural cavity to the atmosphere (*i.e.*, an **open pneumothorax**). Thus, it is important to determine if the lowest palpable rib is the 11th or the 12th. This may be done by counting down from the second rib, the costal cartilage of which is easily located lateral to the **sternal angle** (Figs. 1-1 and 1-11).

Vessels and Nerves of the Pleura. **The parietal pleura** receives its blood supply from the arteries which supply the thoracic body wall (*i.e.*, the **intercostal**, **internal thoracic**, and **musculophrenic arteries**). The costal pleura and the pleura on the peripheral part of the diaphragmatic pleura are supplied by the **intercostal nerves,** whereas the mediastinal pleura and the central part of the diaphragmatic pleura are supplied by the **phrenic nerve**. *The veins of the parietal pleura* join the systemic veins in the neighboring parts of the thoracic wall. Similarly its lymphatic vessels drain into adjacent lymph nodes of the thoracic wall (intercostal, parasternal, posterior mediastinal, and diaphragmatic). These nodes (Fig. 1-20) may in turn drain into the axillary lymph nodes (*i.e.*, nodes in the axilla or armpit).

The visceral pleura receives its arterial supply from the *bronchial arteries*, which are branches of the descending thoracic aorta (Fig. 1-91). Its veins drain into the

Figure 1-35. Drawings of the lungs. *A*, anterior view of a dissection of the lungs and pericardium. *B*, lateral view of the lungs. Observe the three lobes of the right lung and the two lobes of the left. In *A* note that the middle lobe of the right lung lies at the front of the thorax; it is entirely anterior to the midlateral line. Also observe the deficiency of the upper lobe of the left lung, called the cardiac notch, allowing the pericardium to appear. Note the horizontal fissure of the right lung which is complete in *A* and incomplete in *B*.

pulmonary veins and its numerous lymphatic vessels drain into nodes at the hila of the lungs. Its nerve supply is derived from the autonomic nerves innervating the lung which accompany the bronchial vessels (Fig. 1-86).

CLINICALLY ORIENTED COMMENTS

The visceral pleura is insensitive to pain, but *the parietal pleura is very sensitive to pain*, particularly its costal part. Irritation of the costal and peripheral diaphragmatic areas results in local pain and also in **referred pain** along the intercostal nerves to the thoracic and abdominal wall, whereas irritation of the mediastinal and central diaphragmatic areas results in referred pain in the lower part of the neck and over the shoulder. The explanation for this is that the lower neck and shoulder are supplied by the same segments of the spinal cord (C3 to C5) that give origin to the phrenic nerve (Figs. 1-29 and 1-53).

THE LUNGS

The lungs (L. *pulmones*) are the essential **organs of respiration**. During life they are normally light, soft, and spongy. They are very elastic and will shrink to about one-third when the thoracic cavity is opened. During early life they are light pink, but often they are dark and mottled during late life (Figs. 1-36 and 1-37) owing to the accumulation of inhaled dust particles which become trapped in the fixed phagocytes in the lungs over the years.

Each lung has the shape of a half cone and is contained in its own pleural sac within the thoracic cavity (Fig. 1-27). They are separated from each other by the heart and other structures in the mediastinum (Fig. 1-35*A*). The lungs are attached to the heart and the trachea by their roots and the **pulmonary ligaments** (Figs. 1-36 and 1-37); otherwise each lung lies freely within its pleural cavity. *The right lung is larger and heavier than the left* (Fig. 1-35), but the vertical extent of the right lung is less than that of the left because the right dome of the diaphragm is higher (Figs. 1-15 and 1-48). It is also wider than the left lung because the heart and pericardium bulge more to the left.

The hardened lungs in an embalmed cadaver have impressions formed by adjacent structures (*e.g.*, the ribs and costal cartilages), whereas fresh lungs usually do not. These cadaveric markings are helpful reminders of the relationships of the lungs (Figs. 1-36 and 1-37).

CLINICALLY ORIENTED COMMENTS

Healthy lungs always contain air, thus they will float and crepitate (L. *crepo*, to rattle) when squeezed. A diseased lung filled with fluid may not float. The lungs of a stillborn infant are firm and sink when placed in water, whereas those of a liveborn infant will float. *This is of medicolegal significance.*

Lobes and Fissures of the Lungs (Figs. 1-15 and 1-35 to 1-37).

The left lung is divided into superior (upper) and inferior (lower) lobes by a long deep **oblique fissure** which extends from the costal to the medial surface of the lung, both above and below the hilum. The superior lobe has a wide **cardiac notch** on its anterior border, where the lung is deficient owing to the bulge of the heart. This leaves part of the front of the pericardium uncovered by lung tissue. The anteroinferior part of the superior lobe is formed by a small tongue-like projection called the **lingula** (L. tongue). The lingula is embryologically homologous to the middle lobe of the right lung. The inferior lobe of the left lung is larger than the superior lobe and lies below and behind the oblique fissure.

The right lung is divided into superior (upper), middle, and inferior (lower) lobes by oblique and **horizontal fissures**. The horizontal fissure separates the superior and middle lobes and the oblique fissure separates the inferior lobe from the middle and superior lobes. The superior lobe is smaller than in the left lung and the middle lobe is wedge-shaped in outline.

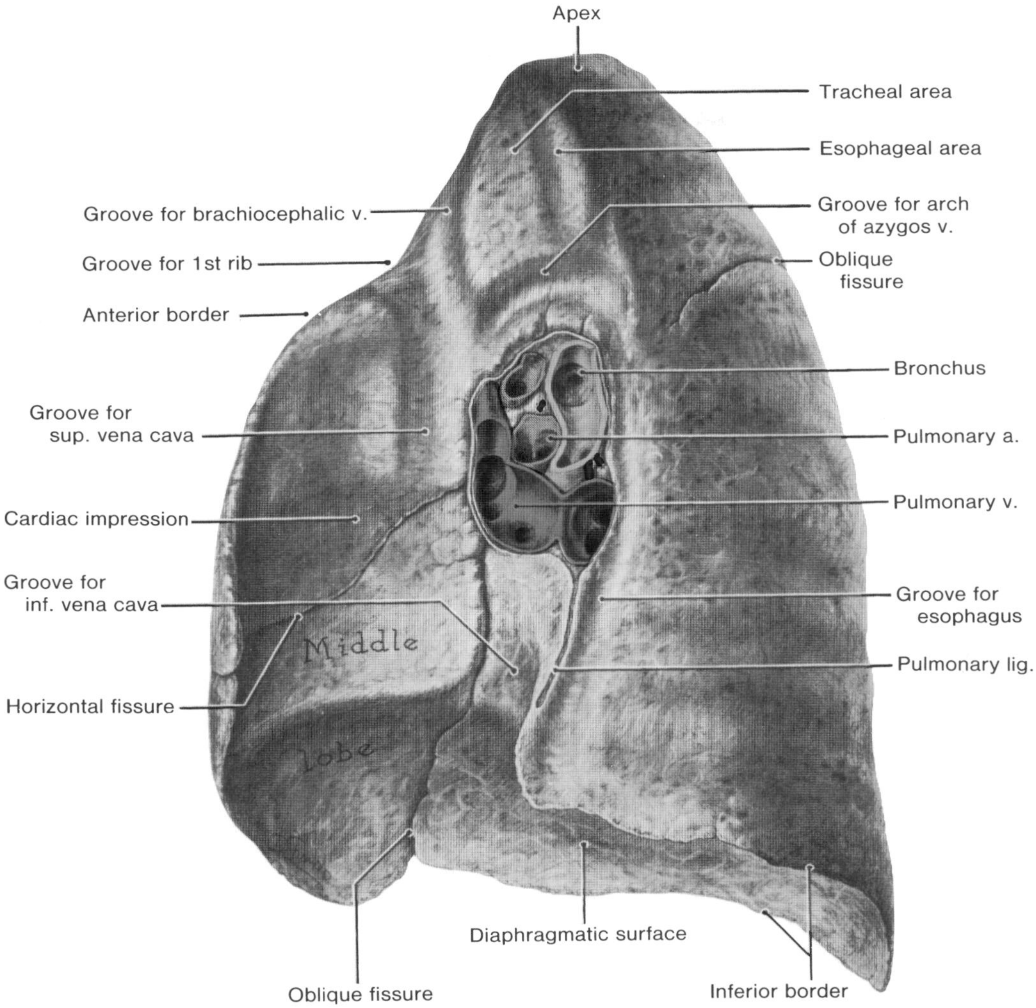

Figure 1-36. Drawing of the mediastinal surface of the *right lung*. Observe that the lung resembles an inflated balloon in that it takes the impressions of the structures with which it comes into contact. Thus, the base is fashioned by the cupola of the diaphragm and the costal surface bears the impressions of the ribs. Note that distended vessels leave their mark, whereas empty vessels and nerves do not. Observe the somewhat pear-shaped root of the lung near the center of the mediastinal surface and the pulmonary ligament descending like a stalk from the root. Note the groove for, or line of contact with, the esophagus throughout the length of the lung, except where the arch of the azygos vein intervenes. This groove passes behind the root and therefore behind the pulmonary ligament, which separates it from the groove for the left vena cava. Observe the oblique fissure, here incomplete, but complete in the lung shown in Figure 1-37. Note the two pulmonary veins, here uniting unusually close to the lung. Note that in this specimen the upper and lower pulmonary veins have united before entering the left atrium.

CLINICALLY ORIENTED COMMENTS

Occasionally extra fissures subdivide the lungs; thus, the left lung sometimes has three lobes. Rarely, the right lung has only two lobes. Often the accessory fissures are incomplete.

A **lobe of the azygos vein** appears in the right lung in about 1% of people. It develops when the apical bronchus grows superiorly, medial to the arch of the azygos

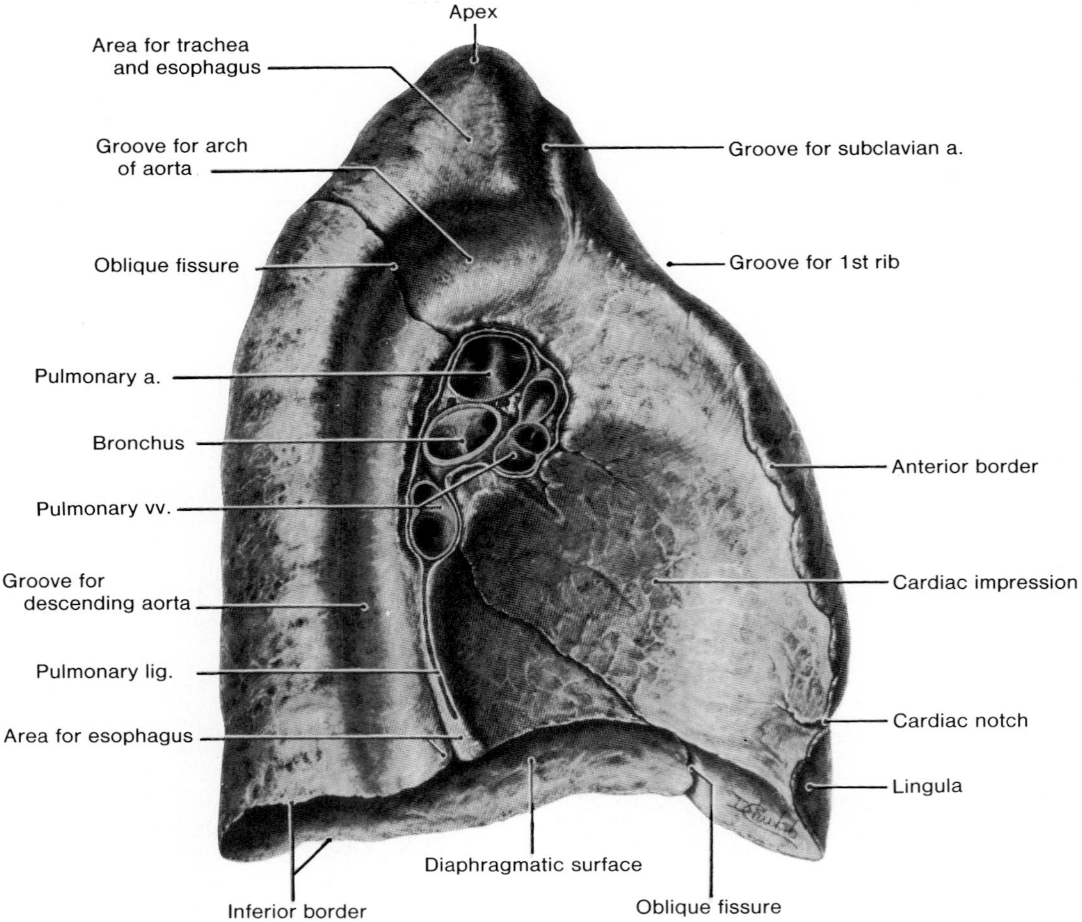

Figure 1-37. Drawing of the mediastinal surface of the *left lung*. Near the center observe the root of the lung and the pulmonary ligament descending from it. Note the lung's site of contact with the esophagus, between the aorta and the lower end of the ligament. Observe the oblique fissure cutting completely through the lung substance. In both the right and left lung roots the artery is above, the bronchus is behind, one vein is in front, and the other is below. In the right root, the bronchus (eparterial) to the upper lobe is the highest structure. The marked groove for the descending aorta was caused by a somewhat arteriosclerotic aorta that had deviated from the midline.

vein instead of lateral to it. As a result, the azygos vein comes to lie at the bottom of a deep fissure in the superior lobe. This fissure with the azygos vein at its lower end produces a linear marking on a radiograph of the chest, which separates the apical part of the lung from the remainder of the superior lobe. The other linear markings seen in normal chest radiographs are produced by pulmonary vessels (Figs. 1-38, 1-58, and 1-59).

Surfaces and Borders of the Lungs (Figs. 1-35 to 1-40). Each lung presents an apex, a base, two surfaces, and three borders.

The Apex. This **rounded superior pole** of each lung extends through the superior aperture of the thorax into the root of the neck, where it lies in close contact with the cupola of the pleura (cervical pleura). Owing to the obliquity of the thoracic inlet, the apex of the lung extends 3 to 5 cm above the anterior part of the first rib. Its summit lies in front of the neck of the first rib, about 2.5 cm above the medial third of the clavicle (Figs. 1-38 to 1-40).

The apex of the lung is crossed by the subclavian artery and vein (Fig. 1-72) and the artery produces a groove in its medial and anterior surfaces (Fig. 1-37). These vessels are separated from the apex of the lung by the cervical pleura and the suprapleural membrane.

The Base. The base or **diaphragmatic**

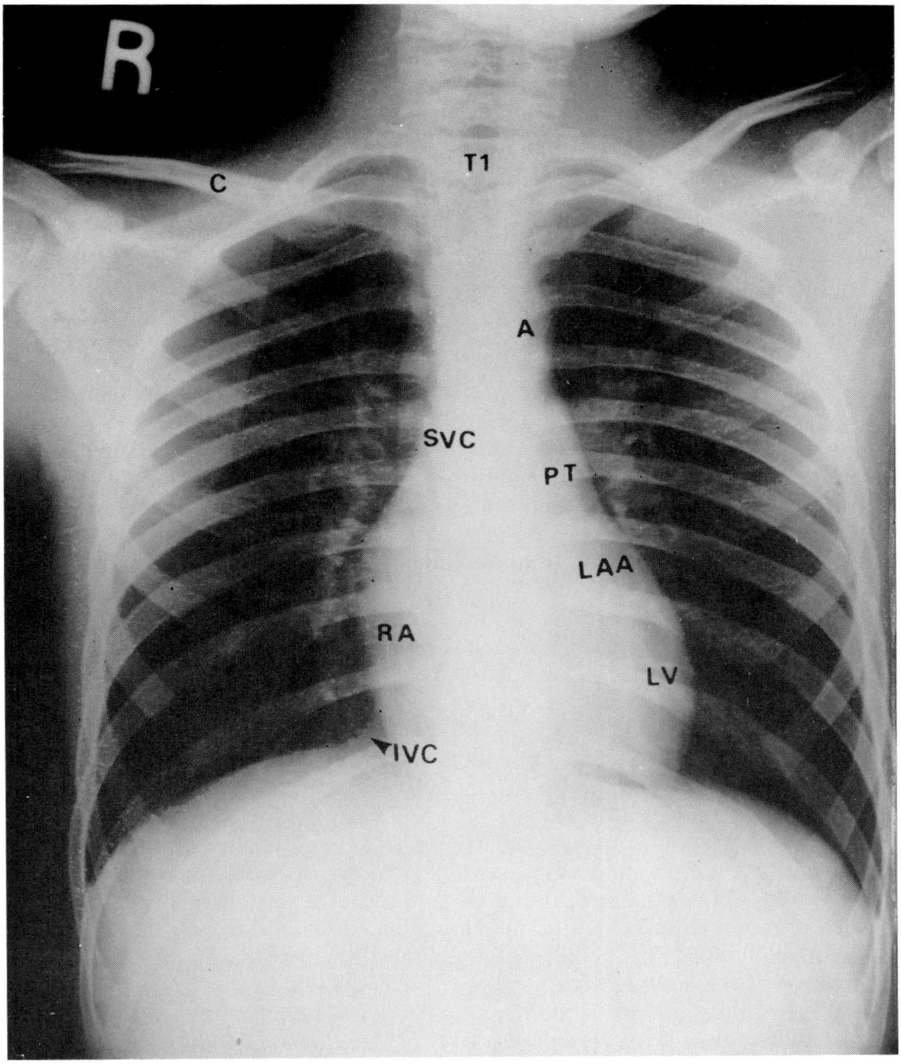

Figure 1-38. Radiograph of the chest, posteroanterior (*PA*) projection. Observe the body of the first thoracic vertebra (*T1*). Follow it laterally to the first rib which curves outward, then medially crossing the clavicle (*C*). Note that the dome of the diaphragm is somewhat higher on the right. Observe that the right mediastinal border is formed by the superior vena cava (*SVC*) and the right atrium (*RA*). In the angle between the right atrium and upper border of the diaphragm, an *arrow* points to the inferior vena cava (*IVC*). Note that the left mediastinal border is formed by the aortic arch (*A*), or "aortic knob," the pulmonary trunk (*PT*), the left auricle or auricular appendage (*LAA*), and the left ventricle (*LV*).

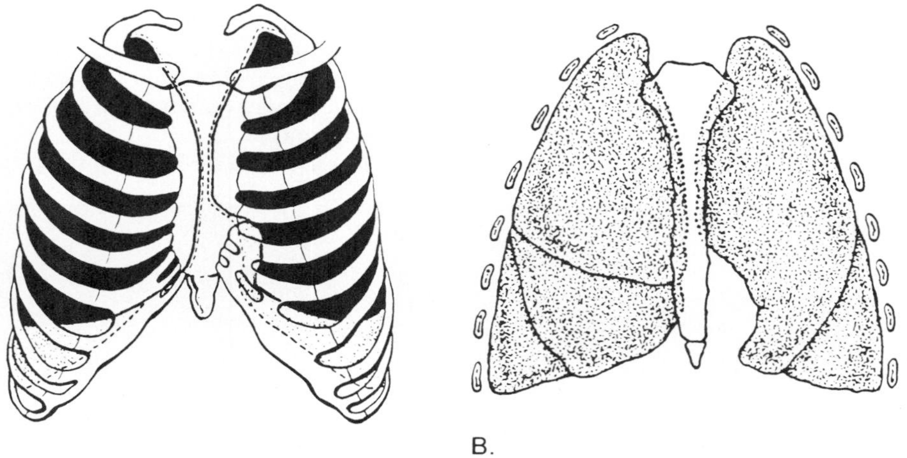

A. B.

Figure 1-39. Drawings illustrating the lungs (*dark line*) and the lines of pleural reflection (*light broken line*). The degree to which the lungs and the pleura diverge from the sternum varies from one person to another.

surface of each lung is concave and semilunar in shape. It rests on the convex surface of the **diaphragm** (Fig. 1-38), which separates the right lung from the liver and the left lung from the liver, stomach, and spleen. The concavity of the base is deeper in the right lung than in the left lung because of the slightly higher position of the right dome of the diaphragm (Fig. 1-48). Laterally and posteriorly the base is bounded by a thin sharp margin which projects into the costodiaphragmatic recess of the pleura (Figs. 1-15 and 1-34).

The Costal Surface (Fig. 1-35). The costal surface of each lung is large, smooth, and convex. It fits against the thoracic wall and includes the bulky posterior part of the lung. It is in contact with the costal pleura and in embalmed cadavers impressions of the ribs are visible on this surface.

The Medial Surface (Figs. 1-36 and 1-37). This surface of the lung is divided into two parts; a vertebral part and a mediastinal part. **The vertebral part** occupies the gutter on each side of the thoracic region of the vertebral column and passes imperceptibly into the costal surface (Fig. 1-32).

The mediastinal part is indented by the heart and great vessels, especially on the left lung. The deep concavity called the **cardiac impression** accommodates the heart and the pericardium. This impression is larger and deeper on the left (Fig. 1-37) than on the right (Fig. 1-36), because the heart projects more to the left than to the right (Fig. 1-38). The **hilum** (hilus) of the lung is where the bronchi, pulmonary vessels, bronchial vessels, lymph vessels, and nerves enter and leave the lung near the center in the mediastinal part. The hilum is surrounded by a sleeve of pleura which is reflected off the lung on to the mediastinum (Fig. 1-36).

The **pulmonary ligament** is the downward extension of this pleural sleeve. The structures entering and leaving the lung form the *root of the lung* (Fig. 1-32) which is attached at the **hilum**.

The Anterior Border (Figs. 1-35 to 1-39). This border is thin and sharp and overlaps the pericardium. It corresponds more or less to the anterior border of the pleura. The anterior border of the left lung has a **cardiac notch** of variable size. Thus, the pericardium in this area is covered only by a double layer of pleura.

The Posterior Border (Figs. 1-32, 1-36, and 1-37). The posterior border of each lung is thick and rounded. It lies in a paravertebral gutter and fits against the thoracic region of the vertebral column.

The Inferior Border (Figs. 1-35 to 1-38). This border limits the base of the lung. It is thin and sharp where it extends into the **costodiaphragmatic recess** (Figs. 1-15 and 1-34) and separates the base of the lung

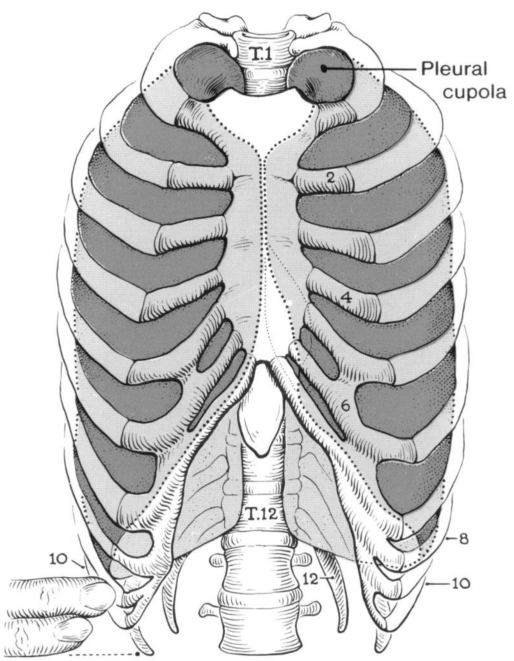

Figure 1-40. Drawing of the thorax illustrating the extent of the pleura. Observe that the pleura rises to, but not above, the neck of the first rib. Note that the right and left sternocostal reflections meet behind the sternum above the level of the second ribs and descend together to the fourth ribs where the left pleura deviates variably to the sixth or seventh rib. These reflections are in the midclavicular line at the 8th rib and in the midlateral line at the 10th rib. Note that the pleura is two fingerbreadths above the margin of the bony thorax and that it descends as the vertebral reflexion on the vertebral bodies of T12 to T1.

from the costal surface. It is blunt and rounded medially where it divides the base from the mediastinal surface.

Surface Markings of the Lungs (Fig. 1-39). The anterior borders of the lungs follow the lines of pleural reflection, except at the cardiac notch below the level of the fourth costal cartilage. The lungs can be outlined on the surface of the thorax using the following landmarks. *These markings are clinically important.*

The apex of the lung is represented by a line drawn superolaterally from the sternoclavicular joint to a point 2.5 cm above the middle third of the clavicle and then drawn inferolaterally to the junction of the middle and medial thirds of the clavicle. The apex of the lung and the pleura are coextensive and the height to which they rise above the clavicle varies slightly from person to person.

The anterior border of the right lung practically corresponds to the anterior border of the right pleura described previously and illustrated in Figures 1-39 and 1-40.

The anterior border of the left lung practically corresponds to the anterior border of the left pleura as far as the level of the fourth costal cartilage. Here, the anterior border of this lung deviates laterally to a point about 2.5 cm lateral to the left border of the sternum to form the cardiac notch. It then turns inferiorly and slightly medially to the sixth left costal cartilage.

The inferior border of both lungs is indicated by a line drawn from the inferior end of the line representing the anterior border that crosses the *6th rib in the midclavicular line*, the *8th rib in the midaxillary line*, the *10th rib in the midscapular line*, and ends about 2.5 cm lateral to the spinous process of the *10th thoracic vertebra*. Remember the numbers 6, 8, and 10 and compare them with the corresponding ones for the inferior border of the pleura. You will find that *the inferior border of the lungs lies two ribs higher than that of the parietal pleura* on each of the three vertical lines just mentioned (Fig. 1-58). In young children the inferior border of the lung is *about one rib higher* than in adults. Understand that the level of the inferior border of the lung varies according to the phase of respiration (Figs. 1-58 and 1-59), and that the surface markings given here represent average levels.

Surface Markings of the Lung Fissures. The **oblique fissure** of the lung is indicated on the surface of the thorax by a line from a point about 2.5 cm lateral to the spinous process of the second thoracic vertebra to the sixth costochondral junction (about 5 cm from the anterior median line). To locate the spinous process of T2, count down from the spinous process of the seventh cervical vertebra. Its process is so prominent when the neck is flexed (Fig. 5-10) that it is called the **vertebra prominens**.

The **horizontal fissure** of the right lung is indicated by a line on the surface of the thorax that runs from the anterior border of the lung along the fourth costal cartilage to the oblique fissure (about 5 cm from the anterior median line). If you place the upper edge of your hand over your right nipple, it will cover most of the middle lobe of the lung.

The Bronchi and the Roots of the Lungs (Figs. 1-15, 1-27, 1-36, 1-37, 1-40, and 1-84). The two **principal (main) bronchi**, one to each lung, pass inferolaterally from the termination of the trachea to the hila of the lungs. Each main pulmonary artery passes transversely into the lung, anterior to its bronchus. The two pulmonary veins on each side (upper and lower) ascend from the hilum of the lung to the left atrium of the heart (Fig. 1-56).

Within the lung *the bronchi divide in a constant fashion in constant directions so that each branch supplies a clearly defined sector of the lung* (Fig. 1-42). Each principal bronchus divides into secondary **lobar bronchi** (two on the left, three on the right), *each of which supplies a lobe* of the lung. Each lobar bronchus then divides into tertiary **segmental bronchi** which supply specific sectors of the lung, called **bronchopulmonary segments** (Figs. 1-41 to 1-46). This term is applied to the largest segments of the lobe.

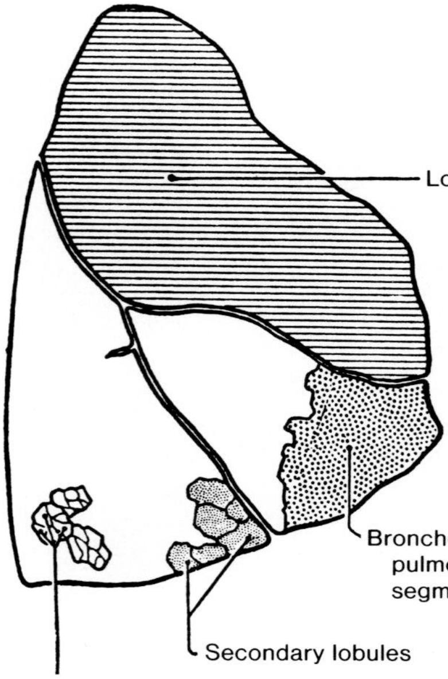

Figure 1-41. Diagram showing the subdivisions of the lung.

CLINICALLY ORIENTED COMMENTS

When the trachea and bronchi are examined with a **bronchoscope**, a projecting keel-like ridge is observed at the inferior end of the trachea marking the origins of the right and left bronchi. It is called the **carina** (L. keel of a ship). Normally the carina is in the median plane and has a fairly definite edge. If the **tracheobronchial lymph nodes** (Figs. 1-47 and 1-85) in the angle between the principal bronchi become enlarged (*e.g.*, owing to the lymphogenous spread of cancer cells from a **bronchogenic carcinoma**), the carina becomes splayed (spread out) and often fixed (Case 1-2). Such morphological changes in the carina are important diagnostic signs for the **bronchoscopist** in assisting with the differential diagnosis of disease of the respiratory system.

The mucous membrane at the carina is one of the most sensitive areas of the tracheobronchial tree and is associated with the **cough reflex**. For example, when a child aspirates (sucks in during inspiration) a peanut he/she chokes and coughs. Once the peanut passes the carina coughing usually stops, but the resulting **chemical bronchitis** (inflammation of the bronchus) caused by substances released from the peanut, and the **atelectasis** (collapse) of the lung beyond the foreign body soon causes difficult breathing **(dyspnea)**. Hence, *the carina is often considered to be the last line of defense* and frequently the violent coughing caused by irritation of it results in expulsion of the aspirated foreign body.

At the bifurcation of the trachea, the right principal bronchus is wider and shorter (Fig. 1-46) and runs more vertically than does the left principal bronchus (Fig. 1-84). This is *the anatomical reason foreign bodies are more likely to enter the right bronchus than the left* and to lodge in it or in one of its branches.

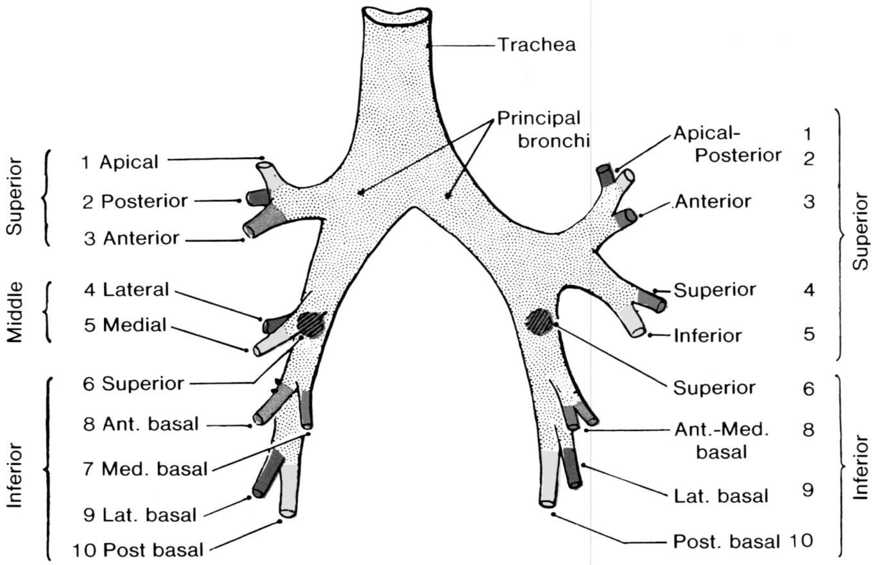

Figure 1-42. Diagram illustrating the tertiary segmental bronchi for correlation with the bronchopulmonary segments shown in Figure 1-43. Observe that the right lung has three lobes and the left two and that there are 10 tertiary or segmental bronchi on the right and 9 on the left. Note that on the left the apical and posterior bronchi arise from a single stem, as do the anterior basal and medial basal.

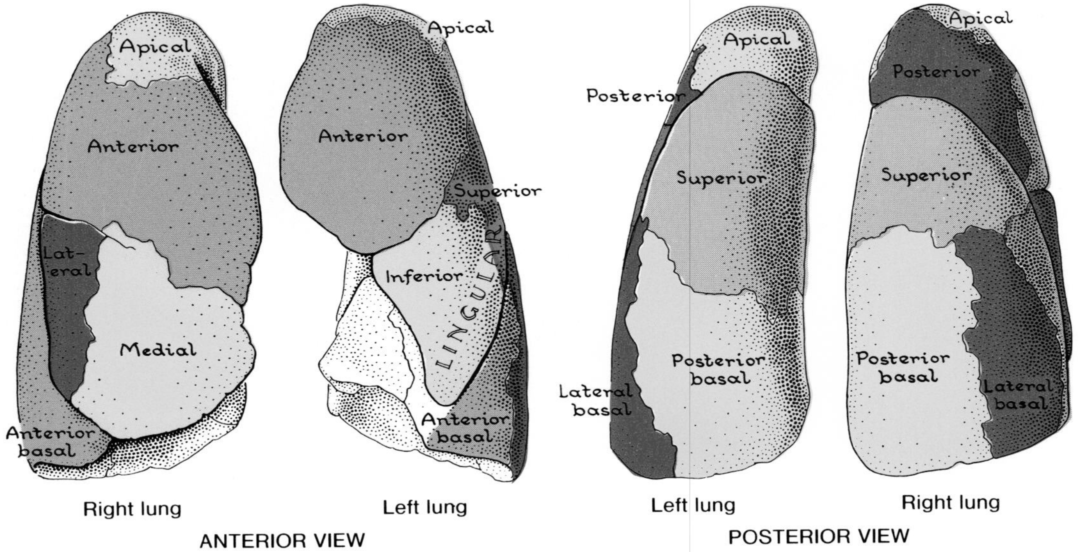

Figure 1-43. Drawings illustrating the bronchopulmonary segments. To prepare these specimens, the tertiary segmental bronchi (Fig. 1-42) of fresh lungs were isolated within the hilum and injected with latex of various colors. Minor variations in the branching of the bronchi result in variations in the surface patterns in different specimens. Understand that a bronchopulmonary segment consists of a tertiary bronchus, the portion of lung it ventilates, an artery, and a vein. These are surgically separable.

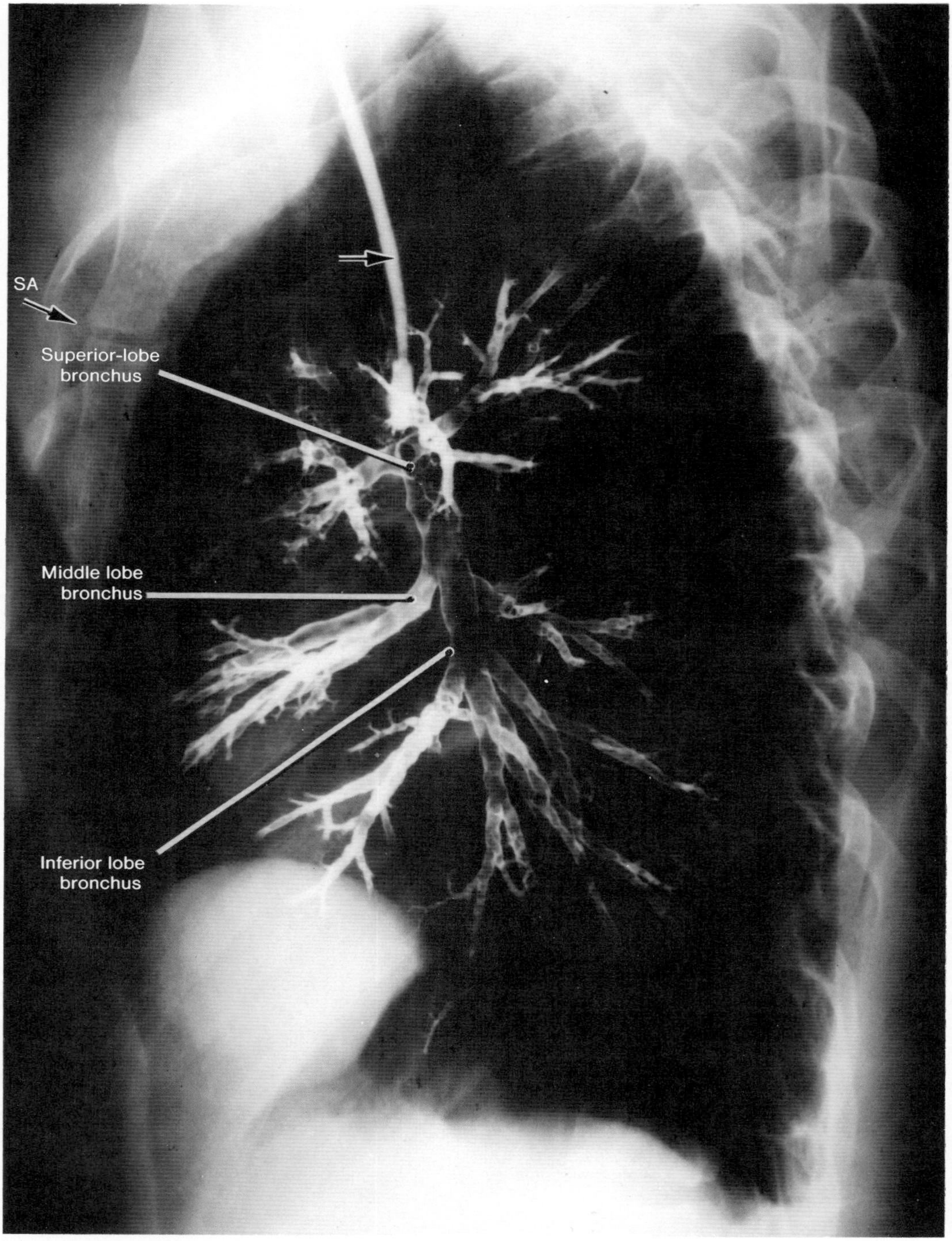

Figure 1-44. Oblique view of the chest showing a bronchogram of the right bronchial tree. The secondary bronchi are labeled. The contrast material was injected via a catheter (*arrow*) after topical anesthesia of the nose, pharynx, larynx, and trachea. The injection was performed under fluoroscopic control so that the patient could be postured in various positions to allow the contrast material to flow into all the secondary and segmental (tertiary) branches. *SA* and *arrow* indicate the sternal angle (see Fig. 1–12).

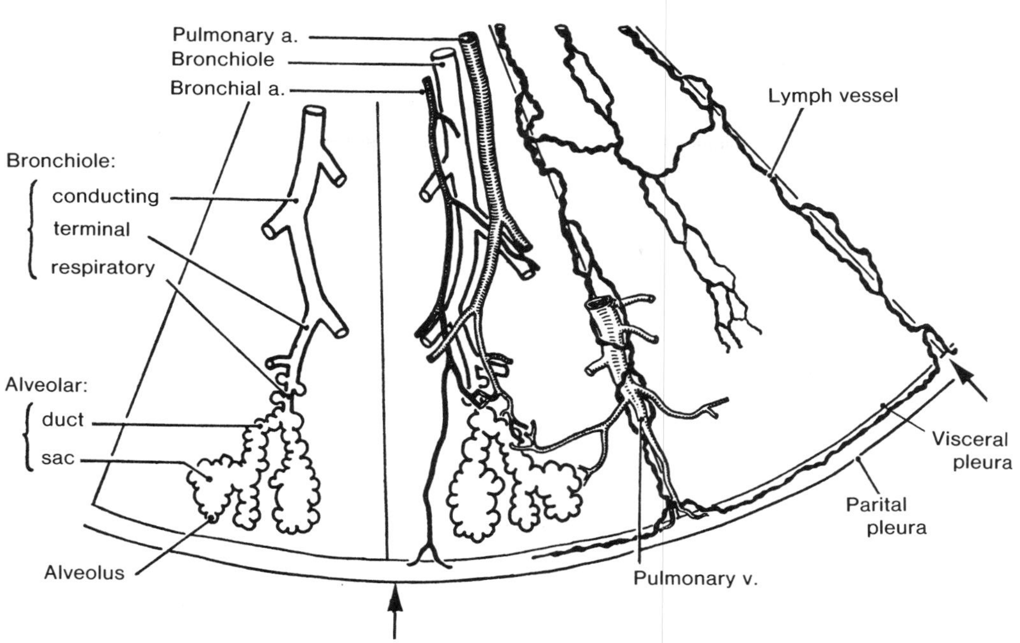

Figure 1-45. Diagrammatic sketch illustrating the structure of a lobule of the lung. The base of a bronchopulmonary segment is between the *arrows*.

Because the left **principal bronchus** lies closer to the pulmonary trunk, the aortic arch, and the descending aorta than does the right principal bronchus (Figs. 1-46 and 1-84), the left one is more difficult to deal with surgically than the right one.

The Bronchopulmonary Segments (Figs. 1-41 to 1-46). Each segment of the lung is pyramidal in shape with its apex pointed toward the root of the lung and its base at the pleural surface. *Each segment has its own segmental bronchus, artery, and vein.* Bronchopulmonary segments are separated from one another by connective tissue septa which are continuous with the visceral pleura. The names of the various bronchopulmonary segments are given in Figures 1-41 and 1-42.

CLINICALLY ORIENTED COMMENTS

Bronchopulmonary segments are of considerable clinical significance. Bronchial and pulmonary disorders (*e.g.*, a tumor or an abscess) may be localized in one of these segments and may be surgically removed without seriously disrupting surrounding lung tissue. Although each **bronchopulmonary segment** is supplied by its own nerve, artery, and vein, it is important to know that during surgical resection (removal) of these segments the planes between them are crossed by branches of pulmonary veins and sometimes by branches of pulmonary arteries (Fig. 1-45). In addition, the **bronchial arteries** run through the interlobular septa to supply the visceral pleura.

Each bronchopulmonary segment is surrounded by connective tissue that is continuous with the visceral pleura. These connective tissue septa, separating the segments, prevent air from passing between segments. Therefore, air in a bronchopulmonary segment whose segmental bronchus is obstructed is absorbed by the blood stream, causing **segmental atelectasis** or collapse.

Malignant tumors and certain infections (*e.g.*, **tuberculosis**) invade the connective tissue septa separating the bronchopulmonary segments and involve adjacent seg-

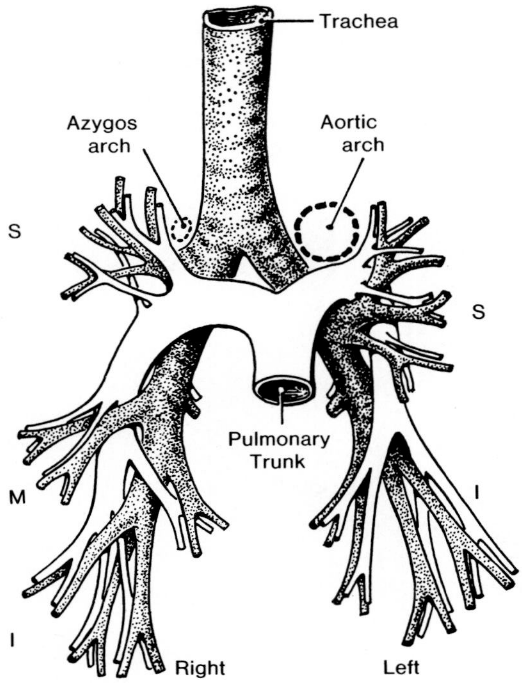

Figure 1-46. Drawing to show the relationship of the pulmonary arteries to the bronchi, anterior view. *S, M,* and *L* indicate branches to the superior, middle, and lower lobes.

ments. In such disorders, surgical resection of several segments, a whole lobe (**lobectomy**) or an entire lung (**pneumonectomy**), may be necessary.

A good knowledge of the branching of the bronchial tree is necessary to determine the appropriate postures for draining infected areas of the lung. For example, when a patient with **bronchiectasis** (dilation of bronchi) is positioned in bed on his/her left side, secretions from the right lung and bronchi flow toward the **carina** of the trachea (the ridge separating the openings of the right and left principal bronchi). As this is a sensitive area, the cough reflex is stimulated and the patient brings up **purulent sputum** (*i.e.*, containing pus), clearing the right bronchial tree. Alternatively, persons with bronchiectasis of the **lingula** of the left superior lobe drain it by lying on the right side. The basal bronchi may be cleared by the patient standing on his/her head for several minutes every morning to promote drainage of the lungs. Thus, there are appropriate positions for optimum drainage of the bronchi when only a few bronchopulmonary segments are involved.

Because oropharyngeal and nasopharyngeal contents containing bacteria may be aspirated into the lungs and cause **pneumonitis** (pneumonia) or a lung abscess in one or more bronchopulmonary segments, the position of very ill and unconscious patients is changed frequently to promote good drainage and aeration of their lungs. In the prone position (face downward), the trachea slopes downward; therefore, the natural supine position one assumes in bed with the head slightly elevated by a pillow is poor for lung drainage.

Tumors may result in blockage of a segmental bronchus, and the subsequent collapse of that part of the lung distal to it, owing to absorption of the air in the bronchopulmonary segment by the blood which is still circulating through it. This can be determined radiographically using a technique known as **bronchography** (Fig. 1-44). Various methods and contrast media are used to visualize the bronchi radiographically. Bronchography requires **topical anesthesia** (produced by direct application of local anesthetic solutions to the pharynx, larynx, and trachea). The contrast medium may be allowed to flow down over the back of the tongue (which has been drawn forward) into the larynx and trachea or a catheter may be introduced into the trachea after complete anesthetization of the throat, larynx, and trachea (Fig. 1-44). Small quantities of the medium are then introduced and the patient is postured in a suitable position to allow the contrast material to flow (by gravity) into the preselected secondary and segmental (tertiary) bronchi.

Only one side is injected at a time because the contrast medium partly obstructs the flow of air to the segmental bronchi which are being visualized. Impaired oxygenation of the blood may occur if both sides are filled with contrast medium at one time. A normal **bronchogram** of the right bronchial tree is shown in Figure 1-44.

The root of the right lung (Figs. 1-32 and 1-36) is enclosed by pleura and is composed of two pulmonary arteries, two pulmonary veins, a bronchus, a bronchial artery, bronchial veins, a pulmonary plexus of nerves, lymph vessels, and lymph nodes enclosed in a connective tissue matrix.

The root of the left lung is similar to the root of the right lung, except that there is only one pulmonary artery and there are usually two bronchial arteries (Figs. 1-37 and 1-84).

Usually the bronchus lies posterior, the artery superior, and the veins inferior. The **right upper bronchus** has a special location that is higher than any other bronchus (Fig. 1-46). It is even higher than the pulmonary artery and for this reason is sometimes called the "**eparterial bronchus.**"

Arteries of the Lung (Figs. 1-36, 1-37, 1-45, 1-46, and 1-86). *The branches of the pulmonary artery distribute venous blood to the lungs for aeration* (changing of venous into arterial blood in the lungs). These branches follow the bronchi and generally lie on their posterior surfaces. Thus, there is a branch to each lobe, bronchopulmonary segment, and lobule of the lung (Fig. 1-41). The terminal branches divide into capillaries which lie in the walls of the **alveoli**, the air sacs where gaseous exchange takes place between the blood and the air (Fig. 1-45).

The bronchial arteries supply the substance of the lung. They are small and pass along the posterior aspect of the bronchi to supply the bronchi as far distally as the **respiratory bronchioles** (ones where gaseous exchange occurs as at alveoli). The two left bronchial arteries arise from the thoracic aorta (Fig. 1-91). The single right bronchial artery arises from the first aortic intercostal artery or from the upper left bronchial artery.

CLINICALLY ORIENTED COMMENTS

Pulmonary thromboembolism (PTE) is a common cause of morbidity (sickness) and mortality (death). (See Case 1-10 for details). An **embolus** (G. a plug) is produced when a **thrombus** (blood clot), fat globules, or air bubbles are carried from a distant site (*e.g.*, from the leg veins following fractures or other injuries of the lower limbs). The thrombus passes through the right side of the heart and passes to a lung via the pulmonary artery. The immediate result of **PTE** is complete or partial obstruction of the pulmonary arterial blood flow to the lung (Case 1-10). **Embolic obstruction** produces a sector of lung which is ventilated but not perfused (*i.e.*, not functioning).

A large embolus may occlude the pulmonary trunk or one of its main branches. The patient suffers **acute respiratory distress** and may die in a few minutes. A medium-sized embolus may block an artery to a bronchopulmonary segment, producing an **infarct** (area of dead tissue). In healthy people a **collateral circulation** (*i.e.*, an indirect or accessory blood supply) often develops so that infarction does not occur owing to the abundant anastomoses (communications) with branches of the bronchial arteries in the region of the terminal bronchioles (Fig. 1-45). In sick people in whom circulation in the lung is impaired (*e.g.*, in a person with chronic congestion of the lungs), embolism commonly results in infarction of the lung.

Because an area of pleura is also deprived of blood, it becomes inflamed (**pleuritis**) and rough. The pleuritis results in **pain** in the side of the chest and the roughness results in a **friction rub** (Case 1-10).

Veins of the Lungs (Figs. 1-36, 1-37, and 1-45). *The pulmonary veins drain oxygenated blood from the lungs to the left atrium of the heart.* Beginning in the pulmonary capillaries, the veins unite into larger and larger vessels which run mainly in the interlobular septa. One main vein drains each bronchopulmonary segment, usually on the anterior surface of the corresponding bronchus. The two pulmonary veins on each side, a superior and an inferior one, open into the posterior aspect of the left atrium (Fig. 1-79). The **superior right pulmonary vein** drains the superior and middle lobes and the **superior left pulmonary vein** drains the superior lobe. The right and left **inferior pulmonary veins** drain the respective inferior lobes.

The bronchial veins drain the larger subdivisions of the bronchi. The right bronchial vein drains into the **azygos vein** (Figs. 1-48 and 1-93). The left bronchial vein drains into the accessory hemiazygos vein or into the left superior intercostal vein (Fig. 1-92).

Lymphatic Drainage of the Lungs (Figs. 1-45, 1-47, and 1-48). *There are two lymphatic plexuses.*

The superficial plexus lies deep to the visceral pleura and the vessels from it drain into the **bronchopulmonary lymph nodes**, located in the hilum of the lung and at the bifurcation of the trachea. They drain the lung tissue and the visceral pleura.

The deep plexus is located in the submucosa of the bronchi and in the peribronchial connective tissue. *No lymph vessels are located in the walls of the pulmonary alveoli.* Lymph vessels from the deep plexus follow the bronchi and the pulmonary vessels to the hilum of the lung where they drain into the **pulmonary nodes**, which are located close to the hilum, and into the **bronchopulmonary nodes** in the hilum. Lymph vessels then pass to **tracheobronchial lymph nodes** which lie around the trachea and the principal bronchi (Figs. 1-47 and 1-85). The lymph then passes to the right and left **bronchomediastinal lymph trunks**, which are formed by the junction of the efferent lymph vessels from the parasternal (Fig. 1-20), tracheobronchial, and anterior mediastinal lymph nodes. These trunks usually terminate on each side at the junction of the subclavian and internal jugular veins (Figs. 1-48 and 1-92). The left trunk may terminate in the **thoracic duct** (Fig. 1-48).

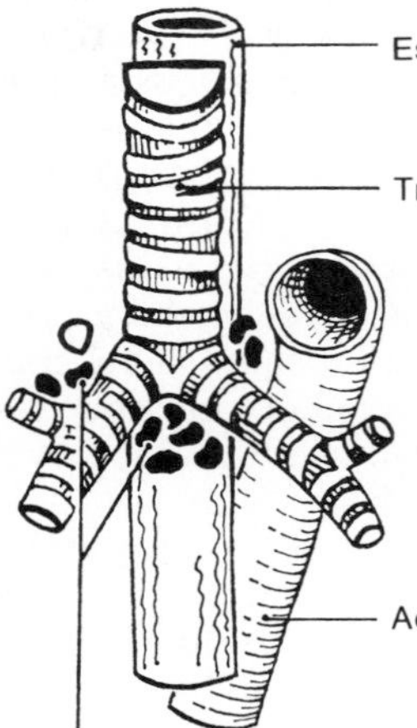

Figure 1-47. Drawing of the tracheobronchial lymph nodes. The deep lymph vessels of the lung follow the bronchial tree and pass through the hilum to these nodes. Efferent vessels from them pass to the bronchomediastinal trunk.

CLINICALLY ORIENTED COMMENTS

Lymph from the lungs carries phagocytes which contain ingested carbon particles that were deposited in the walls of the alveoli from the inspired air. In older people, especially cigarette smokers and/or city dwellers, the surface of the lung has a mottled gray to black appearance (Fig. 1-36) owing to the presence of these particles. The carbon is also carried to the lymph nodes in the hilum of the lung and in mediastinum, giving them a black appearance.

Bronchogenic carcinoma (cancer of a bronchus) is the most common cancer in men and is responsible for about 30% of malignancies. *The major causative factors are cigarette smoking and urban living* (Case 1-2). Because of the arrangement of the lymphatics, these tumors may extend (metastasize) to the pleura, the hila, the mediastinum, and then to distant organs. Involvement of the **phrenic nerve** (closely related, Fig. 1-53), the sole motor nerve to the diaphragm, results in *paralysis of half of the diaphragm.*

The tumor may invade the pleura and produce a **pleural effusion** (fluid in the pleural cavity). This exudate, which can be sampled by a **pleural tap**, may be **sanguineous** (bloody) and/or contain exfoliated malignant (cancer) cells.

Because of the close relationship of the **recurrent laryngeal nerve** to the apex of the lung (Fig. 1-72), this nerve may be involved in apical lung cancers resulting in hoarseness owing to paralysis of a vocal fold (Fig. 9-77).

Involvement of the hilar and mediastinal lymph nodes occurs by **lymphogenous dissemination** (spreading of cancer cells via the lymphatics). Lymph from the entire

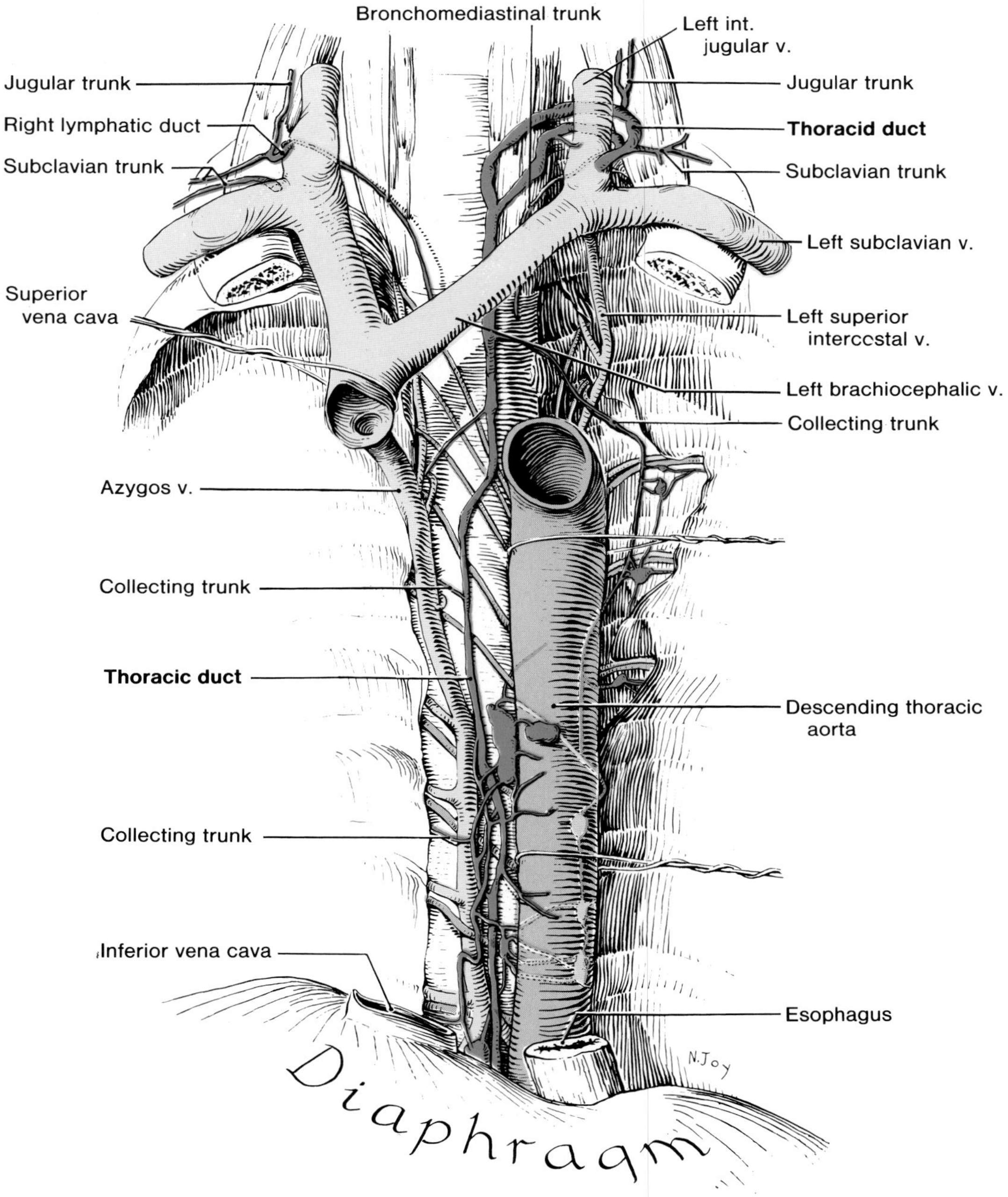

Figure 1-48. Drawing of a dissection of the thoracic duct. Observe that this vessel (1) ascends on the vertebral column between the azygos vein and the descending aorta, and (2) at the junction of the posterior and superior mediastina, it passes to the left and continues its ascent to the neck, where (3) it arches laterally to open near or at the angle of union of the internal jugular and subclavian veins. Observe that the duct here is plexiform in the posterior mediastinum and splits in the neck. It receives branches from the intercostal spaces of both sides via several collecting trunks and also from posterior mediastinal structures. Note that the duct finally receives the jugular, subclavian, and bronchomediastinal trunks. Observe that the right lymphatic duct is very short and is formed by the union of the right jugular, subclavian, and bronchomediastinal trunks. In addition, an accessory subclavian lymph trunk is opening directly into the subclavian vein in this specimen.

right lung drains into the **tracheobronchial nodes** on the right side (Fig. 1-47) and most lymph from the left lung drains into these nodes on the left side, but *some lymph from the inferior lobe on the left also drains into the nodes on the right side.* Thus, tumor cells in the right tracheobronchial lymph nodes can spread from the inferior left lobe by lymphogenous dissemination.

Lymph from the lungs drains into the venous system via the right and left **bronchomediastinal trunks** (Fig. 1-48). Hence, lymph from the lungs may carry cancer cells into the venous system and to the right atrium of the heart. After passing through the pulmonary circulation, the blood returns to the heart for distribution to the body. Common sites of **hematogenous metastasis** (spreading of cancer cells via the blood) from a bronchogenic carcinoma are the brain, bones, lungs, and adrenal glands.

Often the lymph nodes just superior to the clavicle (**supraclavicular lymph nodes**) are enlarged and hard when the patient has a carcinoma of the bronchus or the stomach owing to metastases from the primary tumor. For this reason, the supraclavicular lymph nodes are commonly referred to as **sentinel nodes** because enlargement of them alerts the examiner to the possibility of malignant disease in the thoracic and/or abdominal organs.

The brain is a common site for hematogenous spread of bronchogenic carcinoma. Tumor cells probably enter the systemic circulation by invading the wall of a sinusoid or venule in the lung (Fig. 1-45) and are transported to the brain via the pulmonary veins, the left heart, the aorta, and the cerebral arteries (Figs. 7-89 and 7-90). Once in the brain, the tumor cells probably pass between the endothelial cells lining the capillaries and enter the brain tissue.

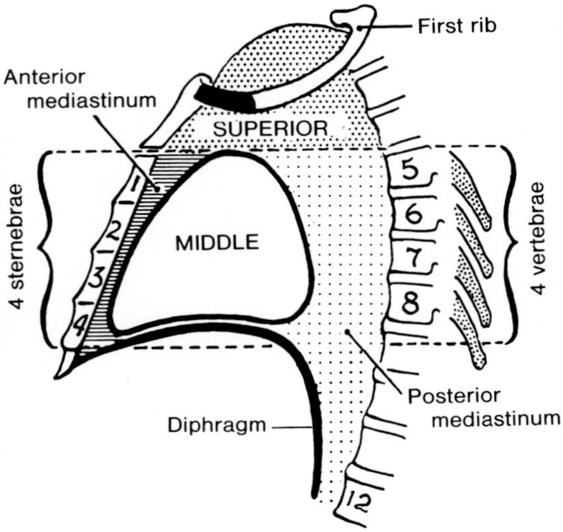

Figure 1-49. Diagram illustrating the four subdivisions of the mediastinum: middle, superior, posterior, and anterior. Observe that a horizontal plane at the level of the sternal angle passes through the intervertebral disc between thoracic vertebrae 4 and 5. Above this imaginary plane lies the superior mediastinum. This plan is especially convenient because it indicates the level of the superior border of the fibrous pericardium and the level of bifurcation of the trachea, *i.e.*, the upper border of the root of the lung. Note the anterior mediastinum, the small portion between the sternum and the pericardium, and the middle mediastinum, which contains the pericardium enclosing the heart and the roots of the great vessels. Examine the posterior mediastinum, the portion behind the pericardium and in front of the bodies of the lower eight thoracic vertebrae. Understand that certain structures traverse the length of the mediastinum (*e.g.*, esophagus, vagus and phrenic nerves, and thoracic duct) and so lie in more than one mediastinal subdivison.

THE MEDIASTINUM

The median region between the two pleural sacs is called the mediastinum (L. a middle septum). It extends from the superior aperture of the thorax to the diaphragm inferiorly (Figs. 1-15 and 1-49) and from the sternum and costal cartilages in front to the anterior surface of the 12 thoracic vertebrae behind. Understand that *the vertebral bodies are not in the mediastinum.*

The mediastinum, lying between the two layers of mediastinal pleura, contains the heart, the great vessels, the remains of the thymus, the distal part of the trachea, the proximal parts of the right and left bronchi, the esophagus, the vagus nerves, the phrenic nerves, and the thoracic duct (Figs. 1-15, 1-34, and 1-48). *These structures are surrounded by loose connective tissue, lymph nodes, and fat.* During life the looseness of the connective tissue and fat and the elasticity of the lungs and pleura enable the mediastinum to accomodate movement and volume changes in the thoracic cavity (*e.g.*, movements of the trachea and bronchi during respiration, pulsations of the great vessels, and volume changes of the esophagus during swallowing).

SUBDIVISIONS OF THE MEDIASTINUM

For purposes of description, the mediastinum is divided by the pericardium (membrane around heart) into *four subdivisions* or parts (Fig. 1-49): middle, superior, posterior, and anterior.

The middle mediastinum is very important because it contains the pericardium (with the adjacent phrenic nerves), the heart, and the roots of the great vessels passing to and from the heart.

The superior mediastinum lies above the other three subdivisions of the mediastinum and is superior to the horizontal line passing from the sternal angle to the lower border of the fourth thoracic vertebra. Thus, it is inferior to the superior thoracic aperture.

The posterior mediastinum is located *posterior to the fibrous pericardium* and the diaphragm and anterior to the bodies of the lower eight thoracic vertebrae.

The anterior mediastinum is the smallest part of the mediastinum and is located *anterior to the fibrous pericardium,* between it and the sternum. Although small in the adult, it is relatively large during the first few months of life because the lower part of the thymus (Figs. 1-80 and 1-81) extends into this region. *In early life the image of the thymus is as wide or wider than that of the heart on chest radiographs.*

Understand that certain structures which pass through the mediastinum (*e.g.*, the esophagus, vagus and phrenic nerves, and thoracic duct) lie in more than one subdivision of the mediastinum.

CLINICALLY ORIENTED COMMENTS

Much of the mediastinum can be visualized and certain minor surgical procedures can be carried out by using a tubular lighted instrument called a **mediastinoscope.**

Mediastinoscopy is commonly done to obtain tissue from the superior and anterior mediastinal and hilar lymph nodes (*e.g.*, to determine if cancer cells have metastasized to them from a bronchogenic carcinoma, Case 1-2). Usually a midline incision is made at the jugular notch and blunt dissection is performed to the area of the tracheal bifurcation and the tracheobronchial lymph nodes (Fig. 1-47).

Mediastinotomy is a less common surgical diagnostic procedure for exploring the mediastinum. A costal cartilage is removed, often the third (Fig. 1-20), the mediastinum explored with a finger, and biopsies taken.

The Middle Mediastinum (Figs. 1-49 to 1-53). The middle mediastinum contains the pericardium and the adjacent phrenic nerves, the heart, and the roots of the great vessels passing to and from the heart. To understand the pericardium, a brief general description of the heart will be given here. The heart is described in detail later.

The heart (Fig. 1-52) is a double, self-

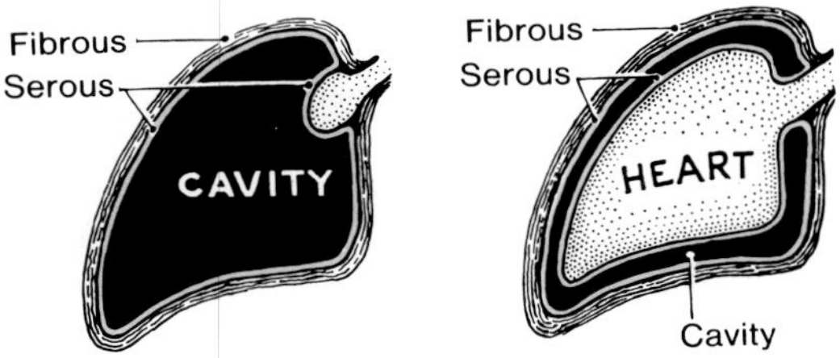

Figure 1-50. Drawings illustrating the scheme of the fibrous and serous pericardia. Observe that the pericardium (pericardial sac) is a double-walled sac enclosing the heart. Its outer surface is fibrous and appears dull. It gradually thins out on the surface of the eight vessels that pierce it (Fig. 1-52). The fibrous layer is lined with serous pericardium. At the roots of the great vessels, the serous pericardium is reflected on to the surface of the heart as the visceral layer (epicardium) of the serous pericardium.

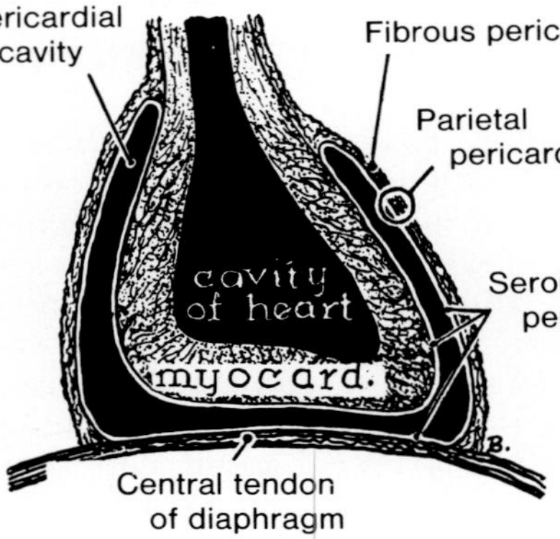

Figure 1-51. Semischematic drawing of the heart to illustrate the pericardium (pericardial sac). Understand that the parietal and visceral layers of the pericardium are separated from one another by only a minimal amount of serous fluid. This enables the heart to move and beat in a frictionless environment. Observe that the visceral pericardium is closely applied to the myocardium (cardiac muscle), where it also is known as the epicardium. Note that the fibrous pericardium adheres to the superior surface of the central tendon of the diaphragm.

adjusting, **muscular pump**, the two parts of which work in unison. At rest each ventricle discharges 5 to 6 liter/min, but it is capable of pumping 36 to 40 liter/min. Its right side receives the venous blood and pumps it to the lungs and its left side receives the oxygenated blood from the lungs and pumps it into the aorta for distribution to various parts of the body. Each side of the heart consists of an **atrium** (L. antechamber) or receiving area which pumps blood into a **ventricle** (L. little belly) or discharging chamber.

The walls of the heart consist of three layers (Fig. 1-51). The outermost layer is the visceral pericardium or **epicardium**. The middle layer is the **myocardium**, composed of **cardiac muscle** which is responsible for the heart's ability to pump. The innermost layer, called the **endocardium**, lines the myocardium.

The Pericardium (Figs. 1-34, 1-35, and 1-49 to 1-54). The pericardium (G. around the heart) or **pericardial sac** is a *double-walled fibroserous sac* that encloses the heart and the roots of the great vessels (aorta and pulmonary trunk). This conical sac is located in the middle mediastinum, *posterior to the body of the sternum and the second to sixth costal cartilages* and anterior to the fifth to eighth thoracic vertebrae (Fig. 1-49).

The pericardium consists of essentially two layers (Fig. 1-50): a strong outer layer composed of tough fibrous tissue called the **fibrous pericardium** and a *double-layered sac* composed of transparent membrane called the **serous pericardium**, which lines the fibrous pericardium and covers the heart.

The Fibrous Pericardium (Figs. 1-34 and 1-49 to 1-54). **The fibrous pericardium** is more or less conical; its truncated **apex** is pierced by the aorta, the pulmonary trunk, and the superior vena cava. The ascending aorta carries the pericardium upward beyond the heart to the level of the sternal angle.

The **base** of the fibrous pericardium rests on and is *fused with the central tendon of the diaphragm*, which separates it from the liver and the fundus of the stomach. Thus, the pericardium is influenced by movements of the diaphragm, in addition to the heart. The central tendon of the diaphragm and the pericardium are pierced by the inferior vena cava posteriorly, on the right side (Fig. 1-34).

The fibrous pericardium extends 1 to 1.5 cm to the right of the sternum and 5 to 7.5 cm to the left of the anterior median line at the level of the fifth intercostal space (Fig. 1-53). It is separated from the sternum and the costal cartilages of the second to sixth ribs by the lungs and the pleurae, except in the anterior median line where it is attached to the posterior surface of the sternum by the superior and inferior **sternopericardial ligaments** and where the bulge of the heart intervenes. Here the lung does not reach as far as the medial margin of the pleural sac (*i.e.*, into the costomediastinal recess, Fig. 1-34). The **cardiac notch** (Fig. 1-35) leaves part of the fibrous pericardium uncovered by lung tissue. This area on the left front of the chest is known as the area of **superficial cardiac dullness**. Being completely devoid of overlying lung, it yields a dull note upon **percussion** (tapping the surface with the finger), espe-

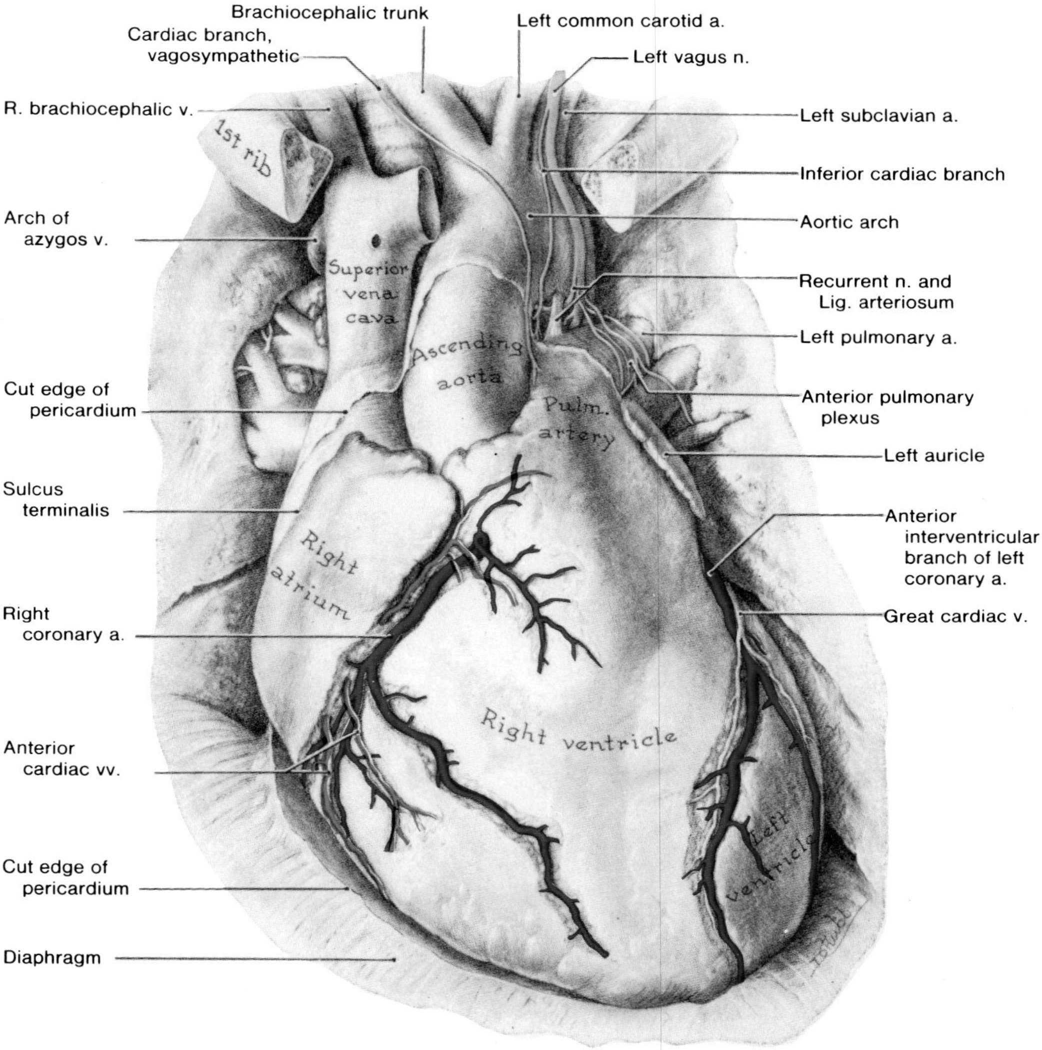

Figure 1-52. Drawing of a dissection of the sternocostal surface of the heart and great vessels, *in situ*. The fibrous pericardium, a cone-shaped sac, is opened. Observe that its apex is continuous with the external coats of the great vessels and that its base is attached to the central tendon of the diaphragm (also see Fig. 1-34). The pericardium or pericardial sac is pierced by eight vessels (two arteries, two caval veins, and four pulmonary veins).

cially in thin persons who are sitting upright.

Owing to its many connections, the pericardium is firmly anchored within the thoracic cavity. This keeps the heart in its normal position within the thoracic cavity (Fig. 1-53).

The Serous Pericardium (Figs. 1-50 and 1-51). **The serous pericardium** lines the fibrous pericardium and covers the heart and a portion of the great vessels. The **myocardium** (middle layer of the heart wall consisting of cardiac muscle) is covered by the *visceral layer of serous pericardium* (often called the **visceral pericardium** or **epicardium**, a word derived from Greek meaning "upon the heart"). This mesothelially covered fibroelastic membrane is

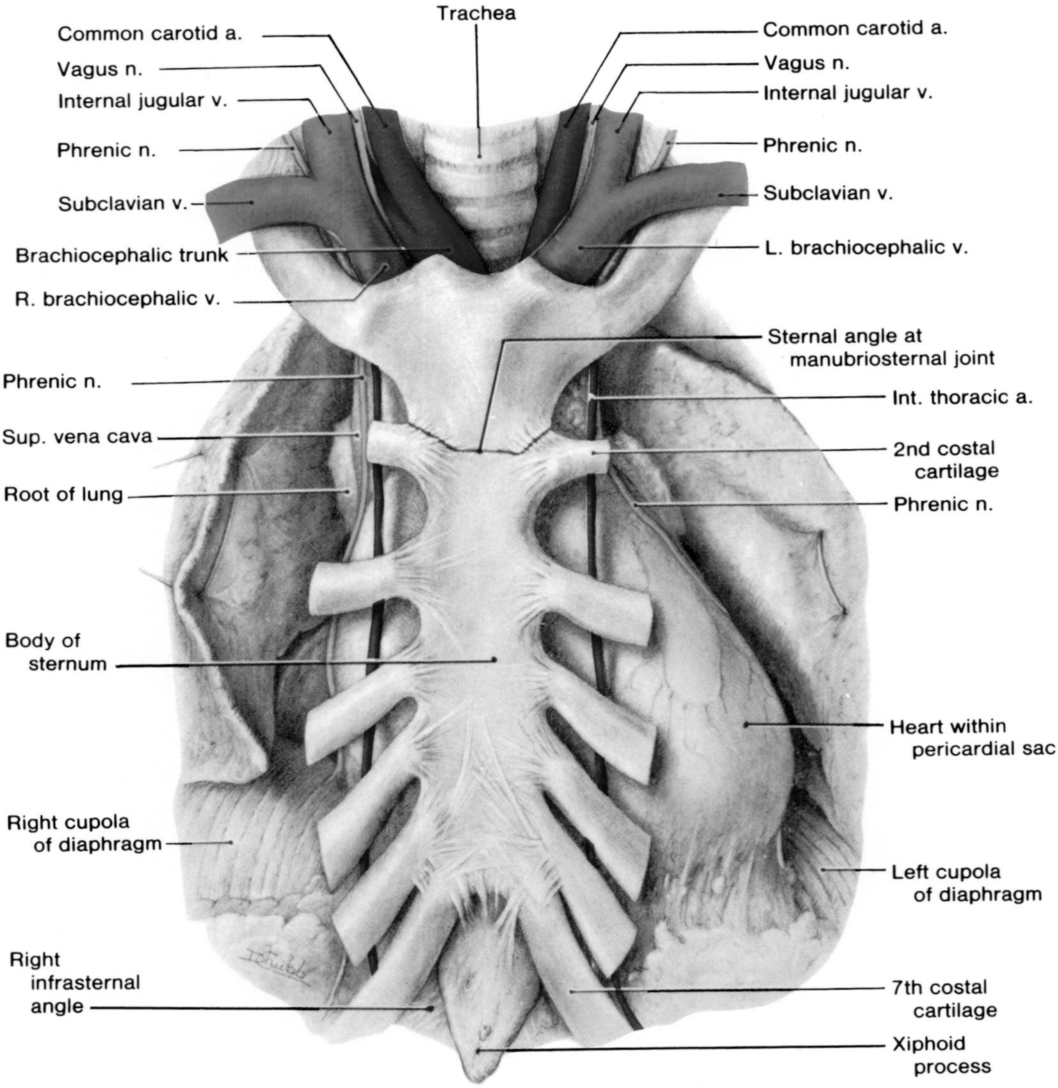

Figure 1-53. Drawing of a dissection that shows the relationship of the pericardial sac to the sternum. Observe that the pericardial sac lies behind the body of the sternum from just above the manubriosternal joint to the level of the xiphisternal joint. Note that about one-third of the heart lies to the right of the median plane and two-thirds to the left; thus, when the sternum is depressed, blood is forced out of the heart into the great vessels. Observe that the internal thoracic arteries lie a fingerbreadth from the borders of the sternum and that the right and left phrenic nerves are applied to the pericardial sac.

bound to and continuous with the fine connective tissue sheaths (**endomysium**) surrounding the myocardial fibers.

Outside the visceral pericardium (epicardium) is another fibroelastic membrane, the *parietal layer of serous pericardium* (often called the **parietal pericardium**). It has an inner lining of mesothelium. The visceral pericardium covers the heart and the great vessels and is reflected from these vessels to become continuous with the parietal pericardium which lines the fibrous pericardium, where the aorta and pulmonary trunk leave the heart and the superior and inferior venae cavae and the pulmonary veins enter the heart. The parietal pericardium is so closely adherent to the fibrous pericardium that they are difficult to separate.

The serous pericardium forms a closed sac (Fig. 1-51). There is a potential space, called the **pericardial cavity**, between the mesothelium lining the visceral and parietal layers of serous pericardium. In healthy

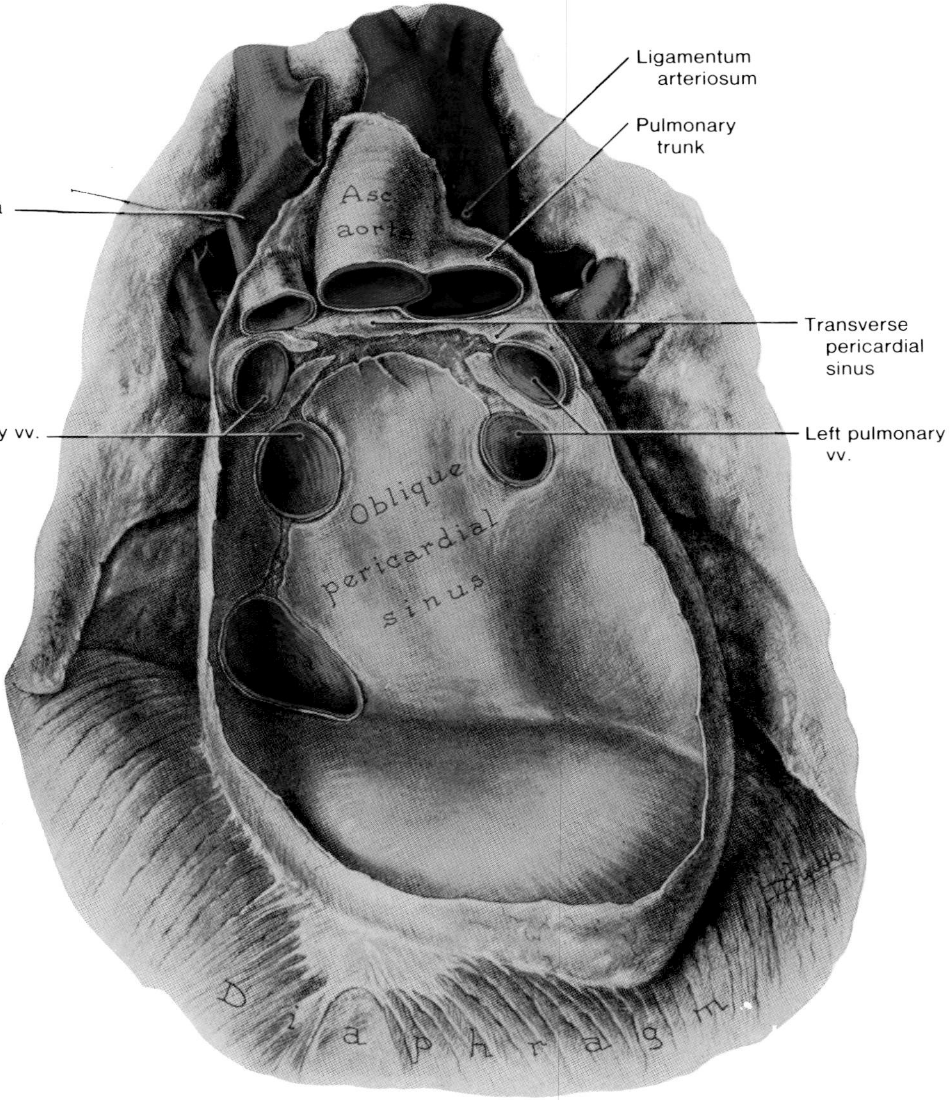

Figure 1-54. Drawing of a dissection of an anterior view of the pericardium or pericardial sac. When the heart was removed, the eight vessels piercing it were severed (two arteries, two caval veins, and four pulmonary veins). Observe that the oblique sinus is circumscribed by five veins and is open below and to the left. Note that the apex of the pericardial sac is near the junction of the ascending aorta and the aortic arch. Examine the superior vena cava, which is partly inside and partly outside the pericardium, and the ligamentum arteriosum, which is entirely outside. The ligamentum arteriosum is the remnant of a fetal vessel (ductus arteriosus). Observe the transverse and oblique pericardial sinuses. The heart removed from this pericardial sac is shown in Figure 1-79.

people this cavity contains up to 50 ml of fluid which is distributed as a capillary film between the opposed mesothelial surfaces. This fluid keeps their contiguous surfaces moist and glistening so that they glide over each other with a minimum of friction during movements of the heart.

The visceral and parietal layers of serous pericardium form as the serous pericardium is invaginated by the heart during early development. You can visualize how this occurred by pushing your fist into a balloon.

Sinuses of the Pericardium (Figs. 1-54, 1-67, and 1-79). The aorta and pulmonary trunk are enclosed by a common sheath composed of visceral pericardium. When the pericardial sac is opened anteriorly, as in Figure 1-54, you can insert your finger behind the aorta and pulmonary trunk in front of the left atrium and the superior vena cava. This passage (aperture), known as the **transverse sinus of the pericardium**, connects the two sides of the pericardial cavity. It is the remnant of an aperture in the dorsal mesocardium of the embryonic heart and lies between the arterial and venous ends of this organ.

As the pulmonary veins and the inferior vena cava penetrate the fibrous pericardium to enter the heart, they bulge into the pericardial cavity. Hence, they are partly covered by serous pericardium, which forms a somewhat inverted U-shaped reflection called the **oblique pericardial sinus** (Figs. 1-54 and 1-79). It is a wide, slit-like recess behind the heart, between the left atrium and the back of the pericardium. A finger inserted into it cannot pass around

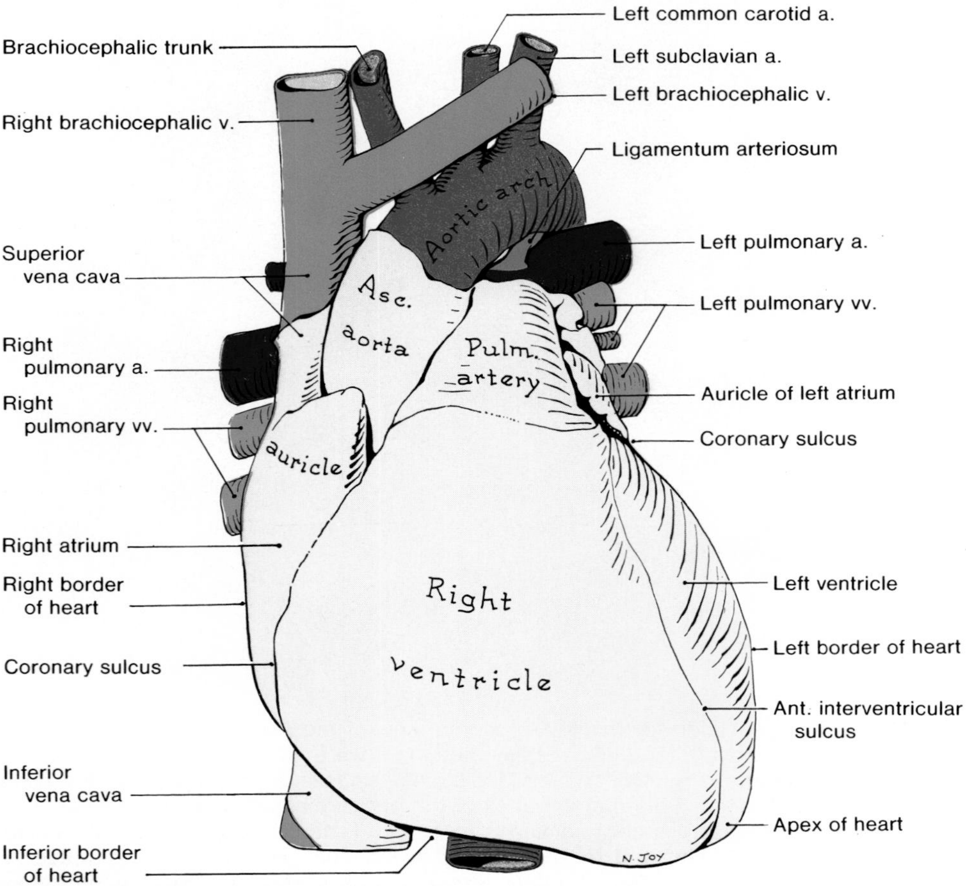

Figure 1-55. Drawing of a dissection of the sternocostal aspect of the heart and great vessels. The pericardium is colored yellow. Observe that the heart resembles a closed right fist in shape and size.

any of the vessels because the oblique sinus is a blind pouch (cul-de-sac) of the pericardial cavity.

Vessels and Nerves of the Pericardium (Figs. 1-19 to 1-21, 1-25, 1-48, 1-53, and 1-92). The arterial supply to the pericardium is derived from the **internal thoracic arteries** via their pericardiacophrenic and musculophrenic branches and from pericardial branches of the bronchial, esophageal, and superior phrenic arteries. *The epicardium is supplied by the coronary arteries* (Fig. 1-75).

The veins are tributaries of the azygos system (Figs. 1-48 and 1-92). There are also pericardiacophrenic veins that enter the internal thoracic veins. Its nerves are derived from the vagus and phrenic nerves and the sympathetic trunks.

CLINICALLY ORIENTED COMMENTS

Acute inflammation of the pericardial sac (**pericarditis**) has many causes. It may be associated with metabolic disorders (*e.g.*, uremia), rheumatic fever, and bacterial, viral, or tuberculous infection. Pericarditis causes **substernal pain**, frequently severe,

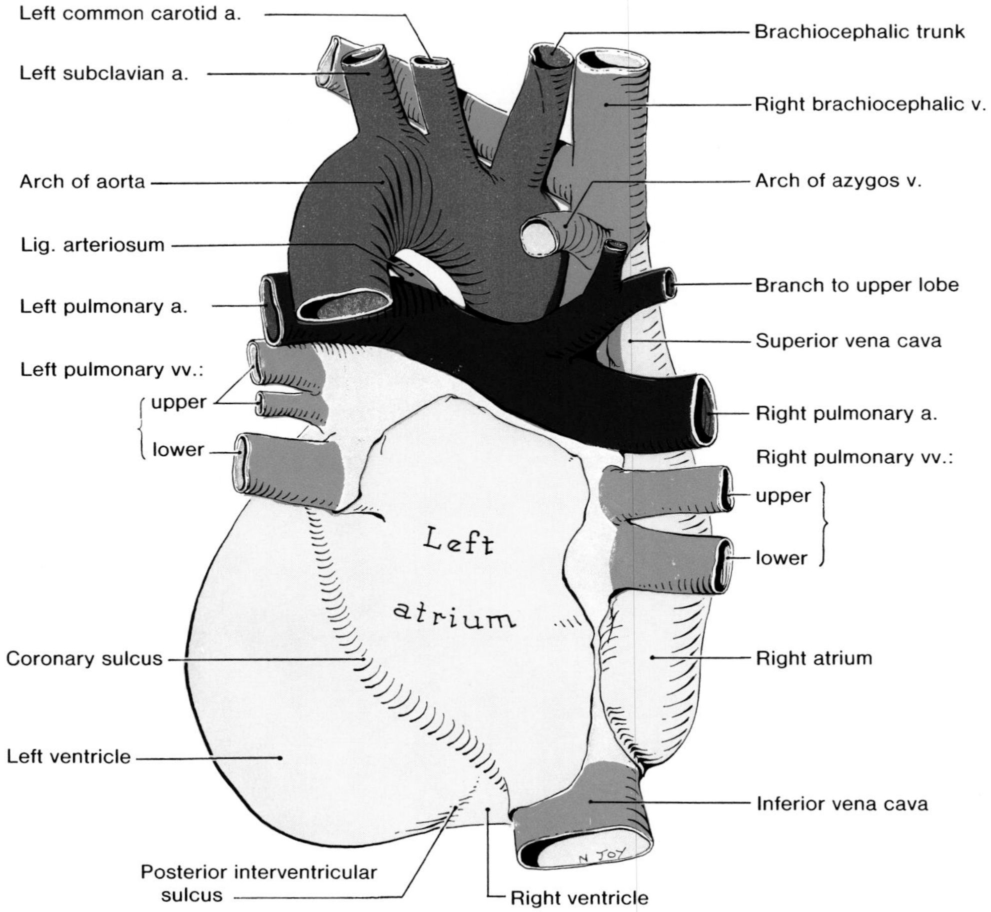

Figure 1-56. Drawing of a dissection of the posterior aspect of the heart and great vessels. The pericardium is colored yellow. Observe the right and left pulmonary veins converging to open into the left atrium. The part of the atrium between them lies to the left of the line of the inferior vena cava and forms the anterior wall of the pericardial cul-de-sac, called the oblique pericardial sinus, which admits two fingers (Fig. 1-54). Note that the aorta arches over the left pulmonary vessels and bronchus, and that the azygos vein arches over the right pulmonary vessels and bronchus.

and often **pericardial effusion** (passage of fluid from the pericardial capillaries into the pericardial cavity). If the effusion is extensive, it may embarrass the action of the heart by compressing the pulmonary veins (as they cross the pericardial sac) and also the atria. This condition, occurring because the fibrous pericardium is inelastic, is called **cardiac tamponade**.

A **pericardial friction rub** is an important physical sign of acute pericarditis. Normally the moist layers of the serous pericardium make no detectable sound during **auscultation** (listening to the sounds produced within the body using a stethoscope). However, inflammation of the pericardium causes the surfaces to become rough and the resulting friction sounds like the rustle of silk (later a leathery sound) through a stethoscope, especially during forced expiration with the patient leaning forward or on his/her hands and knees.

In a **penetrating wound** of the pericardium (*e.g.*, a knife or gunshot wound), the heart is commonly pierced and bleeding occurs into the pericardial cavity (Case 1-3). As the blood accumulates, the heart is compressed (**cardiac tamponade**) and circulation fails correspondingly. The veins of the face and neck become engorged owing to the compression of the superior vena cava as it enters the inelastic pericardium and also to compression of the atria.

Paracentesis of the pericardium (drainage of fluid from the pericardial cavity) is sometimes necessary to relieve the pressure of accumulated fluid on the heart. A wide-bore needle may be inserted through the fifth or sixth intercostal space near the sternum. Care is taken not to puncture the internal thoracic artery (Figs. 1-19 to 1-23). The pericardial sac may also be reached by entering the left infrasternal angle (Fig. 1-53) and passing the needle upward and backward.

The Heart (Figs. 1-38, 1-52, and 1-55 to 1-63). The heart is a *hollow muscular organ* that is somewhat conical in shape and is slightly larger than a clenched fist. It has **four chambers** (two atria and two ventricles), an **apex**, **three surfaces** (sternocostal or anterior, diaphragmatic or inferior, and base or posterior), and **four borders** (right, inferior, left, and superior). The heart lies obliquely in the middle mediastinum within the pericardium. The adjective cardiac is from the Greek *kardia*, meaning heart.

The Apex of the Heart (Figs. 1-52, 1-55, 1-58, and 1-59). The blunt apex is formed by the tip of the left ventricle, which points forward to the left and downward. It is the lowest part of the heart and *lies about four fingerbreadths from the median line in the*

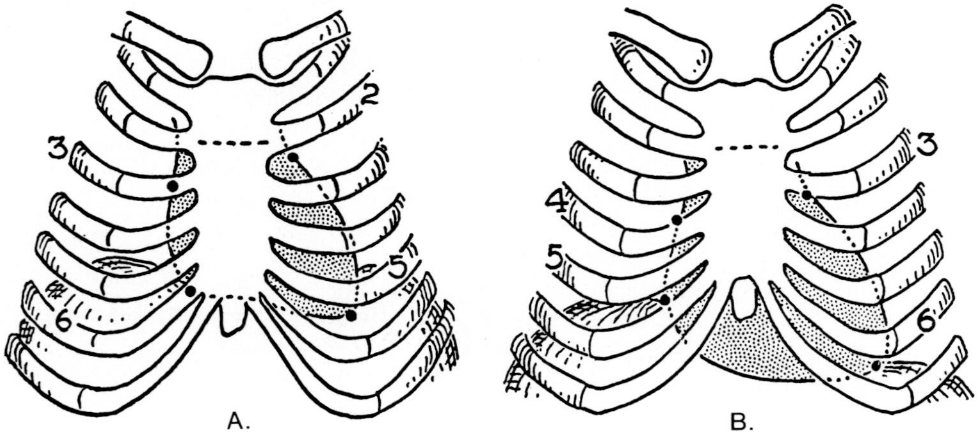

Figure 1-57. Drawings illustrating the surface anatomy of the heart. *A*, in the supine position. Note that the line indicating the inferior border of the heart (Fig. 1-55) passes superficial to the xiphisternal joint. *B*, in the erect position or on erect chest films. Observe that the inferior border of the heart is below the xiphisternal joint. In recumbent persons (*i.e.*, in supine position) the heart approaches the cadaveric position (*A*), but it still lies below the xiphisternal joint.

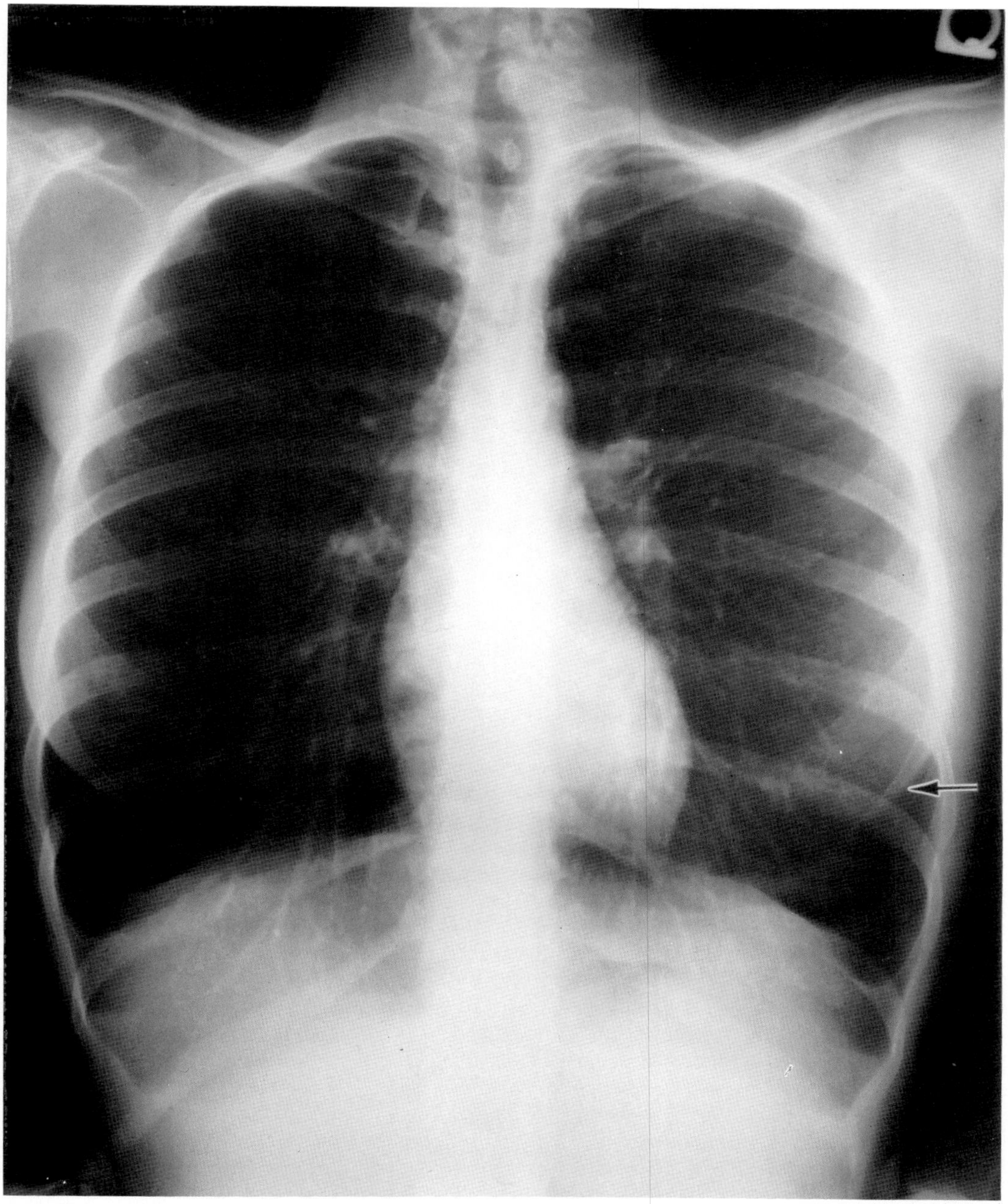

Figure 1-58. Radiograph of the chest *during inspiration*, posteroanterior (PA) view. This is the *common frontal projection* because in it the heart is close to the x-ray film and is magnified less than in an anteroposterior (AP) projection. It also permits the shoulders to be rolled forward, thereby moving the scapulae away from the lungs. The lungs are radiolucent because of the air they contain. In inspiration they contain more air than in expiration; therefore, they are more radiolucent in inspiration. Observe that the ribs are splayed out and widely separated. Note the low position of the diaphragm and the recesses of the pleural cavity that are not filled by the lung. During inspiration the heart appears more vertical because the diaphragm pulls the pericardial sac down; hence, the hila of the lungs are more readily visible. Note the difference between the relation of the left half of the diaphragm and the anterior end of the seventh rib (*arrow*). Compare this radiograph with Figure 1-59, which was taken during expiration.

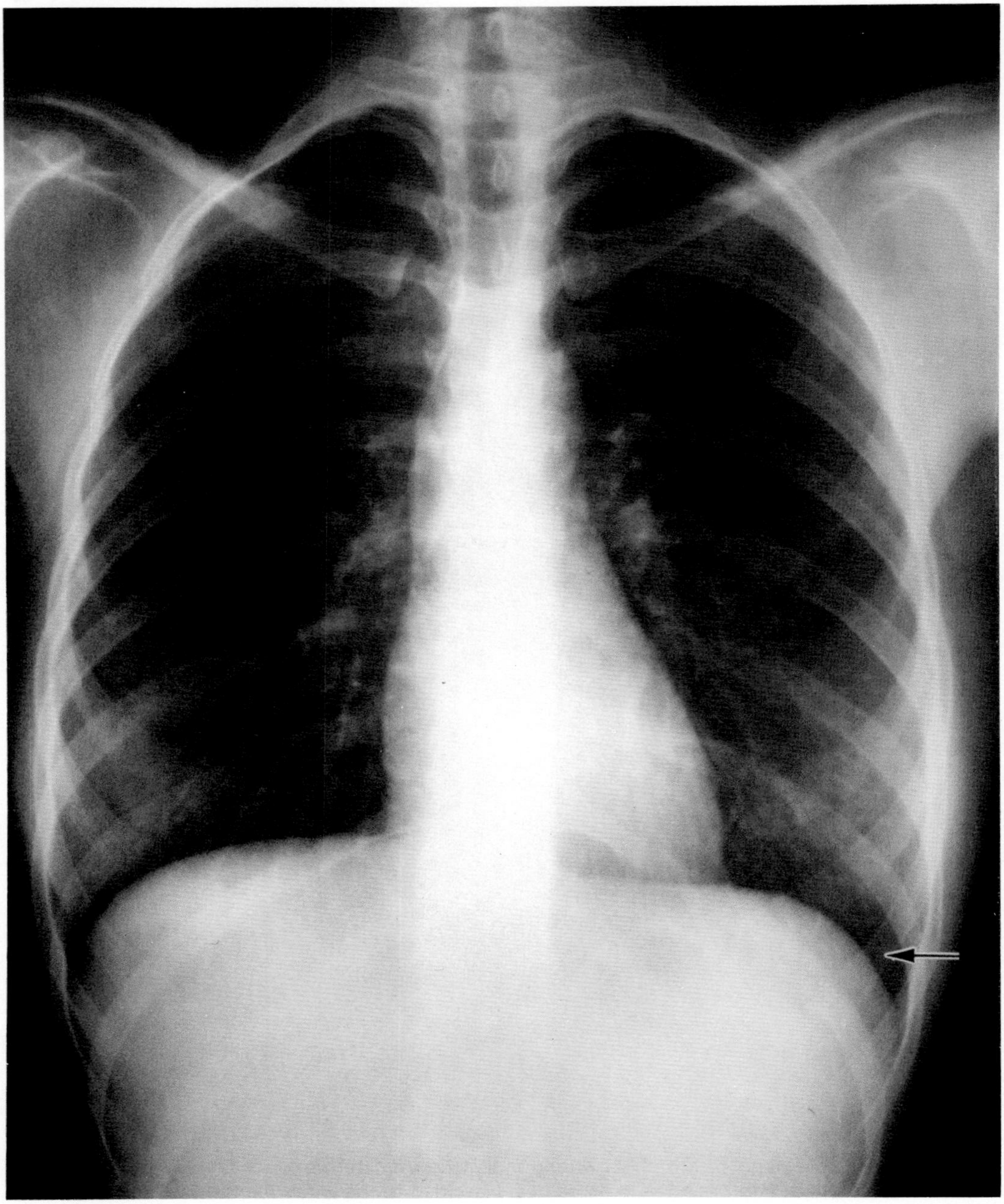

Figure 1-59. Radiograph of the chest *during expiration*, posteroanterior view, of the female shown in Figure 1-58. Observe the high position of the diaphragm and lungs, which are not so translucent because they contain less air. Note that the ribs are closer together. Understand that about one-quarter of the total lung is not visible in these films because it is obscured by the cardiovascular silhouette (shadow) and subdiaphragmatic structures. The *arrow* indicates the seventh rib. Compare this radiograph with Figure 1-58 taken during inspiration. Note that the diaphragm casts dome-shaped shadows on each side (slightly higher on the right). Examine the diaphragm in Figure 1-48.

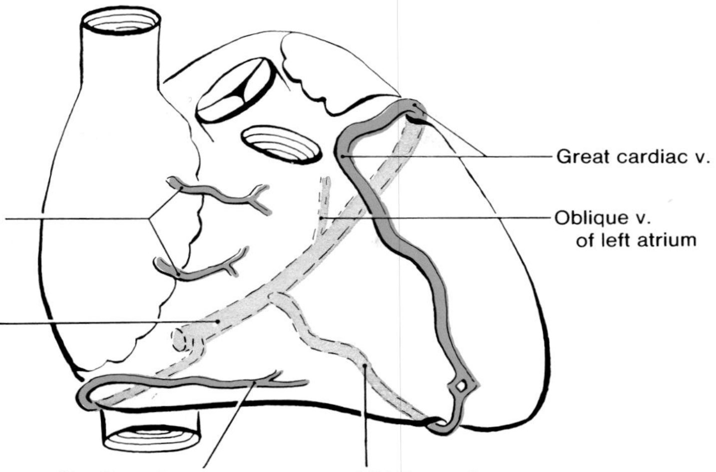

Figure 1-60. Diagram of an anterior view of the cardiac veins. Observe that the coronary sinus, the main vein of the heart, runs from left to right in the posterior part of the coronary sulcus (also see Fig. 1-79). The heart is drained mainly by veins that empty into the coronary sinus and partly by small veins that empty directly into the chambers of the heart. The coronary sinus enters the right atrium (Fig. 1-61).

fifth intercostal space, but its location varies with the person's position and with the phase of respiration (Figs. 1-57 to 1-59).

The Sternocostal (Anterior) Surface of the Heart (Figs. 1-52 and 1-55). This surface is formed mainly by the right ventricle and right atrium. The left ventricle and left atrium lie more posteriorly and form only a small strip on the sternocostal surface.

The Diaphragmatic (Inferior) Surface of the Heart (Figs. 1-56 and 1-79). This surface is usually slightly concave and is formed by both ventricles (mainly the left). It is separated from the liver and stomach by the diaphragm (Fig. 1-34). The posterior interventricular sulcus (groove) divides this surface into a right one-third and a left two-thirds. Frequently you will hear clinicians refer to the right or left diaphragmatic surface of the heart.

The Base (Posterior Surface or "Back") of the Heart (Figs. 1-56 and 1-79). The base of the heart is the posterior or vertebral surface of the heart. It is *formed by the atria*, mainly the left one, and lies opposite the middle four thoracic vertebrae when lying down (Fig. 1-49). The base is separated from the diaphragmatic surface of the heart by the posterior part of the **coronary sulcus**. Understand that *the heart does not rest on its base*; the term derives from the cone shape of the heart, the base being opposite the apex, which points anteriorly.

Borders of the Heart (Figs. 1-52 and 1-55). The heart has four borders: right, inferior, left, and superior. The **right border**, formed by the right atrium, is slightly convex and is almost in line with the superior and inferior venae cavae. The **inferior border** is formed by the right ventricle and slightly by the left ventricle. The **left border** is formed by the left ventricle and very slightly by the left auricle (atrial appendage). The **superior border**, where the great vessels enter and leave the heart, is formed by both atria.

Surface Anatomy of the Heart (Fig. 1-57). Most people know where to feel or hear the apex beat of the heart. It can be felt or heard in the *fifth left anterior intercostal space*, just medial to the midclavicular line (about four fingerbreadths from the median line). In males and immature females this is usually slightly below and medial to the nipple. The location of the nipple is not a reliable guide to the heart's apex in most mature females owing to the variation in the size and pedulousness of the breast. In many people the pulsations of the apex are visible. *In children the heart's apex is*

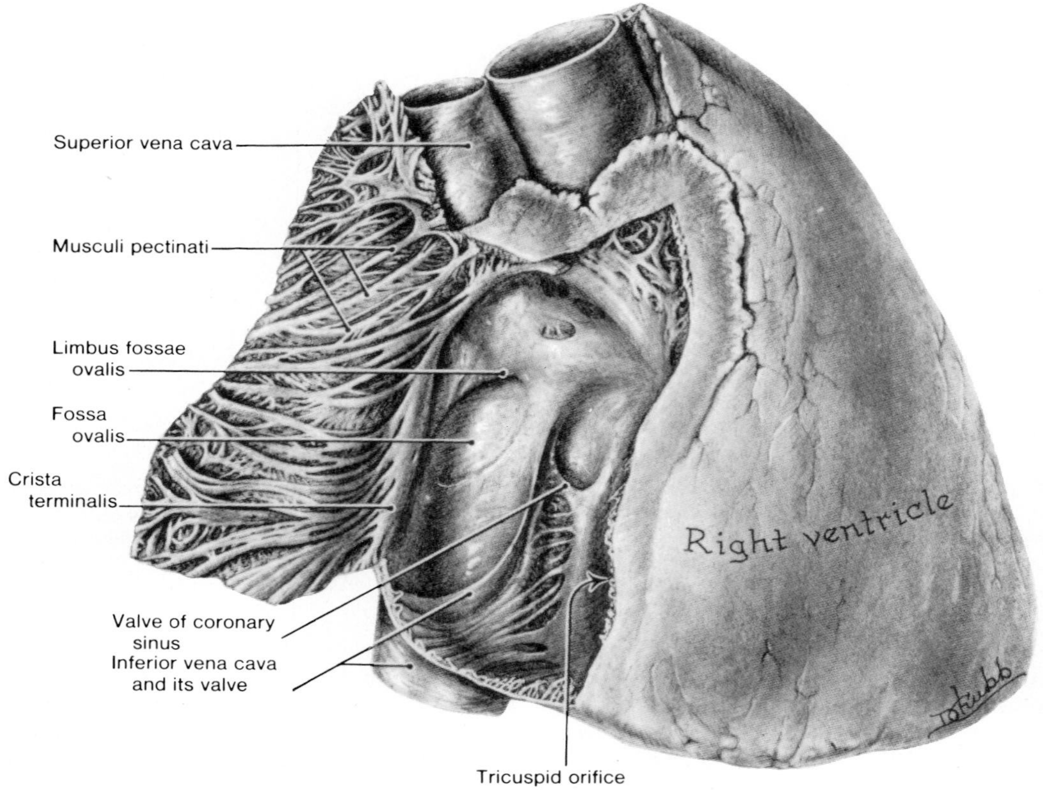

Figure 1-61. Drawing of a dissection of an anterolateral view of the interior of the right atrium. Observe that the smooth-walled part (derived from the absorbed right horn of the embryonic sinus venosus) is separated from the rough-walled part (derived from the primitive atrium) by the vertical ridge known as the crista terminalis. Understand that the crista underlies the sulcus terminalis (Fig. 1-52). Note that the two caval veins and the coronary sinus open into the smooth-walled part. Observe the fossa ovalis and the limbus fossae ovalis which are remnants of the prenatal foramen ovale and its valve. Note that the right atrioventricular (tricuspid) orifice is situated at the anterior aspect of the atrium.

slightly higher and further laterally than in adults. The apex of the heart almost corresponds to the site of the apex beat.

Obviously every doctor needs to know the **surface location of the heart** and the pericardial sac. Their position can be approximated on the chest using **three landmarks** and your fingers. Place a fingertip on each of them (**sternal angle**, right end of **xiphisternal junction**, and the **apex beat**). This gives you a rough indication of the surface location of your heart. However, every doctor must also know how to draw an outline of the heart on someone's chest when they are sitting up or lying in the supine position (on the back). Outline the heart as follows (Fig. 1-57*A*), using a skin pencil (grease pencil or eyebrow pencil).

The right border of the heart is indicated by a line slightly convex to the right, *from the third costal cartilage to the sixth costal cartilage*, a fingerbreadth from the right margin of the sternum.

The inferior border of the heart is represented by a line passing from the inferior end of the right border, *through the xiphisternal joint to the apex beat.*

The left border of the heart is indicated by a line, convex to the left, *from the apex beat to the second intercostal space*, about a fingerbreadth from the left margin of the sternum.

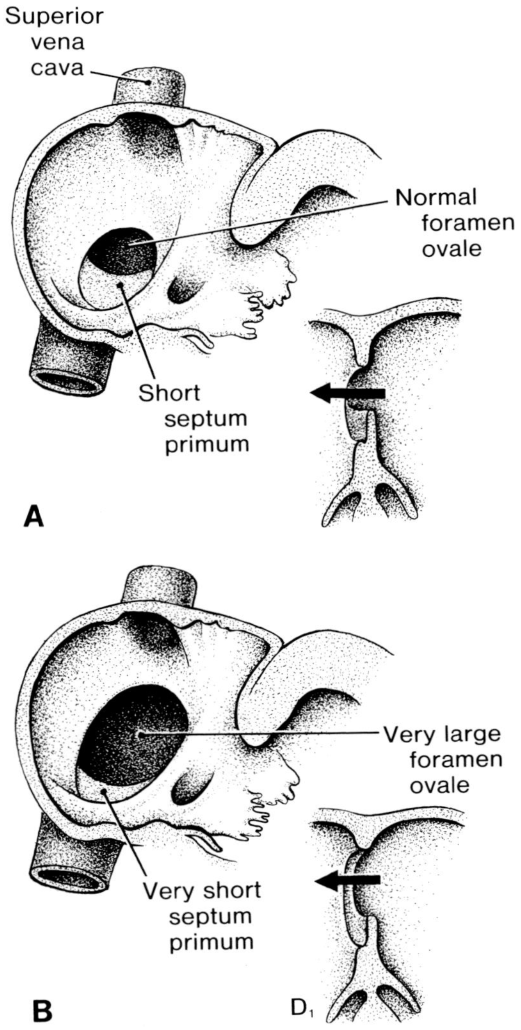

Figure 1-62. Drawings of the right atrial aspect of the interatrial septum, illustrating two common types of ASD. *A*, resulting from excessive absorption of the septum primum during formation of the valve of the foramen ovale. *B*, resulting from excessive absorption of the septum primum (as in *A*) and failure of growth of the septum secundum. The *arrows* indicate the left atrium to right atrium shunt of blood that occurs in these cases.

The superior border of the heart is represented by *a line joining the second left intercostal space to the third right costal cartilage.*

The superior border of the pericardial sac is represented by a line passing through the sternal angle from one side to the other (Figs. 1-53 and 1-57). The borders of this sac are the same as those described for the heart.

Understand that this method for the surface localization of the heart applies only to a person lying in the supine position or to a cadaver. In the erect position and on erect chest films, the heart is slightly lower (Figs. 1-57*B* to 1-59).

After you have outlined the heart on the chest, *visualize the following facts* using Figures 1-52 and 1-55 as a guide: (1) the right ventricle lies partly anterior to the left ventricle and to the right of it; (2) the apex is formed by the tip of the left ventricle; (3) the left border, chiefly by the left ventricle; (4) the superior border, by both atria; (5) the right border, by the right atrium; (6) the inferior border, mainly by the right ventricle; and (7) one-third of the heart is to the right and two-thirds to the left of the median plane.

CLINICALLY ORIENTED COMMENTS

Understand that the preceding surface markings are for the average adult heart and that the heart of any individual may vary slightly from this average and still be *normal for that person.* The surface anatomy of the heart is modified by age, sex, body size and build, respiration, position, and disease of the heart or lungs.

When you learn the clinical art of percussing the heart, you can determine the surface anatomy of a person's heart and compare it with the average learned in anatomy. Later in your course in medicine you will learn how to interpret significant departures from the average. **Percussion** is a commonly used *diagnostic procedure for determining the density* of a part (*e.g.*, the lung or the heart). Verify that the character of the sound changes as you tap different areas of the chest. Place the middle finger of your left hand approximately parallel and to the left of the left border of your heart. Now tap it with the middle finger of your other hand. While percussing, move your finger to the right and note how

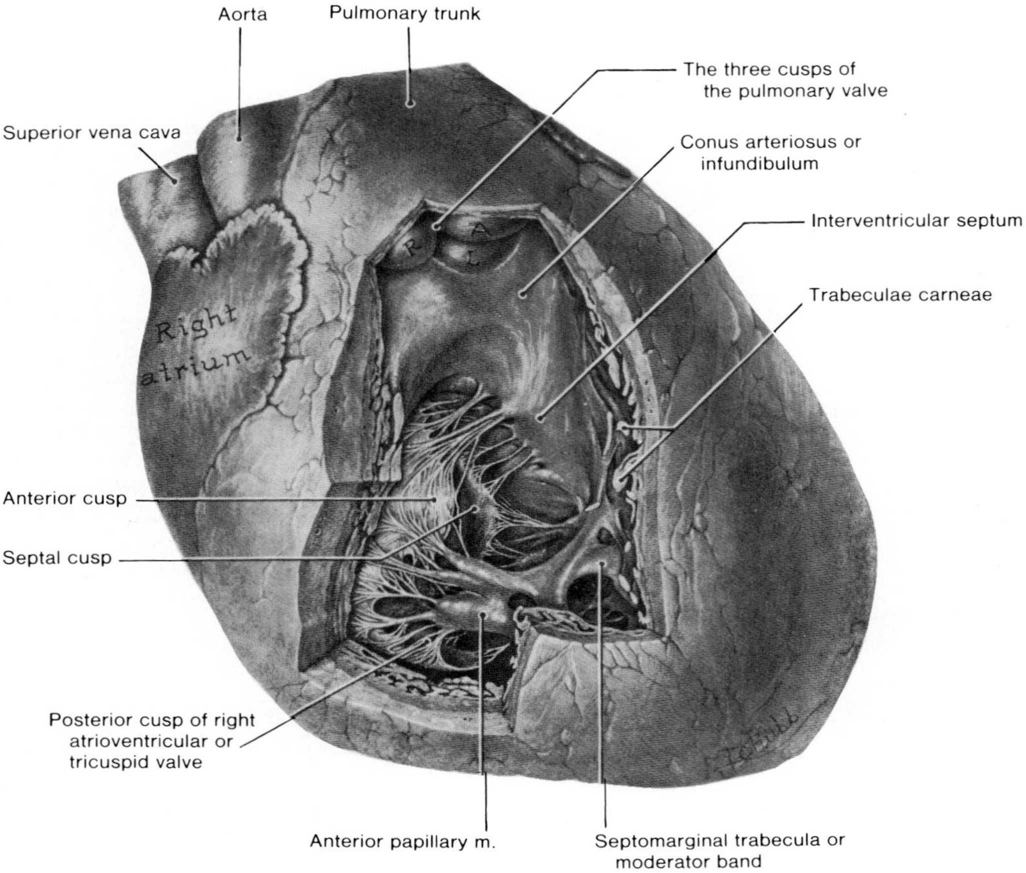

Figure 1-63. Drawing of a dissection of an anterior view of the heart showing the interior of the right ventricle. Observe the entrance to this chamber (right atrioventricular or tricuspid orifice) from the right atrium, situated behind, and the exit (orifice of the pulmonary trunk), situated above. Note the smooth funnel-shaped wall (conus arteriosus) below the pulmonary orifice and the remainder of the ventricle which has rough fleshy trabeculae carneae. Observe the three types of trabeculae: (1) mere ridges, (2) bridges attached only at each end, and (3) finger-like projections called papillary muscles. Note the anterior papillary muscle rising from the anterior wall; the posterior (not labeled) rising from the posterior wall; and a series of small septal papillae arising from the septal wall. Observe the septomarginal trabecula, here very thick, extending from the septum to the base of the anterior papillary muscle and forming a bridge. It contains the right branch (crus) of the atrioventricular bundle (AV bundle), part of the impulse-conducting system of the heart. Note the chordae tendineae (not labeled) passing from the tips of the papillary muscles to the free margins and ventricular surfaces of the three cusps of the tricuspid valve. Understand that each papillary muscle controls the adjacent sides of two cusps.

the sound changes as you move from over your lung to over your heart. By noting the areas of cardiac dullness, you can determine the rough outline of your heart. If it were grossly enlarged you could determine this, but a radiological examination (Fig. 1-58) would be required for a clearer determination of its size and shape.

Radiographic Anatomy of the Heart (Figs. 1-38, 1-58, and 1-59). The heart and great vessels and the blood within them are all of the same order of density. Hence, a frontal chest film shows the contour of the heart and great vessels in the middle mediastinum, called the **cardiovascular silhouette** (cardiac shadow). As the heart and great vessels are full of blood, the cardiovascular silhouette stands out in contrast to the clearer areas occupied by the air-filled lungs.

Because the fibrous pericardium is attached to the diaphragm, the cardiovascular silhouette becomes longer and narrower during inspiration (Fig. 1-58) and shorter and broader during expiration (Fig. 1-59). In an anterior view, the borders of the cardiovascular silhouette from above downward are formed as follows by the heart and great vessels. The *right border* is formed by the superior vena cava, right atrium, and inferior vena cava. The *left border* is formed by the arch of the aorta (producing a prominence known as the aortic knob), the pulmonary trunk, the left auricle (ear-like atrial appendage), and the left ventricle. These structures are less clearly demarcated on radiographs than in fresh hearts because the pleurae and pericardium smooth out the lines of demarcation between adjacent chambers and vessels.

The radiographic appearance of the heart varies in different people (*i.e.,* the "normal heart" may be quite variable in shape). **There are three main types of cardiovascular silhouette:** (1) the *oblique type* is present in most people (Figs. 1-38, 1-58, and 1-59); (2) the *transverse type* is observed in stocky and obese people, pregnant females, and infants; and (3) the *vertical type* is characteristic of thin people with long, narrow chests and low-lying diaphragms.

CLINICALLY ORIENTED COMMENTS

Students and physicians must know the main structures that form the cardiovascular silhouette so that gross abnormalities will be recognized. **Enlargement of the heart** may result from hypertrophy, especially in cases of high blood pressure, in which case the walls grow thicker by increasing the number and size of the cardiac muscle fibers. Enlargement of the heart can also result from dilation. For example, when blood regurgitates from the aorta into the left ventricle, this chamber dilates to accommodate the extra blood. Similarly, when blood regurgitates through a diseased mitral valve back into the left atrium from the left ventricle, the left atrium dilates to accommodate the additional blood.

As stated previously, a complication of pericarditis may be **hydropericardium**, in which the pericardial sac becomes distended with fluid, interfering with the return of blood to the heart. Severe **pericardial effusion** causes an enlargement of the cardiovascular silhouette and differentiation of it from heart enlargement may be difficult.

In the usual chest radiograph, the separate cavities of the heart are not distinguishable, but **angiocardiography** can be used to study the cavities of the heart and the great vessels. When a suitable contrast medium that is miscible with blood is injected via a catheter, the course of the blood can be followed fluoroscopically by either **cineradiography** or by serial x-ray films in various projections.

Most **congenital cardiac defects** can be diagnosed with the aid of cardiac catheterization. The technique of **right cardiac catheterization** consists of passing a radiopaque catheter under sterile conditions into a peripheral vein (*e.g.,* external iliac) and guiding it with the aid of **fluoroscopy** into the great veins, the right heart chambers, or the pulmonary artery. When a measured dose (**bolus**) of contrast material is injected into the right ventricle, it will traverse the pulmonary circulation and enter the left side of the heart. If **congenital cardiovascular abnormalities** are present, the contrast material may pass into an abnormal blood vessel or through a defect. For example, if an **ASD** (atrial septal defect) is present, some contrast material will pass through the defect in the interatrial septum into the left atrium (Fig. 1-62).

In **left cardiac catheterization,** the catheter is inserted into a peripheral artery (*e.g.,* brachial or femoral) and guided by fluoroscopy into the ascending aorta and the left ventricle. Frequently right and left cardiac catheterizations are performed simultaneously. As these methods are not without hazard, they are undertaken only when clearly indicated in the management of persons with heart disease.

During **cardiac fluoroscopy**, the patient is rotated from side to side to detect unusual pulsations, intracardiac calcifications, or abnormal prominences of cardiac chambers or great vessels. Swallowing barium to outline the esophagus allows detection of certain abnormalities of the aortic arch (*e.g.*, retroesophageal subclavian artery and small degrees of enlargement of the left atrium) because the esophagus is normally in contact with the aortic arch and the left atrium.

Chambers of the Heart (Figs. 1-52, 1-55, and 1-56). There are *four chambers* of the heart, two atria and two ventricles. All four of them are visible on the anterior or sternocostal surface. The **coronary sulcus** (atrioventricular groove) encircles most of the upper part of the heart, separating both atria from both ventricles. Similarly, the division of the ventricles is indicated by the anterior and posterior interventricular sulci.

The Right Atrium (Figs. 1-38, 1-52, 1-55, 1-56, 1-61, and 1-63). This chamber *forms the right border of the heart* between the **superior** and **inferior venae cavae.** The right atrium receives venous blood from these vessels and from the coronary sinus. The **coronary sinus** receives blood from the veins that drain the heart (Fig. 1-60).

The right atrium consists of (1) a smooth-walled posterior part, called the **sinus venarum** (sinus of the venae cavae), which receives the venae cavae and the coronary sinus, and (2) a rough-walled anterior part which has internal muscular ridges (**musculi pectinati**) resembling the coarse teeth of a comb. A small conical muscular pouch, called the **auricle** (atrial appendage), projects to the left from the root of the superior vena cava and overlaps the right side of the root of the ascending aorta.

The basis of the two distinctive parts of the right atrium is embryological. The smooth-walled part develops from the absorbed right horn of the embryonic **sinus venosus,** whereas the rough-walled part (including the auricle) develops from the primitive atrium. The two parts are separated externally by a groove called the **sulcus terminalis** (Fig. 1-52) and internally by a vertical ridge called the **crista terminalis** (Fig. 1-61). The crista terminalis and the valves of the inferior vena cava and coronary sinus represent the remains of the valve of the sinus venosus, the right horn of which was absorbed in the right atrium.

The interatrial septum forms the posteromedial wall of the right atrium. A prominent feature of this wall is the **fossa ovalis** (Fig. 1-61), a shallow translucent depression in the septum facing the opening of the inferior vena cava. This thumbprint-sized, oval fossa is a *remnant of the fetal foramen ovale,* through which oxygenated blood from the placenta passed from the inferior vena cava through the right atrium into the left atrium. The floor of the fossa ovalis is formed by tissue derived from the *valve of the foramen ovale,* a derivative of the septum primum.

The opening of the coronary sinus is located between the atrioventricular orifice and the valve of the inferior vena cava. This opening is partly guarded by a thin semicircular valve called the **valve of the coronary sinus**. It probably has no function after birth.

The superior vena cava *returns blood from the upper half of the body* and opens into the superior and posterior part of the atrium, at about the level of the right third costal cartilage (Figs. 1-35 and 1-53). Its valveless orifice is directed downward and forward.

The inferior vena cava opens into the lowest part of the right atrium, almost in line with the smaller superior vena cava. It *returns blood from the lower half of the body.* The valve of the inferior vena cava is a thin fold of variable size that has no function postnatally. Before birth it directed blood from the inferior vena cava toward the foramen ovale.

CLINICALLY ORIENTED COMMENTS

Atrial septal defect (ASD) is a common type of congenital heart defect. The most common form of ASD is persistent or **patent foramen ovale** (Fig. 1-62). Defects in the area of the fossa ovalis are classified as the secundum type of ASD. In clinically significant defects there is a large opening between the right and left atria which usually results from excessive absorption of the septum primum and/or an abnormally large foramen ovale resulting from growth failure of the septum secundum.

Usually the septum primum and the septum secundum fuse after birth so that no opening remains between the right and left atria. In up to 25% of adult hearts a probe can be passed obliquely from one atrium to the other through the upper part of the floor of the fossa ovalis. Although this defect is not considered a pathological occurrence, a **probe patent foramen ovale** may be forced open as a result of other cardiac defects and contribute to functional pathology of the heart. Probe patent foramen ovale results from incomplete adhesion (*i.e.*, imperfect sealing) between the septum primum and the septum secundum.

The Right Ventricle (Figs. 1-52, 1-55, 1-61, and 1-63). This chamber forms the largest part of the sternocostal surface of the heart, a small part of the diaphragmatic surface, and almost all of the inferior border of the heart. Its wall is much thicker than that of the right atrium.

The upper anterior end of the right ventricle tapers into a cone-shaped structure, called the **conus arteriosus,** which gives origin to the pulmonary trunk. Internally this arterial cone has a funnel-shaped appearance; hence, it is also called the **infundibulum** (L. a funnel). The conus arteriosus (infundibulum) is the uppermost part of the right ventricle, lying in front of the root of the aorta and immediately below the root of the pulmonary trunk. Its inner wall is smooth, whereas the rest of the ventricular wall is roughened by a number of irregular muscle bundles (**papillary muscles**) and ridges and bridges (**trabeculae carneae**). The fleshy trabeculae (L. *trabs,* wooden beam + *carneus,* fleshy) project from the ventricular wall, giving it a coarse sponge-like appearance. One of the trabeculae carneae crosses the cavity of the ventricle from the interventricular septum to the base of the anterior papillary muscle. This **septomarginal trabecula,** or moderator band (Figs. 1-63 and 1-64), carries the right branch (crus) of the **atrioventricular bundle** (Fig. 1-71), part of the conducting system of the heart (discussed subsequently).

The papillary muscles are conical projections which have a number of slender fibrous threads (**chordae tendineae**) arising from their apices (Figs. 1-64 and 1-65). The chordae are inserted into the free edges and ventricular surfaces of the cusps (flaps) of the **right atrioventricular valve (tricuspid valve**). As the chordae are attached to adjacent sides of two cusps, they prevent their inversion when the papillary muscles and the ventricle contract. Thus, *the chordae tendineae prevent the cusps of the tricuspid valve from being driven into the right atrium* as the ventricular pressure rises.

There are usually **three papillary muscles** in the right ventricle. The **anterior**

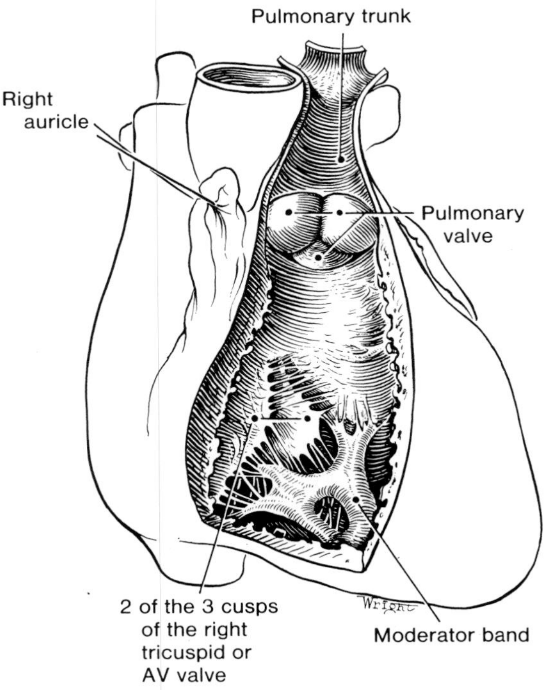

Figure 1-64. Drawing of the interior of the right ventricle and the pulmonary trunk. Observe the tricuspid and pulmonary valves.

papillary muscle, the largest and most prominent of the three, is attached to the anterior wall and its chordae tendineae are attached to the anterior and posterior cusps. The **posterior papillary muscle** is smaller than the anterior papillary muscle and may consist of several parts. It is attached to the inferior wall and its chordae tendineae are attached to the posterior and septal cusps. The **septal papillary muscles,** small and multiple, are attached to the interventricular septum and their chordae tendineae are attached to the anterior and septal cusps.

The papillary muscles contract prior to contraction of the ventricle, tightening the chordae tendineae and drawing the cusps together by the time ventricular contraction begins, thereby preventing ventricular blood from passing back into the right atrium.

The right ventricle is crescentic in cross-section (Fig. 1-66) because the thick muscle of the interventricular septum bulges to the right since the pressure is higher on the arterial side than on the venous side of the heart.

The inflow part of the right ventricle receives blood from the right atrium through the right atrioventricular or tricuspid orifice. It is surrounded by a **fibrous ring** which gives attachment to the cusps of the tricuspid valve. This ring is part of the **fibrous skeleton of the heart** which surrounds both atrioventricular orifices and the pulmonary and aortic orifices (see subsequent description).

The oval right atrioventricular orifice is large enough to admit the tips of three average-sized fingers and is located posterior to the body of the sternum, at the level of the fourth and fifth intercostal spaces.

The right atrioventricular orifice is guarded by **three cusps,** hence the name **tricuspid valve** (Figs. 1-63 to 1-65). The cusps are more or less triangular in outline and are continuous with one another at their bases, which are attached to the **fibrous ring** that surrounds the atrioventricular orifice. Toward the edges they are disposed as **anterior, septal,** and **posterior cusps.** Small secondary cusps may be present which obscure this general arrangement. The valve cusps project into the right ventricle and their edges, to which the chordae tendineae are attached, have a serrated appearance.

When the right atrium contracts, the blood in it is forced through the right atrioventricular orifice into the right ventricle,

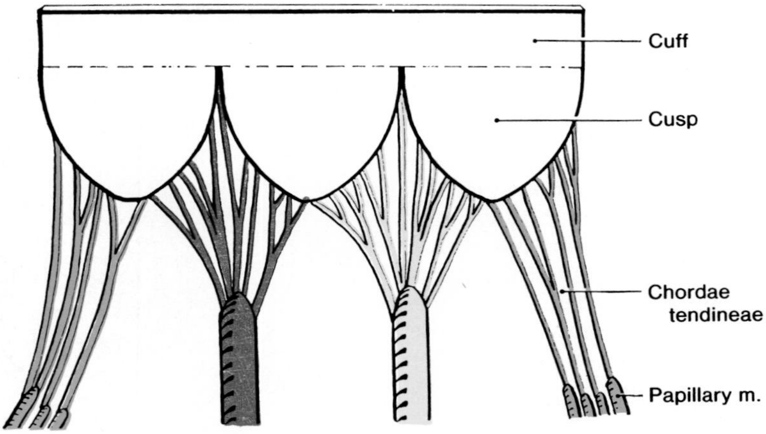

Figure 1-65. Diagram of the right atrioventricular valve spread out. Observe that this valve is composed of three cusps; hence, the name tricuspid valve. Note that the cusps are continuous with one another at their bases. Observe the chordae tendineae or tendinous strands which pass from the margins and ventricular surfaces of the cusps into the apices of papillary muscles. Note that the strands are arranged like the cords of a parachute.

pushing the cusps aside like curtains. When the ventricle contracts, the papillary muscles contract pulling on the chordae tendineae, which prevents the cusps of the tricuspid valve from passing into the right atrium.

The valve of the pulmonary trunk (**pulmonary valve**) guards the pulmonary orifice, which is above the aortic orifice and farther forward (Figs. 1-63 and 1-64). It lies at the apex of the conus arteriosus or infundibulum and is about 2.5 cm in diameter. It is located at about the level of the third costal cartilage at the left side of the sternum. Understand that blood from the right atrium passes through the right atrioventricular orifice and must follow a U-shaped course to pass through the pulmonary orifice.

The pulmonary valve consists of three semilunar valve cusps (*anterior, right,* and *left*), each of which is concave when viewed from above (Fig. 1-67). The cusps are easily pushed aside like curtains and project into the artery, where they lie close to its walls as blood leaves the right ventricle. Following contraction, when the ventricle relaxes, the elastic wall of the artery forces the blood back toward the heart. However, the cusps open up like pockets, ballooning out to completely close the pulmonary orifice, which prevents blood from returning to the ventricle.

Opposite each valve, the wall of the pulmonary trunk is slightly dilated to form a sinus. The blood in these sinuses prevents the cusps from sticking to the wall of the pulmonary artery and failing to shut.

CLINICALLY ORIENTED COMMENTS

In **pulmonary valve stenosis,** the pulmonary valve cusps are fused together to form a dome with a narrow central opening. In **infundibular pulmonary stenosis,** the infundibulum of the right ventricle is underdeveloped. The two types of pulmonary stenosis may occur together or as separate entities. Depending upon the degree of obstruction to blood flow, there is a variable degree of hypertrophy of the right ventricle.

The free margins of the pulmonary valve cusps are thin. If these become thickened and inflexible or damaged owing to disease, the valve will not close completely. As a result, blood can flow back into the right ventricle. This **valvular incompetence** results in a **pulmonic regurgitation** or backrush of blood into the right ventricle under high pressure, which may be heard through a stethoscope as a **heart murmur** (cardiac murmur). The murmur results from vibrations set up in the blood in the pulmonary artery, as a result of turbulent blood flow and formation of eddies (small whirlpools).

The Left Atrium (Figs. 1-38, 1-52, 1-55, 1-56, 1-67, and 1-79). This chamber forms most of the posterior aspect or base of the heart. Its long, tubular **auricle** (atrial appendage) forms the uppermost part of the left border of the heart, which is sometimes visible in radiographs of the heart (Fig. 1-38). The auricle overlaps the root of the pulmonary trunk (Fig. 1-67). **Four pulmonary veins** (two superior and two inferior) enter the sides of the posterior half of the left atrium.

The wall of the left atrium is slightly thicker than that of the right atrium and its interior is smooth, except for a few **musculi pectinati** in the auricle. The smooth-walled part of the atrium formed from the absorption of the primitive pulmonary vein during the embryonic period, whereas the rough-walled part (mainly in the auricle) represents part of the remains of the primitive atrium.

The interatrial septum slopes posteriorly and to the right; hence, much of the left atrium lies posterior to the right atrium.

The left atrioventricular orifice (**mitral orifice**) allows oxygenated blood from the left atrium to pass into the left ventricle. It is smaller than the right atrioventricular orifice and is usually only large enough to admit the tips of two medium-sized fingers. This orifice opens through the lower half of the anterior wall and is located in the lower and anterior part of the left atrium.

CLINICALLY ORIENTED COMMENTS

Thrombi (blood clots) may develop on the walls of the left atrium and in the left auricle in certain types of heart disease. If these clots break off they are free in the systemic circulation and occlude peripheral arteries, large or small depending on the size of the free clot. A thrombus that obstructs or plugs a vessel is called an **embolus.**

Occlusion of a small vessel in the brain usually does little damage owing to the numerous anastomoses (communications) of arteries in the brain, but if a main artery is occluded, an extensive area of the brain is likely to be involved. This results in **embolic stroke** or **cerebrovascular accident (CVA)**, which produces paralysis of the parts of the body previously controlled by the damaged area of the brain.

The mitral valve is the most frequently diseased of the heart valves; **rheumatic fever** used to be a common cause of this type of **valvular heart disease.** Nodules form on the valve cusps which roughens them, resulting in irregular blood flow and a heart murmur that is audible with a stethoscope. Later the diseased cusps undergo scarring and shortening, resulting in a condition called **valvular incompetence.** In these cases the blood in the left ventricle regurgitates into the left atrium, producing a murmur when the ventricles contract.

Further scarring of the cusps results in progressive narrowing of the orifice (**valvular stenosis**). In these cases the blood builds up in the left atrium and the lungs, producing **pulmonary congestion** and a strain on the right side of the heart. In addition, when the atria contract, a murmur is produced as the blood is forced through the narrow valvular orifice just before ventricular contraction.

The Left Ventricle (Figs. 1-38, 1-52, 1-55, 1-56, 1-66, and 1-69). This chamber *forms the apex of the heart,* nearly all of its left border and surface, and the diaphragmatic surface. It forms only a small part of the sternocostal surface. *The large aorta arises from its uppermost part,* anteriorly.

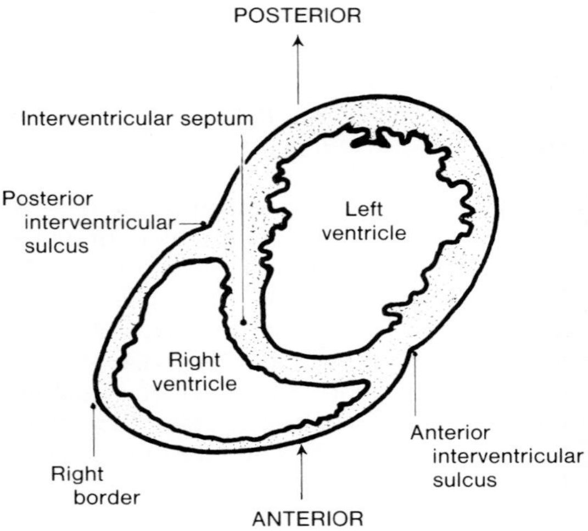

Figure 1-66. Drawing of a horizontal section through the right and left ventricles. The *arrows* indicate the sagittal plane. Observe that the right ventricle is crescentic in cross-section and that the interventricular septum is convex toward this chamber because the pressure is higher on the arterial than on the venous side. Observe that the left ventricular cavity is roughly circular on cross-section. In the normal (not necessarily in the diseased) heart, the left ventricular wall is about three times as thick as the right one.

The cavity of the left ventricle is cone-shaped in outline and is longer than that of the right. It is circular on cross-section. Its muscular wall is 1 to 1.5 cm thick but is much thinner at the apex. In healthy hearts *the wall of the left ventricle is about three times as thick as the wall of the right ventricle.*

The aortic vestibule is the part of the left ventricular cavity just below the aortic valve. The smooth walls of this region are mainly fibrous. The interior of most of the ventricle is covered with a dense mesh of **trabeculae carneae,** which are finer and more numerous than in the right ventricle. The trabeculae carneae are particularly marked in its lower half, except at the very apex where the wall is only about 3 mm thick.

There are *two large papillary muscles,* anterior and posterior. They are larger than in the right ventricle and their chordae tendineae are thicker but less numerous. The **anterior papillary muscle**(s) is attached to the anterior part of the left wall, whereas the **posterior papillary muscle**(s) arises more posteriorly from the inferior wall. The chordae tendineae of each muscle are distributed to the contiguous halves of the two cusps of the left atrioventricular valve.

The left atrioventricular (mitral) valve (Fig. 1-69) has two obliquely set cusps, anterior and posterior; hence, it is occasionally called the *biscuspid valve.* More commonly it is called the **mitral valve** because its flaps are shaped like a bishop's miter (bishop's headdress). The mitral valve is located posterior to the sternum at the level of the fourth left costal cartilage and guards the orifice between the left atrium and the left ventricle.

The two cusps of the mitral valve are attached to the **fibrous ring** which supports the bicuspid orifice. The anterior cusp is the larger. The apices of the cusps project into the left ventricle and, as the papillary muscles contract, the chordae tendineae tighten, preventing the cusps from being forced into the left atrium.

The aortic orifice, about 2.5 cm in diameter, lies in the right posterosuperior

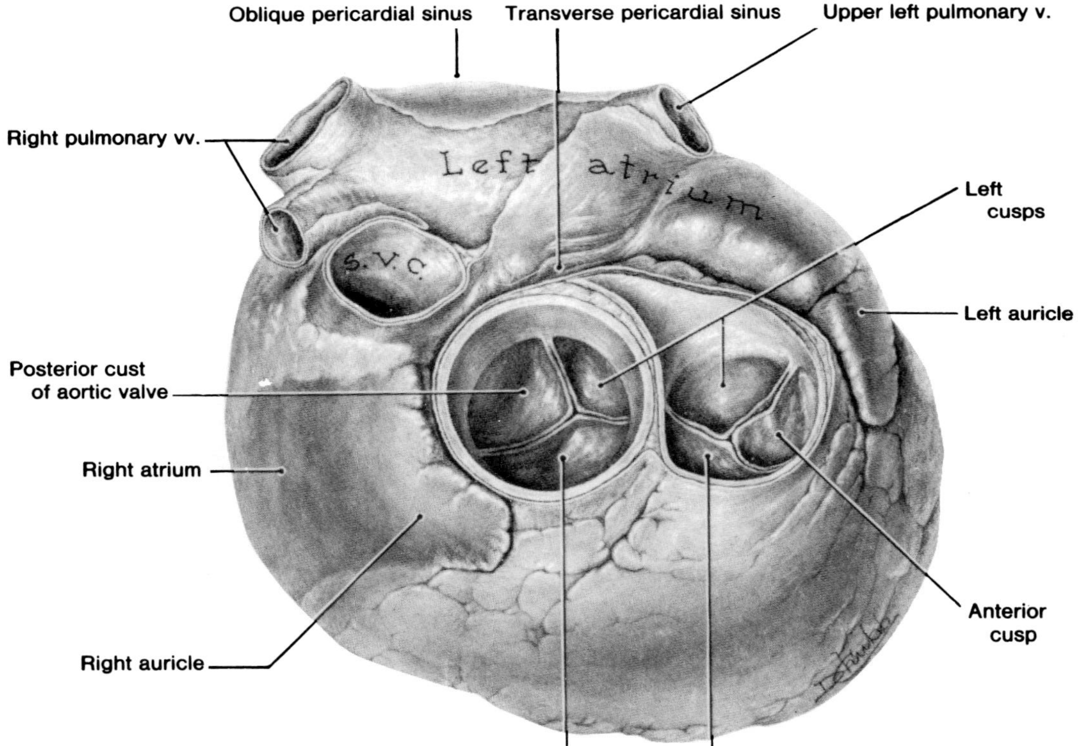

Figure 1-67. Drawing of an excised heart from above showing the aortic and pulmonary valves. Observe that the cusps of these arterial valves are similar. These valves are open only while the ventricles are contracting. Note the anterior position of the ventricles and the posterior position of the atria. Also note that the ascending aorta and the pulmonary trunk, which conduct blood from the ventricles, are placed anterior to the atria and to the superior vena cava and pulmonary veins, which conduct blood to the atria. Observe that the aorta and pulmonary arteries are enclosed within a common tube of serous pericardium and are partly embraced by the auricles of the atria. Examine the transverse pericardial sinus curving behind the enclosed stems of the aorta and pulmonary trunk and in front of the superior vena cava and upper limits of the atria. Note that each of the semilunar valves (aortic and pulmonary) has three cusps.

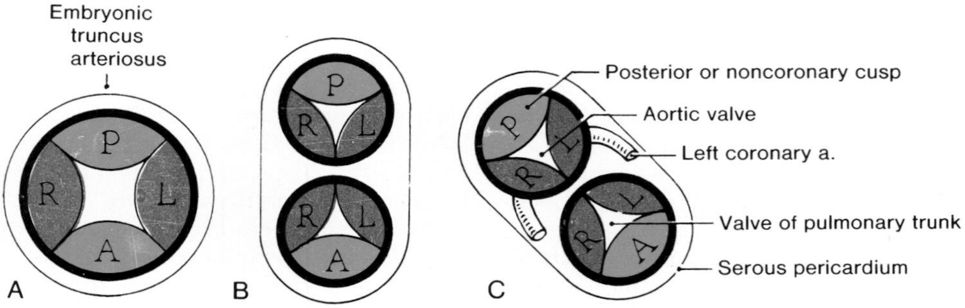

Figure 1-68. Diagrams explaining the embryological basis of the names of the pulmonary and aortic valves. The truncus arteriosus of the embryonic heart with four cusps (*A*) splits to form two valves, each with three cusps (*B*). The heart undergoes partial rotation to the left on its axis resulting in the arrangement of cusps shown in *C*. Inability of the valve to close completely is called insufficiency and results in regurgitation. Fusion of the cusps to each other produces stenosis (a narrowing).

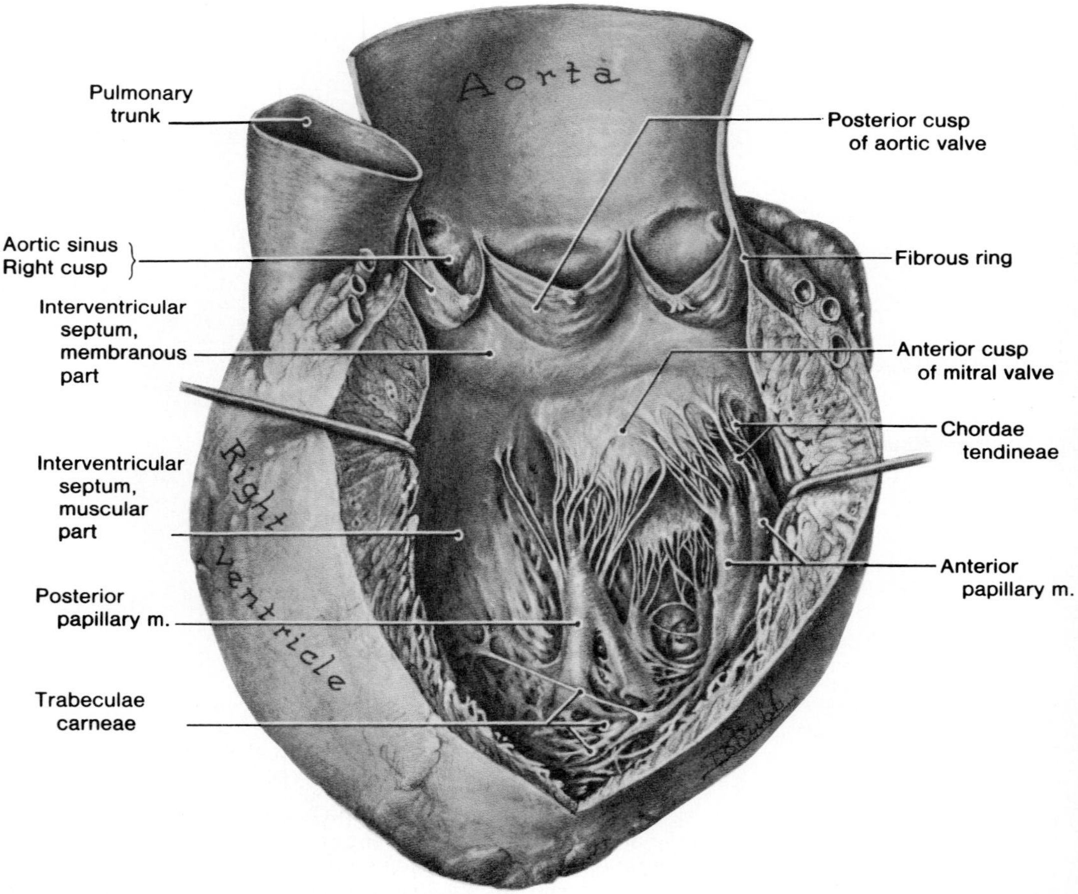

Figure 1-69. Drawing of a dissection of the interior of the left ventricle. Observe the conical shape of this chamber and the entrance (left atrioventricular, bicuspid, or mitral orifice) situated posteriorly. Note that the exit (aortic orifice) is situated superiorly. The ventricular wall is thin and muscular near the apex and thick and muscular above. Observe that the wall is thin and fibrous (nonelastic) at the aortic orifice. Note the trabeculae carneae, as in the right ventricle, forming ridges, bridges, and papillary muscles. Examine the two large papillary muscles, the anterior arising from the anterior wall and the posterior from the posterior wall. Each of these controls (via the chordae tendineae) the adjacent halves of two cusps of the mitral valve. Observe the anterior cusp of the mitral valve intervening between the inlet (mitral orifice) and the outlet (aortic orifice).

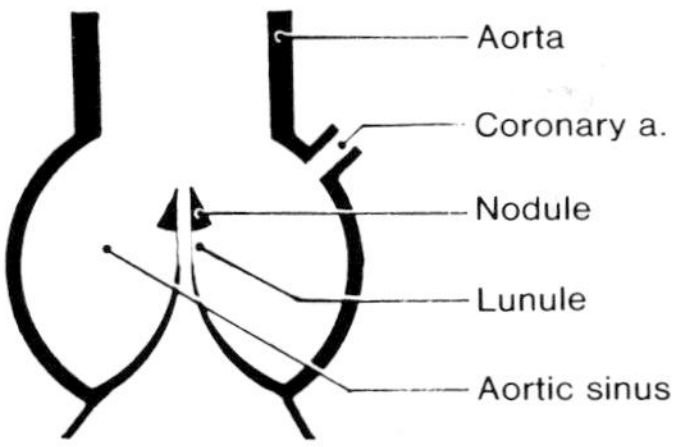

A. Closed, on longitudinal section.

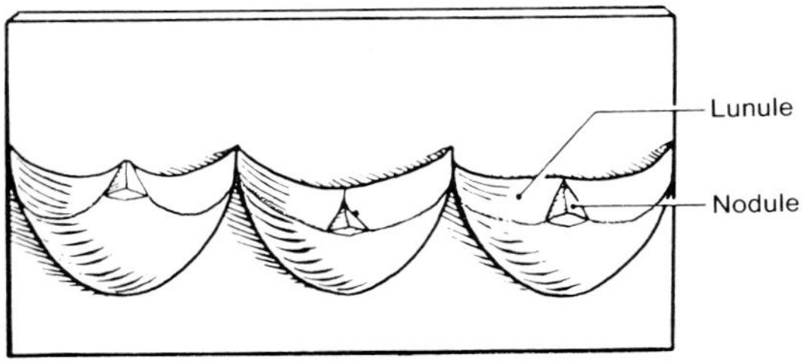

B. Spread out.

Figure 1-70. Diagrams illustrating the aortic valve which, like the valve of the pulmonary trunk (Fig. 1-67), has three semilunar cusps, each with a fibrous nodule at the midpoint of its free edge. When the valve is closed, the nodules meet in the center. Observe that a coronary artery is leaving the aorta from the aortic sinus. The right and left coronary arteries commence at the right and left aortic sinuses (Fig. 1-77).

part of the ventricle. It is also surrounded by a fibrous ring to which the three cusps of the aortic valve are attached.

The aortic valve (Figs. 1-67 to 1-70 and 1-77) is like the pulmonary valve, except that the cusps are thicker and are placed differently. In addition, the **aortic sinuses** above each valve, formed by dilation of the wall of the aorta, are larger. The blood in these aortic sinuses prevents the cusps from sticking to the wall of the artery and failing to close. The aortic valve is located posterior to the left side of the sternum at the level of the third intercostal space.

CLINICALLY ORIENTED COMMENTS

In **aortic valve stenosis** the edges of the valve are usually fused together to form a dome or cone with a narrow opening. This condition may be present at birth (**congenital**) or develop after birth (**acquired**). This valvular stenosis causes extra work for the left ventricle and results in hypertrophy of the left ventricle. A **heart murmur** is also produced.

If the aortic valve is damaged by disease, the valve may not function normally and blood may flow back into the left ventricle. This **valvular incompetence** results in **aortic regurgitation** (a backrush of blood into the left ventricle) that produces a heart murmur and a **collapsing pulse.**

The interventricular septum (Figs. 1-63, 1-66, 1-69, and 1-71) is a strong, *obliquely placed partition between the right and left ventricles.* Its margins correspond with the anterior and posterior interventricular sulci on the surface of the heart (Figs. 1-55 and 1-56); hence, this septum can be mapped out by the courses of the anterior and posterior interventricular arteries (Fig. 1-75). Most of the septum, the **muscular part,** is thick as well as muscular. Its upper oval-shaped part, about the size of a fingernail, is thin, smooth, and fibrous; this **membranous part** is situated just below the attached margins of the right

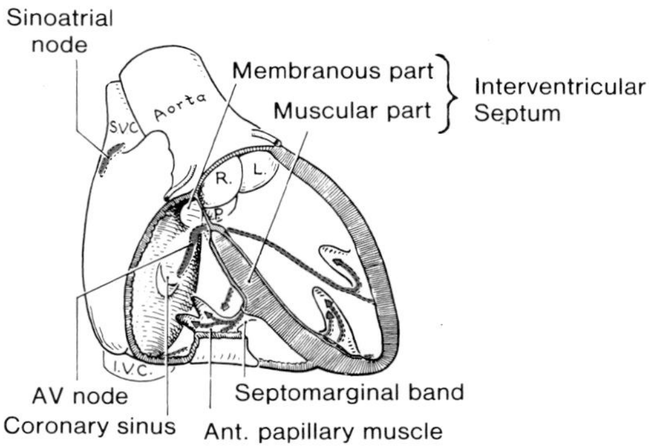

Figure 1-71. Diagram of the impulse-conducting system of the heart. The ventricles have been opened and the tricuspid valve has been removed. Note the sinoatrial node (SA node) at the superior end of the crista terminalis and the atrioventricular node (AV node) in the inferior part of the interatrial septum becoming the AV bundle, which divides into right and left limbs or branches.

coronary and posterior or noncoronary cusps of the aortic valve. The membranous part of the interventricular septum is attached to the fibrous rings surrounding the atrioventricular and arterial orifices.

CLINICALLY ORIENTED COMMENTS

The membranous part of the interventricular septum develops separately from the muscular part of the septum and has a complex developmental origin. Thus, it is the common site of a **ventricular septal defect** (VSD). *VSD, isolated or associated with other cardiac anomalies, is present in about 50% of all congenital abnormalities of the heart.* Isolated VSD accounts for about 23% of all forms of congenital heart disease and ranks first on all lists of cardiac defects. Most cases of VSD (about 70%) result from failure of development of the membranous part of the interventricular septum. The size of the defect varies from 1 to 25 mm.

Surface Anatomy of the Heart Valves. The pulmonary, aortic, mitral, and tricuspid valves lie behind the sternum on an oblique line joining the third left costal cartilage to the sixth right costal cartilage, but this is not of too much clinical interest because the heart sounds produced by these valves are best heard on the chest wall with a stethoscope at other sites.

CLINICALLY ORIENTED COMMENTS

Clinicians' interest in the surface anatomy of the cardiac valves arises from their desire to listen with their stethoscopes to the sounds produced by them. However, the valves are grouped so closely on the oblique line just described that when they are listened to at these sites it is not possible to distinguish clearly the sounds produced at each individual valve. Hence, the valve sounds are listened to over certain **auscultatory areas** which are as wide apart as possible so that the sounds produced at any given valve may be clearly distinguished from those produced at other valves. Because the blood tends to carry the sound in the direction of its flow, each area is situated superficial to the chamber or vessel through which the blood has passed and in a direct line with the valve orifice.

Your clinical teachers will demonstrate how to listen to the various **valve sounds.** For example, the sound produced by the **mitral valve,** located behind the middle of the sternum at the level of the fourth costal cartilage, is listened to superficial to the apex beat of the heart. The sound produced by the **aortic valve** is listened for in the second right intercostal space at the edge of the sternum. That by the **tricuspid valve** is heard over the right half of the inferior end of the body of the sternum, and that produced by the pulmonary valve is audible in the second left intercostal space, just to the left of the sternum.

The Skeleton of the Heart. The **cardiac skeleton**, consisting of dense connective tissue, forms the central support of the heart. Fibrous rings surround the atrioventricular canals and the origins of the aorta and pulmonary trunk. These rings prevent the valve-containing outlets from becoming dilated when the chambers of the heart contract and force blood through them. The various fibrous structures of the cardiac skeleton, together with the membranous part of the interventricular septum, also provide insertion for the fibers of the cardiac musculature.

The Conducting System of the Heart (Fig. 1-71). This system consists of specialized cardiac muscle fibers that initiate the normal heart beat (**SA node**) and coordinate the contractions of the heart chambers. Both atria contract together, as do both ventricles, but atrial contraction occurs first. *This system gives the heart its automatic rhythmic beat.*

The sinoatrial (sinuatrial) node (SA node) *initiates the impulse for contraction.* Its name is a reminder that it was in the wall of the **sinus venosus** during early embryonic development and was absorbed into the right atrium with the sinus venosus. It consists of a small mass of **specialized cardiac muscle fibers** located in the wall of the right atrium at the superior end of the crista terminalis, to the right of the opening of the superior vena cava. The SA node is called the **pacemaker of the heart** because it *initiates the impulse* which spreads through the cardiac muscle cells of both atria causing them to contract. In most people it gives off an impulse about 70 times/min. The rate at which the node produces impulses can be altered by nervous stimulation (sympathetic stimulation speeds it up and vagal stimulation slows it down or even stops it).

The atrioventricular node or AV node is also composed of specialized cardiac muscle fibers. It lies in the posteroinferior part of the interatrial septum, just above the opening of the coronary sinus. The impulses from the cardiac muscle cells of both atria converge on the AV node, which distributes them to the AV bundle. The AV node conducts the impulses slowly, but sympathetic stimulation speeds up conduction and vagal stimulation slows it down.

The atrioventricular bundle (AV bundle), once called the *bundle of His,* is a slender strand that arises from the AV node and runs forward through the right fibrous trigone (part of cardiac skeleton) to the posterior border of the membranous part of the interventricular septum. Here it lies just inferior to the septal cusp of the tricuspid valve. It divides into right and left branches (limbs or **crura**) which straddle the upper border of the muscular part of the interventricular septum. Each limb or crus descends beneath the endocardium, one on each side of the interventricular septum.

The **right branch or crus of the AV bundle** innervates the muscle of the septum, the anterior papillary muscle, and the wall of the right ventricle. The **left branch or crus of the AV bundle** supplies the septum, the papillary muscles, and the wall of the left ventricle.

In summary, the *SA node initiates the impulse for contraction* which is rapidly conducted to the cardiac muscle cells of the atria, causing them to contract. The impulse enters the AV node and is transmitted through the AV bundle and its branches (crura) to the papillary muscles first and then throughout the walls of the ventricles. The papillary muscles contract first, tightening the chordae tendineae and drawing the cusps of the atrioventricular valves together. Next, contraction of the ventricular muscle occurs. The septum and apex contract slightly earlier than the base of ventricles.

CLINICALLY ORIENTED COMMENTS

The progressive passage of impulses over the heart from the SA node can be amplified and recorded as an **electrocardiogram (ECG or EKG)**. The K in EKG is derived from the Greek word *kardia* for the heart. The instrument used for recording the potential of the electrical currents that pass through the heart and initiate its contraction is called an **electrocardiograph.** Electrocardiography gives valuable information concerning the action of the heart and its conduction system. Many heart problems involve abnormal functioning of the impulse-conducting system of the heart; hence, electrocardiograms are of considerable clinical importance in detecting the exact cause of irregularities in heart beat.

Patients with a **massive myocardial infarction** (MI) usually have a *crushing substernal chest pain* and often an abnormal ECG. The nerve impulses from the heart, which are responsible for producing the pain of myocardial infarction, enter the spinal cord through the upper thoracic ganglia of the sympathetic trunk (Figs. 1-25 and 1-74).

Artificial cardiac pacemakers are designed to give off an electrical impulse that will produce ventricular contraction at a predetermined rate. The battery-powered pacemaker, about the size of a pocket watch, is implanted for permanent pacing. An **electrode catheter** connected to it is inserted into a vein and followed with a **fluoroscope** (an instrument for rendering the shadows of x-rays visible when projected on a fluorescent screen). The terminal of the electrode is passed via the vein to the right atrium, through the tricuspid valve to the right ventricle, where it is firmly fixed to the trabeculae carneae on the lining of the walls of the ventricle. Here it makes contact with the endocardium.

Fibrillation of the heart refers to multiple, rapid, circuitous contractions or twitchings of cardiac muscular fibers, rather than of the muscle as a whole.

In **atrial fibrillation** the normal regular rhythmical contractions of the atria are replaced by rapid irregular twitchings of different parts of their walls simultaneously. The ventricles respond at irregular intervals to the dysrhythmic impulses received from the atria, but usually a satisfactory circulation is maintained.

In **ventricular fibrillation** the normal ventricular contractions are replaced by rapid, irregular, twitching movements which do not pump (*i.e.*, do not maintain the systemic circulation, including the coronary circulation). The damaged impulse-conducting system of the heart does not function normally. An irregular pattern of contractions occurs in all areas of the ventricles simultaneously, except in those that

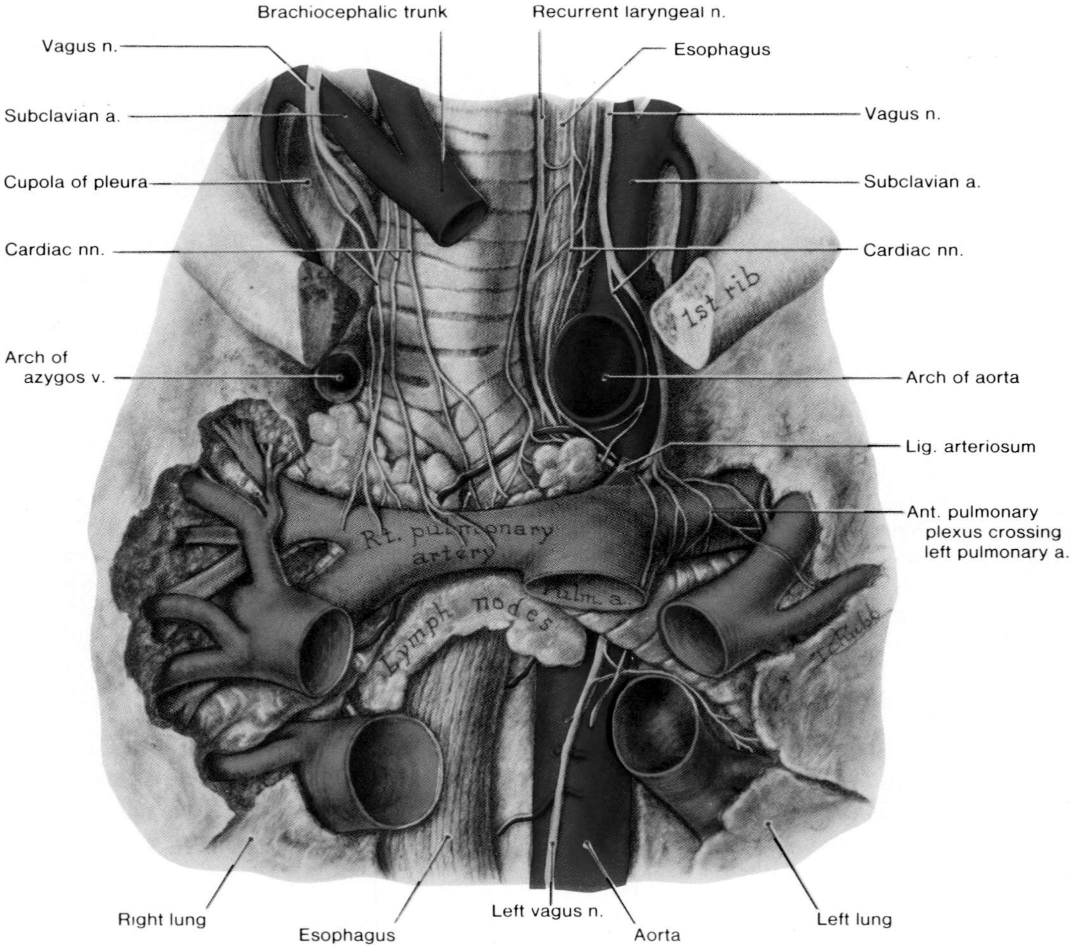

Figure 1-72. Drawing of a dissection of the superior mediastinum. Observe the pulmonary trunk dividing into right and left pulmonary arteries. Note that the right artery is longer and slightly larger than the left artery and crosses below the bifurcation of the trachea, where it is separated from the esophagus by some lymph nodes. Observe the cardiac branches of the vagus and sympathetic nerves forming the cardiac plexus of nerves. Note that the inferior tracheobronchial lymph nodes have fused to form a crescentic mass.

may have been infarcted. **Brain anoxia** (lack of oxygen to the brain) and brain death usually occur before the abnormal heart movements cease.

To defibrillate the heart, an electric shock is given to the heart through the thoracic wall via large electrodes that are often called paddles. This shock causes cessation of all cardiac movements and a few minutes later the heart may begin to beat more normally (regularly). As a result, pumping of the heart is re-established and some degree of systemic (including coronary) circulation results.

The Cardiac Plexus of Nerves (Figs. 1-72 and 1-82). The intrinsic impulse-conducting system of the heart is under the control of the **cardiac nerves of the autonomic nervous system**. This enables the heart to respond to the ever changing physiological needs of the body. *Stimulation through the sympathetic nerves increases the rate and the force of the heart beat.* It also causes dilation of the coronary arteries, resulting in the supply of more oxygen and nutrients to the myocardium. *Stimulation through the parasympathetic nerves slows the rate, reduces the force of the heart beat,* and constricts the coronary arteries. The **vagus** (CN X), the parasympathetic cardiac nerve (Fig. 8-19), supplies three branches on each side. The interlacing plexus of sympathetic and parasympathetic nerves lies on the distal part of the trachea and in front of its bifurcation, posterior to the arch of the aorta. This plexus contains small ganglia near the SA node which belong chiefly to the parasympathetic system.

The cardiac plexus receives nerve fibers from: (1) **the sympathetic trunk** (Fig. 1-25) through all its cervical cardiac branches (except the left superior) and from the cardiac branches of the second, third, and fourth thoracic ganglia of both trunks; and (2) **the vagus nerves** through their cervical cardiac branches (except the left inferior), the thoracic cardiac branch of the right vagus, and the cardiac branches of the recurrent laryngeal nerves.

The central nervous system, via the cardiac plexus, exercises control over the action of the heart and monitors blood pressure and respiration. The cardiac plexus also transmits afferent (sensory) fibers to the vagus from the great vessels and the lungs. These sensory fibers transmit impulses from pressure receptors in the aortic arch, superior vena cava, and elsewhere.

CLINICALLY ORIENTED COMMENTS

The pain of **angina pectoris** and of myocardial infarction commonly radiates from the substernal region and the left pectoral region to the left shoulder and the medial aspect of the arm (Fig. 1-73*A*). This is known as **referred pain.** Less commonly the pain radiates to the right shoulder and arm, with or without concomitant pain on the left side (Fig. 1-73*B* and *C*). All these cutaneous zones of reference for **cardiac referred pain** coincide with the segmental distribution of the sensory fibers that enter the same spinal cord segments as the fibers coming from the heart (Fig. 1-29).

The heart is insensitive to touch, cutting, cold, and heat, but ischemia and the resulting accumulation of metabolic products stimulate pain endings in the myocardium. The afferent pain fibers (dendrites of some neurons in spinal ganglia T1 to T5) run centrally in the middle and inferior cervical branches and thoracic cardiac branches of the **sympathetic trunk** (Fig. 1-25). The axons of these primary sensory neurons enter spinal cord segments T1 to T4 or T5 on the left side. Synaptic contacts may also be made with **commissural neurons** (connector neurons) that conduct impulses to neurons on the right side of comparable areas of the cord. This probably explains why pain of cardiac origin, although usually referred to the left side, may be referred to the right side (Fig. 1-73*C*).

There is no entirely satisfactory explanation for the **referral of heart pain** to the surface of the body, but one view is gaining favor. It postulates that pain impulses from the heart enter the spinal cord via visceral afferent fibers and that some of these fibers synapse with connector neurons, which in turn synapse with cells in the **intermediolateral cell column** in the lateral horn of the spinal cord (Fig. 1-74). Preganglionic fibers from cells in this column then pass out in the ventral roots and synapse with postganglionic neurons in ganglia of the sympathetic trunk. Postganglionic fibers from these neurons terminate in the smooth muscle of blood vessels in the skin. Continued stimulation of this muscle causes spasm of the vessels, which interferes with the disposal of metabolic products in that region. These may serve as stimuli for pain endings in the surrounding area. The pain impulses are carried back to the spinal cord, where they are relayed to higher centers of the brain via the contralateral **spinothalamic tract.** Thus, pain impulses from the heart are interpreted as coming from the skin rather than the heart.

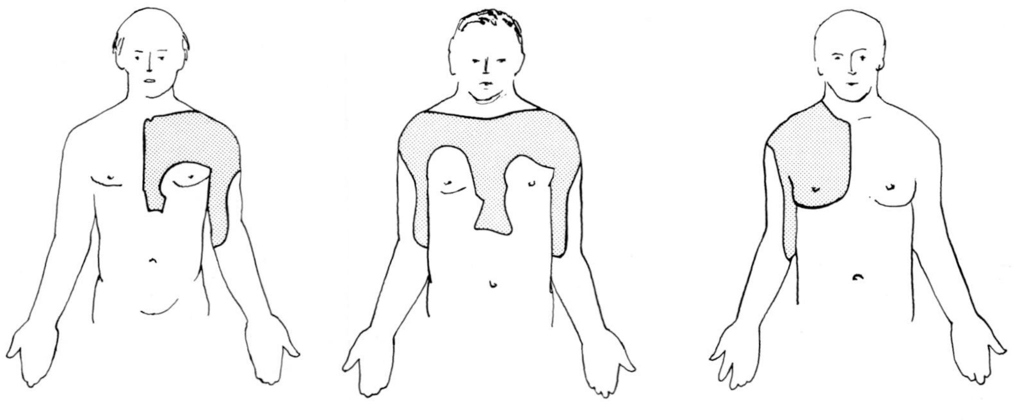

Figure 1-73. Drawings illustrating the common sites of visceral referred pain from the heart. *A,* commonly, substernal discomfort or pain radiates to the left shoulder and the inner aspect of the arm. *B,* less commonly, pain may be referred to both shoulders and arms and to the epigastrium (upper middle part of abdomen). *C,* uncommonly, pain is referred to the right shoulder and the medial aspect of the arm.

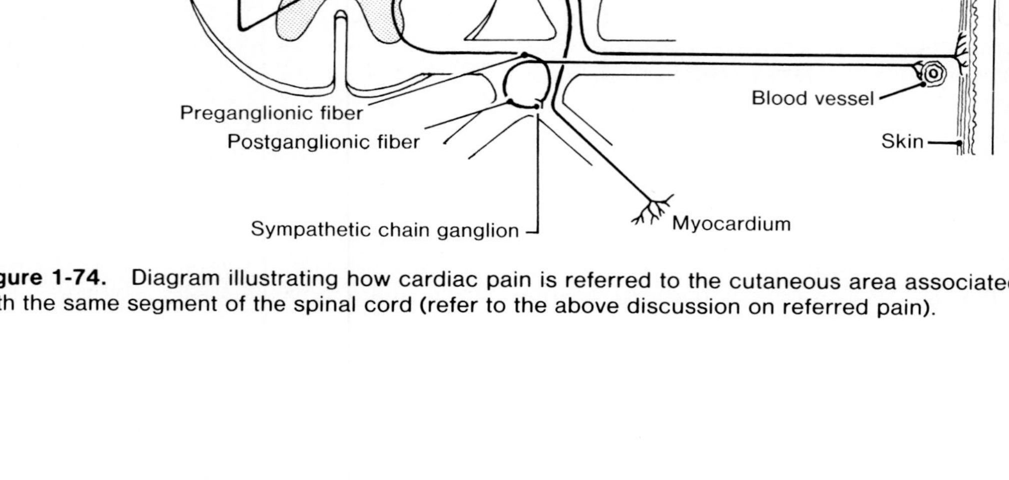

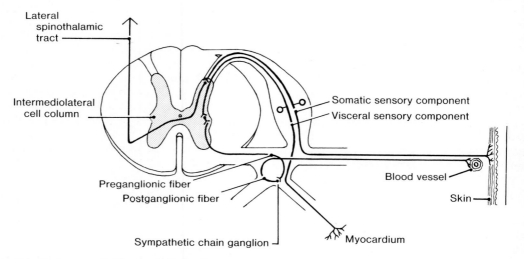

Figure 1-74. Diagram illustrating how cardiac pain is referred to the cutaneous area associated with the same segment of the spinal cord (refer to the above discussion on referred pain).

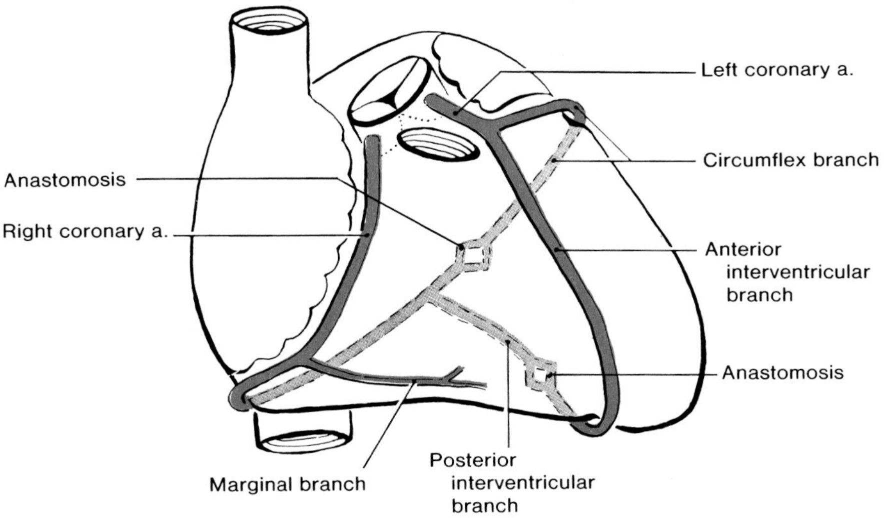

Figure 1-75. Drawing of the coronary arteries. Understand that the coronary circulation is extremely variable in detail. In most cases, the right and left coronary arteries share equally in the blood supply to the heart. In about 15% of hearts, the left coronary artery is said to be dominant in that the posterior interventricular branch comes off the circumflex as in Figure 1-76*A*.

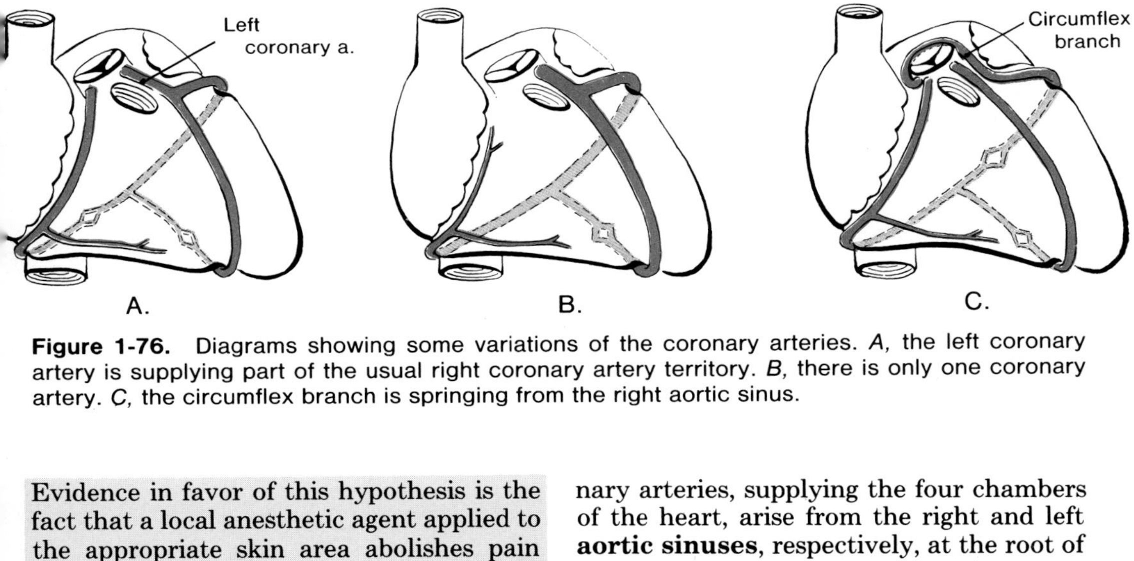

Figure 1-76. Diagrams showing some variations of the coronary arteries. *A,* the left coronary artery is supplying part of the usual right coronary artery territory. *B,* there is only one coronary artery. *C,* the circumflex branch is springing from the right aortic sinus.

Evidence in favor of this hypothesis is the fact that a local anesthetic agent applied to the appropriate skin area abolishes pain that originates in the heart but is referred to the skin.

The Coronary Arteries (Figs. 1-52, 1-68, 1-70, and 1-75 to 1-79). These vessels were called "coronary" (L. *corona,* crown) because they encircle the base of the ventricles like a crown. The right and left coronary arteries, supplying the four chambers of the heart, arise from the right and left **aortic sinuses**, respectively, at the root of the aorta (Fig. 1-77). *There is no sharp line of demarcation between the ventricular distribution of the coronary arteries.* On leaving the aorta, the two coronary arteries pass forward, one on each side of the root of the pulmonary trunk.

Most of the blood in the coronary arteries returns to the chambers of the heart via the **coronary sinus** (Figs. 1-60 and 1-61), but

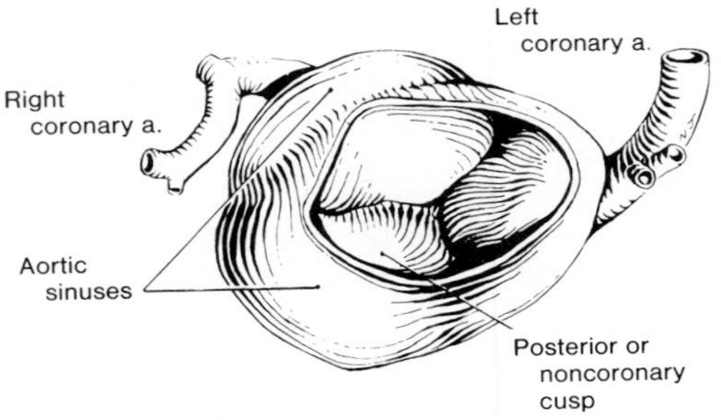

Figure 1-77. Drawing of the ventricular aspect of the closed aortic valve. Observe the coronary arteries arising from the aortic sinuses above the valve. Note that the left coronary is larger than the right.

some small venous channels (**venae cordis minimae and the anterior cardiac veins**) empty directly into its chambers.

The right coronary artery arises from the **right aortic sinus** and passes forward and to the right, emerging between the pulmonary trunk and the right auricle. It then descends in the **coronary sulcus** between the right atrium and the right ventricle to the inferior border of the heart. Here it gives off a **marginal branch** that runs toward the apex. After giving off the marginal branch, the right coronary artery turns to the left in the posterior part of the coronary sulcus, where it gives off its largest branch, the **posterior interventricular branch,** which descends toward the apex in the **posterior interventricular sulcus.** Note that this sulcus, lying on the central tendon of the diaphragm, is really more inferior than posterior. Near the apex, the posterior interventricular branch anastomoses with branches of the anterior interventricular branch of the left coronary artery (Fig. 1-75).

Just before giving off its posterior interventricular branch, the right coronary artery gives off an **AV nodal artery** which enters the posterior part of the atrioventricular sulcus and *passes upward to supply the AV node and the AV bundle.* After giving off its posterior interventricular branch, the right coronary artery continues in the coronary sulcus where it anastomoses with the left coronary artery. *The right coronary artery supplies the right atrium and the right ventricle* and a variable amount of the left atrium and left ventricle.

The left coronary artery arises from the **left aortic sinus** and passes between the left auricle and the pulmonary trunk to reach the **coronary sulcus.** Here it divides into an anterior interventricular branch and a circumflex branch. The **anterior interventricular branch** follows the **anterior interventricular sulcus** to or beyond the apex and anastomoses with the posterior interventricular branch of the right coronary artery. *The anterior interventricular branch supplies both ventricles and the interventricular septum.*

The **circumflex branch** follows the **coronary sulcus** around the left border of the heart to the posterior surface. It terminates to the left of the posterior interventricular sulcus by giving *branches to the left ventricle and left atrium* and anastomosing with the right coronary artery. The circumflex branch gives off a **marginal branch** which follows the left margin of the heart. The circumflex branch supplies the left atrium, the left surface of the heart, and the base of the left ventricle inferiorly.

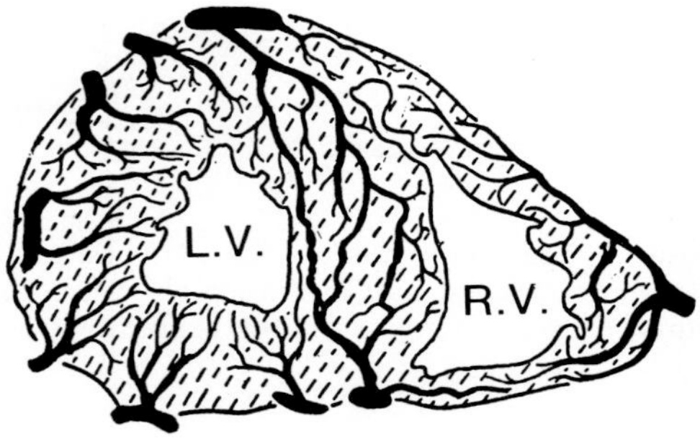

Figure 1-78. Drawing of a transverse section of the ventricles showing the branches of coronary arteries penetrating the heart substance. Note that many anastomoses occur between the vessels in the interventricular septum. When these and other anastomoses become functional, they enlarge. Observe that the right ventricle is crescentic in cross-section, whereas the left ventricle is circular. Note that the left ventricular wall is about three times as thick as the right one.

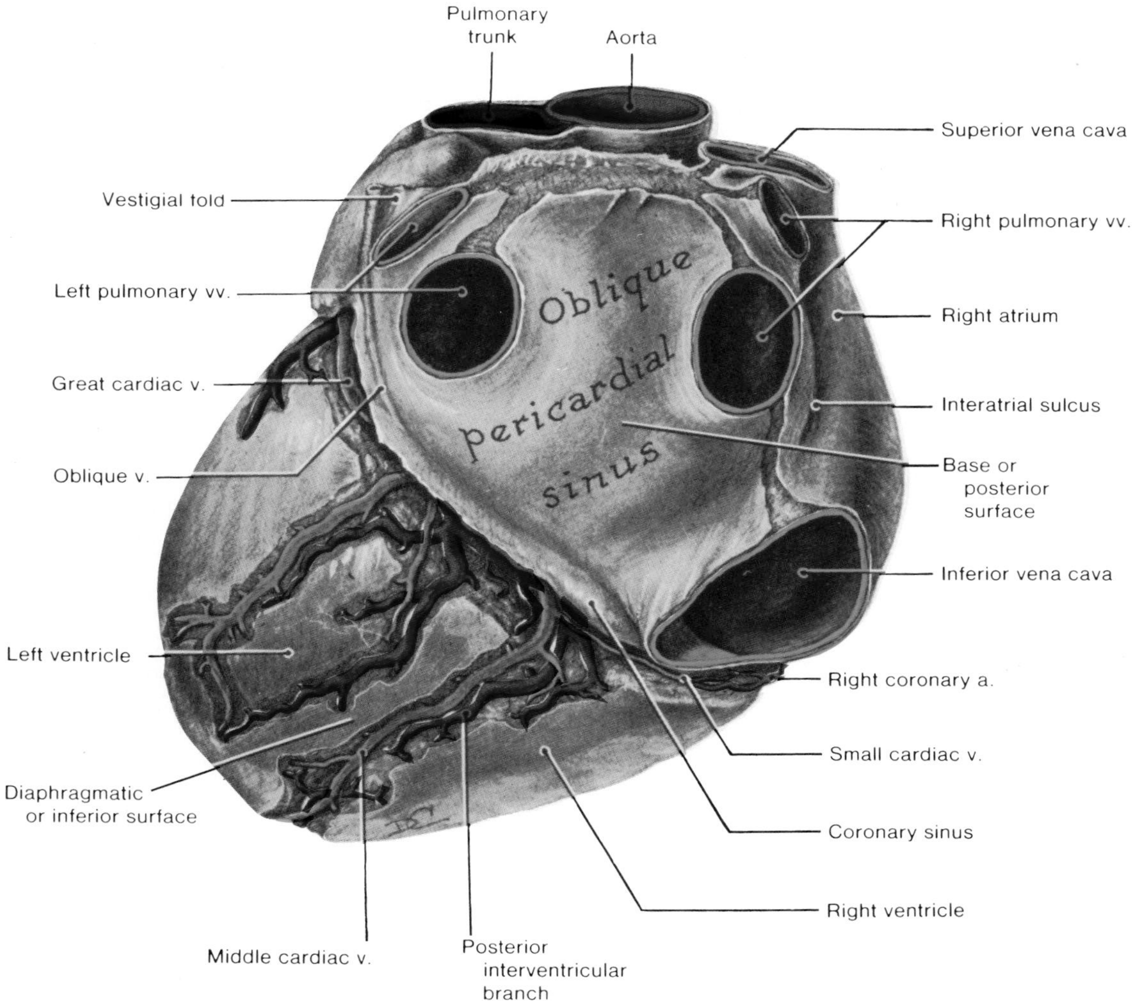

Figure 1-79. Drawing of a dissection of a posterior view of the heart. This heart was removed from the specimen shown in Figure 1-54. Observe that the oblique sinus is circumscribed by five veins. Examine the superior vena cava and the much larger inferior vena cava joining the upper and lower limits of the right atrium. Note that the left atrium forms the greater part of the base or posterior surface of the heart. Observe the coronary arteries, here irregular in that the left one supplies the posterior interventricular branch. Examine the branches of the cardiac veins and note that when they cross branches of the coronary arteries they mostly do so superficially.

CLINICALLY ORIENTED COMMENTS

Variations of the coronary arteries and of their branching patterns are extremely common (Fig. 1-76). In many cases (about one-half), the right coronary artery is dominant, *i.e.*, it crosses to the left side to supply the left ventricular wall and the interventricular septum. In some cases, the left coronary artery, in addition to supplying all of the left ventricle and the interventricular septum, may send branches to the right ventricular wall (left coronary artery dominance; about 20%). In about 30% of cases, the coronary arterial pattern is balanced.

There may be only one coronary artery (Fig. 1-76*B*) and in about 4% of hearts there are accessory coronary arteries.

The branches of the coronary arteries are end arteries in the sense that they supply regions of cardiac muscle without overlap from other large branches (Fig. 1-78). Although there is a rich anastomosis between arterioles, this blood supply is inadequate to supply the requirements of the cardiac muscle when there is a sudden occlusion of a major branch. As a result, the region supplied by the occluded branch becomes infarcted (*i.e.*, rendered virtually bloodless) and soon undergoes **necrosis** (*i.e.*, dies). The area of myocardium that has undergone necrosis is called an **infarct.**

The most common cause of ischemic heart disease is **coronary insufficiency** resulting from **atherosclerosis** of the coronary arteries. The atherosclerotic process, consisting of *lipid accumulations on the inner walls of the coronary arteries,* begins during early adulthood and results in slow narrowing (**stenosis**) of the lumina of these vessels. As coronary atherosclerosis progresses, collateral channels connecting one coronary artery with another expand, permitting adequate perfusion of the heart to continue. Despite this compensatory mechanism, the myocardium may not receive enough oxygen, and when the heart is required to perform increased amounts of work (*e.g.*, during exercise), the inadequate supply of blood to the heart (**myocardial ischemia**) results in retrosternal discomfort and/or pain.

The coronary arteries are frequent sites of arteriosclerosis (G. *sklērosis,* hardness), with resultant narrowing of their lumens to a greater or lesser degree. This reduces blood flow to the various parts of the heart supplied by the two coronary arteries and their branches. Moderate reduction in blood flow may be asymptomatic until a demand for increased work occurs. The narrow artery or arteries cannot supply enough blood to meet the increased demand by the parts of the heart muscle supplied by the narrowed arteries. The result is a characteristic pain on effort called angina pectoris.

Angina pectoris is a clinical syndrome characterized by substernal discomfort that results from myocardial ischemia. Although *frequently a presenting symptom of ischemic heart disease,* it can be produced by aortic valve disease and anemia. Patients commonly describe the discomfort as tightness or squeezing. *The most important feature of angina pectoris is its relation to exertion.* It is relieved by 1 or 2 min of rest and by sublingual **nitroglycerin,** which dilates the coronary arteries.

If the supply of oxygen to the myocardium is cut off (*e.g.*, owing to **coronary occlusion**), the area of muscle concerned dies (undergoes necrosis, infarction). The pain resulting from **myocardial infarction** (MI) is often more severe than with angina pectoris and does not disappear after 1 or 2 min of rest. MI may also follow excessive exertion by a person with stenotic (narrowed) arteries. The straining heart muscle is demanding more oxygen than the stenotic arteries can provide; as a result, an area of myocardium undergoes infarction.

Coronary occlusion (blockage) of any but the smallest branches of one artery usually results in death of the cardiac muscle which it supplies. The damaged muscle is replaced by fibrous tissue and a scar forms. If the nodal or other parts of the impulse-conducting system are affected by the blockage (*e.g.*, of the AV nodal artery), the ventricles may continue to contract at their own rate; (this is called a **heart block**).

The coronary arteries can be visualized by a procedure known as **coronary angiography.** Long narrow catheters with tips of special shape are passed into the ascending aorta via the femoral or brachial artery. Under fluoroscopic control the tip of the catheter is placed just inside the mouth of a coronary artery. A small injection of radiopaque contrast material is made and full-sized radiographs or **cineradiographs** are made to show the lumen of the artery and its branches and any stenotic (narrow) areas that may be present. The procedure is repeated on the other coronary artery. At some time in the procedure, another catheter is passed into the left ventricle and a large injection of contrast material is given as **cineangiograms** are made to show how well the left ventricular wall is functioning. If the patient has had a previous **cardiac infarct** owing to closure of a coronary artery or one of its branches, the infarcted area will not contract because it is composed of scar tissue, not muscle.

In patients with angina pectoris, a procedure called a **coronary bypass** may be carried out. A segment of vein is connected to the aorta or a proximal coronary artery and then to the coronary artery beyond the stenosis.

Veins of the Heart (Figs. 1-52, 1-60, and 1-79). The heart is drained mainly by veins that empty into the **coronary sinus** and partly by small veins (venae cordis minimae and anterior cardiac veins) that open directly into the chambers of the heart, principally those on the right side.

The coronary sinus is the main vein of the heart. It is about 2.5 cm in length and runs from left to right in the posterior part of the coronary sulcus. This sinus is the derivative of the left horn of the embryonic **sinus venosus.** It receives the great cardiac vein at its left end and the middle and small cardiac veins at its right end. *The coronary sinus drains all the venous blood from the heart,* **except** for that carried by the anterior cardiac veins and the venae cordis minimae. It opens into the right atrium (Fig. 1-61), immediately to the left of the inferior vena cava and posterior to the right atrioventricular orifice. The valve of the coronary sinus is variable in size and form and lies to the right of its opening; this remnant of the valve of the sinus venosus is probably of *no functional significance in the adult.*

The great cardiac vein, the main tributary of the coronary sinus, begins at the apex of the heart and ascends in the *anterior interventricular sulcus.* It enters the left end of the coronary sinus and drains the area of the heart supplied by the left coronary artery.

The middle cardiac vein also begins at the apex of the heart but runs in the *posterior interventricular sulcus* to enter the right side of the coronary sinus. The **small cardiac vein** runs in the coronary sulcus and enters the coronary sinus to the right of the middle cardiac vein. The middle and small cardiac veins drain most of the area of the heart supplied by the right coronary artery.

The small **oblique vein of the left atrium** begins over the posterior wall of the left atrium (Fig. 1-60) and descends obliquely to enter the coronary sinus. It is the *adult derivative of the embryonic left common cardinal vein.* In rare cases, two superior venae cavae are present. In these people there is no oblique vein of the left atrium because a left superior vena cava is present and opens into the coronary sinus.

The small **anterior cardiac veins** (two or three) begin over the anterior surface of the right ventricle and cross over the coronary sulcus to end directly in the right atrium.

The **venae cordis minimae** (smallest cardiac veins, Thebesian veins) are minute vessels that begin in the myocardium and open directly into the chambers of the heart, chiefly the atria. Although classified as veins, they may also carry blood to the myocardium.

The Lymphatic Drainage of the Heart (Figs. 1-47, 1-48, and 1-85). The lymphatic vessels of the heart form plexuses adjacent to the endocardium and the epicardium.

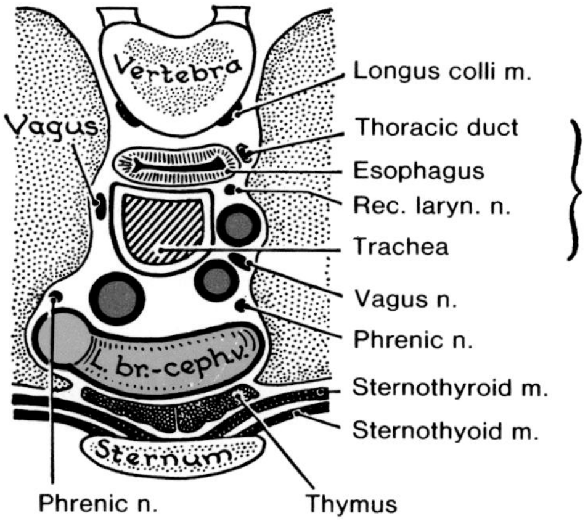

Figure 1-80. Diagram of a cross-section of the superior mediastinum, above the level of the aortic arch. Observe the posterior relations of the thymus and the structures around the trachea.

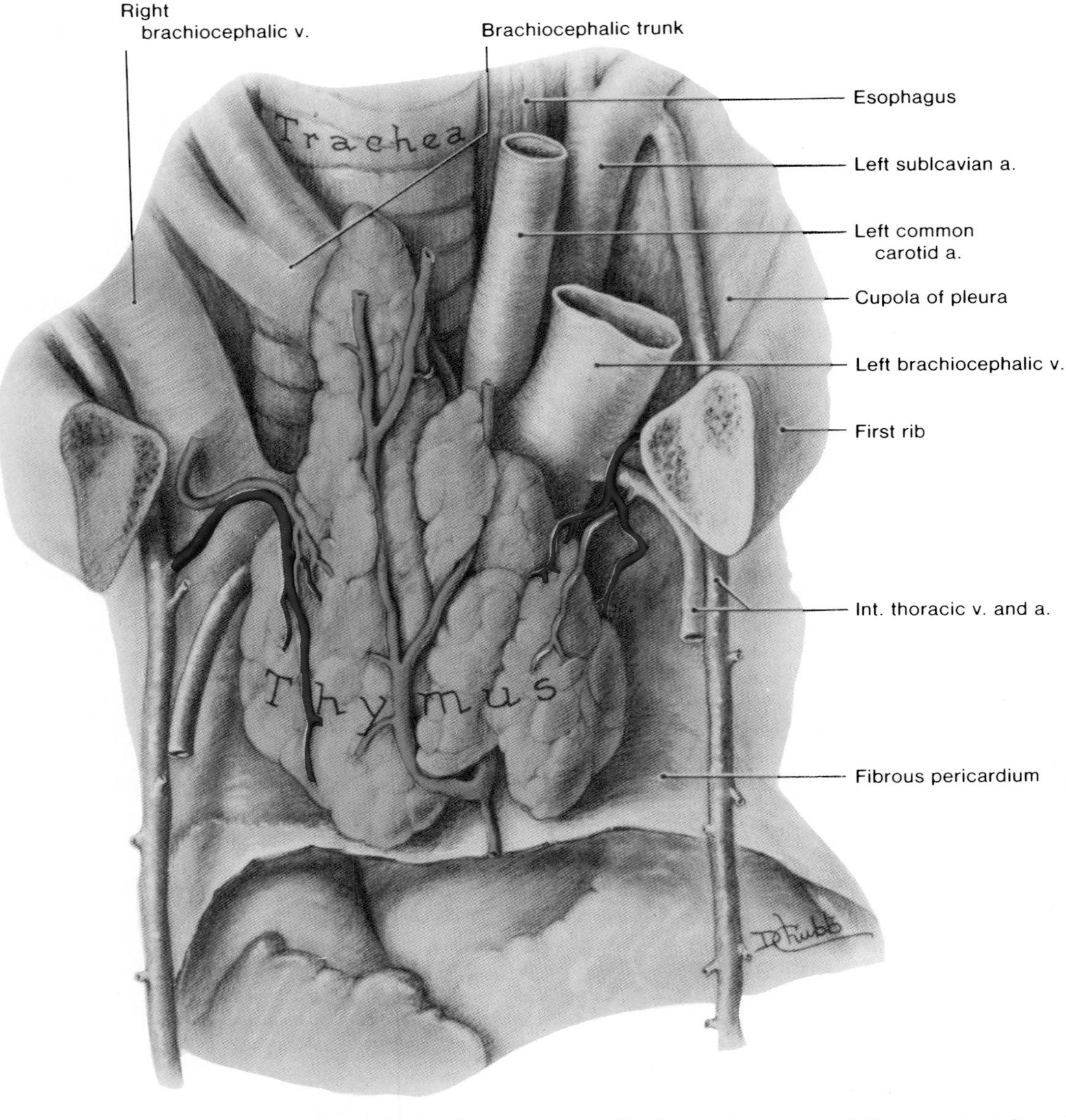

Figure 1-81. Drawing of a dissection of the superior mediastinum of a young adult. In most adults the thymus is difficult to locate. The sternum and ribs have been excised and the pleurae removed. Observe the thymus lying in the superior mediastinum, overlapping the upper limit of the pericardial sac below, and extending upward into the neck, here farther than usual. Note the longitudinal fissure that divides the thymus into two asymmetrical lobes, a larger right and a smaller left. These developmentally separate parts are easily separated from each other by blunt dissection. Observe the blood vessels of the thymus: arteries from the internal thoracic arteries and veins to the brachiocephalic and internal thoracic veins. (See Figs. 1-80 and 1-83 for other views of the thymus).

The efferent vessels follow the coronary arteries and empty into the **mediastinal** and **tracheobronchial lymph nodes.**

The Superior Mediastinum (Fig. 1-49). The superior mediastinum lies between the mediastinal pleurae and superior to the horizontal plane connecting the sternal angle with the lower border of the fourth thoracic vertebrae. Thus, its superior boundary is the superior thoracic aperture (thoracic inlet). Its anterior part is continuous in front of the pericardial sac with the anterior mediastinum; its posterior part is continuous behind the pericardial sac with the posterior mediastinum; and its middle part contains the great vessels entering and leaving the heart (Fig. 1-52).

The main contents of the superior mediastinum are: the thymus, the great veins draining blood to the heart from the upper limbs and the head and neck, the aortic arch and its three branches, parts of the trachea and esophagus and several nerves of which the phrenics and vagi are most prominent.

The Thymus (Figs. 1-80, 1-81, and 1-83). This mass of lymphoid tissue is a prominent feature of the superior mediastinum *in early childhood.* It is a flattened, bilobed structure that has a pink, lobulated appearance during early life. It lies immediately behind the manubrium in the anterior portion of the superior mediastinum and the adjacent part of the anterior mediastinum. In newborn infants it may extend up through the superior aperture of the thorax into the root of the neck in front of the great vessels.

During childhood, particularly as puberty is reached, the thymus begins to diminish in relative size (undergoes involution). *By adulthood it is often scarcely recognizable.* Usually all that can be found are a few thymic nodules in the areolar tissue located in the anterior part of the superior mediastinum.

The blood supply of the thymus is from the inferior thyroid and internal thoracic arteries. Its main veins end in the left brachiocephalic, internal thoracic, and inferior thyroid veins. The **lymph vessels of the thymus** end in the brachiocephalic, tracheobronchial (Fig. 1-47), and parasternal lymph nodes (Fig. 1-20).

CLINICALLY ORIENTED COMMENTS

Because it develops from the ventral parts of the embryonic third pair of **pharyngeal pouches,** in common with the **inferior parathyroid glands** which develop from their dorsal parts (Fig. 9-49), the thymus may retain a fibrous connection with one or both of these cervical endocrine glands. Rarely, one of the inferior parathyroid glands accompanies the thymus into the superior mediastinum.

Thymomas (thymic tumors) are rare, but they may be responsible for vague retrosternal pain, coughing, and dyspnea (shortness of breath) owing to pressure on the trachea. They may compress the superior vena cava, resulting in engorgement of the neck veins. Similarly a retrosternal thyroid gland may enlarge and compress the trachea and esophagus (see thyroid in Chap. 9).

The Brachiocephalic Veins (Figs. 1-48, 1-53, 1-55, 1-56, and 1-80 to 1-82). The brachiocephalic (innominate) veins *arise posterior to the medial ends of the clavicles.* Each is formed by the *union of the internal jugular and subclavian veins.* They have no valves. At the level of the lower border of the first right costal cartilage, the two brachiocephalic veins unite to form the **superior vena cava.** To be specific, this union occurs at the right border of the sternum, posterior to the lower border of the junction of the first right costal cartilage with the sternum. The two brachiocephalic veins represent the union of the veins from the arm (L. *brachium*), the head (G. *kephalē*), and the neck. Each vein receives the internal thoracic, vertebral, inferior thyroid, and highest intercostal veins.

The right brachiocephalic vein (Figs. 1-48, 1-53, and 1-80 to 1-82) is a short vein that *arises behind the right sternoclavicular joint* and descends vertically into the superior mediastinum behind the manubrium, lateral to the arterial brachiocephalic trunk. *The right vagus nerve (CN X) lies between these vessels* and the right phrenic nerve lies posterolateral to the right brachiocephalic vein. This vein joins the left brachiocephalic vein to form the superior vena cava at the right border of the sternum at the lower border of first costal cartilage. In addition to the veins mentioned previously, the right brachiocephalic vein receives the **right lymphatic duct** (Fig. 1-48).

The left brachiocephalic vein (Figs. 1-48, 1-53, and 1-80 to 1-82), about 6 cm long, *arises behind the left sternoclavicular joint* and passes to the right and downward behind the manubrium, where it unites with the right brachiocephalic vein to form the superior vena cava. It is over twice as long as the right brachiocephalic vein because it passes obliquely downward (to the right).

During its descent it crosses the left com-

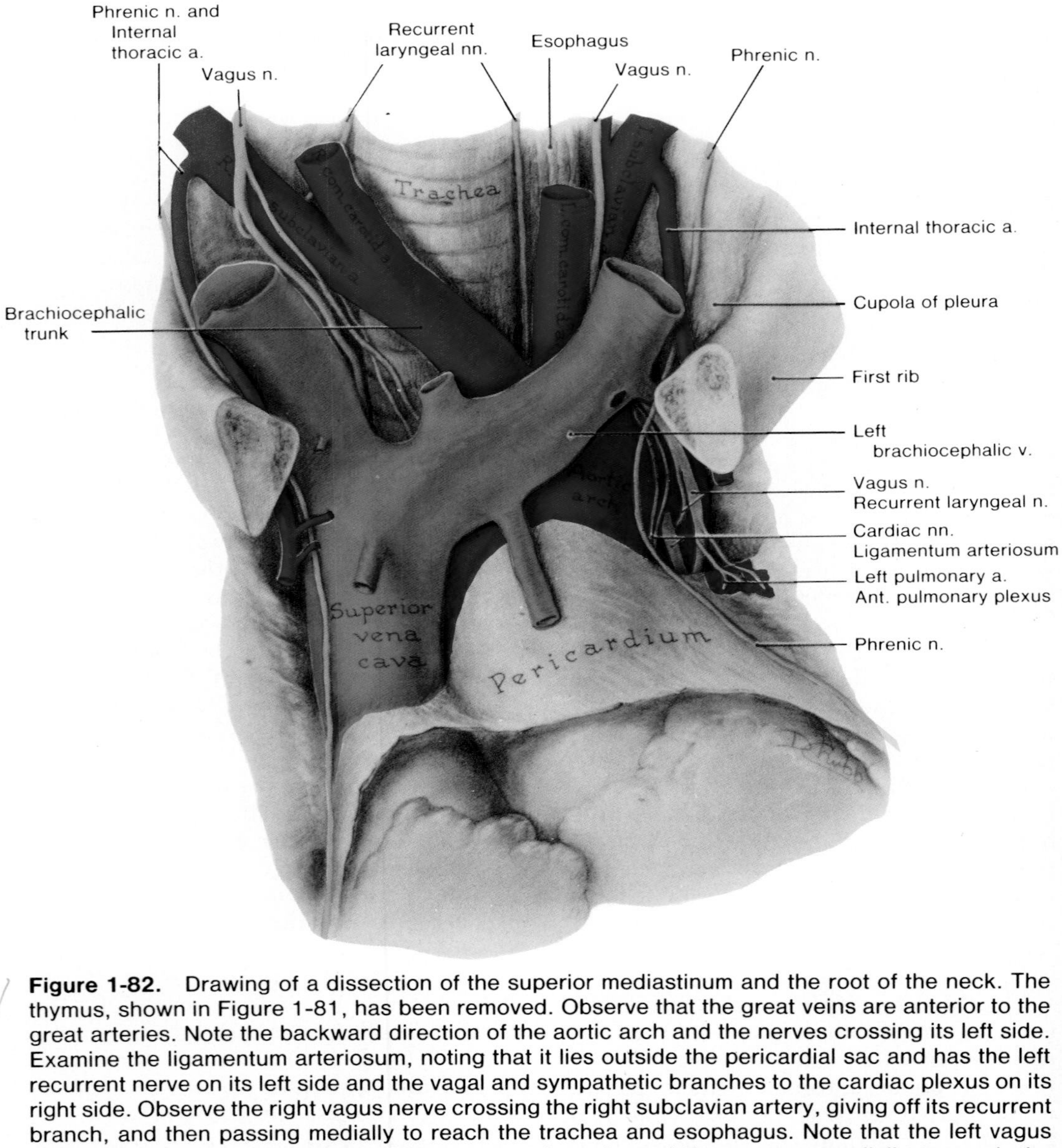

Figure 1-82. Drawing of a dissection of the superior mediastinum and the root of the neck. The thymus, shown in Figure 1-81, has been removed. Observe that the great veins are anterior to the great arteries. Note the backward direction of the aortic arch and the nerves crossing its left side. Examine the ligamentum arteriosum, noting that it lies outside the pericardial sac and has the left recurrent nerve on its left side and the vagal and sympathetic branches to the cardiac plexus on its right side. Observe the right vagus nerve crossing the right subclavian artery, giving off its recurrent branch, and then passing medially to reach the trachea and esophagus. Note that the left vagus crosses the aortic arch, giving off its recurrent branch, and then passes medially to reach the esophagus. Observe that the left phrenic nerve crosses anterior to the vagus nerve.

mon carotid artery, the brachiocephalic trunk, the left vagus nerve, and the left phrenic nerve. The left brachiocephalic vein is separated from the manubrium by the remains of the thymus and the origins of the sternohyoid and sternothyroid muscles (Fig. 1-21).

In addition to the tributaries common to both brachiocephalic veins mentioned previously, the left brachiocephalic vein receives the superior intercostal vein and the **thoracic duct** (Figs. 1-48 and 1-92), the largest lymph vessel in the body.

The Superior Vena Cava (Figs. 1-35*A*, 1-38, 1-48, 1-52 to 1-56, 1-61, 1-64, 1-67, 1-79, 1-82, and 1-83). This large vein, about 7 cm long, *enters the right atrium* vertically from above. It returns blood from everything above the diaphragm (*i.e.*, the head and neck, upper limbs, and thoracic wall), *except the lungs,* the blood from which enters the left atrium. The superior vena cava *forms posterior to the first right costal cartilage* by the union of the right and left brachiocephalic veins. It passes inferiorly and *ends at the level of the third costal cartilage* by entering the right atrium.

In Figures 1-82 and 1-83, observe that the *superior vena cava* lies on the *right side of the superior mediastinum,* anterolateral to the trachea and posterolateral to the ascending aorta. Note that the right phrenic nerve lies between the superior vena cava and the mediastinal parietal pleura, which partly surrounds the right surface of this vessel. *The terminal half of the superior vena cava is in the middle mediastinum,* where it lies beside the ascending aorta in the pericardium (Fig. 1-54). The shadow cast by the superior vena cava is often seen in anteroposterior radiographs of the chest (Fig. 1-38).

The Aortic Arch (Figs. 1-72 and 1-82 to 1-87). This curved continuation of the ascending aorta *begins posterior to the right half of the sternal angle.* It arches upward and posteriorly with an inclination and convexity to the left. It *passes to the left of the trachea and the esophagus,* displacing the trachea to the right, which makes the right principal bronchus almost in line with the trachea (Fig. 1-85). The aortic arch joins the descending aorta on the left of the

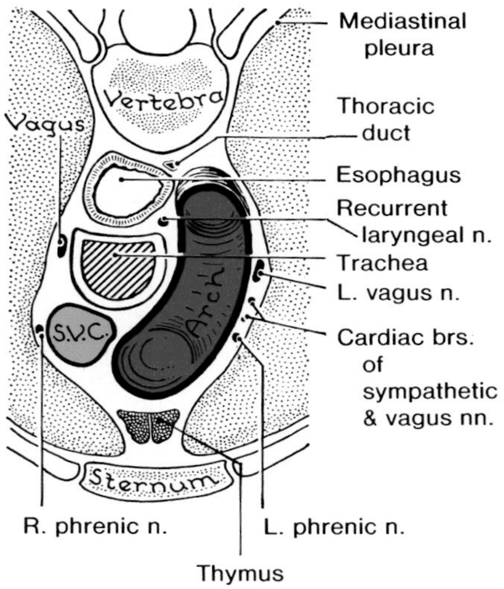

Figure 1-83. Diagram of a cross-section through the superior mediastinum at the level of the aortic arch. Observe the four parallel structures: trachea, esophagus, recurrent laryngeal nerve, and thoracic duct.

intervertebral disc between the fourth and fifth thoracic vertebrae, in the same horizontal plane as its origin from the ascending aorta.

The **terminal part of the aortic arch** may be easily observed in anteroposterior radiographs of the chest (Fig. 1-38). The shadow it casts is often called the **aortic knob** (knuckle). Anteriorly the aortic arch is in contact with the remains of the thymus (Fig. 1-83). The left brachiocephalic vein crosses just above the aortic arch (Fig. 1-82), near the origin of its branches. Further posteriorly, the aortic arch crosses in front of the **phrenic nerve,** the **cardiac branches** of the left vagus and sympathetic nerves (Fig. 1-72), the vagus nerve itself, and the origins of the left common carotid and left subclavian arteries.

The inferior concave surface of the aortic arch curves over the structures passing to the **root of the left lung** (Fig. 1-86), the bifurcation of the pulmonary trunk, the left pulmonary artery, and the left bronchus (Fig. 1-72). The **ligamentum arteriosum** passes from the root of the left pulmonary artery to the inferior concave surface of the aortic arch (Figs. 1-52, 1-72 and 1-86). This

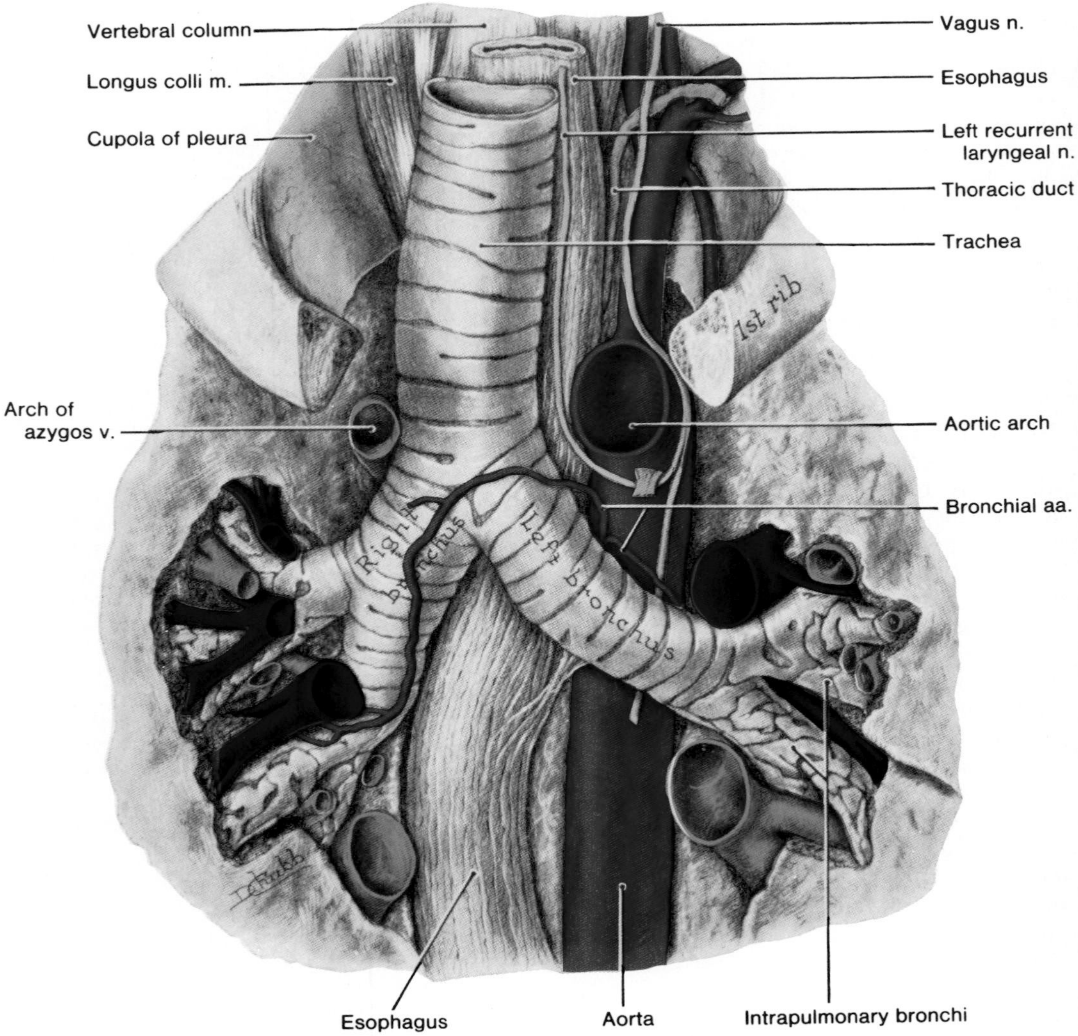

Figure 1-84. Drawing of a deep dissection of the superior mediastinum showing four parallel structures: trachea, esophagus, left recurrent laryngeal nerve, and thoracic duct. Note that this recurrent nerve lies in the angle between the trachea and esophagus and that the thoracic duct is at the side of the esophagus. Observe that the aortic arch runs backward on the left of these four structures and that the arch of the azygos vein passes forward on the right. Examine the trachea inclining to the right and note that the right bronchus is more vertical than the left and that its stem is shorter and wider. This is why foreign bodies usually pass into the right bronchus. Observe the U-shaped rings of the trachea and that the ring at the bifurcation of the trachea is V-shaped.

ligament is the remnant of the **ductus arteriosus,** an embryonic vessel that shunted blood from the left pulmonary artery to the aorta in order to bypass the lungs. The **left recurrent laryngeal nerve** passes posterior to the ligamentum arteriosum and then ascends in a groove between the trachea and the esophagus (Fig. 1-82), medial to the aortic arch.

Branches of the aortic arch (Figs. 1-72, 1-82, and 1-84 to 1-86) supply the head and neck, the upper limbs, and part of the body wall. *The aortic arch has three branches*: the brachiocephalic trunk, the left common

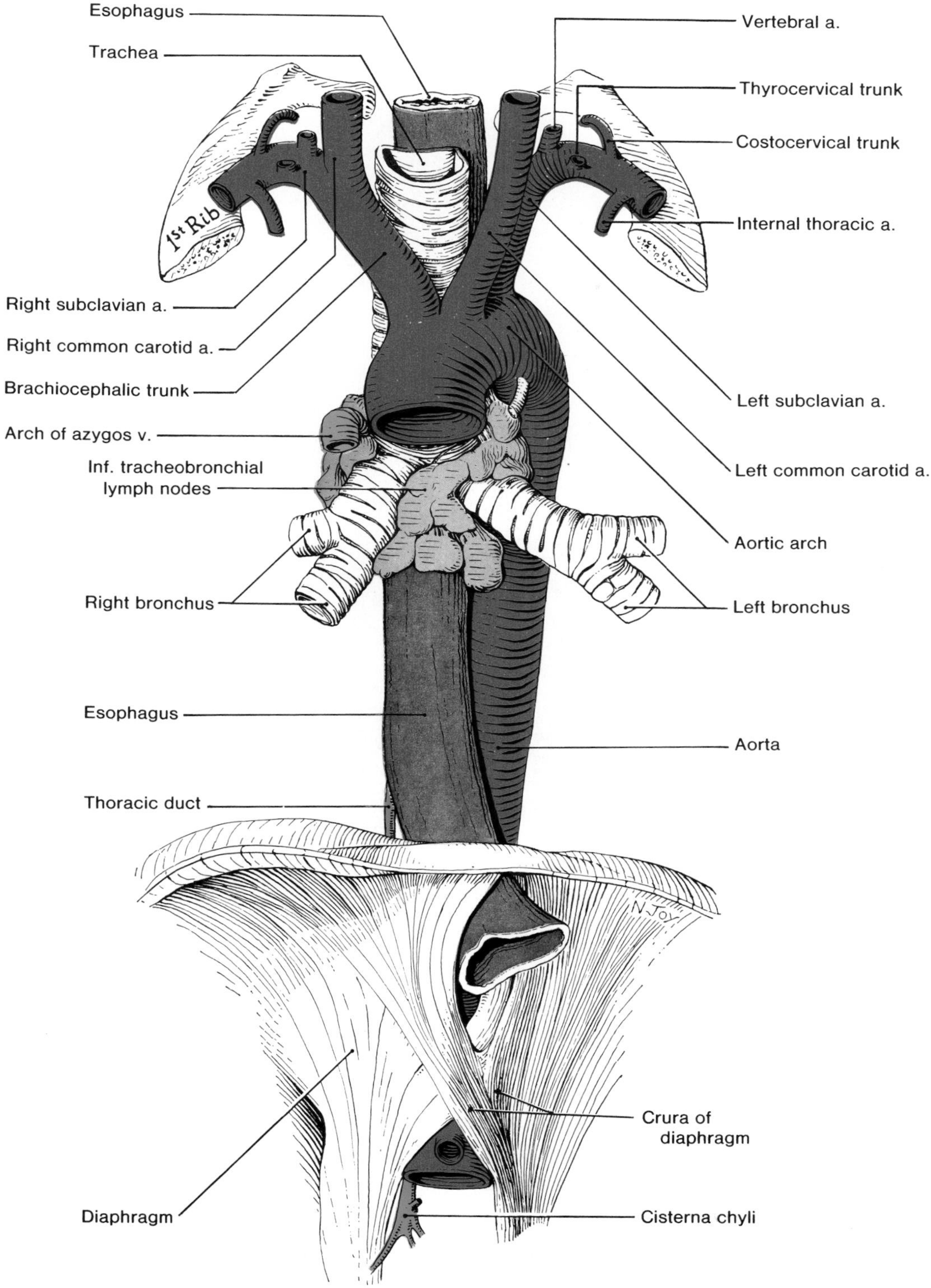

Figure 1-85. Drawing of a dissection of an anterior view of the thoracic parts of the esophagus, trachea, and aorta. Observe that the arch of the aorta curves backward on the left side of the trachea and esophagus and that the arch of the azygos vein arches forward on their right sides. Each of these vessels arches above the root of a lung. Note that the posterior relation of the trachea is the esophagus and that the anterior relations of the thoracic part of the esophagus from above downward are: the trachea (throughout its entire length); the left recurrent laryngeal nerve (Fig. 1-84); the right and left bronchi; the inferior tracheobronchial lymph nodes; the pericardium (removed); and the diaphragm. (See Fig. 1-6 showing the grooves produced in the first rib by the subclavian vessels).

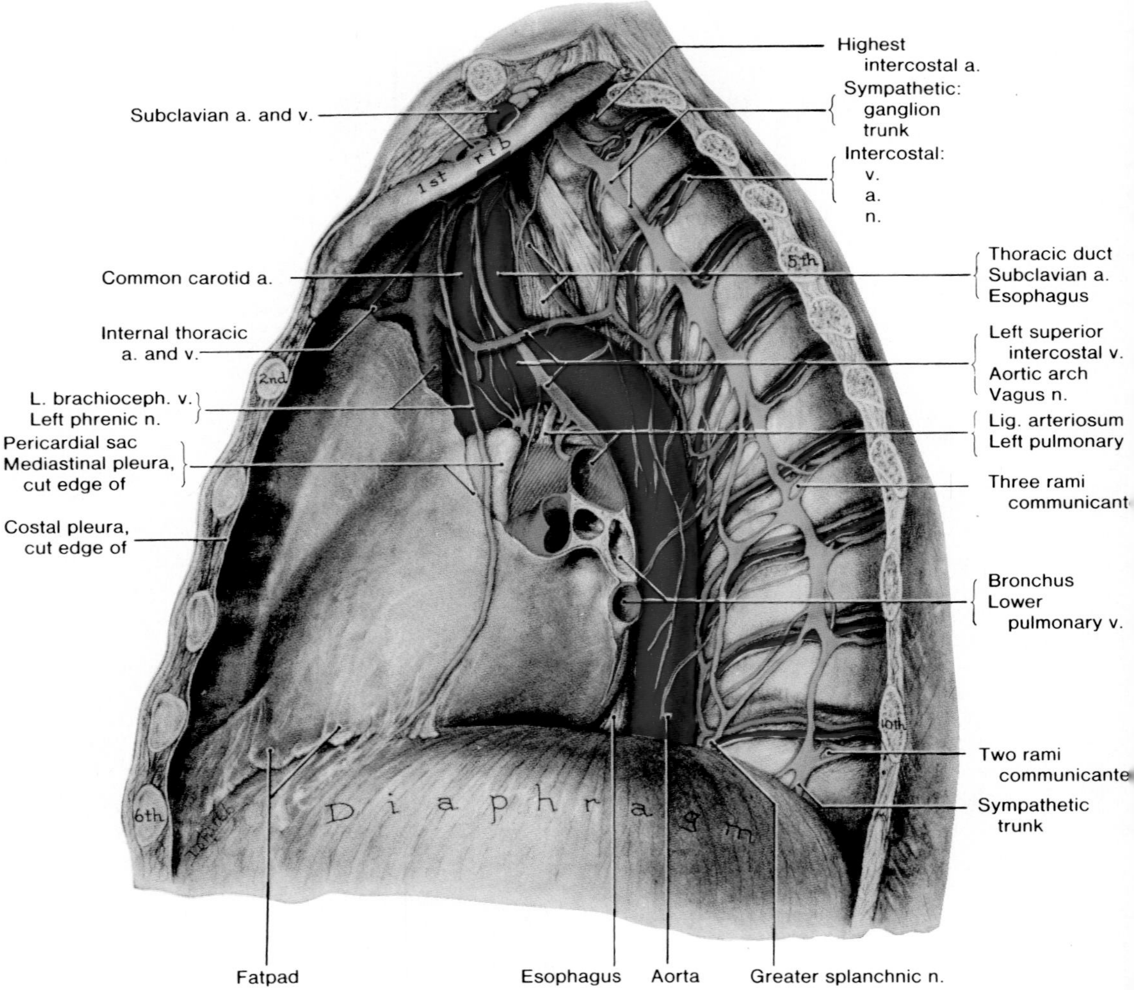

Figure 1-86. Drawing of a dissection of the left side of the mediastinum. The costal and mediastinal pleurae have mostly been removed to expose the underlying structures. Observe that the left side of the mediastinum is the "*red side*" and is dominated by the arch and the descending portion of the aorta, the left common carotid, and the subclavian arteries. Note that the phrenic nerve, freed by removal of the pleura, is passing in front of the root of the lung. Examine the thoracic duct on the side of the esophagus (also see Fig. 1-48). Note that the left vagus nerve on the side of the arteries passes behind the root of the lung sending its recurrent laryngeal branch around the ligamentum arteriosum (the adult derivative of the embryonic ductus arteriosus). Observe that the sympathetic trunk is attached to intercostal nerves by rami communicantes (also see Fig. 1-25).

carotid artery, and the left subclavian artery.

The brachiocephalic trunk is the first and largest of the three branches (Fig. 1-85). It arises from the aortic arch posterior to the center of the manubrium. Here it is anterior to the trachea and posterior to the left brachiocephalic vein (Fig. 1-82). It passes superolaterally to reach the right side of the trachea and the right sternoclavicular joint, where it divides into the right common carotid and right subclavian arteries (Fig. 1-85).

The left common carotid artery arises

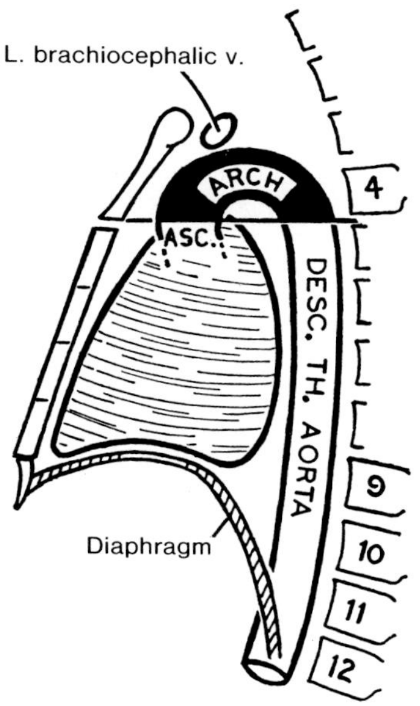

Figure 1-87. Diagram showing the relationships of the ascending aorta (*ASC*), aortic arch, and descending thoracic aorta.

from the aortic arch slightly behind and to the left of the brachiocephalic trunk (Fig. 1-82). It extends upward, anterior to the left subclavian artery, between the left pleura and the trachea. It is at first anterior to and then to the left of the trachea (Fig. 1-85). It enters the neck by passing behind the left sternoclavicular joint (Fig. 1-53).

The left subclavian artery arises from the posterior part of the aortic arch, close to the left common carotid artery (Fig. 1-82). It ascends through the superior mediastinum and lies against the left lung and pleura laterally. In the left lung of a cadaver, the left subclavian usually forms a distinct groove (Fig. 1-37). As it leaves the thorax and enters the root of the neck, it passes behind the left sternoclavicular joint (Fig. 1-53).

CLINICALLY ORIENTED COMMENTS

Because the great arteries and their branches are derived by transformation of the aortic arches of the embryonic branchial arches, abnormalities of them are common.

Several abnormalities of the aortic arch may develop (*e.g.*, double aortic arch and right aortic arch) and several variations in the origins of the branches of the aortic arch occur (Fig. 1-89). A **retroesophageal right subclavian artery** is not uncommon (Fig. 1-88). As it crosses posterior to the esophagus to reach the right upper limb, it may compress the esophagus and cause difficulty in swallowing **(dysphagia)**. In persons with a retroesophageal right subclavian artery, the right recurrent laryngeal nerve does not hook around the right subclavian artery but passes directly from the vagus to the laryngeal muscles.

A **patent ductus arteriosus** (Fig. 1-101) results from failure of the ductus arteriosus to close after birth and become the **ligamentum arteriosum.** It may occur as an isolated abnormality or in association with various heart defects.

Coarctation of the aorta (Fig. 1-99) is a congenital abnormality in which the aortic lumen is constricted, usually below the origin of the left subclavian artery. When the constriction is below the entrance of the ductus arteriosus, the **postductal type,** a collateral circulation develops between the proximal and distal parts of the aorta by way of the intercostal and internal thoracic arteries (Fig. 1-103).

The Vagus Nerves (Figs. 1-53, 1-72, and 1-82 to 1-84). The vagus nerves arise from the medulla of the brain (Fig. 8-20). The thoracic parts of the vagus nerves descend from the neck as posterolateral relations of the common carotid arteries. Each nerve enters the superior mediastinum posterior to the sternoclavicular joint and the brachiocephalic vein.

The right vagus nerve crosses anterior to the origin of the subclavian artery and posterior to the superior vena cava, to run posteroinferiorly on the right surface of the trachea. It divides posterior to the trachea into a number of branches that contribute to the **pulmonary plexuses** and to the **esophageal plexus.** A cardiac branch

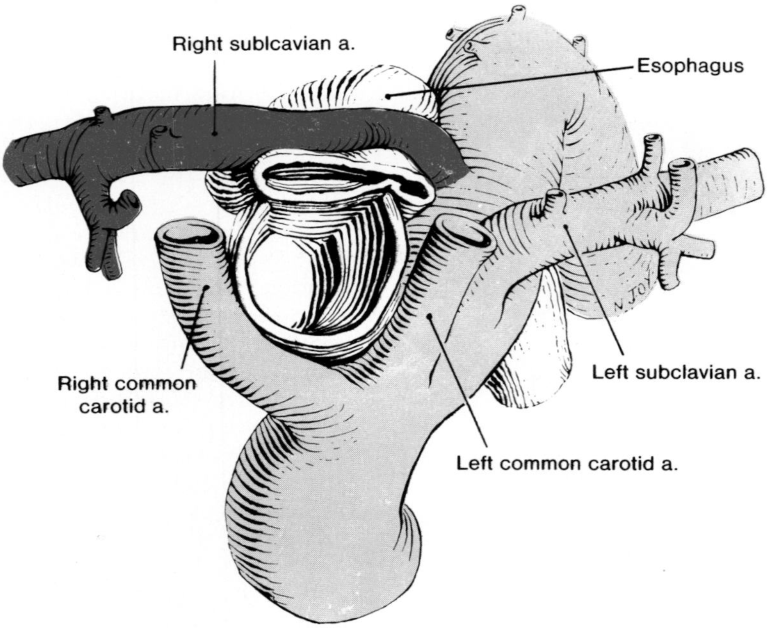

Figure 1-88. Drawing of a dissection of a retroesophageal right subclavian artery. Observe that the artery arises as the last branch of the aortic arch and passes behind the esophagus and trachea. The right recurrent laryngeal nerve (not shown), having no vessel around which to recur, takes a direct course to the larynx. This condition is found in about 1% of people.

arises from the right vagus to the right of the trachea and descends to the **cardiac plexus.** After passing anterior to the subclavian artery, it gives rise to the **right recurrent laryngeal nerve** (Fig. 1-72), which hooks around this artery and ascends into the neck between the trachea and the esophagus (Figs. 8-21 and 9-35).

The left vagus nerve descends from the neck posterior to the left common carotid artery, between it and the left subclavian artery (Fig. 1-82). It descends on the left side of the aortic arch, between the left common carotid and subclavian arteries, and is separated laterally from the phrenic nerve by the left superior intercostal vein (Fig. 1-86). It curves medially at the inferior border of the aortic arch and gives off the **left recurrent laryngeal nerve.** This nerve lies on the left surface of the ligamentum arteriosum and hooks below the aortic arch and ascends through the superior mediastinum in the groove between the trachea and the esophagus (Fig. 9-41). After giving off the left recurrent laryngeal nerve, the left vagus breaks up into the left pulmonary plexus, posterior to the left bronchus. At the lower border of the root of the lung, it emerges as one or more branches which form part of the esophageal plexus (Fig. 1-93).

The Phrenic Nerves (Figs. 1-53, 1-83, 1-86 and 1-102). Each nerve enters the thorax between the subclavian artery and the origin of the brachiocephalic vein. These important nerves are the *sole motor supply to the diaphragm.* They arise from the ventral rami of the third, fourth, and fifth cervical nerves.

The right phrenic nerve traverses the thorax posterolateral to the right brachiocephalic vein and superior vena cava (Fig. 1-82), and descends between the parietal pericardium and the mediastinal pleura. It passes anterior to the lung root and descends to the right of the inferior vena cava to the diaphragm, where it pierces it near the inferior vena caval opening (Fig. 1-34).

The left phrenic nerve descends between the left subclavian and the left com-

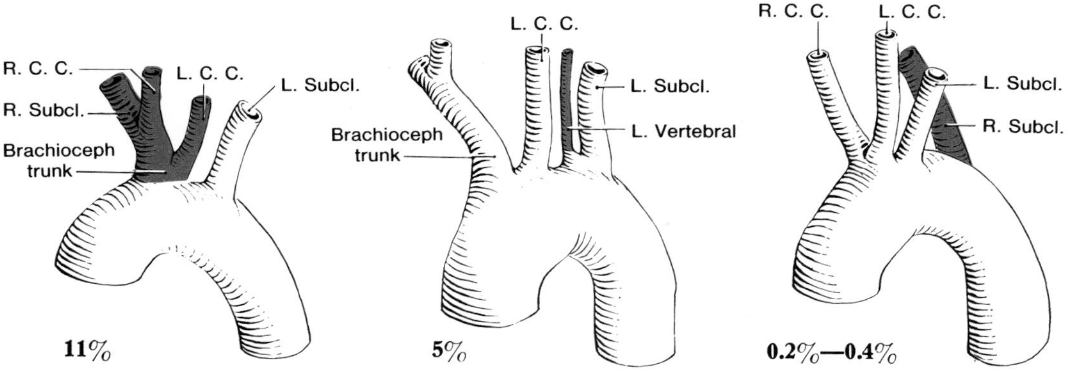

Figure 1-89. Drawings illustrating variations in the origins of the branches of the aortic arch. The approximate incidence of these variations is indicated.

mon carotid arteries and crosses the left surface of the aortic arch (Fig. 1-82). It courses along the pericardium, superficial to the left auricle and ventricle of the heart, and pierces the diaphragm just to the left of the pericardium (Fig. 1-34).

The Trachea (Figs. 1-35*A*, 1-53, and 1-80 to 1-85). The trachea (windpipe) is a wide tube that *begins in the neck* as the continuation of the lower end of the larynx. It descends in front of the esophagus and enters the superior mediastinum a little to the right of the midline, leaving the esophagus exposed on its left side. Its posterior surface is flat where it is applied to the esophagus (Fig. 1-83). It is kept patent by a series of C-shaped bars of cartilage. Its thoracic part is 5 to 6 cm long and ends at the level of the sternal angle by dividing into right and left principal bronchi. This is at the level of the spinous processes of the third and fourth thoracic vertebrae. Here, it lies a little to the right of the midline. During inspiration, the tracheal bifurcation descends to a slightly lower level.

The aortic arch is at first anterior to the trachea and then on its left side (Fig. 1-85). Superior to the aortic arch, the brachiocephalic trunk and the left common carotid artery are at first anterior and then on its right and left sides, respectively. These vessels separate the trachea from the left brachiocephalic vein (Fig. 1-82). The right surface of the trachea is covered with pleura, except where the left vagus and azygos vein intervene. The posterior surface of the trachea lies anterior and a little to the right of the esophagus and the left recurrent laryngeal nerve (Fig. 1-83), which sends branches to both the esophagus and the trachea.

The Esophagus (Figs. 1-34, 1-35*A*, 1-72, and 1-82 to 1-86). The esophagus (gullet) extends from the lower end of the pharynx at the level of the cricoid cartilage (sixth cervical vertebra) to the stomach at the level of the 10th thoracic vertebra. Thus it has cervical, thoracic, and abdominal parts. The esophagus enters the thorax and **superior mediastinum** between the trachea and the vertebral column (Fig. 1-83) and passes posterior to the left principal bronchus to enter the **posterior mediastinum.** It descends behind and to the right of the aortic arch and posterior to the pericardium and the left atrium. It then deviates to the left behind the posterior part of the diaphragm and anterior to the descending thoracic aorta.

The relations of the thoracic part of the esophagus may be summarized as follows.

Its **anterior relations** (Fig. 1-80) in the superior mediastinum are the trachea and the left recurrent laryngeal nerve. In the posterior mediastinum, its anterior relations are the left principal bronchus, the tracheobronchial lymph nodes (Fig. 1-85), the pericardium and left atrium, and finally the diaphragm.

Its **posterior relations** (Figs. 1-83 to 1-85) are the vertebral bodies of T1 to T4, the thoracic duct, the azygos vein, and some right intercostal arteries. At its lower end, the descending aorta lies between the esophagus and the vertebrae (Fig. 1-90).

Its **right side** is close to the mediastinal pleura and lung, except where it is crossed by the azygos vein (Figs. 1-84 and 1-90).

Its **left side** is close to the mediastinal pleura above the aortic arch, except where the thoracic duct and the left subclavian artery intervene. The aortic arch and the descending aorta lie to the left of the esophagus to the level of the seventh thoracic vertebra (Fig. 1-84).

The esophagus has **three "constrictions" in its thoracic part** which may be observed as narrowings of the lumen in oblique radiographs, taken as barium is being swallowed. The full esophagus is compressed by (1) the aortic arch, (2) the left principal bronchus, and (3) where it passes through the diaphragm (Fig. 2-34*A*). *Understand that there are no constrictions in the empty collapsed esophagus;* as the full esophagus expands, the above structures compress its walls. These "constrictions" disappear as the esophagus empties.

CLINICALLY ORIENTED COMMENTS

The impressions formed in the esophagus by the adjacent structures just mentioned are of clinical interest because they indicate where swallowed foreign objects are likely to lodge, and where strictures develop following the accidental drinking of caustic liquids (*e.g.*, lye) because of slower passage of substances through these regions. In addition, carcinoma (**cancer**) **of the esophagus** commonly occurs at its lower end, where it is constricted at the diaphragmatic opening (Fig. 2-34*A*).

The most common congenital abnormality involving the esophagus is **esophageal atresia** (blockage) associated with **tracheoesophageal fistula.** These malformations, occurring in about one in 2500 newborn infants, result from incomplete division of the foregut into respiratory and digestive portions. In the most common type, the upper portion of the esophagus ends as a blind pouch. A fistula (abnormal canal) connects the lower portion of the esophagus with the trachea. As the infant is unable to empty the esophagus downward, saliva and mucous secretions overflow into the larynx and some enters the trachea and bronchi in spite of incessant coughing. If attempts are made to feed the infant, the milk fills the esophageal pouch and then overflows into the trachea.

The Posterior Mediastinum (Fig. 1-49). The posterior mediastinum is the part of the mediastinum located *posterior to the fibrous pericardium,* below the fourth thoracic vertebra. Its lower part lies at a lower level than the anterior high part of the diaphragm, but the posterior mediastinum ends at the level of the posterior lowest part of this musculofascial sheet (Fig. 2-130).

The posterior mediastinum contains: (1) several **longitudinal tubular structures** (thoracic aorta, thoracic duct, azygos and hemiazygos veins, esophagus, and esophageal plexus); and (2) several **transverse tubular structures** (posterior intercostal arteries, thoracic duct as it passes from right to left, certain intercostal veins, and terminal parts of the hemiazygos veins).

The Thoracic Aorta (Figs. 1-48, 1-84 to 1-87, and 1-91). This large vessel is the continuation of the aortic arch. It begins on the left side of the fourth thoracic intervertebral disc and runs on the left sides of the vertebral bodies of T5 to T7 and commonly produces grooves in them. More inferiorly,

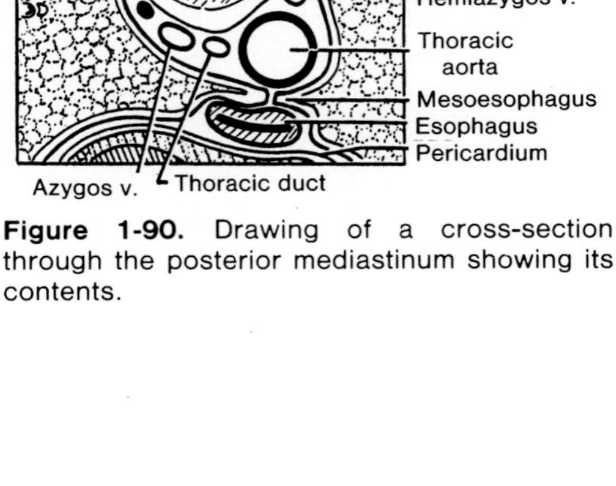

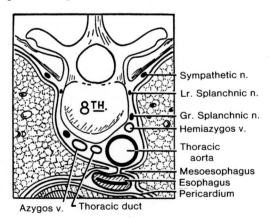

Figure 1-90. Drawing of a cross-section through the posterior mediastinum showing its contents.

it lies anterior to the vertebral bodies of T8 to T12. The aorta descends through the posterior mediastinum against the left pleura with the thoracic duct and the azygos vein to its right. At first it lies posterior to the root of the left lung and then posterior to the pericardium. The aorta enters the abdomen through the most posterior opening in the diaphragm, called the **aortic hiatus** (Figs. 1-48 and 2-130). The thoracic duct and azygos vein lie on its right posterolateral side and accompany it through this hiatus.

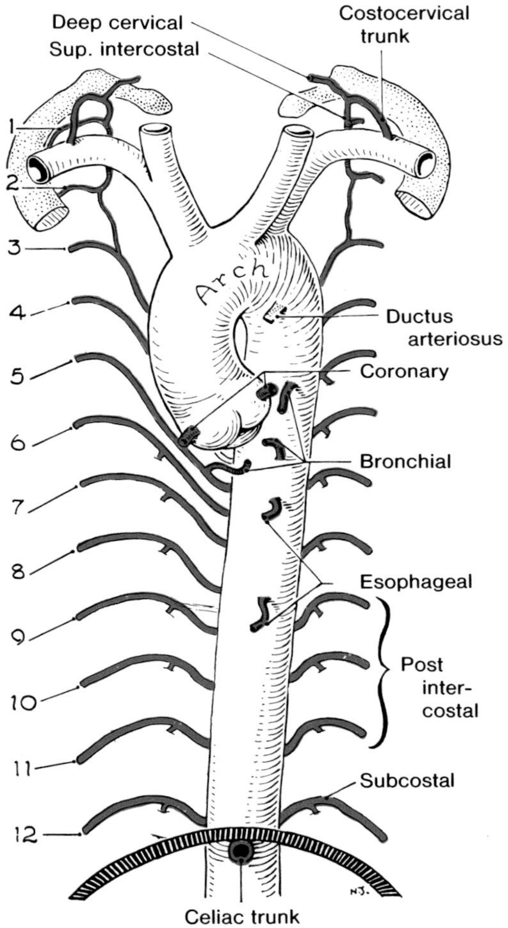

Figure 1-91. Drawing of the thoracic aorta and its branches. Observe that the right bronchial artery arises from either the upper left bronchial or the third right posterior intercostal artery (here the fifth) or the aorta directly. The small arteries to the pericardium, tissues in the posterior mediastinum, and the upper surface of the diaphragm are not shown.

The thoracic aorta gives off **bronchial arteries** to the lungs (Fig. 1-91), one or two esophageal branches, and sends twigs to the pericardium and the diaphragm. It also gives rise to all of the intercostal arteries (except the first two pairs) and one pair of subcostal arteries.

The Thoracic Duct (Figs. 1-34, 1-48, 1-80, 1-83, 1-84 to 1-86, 1-90, and 1-92). This is the **main lymphatic duct** which conveys most of the lymph of the body to the venous system. It drains the **cysterna chyli,** which lies in front of the 12th thoracic vertebra, posterior and to the right of the aorta. The thoracic duct passes superiorly from the cisterna chyli through the aortic hiatus, between the crura of the diaphragm on the right side of the aorta (Fig. 1-85). It reaches the right side of the esophagus and passes superiorly, anterior to the origins of the right posterior intercostal arteries. At about the level of the fifth thoracic vertebra, it deviates to the left, posterior to the esophagus and ascends through the superior mediastinum into the neck. It passes behind the carotid sheath in front of the vertebral artery, and *empties into the venous system at the union of the left internal jugular and subclavian veins* (Fig. 1-48).

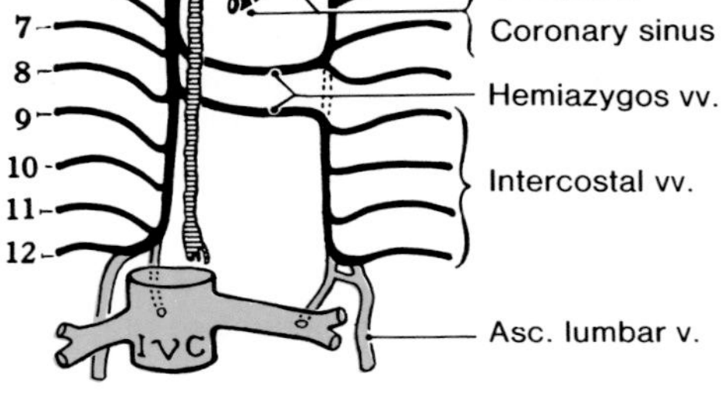

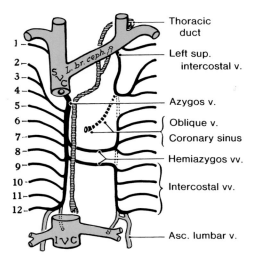

Figure 1-92. Diagram of the azygos system of veins. The thoracic duct and the intercostal veins are also illustrated.

CLINICALLY ORIENTED COMMENTS

If the thoracic duct is cut or torn during an accident, **chyle** escapes from it. This contains a considerable amount of fine fat droplets which gives it a milky appearance. Leakage of chyle may be prevented by tying off the duct. The lymph then returns to the venous system by other lymph channels which join the duct above the ligature. During digestion the thoracic duct is distended with chyle, a product of the small intestine (Fig. 2-103).

The Azygos and Hemiazygos Veins (Figs. 1-48, 1-85, 1-90, 1-92, and 1-93). These

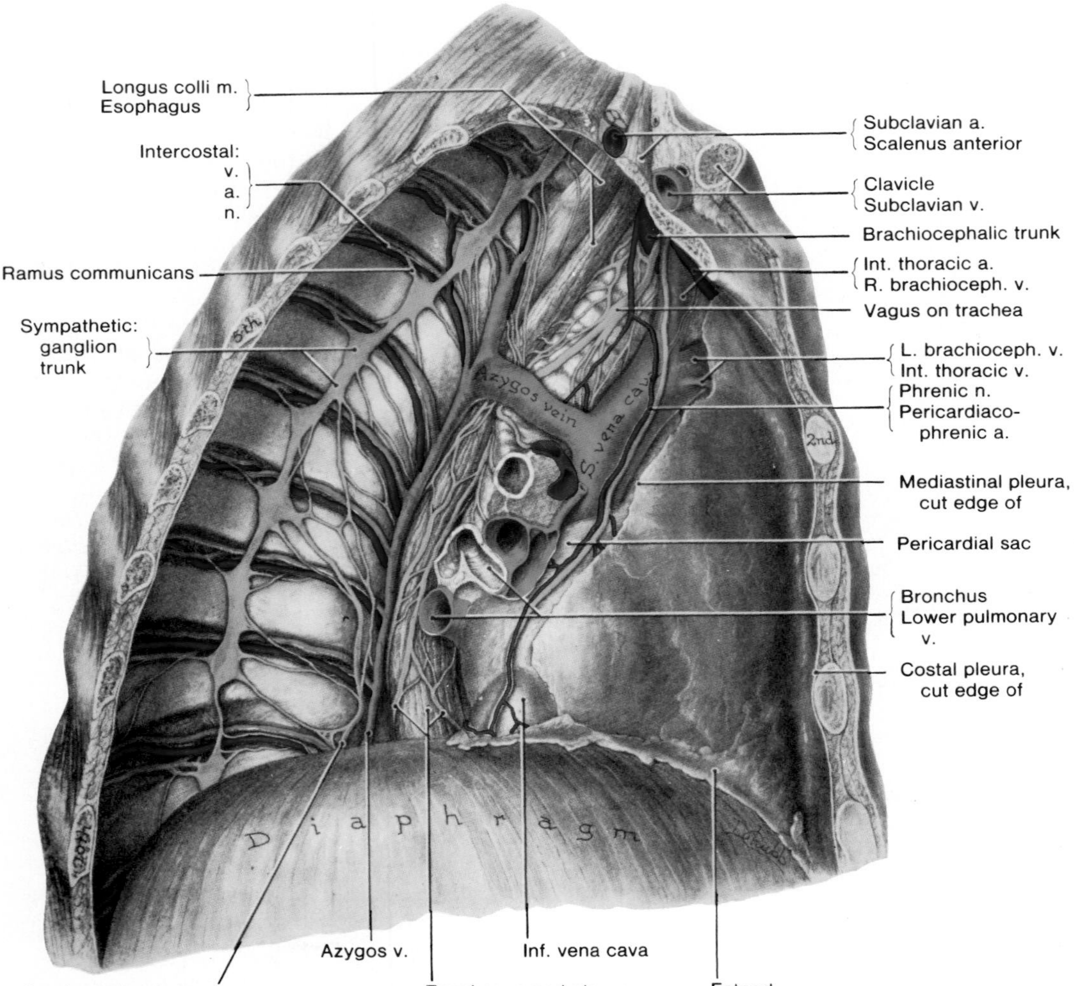

Figure 1-93. Drawing of a dissection of the right side of the mediastinum. Most of the costal and mediastinal pleurae has been removed, exposing the underlying structures. Observe that the right side of the mediastinum is the *blue* side and that it is dominated by the arch of the azygos vein, the superior vena cava, and the right atrium. Note that when the mediastinal pleura is removed, the phrenic nerve is free. Follow its medial relationships to the diaphragm. Observe that the right vagus nerve enters on the trachea, falls back upon the esophagus, and is medial to the azygos arch. Examine the sympathetic trunk and its ganglia, noting that this trunk is lying on the right side of the thoracic vertebral bodies, near their pedicles.

veins are the superior continuation of the ascending lumbar veins in the abdomen. The posterior intercostal veins drain into them and the hemiazygos veins on the left cross over and join the azygos vein on the right, which empties into the superior vena cava (Fig. 1-48).

The azygos vein arches over the root of the right lung (Fig. 1-72), after lying on the vertebrae posterior to the mediastinal pleura throughout its course. In addition to the posterior intercostal veins, the azygos receives the vertebral venous plexus (Fig. 5-64) and the mediastinal, esophageal, and bronchial veins. The azygos vein drains blood from the thoracic wall.

The inferior hemiazygos vein (Fig. 1-92) arises in the abdomen and enters the thorax through the left crus of the diaphragm. It drains the ascending lumbar vein and the inferior intercostal spaces. **The superior hemiazygos vein** drains intercostal spaces 4 to 8. Both these veins cross the midline and enter the azygos vein.

The Esophagus (Figs. 1-85 and 1-90). The relationships of the esophagus in the posterior mediastinum were described with the previous description of this structure. Briefly, it passes from the superior mediastinum and lies on the vertebral bodies down to T10, where it pierces the diaphragm. At its inferior end it lies to the left of the median plane. For a review of its relations in the posterior mediastinum, see Figure 1-90. *Fibers from the vagus nerves* spread out on the esophagus to form an **esophageal plexus** (Fig. 1-93).

The Anterior Mediastinum (Fig. 1-49). The anterior mediastinum is the part of the mediastinum that lies between the body of the sternum anteriorly and the fibrous pericardium posteriorly. This space is continuous with the superior mediastinum at the sternal angle and is limited inferiorly by the diaphragm. *The anterior mediastinum is very narrow above the level of the fourth costal cartilages* owing to the closeness of the right and left pleurae.

The anterior mediastinum contains some loose areolar tissue, fat, lymph vessels, two or three lymph nodes, the sternopericardial ligaments, and a few branches of the internal thoracic artery. In infants and children, the anterior mediastinum may also contain the lower part of the **thymus gland** (Figs. 1-80 and 1-81), which may extend as far inferiorly as the fourth costal cartilages.

JOINTS OF THE THORAX

These joints permit movement of the ribs and the sternum during respiration.

THE COSTOVERTEBRAL JOINTS

Typically the head of a rib articulates with the sides of the bodies of two vertebrae, and the tubercle of a rib articulates with the tip of a transverse process. Hence, there are two articulations of the ribs with the vertebral column. They are the *plane type of synovial joint* which allows gliding movements.

Joints of the Heads of Ribs (Figs. 1-3, 1-4, and 1-94). The head of each typical rib articulates with the demifacets of two adjacent vertebrae and the intervertebral disc between them. The crest of the head is attached to the intervertebral disc by an **intra-articular ligament** which is located within the joint and divides it into two synovial cavities.

An **articular capsule** surrounds each joint and connects the head of the rib with the circumferences of these cavities. The capsule is strongest anteriorly where the **radiate ligament** fans out from the anterior margin of the head of the rib to the sides of the bodies of the two vertebrae and the disc between them.

There are exceptions to this general arrangement just described. The heads of the first and of the last three ribs articulate only with their own vertebral bodies.

The heads of the ribs are connected so closely to the bodies of the vertebrae by ligaments that only slight gliding and rotatory movements occur at the joints of the heads of the ribs.

The Costotransverse Joints (Figs. 1-24, 1-94, and 1-95). The tubercle of a typical rib articulates with the facet at the tip of the transverse process of its own vertebra (Fig. 1-3*B*) to form a synovial joint. These small joints are surrounded by a thin **artic-**

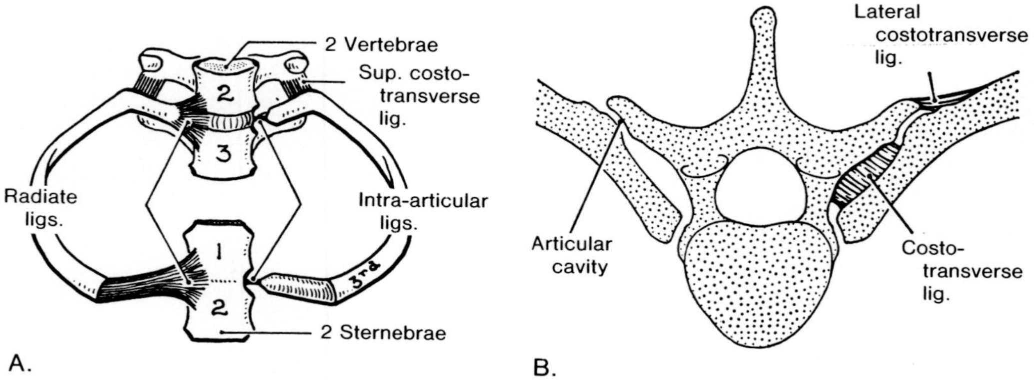

Figure 1-94. Drawings illustrating the costovertebral joints. *A*, compares the articulation at the posterior and anterior ends of a rib and its costal cartilage. *B*, illustrates a costotransverse articulation.

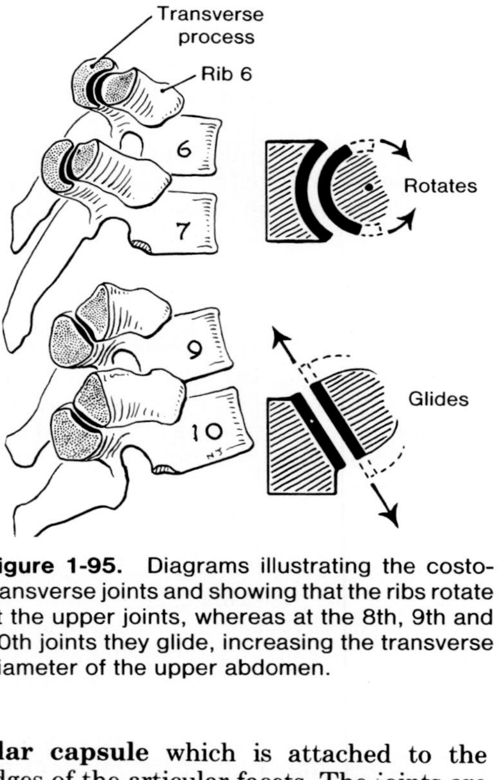

Figure 1-95. Diagrams illustrating the costotransverse joints and showing that the ribs rotate at the upper joints, whereas at the 8th, 9th and 10th joints they glide, increasing the transverse diameter of the upper abdomen.

ular capsule which is attached to the edges of the articular facets. The joints are strengthened on each side by a **lateral costotransverse ligament,** passing from the tubercle of the rib to the tip of the transverse process. In addition, a costotransverse ligament unites the back of the neck of the rib to the anterior surface of the transverse process, and a **superior costotransverse ligament** joins the crest of the neck of the rib to the transverse process above. The aperture between this latter ligament and the vertebral column permits passage of the spinal nerve and the dorsal branch of the intercostal artery.

The last two ribs do not articulate with the transverse process and have freer movement as a result. The strong ligaments binding the costotransverse joints limit their movements to slight gliding (Fig. 1-95). However, the articular surfaces on the tubercles of the upper six ribs are convex and fit into concavities on the transverse processes; hence, some upward and downward movements of the tubercles are associated with rotation of the rib.

THE STERNOCOSTAL JOINTS

Usually seven costal cartilages on each side articulate with the lateral margins of the sternum (Figs. 1-1, 1-10, 1-94, and 1-96). The **first pair of costal cartilages** is directly united to the manubrium by a **synchondrosis** (*i.e.*, united by cartilage).

The **second** to **seventh costal cartilages** articulate with the sternum at **synovial joints,** but the joint cavities are often absent in the lower ones. The thin **articular capsules** of all these joints are strengthened anteriorly and posteriorly by the **radiate sternocostal ligaments,** which pass from the costal cartilages to the anterior and posterior surfaces of the sternum. The joint cavity associated with the second rib is usually divided into two cavities by an intra-articular sternocostal ligament. Some of the other joints may also be double.

THE INTERCHONDRAL JOINTS

These *plane synovial joints* are between the cartilages of the sixth to the ninth ribs (Fig. 1-96). Each of these articulations is enclosed within a fibrous capsule that is lined with a synovial membrane. The joints are strengthened by interchondral ligaments. The joint between the ninth and tenth costal cartilages is united by a fibrous joint.

THE COSTOCHONDRAL JOINTS

Each rib has a cup or pit at its anterior end into which the costal cartilage fits and fuses with the rib (Figs. 1-1 and 1-4). This junction is enclosed by periosteum. No movement occurs at these joints.

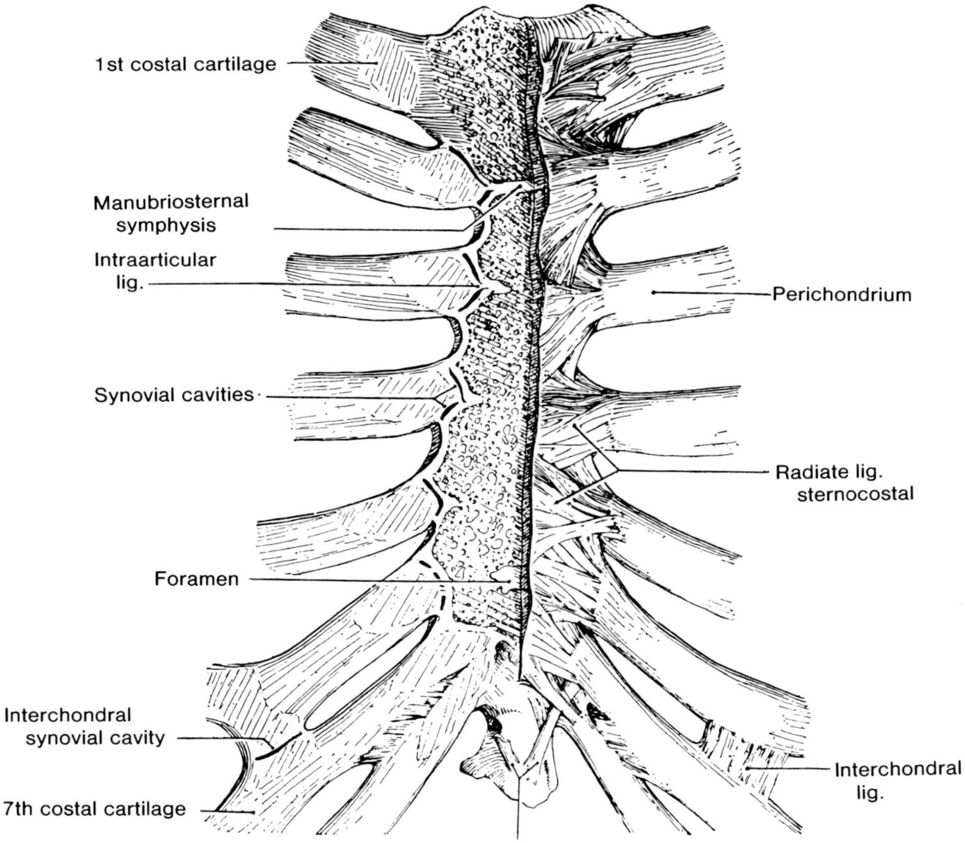

Figure 1-96. Drawing illustrating an anterior view of the sternocostal and interchondral joints. The cortex of the right half of the sternum and of the right costal cartilages has been shaved away. To obtain a specimen of bone marrow, a sternal puncture is made through the thin cortical bone into the area of spongy bone. On the left side, the dissection shows that the fibers of the perichondrium terminate as sternocostal radiate ligaments. Three types of joint are demonstrated here: (1) synchondroses between the first costal cartilages and the manubrium and between the seventh costal cartilage and the sternum (in this case); (2) a symphysis at the manubriosternal joint; and (3) synovial joints at the other sternocostal joints and the interchondral joints. The manubriosternal articulation is at first a synchrondrosis and later a symphysis. (These terms are explained in the *Introduction*; see types of joints).

THE STERNAL JOINTS

The Manubriosternal Joint (Figs. 1-10 and 1-96). This joint is between the manubrium and the body of the sternum and is usually a **symphysis.** The articulating surfaces of these bones are covered by hyaline cartilage and are united by a disc of fibrocartilage. In about 30% of people, the central part of the disc undergoes absorption forming a cavity. The joint is strengthened by anterior and posterior fibers from the periosteum. In most people the manubriosternal joint moves during respiration, but in some people (especially old persons) the manubrium is united to the body of the sternum by bone (Fig. 1-9*C*) and no movement occurs.

The Xiphisternal Joint (Figs. 1-10 and 1-96). This joint is between the xiphoid process and the body of the sternum and is a **symphysis.** This cartilaginous joint usually ossifies after the 40th year and fuses with the body of the sternum, *i.e.*, it becomes a **synostosis** (Fig. 1-9*C*).

PATIENT ORIENTED PROBLEMS

Case 1-1. While having a heated argument with a client, a 48-year-old male lawyer experienced a sudden, heavy, *crushing pain* in his chest (**substernal pain**) and epigastrium that radiated along the medial aspect of his left arm. The client helped him to the chesterfield where the lawyer attempted to relieve the pain by squirming, stretching, and belching. When his secretary noted he was pale, perspiring, and writhing in pain, she called his doctor and an ambulance.

The ambulance attendants administered oxygen and rushed him to the hospital. In view of the patient's history and severe signs of shock, the doctor had the patient taken to the **intensive care unit**, where he was placed under observation with **ECG** monitoring for detection of potential fatal **arrhythmias** (irregularities of the heart rhythm). The patient's blood pressure was low (a sign of shock).

On questioning, the resident learned that the patient had had previous attacks of substernal discomfort (heaviness and pressure) during activity, which he was reluctant to describe as pain. As this discomfort always passed when he rested, he had not complained of it. The resident taking the history recognized these symptoms as a clinical syndrome known as **angina pectoris**, a symptom of **ischemic heart disease** (inadequate perfusion of a portion of the myocardium).

When the resident asked the patient to describe his present chest pain, he said that it was the worst pain he had ever felt and clenched his fist to demonstrate the vise-like nature of the squeezing pain. He said that when the pain struck, he had a feeling of weakness and nausea.

On **auscultation** the resident detected an occasional arrhythmia and the ECG was abnormal. A diagnosis of **acute myocardial infarction** owing to **coronary insufficiency** caused by **coronary atherosclerosis** was made.

Problems. Define acute myocardial infarction and coronary atherosclerosis. Discuss **anastomoses of the coronary arteries** and extracardiac anastomoses and their role in perfusion of the myocardium during slow narrowing (**stenosis**) of a coronary artery. Explain anatomically the referral of the pain from the heart to the left side of the chest, left shoulder, and medial aspect of the arm (**visceral referred pain**). *These problems are discussed on page 111.*

Case 1-2. A 58-year-old man who had lived in an industrial area of Toronto all his life consulted his doctor because he was occasionally coughing up blood (**hemoptysis**) and was having shortness of breath on exertion (**dyspnea on exertion**).

On questioning it was learned that he had been a heavy cigarette smoker for over 40 years and had had a **smoker's cough** for several years. He stated that his cough had been getting worse for the last few months and so had his shortness of breath. He first noticed that his **sputum was blood-streaked** about 3 weeks ago and stated that he experienced vague chest pain on the left side at that time.

Physical examination revealed that his left medial **supraclavicular lymph nodes** (often referred to clinically as prescalene or scalene nodes) were slightly enlarged and more firm than usual. The breath sounds and resonance were diminished on the left side compared with the right side.

The doctor requested chest films. The radiologist reported that there was **obscuration of the left hilum** of the lung by a mass and/or enlargement of the hilum. The normal left mediastinal contours above the hilum could not be recognized, and there was slight radiolucency of the remainder of the left lung. The mediastinum was shifted slightly to the left. He believed that a part of the left lung, at least the upper segments of the upper lobe, were collapsed (**atelectasis**), and this was most likely caused by a tumor in the left upper lobe bronchus with **metastases to the left hilar lymph nodes**.

On examination of the interior of the principal (main) bronchi under local anesthesia with a bronchoscope, the **otolaryngologist** (a physician who specializes in diseases of the ear, nose, and throat) observed a growth obstructing the origin of the left superior lobe bronchus (Fig. 1-42). Through the **bronchoscope** he obtained a biopsy of the tumor. The enlarged supraclavicular lymph nodes were also biopsied for microscopic examination. The pathologist reported **bronchogenic carcinoma** in the bronchial biopsy, but the cervical lymph nodes did not show definite tumor involvement.

Examination of the mediastinum through a suprasternal incision under local anesthesia (**mediastinoscopy**) revealed some enlarged lymph nodes. Through the **mediastinoscope**, the surgeon removed pieces of tissue (biopsies) from the nodes. The pathologist reported that these nodes showed the presence of many tumor cells, a sign that spread (**metastasis**) of the tumor beyond the primary growth had occurred.

In view of the clear evidence of metastases to the lymph nodes, it was decided that the tumor was inoperable; thus, surgical removal of the lung (**pneumonectomy**) was not done.

Problems. Bronchogenic carcinoma (cancer) metastasizes through the lymph (**lymphogenous metastasis**) and the blood (**hematogenous metastasis**). Using your knowledge of the anatomical relations of the lungs, state which structures are likely to be involved by direct extension of a malignant tumor (neoplasm) of the bronchus. Where would you expect tumor cells to spread via the lymph and the blood? What is unusual about the lymph drainage of the left inferior lobe of the lung? Explain the probable anatomical basis for metastasis of tumor cells to the brain. *These problems are discussed on page 112.*

Case 1-3. During an argument with his wife, a 44-year-old inebriated man was *stabbed with a paring knife*, the blade of which was 9 cm long. The knife, penetrating the fourth intercostal space along the left sternal border, produced little external bleeding. By the time he was taken to the emergency room of the hospital, the patient was semiconscious, in shock, and gasping for breath. In a few moments he became unconscious and died.

Problems. Using your knowledge of surface anatomy, what organ(s) would you expect to be punctured by the knife? Where would the blood accumulate? Speculate on the cause of death resulting from the knife wound. *These problems are discussed on page 113.*

Case 1-4. A short thin man with spindly limbs (**gracile habitus**), 42 years of age, complained about recent difficulties in breathing during exercise (**exertional dyspnea**) and fatigue. He stated that other than being physically underdeveloped, he had been well most of his life (**asymptomatic**), until the last year or so when he had had several respiratory infections.

Physical examination revealed a prominent right ventricular cardiac impulse. A moderately loud **midsystolic murmur** (sound caused by turbulent blood flow) was heard over the second and third intercostal spaces along the lower left sternal border.

Radiographs revealed enlargement of the right side of the heart, especially of the outflow tract of the right ventricle, a **small aortic knob** (prominence caused by the aortic arch), **dilation of the pulmonary artery** and its major branches, and increased pulmonary vascular markings. The **ECG** showed changes suggestive of right ventricular hypertrophy.

During **right cardiac catheterization**, the catheter easily passed from the right atrium into the left atrium at about the center of the interatrial septum. Serial samples of blood for determination of oxygen saturation were taken as the catheter was withdrawn from the left atrium into the right atrium and then into the inferior vena cava. These studies revealed **increased oxygen saturation of the right atrial blood** compared with blood in the inferior vena cava. Serial determinations of pressures showed unequal pressures in the atria (slightly higher in the left atrium).

A diagnosis of **atrial septal defect (ASD)** was made. It was classified as the secundum type of defect, the most common type of ASD, with **left atrium to right atrium shunt** of blood.

Problems. Was this man likely born with this defect in his interatrial septum: *i.e.*, **is this a congenital defect?** Where else may defects occur in the interatrial septum? What additional complications do you think might occur in this patient in view of the left to right shunt of blood? Differentiate between ASD and probe patent foramen ovale. *These problems are discussed on page 114.*

Case 1-5. During the routine physical examination of a 15-year-old girl for summer camp, a continuous "**machinery-like" murmur** was heard during auscultation at the second intercostal space near the left sternal edge. On palpation, a continuous thrill (vibration) was felt at the same location. Other physical findings were normal.

Radiographs of the chest revealed *slight left ventricular enlargement* and slight prominence of the pulmonary artery and the aortic knob. An ECG indicated a moderate degree of left ventricular hypertrophy.

On questioning, the girl recalled that she had once been told by a doctor that she had a **heart murmur** but that it was nothing to worry about. She said she had always been well, although she feels that she gets "out of breath" faster than other girls during sports.

Following consultation with her parents and the cardiologist, the family physician decided to conduct further investigations. **Angiocardiography** (radiological study of the heart and great vessels following intracardiac injection of a radiopaque medium) was performed. The radiologist passed a **heart catheter** (a long narrow radiopaque tube) via the femoral vein and inferior vena cava into her right atrium, right ventricle, and pulmonary artery. As he continued, the catheter passed to the left, upward, and backward. A small injection of contrast showed the tip of the catheter to be in the descending thoracic aorta. The catheter was drawn back to the right atrium and a **right angiocardiogram** performed which showed an essentially normal right heart. Another catheter was passed via the femoral artery into the ascending aorta and contrast medium injected into it (**aortography**). The ascending aorta and aortic arch appeared normal, but the left and right pulmonary arteries were opacified, as well as the descending thoracic aorta. The radiologist concluded that there was left to right shunting of blood through a **patent ductus arteriosus**.

Problems. Discuss the location of the ductus arteriosus and its embryological origin, prenatal function, and postnatal closure. What caused the characteristic "machinery-like" murmur and the left ventricular enlargement? How do you think this left to right shunting of blood could be stopped surgically? Based on your anatomical knowledge, what clinical condition do you think might cause **right to left shunting of blood** through the ductus arteriosus. *These problems are discussed on page 115.*

Case 1-6. A healthy 16-month-old boy was "helping" his mother clean up the morning after a cocktail party when he *suddenly started to choke and cough.* Thinking he must have something in his throat, she put her finger in his pharynx but was unable to find anything. As he was now coughing, she held him upside down by his feet and jerked him. Although he seemed to be somewhat better after this, it was not long before he began coughing again. When she observed that he was having difficulty breathing (**dyspnea**), she called her pediatrician who arranged to meet her at the hospital. When asked what the child had been eating when he began to choke, the mother replied, "Nothing! But he could have picked up something that had been dropped onto the floor such as an hors d'oeuvre or a peanut."

On first examination it was obvious that the child was in **respiratory distress** which was characterized by coughing and difficult breathing (**dyspnea**). On subsequent examination, the pediatrician noted limited movement of the right side of the chest. **Auscultation** disclosed reduced breath sounds over the right lung anteriorly and posteriorly. On **percussion** he thought there was slight hyperresonance over the right lung. He requested **fluoroscopic examination of the thorax** and inspiration and expiration chest films.

The radiologist reported that there was *overinflation (hyperinflation) of the middle and inferior lobes of the right lung, with a shift of the heart and mediastinal structures to the left* which decreased on inspiration. In view of these observations, the radiologist suggested that there was likely a **foreign body** lodged in the right intermediate bronchus, inferior to the origin of the superior (upper) lobe bronchus (Fig. 1-42).

Under general anesthesia, the interior of the tracheobronchial tree was examined using an electrically lighted instrument called a **bronchoscope**. A peanut was observed in the right principal bronchus at the site suggested by the radiologist. The **bronchoscopist** removed the peanut with some difficulty, using forceps passed through the bronchoscope. After waking up, the patient breathed better and fluoroscopy showed that both lungs were inflating and deflating normally.

Speaking to the mother later, the pediatrician urged her to keep small objects out of the reach of her child. He explained that inhalation of nuts, beans, and dry watermelon seeds was particularly harmful because they rapidly swell to several times their usual size, causing **bronchial obstruction**.

When asked for details about this condition, the pediatrician made simple sketches (Fig. 1-97) showing how some air can usually go into the lung because the bronchus expands during expiration; however, because the caliber of the bronchus becomes less during expiration, the bronchial wall closes on the peanut, trapping the air distal to it. Thus, the peanut acts like a **check valve** (Fig. 1-97*B*) and the lung beyond the foreign body becomes overinflated with air. He further explained that aspiration of certain materials such as peanuts may cause both a local and a systemic reaction. The *overinflation of a sizeable portion of a lung* may be progressive and compress the rest of the lung and even the other lung (by displacement of the mediastinum) to the point of **respiratory failure** and death. In other cases, the peanut swells and completely obstructs the bronchus, producing **atelectasis** (collapse) of the lung distal to the peanut. In addition, peanuts release substances that induce a **chemical bronchitis** (inflammation of the bronchus) and **pneumonitis** (arachnitic pneumonia).

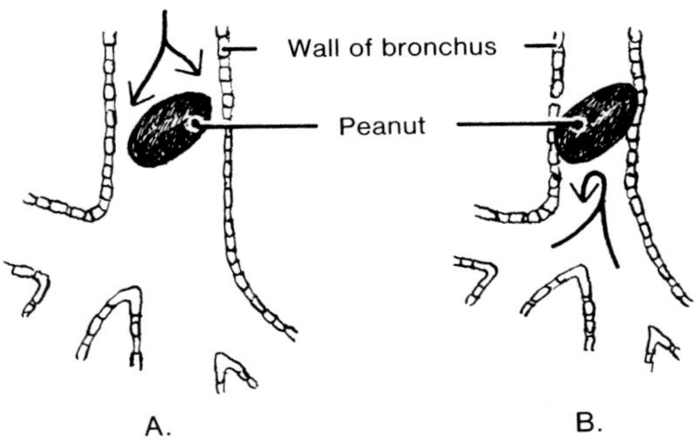

Figure 1-97. Diagram illustrating bronchial obstruction and the check valve action of the peanut. *A*, the bronchus expands during inspiration allowing some air to pass around the peanut into the lung. *B*, the bronchus contracts during expiration preventing little if any air to leave the lung.

Problems. When foreign bodies are aspirated, the right lung is involved more often than the left (3:1). What is the anatomical basis for foreign bodies usually going into the right principal bronchus and involving the middle and inferior lobes of the right lung? If the peanut had not been removed in the present case, the right middle and inferior lobes of the child's lung would later have collapsed (**obstructive atelectasis**). Explain why the lung collapses. What would be the appearance of the atelectatic lobes in a radiograph? What effect would atelectasis have on the position of the heart, other mediastinal structures, and the diaphragm? *These problems are discussed on page 116.*

Case 1-7. A 10-year-old girl, wrapped in a blanket, was carried into the outpatient department by her father. The nurse immediately ushered them into an examining room and called a doctor. As the nurse prepared the child for a physical examination, she observed that the child was shivering (**chills**) and was holding the right side of her chest. She noted that her respirations were rapid (**tachypnea**) but shallow. She had a hacking cough and brought up sputum containing some blood-tinged mucous material. Her temperature was 41.5°C and her pulse rate was 115.

During questioning the doctor learned that the child had had a really bad cold (**upper respiratory tract infection**) for about a week. The mother said that she did not become worried about her child until she developed a chill and a fever with a hacking cough and chest pain.

On percussion of the thorax, the doctor noted dullness over the right lower posterior region of the child's chest. **On auscultation** of her thorax, he noted suppression of breath sounds on the right side and a **pleural rub** (friction caused by rubbing of the inflamed pleurae together).

When asked to describe the pain, the patient said it was a **sharp**, **stabbing pain** that became worse when she breathed in deeply, coughed, or sneezed. When asked where she first felt pain, she placed her hand over her lower chest. When asked where else she experienced pain, she pointed to her umbilical area and to her lower neck and shoulder on the right side. The doctor requested a complete blood count, a sputum culture, and chest films in both prone and upright positions. He told the nurse that he wanted these investigations STAT (L. *statum*, at once).

The patient's white cell count was elevated (**leukocytosis**) and *pneumococci* in large numbers were seen in the sputum. The radiographs revealed an area of consolidation (**airless lung**) in the posterior part of the base of the right lung. There was also a slight shift of the heart and mediastinal structures to the right side.

A diagnosis of **pleurisy** or pleuritis (inflammation of the pleurae) caused by pneumococcal pneumonia or **pneumonitis** (inflammation of the lungs) was made.

Problems. What is the function of the pleurae? Using your knowledge of the nerve supply to the pleurae, explain the referral of pain to the right side of the chest, the periumbilical area, and the right shoulder. Irritation of what abdominal structure causes a similar referral of pain? Explain why a slight shift of the heart and mediastinal structures occurs with pneumonitis. *These problems are discussed on page 117.*

Case 1-8. An anxious mother informed her doctor that recently her 11-month-old infant had been having sudden attacks of shortness of breath (**paroxysmal dyspneic attacks**). She stated that on these occasions he became very restless and turned blue (**cyanosis**) when he gasped for air. She said that these "blue spells," lasting for several minutes, usually followed crying, and then the baby goes to sleep. On close questioning, she revealed that she first oberved these attacks when her son was learning to walk. He would try very hard for a while and then squat down. Also, he would play actively for a short time and then sit or lie down. She said that she did not become concerned about this until *she noticed him turning blue.* She wondered if he was holding his breath or if his lungs were poorly developed.

During the physical examination, the infant began to cry very hard. Gradually, cyanosis developed in the mucous membranes of his lips and mouth and in his fingernails and toenails. Soon his entire skin surface had a dusky, bluish color.

When the mother was able to calm the baby, the doctor continued his examination and noted that the sclerae of his eyes were gray and that the blood vessels at the periphery of his eyes were engorged, giving an appearance of mild **conjunctivitis** (inflammation of the conjunctiva). The blood vessels of the retina were large and dark. He also observed some early **clubbing** (broadening and thickening) of the ends of his fingers and toes, a sign of **arteriovenous shunting**. The baby's pulse was normal, as were his arterial and venous pressures. On auscultation a loud **systolic murmur** was heard over the heart, particularly at the left sternal border.

Radiographic examination of the chest revealed that the hilar areas of the infant's lungs were relatively small and the lungs were very clear. The boot-shaped heart (*coeur en sabot*) was normal-sized, but there was some elevation of the cardiac apex and a concavity in the region of the pulmonary artery. An **ECG** indicated **right ventricular hypertrophy** and right axis deviation.

Cardiac catheterization revealed systolic hypertension in the right ventricle, low pressure in the pulmonary artery, and a sudden change from low to high pressure as the catheter was withdrawn through the pulmonary valve region. These findings indicated obstruction to the right ventricular outflow (**pulmonary stenosis**).

Angiocardiography showed that some of the contrast material injected into the right ventricle passed into the left ventricle, just below the narrow conus arteriosus of the right ventricle. This indicated the presence of a membranous VSD (**ventricular septal defect**). A diagnosis of **tetralogy of Fallot** was made (Fig. 1-98). Although this condition is compatible with life, surgical correction of the defects later in childhood was strongly advised because, without surgery, most patients die by age 20.

Problems. Name the fourth component of the congenital malformation known as tetralogy of Fallot which was not mentioned in the case presentation. Which observation made during **cardiac catheterization** gives a clue to the presence of this defect? Why does cyanosis occur? Give the probable reason for the delay in the development of cyanosis. What is the embryological basis of Fallot's tetralogy? *These problems are discussed on page 117.*

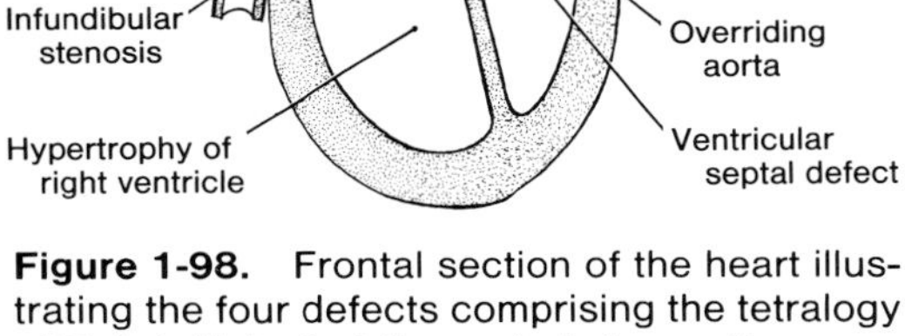

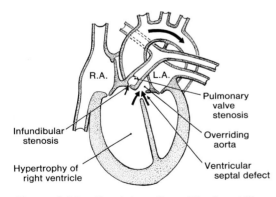

Figure 1-98. Frontal section of the heart illustrating the four defects comprising the tetralogy of Fallot. Note that the aorta is larger than normal and that the pulmonary artery is smaller than normal.

Case 1-9. During the routine examination of the cardiovascular system of one of his classmates as part of a course in clinical (physical) diagnosis, a medical student was surprised to find that his classmate's **femoral pulses** were weak. Believing his technique for taking these pulses was incorrect, he palpated pulsations in the popliteal, posterior tibial, and dorsalis pedis arteries (Chap. 4). As the pulse in these arteries was also weak, he asked his clinical instructor to check his findings. The instructor informed him that his conclusions were correct and suggested that he palpate the femoral and radial pulses simultaneously. When he did this, he found that the femoral pulse appeared later than the radial pulse. He said to his instructor, "I thought that the femoral pulse should appear slightly ahead of the radial pulse." The instructor answered, "You're right. Smith must have a **cardiovascular abnormality**. Check the blood pressure in his arms and legs."

Using his **sphygmomanometer** (instrument for determining blood pressure), he found a considerable elevation of blood pressure in his classmate's brachial (arm) arteries (**hypertension**) and a low pressure in his popliteal arteries (**hypotension**). When he reported these findings, his clinical instructor examined his classmate's heart. On **percussion** he thought that the left ventricle was slightly enlarged. On **auscultation**, he detected a slight systolic **murmur** (vibratory noise) over the student's heart and over his interscapular area, particularly near the medial border of his left scapula. The clinical instructor recommended that the hypertensive student consult a cardiovascular specialist about his blood pressure abnormalities.

On questioning, the student informed the internist that he frequently had **throbbing**

headaches, dizziness (**vertigo**), and nosebleeds (**epistaxis**). The previous findings were confirmed during a thorough physical examination, with emphasis on the cardiovascular system. In addition, pulsations were palpable in the interscapular area and on each side of his sternum along the course of the internal thoracic artery. The internist requested **cardiac fluoroscopy**, chest films, and later an **aortogram** (x-ray study of the aorta after injection of contrast medium).

The radiologist reported that the patient's heart was moderately enlarged owing to left ventricular prominence and that the **aortic knob** was clearly visible. He also reported *notching of the inferior borders of the third to seventh ribs.* He stated that when the patient swallowed barium sulphate emulsion during **fluoroscopy**, the esophagus showed the normal indentations at the levels of the transverse part of the aortic arch and the left main bronchus.

To obtain a clear view of the aorta, the radiologist passed an **arterial catheter** into the patient's axillary artery and guided it with the aid of fluoroscopy into the ascending part of the aortic arch. A series of radiographs was made as a bolus of radiopaque contrast material was injected. The films revealed constriction or **coarctation of the aorta** of severe degree (Fig. 1-99),

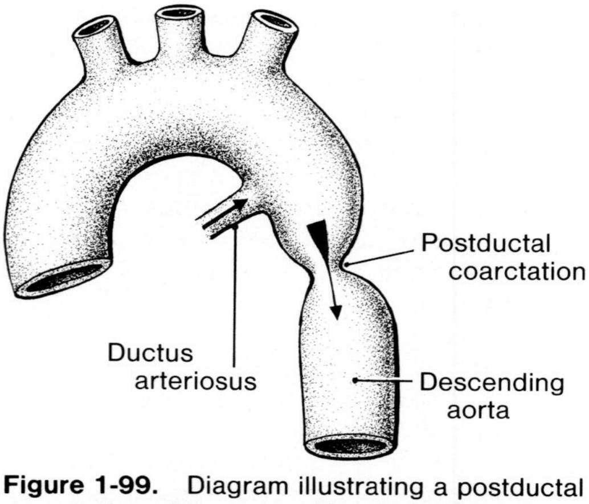

Figure 1-99. Diagram illustrating a postductal coarctation of the aorta. The ductus arteriosus constricts at birth and usually closes in a few days. By the end of the third month, it becomes the ligamentum arteriosum. In uncommon types of coarctation, the ductus arteriosus remains patent.

distal to both the left subclavian artery and the **ligamentum arteriosum**. The aortic arch and its branches showed little or no enlargement, but a well developed collateral circulation was visualized. The internal thoracic arteries were large and tortuous, as were the subscapular and those posterior intercostal arteries that were visible on the radiographs.

The patient was scheduled for **surgical resection of the coarcted segment** of aorta. The results of the operation were good.

Problems. State the probable cause (etiology) of coarctation of the aorta. Discuss the development of **collateral circulation** in this case and explain why the femoral pulse appeared later than the radial pulse. What is the cause of the **notching of the ribs** observed in the chest films? *These problems are discussed on page 118.*

Case 1-10. During a lengthy trip in a car, a 38-year-old woman experienced a pressing **substernal discomfort**, pain in her right chest, and breathlessness (**dyspnea**). She said that she felt sick to her stomach (**nausea**) and that she was going to faint (**syncope**). Believing she may have been having a heart attack, her husband drove her to the closest hospital.

On physical examination, about an hour after the onset of her symptoms, the doctor observed evidence of shock and rapid breathing (**tachypnea**). He also noted swollen, tender veins, particularly in her right thigh and calf in the area drained by the great saphenous vein (Chap. 4), signs and symptoms of **thrombophlebitis**. On questioning he learned that she had painful **varicose veins** in her legs for some time and that they became very painful during her recent long car ride. He also learned that she had been taking birth control pills for about 9 years.

Examination of her lungs revealed a few small, moist **atelectatic rales** (transitory, light cracking sounds) in the right side of her chest. **Auscultation** also revealed a pleural rub on the right side (friction caused by rubbing of inflamed pleurae together).

On cardiac examination the doctor detected **tachycardia** (rapid beating of the heart) and arrhythmia. Her **ECG** suggested some right heart strain. Chest radiographs showed some increase in radiolucency of the right lung.

Fluoroscopy of the lungs revealed poor or absent pulsations in the descending branch of the right pulmonary artery and relative anemia of the right lung which was consistent with the clinical impression of **pulmonary thromboembolism (PTE)**.

Photoscans (scintigrams) were obtained after intravenous injection of radioactive iodinated (^{131}I) human albumin microparticles. The image produced on the **gamma camera** showed practically *no pulmonary blood flow in the right lung*.

To determine the exact site and size of the thrombus, the internist requested **pulmonary angiography**. Radiopaque contrast material, injected into the right ventricle of the heart, revealed a **filling defect** in the right main pulmonary artery at its bifurcation in the right hilum. The left pulmonary artery and its branches were grossly normal.

As the patient was in such critical condition and considered in danger of an **embolus** to the remaining lung, it was felt that immediate prophylactic, life-saving surgery was absolutely necessary. Consequently, surgical *venous interruption* was performed to prevent recurrence of PTE by **plication of the inferior vena cava** (narrowing of the lumen by clips or suture material) below the renal veins.

Problems. Thinking anatomically, how do you think the radiologist injected the contrast material into the right ventricle of the heart? What probably caused the patient's severe substernal discomfort and shoulder pain? Following plication of the patient's inferior vena cava, how was adequate venous drainage of the patient's lower limbs accomplished? *These problems are discussed on page 119.*

DISCUSSION OF PATIENT ORIENTED PROBLEMS

Case 1-1. Acute myocardial infarction is a disease of heart muscle (myocardium), characterized by **necrosis** (death) of ventricular muscle that results from sudden occlusion of a part of the coronary circulation. *This results in dysfunction of the heart as a pump.* If a large branch of a coronary artery is involved, the infarcted area may be so extensive that cardiac function is severely disrupted and death occurs. Myocardial infarction may also result from **excessive exertion** (*e.g.*, running to catch a train) in a person with stenotic (narrowed) coronary arteries. The straining heart muscle is using more oxygen than the stenotic arteries can supply; as a result, the tissue becomes **anoxic** (without oxygen) and soon dies (undergoes necrosis).

The sudden blocking (occlusion) of a coronary artery by an **embolus** composed of a detached clot or its more gradual obstruction by arterial disease or **thrombosis** is a common cause of death in persons 45 years and over. If obstruction of a coronary artery is incomplete, the patient often suffers from **angina pectoris**, a typical substernal pain that is initiated by exertion (*e.g.*, jogging or coitus).

Coronary atherosclerosis (lipid deposits located in the intima of the first 3 to 5 cm of a coronary artery) usually begins early in life and gross evidence of this condition is almost always present in persons over 45 years of age. An **atheroma** is a lipid deposit that produces a swelling on the endothelial surface of the blood vessel. Ulceration of the atheroma results in the release of **atheromatous debris** that is carried along the coronary artery until it reaches the stenotic or narrow part, usually where the vessel bifurcates (divides), and then it stops. Because it blocks the vessel (one type of **coronary embolus**), no blood can pass to the myocardium; thus, myocardial infarction occurs unless a good collateral circulation has developed previously.

Arteriolar anastomoses exist between the terminations of the right and left coronary arteries in the atrioventricular groove and between the interventricular branches around the apex in about 10% of apparently normal hearts (Fig. 1-78). Thus, an important factor in determining whether or not **ischemic heart disease** develops during coronary atherosclerosis is the presence or absence of these anastomoses. The potential for the development of this collateral circulation probably exists in most if not all hearts. In very slow occlusion of a coronary branch, the **collateral circulation** has time to increase so that there will be adequate perfusion of the myocardium and infarction usually does not result. However, when there is sudden blockage of a large coronary branch, some degree of **myocardial infarction** results, but the extent of the area damaged very likely depends on the degree of development of collateral channels that has occurred previously.

If large branches of both coronary arteries are obstructed, there is an **extracardiac collateral circulation** that may be utilized to supply blood to the heart. These collaterals connect the coronary arteries with the **vasa vasorum** in the tunica adventitia of the aorta and pulmonary arteries and with branches of the internal thoracic, bronchial, and phrenic arteries. However, unless these collaterals have dilated in response to pre-existent **ischemic heart disease**, they are unlikely to be able to supply sufficient blood to the heart to prevent myocardial infarction.

The dominant symptom of myocardial infarction is **deep visceral pain**. Afferent pain fibers from the heart run centrally to the middle and inferior cervical branches and the thoracic branches of the sympathetic trunk of the upper thorax and neck. Axons of these primary sensory neurons enter spinal cord segments T1 to T4 or T5 on the left side. Pain of cardiac origin is therefore referred to the left side of the chest and along the inner aspect of the arm and upper forearm (Fig. 1-73*A*), as these are the areas of the body which send sensory impulses to the same segments of the spinal cord that receive cardiac sensation (Fig. 1-29). Radiation of visceral pain to cutaneous areas is called "**referred pain**."

Case 1-2. In view of the anatomical relations of the lungs, some cancers of this organ extend directly into the chest wall, the diaphragm, or the mediastinum and its contents. Involvement of a phrenic nerve in the mediastinum results in **paralysis of half of the diaphragm**. Direct infiltration of the pleura produces **pleural effusion** (escape of fluid from the pleural blood and lymphatic vessels) into the pleural cavity. This exudate may be **sanguineous** (bloody) and may contain exfoliated malignant cells.

Because of the close relationship of the **recurrent laryngeal nerves** to the apices of the lungs, they may be involved in cancer of the lung and produce hoarseness by paralyzing the vocal folds. The left recurrent laryngeal nerve passes around the arch of the aorta to the left of the **ligamentum arteriosum**, the adult derivative of the ductus arteriosus, and then passes superiorly. Although more superior, the right recurrent laryngeal nerve passes around the right subclavian artery and is closely related to the apex of the right lung and the cervical pleura (Fig. 1-72).

If **tumors of the apices of the lungs** invade locally, there may be involvement of the upper thoracic nerves, the thoracic sympathetic chain, and the stellate ganglion. If this occurs, there is likely to be pain in the shoulder and axilla and signs of **Horner syndrome** (**ptosis**, drooping eyelid; **miosis**, pupillary constriction; **anhidrosis**, absence of sweating; and slight **enophthalmos**, recession of the eyeball).

Involvement of the hilar and mediastinal lymph nodes occurs by **lymphogenous dissemination**. The lymph vessels of the lungs originate in superficial (pleural) and deep plexuses (accompanying small blood vessels) (Fig. 1-45). Lymph then drains into **bronchopulmonary lymph nodes** in the hilum (Fig. 1-47), which are often referred to clinically as hilar nodes. As these nodes enlarge, they increase the size of the hilum giving it a lumpy appearance.

The bronchopulmonary lymph nodes drain into inferior and superior groups of tracheobronchial nodes that lie in the angles between the trachea and the bronchi (Fig. 1-72). They form part of the mediastinal group of lymph nodes that are scattered throughout the mediastinum. Clinically, the inferior group of **tracheobronchial nodes** are commonly referred to as *carinal nodes* becomes of their relationship to the **carina** (L., the keel of a boat), the ridge separating the right and left principal bronchi at their junction with the trachea. Splaying and fixation of the carina may be associated with **cancer of a bronchus** when it has metastasized to the carinal nodes. These abnormalities can be seen bronchoscopically and radiologically. Enlarged mediastinal lymph nodes may indent the esophagus and be observed radiologically as the patient swallows a barium sulfate emulsion.

As lymph from vessels in the costal parietal pleura reaches the **parasternal lymph nodes** (Fig. 1-20) via intercostal lymph vessels, lymphogenous metastatic spread of cancer may involve these nodes also. *Lymph from the entire right lung drains into tracheobronchial nodes on the right* side and most lymph from the left lung drains into nodes on the left side, but some lymph from the inferior lobe of the left lung also drains into nodes on the right side. Thus, tumor cells in tracheobronchial lymph nodes on the right side may have spread by lymphogenous dissemination from the left inferior lobe.

Two large lymph trunks, the right and left **bronchomediastinal trunks**, drain lymph from the thoracic viscera and lymph nodes. The right bronchomediastinal trunk may join the **right lymphatic duct** and the left trunk may join the thoracic duct (Fig. 1-48), but more commonly they open independently into the *junction of the internal jugular and subclavian veins* of their own side.

Thus, lymph from the lungs and pleurae containing tumor cells soon enters the venous system and the heart. After passing through the pulmonary circulation, the blood returns to the heart for distribution to the body. Common sites of hematogenous metastasis from bronchogenic carcinoma are the brain, bones, lungs, and adrenal glands.

Often the medial **supraclavicular lymph nodes**, particularly on the left side, are enlarged and hard because they are tumorous (contain malignant cells) when there is carcinoma of the bronchus, stomach, or occasionally other abdominal organs. For this reason, these lymph nodes are often referred to as **sentinel nodes** because enlargement of them alerts the examiner to the possibility of malignant disease from the thoracic and/or abdominal organs.

The anatomical basis for involvement of these nodes is that lymph passes cranially from the thoracic and abdominal viscera via the bronchomediastinal trunks and the **thoracic duct** to reach the venous system (Fig. 1-48). Backflow of lymph from the thoracic duct can pass into the deep supraclavicular nodes, posterior to the sternocleidomastoid muscles. This is probably the reason why nodes on the left side are most commonly involved.

The brain is a common site for hematogenous spread of **bronchogenic carcinoma**. Tumor cells probably enter the blood through the wall of a capillary or venule in the lung and are transported to the brain via the internal carotid artery and vertebral artery systems (Fig. 7-90). Once in the brain the tumor cells probably pass between the endothelial cells of the capillaries and enter the brain.

Although *most cancer cells from the lung are likely transported to the brain via the arterial system*, others may be carried by the venous system. It has been suggested that the constant coughing and **enlarged mediastinal lymph nodes** compress the superior and inferior venae cavae, causing the blood draining the bronchi to reverse its flow and pass via the bronchial veins into the azygos venous system (Fig. 1-92). The **azygos system of veins** drains primarily the thoracic wall. From here, blood and tumor cells pass to the **extradural vertebral plexus of veins** around the spinal dura mater (Fig. 5-64). As this plexus communicates with the **cranial venous sinuses**, tumor cells can be transported to the brain when the patient is lying down because, in this position, the normal negative pressure in the cranial dural venous sinuses becomes equal to the pressure in the vertebral plexus of veins. From the dural venous sinuses the tumor cells pass into the cerebral veins and through their walls into the brain where they establish secondary tumors (**metastases**).

The passage of tumor cells to the veins of the vertebral column also explains the frequency of metastases of tumor cells to vertebrae.

Case 1-3. The knife, entering the fourth intercostal space at the left sternal border (Fig. 1-39*A*), did not penetrate the left lung because of the **cardiac notch** in its sternal border which begins at the fourth costal cartilage. The knife nicked the parietal layer of pleura of the left lung and then passed through the **infundibulum** of the right ventricle and the **aortic vestibule** of the left ventricle, immediately below the aortic orifice (Fig. 1-100).

Blood passed from the wounds in both ventricles into the **pericardial sac**. As blood accumulated in the pericardial cavity, severe compression of the heart (**cardiac tamponade**) and great veins occurred. This pressure increased until it exceeded the pressure in these large veins, thus preventing normal venous return to the heart and outflow of blood from the heart to the lungs and to the systemic circulation. This explains the patient's shock and gasping for breath prior to his death.

Case 1-4. ASD is definitely a congenital abnormality because it is an imperfection in the interatrial septum that developed during embryonic life; thus, it was present at birth (L. *congenitus*, born with). *The common form of ASD is the secundum type* ASD, so classified because it results from abnormal development of the foramen ovale and the septum secundum. The septum primum and the septum secundum normally fuse in such a way that no opening remains between the right and left atrium.

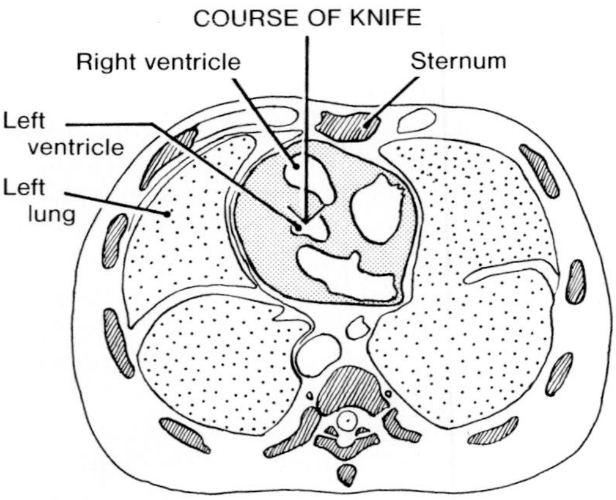

Figure 1-100. Transverse section of the thorax showing the course taken by the knife (*arrow*), passing to the left of the sternum and entering the upper part of the right ventricle and then the left ventricle.

The site of the prenatal opening is represented by the **fossa ovalis** of the adult heart (Fig. 1-61).

Secundum type ASD is more common in females (2:1); the reason for this is not known. The defect is in the region of the fossa ovalis in the right atrium. The ASD probably resulted from an abnormally short valve of the foramen ovale and/or an unusually large foramen ovale (Fig. 1-62).

Primum type ASD, associated with failure of closure of the foramen primum, is next in frequency. The foramen primum is normally a temporary interatrial opening between the growing margins of the septum primum and the endocardial cushions of the embryonic heart. Defects high in the interatrial septum, called the **sinus venosus type ASD**, are uncommon and are associated with incomplete absorption of the right horn of the sinus venosus into the right atrium.

In the present case, the **left to right shunt occurs** because left atrial pressure exceeds that in the right during the major part of the cardiac cycle. *Some of the patient's blood, therefore, makes two circuits through the lungs.* As a result of this shunting, the workload of the right ventricle is increased; thus, its muscular wall hypertrophies. *The cavities of the right atrium, right ventricle, and pulmonary artery are dilated to accomodate the excess amount of blood in them.*

Despite the increase in pulmonary blood flow, most ASD patients are asymptomatic in early life, although there may be some physical underdevelopment, as in the present case. Beyond the fourth decade, many patients develop **pulmonary arterial hypertension** and usually complain of fatigue and dyspnea on exertion. The cause of the pulmonary hypertension is not settled to everyone's satisfaction.

During the first 40 years, a majority of ASD patients have a moderate to good exercise tolerance, despite the fact that the opening in the interatrial septum is 2 to 4 cm in diameter (Fig. 1-62*B*). Usually patients with ASDs do not exhibit **cyanosis** (dark bluish coloration of the skin owing to deficient oxygenation of the blood).

Pulmonary vascular disease (arteriosclerosis) is likely to develop with increased pulmonary artery pressure, particularly if recurrent respiratory infections occur. Severe pulmonary hypertension may eventually result in higher pressure in the right atrium than in the left, reversing the shunt and causing cyanosis, severe disability, and heart failure. In view of the **pulmonary vascular disease** apparent in the present case, the defect would not likely be surgically repaired.

ASD should not be confused with a **patent foramen ovale** resulting from failure of the foramen ovale to close anatomically after birth. The foramen ovale is normally closed functionally at or shortly after birth. In 75 to 80% of normal hearts, the closure is permanent. Anatomical closure results from tissue proliferation and adhesion of the septum primum (valve of the foramen ovale) to the left margin of the septum secundum. The lower edge of the septum secundum forms a rounded fold, the **limbus fossa ovalis** (Fig. 1-61). Even if anatomical closure fails to occur, blood cannot be shunted from the left atrium to the right atrium because of the valvular mechanism of the **probe patent foramen ovale**. A shunt may occur, however, if there are fenestrations (openings) in the valve.

In up to 25% of persons, complete anatomical closure fails to occur; as a result, a potential slit-like opening remains. An isolated **probe patent foramen ovale** is of no clinical significance, as the higher pressure in the left atrium keeps it closed and the defect is not considered to be a pathological occurrence. However, if associated with **pulmonary stenosis** (narrowing of the pulmonary valve) or pulmonary hypertension owing to disease of the lungs (*e.g.*, **emphysema**), the valve may be forced open because of the higher pressure on its right side resulting in a right to left shunt and cyanosis, the consequence of deoxygenated blood getting into the left atrium, *i.e.*, into the systemic arterial flow.

Case 1-5. The **ductus arteriosus** is a fetal vessel that *connects the left pulmonary artery to the aortic arch*, just distal to the origin of the left subclavian artery (Fig. 1-101). Embryologically, the ductus arteriosus *represents persistence of the portion of the left sixth embryonic aortic arch* that joins the left pulmonary artery to the dorsal aorta. At birth the ductus may be equal or larger in diameter than either the pulmonary artery or the aorta.

The **antenatal function of the ductus** is to allow most of the blood in the left pulmonary artery to bypass the uninflated lungs. Because of the relatively high pulmonary vascular resistance to blood flow through the uninflated lungs and the relatively low resistance in the embryonic thoracic and abdominal aorta and umbilical arteries, blood easily flows from the pulmonary artery into the aortic arch and the descending thoracic aorta. The shunting of

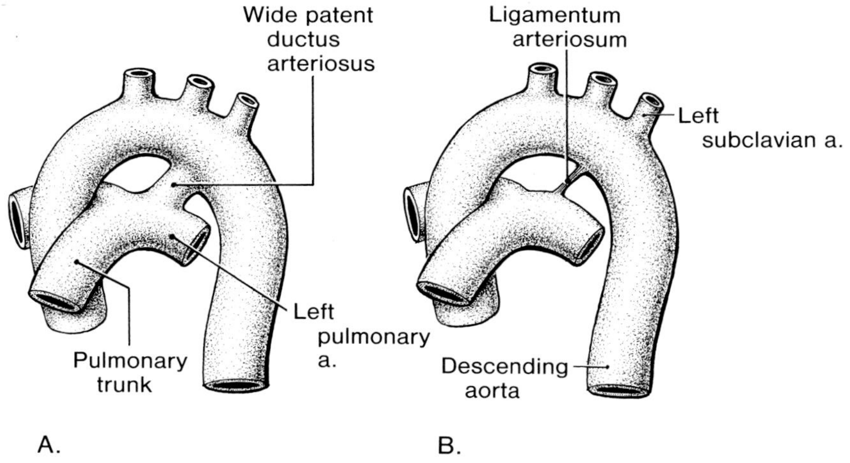

Figure 1-101. Diagram showing *A*, patent ductus arteriosus and *B*, ligamentum arteriosum, the adult derivative of the ductus arteriosus.

blood in this way provides a more direct route for oxygenation of the fetal blood via the umbilical arteries to the placenta.

The ductus arteriosus does not close completely immediately after birth. It may either remain patent or close intermittently for several hours or days. Anatomical closure may take up to 6 weeks. Early functional closure results primarily from contraction of the musculature of the ductus, probably caused by the sudden increase in arterial oxygen tension resulting from inflation of the lungs after birth. Closure of the ductus arteriosus appears to be mediated by **bradykinin**, a substance released from the lungs during the early postnatal period.

Persistent **patency of the ductus arteriosus** after birth is a relatively common congenital cardiac abnormality, occurring about once in every 3,000 births, more often in females than in males. It is the most common malformation associated with **maternal rubella** (German measles) infection during early pregnancy. Although this malformation occurs more frequently as an isolated abnormality, it may coexist with other malformations (*e.g.*, **coarctation of the aorta**).

The typical continuous loud " **machinery-like**" murmur results from turbulent flow of blood from a high pressure vessel (aorta) to a low pressure vessel (pulmonary artery) via the ductus arteriosus. As the pressure gradient exists during both systole and diastole, the murmur is continuous. The left to right shunt increases the workload of the left ventricle. As a result, it enlarges and its walls thicken. The left atrium may also enlarge owing to the increased volume of blood returning from the lungs.

Although a patent ductus arteriosus may result in **cardiac failure** and pulmonary edema in the premature infant, its presence is compatible with survival until adult life in most cases. However, as the leading cause of death in adults with this malformation is cardiac failure and/or **bacterial endocarditis** (inflammation of the endocardium of the heart and its valves and great vessels), ligation or division of the ductus arteriosus is commonly performed.

If severe **pulmonary vascular disease** (arteriosclerosis) develops in a patient with a patent ductus arteriosus, the high pulmonary vascular resistance results in an increase in pressure in the right ventricle and pulmonary artery, causing a reversal of blood flow through the ductus (*i.e.*, right to left). Consequently, unoxygenated blood is shunted from the left pulmonary artery into the aortic arch and descending thoracic aorta. As the ductus enters the aortic arch distal to the origin of the left subclavian artery, the toes (but not the fingers) become **cyanotic** (bluish owing to oxygen deficiency) and **clubbed** (broadened and thickened). The finding of cyanosis in the toes, but not in the fingers, is referred to as **differential cyanosis**.

Case 1-6. As the right principal bronchus is wider, shorter, and more vertical than the left (because the trachea is displaced a little to the right by the arch of the aorta, Fig. 1-84), foreign bodies more frequently pass into the right than into the left principal bronchus. Foreign bodies that are commonly found are nuts, hardware, pins, crayons, and dental material (*e.g.*, part of a tooth).

The right middle and inferior lobes of the right lung are usually involved because (1) the right inferior lobe bronchus is in line with the right principal bronchus (Figs. 1-44 and 1-46), which is almost in line with the trachea, and (2) the foreign body often lodges in the inferior lobe bronchus, above the origin of the middle lobe bronchus.

When there is complete obstruction of a principal bronchus, the entire lung eventually collapses, becoming a nonaerated (atelectatic) lung. Airlessness of the lung(s) owing to failure of expansion, as in the newborn, or absorption of air from the alveoli (collapse), as in the present case, is called **atelectasis**. Collapse of the lung occurs when the gas (air, *i.e.*, oxygen and nitrogen) in the trapped part of the lung is absorbed over the next few hours into the blood perfusing the lung. Depending on the site of obstruction, collapse may involve an entire lung, a lobe, or a **bronchopulmonary segment**. Because the collapsed lung is of soft tissue density, atelectatic lungs, lobes, or segments appear as homogeneous dense shadows on radiographs, in contrast to normal air-filled lung which is relatively lucent and appears dark on films.

When atelectasis of a sizeable segment of lung occurs, the heart and mediastinum are drawn toward the obstructed side and remain there during inspiration and expiration. The diaphragm on the normal side moves normally, whereas on the opposite side it moves much less.

Case 1-7. The **pleurae** (visceral pleura and parietal pleura) are continuous with each other around and below the root of the lung (Fig. 1-32). Normally, these layers are in contact during all phases of respiration. The potential space between them, known as the pleural cavity, contains a capillary film of fluid; thus, the visceral pleura normally slides smoothly on the parietal pleura during respiration, facilitating movement of the lung. When the pleurae are inflamed (**pleuritis**), the pleural surfaces become rough and the rubbing of their surfaces produces friction which is audible as a **pleural rub** (friction rub) during auscultation. Occasionally vibrations produced by rubbing of these roughened pleurae (**fremitus**) can be felt with the hand.

The pleural cavity is not usually visible on radiographs, but when air, fluid, pus, or blood collect between the visceral and parietal layers of pleura, the pleural cavity becomes apparent. If the inflammatory process in the present case had not been treated, an effusion or exudation of serum would have occurred from the blood vessels supplying the pleura. This **pleural exudate** collects in the pleural cavity and is visible on radiographs as a more or less homogeneous density that obscures the normal markings of the lung. Large **pleural effusions** are associated with a shift of the heart and mediastinal structures to the opposite side.

If the inflamed pleurae become infected, pus accumulates in the pleural cavity (**empyema**). A small empyema may be drained by **thoracentesis** during which a wide bore needle is inserted posteriorly through the seventh intercostal space, along the superior border of the eighth rib. *The insertion of the needle close to the superior border of the rib avoids injury to the intercostal nerves and vessels* (Fig. 1-28).

The parietal pleura, particularly its costal part, is very sensitive to pain, whereas the pulmonary pleura is insensitive. Afferent fibers from pain endings in the **costal pleura** and the pleura on the peripheral part of the diaphragm are conveyed through the thoracic wall as fine twigs of the **intercostal nerves**. Irritation of these nerve endings by rubbing of the inflamed pleurae together, particularly during inspiration, produces stabbing pain. Similarly, laughing or coughing may produce paroxysms of pain. The **parietal referred pain** is felt in the thoracic and abdominal walls, the areas of skin innervated by the intercostal nerves. Pain around the umbilicus is explained by the fact that the 10th intercostal nerve supplies the band of skin which includes the umbilicus (Fig. 1-29).

The mediastinal pleura and the pleura on the central part of the diaphragm are supplied by sensory fibers from the phrenic nerve (C3 to C5). Irritation of these areas of pleura, as in the present case, stimulates the nerve endings in the pleura, resulting in pain being referred to the lower part of the neck and over the shoulder. These areas of skin are supplied by the **supraclavicular nerves** (C3, C4) from two of the same segments of the spinal cord that give origin to the phrenic nerve.

Disease of the liver or gall bladder may also irritate the peritoneum covering the diaphragm. The resulting pain is felt in the lower chest if it originates in the periphery of the diaphragm because this area of peritoneum, like the **costal pleura** and the pleura on the peripheral part of the diaphragm, is supplied by sensory fibers from the lower **intercostal nerves** (Fig. 1-102). However, if the central area of the diaphragm is affected, the pain is referred to the shoulder and the lower neck because the peritoneum and pleura related to the central part of the diaphragm are supplied by sensory branches of the phrenic nerves.

The heart and mediastinal structures shift to the affected side in **pneumonitis**, occupying the space created by the slight loss of volume of the consolidated lung tissue resulting from the loss of air from alveoli. If **pleural effusion** or **empyema** occurs, the heart and mediastinal structures are pushed toward the opposite side by the accumulated serum or pus, respectively.

Case 1-8. The fourth component of the tetralogy of Fallot, not named in the case

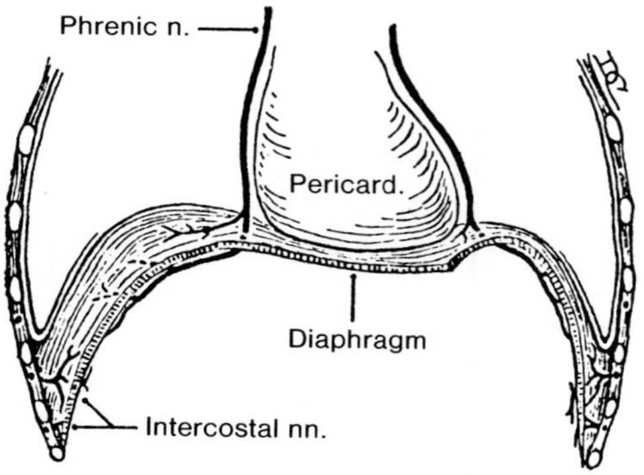

Figure 1-102. Diagram illustrating the nerve supply of the diaphragm. Parts of the pleura and peritoneum related to the diaphragm are supplied by sensory fibers from these nerves.

presentation, is **overriding (dextroposition) of the aorta.** The other three congenital malformations are (1) obstruction to the right ventricular outflow (**pulmonary stenosis**); (2) **VSD**; and (3) **right ventricular hypertrophy** (Fig. 1-98). The overall incidence of Fallot's tetralogy approaches 10% of all forms of congenital heart disease. It is the most common condition accompanied by persistent **cyanosis** (G. dark blue color); hence, the term "**blue baby**" is commonly used. It accounts for about 75% of cases of cyanotic congenital heart disease in persons over 1 year old.

The observation that the VSD was just below the aortic valve is the clue that indicated **dextroposition of the aorta**. The aorta arises directly above the large defect in the interventricular septum and receives blood from both ventricles. Because of the obstruction to pulmonary outflow, blood is shunted across the VSD into the aorta. This results in persistent arterial unsaturation, **cyanosis** (dark bluish coloration of the skin), and **dyspnea** (difficult breathing) on exertion (*e.g.*, during crying and playing).

Cyanosis, one of the characteristic signs of tetralogy, may not be present at birth and may not manifest itself for several months. The absence of cyanosis at birth is probably related to the slow closure of the ductus arteriosus. Under normal conditions, the ductus arteriosus is functionally closed shortly after birth by contraction of its muscular wall, but is not anatomically closed for up to 3 months when the ligamentum arteriosum forms (Fig. 1-101). As the ductus arteriosus obliterates during the first few months after birth, cyanosis may appear gradually or develop suddenly when the infant acquires a severe pulmonary infection.

Tetralogy of Fallot, consisting of *four congenital cardiac defects*, results from abnormalities of bulboventricular growth and septation, particularly underdevelopment of the infundibulum of the pulmonary artery which develops from the bulbus cordis of the embryonic heart.

Case 1-9. Coarctation (L. *coarctare*, to constrict) of the aorta may occur anywhere from the origin of the brachiocephalic artery to the bifurcation of the abdominal aorta, but the constriction nearly always occurs around the ligamentum arteriosum, most often distal to it, in persons over 1 year of age (Fig. 1-99). This **congenital malformation**, occurring about once in 2,000 births, is more common in males than in females (2:1) and is a common cause of heart failure during infancy.

The etiology of coarctation of the aorta is not clearly understood. As the condition is commonly associated with the **Turner syndrome** in females with the XO sex chromosome complement, genetic factors may be involved. Similarly, the embryological basis of coarctation is unclear, except that its presence is related to closure or nonclosure of the **ductus arteriosus**. A current view is that coarctation represents a persistence of the **isthmus of the aorta** that is normally present prenatally, between the left subclavian artery and the ductus arteriosus owing to the passage of little blood through this segment of the aorta. Normally, as the ductus arteriosus closes after birth, the isthmus enlarges until it is the same diameter as the aorta distal to the ductus arteriosus. If this dilation fails to occur, a coarctation of the aorta of the preductal type (or some variant) persists.

The cause of the upper body hypertension seems obvious, but several hypotheses exist, none of which is completely satisfactory. It seems that the blood pressure is elevated in the vessels arising proximal to the coarctation because of the obstruction of blood flow through the descending aorta. The amplitude of pulsation below the coarctation is diminished for the same reason. In addition to this mechanical obstruction, the development of hypertension also appears to be related to humoral factors, probably owing to renal hypotension.

Patients with a coarctation usually do not develop incapacitating symptoms during the first decade of their lives because an extensive **collateral circulation** frequently develops to compensate for the obstruction in the flow of blood to lower parts of the body (Fig. 1-103). Collateral circulation, stimulated by the presence of the coarctation, is largely through branches of vessels arising from the aortic arch that join intercostal arteries distal to the constriction. Branches of the axillary and subclavian arteries anastomose with the posterior intercostal arteries, which connect with the anastomotic network around the scapula (Fig. 6-42). Enlargement of these arteries accounts for the pulsations and **systolic murmurs** over the patient's interscapular area. Similar enlargement of the anastomoses between the internal thoracic arteries and the inferior epigastric arteries explains the presence of pulsations on both sides of the sternum.

The explanation for the delayed femoral pulse is that most blood entering the femoral artery comes via the collateral circulation rather than directly through the descending aorta. The low to normal blood pressure in the lower half of the body associated with hypertension in the upper half is an important sign of coarctation, but this phenomenon is also found in patients with abdominal aortic occlusion resulting from **atherosclerosis** (hardening of the artery characterized by lipid deposits in the intima).

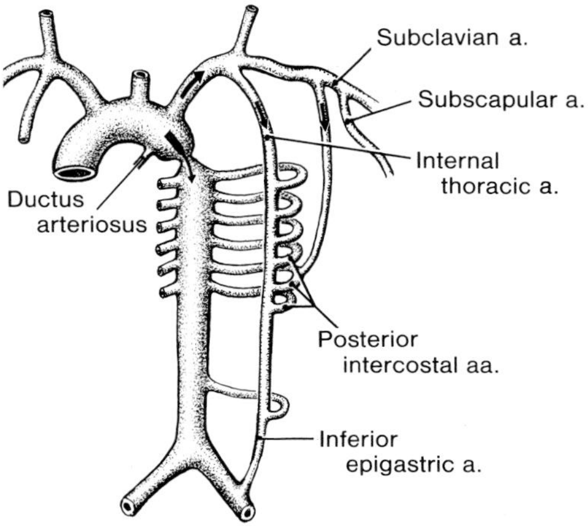

Figure 1-103. Diagrammatic representation of the common routes of collateral circulation that develop in association with coarctation of the aorta.

Notching of the ribs, an important radiological sign of coarctation, is caused by erosion of the ribs in the area of the costal grooves by the dilated intercostal arteries. This process is evident by late childhood and increases with age. Rib notching is also observed in **neurofibromatosis** (a disease characterized by tumors of nerves called neurofibromas) and in a few other conditions.

Although the patient had no incapacitating symptoms, the hypertension was the cause of his frequent headaches, vertigo, and epistaxis. There was radiographic evidence of **cardiomegaly** (cardiac enlargement) and, without operative treatment, he would have a high risk of suffering from **cerebral hemorrhage**, **ruptured aorta** above the coarctation, left **heart failure**, or **bacterial endocarditis**.

Case 1-10. PTE is an important cause of **morbidity** (disease) and **mortality** (death) in patients confined to bed, in pregnant patients, and in patients who have been taking birth control pills for a long time. In the present case, it is probable that the thrombus (clot) was released from the great saphenous vein and transported to the pulmonary circulation where it caused complete or almost complete obstruction of the right pulmonary artery. This lead to the various respiratory and hemodynamic disturbances (*e.g.*, dyspnea, tachypnea, arrhythmias, and tachycardia).

Three factors are involved in thrombus formation (**thrombogenesis**): stasis, abnormalities of the wall of the vessel, and alterations in the blood coagulation system. Various conditions are associated with thromboembolism (*e.g*, pregnancy, fractures of the pelvis or lower limbs, abdominal operations, and the use of oral contraceptives). Possibly the lengthy car trip in a seated position with a safety belt around her abdomen and the birth control pills were contributory factors to **thrombogenesis** in the present case.

Very likely the radiologist visualized the **right** ventricle by the technique of **right cardiac catheterization**. A radiopaque catheter was likely inserted into the left femoral vein, just below the inguinal ligament (Fig. 4-18). It would then have been guided with the aid of **fluoroscopy** into the inferior vena cava, the right atrium, and the right ventricle.

The patient's chest discomfort probably resulted from right heart strain and distention of the left pulmonary artery and its branches. As the right main pulmonary artery was obstructed, most of the blood was going through the left pulmonary artery. When the right lung failed to receive an adequate blood supply, changes very likely resulted in the pleura and pulmonary tissue. In view of the **pleural (friction) rub**, there was likely some **pleuritic chest pain** caused by irritation of nerve endings of pain fibers in the costal pleura. The **parietal referred pain** was felt in the thoracic wall, the area of skin innervated by the intercostal nerves.

When the inferior vena cava is narrowed by plication (L. *plica*, a fold) below the renal veins, adequate venous drainage of the lower limbs is maintained through the collateral lumbar veins which connect with the **azygos system of veins** (Fig. 1-92). The lumbar veins on each side are linked together by an ascending lumbar vein which lies in front of the lumbar transverse processes. This vein begins caudally at the common iliac vein and ends cranially in the azygos (or hemiazygos) vein. The azygos vein joins the superior vena cava (Fig. 1-93).

Although sufficient to permit adequate venous return from lower regions of the body, the plicated inferior vena cava and the **collateral venous circulation** does not prevent the passage of small emboli from reaching the lungs. However, most of these pulmonary emboli are dissolved by the **fibrinolytic system** in about 2 weeks. In some cases, the thrombus is transformed into a linear or plate-like fibrous scar in the lungs.

SUGGESTIONS FOR ADDITIONAL READING

1. Maden, R. E. Cardiopulmonary surgery. In *Basic Surgery*, edited by J. A. McCredie, Macmillan Publishing Co., Inc., New York, 1977.

   This chapter presents a good overview of intrathoracic surgery, describing how pulmonary operations are performed and discussing infectious diseases of the lung (*e.g.*, bronchiectasis). There is also a concise account of tumors of the lung and diseases of the mediastinum. The most important congenital malformations of the heart are also discussed, as is acquired heart disease.

2. Moore, K. L. *The Developing Human, Clinically Oriented Embryology*, Ed. 2, W. B. Saunders Co., Philadelphia, 1977.

   The embryological bases of congenital malformations of the lower respiratory tract and of the heart and great vessels are fully discussed. Review of these accounts will amplify many of the points briefly referred to in the present text (*e.g.*, concerning ASD, VSD, and tetralogy of Fallot).

3. Moore, M. E. *Medical Emergency Manual*, Ed. 2, The Williams & Wilkins Company, Baltimore, 1976.

   This little book presents clearly and succinctly an acceptable approach to the management of patients with chest pain. It explains how doctors begin to evaluate a patient with chest pain and how they discriminate between minor causes of pain and those that are potentially life-threatening.

4. Ross, R. S., Lesch, M., and Braunwald, E. Acute Myocardial Infarction. In *Harrison's Principles of Internal Medicine*, edited by G. W. Thorn, R. D. Adams, E. Braunwald, K. J. Isselbacher, and R. G. Petersdorf, Ed. 8, McGraw-Hill Book Company, New York, 1977.

   Myocardial infarction (MI) is one of several dangerous causes of chest pain. If you read this brief account, you will know the classic characteristics of MI (*e.g.*, crushing anterior chest pain lasting more than 30 minutes that does not disappear with rest). You will also discover that chest pain is not always present with MI.

5. Squire, L. F., Colaiace, W. M., and Strutynsky, N. *Exercises in Diagnostic Radiology*. 1. *The Chest*, W. B. Saunders Co., Philadelphia, 1970.

   This short book presents some of the typical problems faced daily by radiologists. Although the exercises are designed for persons late in their medical training, they will give you some understanding of how radiological diagnoses are made. For example, it shows six chest films and asks, "Do any of the hearts appear enlarged?" It then discusses the answer to the question.

CHAPTER 2

The Abdomen

Abdominal pain is the most common presenting symptom associated with intra-abdominal disease. **Appendicitis** (inflammation of the vermiform appendix) ranks high on the list of diseases leading to hospitalization and is a major cause of abdominal pain; however, any abdominal organ is subject to disease or injury. Rupture of a hollow **gastrointestinal (GI) organ** permits its irritating contents to escape into the peritoneal cavity, producing **peritonitis** (inflammation of the peritoneum, the serous sac lining the abdominal cavity and covering most of the viscera). **GI rupture** may result in free air beneath the diaphragm which can be observed in an upright abdominal radiograph.

Often a doctor's reputation depends on his/her ability to diagnose and treat the common causes of abdominal pain. Some patients requiring an abdominal operation have preoperative chest and/or abdominal radiographs taken because chest films may disclose an unsuspected cause for an abdominal pain (*e.g.*, **pneumonia**), and abdominal films may indicate that rupture of an organ has occurred or disclose a **calculus** (gallstone, urinary stone, or **fecalith** in the appendix, *i.e.*, a concretion formed from feces).

The abdomen is the region between the **thoracoabdominal diaphragm** and the pelvis. The diaphragm forms a roof for the abdominal cavity, but it has no floor; however, *the abdominal cavity is continuous with the pelvic cavity*, which does have a floor (the **pelvic diaphragm**).

The abdominal cavity extends superiorly to about the fifth anterior intercostal space when the person is supine (lying down); hence, *a considerable part of the abdominal cavity lies under cover of the bony thoracic cage.* The abdominal cavity is separated from the thoracic cavity above by the thoracoabdominal diaphragm and joins the pelvic cavity below at the plane of the **superior pelvic aperature** (pelvic inlet).

ANTERIOR ABDOMINAL WALL AND SCROTUM

When a patient's abdomen is examined, the anterior abdominal wall is inspected and palpated. When the abdomen is operated on, the anterior abdominal wall is cut through. Obviously a clear understanding of the structure of this wall is essential knowledge.

ANTERIOR ABDOMINAL WALL

Boundaries (Figs. 2-1 and 2-2). The anterior abdominal wall is bounded *superiorly* by the **xiphoid process** of the sternum and the **costal cartilages** of the 7th to 10th ribs and *inferiorly* on each side by the **iliac crest**, the **anterior superior iliac spine**, the **inguinal ligament**, the **pubic tubercle**, the **pubic crest**, and the **pubic symphysis**.

The infrasternal angle (Fig. 1-53) is formed below the xiphisternal joint by the diverging **costal margins** (Fig. 2-1). Together, the two margins form the **costal arch.**

The inguinal ligament is the inrolled (rolled under) inferior edge of the aponeurosis of the external oblique muscle (Fig. 2-9), the most superficial muscle of the anterior abdominal wall. *It extends from the pubic tubercle to the anterior superior iliac spine.* The **inguinal fold** (Fig. 2-2) overlying it indicates the separation between the anterior abdominal wall and the front of the thigh in thin persons. In obese people,

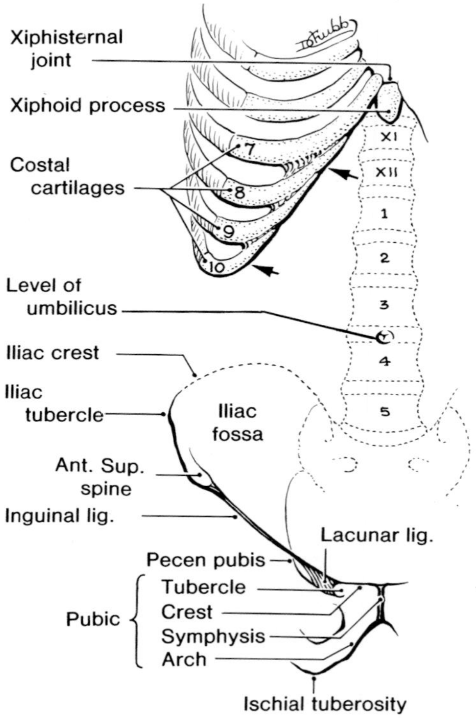

Figure 2-1. Drawing of the skeleton of the abdomen illustrating the boundaries of the anterior abdominal wall. Observe that it is bounded above by the xiphoid process and the costal cartilages of the 7th to 10th ribs and below on each side by the iliac crest, the anterior superior iliac spine, the inguinal ligament, the pubic tubercle, the pubic crest, and the pubic symphysis. The costal margin (*arrows*) is formed by the 7th to 10th costal cartilages; together the two costal margins form the costal arch. Note that the highest point of the iliac crest is at the level of the fourth lumbar vertebra.

the distended abdomen hangs over and conceals the inguinal fold.

Surface Anatomy (Figs. 2-1 to 2-3). The *umbilicus* (navel, belly-button) is the most obvious marking on the abdominal wall of most people. This puckered scar represents the former site of attachment of the **umbilical cord** in the fetus. The position of the umbilicus varies somewhat, depending on such factors as the degree of obesity, the tone of the abdominal muscles, and the distention of the abdomen. In obese people in particular, the position of the umbilicus varies considerably depending on whether they are in the supine or erect position. It is lower in children and old persons and the variation in level may be extreme in obese persons. Usually the umbilicus is inverted and lies at the level of the intervertebral disc between the third and fourth lumbar vertebrae.

The position of the linea alba (L. white line) is indicated by a slight groove or furrow in the anterior median line, which is particularly obvious in thin muscular males (Fig. 2-3). This groove extends from the *xiphoid process* of the sternum to the *symphysis pubis.* Understand that the linea alba is not seen as a white line until the skin is reflected in dissection (Figs. 2-8 to 2-10). The linea alba, deep to the groove in the skin, is a **midline raphe** (G. suture) formed by the fusion of the aponeuroses (tendinous sheets) of the external oblique, internal oblique, and transversus abdominis muscles (Fig. 2-10).

The linea semilunares are slight surface depressions, three or four fingerbreadths to each side of the groove over the linea alba, which indicate the *lateral borders of the rectus abdominis muscles* (Fig. 2-10*A*). To identify these semilunar lines, lie on your back and then sit up without using your arms. This contracts your rectus abdominis muscles, making their lateral margins stand out. These lines are easily visible in persons with good abdominal muscular development (Fig. 2-3). The lineae semilunares form a gentle curve, convex laterally, from the pubic tubercles (Figs. 2-1 and 2-2) to the costal margins at the tip of the ninth costal cartilages. In abdominal operations these lines give a good guide to the lateral borders of the rectus abdominis muscles.

The linea transversae are transverse grooves overlying the **tendinous intersections** of the rectus abdominis muscles (Figs. 2-3 and 2-7). They extend laterally from the linea alba; three or more are visible in muscular persons.

The inguinal ligament extends, with a slight concavity upward, from the anterior superior iliac spine to the pubic tubercle (Figs. 2-1, 2-2, and 2-9). This tubercle may

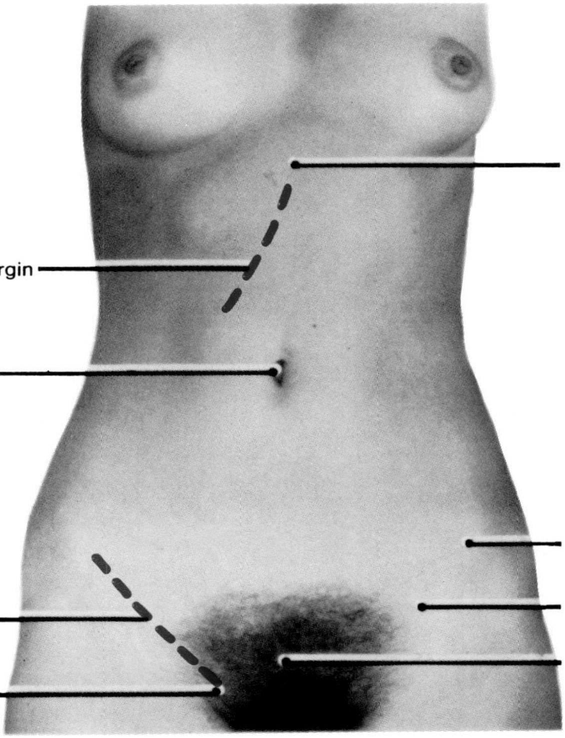

Figure 2-2. Photograph of a 27-year-old woman showing the surface features of her anterior abdominal wall (compare with Fig. 2-1). The costal margin is formed by the upturned costal cartilages of ribs 7 to 10. The pubic symphysis marks the lowest limit of the anterior abdominal wall in the median plane. The inguinal ligament stretches from the pubic tubercle to the anterior superior iliac spine. The shape of the abdomen varies considerably in persons of both sexes and in the same person between the erect and supine positions. The surface features recognizable in the above woman (and in the man shown in Fig. 2-3) may be difficult or impossible to observe or palpate in obese persons. Observe the lateral borders of her rectus abdominis muscles (lineae semilunares, Fig. 2-10*A*).

be felt about 2.5 cm lateral to the symphysis pubis. *To palpate your inguinal ligament,* lie on a table in the supine position and let one leg drop to the floor. You can easily feel your inguinal ligament at its medial end and, if you are thin, you may be able to see it separating your anterior abdominal wall from your thigh. The **inguinal fold** (fold of the groin) over the inguinal ligament in the erect position (Fig. 2-2) forms mainly because there is relatively less subcutaneous fat here compared to that present in the skin of the abdomen and the thigh.

The symphysis pubis is felt as a firm resistance in the anterior midline at the inferior extremity of the anterior abdominal wall (Figs. 2-1, 2-2, and 2-9). In many people the fat covering this cartilaginous joint makes it difficult to palpate.

The pubic crest is felt extending laterally from the symphysis pubis for about 2.5 cm (Fig. 2-1). The crest terminates at the pubic tubercle to which the inguinal ligament attaches.

The iliac crest (Figs. 2-1, 4-7, and 4-8) is easily felt throughout its length, extending posteriorly from the anterior superior iliac spine. It forms the upper tip of the hip region. The **iliac tubercle** (Figs. 2-1 and 4-1) can be palpated about 6 cm posterior to the anterior superior iliac spine.

The epigastric fossa ("pit of stomach") is a small depression in the midline of the

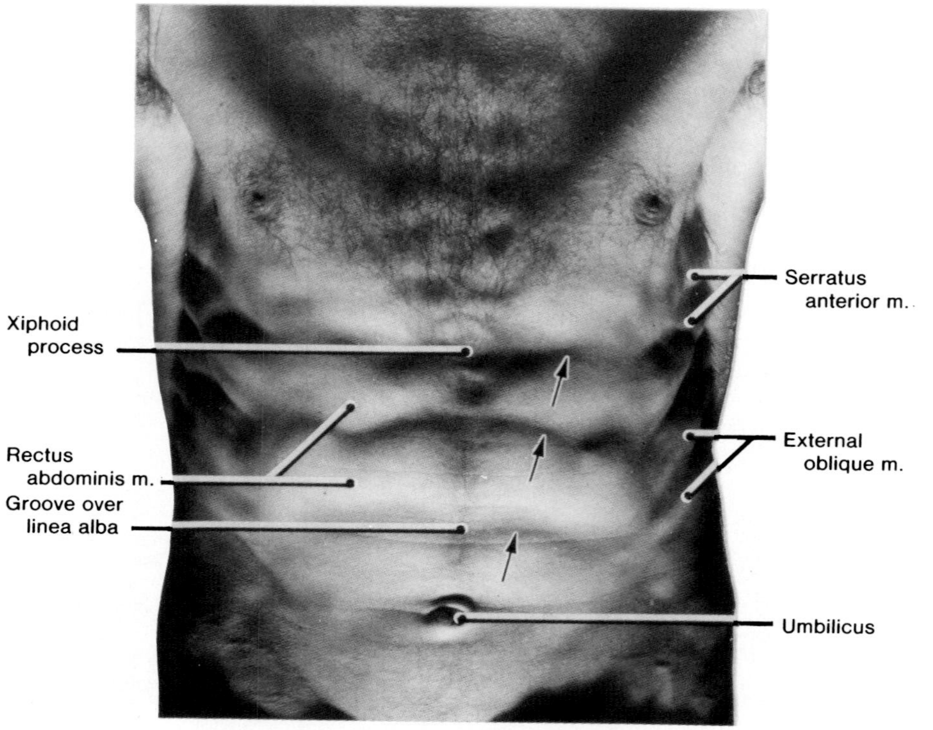

Figure 2-3. Photograph of the anterior abdominal wall of a 46-year-old man showing the surface features. Three tendinous intersections of the rectus abdominis muscle are indicated by *arrows*. Three or more of these intersections are usually present (Fig. 2-7).

uppermost part of the abdomen. It is particularly noticeable when a person is in the supine position because the viscera move backward and laterally, drawing the anterior abdominal wall inward in this region.

Planes and Points of Reference (Fig. 2-4*B*). For clinical purposes, the anterolateral abdominal wall is divided into **nine abdominal regions** by *two vertical* and *two horizontal planes.* These regions are helpful for the localization of a pain or a swelling and for indicating the location of deep structures (*e.g.*, the duodenum).

To relate the various abdominal viscera and other structures to each other and to the surface of the body, *you are urged to use the vertebral column as a scale and refer structures to their vertebral levels.* As will be seen, certain horizontal planes are reliable guides to the vertebral levels.

The Horizontal Planes (Fig. 2-4). Of the various planes described below, *the transpyloric and transtubercular planes are the ones that are commonly used as landmarks* when examining the abdomen. For completeness, the other planes sometimes used are also described.

The transpyloric plane (Fig. 2-4*A*) is a horizontal plane situated midway between the **jugular notch** of the sternum (Figs. 1-10 and 1-11) and the **pubic symphysis.** In most people this plane is *approximately* midway between the xiphisternal joint and the umbilicus. *The transpyloric plane lies at the level of the intervertebral disc between L1 and L2 vertebrae.* It usually passes through the **pylorus** of the stomach (hence its name) in the supine cadaver. *In living persons, the pylorus may lie 2.5 to 8 cm below this plane.* The transpyloric plane also passes through the tips of the ninth costal cartilages, the duodenojejunal junction, the neck of the pancreas, and the hila of the kidneys.

The subcostal plane (Fig. 2-4*B*) joins the lowest point of the costal margin on

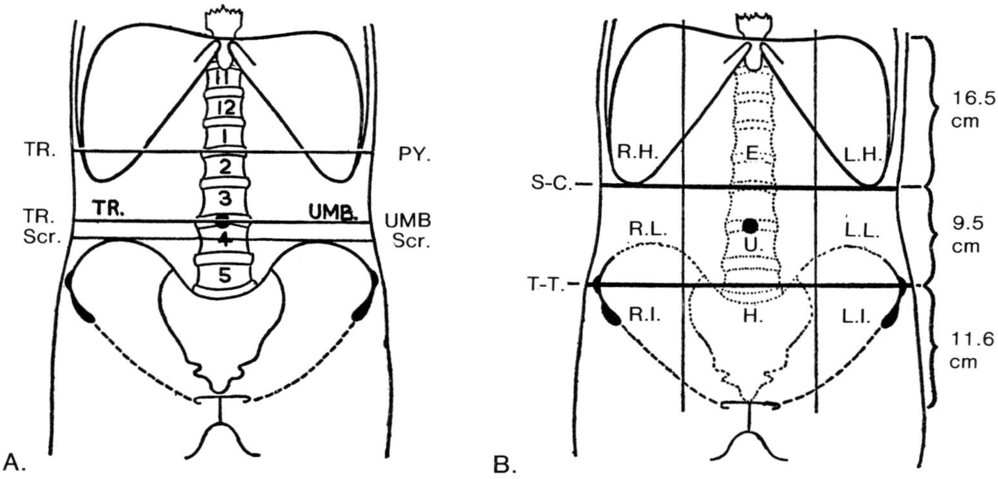

Figure 2-4. Diagrams illustrating various planes and points of reference. *A*, shows three horizontal planes and their relationship to the vertebral column. *TR-PY*, transpyloric plane. *TR-UMB*, transumbilical plane. *Scr*, supracristal plane. *B*, illustrates the nine abdominal regions. *RH*, *LH*, right and left hypochondriac. *RL*, *LL*, right and left lateral or lumbar. *RI*, *LI*, right and left inguinal or iliac. *E*, epigastric. *U*, umbilical. *H*, suprapubic or hypogastric. *S-C*, subcostal plane. *T-T*, transtubercular plane. The vertical planes are the midclavicular lines; each joins the midpoint of the clavicle with the midinguinal point. Note that the midinguinal point is the midpoint between the symphysis pubis and the anterior superior iliac spine and not the midpoint of the inguinal ligament.

each side (*i.e.*, the inferior level of the thoracic cage as seen from the front). Hence, it indicates the inferior margin of the 10th costal cartilages (Fig. 1-1). *The subcostal plane lies at the level of the intervertebral disc between L2 and L3 vertebrae* (Figs. 2-1 and 2-4*B*).

The transumbilical plane (Fig. 2-4*A*) passes through the umbilicus. Because of the variability in the position of the umbilicus, the vertebral level of this plane is somewhat unreliable. However, in spite of this, it is sometimes used because of its convenience. *In persons with a reasonably firm abdominal wall the transumbilical plane indicates the level of the intervertebral disc between L3/L4.*

The transtubercular or **intertubercular plane** (Fig. 2-4*B*) *passes through the iliac tubercles and lies at the level of the body of L5 vertebra.*

The interspinous plane passes through the right and left anterior superior iliac spines and the promontary of the sacrum (Fig. 5-25).

The supracristal (intercristal) plane passes between the highest points of the iliac crests and *lies at the level of the spinous process of L4 vertebra.* This plane is generally used as a landmark on the posterior surface of the body for identifying the individual vertebral spinous processes.

The plane of the **fifth intercostal space** (anteriorly) gives an approximate indication of the level of the upper limit of the abdomen and the dome of the diaphragm (Fig. 2-36) when a person is supine. This space *lies at the level of T10 or T11 vertebrae.*

The Vertical Planes (Fig. 2-4*B*). The two vertical planes commonly used to divide the abdomen into regions are the **midclavicular lines**. They extend downward from the *midpoints of the clavicles to the midinguinal points* (the midpoints of the lines joining the anterior superior iliac spines and the top of the pubic symphysis). They are roughly equivalent to vertical lines from a point midway between the anterior median line and the lateral border of the acromion of the scapula. *The midclavicular lines are sagittal planes* (*i.e.*, they are parallel with the median plane).

Regions of the Abdomen (Fig. 2-4*B*).

The *nine abdominal regions* used for location of the viscera are mapped out using two horizontal (subcostal and transtubercular) planes and two vertical planes, right and left midclavicular lines. The following are the commonly described regions: (1) *in the superior zone*, **epigastric region** (G. *epi*, upon + *gastēr*, stomach) and **right** and **left hypochondriac regions** (G. *hypo*, under + *chondros*, cartilage, *i.e.*, of ribs); (2) *in the middle zone*, **umbilical region** and **right** and **left lumbar** or **lateral regions**; and (3) *in the lower zone*, **hypogastric region** (G. *hypo*, under + *gastēr*, stomach) or **suprapubic region** and **right** and **left iliac** or **inguinal regions**.

Quadrants of the Abdomen (Fig. 2-5). A simple and commonly used clinical method of dividing the abdominal wall for descriptive purposes is to divide it into **four quadrants** (upper and lower right and upper and lower left), using the median plane and the transumbilical plane. These quadrants are useful to clinicians who are stating the position of a pain or a tumor (*e.g.*, the pain of acute **appendicitis** usually starts in the periumbilical region and later localizes to the right lower quadrant).

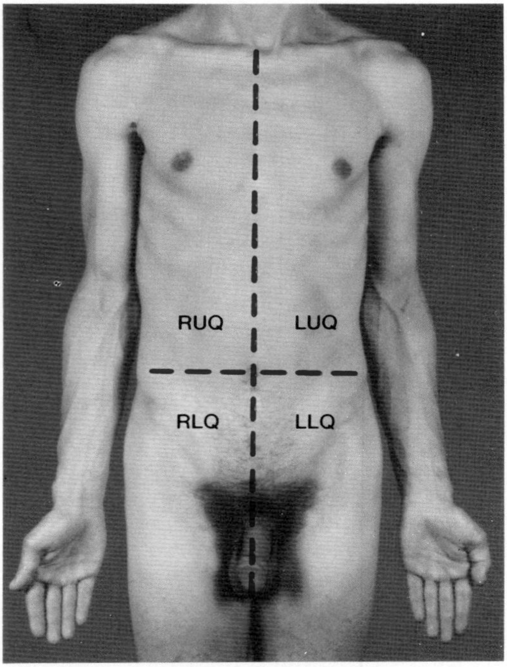

Figure 2-5. Photograph of a 27-year-old man showing division of his abdomen into four quadrants by the median plane and the transumbilical plane. In obese persons the horizontal plane is best made midway between the xiphisternal joint and the symphysis pubis. *RUQ*, right upper quadrant. *LUQ*, left upper quadrant. *RLQ*, right lower quadrant. *LLQ*, left lower quadrant.

Contour of the Abdomen (Figs. 2-2, 2-3, and 2-5). In persons with good abdominal muscular development, the contour of the abdomen is flat from above downward and evenly rounded from side to side. The contour varies in other people. Protuberance of the abdomen is normal in young infants because their GI tracts contain considerable amounts of air. Also their abdominal cavities are still enlarging and their abdominal muscles are gaining strength. The child's liver is relatively large which accounts for some of the abdominal protrusion.

Protrusion of the abdomen in women occurs during pregnancy owing to the **fetus** and expands in both sexes following the deposition of **fat** or the accumulation of **feces**, **fluid**, or **flatus** (gas in the GI tract). Note that five common causes of abdominal protrusion all begin with the letter "**f**." During old age, muscle laxity also contributes to the abdominal protruberance.

CLINICALLY ORIENTED COMMENTS

Abdominal or pelvic tumors and accumulation of fluid in the peritoneal cavity (**ascites**) also result in abdominal enlargement. As this happens the muscles thin out, but the skin grows and the nerves and blood vessels lengthen. Reddish elongate lines called **striae gravidarum** (L. *gravidus*, heavy) may appear in the anterolateral abdominal skin of pregnant and/or obese persons. These striae gradually change into thin scar-like lines called **lineae albicantes** ("stretch marks"). They also appear in the skin of the thighs of obese men and women.

When examining the abdomen, warm hands are used so that the patient's muscles will not become tense. To relax the abdominal wall, patients are examined while lying in the supine position with their hips semiflexed by a pillow under their knees. If this is not done, the deep fascia of the thigh pulls on the deep layer of the superficial fascia of the abdomen and tenses the anterior abdominal wall.

Fascia of the Abdominal Wall. The fascia of the anterior abdominal wall consists of superficial and deep layers, but the deep layer is unremarkable.

The Superficial Fascia (Tela Subcutanea). Over the greater part of the anterior abdominal wall, the superficial fascia consists of one layer containing a variable amount of fat. *In some persons this fat layer is several inches thick* and can be separated from the thin deep fascia by blunt dissection. The superficial fascia of the lower abdominal wall just superior to the inguinal ligament may be divided into (1) a fatty **superficial layer** (Camper's fascia) and (2) a membranous **deep layer** (Scarpa's fascia) containing fibrous tissue and very little fat. The superficial layer is continuous with the superficial fascia of the thigh and the deep layer is continuous with the deep fascia of the thigh, called the **fascia lata** (Fig. 4-19), distal to the inguinal ligament. The deep layer is also continuous with the superficial fascia of the perineum (Colle's fascia) and with that investing the scrotum and penis. This deep layer of superficial fascia fuses with the deep fascia of the abdomen.

CLINICALLY ORIENTED COMMENTS

Surgeons often use the deep membranous layer of the superficial fascia for holding sutures during closure of a skin incision.

Between the deep layer of the superficial fascia and the deep fascia of the abdomen, there is a potential space in which fluid may accumulate. For example, urine may pass through a rupture of the spongy urethra (Fig. 2-114), called **extravasation of urine**, into this space and extend upward into the anterior abdominal wall. Falling astride a fence and car accidents are common causes of a ruptured urethra. (See Case 3-2 at the end of Chap. 3).

The Deep Fascia. Little needs to be said about the deep fascia of the abdominal wall except that it forms a thin layer over the external oblique muscle.

Muscles of Anterior Abdominal Wall (Figs. 2-3 and 2-6 to 2-15). Four muscles form parts of the anterior abdominal wall: **three flat muscles** (external oblique, internal oblique, and transversus abdominis and **one straplike muscle** (rectus abdominis). This straight (L. *rectus*) muscle is enclosed in a sheath produced by the **aponeuroses** (fibrous sheets) of the three flat muscles (Fig. 2-10).

The combination of muscles and aponeuroses in the abdominal wall affords considerable protection to the abdominal viscera, especially when the muscles are in good physical condition. The flat muscles cross each other in a way (somewhat like a three-plied corset) that strengthens the abdominal wall and diminishes the risk of hernial protrusion between separated muscle bundles.

The External Oblique Muscle (Figs. 2-3 and 2-6 to 2-9). This is the largest and most superficial of the three flat abdominal muscles. This large muscle lies on the anterior and lateral parts of the abdomen.

Origin (Fig. 2-6). **External surface of lower eight ribs** (*above costal margin*) by eight fleshy digitations or slips. The upper four fleshy digitations interdigitate with the serratus anterior muscle (Fig. 2-3) and the lower four with the latissimus dorsi muscle (Fig. 2-6). These fleshy digitations unite almost immediately to form a broad, somewhat fan-shaped muscle.

Insertion. Except for the muscle fibers arising from the lower two ribs, which pass almost vertically downward, the fibers of the external oblique radiate downward, forward, and medially. It may help you to remember this if you note that this is the direction taken by your outstretched fingers when put into the pockets of your pants. The most **posteroinferior fibers insert into the iliac crest** (Fig. 2-1), thereby forming a free posterior border.

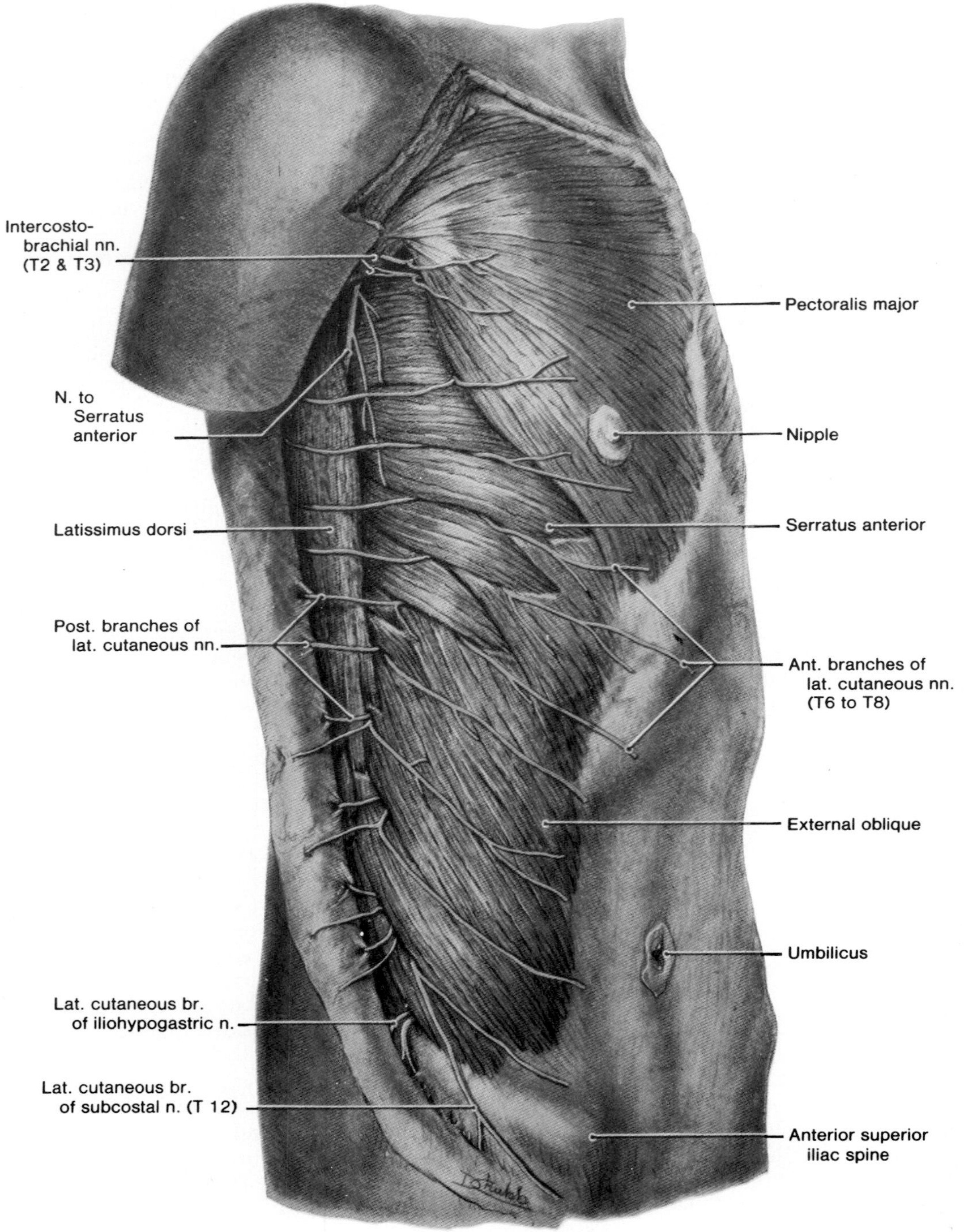

Figure 2-6. Drawing of a lateral view of a superficial dissection of the trunk showing the serratus anterior and external oblique muscles and the lateral cutaneous nerves. Observe that the fleshy fibers of the external oblique originate above the costal margin (Fig. 2-1). Note that the upper four fleshy digitations of the external oblique interdigitate with the serratus anterior and that the lower four interdigitate with the latissimus dorsi muscle. Between the digitations of the external oblique, observe the lateral cutaneous nerves (T7 to T12). The posterior branches of these nerves turn backward over the latissimus dorsi and the anterior branches descend in line with the fibers of the external oblique.

The other muscle fibers end in a broad **aponeurosis**. By means of this aponeurosis, the external oblique reaches the midline, where it fuses with the aponeuroses of the other anterior muscles on its same side and with those on the opposite side to form the **linea alba** (Figs. 2-9 and 2-10), *a tendinous raphe stretching from the xiphoid process to the symphysis pubis*. The aponeurosis is also attached to the upper border of the symphysis pubis and to the pubic crest as far as the pubic tubercle (Figs. 2-1 and 2-9). *The lower turned under part of the aponeurosis of the external oblique forms the inguinal ligament*, which is attached to the anterior superior iliac spine and the pubic tubercle (Fig. 2-1). The **superficial inguinal ring** (Fig. 2-9) lies at the end of a triangular cleft in the external oblique aponeurosis, immediately above the pubic tubercle. This cleft represents a weakness in the aponeurosis and the anterior abdominal wall (p. 145).

The insertion of the external oblique may be summarized as follows. Most of its fibers are inserted via its aponeurosis into the linea alba. Other fibers are inserted into the pubic symphysis, the pubic tubercle, the pecten pubis, and the iliac crest. The lower border of its aponeurosis is infolded to form the inguinal ligament.

Nerve Supply. Ventral rami of **lower six thoracic nerves**.

The Internal Oblique Muscle (Figs. 2-6 to 2-15). This is the middle muscle of the three flat abdominal muscles.

Origin. Posterior layer of thoracolumbar **fascia,** anterior two-thirds of **iliac crest**, and lateral two-thirds of **inguinal ligament**. Its fibers run at right angles to those of the external oblique muscle, fan out from its origins, and radiate upward and forward.

Insertion. Posterior fibers insert into the **costal margin** (cartilages of 7th to 10th ribs); the remaining fibers end in a broad aponeurosis that inserts into the **linea alba** and the **pubis**. The upper fibers of its aponeurosis split to enclose the rectus abdominis muscle (Fig. 2-10) and come together again at the linea alba. The lower fibers of its aponeurosis arch over the spermatic cord as it lies in the **inguinal canal** (Figs. 2-7 and 2-8) and then descend behind the superficial inguinal ring to insert into the **pubic crest** and the adjoining part of the **pecten pubis** (Figs. 2-1 and 4-1). These fibers join with aponeurotic fibers of the transversus abdominis muscle to form the **conjoint tendon** (Fig. 2-11), which turns downward to insert into the pubic crest and the pecten pubis.

Nerve Supply. Ventral rami of **lower six thoracic** nerves and **first lumbar nerves**.

The Transversus Abdominis Muscle (Figs. 2-8, 2-10, and 2-11). The transversus is the deepest of the three flat abdominal muscles.

Origin. Deep surfaces of **costal cartilages of lower six ribs**, where it interdigitates with the origin of diaphragm (Figs. 1-21 and 2-131). It also arises from the **thoracolumbar fascia**, the **iliac crest**, and the lateral third of **inguinal ligament**. The fibers run more or less horizontally, except for the lowermost ones, which pass downward and run parallel to those of the internal oblique muscle. Most of its fibers end in the aponeurosis that contributes to the rectus sheath (Fig. 2-10*C*).

Insertion. **Linea alba** with the aponeurosis of the internal oblique, the **pubic crest**, and the **pecten pubis** via the conjoint tendon.

Nerve Supply. Ventral rami of **lower six thoracic nerves** and **lumbar nerves**.

The Transversalis Fascia (Figs. 2-10C, 2-11, 2-14, and 2-16). This somewhat transparent fascia is the internal investing layer which **lines the entire abdominal wall**. It covers the deep surface of the transversus abdominis muscle and its aponeurosis and is *continuous from side to side deep to the linea alba*. Each part of the fascia transversalis is named according to the structures on which it lies; hence, it is called the **diaphragmatic fascia** on the diaphragm; the **iliac fascia** on the iliacus and **psoas fascia** on the psoas; and the **pelvic fascia** in the pelvis. It is also prolonged into the front of the thigh together with the iliac fascia to form the **femoral sheath** (Fig. 4-19) and through the inguinal canal to form the **internal spermatic fascia**, part of the covering of the spermatic cord (Figs. 2-8, 2-16, and 2-19).

Internal to the transversalis fascia is the

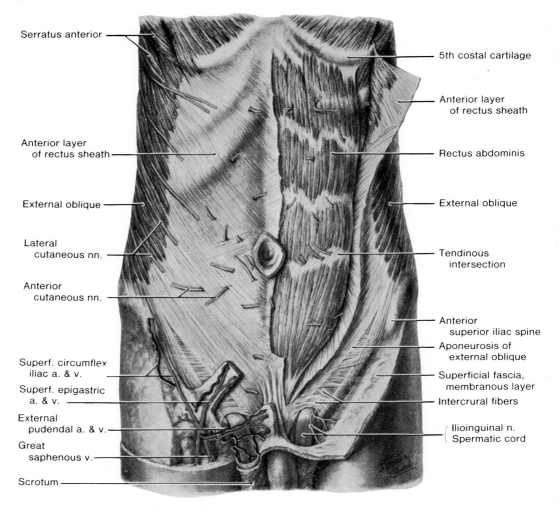

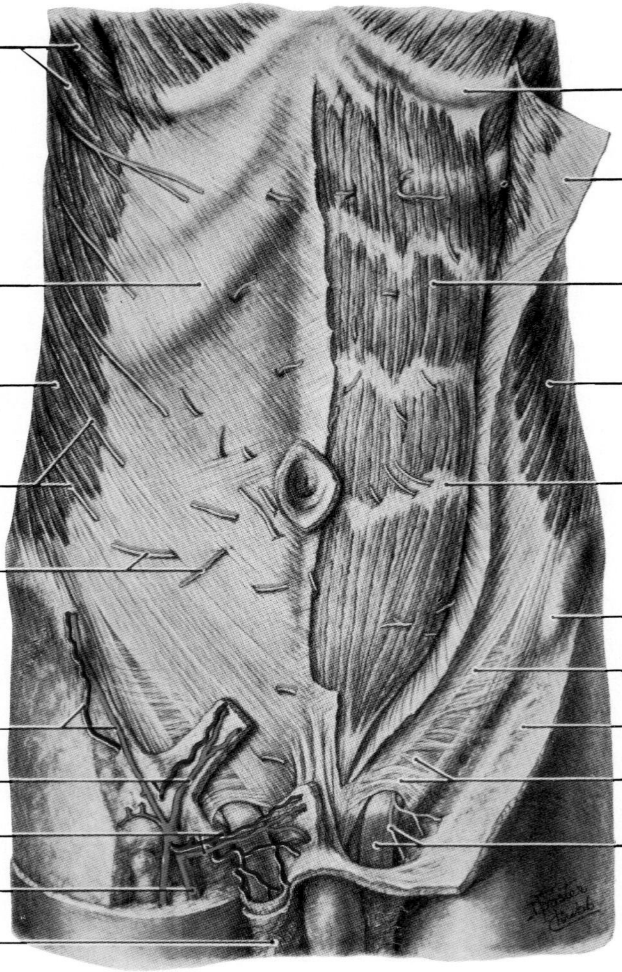

Figure 2-7. Drawing of a dissection of the anterior abdominal wall. The anterior layer of the rectus sheath is reflected on the left side. Observe that the external oblique muscle is aponeurotic medial to a line that curves upward from a point 2.5 cm lateral to the anterior superior iliac spine to the fifth rib. Note that the lateral border of the rectus abdominis muscle curves from the pubic tubercle, through the midpoint between the umbilicus and the anterior superior iliac spine, and across the chest margin to the fifth rib. Observe the anterior cutaneous nerves (T7 to T12) piercing the rectus abdominis muscle and the anterior layer of the rectus sheath. T10 supplies the region of the umbilicus (also see Fig. 2-141). In the superficial layer of the superficial fascia, examine the three superficial inguinal branches of the femoral artery and the three superficial inguinal tributaries of the great saphenous vein. Of these, note that the external pudendal artery and vein cross the spermatic cord. Observe that the membranous deep layer of the superficial fascia blends with the fascia lata of the thigh, a fingerbreadth below the inguinal ligament. Examine the spermatic cord and the ilioinguinal nerve issuing through the superficial inguinal ring.

peritoneum (Fig. 2-16), the extensive serous membrane which lines the abdominal and pelvic cavities. The transversalis fascia is separated from the peritoneum by a variable amount of subperitoneal fat, referred to as **extraperitoneal fatty tissue**.

Actions of the Flat Abdominal Muscles. The anterior abdominal wall is unsup-

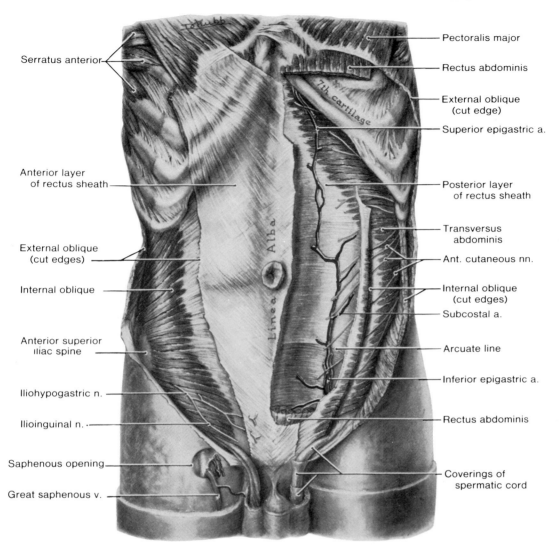

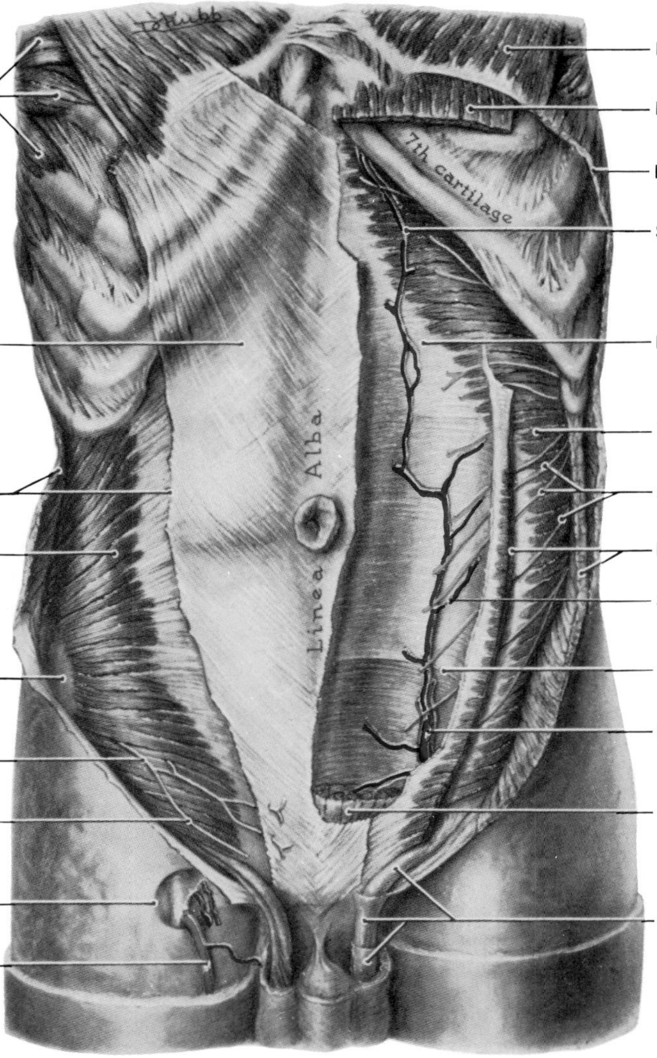

Figure 2-8. Drawing of a deeper dissection than that shown in Figure 2-7. Most of the external oblique muscle is excised on the right side. On the left side, the rectus abdominis is excised and the internal oblique is divided. Observe that the fibers of the internal oblique run horizontally at the level of the anterior superior iliac spine, obliquely upward above this level, and obliquely downward below it. Note the anastomosis between the superior and inferior epigastric arteries which indirectly unites the arteries of the upper limb to those of the lower limb (subclavian to external iliac). Observe that nerves T7 to T12, but not L1, enter the rectus sheath. Of these nerves, note that the upper ones ascend and the lower ones descend. Note that the external oblique is attached a handbreadth above the costal margin, the internal oblique to this margin, and the transversus within the margin.

ported and unprotected by bone; however, *the three flat muscles and their aponeuroses* form a strong but expansible **support** for the viscera and considerable **protection** to the viscera, especially when the muscles are in good condition.

The normal muscle tone of these muscles also plays an *important role in movements of the vertebral column* (flexion, extension, and lateral bending, Fig. 5-9) and the pelvis. These muscles also act when the body is in the supine position and the head and/or

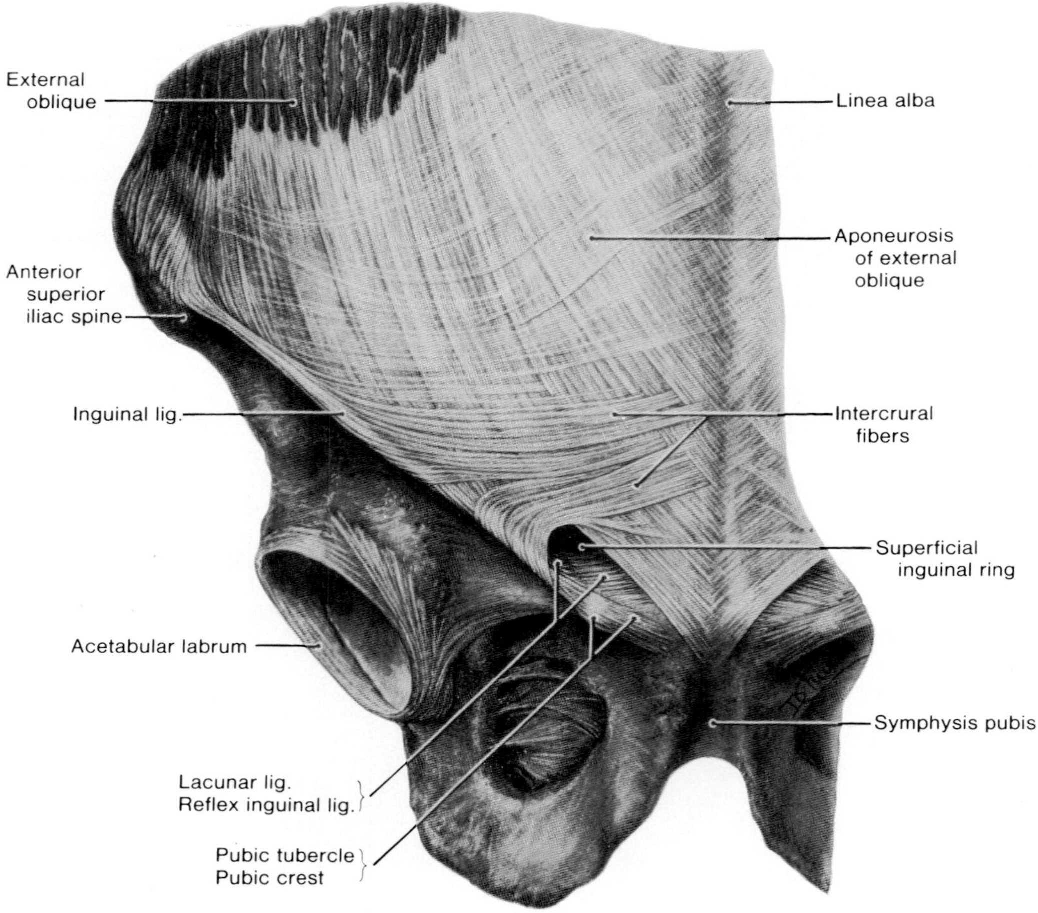

Figure 2-9. Drawing of a superficial dissection of the inguinal region showing the aponeurosis of the external oblique and the superficial inguinal ring. Observe that the linea alba is a ligament uniting the sternum to the symphsis pubis. Note that the intercrural fibers, well developed in this specimen, which prevent the crura of the superficial inguinal ring from spreading. Note that the superficial inguinal ring is triangular in shape and that (1) its central point is above the pubic tubercle, (2) its base is the lateral half of the pubic crest, (3) its lateral crus is the inguinal ligament, and (4) its medial crus is formed by fibers of the external oblique aponeurosis that cross the pubic crest at its midpoint. Observe that behind the superficial inguinal ring, some fibers of the external oblique aponeurosis from the opposite side pass to the pubic crest and the pecten pubis; this is called the reflected inguinal ligament.

legs are raised from the horizontal. These are common exercises used to strengthen the abdominal muscles to reduce the sagging of the abdomen, often caused by excess fat.

Normally there are quiet rhythmic movements of the anterior abdominal wall accompanying respirations. When the diaphragm contracts during inspiration, its dome flattens and descends, increasing the vertical dimension of the thorax (Fig. 1-58). To make room for the abdominal viscera, the anterior abdominal wall expands as its muscles relax. When the thoracic cage and the diaphragm relax, the abdominal wall sinks in passively; however, in the forced expiration that occurs during coughing, sneezing, vomiting, and straining, all four abdominal muscles act strongly.

When the ribs and the diaphragm are

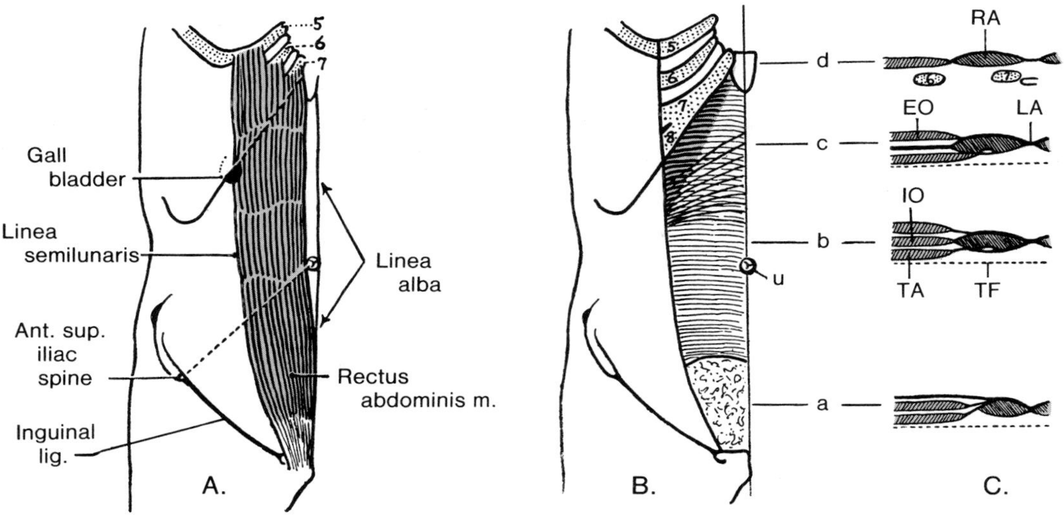

Figure 2-10. Drawings illustrating the rectus abdominis muscle and the rectus sheath. *A*, anterior view of the right rectus abdominis muscle. *B*, the posterior wall of the rectus sheath. *C*, transverse sections of the rectus sheath at four levels. *EO*, external oblique; *IO*, internal oblique; *TA*, transversus abdominis; *RA*, rectus abdominis; *TF*, transversalis fascia. *LA*, linea alba; *U*, umbilicus. The linea alba is a fibrous band stretching from the xiphoid process of the sternum to the symphysis pubis (also see Figs. 2-8 to 2-10). It is wider above than below the umbilicus and forms the central anterior attachment for the muscles of the abdomen. Note that it is formed by the interlacing fibers of the aponeuroses of the right and left oblique and transversus abdominis muscles. Observe that the rectus sheath is formed by the aponeuroses of the three flat abdominal muscles which surround the rectus abdominis.

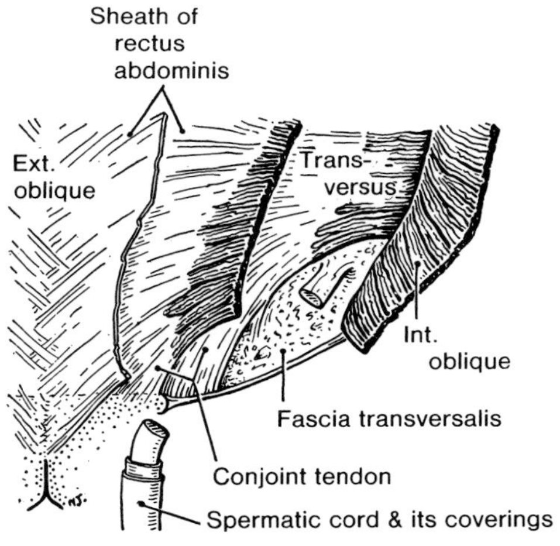

Figure 2-11. Drawing of a dissection of the rectus sheath demonstrating its continuity with the conjoint tendon.

fixed, compression of the viscera by the abdominal muscles raises the intra-abdominal pressure. These actions produce the force required for **defecation** (bowel movement), **micturition** (urination), and **parturition** (childbirth). They also make the trunk rigid, a requirement for pushing or lifting heavy objects.

Acting together, the three flat muscles compress the abdomen (increasing intra-abdominal pressure) and depress the ribs (increasing the vertical diameter of the chest). *Acting separately*, they can move the vertebral column; *e.g.*, contraction of one internal oblique muscle produces a combination of flexion and rotation of the trunk to its side.

The Rectus Abdominis Muscle (Figs. 2-3, 2-7, 2-8, 2-10, 2-11, and 2-15). These long strap muscles are the *principal vertical muscles* of the anterior abdominal wall. One lies on each side of the linea alba and is three times as wide superiorly as it is inferiorly. The lateral borders of the rectus and its sheath are convex and form clinically important surface markings known as the **lineae semilunares**, easily observed on lean persons (Fig. 2-3). *The rectus abdominis muscle is largely enclosed in the rectus*

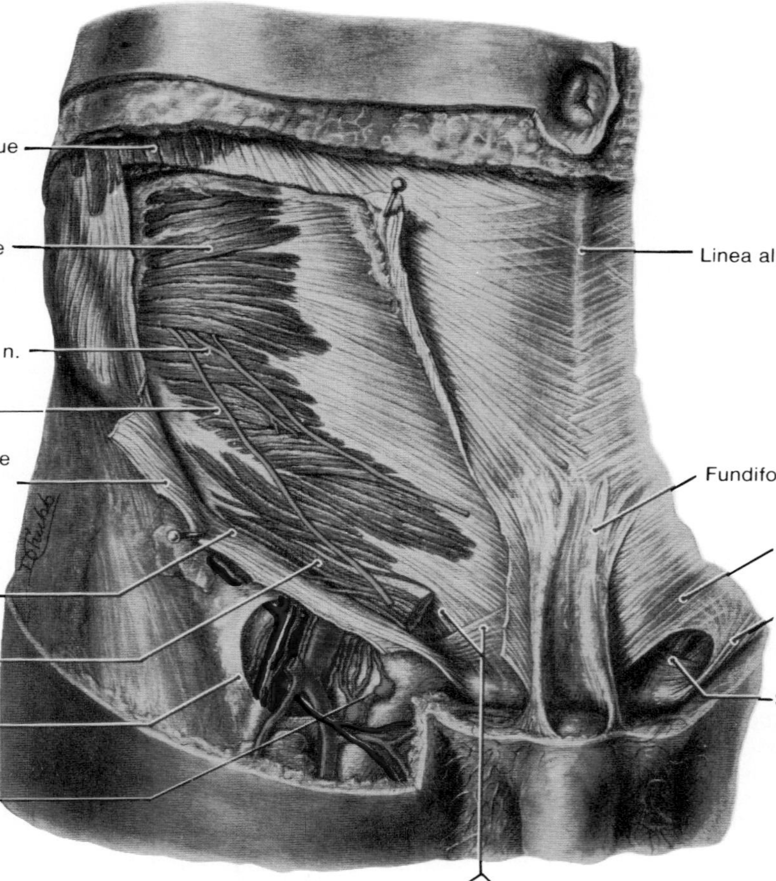

Figure 2-12. Drawing of a dissection of the inguinal region. The external oblique aponeurosis is partly cut away and the spermatic cord is cut short. Observe the laminated, fundiform (suspensory) ligament of the penis descending to the junction of the fixed and mobile parts of the organ. Examine the reflex inguinal ligament which represents the external oblique, lying anterior to the conjoint tendon which represents the internal oblique and transversus abdominis muscles. Note that only two structures course between the external and internal oblique muscles, namely the iliohypogastric and ilioinguinal branches of the first lumbar nerve segment. They are sensory from this point to their terminations. Observe that the fleshy fibers of the internal oblique at the level of the anterior superior iliac spine run horizontally; those from the iliac crest pass mediocranially, and those from the inguinal ligament arch mediocaudally. Note the cremaster muscle covering the cord and filling the arched space between the conjoint tendon and the inguinal ligament. Observe that at the level of the umbilicus, the aponeurosis of the external oblique blends with the aponeurosis of the internal oblique near the lateral border of the rectus, but in the suprapubic region it is free as far as the median plane. Note the numerous lymph vessels (not labeled) streaming cranially around the femoral vessels.

sheath, formed by the aponeuroses of the three flat abdominal muscles (Fig. 2-10).

Origin. Front of **pubic symphysis** and **pubic crest**.

Insertion. Anterior surfaces of **xiphoid process** and the **costal cartilages** (fifth to seventh). The anterior wall of the rectus sheath is firmly attached to the rectus muscle at three or four **tendinous intersections** (Fig. 2-7). When this muscle is tensed

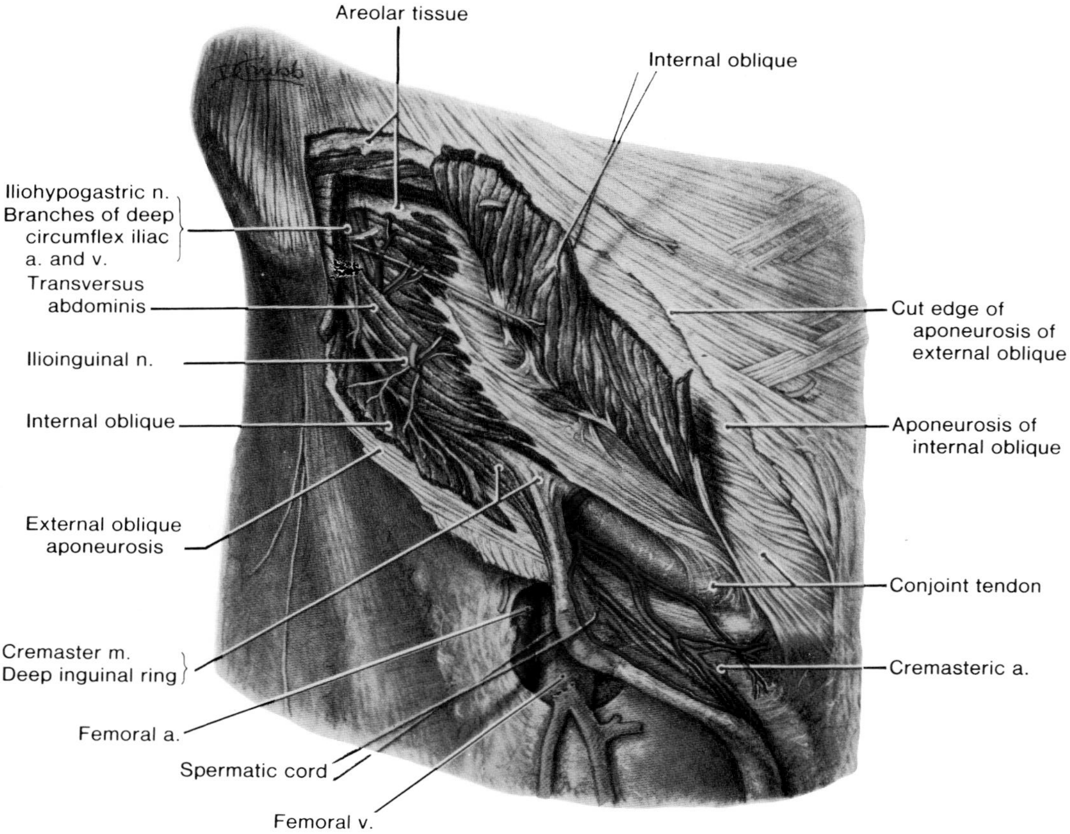

Figure 2-13. Drawing of a dissection of the inguinal region with the internal oblique muscle reflected and the spermatic cord retracted. Observe the transversus abdominis muscle fibers taking, in this region, the same common mediocaudal direction as the fibers of the external oblique aponeurosis and the internal oblique. Note that the transversus abdominis has a less extensive origin from the inguinal ligament than the internal oblique muscle. Observe that the internal oblique portion of the conjoint tendon is attached to the pubic crest and that the transversus portion extends laterally along the pecten pubis. Note that the conjoint tendon is not sharply defined from the fascia transversalis but blends with it. Observe that lumbar segment 1, via the iliohypogastric and ilioinguinal nerves, supplies the fibers of the internal oblique and transversus abdominis and therefore controls the conjoint tendon. Observe that the fascia transversalis is evaginated to form the tubular internal spermatic fascia; the mouth of the tube, called the deep (internal) inguinal ring is situated lateral to the inferior epigastric vessels. Note that the cremasteric artery, a branch of the inferior epigastric, anastomoses with the testicular artery and the artery to the ductus deferens. Observe the cremaster muscle arising from the inguinal ligament.

in well developed males (Fig. 2-3), each stretch of muscle between the tendinous intersections bulges out. The *location of these intersections* are indicated by the grooves between the muscle bulges and are located at the level of (1) the xiphoid process, (2) the umbilicus, and (3) about halfway between these structures. If a fourth intersection is present, it may be above or below the umbilicus. About 6% of people have only two tendinous intersections.

Nerve Supply. Ventral rami of **lower six** or **seven thoracic nerves**.

Actions. **Flexes lumbar region of vertebral column**, **depresses ribs**, and **stabilizes pelvis** during walking. This fixation

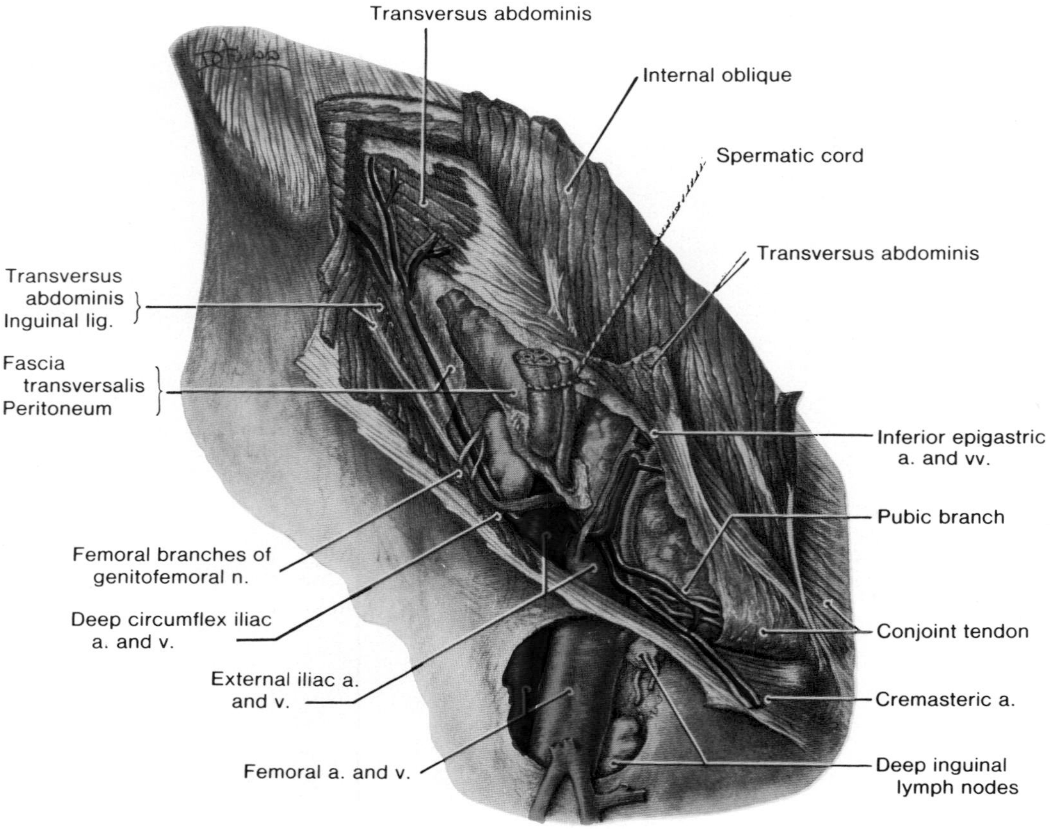

Figure 2-14 Drawing of a deep dissection of the inguinal region. The inguinal part of the transversus abdominis muscle and the fascia transversalis are partly cut away and the spermatic cord is excised. Observe that the lower limit of the peritoneal sac lies some distance above the inguinal ligament laterally but close to it medially. Note the location of the deep inguinal ring, about a fingerbreadth above the inguinal ligament at the midpoint between the anterior superior iliac spine and the pubic tubercle. Observe the proximity of the external iliac artery and vein to the inguinal canal and the three branches of the external iliac artery: the deep circumflex iliac, inferior epigastric, and femoral arteries.

of the pelvis enables the thigh muscles to act effectively. Similarly, during leg lifts from the supine position, the rectus abdominis muscles contract to prevent tilting of the pelvis by the weight of the lower limbs.

The Linea Alba and the Rectus Sheath (Figs. 2-3, 2-8 to 2-10, 2-12, and 2-15). These structures have been mentioned several times previously and briefly described; however, owing to its clinical importance, a more detailed description of the rectus sheath and its relationship to the linea alba is required.

The rectus sheath is the strong, incomplete *fibrous compartment of the rectus abdominis* muscle. It forms as follows. At its lateral margin, the internal oblique aponeurosis splits into two layers, one passing anterior to the rectus muscle and one passing posterior to it (Fig. 2-10*C*). The anterior layer joins with the aponeurosis of the external oblique to form the **anterior wall of the rectus sheath**, and the posterior layer joins with the aponeurosis of the transversus abdominis muscle to form the **posterior wall of the rectus sheath**. The

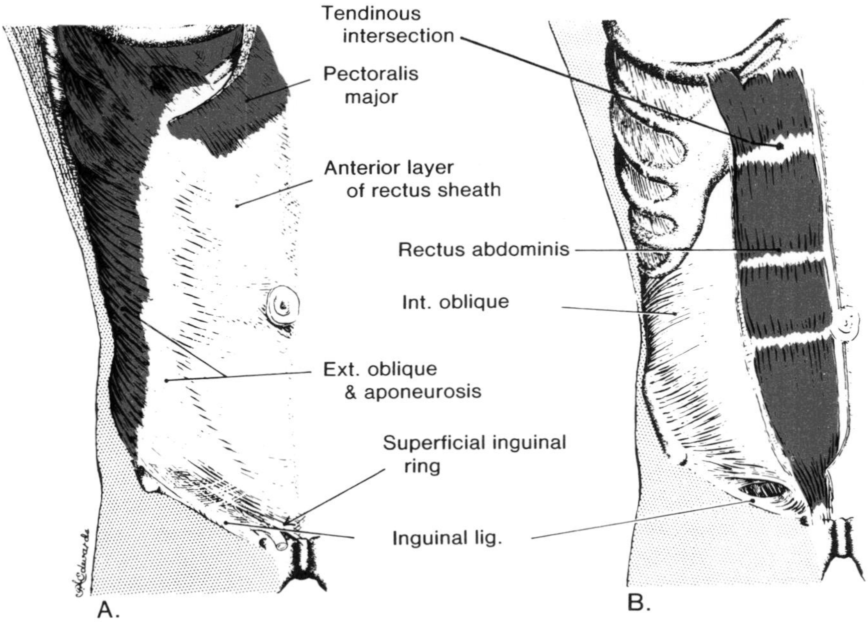

Figure 2-15. Drawing of a dissection of the anterior abdominal wall. *A*, showing the external oblique muscle and its aponeurosis contributing to the anterior wall of the rectus sheath. *B*, showing the internal oblique and rectus abdominis muscles. The right side of the rectus was exposed by removing the anterior wall of the rectus sheath formed by the aponeuroses of the two flat muscles. The anterior layer of the rectus sheath is firmly attached to the rectus muscle at the three tendinous intersections illustrated. The origin and insertion of the rectus muscle is also shown. Observe that the external oblique arises from the *external* surface of the lower ribs and that the internal oblique inserts into the *inferior* surface of the lower ribs.

anterior and posterior walls of the sheath are fused in the anterior median line to form the median raphe, called the **linea alba** (Fig. 2-9).

Above the costal margin, the posterior wall of the rectus sheath is deficient because the transversus abdominis muscle passes internal to the costal cartilages and the internal oblique muscle is attached to the costal margin. Hence, *above the costal margin, the rectus abdominis muscle lies directly on the thoracic wall.*

The lower one-fourth of the rectus sheath is also deficient because here the internal oblique aponeurosis does not split to enclose the rectus muscle (Fig. 2-10*C*). The lower limit of the posterior wall of the rectus sheath is marked by a crescentic border called the **arcuate line** (Fig. 2-8). The position of this line is usuallly midway between the umbilicus and the pubic crest (Fig. 2-1). From this line downward, the aponeuroses of the three flat muscles pass anterior to the rectus muscle to form the anterior layer of the rectus sheath (Figs. 2-8 and 2-10*C*). Here, the rectus muscle is directly in contact posteriorly with the transversalis fascia.

Within the rectus sheath there may be a small triangular muscle, called the *pyramidalis*, which lies on the front of the lower part of the rectus abdominis muscle. It arises from the pubic crest and inserts into the linea alba. Although it tenses the linea alba, the reason for this is unknown. *The pyramidalis muscle is unimportant* and is often absent.

Important structures within the rectus sheath are the **superior** and **inferior epigastric vessels** (Fig. 2-8) and the terminal parts of the lower five **intercostal** and **subcostal vessels** and **nerves** (Fig. 2-131).

Nerves of Anterior Abdominal Wall (Figs. 2-6 to 2-8 and 2-12 to 2-14). The skin

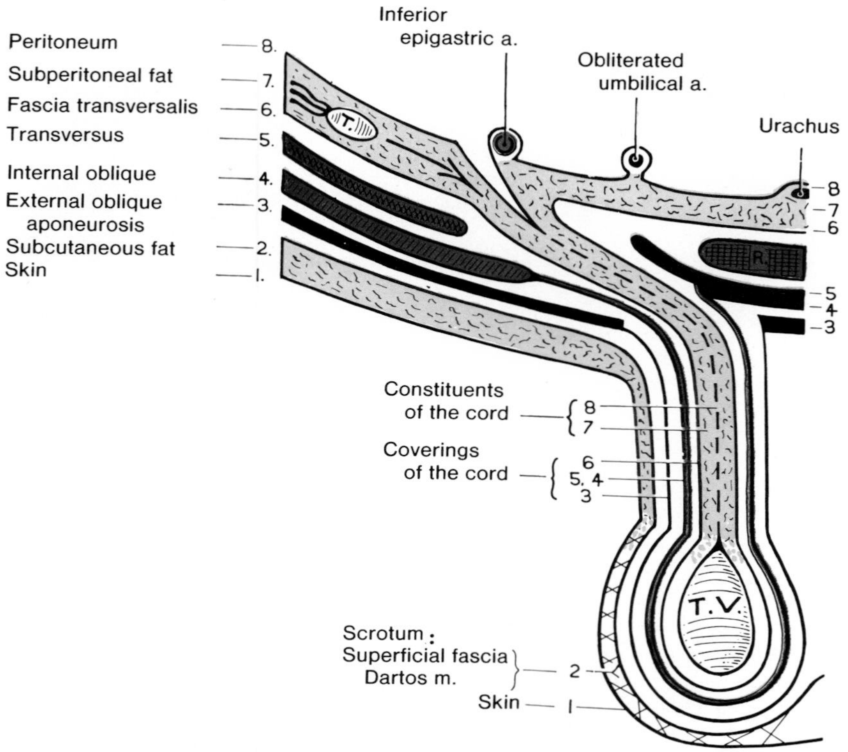

Figure 2-16. Drawing illustrating the scheme of the inguinal canal and the origin of the coverings of the spermatic cord. In this schematic horizontal section, the scrotum and testis are assumed to have been raised to the level of the superficial inguinal ring. The drawing shows the eight layers of the abdominal wall and their three evaginations: the scrotum, the coverings of the spermatic cord, and the constituents of the spermatic cord. T.V., tunica vaginalis of testis. *R,* rectus abdominis.

and muscles of the anterior abdominal wall are supplied almost entirely by the continuation of the **lower intercostal** (T7 to T11) and **subcostal** (T12) **nerves**. The inferior part of the wall is supplied by the first lumbar nerve via the **iliohypogastric** and **ilioinguinal nerves**.

The main trunks of the intercostal nerves pass forward from the intercostal spaces and run between the internal oblique and transversus abdominis muscles (Fig. 2-8). *These nerves supply the abdominal muscles and the overlying skin.* This common nerve supply explains why palpating the abdomen with cold hands is sufficient to cause contraction of the abdominal muscles.

The anterior cutaneous branches of these nerves pierce the rectus sheath a short distance from the median plane and supply the skin of the anterior abdomen (Fig. 2-7). The anterior cutaneous branches of *T7 to T9* supply the skin *superior to the umbilicus* (Fig. 2-141); *T10* innervates the skin at the *level of the umbilicus*; and *T11, T12, and L1* supply the skin *inferior to the umbilicus.* The first lumbar nerve appears just above the inguinal ligament, where it is called the **iliohypogastric nerve** (Fig. 2-8).

CLINICALLY ORIENTED COMMENTS

When incising the anterior abdominal wall during surgery, the *incisions are made through those parts of the wall which give the freest access to the organ(s) concerned with the least disturbance of the nerve supply to the muscles.* Because there are communications between the intercostal nerves in the intercostal spaces and in the anterior abdominal wall, it is possible to cut one or two of the cutaneous nerves without noticeable loss of sensation. It is important to know that *little if any communication occurs between nerves from the lateral border of the rectus abdominis to the midline.* For this reason a transverse incision through this muscle causes the least possible damage to its nerve supply. A vertical incision through the lateral portion of the rectus abdominis muscle (**pararectus incision**) denervates the portion of the muscle medial to the incision (Fig. 2-8). *The rectus abdominis muscle may be divided transversely without serious damage* because when rejoined, a new transverse band forms similar to the normal tendinous intersections, provided the nerve supply is intact. A common incision used by surgeons is a right or left **paramedian incision.** This passes through the anterior layer of the rectus sheath (Fig. 2-7), and the muscle is freed from the sheath and retracted laterally. The posterior layer of the rectus sheath (Fig. 2-8) is then incised to enter the abdominal cavity. In this way, the nerve supply is not interfered with and a strong repair normally results.

Another common incision is the small *muscle-and-aponeurosis-splitting right lower quadrant incision* used for **appendectomy** (Fig. 2-45). The external oblique aponeurosis is split obliquely in the direction of its fibers and retracted. The internal oblique and transversus abdominis musculoaponeurotic fibers, lying at right angles to those of the external oblique (Fig. 2-14), can then be separated parallel to their course. Carefully made, *the entire exposure cuts no musculoaponeuronitic fibers,* so that when the incision is closed the abdominal wall is as strong after the operation as before.

Many incisions are used to penetrate the anterior abdominal wall. The incision used depends on the organ to be reached and the extent of the operation to be performed.

Inflammation of the peritoneum lining the abdominopelvic cavity (**peritonitis**) causes pain in the overlying skin and a *reflex increase in the tone of the abdominal muscles.* Normally, rhythmic movements of the anterior abdominal wall accompany respirations (*i.e.*, the abdomen comes out with the chest). If the abdomen goes in as the chest goes out (**paradoxical abdominothoracic rhythm**) and muscle rigidity is present, it is probable that peritoneal inflammation or pneumonia is present.

Vessels of the Anterior Abdominal Wall (Figs. 2-7, 2-8, 2-13, and 2-14). Small arteries arise from the anterior and collateral branches of the **posterior intercostal arteries** of the 10th and 11th intercostal spaces and from the anterior branch of the **subcostal artery** to supply the muscles of the anterior abdominal wall. They anastomose with the **superior epigastric artery**, with the upper **lumbar arteries**, and with each other.

The main arteries of the anterior abdominal wall are the inferior epigastric and deep circumflex iliac arteries, branches of the **external iliac artery** (Fig. 2-142) *and the superior epigastric artery,* a terminal branch of the **internal thoracic artery** (Figs. 1-20 and 1-21).

The **inferior epigastric artery** runs upward and medially into the rectus sheath (Fig. 2-8). The **deep circumflex iliac artery** runs on the deep aspect of the anterior abdominal wall, parallel to the inguinal ligament (Fig. 2-7) and along the iliac crest between the transversus abdominis and internal oblique muscles. The **superior epigastric artery** enters the rectus sheath from above (Fig. 2-8), just below the seventh costal cartilage, and supplies the anterior abdominal muscles and the skin.

The superficial epigastric (Fig. 2-7) and **lateral thoracic veins** anastomose, thereby uniting the veins of the upper and lower halves of the body. The three superficial inguinal veins end in the **great saphenous vein** of the lower limb (Figs. 2-7, 2-8, and 4-12 to 4-16).

The superficial lymph vessels of the anterior abdominal wall *above the umbilicus* pass to the **axillary lymph nodes** (Figs. 6-10 and 6-47), whereas those *below the umbilicus* drain into the **inguinal lymph nodes** (Figs. 2-12 and 2-14).

Posterior Surface of Anterior Ab-

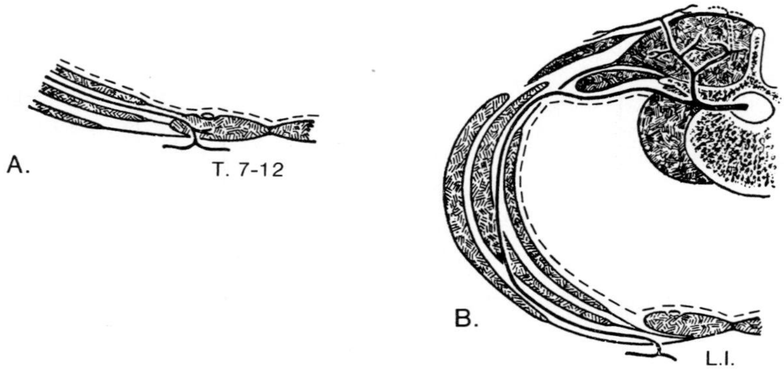

Figure 2-17. Drawings illustrating the course of the ventral (anterior) rami of nerves in the abdominal wall. *A*, lower six thoracic nerves. *B*, first lumbar nerve. ----indicates transversalis fascia (also see Fig. 2-10*C*). Note that the ventral rami of the lower six thoracic nerves run between the internal oblique and transversus abdominis muscles to the lateral margin of the rectus abdominis. Observe that the ventral ramus of the first lumbar nerve pierces the internal oblique and then runs between this muscle and the external oblique to pierce the external oblique aponeurosis.

dominal Wall (Figs. 2-16 and 2-17). The internal surface of the anterior abdominal wall exhibits several folds, some of which contain obliterated fetal vessels that carried blood before birth to and from the placenta. *The term fold is usually used to describe a peritoneal elevation with a free edge.* Most folds are raised by underlying blood vessels and do not provide much strength.

Above the umbilicus there is a median fold of peritoneum, called the falciform ligament (Fig. 2-29), which passes from the umbilical region to the liver. This fold contains the **ligamentum teres** of the liver, the **obliterated umbilical vein.** The umbilical vein carried oxygenated blood from the placenta to fetus before birth. It is usually patent for some time after birth and may be used for **exchange transfusions** during early infancy (*e.g.*, in infants with **erythroblastosis fetalis** or hemolytic disease of the fetus).

Below the umbilicus there are **five umbilical folds** (two on each side and one in the midline)which pass upward toward the umbilicus. The **lateral umbilical folds** are formed by peritoneum covering the previously described **inferior epigastric vessels** (Figs. 2-14 and 2-16). The **medial umbilical folds** are formed by the peritoneum covering the **lateral umbilical ligaments** (obliterated umbilical arteries that carried blood to the placenta for oxygenation before birth). The **median umbilical fold** is formed by the peritoneum covering the **median umbilical ligament**, the remnant of the **urachus** (Figs. 2-16 and 3-17), which developed from the intra-abdominal part of the **allantois**. The median umbilical ligament is attached to the apex of the urinary bladder (Fig. 3-73).

THE INGUINAL REGION

Inferiorly, all the abdominal muscles, chiefly their aponeuroses, contribute to the inguinal ligament and the inguinal canal. As described previously, the lower free edge of the aponeurosis of the external oblique muscle forms a thick band known as the **inguinal ligament** (Fig. 2-9), extending from the anterior superior iliac spine to the pubic tubercle (Fig. 2-1). Fibers are reflected from the medial end of the inguinal ligament to the pecten pubis (Fig. 2-1) to form the **lacunar ligament** (Fig. 2-9).

The Superficial Inguinal Ring (Figs. 2-7, 2-9, and 2-12). Although called a ring, this opening is actually a more or less triangular aperture, the base of which is formed by the pubic bone and the sides by the split in the aponeurosis of the external oblique muscle.

The superficial (external) inguinal ring is for the passage of the **spermatic cord** in the male (Fig. 2-7) and the **round ligament of the uterus** in the female (Fig. 2-23). The central point of the superficial inguinal ring is above the pubic tubercle (Figs. 2-9 and 2-23). Its base is formed by the lateral half of the pubic crest (Fig. 2-1) and its sides are the medial and lateral crura (L. legs). The **lateral (inferior) crus** is formed by the part of the external oblique aponeurosis that attaches to the pubic tubercle via the inguinal ligament (Fig. 2-9). The spermatic cord rests on the inferior part of the lateral crus (Fig. 2-7). The **medial (superior) crus** is formed by the part of the aponeurosis that diverges to attach to the pubic bone and the pubic crest medial to the pubic tubercle (Fig. 2-9). **Intercrural fibers** from the inguinal ligament arch upward and medially across the superficial inguinal ring, preventing the crura from spreading apart (Figs. 2-7 and 2-9).

In living men the superficial inguinal ring can be examined by invaginating the skin of the scrotum with the tip of a finger. By probing gently upward with the finger along the **spermatic cord**, the tip of the finger can be pushed into the superficial inguinal ring without causing pain. In women and children the dimensions of this ring are much less than in adult males and palpation of the superficial ring in them is difficult. In male infants, the superficial inguinal ring does not normally admit the tip of the average adult little finger.

Prenatal Migration of the Testes (Fig. 2-18). To understand the inguinal region and the inguinal canal, an understanding of the migration and **descent of the testes** that occur before birth is essential. The testes develop inside the abdominal cavity deep to the transversalis fascia, between it and the peritoneum, and normally migrate through the **inguinal canals** (Fig. 2-16) into the scrotum just before birth (Fig. 2-18).

The inguinal region is first indicated by a ligament, the **gubernaculum,** which extends from the testis through the anterior abdominal wall and inserts into the inner surface of the scrotum. Later, a finger-like diverticulum of peritoneum called the **processus vaginalis** follows the gubernaculum and evaginates (protrudes through) the anterior abdominal wall. This processus vaginalis carries extensions of the layers of the anterior abdominal wall before it. In males these extensions become the cover-

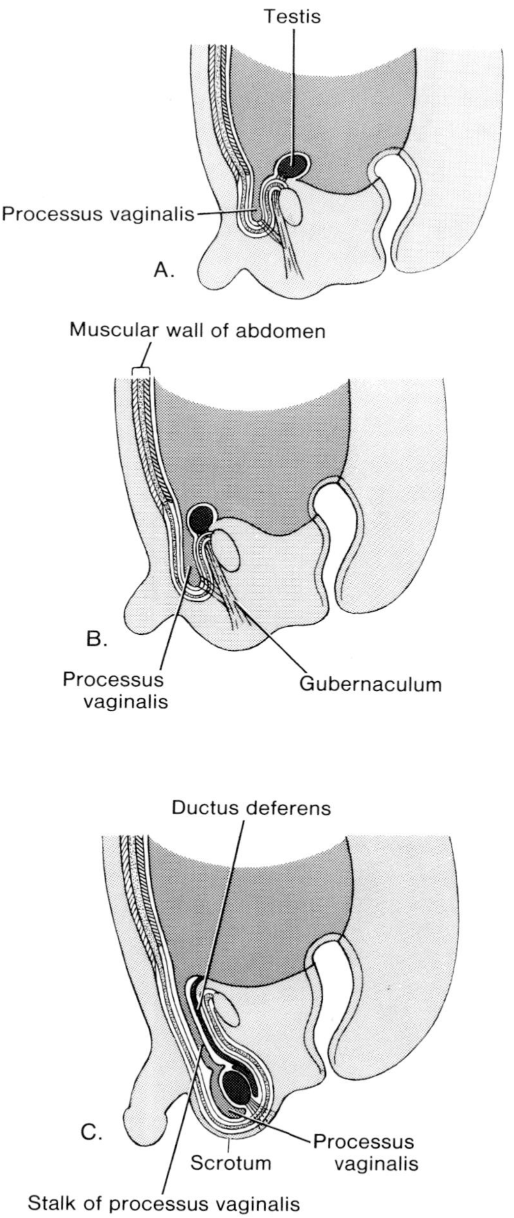

Figure 2-18. Schematic drawings of sagittal sections (28 to 38 weeks) illustrating the formation of the inguinal canals and the descent of the testes. Note that the processus vaginalis evaginates the abdominal wall and carries fascial layers of the abdominal wall before it. Just before birth the testis descends behind the processus vaginalis into the scrotum. Normally this processus obliterates shortly after birth, leaving only the part of it which surrounds the testis, called the tunica vaginalis (see Fig. 2-19*B*).

ings of the spermatic cord (Fig. 2-16). *In both sexes*, the opening produced by the processus vaginalis in the transversalis fascia becomes the **deep inguinal ring** and the opening in the external oblique aponeurosis forms the **superficial inguinal ring.**

Just before birth in males, the testes normally follow the paths (inguinal canals) through the anterior abdominal wall and enter the scrotum. Normally most of the processus vaginalis obliterates shortly after birth, leaving only the part surrounding the testis, which becomes the **tunica vaginalis** (Fig. 2-19*B*).

CLINICALLY ORIENTED COMMENTS

Maldescent of the testis (undescended testis or **cryptorchidism**) is a common abnormality. The testes are undescended at birth in about 3% of fullterm and 30% of premature infants. **Undescended testes** are located in the pelvic cavity or somewhere in the inguinal canal (Fig. 3-110*A*).

Most undescended testes descend during the first few weeks or months after birth. A few more descend at puberty owing to stimulation by testicular androgens (*e.g.*, testosterone). The seminiferous tubules (Fig. 2-19*B*) do not develop fully in testes that remain undescended after puberty and infertility results when the condition is bilateral, but *androgen secretion is usually unimpaired.*

Uncommonly, the gubernaculum attaches in an abnormal location and the testis later follows it through the inguinal canal to the abnormal site. An **ectopic testis** may be located in the perineum, in the pubopenile area, or in the femoral region (Fig. 3-110*B*).

Prenatal Migration of the Ovaries. Although the ovaries migrate from their place of origin in the abdominal cavity to a point just below the pelvic brim, they do not pass through the inguinal canals. The processus vaginalis normally obliterates completely and the **gubernaculum** becomes incorporated into the wall of the uterus, dividing into the **ligament of the ovary** and the **round ligament of the uterus** (Fig. 2-23). The latter one passes through the inguinal canal and attaches to the internal surface of the labium majus (homologous to half of the scrotum in the male).

The Deep Inguinal Ring (Figs. 2-13 and 2-20). This *deficiency in the transversalis fascia* is located just lateral to the **inferior epigastric artery**, immediately superior to the inguinal ligament, and medial to the origin of the transversus abdominis muscle from the inguinal ligament. The deep ring formed when the processus vaginalis evaginated the transversalis fascia (Fig. 2-18). In males, the testis normally passes through this ring during the fetal period.

The margins of the deep inguinal ring are not so sharply defined as those of the superficial inguinal ring. When the external oblique is reflected and the epigastric vessels are displaced, it ceases to exist as a ring; however, from the inner aspect, a dimple in the peritoneum often marks the site of the ring (Fig. 2-16).

Coverings of the Spermatic Cord (Figs. 2-8, 2-11, 2-16, 2-18, and 2-19*A*). The bundle of structures passing to and from the testis (ductus deferens, nerves, and vessels), called the **spermatic cord,** *is covered by three concentric layers of fascia derived from the anterior abdominal wall.* These coverings formed as the processus vaginalis evaginated the abdominal wall and carried part of each of its layers into the scrotum (Fig. 2-18). The coverings are not easily separable from one another, either in a cadaver or in a living man.

The Internal Spermatic Fascia (Figs. 2-16, 2-18, and 2-19*A*). As the processus vaginalis evaginates the **transversalis fascia,** it carries a thin layer of fascia before it that becomes the internal spermatic fascia. It constitutes the filmy *innermost covering of the spermatic cord.* In Figure 2-16 verify that it is continuous with the fascia transversalis.

The Cremaster Muscle and Cremasteric Fascia (Figs. 2-12, 2-13, and 2-19*A*). As the processus vaginalis, with its covering of fascia transversalis (future internal spermatic fascia), evaginates under the edge of the **internal oblique muscle**, it acquires a few

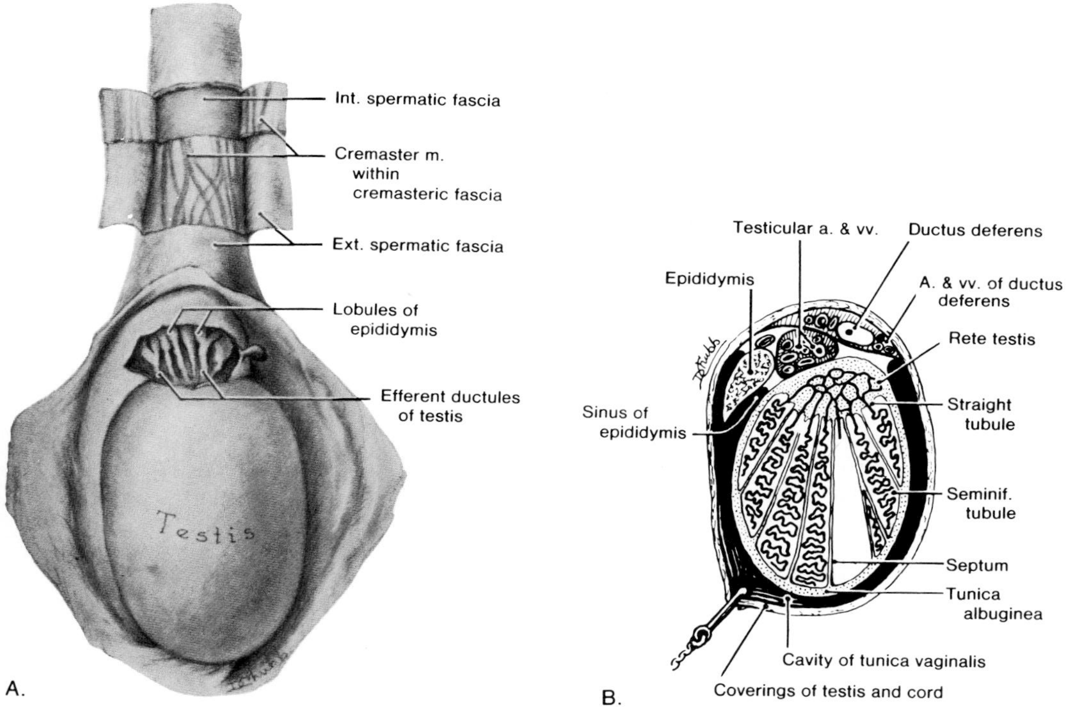

Figure 2-19. *A*, drawing of a dissection of the testis and spermatic cord illustrating, in particular, the coverings of the cord (compare with Fig. 2-16). *B*, drawing of a cross-section of the right testis from above. Observe the cavity of the tunica vaginalis surrounding the testis in front and at the sides and extending between the testis and the epididymis as the sinus of the epididymis. Examine the epididymis lying posterolateral to the testis. It indicates to which side a testis belongs, for it is on the right side of a right testis and on the left side of a left testis. Observe the ductus deferens with its small lumen and thick wall lying posteromedial to the testis. Note the pyramidal compartments for the seminiferous tubules. Each of the 250 compartments contains two or three hair-like seminiferous tubules which join in the mediastinum testis to form the rete testis.

of this muscle's most medial fibers and some investing fascia of the internal oblique muscle. These form the **cremaster muscle** and **cremasteric fascia**, respectively. The areolar cremasteric fascia forms the *middle covering of the spermatic cord*, which contains loops of cremaster muscle (Fig. 2-19*A*). These muscle fibers, which are continuous with the internal oblique, are not usually under voluntary control. They *reflexly draw the testis to a higher position* in the scrotum, particularly in the cold. Contraction of the cremaster muscle (Fig. 2-13) can often be produced by gentle stroking of the skin on the medial aspect of the thigh. This *reflex raising of the testis and scrotum is called* **the cremasteric reflex.** The testis, located outside the body, is sensitive to cold; hence, the cremaster draws it up into the scrotum for warmth and for protection against injury. *The elicitation of the cremasteric reflex is part of every routine physical examination in a male patient.* The afferent fibers of this reflex are carried in the genital branch of the **genitofemoral nerve** (Fig. 2-131). Sensory (afferent) fibers of this nerve supply the skin of the scrotum and the adjacent thigh and its motor fibers supply the cremaster muscle (efferent reflex arc). This reflex involves segments L1 and L2 of the spinal cord.

The External Spermatic Fascia (Figs. 2-16, 2-18, and 2-19*A*). As the **processus vaginalis** evaginates the external oblique aponeurosis and forms the superficial inguinal ring, it carries an extension of the aponeurosis before it which forms the external spermatic fascia. This is the thin *outermost covering of the spermatic cord.* It is attached superiorly to the crura of the superficial inguinal ring (Figs. 2-7 to 2-9) and is continuous with the fascia covering the external oblique muscle.

The Inguinal Canal (Figs. 2-9, 2-12 to 2-14, 2-16, and 2-20). This is an *intermuscular passage immediately superior to the medial half of the inguinal ligament* and parallel with it. It formed during the fetal period as the processus vaginalis evaginated the layers of the anterior abdominal wall (Fig. 2-18). The testis normally descends through it, invaginating the posterior wall of the processus vaginalis just before birth and taking with it the ductus deferens, its blood and lymph vessels, and nerves which become the constituents of the spermatic cord and are covered by the extensions of the abdominal wall.

The inguinal canal **begins at the deep inguinal ring** and **ends at the superficial inguinal ring**. It is 4 to 5 cm long and runs downward and medially from the deep inguinal ring.

The anterior wall of the inguinal canal is formed throughout mainly by the **aponeurosis of the external oblique** muscle. *The posterior wall of the inguinal canal* is formed throughout by the **fascia transversalis**, which is quite thick here and is reinforced medially by the **conjoint tendon** (Figs. 2-12 to 2-14) and the **reflex inguinal ligament** (Figs. 2-9 and 2-12). Between the anterior and posterior walls lies the internal oblique muscle, which is in front of most of the lateral part of the canal and arches over it to join with the aponeurosis of the transversus abdominis to form the conjoint tendon. This tendon lies behind the most medial part of the canal. Hence, the internal oblique lies in front of the deep inguinal ring and, as parts of the conjoint tendon, the two muscles lie behind the superficial inguinal ring (Fig. 2-20).

The inferior epigastric artery (and the obliterated umbilical arteries) run behind the posterior wall of the inguinal canal (Figs. 2-14 and 2-16). *The inferior epigastric artery lies at the medial boundary of the deep inguinal ring* (Fig. 2-26) and pulsations of it form a **useful landmark** during surgery for determining the location of the deep ring. The **floor of the inguinal canal** is formed by the grooved surface of the inguinal ligament (superior surface of lower part of external oblique aponeurosis) and the **lacunar ligament** (Fig. 2-9). The **roof of the inguinal canal** is formed by the arches of the internal oblique and transversus abdominis muscles (Figs. 2-20 and 2-21).

Factors Strengthening the Inguinal Region. The presence of the **inguinal canal produces a potential weak part in the**

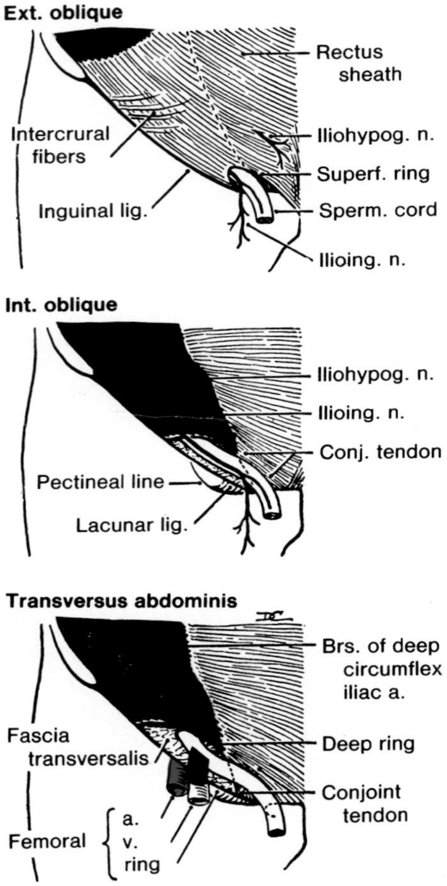

Figure 2-20. Drawings of dissections of the three flat muscles of the anterior abdominal wall below the level of the anterior superior iliac spine and the walls of the inguinal canal. Note that the anterior wall of this canal is formed throughout by the external oblique aponeurosis.

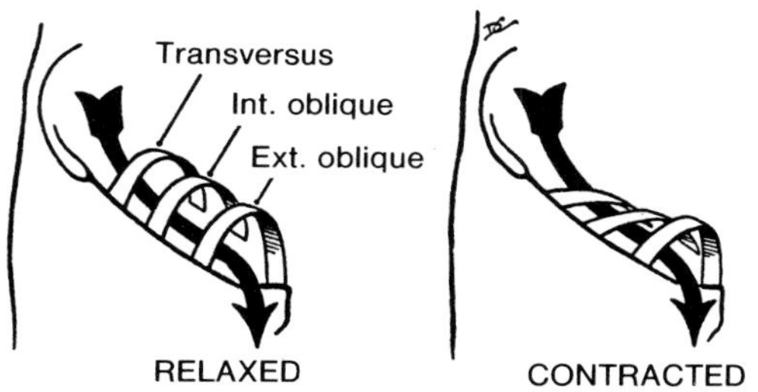

Figure 2-21. Diagrams illustrating "the inguinal arcade." Here the inguinal canal is likened to an arcade of three arches that is transversed by the spermatic cord (represented by the *arrow*). During standing, coughing, or vigorous straining, the anterior abdominal muscles contract and the arched fleshy fibers of the internal oblique and transversus abdominis cause the roof of the canal to become lower and taut. This action is essentially that of a half-sphincter.

lower part of the anterior abdominal wall. The anatomical structure of the canal compensates somewhat for this weakness. *Owing to the obliquity of the inguinal canal, the deep and superficial rings do not coincide*; thus, increases in intra-abdominal pressure act on the deep inguinal ring, forcing the posterior wall against the anterior wall of the canal. This strengthens this potentially weak area of the anterior abdominal wall.

The canal may be likened to an arcade of three arches formed by the three flat muscles (Fig. 2-21). The contraction of the external oblique muscle approximates the anterior wall to the posterior wall. The contraction of the arched fleshy fibers of the internal oblique and transversus abdominis muscles causes them to become taut and straighten. As a result, the roof of the canal is lower and the passage is constricted. During standing there is continuous contraction of the internal oblique and transversus abdominis muscles in the inguinal region. During coughing and straining, when the raised intra-abdominal pressure threatens to force a hernia through the canal, vigorous contraction of the arched fleshy fibers of the internal oblique and transversus abdominis "clamp down," without damaging the cord. The action is that of a half-sphincter.

The superficial inguinal ring has the conjoint tendon immediately behind it and the rectus abdominis muscle behind this tendon. When intra-abdominal pressure rises, the flat muscles of the abdomen all contract, forcing the external oblique aponeurosis against the conjoint tendon, which then pushes against the rectus abdominis. Hence, the conjoint tendon and the rectus abdominis reinforce the posterior surface of the superficial inguinal ring, tending to prevent herniation of the abdominal contents through it.

CLINICALLY ORIENTED COMMENTS

A hernia is a protrusion of a structure, viscus, or organ from the cavity in which it normally belongs. The term is derived from the Greek word meaning offshoot. Laymen refer to a hernia as a rupture, indicating that it is like a blowout caused by force or pressure.

Abdominal hernias are named according to the anatomical location of the protrusion (*e.g.*, inguinal, femoral, hiatal, and umbilical). If the hernia is through the anterior abdominal wall, the structure or viscus is usually covered by peritoneum, which forms a **hernial sac** (see Fig. 2-16 for the anatomical basis for this).

The most common type of hernia is inguinal hernia. Because the scrotum and the layers within it represent an outpouching of the lower anterior abdominal wall (Figs. 2-16 and 2-18), hernias into the scrotum or through the abdominal wall in the inguinal region are particularly common in males. Although the labia majora in females are homologous with the scrotum, they consist mostly of fat (Fig. 2-23); hence, the defect in the abdominal wall is small and *inguinal hernia is much less common in females than in males.* An inguinal hernia typically contains part of a viscus, most commonly part of the small or large intestine (Fig. 2-22*B*). In some cases, even the vermiform appendix passes into an inguinal hernial sac.

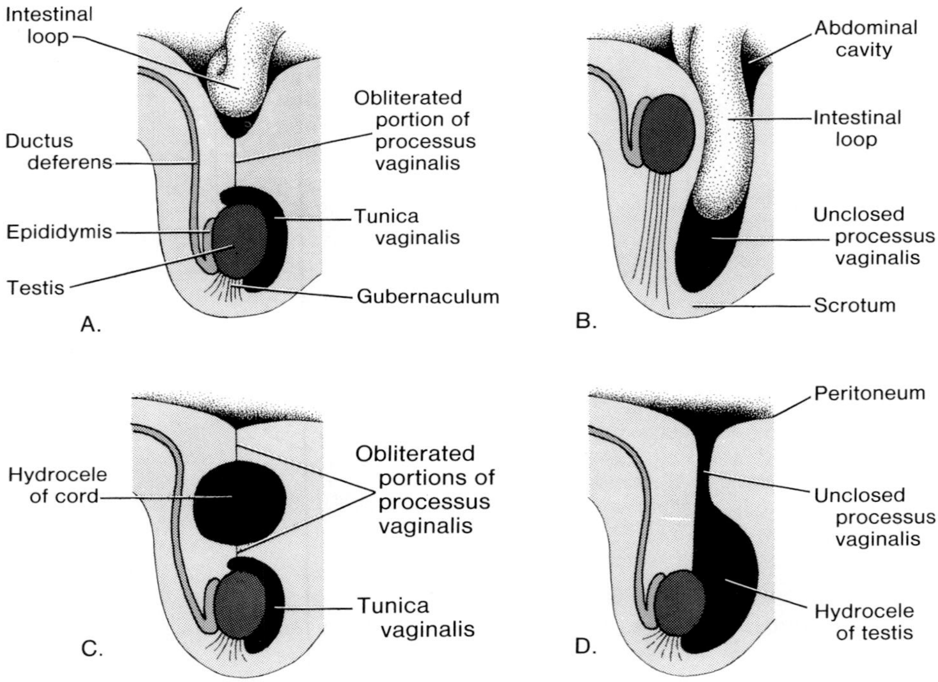

Figure 2-22. Drawings of sagittal sections of the inguinal region of fetuses illustrating the conditions resulting from failure of closure of the processus vaginalis. *A*, incomplete congenital inguinal hernia resulting from persistence of the proximal part of the processus vaginalis. *B*, complete congenital inguinal hernia into the scrotum resulting from persistence of the entire processus vaginalis. Cryptorchidism (undescended testis), a commonly associated malformation, is also illustrated. *C*, large cyst derived from an unobliterated portion of the processus vaginalis. This condition is called a hydrocele of the (spermatic) cord. *D*, hydrocele of the testis and spermatic cord resulting from peritoneal fluid passing into the unclosed processus vaginalis.

There is another weak area in the anterior abdominal wall. It is associated with the passage of the large femoral vessels (Figs. 2-13 to 2-15) behind the inguinal ligament to reach the lower limb. These **femoral hernias** are most common in females and are discussed with the lower limb (see Case 4-8 and Fig. 4-155).

There are two types of inguinal hernia, indirect (oblique) and direct. **Indirect inguinal hernia** is most common and *makes up about 75% of inguinal hernias.* As its name indicates, the hernia takes an indirect or oblique course through the anterior abdominal wall. It follows the route normally taken by the testis just before birth and **leaves the abdominal cavity lateral to the inferior epigastric vessels**, traversing the deep inguinal ring, the inguinal canal, and the superficial inguinal ring *within the spermatic cord.* Hence, it is covered by all three layers of this cord.

Indirect inguinal hernia has an embryological basis and is most common in young males. The evagination of the peritoneum, called the **processus vaginalis**, forms the inguinal canal (Fig. 2-18) and creates the potential passageway for an indirect inguinal hernia. *The hernial sac represents the remains of the processus vaginalis*, which normally obliterates, except for the part that forms the tunica vaginalis (Figs. 2-19B and 2-22*A*). If the processus vaginalis does not undergone obliteration, the hernia is complete and extends into the scrotum or the labium majus (Fig. 2-22*B*). *Indirect inguinal hernia is about 20 times more common in males than in females.* The main reason for this is that the ovary and its vessels do not descend through the

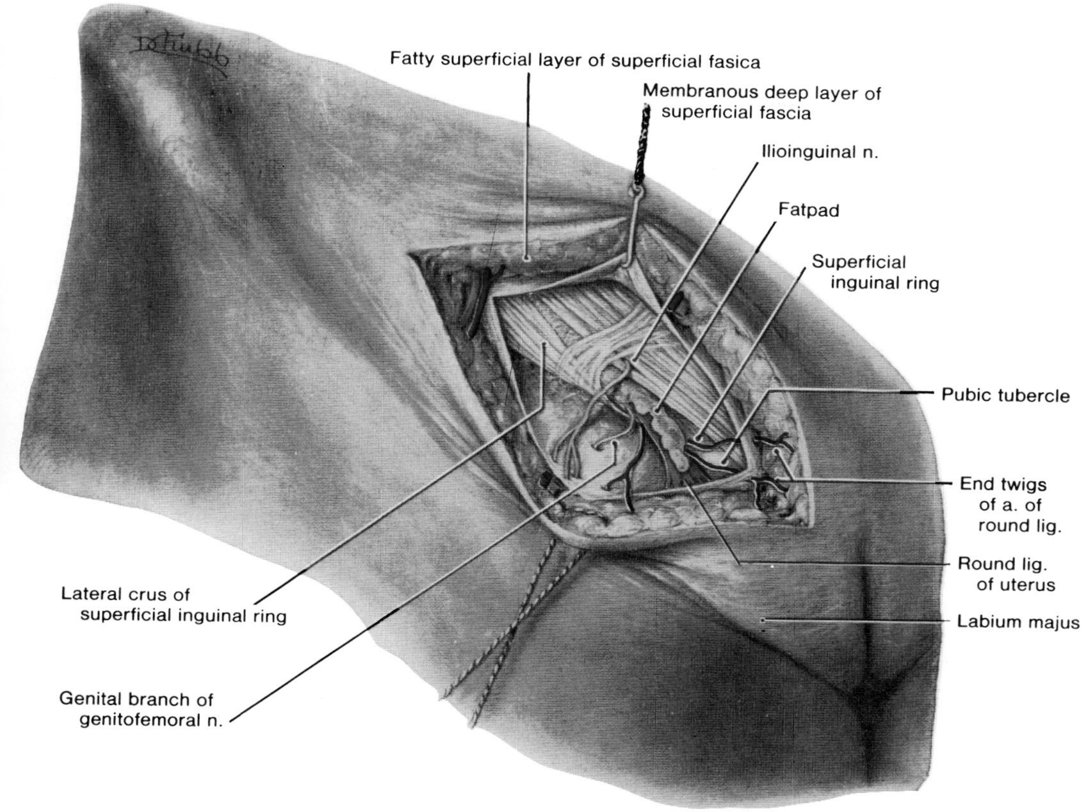

Figure 2-23. Drawing of a dissection of the female inguinal canal. Observe that the superficial inguinal ring is small and that its crura are prevented from spreading by the intercrural fibers. Note the following structures issuing from the superficial inguinal ring: (1) the round ligament of the uterus, (2) a closely applied pad of fat, (3) the genital branch of the genitofemoral nerve, and (4) the artery of the round ligament of the uterus. This artery is homologous with the cremasteric artery in the male, shown in Figure 2-14. Observe that the ilioinguinal nerve in this specimen perforates the medial crus of the superficial inguinal ring.

inguinal canal; hence, the defect in the abdominal wall is not so great as in the male. However, if the processus vaginalis persists in a female, a hernia may follow it through the inguinal canal into the labium majus. A persistent processus vaginalis in the female is known as the *canal of Nuck*.

Direct inguinal hernia *protrudes anteriorly through the posterior wall of the inguinal canal* and **leaves the abdominal cavity medial to the inferior epigastric vessels**. In direct inguinal hernia, the protrusion passes through some part of the **inguinal triangle** (Hesselbach's triangle), usually the lower part. *This triangle is bounded by the inguinal ligament inferiorly, the inferior epigastric artery laterally, and the rectus abdominis muscle medially.* The inguinal triangle lies just posterior to the superficial inguinal ring and marks the area of the posterior wall of the inguinal canal that is formed only by transversalis fascia. Obviously, *the inguinal triangle is a weak area of the anterior abdominal wall.*

In direct inguinal hernia, the hernial sac does not pass through the deep inguinal ring but passes through or around the conjoint tendon and directly to the superficial inguinal ring. If the hernia passes lateral to the conjoint tendon, it pushes before it the peritoneum and the transversalis fascia to emerge through the superficial inguinal ring, either above or below the spermatic cord. If the hernia passes through the fibers of the conjoint tendon it is covered by peritoneum, the transversalis fascia, and the fibers of the conjoint tendon on its way to emerge through the superficial inguinal ring.

Direct inguinal hernia is much less common than indirect inguinal hernia and occurs more often in men than women. It usually results from weakening of the conjoint tendon, a condition that is most common in old persons.

THE SCROTUM AND ITS CONTENTS

The scrotum and the testes are considered here because their development is related to the abdomen. Each half of the scrotum and the layers within it represent outpouchings of the anterior abdominal wall in the inguinal region.

The Scrotum (Figs. 2-16, 2-18, 2-19, and 2-24). The scrotum is a pendulous sac that contains the testes. It *consists of two layers*, **skin** and **superficial fascia**. The thin skin is dark colored and rugose (wrinkled). The superficial fascia is devoid of fat, but contains a sheet of smooth muscle called the **dartos muscle**. Its fibers are united to the skin and contraction of them cause the scrotal skin to wrinkle when cold. This helps to regulate the loss of heat through the skin of the scrotum. *Normal spermatogenesis* (*sperm formation*) *requires a controlled temperature*.

The superficial fascia of the scrotum is continuous anteriorly with the membranous layer of superficial fascia of the anterior abdominal wall (Scarpa's fascia) and posteriorly with the superficial fascia of the perineum (Colle's fascia). The superficial fascia, including the dartos muscle, forms an incomplete scrotal septum that divides the scrotum into right and left halves, one for each testis.

The coverings of testis are continuous with the coverings of the spermatic cord described previously (Figs. 2-16 and 2-19*A*).

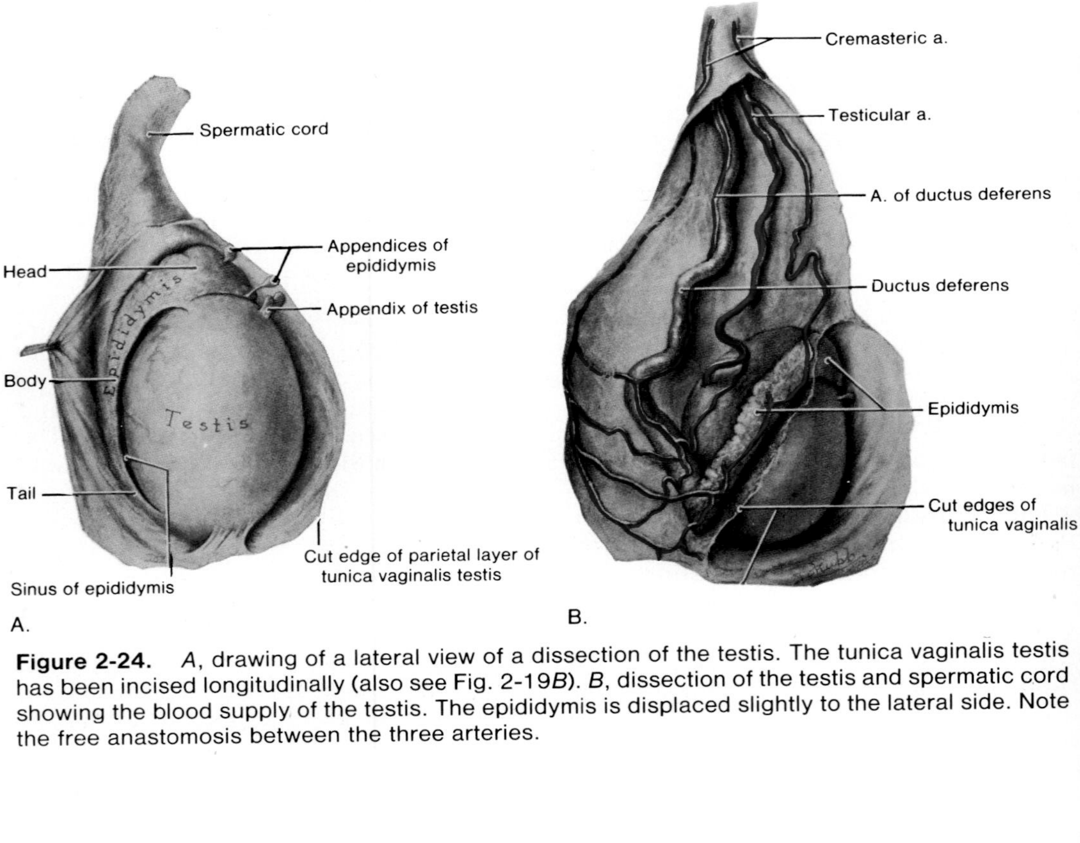

Figure 2-24. *A*, drawing of a lateral view of a dissection of the testis. The tunica vaginalis testis has been incised longitudinally (also see Fig. 2-19*B*). *B*, dissection of the testis and spermatic cord showing the blood supply of the testis. The epididymis is displaced slightly to the lateral side. Note the free anastomosis between the three arteries.

The outermost layer (tunic) of the testis, the **external spermatic fascia**, is continuous with this covering of the spermatic cord which is continuous with the external oblique aponeurosis at the superficial ring. Internal to this layer is the **cremaster muscle** and **cremasteric fascia**, which is primarily fascial in the scrotum. Inside this layer is the **internal spermatic fascia**, which is continuous with this layer covering the spermatic cord and the transversalis fascia. Inside the internal spermatic fascia is the **tunica vaginalis testis** (Fig. 2-19*B*), a derivative of the processus vaginalis (Fig. 2-22*A*). This peritoneal sac (closed serous sac) is applied to the front and sides of the testis. It consists of two layers: (1) the **parietal layer** is superficial and is *adjacent to the internal spermatic fascia*, and (2) the **visceral layer** is *adherent to the testis and the epididymis*, a coiled tubular structure that stores the sperms. Laterally the visceral layer of the tunica vaginalis passes between the testis and the epididymis to form the **sinus of the epididymis** (Figs. 2-19*B* and 2-24*A*). A capillary layer of fluid normally separates the visceral and parietal layers of the tunica vaginalis.

CLINICALLY ORIENTED COMMENTS

The presence of fluid anywhere within the processus vaginalis after birth is called a hydrocele (Fig. 2-22). Infants with an obliterated processus vaginalis may have residual peritoneal fluid in the cavity of their tunica vaginalis testis (**noncommunicating hydrocele**), but this fluid usually absorbs during the first year.

If the processus vaginalis remains open (Fig. 2-22*B* and *D*), peritoneal fluid may be forced into it, forming a **communicating hydrocele**. An indirect inguinal hernia is often associated with this condition (Case 2-3 and Fig. 2-22*B*). The length of the hydrocele depends upon how much of the processus vaginalis remains patent.

Certain pathological conditions (*e.g.*, injury and/or inflammation of the epididymis) may result in an increase in the fluid in the tunica vaginalis, producing **hydrocele** and marked scrotal enlargement (Fig. 2-22*D*). Surgical treatment of this condition may be required.

The Testis (Figs. 2-19, 2-24, and 2-25). The testis is an ovoid gland that is surrounded by a dense layer of connective tissue known as the **tunica albuginea** which is adjacent to the visceral layer of the tunica vaginalis. The male germ cells or **sperms** (spermatozoa) are formed in the several hundred **seminiferous tubules** within lobules formed by septa in the testes. These tubules join to form a network of canals known as the **rete testis**. Small **efferent ductules** (15 to 20) connect the rete testis to the head of the epididymis.

The Epididymis (Figs. 2-19 and 2-24 to 2-26). This *comma-shaped structure* is applied to the superior and posterolateral surfaces of the testis. The **body of the epidid-**

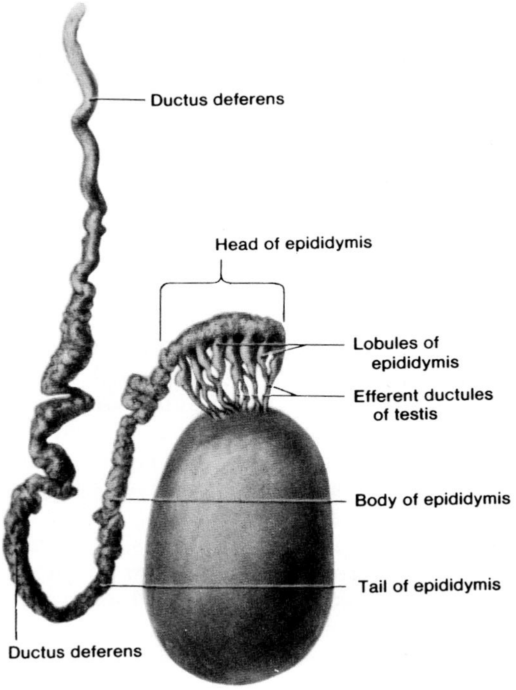

Figure 2-25. Drawing of a testis and epididymis after removal of their coverings. Observe the efferent ductules passing from the rete testis to the epididymis (also see Figs. 2-16 and 2-19).

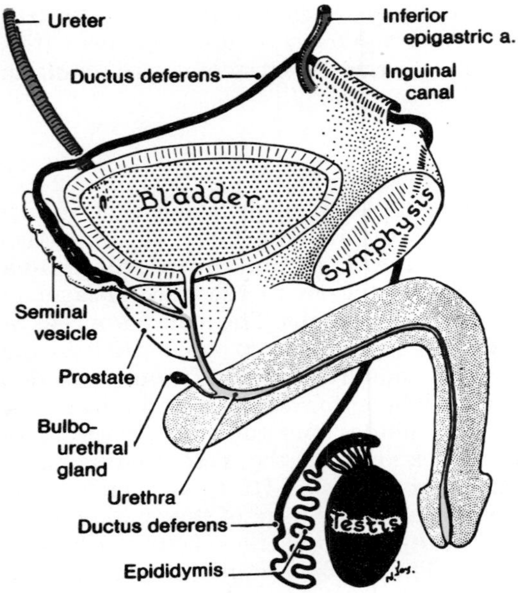

Figure 2-26. Diagram of the male genital system. Note that the ductus deferens begins at the tail of the epididymis. It is incorporated in the spermatic cord (Fig. 2-24), continues upward to the superficial inguinal ring, and passes through the inguinal canal. Note that it joins the duct of the seminal vesicle to form the ejaculatory duct, which opens into the urethra (Fig. 3-76).

ymis consists of the highly convoluted **duct of the epididymis**. The sperms are stored in this duct where they undergo their final stages of maturation as they pass slowly through it. The **tail of the epididymis** is continuous with the **ductus deferens** (vas deferens), the duct which transports the sperms to the **ejaculatory duct** for expulsion into the urethra. The **sinus of the epididymis** is a small recess of the tunica vaginalis (Figs. 2-19*B* and 2-24*A*).

The Spermatic Cord (Figs. 2-13, 2-14, 2-16, 2-19, 2-24, and 2-25). This cord consists of the structures running to and from the testis which are surrounded by the coverings derived from the layers of the anterior abdominal wall. *The spermatic cord begins at the deep inguinal ring, lateral to the inferior epigastric artery,* where its constituents assemble. It passes through the inginual canal and *emerges at the superficial inguinal ring to descend in the scrotum to the testis.* As it emerges from the inguinal canal, it rolls over the pubic tubercle and acquires its covering of external spermatic fascia. Here it can be felt as a firm cord when held between the thumb and the index finger.

Constituents of the Spermatic Cord (Figs. 2-13, 2-14, 2-19, and 2-24). Within the coverings of the spermatic cord are:

1. **Ductus deferens**. This large *duct of the testis* lies in the posterior part of the spermatic cord. It is easily palpable because of its *thick wall,* which contains three layers of smooth muscle.
2. **Arteries**. The **testicular artery** (Figs. 2-24*B* and 2-113) is a long slender vessel that arises from the front of the aorta at the level of the second lumbar vertebra (Fig. 2-55), where the testis started to develop in the embryo. It is the *principal artery supplying the testis and the epididymis.*

   The **artery of the ductus deferens** (Fig. 2-24*B*) is a slender vessel that *arises from the inferior vesical artery* (artery to the urinary bladder) and accompanies the ductus deferens throughout its course. It anastomoses with the testicular artery near the testis.

   The **cremasteric artery** is a small vessel (Fig. 2-24*B*) that *arises from the inferior epigastric artery.* It accompanies the spermatic cord and supplies the cremaster muscle and other coverings of this cord. It also anastomoses with the testicular artery near the testis.
3. **Veins**. *Up to 12 veins* from the posterior surface of the testis *anastomose to form a* **pampiniform plexus**. This unusual name is derived from the Latin word for tendril and was used to denote this *vine-like structure.* This large plexus, forming much of the bulk of the spermatic cord, surrounds the ductus deferens and the arteries in the spermatic cord. It is located within the internal spermatic fascia and *ends in the testicular vein* (Figs. 2-113 and 2-129).
4. **Nerves**. There are sympathetic fibers on the arteries and sympathetic and parasympathetic fibers on the ductus

deferens. The autonomic sensory nerves carry the impulses that result in the excruciating pain and sickening sensation that occur when the testis is hit.

The genital branch of the genitofemoral nerve passes into the spermatic cord and supplies the cremasteric muscle (Figs. 2-19*A* and 2-131).

5. **Lymph vessels.** The testicular lymph vessels, draining the testis and immediately associated structures, pass upward in the spermatic cord and end in the **lumbar lymph nodes** (Figs. 2-27 and 2-134), situated between the common iliac and renal veins. *Understand that the lymph vessels of the scrotum do not ascend in the spermatic cord*; they ascend in the superficial fascia of the scrotum to the superficial *inguinal lymph nodes* (Figs. 2-12 and 4-38).
6. **Remnants of the processus vaginalis.** Normally the cavity of the stalk of the processus vaginalis in the spermatic cord obliterates, leaving only a fibrous thread that soon disappears.

CLINICALLY ORIENTED COMMENTS

Occasionally the processus vaginalis persists throughout the spermatic cord (Fig. 2-22*D*) and may be associated with an **indirect inguinal hernia** (Fig. 2-22*B*; discussed previously). Sometimes isolated remnants of the processus vaginalis persist, and one or more of these may become swollen with fluid and form **hydroceles of the spermatic cord** (Fig. 2-22*C*).

The pampiniform plexus of veins sometimes becomes varicose (dilated and tortuous), producing a condition known as **varicocele** that reminds one of a "bag of worms." This condition, more common on the left side, often results from defective valves in the testicular vein. The **worm-like swelling** disappears when the person lies down. Persons claiming to have two testis on one side usually have a varicocele or testicular tumor. Rarely, a varicocele may result from blockage of the renal vein owing to a tumor of the left kidney. This blockage interferes with drainage of the left testicular vein.

A hematocele of the testis is a collection of blood in the tunica vaginalis testis, often resulting from trauma to the testis that damages the vessels around the testis and the epididymus. A severe injury may produce a **hematoma** (localized mass of blood) within the testis that may rupture through the tunica albuginea (Fig. 2-19*B*).

The difference in the lymphatic drainage of the testis and the scrotum is clinically important. Cancer cells from a **testicular tumor** may spread by lymphogenous dissemination to the **lumbar lymph nodes** (Fig. 2-134), whereas a **skin cancer** of the scrotum may metastasize to the **inguinal lymph nodes** (Fig. 2-12).

Rudimentary structures may be observed around the testis and epididymis (Fig. 2-24*A*). The **appendix of the testis** and the **appendix** (or **appendices**) **of the epididymis** are visible when the tunica vaginalis is opened. These vestigial remnants of the cranial ends of the genital ducts in the embryo are rarely observed, unless pathological changes occur in them, because normally they are tiny structures.

The vesicular **appendix of the testis**, the remnant of the cranial end of the paramesonephric duct (embryonic female genital duct), is attached to the upper pole of the testis. The **appendix of the epididymis**, the remnant of the cranial end of the mesonephric duct (embryonic male genital duct), is attached to the head of the epididymis.

Another vestigial remnant, the **paradidymis**, may be detected when the ductus epididymis is unraveled. If present, it is located between the efferent ductules and the body of the epididymis (Fig. 2-25). The paradidymis forms from embryonic mesonephric tubules that do not become efferent ductules. In most people these unused tubules degenerate.

The ductus deferens (vas deferens) is sometimes ligated bilaterally when **sterilization of the male** is desired. In performing this operation, called a **vasectomy**, the ductus deferens is isolated by approaching it through the upper scrotal wall (Fig. 2-26). Following the operation, sperms no longer pass to the urethra, but the secretions of

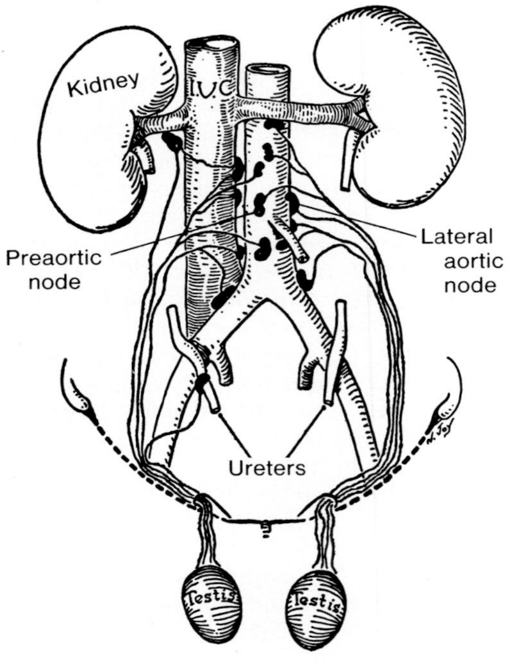

Figure 2-27. Drawing illustrating the lymphatic drainage of the testes. The testicular lymph vessels, *not those of the scrotum*, ascend through the spermatic cord and end in the lumbar lymph nodes which are scattered along the abdominal aorta and the inferior vena cava (also see Fig. 2-134).

the auxillary genital glands (*e.g.*, seminal vesicles) can still be ejaculated.

THE PERITONEUM AND ABDOMINAL VISCERA

THE PERITONEUM

The peritoneum is a thin, translucent, serous membrane which *lines the walls of the abdominal and pelvic cavities* and either completely or partially *covers the organs and other structures contained in these cavities.* It consists of mesothelium and a thin layer of connective tissue. Its **parietal** and **visceral layers** are separated from each other by a *capillary film of serous fluid* which lubricates the peritoneal surfaces, enabling the intra-abdominal organs to move upon each other without friction. The fourth and outermost coat of the wall of the alimentary tube is called the serosa or adventitia. If the viscus is covered with peritoneum, its fourth coat is called the **serosa**; if the viscus is not covered with peritoneum, its fourth coat is called an **adventitia**.

The parietal peritoneum is applied to the walls of the abdominal cavity and the visceral peritoneum covers most of the viscera within it. All of the peritoneum is continuous. It forms two sacs, a greater sac and a lesser sac, but if the peritoneum could be separated from the abdominal walls and the viscera, it would form one large completely **closed sac**, except in the female where the abdominal ostia of the uterine tubes open into it. The cavity of this sac is known as the **peritoneal cavity**. Understand that there is no cavity, but only a *potential space* containing a capillary layer of fluid. During fetal development the various organs invaginated this sac, reducing the embryonic peritoneal cavity to the merest interval between the visceral and parietal layers of peritoneum. It is during this invagination that the viscera receive their covering of visceral peritoneum. *To visualize this process*, push your fist into a partially inflated balloon which contains a few drops of water. The inner wall of the balloon surrounding your fist is comparable to the visceral layer of peritoneum. The outer wall of the balloon is comparable to the parietal layer of peritoneum and the cavity of the balloon represents the peritoneal cavity. Observe that as you push your fist further toward the outer wall, the two walls come into contact and the cavity practically disappears. Note also that at your wrist the two layers form a double fold (**mesentery**) and that they are continuous with each other. This area is also comparable to the **hilum** or stalk through which the blood vessels pass to reach the viscus, represented by your fist.

Remove your fist from the balloon and then push your fingers into it. Visualize them as the various organs packed together within the abdomen. These organs fill the abdomen as your fingers fill the balloon, and the peritoneal cavity surrounds the viscera as the cavity of the balloon surrounds your fingers. Understand from this that the peritoneal cavity normally has a very small volume; however, it may be distended with air or fluid as far as the abdominal walls will permit, just as you could inject air or fluid into the balloon.

CLINICALLY ORIENTED COMMENTS

Under certain pathological conditions, the potential space of the peritoneal cavity may be distended to form an actual space containing several liters of fluid. **Ascites** is *an accumulation of serous fluid in the peritoneal cavity* (**hydroperitoneum**).

When the gut ruptures, gas and intestinal material enter the peritoneal cavity. **Generalized peritonitis** and ileus of the bowel results. **Ileus** is an obstruction of the bowel (intestine) associated with severe **colicky pain**, vomiting, and often fever and dehydration. **Distention of the bowel** occurs with the ileus.

Commonly during dissections, the opposing surfaces of peritoneal membranes are found to be adherent (Fig. 2-52). These **adhesions** (strands of fibrous tissue) probably resulted from inflammatory processes (*e.g.*, peritonitis). If the mesothelium is damaged or removed, adjacent layers of peritoneum may adhere to each other, forming an adhesion. During dissection you can break them down with your fingers.

Terminology. Several terms are used to describe the different parts of the peritoneum. These are mesentery, omentum, peritoneal ligaments, and folds (L. *plicae*).

Mesentery (Fig. 2-28). This is a **double sheet of peritoneum** or suspensory fold which connects an organ with the abdominal wall. Mesenteries are covered on both sides by mesothelium and have a core of loose connective tissue containing a variable number of fat cells and lymph nodes, together with the blood and lymphatic vessels and the nerves passing to and from the viscus. *The most mobile parts of the intestine have a mesentery.* It may help you understand a mesentery if you suspend a rubber tube in a towel. The towel (visceral peritoneum) surrounds the tube (intestine) and passes from it as two parallel layers (mesentery) to your hands (posterior abdominal wall) holding the towel. Between these layers, imagine that there is a variable amount of **extraperitoneal fatty tissue** in which blood and lymphatic vessels and nerves pass to and from the hose (intestine). Where these layers (mesentery) meet your hands (posterior abdominal wall), they become continuous with the parietal peritoneum lining it.

Figure 2-28. Diagrams illustrating the primitive mesentery of the large intestine in various stages of absorption. The extent to which the ascending and descending colons lose their primitive mesenteries varies. The *arrow* indicates the paracolic gutter, where the visceral peritoneum is attached to the parietal peritoneum and where an incision is made during mobilization of the intestine prior to surgery on the duodenum, ascending colon, or descending colon.

Unfortunately, the comparatively simple arrangements suggested by a fist in a balloon and a tube suspended by a towel, while instructive, oversimplify the mesenteries, because several *secondary changes occur during fetal development.* Examples are: (1) two opposed layers of peritoneum fuse, (2) viscera change position after receiving a peritoneal coat, (3) mesenteries disappear after they form (Fig. 2-28), and (4) pouches of peritoneum develop (Fig. 2-38).

The disposition of the peritoneum in the adult is complex, especially to those unfamiliar with its prenatal development. If you do not understand the relatively simple arrangement of the mesenteries in the embryo or you are unfamiliar with the developmental changes and modifications that lead to their disposition in the adult, you are urged to correct this deficiency in your knowledge before proceeding.

Omentum (Figs. 2–29 and 2–36 to 2–38). *This is a mesentery that extends from the stomach to adjacent organs.* For example,

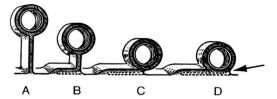

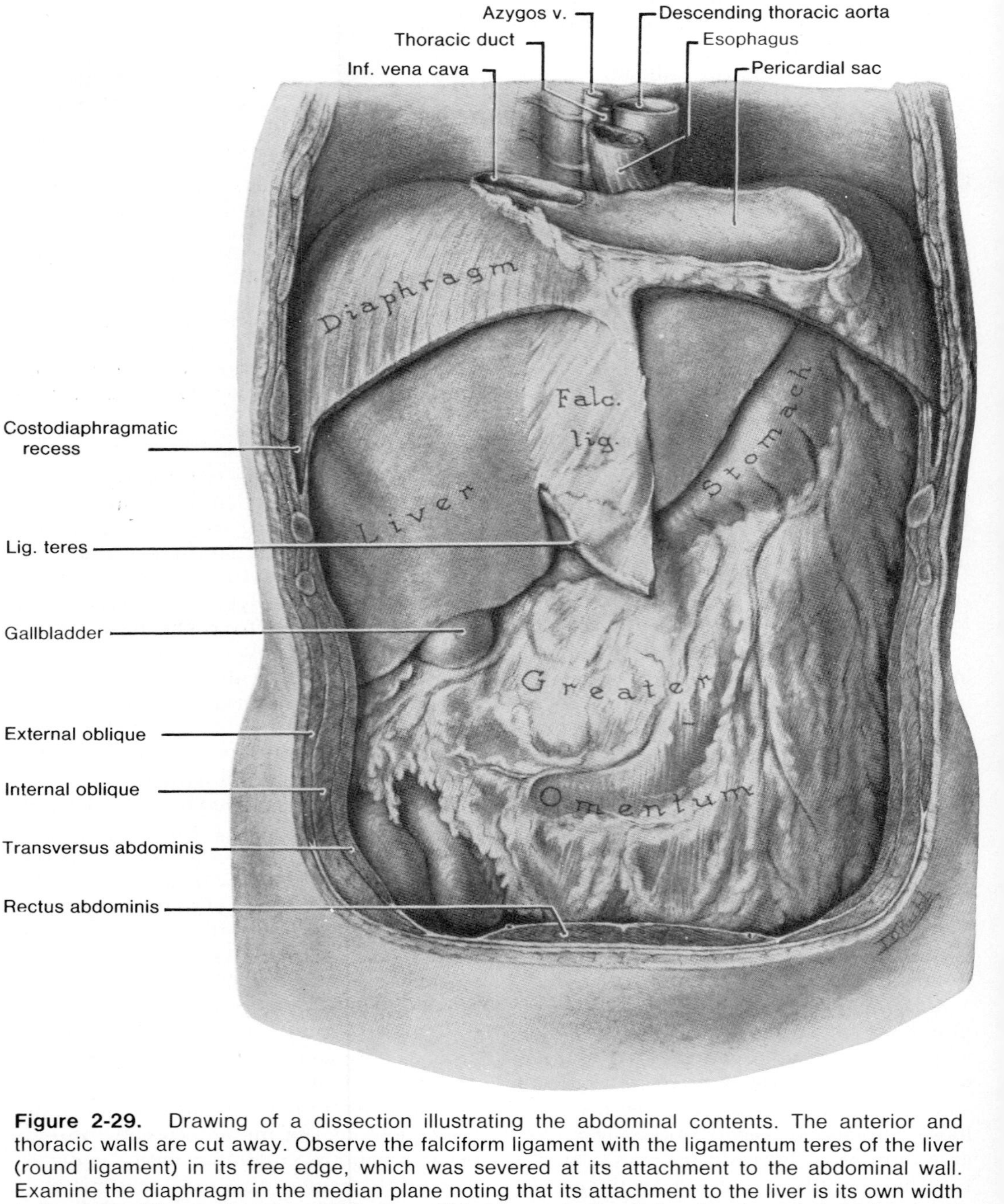

Figure 2-29. Drawing of a dissection illustrating the abdominal contents. The anterior and thoracic walls are cut away. Observe the falciform ligament with the ligamentum teres of the liver (round ligament) in its free edge, which was severed at its attachment to the abdominal wall. Examine the diaphragm in the median plane noting that its attachment to the liver is its own width to the right of the median plane. Note the gallbladder projecting below the sharp, inferior border of the liver and the two recti muscles meeting in the median plane above the pubis. Observe that the internal oblique is the thickest of the three flat abdominal muscles.

the **lesser omentum** joins the lesser curvature of the stomach and the proximal part of the duodenum to the liver. Inspect the abdominal cavity and its contents, observing the fatty peritoneal apron, called the *greater omentum*, that is attached to the greater curvature of the stomach and draped over the intestine like an apron; hence its name (L. *omentum*, caul or veil).

Ligaments. All double layers or folds of peritoneum that are not called mesenteries or omenta are referred to as **peritoneal ligaments**. These lack the connective tissue character and strength of a ligament connecting a muscle to a bone. *Peritoneal ligaments are folds or parts of folds of peritoneum* that run from one viscus to another (*e.g.*, the **gastrolienal ligament** passing from the stomach to the spleen, Fig. 2–39), or from a viscus to the body wall (*e.g.*, **falciform ligament** passing from the liver to the anterior abdominal wall, Fig. 2–29). Ligaments may contain blood vessels.

Folds (Figs. 2–16, 2–40, 2–43, 2–70, and 2–97). **Folds**, or **plicae**, are usually reflections of peritoneum with more or less sharp borders. Often they are formed by peritoneum covering blood vessels and ducts, some of which represent obliterated fetal vessels (Fig. 2–40). In these places the peritoneum is lifted off the body wall. Refer to previous descriptions of the lateral, medial, and median **umbilical folds** on the posterior surface of the anterior abdominal wall.

Retroperitoneal Organs (L. *retro*, back or behind). These organs are *behind the peritoneal sac*, thus they are merely covered in front with peritoneum. *Viscera without free mesenteries are retroperitoneal* (*e.g.*, the duodenum, the ascending colon, and the descending colon).

Peritoneal Recesses (Figs. 2–36 to 2–38 and 2–70). In certain places in the peritoneal cavity, the peritoneum folds to form blind pouches (**culs-de-sacs**) or tubular cavities that are closed at one end and yet have an opening into the main part of the peritoneal cavity. The largest peritoneal recess is the **omental bursa** (lesser sac), which lies behind the lesser omentum and the stomach. It communicates with the general peritoneal cavity (greater sac) via the **epiploic foramen** (foramen of Winslow). See the subsequent description of this clinically important bursa.

The duodenojejunal area often has two or three peritoneal recesses which are produced by accessory peritoneal folds (Fig. 2–70). In the ileocecal area there is usually a **retrocecal recess** where the peritoneal cavity extends upward, posterior to the cecum. *Frequently the vermiform appendix lies in the retrocecal recess* (Fig. 2–44). Often there are one or two **ileocecal recesses** (Fig. 2–43). The superior ileocecal recess opens downward, just above the terminal part of the ileum. The inferior ileocecal recess also opens downward and is produced by the **ileocecal fold** which extends from the front and lower part of the ileum to the **mesentery of the appendix** (Fig. 2–43). At the inferior aspect of the apex of the sigmoid mesocolon (Fig. 2–40), there is often a pocket-like extension of the peritoneal cavity, called the **intersigmoid recess**, that passes upward, posterior to the root of the sigmoid mesocolon.

CLINICALLY ORIENTED COMMENTS

Knowledge of the various peritoneal recesses is clinically important because **internal hernias** may occur in them. A loop of gut, usually the small intestine, may pass into one of these recesses and become strangulated. The intestine becomes twisted around the herniated or trapped loop, resulting in a stoppage or obstruction of the bowel. The patient usually presents with severe colicky pain owing to the **acute obstruction of the bowel**. Operative relief of the obstruction and closure of the hernial defect is required.

Fluid sometimes accumulates in the peritoneal recess and, if excessive, may have to be aspirated (*e.g.*, **culdocentesis** or transvaginal aspiration of fluid from the recess between the uterus and the rectum, called the rectouterine pouch, Fig. 2-32).

The Abdominal Cavity (Figs. 2-30 to 2-33). The abdominal cavity is the larger part of the abdominopelvic cavity, *above the*

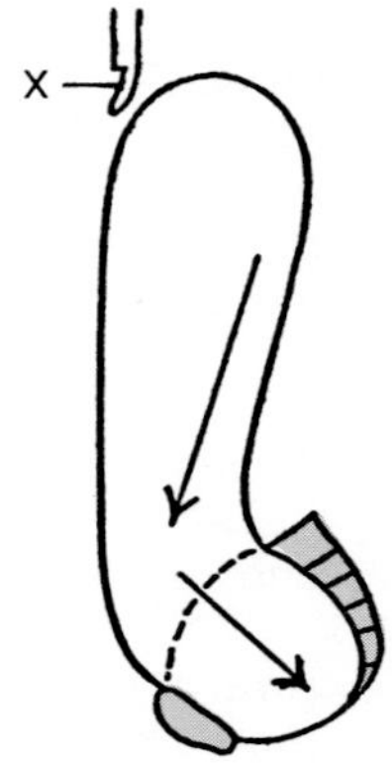

Figure 2-30. Diagram illustrating the abdominal and pelvic cavities as viewed in a median section. ----indicates the plane of the superior aperture (inlet) of the pelvis which divides the abdominopelvic cavity into the abdominal cavity (*top arrow*) and the pelvic cavity (*bottom arrow*). *X*, xiphoid process.

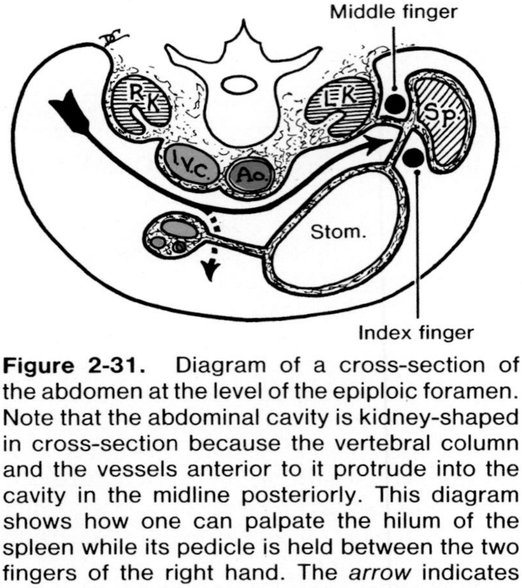

Figure 2-31. Diagram of a cross-section of the abdomen at the level of the epiploic foramen. Note that the abdominal cavity is kidney-shaped in cross-section because the vertebral column and the vessels anterior to it protrude into the cavity in the midline posteriorly. This diagram shows how one can palpate the hilum of the spleen while its pedicle is held between the two fingers of the right hand. The *arrow* indicates the path taken by a finger passed through the epiploic foramen (Fig. 2-36) into the omental bursa to reach the hilum of the spleen. The *broken arrow* is to indicate the passage upward into the superior recess of the omental bursa (see Fig. 2-38). *RK*, *LK*, right kidney, left kidney. *Sp.*, spleen.

superior aperture of the pelvis minor (lesser pelvis). It is limited above by the diaphragm and is continuous below with the pelvic cavity, the smaller part of the abdominopelvic cavity, at the brim of the

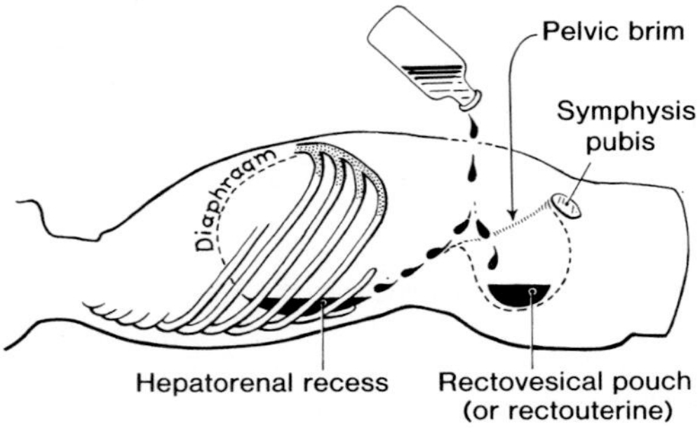

Figure 2-32. Diagram illustrating the two lowest (most dorsal) parts of the peritoneal cavity when a person is in the recumbent or supine position. Serous fluid or blood from ruptured abdominal organs gravitates to the upper abdomen in this position because the paravertebral grooves (gutters) slope posterosuperiorly. The hepatorenal pouch (pouch of Morrison) is in the greater peritoneal sac just to the right of the epiploic foramen (Fig. 2-36). Its medial margin is the right kidney and its superior boundary is the liver. Fluids drain from this pouch into the pelvis via the right parcolic gutter that lies to the right of the ascending colon (Fig. 2-110).

pelvis minor. *Understand that a large part of the abdominal cavity is under cover of the thoracic or rib cage* (Figs. 2-32 and 2-117).

Peritoneum lines the walls of the abdominal cavity; hence, *the peritoneal sac and the peritoneal cavity are within the abdominal cavity* and the pelvic cavity. **The abdominal cavity is completely filled with abdominal viscera** (stomach, intestines, pancreas, liver, gallbladder, spleen, suprarenal glands, kidneys and ureters, blood and lymph vessels, and lymph nodes).

Understand that neither the abdominal cavity nor the peritoneal cavity is actually a cavity. The peritoneal cavity contains only a capillary layer of fluid and the abdominal cavity is occupied by closely packed viscera. Nevertheless, the term cavity is useful for descriptive purposes and is a clinically important concept.

The abdominal cavity is kidney-shaped in cross-section because the vertebral column protrudes into it in the posterior midline (Fig. 2-31). On each side of the vertebral column is a **paravertebral groove** (gutter) containing a kidney, a ureter, and part of the colon. These grooves slope posterosuperiorly so that when fluid accumu-

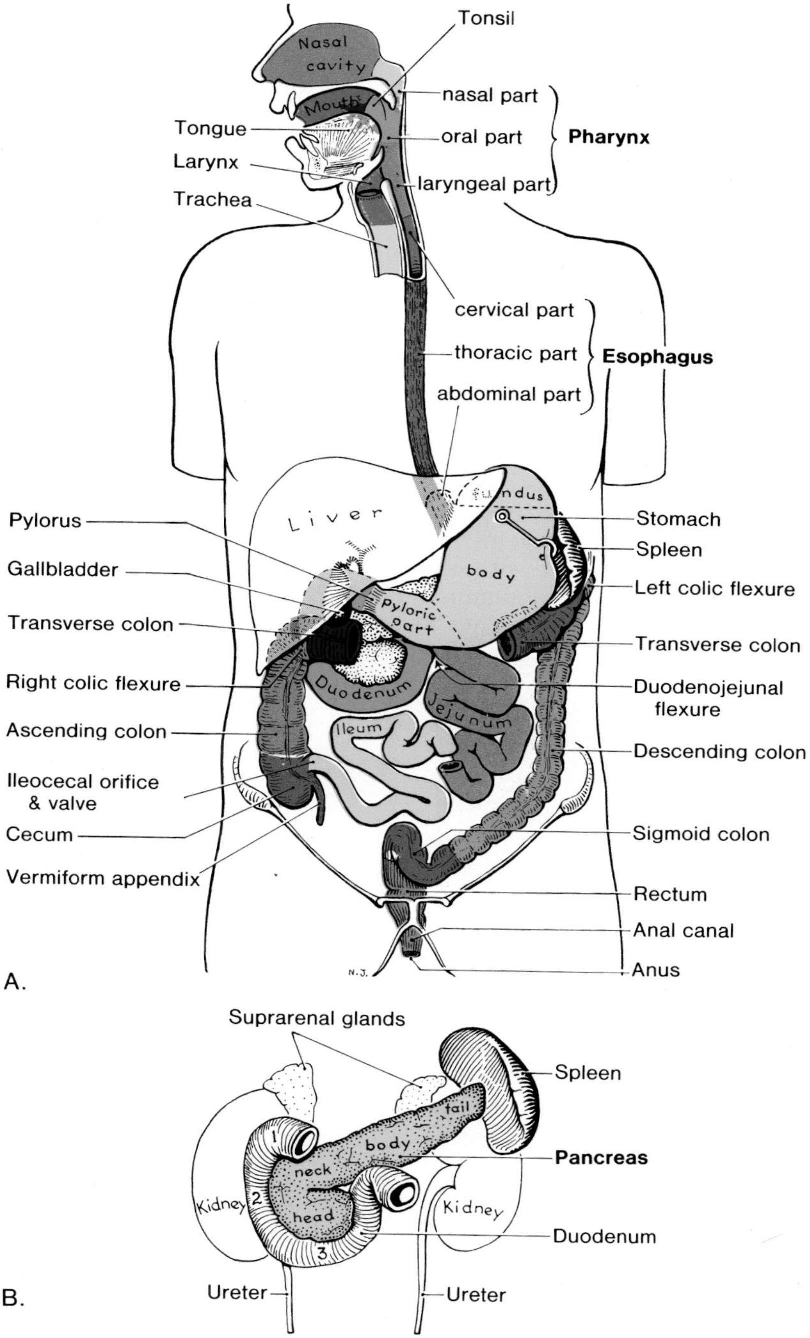

Figure 2-33. Diagram of the digestive system. *A*, shows that it extends from the lips to the anus. In *B*, the spleen, pancreas, and duodenum are drawn after removal of the stomach and the transverse colon. The abdominal viscera are the stomach, intestines, liver, pancreas, spleen, kidneys, and suprarenal glands. Observe that the kidneys, ureters, and suprarenal glands lie on the posterior abdominal wall, where they are retroperitoneal and are enclosed in the fascial lining of the abdominal cavity. Note that other viscera lie anterior to these structures, where they are surrounded to a greater or lesser extent by the peritoneal cavity. The size of the peritoneal cavity appears exaggerated because most of the small intestine is not illustrated.

lates in the peritoneal cavity it follows these grooves (Figs. 2-32 and 2-110) to the upper abdomen when a patient lies in the supine position.

SURVEY OF ABDOMINAL CONTENTS

Before considering the viscera in detail, a survey of the abdominal contents will be given for orientation.

The Liver (Figs. 2-29 and 2-33). The liver is a huge gland (1.2 to 1.6 kg), the largest in the body. Most of the liver lies on the right side of the body because its right lobe is about six times as large as the left. To be more specific, it lies in the right hypochondriac and epigastric regions. Its smooth surfaces are in contact with the diaphragm and with the anterior abdominal wall. The **falciform ligament** attaches it to both of these structures. The main attachment of the diaphragm to the liver, however, is through the **coronary ligaments** (Fig. 2-79). Both the coronary and falciform ligaments are composed of double layers of peritoneum. The liver also contacts the right lateral abdominal wall.

The stomach and the abdominal part of the esophagus are in contact with the left lobe of the liver, whereas the right lobe is in contact with the right colic flexure and the duodenum, close to the gallbladder. The right kidney and suprarenal gland are also in contact with the right lobe of the liver. *Most of the liver is covered with peritoneum*; in Figure 2-29 observe that it occupies most of that part of the abdominal cavity that lies within the thoracic cage (Fig. 2-76).

The Esophagus (Figs. 2-29, 2-33, and 2-34). The esophagus is a fairly straight tube that extends from the pharynx to the stomach. It pierces the diaphragm just to the

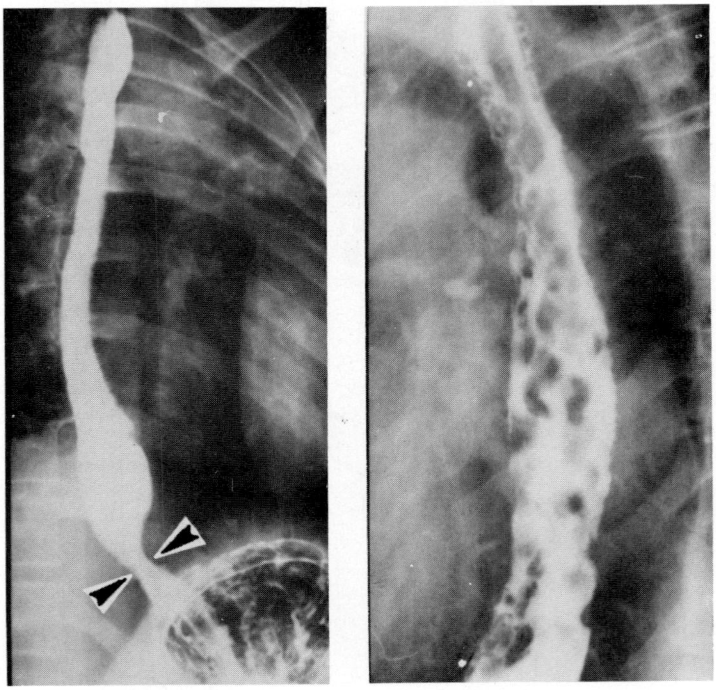

Figure 2-34. Radiographs of the esophagus. *Left*, a normal esophagus after swallowing barium. Note the constriction where it passes through the esophageal hiatus in the diaphragm (*arrows*; also see Fig. 2-130) and its short (1.5 to 2.5 cm) course in the abdomen before entering the stomach at the cardiac orifice. *Right*, abnormal esophagus showing the barium outlining distended veins (esophageal varices) which are encroaching on the lumen. See Case 2-8 for discussion of this abnormality.

left of the midline. The abdominal part of the esophagus, only about 1.5 cm long, grooves the left lobe of the liver and enters the stomach. Here, the esophagus is covered anteriorly and laterally by peritoneum and is accompanied by the **vagal trunks** (CN X), the esophageal branches of the left gastric artery, and the accompanying veins. The vagal trunks arise from the **esophageal plexus** of nerves (Fig. 1-93), which enmeshes the lower thoracic part of the esophagus.

The Stomach (Figs. 2-29, 2-31, 2-33 to 2-39, and 2-48 to 2-51). The stomach is the expanded portion of the alimentary canal between the esophagus and the small intestine. The esophagus enters the stomach at the *cardiac orifice*. The stomach consists of a **fundus**, a **body**, and a **pyloric part**. The **pylorus** is the distal portion of the stomach that opens into the duodenum. *The position and shape of the stomach varies according to the habitus (physical appearance) of a person*, but generally it lies in the left upper quadrant when the person is in the supine or recumbent position. In most people the stomach is J-shaped and its pyloric part lies horizontally or ascends to the proximal part of the duodenum (Fig. 2-33). The lowest part of the greater curvature of the stomach may extend into the pelvis major (part above pelvic brim) in the erect position. Hence, *the position and shape of the stomach vary in different people* and in the same person, depending on its contents and the person's position. The stomach has a complete covering of peritoneum and is connected to other organs by peritoneal ligaments and omenta.

The Lesser Omentum (Figs. 2-36 to 2-39). This *double layer of peritoneum* embraces the abdominal part of the esophagus and connects the lesser curvature of the stom-

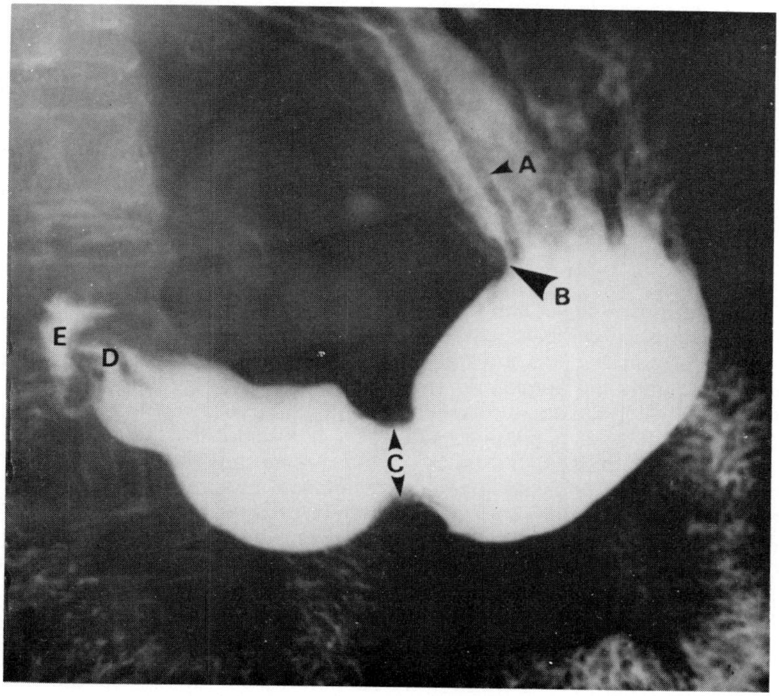

Figure 2-35. Radiograph of the stomach following a barium meal with the patient in the prone (right anterior oblique) position. The barium (*white*) is in a low anterior position in the stomach and the air (*gray* to *black*) is in a high posterior position. Observe *A*, longitudinal ridges of mucous membrane (rugae); *B*, the angular notch (incisura angularis); *C*, a peristaltic wave travelling toward the pylorus; *D*, the pylorus; *E*, the duodenal "cap." Note also the feathery appearance of the barium in the small intestine.

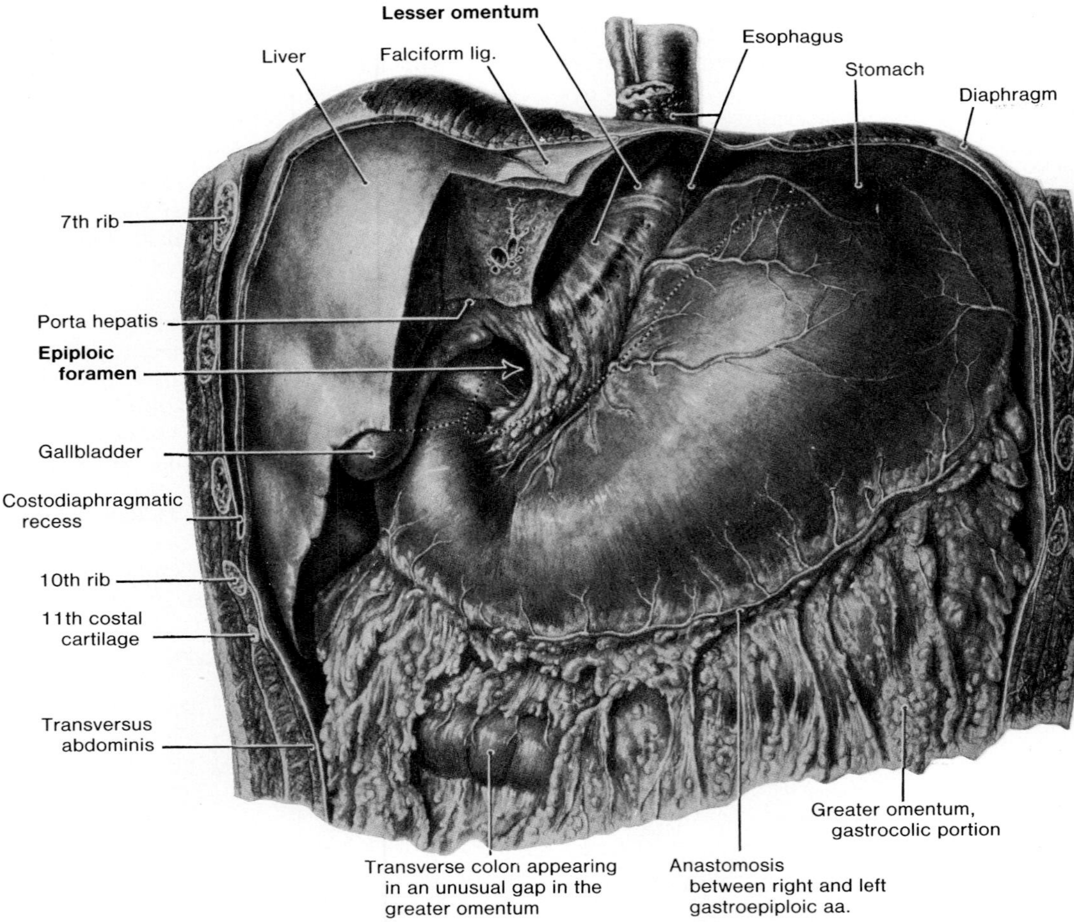

Figure 2-36. Drawing of a dissection of an anterior view of the stomach and the omenta. The stomach is inflated with air and the left part of the liver is cut away. Observe that the pyloric end of the stomach lies inferoposterior to the gallbladder. Note that the first or superior part of the duodenum almost occludes the epiploic foramen. The *arrowhead* indicates the mouth of omental bursa. Observe that the gallbladder, followed cranially, leads to the free margin of the lesser omentum and, hence, acts as a guide to the epiploic foramen lying behind that free margin. Examine the lesser omentum passing from the lesser curvature of the stomach and the first 2 cm of the duodenum to the fissure for the ligamentum venosum and the porta hepatis. This omentum is thickened at its free margin where it forms the anterior lip of the epiploic foramen. Elsewhere the omentum is perforated so that the caudate lobe of the liver is visible through it. Observe the greater omentum hanging from the greater curvature of the stomach and the right cupola (dome) of the diaphragm rising higher than the left cupola.

ach and the first 2 cm of the duodenum to the liver. The lesser omentum lies posterior to the left lobe of the liver and is attached to the liver in the fissure for the **ligamentum venosum** (remnant of fetal ductus venosus) and to the **porta hepatis** (Fig. 2-80). In the interval between the stomach and the liver, the lesser omentum encloses the bile duct (Fig. 2-37). This omentum is a double layered sheet which may be divided into two parts (Fig. 2-39): the **hepatogastric ligament** and the **hepatoduo-**

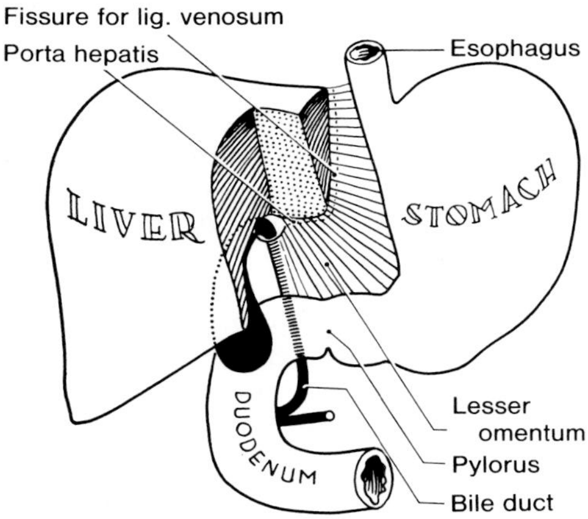

Figure 2-37. Diagram illustrating the attachments of the lesser omentum. Two sagittal cuts have been made through the liver: one at the fissure for the ligamentum venosum, the other at the right limit of the porta hepatis. These two cuts have been joined by a coronal cut. Note that the bile duct occupies the free edge of lesser omentum. Observe that the lesser omentum extends from the lesser curvature of the stomach and the first 2 cm of the duodenum to the fissure for the ligamentum venosum and to the porta hepatis. The part of the lesser omentum attached to the body of the stomach passes to the fissure and that attached to the pyloric part of the stomach and duodenum passes to the porta hepatis.

denal ligament. The lesser omentum ends in a free edge between the porta hepatis and the duodenum. The **portal vein**, the **hepatic artery**, and the **bile duct** *run*

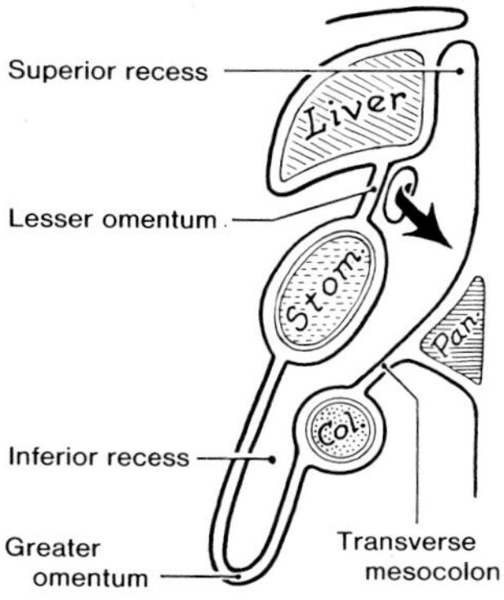

Figure 2-38. Diagram of a median section of the abdomen showing the vertical extent of the omental bursa (lesser sac). The *arrow* passes through the epiploic foramen (mouth of omental bursa). The transverse colon (*Col*), its mesentery, and the greater omentum are also illustrated. The walls of the greater omentum commonly fuse, thereby obliterating the inferior recess of the omental bursa. As a result, the greater omentum is usually composed of four layers of peritoneum.

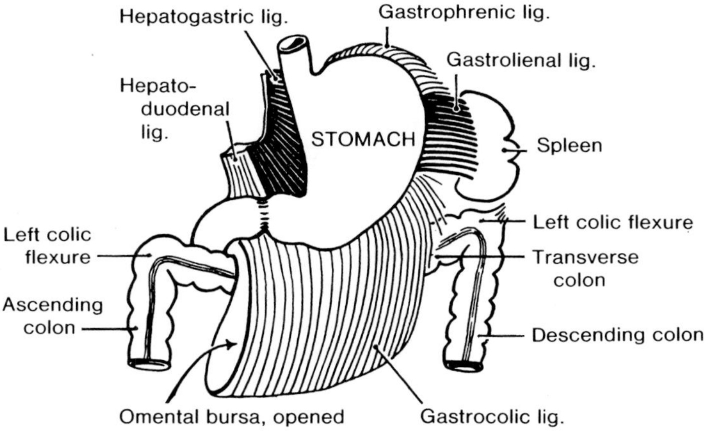

Figure 2-39. Diagram illustrating the two parts of the lesser omentum (hepatogastric and hepatoduodenal ligaments) and the three parts of the greater omentum (gastrophrenic, gastrolienal, and gastrocolic ligaments). *Gaster* is the Greek word for belly (stomach) and is the basis of many medical terms; *e.g.*, gastritis means inflammation of the stomach.

between the layers of the lesser omentum near its free edge (Fig. 2-90).

The Greater Omentum (Figs. 2-29, 2-36, and 2-38 to 2-40). When you cut through the peritoneum of the anterior abdominal wall, the intestines are more or less hidden by this **fatty omental apron** that hangs down over them from the greater curvature of the stomach. Some people believe that it prevents the intestines from adhering to the parietal peritoneum of the anterior abdominal wall. *It has considerable mobility in living persons and can surround an inflamed organ and "wall off" the infection.*

The greater omentum often contains a considerable amount of extraperitoneal tissue and fat and may be short or long enough to reach the pelvic brim. In emaciated persons, the greater omentum may be as thin as a piece of paper, whereas *in obese persons the greater omentum is of considerable thickness and weight.*

After passing downward, the greater omentum loops back on itself (Fig. 2-38), overlying and attaching to the transverse part of the large intestine (**the transverse colon**), which runs across the abdomen just below the stomach (Fig. 2-39). *The greater omentum, extending from the greater curvature of the stomach, may be divided into three parts* (Fig. 2-39): (1) *the lower apron-like part*, called the **gastrocolic ligament**, is attached to the transverse colon. This is the part usually referred to when the term greater omentum is used; (2) *the left part*, called the **gastrolienal (gastrosplenic) ligament**, is attached to the spleen (L. *lien*). This part connects the spleen to the left part of the greater curvature; and (3) *the upper part*, called the **gastrophrenic ligament**, is attached to the diaphragm (G. *phrēn*).

The Small Intestine (Figs. 2-33 and 2-40). The convoluted tube, *extending from the pylorus to the ileocecal valve*, is called the small intestine (bowel). It consists of three parts: **duodenum**, **jejunum**, and **ileum**. *Most digestion occurs in the small intestine.* The length of the small intestine varies in different persons, but the average is 6 to 7 m; resection (excision) of up to one-third of it is compatable with a normal life.

The Duodenum (Figs. 2-29, 2-33, 2-35 to 2-37, 2-39, and 2-40). This first part of the small intestine pursues a horseshoe-shaped or *U-shaped course* from the pylorus around the head of the **pancreas** to become continuous with the jejunum (next part of small intestine). The duodenum (L. *duodeni*, twelve) was given its name because it is about 12 fingerbreadths long.

The position of the duodenum is variable, but it **begins on the right side** of the midline (2 to 3 cm from the median plane) and **ends on the left side** at the duodenojejunal junction (2 to 3 cm to the left of the median plane, just above or below the transpyloric plane, depending upon the person's habitus and the position of their stomach). Consequently, *although about 25 cm long, its two ends are only about 5 cm apart.*

Most of the duodenum is **fixed** and **retroperitoneal**; *i.e., most of it does not have a mesentery*; it lost its primitive mesentery during fetal development and came to lie retroperitoneally against the posterior abdominal wall.

The Jejunum (Figs. 2-33 and 2-40). The jejunum (L. *jejunus*, empty) begins at the duodenojejunal flexure and constitutes *about two-fifths of the small intestine beyond the duodenum.* It tends to lie in the umbilical region and in general runs a tortuous path from the upper left to the lower right of the abdomen.

The Ileum (Figs. 2-33, 2-40, and 2-42). The ileum (L. rolled up, twisted) *comprises the distal three-fifths of the small intestine*, which tends to lie in the hypogastrium and the pelvis. The distal part of the ileum is nearly always in the pelvis, from which it ascends to end in the medial aspect of the cecum. The jejunum and ileum are attached to the posterior abdominal wall by a fan-shaped mesentery, the root of which runs obliquely downward and to the right from the upper left to the lower right quadrant of the abdomen (Figs. 2-98 and 2-99).

The Large Intestine (Figs. 2-33 and 2-39 to 2-42). The large intestine (bowel) consists of the cecum, the vermiform appendix, the colon (ascending, transverse, descending, and sigmoid), the rectum, and the anal canal. The large intestine forms an arch

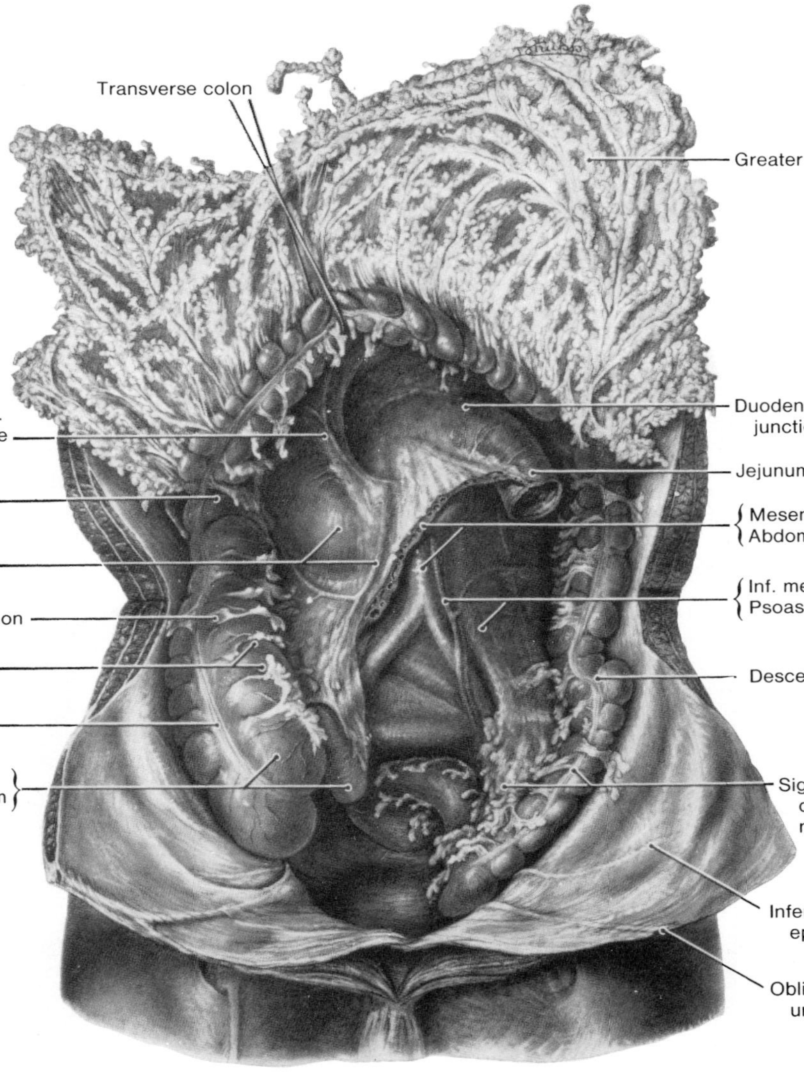

Figure 2-40. Drawing of a dissection of the intestines. The greater omentum is reflected upward and with it the transverse colon and the transverse mesocolon (the mesentery of the transverse colon). The jejunum and ileum are cut away, except their end pieces, and the mesentery is cut short. Observe the duodenojejunal junction, situated to the left of the median plane and immediately below the root of the transverse mesocolon. Note that the first few centimeters of the jejunum descend downward and to the left, anterior to the left kidney, and that the last few centimeters of the ileum ascend upward and to the right out of the pelvic cavity. Of these two parallel pieces of intestine the former is much the larger. Observe that the large intestine forms 3½ sides of a square picture frame around the jejunum and ileum (removed); the missing half-side being between the cecum and the sigmoid colon. Note the following distinguishing features of the large intestine: (1) its position around the small gut; (2) the teniae coli or longitudinal muscle bands; (3) the sacculations or haustra; and (4) the appendices epiploicae. Observe that the right colic flexure, which lies below the liver, is placed at a lower level than the left colic flexure, which lies below the spleen. The vermiform appendix is not present; it was removed at operation.

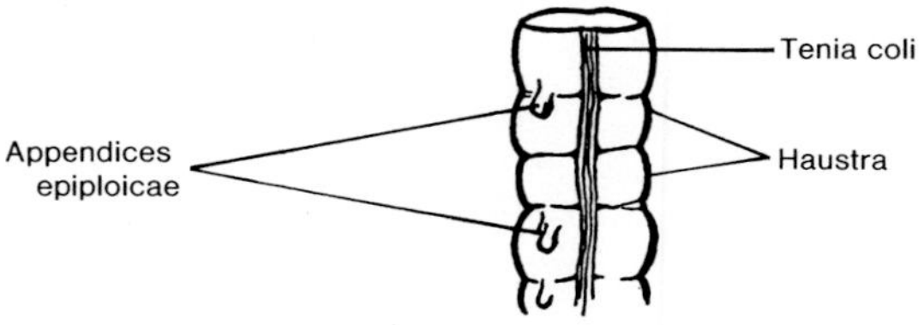

Figure 2-41. Diagram of a segment of colon showing its distinguishing features. Only one of its three teniae coli is visible. Note the sacculations of the wall, called haustra, between these longitudinal bands of muscle. The haustra form because the teniae coli are shorter than the colon to which they are attached. Observe the small projecting sacs of peritoneum filled with fat, known as appendices epiploicae (also see Figs. 2-40 and 2-43). These must not be confued with diverticula of the colon (Case 2-5), which are found most frequently in the sigmoid and left colon. Abnormal outpouchings of the wall of the colon (Fig. 2-149) are present in about 40% of people over 70 years of age.

or almost complete frame for the coils of small intestine and can easily be distinguished from the small intestine by (1) its *three thickened bands of longitudinal muscle*, called **teniae coli**, on its external surface; (2) characteristic sacculations of its wall between the teniae coli, called **haustra**; and (3) small pouches of peritoneum filled with fat, called **appendices epiploicae** (Figs. 2-41 and 2-43).

The Cecum (Figs. 2-33, 2-40, 2-42, 2-43, and 2-96). The cecum (L. *caecus*, blind) is the sac-like blind end of the large intestine, 5 to 7 cm in length, that usually lies in the right iliac fossa. The ileum joins the cecum at the **ileocecal valve**; hence, the cecum is the commencement of the large intestine. The **vermiform appendix**, easily recognizable because of its small caliber, joins the cecum about 2 cm below the ileocecal junction. Usually the cecum is almost en-

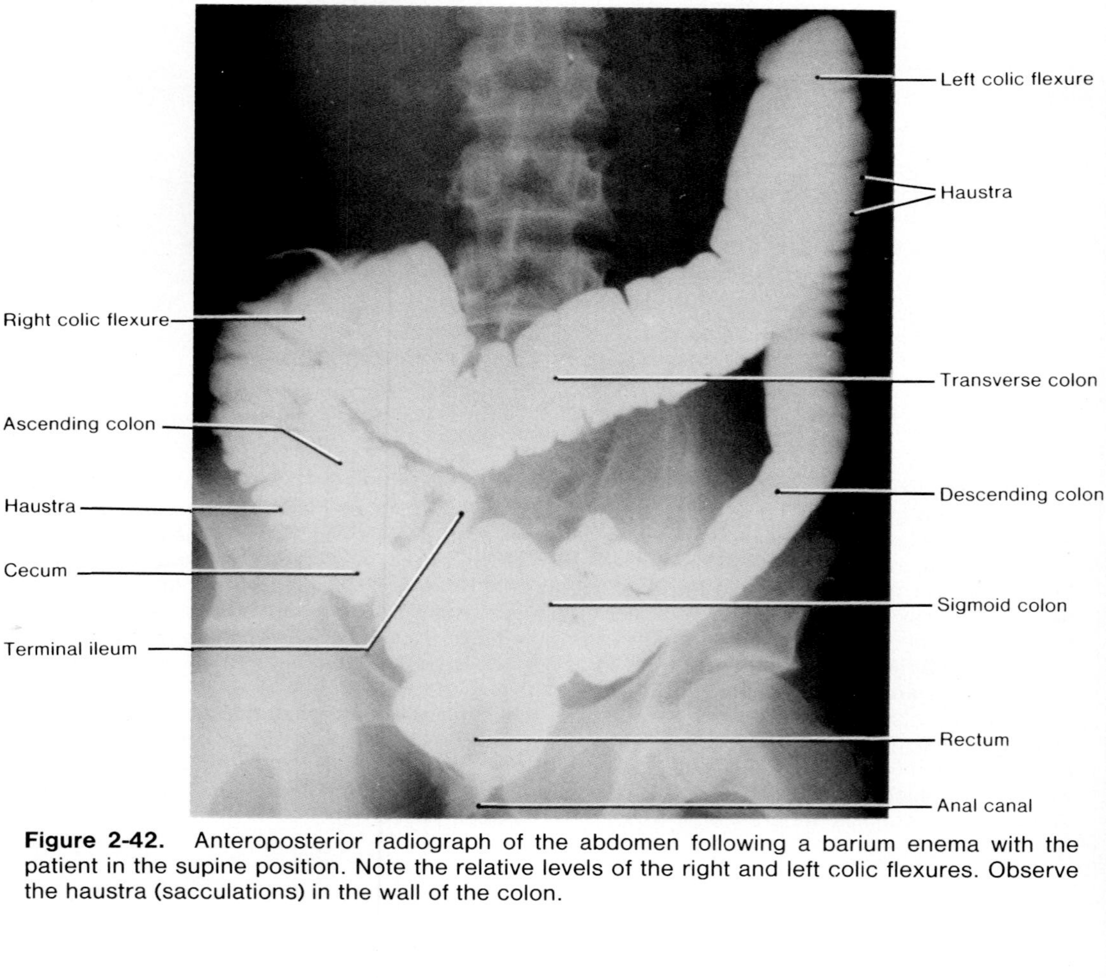

Figure 2-42. Anteroposterior radiograph of the abdomen following a barium enema with the patient in the supine position. Note the relative levels of the right and left colic flexures. Observe the haustra (sacculations) in the wall of the colon.

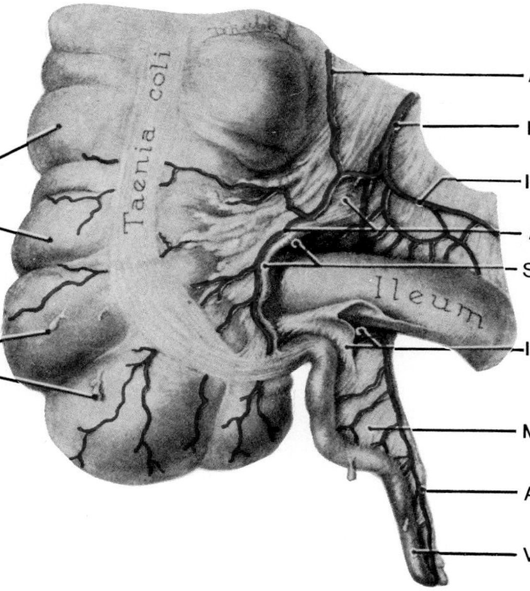

Figure 2-43. Drawing of a dissection of the ileocecal region. Observe the appendix is in one free border of the mesoappendix and the artery is in the other. Note the anterior tenia coli (band of longitudinal muscle fibers) leading to the appendix; this is a guide to the appendix during appendectomy. Observe the inferior ileocecal fold extending from the ileum to the mesoappendix. Although this is often called the "bloodless fold," one should be alert to the possibility of the presence of a small artery in it.

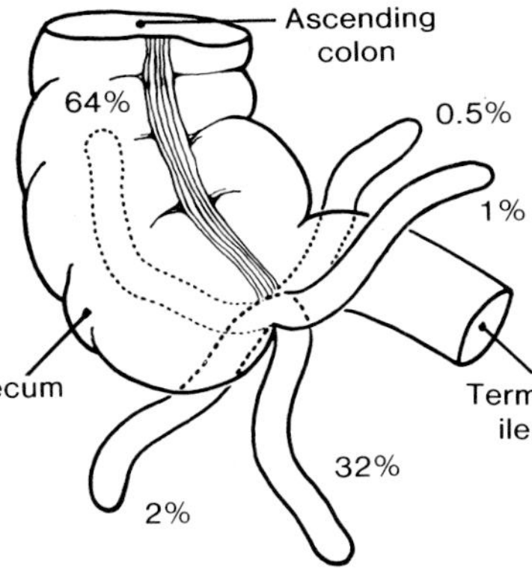

Figure 2-44. Diagram showing the approximate incidence of the various locations of the vermiform appendix. Like the hands of a clock, it may point in any direction. It may be long (20 cm) or short, but most appendices are longer than they appear to be because their proximal parts are buried in the wall of the cecum. Note that in most people (64%) the appendix is found behind the cecum (*i.e.*, retrocecal) in the retrocecal recess. When long enough it may lie behind the lower part of the ascending colon (*i.e.*, retrocolic). When it extends into the pelvis minor (32%), it often lies close to the ovary and the uterine tube in females and to the ureter in both sexes. Very few appendices (1%) are in the position depicted in most textbooks.

tirely enveloped by peritoneum, but it does not form a mesentery. However, the cecum is frequently attached by the peritoneum to the iliac fossa laterally and medially, producing a small pocket or cul-de-sac of the peritoneal cavity, called the **retrocecal recess**. It lies behind the cecum and may extend upward posterior to the inferior end of the ascending colon. Often this recess is deep enough to admit a finger and commonly the vermiform appendix lies in it.

The Vermiform Appendix (Figs. 2-33, 2-43 to 2-45, and 2-96). This is a narrow, worm-shaped (L. *vermis*, worm + *forma*, form) blind tube of variable length (5 to 20 cm). It is longer in the child than in the adult. *The appendix joins the posteromedial aspect of the cecum* 2 cm or less below the ileocecal junction. In the fetus the appendix arises from the inferior end of the

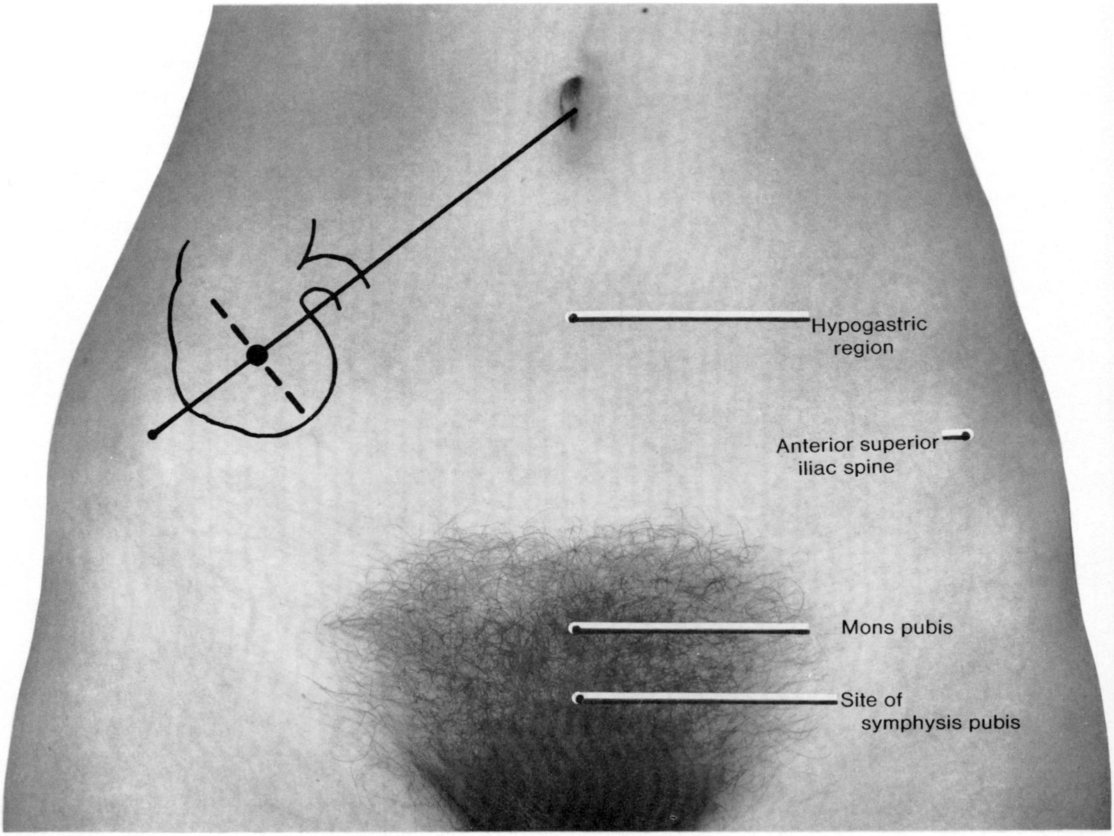

Figure 2-45. Photograph of the abdomen of a 27-year-old woman showing a projection of the cecum and terminal ileum and the location of the base of the appendix as indicated by McBurney's point (*black dot*). Note that this clinically important landmark is at the junction of the lateral and middle thirds of a line joining the anterior superior iliac spine and the umbilicus. McBurney's point indicates where the vermiform appendix usually opens into the cecum (see Fig. 2-43) and where pressure of the finger elicits tenderness in acute appendicitis. The broken line (----) indicates the classical McBurney oblique skin incision centered at McBurney's point. The symphysis pubis is the cartilaginous joint (Fig. 2-1) that is located in the midline between the bodies of the pubic bone. The mons (L. mountain) pubis is a prominence caused by a pad of fatty tissue over the symphysis pubis in the female.

cecum, but differential overgrowth of the lateral cecal wall results in its medial displacement.

The appendix has its own short mesentery called the **mesoappendix** (Fig. 2-43) which connects it to the lower part of the mesentery of the ileum. *The position of the appendix is very variable* (Fig. 2-44). **Usually it is retrocecal or retrocolic**, but it may descend over the brim of the pelvis minor (pelvic or descending appendix). The base of the appendix usually lies deep to **McBurney's point** (Fig. 2-45), which is at the junction of the lateral and middle thirds of the line joining the anterior superior iliac spine to the umbilicus (Fig. 2-10*A*).

The appendicular artery, a branch of the ileocolic artery (Figs. 2-43 and 2-98), represents the entire vascular supply of the appendix. At first it runs in the appendicular mesentery and then it passes distally along the wall of the appendix.

CLINICALLY ORIENTED COMMENTS

Inflammation of the vermiform appendix (**appendicitis**) is the most common cause of an "**acute abdomen**" in most parts of the world. The pain of acute appendicitis (Case 2-4) usually *commences* near the umbilicus (**periumbilical pain**) and *then* passes to the right lower quadrant. In typical cases, fingertip pressure over **McBurney's point** (Fig. 2-45) registers the maximum abdominal tenderness, but in cases of high retrocecal appendix (Fig. 2-44) the maximum tenderness may be as high as the level of the umbilicus.

Although uncommon, *you must keep in mind* that in cases of **malrotation** or **incomplete rotation of the cecum**, the base of the appendix is not located at McBurney's point. *When the cecum is high, the appendix is located in the right subcostal region,* and in these unusual cases, the pain is felt in this region, not in the right lower quadrant.

Acute infection of the appendix may result in **thrombosis of the appendicular artery**, the development of **gangrene** (necrosis owing to obstruction of blood supply), and subsequent **rupture of the appendix**. This results in infection of part or all of the peritoneum (*i.e.*, local or general **peritonitis**) and increased abdominal pain and **abdominal rigidity**.

Appendectomy may be performed through a muscle splitting incision in the right lower quadrant which is centered at McBurney's point (Fig. 2-45). The cecum is delivered into the wound and then the mesentery of the appendix containing the appendicular vessels (Fig. 2-43) is firmly ligated and divided. The base of the appendix is tied, the appendix is excised, and its stump is usually cauterized and then invaginated into the cecum.

The Ascending Colon (Figs. 2-33, 2-39, 2-40, and 2-42). This part of the colon (G. *kolos*, large intestine, hollow), varying from 12 to 20 cm in length, extends upward from the cecum to the **right colic flexure** (hepatic flexure). Its front and sides are covered with peritoneum; usually *it has no mesentery* and is attached to the posterior abdominal wall. Its original fetal mesentery became adherent to the peritoneum of the posterior abdominal wall (Fig. 2-28*D*), but sometimes a short mesentery is retained.

CLINICALLY ORIENTED COMMENTS

Prior to **resection** (surgical excision) of all or part of the ascending colon, it has to be mobilized. The basic principle of **mobilization of the colon** is reconstruction of its primitive mesentery to the stage shown in Figure 2-28*A*. An incision is made along the attachment of the visceral to the parietal peritoneum in the right paracolic gutter and the colon is reflected medially by blunt cleavage of the fused layers of fascia. *During mobilization, neither the vessels supplying the ascending colon nor the ureter and the vessels to the kidney are disturbed* because they lie behind the separated layers of fascia (Fig. 2-28*D*).

The Transverse Colon (Figs. 2-33, 2-36, 2-38 to 2-40, and 2-42). The transverse colon crosses the abdomen transversely from the **right colic flexure** (hepatic flexure) to the **left colic flexure** (splenic flexure), where it bends sharply downward to become the descending colon. The left colic flexure is attached to the diaphragm by the **phrenicocolic ligament** (Fig. 2-52), which also forms a shelf for supporting the spleen.

In Figure 2-42 observe that the left colic flexure is at a more superior level and in a more posterior plane than the right colic flexure. Between these two flexures, the transverse colon is freely movable and forms a loop that is directed downward and forward. *The transverse colon has a mesentery,* the **transverse mesocolon**, which is connected to the inferior border of the pancreas (Fig. 2-38) and to the greater omentum that covers it anteriorly (Fig. 2-36). Because it is freely movable, *the transverse colon is very variable in position*; it may be at the level of the transpyloric plane or it may hang down as far as the pelvic brim in some people.

The Descending Colon (Figs. 2-33, 2-39, 2-40, and 2-42). The descending colon descends from the sharply curved left colic flexure into the left iliac fossa down to the pelvic brim, where it is continuous with the sigmoid colon. In Figure 2-42 observe that the caliber of the descending colon is considerably smaller than that of the ascending colon. *The descending colon has no mesentery.* Its posterior surface is attached to the posterior abdominal wall, but the descending colon can be mobilized surgically in the manner previously discussed for the ascending colon.

The Sigmoid Colon (Figs. 2-33, 2-40, and 2-42). The sigmoid (pelvic) colon forms a loop of variable length (15 to 80 cm) that reminded early anatomists of the Greek letter *sigma.* It has a mesentery (**sigmoid mesocolon**) and therefore considerable freedom of movement. The sigmoid mesentery has a ∧-shaped attachment, upward along the external iliac vessels and then downward from the bifurcation of the common iliac vessels to the front of the sacrum. The **appendices epiploicae** are very long in the sigmoid colon. At the point where the sigmoid mesentery ends (Fig. 2-40), the sigmoid colon is continuous with the rectum.

The Rectum (Figs. 2-33 and 2-42). The rectum (L. *rectus,* straight) is only partially covered with peritoneum and has no mesentery. The lower part of the rectum passes through the pelvic floor to become the anal canal. As the rectum lies in the pelvis, it is described with the other contents of the pelvic cavity in Chapter 3.

The Anal Canal (Figs. 2-33 and 2-42). The rectum ends in the anal canal, *the terminal part of the digestive system.* The anal canal is also described in Chapter 3.

The Kidneys and Suprarenal Glands (Figs. 2-31, 2-33, and 2-68 to 2-71). The two kidneys (L. *renes,* kidneys), one on each side of the vertebral column, lie in the **paravertebral grooves** (gutters) at about the level of vertebrae T12 to L3. Their long axes are almost parallel with the long axis of the body, but *their superior poles are more medial than their inferior poles.* If the inferior poles are close together it always indicates that a malformation of the kidneys and/or of the pelves of the kidneys is present (*e.g.,* horseshoe kidney, Fig. 2-128*A*). Owing to the bulk of the liver, the right kidney usually lies at a slightly lower level than the left. The kidneys lie in a mass of **perirenal fat** posterior to the peritoneum; hence, they are **retroperitoneal.** They can easily be seen and palpated through the parietal peritoneum on the posterior abdominal wall (Fig. 2-70). A **ureter** runs inferiorly from each kidney and passes over the pelvic brim at the bifurcation of the common iliac artery to run along the sidewall of the pelvis to enter the urinary bladder (Fig. 2–26). *the ureter is covered with peritoneum on its anterior surface throughout its entire length in the abdomen* (Fig. 2-134).

Each of the triangular **suprarenal glands** (adrenal glands) lies against the superomedial surface of the corresponding kidney, forming a cap over its superior pole (Fig. 2-33*B*). *Like the kidneys, these endocrine glands are retroperitoneal.*

The Omental Bursa or Lesser Sac of the Peritoneum (Figs. 2-31, 2-38, 2-46, 2-47, and 2–78). The omental bursa (lesser-sac) is a *compartment or recess of the peritoneal cavity* which is located between the stomach and the posterior abdominal wall. It is called a *bursa* (L. purse) because it facilitates movements of the stomach. It develops during the embryonic period as an extension of the peritoneal cavity into the right side of the dorsal mesentery of the stomach (dorsal mesogastrium) and soon expands to the left and inferiorly. Its inferior extension, called the **inferior recess** of the omental bursa (Fig. 2-38), is between the duplicated layers of the gastrocolic ligament of the greater omentum. Occasionally this inferior recess is shut off from the main part of the bursa by adhesions of the layers of the gastrocolic ligament. In some cases, the inferior recess is completely obliterated. The omental bursa also has a **superior recess** which is limited above by the diaphragm and the posterior layer of the **coronary ligament** (Fig. 2-79).

The omental bursa is closed off from the main peritoneal cavity (greater sac of the peritoneum), except for the communication through the **epiploic foramen**, *located posterior to the free edge of the lesser omentum at the upper border of the superior (first) part of the duodenum* (Figs. 2-36 and 2-46).

The boundaries of the epiploic foramen, opening into the upper part of the right side of the peritoneal cavity, are: **anteriorly**, the portal vein, the hepatic artery, and the bile duct (*all in free edge of lesser omentum*); **posteriorly**, the inferior vena cava and the right crus of diaphragm; **superiorly**, the caudate process of liver; and **inferiorly**, the first part of the duodenum and the portal vein, the hepatic artery, and the bile duct on their way to and from the lesser omentum.

The omental bursa is located posterior to the lesser omentum and the stomach (Figs. 2-36 and 2-38). As the stomach lies on the anterior wall of this bursa, it expands and slides on this bursa as it becomes full. As the anterior and posterior walls of the bursa slide smoothly on each other, *the omental bursa gives considerable movement to the stomach*, permitting it to slide freely on it during contraction and distention.

CLINICALLY ORIENTED COMMENTS

A loop of small intestine occasionally passes through the epiploic foramen into the omental bursa and becomes strangulated by the edges of the foramen. As none of the boundaries of this formen can be incised because of the presence of blood vessels, the swollen intestine is usually decompressed by a needle to reduce it so it may be returned through the foramen.

When the cystic artery is severed during **cholecystectomy** (removal of gallbladder), hemorrhage from it can be controlled by compressing the hepatic artery between the index finger in the epiploic foramen and the thumb on its anterior wall.

THE ABDOMINAL VISCERA

General descriptions of the abdominal viscera have been given previously. These organs shall now be described in more detail. The **digestive tract** (Fig. 2-33) consists of a long muscular tube composed of the pharynx, the esophagus, the stomach, and the intestines which *extends from the lips to the anus*. The epithelial lining of the ends of this tube is continuous with the epidermis of the skin. Associated with the digestive tract are large glands (*e.g.*, the liver and the pancreas) that empty their secretions into it.

The Esophagus (Figs. 2-29, 2-33, and 2-34 to 2-37). This *relatively straight muscular tube*, 23 to 25 cm long, is continuous with the lower end of the pharynx. It follows the longitudinal curve of the vertebral column as it descends through the neck and the posterior mediastinum (Chap. 1) to perforate the diaphragm (Fig. 2-130). It ends a little further on by opening into the **cardiac orifice** of the stomach (Fig. 2-48), posterior to the seventh left costal cartilage about 2.5 cm from the midline.

When the esophagus is full, it is constricted in four places: (1) at its beginning in the neck, (2) where it is crossed by the aortic arch, (3) where it is crossed by the left principal bronchus, and (4) where it pierces the diaphragm (Fig. 2-34*A*). An awareness of the sites of these indentations is important clinically when passing instruments along the esophagus (*e.g.*, an **esophagoscope** or a **gastroscope**); otherwise the wall of the esophagus may be damaged at these places. *Understand that these narrowings of the lumen of the esophagus are not anatomical constrictions*; they are visible only when the esophagus is full. The narrowings can be observed in radiographs taken as barium is being swallowed (Fig. 2-34) and they disappear as the esophagus empties.

The abdominal part of the esophagus (Fig. 2-33), 1.5 to 2.5 cm long, is conical in shape. The right border of the esophagus is directly continuous with the lesser curvature of the stomach, but its left border is separated from the fundus of the stomach by the **cardiac notch** (Fig. 2-48).

As the food is previously mixed with saliva, it passes rapidly down the esophagus. Its wall contains only a few mucous glands to supply additional lubrication.

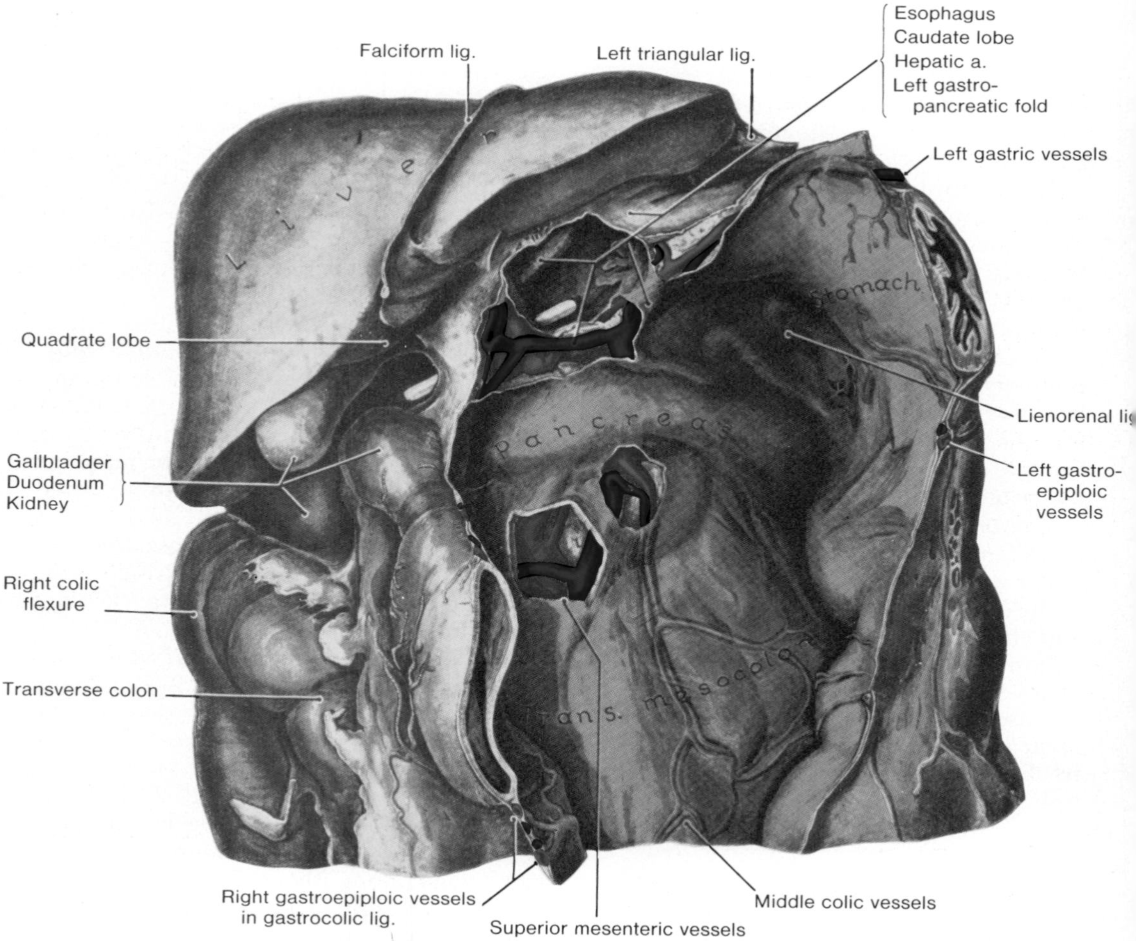

Figure 2-46. Drawing of a dissection of the omental bursa (lesser sac) which has been opened. The anterior wall of the bursa, consisting of the stomach with its two omenta and the vessels along its two curvatures, has been divided vertically and the two parts turned up and to the left and down and to the right. The transverse mesocolon has also been pulled downward somewhat in order to show the full extent of the omental bursa. The *white rod* passes through the epiploic foramen into the omental bursa. Observe the esophagus and the body of the stomach on the left side and the pyloric part and the superior (first) part of the duodenum on the right side. Note that the first part of the duodenum runs backward, upward, and to the right and that the gallbladder and quadrate lobe of the liver are in contact with it above. Observe that the right kidney forms the posterior wall of the hepatorenal pouch and that a white rod has been passed from this pouch through the epiploic foramen into the omental bursa. Examine the pancreas on the posterior wall of the bursa, molded on the vertebral column, and lying roughly horizontally. Note that above the pancreas, the left gastropancreatic fold separates the superior recess, into which the caudate lobe projects, from the splenic recess, which lies to the left.

The Stomach (Figs. 2-29, 2-31, 2-33, 2-35 to 2-39, and 2-46 to 2-52). *The stomach acts as a blender and a reservoir where the digestive juices can act on the food.* The empty stomach is only of slightly larger caliber than the large intestine, but it is capable of considerable expansion and can hold 2 to 3 liters of material. The newborn infant's stomach is about the size of a hen's egg, but it can hold about 30 ml of fluid.

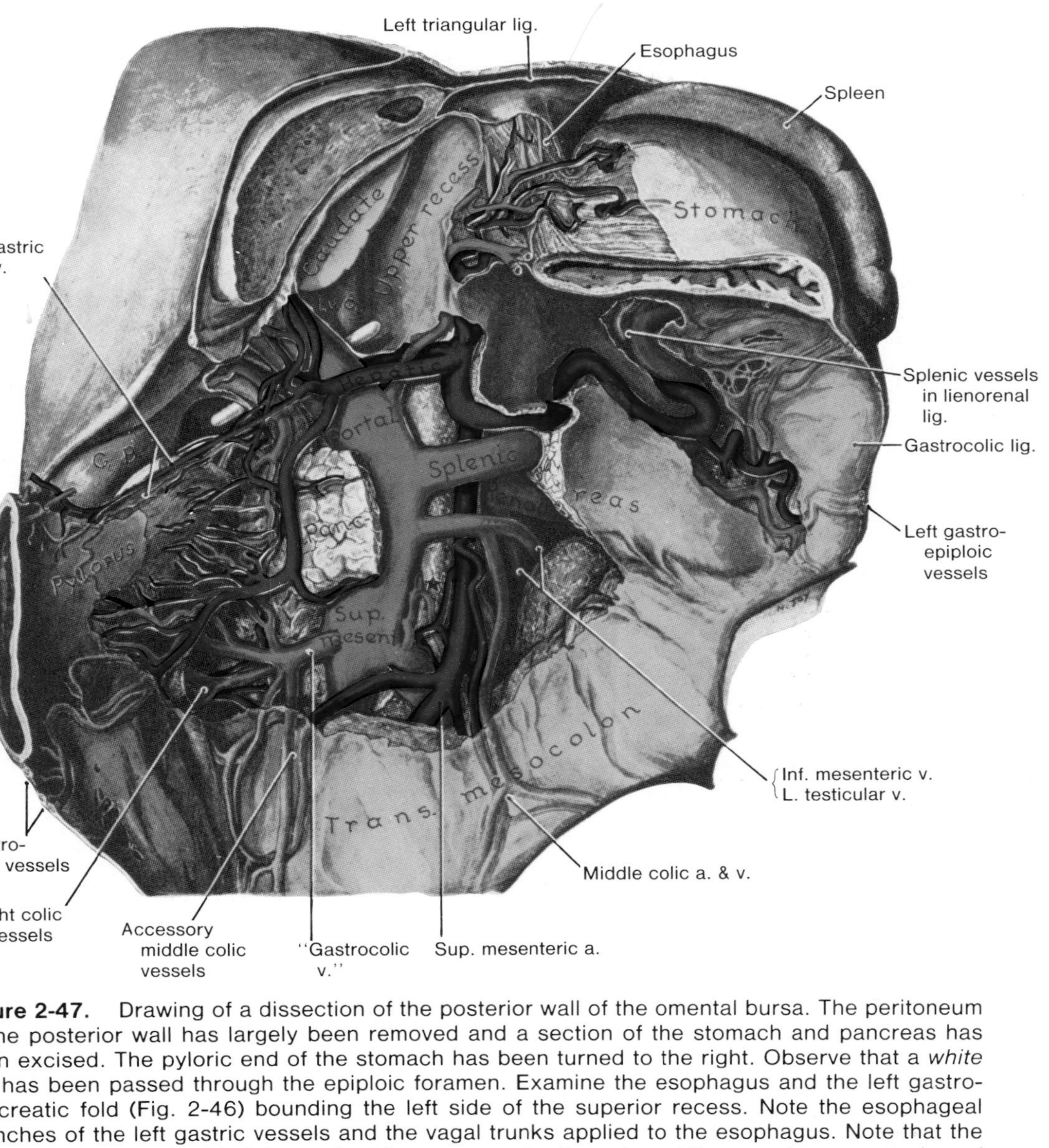

Figure 2-47. Drawing of a dissection of the posterior wall of the omental bursa. The peritoneum of the posterior wall has largely been removed and a section of the stomach and pancreas has been excised. The pyloric end of the stomach has been turned to the right. Observe that a *white rod* has been passed through the epiploic foramen. Examine the esophagus and the left gastro-pancreatic fold (Fig. 2-46) bounding the left side of the superior recess. Note the esophageal branches of the left gastric vessels and the vagal trunks applied to the esophagus. Note that the portal vein is formed behind the neck of the pancreas by the union of the superior mesenteric and splenic veins, with the inferior mesenteric vein joining at or near the angle of union. Here, the left gastric vein joins it. Observe the left renal vein receiving the left testicular vein on a plane dorsal to the splenic vein. The hepatic artery proper is labelled as hepatic (see Fig. 2-83).

Thus, *the stomach is a very distensible organ.*

The lower **esophageal "sphincter"** (cardiac "sphincter") normally prevents regurgitation of material into the esophagus, and the **pyloric sphincter** controls the passage of material into the duodenum. Although the muscularis externis of the esophagus is not thickened sufficiently at the cardiac orifice to justify the anatomical designation "sphincter," there is a physiological sphincter here that is quite efficient in preventing reflux of gastric contents into the esophagus.

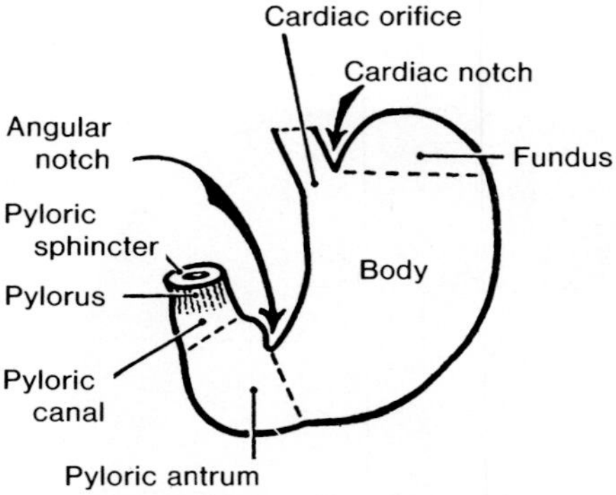

Figure 2-48. Drawing of the anterior surface of the stomach illustrating its parts. An oblique line joining the angular notch or incisura angularis on the lesser curvature to the greater curvature separates the body of the stomach from the pyloric part of the stomach. Another oblique line from an indentation on the greater curvature to the lesser curvature subdivides the pyloric part into a large chamber, the pyloric antrum, and a more tubular part, the pyloric canal, which ends at the pylorus. The pylorus is the area which contains the pyloric sphincter and feels thicker because of this ring of thick muscle. The pylorus is highly mobile because the greater and lesser omenta are attached to it (Fig. 2-36). It may be located anywhere between the first and third lumbar vertebrae, depending upon the person's position (*i.e.*, supine or erect).

The stomach has two curvatures. The **lesser curvature** is continuous with the right border of the esophagus and *forms the right or concave border of the stomach.* The **greater curvature** is continuous with the left border of the esophagus and forms the left or convex border of the stomach. The greater curvature is four to five times longer than the lesser curvature.

The cardiac part of the stomach is a rather indefinite region around the **cardiac orifice** (cardia). The adjective "cardiac" is derived from the Latin word *cardo* for doorhinge; hence the cardiac part is at the "door" or entrance to the stomach. To the left of and superior to the **cardiac orifice** (esophageal opening) is the fundus, a dilation or bulge of the stomach (Fig. 2-48). The fundus rests against the left dome of the diaphragm (Fig. 2-36) and usually contains a bubble of gas (Figs. 2-34 and 2-35).

The body of the stomach continues into the pyloric part and consists of a wider portion, the **pyloric antrum**, and a narrow portion, the **pyloric canal**. The pyloric canal is continuous with the pylorus. The **incisura angularis** or **angular notch** is a sharp angulation of the lesser curvature (Figs. 2-35 and 2-48) which indicates the junction of the body and the pyloric part of the stomach. The **pylorus** (G. gate keeper), the *distal sphincteric region*, is the thickened part of the stomach because it contains an increased amount of smooth circular muscle. The middle layer of this muscle is greatly thickened at the pylorus to form the **pyloric sphincter**, which *controls the rate of discharge of stomach contents* into the duodenum. The pylorus is normally in **tonic contraction** (*i.e.*, it is closed except when emitting the contents of the stomach).

A semisolid **bolus** (L. lump) of food from the esophagus enters the stomach, where it is mixed with and partly digested by the **gastric juices** until it has the consistency of gruel (thin porridge). At irregular intervals the gastric peristalsis passes this semifluid mass of partly digested food, called **chyme** (G. juice), through the pyloric canal (1 to 2 cm long) into the small intestine for further mixing, digestion, and absorption. The stomach is usually empty 2 to 3 hr after eating or sooner if the person lies on the right side because of the left-sided location of the stomach.

The shape of the stomach varies in position and shape in different persons and in the same individual, depending upon its contents and whether the person is in the supine or erect position. *In the supine position, the stomach commonly lies in the left upper quadrant* (epigastric, umbilical, and left hypochondriac regions, Fig. 2-4*B*). In the erect position, the J-shaped stomach moves inferiorly from 1 to 16 cm. In asthenic (weak) persons the body of the stomach may extend into the pelvis major.

The lining mucosa of the empty contracted stomach is thrown into numerous ridges and folds called **rugae** (Figs. 2-35 and 2-49).

The Surface Anatomy of the Stomach (Fig. 2-51). The surface features of the stomach vary greatly because its size and

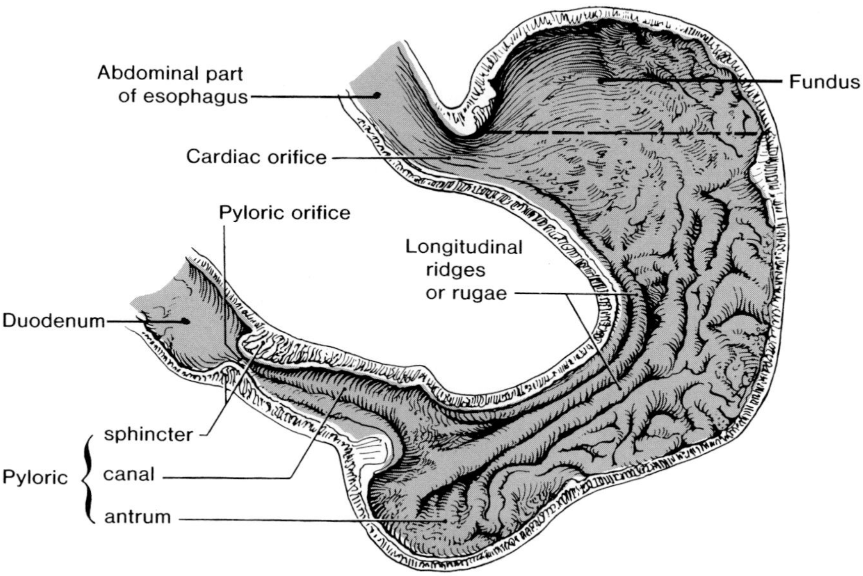

Figure 2-49. Drawing of the mucous membrane of the stomach. Along the lesser curvature observe the longitudinal ridges extending from the esophagus to the pylorus. Elsewhere note that the mucous membrane is rugose when the stomach is empty. The numerous prominent ridges and folds of the lining mucosa are called rugae (L. wrinkles); they tend to disappear or become smaller when the stomach is distended. The rugae are also visible in radiographs of the stomach taken after a barium meal (Fig. 2-35).

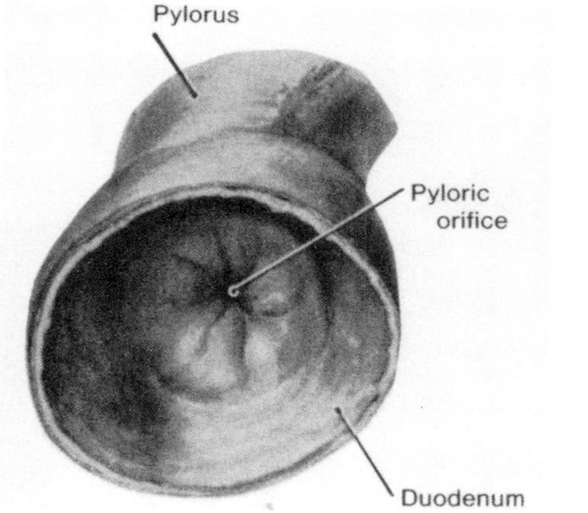

Figure 2-50. Drawing of the pylorus of a stomach and the first or superior part of the duodenum. The pylorus is the thickened part which unites the stomach and the duodenum. Observe that the pyloric orifice of the stomach is narrow. It is surrounded by a thick ring of circular muscle forming the pyloric sphincter which controls the rate of discharge of stomach contents into the duodenum.

position change under a variety of circumstances; hence, it is difficult to draw an outline of the stomach on the surface. However, certain surface features of the stomach are noteworthy and are clinically important.

The cardiac orifice of the stomach is located *posterior to the seventh left costal cartilage*, 2 to 4 cm from the midline, at the level of the 10th or 11th thoracic vertebra. **The highest point of the fundus** of the stomach is located *posterior to the fifth left rib* in the midclavicular line (Fig. 2-36). The **pylorus** of the stomach lies at the level of the **transpyloric plane** which passes through the pylorus (obviously) and the lower part of the body of the first lumbar vertebra (Fig. 2-51).

The normal stomach is not palpable because its walls are flat and rather flabby. **Fluorscopic studies** of the stomach have shown that the cardiac orifice remains nearly stationary, but the level of the pylorus varies from about L1 to L3 in the

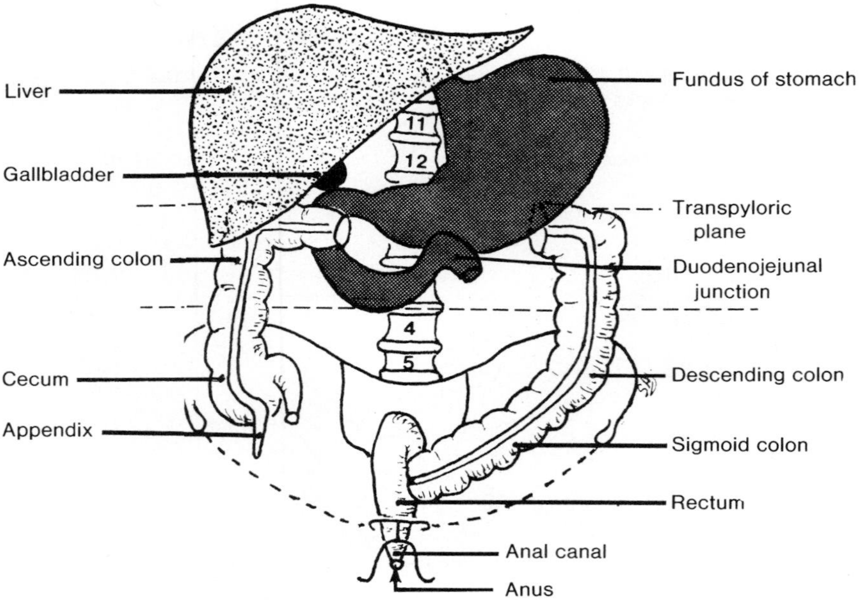

Figure 2-51. Diagram illustrating the surface anatomy of some of the abdominal viscera, particularly their relationship to the vertebral column.

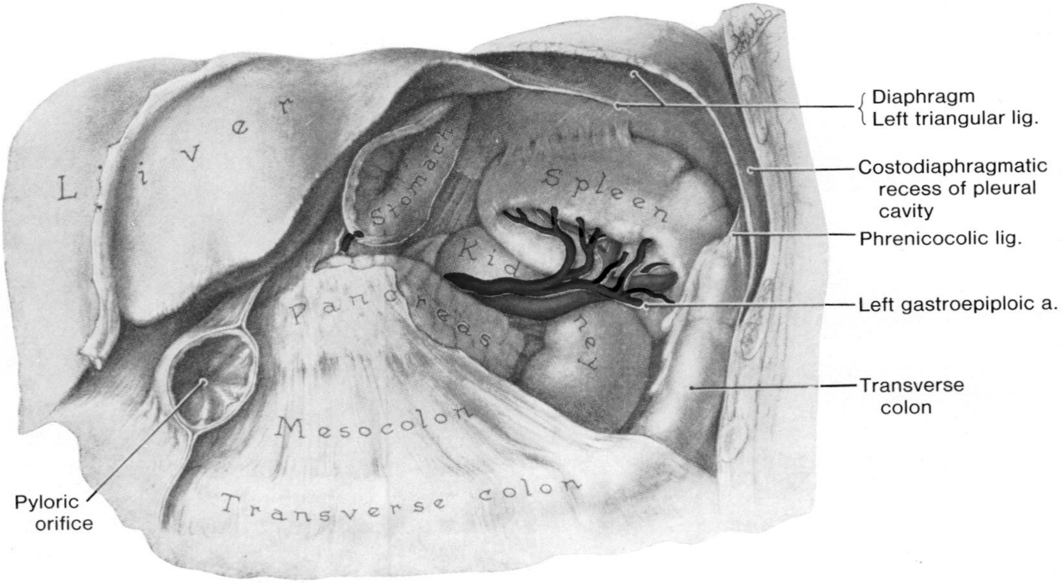

Figure 2-52. Drawing of a dissection of the stomach bed. The stomach is excised and the peritoneum of the omental bursa (lesser sac) covering the stomach bed is largely removed; so is the peritoneum of the greater sac covering the lower part of the kidney and pancreas. In this specimen the pancreas is unusually short and there are adhesions binding the spleen to the diaphragm; these are pathological but not unusual. Observe the lesser omentum attached to the upper border of the pylorus and the greater omentum to its lower border. Note the pleural cavity separating the spleen and the diaphragm from the thoracic wall. Observe the notched superior border of the spleen. (Also see Fig. 2-60).

supine position. In the erect position, *the location of the pylorus varies from about the level of L2 to L4* and is usually on the right side, but occasionally it is in the midline.

CLINICALLY ORIENTED COMMENTS

When the body or the pyloric part of the stomach contains a tumor, the mass may be palpable. In infants with **hypertrophic pyloric stenosis** (see subsequent discussion), the hypertrophied pylorus may be felt, usually as it descends during inspiration, as a small hard mass about the size of an olive (Case 2-10).

Relations of the Stomach (Figs. 2-29, 2-31, 2-33, 2-36 to 2-38, 2-46, 2-47, and 2-52). *The stomach is between the two layers of peritoneum that form the anterior wall of the omental bursa.* The **stomach bed** is formed by the posterior wall of the omental bursa and by the retroperitoneal structures between it and the posterior abdominal wall (*e.g.*, the pancreas). *Superiorly the stomach bed consists of* the **diaphragm**, the **spleen**, the upper pole of the **left kidney**, and the left **suprarenal gland**. *Inferiorly the stomach bed consists of* the **body** and **tail of the pancreas** and the mesentery of the transverse colon, called the **transverse mesocolon.** Understand that the structure of the stomach bed varies somewhat according to the person's position. The above description refers to a person who is recumbent or supine, the usual position of a patient in bed or on the operating table. In radiographs (Fig. 2-35), the position of the stomach usually extends more inferiorly than that found in cadavers (Fig. 2-36).

The fundus of the stomach and a portion of the cardiac part is in contact with the diaphragm behind the lower costal cartilages. In upright radiographs of the chest, there is often a gas bubble below the left dome of the diaphragm (Fig. 1-58). This bubble outlines the curved fundus of the stomach and is also visible in radiographs of the esophagus (Fig. 2-34*A*) and the stomach (Fig. 2-35). Portions of the longitudinal **rugae** are also outlined by gas in radiographs of the stomach. The gas bubble, visible below the left dome of the diaphragm on radiographs, is sometimes in the left colic flexure (Fig. 2-42), but the colon can usually be recognized by the presence of **haustra** (Figs. 2-41 and 2-42).

In Figures 2-29, 2-33, and 2-36 observe that *the anterior surface of the stomach is in contact with* (1) the **diaphragm** in the fundic region, (2) the left lobe of the **liver**, and (3) the **anterior abdominal wall**.

CLINICALLY ORIENTED COMMENTS

Malformations of the stomach are very rare, except for **congenital hypertrophic pyloric stenosis**. This marked thickening of the pylorus affects approximately 1 in every 150 male and 1 in every 750 female infants (Case 2-10). The elongated, thickened pylorus is very hard and *there is severe narrowing (stenosis) of the pyloric canal* owing to hypertrophy of the circular musclar layer. The stomach is usually secondarily dilated. Although the cause of congenital hypertrophic pyloric stenosis is unknown, genetic factors appear to be involved because of its high incidence in both infants of monozygotic (identical) twins.

Although part of the stomach may be herniated through the diaphragm at birth owing to a congenitally large esophageal hiatus, a **thoracic stomach** is rare. Sometimes the stomach may enter the thorax through a large posterolateral defect in the diaphragm (Fig. 2-152). This type of **congenital diaphragmatic hernia** occurs about once in every 2200 newborn infants (see discussion on p. 257).

Much more common are **acquired hiatal hernias**, which occur most often in middle-aged people owing to *weakening and widening of the esophageal hiatus.* A portion of the fundus of the stomach may herniate through the esophageal hiatus into the lower chest. There are two main types.

In **sliding hiatal hernia** (Fig. 2-53*A*), *the gastroesophageal region slides upward into the chest* through the lax esophageal hiatus when the person lies down or bends over. There is often regurgitation of acid from the stomach into the lower esophagus because the clamping action of the crura of the diaphragm on the esophagus is lost.

In **paraesophageal hiatal hernia** or rolling hiatal hernia (Fig. 2-53*B*), which is **far less common**, *the gastroesophageal region remains in its normal position*, but a pouch of peritoneum often containing the fundus of the stomach rolls up or extends through the esophageal hiatus, anterior to the esophagus. In these cases there is no regurgitation because the cardiac "sphincter" is in its normal positon. There may be pain, nausea, vomiting, and **dysphagia** (difficulty in swallowing).

Arteries of the Stomach (Figs. 2-54 to 2-56, 2-61, 2-62, and 2-64). The stomach has a rich blood supply. *Its arteries are derived from all three branches of the celiac trunk* (axis, artery). They are (1) the **left gastric artery**, a branch of the celiac trunk, (2) the **right gastric** and **right gastroepiploic branches** via the common hepatic artery, and (3) the **left gastroepiploic** and **short gastric branches** of the splenic artery.

The celiac trunk is a short artery (1 to 2 cm long) which is the most superior of the three unpaired branches of the abdominal aorta that supply the GI tract and other organs. It arises from the aorta just after it passes through the diaphragm at about the level of the *12th thoracic vertebra*, just above the *transpyloric plane* (Fig. 2-55).

The left gastric artery is a small branch that arises directly from the celiac trunk and passes upward and to the left, across the posterior wall of the omental bursa. It lies in the floor of this bursa, posterior to the parietal peritoneum. The left gastric artery passes from the posterior abdominal wall to the cardiac part of the stomach where it frequently gives rise to the **left hepatic artery**, which passes between the layers of the hepatogastric ligament to supply the left lobe of the liver. It then runs inferiorly between the layers of the lesser omentum (**hepatogastric ligament**) along the lesser curvature (frequently as two branches) to the pylorus. It supplies both surfaces of the stomach and anastomoses with the right gastric artery. It gives rise to ascending **esophageal branches** which supply the esophagus and anastomose with esophageal branches of the aorta in the thorax.

The right and **left gastroepiploic ar-**

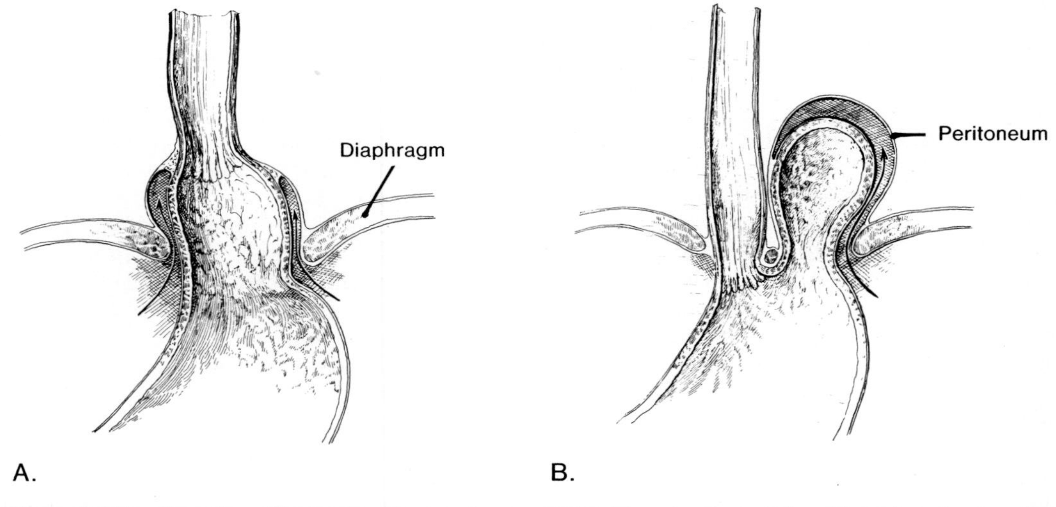

Figure 2-53. Drawings illustrating the two types of hiatal hernia. *A*, a sliding hiatal hernia showing the gastroesophageal junction situated above the esophageal hiatus. *B*, a paraesophageal hiatal hernia with the cardioesophageal junction in its normal position. Note that the pouch of peritoneum extending through the hiatus into the chest contains a portion of the fundus of the stomach.

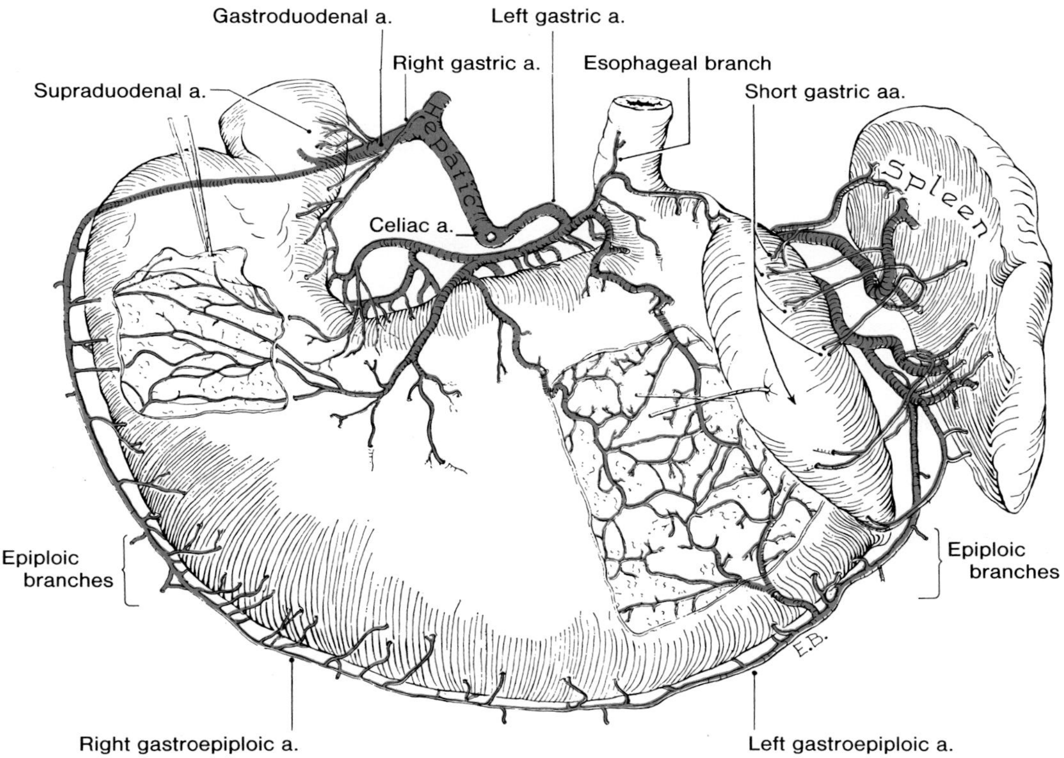

Figure 2-54. Drawing of a dissection of the arteries of the stomach and spleen. (For a simpler illustration of these arteries, see Fig. 2-56.) The serous and muscular coats are removed from two areas of the stomach, thereby revealing the anastomotic networks in the submucous coat. Observe the arterial arch on the lesser curvature which is formed by the larger left gastric artery and the much smaller right gastric artery. Note that the arterial arch on the greater curvature is formed equally by the right and the left gastroepiploic arteries. The anastomosis between their two trunks is attenuated; commonly it is absent. Observe the anastomoses between the branches of the two foregoing arterial arches taking place in the submucous coat two-thirds of the distance from the lesser to the greater curvature of the stomach. Note the four or five tenuous short gastric arteries leaving the terminal branches of the splenic artery close to the spleen. Also observe the left gastroepiloic artery belonging to the short gastric artery series, arising within 2.5 cm of the hilum of the spleen. The vessel labelled *Hepatic* is the common hepatic artery.

teries run along the greater curvature of the stomach, supplying both its surfaces. These branches run between the layers of the greater omentum a short distance from its attachment to the stomach.

The right gastroepiploic artery (Fig. 2-54), a branch of the gastroduodenal, runs to the left and anastomoses with the left gastroepiploic artery. It sends branches to the right part of the stomach, the superior part of the duodenum, and the greater omentum.

The left gastroepiploic artery (Fig. 2-56), a branch of the splenic, runs between the layers of the gastrolienal (gastrosplenic) ligament to the greater curvature of the stomach. It runs to the right within the greater omentum, supplying the stomach and this omentum, and ends by anastomosing with the right gastroepiploic artery.

The short gastric arteries (4 to 5) are also branches of the splenic artery. They pass between the layers of the gastrolienal ligament to the fundus of the stomach,

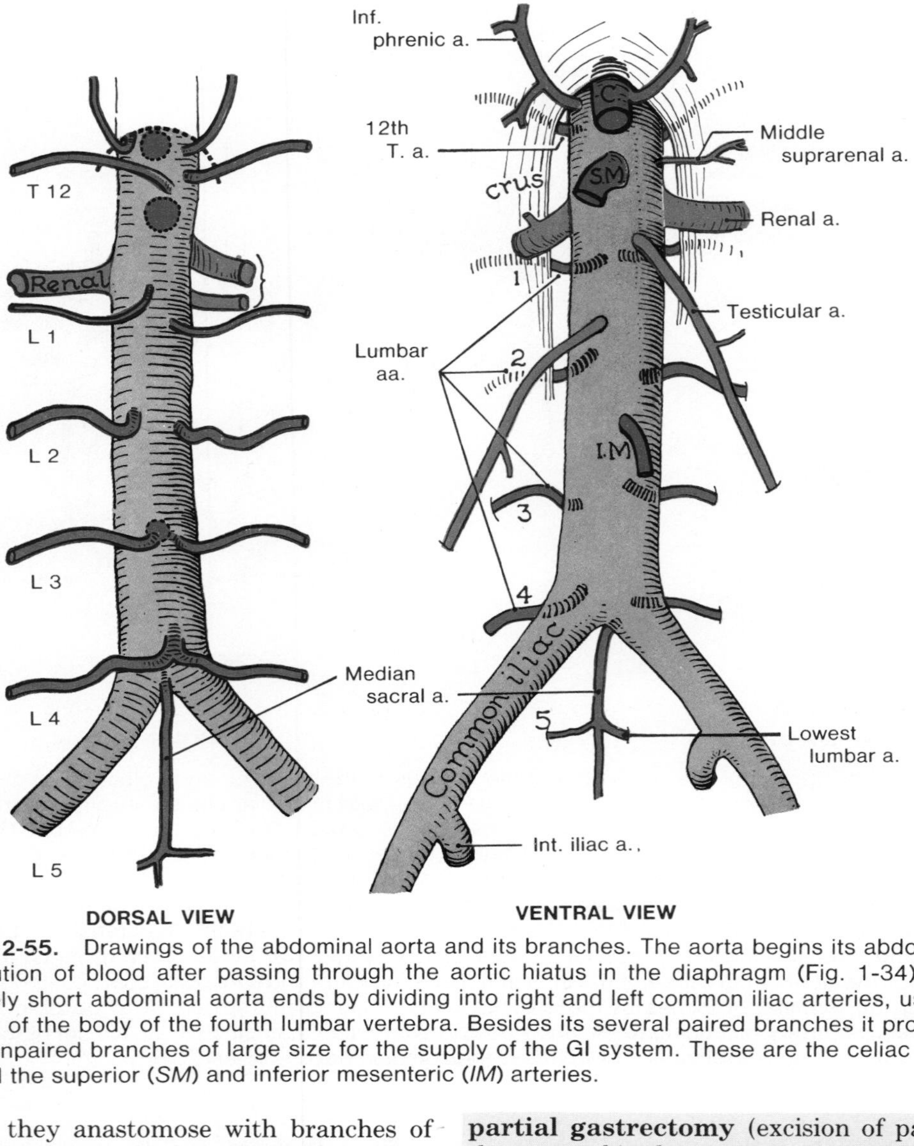

DORSAL VIEW **VENTRAL VIEW**

Figure 2-55. Drawings of the abdominal aorta and its branches. The aorta begins its abdominal distribution of blood after passing through the aortic hiatus in the diaphragm (Fig. 1-34). The relatively short abdominal aorta ends by dividing into right and left common iliac arteries, usually in front of the body of the fourth lumbar vertebra. Besides its several paired branches it provides three unpaired branches of large size for the supply of the GI system. These are the celiac trunk (*C*) and the superior (*SM*) and inferior mesenteric (*IM*) arteries.

where they anastomose with branches of the left gastric and left gastroepiploic arteries.

CLINICALLY ORIENTED COMMENTS

Owing to the anastomoses of the various arteries of the stomach providing a good **collateral circulation**, one or more of the major arteries may be ligated without seriously affecting its blood supply. During a **partial gastrectomy** (excision of part of the stomach), the greater omentum is incised below the right gastroepiploic artery (Fig. 2-54). Even though all the omental branches of this artery are ligated, the greater omentum does not degenerate because the omental branches of the left gastroepiploic artery are still intact.

Veins of the Stomach (Figs. 2-47, 2-57, and 2-85). The veins of the stomach parallel the arteries in position and in course and

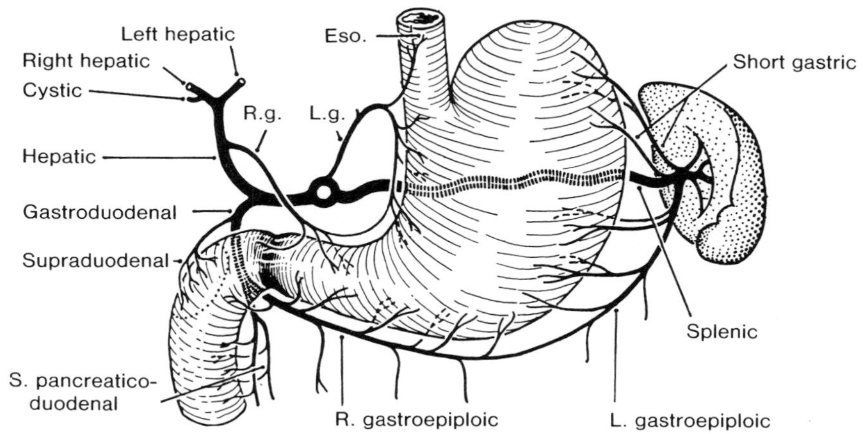

Figure 2-56. Drawing of the esophagus, stomach, duodenum, and spleen showing the branches of the celiac trunk. This very short unpaired artery arises directly from the abdominal aorta (Figs. 2-55 and 2-143*A*), immediately inferior to the diaphragm at the level of the upper part of the first lumbar vertebra.

drain into the **portal system of veins** which enter the liver. The portal vein is formed by the union of the superior mesenteric and splenic veins, posterior to the neck of the pancreas and anterior to the inferior vena cava. *Venous blood from the stomach and other parts of the GI tract enters the liver via the portal vein* and passes through its capillary network before continuing on to the heart (Fig. 2-85).

There is considerable variation in the way the gastric veins drain into the portal system of veins. Usually the **right** and **left gastric veins** drain directly into the portal vein. The **right gastroepiploic** vein usually drains into the superior mesenteric vein, but it may enter the portal vein directly or join the splenic vein. The **left gastroepiploic vein** and the **short gastric vein** drain into the splenic vein or its tributaries.

Lymphatic Drainage of the Stomach (Fig. 2-58). The lymph vessels of the stomach accompany the four main arteries to the stomach along its greater and lesser curvatures. *There are four major areas of lymphatic drainage, each of which has its own regional lymph nodes.* The lymph vessels of the stomach drain lymph from its anterior and posterior surfaces toward its curvatures, where many of the lymph nodes are located.

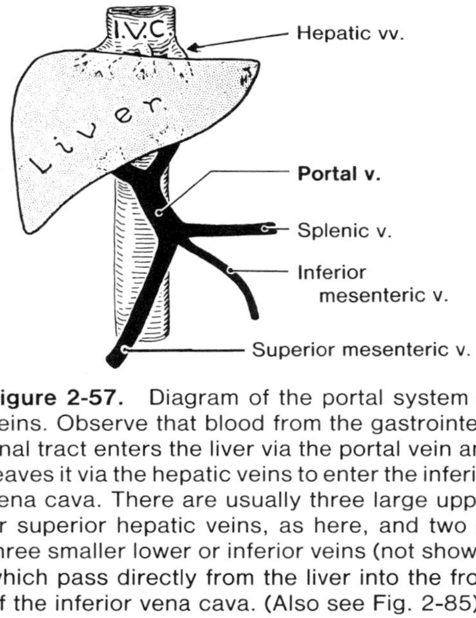

Figure 2-57. Diagram of the portal system of veins. Observe that blood from the gastrointestinal tract enters the liver via the portal vein and leaves it via the hepatic veins to enter the inferior vena cava. There are usually three large upper or superior hepatic veins, as here, and two or three smaller lower or inferior veins (not shown) which pass directly from the liver into the front of the inferior vena cava. (Also see Fig. 2-85).

The largest area of lymphatic drainage is from the lesser curvature and a large part of the body of the stomach into the **left gastric lymph nodes**, which lie along the left gastric artery.

The next largest area of lymphatic drainage is from the right part of the greater curvature and most of the pyloric part of the stomach partly into the **gastroepiploic nodes**, which lie along the right gastroepiploic vessels. Other lymph vessels from this area pass directly into

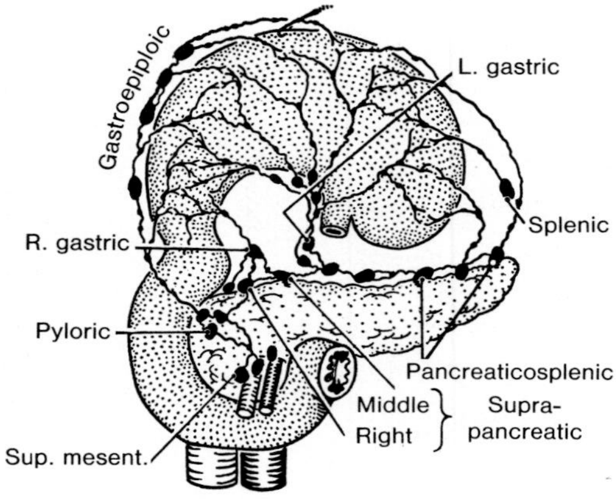

Figure 2-58. Diagram illustrating the lymphatics of the upper abdomen and stomach. The gastric nodes consist of right and left gastric, right gastroepiploic, and pyloric groups. The collecting vessels from the capsule of the spleen end in the pancreaticosplenic lymph nodes.

the *very important* **pyloric nodes**, located on the anterior surface of the head of the pancreas close to the pyloric end of the stomach.

The third area of lymphatic drainage is smaller than the previous two. Lymph vessels from the left part of the greater curvature pass to the **gastroepiploic nodes**, which lie along the left gastroepiploic vessels, and to the pancreaticolienal nodes which lie along the splenic vessels.

The fourth and smallest area of drainage is from the lesser curvature related to the pyloric part of the stomach. Lymph vessels from this area pass to the **right gastric nodes**, which lie along the right gastric artery.

Lymph from all four major groups of lymph nodes drains into the celiac lymph nodes, which are congregated around the origin of the celiac trunk. Lymph from these nodes passes with that from other parts of the GI tract to **cisterna chyli** and the **thoracic duct** (Figs. 1-48 and 2-147).

CLINICALLY ORIENTED COMMENTS

Resection of the stomach for carcinoma involves the *removal of all involved regional lymph nodes*. The **pyloric nodes** on the front of the head of the pancreas are especially important because they receive lymph from the pyloric region of the stomach, where carcinoma is most frequent. As lymph from this region also drains into the **right gastroepiploic nodes** along the right gastroepiploic vessels, they are very frequently involved by carcinoma of the stomach. In more advanced cases, cancer cells spread by lymphogenous dissemination to the **celiac nodes** grouped around the origin of the celiac trunk, because all four major groups of lymph nodes around the stomach drain into them.

Nerves to the Stomach (Figs. 2-59 and 2-127). The **parasympathetic nerve supply** is derived from the anterior and posterior **vagal trunks** (nerves) and their branches. The **sympathetic nerve supply** is mainly from the **celiac plexus** through the plexuses around the gastric and gastroepiploic arteries (Fig. 2-111).

The anterior vagal trunk, derived mainly from the left vagus nerve, enters the abdomen as a single branch (sometimes double or triple) that lies on the anterior surface of the esophagus. It runs toward the lesser curvature of the stomach where it gives off hepatic and duodenal branches that leave the stomach within the hepatoduodenal ligament. The rest of the anterior vagal trunk continues along the lesser curvature of the stomach, giving rise to anterior gastric branches.

The posterior vagal trunk, derived mainly from the right vagus nerve, enters the abdomen on the posterior surface of the esophagus and passes toward the lesser curvature of the stomach. Hence, *both vagal trunks can often be found close to where the left gastric artery reaches the stomach.* The posterior vagal trunk gives off a celiac branch that runs to the celiac plexus and then continues along the lesser curvature, giving rise to posterior gastric branches.

CLINICALLY ORIENTED COMMENTS

The secretion of acid by the parietal cells of the stomach is largely controlled by the vagus nerves; hence, section of the vagus trunks (vagotomy) as they enter the abdo-

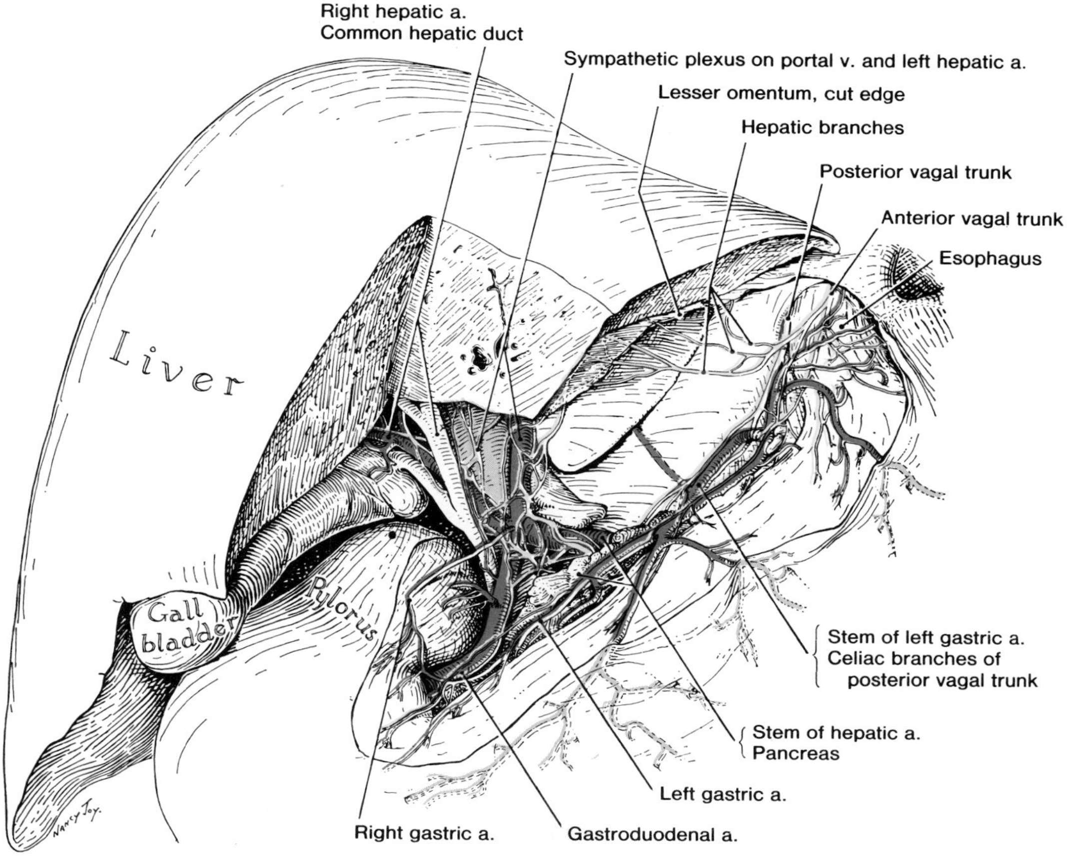

Figure 2-59. Drawing of a dissection of the upper abdomen illustrating the vagus nerves. The nerves to the stomach are branches of the anterior and posterior vagal trunks (nerves). These parasympathetic fibers arrive via the right and left vagus nerves and the sympathetic fibers come via preganglionic fibers from the right and left sympathetic trunks (splanchnic nerves), which synapse in preaortic ganglia. Understand that both kinds of nerves mingle in the rich tangle of nerve plexuses on the front of the aorta, especially around the celiac trunk (celiac plexus). Laymen refer to this as the ''solar plexus.'' Right and left *celiac ganglia* connect with the celiac plexus medially and send large plexuses into the suprarenal glands. Both kinds of fibers are distributed by ''hitchhiking'' on the walls of branches of the abdominal aorta to their destinations. Observe that the posterior and anterior vagal trunks enter on the esophagus and supply gastric branches, and that the celiac branch of the posterior vagal trunk leaves to contribute to the preaortic plexuses. Note the hepatic branches of the anterior vagal trunk are joined by sympathetic fibers from the celiac plexus.

men is sometimes performed to reduce the production of acid in persons with **peptic ulcers** (L. sores) in the stomach or the duodenum (Case 2-1). Excess acid secretion is associated with these lesions of the gastric and/or duodenal mucosa. **Vagotomy** (*division of the vagus nerve*) is often done in conjunction with resection (excision) of the ulcerated area. Often a **selective vagotomy** is done during which only the gastric branches of the vagus are sectioned. This has the desired effect on the acid-producing cells of the stomach without affecting other structures in the abdomen which are supplied by the vagus.

The Spleen (Figs. 2-31, 2-33, 2-39, 2-46, 2-47, 2-52, 2-54, 2-56, and 2-60 to 2-63). The spleen (G. *splēn* and L. *lien*) is a large

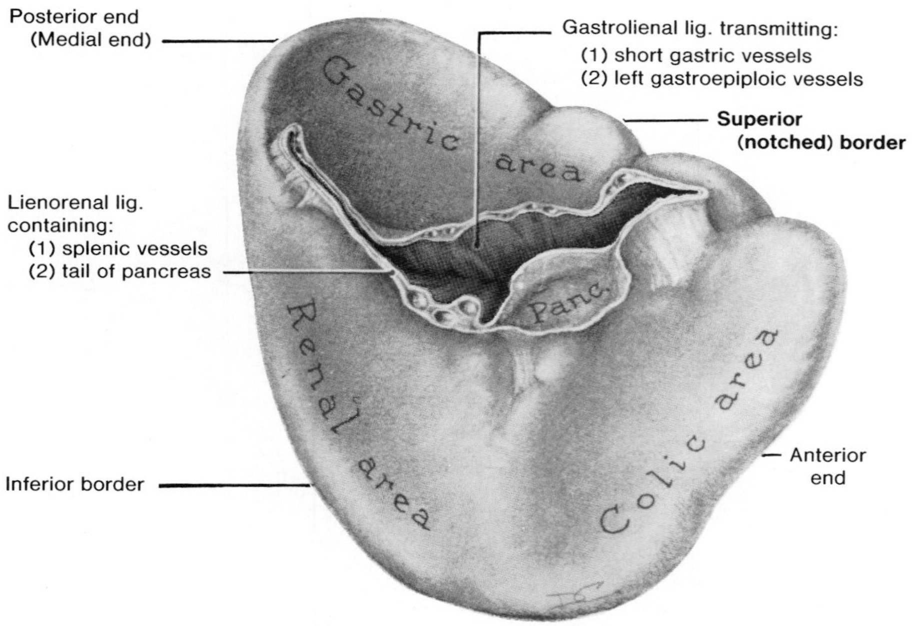

Figure 2-60. Drawing of the visceral surface of the spleen (For orientation, see Fig. 2-52). Observe its "circumferential border" comprising the inferior, superior, and anterior borders and separating the visceral surface from the diaphragmatic surface. Note the notches which are characteristic of the superior border. Examine the left limit of the omental bursa at the hilum of the spleen between the lienorenal and gastrolienal ligaments. Observe that this cadaveric spleen takes the impressions of the structures in contact with it. The large colic area seen here presumably resulted from the colon being full of gas. (See clinical comments on page 185 concerning the notched border).

vascular lymphatic organ in the left upper quadrant. *It is the largest single mass of lymph tissue in the body.* The spleen is described here because of its close relationship to the stomach. It is in contact with the posterior wall of the stomach and is connected to its greater curvature by the gastrolienal ligament.

During life it is soft, purplish, freely movable, and considerably larger than in the cadaveric specimen. It is located in the left hypochondrium, posterior to the stomach and anterior to the superior part of the left kidney. The spleen lies against the diaphragm laterally (Fig. 2-52) which separates it from the pleural cavity. The **diaphragmatic surface of the spleen** is convexly curved to fit the concavity of the diaphragm. *The anterior and superior borders of the spleen are sharp and are often notched.* These notches indicate the lobulated character of the fetal spleen. The posterior and inferior borders of the spleen are rounded.

It is helpful in understanding the peritoneal relations of the spleen to recall that it develops between the two layers of the dorsal mesentery of the stomach (**dorsal mesogastrium**) and that as it enlarges it projects from the left side of this mesentery (Fig. 2-31). As a result, it does not protrude into the omental bursa and is held in position against the lateral part of the left hemidiaphragm by the left wall of the omental bursa. The **gastrolienal (gastrosplenic) ligament**, which is part of the greater omentum, connects the spleen to the greater curvature of the stomach, and the **lienorenal ligament**, containing the splenic vessels and the tail of the pancreas, connects it to the left kidney (Figs. 2-46 and 2-47). Understand that both of these ligaments are parts of the embryonic dorsal mesentery of the stomach. The gastrolienal

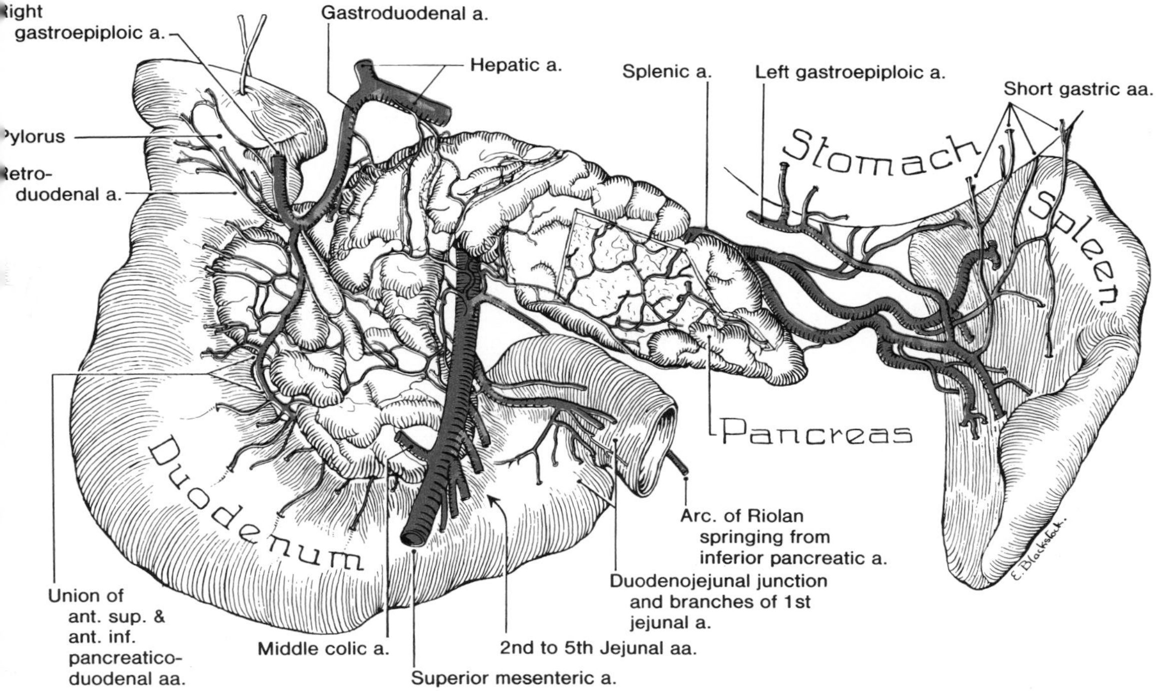

Figure 2-61. Drawing of an *anterior view* of the pancreas, duodenum, and spleen illustrating their blood supply. A slice has been removed from the pancreas. Observe the territory supplied by the hepatic, splenic, and superior mesenteric arteries. Note that several retroduodenal branches spring from the right gastroepiploic artery. Observe that the anterior superior pancreaticoduodenal branch of the gastroduodenal artery and the anterior inferior pancreaticoduodenal branch of the superior mesenteric artery form an arch in front of the head of the pancreas. Note the "arc of Riolan," *an occasional artery* that appears on the posterior abdominal wall and connects the superior mesenteric artery to a branch of the inferior mesenteric artery. Observe the many arteries entering the hilum of the spleen; these are end arteries and do not have significant anastomoses in the substance of the spleen.

and lienorenal ligaments are attached to the **hilum** on the medial aspect of the spleen, where the branches of the splenic artery enter and the tributaries of the splenic vein leave the spleen. Except at the hilum, the spleen is completely surrounded by peritoneum. *The hilum of the spleen is usually intimately related to the tail of the pancreas* (Figs. 2-33 and 2-71).

The spleen varies in size and shape, but it is usually about 12 cm long and 7 cm wide and fits into one's cupped hand. *It normally contains a large amount of blood* and its capsule and trabeculae contain some smooth muscle which enables it to expel some of its blood into the circulation. However, this process is not very efficient in man. The shape of the spleen is affected by the fullness of the stomach and the colon at the left colic flexure. The distended stomach gives the spleen the shape of a segment of orange, whereas when the colon is full the spleen has a tetrahedral appearance (Fig. 2-60).

Surface Anatomy of the Spleen (Figs. 2-68 and 2-117). The spleen is normally under the shelter of the ribs. It lies deep to the 9th, 10th, and 11th ribs and its outer surface is convex to fit these ribs. *It lies approximately parallel to the 10th rib,* which is along its long axis, where it rests on the left colic flexure (Figs. 2-33 and 2-42). *Normally the spleen does not extend below the left costal margin* and its anterior tip usually

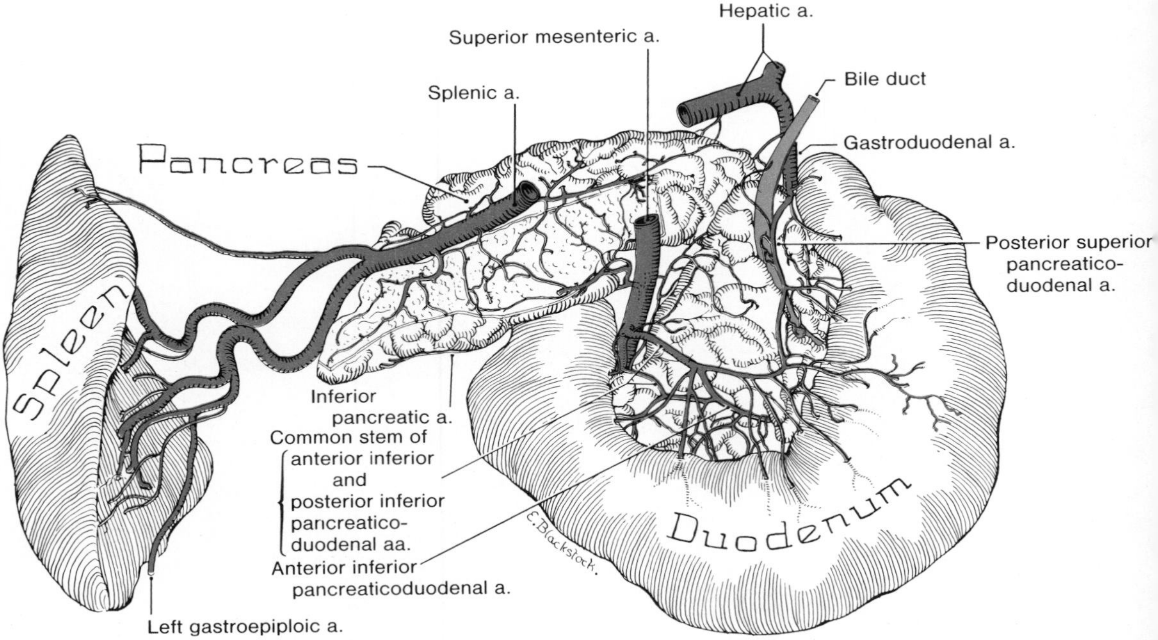

Figure 2-62. Drawing of a *posterior view* of the pancreas, duodenum, and spleen illustrating their blood supply. A slice has been removed from the pancreas. Observe that the posterior superior and posterior inferior branches of the gastroduodenal artery and the superior mesenteric artery form an arch behind the pancreas. Note the two inferior arteries here, as is usual, spring from a common stem. From the arch thus formed, straight vessels called vasa recta duodeni pass to the posterior surface of the second, third, and fourth parts of the duodenum. Observe that the duodenojejunal junction is supplied by the large branching vessel depicted. Examine the fine network of arteries that pervades the pancreas and are derived from: (1) the common stem of the hepatic artery, (2) the gastroduodenal artery, (3) the pancreaticoduodenal arches, (4) the splenic artery, and (5) the superior mesenteric artery.

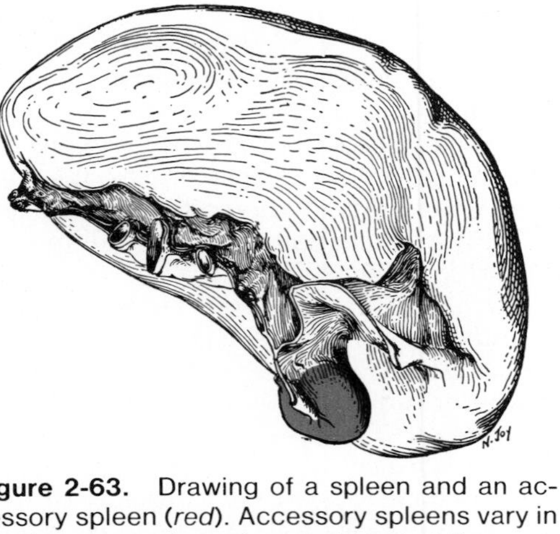

Figure 2-63. Drawing of a spleen and an accessory spleen (*red*). Accessory spleens vary in size from a pea to a plum, but most of them are about 1 cm in diameter and resemble lymph nodes. Like the spleen, they are usually covered with peritoneum. They often lie along the course of the splenic artery or its gastroepiploic branch, but they may be elsewhere. The commonest location is at or near the hilum of the spleen, but some are partially (or wholly) embedded in the tail of the pancreas.

does not extend farther anteriorly than the midaxillary line. The normal spleen is not usually palpable on physical examination. If the spleen can be palpated it is almost surely enlarged.

Arterial Supply of the Spleen (Figs. 2-52, 2-54, 2-56, 2-61, 2-62, and 2-64). The **splenic artery** is the *largest branch of the celiac trunk*. It follows a tortuous course posterior to the omental bursa and anterior to the left kidney and along the superior border of the pancreas. Between the layers of the lienorenal ligament, the splenic artery *divides into five or more branches* which enter the hilum of the spleen, where they ramify throughout its substance to supply the individual elements of the spleen as **end arteries**. The splenic artery also gives rise to pancreatic branches, the short gastric arteries to the fundus of the stomach, and the left gastroepiploic artery.

Venous Drainage of the Spleen (Figs. 2-47, 2-52, 2-57, and 2-85). The **splenic vein** is formed by several tributaries that emerge from the hilum of the spleen. It runs behind the body and tail of the pancreas throughout most of its course and *unites with the superior mesenteric vein* behind the neck of the pancreas to form the **portal vein**.

Lymphatic Drainage of the Spleen (Fig. 2-58). The lymph vessels arise from the capsule and the trabeculae of the spleen and pass along the splenic vessels to drain into the **pancreaticosplenic lymph nodes**.

Nerve Supply of the Spleen (Fig. 2-111). The nerves to the spleen come from the **celiac plexus**. They are distributed mainly to the branches of the splenic artery and are vasomotor in function.

CLINICALLY ORIENTED COMMENTS

When the spleen is diseased it may be 10 or more times its normal size (**splenomegaly**). *Any degree of splenic enlargement is abnormal.* In some cases of splenomegaly, the spleen may fill the left half of the abdomen. *When a spleen is grossly enlarged it projects below the left costal margin.* Its notched superior border (Fig. 2-60) extends forward, downward, and medially so that it faces inferomedially. The notched border is very helpful when palpating an enlarged spleen because when the patient takes a

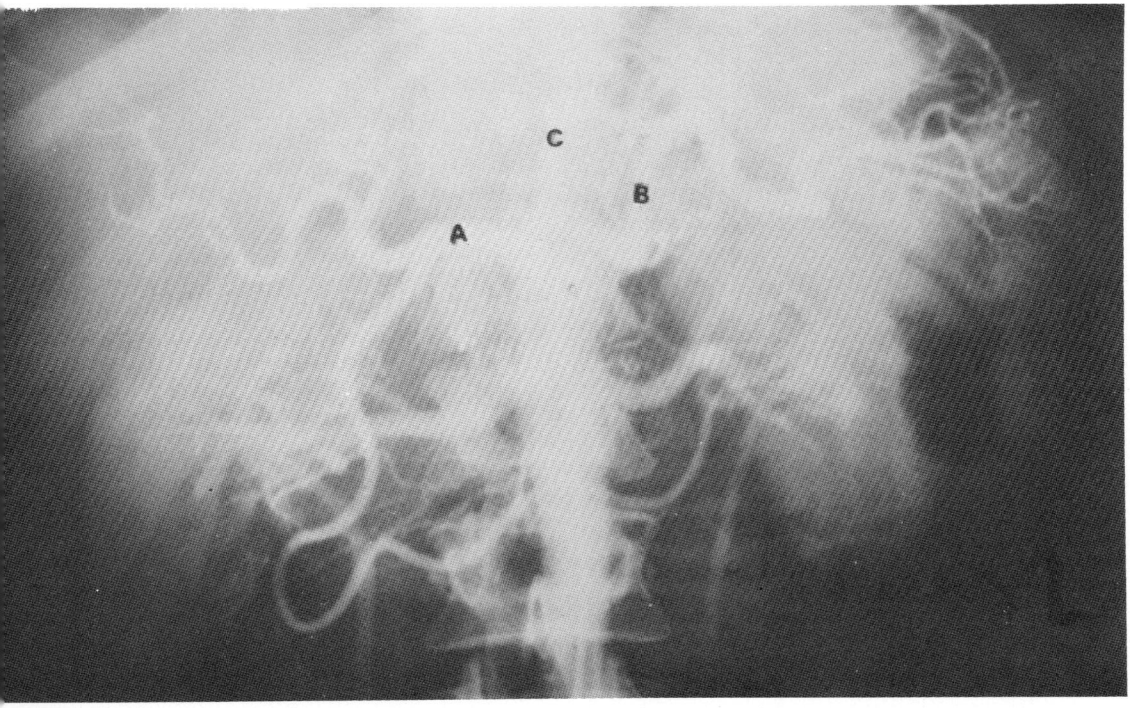

Figure 2-64. A celiac arteriogram. *A*, the common hepatic artery; its right gastroepiploic branch is well shown, following the greater curvature of the stomach; *B*, the tortuous splenic artery; and *C*, the left gastric artery. (If orientation is needed, see Figs. 2-54 and 2-56.) The spleen is barely visible in this radiograph. It may be opacified by superselective catheterization of the splenic artery; a contrast agent is injected and radiographs are taken in the arterial, capillary, and venous phases of circulation through the spleen.

deep breath you can feel this notched edge of the spleen as it moves downward and forward.

Certain conditions (trauma, tumors, and certain hematological diseases) require *removal of the spleen* (**splenectomy**). During this operation, there must be awareness of the intimate relationship of the tail of the pancreas to the hilum of the spleen (Fig. 2-71) to avoid injury to this important digestive gland.

Injuries to the left upper abdomen or left loin may injure the spleen and the structures related to it (*e.g.*, 9th, 10th, or 11th ribs, left diaphragm, and left kidney). Sometimes football players have their spleens ruptured when they are tackled from the left side. In some cases the spleen ruptures spontaneously in patients with infectious mononucleosis, malaria, and septicemia ("blood poisoning") because it is large and friable under these conditions.

Accessory spleens (one or more) occur most commonly near the hilum of the spleen (Fig. 2-63) or they may be embedded partly or wholly in the tail of the pancreas. They may also be found between the layers of the gastrolienal ligament. *Accessory spleens occur in about 10% of people* and usually are about 1 cm in diameter. Awareness of their possible presence is important because if not removed during splenectomy, they may result in persistence of the symptoms which indicated removal of the spleen (*e.g.*, **splenic anemia**).

The relationship of the costodiaphragmatic recess of the pleural cavity to the spleen is clinically important (Figs. 2-36 and 2-52). This *potential cleft* occurs at the level of the 10th rib in the midaxillary line and must be kept in mind when doing a **splenic needle biopsy** and when injecting a radiopaque material into the spleen for visualization of the portal vein (**splenoportography**). If not, the material may enter the pleural cavity.

The Duodenum (Figs. 2-33, 2-36, 2-37, 2-39, 2-40, 2-46, 2-49, 2-61, 2-62, and 2-65 to 2-75). The duodenum, **the first part of the small intestine**, joins the pylorus to the jejunum. It is the *shortest, widest, and most fixed part of the small intestine.* The duodenum forms a **U-shaped loop** (about 25 cm long) which is molded around the head of the pancreas. Its concavity faces upward and to the left. *The duodenum is particularly important because it receives the openings of the bile and pancreatic ducts* (Fig. 2-73). All but the first 2.5 cm of the duodenum lies behind the peritoneum (**retroperitoneal**) and the omental bursa (Fig. 2-46). The horizontal or third part of the duodenum lies astride the vertebral column, in front of the aorta and the inferior vena cava (Fig. 2-71).

For purposes of description, *the duodenum is divided into four parts* which are related to the vertebral column as follows (Figs. 2-68 and 2-71): superior or **first part**, anterolateral to the **body of L1**; descending or **second part**, to the right of the **bodies of L1, L2**, and **L3**; horizontal or **third part**, anterior to **L3**; and ascending or **fourth part**, to the left of the **body of L3** rising as high as L2. Hence, the superior and ascending parts are only about 5 cm apart.

The Superior (First) Part of the Duodenum (Figs. 2-33, 2-35, 2-36, 2-65 to 2-69, and 2-71). The **superior part**, only 2.5 to 3 cm long, is the *most movable of the four parts of the duodenum.* It begins at the pylorus and passes upward, posteriorly, and to the right toward the neck of the gallbladder. In right anterior oblique radiographs, the superior part of the duodenum appears much shorter because of its oblique direction (Fig. 2-35). Radiologists refer to the *beginning* of the first part of the duodenum as the **duodenal cap** or bulb; the term recommended by the Nomina Anatomica for this part is **duodenal ampulla**. *The proximal half of the superior part of the duodenum has a mesentery.* The greater omentum and the hepatoduodenal ligament of the lesser omentum are attached to this part; hence, it is free to move with the stomach. For this reason, *the beginning of the first part of the duodenum (duodenal cap) is often called the free part.* The distal half of the superior part of the duodenum has no mesentery and so is not freely movable. It is attached to the posterior abdominal wall.

The relations of the superior part of the duodenum are: *anteriorly*, peritoneum, gallbladder, and quadrate lobe of liver (Figs. 2-36, 2-46, 2-67, and 2-69); *posteriorly*, bile duct, portal vein, inferior vena cava, and gastroduodenal artery (Figs. 2-37, 2-62, and 2-66); *superiorly*, neck of gallbalder (Figs. 2-36, 2-67, and 2-69); and *inferiorly*, pancreas (Figs. 2-33, 2-65 and 2-69*A*). Because of its close relationship to the gallbladder, the anterior surface of the superior part of the duodenum is commonly stained with bile in the cadaver.

The Descending (Second) Part of the Duodenum (Figs. 2-33, 2-36, 2-37, 2-65 to 2-69, and 2-71). The **descending part is 8 to 10 cm long and has no mesentery**. It *descends retroperitoneally* along the right side of the first, second, and third lumbar vertebrae (Fig. 2-71). In its descent, it passes parallel to the inferior vena cava and to the right of it and lies directly on the medial part of the right kidney (Fig. 2-69*A*).

The principal relations of the descending part of the duodenum are: *anteriorly*, transverse colon, transverse mesocolon, and some coils of small intestine (Figs. 2-40, 2-52, and 2-69); *posteriorly*, hilum of right kidney, renal vessels, ureter, and psoas major muscle (Figs. 2-66 and 2-69*B*); and *medially*, head of pancreas, pancreatic duct, and bile duct.

The **bile duct** and the **main pancreatic duct** enter the posteromedial wall of the duodenum about two-thirds of the way along its length (Fig. 2-73). These two ducts enter the wall obliquely and usually unite to form a short dilated tube known as the **hepatopancreatic ampulla**. This ampulla opens on the summit of the **major duodenal papilla** (Fig. 2-74), located 8 to 10 cm distal to the pylorus (Fig. 2-73). The opening of the major duodenal papilla is guarded by the **sphincter of the hepatopancreatic ampulla**. It encloses and is capable of constricting the ampulla, thereby controlling the discharge of bile and pancreatic secretions into the duodenum. In some cases the bile and pancreatic ducts do not join but open separately on the major duodenal papilla (Fig. 2-74).

The Horizontal (Third) Part of the Duodenum (Figs. 2-33, 2-40, 2-65 to 2-69, and 2-71). The **horizontal part** of the duodenum, about 10 cm long, runs horizontally from right to left across the third lumbar vertebra (Fig. 2-71). *It is adherent to the posterior abdominal wall and is retroperitoneal.*

The principal relations of the horizontal part of the duodenum are: *anteriorly*, superior mesenteric artery and coils of small intestine and their mesentery (Figs. 2-67 and 2-107); *posteriorly*, right psoas major muscle, inferior vena cava, aorta, and right ureter (Fig. 2-69*B*); and *superiorly*, pancreas and superior mesenteric vessels (Figs. 2-67 and 2-71).

The Ascending (Fourth) Part of the Duodenum (Figs. 2-33, 2-40, and 2-65 to 2-71). The **ascending part** of the duodenum is usually short (about 2.5 cm) and ascends to the left of the aorta to the level of the second lumbar vertebra (Fig. 2-71). Here it bends abruptly forward to become continuous with the jejunum at the **duodenojejunal junction** (Figs. 2-40 and 2-70). *The distal end of the duodenum is covered with peritoneum and is movable*; however most of the ascending part of the duodenum is retroperitoneal.

The duodenojejunal flexure is supported by a fibromuscular band called the **suspensory muscle of the duodenum** (ligament of Treitz). The upper part of this slender muscle contains striated muscle, its intermediate part consists of elastic tissue, and its lower part contains smooth muscle. It passes from the superior surface of the ascending (third) part of the duodenum and the duodenojejunal flexure to the right crus of the diaphragm, close to the esophageal opening. *The suspensory muscle of the duodenum supports the duodenojejunal flexure and aids in its fixation* (*i.e.*, it tethers it in place).

The principal **relations of the ascending part of the duodenum** are: *anteriorly*, beginning of root of the mesentery and coils of jejunum (Figs. 2-40 and 2-69*A*); *posteriorly*, left psoas major muscle and left margin of aorta (Figs. 2-40 and 2-69*B*); and *medially*, head of pancreas.

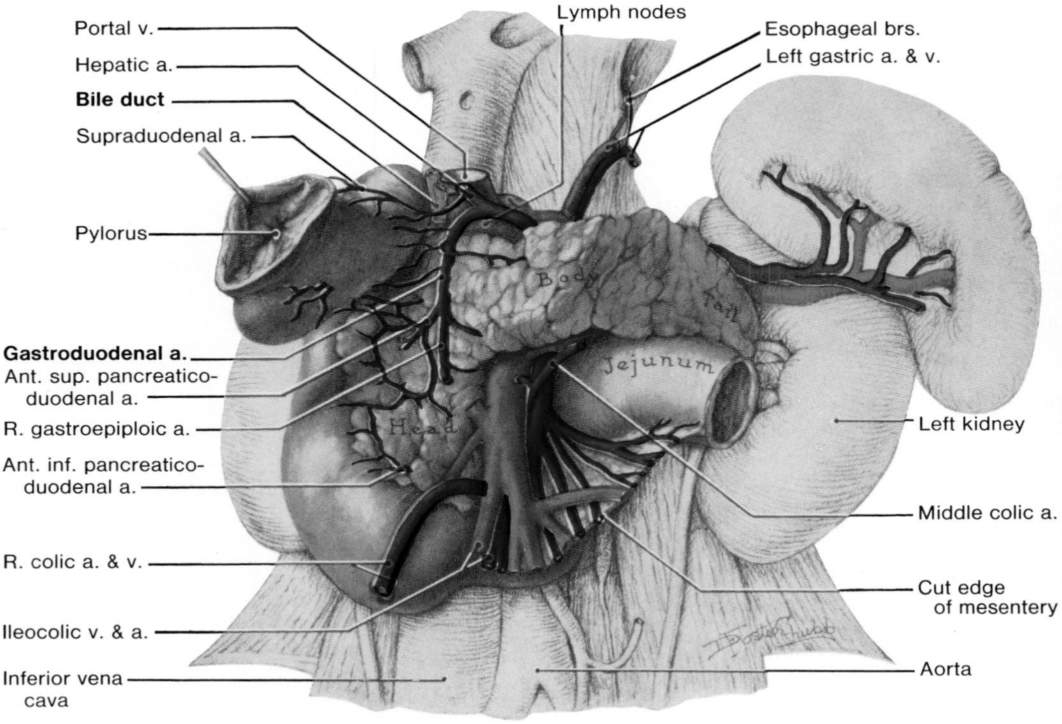

Figure 2-65. Drawing of an *anterior view* of a dissection of the duodenum and pancreas in situ. Observe that the duodenum is molded around the head of the pancreas. Its first or superior part (retracted) is overlapping the pancreas and passing backward, upward, and to the right. Its remaining parts (second to fourth) are overlapped by the pancreas. Note that near the junction of its third and fourth parts, the duodenum is crossed by the superior mesenteric vessels. Observe the pancreas, here very short; usually it touches the spleen and is blunt. Note that it is arched forward because it crosses the vertebral column and the aorta.

CLINICALLY ORIENTED COMMENTS

In **duodenal ulcer**, *one type of peptic ulcer* (see discussion of Case 2-1), the mucosa is eroded to form a crater-like depression that penetrates the duodenal wall to various depths. For a description of the signs and symptoms of a peptic ulcer, consult the history of the patient described in Case 2-1 and Figure 2-148.

Duodenal ulcers are commonly located in the duodenal ampulla or cap (Fig. 2-35), within 5 cm of the pylorus. In some cases the ulcer perforates and gives rise to a local or generalized **peritonitis** (Case 2-1). Fluid from a perforated duodenal ulcer has a tendency to run down the right paracolic gutter to the right iliac fossa (Figs. 2-32 and 2-110). The signs produced in such a patient may somewhat resemble those of a perforated vermiform appendix.

As *the superior part of the duodenum is close to the liver and the gallbladder*, either of them may become adherent to or be ulcerated by a duodenal ulcer. The proximity of the duodenum to the gallbladder also explains the frequency with which adhesions are found in persons who have had attacks of **cholecystitis** (inflammation of the gallbladder, Case 2-7). This close relationship also explains how a gallstone may ulcerate from the fundus of the gallbladder into the duodenum (Fig. 2-67).

Because of the intimate relationship of the pancreas to the duodenum, it may be invaded by a posterior duodenal ulcer. **Ero-**

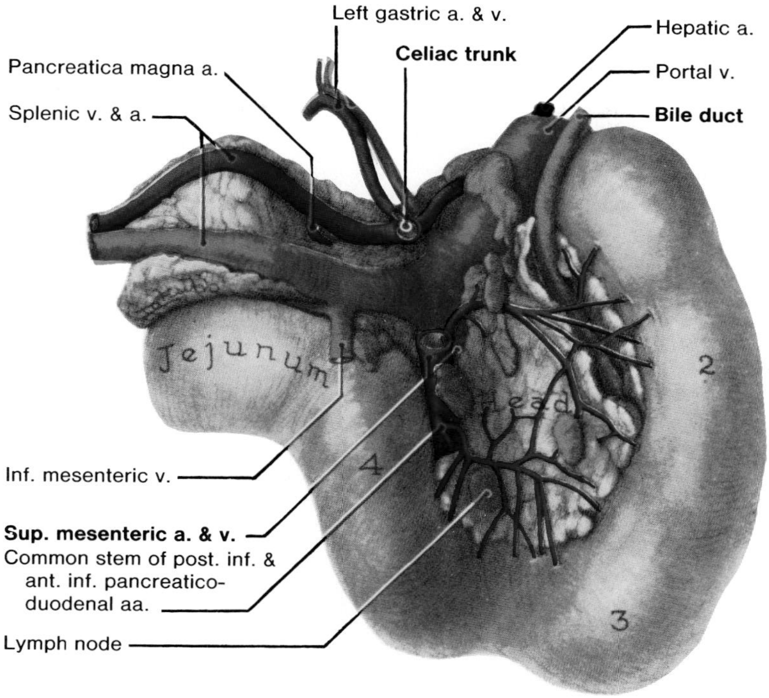

Figure 2-66. Drawing of a *posterior view* of the duodenum, pancreas, and bile duct. This is the reverse of the specimen shown in Figure 2-65. Observe that only the end of the superior (first) part of the duodenum is in view and that the bile duct is descending in a long fissure (opened up) in the posterior part of the head of the pancreas.

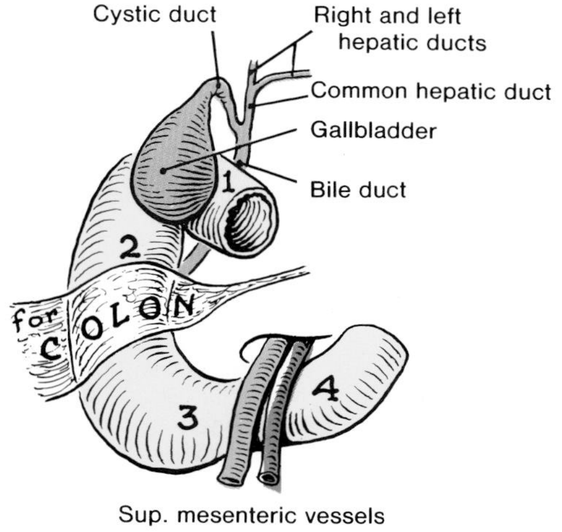

Figure 2-67. Drawing showing the three notable structures that are related anteriorly to the duodenum. The pear-shaped gallbladder is suspended by the cystic duct so that its blind lower end or fundus is its most inferior part.

sion of the gastroduodenal artery, a posterior relation of the superior part of the duodenum (Fig. 2-62), results in **severe hemorrhage**.

During the early fetal period, the duodenum has a mesentery, but it becomes fused to posterior abdominal wall structures owing to pressure of the overlying transverse colon. Because this is a secondary attachment, the duodenum and the closely associated pancreas may be separated from the underlying retroperitoneal viscera (Figs. 2-90 and 2-91) during operations involving the duodenum (*e.g.*, **partial gastrectomy**) without endangering the blood supply of the kidney or the ureter (Fig. 2-124).

Peritoneal Relations and Peritoneal Recesses of the Duodenum (Figs. 2-36, 2-37, 2-

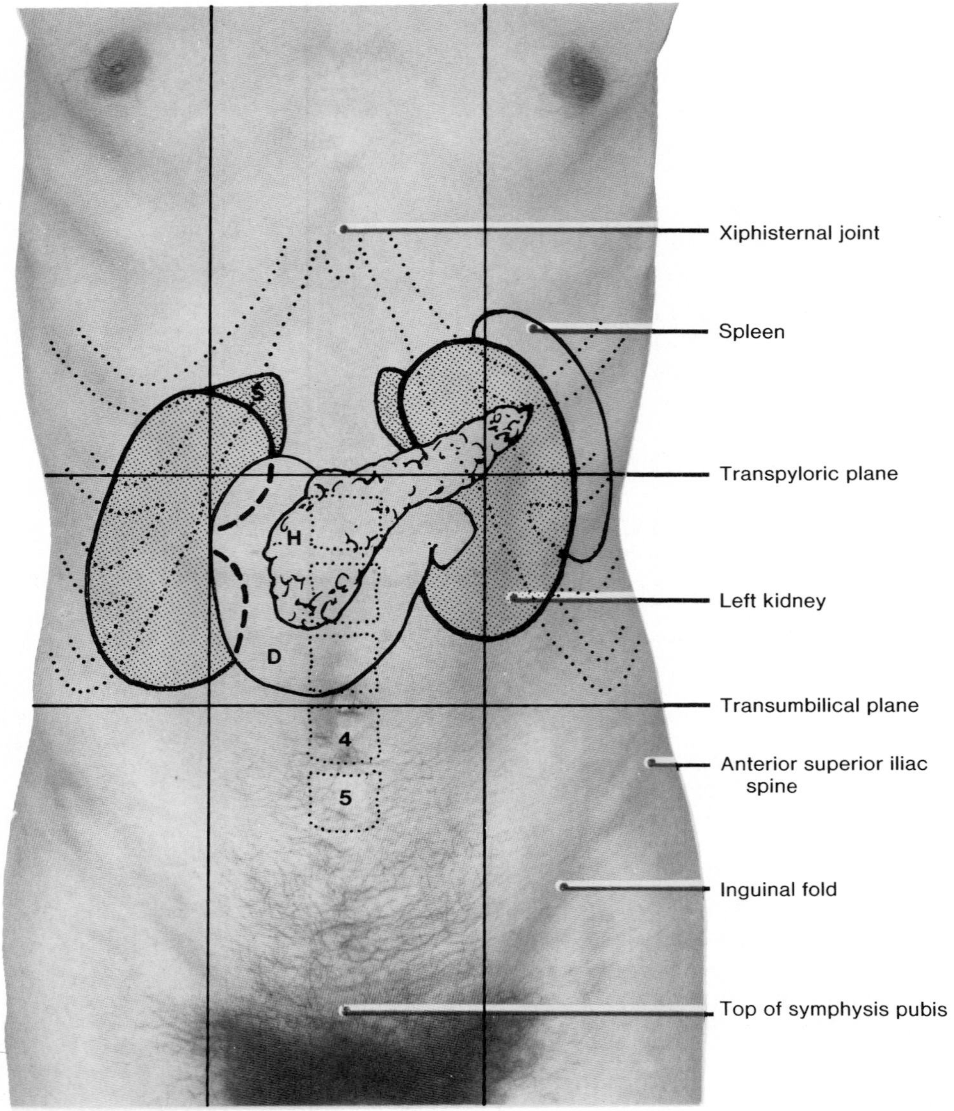

Figure 2-68. Photograph of the abdomen of a 27-year-old man showing the surface projection of the duodenum (*D*), pancreas, kidneys, spleen, and suprarenal glands (*S*). The lower ribs and their costal cartilages and the lumbar vertebrae are also indicated. The right and left vertical planes are erected on the midpoint of the line joining the corresponding anterior superior iliac spine to the top of the symphysis pubis. The transpyloric plane is approximately midway between the xiphisternal joint and the umbilicus. Note that the U-shaped duodenum (*D*) enclosing the head (*H*) of the pancreas, lies entirely above the level of the umbilicus and that its two ends are not very far apart (usually about 2.5 cm).

69, and 2-70). As described previously, the superior part of the duodenum is attached to the liver by the **hepatoduodenal ligament** (part of the lesser omentum). The beginning of this first part is covered by peritoneum in front and behind; thus it is very mobile. The rest of the superior part and all other parts of the duodenum are retroperitoneal, and the posterior aspect of the duodenum is attached to the posterior abdominal wall and to adjacent organs.

Several **accessory peritoneal folds** and

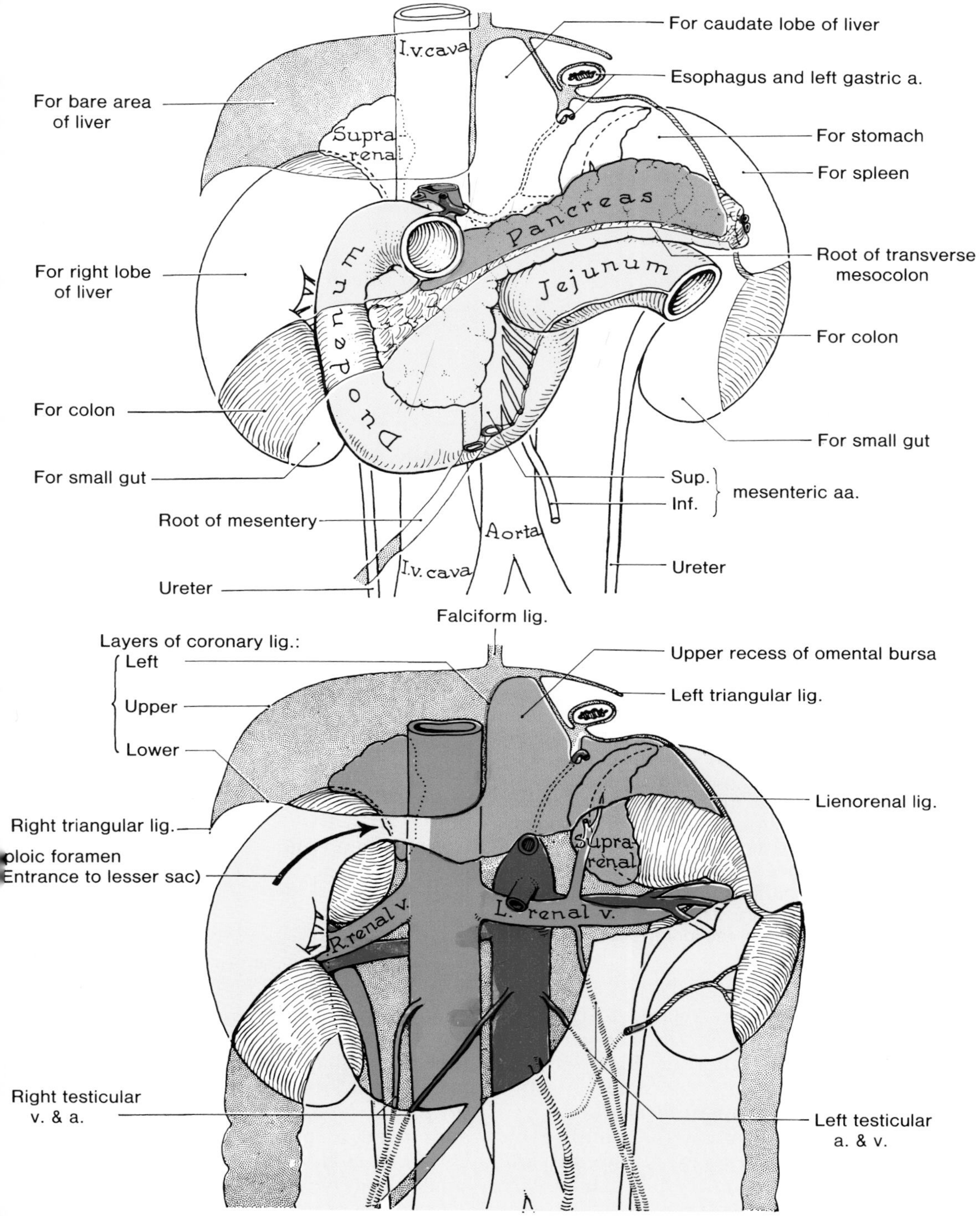

Figure 2-69. Drawings of dissections of the posterior abdominal viscera and their relations. *A*, duodenum and pancreas in situ. *B*, duodenum and pancreas removed. Observe the peritoneal covering (*yellow*) of the pancreas and the duodenum. Examine the colic area of the right kidney, the descending or second part of the duodenum, and the head of the pancreas. Note the line of attachment of the transverse mesocolon to the body and tail of the pancreas and to the colic area of the left kidney. Observe the anterior relations of the kidneys and the suprarenal glands. Note that the right suprarenal gland is at the epiploic foramen. Observe that the three parts of the coronary ligaments are attached to the diaphragm, except where the inferior vena cava, the suprarenal gland, and the kidney intervene.

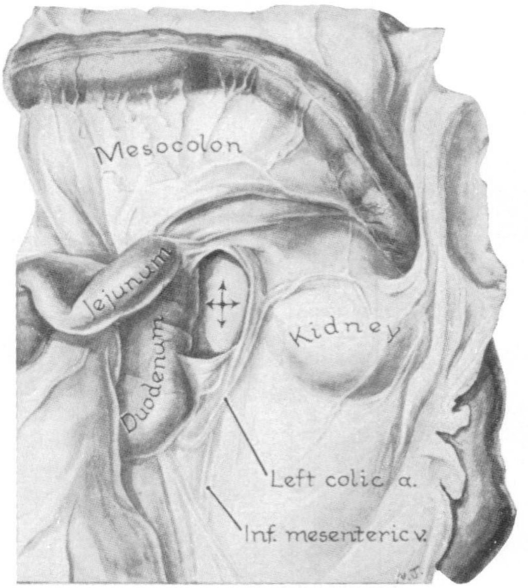

Figure 2-70. Drawing of a dissection of the duodenal folds and recesses (*arrows*). Note their relationship to the duodenojejunal flexure and the *left* kidney. The transverse colon and mesocolon have been reflected upward. The paraduodenal recess (*left arrow*) is located medial to and behind the inferior mesenteric vein, between it and the ascending (fourth) part of the duodenum. Observe the superior duodenal recess (*upper arrow*), guarded by the superior duodenal fold; the inferior duodenal recess (*lower arrow*), guarded by the inferior duodenal fold; and the retroduodenal recess (*right arrow*). The inferior duodenal fold is bloodless, but the superior duodenal fold often contains the inferior mesenteric vein. The paraduodenal fold contains the inferior mesenteric vein and the upper left colic artery.

recesses (fossae) are related to the duodenum, particularly in the region of the **duodenojejunal junction** (Figs. 2-40 and 2-70). This is where the small intestine changes from a retroperitoneal (duodenum) to a peritoneal position (jejunum). From this junction, a **superior duodenal fold** passes upward and to the left. Under it, in about 30% of people, there is a **superior duodenal recess** which opens downward. There is also an **inferior duodenal fold** that extends to the left from the distal part of the duodenum. This fold covers an inferior duodenal recess in about 50% of people and opens upward (Fig. 2-70). Frequently the terminal part of the ascending part of the duodenum is covered with peritoneum on its posterior surface. In these cases there is a **retroduodenal recess** between the superior and inferior duodenal recesses. Ocassionally a **paraduodenal fold** is raised by the inferior mesenteric vein and a **paraduodenal recess** may be present behind it, particularly in infants. It is on the left side of the duodenojejunal junction and opens to the right. All the duodenal recesses may unite with each other to form one sac of peritoneum.

CLINICALLY ORIENTED COMMENTS

The pocket-like duodenal recesses are of surgical importance because they may become sites of intraperitoneal or **internal hernias**. A loop or a large amount of small intestine may enter a recess and become constricted (strangulated) by the peritoneal fold at the entrance to the recess. The common type of this *very rare internal hernia* is into the paraduodenal fossa and is called a **paraduodenal hernia**. As the periteoneal fold guarding the recess usually has to be cut to relieve the stangulation and to remove the herniated bowel, it is important to know that *the paraduodenal fold is vascularized,* and contains the inferior mesenteric vein and the upper left colic artery.

Arterial Supply of the Duodenum (Figs. 2-54, 2-56, 2-61, 2-62, 2-65, and 2-66). The duodenum is derived from the foregut and the midgut; thus it is supplied by the **foregut** (celiac) and the **midgut** (superior mesenteric) arteries. *The main blood supply to the duodenum* is from the **superior** and **inferior pancreaticoduodenal arteries**, branches of the gastroduodenal and superior mesenteric arteries, respectively. The *proximal half* of the duodenum is supplied by the **superior pancreaticoduodenal artery** and the *distal half* is supplied by the **inferior pancreaticoduodenal artery**. These anastomose to form anterior and posterior arterial arcades (L. *arcus,* arc, bow) which lie in the angle between the duodenum and the pancreas (Fig.

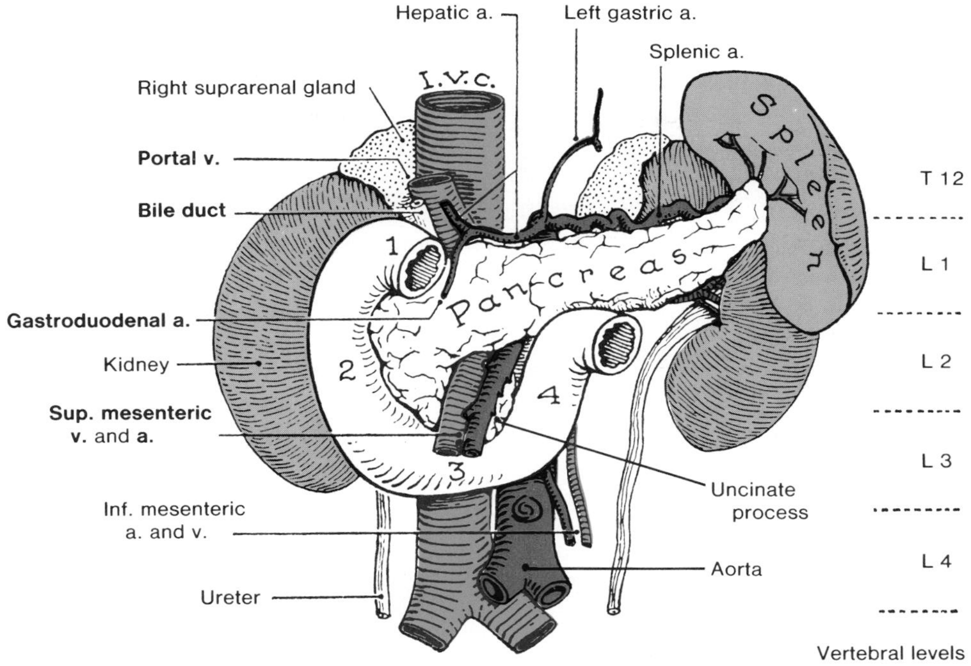

Figure 2-71. Drawing of an anterior view of a dissection of the abdominal viscera and vessels. Note that the pancreas resembles the letter J set obliquely and that the uncinate process of the head of the pancreas projects medially behind the superior mesenteric vessels. For a view of the posterior relations of the pancreas and duodenum, see Figure 2-67*B*.

2-65). The superior part of the duodenum may, in addition, receive blood from (1) the **supraduodenal artery**, a branch of the hepatic artery proper, (2) the **right gastric**, (3) the **right gastroepiploic**, and (4) the **gastroduodenal** (retroduodenal) arteries. These vessels often anastomose with each other.

Venous Drainage of the Duodenum (Figs. 2-65, 2-66, 2-85, and 2-91). In general, the veins of the duodenum follow the arteries and drain into the **portal venous system**. *Most veins drain into the superior mesenteric vein,* but some enter the portal vein directly. There are numerous small veins on the anterior and posterior surfaces of the superior part of the duodenum, some of which drain into the superior pancreaticoduodenal veins. One of the anterior veins, called the **prepyloric vein** (of Mayo), drains into the right gastric vein and is clinically important because it is used by surgeons as a guide to the gastroduodenal junction.

Lymphatic Drainage of the Duodenum (Figs. 2-58, 2-65, and 2-66). The **lymph vessels** on the anterior and posterior surfaces of the duodenum anastomose freely with each other within the duodenum. *The anterior efferent vessels follow the arteries and drain upward* via pancreaticoduodenal lymph nodes to gastroduodenal lymph nodes and finally to the **celiac lymph nodes**. *The posterior efferent vessels pass behind the head of the pancreas and drain downward* into the **superior mesenteric lymph nodes** (Fig. 2-109), located around the origin of the superior mesenteric artery.

Nerves of the Duodenum (Figs. 2-59 and 2-111). The **sympathetic** and **parasympathetic nerves** are derived from the **celiac** and **superior mesenteric plexuses** located on the arteries with corresponding names.

The Pancreas (Figs. 2-33, 2-38, 2-46, 2-47, 2-52, 2-58, 2-65, 2-66, and 2-71). The pancreas (G. all flesh) is an unpaired diges-

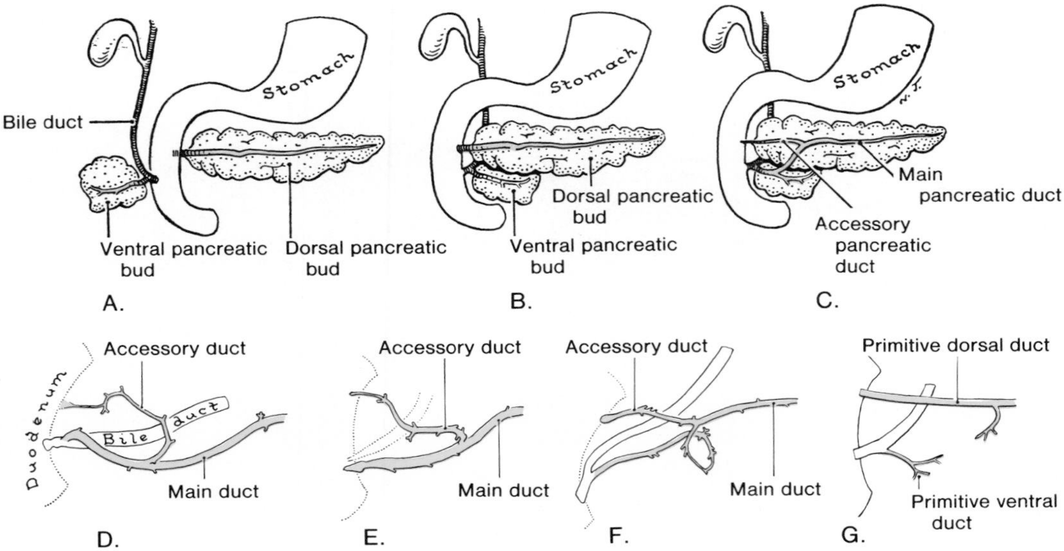

Figure 2-72. Drawings illustrating development of the pancreas and the embryological basis of the variability in the anatomy of the pancreatic ducts. *A*, the smaller ventral pancreatic bud arises in common with the bile duct and the larger dorsal pancreatic bud arises independently from the duodenum, cranial to the ventral bud. *B*, the descending part of the duodenum rotates on its long axis which brings the ventral pancreatic bud and the bile duct behind the dorsal pancreatic bud. *C*, a connecting segment unites the dorsal duct to the ventral duct, whereupon the duodenal end of the dorsal duct tends to atrophy and the direction of flow within it is reversed. *D*, in about 44% of people the accessory pancreatic duct loses its connection with the duodenum. *E*, in about 10% of people the accessory pancreatic duct opens into the duodenum and is large enough to relieve an obstructed main pancreatic duct (see clinically oriented comments on the pancreas). *F*, in about 20% of people the accessory duct is small and might substitute for the main duct. *G*, in about 9% of people the main duct (primitive dorsal duct) has no connection with the duct draining the head.

tive gland which produces (1) an external secretion (**pancreatic juice**) that enters the duodenum via the pancreatic duct and (2) internal secretions (**glucagon** and **insulin**) that enter the blood. Some laymen refer to the pancreas as the stomach or abdominal sweetbread.

The pancreas is located in the epigastric and left hypochondriac regions (Fig. 2-68). It lies across the bodies of the upper lumbar vertebrae (Fig. 2-71), with its right side (head) mostly below the transpyloric plane and its left side (tail) slightly above this plane (Fig. 2-68). The pancreas lies posterior to the omental bursa, where it *forms a major portion of the stomach bed* (Figs. 2-46 and 2-52). In living persons the pancreas is a long (12 to 15 cm), soft, lobulated, fleshy (hence its name), greyish-pink or yellowish gland. For descriptive purposes, it is divided into **four parts**: a *head*, a *neck*, a *body*, and a *tail* (Fig. 2.33*B*).

The head of the pancreas is located within the curve of the duodenum. It has a prolongation, called the **uncinate process** (L. hook-shaped), which projects upward and to the left. *The head of the pancreas rests posteriorly on the inferior vena cava, the right renal vessels, and the left renal vein* (Figs. 2-69*B* and 2-71). The hook-shaped uncinate process projects medially behind the superior mesenteric vessels and rests against the aorta posteriorly (Fig. 2-71). The **bile duct** lies in a groove on the upper posterior surface of the head of the pancreas (Fig. 2-66) and sometimes is embedded in it. The posterior surface of the head is also related to the *right crus of the diaphragm* (Fig. 2–130).

The neck of the pancreas (Fig. 2-33*B*)

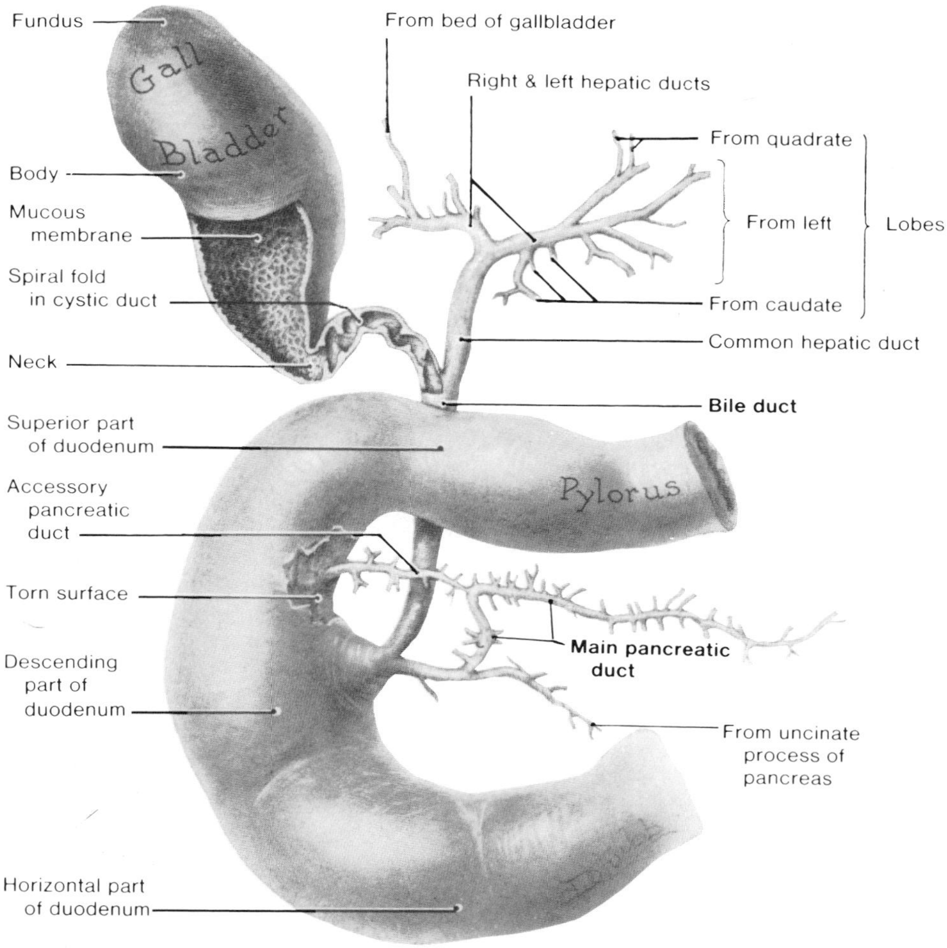

Figure 2-73. Drawing of an anterior view of a dissection of the extrahepatic bile passages and the pancreatic ducts. The right hepatic duct collects from the right lobe of the liver and the left hepatic duct collects from the left, quadrate, and caudate lobes. The common hepatic duct unites with the cystic duct to form the bile duct. Observe that the mucous membrane of the gallbladder has a honeycomb surface. Note that the cystic duct is sinuous and that its mucous membrane forms a spiral fold (spiral valve). Note that the bile duct, after descending behind the superior (first) part of the duodenum and the accessory pancreatic duct, is joined by the main pancreatic duct; these open on the major duodenal papilla (Fig. 2-74). Observe that the main pancreatic duct with its tributaries resembles a herring bone, and that the common hepatic duct with its tributaries resembles a deciduous tree. Note that the accessory pancreatic duct is joined to the main pancreatic duct, as it usually is (see Fig. 2-72*D* to *F*). Observe that the pancreas invades the duodenal wall around the accessory pancreatic duct, because when removed it lacerates the duodenum. In about 5% of people, the bile and main pancreatic ducts open separately on the major duodenal papilla (Fig. 2-74).

is continuous with the upper left portion of the head and *merges imperceptibly into the body*. It is the somewhat constricted segment, about 2 cm long, that is grooved posteriorly by the superior mesenteric vessels (Fig. 2-66). Its anterior surface is covered with peritoneum and is adjacent to the pylorus (Fig. 2-65). *The superior mesen-*

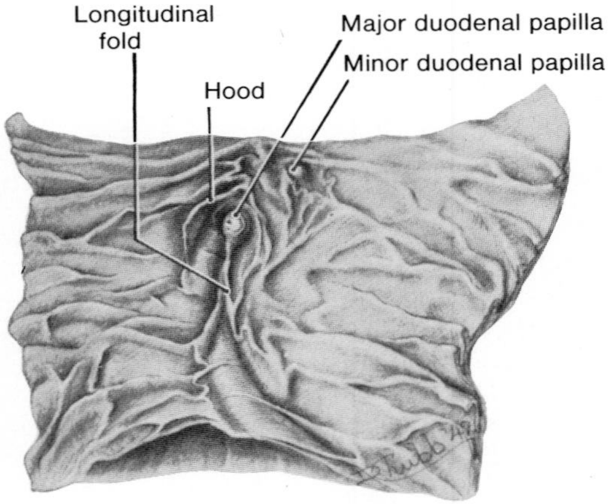

Figure 2-74. Drawing of the interior of the descending (second) part of the duodenum. Observe that the mucous membrane is thrown into circularly or spirally disposed folds called plica circulares; these begin about 2 cm from the pylorus. Observe that the major duodenal papilla (of Vater) projects into this part of the duodenum on the concave border, 8 to 10 cm from the pylorus. On its tip is the orifice of the bile duct and below it, the orifice of the main pancreatic duct, but usually these two ducts open together (Fig. 2-88). A hood is thrown over the major papilla and a longitudinal fold descends from it. Note that the minor duodenal papilla, into which the accessory pancreatic duct opens (Fig. 2-73), is about 2 cm anterosuperior to the major duodenal papilla.

teric vein is joined by the splenic vein behind the neck of the pancreas to form the portal vein (Figs. 2-57, 2-66, and 2-85).

The body of the pancreas extends upward and to the left across the aorta and the upper lumbar vertebrae, behind the omental bursa (Fig. 2-46). It is somewhat triangular in cross-section and has *three surfaces*: **anterior**, **posterior**, and **inferior**. *The anterior surface is covered with peritoneum* (Fig. 2-69*A*) and forms part of the bed of the stomach, where it provides attachment for the transverse mesocolon (Figs. 2-38, 2-52, and 2-69*A*). *The posterior surface is devoid of peritoneum (Fig. 2-69B)*, is in contact with the aorta, the superior mesenteric artery, the left suprarenal gland, the left kidney and its vessels, and is *intimately related to the splenic vein* (Fig. 2-66). The inferior border of the body separates the posterior surface from the **inferior surface**. The body has a small projection, the **omental tuber**, from its superior border which contacts the lesser omentum, immediately inferior to the celiac trunk.

The tail of the pancreas (Fig. 2-65) is thick, narrow, and blunt and passes within the two layers of the **lienorenal ligament** with the splenic vessels. Its tip usually comes into contact with the hilum of the spleen (Fig. 2-71).

Ducts of the Pancreas (Figs. 2-72 to 2-74). The pancreas develops from two outgrowths, called the **dorsal** and **ventral pancreatic buds**, which normally fuse in such a way that their ducts communicate. Usually the duct of the ventral pancreatic bud forms the duodenal end of the **main pancreatic duct** and the proximal part of the dorsal pancreatic duct forms the rest. Frequently the duodenal end of the dorsal pancreatic duct also persists and forms an accessory pancreatic duct.

The main pancreatic duct (Fig. 2-73) *begins in the tail of the pancreas* and runs through the substance of the gland near its posterior surface. When joined by the portion of the duct in the head and the uncinate process, the main duct becomes **Y-shaped**. The stem of the duct turns downward in the head and comes into *close relationship with the bile duct*, which lies to the right. The two ducts pierce the posteromedial wall of the descending (second) part of the duodenum obliquely near its middle. *Usually the pancreatic and bile ducts unite* to form a short dilated duct called the **hepatopancreatic ampulla** (ampulla of Vater), but in about 5% of people they open separately into the duodenum. The hepatopancreatic ampulla opens into the summit of the **major duodenal papilla** (Figs. 2-74 and 2-88).

The circular muscle around the lower part of the bile duct is thickened to form a **choledochal sphincter** (sphincter of the bile duct). There is a similar sphincter around the terminal part of the main pancreatic duct, called the **pancreatic duct sphincter**, and another around the hepatopancreatic ampulla called the **hepatopancreatic sphincter** (sphincter of Oddi).

The accessory pancreatic duct is quite variable (Fig. 2-72 *D* to *G*); it drains the upper part of the head and its lower ante-

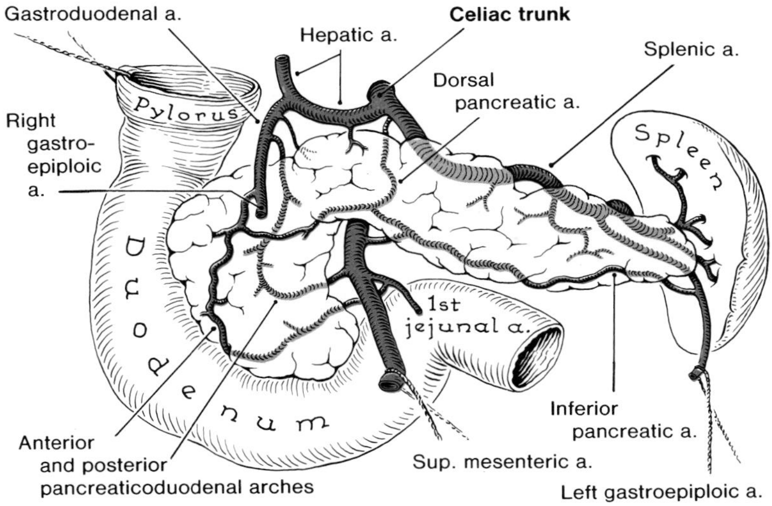

Figure 2-75. Diagram of the blood supply to the pancreas. The rich supply to this important gland is at the junction of the celiac trunk and the superior mesenteric artery (Fig. 2-55). Observe that the head and tail of the pancreas are supplied by several branches from the splenic artery and that the head is supplied by the anterior and posterior superior pancreaticoduodenal arteries from the gastroduodenal artery, and from the anterior and posterior inferior pancreaticoduodenal arteries from the superior mesenteric artery. Note the anastomoses between the branches of the superior and inferior pancreaticoduodenal arteries.

rior part. Usually it is connected to the main pancreatic duct, but in about 9% of people it is a completely separate duct (Fig. 2-72*G*) which opens into the duodenum at the summit of the **minor duodenal papilla** (Fig. 2-74). This papilla is about 2.5 cm above and anterior to the opening of the main pancreatic duct into the major duodenal papilla.

Vessels and Nerves of the Pancreas (Figs. 2-56, 2-58, 2-61, 2-62, 2-65, 2-66, and 2-75). *The arteries of the pancreas* are derived from the **splenic artery** and the **pancreaticoduodenal arteries**. Up to 10 small branches from the splenic artery supply the body and tail of the pancreas. The **superior pancreaticoduodenal artery** from the *gastroduodenal artery* and the **inferior gastroduodenal artery** from the *superior mesenteric artery* supply the head. The superior and inferior pancreaticoduodenal arteries anastomose with each other.

The veins of the pancreas open into the portal, splenic, and superior mesenteric veins, but most of the veins draining the pancreas empty into the **splenic vein**.

The lymph vessels of the pancreas (Figs. 2-58, 2-65, and 2-66) follow the course of the blood vessels to end in (1) the **pancreaticosplenic nodes** along the superior border of the pancreas, (2) the **pyloric nodes** to the right, and (3) the **lumbar** and **celiac nodes** around the superior mesenteric and celiac arteries. *Most lymph vessels from the spleen end in the pancreaticosplenic nodes* (Fig. 2-58).

The nerves of the pancreas are derived from the vagus and splanchnic (visceral) nerves. The sympathetic and parasympathetic nerve fibers reach the gland by passing along the arteries from the **celiac** and **superior mesenteric plexuses** (Fig. 2-111).

CLINICALLY ORIENTED COMMENTS

Because the main pancreatic duct usually joins the bile duct as it pierces the duodenal wall to form the short **hepatopancreatic ampulla**, *a gallstone passing down the extrahepatic bile passages* (Fig. 2-73) *may become lodged* in the constricted distal end of this ampulla, where it opens on the **ma-**

jor duodenal papilla (Fig. 2-88). In this case, both the biliary and the pancreatic duct systems are blocked. Neither bile nor pancreatic juice can enter the duodenum, but bile may back up and enter the pancreatic duct.

A similar reflux of bile may occur owing to **spasm of the hepatopancreatic sphincter**. Normally the pancreatic duct sphincter prevents the reflux of bile into the pancreatic duct; however, if their common duct (hepatopancreatic ampulla) is closed, the weak pancreatic duct sphincter may be unable to withstand the excessive pressure. *Reflux of bile into the pancreatic duct* is thought to be one cause of **pancreatitis** (inflammation of the pancreas). Swelling of the head of the pancreas occludes the main pancreatic duct and soon results in pancreatitis involving the body and tail of the pancreas.

If the accessory pancreatic duct connects with the main pancreatic duct (Fig. 2-72), and opens into the duodenum it may compensate for an obstructed main duct or spasm of the hepatopancreatic sphincter.

Pancreatic injury may occur whenever there is sudden forceful compression of the upper abdomen, as occurs in an auto accident when a person is thrown forward against the steering wheel. However, the pancreas is damaged in only 2 to 3% of all abdominal injuries. Because the pancreas lies transversely across the posterior abdominal wall, the vertebral column acts like an anvil and the traumatic force may rupture the pancreas. **Rupture of the pancreas** frequently tears the duct system, allowing pancreatic juice to enter the substance of the gland and the adjacent tissues (retroperitoneal and intraperitoneal). *Digestion of tissues by pancreatic juice is very serious* and *painful and may be fatal.*

Owing to the posterior relations of the head of the pancreas (Figs. 2-65 and 2-66), cysts or tumors of it may cause symptoms by pressing on the portal vein, the bile duct, or the inferior vena cava. Pressure on the portal vein may cause **ascites**, an accumulation of serous fluid in the peritoneal cavity. *Cancer of the head of the pancreas frequently results in obstruction of the bile duct and/or the hepatopancreatic ampulla*, resulting in the retention of bile pigments and staining of most tissues of the body. **Jaundice** (F. *jaune*, yellow) is the name given to the *yellow or bronze color of the skin*, the mucous membranes, and the conjunctiva that results. **Cancer of the body of the pancreas** is often not diagnosed until the tumor is large and has infiltrated the somatic nerves of the posterior abdominal wall (Fig. 2-122), producing mid-back pain. An extensive growth in the body of the pancreas may cause **inferior vena caval obstruction** (Fig. 2-71).

The neck of the pancreas is below and behind the pylorus (Fig. 2-65); hence, tumorous enlargement of this region may cause obstruction of the pylorus.

In rare cases, the two primordia of the pancreas (Fig. 2-72*A*) may completely surround the descending or second part of the duodenum, forming an **anular pancreas** (L. *anus*, ring). This may produce duodenal obstruction during the perinatal period or later if inflammation or malignant disease develops in this ring-like pancreas.

The Liver (Figs. 2-29, 2-33, 2-36 to 2-38, 2-46, 2-47, 2-51, 2-52, 2-57, 2-69, and 2-75 to 2-82). The liver (L. *hepar*) is a huge glandular organ belonging to the GI system. It is the *largest gland in the body*, accounting for about 2% of the body weight in an adult and 5% in a newborn infant. As it is relatively larger in young infants, it produces most of the prominence of their abdomens. In adults the liver still occupies much of the right upper quadrant of the abdomen.

The liver receives venous blood returning from the GI tract through the **portal vein** (Fig. 2-85) which is laden with the products of digestion. In addition to its many metabolic activities, *the liver is a storehouse for glycogen and secretes bile.* Bile is an important agent in digestion, especially of fats. **Liver bile** passes via the hepatic ducts and the cystic duct to the **gallbladder** (Fig. 2-83), where it is concentrated by absorption of water and inorganic salts and stored. When fat-containing **chyme** enters the duodenum from the stomach, a hormone (**cholecystokinin**) released by the upper GI tract stimulates contraction of the gallbladder, forcing con-

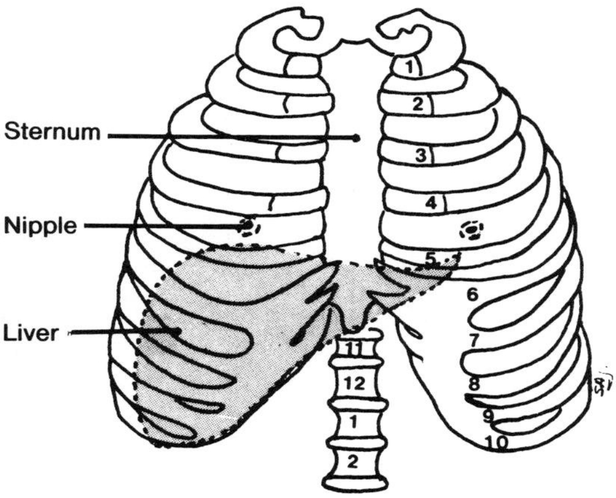

Figure 2-76. Drawing of the thoracic cage showing the location of the liver. Observe that the oblique inferior border of the liver extends from the tip of the right 10th costal cartilage across the tip of the xiphoid process to a point just below the left nipple. Note that it occupies almost the whole of the right hypochondrium, much of the epigastrium, and extends into the left hypochondrium. Although the inferior border of the liver may lie below the right costal margin, the normal liver is so soft that it is usually not easily palpable.

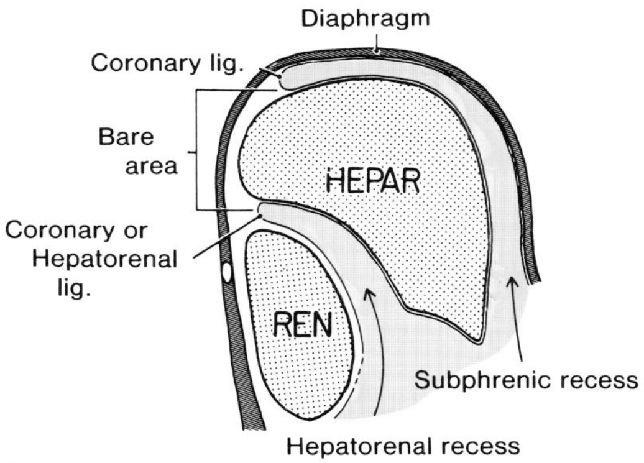

Figure 2-77. Diagram of a sagittal or paramedian section through the diaphragm, liver, and right kidney (L. *ren*) showing that the bare area of liver (L. *hepar*) is situated between the dorsal ends of two peritoneal recesses or pouches. Note that the diaphragmatic surface of the liver is dome-shaped and conforms to the concavity of the dome of the diaphragm.

centrated **gallbladder bile** into the duodenum along with some liver bile already in the bile duct. It is clinically important to distinguish between liver bile and the more concentrated gallbladder bile.

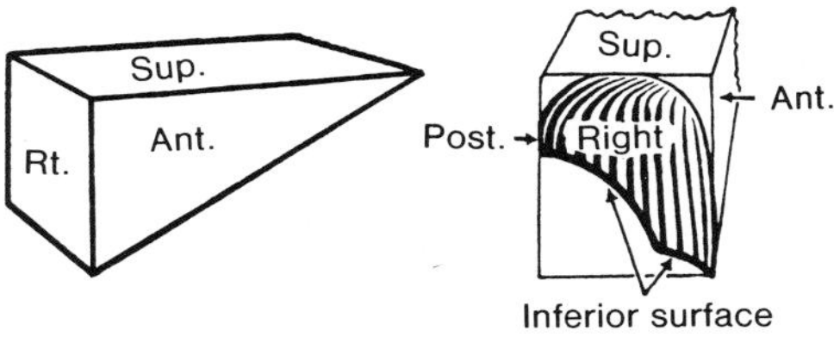

Figure 2-78. Diagram illustrating the general shape of the liver and its surfaces. When hardened by embalming, the inferior or visceral surface of the liver faces downward, to the left, and backward.

Surface Anatomy and Position of the Liver (Figs. 2-46, 2-47, 2-51, 2-52, 2-56, 2-59, 2-76 to 2-82, and 2-117). *In living persons the liver is a soft pliable organ* that is molded by the structures related to it. It conforms to the cavity of the right dome (cupola) of the diaphragm and *rises to its highest point behind the fifth rib,* just below the nipple. The liver is located in the upper and right parts of the abdominal cavity, occupying almost all of the *right hypochondrium* and much of the *epigastrium* and extending into *the left hypochondrium.* It is somewhat triangular in shape with its base at the right and its apex toward the left.

The liver moves with respiration because it is connected to the diaphragm; it also *shifts its position with any postural change that affects the diaphragm.* In addition, its position varies according to a person's body type (described below). In nearly all people, *the major part of the liver lies on the right side under cover of ribs 5 to 10* (Fig. 2-76) and the diaphragm (Figs. 2-29 and 2-117). It extends above the level of the inferior border of the lung on the right side. During infancy and childhood, and in some adults, the liver extends slightly below the costal margin. *In thin people with narrow chests, most of the liver lies to the right* of the midline and its lower right corner may reach the iliac crest. *In plump people with broad chests, the liver extends much more to the left* of the median plane and the slope of its inferior border is much less.

Surfaces and Borders of the Liver (Figs. 2-77 to 2-80). The liver has *two surfaces,* **diaphragmatic** and **visceral**, but the extensive diaphragmatic surface may be subdivided into superior, anterior, right, and

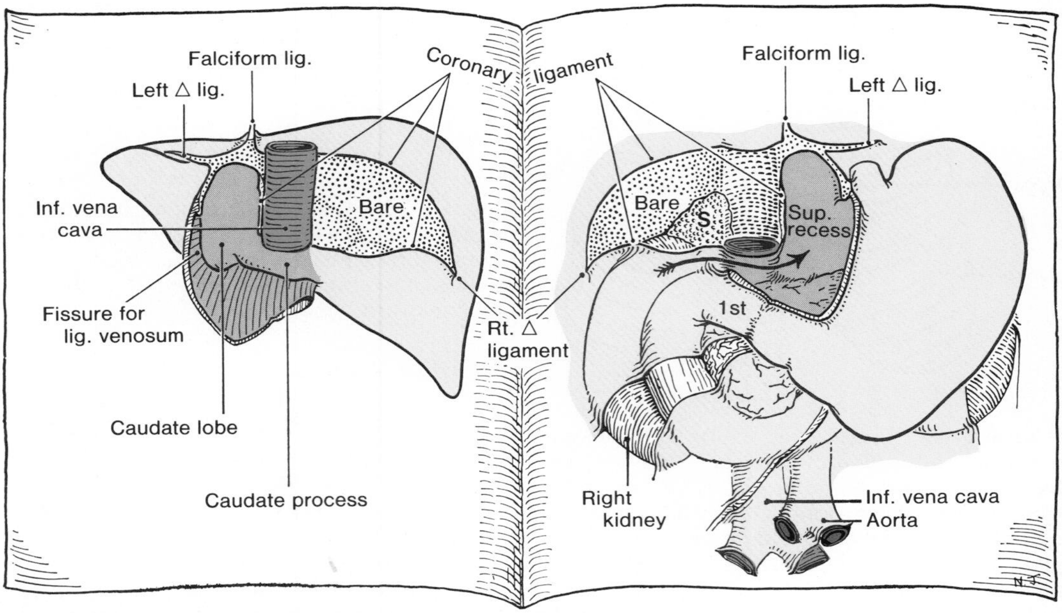

Figure 2-79. Diagram illustrating the peritoneal ligaments of the liver. The attachments of the liver are cut through and the liver is turned to the right side of the cadaver, as you would turn the page of a book. Hence, the posterior aspect of the liver is shown on the left and its posterior relations on the right. On the right diagram, observe the *arrow* passing from the greater sac of peritoneum (*yellow*) into the upper recess of the lesser sac of peritoneum or omental bursa (*orange*). Note that most of the upper or superior recess of the omental bursa lies to the left of the median plane of the body. Observe that the descending thoracic aorta lies dorsal to the liver and the superior recess. Note that the inferior vena cava occupies the left or medial limit of the *bare area* of the liver. Observe that the bare area is triangular; hence the so-called coronary ligament surrounding it is not a crown (L. *corona*) but is three-sided. Its left side or base is between the inferior vena cava and the caudate lobe of the liver and can be palpated when the right index finger is inserted into the superior recess. Its apex is at the right triangular ligament, where the cranial and caudal layers of the coronary ligament meet. The lower or caudal layer of the coronary ligament is reflected from the liver onto the diaphragm, the right kidney, and the right suprarenal gland(*S*). It is often called the hepatorenal ligament. Followed medially, this layer crosses the inferior vena cava at the epiploic foramen and turning cranially becomes the left or basal layer of the ligament.

posterior parts. The diaphragmatic and visceral surfaces are separated from each other by the **sharp inferior border**, except posteriorly.

The diaphragmatic surface of the liver is smooth and dome-shaped because it *conforms to the concavity of the inferior surface of the diaphragm* (Figs. 2-29, 2-36, and 2-77). Its superior, anterior, right, and posterior parts combine to form a curved surface that is applied to the diaphragm. The **superior part** is under the dome of the diaphragm and is adapted to its curvature. The diaphragm separates this part of the liver from the structures in the thorax (lungs, pleura, heart, and pericardium). The superior part is covered wih peritoneum, except posteriorly at the edge of the bare area (Figs. 2-77 and 2-79). The **anterior part** is somewhat triangular and is in contact with the diaphgram, the costal margin, the xiphoid process, and the anterior abdominal wall. The large **posterior** and **right parts** of the diaphragmatic surface are in contact with the diaphragm and the lower ribs. The posterior part includes most of the bare area that is between the reflections of the **coronary ligament** (Figs. 2-77 and 2-79). *In the bare area, the naked liver is in contact with the diaphragm* and the

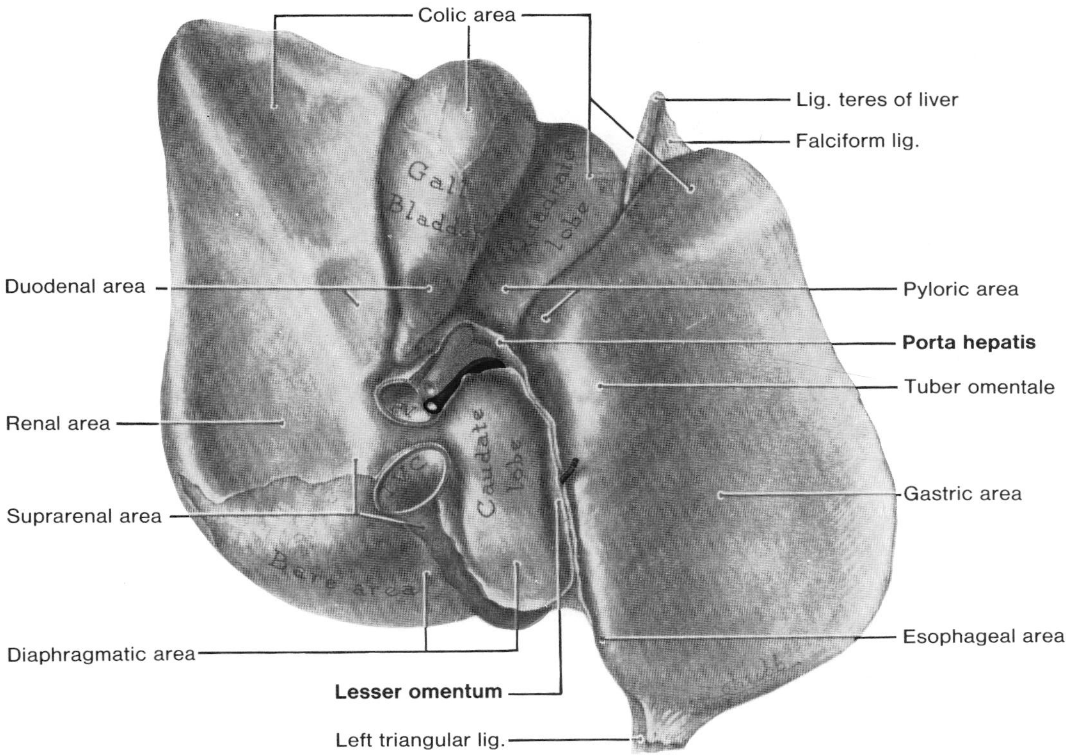

Figure 2-80. Drawing of a dissection of the inferior and posterior surfaces of the liver. To get this view, stand on the right side of a cadaver and face the head; divide the attachments of the liver and raise its sharp inferior border. Observe the visceral areas: (1) for the esophagus, stomach, pylorus, and duodenum; (2) for the transverse colon; and (3) for the right kidney and the right suprarenal gland. The gallbladder rests on the transverse colon and on the duodenum (see Fig. 2-36). Examine the posterior surface comprising (1) the bare area occupied on its left by the inferior vena cava, (2) the caudate lobe, and (3) the groove for the esophagus. Note that the caudate lobe is separated from the quadrate lobe by the porta of the liver and is joined to the right lobe by the caudate process (not labelled), which is squeezed between the inferior vena cava and the portal vein. Examine the cut edge of the peritoneum. At the right end of the bare area, the right triangular ligament (not labelled) bifurcates into the upper and lower layers of the coronary ligament. The lower layer crosses the renal and suprarenal areas and, after passing in front of the inferior vena cava, turns cranially as the left layer or base of the coronary ligament. Followed to the left, this layer of peritoneum forms the upper limit of the upper or superior recess and then turns caudally as the posterior layer of the lesser omentum. This omentum is attached to the fissure for the ligamentum venosum and to the porta hepatis. This specimen contains an accessory hepatic artery, a branch of the left gastric artery.

inferior vena cava occupies a sulcus in the left part of the **bare area** (Figs. 2-79 to 2-81), just to the right of the median plane.

The visceral surface of the liver (Figs. 2-80 to 2-83) is directed downward, backward, and to the left. It is separated from the diaphragmatic surface of the liver by the **inferior border**. *Under cover of this surface are*: (1) the upper right portion of the anterior surface of the **stomach**; (2) the superior (first) part of the **duodenum**; (3) the **lesser omentum** (Figs. 2-36 to 2-38); (4) the **gallbladder**; (5) the **right colic flexure**; and (6) many associated **vessels** and **nerves**. The visceral surface is covered with peritoneum, except at the gallbladder and the porta hepatis (Fig. 2-80).

There are many irregularities on the inferior surface. It contains an **H-shaped group of deep fissures and wide sulci**

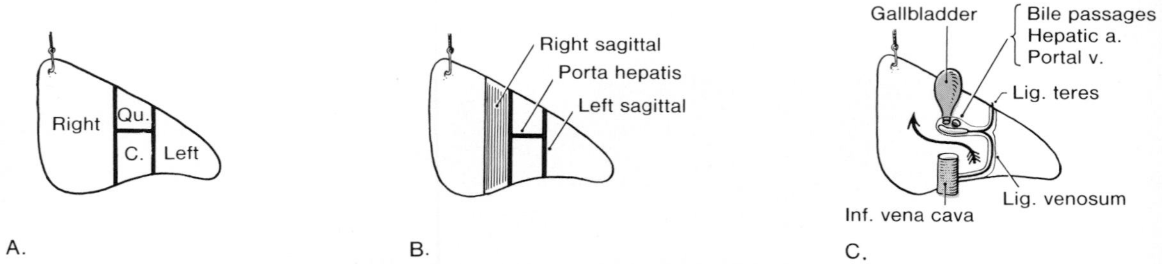

Figure 2-81. Diagrams of the liver which is hooked upward to show the features of its inferior surface. *A*, illustrates its four lobes: right, quadrate, caudate, and left. *B*, demonstrates the H-shaped deep fissures and wide sulci defining the lobes. *C*, shows the occupants of the fissures and sulci. The *arrow* traverses the epiploic foramen and passes into the omental bursa (see Fig. 2-79).

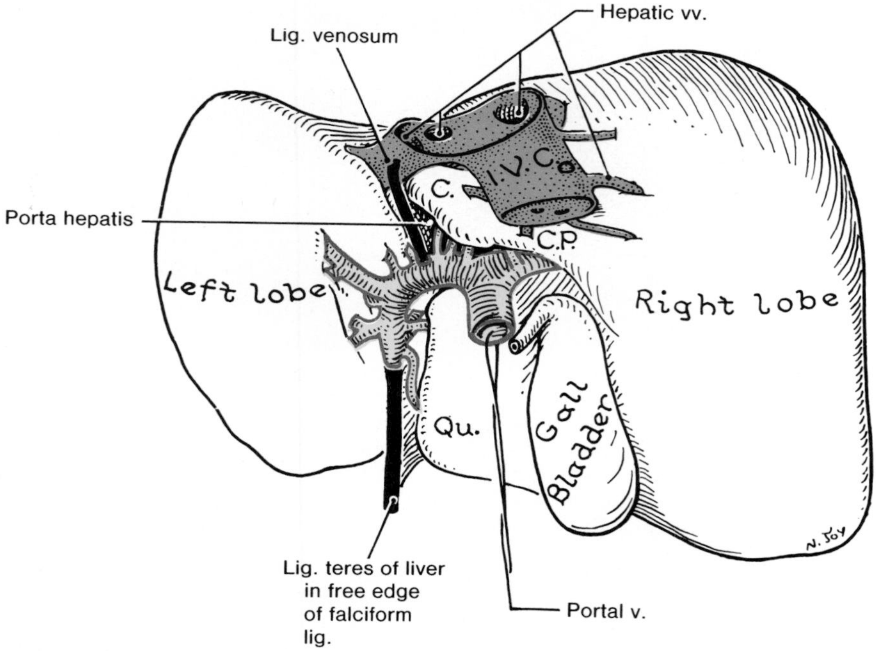

Figure 2-82. Drawing of a posteroinferior view of the liver showing its veins. Observe the branches of the portal vein (*yellow*) entering the liver and the three large and several small hepatic veins (*blue*) leaving the liver to join the inferior vena cava. *C*, caudate lobe; *CP*, caudate process; *Qu*, quadrate lobe.

which define the four lobes of the liver. The crossbar of the H is the **porta hepatis** (Figs. 2-80 and 2-81). *The porta (L. gate) or hilum is a deep transverse fissure, about 5 cm long, that contains the* **portal vein**, the **hepatic artery proper**, the **hepatic nerve plexus**, the **hepatic ducts**, and **lymphatic vessels**. The left sagittal limbs of the H are deep fissures containing the **ligamentum teres** (umbilical vein in fetuses and newborn infants) and the **ligamentum venosum** (ductus venosus in fetuses and newborn infants). The right sagittal limbs of the H are fossae for the gallbladder and the inferior vena cava.

Lobes of the Liver (Figs. 2-46, 2-47, and 2-81 to 2-83). For descriptive purposes the liver is divided into a **large right lobe** and a **smaller left lobe** by the **falciform ligament** (Fig. 2-46). The right lobe is subdivided into a **quadrate lobe**, lying between the gallbladder and the falciform ligament,

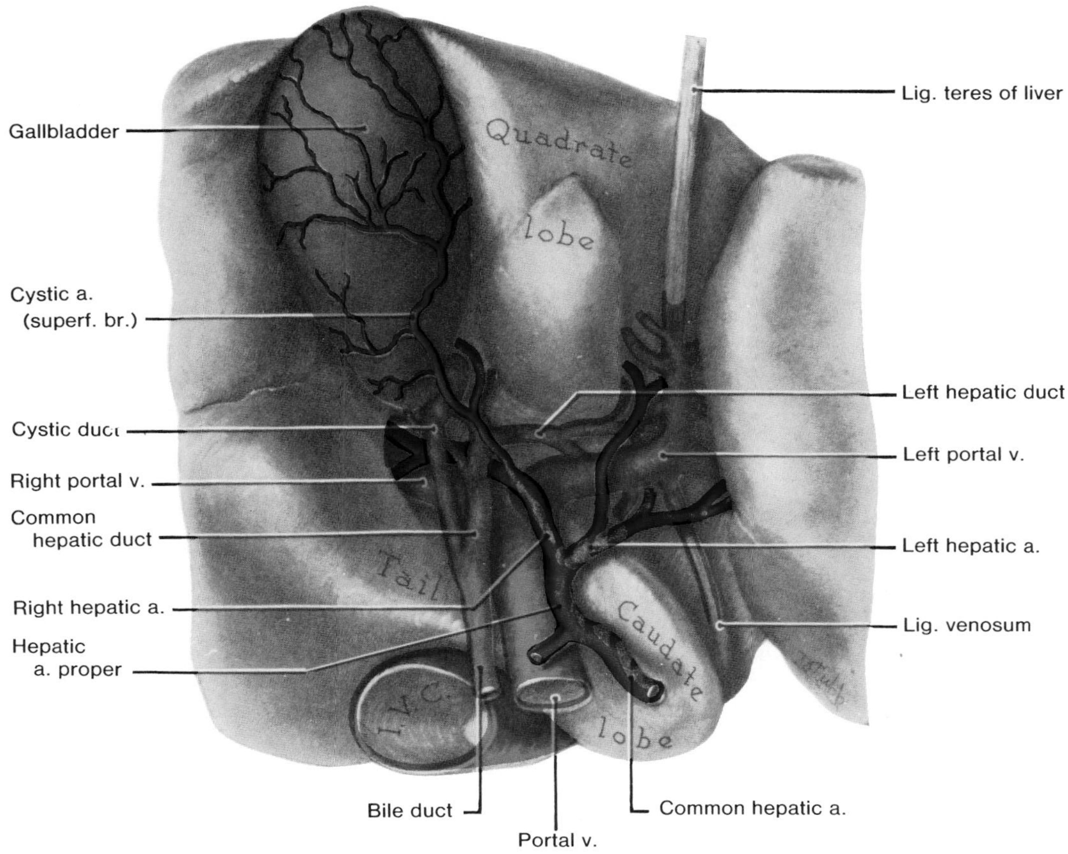

Figure 2-83. Drawing of the inferior surface of the liver showing the porta hepatis and the cystic artery. Observe that the tail of the caudate lobe, called the caudate process, forms the superior boundary of the epiploic foramen and lies between the upper end of the portal vein and the inferior vena cava. The structures entering the liver at the porta hepatis are sometimes referred to clinically as the hepatic pedicle. Note the relation of the structures as they ascend to the porta hepatis: duct to the right, artery to the left, and vein behind. Observe the order of the structures at the porta hepatis: duct, artery, vein from before backward. Note that the left portal vein and the left hepatic artery supply the quadrate and caudate lobes en route to the left lobe and that they are accompanied by the tributaries of the left hepatic duct. Examine the ligamentum teres passing to the left portal vein and the ligamentum venosum arising opposite it and ascending to the inferior vena cava (as in Fig. 2-82). Observe the cystic artery springing from the right hepatic artery and dividing into superficial and deep branches which arborize on the respective surfaces of the gallbladder. Note that the cystic duct is sinuous at its origin.

and a **caudate lobe**, lying between the inferior vena cava and the fissure for the ligamentum venosum (Fig. 2-81*A*). *The quadrate lobe is separated from the caudate lobe by the porta hepatis* (Fig. 2-82).

Although for purposes of description the quadrate and caudate lobes are considered to be part of the right lobe, it must be understood that according to internal morphology, based mainly on the distribution of blood vessels, they belong to the left lobe of the liver. Thus, *the right and left halves of the liver are functionally separate. Each half receives its own arterial and portal venous supply and has its own venous drainage.* There is little (if any) overlap between the two halves. Similarly, the **right hepatic duct** drains bile from the right half of the liver and the **left hepatic duct** drains it from the left half of the liver.

The pattern of blood vessel distribution also forms a basis for dividing the liver into **hepatic segments** (Fig. 2-86). These segments are of surgical significance.

The caudate lobe (Fig. 2-47) is the lobe with a tail (L. *cauda*), called the **caudate process** (Fig. 2-82). This narrow isthmus of liver bounds the epiploic foramen above (Fig. 2-47) and connects the caudate lobe to the visceral surface (Fig. 2-80).

Peritoneal Relations of the Liver (Figs. 2-29, 2-36 to 2-38, 2-79, and 2-80). The liver is **almost entirely covered with peritoneum** and so it presents a smooth glistening appearance in the fresh state. Its peritoneal relationships are not difficult when the development of the liver is clearly understood. The liver grows between the two layers of the **ventral mesentery** and much of this double-layered sheet becomes the peritoneal covering (**visceral peritoneum**) of the liver. The remainder of the ventral mesentery forms the **lesser omentum** (Figs. 2-36 and 2-37) and the **falciform ligament** (Fig. 2-29). The various reflections of peritoneum from the liver constitute its ligaments. The passage of the **embryonic umbilical vein** from the umbilicus to the liver produces a sickle-shaped fold, the **falciform ligament**, that connects the liver to the anterior abdominal wall and to the diaphragm from the umbilicus to the dome of the structure. The line of attachment of the double-layered falciform ligament to the liver is the line of division of the organ into *anatomical* right and left lobes. Along this line the two layers of the falciform ligament separate to enclose the liver, forming the **visceral peritoneum of the liver**. The falciform ligament encloses a few small *paraumbilical veins* (Fig. 2-112) and the umbilical vein in its free border during prenatal life. Several weeks after birth the umbilical vein obliterates close to the umbilicus, but it usually remains patent in the free edge of the falciform ligament as far as the left branch of the portal vein. *The obliterated portion of the umbilical vein is known as the ligamentum teres* (round ligament) of the liver. On the visceral surface (Figs. 2-80 and 2-81*C*), the layers of the falciform ligament reflect onto the liver along the line of the fissure for the ligamentum teres, as far as the **porta hepatis**. At the superior end of the falciform ligament, its two layers separate from each other, exposing a hand-sized triangular area on the superior surface of the liver. This is called the **bare area** because it is *devoid of peritoneum.* Here, the two peritoneal layers diverge laterally and are reflected onto the diaphragm to form the **coronary ligament** (Fig. 2-79). Because the liver is applied directly to the diaphragm in the bare area, *the right and left layers of this ligament are spread apart and surround the bare area.* In the fetus the coronary ligament surrounds the superior extremity of the liver like a crown (L. *corona*), hence its name. However, when the liver becomes relatively larger than that in the young fetus, the coronary ligament surrounds only the triangular bare area. *The right reflection of the falciform ligament constitutes the anterior layer of the coronary ligament.* It passes to the right and then bends sharply at the right triangular ligament to become the posterior layer of the coronary ligament. *The left reflection of the falciform ligament forms the left triangular ligament,* which becomes continuous with the posterior layer of the coronary ligament.

From the **porta hepatis** the peritoneal reflections pass to the lesser curvature of the stomach and the first part of the duodenum as the lesser omentum. *The left triangular ligament (posterior layer) is continuous with the lesser omentum* (Fig. 2-79). The portion of the lesser omentum extending between the liver and the stomach is called the **hepatogastric ligament** and that portion between the liver and the duodenum is called the **hepatoduodenal ligament**. *Near the free edge of the lesser omentum,* the two layers enclose the hepatic artery, the portal vein, the bile duct, a few lymph nodes and vessels, and the hepatic plexus of nerves.

Blood Vessels and Nerves of the Liver (Figs. 2-46, 2-47, 2-56, 2-57, and 2-82 to 2-86). The liver has a *double blood supply* from the **hepatic artery** (30%) and the **portal vein** (70%). The hepatic artery carries oxygenated blood to the liver and the portal vein carries venous blood containing the products of digestion absorbed from the GI tract. The arterial blood is conducted to the **central vein** of each liver lobule via the sinusoids of the liver. The central veins drain into the hepatic veins which open into the inferior vena cava (Figs. 2-85 and 2-86).

The common hepatic artery arises from the **celiac trunk** and passes forward to the right in the posterior wall of the omental bursa (Fig. 2-46). *It runs inferior to the epiploic foramen* to reach the superior (first) part of the duodenum. After giving off the gastroduodenal artery, it passes between the layers of the lesser omentum as the **hepatic artery proper** (Fig. 2-87). This artery ascends in the free edge of the lesser omentum anterior to the portal vein and to the left of the bile duct. Near the porta hepatis the hepatic artery proper divides into right and left terminal branches, called the **right** and **left hepatic arteries.** However, *in about 11% of cases the left hepatic artery arises from the left gastric artery* in the vicinity of the gastroesophageal junction (Fig. 2-84) and passes between the layers of the upper part of the lesser omentum to the left lobe of the liver. The **cystic artery**, supplying the gallbladder, usually arises from the right hepatic artery just above the cystic duct.

The portal vein, supplying most of the blood to the liver, **is formed behind the neck of the pancreas by the union of the superior mesenteric and splenic veins** (Figs. 2-57 and 2-85). The portal vein runs in the free right edge of the lesser omentum posterior to the bile duct and the hepatic artery and anterior to the epiploic foramen. At the right end of the porta hepatis it terminates by dividing into two branches (right and left), each of which supplies about half of the liver.

The hepatic veins draining blood from the liver are formed by the union of the central veins of the lobules of the liver (Fig. 2-86). *They open into the inferior vena cava just below the diaphragm* (Figs. 2-57 and 2-82). There are upper and lower groups of hepatic veins which open into the inferior vena cava just below the diaphragm (Figs. 2-57 and 2-82). The upper group may consist of only right and left veins, but usually there is a middle vein from the caudate lobe. All of these are large vessels. The lower group consists of 6 to 18 small veins which drain blood from the right and caudate lobes of the liver.

The lymph vessels of the liver pass in several directions: (1) those from the superior and anterior parts of the *diaphragmatic surface* of the liver pass through the falciform ligament to the lower **parasternal lymph nodes** (Fig. 1-20); (2) those from the *inferior surface* and *deep parts of the liver* drain into the **hepatic lymph nodes** in the porta hepatis, into the lymph nodes around the hepatic artery, and into the **gastric lymph nodes** via the lesser omentum; and (3) those from the *bare area* drain into the **middle diaphragmatic lymph nodes** on the thoracic surface of the diaphragm and also into the **celiac lymph nodes**. *Most of the lymph from the liver eventually drains into the thoracic duct* (Fig. 1-48). It has been estimated that one-quarter to one-half of the lymph reaching this *large trunk of the lymph vessels* of the body is derived from the liver.

The nerves of the liver (Fig. 2-59) are numerous and contain both *sympathetic* and *parasympathetic* (vagal) fibers. These nerves reach the liver by way of a very extensive **hepatic plexus**, the largest derivative of the celiac plexus (Figs. 2-111 and 2-127), which also receives filaments from the **left** and **right vagus** and **right phrenic nerves**. The hepatic plexus accompanies the hepatic artery and the portal vein and their branches and enters the liver at the porta hepatis.

CLINICALLY ORIENTED COMMENTS

Variations in the origin and the course of the hepatic arteries are common (Fig. 2-84) and knowledge of them is important to the surgeon.

Liver tissue for diagnostic purposes may be obtained by **liver biopsy**. The needle puncture is commonly made through the right seventh, eighth, or ninth intercostal space in the midaxillary line (Fig. 2-36) while the patient is holding his/her breath in full expiration to reduce the costodia-

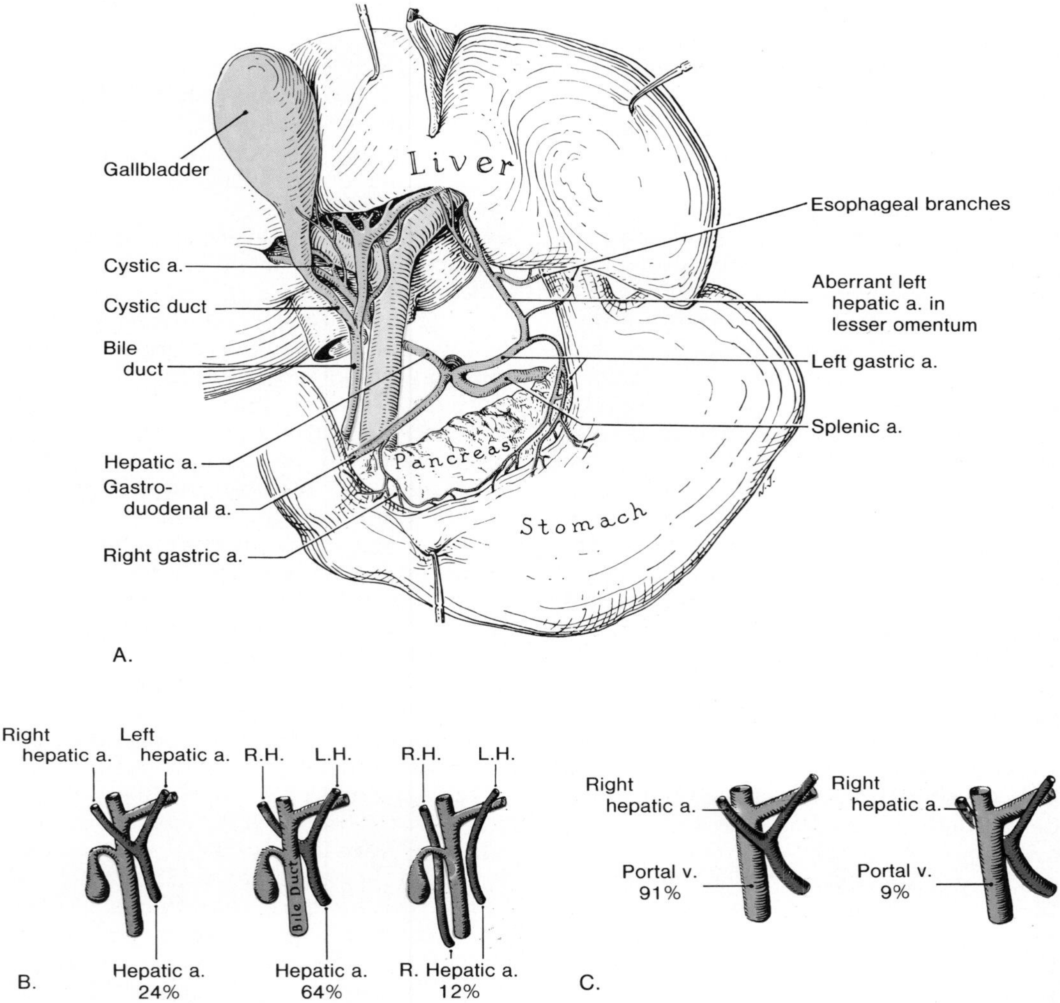

Figure 2-84. Drawings of variations in the hepatic arteries which are common and are important to the surgeon. *A*, aberrant left hepatic artery. The left hepatic artery was entirely replaced by a branch of the left gastric artery, as in this specimen, in 11.5% of 200 cadavers, and in another 11.5% it was partially replaced. *B*, right hepatic artery variants. In a study of 165 cadavers, three patterns were observed: in 24%, the right hepatic artery crossed ventral to the bile passages; in 64%, the right hepatic artery crossed dorsal to the bile passages and in 12%, the aberrant artery arose from the superior mesenteric artery. *C*, the artery crossed ventral to the portal vein in 91% of 165 specimens and dorsal in 9%.

phragmatic recess (Figs. 2-29, 2-36, and 2-113) and to lessen the possibility of damaging the lung and contaminating the pleural cavity.

The liver is a common site of metastatic carcinoma from the GI tract or from any region drained by the portal vein (Fig. 2-85). Cancer cells may also travel to it from the thorax or the breast owing to communications between thoracic lymph nodes and the lymph vessels draining the bare area of the liver.

Normally the liver is a soft mass with a jelly-like consistency, almost all of which is protected by the rib cage (Fig. 2-76). In some normal people the inferior edge of the

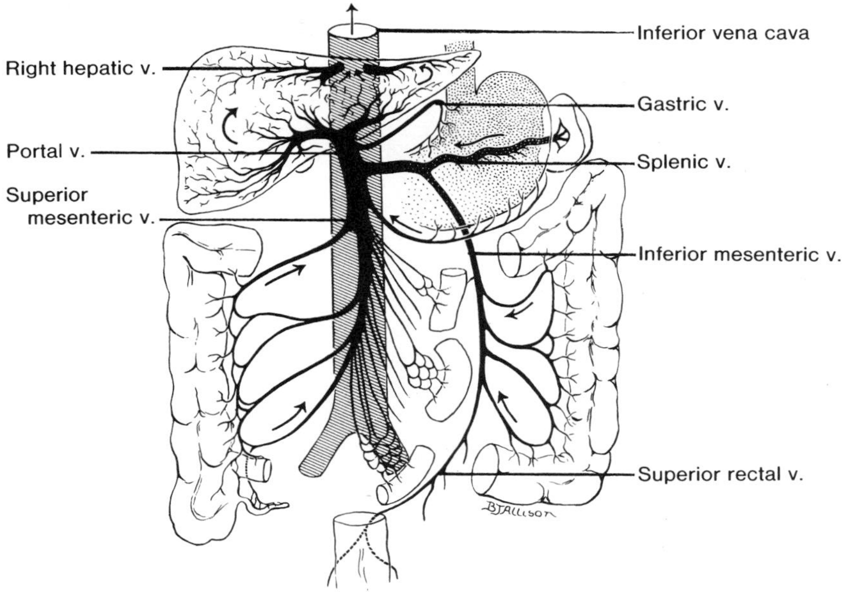

Figure 2-85. Scheme of the portal circulation. Understand that the portal vein drains only the gastrointestinal tract and its unpaired glands, the liver of course excepted. It returns to the liver the blood delivered by the celiac, superior mesenteric, and inferior mesenteric arteries to these parts. The portal vein is formed between the head and neck of the pancreas by the union of the splenic, the superior mesenteric, and the inferior mesenteric veins. It ascends to the right end of the porta hepatis, where it divides into the right and left portal veins. The right vein enters the right lobe and the left vein passes transversely to the left end of the porta hepatis to supply the caudate, quadrate, and left lobes. There are no functioning valves in the portal system.

liver may be palpable 1 to 2 cm below the right costal margin; hence, a palpable edge of the liver does not by itself indicate liver enlargement (**hepatomegaly**). Large livers are associated with carcinoma (primary or metastatic), congestive heart failure, fatty infiltration, and Hodgkin's disease.

In **cirrhosis of the liver** (Case 2-8), there is progressive *destruction of hepatocytes* and replacement of them by fibrous tissue. This tissue surrounds the intrahepatic blood vessels and biliary radicles, impeding circulation of blood through the liver. The consistency of the liver is very firm owing to the large amounts of fibrous tissue. The surface of the liver has a nodular appearance, accounting for usage of the term "*hob-nail liver.*" There is often a reddish yellow or tawny color to the liver, hence the name **cirrhosis** (G. *kirrhos*, tawny, orange colored + *osis*, condition).

Inflammation of the peritoneum (*peritonitis*) may result in the formation of localized **abscesses** (collections of pus) in various parts of the peritoneal cavity. One dangerous site is in a **subphrenic recess** (Fig. 2-77), located between the diaphragmatic surface of the liver and the diaphragm. **Subphrenic abscesses** occur much more frequently on the right side because of the frequency of ruptured appendices, duodenal ulcers, and gallbladders. As the right and left subphrenic recesses are continuous with the **hepatorenal recesses** (Figs. 2-32, 2-77, and 2-90), pus in a **subphrenic abscess** may drain into one of these recesses when the patient is supine, because in this position the hepatorenal recesses are the lowest parts of the peritoneal cavity. *Pus in a hepatorenal recess may be drained through a posterior incision* above the 12th rib (for the anatomical basis of this procedure, see Fig. 2-32).

The Biliary Ducts and Gallbladder (Figs. 2-29, 2-33, 2-36, 2-73, and 2-80 to 2-95). **Bile** is secreted by the hepatic cells

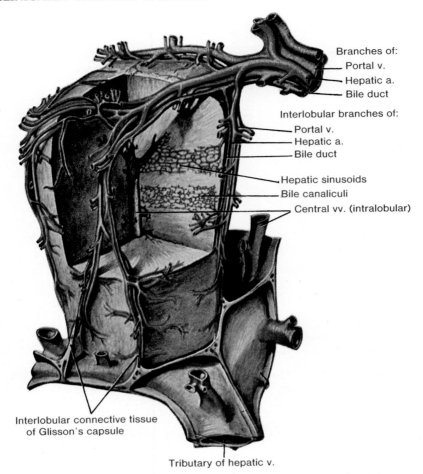

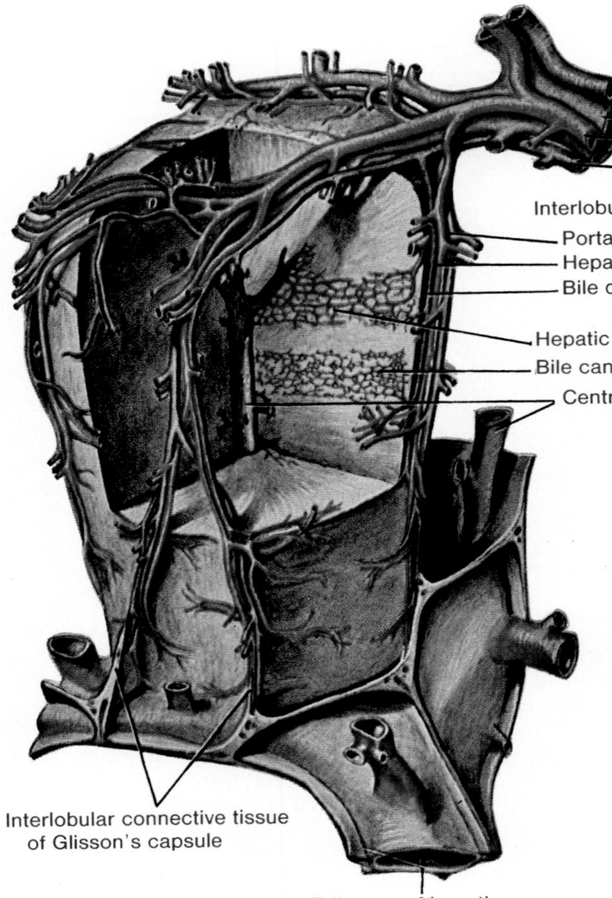

Figure 2-86. Reconstruction of a liver lobule. A portion of the lobule is cut away to show the hepatic sinusoids and the bile canaliculi. (Redrawn and slightly modified from Braus, after a reconstruction by A. Vierling).

into the **bile canaliculi**; these are the smallest branches of the intrahepatic duct system (Fig. 2-86). Most of the canaliculi drain into small **interlobular bile ducts**. Each interlobular duct joins with others to form progressively larger ducts; eventually, **right** and **left hepatic ducts** are formed which emerge from the porta hepatis. The right hepatic duct drains approximately the right half of the liver and the left hepatic duct drains approximately the left half of the liver. The areas drained by these ducts are the same as those supplied by the right and left branches of the hepatic artery and the portal vein.

Shortly after leaving the porta hepatis, the right and left hepatic ducts unite to form the **common hepatic duct** (about 4 cm in length). It passes downward and to the right, between the layers of the lesser omentum, where it is joined on the right side by the **cystic duct** from the gallbladder to form the **bile duct** (Figs. 2-88 and 2-89). This duct is 8 to 10 cm long and 5 to 6 mm in diameter.

During the first part of its course to the duodenum, *the bile duct passes in the free edge of the lesser omentum with the hepatic artery and the portal vein* (Fig. 2-90). It runs downward, anterior to the **epiploic**

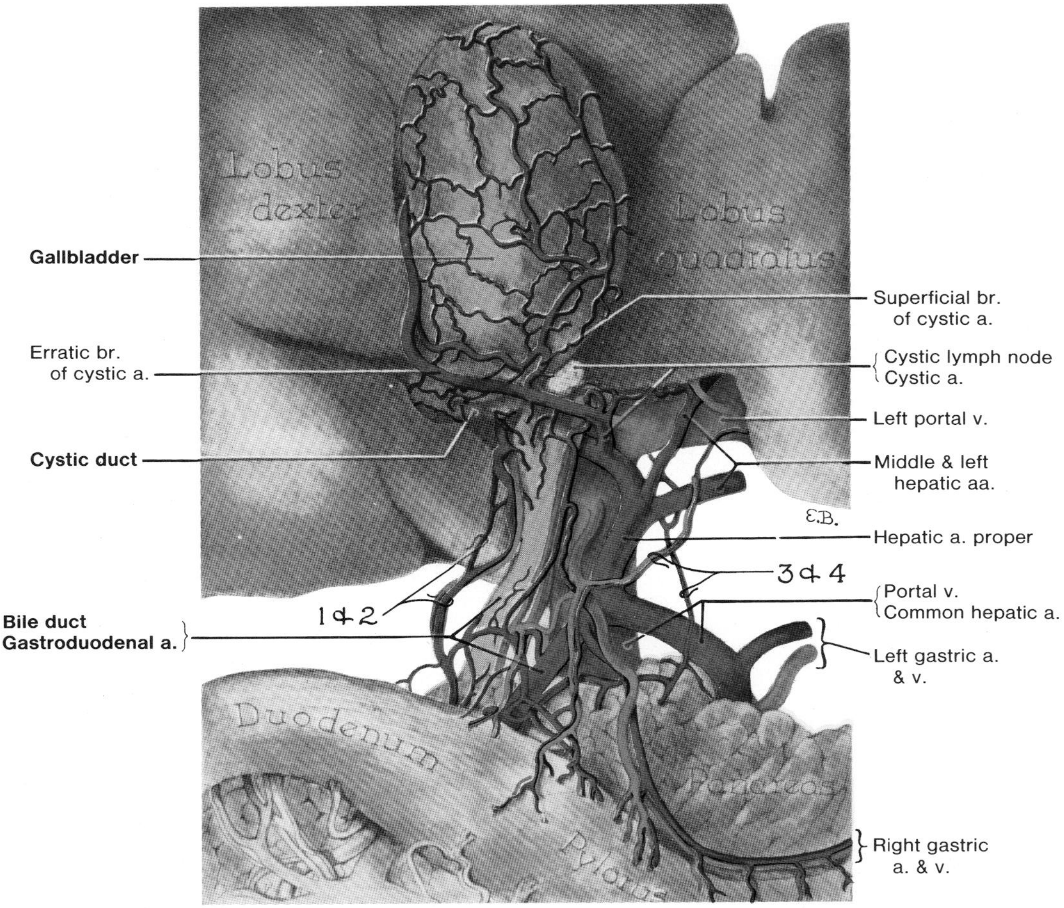

Figure 2-87. Drawing of a dissection of the gallbladder, the bile passages, and the related blood vessels. The liver is reflected upward with the gallbladder and the duodenum is pulled down. Observe the network of arteries on the gallbladder and that most of the smaller arteries lie on a deeper plane than the larger arteries. Note the large erratic deep branch of the cystic artery crossing superficial to the neck of the gallbladder. Examine the many fine sinuous arterial twigs supplying the bile passages and springing from the nearby arteries. Observe that the right gastric artery arises from the gastroduodenal artery. Note that there are five anastomotic arteries capable of bringing blood from various gastric and pancreatic arteries to the porta hepatis; four of these have been retracted and one of them passes to the left lobe.

foramen (Figs. 2-36 to 2-38), where it is in front of the right edge of the portal vein and on the right of the hepatic artery (Fig. 2-87). The bile duct then *passes posterior to the superior or first part of the duodenum and the head of the pancreas* (Figs. 2-65 to 2-67, and 2-73), occupying a groove in the posterior part of the head or embedded in it. As it runs behind the duodenum, *the bile duct lies to the right of the gastroduodenal artery* (Figs. 2-65 and 2-87). At the left side of the descending or second part of the duodenum, the bile duct comes into contact with the pancreatic duct and the two of them run obliquely through the wall of the duodenum, where they usually unite (Figs. 2-72*D* and 2-73) to form the **hepatopancreatic ampulla** (Fig. 2-88). In about 9% of people, the bile and pancreatic ducts do not unite to form an ampulla and

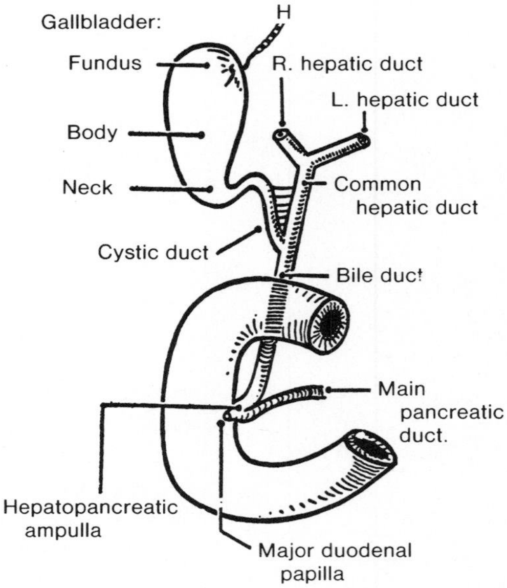

Figure 2-88. Diagram showing the extrahepatic parts of the biliary system and the relationship of the bile and pancreatic ducts. The gallbladder has been pulled upward with a hook (*H*). See Figures 2-67 and 2-89 for its normal relationship to the duodenum. Observe that the cystic duct joins the common hepatic duct to form the bile duct. Note that the bile duct runs behind the superior part of the duodenum and passes obliquely through the duodenal wall, where it is joined by the main pancreatic duct. Usually the two ducts empty into a common channel, the hepatopancreatic ampulla, which empties into the duodenum at the apex of the major duodenal papilla (also see Fig. 2-74).

open separately into the duodenum (Figs. 2-72*G* and 2-74). Usually the distal constricted end of the ampulla opens into the descending part of the duodenum at the summit of the **major duodenal papilla**, 8 to 10 cm from the pylorus (Fig. 2-73).

The circular muscle around the distal end of the bile duct is thickened to form the **choledochal sphincter** or the bile duct sphincter (G. *cholēdochus*, containing bile). This sphincter consists of a funnel-shaped muscular sheath that surrounds the bile duct, just before and after it penetrates the duodenal wall. There is also a sphincter around the hepatopancreatic ampulla called the **sphincter of the hepatopancreatic ampulla** (sphincter of Oddi). This sphincter controls the discharge of bile and pancreatic juice into the duodenum. When the choledochal sphincter contracts, bile cannot enter the ampulla and/or the duodenum; hence, it backs up and passes along the **cystic duct** into the gallbladder for concentration (by absorption of water) and storage.

CLINICALLY ORIENTED COMMENTS

As the distal constricted end of the hepatopancreatic ampulla is the narrowest part of the biliary passage, it is a common site for impaction of a gallstone. Stones in the ampulla can usually be removed

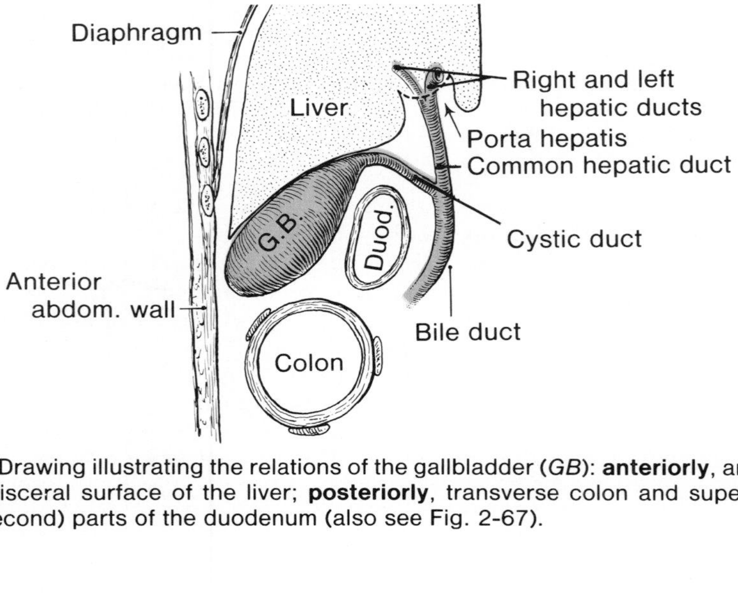

Figure 2-89. Drawing illustrating the relations of the gallbladder (*GB*): **anteriorly**, anterior abdominal wall and visceral surface of the liver; **posteriorly**, transverse colon and superior (first) and descending (second) parts of the duodenum (also see Fig. 2-67).

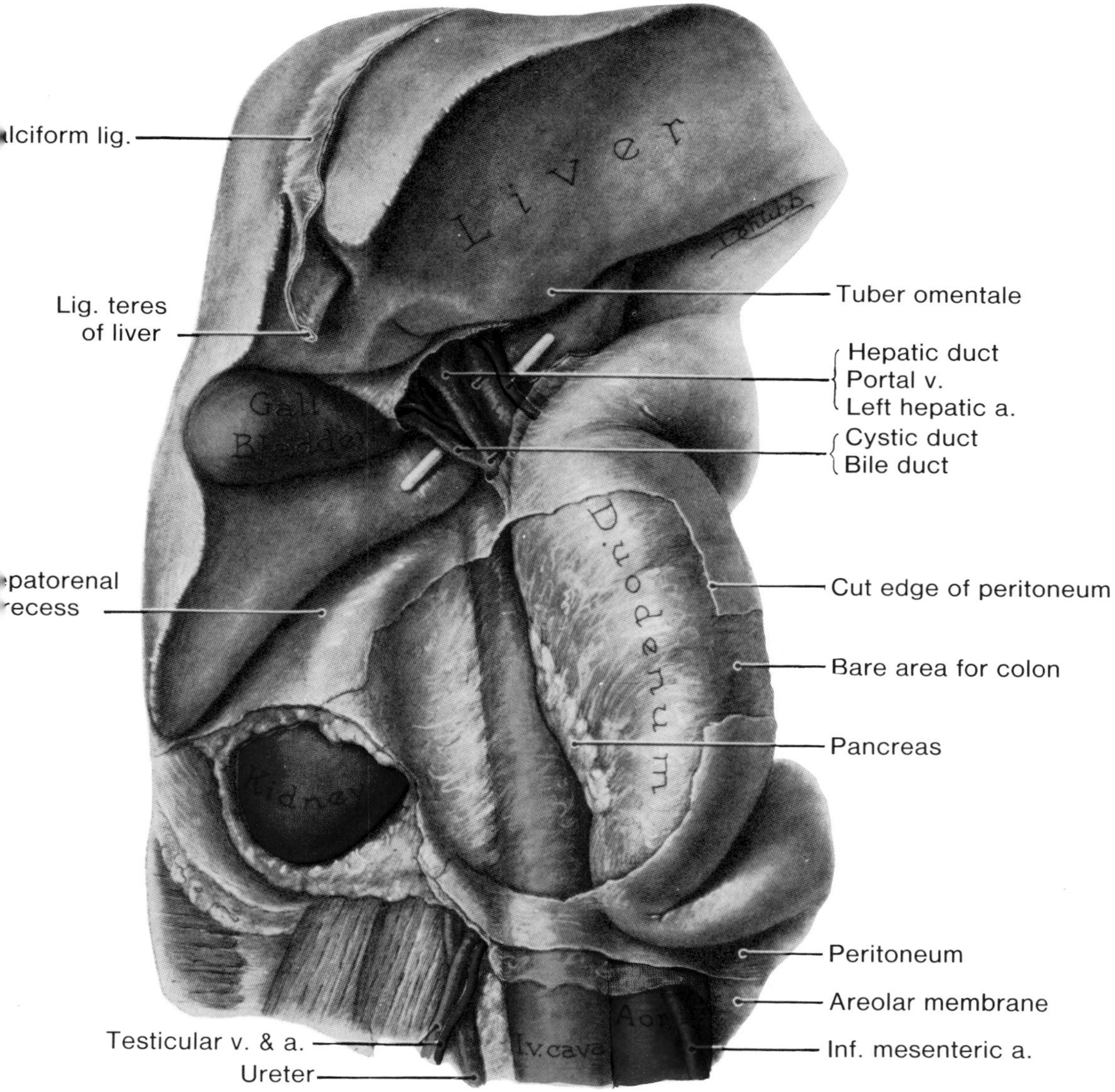

Figure 2-90. Drawing of a dissection illustrating how the duodenum is mobilized to expose the bile duct. (A further dissection is shown in Fig. 2-91.) The lesser omentum has been removed and the transverse colon has been separated from the front of the descending part of the duodenum and turned down. The peritoneum has been cut along the right convex border of the descending part of the duodenum and this part of the duodenum has been swung forward like a door on a hinge. Observe the three main structures that were exposed when the anterior wall of the lesser omentum was removed: the portal vein is posterior, the hepatic artery ascends from the left, and the bile passages descend to the right. Note that in this specimen the right hepatic artery springs from the superior mesenteric artery.

through an incision in the supraduodenal part of the bile duct (Figs. 2-67 and 2-87). Sometimes the duodenum and the head of the pancreas have to be mobilized, as shown in Figures 2-90 and 2-91, to expose the duct in its retropancreatic position.

Blockage of the bile duct may cause severe pain (**biliary colic**) in the right upper quadrant of the abdomen; however, in 10 to 15% of patients pain is not a prominent feature. Understand that *it is not the stone that causes the pain, but the distention of*

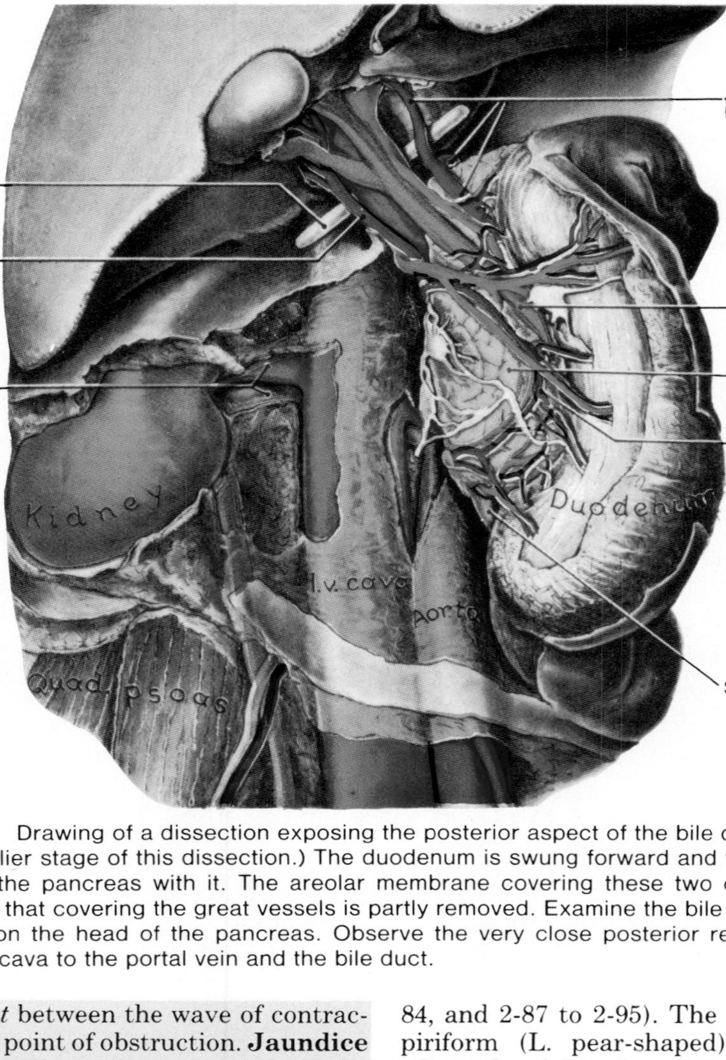

Figure 2-91. Drawing of a dissection exposing the posterior aspect of the bile duct. (See Fig. 2-90 for an earlier stage of this dissection.) The duodenum is swung forward and to the left, taking the head of the pancreas with it. The areolar membrane covering these two organs is largely removed and that covering the great vessels is partly removed. Examine the bile duct descending in a groove on the head of the pancreas. Observe the very close posterior relationship of the inferior vena cava to the portal vein and the bile duct.

the bile duct between the wave of contraction and the point of obstruction. **Jaundice** (see previous discussion) may occur if the blockage has been present for some time; often it is intermittent. **Extrahepatic bile duct obstruction** may also result from extramural or intramural causes (*e.g.*., cancer).

Accessory hepatic ducts are common (Fig. 2-95*D* to *F*) and awareness of their possible presence is of surgical importance. In some cases the cystic duct opens into one of these accessory ducts rather than the common hepatic duct.

The Gallbladder (Figs. 2-29, 2-33, 2-36, 2-46, 2-47, 2-51, 2-59, 2-67, 2-73, 2-80 to 2-84, and 2-87 to 2-95). The gallbladder is a piriform (L. pear-shaped) sac that *lies along the right edge of the quadrate lobe of the liver in a shallow fossa on the visceral surface of the liver.* **The gallbladder concentrates the bile secreted by the liver** by absorption of water by its epithelium. It **stores the bile** in the intervals between active phases of digestion. Although it is only 7 to 10 cm in length and about 4 cm in diameter, the gallbladder has a capacity of 30 to 60 ml. For descriptive purposes it is divided into a *fundus, body,* and *neck* (Figs. 2-73 and 2-88).

The fundus of the gallbladder is *the wide blind end which projects from the inferior border of the liver* (Fig. 2-29). *It is located at approximately the tip of the*

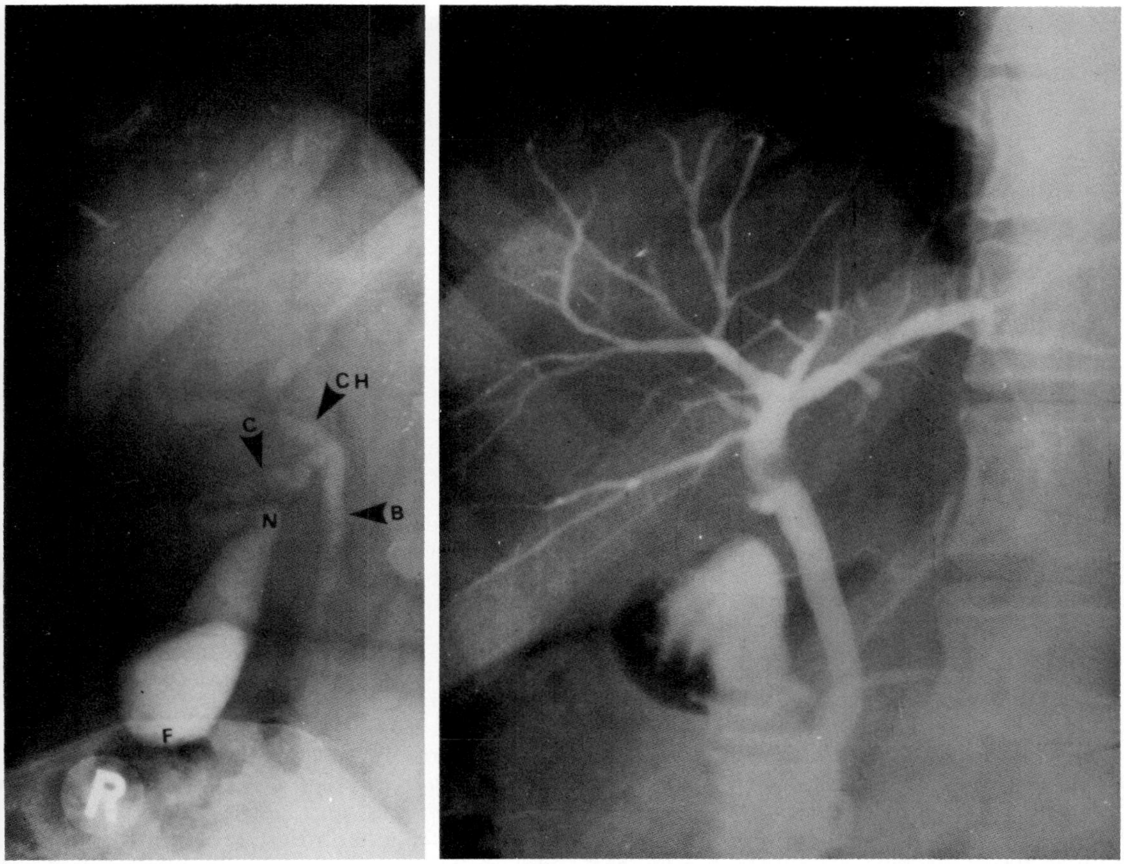

Figure 2-92. Radiographs of the biliary passages. *On the left*, a cholecystogram of the gallbladder and the biliary passages which are visualized with contrast medium. Observe the body, fundus (*F*), and neck (*N*) of the gallbladder and the cystic (*C*), common hepatic (*CH*), and bile (*B*) ducts. The spiral fold (valve) of the cystic duct gives it a tortuous appearance. *On the right*, following cholecystectomy (excision of the gallbladder), contrast medium has been injected via a T tube into the bile pasages.

ninth costal cartilage in the midclavicular line, where the linea semilunaris meets the costal margin (Figs. 2.10 and 2-36). It is directed downward, forward, and to the right where it comes into relationship with the posterior surface of the anterior abdominal wall and the descending part of the duodenum (Figs. 2-67 and 2-89).

The body is the *main part of the gallbladder* which is directed upward, backward, and to the left from the fundus. *It lies in contact with the visceral surface of the liver* to which it is attached by areolar tissue. It also contacts the right part of the transverse colon (Fig. 2-80) and the superior part of the duodenum (Fig. 2-89).

The neck of the gallbladder (Fig. 2-88), narrow and tapered, is directed toward the porta hepatis (Fig. 2-36). It makes an S-shaped bend and is somewhat constricted as it becomes continuous with the **cystic duct** (Fig. 2-92). It is twisted in such a way that its mucosa is thrown into a **spiral fold.** *The neck of the gallbladder serves as a guide to the epiploic foramen*, which lies immediately to its left (Fig. 2-36) behind the free margin of the lesser omentum.

The peritoneum on the visceral surface of the liver usually passes over the body of the gallbladder; thus its deep or anterior surface is attached to the visceral surface of the liver by areolar connective tissue.

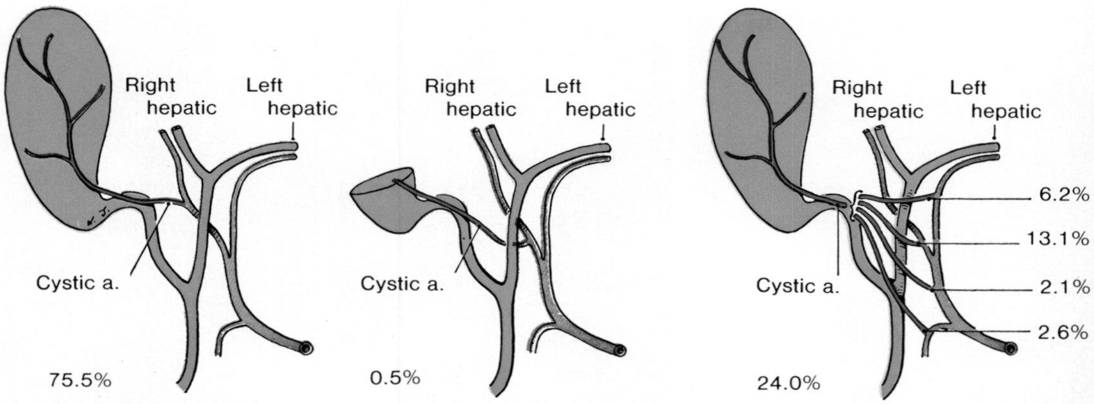

Figure 2-93. Drawings illustrating some variations in the origin and course of the cystic artery. The cystic artery usually (about 75%) arises from the right hepatic artery in the angle between the common hepatic duct and cystic duct. However, when it arises on the left of the bile passages, it usually crosses anterior to these passages. (These diagrams are based on the study of 580 cases.) The right-hand diagram is a *composite* of the variations of the cystic artery passing in front of the common hepatic duct. Because of the above variations, the arterial supply to the gallbladder must be clearly visualized before removal. Otherwise, the right hepatic artery may be inadvertently ligated. If this is done, half of the liver will probably degenerate.

The fundus of the gallbladder is almost completely covered with peritoneum. Occasionally the gallbladder is completely invested with peritoneum and may even be connected to the liver by a short mesentery.

The Cystic Duct (Figs. 2-67, 2-73, 2-83, 2-84*A*, 2-88 to 2-90, and 2-93). The cystic duct, 2 to 4 cm long, *first* runs upward and to the left from the gallbladder, *then* it turns posteriorly and *finally* downward to join the **common hepatic duct**, forming the **bile duct**. Occasionally the cystic duct joins the right hepatic duct (Fig. 2-95*B*) or the common hepatic duct (Fig. 2-95*D*).

The cystic duct runs between the layers of the lesser omentum, usually parallel to the common hepatic duct, before joining it just below the porta hepatis (Fig. 2-90). The mucous membrane of the cystic duct is thrown into a **spiral fold** (of Heister) with a core of smooth muscle (Figs. 2-73 and 2-92). This fold is continuous with a similar one in the neck of the gallbladder and coils along the cystic duct, giving it the tortuous *appearance of a spiral valve.* **The spiral fold keeps the cystic duct constantly open** so that (1) bile can easily pass into the gallbladder when the bile duct is closed by the choledochal sphincter and/or the hepatopancreatic sphincter, or (2) bile can pass in the opposite direction into the duodenum when the gallbladder contracts. A hormonal mechanism is involved in gallbladder contraction. *Eating fat is particularly effective in producing gallbladder contraction.* While digesting fatty food, a hormone called **cholecystokinin** is produced by the intestinal mucosa which passes to the gallbladder and causes it to contract and release bile into the cystic and bile ducts.

Vessels and Nerves of the Extrahepatic Bile Passages and the Gallbladder (Figs. 2-56, 2-59, 2-62, 2-83, 2-87, 2-93, and 2-94). The gallbladder is supplied by the **cystic artery**, which commonly arises from the right hepatic artery in the angle between the common hepatic duct and the cystic duct. *Variations in the origin and course of the cystic artery are common* (Fig. 2-93).

The **veins** draining the bile passages and the neck of the gallbladder join veins which connect the gastric, duodenal, and pancreatic veins partly to the liver directly and partly via a portal vein. The veins of the fundus and body plunge directly into the liver (Fig. 2-94).

The **lymph vessels** pass to the **cystic lymph node** at the neck of the gallbladder (Fig. 2-87) and to the **node of the epiploic**

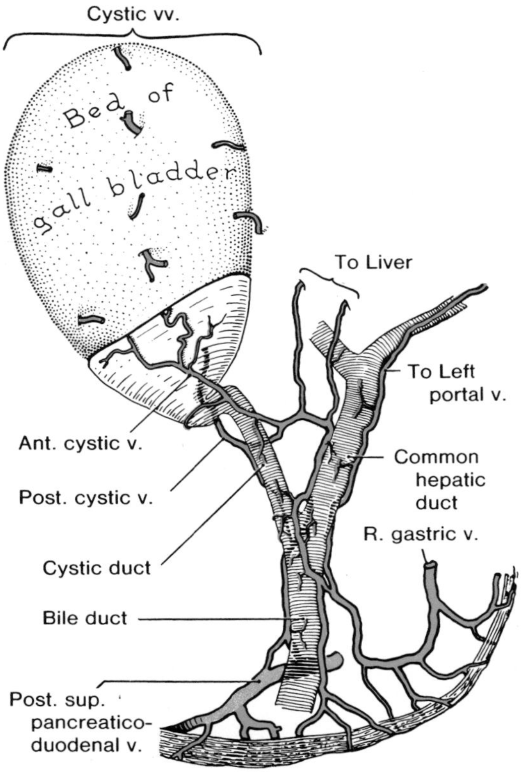

Figure 2-94. Drawing of the veins of the extrahepatic bile passages and the gallbladder. Observe that the venous twigs draining the passages and the neck of the gallbladder join veins which connect the gastric, duodenal, and pancreatic veins partly to the liver directly and partly via a portal vein. The veins of the fundus and the body of the gallbladder plunge directly into the liver.

foramen. From these nodes lymph passes to the hepatic nodes and then to the celiac nodes.

The **nerves** to the gallbladder pass along the cystic artery from the **celiac plexus** (sympathetic, Fig. 2-111), the **vagus** (parasympathetic), and the **right phrenic nerve** (sensory).

The bile duct is supplied by several arteries (Figs. 2-87 and 2-91): (1) the distal or *retroduodenal part* is supplied by the **posterior superior pancreaticoduodenal artery** (Fig. 2-62); (2) the *middle part* is supplied by the **right hepatic artery**; and (3) the *proximal part* is supplied by the **cystic artery** (Fig. 2-87). The supraduodenal branches of the gastroduodenal artery (Figs. 2-54 and 2-56) also give branches to the bile duct as it passes behind the superior or first part of the duodenum (Fig. 2-88). *There is considerable variation in the arrangement of these vessels.*

The **veins** from the proximal part of the bile duct and the hepatic ducts generally enter the liver directly (Fig. 2-94). They are connected below with the posterior superior pancreaticoduodenal vein. Veins from the distal part of the bile duct drain into the portal vein (Fig. 2-85).

The lymph vessels of the bile duct pass to the cystic node (Fig. 2-87), the node of the epiploic foramen, the hepatic nodes, and the **celiac nodes** (Fig. 2-58).

CLINICALLY ORIENTED COMMENTS

After the gallbladder is removed at operation, a procedure called **cholecystectomy** (Case 2-7), the hepatic ducts and the bile duct often dilate in order to store bile.

Variations in the arterial supply of the liver, gallbladder, and extrahepatic bile passages are very common (Figs. 2-84 and 2-93). *The pattern described in most textbooks occurs in about one-third of people.* Most errors in gallbladder surgery result from failure to appreciate the common variations in the anatomy of the biliary system. Before dividing any structures and removing the gallbladder, surgeons clearly identify all three biliary ducts, including the cystic and hepatic arteries. *Hemorrhage during cholecystectomy may be controlled by compressing the hepatic artery in the anterior wall of the epiploic foramen* (Fig. 2-91). **Practice this in a cadaver!** Put one finger in the epiploic foramen and your thumb on its anterior edge (right edge of the lesser omentum) and pinch. This procedure stops the bleeding so the torn artery can be ligated.

The gallbladder and cystic duct have the radiolucency of water and only a few gallstones (about 30%) produce radiodense shadows on plain radiographs of the abdomen. To visualize the gallbladder and its contents radiographically, a technique

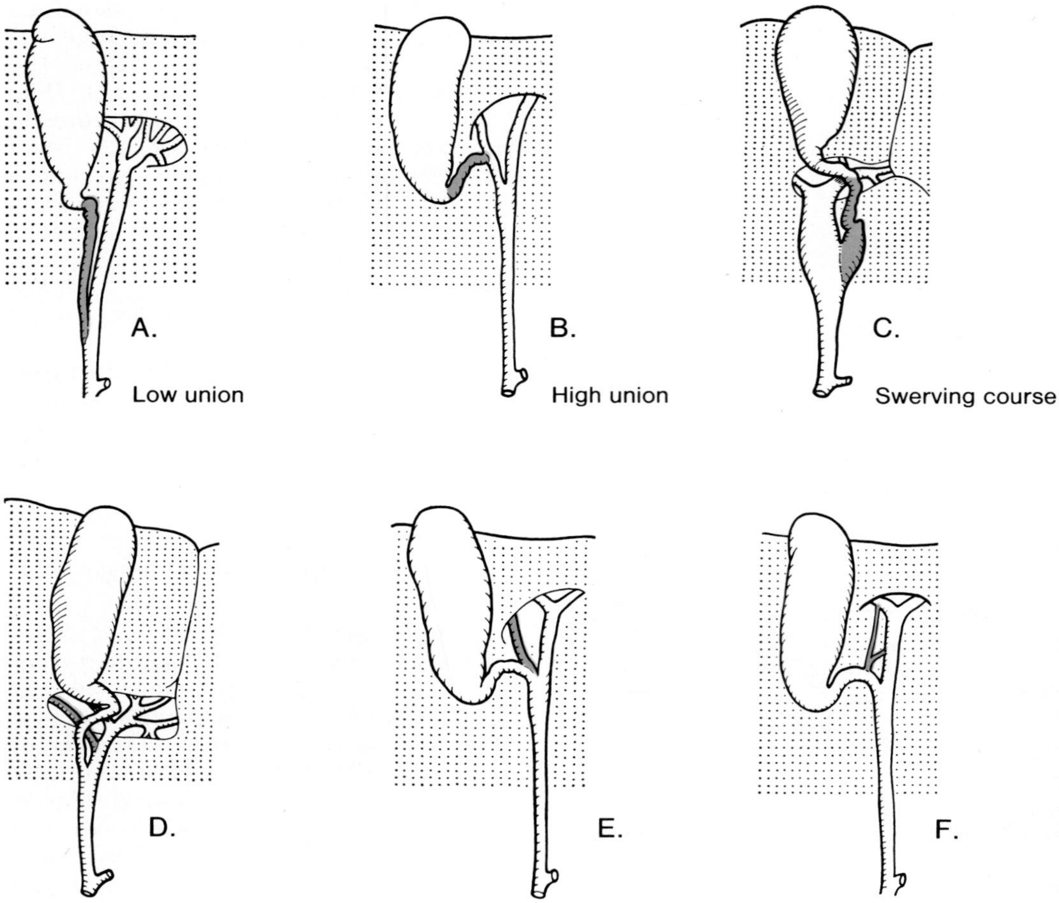

Figure 2-95. *A* to *C*, drawings illustrating variations in the length and the course of the cystic duct. The cystic duct usually lies on the right of the common hepatic duct and joins it just above the superior part of the duodenum, but this varies as shown here. *D* to *E*, drawings showing some varieties of accessory hepatic ducts (*green*) which are common. Of 95 gallbladders and bile passages injected in situ with melted paraffin wax and then dissected, 7 had accessory hepatic ducts in positions of surgical danger. Of these *D*, four joined the common hepatic duct near the cystic duct, *E*, two joined the cystic duct, and *F*, one was an anastomosing duct.

called **oral cholecystography** is commonly used. Patients are given a contrast medium by mouth after a fat-free evening meal. The **contrast material** is absorbed by the small intestine, carried to the liver by the portal venous system, and secreted from the blood into the dilute liver bile. The bile passes to the gallbladder where water is absorbed from it if it is not diseased. The resulting **gallbladder bile** is sufficiently concentrated (10 to 12 times) to be radiopaque. Radiolucent gallstones produce negative images in the opacified gallbladder bile.

Following these studies, the patient *may* be given a fatty meal to cause contraction of the gallbladder, forcing the radiopaque bile into the cystic and bile ducts. Usually these ducts can be visualized radiographically 15 to 20 min after ingestion of the fatty meal.

Using **cholecystography**, it has been shown that the form and position of the gallbladder vary in normal individuals. In short persons with good muscular development (**hypersthenic physical type**), the gallbladder tends to be broad and to lie high up and laterally, opposite the first lumbar vertebra. In tall slender persons with poor muscular development (**asthenic physical type**), the gallbladder tends to be narrow and appears to lie closer to the vertebral column, as low as the fourth lumbar vertebra.

If the gallbladder cannot be visualized or is poorly visualized by **oral cholecystography**, the contrast material may be given intravenously (**intravenous cholangiography**). Sometimes the gallbladder can be visualized by this technique. *If the biliary duct system is obstructed*, it is usually dilated and contrast material may be injected directly into a duct via a slender needle passed through the skin toward the porta hepatis. This technique is called **transhepatic cholangiography.**

Radiographic studies of the gallbladder may also reveal congenital abnormalities such as double gallbladder (very rare), folded gallbladder (present in about 15% of people), and abnormal position of the gallbladder.

The junction of the cystic and common hepatic ducts varies. When the junction is low (Fig. 2-95*A*), the two ducts may be closely connected by fibrous tissue, making it difficult to clamp the cystic duct without injuring the hepatic or bile ducts. Failure to recognize a high union of the cystic duct (Fig. 2-95*B*) would result in no drainage of bile from the left half of the liver if the left hepatic duct was ligated.

Occasionally there are narrow channels (**accessory hepatic ducts**) running from the right lobe of the liver into the anterior surface of the body of the gallbladder. As they carry bile directly from the liver to the gallbladder, they are a cause of **bile leakage** after cholecystectomy. This is usually controlled by cauterizing the gallbladder bed and then sewing a patch taken from the greater omentum over it.

From the right wall of the neck of the gallbladder, a dilation may be present called **Hartmann's pouch**. It projects downward and backward toward the duodenum. *Gallstones frequently lodge in this sac* and if inflamed it may adhere to the cystic duct. As it is almost always present when the gallbladder is dilated, it is used as a point of traction for making identification of the cystic duct easier.

The Jejunum and Ileum (Figs. 2-33, 2-40, 2-42, and 2-96). The jejunum and ileum are *the greatly coiled parts of the small intestine.* The jejunum is continuous with the ascending (fourth) part of the duodenum at the duodenojejunal flexure (Fig. 2-70), and the ileum joins the cecum at the ileocecal valve (Fig. 2-96). The term **jejunoileum** is occasionally used for these parts of the small intestine because *there is no clear line of demarcation between the jejunum and the ileum*, but the character of the small intestine does change gradually. The jejunum and ileum are 6 to 7 m long, the upper two-fifths of which is considered to be jejunum.

As *intestinal localization is of surgical importance*, the gross characteristics of the jejunum and the ileum will be described. The jejunum is often empty, hence its name (L. *jejunus*, empty). It is *thicker, more vascular, and redder in living persons than is the ileum.* Most of the jejunum usually lies in the umbilical region of the abdomen, whereas the ileum occupies much of the hypogastric and pelvic regions. The terminal part of the ileum usually lies in the pelvis and ascends over the right psoas major muscle and the right iliac vessels to enter the cecum (Figs. 2-42 and 2-96). The **circular folds** or **plicae circulares** of the mucous membrane are large and well developed in the upper jejunum (Fig. 2-97), whereas they are small in the upper ileum and absent in the terminal ileum. When the living jejunum is grasped between the forefinger and thumb, *the plicae circulares can be distinctly felt through the wall of the upper jejunum.* As they are low and sparse in the upper ileum and absent in the lower ileum, it is possible to distinguish the upper from the lower part of the jejunum and ileum.

The Mesentery of the Jejunum and Ileum (Figs. 2-40, 2-69, 2-98, 2-99, 2-101, and 2-102). The jejunum and ileum are

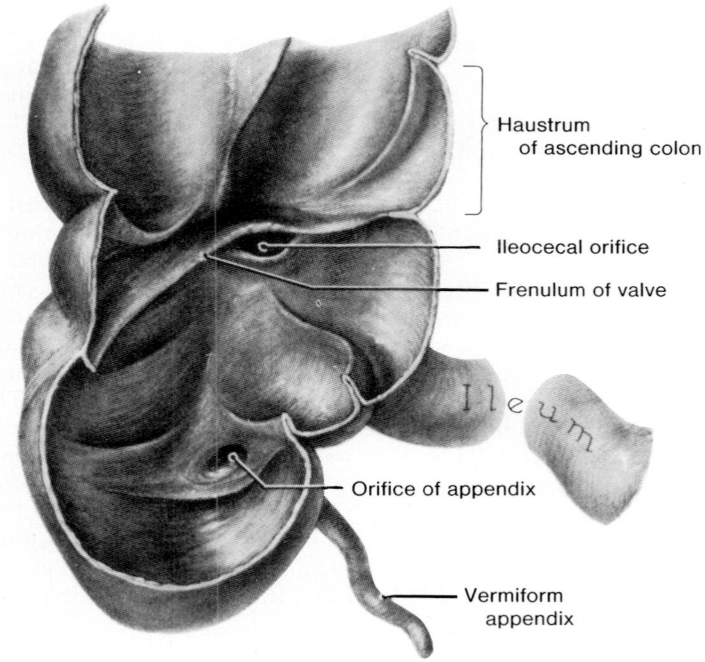

Haustrum of ascending colon
Ileocecal orifice
Frenulum of valve
Ileum
Orifice of appendix
Vermiform appendix

Figure 2-96. Drawing of the interior of a dried cecum. This cecum was filled with air until dry and then opened and varnished. Observe the ileocecal valve guarding the iliocecal orifice. Note that its upper lip overhangs its lower lip. Note the folds or frenula running horizontally from the commissures of the lips and the slight fold closing the upper part of the orifice of the appendix.

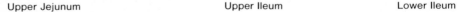

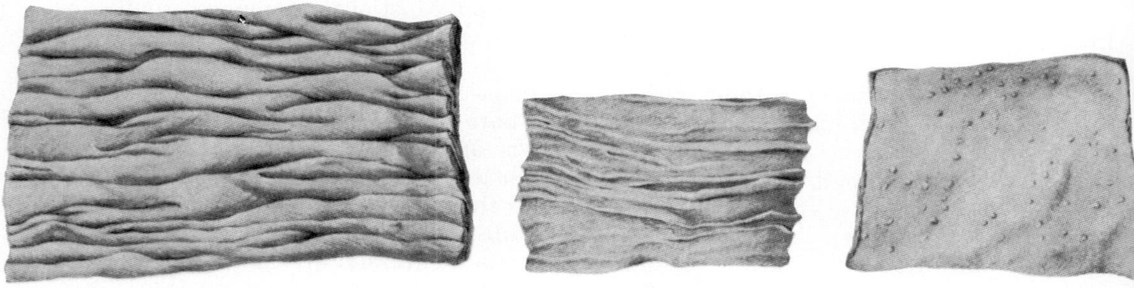

Upper Jejunum
Upper Ileum
Lower Ileum

Figure 2-97. Drawing of the interior of the jejunum and ileum. Observe that the permanent circular folds or plicae semilunares are: large, tall, and closely packed in the upper jejunum; low and sparse in the upper ileum; and absent in the lower ileum. Note that the caliber of the ileum is reduced compared with the jejunum. Observe the solitary lymph nodules which stud the wall of the lower ileum. Occasionally, aggregated lymph nodules (Peyer's patches) are found on the antimesenteric wall of the ileum, especially near its junction with the colon.

suspended from the posterior abdominal wall by a fan-shaped mesentery. The vertebral border or **root of the mesentery**, attached to the posterior abdominal wall, is about 15 cm long. It is directed obliquely downward and to the right *from the left side of the second lumbar vertebra to the right sacroiliac joint.* Between these two points, **the root of the mesentery crosses** (1) the *third or horizontal part of the duodenum*, (2) the *aorta*, (3) the *inferior vena cava*, (4) the *psoas major muscle*,

(5) the *right ureter*, and (6) the *right testicular or ovarian vessels.*

The mesentery consists of two layers of peritoneum, between which are the jejunal and ileal blood vessels, lymph nodes and vessels, nerves, and extraperitoneal fatty tissue. *The jejunal mesentery contains less fat than that of the ileum; thus the* **arterial arcades** (Figs. 2-101 and 2-102) *are easier to observe.* This anatomical characteristic helps the surgeon to differentiate the jejunum from the ileum at the operating table. Another method used by surgeons is passing their fingers down the mesentery to its root. By passing the fingers to the right or left along the root of the mesentery, the proximal and distal ends of the jejunum and ileum may be determined.

The Vessels and Nerves of the Jejunum and Ileum (Figs. 2-55, 2-98 to 2-103, and 2-143). The **arteries** to the jejunum and ileum arise from the **superior mesenteric artery**. This is the second of the unpaired branches of the abdominal aorta, the celiac trunk being the first (Figs. 2-55 and 2-143*A*). *The superior mesenteric artery usually arises from the aorta at the level of the first lumbar vertebra*, about 1 cm below the celiac trunk and posterior to the body of the pancreas and the splenic vein. It descends across the left renal vein, the uncinate process of the pancreas, and the horizontal or third part of the duodenum to enter the mesentery (Fig. 2-71). It runs obliquely in the root of the mesentery to the right iliac fossa, sending branches to the intestines (Fig. 2-98). Its last branch anastomoses with a branch of the ileocolic artery. The *superior mesenteric artery and its branches are surrounded by a plexus of sympathetic and parasympathetic nerve fibers* (Figs. 2-111 and 2-127). Each plexus is named after the vessel it surrounds.

The **15 to 18 jejunal and ileal branches** arise from the left side of the superior mesenteric artery and pass between the two layers of the mesentery. These arteries unite to form loops or arches called **arterial arcades** (Figs. 2-100 to 2-102) from which **vasa recta** (L. straight vessels) arise. *The vasta recta do not anastomose within the mesentery*; hence, "windows" appear between the vessels (Fig. 2-101). The vasa recta pass from the arcades to the mesenteric border of the intestine, where they pass more or less alternately to opposite sides. *There are many anastomoses in the wall of the intestine* (Figs. 2-101 and 2-102). The vascularity of the wall is greater in the jejunum than in the ileum, but the *arterial arcades are shorter and more complex in the ileum.* These vascular differences are also used by surgeons to differentiate the ileum from the jejunum at the operating table.

The superior mesenteric vein drains the jejunum and ileum (Fig. 2-85). It accompanies the superior mesenteric artery, lying anterior and to its right in the root of the mesentery (Fig. 2-105). It crosses the horizontal or third part of the duodenum and the uncinate process of the pancreas (Fig. 2-71) before terminating behind the neck of the pancreas by uniting with the splenic vein to form the portal vein (Fig. 2-57). The tributaries of the superior mesenteric vein have an arrangement similar to the branches of the superior mesenteric artery and they drain the same area supplied by the artery.

The lymphatics in the intestinal villi, called **lacteals** (L. *lactis*, milk), empty their milk-like fluid into a plexus of lymph vessels in the wall of the jejunum and ileum (Fig. 2-103). The lymph vessels then pass between the two layers of the mesentery to the 100 to 150 **mesenteric lymph nodes** (Figs. 2-102 and 2-109). *The mesenteric lymph nodes are in three locations*: (1) close to the wall of the intestine, (2) amongst the arterial arcades, and (3) along the upper part of the trunk of the superior mesenteric artery. *Lymph vessels from the terminal ileum follow the ileal branch of the ileocolic artery to the ileocolic lymph nodes* (Fig. 2-109).

The nerves of the jejunum and ileum are derived from the **vagus** and the **splanchnic (visceral) nerves** through the celiac ganglion and the plexuses around the superior mesenteric artery (Figs. 2-111 and 2-127). The superior mesenteric nerve plexus receives its parasympathetic fibers from the celiac division of the **posterior vagal trunk** and its sympathetic fibers from the **superior mesenteric ganglion**.

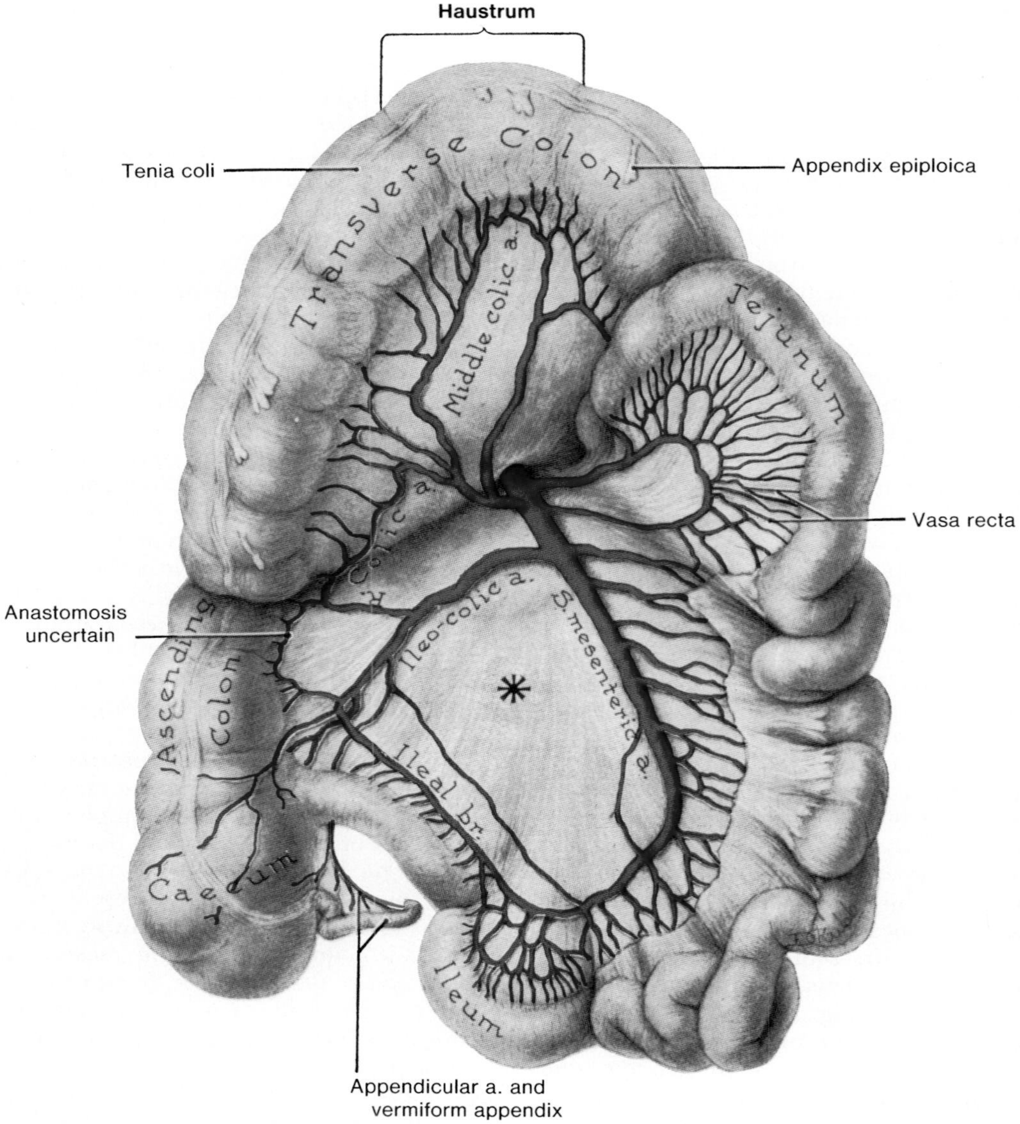

Figure 2-98. Drawing of a dissection demonstrating the *superior mesenteric artery*. The peritoneum is partly stripped off. Observe the extensive field of supply of the superior mesenteric artery. Note that it ends by anastomosing with one of its own branches, the ileal branch of the ileocolic artery. Examine the branches of the superior mesenteric artery: (1) *from its left side*, 12 to 20 jejunal and ileal branches which anastomose to form arcades from which vasa recta pass to the small intestine; and (2) *from its right side*, the middle colic, the ileocolic, and commonly, but not here, an independent right colic artery. These anastomose to form a **marginal artery** (labelled in Fig. 2-107) from which vasa recta pass to the large intestine; (3) the two inferior pancreaticoduodenal arteries (not in view but seen in Fig. 2-66) arise from the main artery either directly or in conjunction with the jejunal branch. Note the teniae coli, sacculations or haustra, and appendices epiploicae, which distinguish the large intestine from the smooth-walled small intestine. The *asterisk* indicates the area of the mesentery between the superior mesenteric and ileocolic arteries which is almost avascular and liable to break down and produce a hole through which the other coils of small intestine may herniate. This is one type of *internal hernia*.

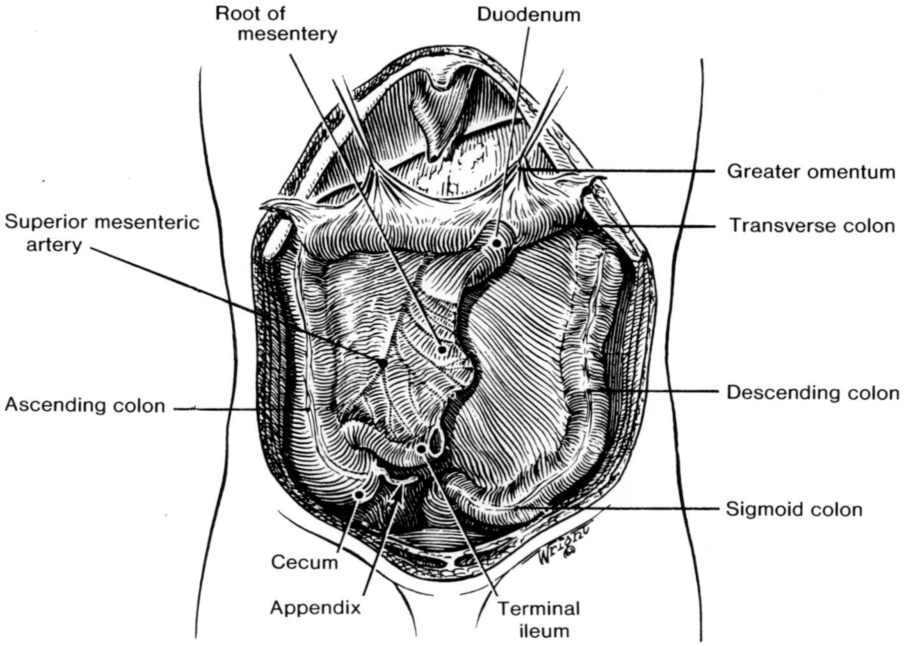

Figure 2-99. Drawing illustrating the root of the mesentery. The jejunum and ileum are removed. Note that the root of the mesentery extends in an oblique manner from the left side at the level of the second lumbar vertebra to the right sacroiliac joint, a distance of about 15 cm.

CLINICALLY ORIENTED COMMENTS

Congenital malformations resulting from abnormal rotation of the midgut during the prenatal period are not uncommon. Sometimes the intestinal loops fail to return to the abdominal cavity from the umbilical cord during the 10th fetal week. This hernia or **omphalocele** may consist of a single loop of intestine or may contain most of the GI tract. The wall of the hernial sac is formed by the **amnion** covering the umbilical cord.

Sometimes the intestines return to the abdominal cavity during the fetal period, but there is incomplete closure of the anterior abdominal wall in the umbilical region. As a result, an intestinal loop herniates in the umbilical cord again, forming a **congenital umbilical hernia**, often no larger than a cherry.

Abnormal rotation and lack of fixation of the midgut loop sometimes occurs when it returns to the abdominal cavity. *Incomplete rotation usually results in nonfixation of the mesentery*, and the entire midgut loop may hang from a narrow pedicle. This sometimes results in twisting of the intestine and the superior mesenteric vessels. This twisting, called a **volvulus** (L. *volvo*, to roll), may render the small intestine **ischemic** (deficient in blood) and even **necrotic** (dying tissue). Rupture of its wall may occur if the condition is not corrected promptly after symptoms of intestinal obstruction begin. The irregularities resulting from malrotation and improper fixation are numerous (*e.g.*, **left-sided appendix**), but the surgeon with a sound knowledge of the normal stages of intestinal rotation has little difficulty understanding the embryological basis of the congenital abnormality.

Meckel's diverticulum (Fig. 2-104) is one of the most common malformations of the digestive tract. It represents the *remnant of the proximal part of the embryonic yolk stalk* (vitelline duct). A Meckel's diverticulum is of clinical significance because it sometimes becomes inflamed and causes symptoms mimicking appendicitis.

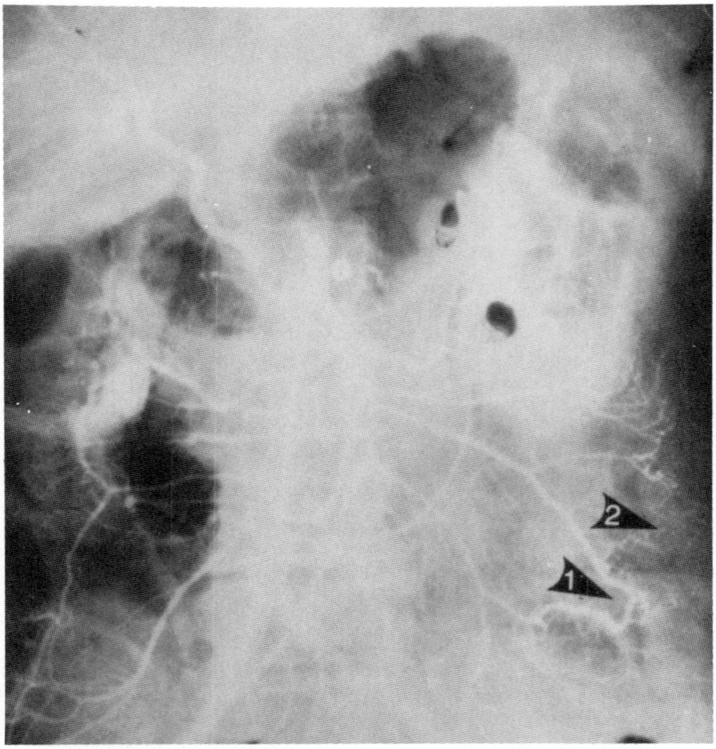

Figure 2-100. Arteriogram of the superior mesenteric artery. Branches of the celiac trunk are also prominent in this radiograph. Observe in particular, examples of anastomotic loops or arterial arcades (*1*) and vasa recta (*2*). *Compare with Figure 2-98*. The superior mesenteric artery supplies all of the small intestine, except the proximal part of the duodenum. It also supplies the large intestine to near the left colic flexure. Superior mesenteric arteriograms are useful for determining if any of the branches of the artery are occluded.

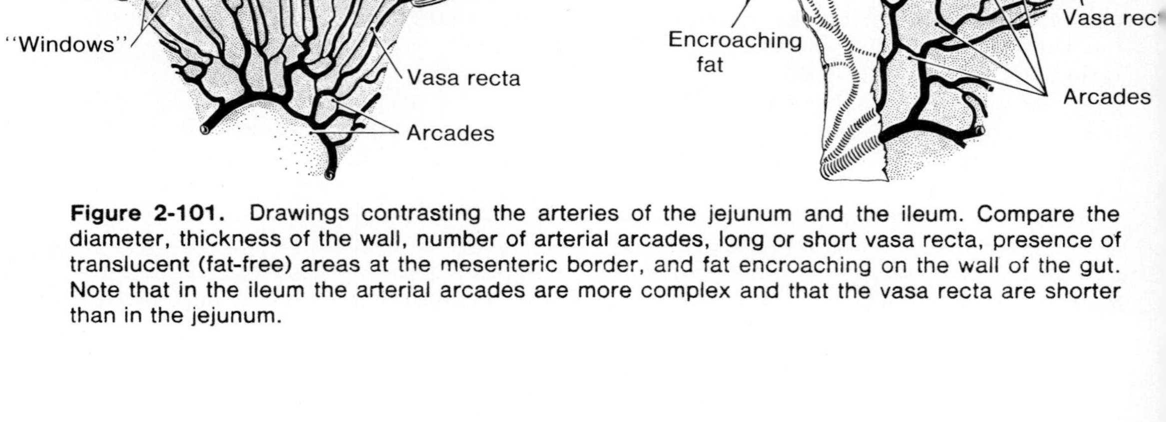

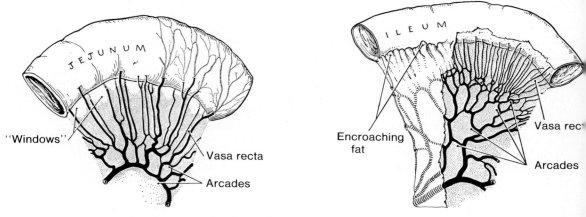

Figure 2-101. Drawings contrasting the arteries of the jejunum and the ileum. Compare the diameter, thickness of the wall, number of arterial arcades, long or short vasa recta, presence of translucent (fat-free) areas at the mesenteric border, and fat encroaching on the wall of the gut. Note that in the ileum the arterial arcades are more complex and that the vasa recta are shorter than in the jejunum.

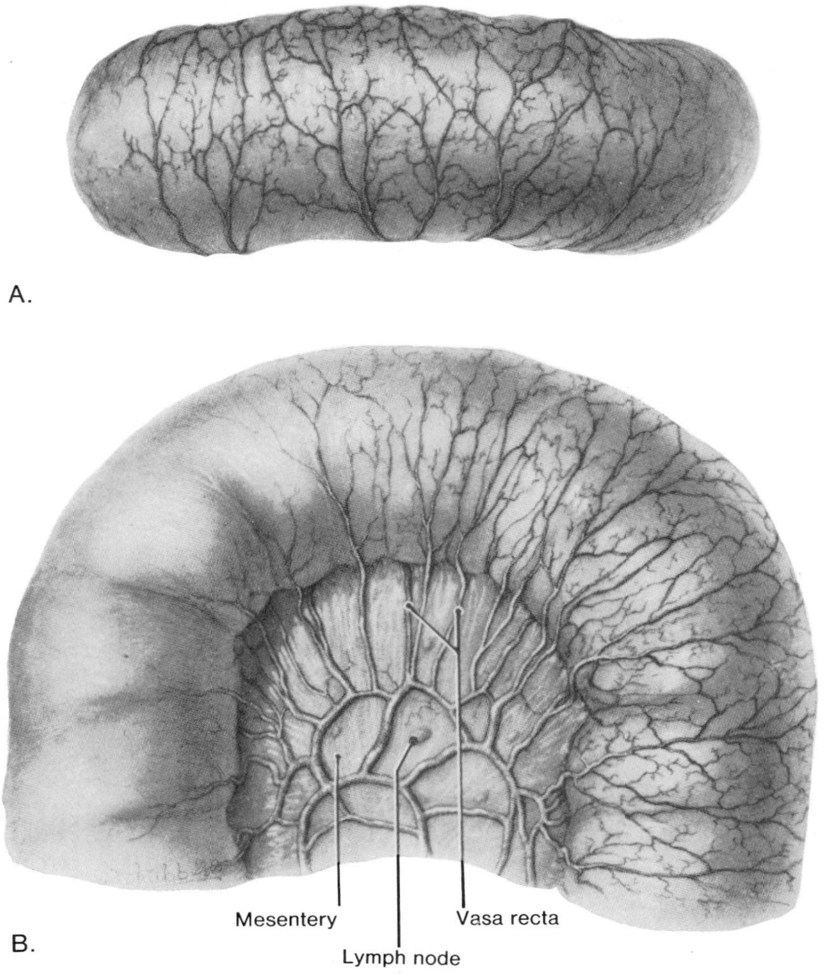

Figure 2-102. Drawings illustrating the blood supply of the small intestine. *A*, antimesenteric border. *B*, segment of jejunum with its mesentery and arteries. Observe the series of anastomotic arterial arches in the mesentery. Note that the vasa recta proceed from the arches to the mesenteric border of the intestine and then pass more or less alternately to opposite sides of the intestine. Examine the arborizations of the vasa recta in the wall of the intestine and the fine anastomoses effected between adjacent arborizations. Observe the efficient anastomoses across the antimesenteric border. Note the mesenteric lymph nodes. Enlargement of these nodes occurs in many diseases of the intestine.

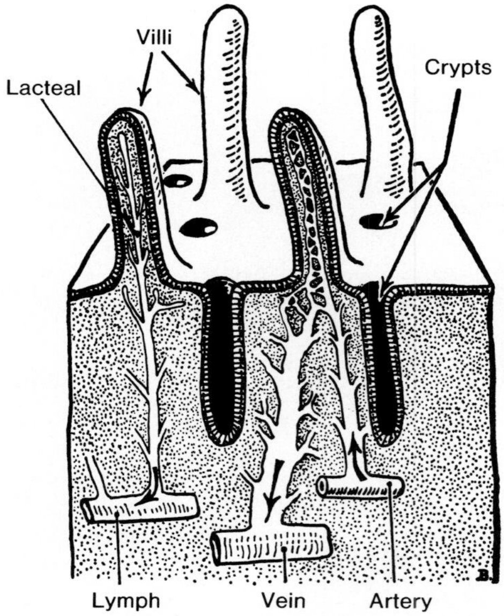

Figure 2-103. Three-dimensional diagram of a microscopic piece of small intestine. The villi are drained by both veins and lymphatics. Small fat particles pass between the endothelial cells into the lymphatic capillaries called lacteals. The milk-like lymph then passes to a lymph vessel in the wall of the intestine.

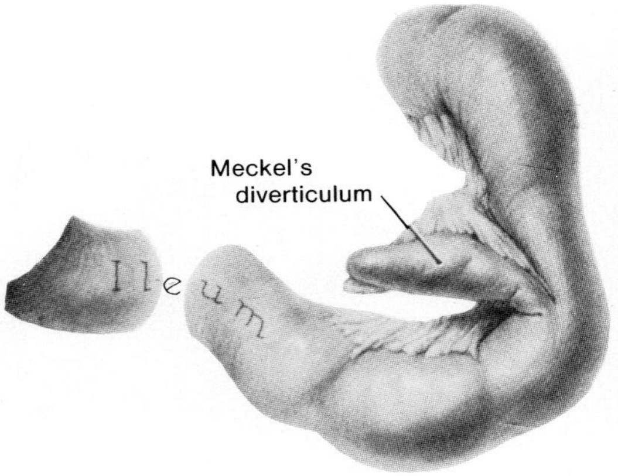

Figure 2-104. Drawing of the ileum illustrating a Meckel's diverticulum. This outpouching of the ileum, found in 2 to 4% of people, is the remains of the embryonic yolk stalk. It projects from the antimesenteric border of the ileum. Inflammation of this diverticulum may simulate appendicitis.

The wall of the diverticulum contains all layers of the ileum and may contain patches of gastric-type epithelium and pancreatic tissue. The gastric mucosa often secretes acid, producing ulceration and bleeding of the diverticulum. *Typically, a Meckel's diverticulum is a finger-like blind pouch,* 3 to 6 cm long, projecting from the antimesenteric border of the ileum, within 50 cm of the ileocecal junction. A Meckel's diverticulum may be connected to the umbilicus by a fibrous cord or a fistula (persistent yolk stalk or vitilline duct).

Occlusion of a series of vasa recta (arteries or veins) results in poor nutrition or drainage of the part of the intestine concerned. A thrombosis of a vein or an embolus in an artery *may* lead to necrosis of the segment of bowel concerned and **ileus** of the paralytic type. If the condition can be diagnosed early enough (*e.g.*, using a **superior mesenteric arteriogram**, Fig. 2-100), the obstructed portion of the vessel may be cleared surgically. Owing to the many anastomoses of blood vessels, blockage of a single vessel or group of vessels is not usually followed by **gangrene** of the mesentery or the intestine.

The Large Intestine (Figs. 2-33, 2-40 to 2-43, 2-52, 2-98, and 2-105 to 2-109). General features of the large intestine have been described previously. The large intestine, about 1.5 m long, extends from the cecum in the right iliac fossa to the anus in the perineum. Although in general larger in diameter than the small intestine, it may not always be. Hence, its characteristic distinguishing features must be noted (Figs. 2-41 to 2-43): **teniae coli**, **haustra**, and **appendices epiploicae** (see previous description on page 164).

The Cecum and Vermiform Appendix (Figs. 2-33*A*, 2-43 to 2-45, 2-51, 2-96, 2-98, and 2-105). The cecum is a blind sac, continuous with the ascending colon, into which the terminal ileum and the vermiform appendix enter posteromedially. The ileum enters the cecum obliquely and is partly invaginated into it, forming lips or folds above and below the **ileocecal orifice** which constitute the **ileocecal valve**. These lips meet medially and laterally to form ridges, called the **frenula** of the ileocecal valve (Fig. 2-96). When the cecum

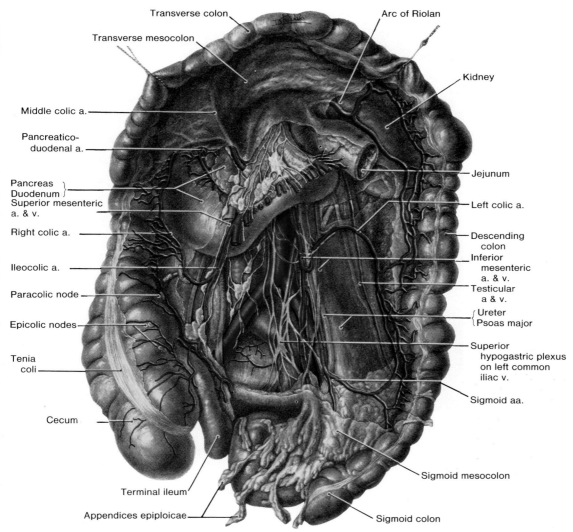

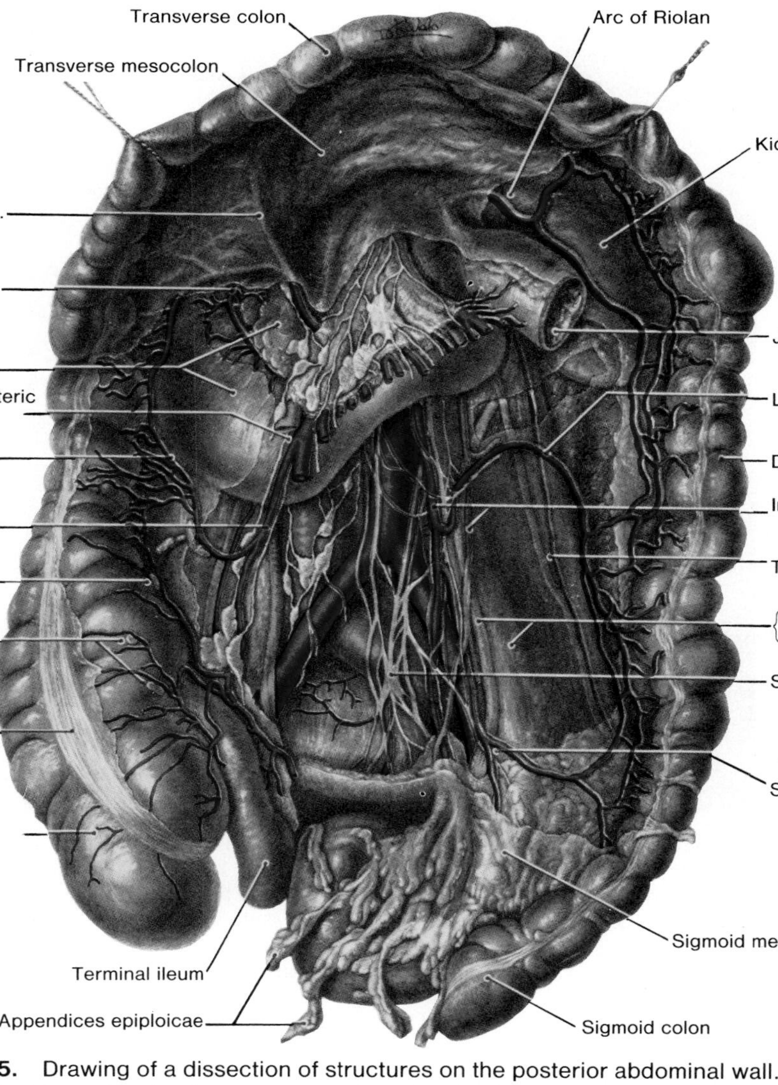

Figure 2-105. Drawing of a dissection of structures on the posterior abdominal wall. Observe the jejunal and ileal branches (cut) passing from the left side of the superior mesenteric artery and the right colic artery, here, as commonly, a branch of the ileocolic artery. Note the accessory artery, called the arc of Riolan, which connects the superior mesenteric artery to the left colic artery. On the right side observe the small epicolic lymph nodes on the colon, the small paracolic nodes beside the colon, and the lymph nodes along the ileocolic artery which drain into the main nodes ventral to the pancreas. Note that the intestines and the intestinal vessels lie on a plane anterior to that of the testicular vessels, and that these in turn lie anterior to the plane of the kidney, its vessels, and the ureter. Observe that the right and left ureters are asymmetrically placed in this specimen. Examine the superior hypogastric plexus (presacral nerve) lying within the fork of the aorta and ventral to the left common iliac vein, the body of the fifth lumbar vertebra, and the fifth intervertebral disc.

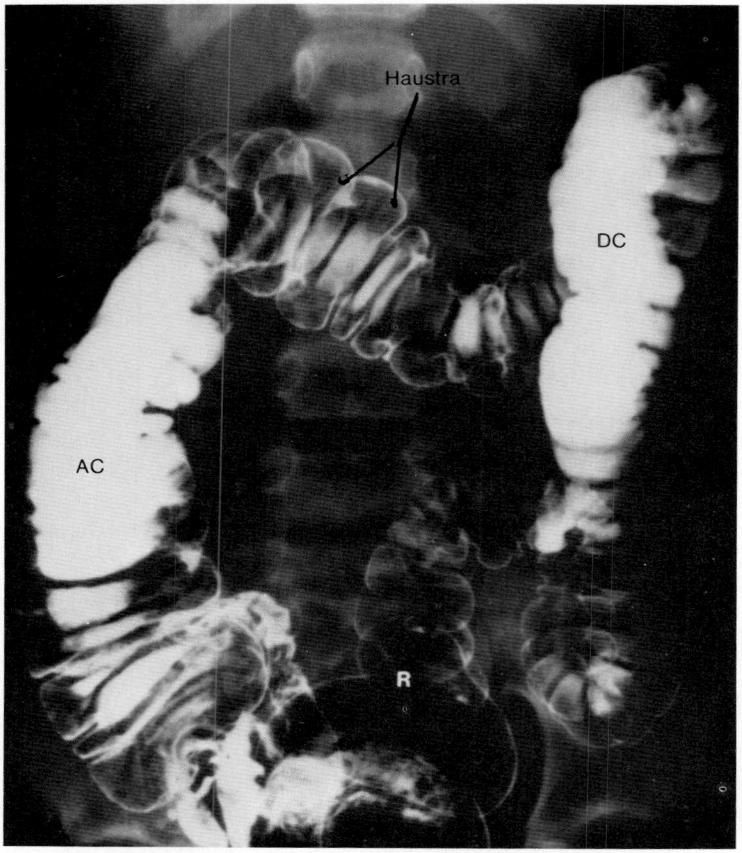

Figure 2-106. Radiograph of the large intestine. (If orientation is needed, see Figs. 2-33*A* and 2-42). After evacuating the barium introduced by a barium enema, the colon was inflated with air and a radiogaph was made in the supine position. Observe that the barium clinging to the walls of the air-filled parts of the colon gives a good view of the hausta. As the colon seldom can be completely evacuated, as in this patient, parts of the right and left colon are still filled with the barium sulphate emulsion (*white areas*). *AC*, ascending colon. *DC*, descending colon. *R*, rectum.

is distended the frenula tighten, drawing the lips of the valve together. However, as the circular muscle is poorly developed in these lips, *the ileocecal valve has little sphincteric action.* Following a barium enema, barium commonly enters the terminal ileum (Fig. 2-42); hence, it probably is unable to prevent reflux of the normal cecal contents into the ileum. Contraction of the circular muscle of the terminal ileum is probably more important in preventing excessive reflux of material.

The cecum and appendix are supplied by the **ileocolic artery** (Figs. 2-40, 2-43 and 2-98), a branch of the superior mesenteric artery. The **ileocolic vein**, a tributary of the superior mesenteric vein, drains blood from the cecum and appendix (Fig. 2-85). **Lymph vessels** from the cecum and appendix pass to lymph nodes in the mesentery of the appendix and to those along the ileocolic artery (Fig. 2-109). The **nerves** are derived from the **superior mesenteric plexus** (Fig. 2-111).

The Ascending Colon (Figs. 2-33*A*, 2-39, 2-40, 2-42, 2-51, 2-98, 2-105, 2-106, 2-109, and 2-119). The ascending colon, 12 to 20 cm long, is narrower than the cecum. *It extends from the ileocecal valve to the right colic flexure*, where it lies between the inferior surface of the liver and the front of the right kidney. It ascends retroperitoneally on the posterior abdominal wall in the right **paravertebral groove**

(Fig. 2-110). It is separated from the muscles posteriorly by the kidney and the nerves of the posterior abdominal wall (Figs. 2-113 and 2-134). It is usually separated from the anterior abdominal wall by coils of small intestine and the greater omentum (Fig. 2-29).

The ascending colon is covered by peritoneum on its front and sides, which attach it to the posterior abdominal wall. On the lateral side of the ascending colon, the peritoneum forms a trench called the **right paracolic gutter** (Figs. 2-28 and 2-110). The depth of this gutter depends on how much gas the ascending colon contains. Fluid in the right **hepatorenal recess** (Fig. 2-32) passes along the right paracolic gutter to the **rectouterine** or **rectovesical pouch** when the person is in an inclined position (*Fowler's position*).

The ascending colon and right colic flexure are supplied by the **ileocolic** and **right colic arteries**, branches of the superior mesenteric artery (Fig. 2-98). The **ileocolic** and **right colic veins**, tributaries of the superior mesenteric vein, drain blood from the ascending colon. The **lymph vessels** of the ascending colon pass to the *paracolic lymph nodes* (Fig. 2-105) and end in the *superior mesenteric lymph nodes* (Fig. 2-109). The nerves are derived from the **superior mesenteric plexus** (Fig. 2-111).

The Transverse Colon (Figs. 2-36, 2-38 to 2-40, 2-42, 2-51, 2-52, 2-98, 2-99, 2-105 to 2-107, and 2-109). The transverse colon, 40 to 50 cm long, is the *largest and most mobile part of the colon.* It **extends between the right and left colic flexures**, forming a loop that is directed downward and forward. In some people it drops as low as the pelvis when they are in the erect position. The transverse colon is suspended posteriorly by the **transverse mesocolon**, a broad fold of peritoneum that passes forward from the pancreas (Figs. 2-38, 2-46, and 2-52). The transverse mesocolon is fused to the posterior surface of the greater omentum (Figs. 2-36 and 2-46).

The transverse colon is supplied mainly by the middle colic artery, a branch of the **superior mesenteric artery**, but it also receives blood from the **right** and **left colic arteries** (Fig. 2-98). *The left colic is a branch of the inferior mesenteric artery.* Blood is drained from the transverse colon via the **superior mesenteric vein** (Fig. 2-85). The **lymph vessels** of the transverse colon end in the **superior mesenteric lymph nodes** after traversing nodes located along the middle colic artery (Fig. 2-109).

The nerves on the right and middle colic arteries are derived from the **superior mesenteric plexus** (Fig. 2-111) and transmit sympathetic and vagal nerve fibers, whereas those on the left colic artery are derived from the **inferior mesenteric plexus** and carry sympathetic and pelvic parasympathetic fibers.

The Descending Colon (Figs. 2-33, 2-39, 2-40, 2-42, 2-51, 2-85, 2-99, 2-105 to 2-110, and 2-113). The descending colon passes inferiorly from the left colic flexure to the brim of the pelvis, where it *joins the sigmoid colon.* It is usually narrower than other parts of the colon and, like the ascending colon, it **lies retroperitoneally**. The descending colon passes inferiorly anterior to the lateral border of the left kidney and the transversus abdominis and quadratus lumborum muscles to the left iliac fossa. It then curves medially and downward over the iliacus and psoas major muscles as it *joins the sigmoid colon.*

The descending colon is supplied by the **left colic** and **upper sigmoid arteries** (Fig. 2-107), branches of the inferior mesenteric artery. The **inferior mesenteric vein** drains the descending colon (Fig. 2-85). The **lymph vessels** from the descending colon pass to the lymph nodes along the left colic arteries and then to the **inferior mesenteric lymph nodes** around the inferior mesenteric artery (Fig. 2-109); however, those from the left colic flexure also drain to the **superior mesenteric lymph nodes** by vessels that accompany the superior mesenteric vein.

The Sigmoid Colon (Figs. 2-33, 2-40, 2-42, 2-51, 2-105 to 2-110, and 2-113). This **S-shaped part** of the colon varies in length from 15 to 80 cm but averages about 30 cm. The sigmoid (pelvic) colon extends from the descending colon to the third piece of the sacrum, where it *joins the rectum.* It is suspended from the pelvic wall by a $\wedge$-shaped mesentery, the **sigmoid mesocolon** (Fig. 2-105). The center of the sigmoid

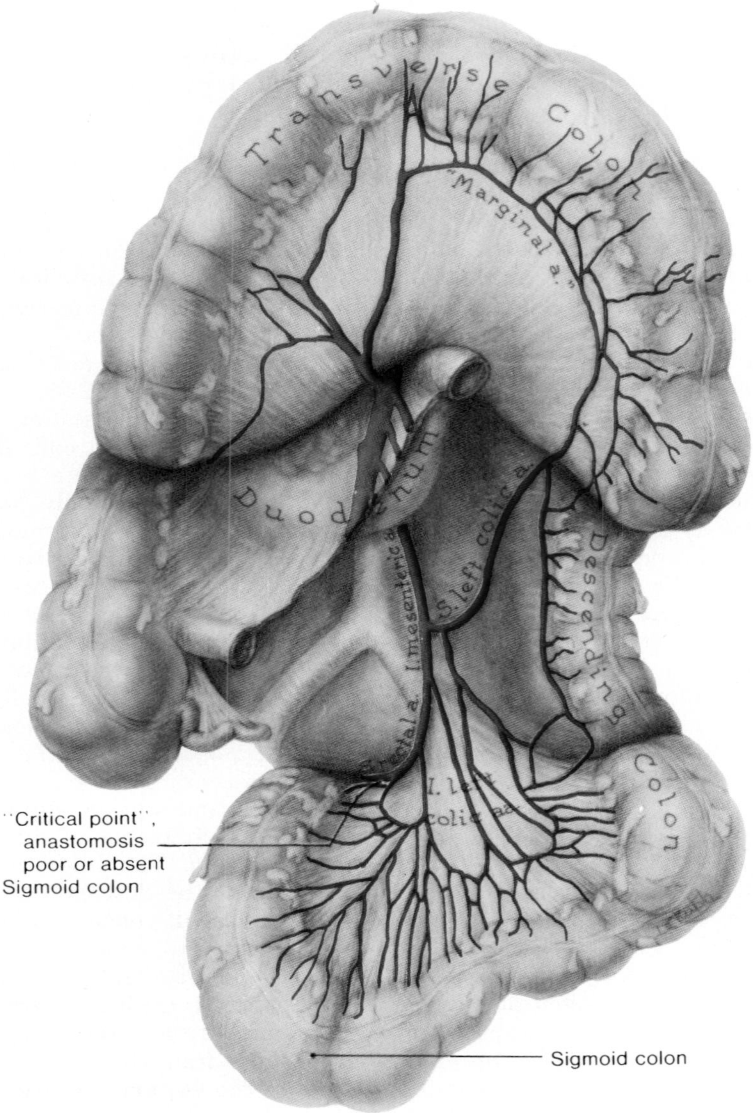

Figure 2-107. Drawing of a dissection illustrating the inferior mesenteric artery. The mesentery has been cut at its root and discarded with the jejunum and ileum. Observe the inferior mesenteric artery arising behind the duodenum, above the bifurcation of the aorta. On crossing the left common iliac artery, it becomes the superior rectal artery. Note its branches: (1) a superior left colic artery and (2) several sigmoid arteries (inferior left colic arteries) springing from its left side. In this specimen, the two lowest sigmoid arteries spring from the superior rectal artery. The point at which the last artery to the colon leaves the artery to the rectum is known as the "critical point of Sudeck."

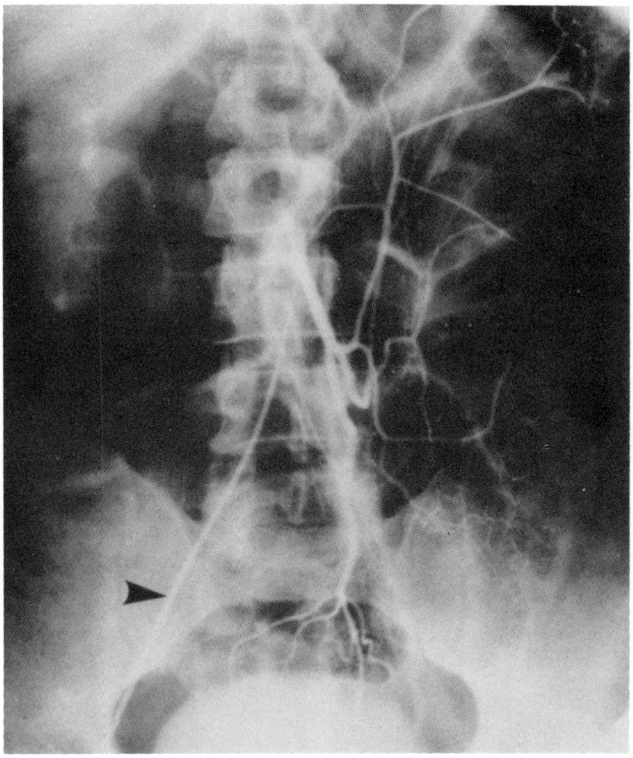

Figure 2-108. Arteriogram of the inferior mesenteric artery. (Compare with Fig. 2-107). Observe the left colic artery, the sigmoid arteries, and the termination of the inferior mesenteric artery as the superior rectal artery. An *arrow* points to an arterial catheter which was inserted percutaneously into the femoral artery, just inferior to the inguinal ligament (see Figs. 2-13 and 4-32).

colon is its longest part. *The apex of this mesentery lies anterior to the left ureter* and the division of the left common iliac artery. **The sigmoid colon forms a loop,** the shape and position of which depends upon how full it is. Usually it lies relatively free within the pelvis minor, below the small intestine (Fig. 2-33*A*). Posterior to the sigmoid colon are the left external iliac vessels, the left sacral plexus, and the left piriformis muscle (Fig. 2-113).

The two to three **sigmoid arteries** supply the lower part of the descending colon and the sigmoid colon. The **inferior mesenteric vein** returns blood from the sigmoid colon (Fig. 2-85). **Lymph vessels** from the sigmoid colon pass to lymph nodes on the branches of the left colic arteries and end in the **inferior mesenteric lymph nodes** around the inferior mesenteric artery (Fig. 2-109).

The Rectum and The Anal Canal (Figs. 2-33, 2-42, 2-51, 2-106, and 2-109). Brief descriptions of these regions of the large intestine have been given on page 168. Detailed descriptions are given in Chapter 3 on the pelvis.

CLINICALLY ORIENTED COMMENTS

A chronic disease of the colon of unknown origin, called **ulcerative colitis,** is characterized by severe *inflammation and ulceration of the colon and rectum.* In some of these patients, a **total colectomy** is

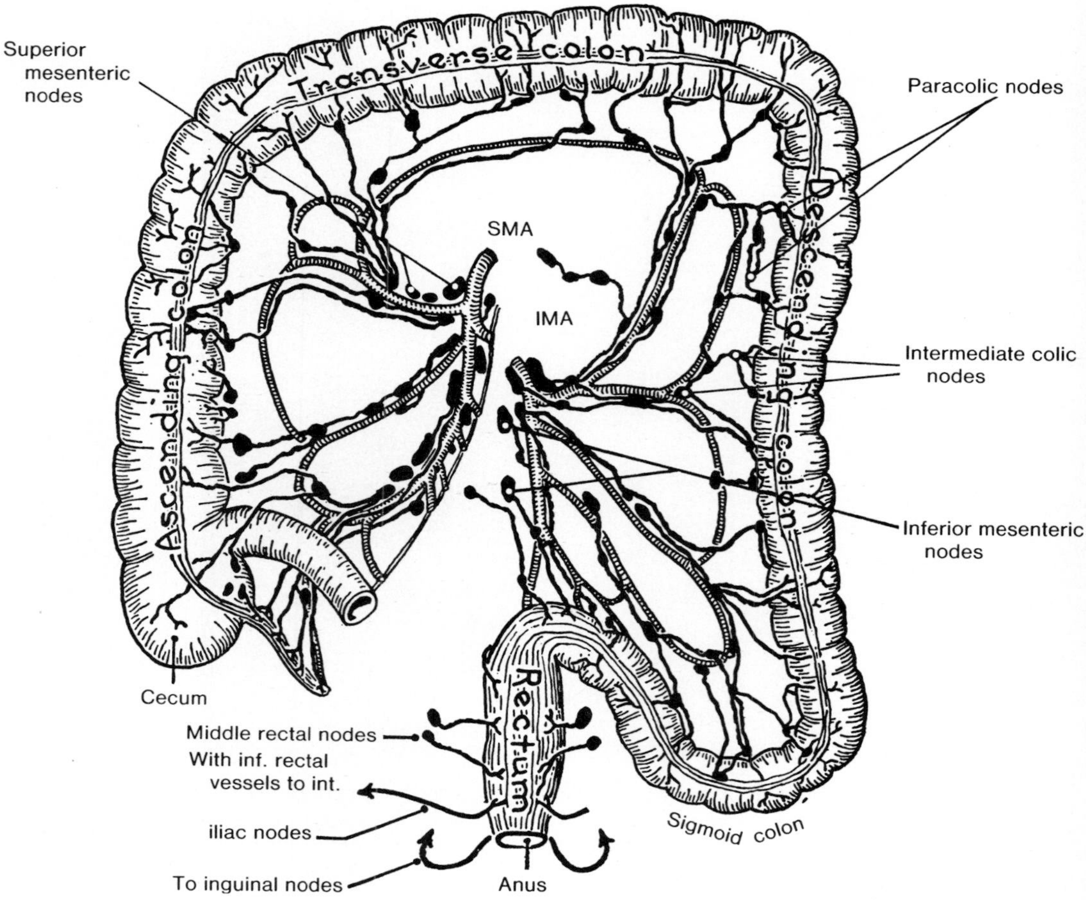

Figure 2-109. Diagram illustrating the lymphatics of the large intestine. The lymph nodes of the colon are in four groups: (1) *epicolic nodes* on the wall of the gut (Fig. 2-105); (2) *paracolic nodes* along the medial borders of the ascending and descending colon; (3) *intermediate nodes* along the right, middle, and left colic arteries; and (4) *terminal colic nodes* near the main trunks of the superior (*SMA*) and inferior (*IMA*) mesenteric arteries.

performed during which the terminal ileum, ascending, transverse, descending, and sigmoid colon, as well as the rectum and anal canal, are removed. A permanent **ileostomy** is then constructed to establish an opening between the ileum and the skin of the anterior abdominal wall. In **subtotal colectomy**, the rectum and anal canal are preserved and the ileum is joined to the rectum by an *end-to-end anastomosis*.

Colostomies establish an opening (G. *stoma*, mouth) between the colon and the skin of the anterior abdominal wall, creating a temporary **fecal fistula** or a permanent **artificial anus.** The most mobile parts of the colon are used; thus the usual colostomies are: *cecostomy*, *transverse colostomy*, and *sigmoidostomy*). The type of colostomy constructed depends upon which part of the colon has been resected. When parts of the colon are resected, it must be ensured that an adequate blood supply to the remaining segments is preserved. Failure to do so would result in **necrosis** of the segment of intestine concerned.

Herniations (diverticula) of the mucosa through the muscularis mucosae of the sigmoid colon are common. This con-

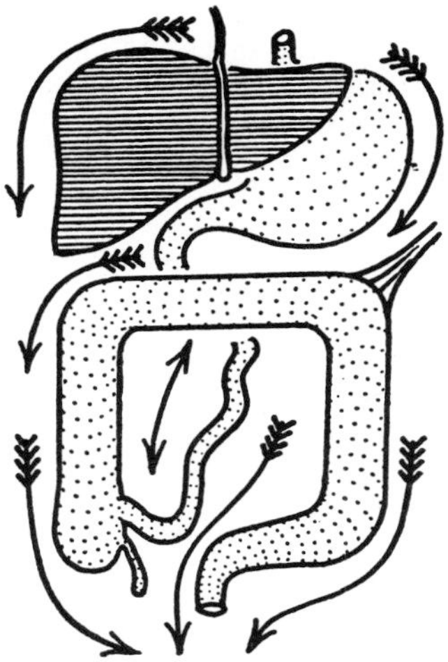

Figure 2-110. Diagram illustrating the peritoneal gutters which can conduct fluid (*e.g.*, ascites, inflammatory material, blood, bile, etc.,) from one part of the peritoneal cavity to another. The right lateral or paracolic gutter to the right of the ascending colon may conduct fluid from the omental bursa via the hepatorenal pouch (Fig. 2-32) into the pelvis. The left lateral or paracolic gutter to the left of the descending colon is closed cranially by the phrenicocolic ligament (Fig. 2-52). The gutter to the right of the mesentery is closed cranially and caudally. The gutter to the left of the mesentery opens widely into the pelvis.

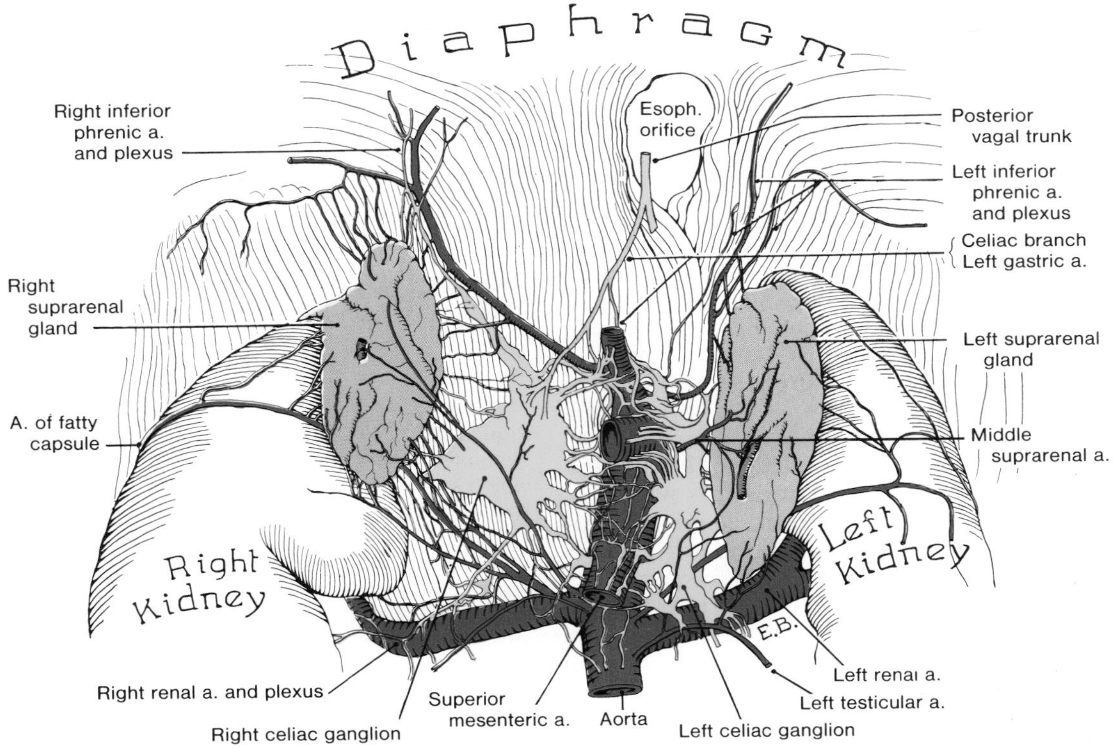

Figure 2-111. Drawing of a dissection showing the celiac trunk, plexus, and ganglia, and the suprarenal glands. Observe the celiac plexus of nerves surrounding the celiac trunk (not labelled) and connecting the right and left celiac ganglia. Note a stout branch from the posterior vagal trunk descending along the stem of the left gastric artery and conveying vagal (parasympathetic) fibers to the celiac ganglia. Examine the nerves extending along the arteries to the viscera and down the aorta. The nerves to the suprarenal glands are mostly preganglionic.

dition, known as **diverticulosis**, can be observed in about 10% of persons over 40 years of age who have barium enemas for radiological studies (Fig. 2-149). When one or more of the diverticula become inflamed, the condition is known as **diverticulitis**. For the usual signs and symptoms of this condition, see Case 2-5.

The Portal Vein and the Portal-Systemic Anastomoses (Figs. 2-57, 2-85, and 2-112). *The Portal vein drains the abdominal and pelvic parts of the GI system,* except for the distal part of the anal canal. It also drains blood from the spleen, pancreas, and gallbladder. The portal vein is formed posterior to the neck of the pancreas by the *union of the splenic and superior mesenteric veins.* The inferior mesenteric vein opens into (1) the splenic vein (Fig. 2-85), (2) the junction of the splenic and superior mesenteric veins (Fig. 2-57), *or* (3) the superior mesenteric vein (Fig. 2-47); thus, *the portal vein carries blood from three major veins.* The course of the portal vein in the free edge of the lesser omentum (Fig. 2-90) has been discussed.

At the **porta hepatis** (Fig. 2-83), *the portal vein divides into right and left branches* which empty their blood into the **hepatic sinusoids** (Fig. 2-86). This blood contains the products of digestion of carbohydrates, fats, and protein from the intestine and the products of red cell destruction from the spleen.

The Portal-Systemic Anastomoses (Fig. 2-112). **In several locations the portal venous system communicates with the systemic venous system.** *These anastomoses are very important clinically.* When the portal circulation is obstructed (*e.g.*, owing to liver disease) blood from the GI tract can still reach the right side of the heart (Fig. 2-144) through the inferior vena cava via a number of **collateral routes**. The portal vein and its tributaries have no valves; hence, blood can flow from the obstructed liver to the inferior vena cava through these alternate routes. In **portal hypertension** venous pressure in the portal venous system is increased; consequently, some blood in the portal venous system may reverse its direction and pass through the portal-systemic anastomoses into the systemic venous system. This causes the veins in the portal-systemic

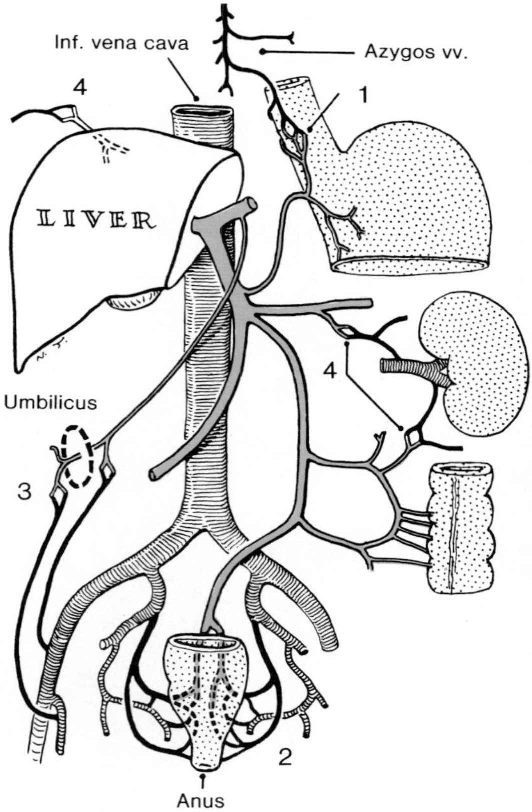

Figure 2-112. Diagram illustrating the portal-systemic anastomoses (porta-caval system) which provide a collateral portal circulation or bypass in cases of obstruction in the liver or the portal vein. In this diagram, portal tributaries are *blue*, systemic tributaries are *striped*, and communicating veins are *black*. In portal hypertension (as in hepatic cirrhosis), the anastomotic veins become varicose (large and tortuous) and may rupture. The sites of anastomosis shown are: (*1*) *between the esophageal veins* (when dilated these veins are called esophageal varices) (*2*) *between the rectal veins* (when dilated these veins are called hemorrhoids); (*3*) *paraumbilical veins* (when dilated these veins may produce the "caput medusae," see Case 2-8); and (*4*) twigs of *colic* and *splenic veins with renal veins* and veins of the bare area of the liver with the right internal thoracic vein.

anastomotic areas to dilate and become varicose.

The following are the portal-systemic anastomotic areas (Fig. 2-112).

1. *In the gastroesophageal region,* the esophageal tributaries of the **left gastric vein** anastomose with the **esophageal veins**, which empty into the **azygos vein** (Figs. 1-48 and 2-146).
2. *In the anorectal region,* the **superior rectal vein** (a tributary of the inferior mesenteric vein) anastomoses with the **middle** and **inferior rectal veins**, which are tributaries of the internal iliac and internal pudendal veins, respectively.
3. *In the paraumbilical region,* the **paraumbilical veins** in the falciform lig-

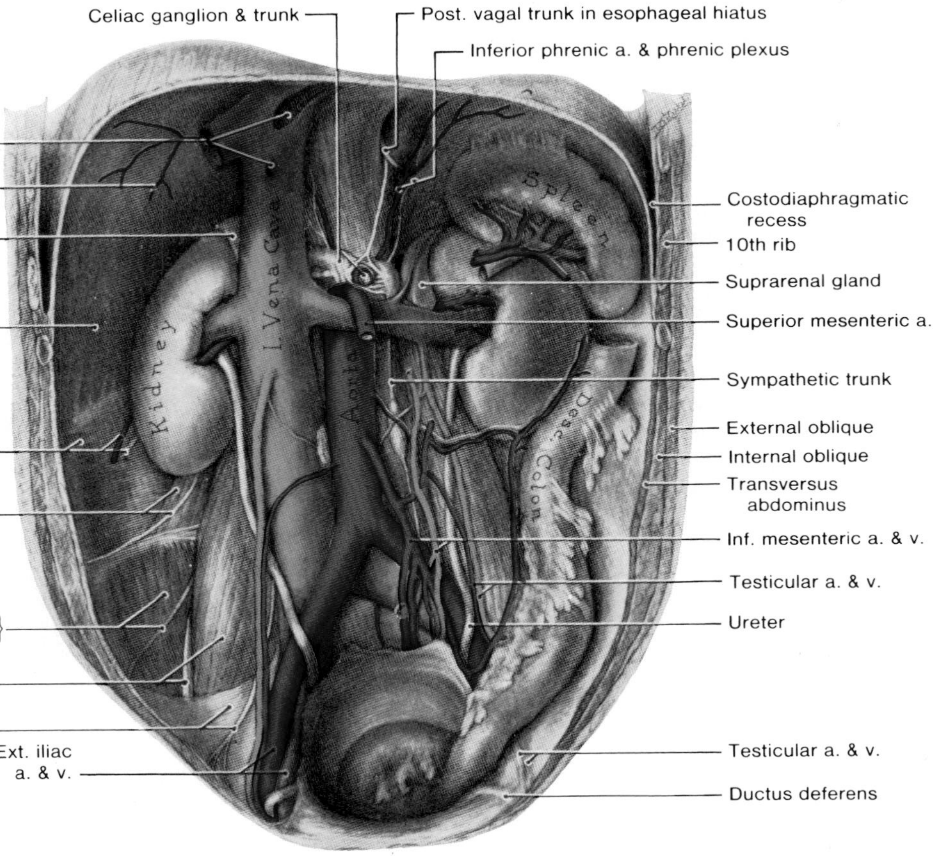

Figure 2-113. Drawing of a dissection showing the great vessels, the kidneys, the ureters, and the suprarenal glands. Most of the fascia has been removed from the posterior abdominal wall. Note that the abdominal aorta is shorter than the combined common and external iliac arteries, and that the superior mesenteric artery arises just below the celiac trunk. Observe that the inferior mesenteric artery arises about 4 cm above the aortic bifurcation and crosses the left common iliac vessels to become the superior rectal artery. Note that the kidneys lie anterior to the diaphragm, the transversus aponeurosis, the quadratus lumborum, and the psoas major. Observe that the ureter crosses the external iliac artery just beyond the common iliac bifurcation and that the testicular vessels cross ventral to the ureter, and at the deep (internal) ring they pass with the ductus deferens into the inguinal canal. The ureter in living persons can be readily identified by its thick muscular wall, which undergoes worm-like movements when it is gently stroked or squeezed. The ureter during its abdominal and upper pelvic course adheres to the parietal peritoneum and remains with it when the peritoneum is dissected upward.

ament anastomose with subcutaneous veins in the anterior abdominal wall.

4. *In the retroperitoneal region*, tributaries of the **splenic** and **pancreatic veins** anastomose with the **left renal vein**. Short veins also connect the splenic and colic veins to **lumbar veins** of the posterior abdominal wall. The **veins of the bare area** of the liver also communicate with the veins of the diaphragm and the right internal thoracic vein.

CLINICALLY ORIENTED COMMENTS

In patients with **portal hypertension**, the abnormal increase in pressure in the portal vein and its tributaries is often caused by **cirrhosis of the liver**, a disease characterized by progressive destruction of hepatic parenchymal cells with replacement by fibrous tissue (Case 2-8) or from involvement of the portal vein outside the liver. *Portal hypertension and the diseases causing it are serious conditions*, but the symptoms are modified by the portal-systemic anastomoses providing alternative pathways for the blood to flow. Because *there are no functionally competent valves anywhere in the portal venous system*, the increase in portal pressure is reflected throughout the system. Blood tends to be diverted into the systemic venous system in the regions where **portal-systemic anastomoses** occur (Fig. 2-112). The veins in these areas tend to become dilated and tortuous and are called varicose veins. **Varicose veins** in the region of the anal canal are called **hemorrhoids** or piles. Varicose veins in the gastroesophageal region are called **esophageal varices**. The veins in both locations may become so dilated that their walls rupture, resulting in **hemorrhage**. *Bleeding from esophageal varices is often severe and may be fatal.*

In severe cases of portal obstruction (Case 2-8), even the *paraumbilical veins may become varicose* (Fig. 2-150) and appear like snakes under the skin. This condition is referred to as **caput medusae** because of its resemblance to the serpents on the head of Medusa, a character in Greek mythology.

The common way of reducing portal pressure is to divert blood from the portal venous system to the systemic venous system by creating a communication between the portal vein and the inferior vena cava. This **portacaval anastomosis** may be done where these vessels lie close to each other posterior to the liver (Figs. 2-83 and 2-91). Another way is to join the splenic vein to the left renal vein (**splenorenal anastomosis**) following removal of the spleen (*splenectomy*). Various other anas-

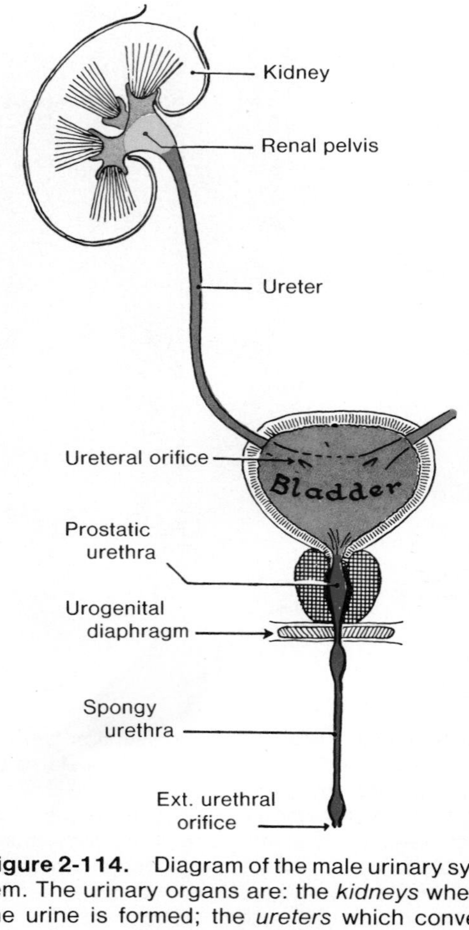

Figure 2-114. Diagram of the male urinary system. The urinary organs are: the *kidneys* where the urine is formed; the *ureters* which convey the urine to the urinary bladder; the *urinary bladder* where the urine is temporarily stored; and the *urethra* through which the urine passes to the exterior. The membranous urethra is the part surrounded by the urogenital diaphragm.

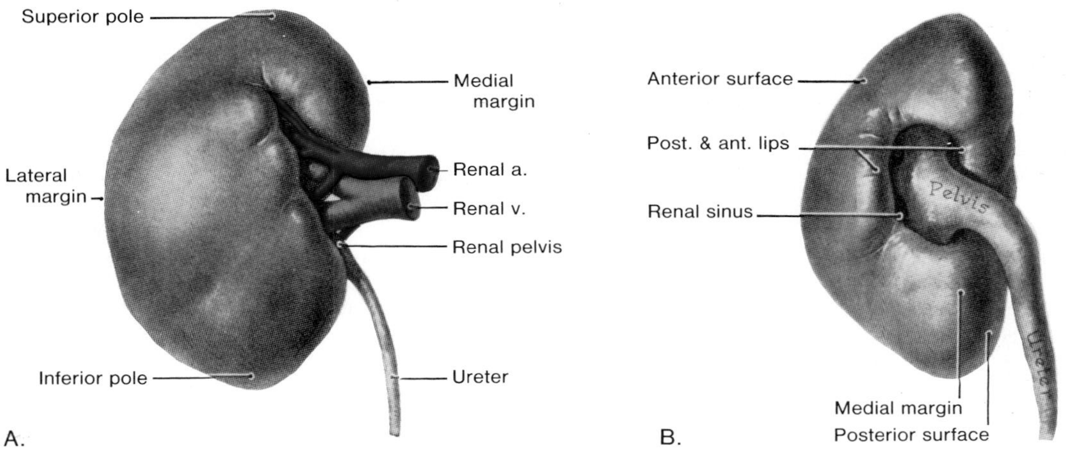

Figure 2-115. Drawings of the right kidney. *A*, anterior view. Examine the order of the structures at the hilum (entrance to the renal sinus) from before backward: vein, artery, duct (pelvis or ureter). Note that a branch of the artery crosses behind the pelvis. *B*, anteromedial view showing the renal sinus. Observe that the sinus is a considerable space making up a large part of the interior of the kidney. Note that it contains the greater part of the renal pelvis, the calyces (Fig. 2-116), the blood and lymph vessels, and the nerves of the kidney. There are also variable amounts of fat in the renal sinus, sometimes a rather large amount (Fig. 2-116*B*).

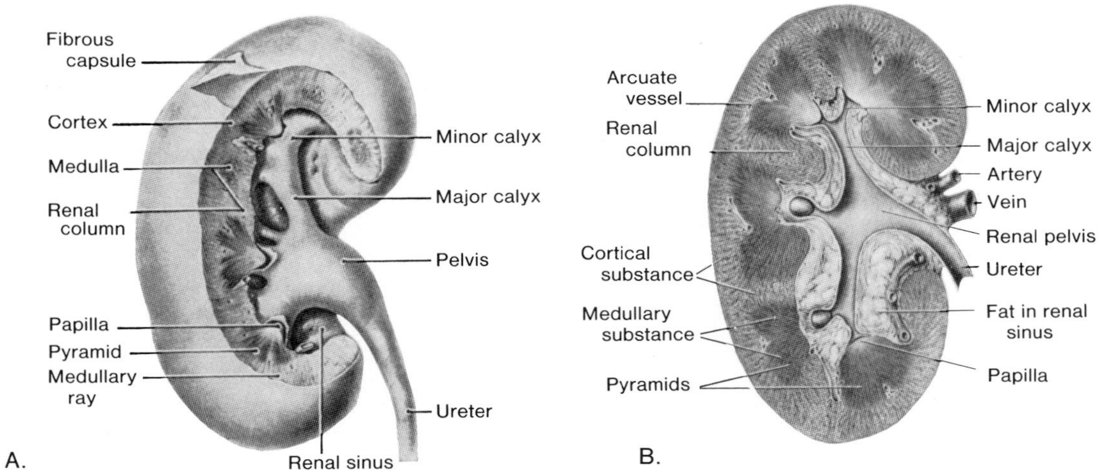

Figure 2-116. *A*, drawing of a right kidney from which the anterior lip of the renal sinus (Fig. 2-115) is cut away to show the structure of the kidney. Observe that the outer one-third of the renal substance is cortex and the inner two-thirds is medulla. Note that the cortical tissue (composed of glomeruli and convoluted tubules) is granular on section and extends as renal columns through the medulla to the renal sinus. The medulla contains 7 to 14 pyramids which are striated because of the visible collecting tubules they contain. Each pyramid ends as a papilla on which a dozen or more of the largest collecting tubules open. One to four papillae project into each minor calyx. Usually there are from 8 to 18 renal papillae and 7 to 15 minor calyces. Several minor calyces unite to form a major calyx. There are usually two major calyces, an upper and a lower, but often there are also one or two middle calyces. *B*, longitudinal section of the kidney.

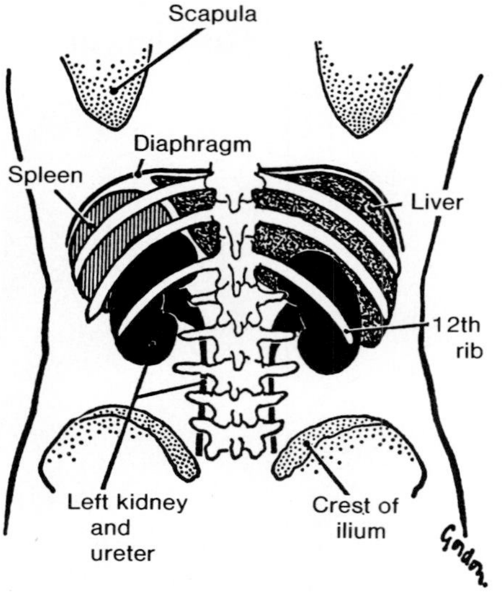

Figure 2-117. Diagram illustrating the surface anatomy of the back of a person lying in the prone position. Observe that the kidneys lie on each side of the vertebral column from T12 to L3 vertebrae and that the right kidney is slightly lower than the left one owing to the bulk of the right lobe of the liver. In the erect position the kidneys drop to a somewhat lower level. Note that the superior poles of the kidneys are protected by the 11th and 12th ribs and the inferior poles are about a fingerbreadth above the crest of the ilium. Observe that the ureters arise from the renal pelves in the hila, which lie near the transpyloric plane and descend anterior to the tips of the transverse processes of L2 to L5 vertebrae.

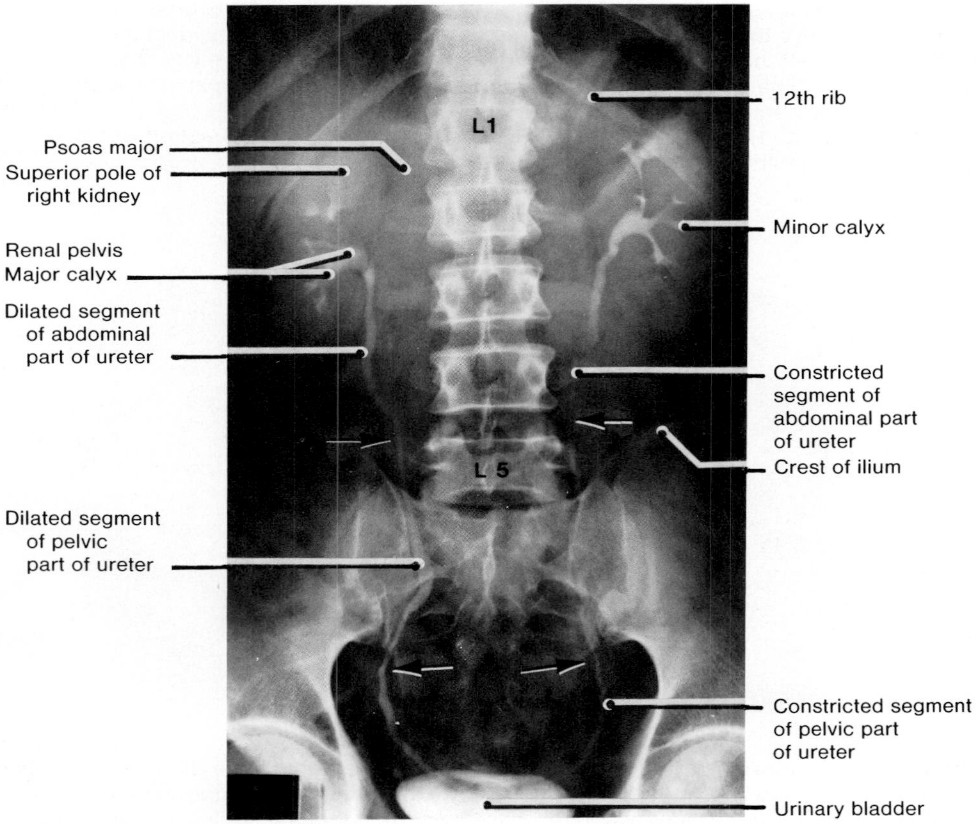

Figure 2-118. Intravenous urogram (pyelogram). The contrast medium was injected intravenously and was concentrated and excreted by the kidneys. This anteroposterior projection shows the calyces, renal pelves, and ureters outlined by the contrast medium filling their lumina. Note the difference in shape and level of the renal pelves and the constrictions and dilations in the ureter resulting from peristaltic contractions of their smooth muscle walls. Observe the relation of the ureters to the transverse processes of L3 to L5 vertebrae. The *arrows* indicate narrowings of the lumen resulting from peristaltic contractions. (courtesy of Dr. John Campbell, Sunnybrook Medical Centre, Toronto).

tomoses between the portal and systemic venous systems are sometimes created.

The Kidneys and Ureters (Figs. 2-31, 2-33*B*, 2-46, 2-52, 2-65, 2-68 to 2-71, 2-90, 2-91, 2-113 to 2-119, 2-123 to 2-128, and 2-134). The kidneys remove excess water, salts, and products of protein metabolism from the blood and maintain its pH. These substances removed from the blood, called urine, are conveyed to the **urinary bladder** by the **ureters** (Fig. 2-114). The adjectives *renal* and *nephric* are derived from the Latin word *renis* and the Greek word *nephros* for the kidney. Many other terms are derived from these roots.

Position, Form, and Size of the Kidneys. Each kidney lies posterior to the peritoneum (**retroperitoneally**) on the posterior abdominal wall. These bean-shaped **urinary organs** *lie alongside the vertebral column*, against the psoas major muscles (Figs. 2-113 and 2-119). They occupy the

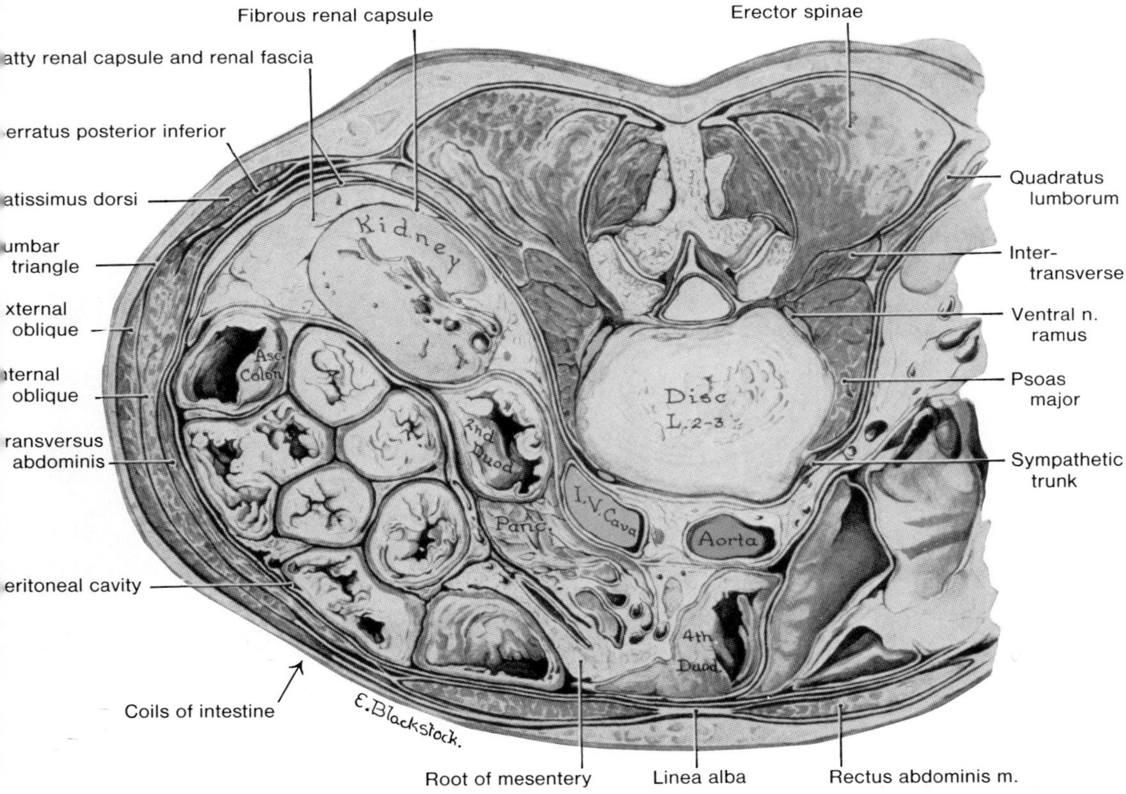

Figure 2-119. Drawing of a transverse section through the abdomen at the level of the disc between L2 and L3 vertebrae and between their transverse processes. Observe that the anterior aspect of the verebral column is nearer to the anterior surface of the body than to the posterior surface in this thin recumbent cadaver. Note that the ascending colon with an appendix epiploica, having no mesentery, is bare posteriorly. Observe that the anterior and posterior surfaces of the kidney do not face anteriorly and posteriorly but ventrolaterally and dorsomedially. Examine the fatty renal capsule (perirenal fat) massed along the borders of the kidney and leaving the anterior surface close to the peritoneum. Note that little fatty tissue lies anterior to the kidney. Observe that the second or descending part of the duodenum overlaps this surface of the kidney. Note the sympathetic trunk lying along the anterior border of the psoas muscle and on the right side behind the inferior vena cava. The linea alba is band-like above the umbilicus but is linear below it, as shown here.

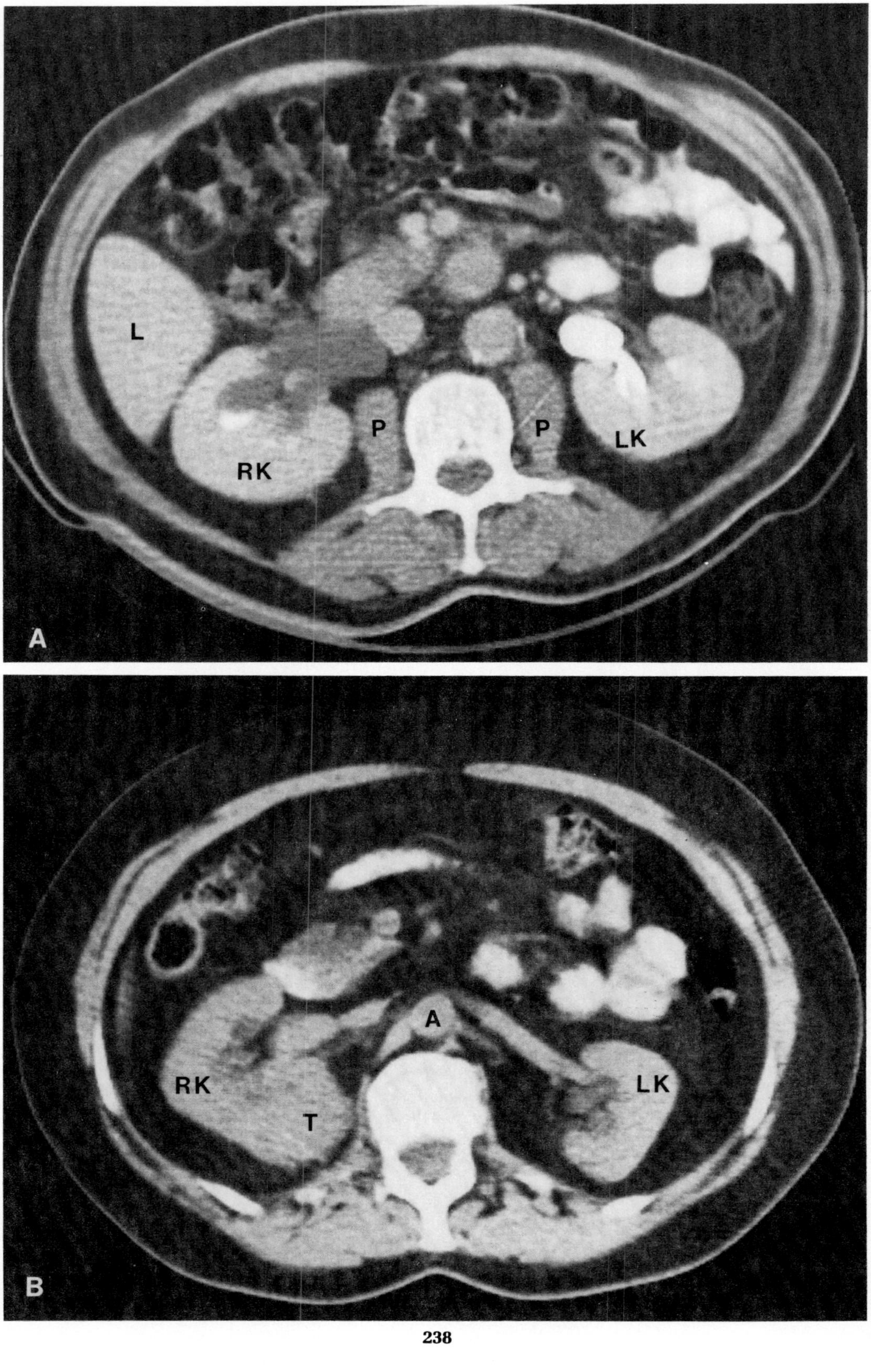
L
P
P
RK
LK
A
A
RK
LK
T
B

upper parts of the **paravertebral grooves** (gutters), anterior to the diaphragm. Their long axes are almost parallel to the long axis of the body and to the lateral border of the psoas muscle (Figs. 2-113 and 2-120*A*). *The superior parts of the kidneys are protected by the bony thorax* and are tilted so that their superior poles are nearer the midline than their inferior poles (Fig. 2-117). Owing to the large size of the right lobe of the liver, the right kidney lies at a slightly lower level than the left kidney.

Fresh adult kidneys are reddish-brown in color and measure about 10 cm in length, 5 cm in width, and 2.5 cm in thickness. The left kidney is often somewhat longer than the right kidney. The lobes of the kidney are demarcated on the surface of fetal and infantile kidneys. This external evidence of the lobes usually disappears by the end of the first year.

Each kidney is ovoid in outline, but its medial margin is deeply indented, giving it a somewhat bean-shaped appearance. At this concave middle part of each kidney there is a vertical cleft, called the **renal hilum**, through which the renal artery enters and the renal vein and the renal pelvis leave the kidney. The hilum leads into a space within the kidney called the **renal sinus**, which is about 2.5 cm deep. The renal sinus is occupied by *the renal pelvis, the renal calyces, the renal vessels and nerves, and varying amounts of adipose tissue* (Figs. 2-115 and 2-116).

CLINICALLY ORIENTED COMMENTS

In rare instances evidence of the fetal lobes may be visible in adult kidneys (Fig. 2-128*B*). It appears as several indentations along the lateral margin of the kidney which correspond to the renal pyramids of the medulla. The indentations are usually bilateral.

Occasionally the left kidney is somewhat triangular in shape, probably as the result of molding by the spleen. The superior pole of the kidney is narrow and the inferior pole is wide, giving the kidney a *humpback appearance.* This variation of kidney form, often called a **dromedary kidney**, has no clinical significance.

Surface Anatomy of the Kidneys (Figs. 2-68 and 2-117). In very muscular and/or obese people, the kidneys may be impalpable. In thin adults with poorly developed abdominal musculature, *the inferior pole of the right kidney is usually palpable by bimanual examination in the right lumbar region* as a firm, smooth, somewhat rounded mass that descends during inspiration. The normal left kidney is usually not palpable. When the kidney is enlarged (*e.g.*, owing to a tumor, Fig. 2-120*B*) or is abnormally mobile, it can usually be felt as it slides between the opposed fingers of the examiner's hands.

Figure 2-120. CT scans (computerized tomographic x-ray scans) of the upper abdomen, showing the cross-sectional radiographic anatomy of living patients. These sections are visualized as if you were looking at cross-sections of the abdomen from below, with the right side to your left. The images of the vertebrae indicate the anterior and posterior surfaces. *A*, fairly normal patient who has had a contrast agent injected intravenously a few minutes previously. There is slight *hydronephrosis* (dilation of the renal pelvis and calyces) of the right kidney (*RK*). In a right calyx, observe the layer of heavier opacified urine posterior to the lighter, less dense urine in the dilated calyx. On the left (*LK*), note a normal calyx and renal pelvis filled with opacified urine (*white*). The renal pelvis seems to lie more outside the kidney than you might expect, but this is normal. Observe the psoas muscles (*P*) medial to the kidneys on the sides of the vertebra (compare with Fig. 2-119). Note the tip of the right lobe of the liver (*L*). *B*, patient with a malignant tumor (*T*) of the right kidney (*RK*). This scan was made at a slightly higher level than in *A*. Note that the psoas muscle is not visible. The soft tissues at the sides of the vertebra are the crura of the diaphragm (Fig. 2-130). Observe the renal artery to the left kidney (*LK*) passing to the aorta (*A*). Note the much larger renal vein lying anterior to the artery. The liver is not visible because (1) the tumor has pushed it up, (2) the patient's habitus is different from the one shown in *A* and the liver is relatively higher, or (3) the patient has a small diseased liver.

The levels of the kidneys change during respiration and with changes in posture. Each kidney moves about 3 cm in a vertical direction during full movement of the diaphragm that occurs with deep breathing. **The hila of the kidneys lie in the neighborhood of the transpyloric plane** (Fig. 2-68), about three fingerbreadths (5 cm) from the median plane. In the erect position, *the transpyloric plane passes through the superior part of the hilum of the left kidney and the inferior part of the hilum of the right kidney.* As the usual approach to the kidney is from the back (Fig. 2-123), it is helpful to know that its inferior pole is about a fingerbreadth above the crest of the ilium and its superior pole is above the 12th rib (Fig. 2-117).

Surfaces and Margins of the Kidneys (Fig. 2-115). Each kidney has *anterior* and *posterior surfaces, medial* and *lateral margins* (borders), and *superior* and *inferior poles* (ends, extremities). **The lateral margin is convex** and **the medial margin is indented** or concave where the renal sinus and renal pelvis are located.

Structure of the Kidneys (Figs. 2-115, 2-116, and 2-119). The kidneys are closely invested by a thin but strong **fibrous capsule** of dense collagenous fibers. This capsule gives the fresh kidney a glistening appearance. It strips easily from a normal kidney. It passes over the **lips of the hilum** (Fig. 2-115*B*) to line the renal sinus and become continuous with the walls of the calyces. The kidney and its capsule are surrounded by fat, but it is sparce on the anterior surface. This **perirenal fat** is less dense (lower specific gravity than the kidney); thus an outline of the kidney is usually visible in radiographs (Fig. 2-118).

The renal pelvis is the superior *expanded end of the ureter.* It is surrounded by the fat, vessels, and nerves in the renal sinus (Fig. 2-116*B*). The word *pelvis* is derived from the Greek word *pyelos*, meaning a tub or basin; hence, a **pyelogram** (Fig. 2-118) is a radiograph of the renal pelvis and ureter and **pyelonephritis** indicates an inflammation of the renal pelvis and the kidney. Within the renal sinus, the renal pelvis divides into two or three wide, funnel-like tubes called **major calyces** (G. cups of flowers). Each major calyx is subdivided into 7 to 14 **minor calyces**. The urine empties into a minor calyx from the collecting tubules which pierce the tip of a **renal papilla** obliquely. It then passes through the major calyx, the renal pelvis, and the ureter.

The Ureters (Figs. 2-113 to 2-118). The ureters are the muscular ducts that carry the urine to the urinary bladder by **peristaltic waves** that occur in their walls. Each ureter begins in the renal pelvis, its funnel-shaped superior end.

The abdominal part of the ureter is about 12.5 cm long and 5 mm wide; its total length is about 25 cm. It is an expansile, thick-walled muscular tube with a narrow lumen (Fig. 2-118). *The ureter is retroperitoneal throughout its entire length.* It adheres closely to the peritoneum and is usually lifted with it. As it is pale colored and somewhat resembles a blood vessel, it is in danger during surgery in the lower abdomen and the pelvis. It is slightly constricted where it joins the renal pelvis. The ureter descends almost vertically along the psoas major (Fig. 2-121), anterior to the tips of the transverse processes of L2 to L5 vertebrae (Fig. 2-117). In Figure 2-134 note that as the **right ureter** descends toward the pelvic brim, it lies in close relationship to the **inferior vena cava**, the paracaval **lumbar lymph nodes**, and the **sympathetic trunk**. In Figure 2-113, observe that the ureter crosses the brim of the pelvis and the external iliac artery, just beyond the bifurcation of the common iliac artery. Also note that it passes posterior to the testicular vessels.

CLINICALLY ORIENTED COMMENTS

Rapid, excessive distention of the ureter causes severe rhythmic pain (**ureteric colic**). Frequently the colic results from a **ureteric calculus** (L. a pebble) that is usually composed of calcium oxalate, calcium phosphate, and/or uric acid. *Urinary calculi or stones may be located in the calyces, the renal pelvis, the ureter, or the* *urinary bladder.* Calcium-containing stones are radiopaque, whereas those composed of uric acid are radiolucent.

Ureteric stones may cause complete or intermittent obstruction of urinary flow. The obstruction may occur at the **ureteropelvic junction** or anywhere along the ureter, but most often it occurs (1) where the ureter crosses the iliac vessels and the brim of the pelvis and (2) where it passes obliquely through the wall of the urinary bladder.

Ureteric colic may produce a sharp, stabbing pain which follows along the course of the ureter *i.e., from the loin* (between the ribs and the pelvis) *to the groin* (inguinal region) as the stone is gradually forced down the ureter by peristalsis or **hyperperistalsis**. In males, the pain is frequently also referred to the scrotum and in females it may radiate to the labia majora (Fig. 2-23). The ureter is supplied with pain afferents that are included in the **lowest splanchnic nerve**. Impulses enter via T12 and L1 segments, which explains why the spasmodic and agonizing pain is referred to the loin and the groin, the cutaneous areas supplied by T12 and L1 (Fig. 2-141).

To study the kidneys, ureters, and urinary bladder, a radiopaque contrast medium is injected intravenously (**intravenous urography**) and serial radiographs (*urograms*) are taken at intervals (Fig. 2-118), usually with the patient in different positions. The length of the two kidneys, as determined radiologically, should be within 1.5 cm of each other and their contours should be smooth. Various abnormalities of the kidney and ureter may be detected radiologically, *e.g.*, **duplications of the upper urinary tract** (Fig. 2-128, *C* and *E*), usually of the upper part of the ureter and pelvis. Bulges on the renal surface representing tumors or cysts, depression on the renal surface representing scars, and displacements by retroperitoneal masses can also be detected radiographically. **Acute obstruction of one ureter** results in an abnormally dense and persistent kidney shadow on that side during the first few minutes (**nephrogram phase**) after the injection of contrast material. *Opacification of the renal calyces and pelvis is delayed and poor compared to the normal side* (Fig. 2-120*A*). Obstruction of the lower urinary tract, *e.g.*, resulting from hypertrophy and/or cancer of the prostate gland, is usually chronic. In such cases, **urography** usually shows dilation and poor opacification of the upper urinary tract.

In **retrograde urography** (pyelography), the contrast medium is injected through a catheter that is inserted via a **cystoscope** into the urinary bladder and the ureter. The contrast medium is usually injected when the tip of the catheter enters the renal pelvis. Retrograde studies, although not commonly used, are helpful when visualization of the upper urinary tract is poor during **intravenous urography** (pyelography) (Fig. 2-118). The passage of a catheter into the ureter is also useful for locating the position of a stone in the ureter during surgery.

Renal Fascia and Renal Fat (Fig. 2-119). The kidney, invested by a smooth **fibrous renal capsule**, is embedded in a substantial mass of perirenal fat that constitutes a **fatty renal capsule**. Very little fatty tissue lies anterior to the kidney. This fatty capsule is in turn covered by fibroareolar tissue called the **renal fascia**. Thus, *the renal fascia encloses the kidney, its surrounding fibrous and fatty capsules, and the suprarenal gland.* The coverings help to maintain these organs in position.

The renal fascia is adherent to the parietal peritoneum, and for this reason the kidney is easily lifted from the posterior abdominal wall in a retroperitoneal approach (Fig. 2-134). Superiorly the renal fascia is continuous with the fascia on the inferior surface of the diaphragm (**diaphragmatic fascia**). Medially the anterior layers of the right and left sides blend with each other anterior to the abdominal aorta and inferior vena cava. The posterior layer of renal fascia fuses medially with the fascia over the psoas major muscle (Figs. 2-118 and 2-138). The layers of renal fascia are loosely united inferiorly and may be easily separated below the kidney. At body temperature the perirenal fat is soft; hence, *the kidneys move slightly up and down* *during respiration* because they lie in contact with the diaphragm. It has been determined radiographically that *the normal renal mobility is about 3 cm* or roughly the height of one vertebral body.

The encasement of the kidney in fat is an important factor in anchoring it in position. The amount of fat in the fatty capsule varies with the individual. The fat outside the renal fascia, called the **pararenal fat**, is located between the peritoneum of the posterior abdominal wall and the renal fascia. In emaciated cadavers there may be very little fat around the kidneys.

CLINICALLY ORIENTED COMMENTS

Gases (O_2 or CO_2) injected into the extra-peritoneal tissue of the pelvis will rise to the level of the kidneys and diffuse amongst the extraperitoneal pararenal fat in 1 to 2 hr. Radiologists sometimes utilize this knowledge to outline the kidney and the suprarenal gland with gas for visualization of these structures. For **insufflation of gases** around the renal and suprarenal areas, the needle is inserted through the sacral hiatus (Fig. 5-25) or supra pubically (above pubic arch). *As gas embolism may occur during this technique*, this procedure has been replaced by CT scanning (Fig. 2-120).

If the fatty renal capsule is thin or absent, as occurs in emaciated patients, the kidneys are difficult to see radiologically, because the perirenal fat does not produce an outline of the kidney as in Figure 2-118. When this fatty capsule is absent, *the kidney may descend to an abnormally low level*, where it is supported primarily by the renal vessels. This downward displacement of the kidney is called **nephroptosis** (G. *ptōsis*, a falling). In **hypermobility of the kidney** ("floating kidney"), the organ moves up and down within the renal fascia in a vertical plane more than is normal. It does not move from side to side. In excessively low positions the ureter may be kinked, *possibly* resulting in some obstruction to the downflow of urine to the urinary bladder.

Blood from an injured kidney or pus from a **perinephric abscess** distends the renal fascia and may force its way inferiorly into the pelvis, between the anterior and posterior layers of pelvic fascia. The attachment of the renal fascia in the midline prevents extravasation or spread of blood and/or pus to the opposite side.

Relations of the Kidneys (Figs. 2-111, 2-113, 2-117, and 2-119 to 2-124). **Posteriorly, each kidney lies on muscle.** The posterior surface of the superior pole is related to the **diaphragm** which separates it from the pleural cavity and the 12th rib. More inferiorly it is related posteriorly to the **quadratus lumborum** muscle, sometimes encroaching slightly on the **psoas major** muscle medially and the **transversus abdominis** muscle laterally. *The subcostal nerve and vessels and the iliohypogastric and ilioinguinal nerves descend diagonally across the posterior surface of the kidney* (Figs. 2-113 and 2-121).

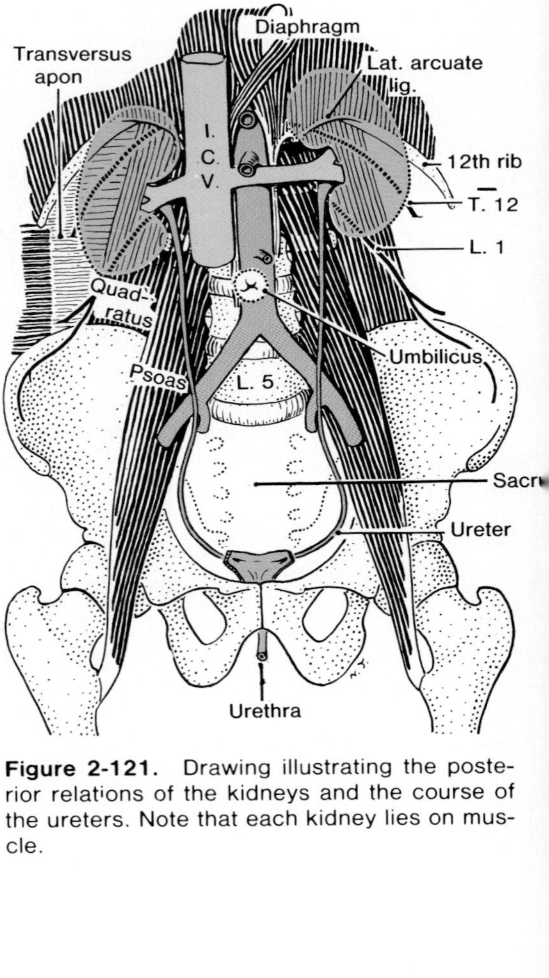

Figure 2-121. Drawing illustrating the posterior relations of the kidneys and the course of the ureters. Note that each kidney lies on muscle.

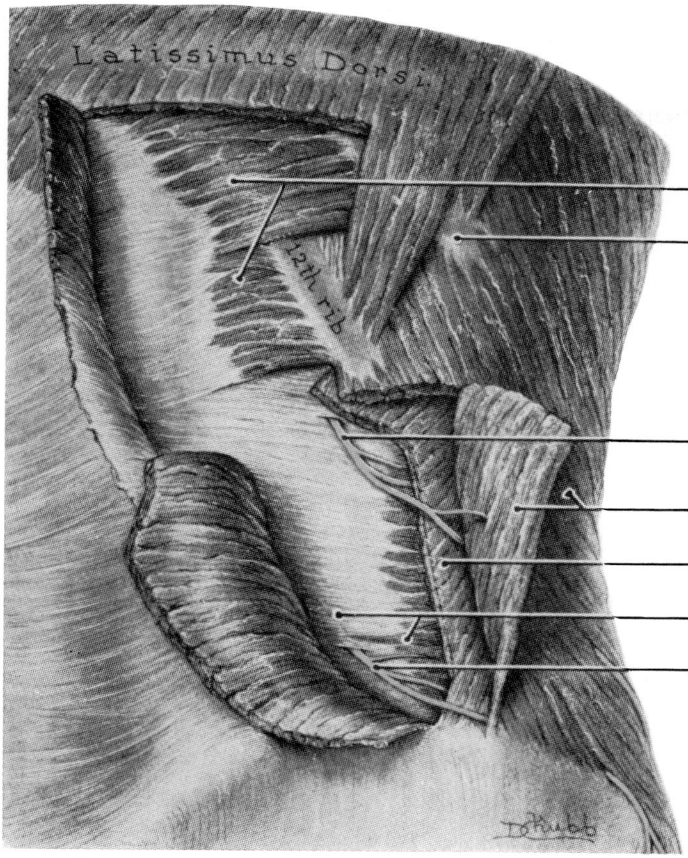

Figure 2-122. Drawing of a posterolateral view of the right posterior abdominal wall. The external oblique muscle has been incised and turned laterally and the internal oblique muscle incised and turned medially, exposing the transversus abdominis muscle and its posterior aponeurosis. Observe the subcostal (T12) and iliohypogastric (L1) nerves which give off motor twigs and lateral cutaneous (iliac) branches and continue forward between the internal oblique and the transversus abdominis muscles.

Anteriorly, the relations of the kidneys differ on the two sides, except that the anterior aspect and medial aspect of *the superior pole of each kidney is covered by the corresponding suprarenal gland* (Fig. 2-111). The superior pole of the **right kidney** is related to the **inferior surface of the liver** (Figs. 2-69 and 2-80). Except for the superior pole, the right kidney is separated from the liver by the **hepatorenal recess** (Figs. 2-32, 2-77, and 2-90). More inferiorly the second or **descending part of the duodenum** passes across the hilum of the kidney (Figs. 2-33*B*, 2-69*A*, 2-90, and 2-119. The **right colic flexure** lies anterior to the lateral border and the inferior pole of the right kidney (Figs. 2-42, 2-46, and 2-69). In Figure 2-69 observe that *the suprarenal, duodenal, and colic areas of the kidney are not covered by peritoneum.* Part of the small intestine lies across the inferior pole of the right kidney, but it is separated from it by a thin film of fluid in the peritoneal cavity (Fig. 2-119).

The anterior relations of the left kidney (Fig. 2-69) are the left **suprarenal gland**, the **stomach**, the **spleen**, the **pancreas**, the **jejunum**, and the **descending colon**. The gastric, splenic, and jejunal areas are covered by peritoneum. The left kidney, along with the pancreas and the spleen, is in the **stomach bed** (Fig. 2-52), where it is

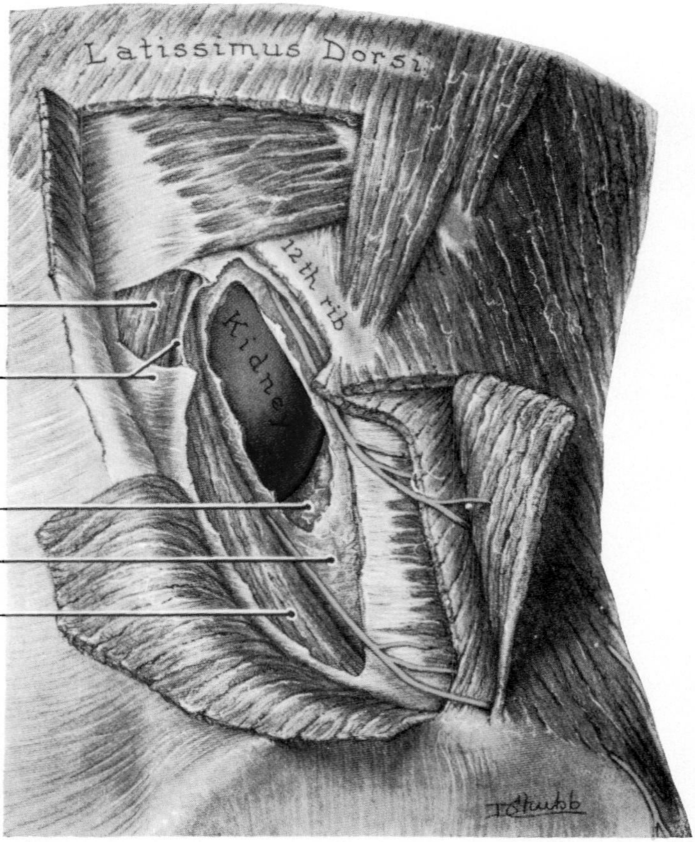

Figure 2-123. Drawing of a posterolateral view of a deeper dissection of the right posterior abdominal wall than that illustrated in Figure 2-122. Observe that on dividing the posterior aponeurosis of the transversus abdominis muscle between the subcostal and iliohypogastric nerves and lateral to the oblique lateral border of the quadratus lumborum muscle, the retroperitoneal fat surrounding the kidney is exposed. The renal fascia is within this fat. The portion of fat inside the renal fascia is termed the *fatty renal capsule* (perirenal fat); the fat outside the renal fascia is *pararenal fat* (also see Fig. 2-119).

covered by the posterior wall of the omental bursa.

CLINICALLY ORIENTED COMMENTS

The close relationship of the kidney to the psoas major muscle explains why extension of the thigh may increase pain resulting from inflammation in the pararenal region.

The common surgical approach to the kidney is the lumbar renal or retroperitoneal approach. **Lumbar nephrectomy** (removal of a kidney via the retroperitoneal lumbar route) is indicated when contamination of the peritoneal cavity is likely (*e.g.*, if there is **inflammatory renal disease** and/or **renal calculi**). The lumbar approach to the kidney is illustrated in Figures 2-121 and 2-122. During this surgery the subcostal, iliohypogastric, and ilioinguinal nerves are vulnerable to injury. The transabdominal approach to the kidney is used for surgery of the renal vessels or the ureter (Fig. 2-134).

Renal transplantation is now an established operation for the treatment of se-

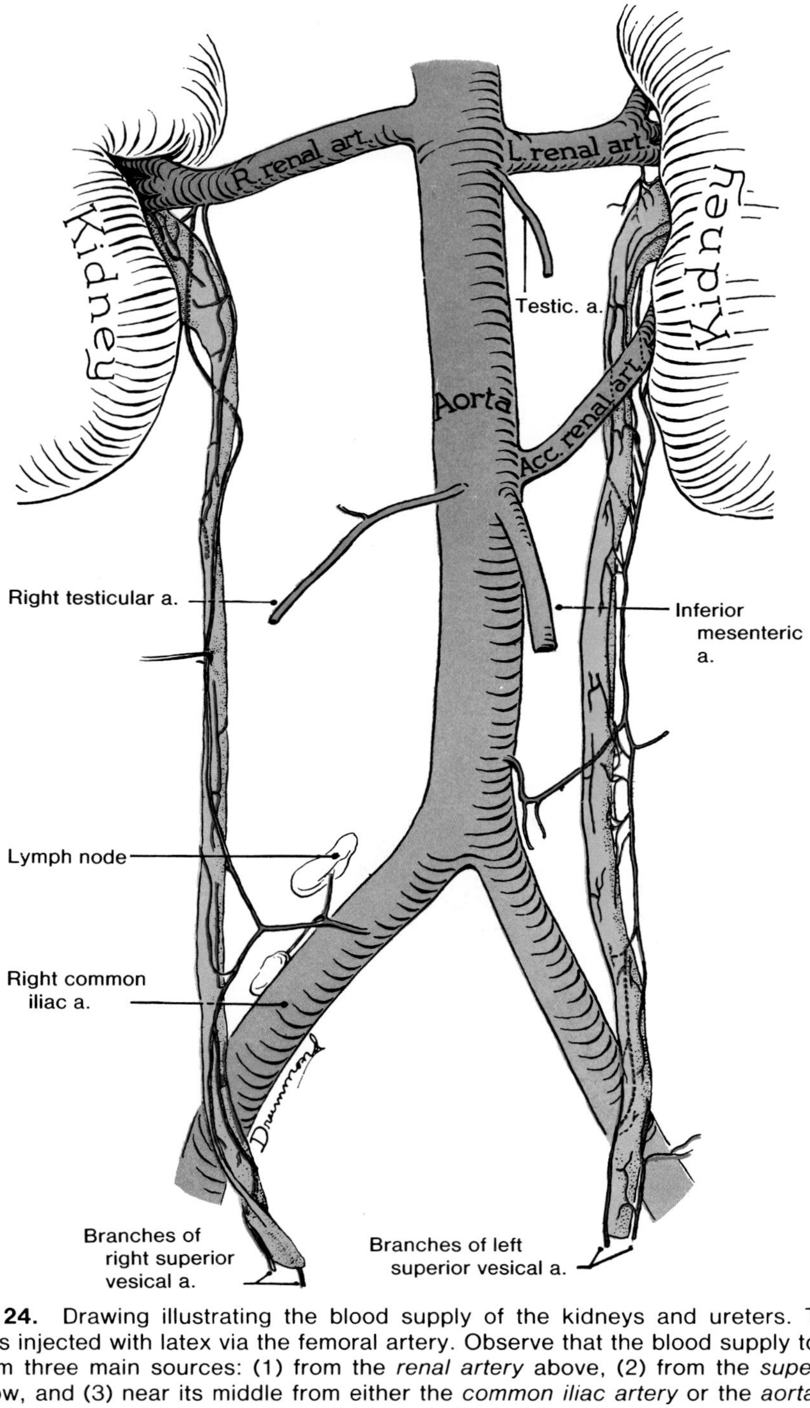

Figure 2-124. Drawing illustrating the blood supply of the kidneys and ureters. The arterial system was injected with latex via the femoral artery. Observe that the blood supply to the ureter comes from three main sources: (1) from the *renal artery* above, (2) from the *superior vesical artery* below, and (3) near its middle from either the *common iliac artery* or the *aorta*. Note that these branches approach the ureter from the medial site. In this specimen an accesory renal artery also supplies branches, and in some people the testicular artery also contributes a branch. Examine the excellent *anastomotic chain* made by these long, tenuous branches.

lected cases of chronic **renal failure**. A long survival of a *kidney transplant* is most likely when the kidney is obtained from a monozygotic (identical) twin.

Vessels and Nerves of the Kidneys and Ureters (Figs. 2-55, 2-69*B*, 2-111, 2-113, 2-115*A*, 2-120, and 2-124 to 2-129). The **renal arteries** are large vessels that arise from the aorta at right angles at the level of the intervertebral disc between L1 and L2 vertebrae. Typically each renal artery divides close to the hilum into *five segmental arteries.* Most of these pass anterior to the pelvis of the kidney (Fig. 2-125), but one or two pass posterior to it. *Based on the arterial distribution,* segments of the kidney are described (Fig. 2-125*B*), each of which is supplied by a **segmental artery**. The initial branches of the segmental arteries are called **lobar arteries**. Each of these divides into **interlobar arteries** (Fig. 2-126), which enter the kidney and ascend at the sides of the pyramids. The interlobar arteries become **arcuate arteries**, which pass between the cortex and medulla of the kidney. The arcuate arteries give rise to **interlobular arteries** from which numerous side branches called **intralobular arteries** arise. Each of these branches into one or more afferent **glomerular arteries**.

The blood supply to the ureter comes from several arteries; usually there are three main sources as shown in Figure 2-124, but **branches to the ureter** may arise from the following arteries (*main sources appear in bold face*): **renal**, testicular or ovarian, **aorta**, internal and **common iliac**, and **vesical** or **uterine** arteries. Usually these long branches form such an excellent anastomotic chain that some of the

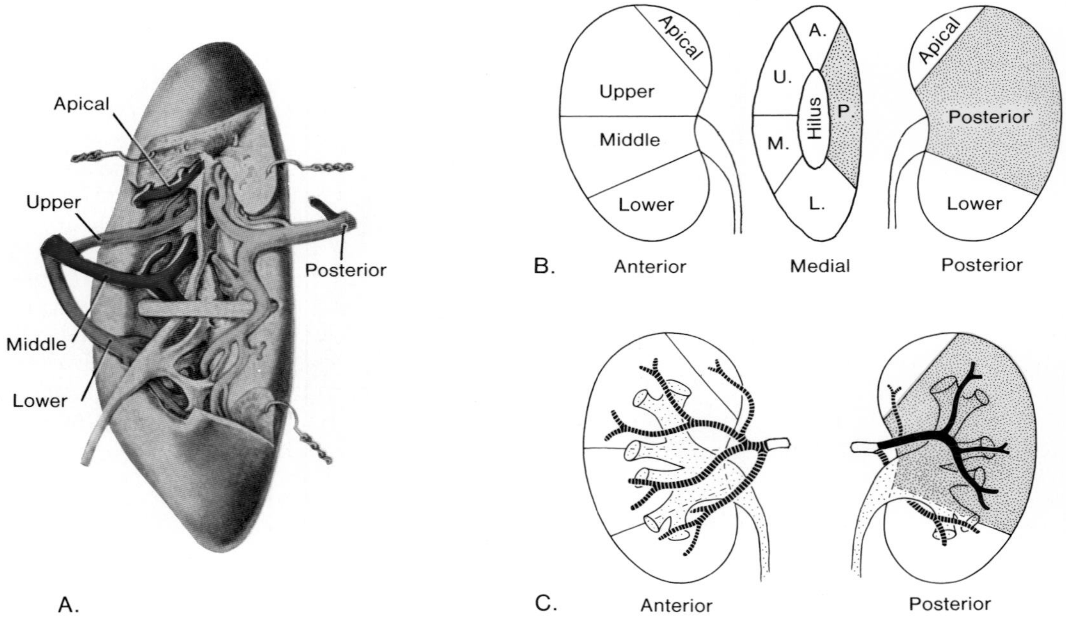

Figure 2-125. Drawings of the kidneys illustrating their arterial supply. *A*, drawing of the branches of the renal artery within the renal sinus. Typically, as shown, there are five segmental arteries. The posterior lip of the sinus has been incised, above and below, near the limits of the territory of the posterior segmental artery. *B*, diagram of the segments of the kidney. According to its arterial supply the kidney has five segments: (1) apical (superior); (2) superior (anterosuperior); (3) middle (anteroinferior); (4) lower or inferior; and (5) posterior. *C*, diagram of the segmental arteries supplying the segments of the kidney shown in *B*. Only the apical and inferior arteries supply the whole thickness of the kidney. Note that the posterior artery crosses cranial to the renal pelvis to reach its segment.

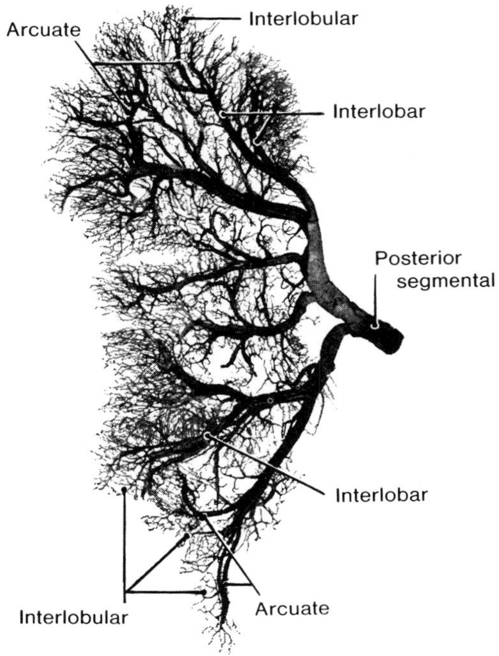

Figure 2-126. Drawing of a corrosion specimen of a segmental artery of the kidney. Note that the interlobar arteries are *end arteries*; hence, obstruction of one of these vessels leads to necrosis (death) of the part of the kidney supplied by it. This area of dead tissue is referred to as a *renal infarct*.

branches may be ligated without interfering with the blood supply of the ureter. In some cases, the longitudinal anastomosis along the ureter is poor owing to the wide spacing of the vessels supplying it.

The renal veins lie anterior to the arteries and *the left renal vein passes anterior to the aorta*, just inferior to the origin of the superior mesenteric artery (Fig. 2-113). Each renal vein joins the inferior vena cava (Fig. 2-129).

The nerve supply of the kidney and ureter is via the **renal plexus** (Figs. 2-113 and 2-127), consisting of sympathetic and parasympathetic fibers. The renal plexus is supplied by fibers from the lesser and lowest **splanchnic nerves** which pass along the renal artery to supply the kidney.

The lymph vessels of the kidney follow the renal vein and drain into the lateral **aortic lymph nodes** (Figs. 2-27 and 2-134). *Lymph vessels from the upper part of the ureter* may join those of the kidney or pass directly to the lateral **aortic lymph nodes**. *Lymph vessels from the middle part of the ureter* usually drain into the **common iliac nodes**, whereas lymph *vessels from the lower part of the ureter* drain into the common, external, or internal **iliac lymph nodes.**

CLINICALLY ORIENTED COMMENTS

The renal pelvis and calyces will accommodate about 8 ml of fluid. If more than this amount of radioopaque contrast material is injected into them during **retrograde urography** (see the previous comments on this technique), the excessive pressure may tear the epithelial junction of the minor calyces with the papillae (Fig. 2-116), allowing the material to enter the adjacent renal veins. This is undesirable but not a serious occurrence.

The embryonic kidneys develop in the pelvis and normally ascend to their final position in the abdomen. During this ascent the kidneys receive their blood supply from successively higher sources. Usually the lower vessels degenerate as the upper ones develop. Failure of degeneration of some of these vessels results in **multiple renal arteries** (Fig. 2-128*B*). Variations in the number of renal arteries and in their position with respect to the renal veins are common. Supernumerary arteries, usually two or three, are about twice as common as supernumerary veins, and they usually arise at the level of the kidney.

When first formed in the pelvis the two kidneys are close together. In 1 in about 600 persons, the kidneys are fused across the midline; usually it is the inferior poles that are fused to form a **horseshoe kidney** (Fig. 2-128*A*). The large U-shaped kidney usually lies at the level of the lower lumbar vertebrae because normal ascent was prevented by the root of the inferior mesenteric artery. *Horseshoe kidney usually produces no symptoms,* but there may be associated abnormalities of the renal pelvis and kidney which may favor development of an obstruction and/or infection.

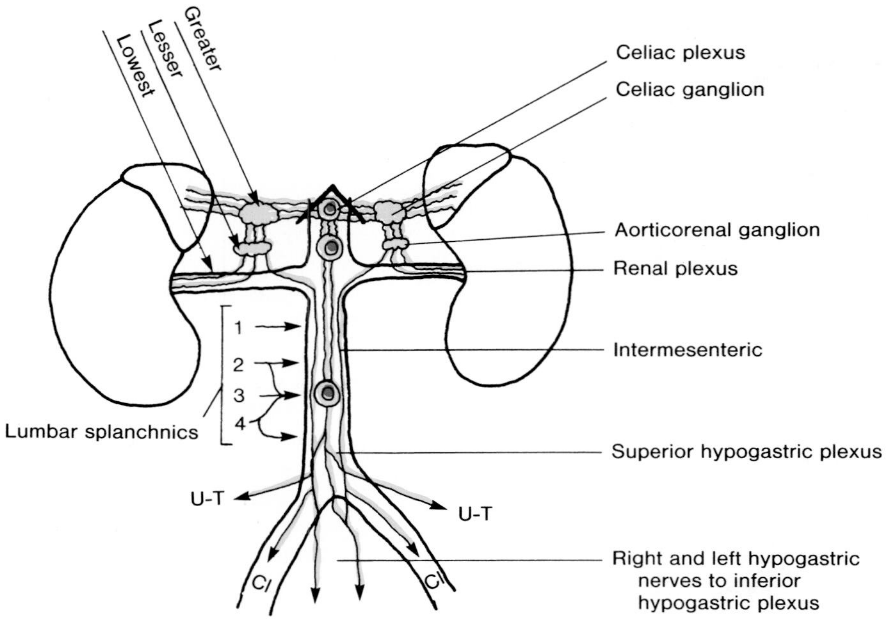

Figure 2-127. Diagram illustrating the autonomic supply to the abdomen and pelvis. Both sympathetic and parasympathetic fibers are delivered via a complex tangle of nerves around the abdominal and pelvic arteries. This network is variable, difficult to dissect, peculiarly named, and described differently by different authors. The above simplified plan is for orientation. Observe the interconnected plexuses on the abdominal arteries. Note that the stems of the celiac, superior mesenteric, and inferior mesenteric arteries are surrounded by nerve fibers. Observe that the sympathetic fibers here synapse *outside* the sympathetic trunk in ganglia, some of which are small and scattered but two of which are large and named: celiac and aorticorenal. The *arrows* show the source of sympathetic input: greater, lesser, lowest, and four lumbar splanchnic nerves. Although paired, they are shown here only on one side. Note that the superior hypogastric plexus supplies the ureteric and testicular (*U-T*) plexuses and a plexus on each of the common iliac arteries (*CI*). The parasympathetic nerve supply is not shown here. Branches of the vagus nerve are distributed to the foregut and the midgut. Pelvic splanchnic nerves join the lower part of the nerve network shown and supply the hindgut and pelvic viscera. The term "splanchnic" simply means "viscera." There are three types of splanchnic nerve as listed below:

Names	Type	Origin
1. Thoracic (greater, lesser and lowest)	Sympathetic	Branches of thoracic sympathetic ganglia 5 to 12.
2. Lumbar splanchnics	Sympathetic	Branches of the four lumbar sympathetic ganglia
3. Pelvic splanchnics	Parasympathetic	Branches of ventral rami of sacral spinal nerves, S2, S3, (S4).

Sometimes the embryonic kidney on one or both sides fails to ascend into the abdomen (Fig. 2-128*D*) and lies in the hollow of the sacrum. This ectopic **pelvic kidney** should not be mistaken for a **pelvic tumor**. In addition, it may be injured or cause obstruction to the passage of the infant's head during childbirth. *Pelvic kidneys do not receive their blood supply from the usual source* but from arteries that arise from one of the following: the inferior end of the aorta, the iliac artery, or the median sacral artery.

Duplication of the abdominal part of the ureter and of the renal pelvis are common (Fig. 2-128*C* and *E*), but a supernumerary kidney is rare. These abnormalities result from division of the **metanephric diver-**

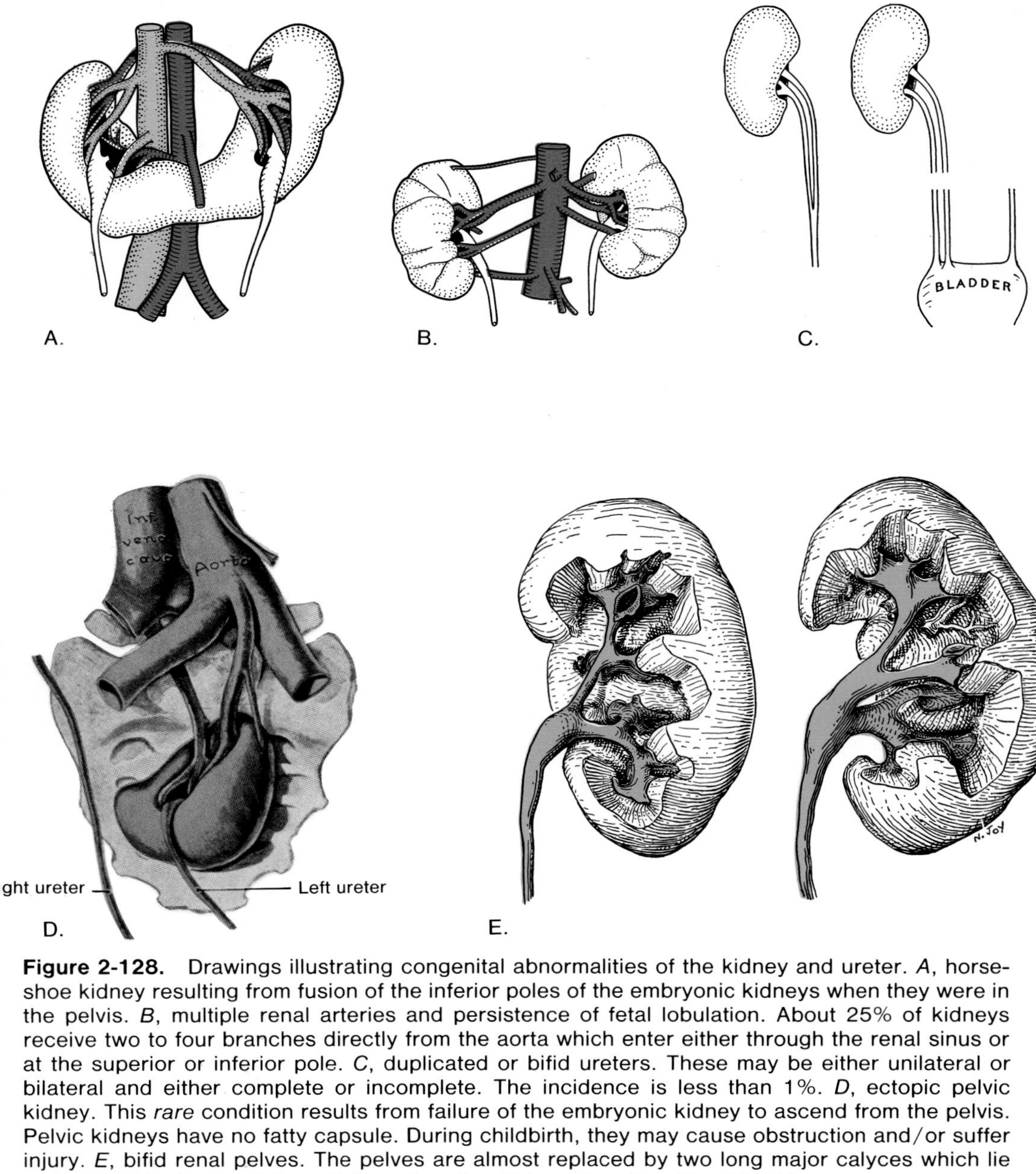

Figure 2-128. Drawings illustrating congenital abnormalities of the kidney and ureter. *A*, horseshoe kidney resulting from fusion of the inferior poles of the embryonic kidneys when they were in the pelvis. *B*, multiple renal arteries and persistence of fetal lobulation. About 25% of kidneys receive two to four branches directly from the aorta which enter either through the renal sinus or at the superior or inferior pole. *C*, duplicated or bifid ureters. These may be either unilateral or bilateral and either complete or incomplete. The incidence is less than 1%. *D*, ectopic pelvic kidney. This *rare* condition results from failure of the embryonic kidney to ascend from the pelvis. Pelvic kidneys have no fatty capsule. During childbirth, they may cause obstruction and/or suffer injury. *E*, bifid renal pelves. The pelves are almost replaced by two long major calyces which lie entirely within the renal sinus (*left*) and partly within and partly without (*right*).

ticulum (ureteric bud), the primordium of the ureter and renal pelvis. The extent of ureteral duplication depends on how complete the division of the ureteric bud is. Incomplete division of the bud results in the formation of a **bifid ureter** or renal pelvis.

The Suprarenal Glands (Figs. 2-33*B*, 2-68, 2-69, 2-71, 2-113, 2-127, and 2-140). The paired suprarenal (adrenal) glands, 3 to 5 cm long, *lie on each side of the vertebral column and against the superomedial surface of the corresponding kidney.* When fresh they are yellowish in color owing to

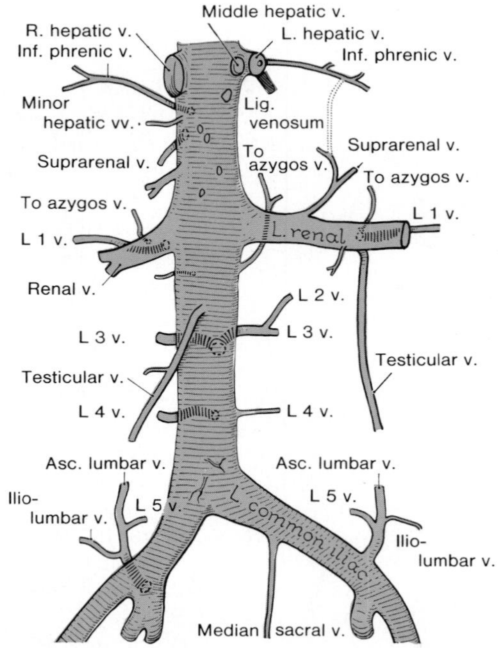

Figure 2-129. Drawing of the inferior vena cava and its tributaries. This is the widest vein in the body. It drains blood from the lower limbs, most of the abdominal wall, the urogenital system, and the suprarenal glands.

the presence of lipoid substances in them. *Each suprarenal gland is enclosed with the kidney within the renal fascia.* A little fatty connective tissue separates it from the superior pole of the kidney; hence, it can be easily separated from this organ. The shape and relations of the suprarenal glands differ on the two sides.

The Right Suprarenal Gland. This gland is *pyramidal in shape* with its apex upward and its base on the kidney. It lies between the diaphragm posteromedially and the inferior vena cava anteromedially. The **bare area of the liver** is anterior to it (Fig. 2-79) and the kidney is inferior to it. Superiorly the gland lies on the bare area of the liver (Fig. 2-69*A*). Its inferior end is covered by peritoneum reflected onto it from the liver. Its hilum is on its anterior surface and from it the right suprarenal vein leaves to drain into the inferior vena cava (Fig. 2-129).

The Left Suprarenal Gland. This gland is *semilunar in shape* and extends further down the medial margin of the kidney than does the right gland (Fig. 2-69*B*). It is *related anteriorly to the stomach and pancreas and posteriorly to the diaphragm.* Its hilum is also anterior and from it the left suprarenal vein leaves to drain into the left renal vein (Fig. 2-129).

Structure of the Suprarenal Glands. A sectioned, fresh suprarenal gland shows two distinct regions, an outer **cortex** and an inner **medulla**. These regions are distinct embryologically, structurally, and functionally. Each gland is surrounded by a tough connective tissue capsule. The cortex, the major part of the gland, secretes a considerable number of steroid hormones and is essential to life. The medulla, *derived from the neural crest*, secretes **adrenaline** and noradrenaline. It is not essential to life because these hormones are also secreted by postganglionic sympathetic nerve fibers.

Vessels and Nerves of the Suprarenal Glands (Figs. 2-55, 2-69, 2-111, 2-113, 2-127, 2-129, and 2-140). The suprarenal glands have an **abundant arterial supply** from *three sources.* Each gland has a direct branch from the **aorta** (up to 10) and also receives branches from the **inferior phrenic** (up to 27) and **renal** (up to 30) arteries. Although each gland may receive over 60 arteries, it is drained by a *single, large, central vein.* The right suprarenal vein drains into the superior vena cava, whereas the left suprarenal vein joins the left renal vein (Fig. 2-129).

Each suprarenal gland also has a **rich nerve supply**, mainly from preganglionic sympathetic fibers from the splanchnic nerves and the celiac plexus (Figs. 2-111 and 2-127). These nerve fibers pass through the hilum into the medulla of the gland. Apparently the cortex receives no nerve supply. Many **lymph vessels** leave these glands and end in the **aortic lymph nodes** (Figs. 2-27 and 2-134).

THE DIAPHRAGM AND POSTERIOR ABDOMINAL WALL

THE DIAPHRAGM

The diaphragm (G. *dia*, through, across + *phragma*, a partition) is a *musculotendinous partition separating the thoracic and abdominal cavities* (Figs. 2-29 and 2-130). The diaphragm, **the principal muscle of respiration**, closes the inferior thoracic aperture (thoracic outlet); hence, *it forms the dome-shaped roof of the abdomen and the floor of the thorax.* It is pierced by the structures passing between the thorax and the abdomen (Figs. 2-36 and 2-132). As it **rises and falls during respiration**, it *alternately decreases and increases the vertical dimension of the thoracic cavity.* The heart lies on the central part of the diaphragm and slightly depresses it (Fig. 2-133). For descriptive purposes, the cup-shaped right and left sides of the diaphragm are referred to as the **hemidiaphragms** (cupolae, domes, leaves). *All four terms refer to the halves of the diaphragm.*

Structure of the Diaphragm (Figs. 1-34, 2-29, 2-36, and 2-130 to 2-132). The diaphragm is composed of a **muscular portion** consisting of a sheet of radiating muscle fibers, extending from the inferior border of the thorax and the upper lumbar vertebrae, and converging on a trefoil-shaped **aponeurotic portion** called the **central tendon.**

The Central Tendon (Figs. 1-34 and 2-130). The central tendon is *a strong aponeurosis with interlacing tendinous fibers.* **All muscle fibers of the diaphragm converge on the central tendon.** It is incompletely divided into three leaves (*i.e.*, it is trefoiled) which give it a C-shaped appearance somewhat like a boomerang. The middle leaf (lobe) is anterior and intermediate in size, whereas the right lateral one is the largest and the left lateral leaf is the smallest. The right and left leaves curve posteriorly in the corresponding halves of the diaphragm. *The middle leaf of the central tendon lies just below the heart* (Figs. 1-34, 1-52 to 1-54, 2-29, and 2-133). The heart is held closely to the diaphragm because the **fibrous pericardium** (the fibrous sac enclosing the serous pericardium and the heart) is fused with the central tendon. The central tendon has no bony attachments. The *foramen for the inferior vena cava* is in the right side of the middle leaf (Figs. 2-130 and 2-132).

The Muscular Portion (Figs. 2-113 and 2-130 to 2-133). The muscular part **inserts into the central tendon** and is *divided into three parts* according to the origin of its fibers.

1. **The sternal part** consists of two *small muscular slips* that arise from the posterior aspect of the **xiphoid process** of the sternum and pass backward to insert into the central tendon. In the cadaver the sternal part often appears to ascend from its origin because of the postmortem relaxation of the diaphragm. On each side of these small muscle slips there is a small anterolateral gap or hiatus known as the **sternocostal hiatus** (foramen of Morgagni). The superior epigastric branch of the **internal thoracic artery** (Fig. 1-21), its **venae comitantes** (accompanying veins), and some **lymph vessels** from the abdominal wall and the superior surface of the liver pass through the sternocostal hiatus (Fig. 2-130).
2. **The costal part** consists of *wide muscular slips* arising from the internal surface of the **lower six ribs** at the costal margin. *They interdigitate with the slips of the transversus abdominis muscles* at their costal attachments (Figs. 1-21 and 2-131). The costal parts of the muscular portion of the diaphragm form the right and left hemidiaphragms or domes that are visible on radiographs of the chest (Figs. 1-38, 1-58, and 1-59).
3. **The lumbar part** (vertebral part) arises from the lumbar vertebrae by **two crura** and from the **arcuate ligaments.** The diaphragm has two musculotendinous crura (L. legs) which are *attached on each side of the aorta to the anterolateral surfaces of the upper two (left) or three (right)* lumbar vertebrae and the intervening intervertebral discs. The crura blend with the **anterior longitudinal ligament** of the vertebral column (Fig. 2-131). The **right crus** is broader and longer than the **left crus**. *The fibers of the right crus surround the esophageal hiatus.*

There are three arcuate ligaments (Figs. 2-130, 2-131, and 2-134) which give rise to fibers of the diaphragm.

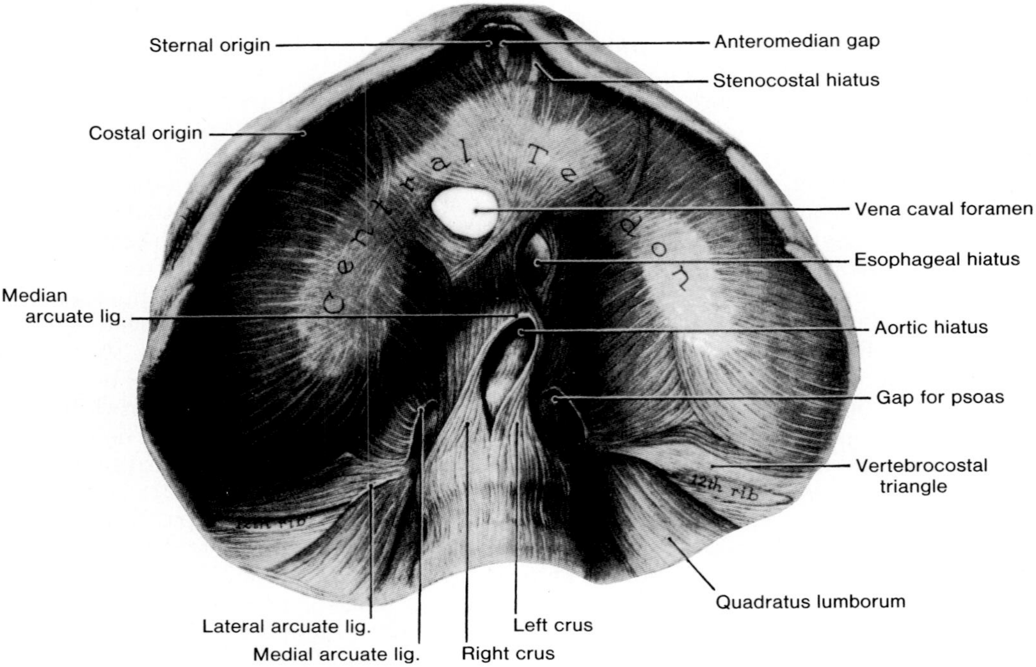

Figure 2-130. Drawing of the diaphragm as viewed from below. Observe the trefoil-shaped, aponeurotic insertion called the *central tendon* and the fleshly fibers of the sternal, costal, and lumbar origins that converge on this tendon. Examine the three large openings in the diaphragm: (1) the vena caval foramen in the central tendon; (2) the esophageal hiatus (almost a canal) surrounded by fibers of one or both crura; and (3) the aortic hiatus lying behind the diaphragm in the median plane. Observe the right and left crura on the sides of the aortic hiatus which are united above by a fibrous arch, the median arcuate ligament. Note the thickenings of the psoas and quadratus lumborum fasciae, called the medial and lateral arcuate ligaments. These structures give origin to the diaphragm. In this cadaver the diaphragm does not arise from the left arcuate ligament; hence, the vertebrocostal triangle consists only of an areolar membrane separating the kidney and its pararenal fat from the pleura.

The median arcuate ligament is a tendinous band that unites the medial sides of the two crura. It passes over the anterior surface of the aorta and gives origin to some fibers of the right crus of the diaphragm (Figs. 2-130 and 2-131). The median arcuate ligament is often poorly defined.

The medial arcuate ligament (medial lumbosacral arch) on each side is a thickening of the anterior layer of the thoracolumbar fascia over the superior part of the psoas major muscle. It forms a fibrous arch that runs from the crus of the diaphragm, superficial to the psoas major muscle, and attaches to the transverse process of the first lumbar vertebra.

The lateral arcuate ligament (lateral lumbosacral arch) on each side is also a thickening of the anterior layer of the thoracolumbar fascia over the superior part of the quadratus lumborum muscle, which forms a fibrous arch running from the transverse process of the first lumbar vertebra to the 12th rib. Above the lateral arcuate ligament, the muscular portion of the diaphragm is often thin, especially above the left kidney, because the lateral arcuate ligament does not reach the tip of the 12th rib. This triangular deficiency, known as the **vertebrocostal triangle**, consists only of an areolar membrane separating the left kidney from the pleura. This triangular area is the *usual site for a diaphragmatic hernia* and an eventration of the diaphragm (see subsequent clinically oriented comments).

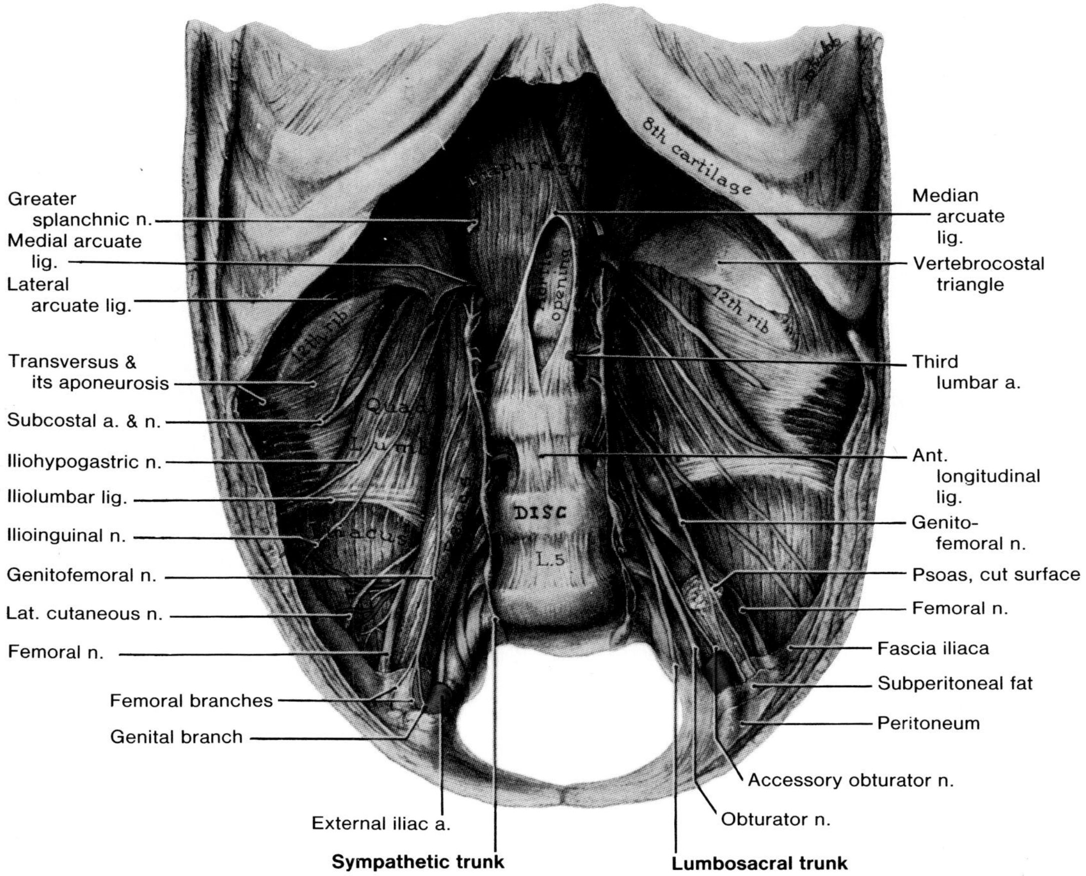

Figure 2-131. Drawing of a dissection of the posterior abdominal wall showing the lumbar plexus. Most of the fascia has been removed from the posterior wall. *Examine the muscles.* Note that most of the left psoas major muscle has been removed to show the lumbar plexus and that the transversus abdominis becomes aponeurotic on a line dropped from the tip of the 12th rib. Observe that the quadratus lumborum has an oblique lateral border and that its fascia is thickened to form the lateral arcuate ligament above and the iliolumbar ligament below. Note that the iliacus lies below the iliac crest and that the psoas major rises above the crest and extends above the medial arcuate ligament, which is thickened psoas fascia. Next *examine the nerves.* Observe that the subcostal nerve (T12) passes behind the lateral arcuate ligament and runs at some distance below the 12th rib with its artery. Note that the next four nerves appear at the lateral border of the psoas major muscle and that of these, the iliohypogastric (T12, L1) takes the characteristic course shown here. The ilioinguinal (L1) and the lateral femoral cutaneous nerve (L2, L3) are variable; the femoral (L2, L3, L4) descends in the angle between the iliacus and the psoas major muscles. Observe that the genitofemoral nerve (L1, L2) pierces the psoas major and its fascia anteriorly. Note that the obturator nerve (L2, L3, L4) and a branch of L4 that joins with L5 to form the lumbosacral trunk appear at the medial border of the psoas major and cross the ala of the sacrum to enter the pelvis. Now examine the *sympathetic trunk.* Observe that it enters the abdomen with the psoas major muscle from behind the medial arcuate ligament and descends on the vertebral bodies and the intervertebral discs, following closely the attached border of the psoas major to enter the pelvis. Note that its rami communicantes run dorsally with or near the lumbar arteries to join the lumbar nerves.

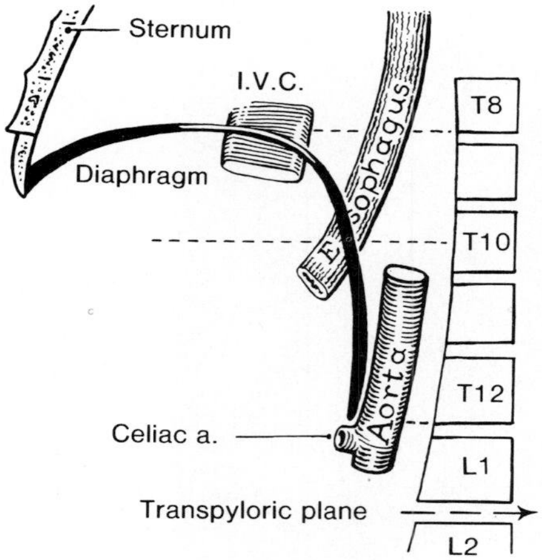

Figure 2-132. Diagram showing the three openings in the diaphragm and their vertebral levels. (Compare with Fig. 2-130). Observe that the higher the vertebral level, the more anterior is the hiatus or opening in the diaphragm. The vertebral levels are **T8, T10**, and **T12** for the inferior vena cava, esophagus, and aorta, respectively.

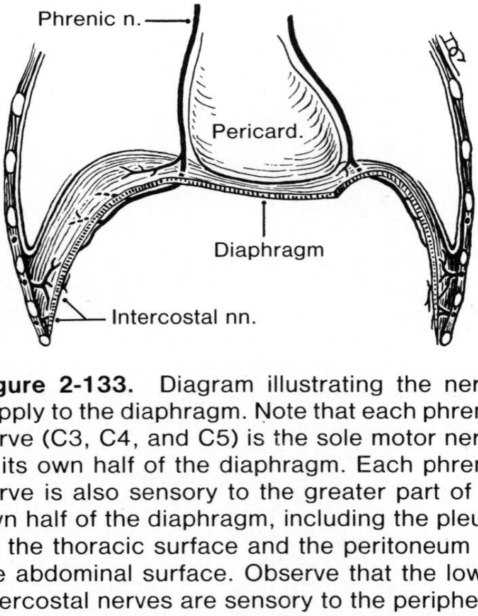

Figure 2-133. Diagram illustrating the nerve supply to the diaphragm. Note that each phrenic nerve (C3, C4, and C5) is the sole motor nerve to its own half of the diaphragm. Each phrenic nerve is also sensory to the greater part of its own half of the diaphragm, including the pleura on the thoracic surface and the peritoneum on the abdominal surface. Observe that the lower intercostal nerves are sensory to the peripheral fringe of the diaphragm. The pericardial sac contains the heart (also see Fig. 1-53).

Foramina in the Diaphragm (Figs. 1-34, 1-85, and 2-130 to 2-132). *There are three major foramina* (openings, apertures) in the diaphragm.

The Vena Caval Foramen (Figs. 1-48 and 2-130). The opening for the inferior vena cava is in the right side of the middle leaf of the central tendon of the diaphragm. It is located approximately *at the level of the disc between the eighth and ninth thoracic vertebrae,* 2 to 3 cm to the right of the median plane (Fig. 2-132). It is the highest of the three large openings in the diaphragm. *The inferior vena cava is adherent to the margin of the vena caval foramen*; thus, when the diaphragm contracts during inspiration, it pulls the vena caval foramen open and stretches and dilates the inferior vena cava. These changes facilitate the flow of blood through it from the abdomen to the thorax. *Some branches of the right phrenic nerve and some lymph vessels from the liver pass through the vena caval foramen.* Sometimes the right hepatic vein passes through this foramen before it drains into the inferior vena cava.

The Esophageal Hiatus (Figs. 1-85 and 2-130). The esophagus passes obliquely through this oval hiatus in the muscular portion of the diaphragm, just posterior to the central tendon. *It is located in the right crus of the diaphragm,* 2 to 3 cm to the left of the median plane, approximately *at the level of the 10th thoracic vertebra* (Fig. 2-132). It also transmits the **anterior** and **posterior vagal trunks** (Fig. 2-111) and the esophageal branches of the **left gastric vessels** (Fig. 2-56). When the portal vein is obstructed, these veins provide a clinically important alternate route for drainage of portal venous blood (see previous discussion of portal-caval anastomoses and Fig. 2-112). *The esophagus is circled by the fleshy fibers of the right crus* as they swing across the midline. These fibers constrict the distal end of the esophagus during inspiration, helping to prevent the reflux of gastric contents into the esophagus. This constriction can be easily observed during barium studies of the esophagus (Fig. 2-34).

The Aortic Hiatus (Figs. 1-85 and 2-130). The aorta does not pierce the diaphragm but *passes posterior to the median arcuate ligament and anterior to the 12th thoracic vertebra* (Fig. 2-132) just to the left of the midline (Fig. 2-130). The aorta is unaffected by contraction of the diaphragm because it lies behind it. The aortic hiatus also trans-

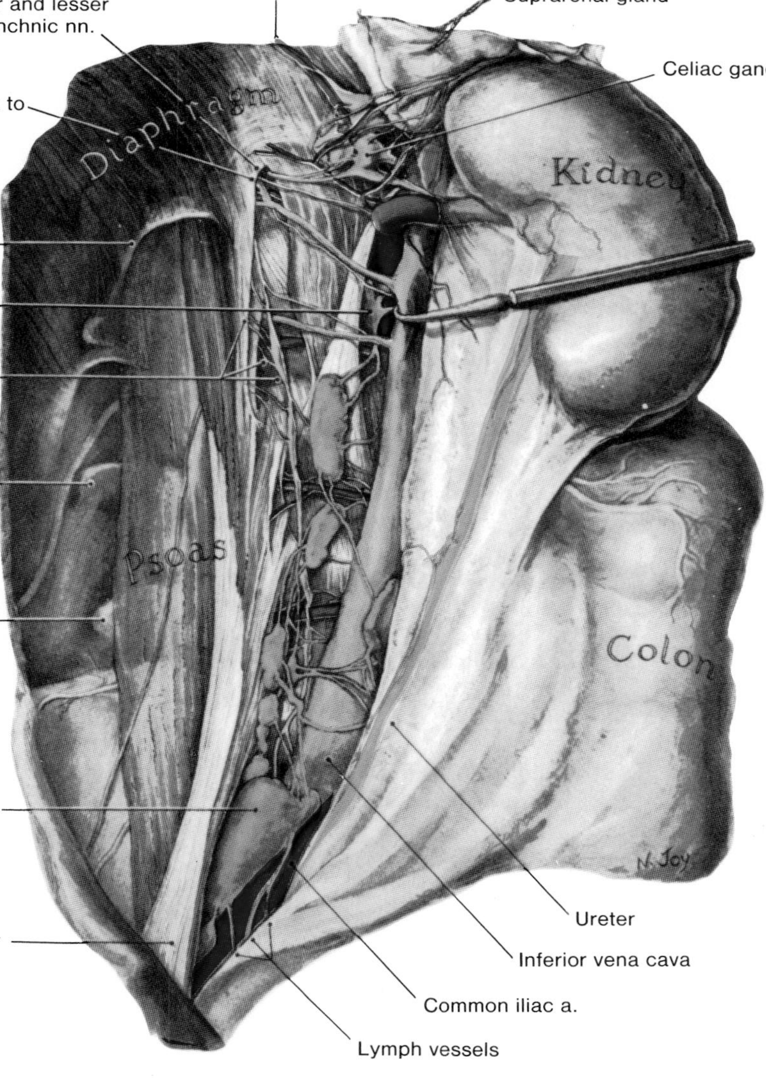

Figure 2-134. Drawing of a dissection of the posterior abdominal wall showing the right celiac ganglion, the splanchnic nerves, and the sympathetic trunk. The right suprarenal gland, kidney, ureter, and colon are turned to the left like the page of a book so that the posterior surface of the right kidney is facing you. The inferior vena cava is pulled medially and the third and fourth lumbar veins are removed. Observe that there is a psoas minor muscle in this specimen. Note the wide cleft in the right crus of the diaphragm (not labelled) through which pass both splanchnic nerves, the sympathetic trunk, and a communicating vein. Observe the greater splanchnic nerve ending in the celiac ganglion. Usually the greater splanchnic nerve pierces the crus at the level of the celiac trunk (Fig. 2-131). The lesser splanchnic nerve passes inferolateral to this and the sympathetic trunk enters with the psoas major muscle. Examine the sympathetic trunk lying on the bodies of the vertebrae, the lumbar vessels alone intervening, and descending along the anterior border of the psoas major muscle. Note that the trunk is slender where it enters the abdomen and that its ganglia are ill defined. Observe that about 11 rami communicantes join it posterolaterally and about 6 visceral branches or lumbar splanchnic nerves, leave it anteromedially. Examine the right lumbar lymph nodes and lymph vessels (*green*) draining into the cisterna chyli (also see Fig. 1-85).

mits the **thoracic duct** (Fig. 2-147), the **azygos vein**, and **lymph vessels** descending from the thorax to the **cysterna chyli** (Figs. 1-85, 2-134, and 2-147).

Other Structures Passing Through or Around the Diaphragm (Figs. 2-131, 2-132, and 2-134). The **right phrenic nerve** passes through the *central tendon* of the diaphragm, either through the vena caval foramen or just lateral to it (Fig. 1-53). The **left phrenic nerve** passes through the *muscular portion of the diaphragm* in front of the central tendon, just lateral to the pericardium of the heart (Fig. 2-133).

The **superior epigastric vessels** (Fig. 2-8) pass through the *sternocostal hiatus*, the interval between the sternal and costal origins of the muscular part of the diaphragm (Fig. 2-130). The **musculophrenic vessels** perforate the diaphragm near the ninth costal cartilage.

The lower five **intercostal nerves** pass between the muscle slips of the diaphragm arising deep to the costal cartilages of the lower six ribs. The **subcostal nerves** and **vessels** pass through the diaphragm *posterior to the lateral arcuate ligament* (Fig. 2-131). The **sympathetic trunks** pass through the diaphragm *posterior to the medial arcuate ligaments. The* **splanchnic nerves** pierce the crura (Fig. 2-131) and the **hemiazygos** vein passes through the left crus.

Vessels and Nerves of the Diaphragm (Figs. 2-55, 2-111, and 2-133). The main arteries supplying the diaphragm are the **phrenic arteries** which arise from the front of the aorta and two branches of the internal thoracic artery, the **musculophrenic** and the **pericardiophrenic**. Each pericardiophrenic artery accompanies a phrenic nerve between the pleura and the pericardium to the diaphragm.

There is an extensive network of lymph vessels on the thoracic and abdominal surfaces of the diaphragm. These drain into the phrenic or **diaphragmatic lymph nodes** located on the thoracic surface of the diaphragm. Lymph vessels from the **bare area of the liver**, which is in direct contact with the diaphragm, also drain into middle diaphragmatic lymph nodes on the thoracic surface of the diaphragm. Lymph from these nodes drains into the *parasternal, middle phrenic, and posterior mediastinal lymph nodes* (Figs. 1-20 and 1-48). A few lymph vessels from the abdominal surface of the diaphragm drain into the **lumbar lymph nodes** (Fig. 2-134).

The motor supply to the diaphragm is from the phrenic nerves (Fig. 2-133) which arise from the ventral rami of C3, C4, and C5 (chiefly C4). *The phrenic nerve is the sole motor supply to the diaphragm,* but it also contains sensory fibers. The contribution to the phrenic nerve from the ventral ramus of C5 may be derived as a branch from the **nerve to the subclavius muscle** (Fig. 6-24). This is called the **accessory phrenic nerve**. *The high level of origin of the phrenic nerves from the cervical segments results from the caudal migration of the developing diaphragm relative to the vertebral column.* In addition to the sensory nerve supply from the phrenic nerves, the diaphragm receives sensory fibers from the **intercostal nerves** (Fig. 2-133). They supply the peripheral fringes of the diaphragm that develop from the lateral body walls (Fig. 2-135).

Actions of the Diaphragm. *The diaphragm is the chief muscle of inspiration.* During inspiration its muscular portion contracts, drawing its central tendon downward and forward. As the dome of the diaphragm moves downward it pushes the abdominal viscera before it. This **increases** *the volume of the thoracic cavity* and **decreases** *the intrathoracic pressure*, resulting in air being taken into the lungs. In addition, the volume of the abdominal cavity is somewhat decreased and the intra-abdominal pressure is somewhat raised because **the anterior abdominal wall moves reciprocally with the diaphragm**.

Diaphragmatic movements are also important in the circulation of blood because the increased abdominal pressure and decreased thoracic pressure accompanying contraction of the diaphragm are helpful in returning blood to the heart. When the diaphragm contracts, compressing the abdominal viscera, blood in the inferior vena cava is forced upward into the heart. This movement is facilitated by the enlargement of the vena caval foramen and the dilation of the inferior vena cava that occurs when the diaphragm contracts (see previous discussion).

The diaphragm is an important muscle in abdominal straining. It assists the anterior abdominal muscles in raising the intra-abdominal pressure during **micturition** (urination), **defecation** (bowel movements), and **parturition** (childbirth). **During these processes, a person often inspires deeply, closing the glottis (the opening in the larynx or organ of voice production). This traps air in the respiratory tract and** prevents the diaphragm from rising. A grunt is produced when some air escapes from the respiratory tract. A different sound is heard when air escapes from the GI tract.

The diaphragm is used during weight lifting. A person about to lift a heavy object also takes a deep breath to raise intra-abdominal pressure by the mechanism described in the previous paragraph. *Increased intra-abdominal pressure gives additional support to the vertebral column* and helps to prevent its flexion. Persons with diarrhea and/or incontinence are advised not to lift weights for obvious physiological reasons.

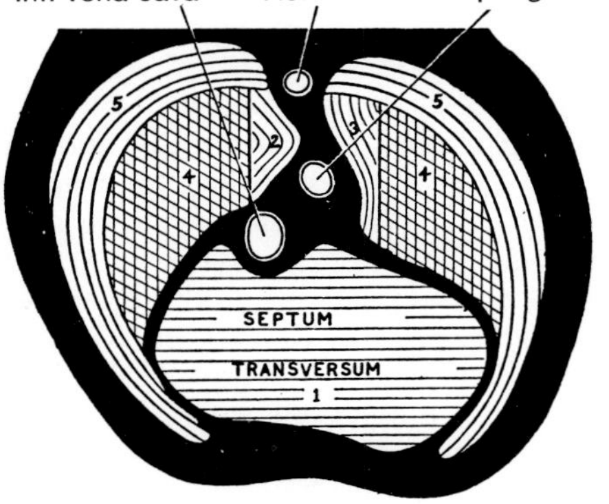

Figure 2-135. Diagram illustrating the composite origin of the diaphragm, viewed from below. The structures from which the diaphragm developed are: *1* = septum transversum; *2,3* = dorsal mesentery; *4* = pleuroperitoneal membrane; *5* = body wall. The septum transversum forms the central tendon. The pleuroperitoneal membranes (*4*) fuse with the dorsal mesentery of the esophagus (*2,3*) and with the septum transversum. Failure of a pleuroperitoneal membrane, usually on the left, to unite with the crural part of the diaphragm (formed from the dorsal mesentery of the esophagus) results in the pleural and peritoneal cavities remaining in communication and in herniation of abdominal contents into the thoracic cavity. (Fig. 2-152).

Position of the Diaphragm (Figs. 1-34, 1-38, 1-53, 1-58, 1-59, 2-29, 2-36, and 2-130 to 2-133). *It is clinically important to acquire a three-dimensional concept of the diaphragm,* particularly for viewing radiographs of the thorax and abdomen. The posterior attachment of the dome-shaped diaphragm is considerably lower than its anterior attachment; hence there is much of it that cannot be seen in posteroanterior radiographs. Normally the right hemidiaphragm bulges higher into the thorax than does the left hemidiaphragm (Fig. 2-133). Moreover, *the level of the diaphragm on both sides varies in relation to the ribs and the vertebrae according to* (1) *the phase of respiration* (compare Figs. 1-58 and 1-59), (2) the posture assumed, and (3) the size and degree of distention of the abdominal viscera. The diaphragm is highest when a person is supine (particularly when the head is lower than the feet) because the abdominal viscera push the diaphragm upward into the thorax. The diaphragm assumes a lower level when the person is sitting or is in an erect position. This explains why patients with **dyspnea** (difficult breathing) prefer to sit up rather than lie down. When a person lies on one side, the hemidiaphragm next to the bed or table rises to a higher level owing to the upward push of the viscera on that side.

CLINICALLY ORIENTED COMMENTS

The diaphragm develops from four different sources, as illustrated in Figure 2-135. Failure of fusion of these parts occurs about once in every 2200 fetuses and results in **congenital diaphragmatic hernia** (Fig. 2-152), usually on the left side. Defective formation and/or fusion of the left pleuroperitoneal membrane with other parts of the diaphragm is the usual cause of developmental defects in the diaphragm. *A posterolateral defect occurs five times more often on the left side than on the right* and is located at the periphery of the diaphragm in the region of the **vertebrocostal triangle** (Fig. 2-130). The intestines and occasionally other abdominal viscera pass through this **posterolateral defect** (foramen of Bochdalek) into the thoracic cavity. Radiographs of the chest reveal gas-filled loops of bowel in the left pleural cavity and displacement of the thoracic viscera. The herniated bowel prevents inflation of the lung when the baby is born. After a few minutes or hours, the infant swallows air, which distends the gut somewhat, and the underinflated lung is then compressed. These conditions frequently result in the infant suffering **severe respiratory distress**. When the hernia is detected, the herniated viscera are replaced into the abdominal cavity and the defect in the diaphragm is closed surgically. *Expansion of the hypoplastic lung may take several days.*

When muscle fails to grow into the pleuroperitoneal membrane in the region of the **vertebrocostal triangle**, only an areolar membrane separates the kidney and other abdominal viscera from the thoracic cavity (Figs. 2-130 and 2-131). *This creates a potential site for eventration.* If this occurs, the abdominal viscera herniate into the thoracic cavity, but they are covered by the thin areolar membrane that closed the vertebrocostal triangle. This condition, also more common on the left, is called **eventration of the diaphragm** (extreme elevation of half or part of the diaphragm). This abnormality may be present at birth or develop later in life. Eventrations may also occur through a very thin part of the central tendon.

A rare type of hernia is through the **sternocostal hiatus** (foramen of Morgagni) for the superior epigastric vessels (Fig. 2-130). This uncommon type of hernia usually occurs on the right because of the attachment of the pericardium to the diaphragm on the left (Figs. 1-30 and 1-53).

Acquired hiatal herniae are common. This condition develops in people around middle age in whom *weakening* and *widening of the esophageal hiatus* has occurred (see previous discussion of this type of hernia on page 175 and Fig. 2-53).

Section of the phrenic nerve in the neck results in complete paralysis and atrophy of the muscle of the corresponding half of the diaphragm, except in persons who have an **accessory phrenic nerve** supplying motor fibers distal to the lesion. *Paralysis of a hemidiaphragm can be recognized radiographically by its permanent elevation and paradoxical movement.* Instead of descending on inspiration, it is forced upward by the increased intra-abdominal pressure secondary to descent of the unparalyzed opposite hemidiaphragm.

Because there are many communications between the lymphatics on the abdominal surface of the diaphragm with those on its thoracic surface and with the lymphatics in the thorax, a **subphrenic abscess** (discussed on page 207) or collection of pus in the **subphrenic recess** (Fig. 2-77) may lead to **pleuritis** (inflammation of the pleura). Similarly, **empyema** or pus in the pleural cavity, called *pyothorax*, may lead to development of a subphrenic abscess.

THE POSTERIOR ABDOMINAL WALL

The posterior abdominal wall is composed principally of **muscles** and **fascia** attached to the vertebrae, the ossa coxae (hip bones), and the ribs. There are also important **nerves**, **vessels**, and **lymph nodes** on the posterior abdominal wall.

Muscles of the Posterior Abdominal Wall (Figs. 2-113, 2-119 to 2-123, 2-130, 2-131, 2-134, and 2-136 to 2-138). The diaphragm and its crura, which could be included under this heading, have been described. *There are three paired muscles of the posterior wall that are clinically important*: **psoas major**, **iliacus**, and **quadratus lumborum**. As the psoas major and the iliacus muscles form a functional unit, they are often referred to as the **iliopsoas muscle**, *the most powerful flexor of the thigh.* These muscles are attached to the femur and act on the hip joint; hence, they are also described with the lower limb (Chap. 4).

The Psoas Major Muscle (Figs. 2-113, 2-118 to 2-121, 2-131, 2-134, 2-138, 4-19, and 4-20). This long, thick, fusiform muscle *lies* *lateral to the sides of the lumber region* of the vertebral column. Psoas is a Greek word meaning *the muscle of the loin.* Butchers refer to the psoas muscle in animals as the tenderloin.

Origin. **Transverse processes** and upper and lower borders of sides of **bodies of L1 to L5** vertebrae and associated **intervertebral discs of T12 to L5** vertbrae. It descends along the brim of the pelvis and enters the thigh by passing posterior to the inguinal ligament.

Insertion (Fig. 4-30). **Lesser trochanter of femur.**

Nerve Supply. Ventral rami of **lumbar nerves L2 to L4.**

Actions. **Flexes thigh** at hip joint. *Acts with iliacus muscle as part of iliopsoas* muscle. **Bends vertebral column forward,** (*e.g.,* when sitting up from supine position). **Bends (flexes) lumbar region laterally.** This action is used to maintain the balance of the trunk when sitting.

The Iliacus Muscle (Figs. 2-113, 2-131, 4-19, and 5-40). This large triangular sheet of muscle *lies along the lateral side of the lower part of the psoas* major muscle.

Origin. Upper part of **iliac fossa.** Its fibers pass inferomedially behind the inguinal ligament. Most of them attach to the side of the psoas tendon and the two muscles are then called the iliopsoas muscle.

Insertion (Fig. 4-30). With psoas major into **lesser trochanter of femur,** and to femur just inferior to trochanter.

Nerve Supply. **Femoral** nerve (L2, L3).

Actions. Acting with psoas major, **flexes thigh** at hip joint. *The iliopsoas muscle is the most powerful flexor of the thigh.*

The Psoas Minor Muscle (Figs. 2-134 and 4-23*A*). This small *weak muscle* with a short belly and a long tendon is present in about 60% of cadavers. It lies in front of the psoas major in the abdomen. This muscle is well developed in cursory animals (*e.g.,* the cheetah). *It appears to be an unimportant muscle in man.*

Origin. Sides of **bodies of T12** and **L1** vertebrae and the disc between them.

Insertion (Fig. 4-1). **Pecten pubis** and **iliopubic eminence.**

Nerve Supply. Ventral ramus of **first lumbar nerve.**

Action. **Weak flexor of pelvis** and **lumbar region** of vertebral column.

CLINICALLY ORIENTED COMMENTS

When the neck of the femur breaks, a common injury in elderly persons (see Case 4-1), the iliopsoas muscle rotates the femur outward so that the foot lies with the toes pointing laterally (Fig. 4-157). This is an *important clinical sign* of a **fracture of the femoral neck.** A fracture of the femoral body would give the limb a similar appearance because lateral rotation would be produced by the adductor muscles (see Chap. 4).

The iliopsoas muscle has extensive and clinically important relations (Figs. 2-113 and 2-134). If the kidneys, ureters, cecum, appendix, sigmoid colon, pancreas, lumbar lymph nodes, or nerves of the posterior abdominal wall are diseased, *movements of the iliopsoas muscle may be accompanied by pain.* As it lies along the vertebral column and crosses the sacroiliac joint, disease of the intervertebral and **sacroiliac joints** may cause **spasm of the iliopsoas** muscle, a *protective reflex.*

Although there has been a great fall in the prevalance of *tuberculosis* in North America in recent years, this infection still occurs and may spread via the blood (**hematogenous spread**) to the vertebrae, particularly during childhood. An **abscess** (collection of pus) caused by tuberculosis in the lumbar region of the vertebral column tends to spread from the vertebrae into the psoas major muscle (**psoas abscess**). As a consequence the psoas fascia (Fig. 2-138) thickens to form a strong stocking-like tube. The pus then *tracks* (passes) inferiorly along the psoas major muscle within this fascial tube over the pelvic brim and deep to the inguinal ligament. The pus *points* (surfaces) in the **femoral triangle** (Fig. 4-18) in the upper thigh region. *The presence of a swelling in the femoral triangle may be an early sign of tuberculosis in the lumbar vertebrae.* Infected material (pus) may also travel from the thoracic region of the vertebral column to the inguinal region via the long *psoas fascial tube.*

The lower **iliac fascia** (Fig. 4-19) is often tense and raises a fold that passes to the inner aspect of the iliac crest (Fig. 2-113). The upper iliac fascia is loose and may form a pocket, sometimes called the **fossa iliacosubfascialis**, behind the above mentioned fold into which a portion of bowel may become trapped (cecum and/or appendix on the right and sigmoid colon on the left).

The Quadratus Lumborum Muscle (Figs. 2-113, 2-119, 2-121, 2-123, 2-131, 2-136, and 2-138). This is a thick **quadrilateral** (hence its name) muscular sheet. *It lies adjacent to the transverse processes of the lumbar vertebrae* and is broader inferiorly.

Origin (Figs. 2-131 and 2-136). **Iliolumbar ligament**, adjacent part of **iliac crest**, and lower two to four **lumbar transverse processes**.

Insertion (Figs. 2-136 and 2-138). Medial part of anterior surface of **12th rib** and tips of **transverse processes of L1 to L4** vertebrae. It narrows as it ascends behind the inferior margin of the diaphragm, *i.e.*, posterior to the lateral arcuate ligament.

Nerve Supply. Ventral rami of T12 (**subcostal nerve**) and **upper lumbar nerves** (usually L1 to L4).

Actions. **Fixes 12th rib** in relation to the pelvis, holding it down against the traction exerted by the diaphragm when it contracts during inspiration. It is a **muscle of inspiration** because it increases the vertical diameter of the thorax. *Acting alone*, it bends the trunk toward the same side (*i.e.*, laterally bends or laterally flexes it). *Acting together*, the two muscles help to extend the lumbar region of the vertebral column and to give it lateral stability.

The Transversus Abdominis Muscle (Figs. 1-21, 2-113, 2-122, and 2-136). This is the third and *innermost of the three flat muscles of the anterior abdominal wall.* It was described previously with these muscles. In Figure 2-134 note that the aponeurosis of the transversus abdominis muscle runs horizontally, posterior to the oblique borders of the quadratus lumborum muscle.

Fascia of the Posterior Abdominal Wall (Figs. 2-113, 2-123, 2-130, 2-137, and 4-19). Each of the muscles forming the greater part of the posterior abdominal wall is enclosed in fascia.

The Iliac Fascia (Figs. 2-131, 4-18, and 4-19). The iliac fascia **covers the psoas and iliacus muscles**. Although thin superiorly, it thickens inferiorly as it approaches the inguinal ligament. The part of the iliac fascia covering the psoas major muscle is one sheet that is *attached medially to the lumbar vertebrae and the pelvic brim* (Figs. 2-136 and 2-138). This fascial sheet is fused laterally with the anterior layer of the thoracolumbar (lumbar) fascia and, inferior to the iliac crest, it is continuous with the part of the iliac fascia covering the iliacus muscle. The part of the iliac fascia over the psoas major muscle also blends with the fascia covering the quadratus lumborum muscle. Superiorly this part of the iliac fascia is thickened to form the **medial arcuate ligament** of the diaphragm (Figs. 2-130 and 2-131).

The iliac fascia continues downward into the thigh (Fig. 4-19). The dense part of the iliac fascia covering the iliacus muscle is attached to the iliac crest and to the pelvic brim (Figs. 2-134 and 4-19) and is continuous with the transversalis fascia (Figs. 2-14 and 2-16). The posterior margin of the transversalis fascia is attached to the inguinal ligament and is there continuous with the iliac fascia as it passes into the thigh.

The Quadratus Lumborum Fascia (Figs. 2-123, 2-130, 2-131, 2-136, and 2-138). The fascia covering the quadratus lumborum muscle is the dense membranous layer that is continuous laterally with the anterior layer of the **thoracolumbar fascia**. *The fascia of the quadratus lumborum is attached to the anterior surfaces of the transverse processes of the lumbar vertebrae, the iliac crest, the 12th rib, and the fascia of the transversus abdominis muscle.* The fascia of quadratus lumborum is thickened to form the **lateral arcuate ligament** superiorly and is adherent to the **iliolumbar ligament** inferiorly (Fig. 2-131).

The Thoracolumbar Fascia (Figs. 2-122, 2-123, 2-136, 2-137, and 2-138). The thoracolumbar (lumbar) fascia is an extensive sheet of fascia covering the deep muscles of the back (Fig. 5-44). *The lumbar part of the thoracolumbar fascia extends between the 12th rib and the iliac crest.* Laterally it is

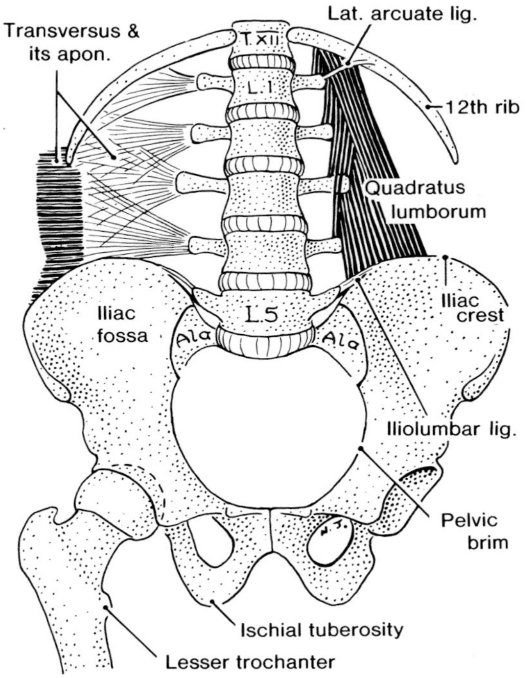

Figure 2-136. Diagram illustrating some muscles of the posterior abdominal wall. Note that the quadratus lumborum, a four-sided muscle, lies adjacent to the transverse processes of the lumbar vertebrae and that it is broader below than above. It bends (flexes) the lumbar region of the vertebral column laterally and fixes the 12th rib, preventing it from rising with the other ribs. In this way it helps to elongate the thorax during deep inspiration.

attached to the internal oblique and transversus abdominis muscles. It **splits into three layers** medially. The quadratus lumborum muscle lies between the anterior and middle layers (Fig. 2-138).

The deep back muscles are enclosed between the middle and posterior layers of the thoracolumbar fascia (Fig. 2-138). The thin **anterior layer** of thoracolumbar fascia (forming the fascia covering the quadratus lumborum) is attached along with the psoas fascia to the anterior surfaces of the lumbar transverse processes. *The thick* **middle layer** *is attached to the tips of the transverse processes. The dense* **posterior layer** *is attached to the spinous processes of the lumbar and sacral vertebrae and to the* supraspinous ligament (Fig. 5-34).

Nerves of the Posterior Abdominal Wall (Figs. 2-111, 2-113, 2-119, 2-121 to 2-123, 2-127, 2-131, and 2-137). There are *two types of nerves* in the posterior abdominal wall; **somatic nerves of the lumbar plexus** and its branches (Fig. 2-131), and visceral or **splanchnic nerves of the autonomic nervous system** (Figs. 2-127 and 2-131).

The five lumbar nerves pass from the spinal cord through the intervertebral foramina below the corresponding vertebrae and divide into dorsal and ventral primary rami. Each ramus contains both sensory and motor fibers. The **dorsal primary rami** pass posteriorly to supply the muscles and skin of the back (Fig. 2-137), whereas the **ventral primary rami** extend into the posterior part of the psoas major muscle. Here they are connected to the sympathetic trunk by **rami communicantes** (Figs. 2-131 and 2-134) and give branches to the psoas major, quadratus lumborum, and intertransverse muscles (Fig. 2-138). *The ventral rami of L1 to L3 nerves and the upper branch of L4 form the* **lumbar plexus** (Figs. 2-131 and 2-139). The lower branch of L4 and the whole of L5 form the **lumbosacral trunk** (Fig. 2-131), which descends to the **sacral plexus** (Fig. 2-139).

The subcostal nerve is the ventral ramus of **T12**. It *passes below the lateral arcuate ligament* of the diaphragm, about 1 cm caudal to the 12th rib (Fig. 2-131). Usually it sends a branch to the ventral ramus of the first lumbar nerve and then runs inferolaterally across the anterior surface of the quadratus lumborum muscle. It pierces the transversus abdominis muscle and runs in the anterior abdominal wall between this muscle and the internal oblique. The subcostal nerve (T12) supplies the abdominal wall inferior to the umbilicus and superior to the pubic symphysis (Figs. 2-45 and 2-141).

The Lumbar Plexus of Nerves (Figs. 2-131 and 2-139). **The lumbar plexus is formed within the psoas major muscle**, anterior to the transverse processes of the lumbar vertebrae. Hence, the origin of the nerves contributing to it can be studied only when this muscle is carefully removed. These *nerves pass through the psoas major*

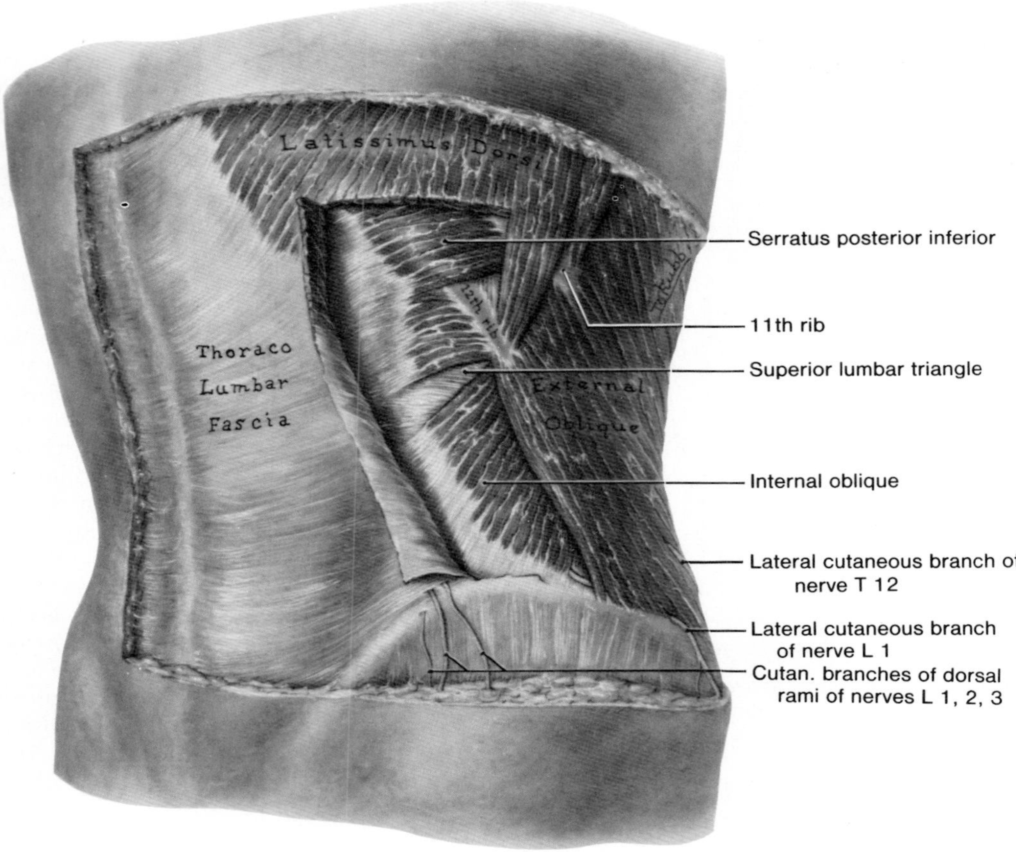

Figure 2-137. Drawing of a dissection of a posterolateral view of the posterior abdominal wall. The latissimus dorsi muscle is in the part reflected. Observe that the external oblique muscle has an oblique, free posterior border which extends from the tip of the 12th rib to the midpoint of the iliac crest. Examine the small triangular space between the external oblique, the latissimus dorsi, and the iliac crest. This is the (inferior) lumbar triangle. Observe that the internal oblique muscle extends behind the external oblique and forms the floor of the lumbar triangle, creeping up on the lumbar fascia. Note that the internal oblique has a triangle between it and the serratus posterior inferior muscle. This is the "superior lumbar triangle."

at different levels. The plexus is formed by the **ventral rami of the first three lumbar nerves with the upper part of the fourth lumbar nerve.** In many people (at least 50%) there is a *contribution from the subcostal nerve* (the large ventral ramus of T12). All five ventral rami receive gray rami communicantes from the sympathetic trunk, and the upper two send white rami communicantes to the sympathetic trunk. The rami communicantes are discussed more fully in a subsequent section.

The largest and most important branches of the lumbar plexus are the femoral and obturator nerves, which are derived from the same spinal cord segments.

The obturator nerve (L2, L3, and L4) descends through the psoas major muscle, leaving the medial border of this muscle at the brim of the pelvis (Fig. 2-131). It pierces the psoas fascia, crosses the sacroiliac joint, passes lateral to the internal iliac vessels and the ureter, and enters the pelvis minor. Here it lies in the extraperitoneal fat where it is liable to be injured in operations designed to remove the pelvic lymphatics. *It leaves the pelvis by passing through the obturator foramen into the thigh.* (Also see

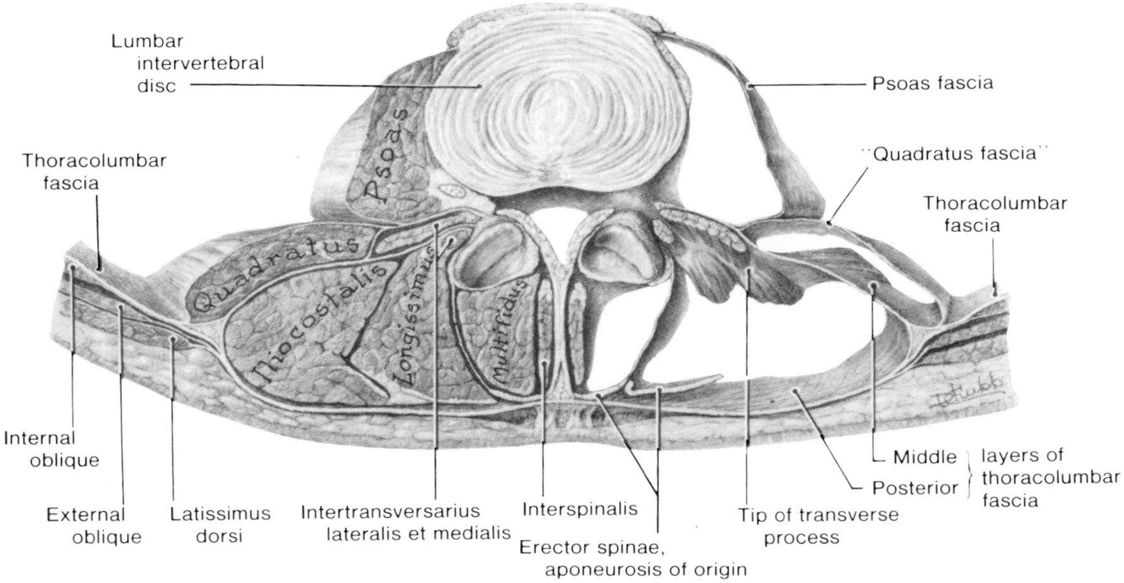

Figure 2-138. Drawing of a dissection of the muscles of the back in a cross-section of the upper lumbar region. On the *right side* the empty sheaths are seen. Observe the anterior, middle, and posterior layers of the thoracolumbar (lumbar) fascia which enclose the deep muscles of the back. Note that the posterior layer is reinforced by the latissimus dorsi and at a higher level by the serratus posterior inferior. Observe the fascial layers covering the quadratus lumborum and psoas muscles. Note that the ends of the intertransversarius, longissimus, and quadratus lumborum muscles are attached to a transverse process.

discussion of this nerve in Chap. 3 and Figs. 3-58 and 3-59).

The femoral nerve (L2, L3, and L4) pierces the psoas major muscle, runs downward and laterally within it to emerge between the psoas major and the iliacus (Fig. 4-131), just above the inguinal ligament. It enters the thigh lateral to the femoral artery and the femoral sheath (Figs. 4-18 and 4-20). In the abdomen it *supplies the psoas and iliacus muscles.* (See Chap. 4 for its distribution in the thigh).

The ilioinguinal and iliohypogastric nerves are both derived from **L1**, often by a common stem. *They enter the abdomen behind the medial arcuate ligament* of the diaphragm (Fig. 2-131) and **pass inferolaterally in front of the quadratus lumborum** muscle. Often the two nerves do not separate until they are under cover of the transversus abdominis muscle. They pierce the transversus abdominis muscle near the **anterior superior iliac spine** and then the internal and external oblique muscles to *supply the skin of the suprapublic and inguinal regions.* Both nerves also supply branches to the abdominal musculature. **The iliohypogastric nerve (L1)** sends a *lateral branch* to supply the *skin of the gluteal region* (Fig. 4-49) and an *anterior branch* to the *skin of the hypogastric region* (Figs. 2-6 and 2-8). **The ilioinguinal nerve (L1)** passes through the superficial inguinal ring and supplies the *skin of the groin and the scrotum or labium majus* (Fig. 2-7).

The genitofemoral nerve (L1 and L2) pierces the iliac fascia and the anterior surface of the psoas major muscle (Figs. 2-131 and 4-19). It runs inferiorly in the muscle and divides lateral to the common and external iliac arteries into *two branches,* **femoral** and **genital**.

The genital branch of the genitofemoral nerve runs to the deep inguinal ring and *transverses the inguinal canal,* supplying the **cremaster** and **dartos muscles** (Fig. 2-12) and the *skin of the scrotum* or the

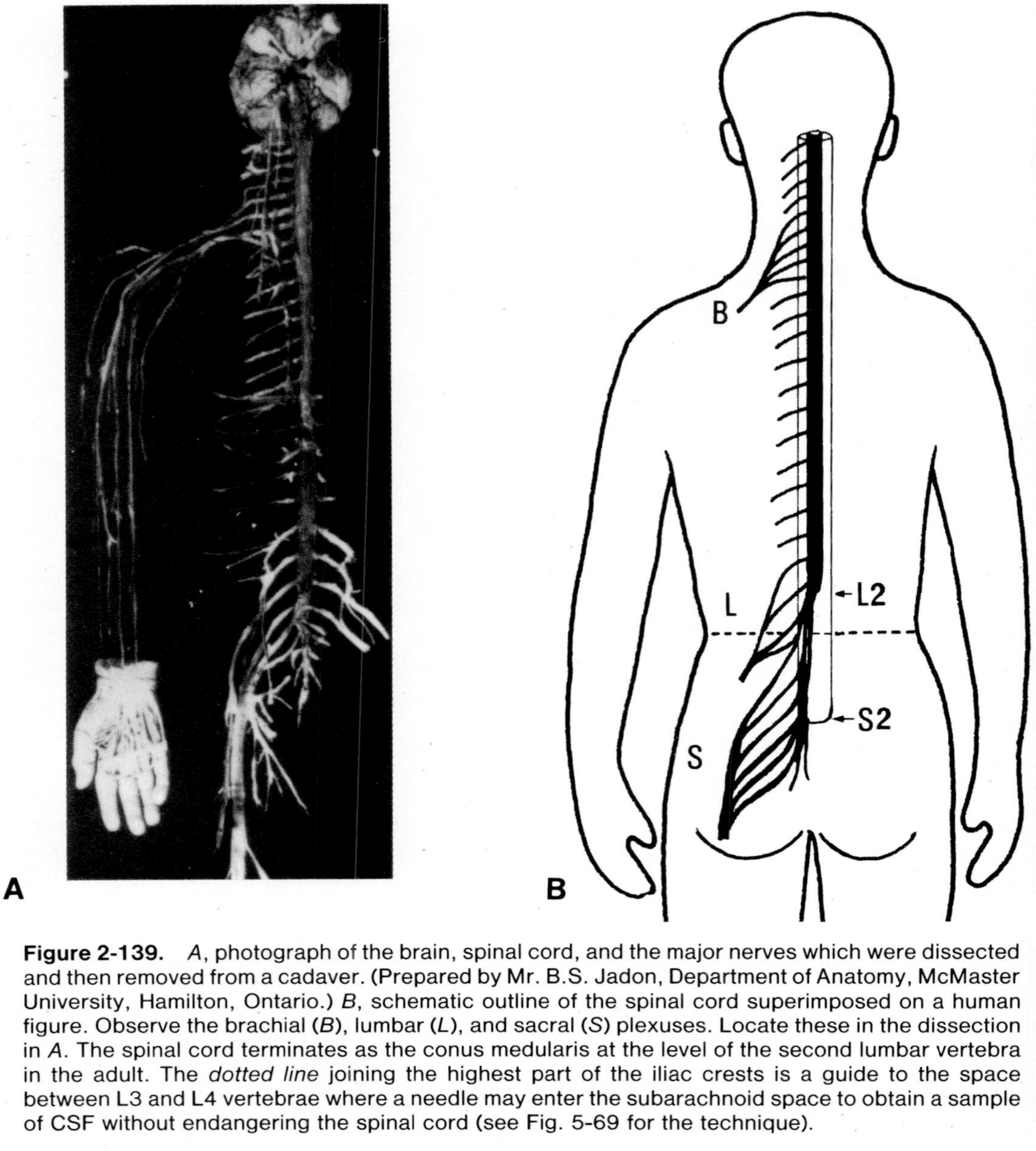

Figure 2-139. *A*, photograph of the brain, spinal cord, and the major nerves which were dissected and then removed from a cadaver. (Prepared by Mr. B.S. Jadon, Department of Anatomy, McMaster University, Hamilton, Ontario.) *B*, schematic outline of the spinal cord superimposed on a human figure. Observe the brachial (*B*), lumbar (*L*), and sacral (*S*) plexuses. Locate these in the dissection in *A*. The spinal cord terminates as the conus medularis at the level of the second lumbar vertebra in the adult. The *dotted line* joining the highest part of the iliac crests is a guide to the space between L3 and L4 vertebrae where a needle may enter the subarachnoid space to obtain a sample of CSF without endangering the spinal cord (see Fig. 5-69 for the technique).

round ligament of the uterus and the *skin of the labium majus* (Fig. 4-14).

The femoral branch of the genitofemoral nerve passes on the lateral side of the femoral artery beneath the inguinal ligament, within the **femoral sheath** (Fig. 4-16). It pierces the anterior wall of this sheath to supply *skin over the femoral triangle* (Fig. 4-24).

The lateral femoral cutaneous nerve (L2 and L3) passes through the psoas major muscle, emerging above the **iliac crest** (Figs. 2-113 and 2-131). It runs inferolaterally on the iliacus muscle and enters the thigh behind or through the inguinal ligament, just medial to the anterior superior iliac spine (Figs. 2-14 and 4-19). It *supplies skin over the anterior and lateral parts of the thigh.*

The Lumbosacral Trunk (L4 and L5).

This large flat trunk is *formed by the lower part of the ventral ramus of the fourth lumbar nerve and the ventral primary ramus of L5.* **The L4 component** descends through the psoas major muscle (Fig. 2-131) on the medial part of the transverse process of L5 vertebra and then passes over the **ala of the sacrum** (Fig. 4-136), to which it is closely applied (Fig. 2-131), to join the **first sacral nerve**.

CLINICALLY ORIENTED COMMENTS

The iliohypogastric nerve is in danger during an appendectomy (Case 2-4). It may be injured during the **McBurney incision** (Fig. 2-45) as it passes between the external and internal oblique muscles (Fig. 2-12) in the anterior abdominal wall. If this nerve is inadvertently severed, the resulting weakness of the muscles in the region of the inguinal canal may subsequently result in the development of a **direct inguinal hernia** (Case 2-9).

In persons in whom the lateral cutaneous nerve of thigh passes through the inguinal ligament, the nerve may be compressed and irritated at this site, particularly in obese persons owing to the pressure of the bulging abdomen. This condition, called **meralgia paraesthetica**, is characterized by numbness and tingling on the outer side of the lower part of the thigh which can usually be relieved by flexing the thigh.

The Autonomic Nervous System (Figs. 1-25, 1-26, 2-59, 2-111, 2-113, 2-127, 2-131, 2-134, and 2-140). *The efferent nerves of the viscera are part of the autonomic nervous system.* It was given this name because it is concerned with involuntary activity as distinct from the nerves supplying muscles which control voluntary movement. *The autonomic nervous system has two parts,* **sympathetic** and **parasympathetic**, which are anatomically separate and mostly functionally reciprocal. The autonomic nerves emerge from the spinal cord (Fig. 1-26) and the brain stem (medulla, pons, and midbrain) as fibers of certain spinal nerves.

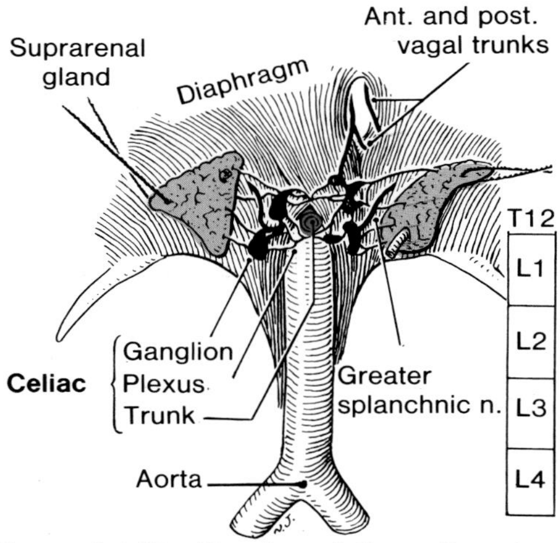

Figure 2-140. Drawing of the celiac plexus and its ganglia located around and on each side of the celiac trunk, a short artery that arises from the abdominal aorta at the level of the 12th thoracic vertebra (*T12*). Note that the celiac plexus and its ganglia are located at the level of the upper part of the first lumbar vertebra. (Also see Fig. 2-111).

The sympathetic and parasympathetic nerves are distributed to the abdominal viscera by a rich tangle of nerve plexuses and ganglia along the front of the abdominal aorta (Figs. 2-105 and 2-127). *The principal part of this system is the celiac (solar)* plexus and its ganglia located on each side of the celiac trunk, at the level of the upper part of the first lumbar vertebra (Fig. 2-111).

The Sympathetic Nerves. The thoracic splanchnic (visceral) nerves are the main source of sympathetic nerves in the abdomen (Fig. 2-127). *The greater, lesser, and lowest splanchnic nerves are branches of thoracic sympathetic ganglia 5 to 12.* The splanchnic nerves (Fig. 2-131) are **preganglionic fibers** which come from the spinal cord via **white rami communicantes** (Fig. 1-26) and *pass through the sympathetic ganglia without stopping.* They end in the celiac and aorticorenal ganglia, from which they are relayed as unmyelinated postganglionic fibers.

The greater splanchnic nerve (Figs. 2-131 and 2-134) is usually formed by branches that run anteroinferiorly on the bodies of the vertebra from the **fifth to the ninth sympathetic ganglia**. It runs caudally just lateral to the azygos vein, *pierces* *the crus of the diaphragm* (Fig. 1-131), and **ends in the celiac ganglion** (Figs. 2-111, 2-127, and 2-140).

The lesser splanchnic nerve usually arises from the **9th** and **10th sympathetic ganglia** and runs caudally, lateral to the greater splanchnic nerve, and *pierces the crus of the diaphragm*. It ends in the lower part of the celiac ganglion, also called the **aorticorenal ganglion** (Fig. 2-127).

The lowest splanchnic nerve is formed by branches from the **11th** and/or **12th sympathetic ganglion**. It pierces the crus of the diaphragm near to or with the lesser splanchnic nerve and *ends in the renal plexus* (Figs. 2-111 and 2-117).

The Abdominal Sympathetic Trunks (Figs. 2-113, 2-119, 2-131, 2-134, and 2-147). *The paired sympathetic trunks receive their preganglionic fibers from white rami communicantes* arising in the spinal cord (Fig. 1-26). Each trunk consists of a series of ganglia (11 or 12 in the thorax and 5 in the abdomen) connected by nerve fibers. Each trunk lies on the anterolateral surfaces of the vertebrae and enters the abdomen by passing *posterior to the medial arcuate ligament* (Fig. 2-131) or through the crura of the diaphragm (Fig. 2-134). It then descends anterior to the psoas major muscle or in a groove between it and the vertebral bodies. *The right sympathetic trunk lies posterior to the inferior vena cava, the lumbar lymph nodes,* and *the right ureter* (Fig. 2-134). This relationship is surgically important. Both trunks pass anterior to the small lumbar vessels supplying the posterior abdominal wall (Fig. 2-131) and then *posterior to the common iliac vessels* to enter the pelvis (Fig. 2-134). The two trunks unite in the median **ganglion impar** on the coccyx (Fig. 3-64).

The medial branches passing from the lumbar sympathetic ganglia are called the **lumbar splanchnic nerves** (Fig. 2-127). Usually their synapses are in the superior or inferior mesenteric ganglia. They pass to the **intermesenteric** (aortic) or **hypogastric plexuses** (Fig. 2-127). Branches from these plexuses pass along the arteries to the viscera.

The Abdominal Autonomic Plexuses (Figs. 2-111, 2-113, 2-127, and 2-134). These plexuses surround the abdominal aorta and its major branches. *They receive parasympathetic fibers from the vagus nerve and the sacral parasympathetic outflow. The sympathetic fibers are derived from the greater, lesser, and lowest splanchnic nerves and from the lumbar splanchnic nerves* (Fig. 2-127). The plexuses are named according to the arteries they surround or accompany (*e.g.*, celiac and aorticorenal). Collections of nerve cells (sympathetic ganglia) are scattered amongst the celiac and intermesenteric plexuses (Figs. 2-111 and 2-127). *The parasympathetic ganglia are in the walls of the viscera, e.g.*, the myenteric plexus (of Auerbach) in the muscular coat of the stomach and intestines.

The intermesenteric plexus (aortic plexus) consists of 4 to 12 nerves on the anterior and anterolateral aspects of the aorta (Fig. 2-127), *between the superior and inferior mesenteric arteries.* The intermesenteric plexus **receives contributions from the first two lumbar splanchnic nerves** and gives rise to renal, testicular (or ovarian), and ureteric branches. Occasionally it gives off branches to the duodenum, pancreas, aorta, and inferior vena cava.

The superior hypogastric plexus (presacral plexus) is continuous with the intermesenteric plexus (Fig. 2-127). It lies anterior to the inferior part of the aorta, its bifurcation, and the median sacral vessels. It *receives the lower two lumbar splanchnic nerves* and divides into **right** and **left hypogastric nerves** which pass to the inferior hypogastric plexus. The superior hypogastric plexus supplies **ureteric** and **testicular plexuses** and a plexus on each common iliac artery (Fig. 2-127).

The inferior hypogastric plexuses (Fig. 3-93) are *formed by the right and left hypogastric nerves.* There are small sympathetic ganglia within these plexuses which surround the corresponding internal iliac artery. Each plexus receives small branches from the upper sacral sympathetic ganglia and the **sacral parasympathetic outflow** from S2 to S4 (pelvic splanchnic nerves). Extensions of the inferior hypogastric plexus send autonomic fibers along the blood vessels which form visceral plexuses on the walls of the pelvic viscera (*e.g.*, the rectal plexus and the vesical plexus).

Afferent Fibers in Sympathetic Nerves. Although the sympathetic nerves are motor, they also carry some sensory fibers from sense organs in the viscera. These fibers pass toward the spinal cord via the splanchnic nerves (Fig. 2-127) as far as the sympathetic trunk (Fig. 2-131). They then pass up or down this trunk to reach the level of the spinal cord, which is to convey the impulses conducted by them to the central nervous system. They then *leave the sympathetic trunk in a white ramus communicans* (Figs. 1-26 and 2-134) and enter a spinal nerve and then the spinal cord via its dorsal root. *The cell bodies of the visceral sensory fibers are in the dorsal root ganglion.*

Afferent Fibers in Parasympathetic Nerves. Although **the parasympathetic nerves are visceral efferent** (*i.e.*, motor to smooth muscle and glands), the viscera supplied by them contain sense organs and the afferent (sensory) fibers from them pass back to the central nervous system in the parasympathetic nerves. *All the sensory fibers have their cell bodies in the sensory ganglion of the nerve supplying the viscus with parasympathetic fibers* (*e.g.*, in the sensory ganglion of the vagus or 10th cranial nerve and in the dorsal root ganglia of S2, S3, and S4 nerves).

CLINICALLY ORIENTED COMMENTS

Pain arising from an abdominal viscus varies from dull to very severe and is poorly localized. It radiates to the part of the body served by somatic sensory fibers associated with the same segment of the spinal cord which receives visceral sensory fibers from the viscus concerned (Fig. 2-141). This is referred to as **visceral referred pain**. Hence, a knowledge of the segmental origin of the sensory nerve fibers of each of the viscera is helpful in interpreting pain referred to the abdominal wall by a diseased viscus. A few examples will illustrate this important clinical principle.

Pain emanating from the **stomach** (*e.g.*, gastric ulcer) is referred to the **epigastric region** because the stomach is supplied by pain afferents which reach the seventh and eighth thoracic segments of the spinal cord via the *greater splanchnic nerve.* The pain is interpreted by the brain as if the irritation occurred in the area of skin supplied by the dorsal (sensory) roots of the seventh to ninth thoracic nerves (Fig. 2-141).

The impulses arising from an inflamed **vermiform appendix** pass centrally in the lesser splanchnic nerve on the right side. *The visceral pain is referred* **initially** *to the umbilical region* (Case 2-4), which lies in the T10 dermatome. *Pain is* **later** *referred to the lower right quadrant* if the parietal peritoneum in contact with the appendix becomes inflamed. Abdominal pain arising from the parietal peritoneum is of the somatic type and is usually severe. It can be precisely located to the site of origin. The anatomical basis for this is that *the parietal peritoneum is supplied by somatic sensory fibers through the thoracic nerves,* whereas the appendix is supplied by visceral sensory fibers.

An inflamed parietal peritoneum is extremely sensitive to stretching. Hence, when pressure is applied to the abdominal wall over the site of inflammation (*e.g.*, **McBurney's point**, Fig. 2-45 and Case 2-4) and suddenly removed, extreme local pain is usually felt. As the inflamed parietal peritoneum is stretched by pressure and then rebounds, pain is produced. This is called **rebound tenderness**. For other examples of referred pain see Cases 1-1, 1-7, 2-1, 2-2, 2-5, and 2-7).

The treatment of some patients with arterial disease in the lower limbs may occasionally include the surgical *removal of two or more lumbar sympathetic ganglia* with division of their rami communicantes. This operation is called a **lumbar sympathectomy**.

Surgical access to the sympathetic trunks is commonly through a lateral **extraperitoneal approach** because *they lie retroperitoneally in the extraperitoneal fatty tissue.* The muscles of the anterior abdominal wall are split and the peritoneum is swept medially and forward to expose the medial edge of the psoas major

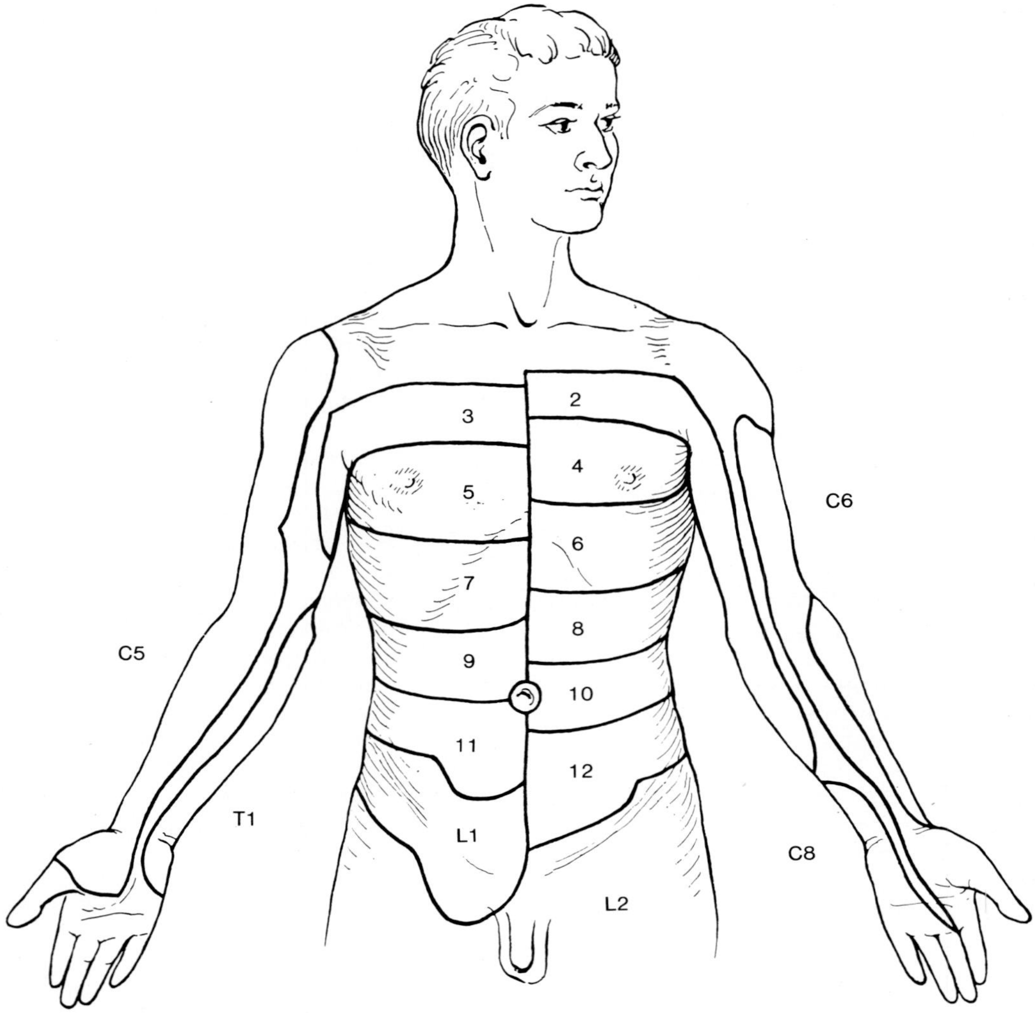

Figure 2-141. Drawing illustrating the *dermatomes* of the upper parts of the body. *A dermatome is an area of skin supplied by the dorsal (sensory) root of a spinal nerve.* These dermatomes were determined by plotting (1) the areas of vasodilation that resulted on stimulation of individual dorsal nerve roots and (2) the areas of "remaining sensibility" after cutting three roots above and three roots below a given nerve root. The areas plotted represent the average finding for each dorsal root based on pain sensation. Note that there is considerable overlapping of contiguous dermatomes; that is, each segmental nerve overlaps the territories of its neighbors. Consequently, no anesthesia results unless two or more consecutive dorsal roots have lost their functions.

muscle, along which the sympathetic trunk lies (Fig. 2-119). As the left trunk is slightly overlapped by the aorta (Fig. 2-113), and sometimes by a **persisting left inferior vena cava** (Fig. 2-145), and the right sympathetic trunk is covered by the inferior vena cava (Figs. 2-119 and 2-134), the surgeon has to retract these structures medially to expose the sympathetic trunks. They usually lie in the groove between the psoas major muscle laterally and the lumbar vertebral bodies medially, but they are often obscured by fat and lymphatic tissue (Fig. 2-134).

Identification of the sympathetic trunks is not easy and great care is taken not to remove inadvertently pieces of the genitofemoral nerve (Fig. 2-131), the lumbar lymphatics (Fig. 2-134), or the ureter. The intimate relationship of the sympathetic trunks to the aorta and the inferior vena cava (Figs. 2-119 and 2-134) also make these large vessels vulnerable to injury during a lumbar sympathectomy.

Vessels of the Posterior Abdominal Wall (Figs. 2-113, 2-119, 2-124, 2-129, 2-131,

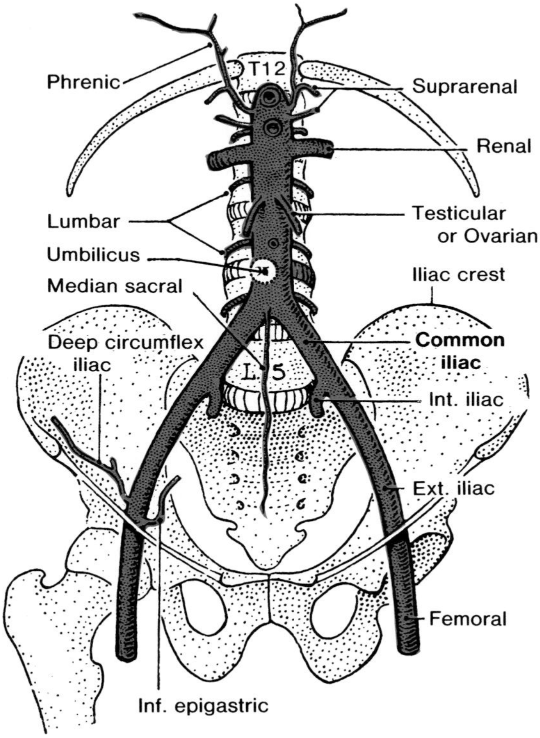

Figure 2-142. Drawing of the abdominal aorta showing its branches. It is only about 13 cm in length. Observe the stems of the celiac, superior mesenteric, and inferior mesenteric arteries. (For a better view of them, see Fig. 2-143). Note that the abdominal aorta begins in the median plane in front of the lower border of the body of *T12* vertebra and ends at the level of the body of *L4* vertebra by dividing into two common iliac arteries. Note that this division occurs slightly to the left and below (about 1 cm) the level of the umbilicus (*U*). It is very unusual for the median sacral artery to arise from the anterior surface of the aorta as here. (See Fig. 2-55 for its usual origin.)

2-132, 2-134, and 2-142 to 2-147). The arteries of the posterior abdominal wall arise from the **abdominal aorta**, except for the subcostal arteries. The veins are tributaries of the **inferior vena cava**, except for the left testicular or ovarian vein which enters the renal vein.

The Subcostal Arteries (Figs. 1-91, 2-8, 2-113, and 2-131). These are the *last branches of the descending thoracic aorta.* They were given their name because they are *situated below the 12th rib.* Each artery runs laterally over the body of the 12th thoracic vertebra and posterior to the splanchnic nerves, the sympathetic trunk, the pleura, and the diaphragm. *Each subcostal artery enters the abdomen behind the lateral arcuate ligament* (Fig. 2-131), passing with the subcostal nerve (T12) below the lower border of the 12th rib. They then run anterior to the quadratus lumborum muscle and posterior to the kidney (Figs. 2-113 and 2-121) before piercing the aponeurosis of origin of the transversus abdominis muscle to run between that muscle and the internal oblique. The subcostal arteries anastomose anteriorly with the inferior epigastric and lower intercostal arteries (Fig. 2-8) and posteriorly with the lumbar arteries (Fig. 2-55).

The Abdominal Aorta (Figs. 2-55, 2-91, 2-113, 2-119, 2-121, 2-124, 2-140, and 2-142 to 2-144). The **abdominal aorta** is the direct continuation of the descending thoracic aorta. It **begins** *at the aortic hiatus in the diaphragm at the level of the intervertebral disc between T12 and L1 vertebrae* and **ends** *at about the level of the fourth lumbar vertebra by dividing into the two common iliac arteries.* **The relations of the abdominal aorta** are important, particularly to surgeons (*e.g.*, when excising part of the aorta, a procedure called **aortectomy**).

Anteriorly, the abdominal aorta is related to the **celiac trunk** and its branches, the **celiac plexus** (Fig. 2-111), the **omental bursa** (Figs. 2-47 and 2-79), the **pancreas**, the left **renal vein** (Fig. 2-69*B*), the ascending (third) part of the **duodenum** (Fig. 2-71), the **root of the mesentery** (Fig. 2-69*A*), and the **intermesenteric (aortic) plexus** of nerves (Fig. 2-127).

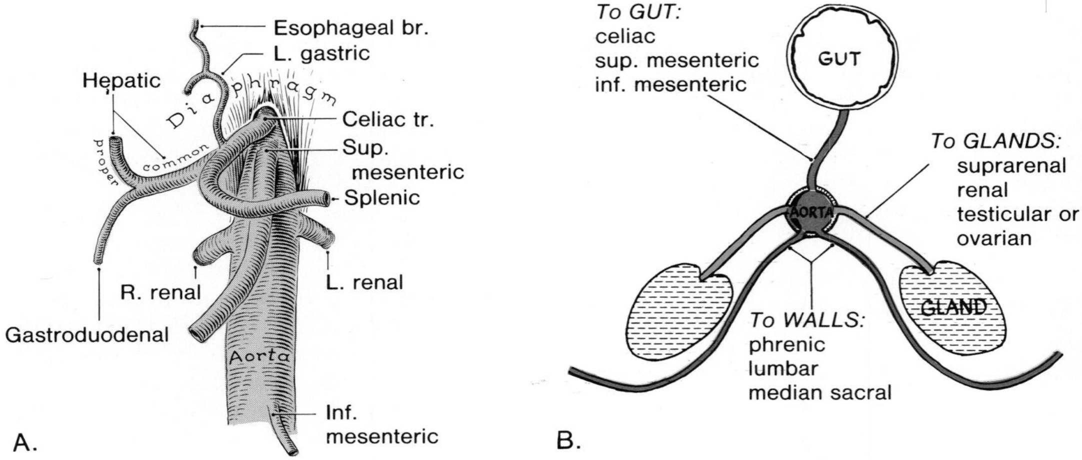

Figure 2-143. Drawing of the abdominal aorta illustrating its branches. *A*, note that the abdominal aorta begins where the diaphragm rests on the celiac trunk at the level of the intervertebral disc between T12 and L1 vertebra (also see Fig. 2-142). *B*, shows three of the four types of branches of the aorta: (1) unpaired visceral branches to the gut; (2) paired visceral branches to the glands; and (3) paired parietal branches to the walls. The fourth type (unpaired parietal) is represented by the median sacral artery (see Figs. 2-55 and 2-142).

Posteriorly, the abdominal aorta descends in front of the bodies of **L1 to L4 vertebrae**, the **intervertebral discs** between them, and the corresponding part of the **anterior longitudinal ligament** (Fig. 2-131).

On the right, the abdominal aorta is related superiorly to the **cisterna chyli** (Fig. 2-147), the **thoracic duct** (Figs. 1-85 and 2-147), and the **right crus** of the diaphragm (Figs. 2-121 and 2-130). Inferiorly, it is in direct contact with the **inferior vena cava** (Figs. 2-113 and 2-144).

On the left, the abdominal aorta is related superiorly to the **left crus** of the diaphragm (Fig. 2-121) and the **left celiac ganglion** (Fig. 2-111). The **duodenojejunal flexure** is on its left (Fig. 2-40), opposite the second lumbar vertebra (Fig. 2-71), and the abdominal sympathetic trunk courses along its left side (Figs. 2-113, 2-119, and 2-147).

The surface anatomy of the abdominal aorta may be represented by a broad band, about 2 cm wide, extending from a midline point about a fingerbreadth (2.5 cm) above the **transpyloric plane** to a point slightly (1.5 cm) inferior and to the left of the **umbilicus** (Fig. 2-142). This inferior point indicates the bifurcation of the aorta into the left and right common iliac arteries. Also, *the aortic bifurcation is to the left of the midpoint of the line joining the highest points of the iliac crests* seen from the front (Fig. 2-142). This line is very helpful when examing obese persons in whom the umbilicus is usually not a reliable landmark. When the anterior abdominal wall is relaxed, particularly in children and thin adults, the lowest part of *the abdominal aorta may be readily compressed against the body of the fourth lumbar vertebra* by firm pressure on the anterior abdominal wall, just above the umbilicus. The pulsations of the aorta can easily be felt; however, too much pressure should not be applied or else the pulsations will be obliterated.

The branches of the abdominal aorta may be grouped into **four types**: (1) *unpaired visceral branches*; (2) *paired visceral branches*; (3) *paired parietal branches*; and (4) an *unpaired parietal branch*.

The unpaired visceral branches (Fig. 2-143) are the *celiac trunk*, the *superior mesenteric artery*, and the *inferior mesenteric artery*. They arise from the anterior surface of the aorta at the following verte-

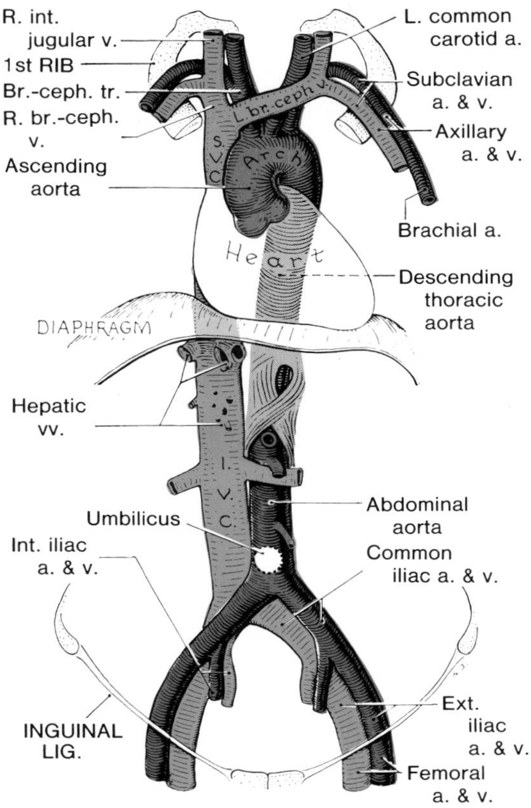

Figure 2-144. Diagram of the great arteries and veins. The abdominal aorta, a continuation of the thoracic aorta, *begins* in the median plane at the aortic hiatus of the diaphragm (Fig. 2-130) and *ends* by dividing into two common iliac arteries. Observe that the inferior vena cava begins a little below and to the right of the bifurcation of the aorta by the union of the two common iliac veins which lie posterior to their respective arteries.

bral levels (Figs. 2-71, 2-132, and 2-142): the **celiac trunk (T12)**; the **superior mesenteric artery (L1)**; and the **inferior mesenteric artery (L3)**. These important arteries have been discussed previously.

The paired visceral branches arise from the lateral surfaces of the aorta at the following vertebral levels (Figs. 2-55 and 2-142): (1) the **middle suprarenal arteries (L1)**, one or more on each side, arise close to the origin of the superior mesenteric artery (Figs. 2-55 and 2-111). They run laterally on the crura of the diaphragm to the

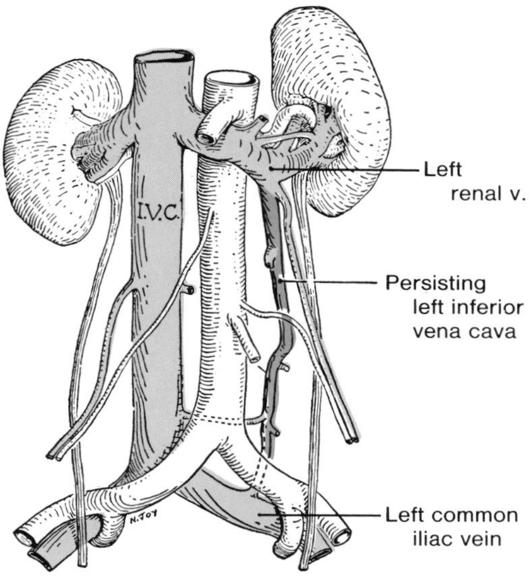

Figure 2-145. Drawing of a dissection of a persisting left inferior vena cava which joins the left common iliac vein to the left renal vein. This occasional vein may be small, as in this specimen, or it may be large. This abnormal vessel results from persistence of the left embryonic sacrocardinal vein which normally disappears. The possible presence of this vessel is of surgical significance during left lumbar sympathectomy because it may cover the sympathetic trunk.

suprarenal glands; (2) the **renal arteries (L1)** arise just below the superior mesenteric artery (Figs. 2-55*B*, 2-111, and 2-143*A*). Occasionally there is an *accessory renal artery*, particularly on the left side (Fig. 2-124); (3) the **testicular** or **ovarian arteries (L2)** are long slender vessels that arise from the aorta, usually a short distance below the renal arteries (Figs. 2-55 and 2-124). They pass inferiorly either anterior (Fig. 2-113) or posterior (Fig. 2-105) to the inferior vena cava on the right side across the psoas major muscle, but adherent to the parietal peritoneum (Fig. 2-113). At the pelvic brim the **testicular artery** passes through the deep inguinal ring to *enter the inguinal canal* and become part of the **spermatic cord** (Fig. 2-27). The **ovarian artery** follows a similar course through the abdomen but crosses the proximal ends of the external iliac vessels to enter the pelvis minor, where it runs in the **infundibulo-**

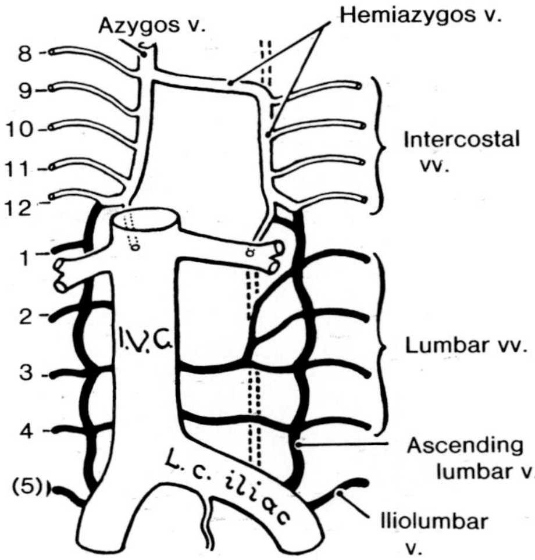

Figure 2-146. Diagram showing the azygos, hemiazygos, ascending lumbar, and lumbar veins. Observe that the ascending lumbar vein is a long vessel that connects the segmental veins and terminates in the subcostal vein. For other views of the azygos vein, see Figures 1-48 and 1-92.

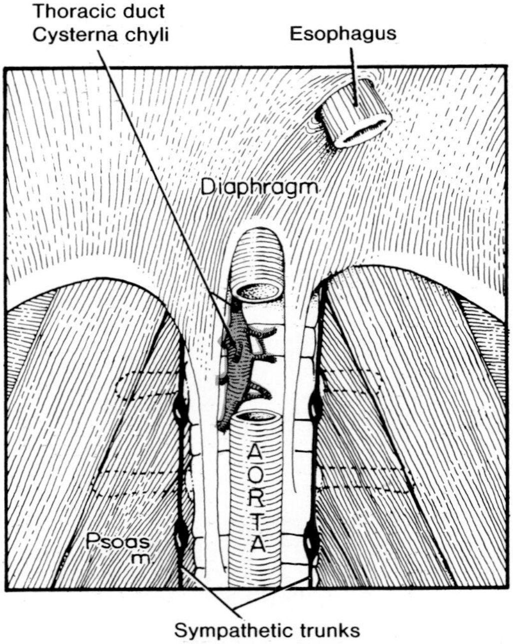

Figure 2-147. Drawing illustrating the cysterna chyli, the principal feature of the lymphatic system of the posterior abdominal wall. It lies on the upper two lumbar vertebrae, posterolateral to the aorta, and may be hidden by the right crus of the diaphragm (Fig. 2-130). About 5 cm long, the cysterna chyli somewhat resembles the dilated portion of a vein. Its diameter is slightly less than that of a lead pencil. Observe that it receives five or more lymph trunks.

pelvic ligament to reach the **broad ligament** and supply the ovary (Fig. 3-71).

The paired parietal (somatic) branches arise from the posterolateral surfaces of the aorta (Fig. 2-55). The **inferior phrenic arteries** (Figs. 2-111 and 2-113) arise just below the diaphragm and pass superolaterally over the crura of the diaphragm. Each of them gives rise to several **superior suprarenal arteries** (Fig. 2-111) and then spreads out on the inferior surface of the diaphragm.

The lumbar arteries (Fig. 2-55) arise from the posterolateral surface of the abdominal aorta. There are *four pairs of lumbar arteries,* each pair passing around the sides of the upper four lumbar vertebrae (Fig. 2-131). *They pass posteromedial to the sympathetic trunks and,* **on the right**, *run posterior to the inferior vena cava* (Fig. 2-134). The lumbar arteries divide between the transverse processes of the lumbar vertebrae into anterior and posterior branches. **Each anterior branch** passes deep to the quadratus lumborum muscle and then *around the abdominal wall between the internal oblique and transversus abdominis muscles, where they anastomose in the posterior part of the rectus abdominus muscle with the inferior epigastric arteries* (Fig. 2-8). The anterior branches supply the anterolateral walls of the lower half of the abdomen.

Each posterior branch passes posteriorly, lateral to the articular processes, and *supplies the spinal cord, the cauda equina, the spinal meninges* (Figs. 5-62 and 5-63), *the erector spinae muscles, and the overlying skin.* The **spinal arteries** arise from the posterior branches of the lumbar arteries and pass through the intervertebral foramina to supply the vertebrae. Important branches of the spinal arteries, called **radicular arteries**, join either the anterior or posterior spinal arteries (Fig. 5-62). The largest of the radicular arteries, called the **great radicular artery** or **arteria radicularis magna** (spinal artery of

Adamkiewicz), joins the inferior half of the anterior spinal artery and *supplies most of the blood to the inferior part of the spinal cord,* including the **lumbosacral enlargement**.

The unpaired parietal artery is the **median sacral artery** (Figs. 2-55 and 2-142). This tiny vessel, originally the dorsal aorta in the sacral region of the embryo, typically arises from the posterior surface of the aorta just proximal to its bifurcation (Fig. 2-55). It descends in the midline anterior to L4 and L5 vertebrae, usually giving off a small lumbar artery on each side called the **lowest lumbar artery** or arteria lumbalis ima (Fig. 2-55). Their distribution is similar to that of the lumbar arteries.

CLINICALLY ORIENTED COMMENTS

The abdominal aorta and its branches can be studied radiologically by injecting a radiopaque contrast medium into them (Figs. 2-100 and 2-108). When the distal part of the abdominal aorta and/or the external iliac artery are not occluded, a catheter is passed into a femoral artery just below the inguinal ligament (Fig. 4-18) using the *Seldinger technique.* A **percutaneous puncture of the femoral artery** (Fig. 2-142) is made with a size 16 needle. A spring wire guide is passed through the needle and up the external iliac artery for several cm. The needle is then slipped off, leaving the guide in the artery. Next, a size 16 plastic catherer with a curved tip is threaded on the guide up to the artery wall. With a rotary motion, the catheter and guide are advanced into the lumen of the artery. The guide is then withdrawn, leaving the catheter in the artery. *Seldinger was a medical student when he devised this technique.* Under fluoroscopic control the catheter is then passed to the desired level of the aorta for injection of the contrast medium to show it and its branches, or it can be manipulated until it is in an aortic branch for **selective angiography** of one branch only (Figs. 2-64, 2-100, and 2-108).

When there is **atherosclerosis** (narrowing of the aorta and/or the iliac arteries owing to lipid deposits in their walls), the Seldinger technique may not be feasible. In *some* of these cases, the abdominal aorta is injected with contrast material by *direct needle puncture.* For this **translumbar aortography**, the level of puncture is from L1 to L3 vertebrae. It is sometimes performed at T12/L1 level because of the constancy of the position of the aorta at this level in the **aortic hiatus** of the diaphragm (Fig. 2-131). The needle puncture is commonly made 1 cm below the 12th rib, 6 to 8 cm to the left of the midline. Examine Figure 2-119, noting that to pierce the aorta the needle has to be directed anteromedially at about a 60° angle.

A common site for **atheromatous occlusion** (blockage owing to lipid deposits in the intima of arteries) is one of the common iliac arteries, just distal to the bifurcation of the aorta (Fig. 2-142). Patients with this **arteriosclerotic occlusive disease** complain of calf, thigh, or hip pain on exertion (**claudication**). *This pain disappears when they rest.* Sometimes this condition is treated by inserting a **prosthetic graft** into the artery which bypasses the obstructed area. Similarly a localized dilation or **aneurysm of the abdominal aorta** (Fig. 5-76) distal to the renal arteries may be resected and replaced by a prosthetic graft (Case 5-8).

During certain surgical procedures in the abdomen, it may be necessary to ligate or to retract for several minutes one or more lumbar arteries. When doing this, it must be kept in mind that the **arteria radicularis magna** (spinal artery of Adamkiewicz) supplying the lower two-thirds of the spinal cord may arise from one of the lumbar arteries. The origin of this **large artery** varies, but it *commonly arises from one of the lower intercostal or upper lumbar arteries.* In most cases it arises on the left-hand side and joins or forms the lower half of the anterior spinal artery (Fig. 5-62). It usually gives off a small branch that anastomoses with the posterior spinal artery. *Prolonged pressure on or ligation of the lumbar artery giving rise to the arteria radicularis magna leads to* **circulatory impariment** *of the inferior part of the* *spinal cord, which may result in an area of necrosis* (**infarction**). This could result in **paralysis of the lower limbs (paraplegia**) and loss of all sensation inferior to the infarcted areas (see discussion of Case 5-8 at the end of Chap. 5)

Prior to replacing part of the abdominal aorta with a prosthetic graft, **angiograms** (radiographs of blood vessels) are often made to determine the origin of the arteria radicularis magna. If it arises from a lumbar artery, provision has to be made for an adequate supply of blood to the spinal cord if it is necessary to ligate the lumbar artery from which it arises.

The Inferior Vena Cava (Figs. 2-71, 2-90, 2-113, 2-119, 2-121, 2-129, 2-134, and 2-144). *The inferior vena cava is the largest vein in the body.* It returns blood from the lower limbs, most of the abdominal walls, and the abdominopelvic viscera. Blood from the abdominal viscera passes through the **portal system** and the liver (Fig. 2-85) before entering the inferior vena cava via the **hepatic veins** (Fig. 2-82).

The inferior vena cava *begins anterior to the fifth lumbar vertebra* by the **union of the common iliac veins**, below the bifurcation of the aorta and the proximal part of the right common iliac artery (Fig. 2-144). *It ascends to the right of the median plane, pierces the central tendon of the diaphragm* (**vena caval foramen**, Fig. 2-130) *at the level of the eighth thoracic vertebra* (Fig. 2-132), and *enters the right atrium* of the heart (Fig. 2-144).

The relations of the inferior vena cava are noteworthy. *Posteriorly*, from below upward, it lies on the bodies of **L5 to L3 vertebrae** (Fig. 2-71), the **right psoas major muscle** (Fig. 2-113), the **right sympathetic trunk** (Figs. 2-119 and 2-134), the **right renal artery**, the **right suprarenal gland**, the **right celiac ganglion** (Fig. 2-113), and the **right crus** of the diaphragm as it passes to the vena caval foramen (Fig. 2-130) in the central tendon of the diaphragm.

Anteriorly, the relations of the inferior vena cava are the **peritoneum** (Fig. 2-69*B*), the **superior mesenteric vessels** in the root of the mesentery (Fig. 2–71), and the horizontal or **third part of the duodenum** and the head of the **pancreas**, with the portal vein and the bile duct intervening (Fig. 2-65).

Superior to the first part of the duodenum, the inferior vena cava lies in the posterior boundary of the epiploic foramen (Figs. 2–90 and 2–91). It then enters a groove on the inferior surface of the liver between the right and caudate lobes (Figs. 2–79 to 2–83). *To the left* of the inferior vena cava is the **aorta** (Fig. 2–144); *to its right* are the right **ureter** and **kidney** and the descending or second part of the **duodenum** (Figs. 2–119 and 2–134).

The tributaries of the inferior vena cava (Fig. 2–129) are: (1) the *common iliac veins*; (2) the third and fourth *lumbar veins*; (3) the right *testicular* or *ovarian vein*; (4) the *renal veins*; (5) the *azygos vein*; (6) the right *suprarenal vein*; (7) the *inferior phrenic veins*; and (8) the *hepatic veins.*

The **right** and **left common iliac veins** are formed by the *union of the external and internal iliac veins* (Fig. 2–144), and through them the inferior vena cava returns blood from the lower limbs and most of the pelvis.

The **right testicular** or **ovarian vein** and the **right suprarenal vein** usually drain into the inferior vena cava, whereas *these veins on the left side usually drain into the left renal vein* (Fig. 2–129).

The renal veins draining into the inferior vena cava at the *level of L2 vertebra* lie anterior to the corresponding renal artery (Fig. 2–113). The right renal vein receives few if any tributaries other than those from the kidney, whereas *the left renal vein also drains blood from the left suprarenal gland and the testis or ovary.*

The azygos and hemiazygos veins (Figs. 1–48, 1–92, 2–129, and 2–146) usually commence in the abdomen. *The azygos vein commonly arises from the inferior vena cava at the level of the renal vein*, but it may begin as the continuation of the right subcostal vein or from the junction of that vein and the right ascending lumbar vein. It enters the thorax through the **aortic hiatus** or the right crus of the diaphragm (Fig. 2–130). *The inferior hemiazygos vein arises from the posterior surface of the left* *renal vein*, but it may also arise from the union of the left subcostal and the left ascending lumbar vein (Fig. 2–146).

The right suprarenal vein (Figs. 2–111 and 2–129) is short and drains into the posterior aspect of the superior vena cava, whereas the **left suprarenal vein** is long and *usually drains into the left renal vein*, but it may drain into the inferior vena cava.

The inferior phrenic veins drain blood from the abdominal surface of the diaphragm. The right inferior phrenic vein generally empties into the inferior vena cava, whereas *the left inferior phrenic generally joins the left suprarenal vein.*

The hepatic veins (Figs. 2–57, 2–85, and 2–129) are short trunks, discussed previously, which open into the inferior vena cava, just as it passes through the diaphragm (Fig. 2–130). The right hepatic vein sometimes passes through the vena caval foramen before entering the inferior vena cava.

The lumbar veins consist of four or five segmental pairs (Figs. 2–129 and 2–146). Their dorsal branches drain the back and communicate with the **vertebral venous plexuses** (Fig. 5–64). The mode of termination of the lumbar veins varies. They may drain separately into the inferior vena cava or the common iliac vein (Fig. 2–129), but they are generally united on each side by a vertical connecting vein, the **ascending lumbar vein** (Figs. 2–146 and 5–64), which lies posterior to the psoas major muscle. Each ascending lumbar vein passes behind the medial arcuate ligament (Fig. 2–134) to enter the thorax. *The right ascending lumbar vein joins the right subcostal vein to form the azygos vein* (Figs. 1–52 and 2–146), whereas the left ascending lumbar vein unites with the left subcostal vein to form the **hemiazygos vein**.

CLINICALLY ORIENTED COMMENTS

There are three collateral routes available for venous blood to pass to the right side of the heart if the inferior vena cava becomes obstructed or if ligation of the inferior vena cava is necessary. In such cases an extensive collateral venous circulation is soon established owing to enlargement of superficial and/or deep veins.

The first route is via various anastomoses in the pelvis and the abdomen which enable blood to reach the **superficial** and **inferior epigastric veins** (Fig. 2–7) and to ascend in them to the thoracoepigastric and superior epigastric veins and the superior vena cava.

The second route by which venous blood can travel is via tributaries of the inferior vena cava that anastomose with the **vertebral system of veins** (Fig. 5–64). This system of veins, passing *within the vertebral canal and the vertebral bodies*, can also provide a route for metastasis of cancer cells to the vertebral bodies or to the brain from an abdominal or pelvic tumor (*e.g.*, of the kidney, Fig. 2–120*B*).

The third route is via the **lateral thoracic vein** which connects the circumflex iliac veins with the axillary vein (Fig. 2–7).

Sometimes the inferior vena cava is ligated or plicated (folded to reduce its size) in order to prevent **pulmonary emboli** following thrombosis of the veins in the pelvis or lower limbs from reaching the lungs and producing **pulmonary infarcts** (areas of necrotic tissue; see Case 1–10). Surgical exposure of the inferior vena cava may be by a transperitoneal or an extraperitoneal approach from the right side of the abdominal wall (Fig. 2–134).

The inferior vena cava and the common iliac veins are vulnerable to injury during operative procedures for repairing a **herniated nucleus pulposis** of an intervertebral disc (see Case 5–3 and Fig. 5–80). As these vessels lie anterior to the fifth intervertebral disc (Figs. 2–71 and 2–142), they could be injured by a **rongeur** (F. *ronger*, to gnaw) that is unintentionally pushed through the L4/L5 intervertebral disc during removal of its herniated nucleus pulposis. A rongeur is a strong biting forceps used for gouging away bone or for removing herniated intervertebral discs.

Lymphatic Drainage of the Posterior Abdominal Wall (Figs. 1–85, 2–105, 2–109, 2–124, 2–134, and 2–147). The lymph nodes of the posterior abdominal wall lie along the iliac vessels, the aorta, and the inferior vena cava.

The external iliac lymph nodes are scattered along the corresponding vessels. Inferiorly, *the medial lymph nodes receive lymph from the lower limbs and the pelvic viscera*, whereas *the lateral lymph nodes receive lymph from the areas supplied by the inferior epigastric and deep circumflex iliac vessels.*

The common iliac lymph nodes, scattered along the common iliac vessels, *receive lymph from the external and internal iliac lymph nodes.* The medial group of common iliac lymph nodes also drains lymph directly from the pelvis. *Lymph from the common iliac lymph nodes passes to the lumbar lymph nodes.*

The lumbar lymph nodes (Fig. 2–134) lie along the abdominal aorta and the inferior vena cava. They receive lymph directly from the posterior abdominal wall, the kidneys and ureters, the testes or ovaries, and the uterus and uterine tubes. They also receive lymph from the descending colon, the pelvis, and the lower limbs through the inferior mesenteric and common iliac lymph nodes. *Efferent vessels from these large lymph nodes form the right and left lumbar lymph trunks.*

The Cysterna Chyli (Figs. 1–48, 1–85, 2–134, and 2–147). The sac-like cysterna chyli, about 5 cm long and 6 mm wide, is *located between the origin of the abdominal aorta and the azygos vein.* It lies on the right sides of the bodies of the first two lumbar vertebrae and is *usually located posterior to the right crus of the diaphragm.*

The thoracic duct, which begins in the cysterna chyli, ascends through the **aortic hiatus** in the diaphragm into the thorax (Fig. 1–45) to open near or at the angle of union of the internal jugular and subclavian veins.

The cisterna chyli receives lymph from the right and left lumbar lymph trunks, the intestinal trunk (draining the liver, stomach, pancreas, spleen, and small bowel), and a pair of vessels that descend from the lower intercostal lymph nodes. Lymph from the digestive tract first passes to the lymph nodes close to the viscera (Figs. 2–58, 2–65, and 2–109). It then passes along vessels that follow the major blood vessels to the **mesenteric lymph nodes** (Fig. 2–109) and from them into the preaortic lymph nodes (Fig. 2–27).

PATIENT ORIENTED PROBLEMS

Case 2-1. A 32-year-old accountant complained to his doctor about a steady, gnawing, **burning pain** of about 2 weeks duration in the "pit of his stomach" (**epigastric region**). On careful questioning it was revealed that the pain usually began about 2 hr after the patient eats and then disappears when he eats again or drinks a glass of milk. He said that he did not become overly concerned about this pain until it started to awake him in the middle of the night.

Except for *mild tenderness in the right upper quadrant* just lateral to his xiphoid process, the physical examination was normal. Suspecting a **peptic ulcer**, the doctor ordered plain radiographs of the patient's abdomen and upper GI studies (gastrointestinal series of x-ray examinations with **fluoroscopy** and films during and after the swallowing of a barium sulphate emulsion, often called a **barium meal**).

The plain radiographs were normal, but the GI studies showed the presence of an **active ulcer** (lesion of the mucosa caused by loss of tissue, usually associated with inflammation) in a moderately deformed **duodenal cap** (the superior or first part of the duodenum as seen radiographically (Fig. 2-35). A diagnosis of active **duodenal ulcer** was made (Fig. 2-148).

The patient responded fairly well to medical treatment (*e.g.*, antacids, frequent bland feedings, and abstinence from smoking and drinking alcohol). Although the patient curtailed his responsibilities for 2 months, he again began to work long hours, to smoke heavily, and to consume excessive amounts of coffee and alcohol. His symptoms became worse again and vomiting sometimes occurred when the pain was severe. This gave him some relief from the pain.

One evening the patient developed a sud-

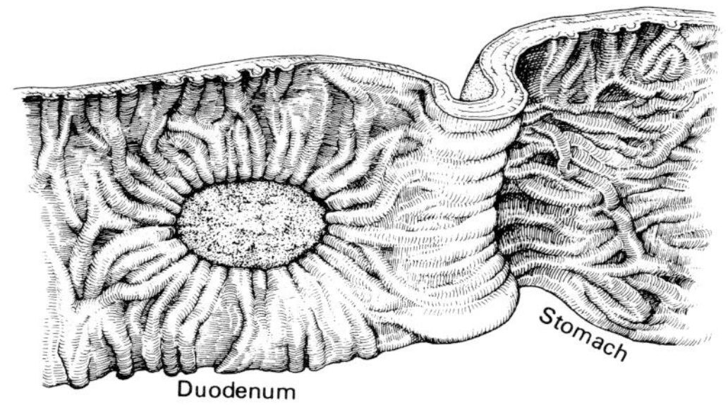

Figure 2-148. Drawing illustrating a peptic ulcer of the duodenum. About 80% of peptic ulcers occur in the duodenum, usually within 3 cm of the pylorus. Peptic ulcers also occur in the stomach.

den upper abdominal pain, vomited, and fainted. He was rushed to the emergency room of the hospital. Examination revealed extreme pain and **rigidity** of the abdomen and **rebound tenderness** (sharp pain elicited when the depressed palpating hand is quickly removed). Maximum tenderness was higher than would be expected in **acute appendicitis**. On questioning, the patient revealed that his ulcer had been "acting up" lately and that he had noticed blood in his vomitus (**hematemesis**).

Emergency surgery was performed and a duodenal ulcer which had perforated was found. There was a generalized **chemical peritonitis** resulting from the escape of bile and the contents of the GI tract into the peritoneal cavity.

Problems. Define **peptic ulcer**, with special emphasis on duodenal ulcer. What structures, closely related to the first part of the duodenum, might be eroded by a **perforated duodenal ulcer**? Name the congenital malformation of the ileum in which peptic ulcers commonly develop. Explain the anatomical basis for abdominal pain in the right upper and lower quadrants. What nerves might be cut during surgical procedures to reduce the secretion of acid by the parietal cells of the stomach. *These problems are discussed on page 282.*

Case 2-2. On the way home from work, a 42-year-old office worker suddenly experienced a sharp, **lancinating pain** in his right **loin** (the area of the side and back between the false ribs and the pelvis). The pain was so excruciating that he doubled up and moaned in agony. A fellow worker helped him to the emergency room of the hospital.

When the doctor asked him to describe the onset of pain, the patient said that he first felt a slight pain and then it gradually increased (**exacerbation of pain**) until it was so severe that it brought tears to his eyes. He said that this unbearable pain lasted for several minutes and then suddenly eased. He explained that the pain comes and goes but seemed to be moving down toward his groin (**inguinal region**).

During the physical examination, the doctor noted that the patient's abdomen moved with his respirations and that there was some **tenderness** and slight **guarding** (abdominal muscle spasm) in the right lower quadrant of his abdomen, but there was no rigidity. While palpating the tender area as deeply as possible, the doctor suddenly removed his hand. Instead of wincing, the patient seemed relieved that the probing had stopped (**absence of rebound tenderness**). By this time the patient reported that he felt the pain in his right groin and testis and along the medial side of his thigh. The doctor found that the right testis was unusually tender and was retracted. When asked to produce a urine sample, the patient stated that it was difficult and painful for him to urinate (**dysuria**). The nurse reported that his urine sample contained blood (**hematuria**). Although the doctor was quite certain that the diagnosis was **ureteral (ureteric) colic**, he ordered plain radiographs of the abdomen. It was reported that a small calcified object, compatible with a **ureteral calculus** (stone), was visible in the region of the lower end of the right ureter.

Problems. What probably caused the patient's attack of **excruciating pain**? At what other sites would a ureteral calculus apt to become lodged? Explain the intermittent exacerbation of pain and the course taken by the pain from his loin to his groin. Briefly discuss **referred pain** from the ureter. Explain the anatomical basis of the absence of rebound tenderness in the abdomen in cases of ureteric colic. *These problems are discussed on page 283.*

Case 2-3. A 14-year-old boy suffered

pain in his right groin while attempting to lift a heavy weight. As soon as he noticed a lump in the region where he felt pain, he decided to lie down. The bulge soon disappeared and he went home. On the way, he blew his nose very hard and again experienced pain and felt the swelling in his right groin. Fearing that he may have developed a rupture, his father called the family doctor.

During the physical examination, the doctor inserted the tip of his little finger through the **superficial (external) inguinal** ring and along the inguinal canal toward the **deep (internal) ring.** Nothing was felt until he asked the patient to cough; he then felt an impulse with the tip of his finger. *When the patient was in a horizontal position the bulge disappeared*, but on straining, a plum-sized bulge appeared in the right inguinal region which was palpable below the superficial inguinal ring and *medial to the pubic tubercle.* A diagnosis of complete **indirect inguinal hernia** was made.

Problems. Define the condition called indirect inguinal hernia. *Explain the embryological basis of this kind of hernia.* What layers of the spermatic cord cover the hernial sac? What structures are endangered during an operation for repair of an indirect inguinal hernia? *These problems are discussed on page 284.*

Case 2-4. A 22-year-old married female medical student woke up one morning not feeling as well as usual; she was **anorexic** (no appetite) and had crampy abdominal pains. As this coincided with the time of her menses or monthly period (L. *mensis*, month), she thought at first that these cramps were the beginning of her usual painful menstruation (**dysmenorrhea**). Because she had missed her last menstrual period, she also thought that she might be having early symptoms of a ruptured **ectopic pregnancy**. She had a slight fever and felt dizzy and uncomfortable owing to the cramps so she decided to stay in bed. *The pain soon localized around her umbilicus.* By evening the site of pain shifted to the right lower quadrant of her abdomen and she suspected **acute appendicitis**. As she was in considerable pain, her husband decided to take her to the hospital.

On examination it was found that she had a slight elevation of temperature (38°C), an increased pulse rate, and an abnormally high white blood cell count (**leukocytosis**). When asked to indicate where the pain began, she circled her umbilical area. When asked where she now felt pain, she put her finger on **McBurney's point** in the right lower quadrant (Fig. 2-45).

During gentle palpation of her abdomen, the doctor detected localized rigidity (muscle spasm) and tenderness in her right lower quadrant. When the doctor suddenly removed her palpating hand from the area of McBurney's point, the patient winced in pain (**rebound tenderness**). On rectal examination, there was slight right-sided tenderness in her **rectouterine pouch**. As these findings were highly suggestive of acute appendicitis, an immediate operation for excision of her vermiform appendix was performed (**appendectomy**).

Problems. What type of incision would the surgeon most likely have made to expose the vermiform appendix? Why is this a good incision anatomically? *How would you locate McBurney's point.* What part of the appendix is usually deep to this point? *Based on your knowledge of dissection, how do you think the appendix would be exposed*? Where is the appendix most likely to be located? What position of an inflamed appendix might give rise to pelvic or rectal pain? Discuss **referred pain** from the vermiform appendix. If this patient had had her appendix removed previously, what other appendage of the small intestine (congenital abnormality) could give signs and symptoms similar to appendicitis? *These problems are discussed on page 285.*

Case 2-5. A 67-year-old woman complained to her doctor about **pain in her abdomen** and **constipation** of 2 days' duration. She stated that the pain was most severe when she attempted to have a bowel movement. When asked to show where she experienced most pain, she placed her hand on the **lower left quadrant** of her abdomen. When asked to indicate where she first felt pain, she pointed to the area below her umbilicus (**hypogastrium**).

There was some distention of her abdomen which was thought to result from an accumulation of gas and feces above an

obstruction in the sigmoid colon. During palpation of the abdomen with the flat of the hand, **localized rigidity of the abdominal muscles** and tenderness were demonstrated in the left lower quadrant. When the palpating hand was pressed into the abdominal wall over her sigmoid colon and rapidly released, the patient winced in pain (**rebound tenderness**). Rectal examination revealed tenderness in the left side of her **rectouterine pouch.**

The doctor admitted the patient to hospital and ordered an emergency **barium enema.** The barium sulphate emulsion was given rectally under low pressure with the patient on her left side. The radiologist reported that the rectum and lower sigmoid colon (pelvic colon) were normal, except for a few small round outpouchings (**diverticula**) from the wall of the lower sigmoid colon (Fig. 2-149). He also reported an obstruction of the middle portion of the sigmoid colon and that there was much gas and fecal material above this region. Two of the diverticula at the obstructed region of the colon were pointed, that is, not rounded like the others. The radiologist concluded that the patient had **diverticulosis** and **diverticulitis** and that the obstruction of the sigmoid colon was more likely caused by diverticulitis and local peritonitis than by an **anular carcinoma** of the colon.

Problems. Differentiate between **diverticulosis** and **diverticulitis.** Do you think left lower quadrant pain could result from appendicitis? If so, explain how the appendix could be located on the left side? *These problems are discussed on page 286.*

Case 2-6. A 58-year-old obese man with a history of heartburn, indigestion (**dyspepsia**), and belching after heavy meals complained to his doctor about recent **epigastric** and **retrosternal pain.** He stated that the pain behind his breastbone (sternum) developed recently and that it was most severe after dinner when he lies or stoops down. Fearing these might be heart pains (**angina pectoris**), his wife insisted that he consult a doctor.

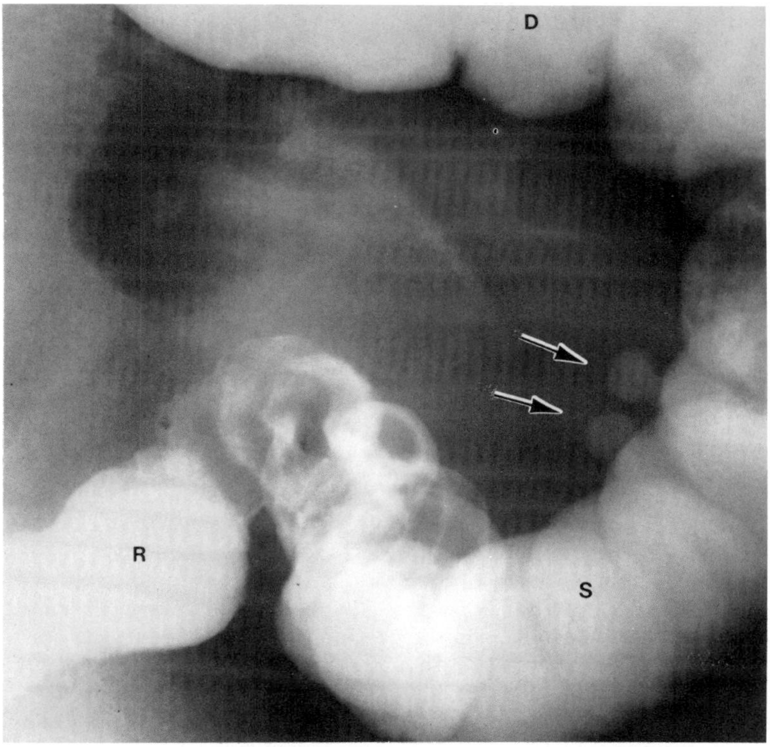

Figure 2-149. Radiograph of the descending colon (*D*), sigmoid colon (*S*), and rectum (*R*) taken following a barium enema. Note the diverticula (*arrows*) of the sigmoid colon.

When asked if he had noticed any other abnormalities, he stated that he often brought up (regurgitates) small amounts of sour or bitter-tasting substances (**gastroesophageal reflux**) into his mouth, particularly when he stooped to tie his shoes. He also reported that he recently had been having bouts of hiccups (hiccoughs) and that he occasionally had difficulty swallowing (**dysphagia**). He said that these symptoms were similar to those of his brother who had a **peptic ulcer**.

An **ECG** (electrocardiogram), a graphic record of the electrical activity of the heart, showed no evidence of heart disease. Plain radiographs of the abdomen were negative, but **fluoroscopic examination** with the patient standing erect behind a fluoroscope showed a round space filled with gas and fluid in the lower part of the patient's posterior **mediastinum**. Most of these examinations are done using an image amplifier in order to reduce the radiation dose. On swallowing a barium sulphate emulsion, the barium was seen to enter this space, identified as *the gastroesophageal region of the stomach*. There was no radiological evidence of gastric or duodenal ulcers. A diagnosis of **sliding hiatal hernia** (Fig. 2-53) was made.

Problems. Define **diaphragmatic hernia**. Discuss the embryological basis of congenital diaphragmatic hernia. Is a **hiatal hernia** usually present at birth or is it an acquired condition? What caused the patient's epigastric and retrosternal pain and hiccups? Based on your anatomical knowledge, what structures do you think would be endangered in the surgical repair of a hiatal hernia? *These problems are discussed on page 286.*

Case 2-7. A fair, fat, flatulent, 40-year-old woman with five children was rushed to hospital with **severe colicky pain** in the right upper quadrant of her abdomen. When asked where she first felt pain, she pointed to the upper middle part of her abdomen (**epigastrium**). When asked where the pain went (was referred), she ran her fingers under her right ribs (**hypochondrium**) and around her right side to her back, stating that the pain was felt near the lower end of her shoulder blade (*i.e.*, the inferior angle of her scapula).

On questioning, she said the sharp midline pain followed a heavy meal containing several fatty foods, after which she felt nauseated and vomited. Gradually there was an increase (**exacerbation**) in pain; when it became excruciating, her husband rushed her to the hospital.

During gentle palpation of her abdomen, the doctor noted **rigidity** and **tenderness** in the right upper quadrant of her abdomen, especially during inspiration. The radiologist reported that plain radiographs of her abdomen showed that there was *probably a small stone in her cystic duct*. In view of this observation and her symptoms, a diagnosis of **biliary colic** (intense pain from impaction of a gallstone in the cystic duct) was made. A **cholecystectomy** (removal of gallbladder and cystic duct) was performed and a sound (metal probe) was passed down her common bile duct and up her hepatic ducts to remove any stones that may have been lodged in them.

Problems. Why was the radiologist not able to state clearly that the stone was in the cystic duct? What is a gallstone? Explain the anatomical basis of the patient's pain in (1) the epigastric region, (2) the right hypochondrium, and (3) the infrascapular region. Does peritoneum separate the gallbladder from the liver? What structures are endangered during cholecystectomy? *These problems are discussed on page 288.*

Case 2-8. A 54-year-old mechanic was admitted to the hospital because of epigastric pain and vomiting of blood (**hematemesis**). It was obvious that he had been drinking heavily.

On examination, it was noted that *the blood in his vomitus was bright red.* On questioning, it was learned that the patient had exhibited upper gastrointestinal bleeding on previous occasions, but never so profusely. *His blood pressure was low and his pulse rate was high.*

Although the patient stated that he was not a heavy drinker, his wife said that he usually drank at least 12 beers a day. The patient's skin and conjunctivae were slightly yellow (**jaundiced**). His eyes appeared to be slightly sunken. **Spider nevi** or **angiomas** (branching arterioles) were present on his cheeks, neck, shoulders, and upper arms. His abdomen was large and there was protrusion and downward displacement of his umbilicus (Fig. 2-150). Palpation of the patient's abdomen revealed some enlargement of the liver (**hepatomegaly**) and of the spleen (**splenomegaly**). The large size of the abdomen resulted from the hepatomegaly, the splenomegaly, and **ascites** (accumulation of serous fluid in the peritoneal cavity).

Several bluish, dilated varicose veins radiated from his umbilicus, forming a **caput medusae** (Fig. 2-150). During a **proctoscopic examination** (inspection of the rectum and anal canal with a proctoscope), **internal hemorrhoids** were observed. On questioning, the patient said that he sometimes saw blood in his bowel movements (**feces, stools**) and at other times his stools were black and shiny. A diagnosis of **alcoholic cirrhosis of the liver** was made.

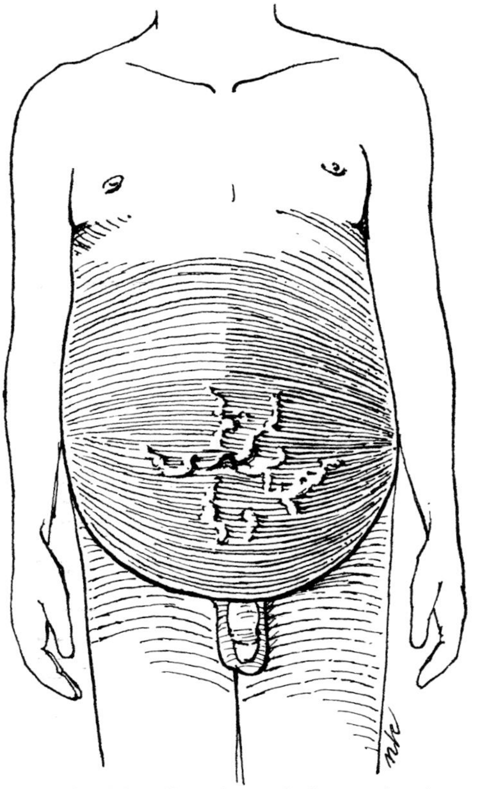

Figure 2-150. Drawing of the patient's enlarged abdomen owing to ascites. Note the slight downward displacement of the umbilicus and the varicose veins radiating from his umbilicus (caput medusae).

Problems. Briefly define hepatic cirrhosis. *Discuss anatomically* the basis of the patient's hematemesis, hemorrhoids, bloody stools, and caput medusae. What is the likely cause of the **ascites** and **splenomegaly**? Thinking anatomically, how would you suggest that blood pressure in the portal system could be reduced? *These problems are discussed on page 289.*

Case 2-9. The presenting complaint of a 54-year-old man was an *oval swelling in his left groin* (Fig. 2-151). He stated that this painless swelling enlarged when he coughed and disappeared when he lay down.

During examination of the patient in the standing position, the doctor put his little finger through the patient's left **superficial inguinal ring**. He got the sensation that his finger was going directly back into the abdomen, rather than along the inguinal canal. *When the patient coughed, the doctor felt a mass strike the pad of his finger, which was against the posterior wall of the inguinal canal.* When the patient was asked to lie down, the mass reduced itself immediately. The doctor then placed his fingers over he **inguinal triangle** Hesselbach's triangle) and instructed the patient to hold his nose and blow it. The doctor felt a mass protruding from the lower portion of this triangle. A diagnosis of **direct inguinal hernia** was made.

Problems. Explain what is meant by the

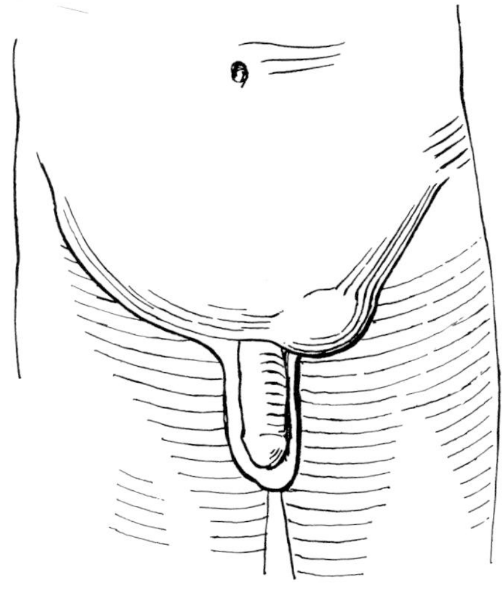

Figure 2-151. Illustration of the direct inguinal hernia protruding through the inguinal triangle.

term direct inguinal hernia. *How does it differ from an indirect (oblique) inguinal hernia*? Does a direct inguinal hernia have an embryological basis? What is the relationship of a direct inguinal hernia to the **inferior epigastric artery**? Is this relationship different from that of indirect inguinal hernia? Inadvertent injury to which nerves of the abdominal wall during surgery may predispose to the development of inguinal hernia? *These problems are discussed on page 289.*

Case 2-10. During the 2nd week after birth, a male infant began expelling the contents of his stomach with great force (**projectile vomiting**). His mother reported that his vomiting occurred during or shortly after his feeding. She also said that the baby become hungry right away and would take another feeding immediately.

The pediatrician who had cared for the infant since birth noted that the infant had a weight loss and was somewhat dehydrated. As the baby was obviously hungry, the doctor asked the mother to feed him. As she did this, he palpated the infant's abdomen. He was unable to palpate the baby's pylorus. *Before the baby finished feeding, he vomited, projecting the vomitus several feet.* The pediatrician noted that the vomitus consisted only of gastric contents and was neither blood-tinged nor bile-stained. Suspecting a partial obstruction of the GI tract, most likely in the pyloric region, the pediatrician requested radiographic studies.

The nurse fed the infant a bottle of his formula containing some barium. During the radiographic examination, the radiologist noted delayed emptying of the infant's stomach, vigorous peristaltic activity, and a narrowed elongated pyloric canal.

A diagnosis of **congenital hypertrophic pyloric stenosis** was made and the infant was scheduled for surgery. At operation the surgeon noted that the infant's pylorus was the size and consistency of a medium-sized olive. He incised the pyloric musculature and separated it longitudinally down to the mucosa (**pyloromyotomy**).

Problems. Define **pyloric stenosis**. What do the adjectives *congenital* and *hypertrophic* imply? What is the embryological basis of this GI anomaly? Is pyloric stenosis a common condition? Is its incidence sex related? If the infant's vomitus had been bile stained, where would you think the obstruction might be? *These problems are discussed on page 290.*

DISCUSSION OF PATIENT ORIENTED PROBLEMS

Case 2-1. A **peptic ulcer** is an ulceration of the mucous membrane of the stomach or the duodenum and occurs only in tissues in contact with gastric juice. Ulcers are common in the stomach (**gastric ulcers**) and in the duodenum (**duodenal ulcers**), but about 80% of peptic ulcers occur in the duodenum. Ulcers are usually found within 3 cm of the pylorus and occur more commonly in males. The depth of the ulcer varies from a shallow erosion of the mucosa to complete penetration of the wall of the duodenum (**perforated duodenal ulcer**). Both gastric and duodenal ulcers tend to bleed. Sometimes organs and vessels adjacent to the duodenum, usually the pancreas, become adherent to an ulcer and are eroded; *e.g.*, a posterior penetrating ulcer may erode the gastroduodenal artery or one of its branches. This causes sudden massive hemorrhage, which may be fatal.

Peptic ulcers may occur in a **Meckel's diverticulum**, a remnant of the yolk stalk attached to the ileum which is present in about 2% of persons (Fig. 2-104). *Gastric tissue may be present in the wall of the diverticulum* and may secrete acid that causes ulcer formation. Hemorrhage is a common complication of a Meckel's diverticulum, particularly in males 10 years and under. A Meckel's diverticulum is not often visualized in a GI series, but those that are bleeding and contain gastric tissue can be detected by radioisotope studies (**scintigram** of the abdomen).

Pain is the distressing symptom of peptic ulceration, varying from a slight discomfort to a boring, gnawing ache. Some authorities attribute the pain to the contact of hydrochloric acid with the ulcerated surface; others believe the pain results from contractions of the stomach. It seems certain that pain occurs when there is marked **inflammatory reaction** or penetration of surrounding organs (*e.g.*, the pancreas). Pain resulting from a gastric ulcer is referred to the epigastric region because the stomach is supplied with pain afferents that reach the seventh and eighth thoracic segments through the greater splanchnic branch of the sympathetic trunk. *Pain resulting from a peptic ulcer is referred to the anterior abdominal wall above the umbilicus* because both the duodenum and this area of skin are supplied by the ninth and tenth thoracic nerves (Fig. 2-141).

When a duodenal ulcer perforates there may be pain all over the abdomen. Sometimes the peritoneal gutter associated with the ascending colon (right lateral or **right paracolic gutter** may act as a watershed and direct the escaping inflammatory material into the right iliac fossa (Fig. 2-110). The leakage of duodenal contents through such a perforation leads to acute **chemical peritonitis**. This explains why pain from an anterior perforation of a duodenal ulcer may cause right upper and lower quadrant pain. In such cases, the differential diagnosis between a perforated duodenal ulcer and a perforated appendix may be difficult.

As the **vagus nerves** largely control the secretion of acid by the parietal cells of the stomach, and as excess acid secretion is associated with peptic ulcers, section of the vagus nerves (**vagotomy**) as they enter the abdomen is sometimes performed to reduce acid production. Vagotomy is often performed in conjunction with **resection** (excision) of the ulcerated area and the acid-producing part of the stomach. Often only the gastric branches of the vagus nerves are cut (**selective vagotomy**), thereby avoiding adverse effects on other organs (*e.g.*, dilation of the gallbladder).

Case 2-2. The patient's initial attack of excruciating pain was almost certainly caused by *passage of the stone* from his funnel-shaped renal pelvis into the upper end of his right ureter, a narrow cylindrical tube (Fig. 2-124). Stones that are larger than the lumen of the ureter (3 mm) cause considerable pain when they attempt to pass through it. The *pain moves from loin to groin* as the stone passes along the ureter and the pain ceases when it passes into the urinary bladder, although tenderness along the course of the ureter often persists for some time. During a subsequent micturition, the stone passes through the urethra (Fig. 2-114).

The patient very likely would experience severe pain when the stone was temporarily held up owing to angulation of the ureter as it crosses the brim of the pelvis minor and when it became wedged in the ureter, where it passed through the wall of the urinary bladder. At the lower end of the ureter, there is a definite **narrowing of the lumen**; thus it is a common site of obstruction.

The **ureteral pain (colic)** results from passage of the stone through the ureter. As the ureter is a muscular tube in which peristaltic contractions normally convey urine from the kidney to the urinary bladder, *pain results from distention of the ureter by the stone and the urine that is unable to pass by it.* The smooth muscular coat of the ureter normally undergoes peristaltic contractions from above downward. As the peristaltic wave approaches the obstruction, forceful smooth contraction causes excessive dilation of the ureter between the wave and the stone. It is the **ureteral distention** that produces the lancinating pain, and **exacerbation of pain** occurs as distention increases. Thus, *there is some easing of pain between peristaltic waves.* Consequently the peristaltic contractions of the ureter explain the intermittent exacerbation of pain.

The afferent pain fibers supplying the ureter are included in the **lesser splanchnic nerve** (Figs. 2-127 and 2-134). Impulses also enter the first and second lumbar segments of the spinal cord and the pain is felt in the cutaneous areas innervated by the lower intercostal nerves (T11, T12), the **iliohypogastric** and **ilioinguinal nerves** (L1), and the genitofemoral nerve (L1, L2). These are the same regions of the spinal cord that supply the ureter (T11 to L2); hence, the pain commences in the loin and radiates downward and forward to the groin and the scrotum (Fig. 2-141). The retraction of the testis by the cremaster muscle and the pain along the medial part of the front of the thigh in the present case indicates that the genital and femoral branches of the **genitofemoral nerve** (L1, L2) were involved.

As discussed, *ureteral colic is caused by ureteral distention which stimulates pain afferents in its wall.* As there was **no peritonitis** (inflammation of the abdominal peitoneum), there was **no rigidity** and **no rebound tenderness**. When peritonitis is present, pressing the hand into the abdominal wall and rapidly releasing it causes pain when the abdominal musculature springs back into place, carrying the inflamed peritoneum with it. Hence, the **rebound test** is useful in the differentiation of ureteral colic from **appendicitis** and **intestinal colic**.

Case 2-3. *An indirect inguinal hernia is an outpouching of the peritoneal sac* that enters the deep inguinal ring, traverses the inguinal canal and (if complete) exits through the superficial inguinal ring and enters the scrotum. *It is referred to as an indirect hernia because it pursues an oblique course through the anterior abdominal wall and the inguinal canal.* A direct inguinal hernia does not pass through the deep inguinal ring; it protrudes through the anterior abdominal wall medial to the deep ring and the inferior epigastric artery.

The embryological basis of an indirect inguinal hernia is persistence of the **processus vaginalis**, a diverticulum or outpouching of the peritoneum which pushes through the abdominal wall and forms the inguinal canal (Fig. 2-18) in preparation for later descent of the testis through it. The processus vaginalis evaginates all layers of the abdominal wall before it, and in males they become the coverings of the spermatic cord. *The opening produced in the transversalis fascia by the processus vaginalis becomes the deep inguinal ring* and the opening it forms in the aponeurosis of the external oblique becomes the superficial inguinal ring. *In females, the entire processus vaginalis normally disappears*, whereas in males the lower portion persists and becomes the **tunica vaginalis** (Fig. 2-19*B*). If the stalk of this processus does not obliterate after birth, a loop of intestine may herniate into it and enter the scrotum (Fig. 2-22*B*) or the labium majus.

The persistent **hernial sac** (processus vaginalis) may vary from a short one not extending beyond the superficial ring to one that extends into the scrotum (or the labium majus), where it is continuous with the tunica vaginalis.

A persistent processus vaginalis predisposes to indirect inguinal hernia by creating a weakness in the anterior abdominal wall and a hernial sac into which abdominal contents may herniate if the intra-abdominal pressure becomes very high, as occurs during straining while lifting a heavy object. *The obliquity of the inguinal canal and the contraction of the abdominal muscles usually prevent herniation of abdominal contents* during rises of intra-abdominal pressure that occur during coughing, straining, or nose blowing. When infants become more active at 2 to 3 months, increases in intra-abdominal pressure, as occur during crying and coughing, may force part of the greater omentum and/or an abdominal organ, usually a loop of bowel, into the **patent processus vaginalis**. The hernial sac then appears as a bulge in the inguinal region extending into the scrotum or labium majus. The herniated gut in the sac may become constricted, resulting in interference with its blood supply and formation of a **strangulated hernia**.

Once the deep ring has become enlarged by a herniation of abdominal contents, coughing may cause herniation to occur again. This is the basis of the test done during physical diagnosis, where the examiner's finger is inserted through the superficial ring into the inguinal canal and the patient is asked to cough.

In males, the testis and spermatic cord normally pass through the inguinal canal before birth. The spermatic cord and testis are therefore covered by extensions of the abdominal wall. *Passage of the spermatic cord through the inguinal canal enlarges the canal and weakens the entrance to it* (the deep ring). This explains why indirect hernia is more common in males (about 20:1). The hernial sac lies within the coverings of the spermatic cord; thus, it is covered by internal spermatic fascia and the cremaster muscle and cremasteric fascia. As the testis passed posterior to the processus vaginalis, descending through the inguinal canal before or shortly after birth, *the ductus deferens lies immediately posterior to the hernial sac.*

During the surgical repair of an indirect inguinal hernia, the genital branch of the **genitofemoral nerve** is endangered because it traverses the canal in both sexes and exits through the **superficial ring** (Fig. 2-9). The ilioinguinal nerve may also be injured. This nerve supplies the skin of the superomedial area of the thigh, the skin over the root of the penis, and the upper part of the scrotum with sensory fibers. In the female, it supplies the same area of the thigh, the skin covering the mons pubis, and the adjoining part of the labium majus. If this nerve is injured, anesthesia of these areas of skin will likely result. If the nerve is constricted by a suture, **postoperative neuritic pain** may also occur in these areas.

Injury to the **external iliac artery** or to the inferior epigastric artery, one of its two main branches, is uncommon during the repair of an inguinal hernia, but their relationship to the deep ring makes them liable to injury, *e.g.*, by a suture that is placed too deeply. Serious extraperitoneal bleeding can result from an unrecognized tear of these vessels.

As the **ductus deferens** lies immediately posterior to the hernial sac, it may be damaged when the sac is freed, ligated, and excised. As the hernial sac is within the spermatic cord, the **pampiniform plexus** of veins and the internal spermatic artery may also be injured, resulting in impairment of circulation to the testis. Injury to the ductus deferens or to the vessels of the spermatic cord may result in **atrophy of the testis** on that side.

Case 2-4. The type of skin incision used for an appendectomy depends on the type of patient and the certainty of the diagnosis. Usually the McBurney or **gridiron incision** is made (Fig. 2-45), which is an oblique or almost transverse one that follows *Langer's lines* (cleavage lines of the skin). The center of the incision is at **McBurney's point**, which is at the junction of the lateral and middle thirds of the line joining the anterior superior iliac spine and the umbilicus (Fig. 2-45). In most cases, this point overlies the base or origin of the appendix from the cecum.

Following incision of the skin and the superficial fascia, *the aponeurosis of the external oblique muscle* (Fig. 2-9) *is incised in the direction of the fibers of this muscle* (downward, forward, and medially). The other two muscles of the anterior abdominal wall (internal oblique and transversus abdominis) are then split (not cut) in the direction of their fibers; this lessens the chances of injuring the nerves supplying them. Next the transversalis fascia and the parietal peritoneum are incised to expose the cecum. *The base of the appendix is indicated by the point of convergence of the three teniae coli* (Fig. 2-43).

The vermiform appendix varies in length and in position (Fig. 2-44). It usually lies behind the cecum and, if long enough, behind the lower part of the ascending colon (**retrocecal appendix** or **retrocolic appendix**), but it may descend over the brim of the pelvis minor (pelvic appendix). In the female, a **pelvic appendix** lies close to the right uterine tube and ovary.

The variations in length and position of the appendix may give rise to varying signs and symptoms in appendicitis. For example, the site of maximum tenderness in cases of retrocecal appendix may be just superomedial to the anterior superior iliac spine, even as high as the level of the umbilicus. **Subhepatic cecum** and appendix are uncommon. This unusual condition results from incomplete rotation of the gut during the fetal period. *In these cases the site of pain is likely to be in the right upper quadrant* of the abdomen.

If the appendix is long (10 to 15 cm) and extends into the pelvis minor, the site of pain in a female might suggest peritoneal irritation resulting from a ruptured **ectopic pregnancy**. As the appendix crosses the psoas major muscle, the patient often flexes the right thigh to relieve the pain. Thus, *hyperextension of the thigh (psoas test) causes pain because it stretches the muscle and its inflamed fascia.* Tenderness on the right side during a rectal examination may indicate an inflamed pelvic appendix.

Initially, the pain of typical acute appendicitis is referred to the periumbilical region of the abdomen; later, the site of pain usually shifts to the right lower quadrant. Afferent nerve fibers from the appendix are carried in the lesser splanchnic nerve and impulses enter the 10th thoracic segment of the spinal cord (Fig. 2-141). As impulses from the skin in the periumbilical region are also sent to this region of the spinal cord, the pain is interpreted as somatic rather than **visceral**, apparently because impulses of cutaneous origin are more often received by the thalamus. *The shift of pain to the right lower quadrant is caused by irritation of the parietal peritoneum,* usually on the posterior abdominal wall. Afferent fibers from this region of peritoneum and skin are carried in the lowest intercostal, the subcostal, and the first lumbar nerves. The pain during palpation results from stimulation of pain receptors in the skin and the peritoneum, whereas the increased tenderness detected in the right side of the **rectouterine pouch** (rectovesical pouch in the male) is caused by irritation of the parietal peritoneum in this pouch. When the abdominal wall is depressed and then allowed to rebound, the patient usually winces because, as the abdominal muscles spring back into place, the inflamed peritoneum is carried with it.

If the patient had previously had her appendix removed, an inflamed **Meckel's diverticulum** could give rise to signs and symptoms similar to appendicitis. This ileal diverticulum is one of the most common abnormalities of the intestinal tract, occurring in 2 to 4% of people (Fig. 2-104). A *Meckel's diverticulum represents the remnant of the proximal portion of the yolk stalk* and appears as a finger-like projection (usually 3 to 6 cm long) from the antimesenteric border of the ileum, 40 to 50 cm from the ileocecal junction.

Case 2-5. True **diverticula of the colon**, consisting of all layers of the bowel, are rare, but false diverticula, or *herniations of the mucosa through the muscularis mucosae, are observed in about 10% of persons over 40 years of age* who have had barium enemas for radiological studies. These small herniations, apparently developing along the course of the terminal blood vessels that penetrate the muscles of the intestinal wall, are **most common in the sigmoid colon** (Fig. 2-105).

When one or more of these diverticula become inflamed, the condition is known as **diverticulitis**. The initial causes of the inflammation are usually mechanical, *e.g.*, blockage of the neck of a diverticulum by bowel contents; later the diverticulum becomes infected and **peritonitis** develops.

Diverticulitis has been called "left-sided appendicitis" because it produces symptoms on the left similar to those produced on the right by appendicitis.

In extremely rare cases, the vermiform appendix is located in the lower left quadrant of the abdomen. This condition exists when there is **situs inversus viscerum** (transposition of the viscera). *During rotation of the midgut in the embryonic period, the midgut loop rotates in a clockwise instead of counterclockwise direction.* This condition sometimes occurs in one of a pair of identical twins who exhibit the phenomenon of mirror imaging (e.g., one twin is right-handed and the other left-handed).

Case 2-6. *Diaphragmatic hernia is a herniation of abdominal viscera into the chest through an opening in the thoracoabdominal diaphragm.* A **congenital diaphragmatic hernia** is present in about one of 2220 infants and results from *defective formation and/or fusion of a pleuroperitoneal membrane* with the dorsal mesentery of the esophagus and the septum transversum during development of the diaphragm (Fig. 2-135). As a result there is a **posterolateral defect in the diaphragm**, usually on the left (Fig. 2-152), through which abdominal organs, usually the intestines, herniate into the chest.

Hiatal hernia is common, particularly in older people. Usually the gastroesophageal region of the stomach herniates through the esophageal hiatus in the diaphragm into the lower chest. Although *hiatal hernia is usually acquired*, a congenitally enlarged esophageal hiatus may be a predisposing factor. The esophageal hiatus is in the muscular part of the diaphragm.

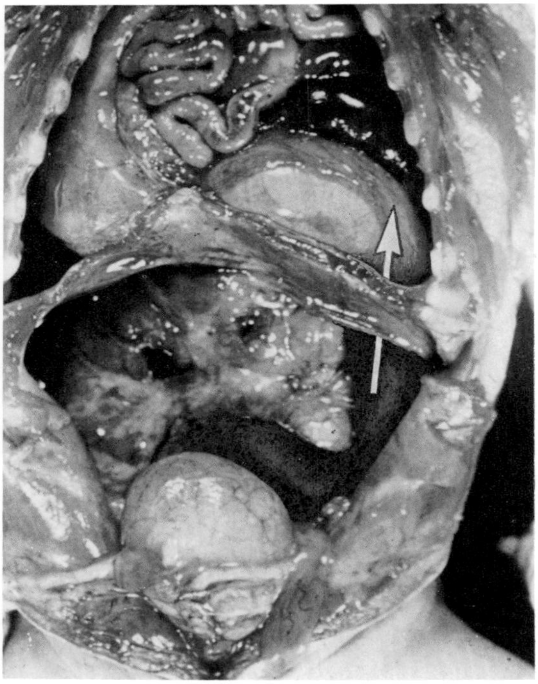

Figure 2-152. Photograph of an infant's thorax and abdomen taken at autopsy. The *arrow* is passing through a large posterolateral defect in the diaphragm. The liver has been removed. Note the intestines in the thorax.

Understand that the right crus passes to the left of the midline; hence, the esophageal hiatus and hernia are to the left of the midline even though they are within the right crus. In most cases, herniation appears after 50 years of age and results from **widening of the esophageal hiatus** owing to weakening of muscle fibers of the right crus of the diaphragm and of the fascia connecting the esophagus to the diaphragm, sometimes termed the phrenoesophageal ligament.

There are two main types of hiatal hernia (1) *sliding hiatal hernia* and (2) *paraesophageal hernia*, but some hernias present characteristics of both types and are referred to as *mixed hiatal hernias*.

Sliding hiatal hernia (Fig. 2-53*A*) is the most common type (up to 10 times more common than the paresophageal and mixed types combined). In sliding hiatal hernia, as in the present case, **the gastroesophageal junction herniates into the chest**. The hernial sac consists of parietal peritoneum in front and the anterior wall of the stomach behind.

Paraesophageal hiatal hernia is much less common than sliding hiatal hernia, but it is more common in women than in men (10 to 1). In this type, **the gastroesophageal junction remains in the normal position**, but a pouch of peritoneum herniates through the esophageal hiatus into the lower chest. *Usually the hernial sac contains a portion of the fundus of the stomach* (Fig. 2-53*B*).

Some authorities believe that the sac of peritoneum protrudes through the hiatus before birth, in much the same way as a persistent processus vaginalis protrudes through the inguinal canal and predisposes to indirect inguinal hernia.

The thoracic region of the vertebral column becomes shorter with age owing to **dessication of the intervertebral discs**, and the abdominal fat generally increases during middle age. Both of these occurrences favor development of hiatal hernia.

Most of the present patient's complaints (heartburn, belching, regurgitation, and epigastric pain) can be attributed to irritation of the esophageal mucosa by the **reflux of gastric juice** into the esophagus and herniated pouch of the stomach. The irritant effect of the gastric juice produces **esophageal spasm** (involuntary muscular contractions of the esophagus), resulting in **dysphagia** (difficulty in swallowing) and **retrosternal pain**. Pain endings in the esophagus are stimulated by the forcible contractions of the smooth muscle in esophageal wall occurring during spasm. *Pain of gastroesophageal origin is referred to the epigastric and retrosternal regions*, the cutaneous zones of reference for these regions of the viscera. The patient's **hiccups** are caused by **spasmodic contractions of the diaphragm**, which result from pressure created by the hernia. Probably enlargement of the esophageal hiatus stimulates fibers of the phrenic nerves supplying the diaphragm (Fig. 2-133).

An incidence of hiatal hernia as high as 70% has been reported in routine radiographic studies, but in most cases these abnormalities are relatively asymptomatic (*i.e.*, produce only heartburn and mild indigestion). Most hiatal hernias either require no treatment or can be managed medically by decreasing **gastroesophageal reflux** (*e.g.*, through weight reduction).

As the **esophageal hiatus** also transmits the **vagus nerves** and the **esophageal branches of the left gastric vessels**, these structures as well as the esophagus must be protected from injury during surgical repair of hiatal hernias.

Case 2-7. The radiologist was unable to identify the presumed stone in the cystic duct because it was small and not faceted or laminated. This is typical of the **nidus** (L. nest) around which other substances are deposited to produce a larger, more typical gallstone. In addition, a small calcification in this region might be in some other structure, such as a lymph node in the porta hepatis.

Obese middle-aged women, such as the present patient, who have had several children (**multipara**), are most prone to gallbladder disease, but tall thin men, virgin women, and children may also develop the disease. Thus, the common aphorism "*forty*, *flatulent*, *female*, *fertile*, and *fat*" describes some patients, but it does not characterize all patients with gallstones. Over 20 years of age, stones are more common in females, but this is not necessarily so after 50 years of age. *In about 50% of persons, gallstones are "silent" (asymptomatic).* A gallstone is a concretion in the gallbladder, cystic duct, or bile duct, composed chiefly of cholesterol crystals.

The pain is severe when a stone is lodged in the cystic or bile duct. The patient's sudden severe pain in the epigastric region (**biliary colic**) was caused by a gallstone wedged in the cystic duct. It has been suggested that colicky pain is initially felt in the midline because the primitive gut, from which the gallbladder and intestines are derived, is originally in the midline. Although appealing, there is no good experimental evidence to support this hypothesis. *The pain referred to the right upper quadrant and scapular region results from inflammation of the gallbladder and distention of the cystic duct.* The nerve impulses pass centrally in the greater splanchnic nerve on the right side (Fig. 2-134) and enter the spinal cord through the dorsal roots of the seventh and eighth thoracic nerves. This **visceral referred pain** is felt in the right upper quadrant of the abdomen and in the right infrascapular region because the source of the stimuli entering this region of the cord is wrongly interpreted as cutaneous (Fig. 2-141).

Often the inflamed gallbladder irritates the peritoneum covering the diaphragm, resulting in a **parietal referred pain** in the lower chest wall if peripheral parts of the diaphragm are involved, as this area of peritoneum is supplied by **lower intercostal nerves**. In other cases, the peritoneum covering the diaphragm is irritated and the pain is referred to the shoulder region because this area of peritoneum is supplied by the **phrenic nerve** (C3, C4, and C5 segments of the spinal cord, Fig. 2-141). The skin of the shoulder region is supplied by the **supraclavicular nerves** (C3 and C4), the same segments of the cord that receive pain afferents from the central portion of the diaphragm.

Although the stone in the cystic duct is radiopaque, *only one in five gallstones contain enough calcium to be visible on plain radiographs* of the abdomen. **Cholecystokinin** liberated by fat entering the duodenum causes contraction of the gallbladder. In the present case, it is very likely that the patient's gallbladder contracted vigorously after her fatty meal, squeezing a stone into her cystic duct. **Acute cholecystitis** is associated with a gallstone impacted in the cystic duct in a high percentage of cases. *Sudden distention of the gallbladder compromises its blood and lymphatic supply.*

Usually peritoneum does not separate the gallbladder from the liver. The gallbladder lies in a fossa on the inferior surface of the right hepatic lobe (Fig. 2-83) and the peritoneum on this surface of the liver passes over the inferior surface of the gallbladder, leaving the superior surface attached to the liver by connective tissue.

The **abdominal rigidity** detected in the present case resulted from *involuntary contraction of the muscles of the anterior abdominal wall*, particularly the rectus abdominis. This muscle spasm is a reflex response to stimulation of nerve endings in the peritoneum associated with the gallbladder.

Anatomical variations in the gallbladder and the cystic duct and in the arteries supplying them are very common (Figs. 2-93 and 2-95). Because of this, surgeons must determine the existing anatomical pattern and identify the cystic bile, and hepatic ducts and the cystic and hepatic arteries before dividing the cystic duct and its artery. *Important variations occur in the length and course of the cystic duct* (Fig. 2-95*A* to *C*). If these abnormalities are not recognized, the bile duct may be mistaken for the cystic duct and be ligated and divided. This results in severe **jaundice** (F. *jaune*, yellow) and death if it is not reopened.

Variations in the origin and course of the cystic artery occur in up to 25% of persons (Fig. 2-93). As there may be accessory cystic branches from the hepatic arteries, unexpected hemorrhage may occur during cholecystectomy. A more serious complication is postoperative hemorrhage following unrecognized injury during surgery to an abdominal blood vessel.

Case 2-8. *Hepatic cirrhosis is a disease of the liver characterized by progressive destruction of hepatic parenchymal cells* (hepatic cells or hepatocytes) that are replaced by fibrous tissue (**fibrosis**) which contracts and hardens like scar tissue elsewhere. The new fibrous tissue surrounds the intrahepatic blood vessels and biliary radicles (roots). As this process advances, the circulation of blood through the branches of the portal vein and bile through the **biliary radicles** in the liver is impeded (Fig. 2-86). As the pressure in the portal vein rises (**portal hypertension**), the liver becomes more dependent on the hepatic artery for its blood supply, and blood pressure in the portal vein rises, reversing blood flow in the normal **portacaval anastomoses** so that portal blood enters the systemic circulation (Fig. 2-112). As these anastomotic veins seldom possess valves, they can conduct blood in either direction. This causes enlargement (**varicose veins**) in these anastomoses at the lower end of the esophagus (**esophageal varices**), the lower end of the rectum and anal canal (**hemorrhoids** or piles), and around the umbilicus (**caput medusae**). Because of pressure during swallowing and defecation, the esophageal varices and hemorrhoids, respectively, may rupture, resulting in **bloody vomitus** and/or bleeding from the anus. The bloody stools result from bleeding of the enlarged hemorrhoids. *When the stool is black it is the result of upper GI tract blood being acted upon by the gastric juices* and passing into the lower GI tract.

Internal hemorrhoids are varicosities of the tributaries of the **superior rectal vein** (hemorrhoidal vein). Blood may also pass in a retrograde direction in the paraumbilical veins, which are small **tributaries of the portal vein**, via the vein in the ligamentum teres. In **portal hypertension** these vessels may (but rarely) become varicose, forming a radiating pattern at the umbilicus, called a **caput medusae** (Fig. 2-150), owing to its resemblance to the snakes adorning the head of Medusa, a mythological character.

In **cirrhosis of the liver**, the ramifications of the portal vein are compressed by the contraction of the fibrous tissue in the portal canals. As a result, *there is increased pressure in the splenic and superior and inferior mesenteric veins.* Fluid is forced out of the capillary beds drained by these veins into the peritoneal cavity. This *accumulation of fluid in the peritoneal cavity* is called **ascites**.

The spleen usually enlarges (**splenomegaly**) because of increased pressure in the splenic vein. As there are *no valves in the portal system*, pressure in the splenic vein is equal to that in the portal vein. A common method of reducing portal pressure is by diverting blood from the portal vein to the inferior vena cava through a surgically-created anastomosis (**portacaval anastomosis**). Similarly, the splenic vein may be anastomosed to the left renal vein (**splenorenal anastomosis**).

Case 2-9. A **direct inguinal hernia** enters the inguinal canal through its posterior wall, whereas an **indirect inguinal hernia** enters the inguinal canal at the deep inguinal ring. *Direct inguinal hernia is much* *less common than indirect inguinal hernia* and both types occur more often in men than in women. Usually a direct inguinal hernia is acquired and occurs in men over 40 years of age.

The sac of a direct hernia, formed by peritoneum behind the anterior abdominal wall, protrudes through some part of the **inguinal triangle**. This triangle is bounded *medially* by the **lateral border of the rectus abdominus** muscle, *inferiorly* by the **inguinal ligament**, and *laterally* by the **inferior epigastric artery**. The hernia may protrude through the anterior abdominal wall and escape from the abdomen on the lateral side of the conjoint tendon to enter the inguinal canal. In this case, the hernial sac is covered by transversalis fascia, cremaster muscle and fascia, and external spermatic fascia. Occasionally the hernial sac is forced through the fibers of the **conjoint tendon** to enter the lower end of the inguinal canal. In this case, it is covered by transversalis fascia, conjoint tendon, and external spermatic fascia. Direct hernias usually protrude anteriorly through the lower part of the **inguinal triangle** and extend toward the superficial inguinal ring, but they rarely pass through this ring and enter the scrotum or the labium majus.

A direct hernia is acquired and results from some type of *weakness of the anterior abdominal wall, e.g.*, of the transversalis fascia with atrophy of the conjoint tendon. There is no known embryological basis for this type of hernia. The type of inguinal hernia (direct or indirect) can often be determined by the relationship of the hernial sac to the inferior epigastric artery. The pulsations of this artery can usually be felt by the tip of the examiner's finger in the inguinal canal. *In direct hernia, the neck of the hernial sac is in the inguinal triangle and lies* **medial** to the inferior epigastric artery, whereas *in indirect hernia the neck of the hernial sac is in the deep inguinal ring and lies* **lateral** to the inferior epigastric artery.

As the lower intercostal nerves and the **iliohypogastric** and **ilioinguinal nerves** from the first lumbar nerve supply the abdominal musculature (Fig. 2-8), injury to any of them during surgery or an accident could result in weakening of muscles in the inguinal region, predisposing to development of direct inguinal hernia. In addition, the **ilioinguinal nerve** gives motor branches to the fibers of the internal oblique which are inserted into the lateral border of the conjoint tendon. Division of this nerve paralyzes these fibers and relaxes the conjoint tendon and may predispose to the appearance of a direct inguinal hernia.

Case 2-10. Pyloric stenosis is a progressive *narrowing of the pyloric canal.* Often there is also narrowing of the lower part of the pyloric antrum. The adjective *congenital* indicates that the condition is present at birth, although the onset of **projectile vomiting** (a characteristic clinical manifestation) is rarely present before 1 week of age. Although *the cause of pyloric stenosis is not known*, a hereditary basis is suspected because of the high incidence of the condition in both of monozygotic (identical) twins, in contrast to the relative infrequency in both of dizygotic (nonidentical) twins.

The adjective **hypertrophic** indicates there is an *overgrowth or general increase in the size of a part*, in this case, of the pylorus. The embryological and pathological basis of pyloric stenosis is narrowing of the pyloric canal owing principally to hypertrophy of the circular muscle layer of the pylorus. Normally the circular fibers form a uniform layer over the whole stomach but are most abundant in the pylorus, where they aggregate to form the pyloric sphincter. When these muscle fibers become enlarged they narrow the pyloric canal. In these infants, *the pylorus is enlongated and thickened* to as much as twice its usual size and has an almost cartilaginous consistency.

Congenital pyloric stenosis is a very common condition. It affects about 1 in every 150 males and 1 in every 750 females and tends to occur in firstborn children.

If the infant's vomitus had been bile-stained, obstruction most likely in the duodenum would have been strongly suspected. The vomitus contains bile if the obstruction is distal to the **hepatopancreatic ampulla** (Fig. 2-88), as it usually is.

SUGGESTIONS FOR ADDITIONAL READING

1. Anson, B. J., and McVay, C. B. *Surgical Anatomy*, Ed. 5, vol. 1, W. B. Saunders Co., Philadelphia, 1971.

This classical textbook gives good accounts of the various *types of abdominal incision* and discusses the anatomical basis for them. There is a *well-illustrated account of hernias* and how they are repaired. Various methods of anastomosing the stomach to the intestine after partial gastric section are also described. *Kidney transplantation is discussed* with emphasis on the importance of understanding the renal vascular variations and abnormalities of the upper urinary tract.

2. Healey, J. E. *A Synopsis of Clinical Anatomy*, W. B. Saunders, Co., Philadelphia, 1969.

This book gives a good account of the *clinical applications of gross anatomy*. It is particularly well illustrated and has a good account of the *embryology of the GI tract*. Areas are pointed out where surgical injury can occur, *e.g.*, he states "Surgical injury to the ductal system is far too frequent and often tragic. Awareness of the anatomic variations encountered in gallbladder surgery will prevent many such accidents."

3. Lowenfels, A. B. *Companion Guide to Surgical Diagnosis*, The Williams & Wilkins Company, Baltimore, 1975.

This small monograph *reviews common diagnostic problems encountered in surgical patients*. Emphasis is placed on a systematic approach to data gathering. There are good accounts of the types of *abdominal hernia*, *abdominal incisions*, *wound drainage*, *abscesses*, *fistulas*, abdominal injuries, the acute abdomen, intestinal obstruction, and abdominal masses.

4. Moore, K. L. *The Developing Human, Clinically Oriented Embryology*, Ed. 2., W. B. Saunders Co., Philadelphia, 1977.

In order to appreciate the normal relationships of the abdominal viscera and the many anatomical variations and congenital abnormalities which may occur, a good knowledge of the mechanisms of the development and rotation of the embryonic gut is imperative. Although the main points are mentioned in the present text, the embryological processes are discussed and illustrated in greater detail in the author's embryology book.

5. Sparberg, M. Examination of the abdomen, In *A Primer of Clinical Diagnosis*, edited by W. B. Buckingham, M. Sparberg, and M. Brandfonbrenner, Harper & Row Publishers, Inc., New York, 1971.

The technique of examining a patient's abdomen is clearly described and illustrated. The various types of palpation and the abnormalities noted on palpation are described and discussed. Hepatomegaly, splenomegaly, gallbladder enlargement, kidney enlargement, aortic enlargement, and enlargement of the stomach, colon, pancreas, and umbilicus are discussed. Bowel sounds, *rebound tenderness, guarding, paralytic ileus*, and other clinical terms are defined.

6. Squire, L. F., Colaiace, W. M., and Strutynsky, N. *Exercises in Diagnostic Radiology. 2. The Abdomen*, W. B. Saunders Co., Philadelphia, 1971.

This short book of exercises includes radiographs of groups of three patients presenting with the same symptom or symptom complex. This will give you some idea of the daily diagnostic problems faced by the radiologist.

CHAPTER 3

The Perineum and Pelvis

THE PERINEUM

In the anatomical position the perineum is a narrow area between the thighs and the gluteal region, but when the thighs are abducted (Fig. 3-1) *the perineum is a diamond-shaped region extending from the symphysis pubis to the tip of the coccyx* (Figs. 3-2 to 3-6). The perineum is best examined and dissected with the person in the **lithotomy position** (Fig. 3-1). The perineum includes the openings of the *anal canal* (**anus**) and of the *urogenital system* (**vagina** and/or **urethra**).

The male perineum (Fig. 3-4) is of special importance to certain surgical specialists, *e.g.*, **proctologists** (surgeons who deal with the rectum and anus and their diseases) and **urologists** (surgeons who are concerned with the urogenital organs). The relationship of the male perineum to the urethra, prostate, seminal vesicles, urinary bladder, rectum, and anal canal is essential knowledge for all doctors.

The female perineum (Fig. 3-3) is of special importance to **obstetricians**, specialists who care for women during pregnancy and parturition (childbirth); **gynecologists** (G. *gyne*, women + *logos*, study), who deal with diseases peculiar to women; and urologists and proctologists (defined previously). *Knowledge of clinically oriented anatomy, including the bony landmarks of the pelvis, is a prime requisite for the clinical management of parturition* and many diseases involving the bladder, urethra, vagina, rectum, and anal canal. **The perineum refers to the skin and subcutaneous structures that close the inferior pelvic aperture** (pelvic outlet) at the inferior end of the trunk between the thighs (Figs. 3-1 to 3-4).

The boundaries of the perineum (Figs. 3-2 to 3-12, 3-39, 4-1, and 4-47) are: (1) the *symphysis pubis*; (2) the *inferior pubic rami*; (3) the *ischial rami*; (4) the ischial tuberosities; (5) the *sacrotuberous ligaments*; and (6) the *coccyx*.

The perineum contains the *anus*, the root of the *scrotum* and the *penis* (male external genitalia) or the *vulva* (female external genitalia). Hence the *perineum includes two parts*, the anal triangle (region) and the urogenital triangle (region). The **anal triangle** is posterior to the line joining the midpoints of the two *ischial tuberosities* (Figs. 3-5 and 3-9*B*) and the **urogenital triangle** is anterior to this line. The anal region is similar in both sexes, but the urogenital region is quite different in the male and the female. However, many homologies (G. *homos*, the same + *logos*, study) are recognizable because *they are derived from the same primordia* (embryonic structures). You should be aware that in obstetrics and gynecology, the term perineum is often used when referring only to the skin and subcutaneous structures between the vaginal orifice anteriorly and the anus posteriorly (Figs. 3-3 and 3-39).

The inferior pelvic aperture (Fig. 3-9) is closed except where it transmits the urethra and the anal canal (Fig. 3-6); *in the female* it also transmits the vagina (Fig. 3-3). The anterior half of the inferior pelvic aperture is closed by the **urogenital diaphragm** (Figs. 3-10, 3-13, and 3-16) and the posterior half is closed by the **levatores ani muscles** (Figs. 3-12 and 3-17). The levatores ani muscles run posteroinferiorly from the anterolateral walls of the pelvis minor and meet one another in the median plane from the posterior margin of the urogenital diaphragm to the coccyx.

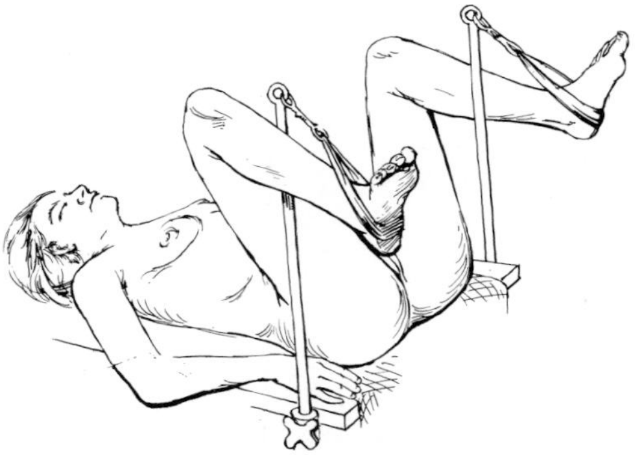

Figure 3-1. Drawing of a woman in the lithotomy position (dorsosacral position), which is used for doing pelvic examinations and delivering babies. The feet are held by straps (as here) or by metal stirrups. The essentials of this position are: (1) the patient is on her back, (2) her lower limbs are flexed at the knees and hips, and (3) her thighs are abducted. In this position the perineum appears as illustrated in Figure 3-39. The term *lithotomy* is derived from a Greek term referring to the *cutting for stones*. This position was originally designed for the cutting for a calculus or stone in the urinary bladder which was made to project into the perineum by means of a finger in the rectum.

The two levatores ani muscles and the two coccygeus muscles form the pelvic diaphragm (Fig. 3-13), which closes the inferior pelvic outlet somewhat like a funnel would if it were dropped into the pelvic cavity (Fig. 3-55). **The pelvic diaphragm divides the pelvic cavity into two parts**: (1) a superior part containing the pelvic viscera, and (2) an inferior part containing mainly fat called the **ischiorectal fossae** (Figs. 3-2 and 3-3). The pelvic diaphragm forms the V-shaped floor of the pelvic cavity and the $\wedge$-shaped roof of each ischiorectal fossa (Fig. 3-13).

THE UROGENITAL DIAPHRAGM

The urogenital diaphragm is a thin sheet of striated muscle stretching between the two sides of the pubic arch, which is formed by the converging **ischiopubic rami.** The urogenital diaphragm covers the anterior part of the inferior pelvic aperture (Figs. 3-9 and 3-10), as you can do with your hand on a dried pelvis. The most anterior and the most posterior fibers of the urogenital diaphragm (*deep transversus perinei muscle*) run transversely (Fig. 3-16), whereas its middle fibers (*sphincter urethrae muscle*) encircle the urethra.

The Sphincter Urethrae Muscle (Figs. 3-14 to 3-16*C*). The sphincter urethrae *is composed of transverse muscle fibers.* It arises from the medial surface of **inferior pubic ramus**. Its fibers pass medially toward the urethra, where they meet the fibers from the opposite side. *The sphincter urethrae encircles the membranes urethra in the male and the superior half of the urethra in the female.* The inferior half of the sphincter urethrae in the female blends with the anterolateral walls of the vagina (Fig. 3-15).

Nerve Supply. Perineal branch of **pudendal** nerve (S2, S3, and S4).

Action. **Constricts urethra**. This is the *voluntary sphincter of the urethra.*

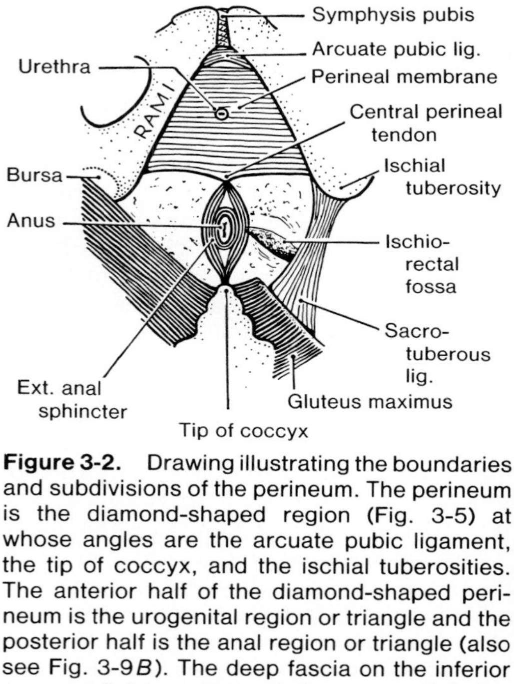

Figure 3-2. Drawing illustrating the boundaries and subdivisions of the perineum. The perineum is the diamond-shaped region (Fig. 3-5) at whose angles are the arcuate pubic ligament, the tip of coccyx, and the ischial tuberosities. The anterior half of the diamond-shaped perineum is the urogenital region or triangle and the posterior half is the anal region or triangle (also see Fig. 3-9*B*). The deep fascia on the inferior or superficial surface of the urogenital diaphragm is thickened to form the dense perineal membrane (also see Figs. 3-11 and 3-14). It is continuous with the deep layer of fascia anteriorly and posteriorly (Fig. 3-10). Observe that the perineal membrane is pierced by the urethra; in the female the vagina also pierces this perineal membrane (Figs. 3-3 and 3-16).

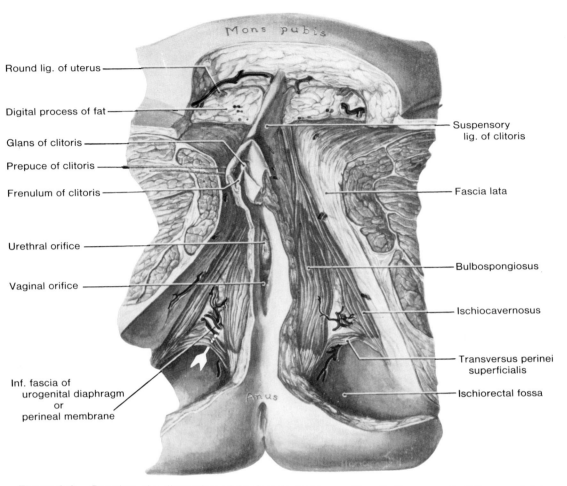

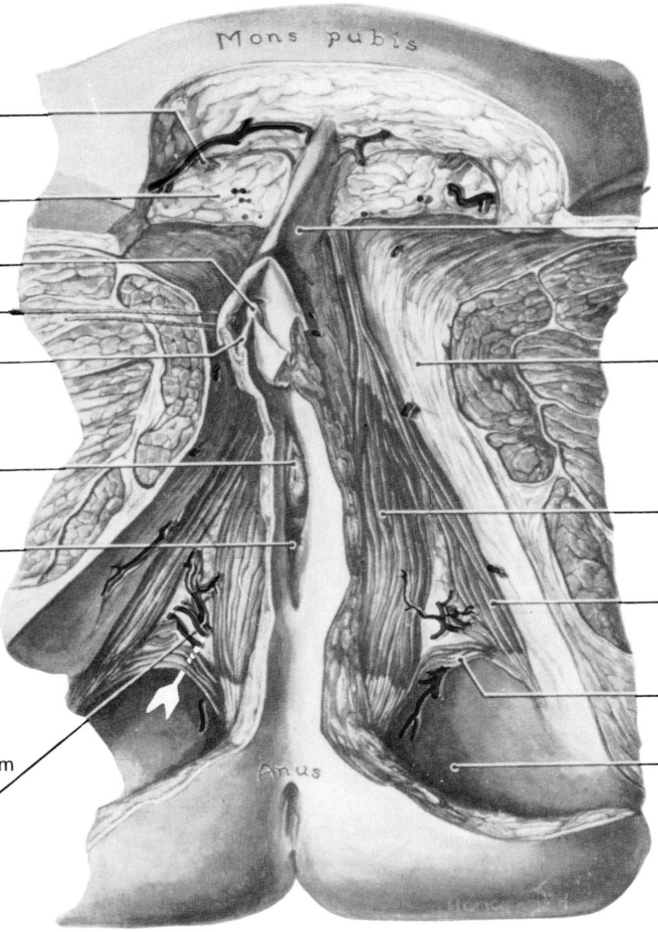

Figure 3-3. Drawing of a dissection of the female perineum. Usually the mons (L. little mountain) pubis, a prominence caused by a pad of fatty tissue over the symphysis pubis in the female (Fig. 3-8), is covered by a triangular mat of pubic hair (Fig. 2-45). Observe the thickness of the superficial fatty tissue at the mons pubis and the encapsulated digital process of fat deep to this. Note that the suspensory ligament of the clitoris descends from the linea alba and the symphysis pubis. Examine the prepuce of the clitoris, which forms a hood over the clitoris and the anterior ends of the labia minora uniting to form the frenulum of the clitoris. Observe the three muscles on each side: bulbospongiosus, ischiocavernosus, and transversus perinei superficialis, which, when slightly separated, reveal the inferior fascia of the urogenital diaphragm or perineal membrane. The bulbospongiosus overlies the bulb of the vestibule. Note that the vestibule and the orifice of the vagina separate the muscles of the two sides. Observe the pinpoint orifices of the right and the left paraurethral ducts below the urethral orifice. Examine the ischiorectal fossa lateral to the anus and the levator ani muscle (also see Figs. 3-2 and 3-13). The anterior recess of this wedge-shaped fascial space is indicated on the left by the tail or feather of the *white arrow*. The arrowhead (invisible) is lying in the anterior recess deep to the perineal membrane; *i.e.*, the anterior recess passes superior to the urogenital diaphragm.

The Deep Transversus Perinei Muscle (Figs. 3-11, 3-12, and 3-16*C*). The transverse muscle fibers *posterior to the urethra* are called the deep transversus perinei or **deep transverse perineal muscle.** It *arises from the medial surface of the ramus of the ischium*, runs transversely, and *inserts into the central perineal tendon.* In

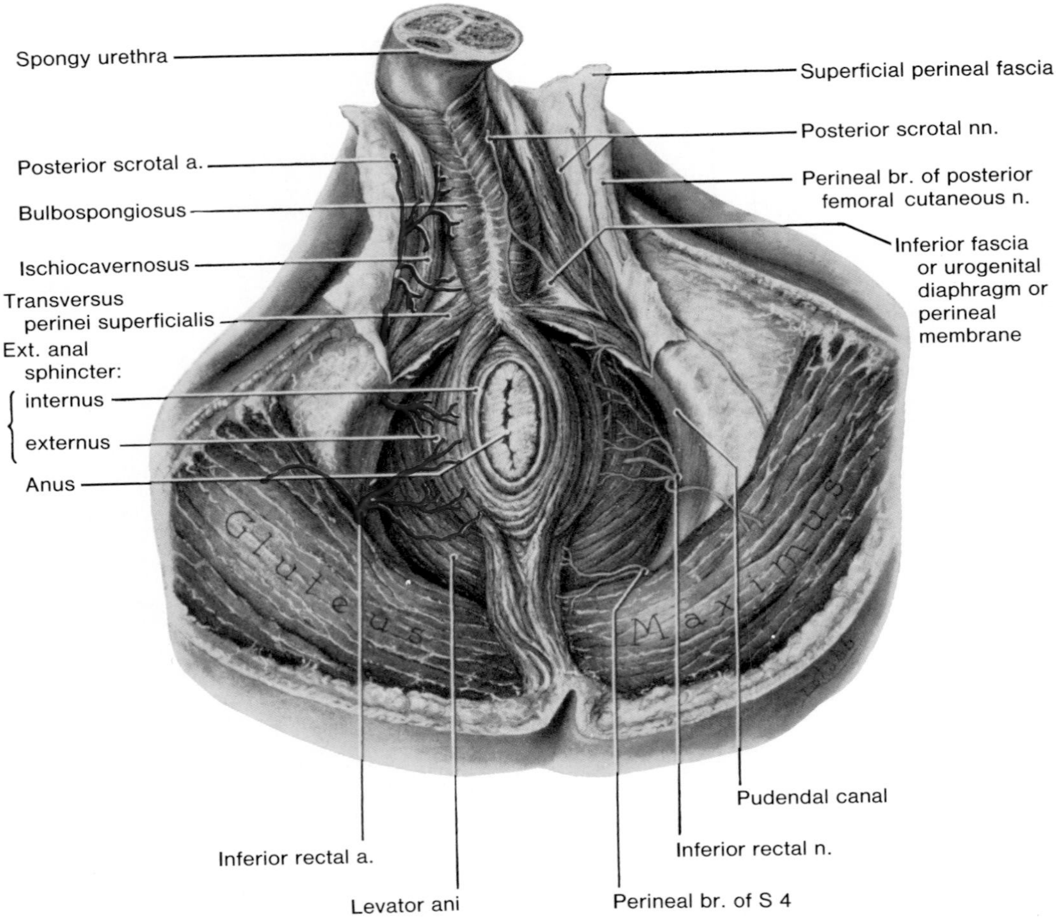

Figure 3-4. Drawing of a dissection of the male perineum. In the anal region or triangle, observe the anal orifice (anus) at the center surrounded by the external anal sphincter and an ischiorectal fossa on each side. Note that the superficial fibers of the external anal sphincter anchor the anus in front to the perineal body (central tendon of the perineum) and behind to the coccyx, here to the skin. Examine the ischiorectal fossa filled with fat, which is bounded (1) *medially* by the levator ani and external anal sphincter muscles, (2) *laterally* by the obturator internus fascia, (3) *behind* by the gluteus maximus muscle overlying the sacrotuberous ligament, and (4) *in front* by the base of the perineal membrane. The apex or roof of the anal triangle is where the medial and lateral walls meet; its base, or floor, formed by tough skin and deep fascia, is removed. Observe the inferior rectal nerve leaving the pudendal canal and, with the perineal branch of S4, supplying the external anal sphincter. Its cutaneous twigs to the anus are removed. The branch turning around the gluteus maximus is replacing the perforating cutaneous nerve. In the urogenital region or triangle, observe that the superficial perineal fascia is (1) incised in the midline, (2) freed from its attachment to the base of the perineal membrane, and (3) reflected. Observe the cutaneous nerves and artery in the superficial perineal space (pouch) and examine the three paired superficial perineal muscles: bulbospongiosus, ischiocavernosus, and transversus perinei superficialis. Note the exposed triangular portion of the perineal membrane or inferior fascia of the urogenital diaphragm.

the female some of its fibers are also inserted into the vaginal wall.

Nerve Supply. Perineal branch of **pudendal** nerve (S2, S3, and S4).

Actions (Fig. 3-12). **Steadies central perineal tendon**, thereby *contributing to the general supportive role of the perineum.*

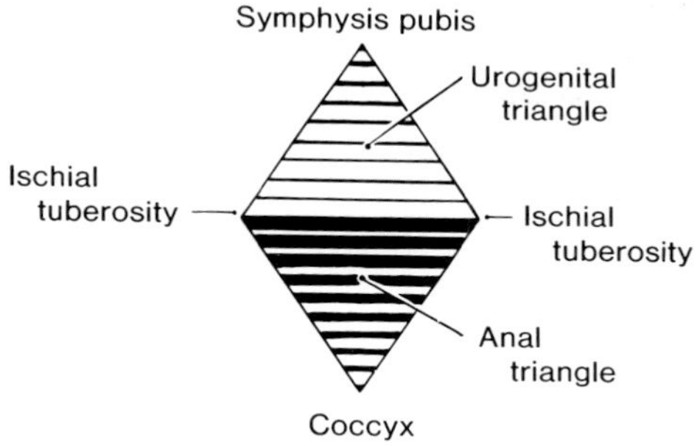

Figure 3-5. Diagram illustrating the diamond-shaped perineum or perineal region, extending from the symphysis pubis to the coccyx. (For orientation see Figs. 3-1, 3-2, and 3-9). Note that a transverse line between the right and left ischial tuberosities divides the perineum into two triangular areas, the urogenital region or triangle anteriorly and the anal region or triangle posteriorly.

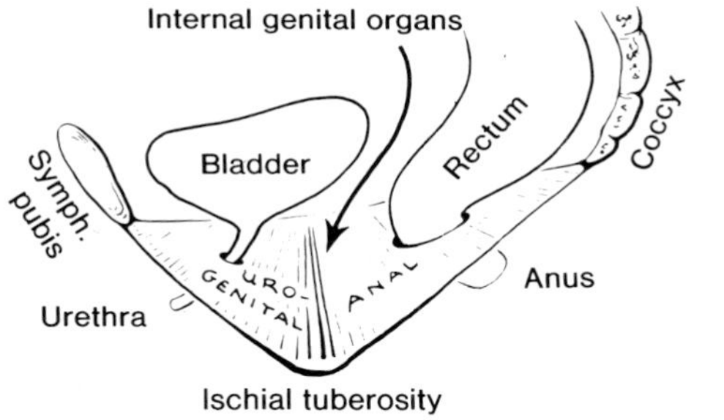

Figure 3-6. Schematic median section of the male pelvis showing the urethra passing through the urogenital triangle and the terminal part of the digestive system traversing the anal triangle of the diamond-shaped perineum (Figs. 3-2 and 3-5). Note that the urogenital triangle faces anteroinferiorly, whereas the anal triangle faces posteroinferiorly (also see Fig. 3-10). Hence, the anal canal makes a right angle curve at its junction with the rectum (also see Fig. 3-61).

The Central Perineal Tendon or Perineal Body (Figs. 3-2 and 3-12). *This fibromuscular node is a small, wedge-shaped mass of fibrous tissue located at the center of the perineum,* between the anal canal and the bulb of the penis or the vagina (Figs. 3-12 and 3-39). The central perineal tendon indicates where the **urorectal septum** divided the *cloacal membrane* in the embryo during partitioning of the cloaca into the rectum and the urogenital sinus (Fig. 3-28B).

The central perineal tendon is the landmark of the perineum, which gives attachment to the transverse perineal muscles, the bulbospongiosus, some fibers of the external anal sphincter, and the levatores ani muscles of both sides. Hence, *several muscles converge to insert into the central perineal tendon.*

CLINICALLY ORIENTED COMMENTS

The central perineal tendon is a particularly important structure in the female. Tearing or stretching of it during parturition removes support from the inferior part of the posterior wall of the vagina. As a result, **prolapse of the vagina** through the vaginal orifice may occur. When a tear of the perineum including the central perineal tendon appears inevitable during childbirth, an incision is often made in the perineum because *a clean surgical incision is preferable to a jagged tear.* This relaxing or appeasing incision is called an **episiotomy** (Fig. 3-44). In a *median episiotomy* (midline episiotomy), the incision passes posteriorly from the frenulum of the labia minora or **fourchette** (Fig. 3-12) through the vaginal mucosa and the central perineal tendon. The incision does not reach the external anal sphincter and the rectum. In cases where there is a possibility of the incision tearing posteriorly and involving the anal sphincter, a *mediolateral episiotomy* is often done (see discussion of Case 3-1 for details).

The Perineal Fascia and Perineal Pouches (Figs. 3-3, 3-4, 3-10, and 3-16). The urogenital diaphragm, like other muscles, is surrounded by deep fascia. The perineal fascia consists of two sheets, the *inferior and superior fasciae of the urogenital diaphragm.* The deep fascia on the inferior (superficial) surface is especially thickened and is called the **inferior fascia of the urogenital diaphragm** or, more often, by its shorter name, the **perineal membrane** (Figs. 3-2 to 3-4, 3-10, 3-11, and 3-16*D*). This fascia is continuous with the deep layer of fascia anteriorly and posteriorly and is also attached laterally to the

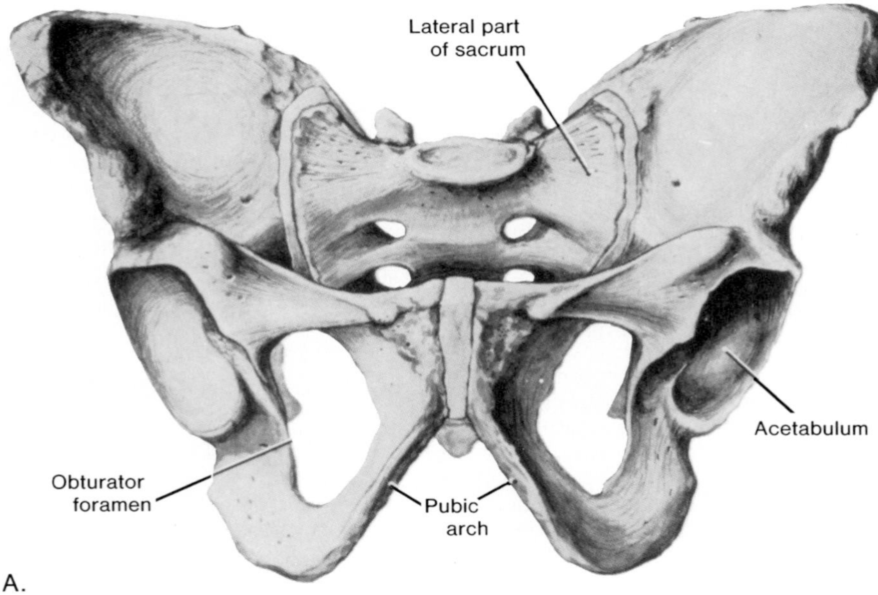

A.

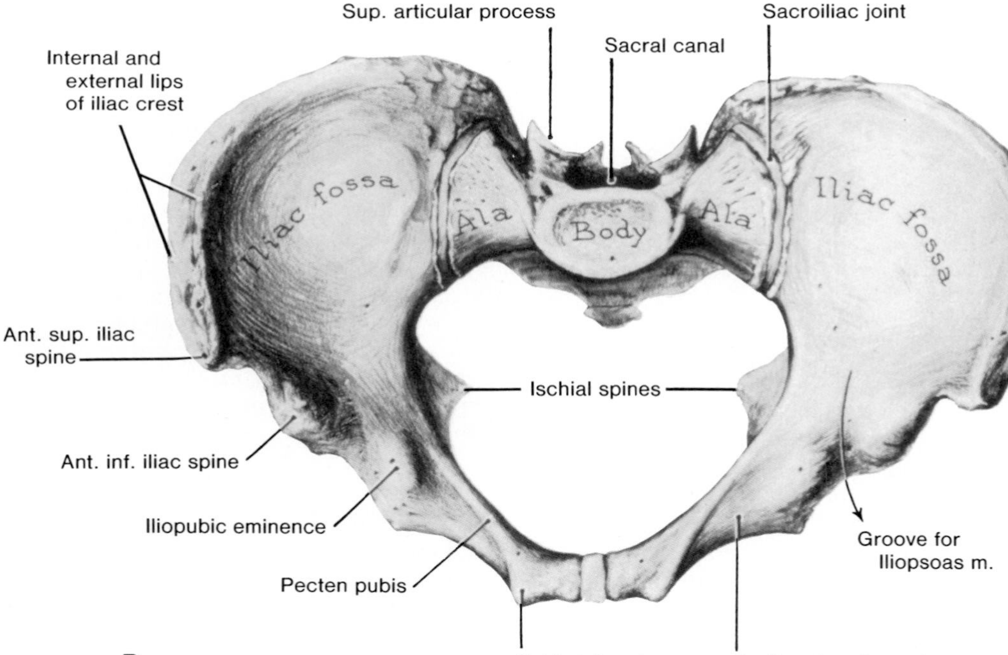

B.

Figure 3-7. Drawings of the *male pelvis*. *A*, anterior view. *B*, superior view. The *pelvis major* (greater pelvis, false pelvis) is formed by the iliac fossae and the alae of the sacrum. The *pelvis minor* (lesser pelvis, true pelvis) is formed by the inner surface of the ischium, the pubis, some ilium, the sacrum, and the coccyx. The groove betwen the anterior inferior iliac spine and the iliopubic eminence conducts the iliopsoas muscle from the pelvis major to the thigh. Three bones, separated by three joints, share in the formation of the pelvic brim. The bones are the two ossa coxae, or hip bones, and the sacrum. The joints are the symphysis pubis and the two sacroiliac joints (Fig. 3-49). Compare Figures 3-7*A* and 3-8*A*, noting that the pubic arch in the male (70°) is much narrower than that in the female (90°).

pubic arch (Fig. 3-11). The superior fascia of the urogenital diaphragm is indistinct.

The superficial perineal fascia (Fig. 3-4) or the membranous layer of the subcutaneous connective tissue of the perineum, *formerly called Colles' fascia* (Fig. 3-10*A*), is continuous with the membranous layer of the subcutaneous connective tissue of the lower anterior abdominal wall, *formerly called Scarpa's fascia.* The superficial perineal fascia is attached to (1) the **fascia lata** enveloping the muscles of the thigh, (2) the **pubic arch**, and (3) the base of the **perineal membrane**. Anteriorly the superficial perineal fascia is prolonged over the penis and scrotum (Figs. 3-4 and 3-10*B*), thereby forming a covering for the testes and the spermatic cords.

The Superficial Perineal Space or Pouch (Figs. 3-10 and 3-16). This is the *fascial space between the superficial perineal fascia and the perineal membrane.* **In the male** the superficial perineal space contains the root of the penis and the muscles associated with it, the proximal part of the spongy urethra, and branches of the internal pudendal vessels and the pudendal nerves. **In the female** the superficial perineal space contains the superficial transversus perinei, the ischiocavernous, and the bulbospongiosus muscles and the *greater vestibular glands* (Fig. 3-42).

CLINICALLY ORIENTED COMMENTS

If the urethra ruptures into the **superficial perineal space** or pouch (Case 3-2), *the attachments of the perineal fascia determine the direction of flow of the extravasated (escaping) urine.* Hence, it may pass into the areolar tissue in the scrotum, around the penis, and upward into the anterior abdominal wall (Fig. 3-10*B*). The urine cannot pass into the thighs because the deep layer of the superficial fascia of the anterior abdominal wall blends with the fascia lata enveloping the thigh muscles (Fig. 4-19) just distal to the **inguinal ligament**. In addition, the urine cannot pass posteriorly into the anal triangle because the two layers of fascia are continuous with each other around the superficial perineal muscles.

The Deep Perineal Space or Pouch (Figs. 3-10*B*, 3-11, 3-16, and 3-17). This is the fascial *space enclosed by the superior and inferior fasciae of the urogenital diaphragm.* **In the male** this space is occupied by the *membranous urethra*, the *sphincter urethrae*, the *bulbourethral glands*, and the *deep transversus perinei muscles* (Fig. 3-16*C*). **In the female** the deep perineal space is occupied by *part of the urethra*, the *sphincter urethrae*, the inferior *part of the vagina*, and the *deep transversus perinei muscles.* The deep perineal space in both sexes also contains the blood vessels and nerves associated with the structures within it.

THE ANAL REGION

The anal region of the perineum (Figs. 3-2 to 3-6), often called the **anal triangle**, is bounded *posteriorly* by the tip of the **coccyx** and *anteriorly* by the line joining the **ischial tuberosities** (Figs. 3-2, 3-5, and 3-9). This region is related anteriorly to the posterior border of the **urogenital diaphragm** (Fig. 3-16) and posterolaterally to the **sacrotuberous ligaments** (Figs. 3-2 and 3-18). Overlying the anal region is the *gluteus maximus* muscle (Figs. 3-1, 3-23, and 4-45).

The anal region contains the anal orifice or anus, the external anal sphincter, and the ischiorectal fossae (Figs. 3-2, 3-13, and 3-19). The anal canal passes through the floor of the pelvis (Fig. 3-6) and opens on the surface of the perineum as the anus (Figs. 3-2 to 3-6). The Latin word *anus* means a ring. The skin around the anus contains large sebaceous glands and sweat glands and is pigmented. The **perianal skin** is thrown into radiating folds, giving it a characteristic puckered appearance. These folds are produced by the pull of the underlying **fibroelastic septa** (Fig. 3-19).

The Sphincter Ani Externus Muscle (Figs. 3-2, 3-4, 3-12, 3-14, and 3-19 to 3-22). *The large external anal sphincter is under voluntary control.* It surrounds the inferior

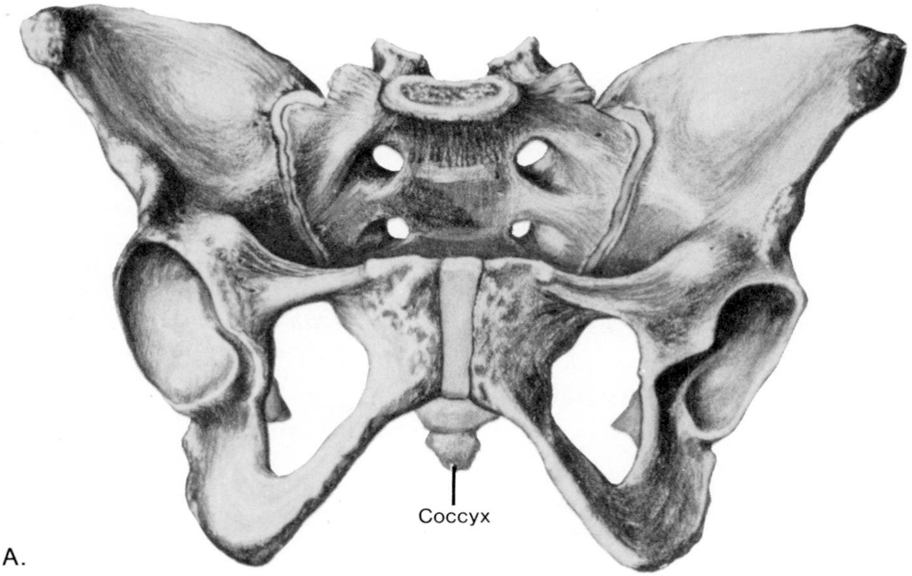
Coccyx

A.

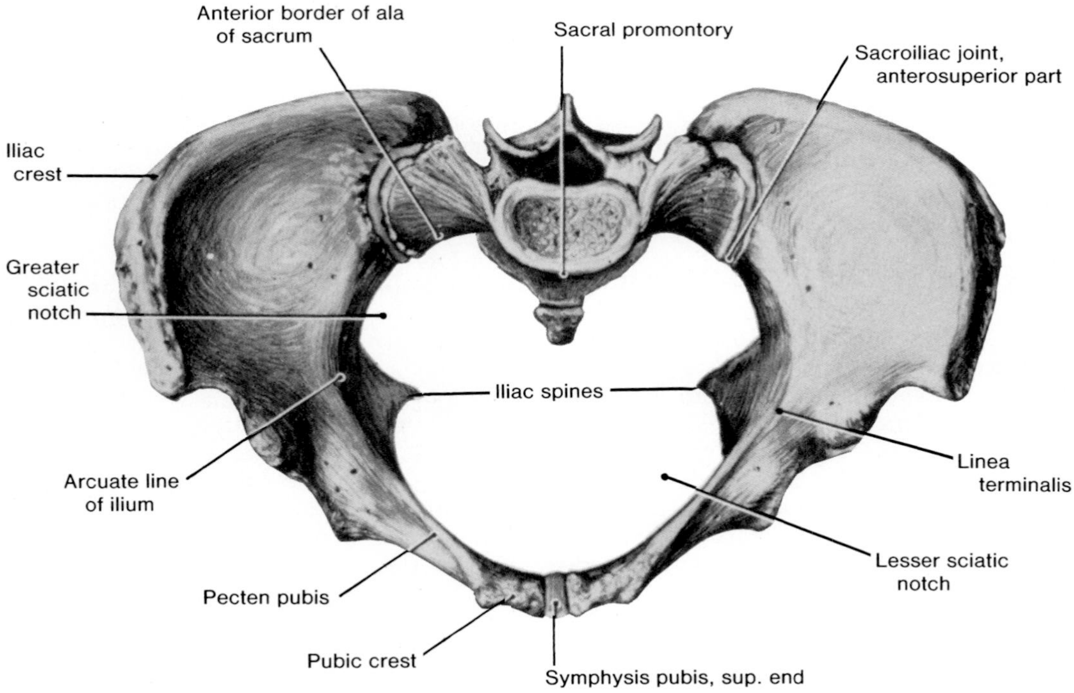
Anterior border of ala of sacrum
Sacral promontory
Sacroiliac joint, anterosuperior part
Iliac crest
Greater sciatic notch
Iliac spines
Linea terminalis
Arcuate line of ilium
Lesser sciatic notch
Pecten pubis
Pubic crest
Symphysis pubis, sup. end

B.

end of the anal canal and lies in the perineum. It forms a broad band on each side of the anal canal (2 to 3 cm wide) which *consists of three parts: subcutaneous, superficial,* and *deep,* but they are not distinctly separated from each other. Many branches of the inferior rectal (hemorrhoidal) vessels and nerve pass between the superficial and deep parts of this muscle (Fig. 3-4). *In general the fibers of the external anal sphincter run from the central perineal tendon to the anococcygeal ligament* (Figs. 3-2, 3-12, 3-22, and 3-57).

The subcutaneous part of the external anal sphincter (Figs. 3-14 and 3-19*A*) is slender and surrounds the anus. These subcutaneous fibers have no bony attachments but cross anterior and posterior to the anus.

The superficial part of the external anal sphincter (Figs. 3-14 and 3-19*A*) is elliptical or oval in shape. Its fibers extend anteriorly from the tip of the coccyx and the **anococcygeal ligament** (Fig. 3-22) around the anus to the central perineal tendon (Fig. 3-12), mooring the anus to the median plane.

The deep part of the external anal sphincter (Figs. 3-14 and 3-19*A*) *surrounds the anal canal like a collar.* Some of these fibers cross to join the opposite **superficial transverse perineal muscle**. It arises from the central perineal tendon (Fig. 3-12) and fuses with the puborectalis part of the levator ani (Fig. 3-19*A*). Superiorly it blends with the levator ani and is not always sharply defined from it.

Nerve Supply. Perineal branch of **fourth sacral** nerve and **inferior rectal** nerves.

Actions. **Closes anus** (subcutaneous and superficial parts) and **draws anal canal forward**, thereby increasing *the anorectal angle* (the angle between the anal canal and the rectum). The deep part of the external anal sphincter is assisted in this action by the **puborectalis muscle**, part of the levator ani, which forms the sling occupying the anorectal angle (Fig. 3-61).

The Ischiorectal Fossa (Figs. 3-2, 3-12, 3-13, 3-17, 3-20, 3-23, and 3-24). *On each side of the anal canal* and rectum there is a large *wedge-shaped, fascia-lined space* called the ischiorectal fossa. *It is located between the skin of the anal region and the pelvic diaphragm and is filled with areolar tissue and fat* (Fig. 3-23). Because this fat is fluid at body temperature, *the ischiorectal fossae permit the rectum to distend* and to empty during the passage of feces. The **apex** or roof of each wedge-shaped fossa lies superiorly, under the pelvic diaphragm where the levator ani muscle arises from the obturator fascia (Figs. 3-13, 3-23, and 3-24). The apex is located about 6 cm superior to the ischial tuberosity. The **base** or floor of the wedge-shaped ischiorectal fossa is formed by the skin and deep fascia of the perineum. *Anteriorly* the ischiorectal fossa continues superior to the urogenital diaphragm as the **anterior recess** of the ischiorectal fossa (Fig. 3-3). This space is filled with loose areolar tissue. There is also a **posterior recess** lateroposteriorly where the gluteus maximus muscle overhangs the ischiorectal fossa (Fig. 3-25). *The ischiorectal fossae of the two sides communicate with each other over the anococcygeal ligament* (Fig. 3-22). *Posteriorly* each fossa is continuous with the **lesser sciatic foramen**, superior to the sacrotuberous ligament (Fig. 3-18).

Boundaries of the Ischiorectal Fossa (Figs. 3-2, 3-13, 3-17, 3-18, 3-20, 3-23, and 3-24). The ischiorectal fossa is bounded *laterally* by the **ischium** and the inferior part of the obturator internus (Figs. 3-13, 3-23,

Figure 3-8. Drawings of the *female pelvis*. *A*, anterior view. *B*, superior view. Observe the following features: (1) the wide angle of the pubic arch; (2) the relative breadth of the alae to the body of the sacrum; and (3) the shape and dimensions of the linea terminalis (terminal line), which is part of the pelvic brim. Each linea terminalis (half of pelvic brim) includes the sacral promontory, the arcuate line of the ilium, the pecten pubis, and the pubic crest. Often the arcuate line and the pecten pubis are called the ilipectineal line. The lineae terminales (pelvic brim) surround the superior aperture of the pelvis (pelvic inlet). Each line extends from the promontory of the sacrum posteriorly to the symphysis pubis anteriorly. The bony pelvis is divided into the pelvis major above the lineae terminales and the pelvis minor below these lines. The pelvis major is related to the inferior part of the abdominal cavity and consists chiefly of the iliac fossae. The pelvis minor, the lowest part of the abdominopelvic cavity (Fig. 2-30), contains the pelvic viscera.

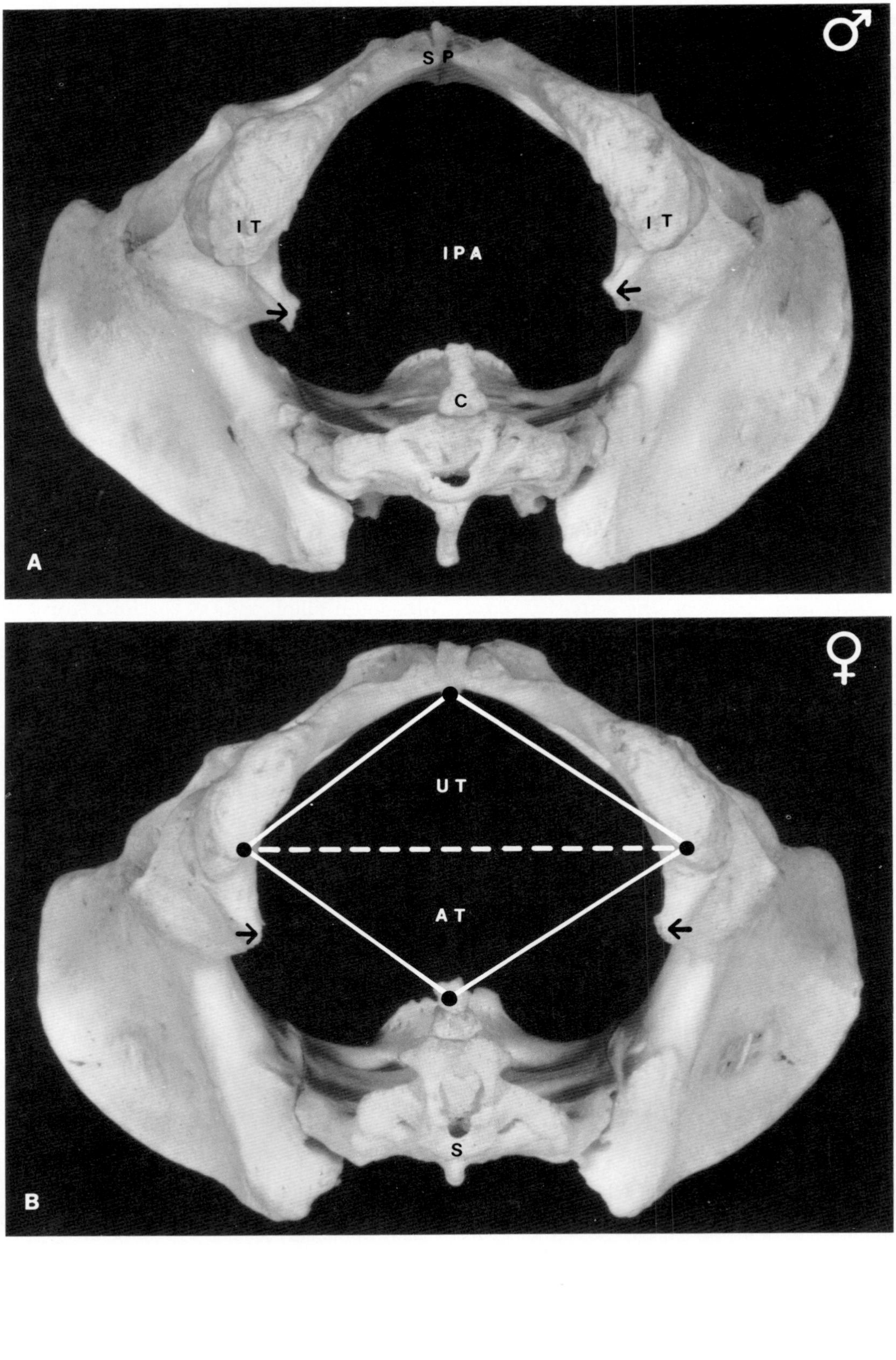
♂
S P
I T
I T
I P A
C
A
♀
U T
A T
S
B

and 3-24); *medially* by the **rectum** and **anal canal** to which the levator ani and sphincter ani externus muscles are applied (Figs. 3-4, 3-23, and 3-24); *posteriorly* by the **sacrotuberous ligament** (Figs. 3-18 and 3-21) and the overlying **gluteus maximus muscle** (Figs. 3-2, 3-18, and 3-23); and *anteriorly* by the base of the **urogenital diaphragm** and its fasciae (Figs. 3-4 and 3-13).

Contents of the Ischiorectal Fossa (Figs. 3-2 to 3-4, 3-17, 3-20, 3-23, and 3-24). This wedge-shaped fascial space is *filled with soft fat*, called the **ischiorectal pad of fat**, which is traversed by many tough, fibrous bands and septa (Fig. 3-19). *This pad of fat supports the anal canal* but is readily displaced to allow feces to pass through this terminal part of the digestive tract.

The ischiorectal fossa also contains the *internal pudendal vessels* and the *pudendal nerve*. The adjective **pudendal** is derived from the Latin verb *pudere*, meaning something of which to be ashamed. These structures run forward on the lateral wall of the fossa in a fibrous canal called the **pudendal canal** (Figs. 3-4, 3-13, 3-23, and 3-26). Far posteriorly these vessels and the nerve give off the **inferior rectal** (hemorrhoidal) **vessels** and **nerve** which pass forward and medially through the ischiorectal fossa on their way to the anal region (Fig. 3-4). These structures become more and more superficial as they pass toward the surface to **supply the external anal sphincter** and the skin around the anus.

Two other cutaneous nerves, the perforating branch of the second and third sacral nerves and the perineal branch of the fourth sacral nerve also emerge through the ischiorectal fossa (Fig. 3-4).

CLINICALLY ORIENTED COMMENTS

The ischiorectal fossa is occasionally the site of infection which may result in the formation of an **ischiorectal abscess** (collection of pus in the ischiorectal fossa). These abscesses are annoying and painful. The fat in the fossa, being near the rectum, is liable to infection. This infection may reach the ischiorectal fossa (1) following **cryptitis** (inflammation of the crypts that are now called anal sinuses), (2) from downward extension of a **pelvirectal abscess**, (3) following a tear in the anal mucous membrane, or (4) from a penetrating wound in the anal region.

Diagnostic signs of an ischiorectal abscess are fullness and tenderness between the anus and the ischial tuberosity (Case 3-3 and Fig. 3-2 and 3-99). *An ischiorectal abscess may spontaneously open into* (1) *the anal canal,* (2) *the rectum,* (3) *the skin in the perineum* near the anus, or (4) into all these places (Fig. 3-99). Usually these abscesses are opened for free drainage. The two ischiorectal fossae communicate with each other posterior to the anal canal **(deep postanal space)** and around the external anal sphincter. This space lies between the superficial and deep parts of this sphincter (Figs. 3-14 and 3-19*A*). Consequently, *an*

Figure 3-9. Photographs of male (♂) and female (♀) pelves showing their inferior pelvic apertures (pelvic outlets). These are closed in living persons by the soft tissues of the perineum (Figs. 3-2 to 3-4). Observe the difference in the size of the inferior pelvic aperture (*IPA*) in the male (*A*) and the female (*B*). This is the view of the pelvis that the obstetrician visualizes in his/her "mind's eye" when the patient is in the lithotomy position (Figs. 3-1 and 3-39). In living persons the inferior pelvic aperture is closed by the perineum, the diamond-shaped region between the upper parts of the thighs and the lower parts of the buttocks (Figs. 3-3 and 3-4). Note that at the angles of the inferior pelvic aperture are the symphysis pubis (*SP*), the coccyx (*C*), and the ischial tuberosities (*IT*). (Compare with the diagram shown in Fig. 3-5.) Note that the *broken transverse white line* between the right and left ischial tuberosities (*IT*) divides the diamond-shaped perineum into two triangles or regions, the urogenital triangle (*UT*) and the anal triangle (*AT*). The *arrows* indicate the ischial spines to which the sacrospinous ligaments are attached (Figs. 3-18 and 3-46). Note that the sacrum (*S*) is wedged between the iliac bones. In living persons it is held there by powerful interosseous and dorsal sacroiliac ligaments (Fig. 3-102).

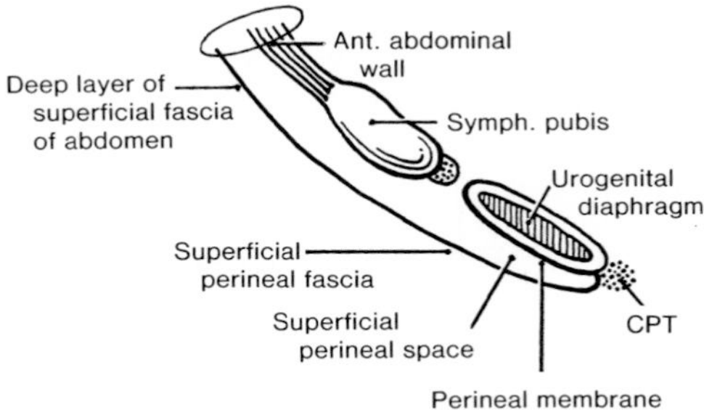

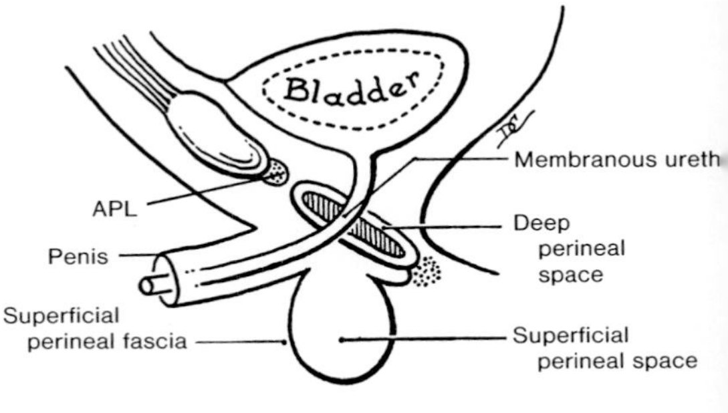

Figure 3-10. Schematic drawings of midline sections showing the urogenital diaphragm and the perineal spaces (pouches). Understand that the superficial perineal fascia (Colles' fascia) is a continuation of the deep or membranous layer (Scarpa's fascia) of the superficial fascia of the abdomen. *CPT*, central perineal tendon (perineal body); *APL*, arcuate pubic ligament (see Fig. 3-2).

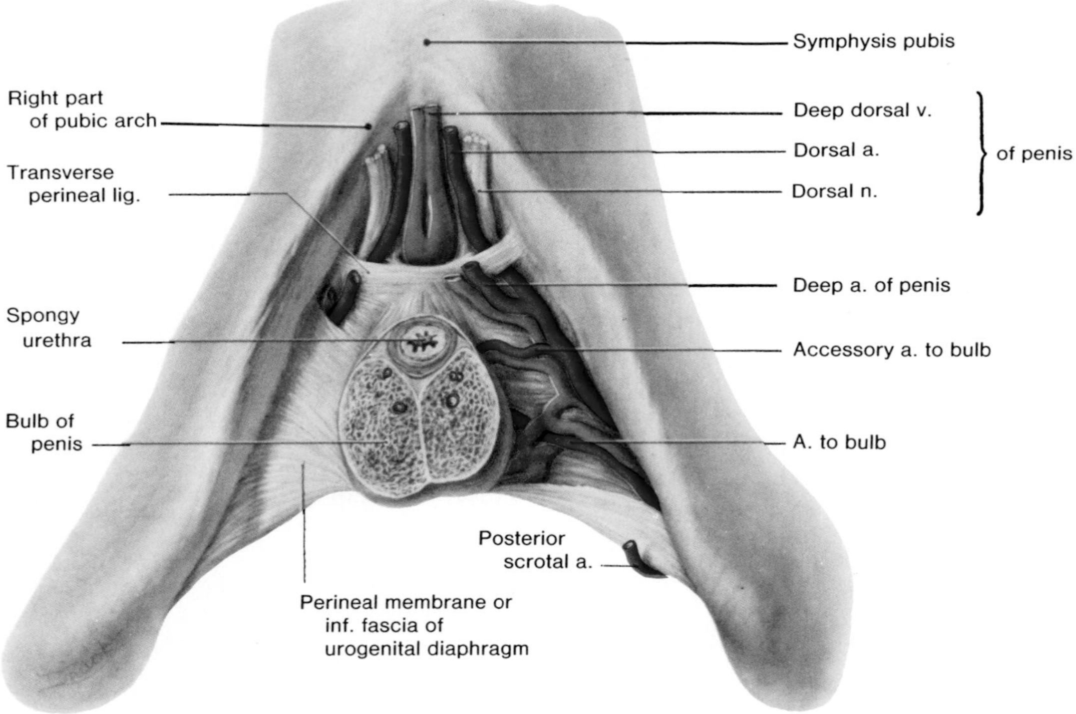

Figure 3-11. Drawing of a dissection of the deep perineal space of a male. The crura of the root of the penis (see Fig. 3-32) have been removed. On the *right* the perineal membrane or inferior fascia of the urogenital membrane is in part removed and the deep perineal space is thereby opened. Observe the fibers of the perineal membrane converging on the bulb of the penis and mooring it to the pubic arch. Note that the urethra is bound to the dorsum of the bulb of the penis. Examine the septum in the bulb, indicating its bilateral origin. Observe the artery to the bulb (here double); the artery to the crus, called the deep artery; and the dorsal artery which ends in the glans penis. Note the deep dorsal vein, originally double, which ends in the prostatic plexus.

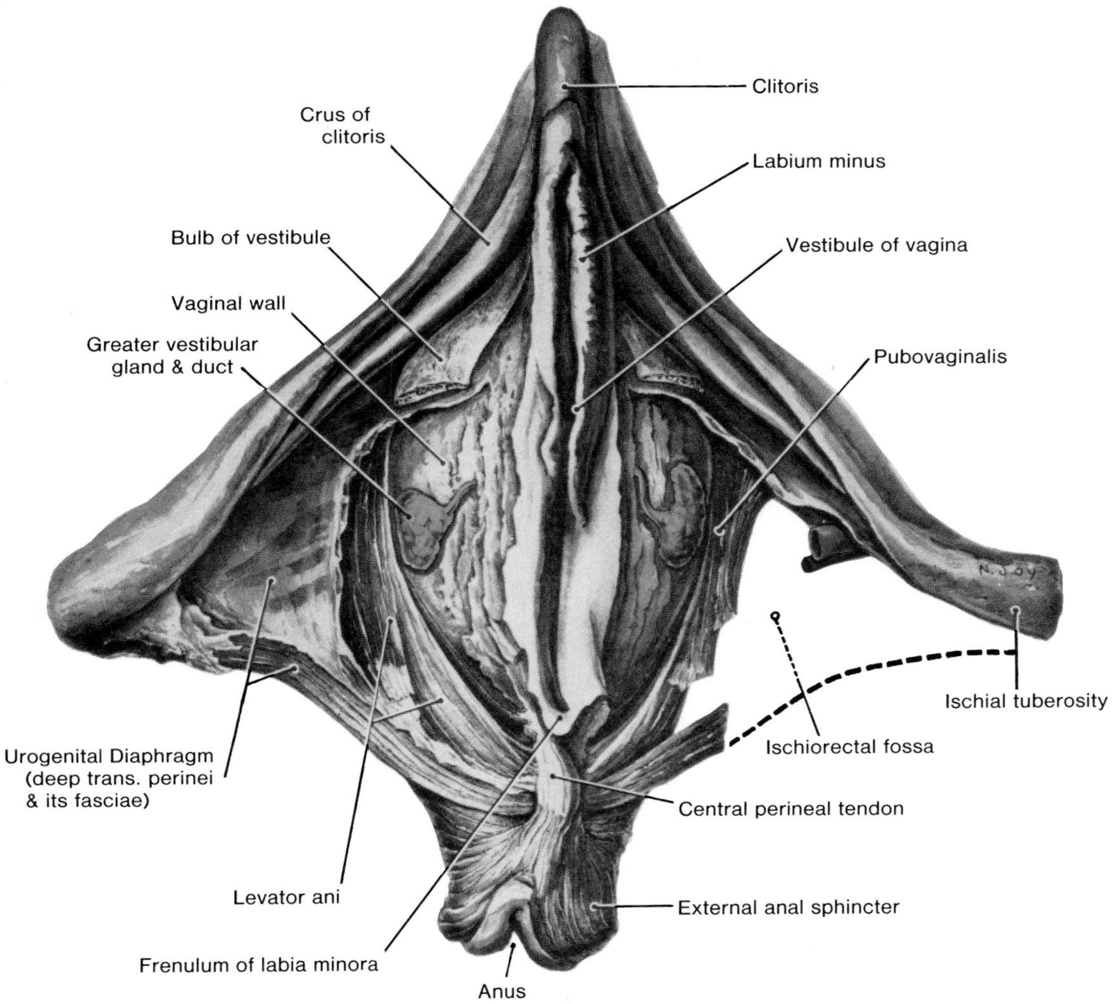

Figure 3-12. Drawing of the female perineum showing the urogenital diaphragm. The bulbs of the vestibule are cut short. The urogenital diaphragm and its fasciae are partly cut away on the right side and are extensively cut away on the left. Examine the urogenital diaphragm, a sheet of striated muscle, mainly deep transversus perinei, placed between a superior and an inferior sheet of fascia and having two parts: (1) a posterior part which is a strong fleshy band that meets its fellow in the central tendon of perineum (perineal body) and (2) an anterior part which is more areolar than fleshy. Medially, the diaphragm and its fasciae have been raised from the sloping inferior surface of the levator ani muscle and detached from the sloping outer wall of the vagina with which it fuses. Observe the anterior parts of the levatores ani muscles (pubovaginales) meeting behind the vaginal orifice. Examine the greater vestibular glands and the bulbs of the vestibule applied to the sides of the vagina, medial to the anterior borders of the levatores ani muscles. Note the laminated nature of this part of the wall of the vagina. It is laminated because several layers of fascia fuse with it and lose their identity in it, namely, the superficial perineal fascia, the diaphragm and its fasciae, and the fasciae of the levatores ani muscles.

abscess in one ischiorectal fossa may spread to the other one and involve a semicircular area around the posterior aspect of the anus.

The Pudendal Canal (Figs. 3-4, 3-13, 3-23, and 3-26). The pudendal canal is *a fibrous tunnel on the lateral wall of the ischiorectal fossa* through which the pu-

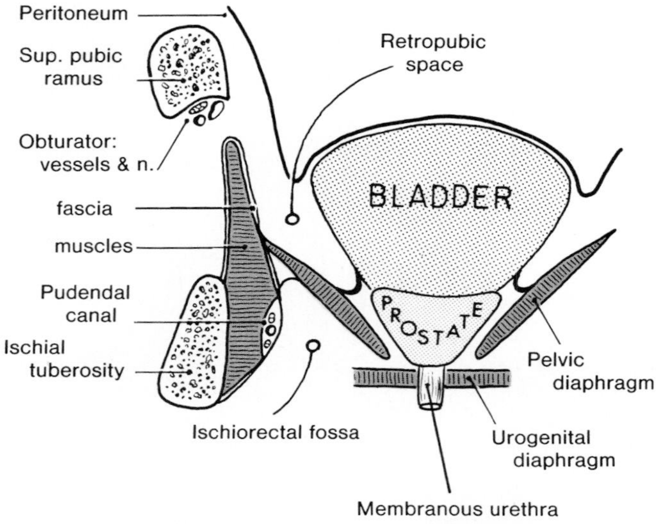

Figure 3-13. Diagrammatic coronal section of the pelvis illustrating the main part of the funnel-shaped pelvic diaphragm formed mainly by the two levatores ani muscles. The pelvic diaphragm forms the floor of the abdominal and pelvic cavities and consists of the paired levatores ani and coccygeus muscles (Fig. 3-3) together with their superior and inferior fasciae. The rectum is anchored to the pelvic diaphragm in the middle (Fig. 3-2). Observe that only the pelvic diaphragm (levator ani portion) intervenes between the ischiorectal fossa and the retropubic space. The urogenital diaphragm is formed basically by the sphincter urethrae muscle (Fig. 3-14), which is attached to the rami of the pubis and ischium (conjoint ramus).

dendal vessels and the pudendal nerve pass. They run forward and medially in the lateral wall of the **ischiorectal fossa** to the anal canal. *The pudendal canal begins at the posterior border of the ischiorectal fossa and runs from the lesser sciatic notch, adjacent to the ischial spine, to the posterior edge of the urogenital diaphragm.* The pudendal canal, sometimes referred to as Alcock's canal by clinicians, is *formed by a splitting of the thickened inferior portion of the obturator fascia* (Fig. 3-13) which forms the lateral wall of the ischiorectal fossa and covers the obturator internus muscle (Fig. 3-23).

There are three structures at the posterior end of the pudendal canal: the **internal pudendal artery**, the **internal pudendal vein**, and the **pudendal nerve** (Figs. 3-24 and 3-26). These structures course along the ischiopubic ramus toward the urogenital diaphragm. *The pudendal nerve supplies most of the innervation to the perineum.* Toward the distal end of the pudendal canal, the pudendal nerve splits to form the **dorsal nerve of the penis** (or **clitoris**) and the **perineal nerve** (Figs. 3-11, 3-26, and 3-42). These nerves run anteriorly on each side of the internal pudendal artery. The **perineal nerve** gives off scrotal or labial branches (Fig. 3-26) and continues to supply the muscles of the urogenital diaphragm (Fig. 3-27). The *dorsal nerve of the penis (or clitoris)*, a sensory nerve, runs through the deep perineal space (deep pouch, Figs. 3-10*B* and 3-26) to reach its area of supply.

The inferior rectal vein passes from the inferior end of the anal canal to empty into the internal pudendal vein in the pudendal canal. This vein forms anastomoses (communications) with the superior rectal veins of the *portacaval system* (Fig. 2-112).

THE UROGENITAL REGION

Developmental Note. It is helpful when studying the urogenital regions of male and female perinea to know that they develop from common beginnings or primordia. Furthermore, *both the urinary and genital systems develop from the intermediate mesoderm and the cloaca* of the early embryo.

A septum of mesoderm, the **urorectal septum**, divides the cloaca into an anterior or urogenital part and a posterior or rectal part. As mentioned previously, *the central perineal tendon (perineal body) indicates where the urorectal septum divides the cloacal membrane into urogenital and anal membranes.* The urorectal septum also divides the **cloacal sphincter** into anterior and posterior parts. The posterior part becomes the external anal sphincter and the anterior part becomes the superficial transversus perinei, the bulbospongiosus, the ischiocavernosus, and the urogenital diaphragm (Fig. 3-16). Knowing this makes it clear why one nerve, *the pudendal nerve, supplies all the muscles into which the cloacal sphincter divides* (Fig. 3-28).

The external genitalia of both sexes also have a common origin. In the male the bilateral primordia fuse in the midline forming the scrotum and the penis with the urethra enclosed within it. In the female these primordia normally do not fuse, but *the parts of the male and female genital organs are homologous* (*e.g.*, penis and clitoris, scrotum and labia majora).

The Male Perineum (Figs. 3-4, 3-14, 3-16, 3-17, 3-20, 3-21, 3-26, and 3-31).

Structures in the Superficial Perineal Space in Males (Figs. 3-10 and 3-16). The superficial perineal space (pouch) is the **fascial space between the superficial perineal fascia** (Colles' fascia) **and the**

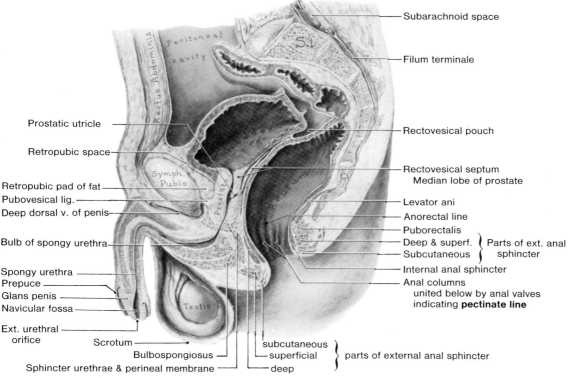

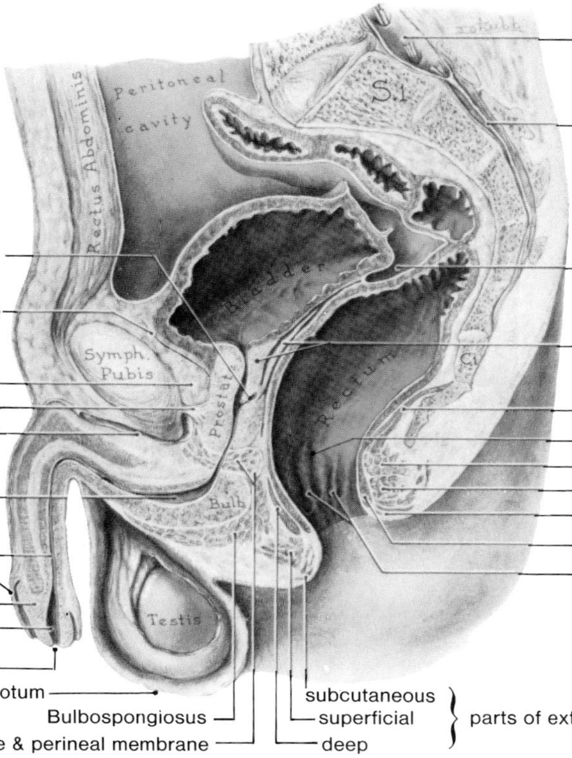

Figure 3-14. Drawing of a median section of the *male pelvis*. Observe (1) the urinary bladder slightly distended and resting on the rectum; (2) the prostatic urethra descending vertically through a somewhat elongated prostate and showing the prostatic utricle opening on to its posterior wall; (3) the short membranous urethra passing through the deep perineal space; (4) the spongy urethra with a dilation in the bulb and another in the glans; and (5) the bulbospongiosus muscle which by contracting empties the urethra. Note that the involuntary internal anal sphincter muscle does not descend so far as the voluntary external anal sphincter muscle and is separated from it by an areolar layer. Examine the two layers of rectovesical septum (fascia) in the median plane between the bladder and the rectum. Note that on each side it contains the ductus deferens, the seminal vesicle, and the vesical vessels. Observe the peritoneum passing from the abdominal wall above the symphysis pubis to the distended bladder, over the bladder to the bottom of the rectovesical pouch, and up the anterior aspect of the rectum.

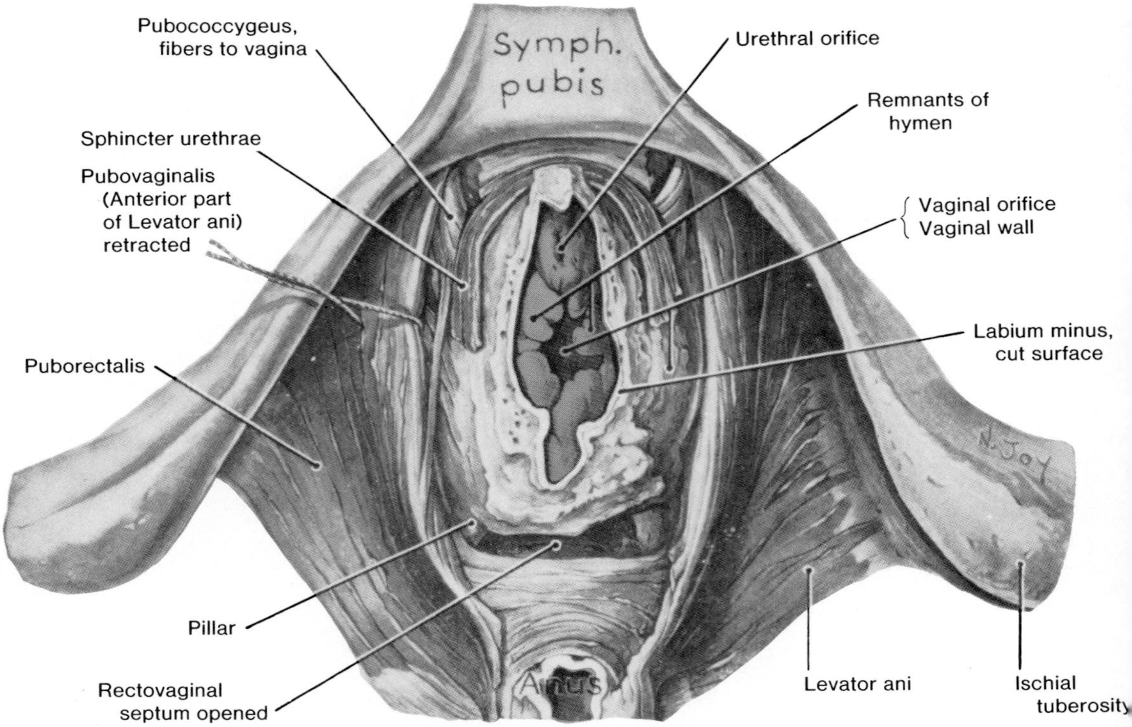

Figure 3-15. Drawing of a dissection of the female perineum. Examine the sphincter urethrae muscle arising from the inferior pubic ramus. Its fibers run medially and encircle the lower end of the urethra as in the male and other fibers cross each other between the urethra and the vaginal orifice. Some of these fibers are attached to the wall of the vagina. Observe the fragments of the torn hymen around the margins of the vaginal orifice; these tags or rounded elevations are called hymeneal caruncles.

inferior fascia of the urogenital diaphragm (perineal membrane). It contains the *root of the penis* (Figs. 3-31 and 3-32) and the *muscles associated with this organ* (Fig. 3-4), the proximal part of the *spongy urethra* (Fig. 3-11), and branches of the *internal pudendal vessels* and *pudendal nerves.*

Structures in the Deep Perineal Space in Males (Figs. 3-10, 3-16, and 3-17). The deep perineal space (pouch) is the fascial space enclosed by the **superior** and **inferior fasciae of the urogenital diaphragm.** It contains the sphincter urethrae and the deep transversus perinei muscles, the bulbourethral glands (Fig. 3-17), and the **membranous urethra** (Figs. 3-10, 3-32, and 3-33). It also contains the *internal pudendal artery, branches of the perineal nerve* supplying the sphincter urethrae and deep transversus perinei muscles, and the *dorsal nerve of the penis* (Fig. 3-26).

The Scrotum (Figs. 2-19, 2-26, 3-14, 3-26, and 3-29). The contents of the scrotum, the **testis** and its coverings, were described in Chapter 2 because the scrotum is a cutaneous pouch that develops from the skin of the anterior abdominal wall. It is a *cutaneous and fibromuscular sac* which is situated posteroinferior to the penis and inferior to the symphysis pubis. *The scrotum is formed by the fusion of the labioscrotal swellings* (Fig. 3-29). The bilateral formation of the scrotum is indicated by the more darkly pigmented midline **scrotal raphe** which continues anteriorly on the the ventral (under) surface of the penis and posteriorly along the median line of the perineum to the anus. The scrotum is composed of skin and the underlying closely associated

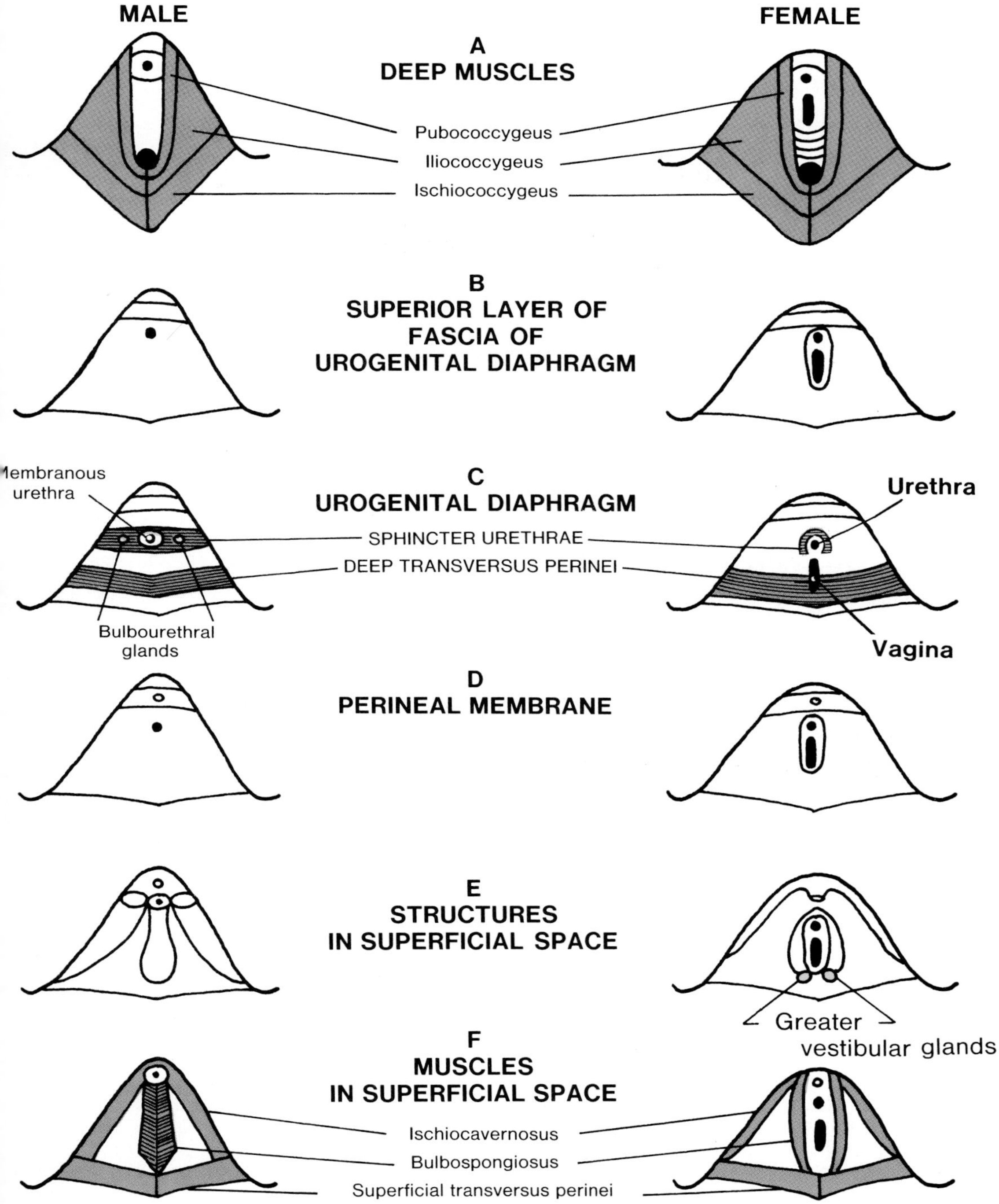

Figure 3-16. Schematic diagrams illustrating the layers of the perineum in the male and female and showing the layers of the perineum built up from deep to superficial. In *A* the angle between the two ischiopubic rami is almost filled by the three coccygeus muscles. The urethra (and vagina in the female) peers through anteriorly, the rectum posteriorly. A superior layer of fascia *B* and an inferior layer of fascia (the perineal membrane) *D* enclose a deep perineal space or pouch *C* containing two muscles and, *in the male*, the bulbourethral (Cowper's) glands. The "sandwich" formed by the two layers of fascia and the contents of the deep space (pouch) comprise the urogenital diaphragm. Observe that the superficial and deep layers of perineal fascia are attached to the ischiopubic ramus and to the posterior margin of the urogenital diaphragm; hence, they enclose the superficial perineal space (pouch) which contains the structures shown in *E* and the muscles shown in *F*. *In the female* the greater vestibular (Bartholin's) glands lie behind the bulb of the vestibule (Fig. 3-42).

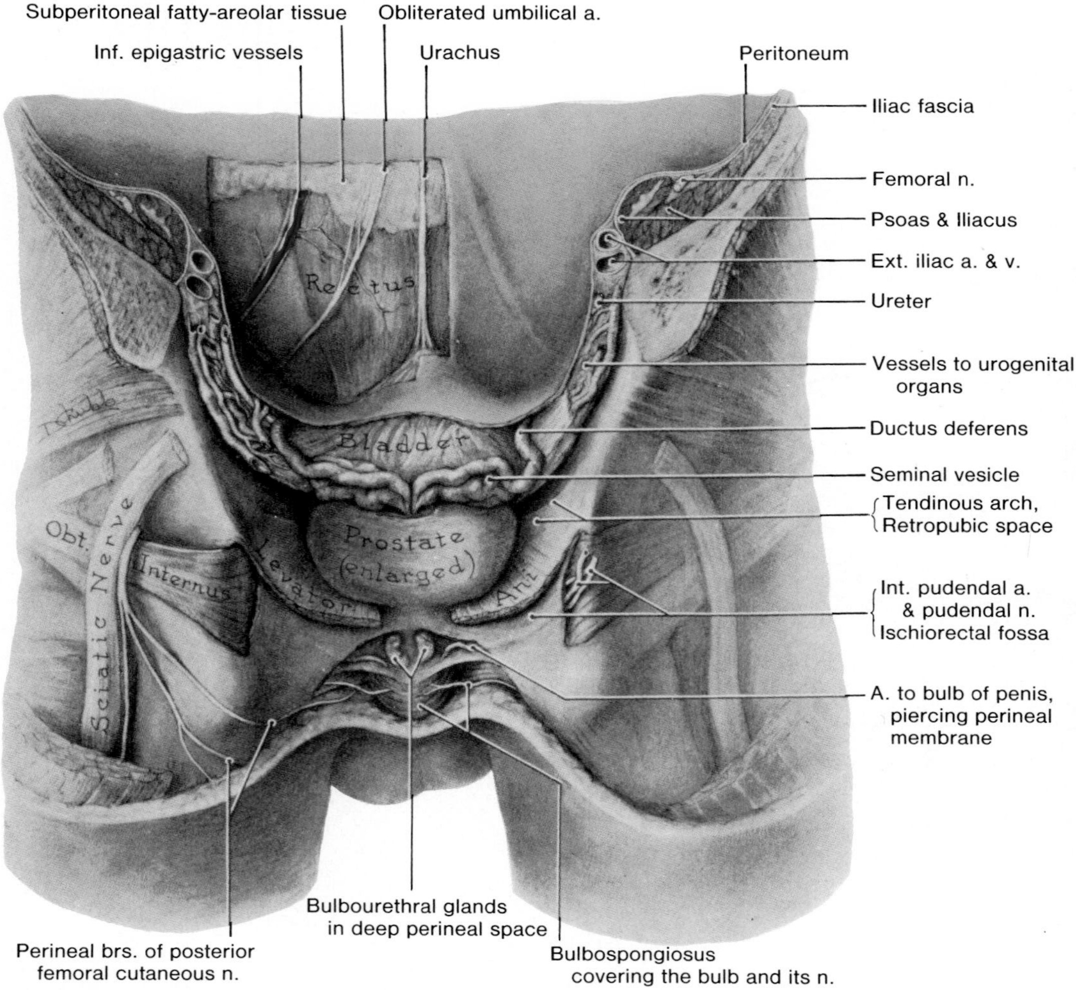

Figure 3-17. Drawing of a coronal section of the male pelvis just anterior to the rectum. This is a view of the anterior part of the pelvis from behind. Observe the inferior epigastric artery and its venae comitantes entering the rectus sheath (also see Fig. 2-8). Note that the obliterated umbilical artery and the urachus, like the urinary bladder, are in the subperitoneal fatty-areolar tissue (also see Fig. 2-16). Examine the femoral nerve lying between the psoas and iliacus muscles, outside the psoas fascia, which is attached to the pelvic brim. Note that the external iliac artery and vein lie inside this fascia. Observe that the ductus deferens and the ureter are both subperitoneal. Near the bladder note that the ureter is accompanied by a leash of vesical vessels enclosed in rectovesical fascia. Examine the levator ani and its fascial coverings separating the retropubic (prevesical) space from the ischiorectal fossa (also see Fig. 3-16). Observe the free anterior borders of the levatores ani which are the width of the scalpel handle apart. Examine the bulbourethral glands and the artery to the bulb lying above the perineal membrane (inferior fascia of the urogenital diaphragm), *i.e.*, in the deep perineal space. Note that the obturator internus muscle makes a right-angled turn as it escapes from its osseofascial pocket.

dartos muscle (Fig. 2-16). The dartos, firmly attached to the skin, consists largely of smooth muscle fibers which contract under the influence of cold, exercise, and sexual stimulation. In old men the dartos muscle loses its tone; hence, the scrotum tends to be smooth and hangs down further.

The blood supply of the scrotum (Figs. 3-

65 and 3-66) is via the **external pudendal arteries** (anterior aspect of scrotum) and the **internal pudendal arteries** (posterior aspect of scrotum). Branches of the testicular and cremasteric arteries also supply the scrotum. The **scrotal veins** accompany the arteries and join the external pudendal veins.

The nerve supply of the scrotum is as follows. The anterior part of the scrotum is supplied by the **ilioinguinal nerve** (Figs. 2-7, 4-14, and 4-16) and its posterior part the scrotum is supplied by the medial and lateral scrotal branches of the **perineal nerve** (Fig. 3-26) and by the perineal branch of the **posterior femoral cutaneous nerve** (Fig. 3-17).

The lymphatics of the scrotum drain into the **superficial inguinal lymph nodes** (Figs. 3-85 and 4-38).

The Penis (Figs. 2-26, 3-4, 3-11, 3-14, 3-20, and 3-29 to 3-38). The penis (L. tail) is the *organ of copulation* in the male and serves as the common outlet for urine and

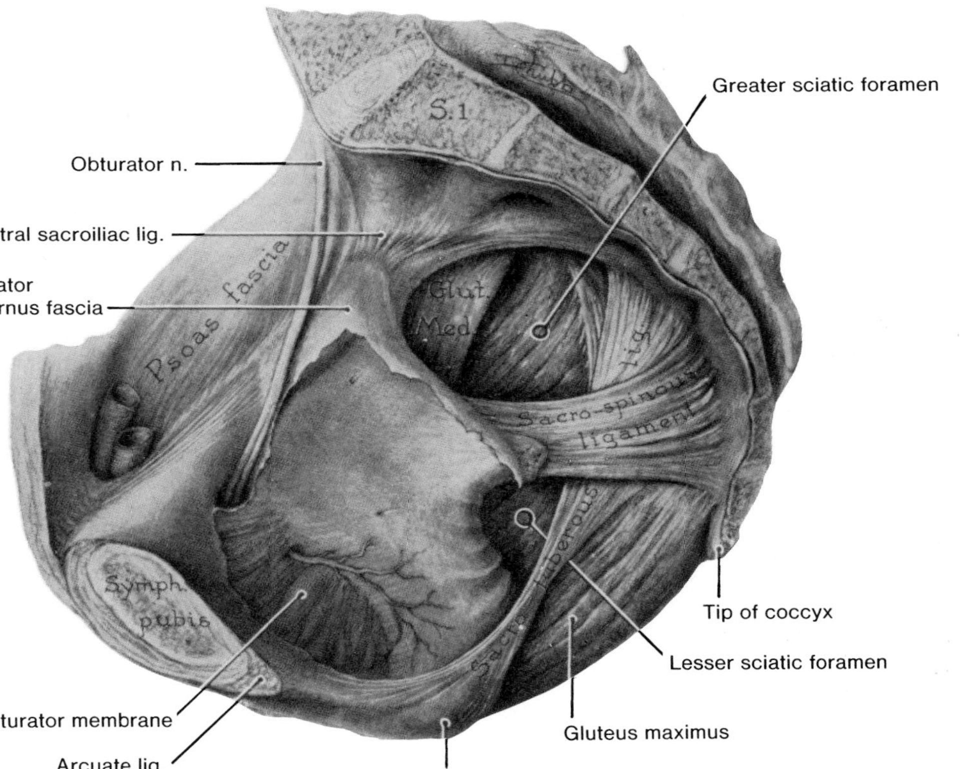

Figure 3-18. Drawing of a dissection showing the bony and ligamentous walls of the pelvis minor (*female specimen*). The pubis is in front and the sacrum and coccyx are behind. Observe that posterolaterally the coccyx and lower part of the sacrum are connected to the ischial tuberosity by the sacrotuberous ligament and to the ischial spine by the sacrospinous ligament. Note that part of the sacrum is joined to the ilium by the ventral sacroiliac ligament. Anterior to the sacrotuberous ligament are the greater and lesser sciatic foramina, the one being above and the other below the sacrospinous ligament. Note that anterolaterally the fascia covering the obturator internus muscle is snipped away and the obturator interus is removed from its osseofascial pocket, thereby exposing the ischium and the obturator membrane. The mouth of this pocket is the lesser sciatic foramen through which the obturator internus escapes from the pelvis. The grooves made by its tendon are conspicuous. Observe that the obturator internus fascia is attached along the line of the obturator nerve superiorly, to the sacrotuberous ligament inferiorly, and to the posterior border of the body of the ischium posteriorly.

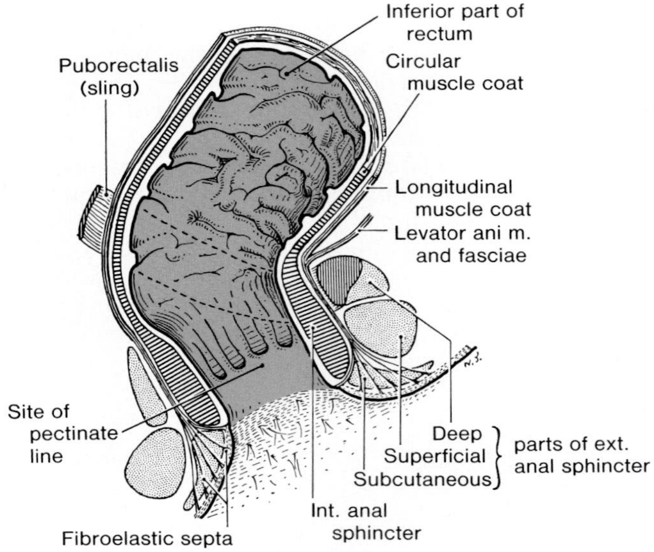

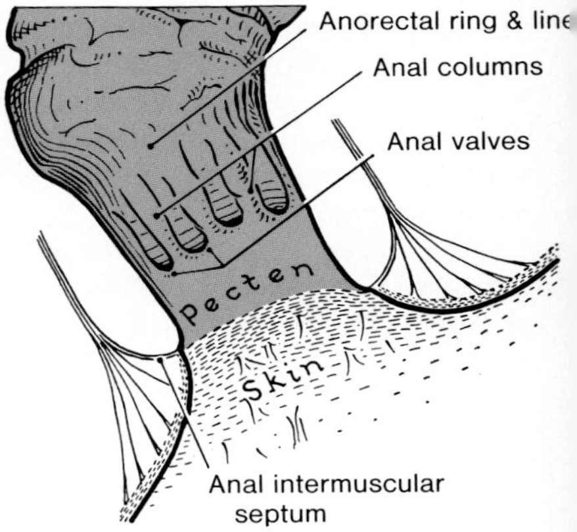

Figure 3-19. Drawings of median sections of the lower rectum and the anal canal. In *A* observe that the anal canal, about 3 cm long, extends posteroinferiorly from the distal end of the rectum. Note that the thickened inferior part of the inner circular muscular layer forms an *involuntary* internal anal sphincter. Examine the large *voluntary* external sphincter forming a broad band on each side of the anal canal. Observe that it has three parts and that its deep part is associated with the puborectalis muscle posteriorly (also see Fig. 3-61). The puborectalis is part of the levator ani muscle. In *B* examine the anal columns, noting that they are vertical folds of mucosa containing twigs of the superior rectal artery and vein. Varicosity of these veins produces *internal hemorrhoids*. Note that the inferior ends of the anal columns are joined by crescentic folds called anal valves. The concavities of the valves (*black*) are called anal sinuses (crypts). The comb-shaped inferior limit of the anal valves forms the *pectinate line* (L. *pecten*, comb). This line indicates the approximate former site of the *anal membrane* which normally ruptures toward the end of the embryonic period.

semen (seminal fluid). *It is composed of three cylindrical bodies* (L. *corpora*) *of erectile or cavernous tissue* that are bound together by loose connective tissue called the **fascia penis**.

The skin of the penis is very thin, dark in color, and loose. Two of the three erectile bodies, the **corpora cavernosa penis**, are arranged side by side in the dorsal part of the organ. The **corpus spongiosum penis** (corpus cavernosum urethrae) lies ventrally in the median plane. The corpora cavernosa are fused with each other in the median plane, except posteriorly where they separate to form two **crura** (L. legs) which are attached on each side to the pubic arch (Figs. 3-31 to 3-34). *The crura support the corpus spongiosum penis* lying between and inferior to them (Fig. 3-31). The penis consists of a root and a body (shaft). The surface of the penis, which faces posterosuperiorly when the penis is erect, is called the *dorsum of the penis* (Fig. 3-30). The other aspect is referred to as the ventral or *urethral surface*.

The root of the penis is the attached portion (Figs. 3-30 to 3-34) which is *located in the superficial perineal space* or pouch (Fig. 3-10*B*), between the inferior fascia of the urogenital diaphragm (perineal membrane, Fig. 3-11) superiorly and the deep perineal fascia inferiorly. *The root of the penis consists of the two crura, the bulb of the penis, and the muscles associated with them.* The **bulb of the penis** is located between the two crura in the superficial perineal space (Figs. 3-17 and 3-32). The enlarged posterior part of the bulb is penetrated above by the urethra (Figs. 3-10*B*, 3-11, and 3-33).

The body of the penis is the *free pendulous part* which is covered by skin (Figs. 3-14 and 3-30). It consists of the corpora cavernosa and the corpus spongiosum (Fig. 3-37). *The dorsum of the penis faces anteriorly when the penis is flaccid* and the ventral surface or urethral aspect faces posteriorly. Hence, the anatomical position of the penis is erect. The median **penile raphe** on its ventral surface is continuous with the scrotal raphe (Fig. 3-29). *The penile raphe indicates where the urogenital folds fused during the fetal period.*

The spongy (cavernous, penile) part of the urethra runs within the corpus spongiosum penis; hence, the **spongy urethra** is the longest part (Figs. 3-14 and 3-35 to 3-38). Distally the corpus spongiosum penis joins to form the conical **glans penis**, the concavity of which covers the free blunt ends of the corpora cavernosa (Figs. 3-32 and 3-33). The prominent margin of the

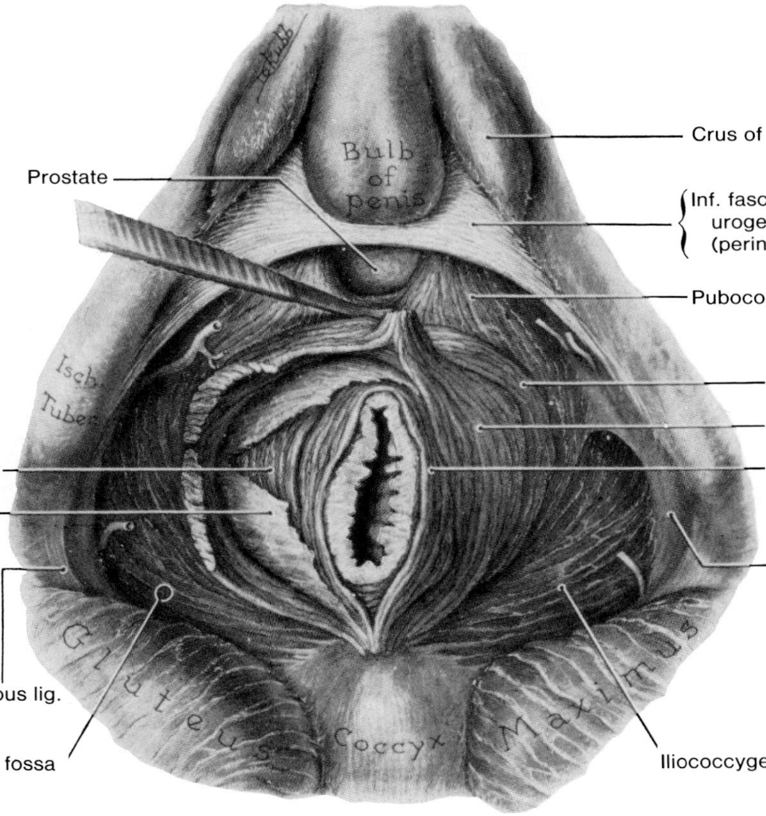

Figure 3-20. Drawing of a dissection of the external anal sphincter (sphincter ani externus muscle). Observe the three parts of this *voluntary sphincter*: (1) subcutaneous, encircling the anal orifice; (2) superficial, anchoring the anus in the median plane to the central perineal tendon in front and to the coccyx behind; and (3) deep, forming a wide encircling band. *On the left* of the figure, the superficial and deep parts of the sphincter are reflected and the underlying sheet, consisting of areolar tissue, levator ani fibers, and an outer longitudinal muscular coat of the gut, is cut in order to reveal the inner circular muscular coat of the gut which is thickened to form the *involuntary internal anal sphincter*. Examine the anterior free borders of the levatores ani muscles meeting in front of the anal canal and pressed backward in order to expose the prostate. *On the right* of the figure, observe the remains of the "false roof" of the ischiorectal fossa, *i.e.*, a layer of fascia that stretches from the obturator internus fascia to the thin fascia covering the levator ani muscle.

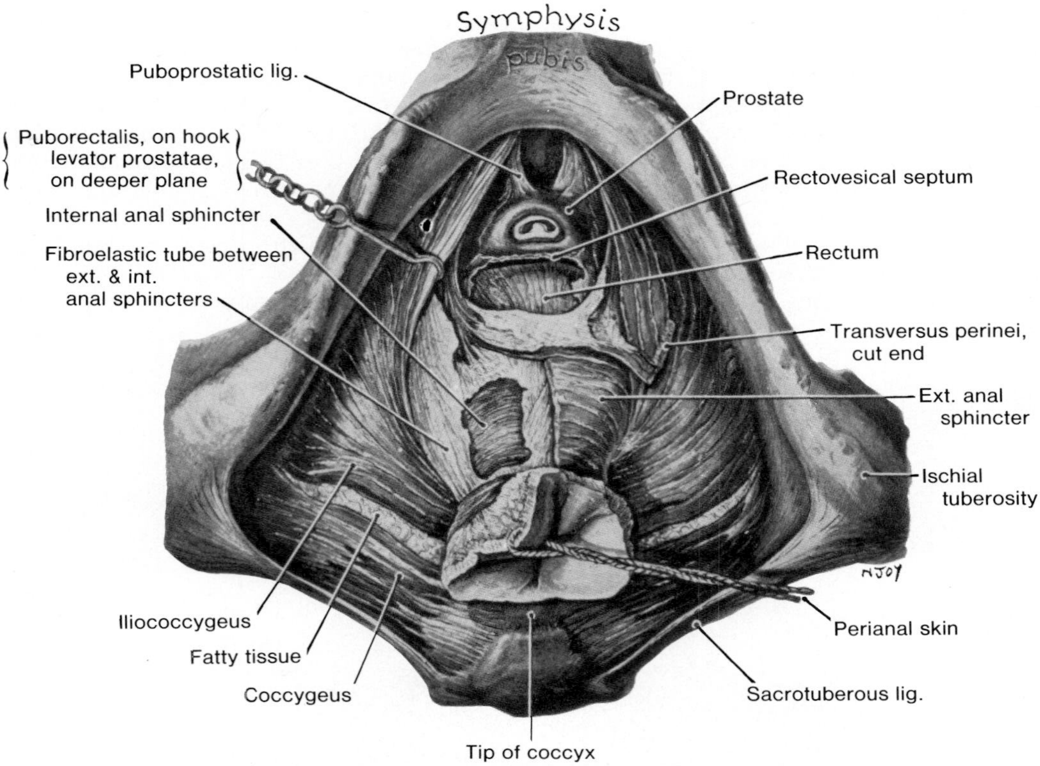

Figure 3-21. Drawing of a dissection of the levatores ani and coccygeus muscles and of an exposure of the prostate from the perineum. The urogenital diaphragm and its fasciae have been removed. *Observe that the anal canal is guarded by two sphincters*: (1) the internal anal sphincter being a continuation of the circular muscle coat of the gut is smooth muscle and (2) the external anal sphincter extending below the internal anal sphincter and having three parts is striated muscle. Examine the puborectalis, the sling-like muscle uniting with the external anal sphincter behind and at the sides (also see Fig. 3-61). The rectovesical septum (rectovesical fascia, Denonvillier's fascia) is a fascial septum which passes from the central perineal tendon (perineal body) to the peritoneum on the floor of the rectovesical pouch. It lies between the lower portion of the rectum and anal canal posteriorly and the prostate and seminal vesicles anteriorly (Fig. 3-76).

glans penis, called the **corona of the glans** (Figs. 3-30, 3-33, and 3-35), projects backward beyond the ends of the corpora cavernosa penis. The corona of the glans overhangs an obliquely grooved constriction called the **neck of the penis**. The slit-like opening of the spongy urethra, called the **external urethral orifice**, is near the tip of the glans penis (Figs. 3-14, 3-30, 3-35, and 3-36). The skin and fasciae of the penis are prolonged as a free fold or *double layer of skin*, called the **prepuce** (L. *praeputium*, foreskin), which covers the glans penis for a variable extent (Figs. 3-14 and 3-35). A median fold, called the **frenulum of the prepuce**, passes from the deep layer of the prepuce to a point just below the external urethral orifice (Fig. 3-35).

The weight of the body of the penis is supported by two ligaments which are continuous with the fascia of the penis (Fig. 3-34). The **fundiform ligament** (L. sling-like) of the penis arises from the inferior part of the *linea alba* (Fig. 2-12) and splits into two parts which pass on each side of the penis. The **suspensory ligament** of the penis (Fig. 3-34) is a condensation of superficial fascia in the form of a thick, triangular fibroelastic band. It *arises from the anterior surface of the symphysis pubis* and passes downward, splitting to form a sling which attaches to the deep fascia of the dorsum and sides of the body of the penis at the junction of its fixed and mobile parts (*i.e.*, where it bends in the flaccid state, Figs. 3-14, 3-30, and 3-34).

CLINICALLY ORIENTED COMMENTS

The prepuce is usually sufficiently elastic to permit it to be retracted over the glans penis; however, in some cases it is not and

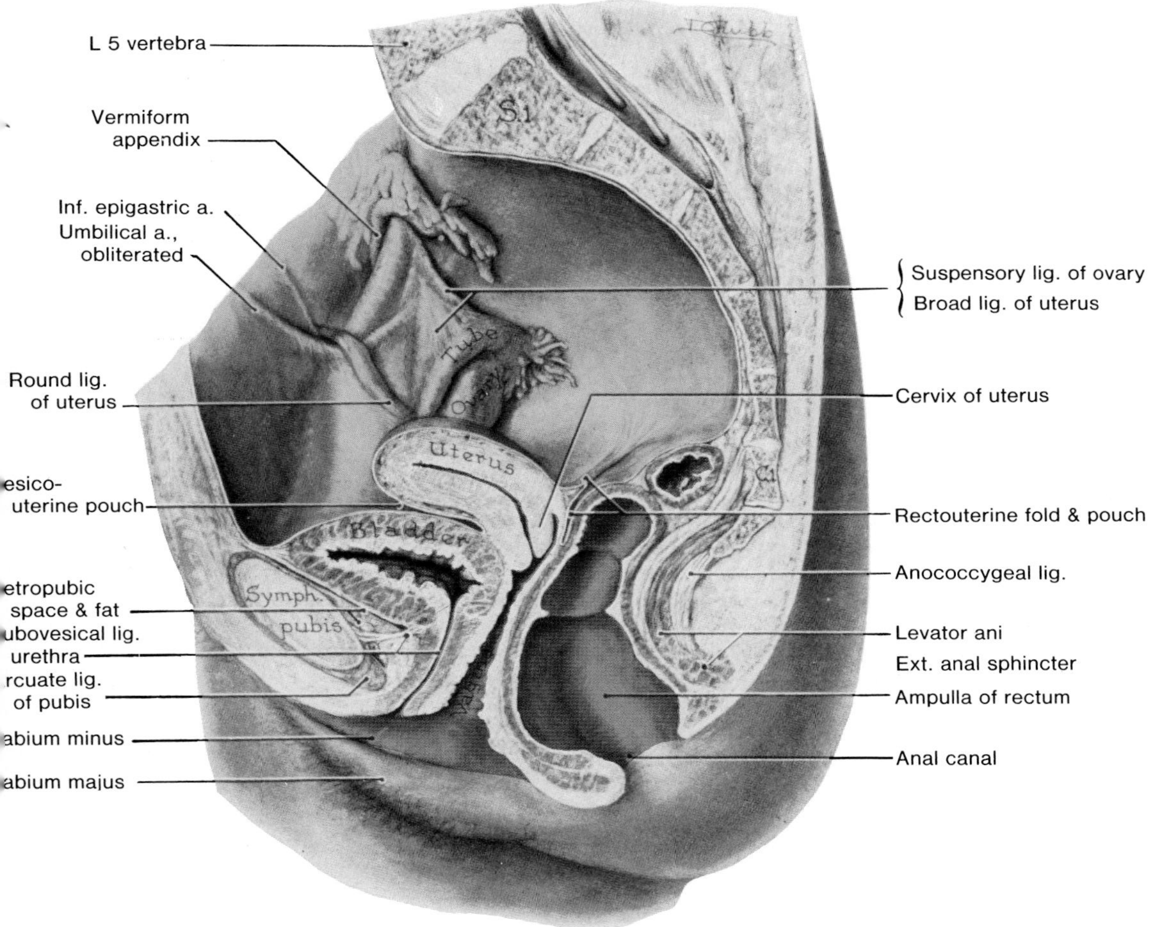

Figure 3-22. Drawing of a median section of the *female pelvis*. The lower parts of the rectum and vagina are slightly distorted owing to the insertion of plugs of cotton wool in them (not shown) before embalming. The uterus was sectioned in its own median plane and depicted as though this coincided with the median plane of the body, which is seldom the case. Observe the uterine tube and the ovary in their virginal positions on the side wall of the pelvis, *i.e.*, in the angle between the ureter and the umbilical artery and medial to the obturator nerve and vessels. Examine the uterus which is bent on itself at the junction of its body and cervix. Note the cervix opening on the anterior wall of the vagina and having a short, round, anterior lip and a long, thinner, posterior lip. Observe the ostium (external os) of the uterus (also see Fig. 3-87) at the level of the upper end of the symphysis pubis and the anterior fornix of the vagina, 1.25 cm or more from the vesicouterine pouch. Examine the posterior fornix covered with 1.25 cm or more of the rectouterine pouch, which is the lowest part of the peritoneal cavity when the person is erect. Observe that the urethra, the vagina, and the rectum are parallel to one another. Note that the uterus is nearly at right angles to them when the bladder is empty.

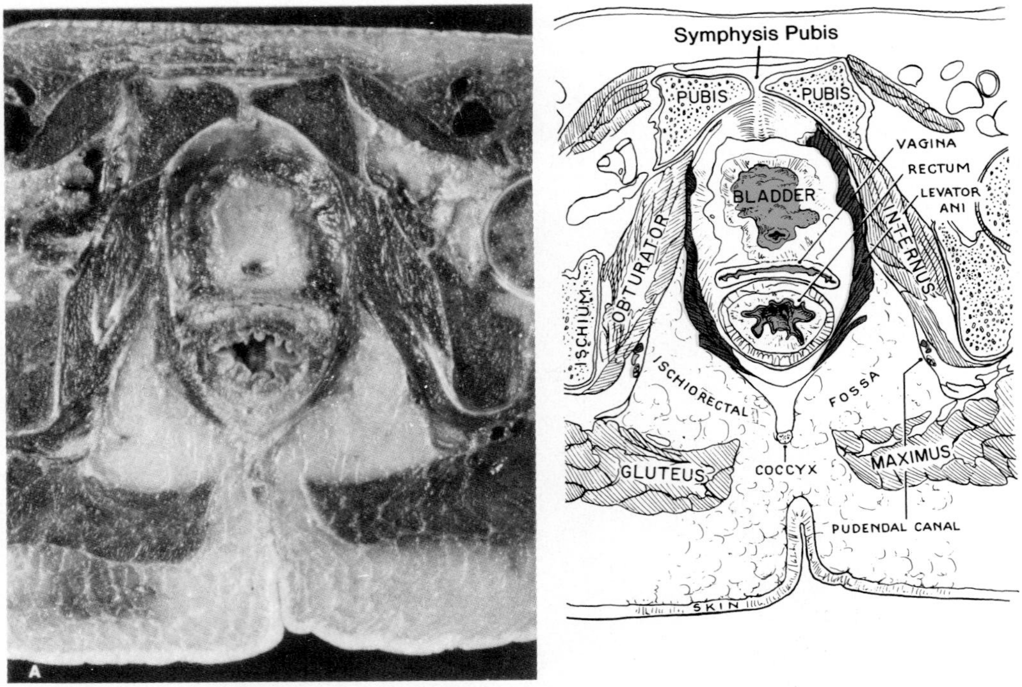

Figure 3-23. Horizontal section of the female pelvis. *A*, photograph. *B*, explanatory drawing. Examine the ischiorectal fossae noting that they are wedge-shaped fascial spaces, one on each side of the rectum and the anal canal (Fig. 3-24). Observe that they are filled with fat which allows the rectum to become distended and to empty. Note that each fossa is bounded *laterally* by the ischium (from which the obturator internus muscle arises); *medially* by the rectum (anal canal inferiorly) to which the levator ani and external anal sphincter are applied; *posteriorly* by the sacrotuberous ligament and the overlying gluteus maximus muscle; and *anteriorly* by the base of the urogenital diaphragm (Fig. 3-13) and its fasciae.

fits tightly over the glans and cannot be retracted, a condition called **phimosis** (F. *phimos*, a muzzle). As there are modified sebaceous glands in the inner surface of the prepuce, the secretions from them usually accumulate in persons with phimosis and may cause irritation. In some persons there is a narrow **preputial opening**, and retraction of the prepuce over the glans penis constricts the neck of the penis so much that interference with the drainage of blood and tissue fluid from the glans occurs. In patients with **paraphimosis** (constriction of the glans penis by the prepuce), the glans enlarges so much that the prepuce cannot be retracted over it. Circumcision is commonly performed in such cases. **Balanitis** (G. *balanos*, acorn + *itis*, inflammation), the term for inflammation of the glans penis, may also result from irritation (*e.g.*, urine contaminated with bacteria).

Circumcision (L. *circumcido*, to cut around) is the operation of removing part or all of the prepuce (Fig. 3-30). This is the most commonly performed operation on male infants in North America. It is usually done on the 3rd or 4th day after birth but is performed on the 8th day by Jews as a religious rite.

The structure of the penis has a spongy form because it is composed mainly of cavernous **erectile tissue** (Fig. 3-37), consisting of interlacing and intercommunicating **cavernous spaces** that are lined by an endothelium which is continuous with that of the veins draining the spaces. *The cavernous spaces are separated by fibrous trabeculae and are filled with blood during an erection*, but many of them are empty when the penis is flaccid (Figs. 3-14 and 3-30).

The principal arteries to the penis are (1) the **dorsal arteries** (Figs. 3-31, 3-35, and 3-37), which run in the interval between the corpora cavernosa penis *on each side of the deep dorsal vein*; and (2) the **deep arteries**, which run within each of the corpora cavernosa penis. *The dorsal and deep arteries of the penis are branches of the internal pudendal arteries* which arise in the pelvis from the **internal iliac arteries** (Figs. 3-27 and 3-66).

The deep arteries of the penis are the principal vessels that supply the cavernous spaces and that are involved in an erec-

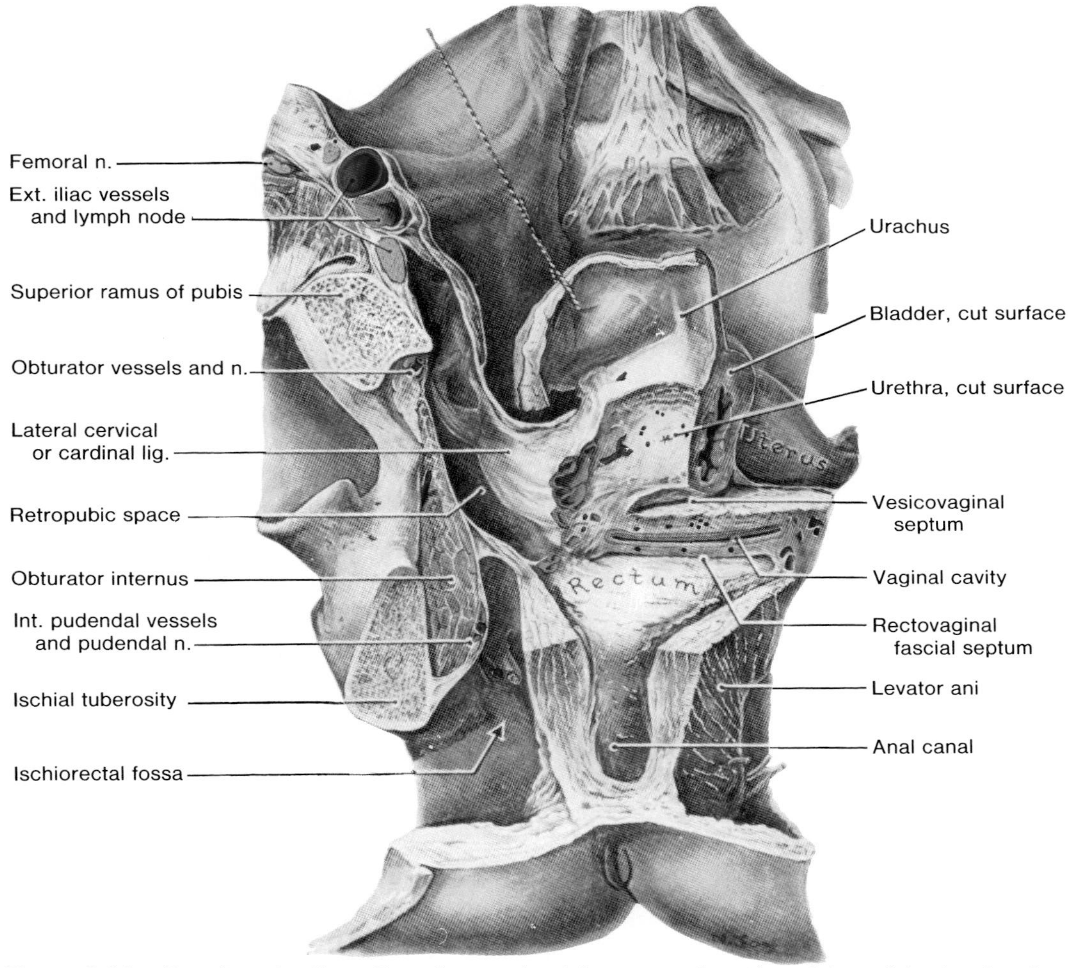

Figure 3-24. Drawing of a dissection of approximately a coronal section of the pelvis showing the suspensory and supporting mechanism of the vagina. The neck of the bladder and the vagina are cut transversely; the bladder is divided sagittally and is rotated backward. Observe that the partition separating the retropubic space from the ischiorectal fossa is formed merely by the thin origin of the levator ani muscle from the obturator internus fascia and its areolar coverings. Note (1) the rectum supporting the posterior wall of the vagina; (2) the posterior wall supporting the anterior wall; and (3) the anterior wall supporting the bladder. Observe the dense areolar tissue within which the vesicovaginal plexus of veins passes posterosuperiorly to join the internal iliac veins. This acts as a suspensory ligament for the cervix and vagina and is called the cardinal ligament. This ligament blends with the fascia that encapsules the vagina and with adjacent fasciae. Note that anteriorly the fascia encapsuling the vagina blends with the vescial fascia and adheres intimately to the urethra; posteriorly it is attached loosely to the rectal fascia.

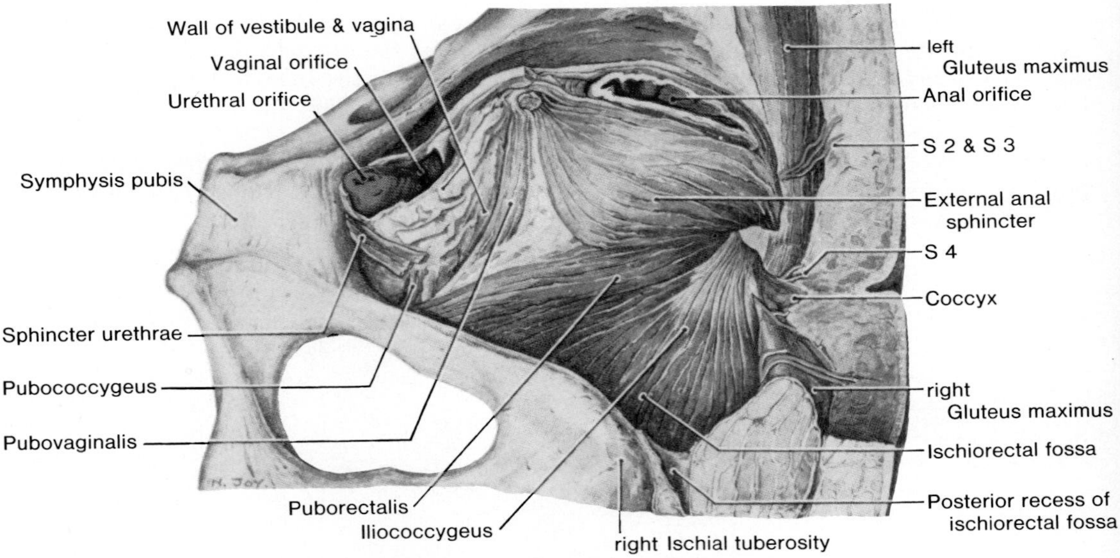

Figure 3-25. Drawing of a dissection of an obliquely tilted lateral view of the pelvis showing one levator ani muscle. Observe the sphincter urethrae muscle resting like a saddle on the urethra and straddling the vagina. Examine the parts of the levator ani: pubococcygeus, puborectalis, and iliococcygeus muscles. The pubovaginalis muscle is formed by anterior fibers of the levator ani that meet behind the vaginal orifice. The puborectal fibers of opposite sides meet in the anorectal junction to form the puborectal sling (Fig. 3-61). The iliococcygeus meets its fellow in an aponeurosis between the rectum and the coccyx (Fig. 3-57).

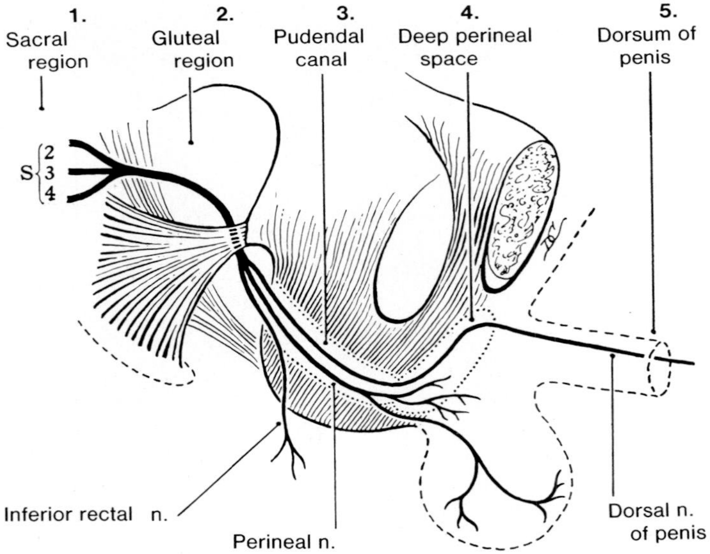

Figure 3-26. Diagram of the *pudendal nerve*. Note the five regions in which it runs and the three divisions into which it divides. Observe the pudendal canal for the pudendal nerve and the internal pudendal vessels (not illustrated here; see Figs. 3-13 and 3-23). Observe that the thickened inferior portion of the fascia of the obturator internus muscle in the ischiorectal fossa splits to form the fibrous pudendal canal. Observe that the dorsal nerve of the penis runs through the deep perineal space or pouch to reach the penis (also see Fig. 3-35).

tion. They give off numerous branches that open directly into these spaces. When the penis is flaccid most of these arterial branches have a spiral course; hence, they are called **helicine arteries** (G. *helix*, a coil). Blood from the cavernous spaces is drained by a **plexus of venules** to the deep dorsal vein located in the *tunica albuginea* (Figs. 3-31 and 3-37). The smooth muscle of the helicine arteries and the trabeculae is supplied both by sympathetic and parasympathetic fibers.

The basis of an erection is that when a male is stimulated erotically, *the smooth*

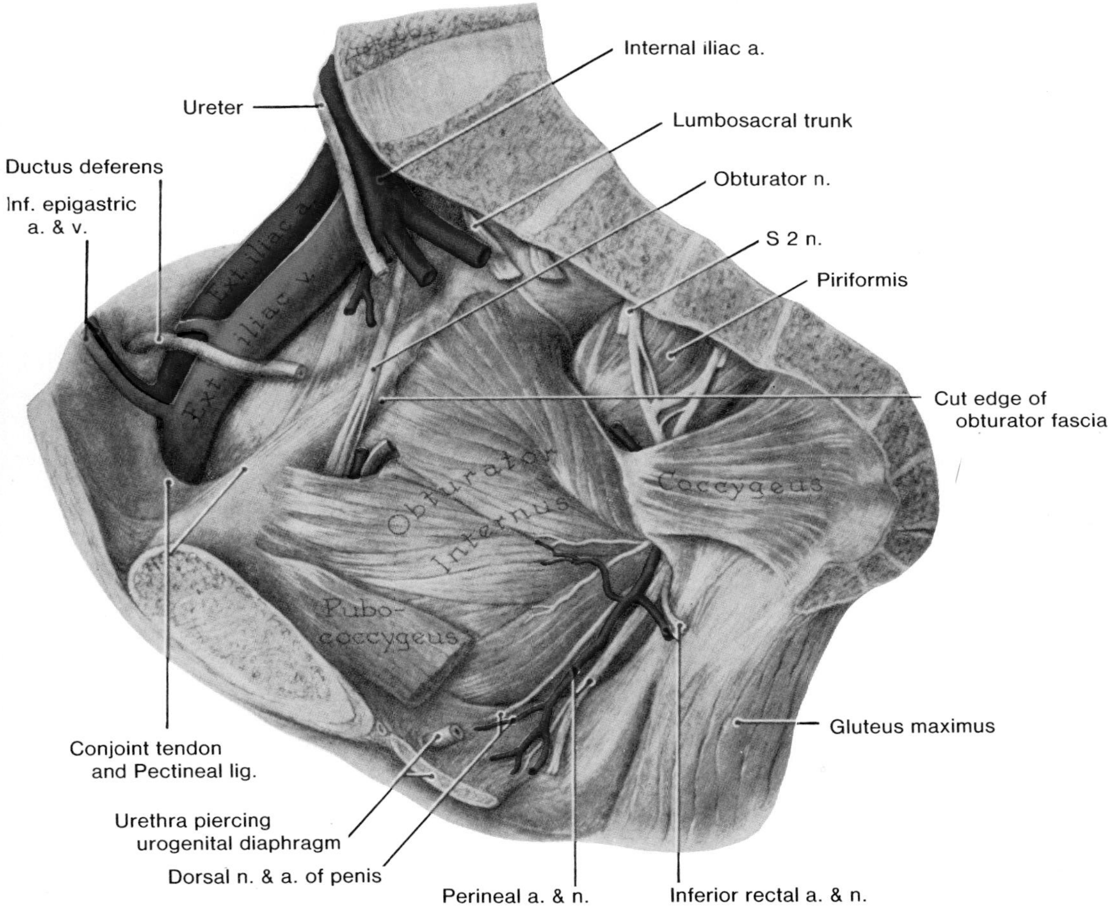

Figure 3-27. Drawing of a dissection of the muscles of the pelvis minor (*male specimen*). Observe the obturator internus muscle padding the side wall of the pelvis and escaping through the lesser sciatic foramen; its nerve is also visible. Examine the cut edge of the obturator fascia which is attached to the pelvic brim (also see Fig. 3-59). The obturator nerve is running in the extraperitoneal fat, medial to the obturator fascia. Note the piriformis muscle padding the posterior wall of the pelvis and escaping through the greater sciatic foramen. Observe the coccygeus muscle concealing the sacrospinous ligament and the pubococcygeus muscle. It is the chief and strongest part of the levator ani muscle springing from the body of the pubis. Examine the obturator nerve, artery, and vein escaping through the obturator foramen. Note the internal pudendal artery and the pudendal nerve making an exit through the greater sciatic foramen, re-entering through the lesser sciatic foramen, and taking a forward course (in the pudendal canal) within the obturator internus fascia to the urogenital diaphragm. In the pelvis major, observe the ductus deferens and the ureter descending across the external iliac artery and vein and the psoas fascia and the pelvic brim to enter the pelvis minor or true pelvis.

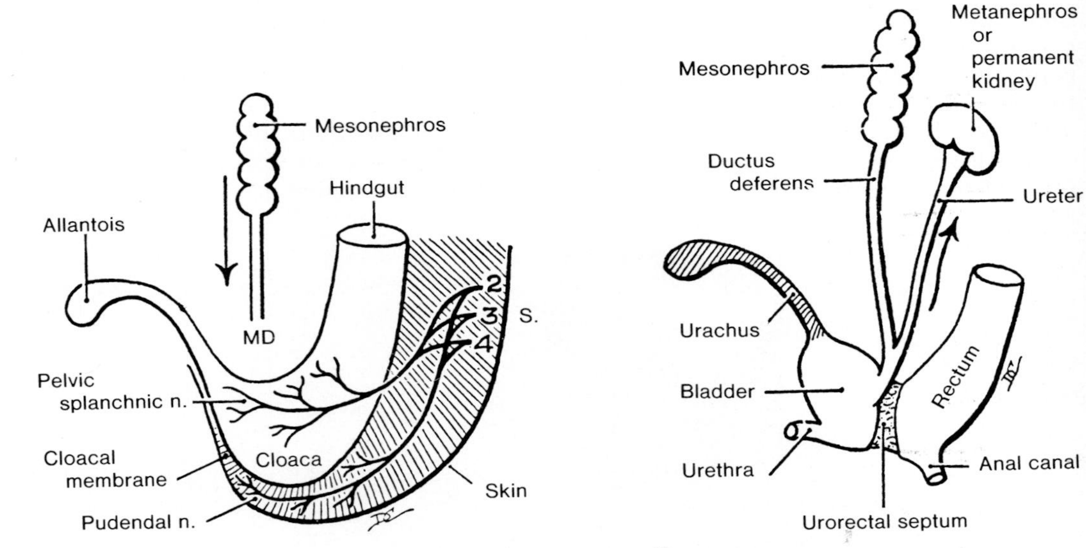

A. B.

Figure 3-28 Drawings illustrating early development of the perineal region. *A*, 4 weeks showing the nerve supply of the cloaca. *B*, 7 weeks showing the connections and subdivisions of the cloaca. The urorectal septum, a mesodermal partition, has now divided the cloaca into urogenital and rectal portions. The central perineal tendon of the adult perineum indicates where the urorectal septum united with the cloacal membrane. As the urinary bladder develops from the urogenital sinus, the inferior ends of the mesonephric duct (*MD*, future ductus deferens) and ureter become absorbed into the base (future trigone) of the bladder (Fig. 3-72). As a result, the orifices of the ducts obtain separate openings.

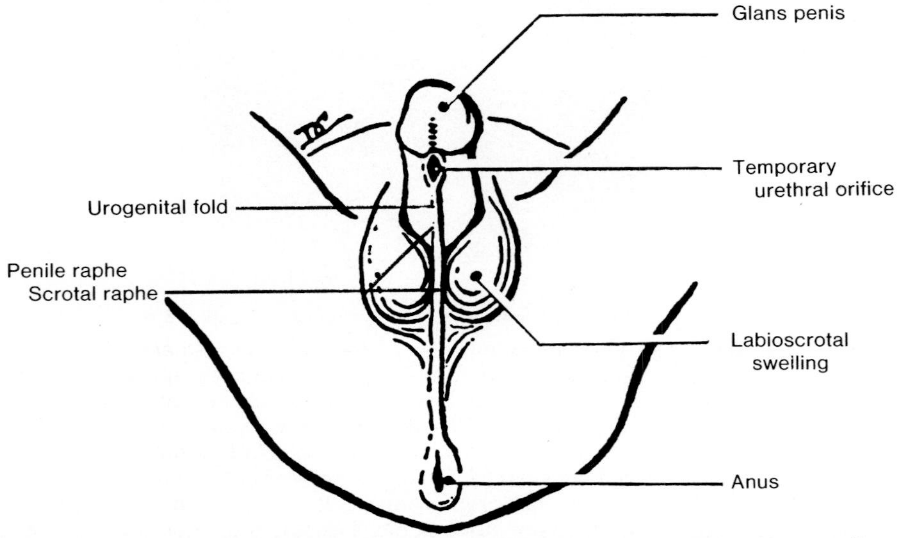

Figure 3-29. Drawing of the developing male external genital organs. The labioscrotal swellings have fused in the midline ventral to the fused urogenital folds. A scrotal raphe marks the site where this fusion occurred. The urogenital folds are fusing and enclosing the urethra in the penis. The site of fusion of these folds is indicated by a dark line called the penile raphe. Should development be arrested at the stage shown here, a condition known as *hypospadias* would exist; *i.e.*, the urethral orifice would be on the ventral or under surface of the penis instead of at the tip of the glans penis (see Fig. 3-79).

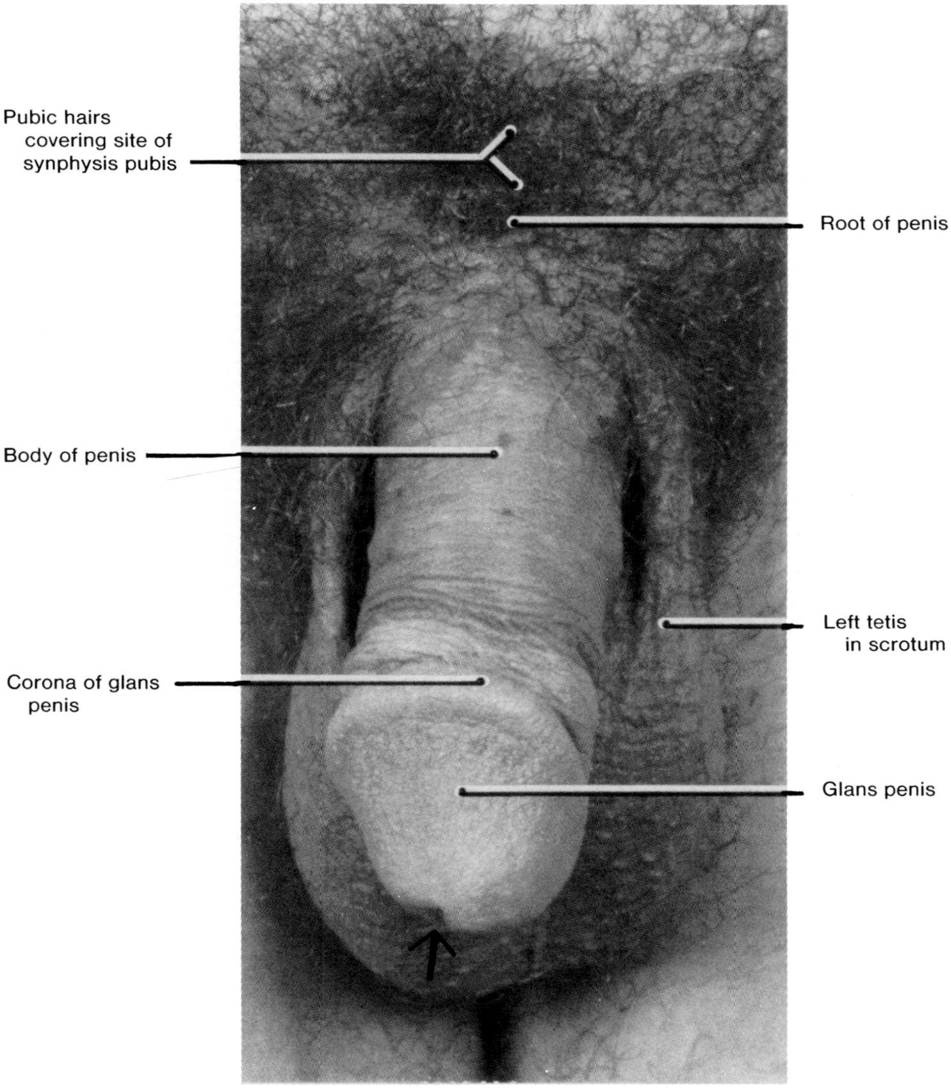

Figure 3-30. Photograpn ot tne penis and scrotum of a 27-year-old man (actual size). The glans (L. acorn) penis is bare because the prepuce was removed by circumcision during infancy. The *arrow* indicates the external urethral orifice. The dorsum of the penis (shown here) faces forward when the organ is in the flaccid state as here. Observe that the penile skin is thin and has no hairs except near its root. In the anatomical (erect) position the dorsum of the penis faces the anterior abdominal wall. Note that the right testis is lower than the left one. This is common in left-handed persons as in this case, but in most men the left is lower than the right. The length of the erect penis varies, but it is usually 15 to 16 cm long and about 3.75 cm in diameter. Many mammals, but not man, possess a bone or cartilage rod in the penis.

muscle of the trabeculae and the helicine arteries relaxes owing to **parasympathetic stimulation**. As a result, these arteries straighten out and their lumina enlarge, *allowing blood from them to flow freely into the cavernous spaces*. Soon **the blood engorges and dilates** the **cavernous spaces**, compressing the venous plexuses at the periphery of the corpora cavernosa. As a result, *the corpora become rigid and enlarged and the penis erects*. The corpus spongiosum penis (Figs. 3-31 to 3-33

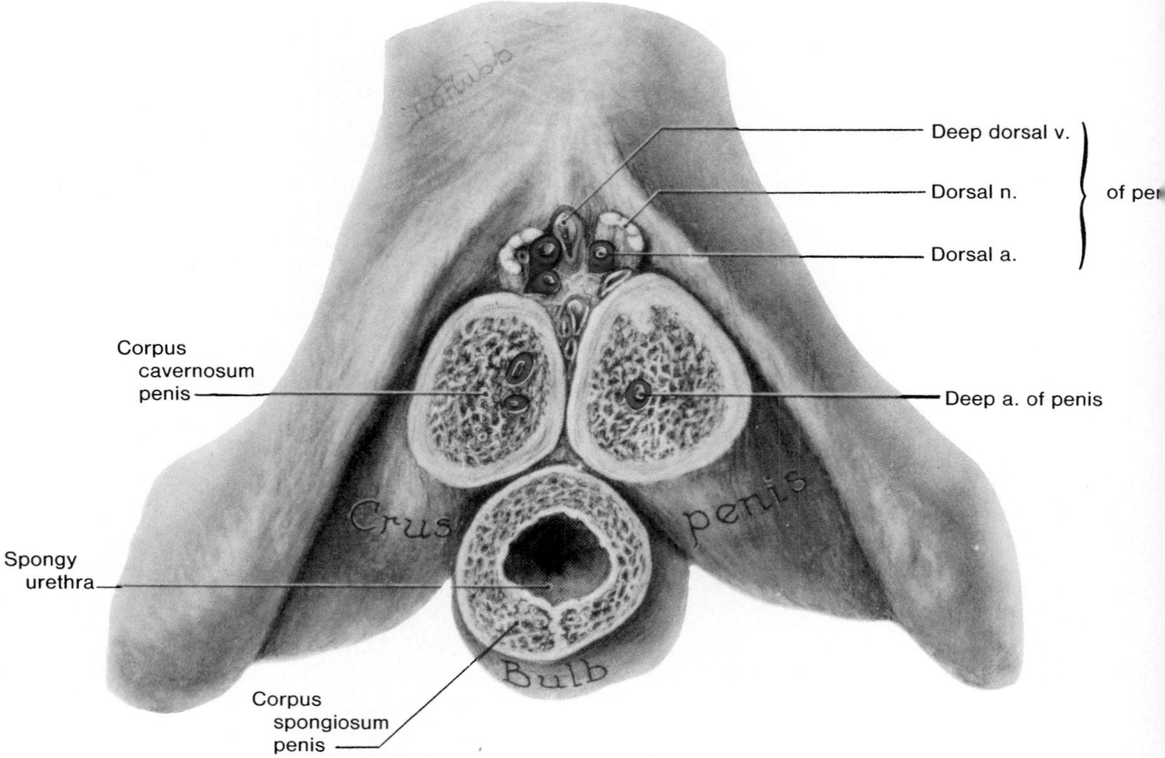

Figure 3-31. Drawing of a section across the root of the penis. Observe that the urethra is dilated within the bulb of the penis, the expanded proximal part of the corpus spongiosum of the penis (Fig. 3-32). Note that the substance of the penis consists essentially of three cylindrical bodies of erectile tissue, two corpora cavernosa and one corpus spongiosum (corpus cavernosum urethrae). The fibrous tissue that binds these cylindrical bodies together and the penile skin are not shown (see Figs. 3-35 and 3-37).

and 3-37) does not become so rigid as the corpora cavernosa penis because its sheath is more elastic. Consequently, the spongy urethra within the corpus spongiosum remains patent, allowing for passage of semen during ejaculation. Following **orgasm** (climax of sexual act) or the passage of erotic thoughts, the penis gradually returns to its flaccid state, a process called **detumescence**. This results from sympathetic stimulation which causes constriction of the smooth muscle in the helicine arteries and the trabeculae. As a result, the excess blood is slowly drained from the penis via the **deep dorsal vein** of the penis (Fig. 3-37).

The dorsal nerve of the penis (Figs. 3-26, 3-27, 3-31, and 3-35) is one of the two terminal branches of the pudendal nerve; the perineal nerve is the other. *The dorsal nerve of the penis arises in the pudendal canal* (Figs. 3-13, 3-23, and 3-26) *and passes forward into the deep perineal space* (pouch). It then passes to the dorsum of the penis where it runs lateral to the arteries and supplies both the skin and the glans penis (Fig. 3-35). The penis is richly provided with a great variety of sensory nerve endings; thus it is very sensitive.

The Superficial Perineal Muscles (Figs. 3-4, 3-16, 3-17, and 3-20). The superficial perineal muscles lie in the superficial perineal space (pouch) which is bounded inferiorly by the superficial perineal fascia and superiorly by the inferior fascia of the urogenital diaphragm (perineal membrane). *The perineal nerve* (Fig. 3-26) *supplies all three of the superficial perineal muscles.*

The superficial transverse perineal muscles are slender, narrow, muscular strips which pass transversely, anterior to

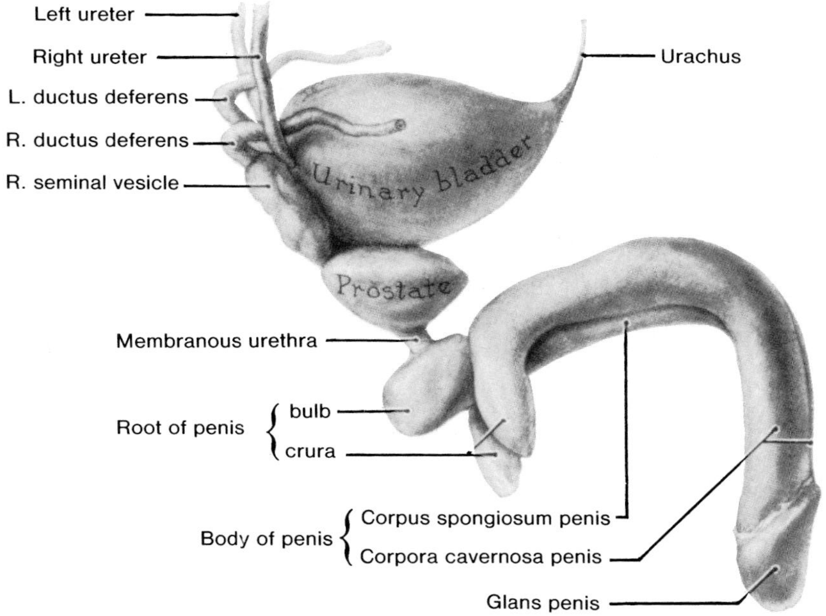

Figure 3-32. Drawing of the inferior parts of the male genital and urinary tracts (also see Fig. 3-30). Observe that the two corpora cavernosa and the corpus spongiosum form the body (shaft) of the penis which has an expanded terminal part called the glans penis. As the corpus spongiosum penis contains the urethra, it used to be called the corpus cavernosum urethrae.

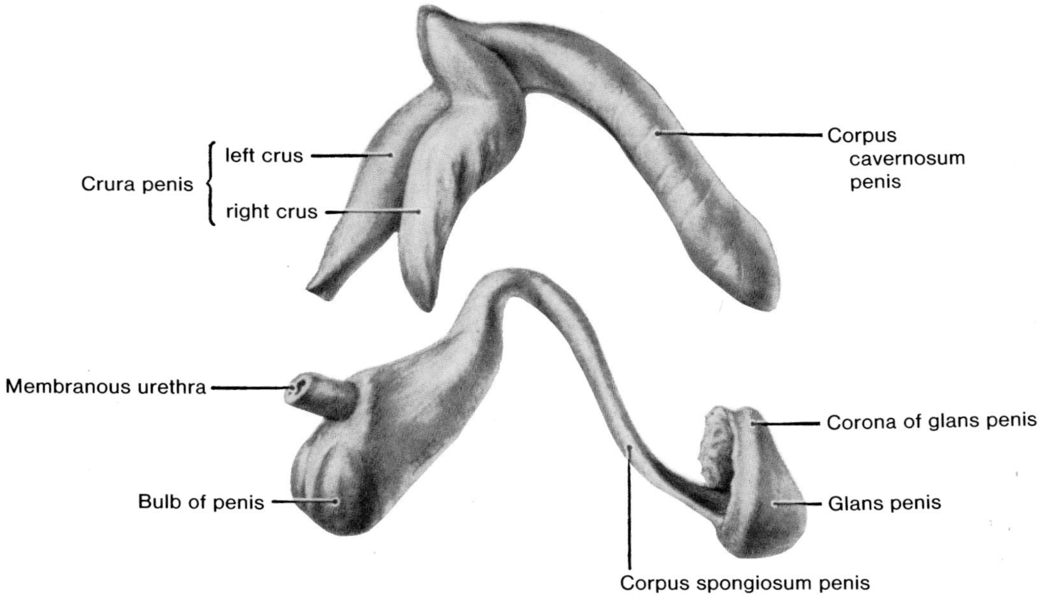

Figure 3-33. Drawing of the parts of a dissected penis. The corpus spongiosum penis is separated from the corpora cavernosa penis; however, their natural flexures are preserved. Observe that the corpora cavernosa penis are bent where the penis is slung by the suspensory ligament of the penis (Fig. 3-34) and that they are grooved by the encircling vessels (Fig. 3-35). The corpus spongiosum penis is enlarged below the urethra posteriorly to form the bulb of the penis and above the urethra anteriorly to form the glans penis. The glans fits like a cap on the blunt ends of the corpora cavernosa penis.

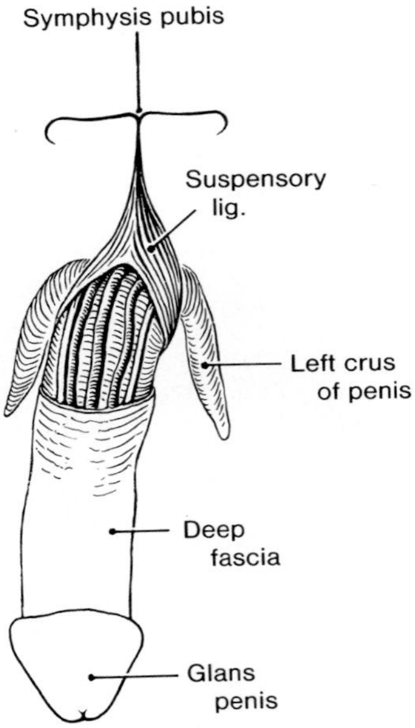

Figure 3-34. Drawing of the penis illustrating its suspensory ligament. The skin and the superficial dorsal vein have been removed. The suspensory ligament is a fibroelastic structure which spreads out from the anterior surface of the symphysis pubis and fuses with the deep fascia on the dorsum and sides of the penis. Note that the deep dorsal vessels and nerves lie deep to the suspensory ligament.

the anus. *Each muscle extends from the ischial tuberosity to the central perineal tendon* (Fig. 3-4); it probably helps to fix this wedge-shaped mass of fibrous tissue.

The bulbospongiosus muscle (Figs. 3-4, 3-10, 3-16*F*, 3-17, and 3-38) lies in the median plane of the perineum, anterior to the anus. It consists of two symmetrical parts that are united by a **median tendinous raphe** below the bulb of the penis. *The bulbospongiosus arises from this median raphe and the central perineal tendon* (perineal body). **The paired bulbospongiosi form a sphincter** which compresses the bulb and the corpus spongiosum of the penis, thereby emptying the spongy urethra of residual urine and/or semen. *Its anterior fibers also assist with erection of the penis by compressing the deep dorsal vein* of the penis, thereby impeding venous drainage of the cavernous spaces and helping to promote enlargement and turgidity of the penis.

The ischiocavernosus muscles (Figs. 3-4 and 3-16*F*) cover the crura of the corpora cavernosa penis (Fig. 3-32). *Each muscle arises from the inner surface of the ischial tuberosity and the ramus of the ischium* and runs forward on the crus of the penis to be *inserted into the sides and under the surface of the crus.* The ischiocavernosus muscles **force blood from the cavernous spaces** in the crura of the bulb into the distal parts of the corpora cavernosa penis, thereby increasing the turgidy of the organ. Contraction of the ischiocavernosi also compresses the deep dorsal vein of the penis as it leaves the crus of the penis (Fig. 3-31), thereby cutting off the venous return from the penis.

The Female Perineum (Figs. 3-3, 3-12, 3-15, 3-16, 3-22, 3-24, and 3-39 to 3-43). The female urogenital region differs markedly from the corresponding region of the male. The urethra is enclosed in the anterior wall of the vagina, not within the clitoris. In addition the vagina pierces the urogenital diaphragm. Despite the obvious differences in the sexes, the urogenital structures develop from the same primordia. As a result the muscles, nerves, and vessels of the female perineum are almost identical with those of the male. *The female external genital organs are known collectively as the vulva or the female pudendum.* **The vulva comprises** the *mons pubis*, the *labia majora*, the *labia minora*, the *vestibule of the vagina*, the *clitoris*, the *bulb of the vestibule*, and the *greater vestibular glands.*

Structures in the Superficial Perineal Space in Females (Figs. 3-10 and 3-16). As in the male, the superficial perineal space (pouch) is the fascial space between the superficial perineal fascia (Colles' fascia) and the inferior fascia of the urogenital diaphragm (perineal membrane). It contains the **superficial transversus perinei**, the **ischiocavenosus**, the **bulbospongiosus** muscles, and the **greater vestibular glands**.

Structures in the Deep Perineal Space in Females (Figs. 3-10 and 3-16). The deep perineal space (pouch) is the fascial space enclosed by the superior and inferior fasciae of the urogenital diaphragm. It contains the **urethra**, the inferior part of the **vagina**, and the **deep transversus perinei** muscles. It also contains the *internal pudendal vessels*, the *dorsal nerve of the clitoris*, and the branches of the *perineal nerve* supplying the sphincter urethrae and deep transversus perinei muscles.

The Mons Pubis (Figs. 2-45, 3-3, and 3-39). The mons (L. mountain) pubis is a **rounded eminence lying anterior to the the symphysis pubis**. It is formed mainly by *a pad of fatty tissue* beneath the skin and become covered with coarse **pubic hairs** (Fig. 2-45) at *puberty* (12 to 15 years). The abrupt discontinuation of this triangular mat of pubic hair at its superior boundary is a female characteristic.

The Labia Majora (Figs. 3-22, 3-39, 3-41, and 3-72). The labia (L. lips) majora are two large folds of skin filled largely with subcutaneous fat which run downward and backward from the mons pubis. *Embryologically, the labia majora are homologus to the scrotum of the male.* After puberty their outer aspects are covered by pigmented skin that contains sebaceous and sweat glands and is covered by coarse hairs (Fig. 3-39). Their moist internal aspects also contain hair follicles and sebaceous glands, but the hairs are delicate.

The **pudendal cleft** or rima pudendi is the slit (L. *rima*) or *opening between the labia majora* into which the vestibule of the vagina opens. Anteriorly the labia majora meet across the midline at the **anterior labial commissure** (Fig. 3-39). Posteriorly the labia majora do not actually join, but a slight transverse fold of the skin called the **posterior labial commissure** unites them. The *round ligament of the uterus* (Fig. 3-89) passes through the inguinal canal and *enters the labium majus where it ends as a branching band of fascia* that is attached to the skin (Figs. 3-3 and 3-41).

The Labia Minora (Figs. 3-12, 3-22, 3-39, 3-41, and 3-72). The labia minora are two

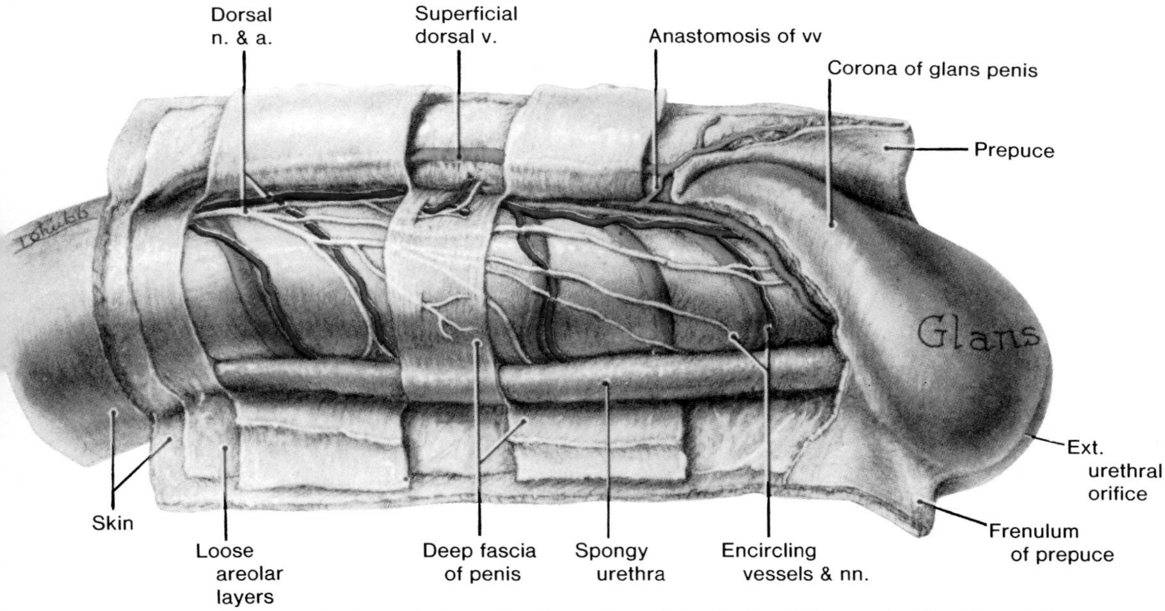

Figure 3-35. Drawing of a lateral view of a dissection of the body of the penis. The three tubular envelopes or coverings of the penis are reflected. Observe that the penile skin is folded upon itself to form the prepuce. Note the loose, laminated, subcutaneous areolar tissue (dartos muscle and fascia), called the superficial fascia of the penis, which is carried forward into the prepuce. Observe that the superficial dorsal vein begins in the prepuce and anastomoses with the deep dorsal vein from the glans; it ends in the superficial inguinal veins. Examine the deep fascia of the penis (Buck's fascia) which ends at the glans penis. Observe the large encircling tributaries of the deep dorsal vein, the thread-like companion arteries, and the numerous oblique nerves. Note the vessels and nerves at the neck of the penis passing into the glans.

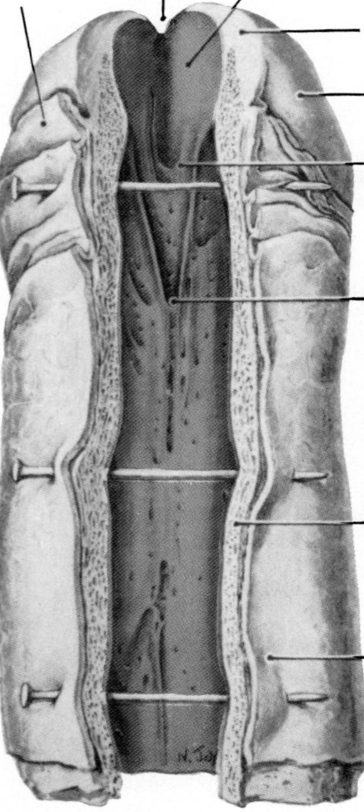

Figure 3-36. Drawing of part of the body of a penis in which a longitudinal incision has been made on its ventral or urethral surface and carried through the floor of the urethra. Hence, the view is of the dorsal surface of the interior of the urethra. The prepuce is retracted. Observe the interior of the spongy portion of the urethra and that the urethra is expanded within the glans penis to form the navicular fossa. Observe the orifices of the numerous urethral glands. Note the large recess (lacuna magna) which may impede the passage of a catheter along the urethra.

thin delicate folds of fat free, hairless skin. Sebaceous and sweat glands open on both surfaces. *The labia minora lie between the labia majora*, and their lateral surfaces are in contact with the smooth moist internal surfaces of the labia majora. Although the internal surface of each labium majus consists of thin skin, it has the pink color typical of a mucous membrane. *The labia minora enclose the vestibule of the vagina and lie on each side of the vaginal orifice* (Figs. 3-3, 3-12, and 3-39). In young females and **virgins** (women who have not engaged in *sexual intercourse*), the labia minora are usually covered by the labia majora, but in **parous women** (ones who have borne children) they may protrude (Fig. 3-39).

The labia minora extend posteriorly from the clitoris for about 4 cm and their medial surfaces are in contact with each other. Posteriorly the labia minora may be united by a small fold of the skin, called the frenulum pudendi or **frenulum of the labia minora**. Some obstetricians and gynecologists refer to this frenulum (L. small bridle) as the *fourchette* (F. fork). The frenulum of the labia minora, usually recognizable in young women, is frequently torn during childbirth.

The Vestibule of the Vagina (Figs. 3-12, 3-39, and 3-41). The vestibule (L. *vestibulum*, antechamber or entrance court) of the vagina is *the space or cleft between the labia minora*. The orifices of the **urethra**, the **vagina**, and the ducts of the **greater vestibular glands** (Bartholin's glands) are located in the vestibule of the vagina.

The external urethral orifice is located 2 to 3 cm posterior to the clitoris and immediately *anterior to the vaginal orifice* (Fig. 3-3). On each side of the urethral orifice are the openings of the **paraurethral glands** (Skene's ducts or glands), which are homologous to the prostate in the male. The external urethral orifice is usually a median slit which has prominent margins that are in contact with each other.

The vaginal orifice, also a median cleft, is much larger than the urethral orifice and is located inferior and posterior to it. The size and appearance of the vaginal orifice depend upon the condition of the **hymen**, a thin incomplete fold of mucous membrane surrounding this opening (Fig. 3-15). The **greater vestibular glands** are located on each side of the vestibule (Figs. 3-12 and 3-42), posterolateral to the vaginal orifice and external to the hymen. There are several small **lesser vestibular glands** on each side of the vestibule which open on each side between the urethral and vaginal orifices.

CLINICALLY ORIENTED COMMENTS

In most virgins the vaginal orifice is partially closed by the hymen, which is variable in size and shape. Pelvic examinations, sexual intercourse, and trauma may

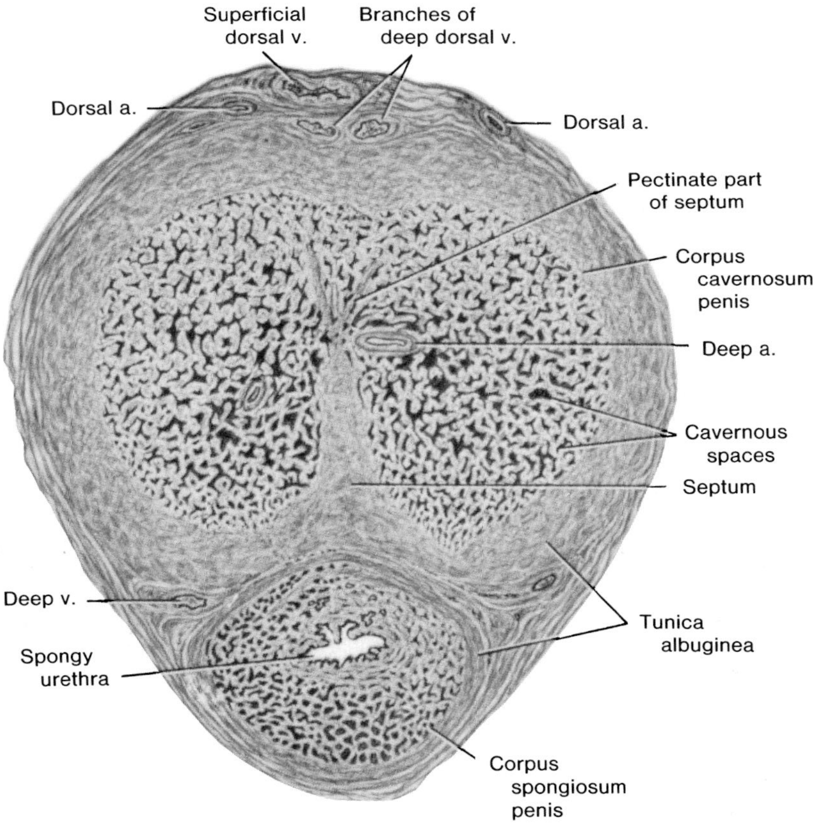

Figure 3-37. Drawing of a cross-section of the body of the penis of an adult male from which the skin has been removed. The section is at the junction of the proximal two-thirds and the distal one-third of the body of the penis. Observe that the corpora cavernosa consist of a mass of cavernous erectile tissue enclosed in a dense sheath of white fibrous tissue called the tunica albuginea. Note that the tunicae albugineae fuse medially to form an incomplete median septum; hence, the cavernous erectile tissue of the two corpora is continuous. ×4.5.

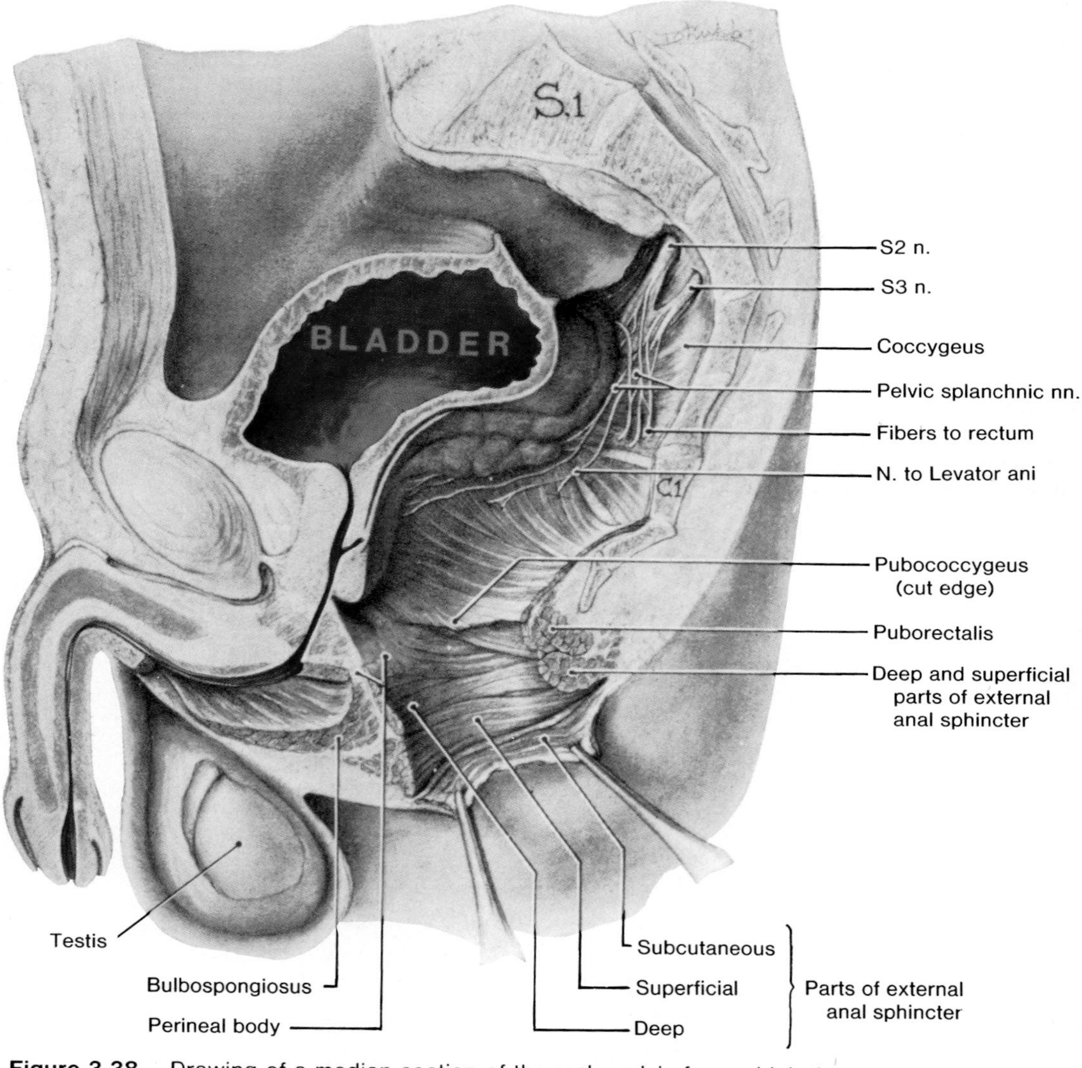

Figure 3-38. Drawing of a median section of the male pelvis from which the rectum, anal canal, and bulb of the penis (shown in Fig. 3-14) have been removed. Examine the external anal sphincter and the levatores ani muscles. Observe the subcutaneous fibers of the external anal sphincter which are reflected with forceps; the superficial fibers mingling posteriorly with deep fibers; and the deep fibers mingling with the puborectalis muscle which forms a sling that occupies the anorectal angle between the anal canal and the rectum (also see Fig. 3-61). Note that the pubococcygeus is divided to allow for the removal of the anal canal to which it is in part attached.

tear the hymen, resulting in varying amounts of bleeding. Following parturition the vaginal orifice is enlarged and the hymen may be represented by only a few tags or rounded elevations of mucous membrane, called **hymeneal caruncles** (Fig. 3-15).

In the virginal state the aperture in the hymen varies from a pinpoint in size to one admitting one or two fingers. At the initial sexual intercourse the hymen usually lacerates in several places. In some cases it may fail to rupture, resulting in difficult and/or painful intercourse known as **dyspareunia** (G. *dyspareunos*, badly mated). In cases where the hymeneal aperture is very small, conception may occur as the result of semen being propelled into the vagina rather than being deposited there by the penis.

In some young women the hymen has no aperture, a persistent fetal condition known as **imperforate hymen**. In these cases there is no communication between the vagina and its vestibule. With the onset of **menses** (menstrual bleeding), there is an accumulation of menstrual blood in the vagina (**hematocolpos**).

The Clitoris (Figs. 3-3, 3-12, and 3-39 to 3-43). The clitoris, usually 2 to 3 cm in length, is homologous with the penis in the male. This small *cylindrical organ is composed of erectile tissue and is capable of enlargement* as a result of engorgement with blood (see the previous description of the basis of an erection in the male). It consists of two crura, two corpora cavernosa, and a glans and is suspended by a suspensory ligament as in the male (Fig. 3-3). Like the glans penis, the glans clitoridis is covered by a very sensitive epithelium. *The clitoris has no corpus spongiosum and is entirely separate from the urethra.*

The clitoris is located between the anterior ends of the labia minora (Figs. 3-39 and 3-41), which divide to enclose it. The parts of the labia minora passing anterior to the clitoris form the **prepuce of the clitoris** (Figs. 3-3 and 3-39), whereas the parts passing posterior to it form the **frenulum of the clitoris**.

The Bulbs of the Vestibule (Figs. 3-12 and 3-42). The bulbs of the vestibule consist of *two elongated masses of erectile tissue, about 3 cm in length, lying along the sides of the vaginal orifice deep to the bulbospongiosus muscle* (Fig. 3-3). These bulbs, connected to the glans clitoridis by a few

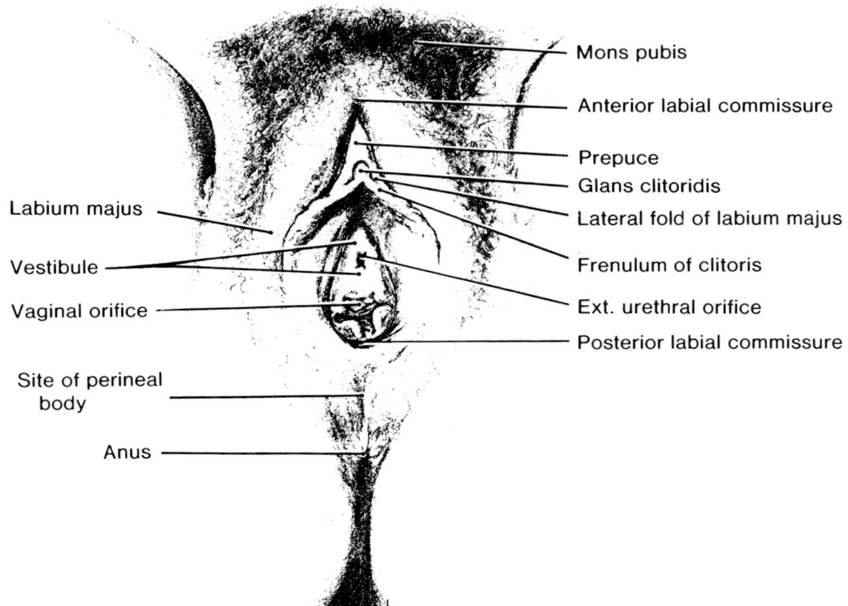

Figure 3-39. Drawing of the female perineum of a *parous woman* as seen in the lithotomy position (Fig. 3-1). The external genitalia occupy the urogenital region or triangle (Fig. 3-9). The feature of the anal region or triangle is the anus. The labia minora are spread to show the space known as the vestibule of the vagina which leads to both the urethral and vaginal orifices. The adjective *parous* is derived from the Latin verb *pario*, to bear; hence, parous indicates that the woman has given birth to an infant or infants. Examine the different parts of the external genitalia, known collectively as the vulva or pudendum. In obstetrics and gynecology the term perineum is often restricted to the region between the anal and vaginal orifices.

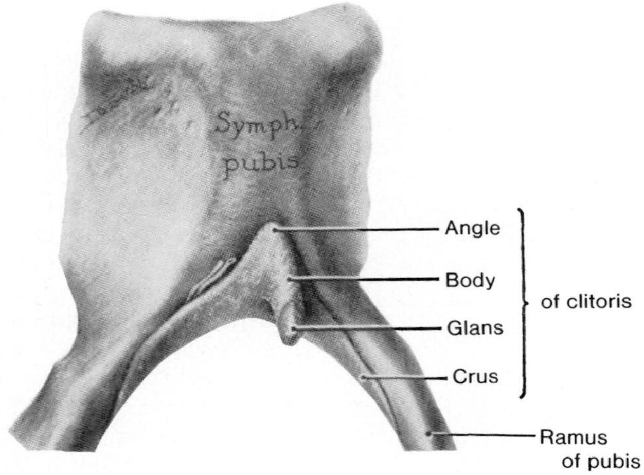

Figure 3-40. Drawing of a dissection of the clitoris, the homologue of the penis. Compare its parts with those of the penis (Figs. 3-32 and 3-33). The clitoris is composed basically of two corpora cavernosa similar to those in the penis, but it contains no corpus spongiosum and *the urethra does not enter it*. During sexual arousal the clitoris becomes erect by a mechanism similar to that described for erection of the penis. Observe that the clitoris, like the penis, arises by two crura from the internal surface of the pubic and ischial rami. In the flaccid state (Fig. 3-39), the prepuce almost completely covers the clitoris in most women.

veins, are homologous to the bulb of the penis and the corpus spongiosum penis (Fig. 3-32). *Their posterior ends are in contact with the greater vestibular glands* (Fig. 3-42).

The Greater Vestibular Glands (Figs. 3-12, 3-16*E*, and 3-42). The two **greater vestibular glands** (major vestibular glands, Bartholin's glands) are *located in the superficial perineal space, one on each side just posterior to the bulb of the vestibule* and partly under the cover of its posterior part. These small, reddish-yellow (*in vivo*), rounded or ovoid *tubuloalveolar glands*, secrete lubricating mucous into ducts which empty into the grooves between the labium minora and the attached margin of the hymen (Figs. 3-12 and 3-42). *The greater vestibular glands are homologous with the bulbourethral glands of the male.*

CLINICALLY ORIENTED COMMENTS

The greater vestibular glands normally are not palpable but become readily so when infected. Infection of the greater vestibular glands (**Bartholinitis**) may result from a number of pathogenic organisms. Infected glands may enlarge to a diameter of 4 to 5 cm and impinge against the wall of the rectum.

Vessels and Nerves of the Female External Genitalia (Figs. 3-42 and 3-43). The *rich arterial supply* to these structures is from two **external pudendal arteries** and one **internal pudendal artery** on each side. The *labial arteries* are branches of the internal pudendal artery. The **nerves to the vulva** are branches of the *ilioinguinal nerve* (Fig. 4-14), the genital branch of the *genitofemoral nerve*, the perineal branch of the *femoral cutaneous nerve of the thigh* (Fig. 4-49), and the *perineal nerve*. As the labia majora are homologous to the scrotum, their nerves are similar to those supplying the scrotum (Fig. 3-26). The **labial veins** are tributaries of the internal pudendal veins and venae comitantes of the internal pudendal artery (Fig. 3-43).

CLINICALLY ORIENTED COMMENTS

Because of the rich arterial supply to the labia major and minora, hemorrhage from

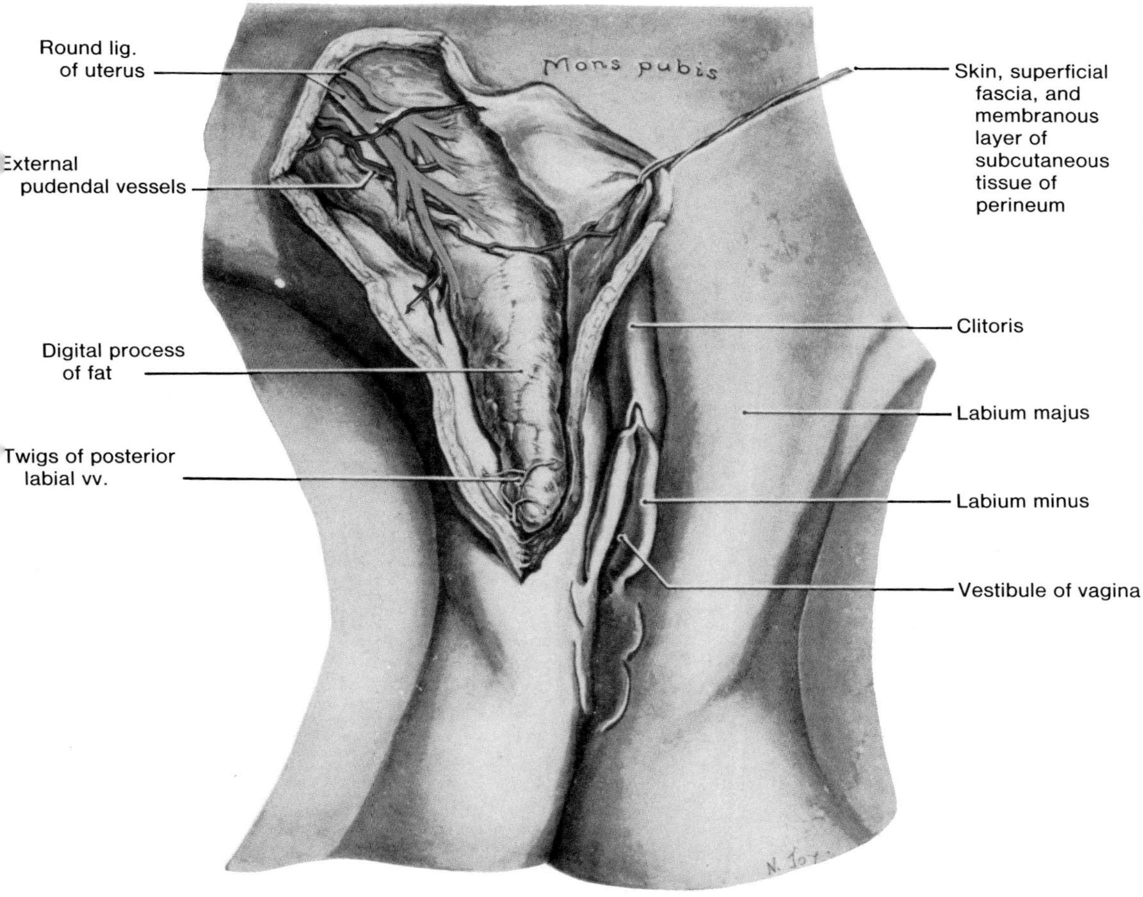

Figure 3-41. Drawing of superficial dissection of the right labium majus. Observe the long digital process of fat lying deep to the subcutaneous fatty tissue and descending far into the labium majus. Note the thin transparent veil of areolar tissue that encloses this process through which its lobulated nature is apparent. Observe the round ligament of the uterus, noting that it ends as a branching band of fascia which spreads out in front of the digital process. Note the external pudendal vessels crossing the process of fat. Examine the vestibule of the vagina, the region between the labia minora and external to the hymen; it includes the orifices of the urethra and the vagina (Fig. 3-3).

injuries to them may be severe. During parturition painful labor often occurs and the most anguish is often felt when the fetal head passes through the vulva owing to stretching of its parts. To relieve pain, **pudendal block anesthesia** may be performed by injecting a local anesthestic agent into the tissues surrounding the pudendal nerve (Fig. 3-111). The injection is usually made where the pudendal nerve crosses the lateral aspect of the sacrospinous ligament (Fig. 3-18), near its attachment to the ischial spine (Fig. 3-43).

To ease delivery of a fetus and to avoid laceration of the perineum, an **episiotomy**, or relaxing incision, is frequently made in the perineum. This enlarges the distal end of the birth canal and prevents serious damage to the perineal structures, especially the rectum and the external anal sphincter. **Two types of episiotomy** are commonly used, median and mediolateral (Fig. 3-44). In a *median episiotomy* the scissor cut is in the midline or median plane of the perineum (Fig. 3-44*A*), beginning at the frenulum of the labia minora (fourchette) and passing posteriorly through the skin, the vaginal mucosa, and the central perineal

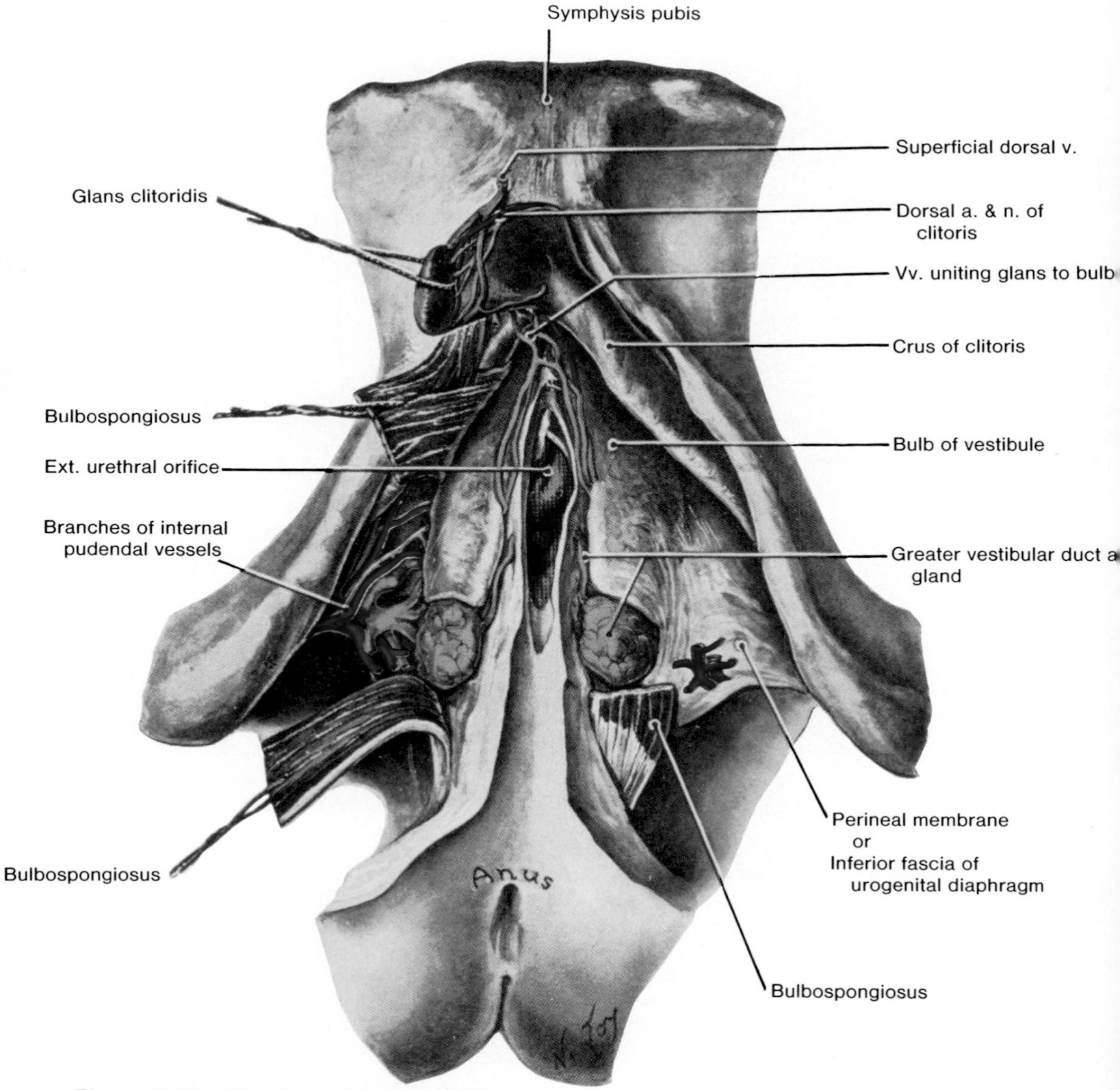

Figure 3-42. Drawing of a dissection of the female perineum. On the *right side* the perineal membrane is removed. Observe the paired bulbospongiosus muscles which are divided and reflected on the right side and largely excised on the left side. Note that the glans clitoridis is pulled over to the right side to show the dorsal vessels and nerve of the clitoris running to it. Observe the bulb of the vestibule (paired right and left), one on each side of the vestibule of the vagina. This differs from the bulb of the penis which is unpaired (Fig. 3-33). Note the veins connecting the bulbs of the vestibule to the glans of the clitoris. Observe the greater vestibular gland situated at the posterior blunt end of the bulb and like it, covered by the bulbospongiosus muscle. Note that this gland has a long duct which opens into the vestibule of the vagina. Examine the perineal membrane (*left side*) to which the bulb is fastened. On the *right side* the membrane is cut away to illustrate the vessels of the bulb and the dorsal nerve and vessels of the clitoris within the deep perineal space.

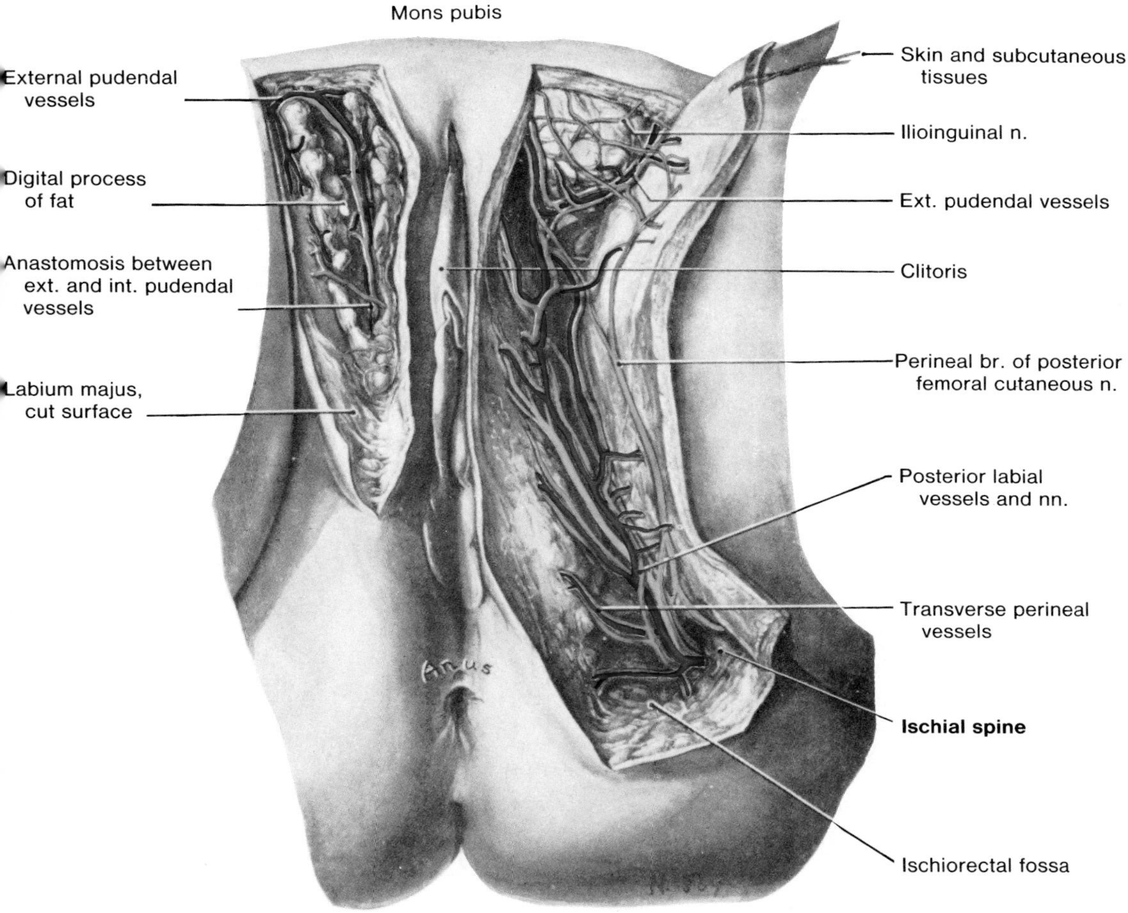

Figure 3-43. Drawing of a dissection of the labia majora demonstrating their vessels and nerves. *On the left* the lobulated digital process of fat has been opened to show the anastomotic vessels which unite the external to the internal pudendal vessels running through its long axis like a core. *On the right* the digital process of fat is largely removed. Observe that the posterior labial vessels and nerves (S2 and S3) are joined by the perineal branch of the posterior cutaneous nerve of the thigh (S1, S2, and S3) and run forward almost to the mons pubis. Here the vessels anastomose with the external pudendal vessels and the nerves meet the ilioinguinal nerve (also see Fig. 2-23). Note that there is a gap here in the numerical sequence of the nerve segments, accounted for by the fact that L2, L5, and S1 are drawn into the lower limb with the result that L1 is succeeded by S2 (see Fig. 4-160).

tendon. *The incision stops well short of the external anal sphincter* and the rectum. Some obstetricians are reluctant to do a median episiotomy, fearing it may tear or extend posteriorly and involve the external anal sphincter and/or the rectum. In the other type of perineal incision, a **medio-lateral episiotomy** (Fig. 3-44*B*), the cut is made on the right or left side, beginning at the midpoint of the frenulum of the labia minora (Fig. 3-12) and extending at a 45° angle toward the ischiorectal fossa and the

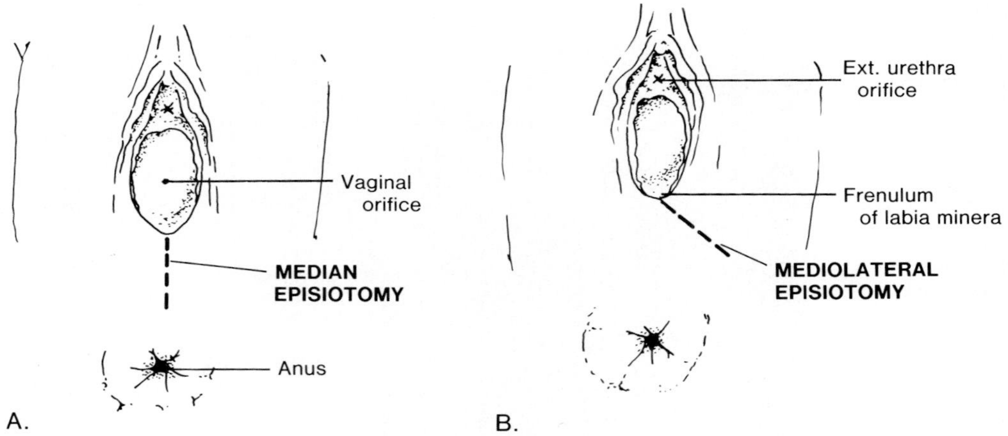

Figure 3-44. Sketches illustrating the main types of episiotomy. (If orientation is required, see Figs. 3-12 and 3-39). *A*, *median episiotomy* (midline episiotomy). The incision passes posteriorly from the frenulum of the labia minora (fourchette) toward the anus, dividing the central perineal tendon (perineal body) in the midline (see Fig. 3-39). *B*, *mediolateral episiotomy*. The incision is at a 45° angle from the midline of the frenulum of the labia minora and passes toward the ischial tuberosity (Fig. 3-46*B*).

ischial tuberosity. *The incision passes through* (1) the posterior vaginal wall, (2) the perineal skin, (3) the bulbospongiosus muscle (Fig. 3-3), (4) the superficial transversus perinei muscle (Fig. 3-16*F*), (5) the perineal membrane (Fig. 3-3), and (6) the deep transversus perinei muscle (Fig. 3-12). *The incision is usually stopped short of the levator ani* because of the important role of this muscle in supporting the pelvic floor (see subsequent discussion of the levatores ani and the pelvic diaphragm and Case 3-1).

THE PELVIS

The pelvis is the lower basin-shaped division of the abdominopelvic cavity (Fig. 2-30). *Pelvis* is the Latin word for *basin* and here refers to the basin-like appearance of the pelvic cavity (Figs. 3-7, 3-8, and 3-45). *The skeleton of the pelvis is referred to as the bony pelvis.* When the term pelvis is used without qualification, it is generally the bony pelvis that is meant.

THE BONY PELVIS

The skeleton of the pelvis, *i.e.*, the bony pelvis, is **formed by** the *two ossa coxae* or hip bones (innominate bones) anteriorly and laterally and by the *sacrum* and *coccyx* posteriorly (Figs. 3-7 to 3-9 and 3-45 to 3-49). *The sacrum and coccyx are parts of the vertebral column* (Fig. 5-1) which are interposed dorsally between the two hip bones.

The os coxae or hip bone (Fig. 3-47) is a large, irregularly shaped bone which *consists of three parts*: the *ilium*, *ischium*, and *pubis*. These three parts meet at the **acetabulum**, the cup-shaped cavity for the head of the femur (Figs. 3-7*A*, 3-46, and 3-49). *In infants and children the three parts of the hip bone are not fused* with each other (Fig. 4-4). Fusion occurs at 15 to 17 years and the bones are firmly joined in the adult (Fig. 3-47). *The ilium, ischium, and pubis are fully described in Chapter 4 on the lower limb* (Figs. 4-1 to 4-4 and 4-8).

The components of the bony pelvis (ossa coxae or hip bones, sacrum, and coccyx) are bound together by dense ligaments (Fig. 3-46). *These four bones are united by four articulations* or joints: **two synovial joints** (the *sacroiliac joints*, Figs. 3-7*B*, 3-8*B*, 3-45*A*, and 4-49) and **two symphyses** (the *symphysis pubis* or pubic symphysis, Figs. 3-8, 3-9, 3-45, and 3-46, and the *sacrococcygeal joint*). The bones involved in the last two joints are connected by a fibrocartilaginous disc as well as by ligaments. These joints of the pelvis are discussed on pages 404 to 407.

For descriptive purposes the pelvis is divided into a **pelvis major** (greater pelvis, false pelvis) and a **pelvis minor** (lesser pelvis, *true pelvis*). Some obstetricians refer to the pelvis minor of the female as the "obstetric pelvis." *The dividing line between the pelvis major and the pelvis minor is an oblique plane that passes through the sacral promontary posteriorly and the lineae terminales* laterally and anteriorly (Fig. 3-8*B*). The **pelvic brim,** surrounding the superior pelvic aperture or pelvic inlet, extends from the **sacral promontory** posteriorly to the top of the **symphysis pubis** anteriorly. The *three parts of the pelvic brim* are (Figs. 3-8*B* and 3-45): (1) anterior border of ala of sacrum (*sacral part*); (2) arcuate line of ilium (*iliac part*); and (3) pecten pubis and pubic crest (*pubic part*).

Main Sex Differences Between Male and Female Pelves (Figs. 3-7 to 3-9, 3-45, 3-46, and 3-49). The pelves of males and females are different in several respects related mainly to the heavier build and the stronger muscles in the male and to the adaption of the female pelvis for childbearing. *The general structure of the male pelvis is heavy and thick and it has more prominent bone markings* than does the female pelvis. In general **the female pelvis is wider and shallower and has larger superior and inferior pelvic apertures** because it surrounds and limits the size of the birth canal (cervix of uterus and the vagina, Fig. 3-22). Using typical male and female pelves (Figs. 3-7 and 3-8), **observe that in females** (1) the hip bones are farther apart owing to the broader sacrum, which explains the relatively wider hips of females; (2) the ischial tuberosities are farther apart because of the greater subpubic angle of the pubic arch (compare Figs. 3-7*A* and 3-9*A* with Figs. 3-8*A* and 3-9*B*); and (3) the sacrum is less curved, which increases the size of the inferior pelvic aperture or pelvic outlet (Figs. 3-9 and 3-46).

CLINICALLY ORIENTED COMMENTS

Although there are usually clear-cut anatomical differences between male and female bony pelves, the pelvis of any person may have anatomical features distinctive of the opposite sex. The diagnosis of pelvic type (Fig. 3-50) is made on overall architecture and not on the appearance of the superior pelvic aperture alone. The presence of certain male characteristics in the female pelvis may offer hazards to successful pelvic delivery of a fetus. This is discussed subsequently.

The Pelvis Major (Figs. 3-7, 3-8, 3-45, and 3-49). The pelvis major (greater pelvis, false pelvis) *lies above the superior pelvic aperture* and the lineae terminales. It is formed on each side by the ala of the sacrum and the concave, fan-shaped iliac fossa and posteriorly by the base of the sacrum. The cavity of the pelvis major is part of the abdominal cavity; hence, it contains abdominal viscera (*e.g.*, the terminal ileum and the sigmoid colon, Figs. 2-33 and 3-49). *The pelvis major is bounded anteriorly by the abdominal wall, laterally by the iliac fossae, and posteriorly by L5 and S1 vertebrae.* Hence, its anterior wall is markedly longer than its posterior wall.

The Pelvis Minor (Figs. 3-7, 3-8, 3-45, and 3-49). The pelvis minor (lesser pelvis, true pelvis) *lies below the superior pelvic aperture* and the lineae terminales and is of great obstetric importance. It is limited superiorly by the **superior aperture of the pelvis** (pelvic inlet) and inferiorly by the **inferior aperture of the pelvis** (pelvic outlet). During life *the pelvis minor contains the pelvic viscera* (urinary bladder, rectum, and parts of the urogenital organs), blood vessels, lymphatics, and nerves.

The cavity of the pelvis minor (pelvic cavity proper) is short and curved and when filled with soft tissues forms a basin that is tilted anteroinferiorly in the anatomical position (Figs. 3-45 and 3-48*B*). *The posterior wall of the cavity of the pelvis minor is notably longer than its anterior wall.* **The posterior wall** is formed by the concave anterior or *pelvic surface of the sacrum* and by the *coccyx* (Fig. 3-45*B*). **The anterior wall** is formed by the *symphysis pubis*, the *body of the pubis*, and the *pubic rami* (Figs. 3-8*B*, 3-45, 3-47, and 3-49). The quadrangular sides of the pelvis minor are formed by the pelvic aspects of the ilium and is-

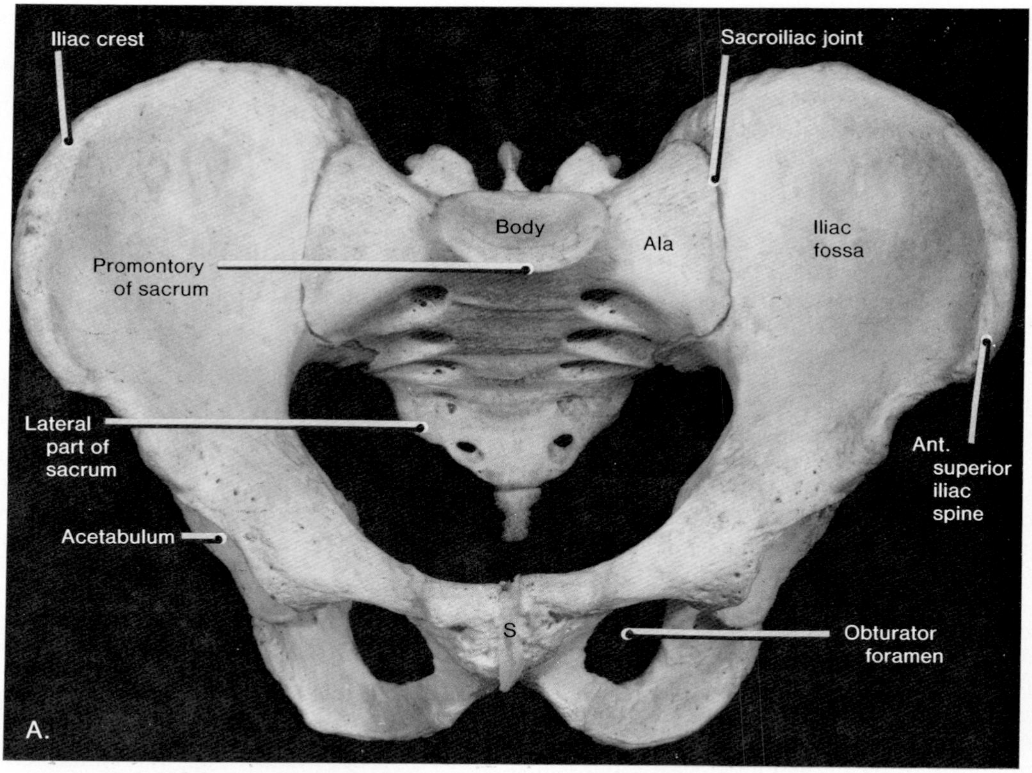

Iliac crest
Sacroiliac joint
Body
Ala
Iliac fossa
Promontory of sacrum
Lateral part of sacrum
Ant. superior iliac spine
Acetabulum
S
Obturator foramen
A.

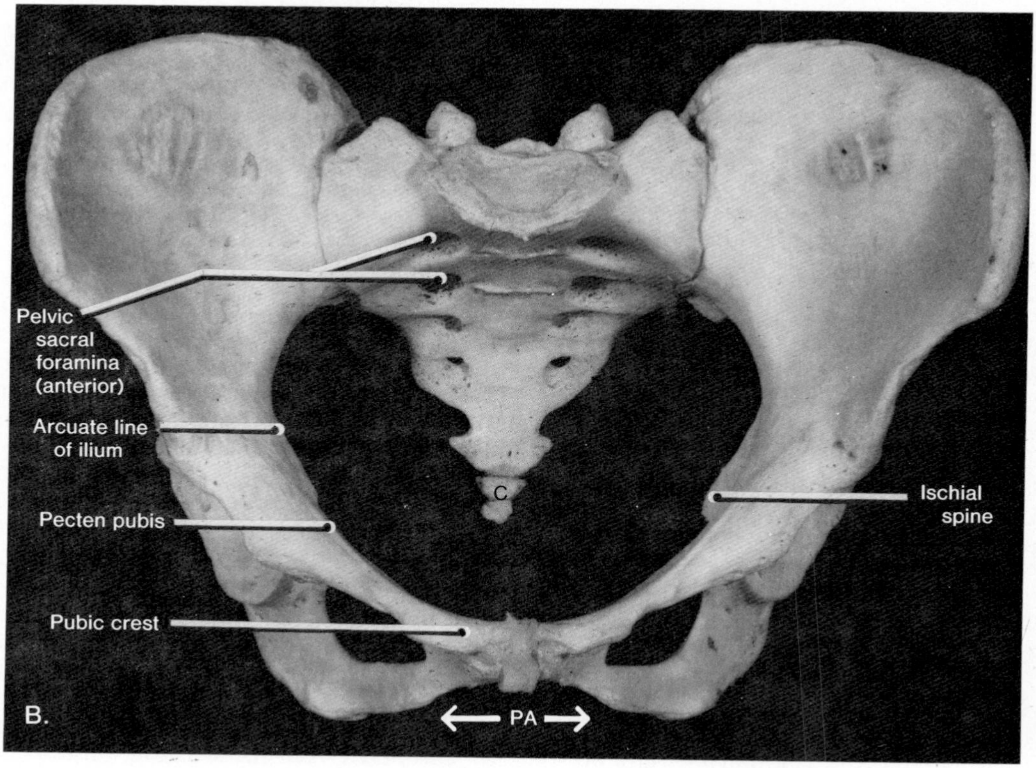

Pelvic sacral foramina (anterior)
Arcuate line of ilium
C
Ischial spine
Pecten pubis
Pubic crest
B.
PA

chium. The **ischial spines** project medially and slightly upward from this surface of the pelvis *when the pelvis is in the anatomical position.* The **sacrospinous ligaments** are attached to the ischial spines and the inferolateral border of the sacrum.

The superior pelvic aperture (pelvic inlet) of the pelvis minor is *variable in contour*. It is heart-shaped in males and in some females (Figs. 3-45*A* and 3-50*C*), but in most females it is larger than in males and is rounded or oval in contour. The superior pelvic aperture is encroached upon by the sacral promontory (Figs. 3-8*B* and 3-45*A*).

The periphery of the superior pelvic aperture is indicated by the lineae terminales (terminal lines) and is often referred to as the **pelvic brim** (Figs. 3-51 and 3-52). Each linea terminalis begins at the top of the symphysis pubis and is formed by (1) the **pubic crest**, (2) the **pecten pubis**, and (3) the **arcuate line** of the ilium.

CLINICALLY ORIENTED COMMENTS

The superior pelvic aperture is routinely measured for obstetric reasons during a pelvic examination (Fig. 3-52). Do not try to memorize these measurements at this time.

The anteroposterior (AP) diameter (true conjugate) of the superior pelvic aperture is the measurement from the *midpoint of the superior border of the symphysis pubis to the midpoint of the sacral promontory* (Fig. 3-52*B*). The average figure is 11.2 cm in females. In the **android type of pelvis** (Fig. 3-50*C*), this measurement is about 10.0 cm.

The diagonal conjugate diameter of the pelvis is the measurement from the *midpoint of the inferior border of the symphysis pubis to the midpoint of the sacral promontory* (Fig. 3-45*A*). Usually the diagonal conjugate measurement is 1.5 cm more than the AP or true conjugate measurement. The AP diameter is determined by inserting the index and middle fingers into the vagina until the middle finger touches the sacral promontory and the upper edge of the index finger is against the inferoposterior border of the symphysis pubis. The AP diameter of the pelvis can be estimated by measuring the distance between the fingers and subtracting 1.5 cm. If one's middle finger cannot reach the sacral promontory, the pelvis is usually considered to be large enough for normal childbirth.

The transverse diameter of the superior pelvic aperture is its greatest width, measured transversely from the linea terminalis on one side to this line on the opposite side. The average figure is 13.1 cm in females. In android pelves (Fig. 3-50*C*), this measurement is 12.5 cm or less.

The oblique diameter of the superior pelvic aperture is measured from one **iliopubic eminence** (Figs. 3-7*B* and 3-47) to the opposite **sacroiliac joint**. The average oblique diameter in females is 12.5 cm. In the android type of pelvis (Fig. 3-50*C*), this measurement is about 12.0 cm. In some cases pelvic measurements are made using radiographs (Fig. 3-49).

A general idea of the shape and position of the sacrum can be developed by palpating the sacral concavity during a **pelvic examination**. The *ischial spines* (Figs. 3-7*B*, 3-45*B*, and 3-47) can also be palpated and a general concept of their prominence can be obtained.

The midplane (interspinous) diameter of the pelvis (plane of least pelvic dimension

Figure 3-45. Photographs of male (*A*) and female (*B*) bony pelves from the front, in the anatomical position (*i.e.*, the anterior superior iliac spines and the superior end of the symphysis pubis (*S*) lie in the same coronal plane; also see Fig. 3-48*B*). Observe that the superior pelvic aperture (pelvic inlet) is larger in the female. This aperture (outlined by the pelvic brim) is the boundary between the pelvis major and the pelvis minor, the true or "obstetric" pelvis. Pelves are classified according to the shape of the superior pelvic aperture (see Fig. 3-50). Note that the pubic arch (*PA*) is very wide in the female pelvis; consequently, the subpubic angle in the female is much wider than in the male (also examine Figs. 3-7*A* and 3-8*A*). When the vagina will admit three fingers placed side by side in the subpubic angle the pelvis is considered adequate to permit proper extension of the fetal head after it has passed through the inferior pelvic aperture (pelvic outlet).

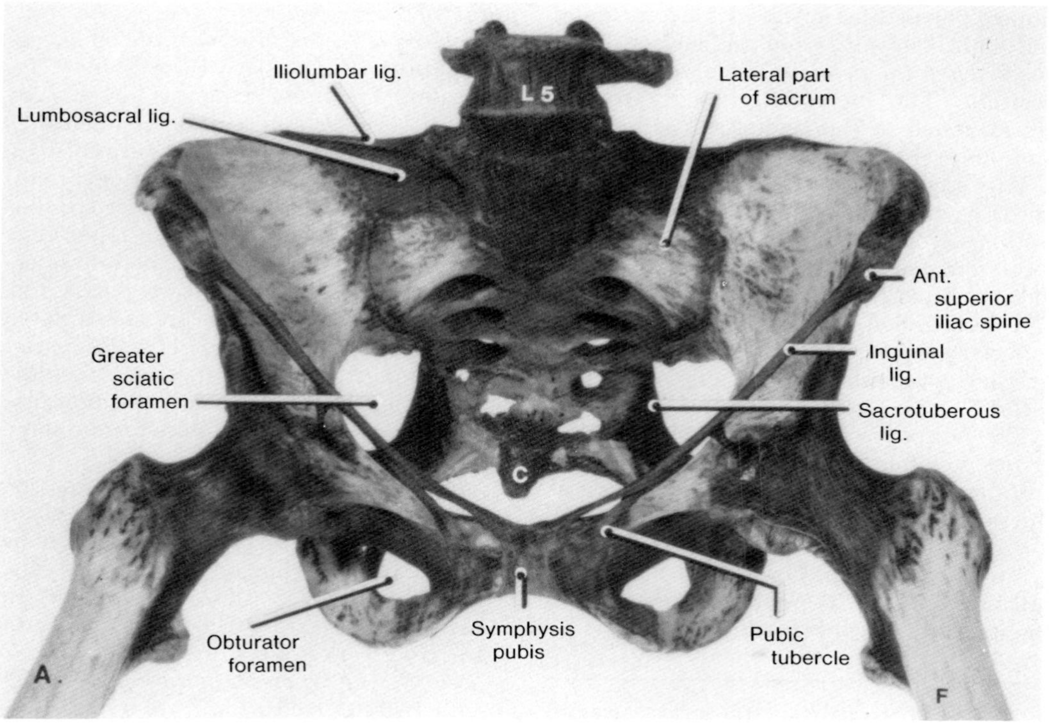
Iliolumbar lig.
L5
Lateral part of sacrum
Lumbosacral lig.
Ant. superior iliac spine
Greater sciatic foramen
Inguinal lig.
Sacrotuberous lig.
C
Obturator foramen
Symphysis pubis
Pubic tubercle
A.
F

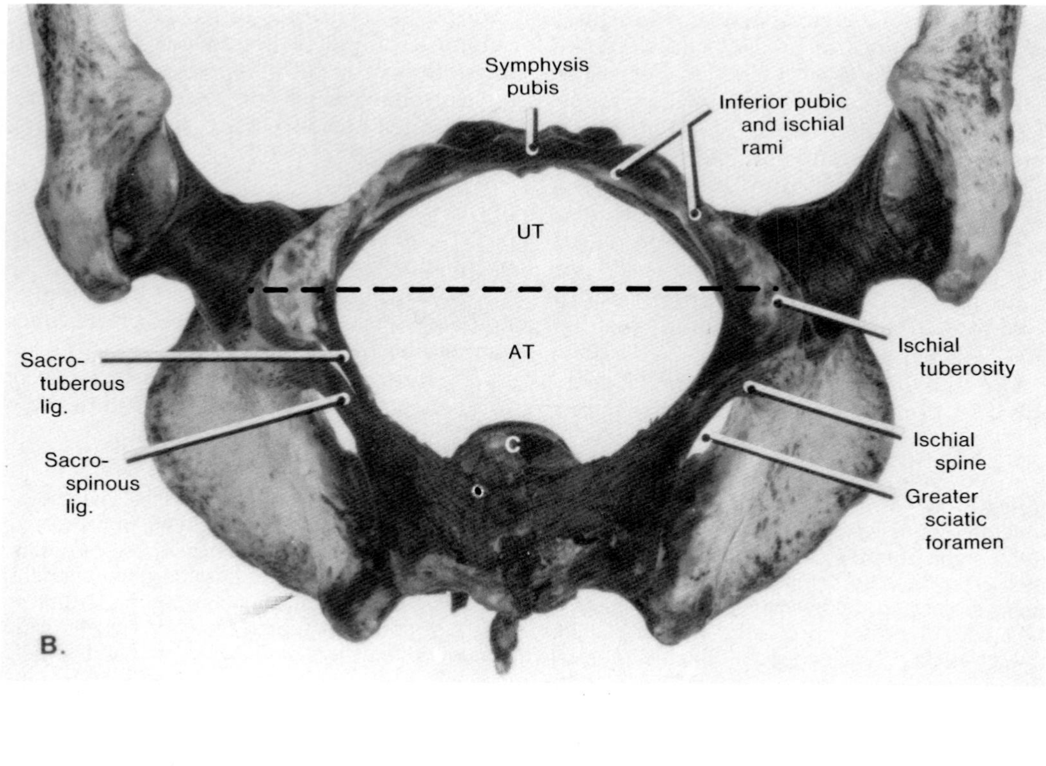
Symphysis pubis
Inferior pubic and ischial rami
UT
AT
Ischial tuberosity
Sacro-tuberous lig.
Sacro-spinous lig.
C
Ischial spine
Greater sciatic foramen
B.

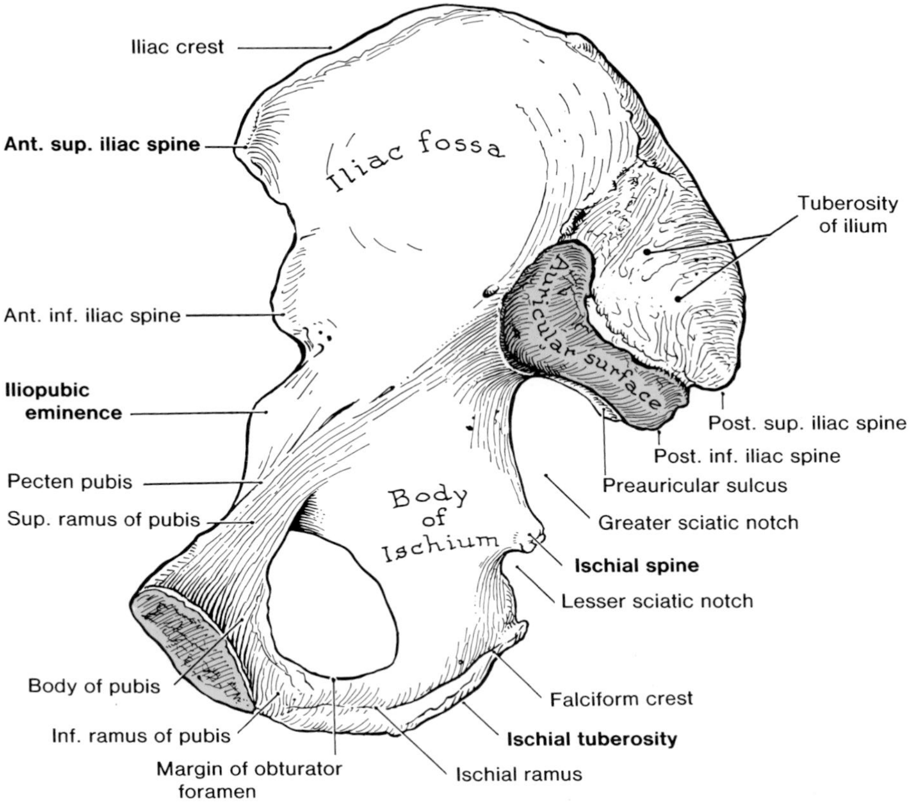

Figure 3-47. Drawing of the medial aspect of the right os coxae or hip bone. This bone consists of three parts, the *ilium*, the *ischium*, and the *pubis*, which are fused together in adults. Fusion of these bones occurs around the 16th year. (For a drawing of the os coxae of a child, see Fig. 4-4). Note that the ilium is fan-shaped. The spread of the fan is called the *ala* (L. wing) and its broad handle is called the body. The iliac crest is the rim of the fan and the iliac fossa is the concavity of the ala (see Fig. 4-7 for the surface features of this bone).

Figure 3-46. Photographs of a bony female pelvis with the femora (*F*) of the lower limbs and the ligaments of the pelvis and the hip joint attached. *A*, *anterior view*. Observe the inguinal ligament extending from the pubic tubercle to the anterior superior iliac spine (also see Figs. 4-18 to 4-20). Note the strong iliolumbar ligament which unites the transverse process of L5 vertebra to the internal lip of the iliac crest (also see Fig. 3-7*B*). Its inferior fibers attach to the lateral part of the sacrum as the lateral lumbosacral ligament. *B*, *inferior view* showing the inferior pelvic aperture as visualized by the obstetrician when the patient is in the lithotomy position (Fig. 3-1). The perineum fills this large aperture (Figs. 3-2 and 3-3), which lies between the upper parts of the thighs and the lower parts of the buttocks (see Figs. 3-3 and 3-39). Here, the diamond-shaped perineal region (Fig. 3-5) is divided by a transverse *broken line* (-----) passing through the ischial tuberosities immediately anterior to the anus into (1) an anterior urogenital region or triangle (*UT*) and (2) a posterior anal region or triangle (*AT*). Examine the sacrotuberous ligaments which have a wide origin from the dorsal surfaces of the sacrum and coccyx (*C*) and from both posterior superior iliac spines (Fig. 3-45). Note that they pass to the upper medial impressions on the ischial tuberosities and extend along their medial margins.

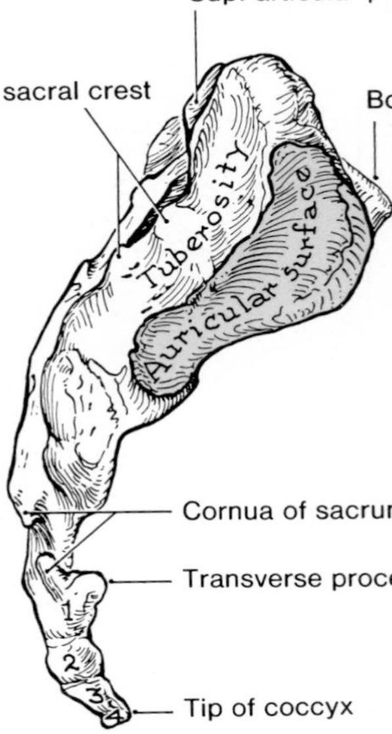

A.

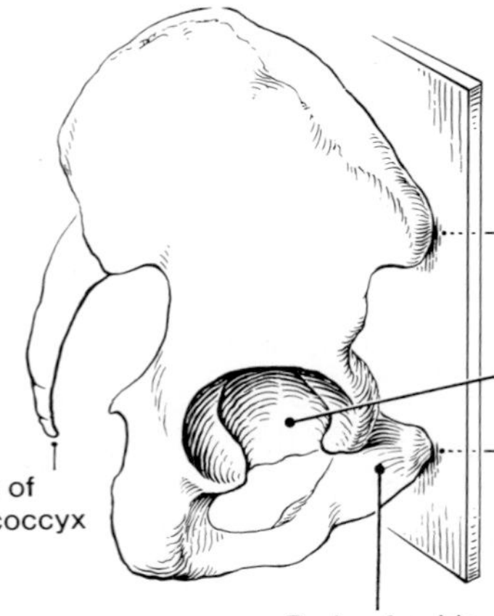

B.

Figure 3-48. *A*, drawing of the right lateral aspect of the sacrum and coccyx. (For other illustrations of these bones, see Figs. 5-24 and 5-25). *B*, drawing of the lateral aspect of the right os coxae or hip bone and coccyx demonstrating that in the anatomical position the anterior superior iliac spine and the superior margin of the symphysis pubis lie in a coronal plane, as though against a wall as illustrated. Note that the tip of coccyx is on a level with the superior half of the body of the pubis.

between the ischial spines) cannot be measured, but it *may be estimated by palpating the sacrospinous ligament during a vaginal examination* (Figs. 3-18 and 3-46*B*). Its length is equal to about half the midplane diameter (about three fingerbreadths). The average measurement of the midplane diameter is 10 cm or more. Obviously *the ischial spines may be a barrier to the passage of the fetal head* during childbirth if they are closer than 9.5 cm.

The inferior pelvic aperture (pelvic outlet) of the pelvis minor does not have a smooth contour (Figs. 3-9 and 3-46*B*) because it is bounded posteriorly by the *coccyx* and the *sacrum*, anteriorly by the *symphysis pubis*, and laterally by the *ischial tuberosities*. The plane of the inferior pelvic aperture makes an angle of 10 to 15° with the horizontal when the pelvis is in the anatomical position (Figs. 3-45 and 3-48*B*).

Observe the two large **sciatic notches** between the sacrum and the coccyx and the ischial tuberosities (Figs. 3-8*B* and 3-47). Note that they are divided into **greater** and **lesser sciatic foramina** by the sacrotuberous and sacrospinous ligaments (Figs. 3-18 and 3-46). These dense ligaments give the inferior pelvic aperture a diamond shape. In Figures 3-9 and 3-46 examine the periphery of the inferior pelvic aperture. The transverse distance between the ischial tuberosities (**intertuberous distance**) in the female pelvis is usually 10 cm or more. This distance can be measured by placing the clenched fist between the **ischial tuberosities**. The distance across the knuckles (excluding the thumb) of the average male hand is 9 to 10 cm.

The anteroposterior (AP) diameter of the inferior pelvic aperture is usually about 11.5 cm. This is measured from the inferior margin of the pubis to the tip of the sacrum (*i.e.*, at the sacrococcygeal joint).

In Figures 3-7 to 3-9, 3-45, and 3-49 examine the **pubic arch**. *Note that the subpubic angle is narrow in the male and wide in the female.* Also observe that this angle in the female is rounded (Fig. 3-8*A*). Verify that the subpubic angle of a male pelvis is about one fingerbreadth (Figs. 3-7*A* and 3-45*A*), whereas this angle in most females accommodates three average fingers. (Figs. 3-8*B* and 3-45*B*).

CLINICALLY ORIENTED COMMENTS

In forensic medicine the bony pelvis is a reliable indicator of sex; even parts of a pelvis may give good clues as to the sex of the person from whom it came.

To pass through the birth canal (cervix and vagina, Fig. 3-22) from the superior pelvic aperture to the inferior pelvic aperture, the fetal head must make almost a 90° turn to follow the *pelvic axis* (Fig. 3-53).

The gynecoid pelvis (Fig. 3-50*D*) has a wide, circular superior pelvic aperture with a wide subpubic arch and widely-spaced ischial spines (Figs. 3-9 and 3-46). *Usually a woman with a gynecoid pelvis has a reasonably uneventful delivery.*

The android pelvis (Fig. 3-50*C*) has a heart-shaped superior pelvic aperture and somewhat resembles the male pelvis (Fig. 3-45*A*). The ischial spines are usually quite prominent and the subpubic angle is narrow. In these cases the fetal head has difficulty engaging or entering the superior pelvic aperture; as a result, labor is likely to be difficult. *Android pelves are about twice as common in white females as in non-whites.*

The anthropoid pelvis, or ape-like pelvis (Fig. 3-50*A*), is fairly common (about 23% of females). Its sides are long and narrow and the AP diameter of the superior pelvic aperture is greater than the transverse diameter. The sacrum is also long; consequently the pelvic cavity is deep. The subpubic angle is narrow and the ischial spines are prominent. *Difficulty in delivery*

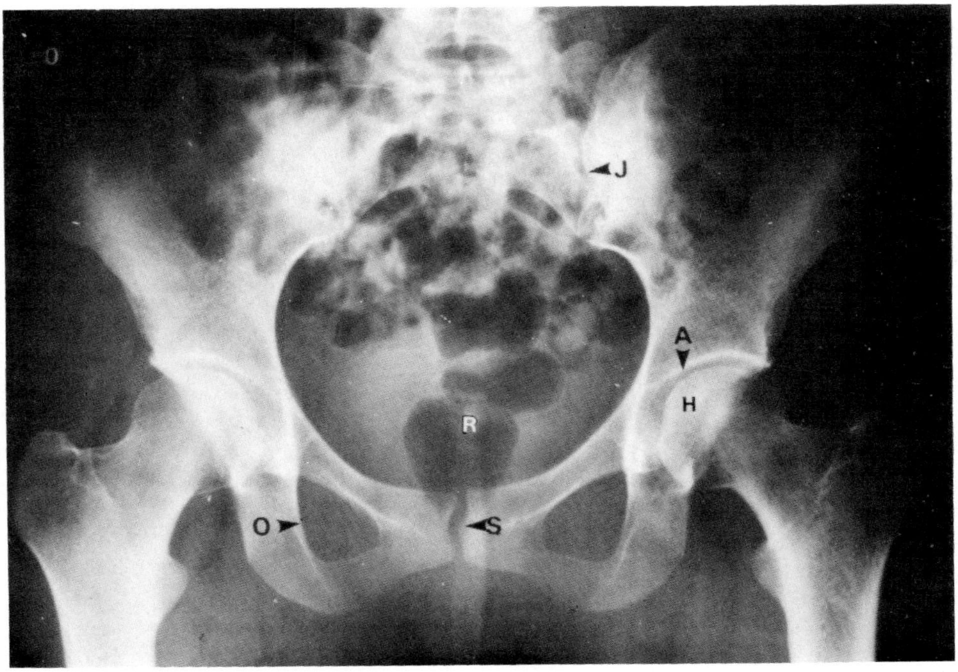

Figure 3-49. Anteroposterior (*AP*) radiograph of the female pelvis. Note that there is a considerable amount of air in the rectum (*R*). The *arrows* point to the symphysis pubis (*S*), the sacroiliac joint (*J*), the roof or superior surface of the cup-shaped acetabulum (*A*), and the margin of the obturator foramen (*O*). *H* indicates the part of the head of the femur which is overlapped by the anterior and posterior parts of the acetabulum. (For details of the hip joint, see Chap. 4 and Figs. 4-41, 4-113, and 4-117).

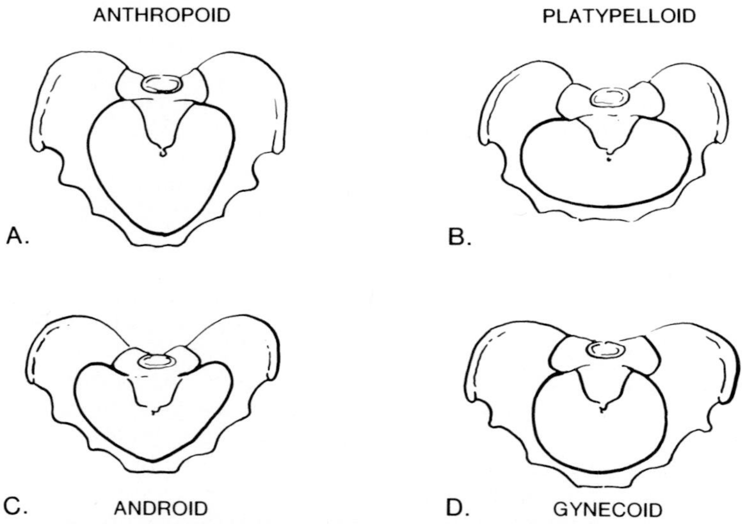

Figure 3-50. Drawings illustrating the four types of pelvis. The types shown in *A* and *C* are most common in males, whereas those illustrated in *C* and *D* are common in females. *B* is uncommon in both sexes. *A*, **anthropoid pelvis** (present in some males and in about 23.5% of females). Note that the AP diameter of the superior pelvic aperture is greater than the transverse diameter. *B*, **platypelloid pelvis** (rare in males; present in about 2.5% of females). Observe that the pelvis is flat because its transverse diameter is greater than its anteroposterior diameter. *C*, **android pelvis** (present in most males and in about 32.5% of females). Note that the superior pelvic aperture has a wide transverse diameter, but the posterior part of the aperture is narrow with an almost triangular anterior segment. Observe that the superior pelvic aperture has the shape of a "heart" or a valentine. *D*, **gynecoid pelvis** (present in about 42% of females). This is the most common type of pelvis in females and is the most roomy obstetrically.

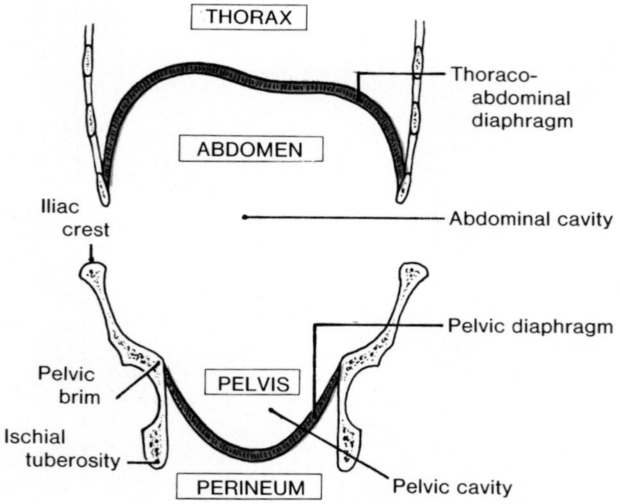

Figure 3-51. Drawing of the thoracoabdominal diaphragm (*the diaphragm*) and the pelvic diaphragm in coronal section. The perineum is the region caudal (inferior) to the pelvic diaphragm. The pelvic cavity is that part of the abdominal cavity enclosed within the pelvis minor or true bony pelvis. The pelvic brim surrounds the pelvic inlet or superior pelvic aperture. The pelvic diaphragm is formed by the two levatores ani and the two coccygeus muscles (Figs. 3-55 and 3-57). When the term diaphragm is used without qualification, it is usually the thoracoabdominal diaphragm that is meant.

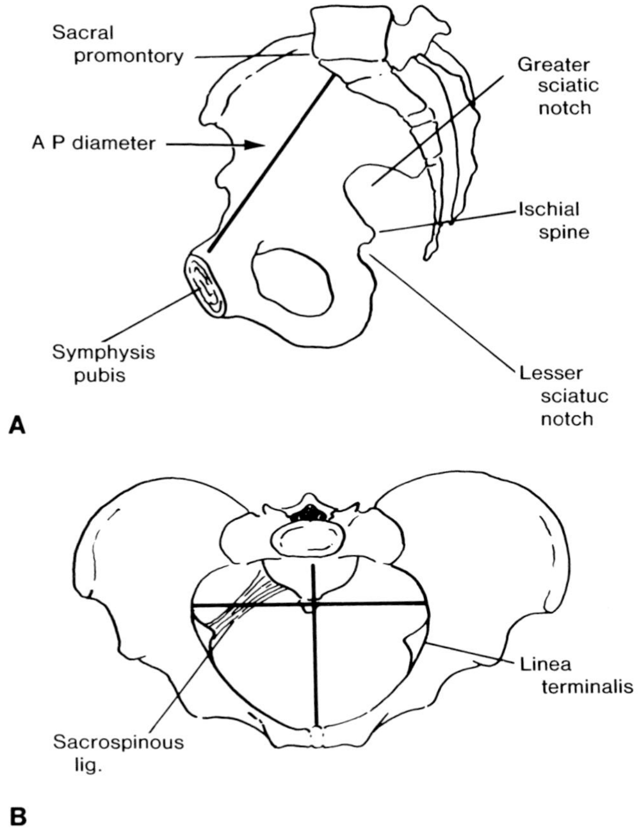

Figure 3-52. Drawings of the female pelvis illustrating the anteroposterior (AP) and transverse diameters of the superior pelvic aperture. These pelvic planes are useful as obstetrical measurements. Observe that the transverse diameter of the superior pelvic aperture is greater than its AP diameter. A pelvis in which any major plane is reduced below normal is called a *contracted pelvis.*

may be encountered owing to the narrowness of the transverse diameter of the superior pelvic aperture.

The platypelloid pelvis (Fig. 3-50*B*) is a flattened type of pelvis which fortunately is present in only about 2.5% of females. The adjective *platypelloid* is derived from the Greek words *platys*, meaning broad or flat, and *pellis*, meaning bowl. Hence, it resembles a shallow, flat bowl; in addition the sacrum is shorter than usual. *The AP diameter of the superior pelvic aperture is short and the transverse diameter is long.* In patients with this type of pelvis, there may be difficulty with the fetal head engaging in the superior pelvic aperture. In some cases, delivery of the fetus by **cesarean section** may be necessary. This is an incision through the anterior abdominal wall and the anterior wall of the uterus through which the fetus is removed. *This operation was named not because it was performed at the birth of Julius Caesar*, but because it was included under *lex cesararea* (Roman law).

The bony pelvis is able to resist considerable trauma. Violent injuries are required to fracture the adult pelvis (*e.g.*, automobile accidents, Fig. 3-54). Lateral parts of the hip bone or os coxae are the strongest. *Pelvic weak areas* are (1) the sacroiliac region, (2) the ala of the ilium, and (3) the pubic rami. *Fractures of the pelvis in the pubo-obturator area are relatively common* and are often complicated because of their relationship to the urinary bladder. (See Case 3-6 and Fig. 3-105.)

Anteroposterior compression of the pel-

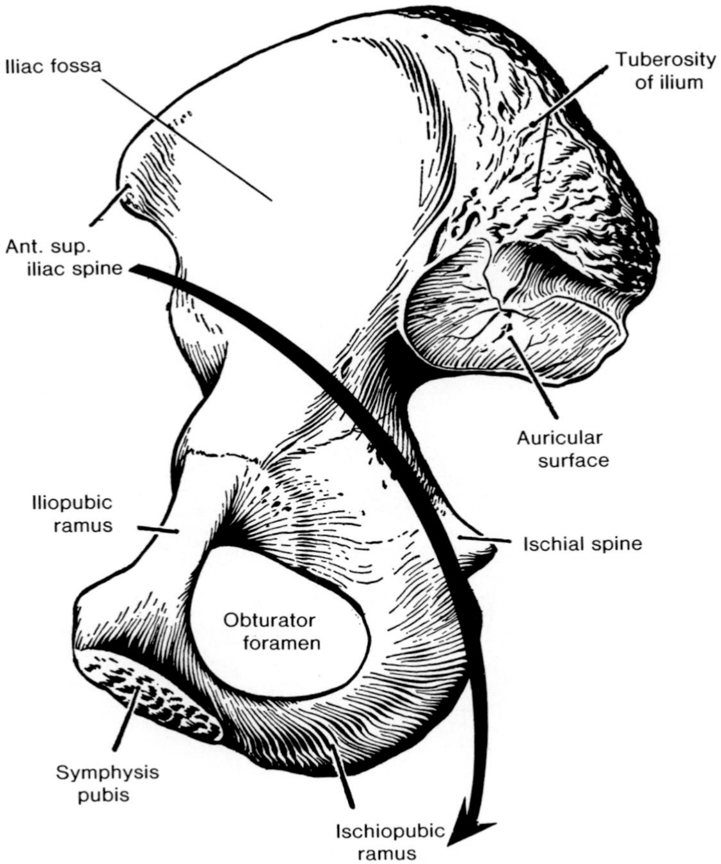

Figure 3-53. Drawing of the medial or internal surface of the right hip bone (os coxae). The *black arrow* indicates the pelvic axis and the path taken by the fetal head during its passage through the birth canal (see Fig. 3-106). Using this drawing, examine a female bony pelvis verifying that in passing through the birth canal (cervix and vagina, Fig. 3-22) from the superior pelvic aperture to the inferior pelvic aperture, the fetal head must make a turn of about 90° to follow the path of the pelvic axis.

vis occurs during "squeezing accidents" and commonly fractures the pubic rami. In severe cases adjacent bones may also be broken. When the pelvis is compressed from the side, the acetabula and the ilia are squeezed toward each other and may be broken. Some fractures of the pelvis result from a tearing away of bone by the posterior ligaments associated with the **sacroiliac joints** (Figs. 3-46*B* and 3-102).

In falls on the feet or on the ischial tuberosities, (1) the pubic arch of the pelvis may be fractured, (2) the acetabula may be injured, and (3) the femora may be driven through the acetabular fossae (Figs. 3-49 and 3-54) into the pelvis, injuring the pelvic organs. In persons under 17 years, the acetabula may fracture into their three developmental parts (Fig. 4-4) or the acetabular margins may be torn away.

Direct violence may also fracture the sacrum, the iliac crest, or any other part of the bony pelvis. *Pelvic fractures are often complicated by damage to the pelvic viscera* (*e.g.,* rupture of the bladder and/or urethra) or to the large pelvic vessels, resulting in extensive internal hemorrhage. (See Case 3-6 and Fig. 3-105.)

The Vertebropelvic Ligaments (Figs. 3-18 and 3-46). The parts of the bony pelvis are bound together by dense ligaments. The ilium is united to L5 vertebra by the *ilio-*

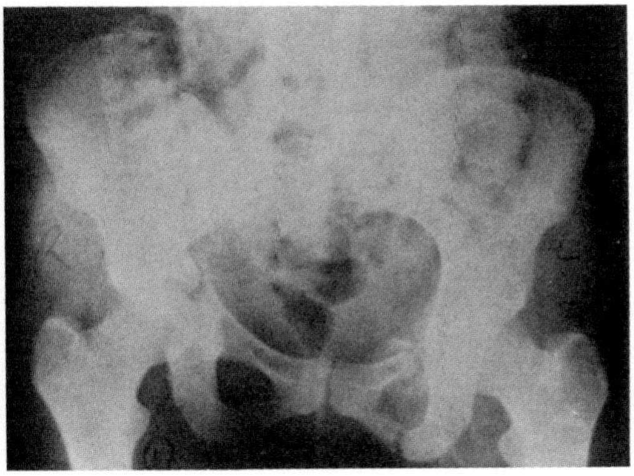

Figure 3-54. Radiograph of the pelvis of a 44-year-old woman who was involved in a serious automobile accident. Observe the vertical fracture of the ilium just lateral to the right sacroiliac joint. Also note that the superior and inferior pubic rami are fractured on the left side and that there is a fracture of the right acetabulum. The right segment of the fractured pelvis, which has shifted upward, was free to move forward and inward.

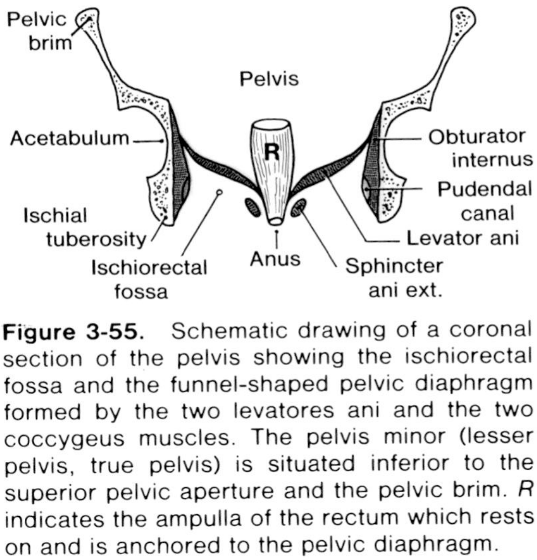

Figure 3-55. Schematic drawing of a coronal section of the pelvis showing the ischiorectal fossa and the funnel-shaped pelvic diaphragm formed by the two levatores ani and the two coccygeus muscles. The pelvis minor (lesser pelvis, true pelvis) is situated inferior to the superior pelvic aperture and the pelvic brim. *R* indicates the ampulla of the rectum which rests on and is anchored to the pelvic diaphragm.

lumbar ligaments and the sacrum is joined to the ischium by the *sacrotuberous* and *sacrospinous ligaments.*

The iliolumbar ligament (Fig. 3-46), strong and triangular, connects the tip and the lower and anterior part of each transverse process of L5 vertebra to the internal lip of each iliac crest posteriorly (Fig. 3-7*B*). Occasionally this ligament is also attached to L4 vertebra. The lower fibers of the iliolumbar ligament are attached to the lateral part of the sacrum; this band is called the **lateral lumbosacral ligament**. *The iliolumbar ligaments are important because they* (1) limit axial rotation of L5 vertebra on the sacrum and (2) *assist the vertebral articular processes in preventing forward gliding of L5* vertebra on the sacrum.

The sacrotuberous ligament (Figs. 3-3, 3-18, 3-21, and 3-46), as its name indicates, *passes from the sacrum to the ischial tuberosity*. It has a wide origin from the dorsal surfaces of the sacrum and the coccyx and the posterior superior iliac spines. Its fibers run inferolaterally to be attached into the upper medial impression on the ischial tuberosity and extend along its medial margin.

The sacrospinous ligament (Figs. 3-18, 3-46, and 4-115), thin and triangular, *extends from the lateral margin of the sacrum and coccyx to the ischial spine.* It is related anteriorly to the coccygeus muscle and some anatomists consider it to be the fibrous degenerated part of this muscle. The sacrum is wedged between the iliac bones (Figs. 3-7, 3-8, and 3-49) and is held in position by the powerful **interosseous** and **dorsal sacroiliac ligaments** (Figs. 3-101 and 4-44). These important ligaments are discussed subsequently with the sacroiliac joints.

The sacrotuberous and sacrospinous ligaments bind the sacrum to the ischium and resist backward rotation of the inferior end of the sacrum. They also hold the posterior part of the sacrum down, thereby preventing the body weight from depressing its anterior part around the sacroiliac joints (Figs. 3-7*B* and 3-102). The sacrotuberous and sacrospinous ligaments permit some movement of the sacrum, which gives resilience to this region when sudden weight increases are applied to the vertebral column (*e.g.*, when landing on the feet during a fall).

CLINICALLY ORIENTED COMMENTS

Progressively during pregnancy, the vertebropelvic ligaments relax and move-

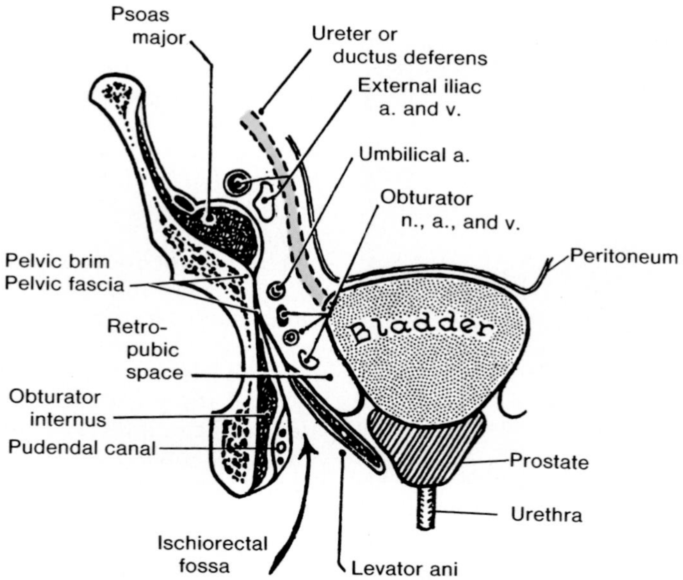

Figure 3-56. Diagrammatic drawing of the side wall of the male pelvis in coronal section. Observe that the intrapelvic surfaces of the muscles lining the walls of the pelvic cavity are covered with pelvic fascia and that this fascia is firmly attached to the pelvic brim surrounding the superior pelvic aperture (pelvic inlet).

ments between the vertebral column and the pelvis become freer. Furthermore, the symphysis pubis relaxes owing to a hormone called **relaxin** and the distance between the pubic bones increases considerably. These changes facilitate passage of the fetus through the birth canal during parturition.

MUSCLES OF THE LATERAL PELVIC WALLS

The walls of the pelvic cavity are lined in part with muscles (Figs. 3-55 to 3-58); however, *no muscles cross the pelvic brim* which surrounds the superior pelvic aperture (pelvic inlet). The muscles of the lateral pelvic walls (piriformis and obturator internus) pass from the pelvis into the gluteal region, where they form part of the muscle group which rotates the thigh at the hip joint (Figs. 4-44 and 4-47).

The Piriformis Muscle (Figs. 3-27, 3-57, 3-58, 4-30, 4-45 to 4-47, and 4-52). *This small pear-shaped muscle* (L. *pirum*, pear + *forma*, form) *occupies a key position in the gluteal region* (see Chap. 4). The piriformis is located partly within the pelvis minor (on its posterior wall) and partly posterior to the hip joint.

Origin (Figs. 3-27, 3-57, and 3-58). Anterior aspect of second, third, and fourth **lateral masses of sacrum** and **sacrotuberous ligament**.

Insertion (Figs. 4-30 and 4-44). Upper border of **greater trochanter of femur**. *It leaves the pelvis via the greater sciatic foramen* (Figs. 3-18 and 4-44) and passes posterior to the head of the femur to reach its insertion. Within the pelvis *the piriformis forms a muscular bed* (Fig. 3-58) *for the sacral plexus* of nerves.

Nerve Supply (Fig. 3-58). Branches of ventral rami of **first** and **second sacral** nerves.

Actions. **Laterally rotates thigh** when hip joint is extended and **abducts thigh** when hip joint is flexed. *Assists in holding head of femur in acetabulum.*

The Obturator Internus Muscle (Figs. 3-27, 3-55, 3-56, and 4-45 to 4-47). This *thick, fan-shaped muscle* of the hip and thigh (Chap. 4) is situated partly within the pelvis minor and partly posterior to the hip joint. It covers most of the side wall of the pelvis minor.

Origin (Fig. 3-55). Almost entire internal

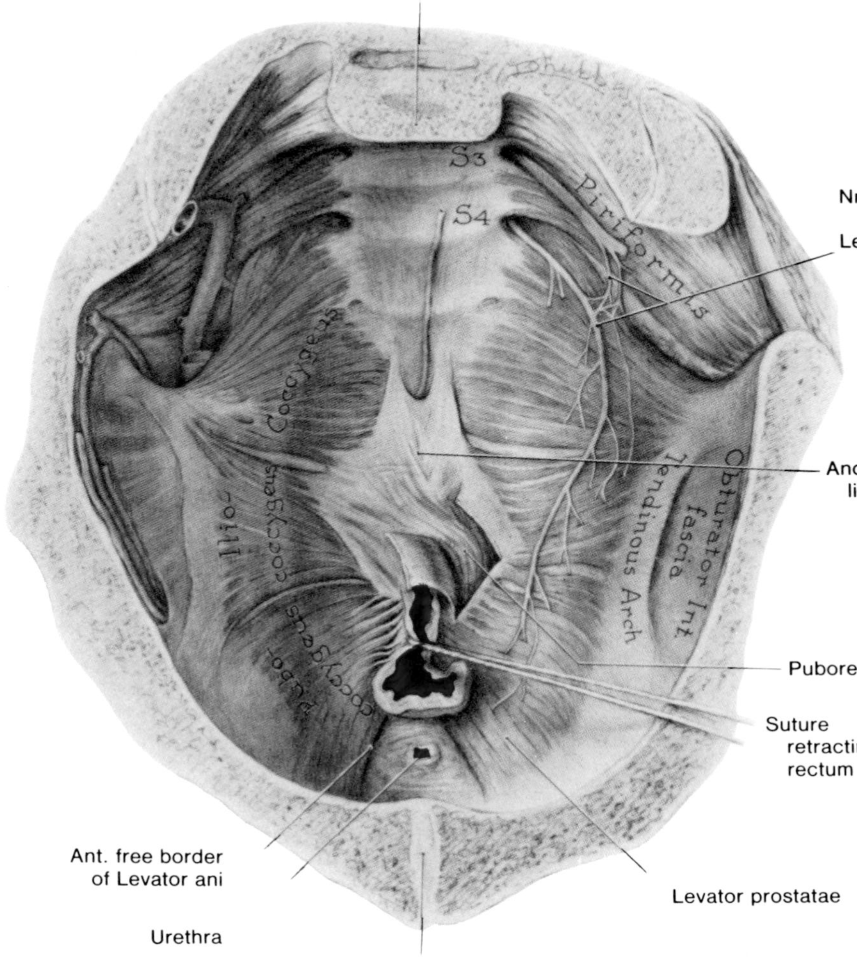

Figure 3-57. Drawing of a dissection of the floor of the male pelvis *from above.* The pelvic viscera are removed and the bony pelvis is sawn through transversely. Observe the pubococcygeus, the part of the levator ani muscle arising mainly from the pubic bone, the coccyygeus arising from the ischial spine, and the iliococcygeus arising from the tendinous arch in between. The pubococcygeus is strong, the iliococcygeus is weak, and the coccygeus is largely transformed into the sacrospinous ligament (Fig. 3-18). Note that the urethra passes between the anterior borders of the pubococcygei and that the rectum perforates the pubococcygei: thus (1) the anterior fibers of the muscles of opposite sides meet and unite in the central perineal tendon (perineal body) in front of the rectum; (2) the posterior fibers unite behind the rectum in an aponeurosis that extends backward to the anterior sacrococcygeal ligament; (3) the middle fibers blend with the outer wall of the anal canal and pass between the internal and external sphincters of the anus; and (4) on the left side this aponeurosis is reflected to show the puborectalis (also see Fig. 3-61). Examine the branches of S3 and S4 nerves supplying the levator ani and the coccygeus muscles. (The pudendal nerve, via its perineal branch, also supplies the levator ani).

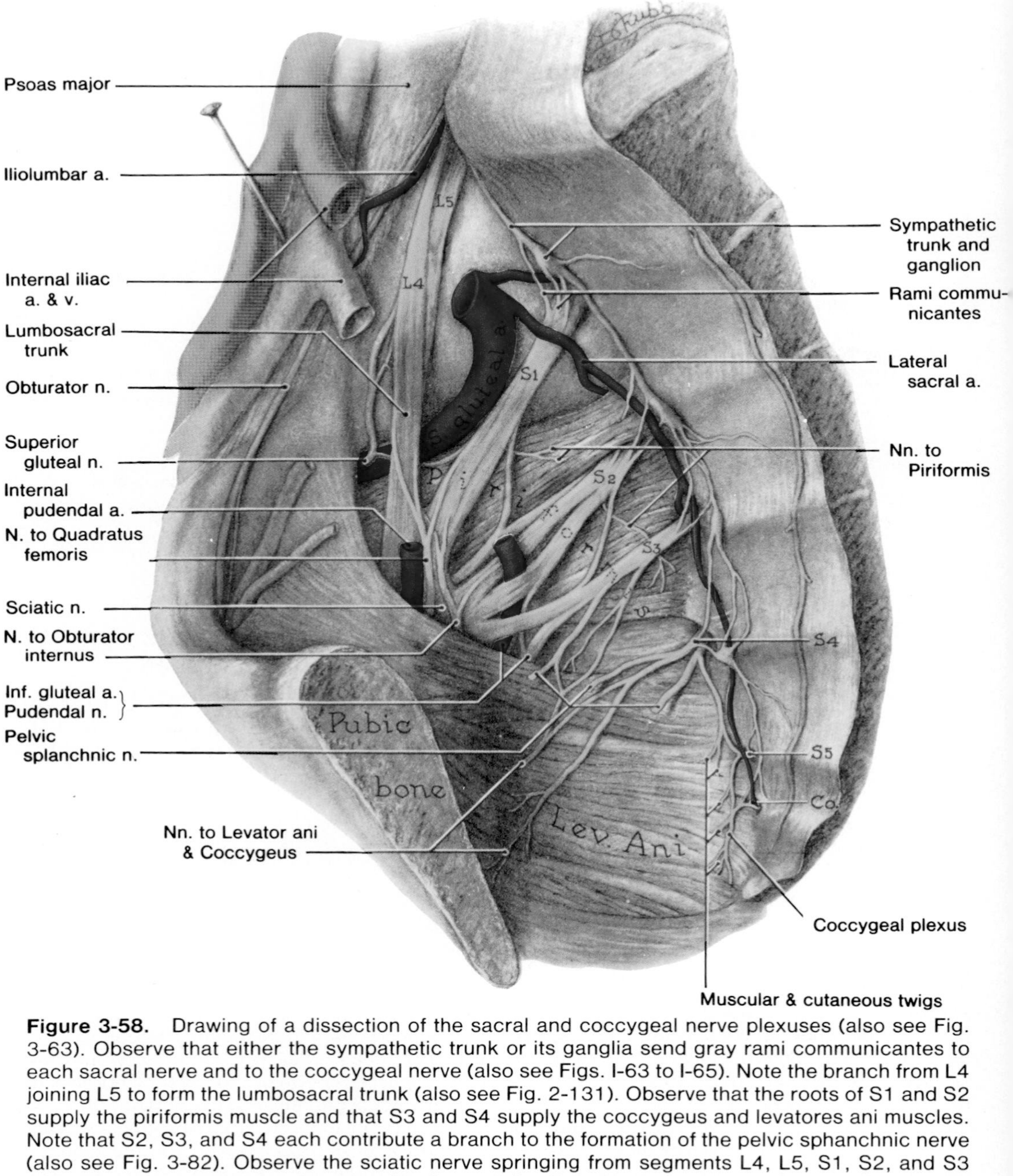

Figure 3-58. Drawing of a dissection of the sacral and coccygeal nerve plexuses (also see Fig. 3-63). Observe that either the sympathetic trunk or its ganglia send gray rami communicantes to each sacral nerve and to the coccygeal nerve (also see Figs. I-63 to I-65). Note the branch from L4 joining L5 to form the lumbosacral trunk (also see Fig. 2-131). Observe that the roots of S1 and S2 supply the piriformis muscle and that S3 and S4 supply the coccygeus and levatores ani muscles. Note that S2, S3, and S4 each contribute a branch to the formation of the pelvic sphanchnic nerve (also see Fig. 3-82). Observe the sciatic nerve springing from segments L4, L5, S1, S2, and S3 and the pudendal nerve arising from S2, S3, and S4. Examine the coccygeal plexus (*CO*) formed from S4 and S5. Note the iliolumbar artery accompanying L5 nerve; the branches of the lateral sacral artery accompanying the sacral nerves; and the superior gluteal artery passing backward between L5 and S1 nerves (its position is not constant).

surface of **anterolateral wall of pelvis minor**, including the margins of the **obturator foramen** and the **obturator membrane**.

Insertion (Fig. 4-30). Medial surface of **greater trochanter of femur**. From its wide origin, the fibers of the obturator internus converge on a strong tendon which *passes through the lesser sciatic foramen* (Fig. 4-47) and makes a right angle turn around the lesser sciatic notch to enter the gluteal region and pass to its insertion.

Nerve Supply (Figs. 3-58 and 4-52). **Nerve to obturator internus** (L5 and S1).

Actions. **Laterally rotates thigh** when hip joint is flexed (see Chap. 4). **Assists in holding head of femur in acetabulum.**

MUSCLES OF THE PELVIC FLOOR

The two levatores ani muscles and the two coccygeus muscles, with their superior and inferior investing fasciae, **form the funnel-shaped pelvic diaphragm** (Figs. 3-13, 3-17, and 3-55 to 3-57). *The pelvic diaphragm forms the fibromuscular floor of the confluent abdominopelvic cavities* (Figs. 2-30, 3-13, and 3-17) *and supports the contents of the pelvis.*

The Levator Ani Muscle (Figs. 3-4, 3-13 to 3-15, 3-17, 3-23, 3-24, and 3-55 to 3-60). *This pair of broad, thin curved sheets of muscle forms the largest and most important part of the clinically significant pelvic diaphragm.* The levatores ani muscles stretch between the pubis anteriorly and the coccyx posteriorly and from one side wall of the pelvis to the other.

The levatores ani muscles form most of the floor of the pelvic cavity which separates this cavity from the ischiorectal fossae. The funnel-shaped muscular floor (pelvic diaphragm) is perforated by the **urethra** and the **anal canal** *in the male* (Figs. 3-6, 3-13, 3-21, and 3-38) and by the **urethra,** the **vagina,** and the **anal canal** *in the female* (Figs. 3-15 and 3-23).

Origin (Figs. 3-56 to 3-59). Linear origin from **pelvic surface of body of pubis to ischial spine.** Between these bony attachments, it arises from a **tendinous arch** formed by *a thickening of the parietal pelvic fascia* covering the obturator internus muscle.

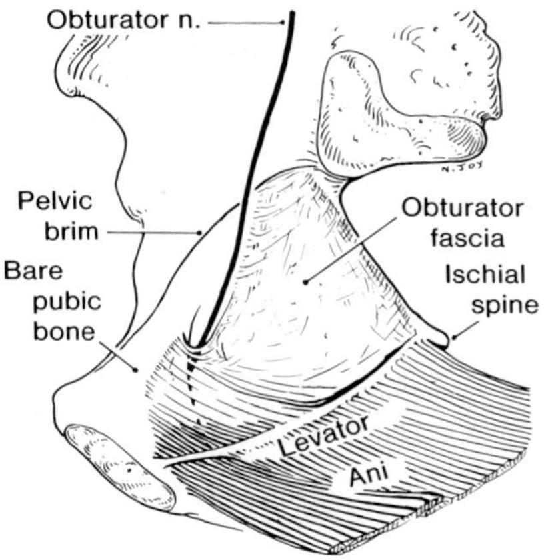

Figure 3-59. Drawing of the side wall of the pelvis illustrating the origin of the levator ani muscle from the body of the pubis, the ischial spine, and the tendinous arch in between these points. The tendinous arch is a thickened band in the obturator fascia.

Insertion (Figs. 3-12, 3-22, and 3-60). The two muscles, one on each side, converge and are inserted together into (1) the **central perineal tendon** (perineal body), (2) the **wall of the anal canal,** (3) the **anococcygeal ligament** (body, raphe), and (4) the **coccyx.** The anterior fibers of both levatores ani muscles pass horizontally backward, inferior to the prostate, to end in the central perineal tendon. These fibers constitute the **levator prostatae muscle** (Figs. 3-21 and 3-57). *In the female* these anterior fibers cross the sides of the vagina before ending in the central perineal tendon. These fibers constitute the **pubovaginalis muscle** which forms an important *sphincter of the vagina* (Figs. 3-12 and 3-15).

For descriptive purposes it is convenient to describe **three parts of the levator ani muscle** (*pubococcygeus, puborectalis,* and *iliococcygeus*). Of these the pubococcygeus and the puborectalis are the most important.

The pubococcygeus muscle (Figs. 3-15, 3-16, 3-20, 3-57, and 3-60) is the part of the levator ani that *arises from the pubis* and runs posteromedially to insert into the

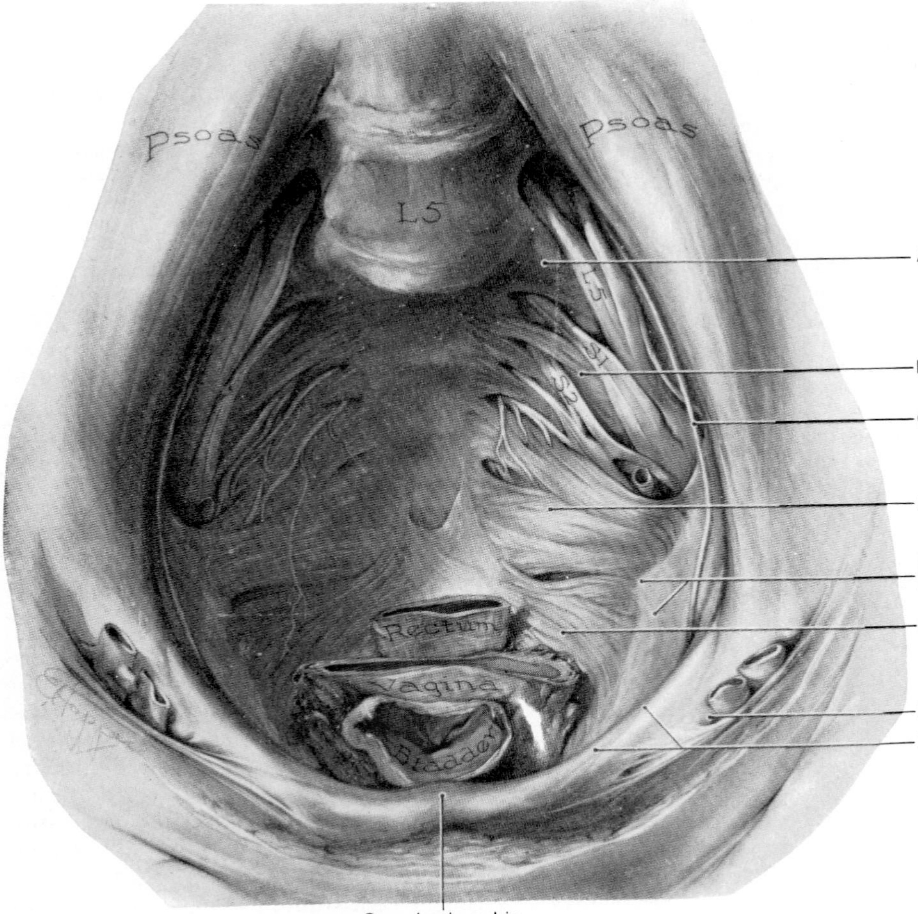

Figure 3-60. Drawing of a dissection of the *floor of the female pelvis.* Note the relative positions of the bladder, vagina, and rectum. Observe the muscles of the pelvic floor (levatores ani and coccygeus). See Figure 3-57 for a view of the floor of the male pelvis and the muscles forming it. Observe the obturator nerve derived from nerves L2, L3, and L4 running along the side wall of the pelvis to enter the thigh through the obturator foramen. Note the femoral ring, the doorway into the femoral canal, and the site of femoral hernia (also see Fig. 4-40).

anococcygeal ligament and into the pelvic surface and sides of the coccyx. *The anococcygeal ligament* (Fig. 3-22) *is the median fibrous intersection of the pubococcygeus muscles from the two sides, located between the anal canal and the tip of the coccyx.* As it courses downward and medially in the female, the pubococcygeus encircles the urethra, the vagina, and the anus and merges into the central perineal tendon (Fig. 3-12).

The puborectalis muscle (Figs. 3-14 to 3-16, 3-19*A*, 3-21, 3-38, and 3-57) is the part of the levator ani that *lies medial to but at a lower level than the pubococcygeus.* Like the pubococcygeus muscle, it arises from the pubis and passes backward; however, instead of inserting into the coccyx, *the muscles from the two sides loop around the posterior surface of the anorectal junction, forming a U-shaped rectal sling* (Fig. 3-61).

The iliococcygeus muscle (Figs. 3-16*A*, 3-21, 3-25, and 3-57) is *the thin part of the levator ani* that arises from the **tendinous arch** of the parietal pelvic fascia and the **ischial spine.** The muscle on each side passes medially and posteriorly to insert

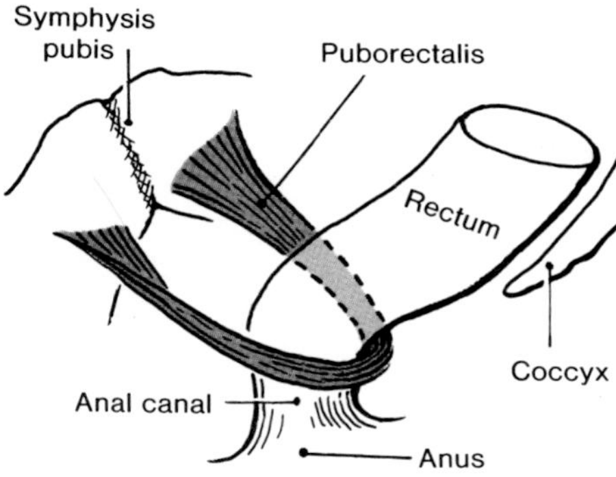

Figure 3-61. Diagram illustrating how the puborectalis muscle, a part of the levator ani, forms a *U-shaped sling* which helps to hold the inferior part of the rectum forward. The puborectal sling keeps the anorectal angle closed, except during defecation, when it relaxes, allowing the anorectal junction to straighten, while other fibers draw the anal canal over the feces that are being expelled. The anorectal junction is indicated by the sharp backward bend of the canal. The rectum is about 12 cm long and the anal canal about 3 cm. The anal canal ends at the anus (also see Fig. 3-19).

into the **coccyx** (Fig. 3-21) and the **anococcygeal ligament** (Fig. 3-22).

Nerve Supply (Fig. 3-57). Fibers from the **third** and **fourth sacral** nerves which enter its pelvic surface and the **inferior rectal** nerve which enters its perineal surface.

Actions. With the coccygeus muscle, all parts of the levatores ani muscles form the **pelvic diaphragm**, which constitutes the pelvic floor. *The muscular pelvic diaphragm supports the pelvic viscera and resists the downward thrust accompanying increases in the intra-abdominal pressure* (*e.g.*, as occurs in forced expiration and coughing). *Acting together* the two levatores ani muscles, forming the most important part of the pelvic diaphragm, **raise the pelvic floor**, thereby assisting the anterior abdominal muscles (Fig. 2–7) in compressing the abdominal contents. This action is an important part of forced expiration, coughing, vomiting, urinating, and fixation of the trunk during strong movements of the upper limbs (*e.g.*, when lifting a heavy object).

The part of the levator ani that inserts into the **central perineal tendon** supports the prostate (*levator prostatae* (Fig. 3–21) and the posterior wall of the vagina (*pubovaginalis*, Fig. 3–15). When the part of the levator ani that inserts into the wall of the anal canal and the central perineal tendon (puborectalis) contracts, it *raises the anal canal over a descending mass of feces*, thereby aiding the process of defecation. **The puborectalis** part of the levator ani (Figs. 3–19*A* and 3–61) *holds the anorectal junction forward*, thereby increasing the angle between the rectum and the anal canal. This prevents passage of feces from the rectum into the anal canal when defecation is not desired or is inconvenient. *The anorectal angle supports most of the weight of the fecal mass*, thereby relieving much pressure on the **external anal sphincter** (Figs. 3–14 and 3–19*A*).

During parturition (childbirth) the levatores ani muscles support the fetal head while the cervix (neck of the uterus, Fig. 3–22) is dilating to permit delivery of the baby (Fig. 3–105).

The Coccygeus Muscle (Figs. 3–21, 3–27, 3–57, and 3–60). This triangular sheet of muscle lies against the posterior part of the iliococcygeus part of the levator ani muscle and is continuous with it. *The coccygeus forms the posterior and smaller part of the pelvic diaphragm.* On its external surface the coccygeus blends with the **sacrospinous ligament** (refer to Figs. 3–18 and 3–27).

Origin (Figs. 3–57 and 3–60). **Ischial spine**.

Insertion (Figs. 3–21 and 3–27). Lateral margins of **fifth sacral vertebra** and **coccyx**.

Nerve Supply (Fig. 3–57). Branches from ventral rami of **fourth** and **fifth sacral** nerves.

Actions. Forms lowest part of posterior wall of pelvis minor and posterior part of pelvic diaphragm. It probably **supports the coccyx** (tailbone) and **pulls it forward** after it has been pressed back during childbirth and defecation. In many mammals it is involved in movements of the tail.

CLINICALLY ORIENTED COMMENTS

Labor and childbirth may injure the supporting structures of the bladder, ure-

thra, vagina, and rectum. The **pubococcygeus** muscle is obstetrically important because it encircles the urethra, vagina, and anus and supports them. A **median episiotomy** (Fig. 3–44*A*) involves the superficial transversus perinei muscle, the central perineal tendon, and often the pubococcygeus muscle. In **mediolateral episiotomy** (Fig. 3–44*B*) some of the same structures are involved in addition to the bulbocavernosus muscle and *possibly* the deep transversus perinei muscle (Case 3–1).

Injuries to the pelvic fascia and the pubococcygeus muscle in particular may result in **cystocele** (herniation of the urinary bladder, Fig. 3–62). When the urethra is also involved, the condition is called **cystourethrocele** or urethrocystocele. Herniation of the rectum (**rectocele**) results from damage to the middle third of the vagina and to the pelvic diaphragm (Fig. 3–23).

Episiotomy is performed to enlarge the external opening of the birth canal and to prevent serious damage to the structures supporting the bladder, urethra, and rec-

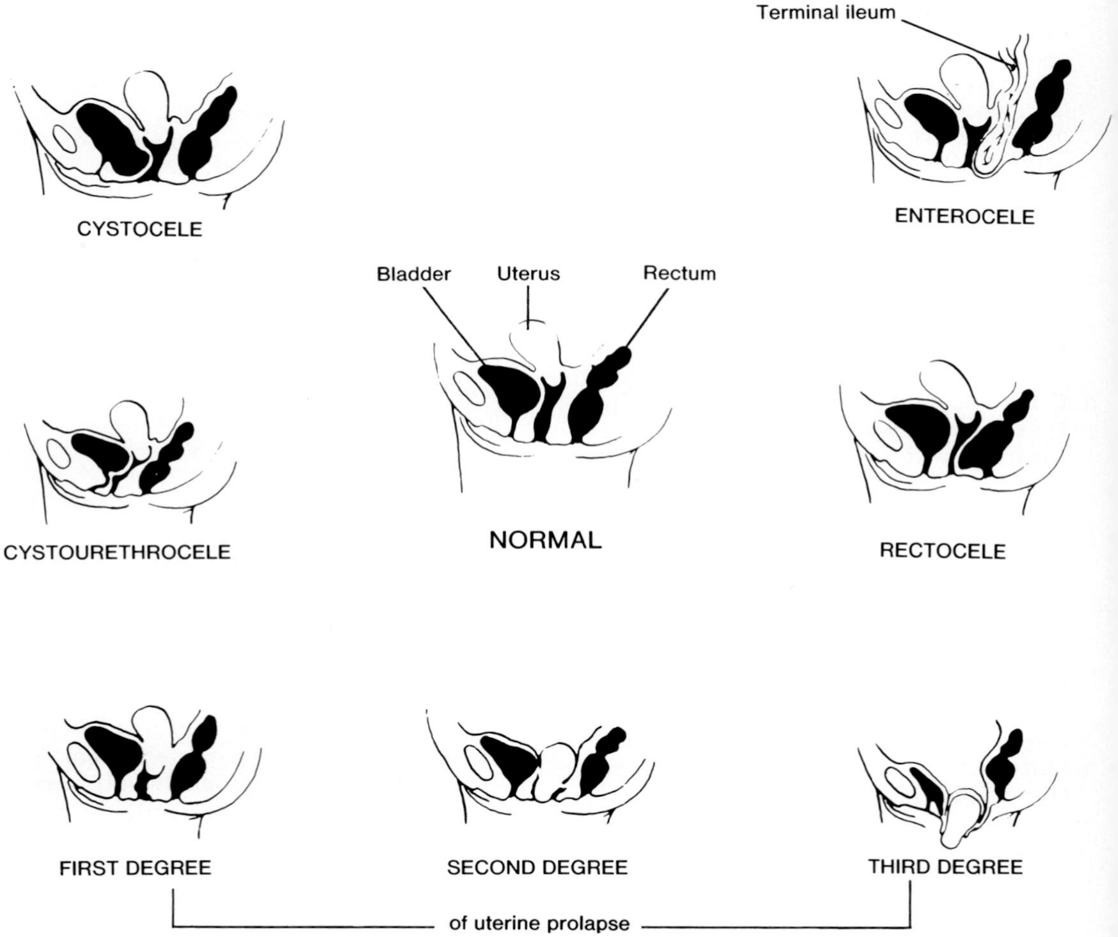

Figure 3-62. Drawings of sagittal views of the female pelvis illustrating various abnormalities of the pelvic viscera resulting from relaxation and weakening of the pelvic floor following injuries that occur during labor and delivery of a fetus. The most commonly encountered abnormalities are cystocele (herniation of bladder), cystourethrocele (herniation of bladder and urethra), and rectocele (herniation of rectum). In third degree uterine prolapse, the cervix of the uterus protrudes through the vaginal orifice and the labia.

tum which may lead to cystocele and rectocele (Fig. 3–62). A patient with a rectocele often complains of inability to have a bowel movement without putting her fingers in her vagina to support the anterior wall of the rectum.

Urinary stress incontinence may accompany pelvic relaxation and cystocele. Stress incontinence is a disease characterized by dribbling of urine whenever the intra-abdominal pressure is raised (*e.g.*, during coughing, sneezing, and lifting). This condition, common in parous women, often results from *weakening of the supporting structures of the bladder and the urethra.* These supports are stretched and occasionally lacerated during parturition. *Weakening of the vesicourethral junction* occurs in these patients so that they are unable to prevent dribbling of urine when the intra-abdominal pressure rises.

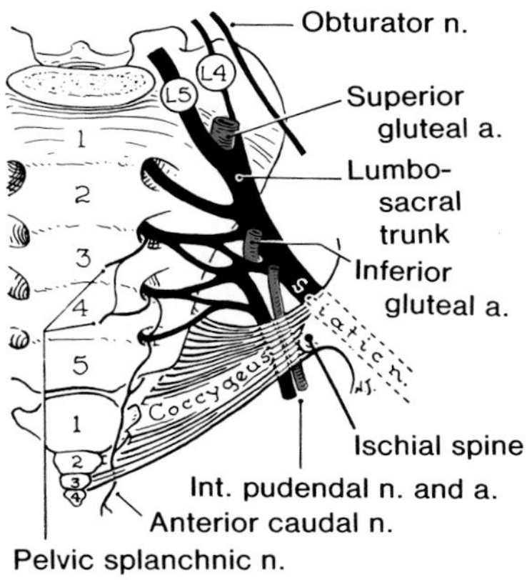

Figure 3-63. Drawing of the sacral plexus illustrating its relationship to the pelvic arteries. Observe that the sacral plexus is pierced by the superior and inferior gluteal arteries which run dorsally, whereas the pudendal artery continues downward and forward toward the ischial spine.

NERVES OF THE LATERAL WALL OF THE PELVIS MINOR

The piriformis muscle, described previously, *pads the posterior wall of the pelvis* (Fig. 3–27) *and forms a bed for the sacral and coccygeal nerve plexuses* (Fig. 3–58). The ventral nerve rami S2 and S3 emerge between digitations of the piriformis.

The lumbosacral trunk, a thick cord formed by the ventral nerve rami of L4 and L5, joins S1 as it passes inferiorly, anterior to the ala of the sacrum, to join the sacral plexus (Figs. 2–131, 3–58, and 3–63). It descends obliquely over the *sacroiliac joint*, and passes into the pelvis posterior to the pelvic fascia. It then crosses above the superior gluteal vessels (Fig. 3–58) to join the first sacral ventral nerve which lies on a bed formed by the piriformis muscle.

The Sacral Plexus (Figs. 2–139, 3–58, and 3–63). *This large plexus of nerves is located in the pelvis minor*, where it is closely related to the anterior surface of the piriformis muscle. *The sacral plexus is formed by the lumbosacral trunk and the ventral rami of the first three and the descending part of the fourth sacral nerves.* The main nerves of the sacral plexuses lie *external to the parietal pelvic fascia* (discussed subsequently). Except for the nerve to the piriformis muscle (S2), the perforating cutaneous nerves (S2, S3), and those to the pelvic diaphragm (Fig. 3–58), *all branches of the sacral plexus leave the pelvis through the greater sciatic foramen* (Figs. 3–18 and 4–44).

The sciatic nerve is formed by the ventral rami of L4 through S3, which converge on the front of the piriformis muscle. *The sciatic, the largest nerve in the body, passes through the greater sciatic foramen inferior to the piriformis* muscle (Figs. 4–47 and 4–52), along with the **inferior gluteal nerve** (L5, S1, and S2), which supplies the gluteus maximus muscle. In the back of the thigh *the sciatic nerve divides into tibial and common peroneal nerves* (see Chap. 4 for details on these nerves).

The pudendal nerve, described previously with the perineum, arises by separate branches from *ventral rami S2, S3, and S4.* It accompanies the internal pudendal artery (Figs. 3–58 and 3–63) and leaves the pelvis between the piriformis and coccygeus muscles, *hooking around the sacrospinous ligament to enter the perineum through the lesser sciatic notch.* Here it is *distributed to the muscles of the perineum*, including the **external anal sphincter**, and *ends as the dorsal nerve of the penis or clitoris*

(Fig. 3–26). The **superior gluteal nerve** (L4, L5, and S1) leaves the pelvis via the greater sciatic foramen superior to the piriformis muscle (Fig. 4–47). It supplies the gluteus medius and minimus and the tensor fasciae latae (see Chap. 4 for details).

Other components of the sacral plexus (Fig. 3–58) include twigs to the piriformis muscle (S1, S2, S3, and S4); (2) twigs to the pelvic diaphragm (S3 and S4); (3) the nerve to the quadratus femoris (L4, L5, and S1); and (4) the nerve to the obturator internus (L5, S1, and S2).

CLINICALLY ORIENTED COMMENTS

Injuries to the sacral plexus are uncommon; however, the sacral plexus and the lumbosacral trunk may be compressed by **pelvic tumors**. This compression usually causes pain in the lower limbs and, when associated with malignant pelvic tumors, it may be excruciating. Similarly a *fetal head may compress nerves of the sacral plexus*, producing aching pains in the lower limbs. Lesions of the ventral rami forming the sacral plexus give rise to disabilities that have a segmental distribution (Fig. 4–160).

The Obturator Nerve (L2, L3, and L4). This nerve is not from the sacral plexus; it *arises from the lumbar plexus in the abdomen* (Figs. 2–131 and 3–64) and enters the pelvis minor. It runs along its side wall *in the extraperitoneal* fat, dividing it into anterior and posterior parts (Fig. 3–59). This nerve will be described in detail later.

The Coccygeal Plexus (Fig. 3–58). This small plexus is usually unimportant. It is formed by the ventral rami of S4 and S5 and the coccygeal nerve and lies on the pelvic surface of the coccygeus muscle. It supplies this muscle, part of the levator ani muscle, and the sacrococcygeal joint and then pierces the coccygeus muscle to supply the skin in the region of the coccyx.

THE PELVIC FASCIA

The pelvic fascia (Figs. 3–14, 3–17, 3–24, and 3–56) *lines the pelvic cavity* as far inferiorly as the ischiopubic rami and is attached to the periosteum just below the **linea terminales** (pelvic brim). The fascia extends onto the superior surface of the **pelvic diaphragm** (levatores ani and coccygeus muscles) and is attached to such pelvic viscera as the urethra, vagina, prostate, and rectum.

The fascial lining of the abdominal and pelvic cavities is continuous, but it is **anchored at the lineae terminales** (Fig. 3–56) and is separated from the parietal peritoneum by extraperitoneal fat (Fig. 2–17). In addition to enclosing these cavities, the fascial lining encloses the pelvic viscera and the great vessels. Superiorly the pelvic fascia is continuous with the **transversalis fascia**, the fascia lining the deep surface of the transversalis muscle (Fig. 2–14). However, the pelvic fascia is anchored to the periosteum on the posterior aspect of the body of the pubis. *This attachment prevents the spread of infection from the anterior abdominal wall into the pelvis.*

The pelvic fascia is divided into two layers for descriptive purposes: (1) *the parietal pelvic fascia* forming the fascial sheaths of the pelvic muscles and (2) *the visceral pelvic fascia* forming the fascial coverings or sheaths of the pelvic viscera (Figs. 3–17, 3–24, and 3–56).

The parietal pelvic fascia covers the pelvic surfaces of the obturator internus, the piriformis, the coccygeus, the sphincter urethrae, the deep transversus perinei, and the levatores ani muscles (Figs. 3–17, 3–24, and 3–56). The fascia covering the obturator internus muscle, called the **obturator fascia** (Figs. 3–18, 3–20, 3–56, and 3–60), is thicker than other parts of the parietal pelvic fascia and is separated superiorly from the **psoas fascia** (Figs. 3–18 and 4–19) by its attachment to the periosteum just below the lineae terminales and the pelvic brim.

As described previously, the levator ani muscle arises from a *thickening of the obturator fascia*, known as the **tendinous arch** (arcus tendineus), that stretches between the body of the pubis and the ischial spine (Figs. 3–17 and 3–57). *Superior to the tendinous arch the obturator fascia is thick and tough*, whereas inferior to it the fascia is thin and lines the lateral wall of

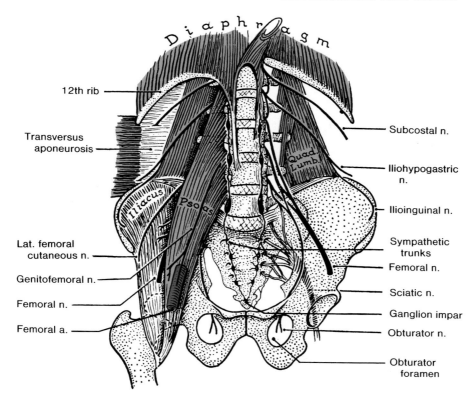

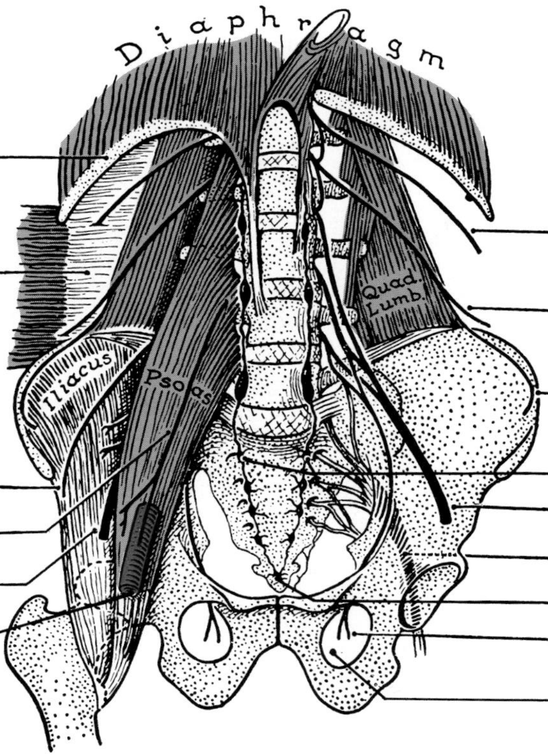

Figure 3-64. Drawing of the lumbar plexus and the muscles of the posterior abdominal wall. Observe the obturator nerve (L2, L3, and L4) coursing along the side wall of the pelvis to the superior part of the obturator foramen. On the right side, observe that this nerve appears from under cover of the medial border of the psoas major muscle and pierces the psoas fascia. Observe that the sympathetic trunks follow the anterior borders of the psoas muscles and lie on the bodies of the vertebrae. Note that in the pelvis each trunk has four ganglia and that they converge on the front of the sacrum and end in a small ganglion called the ganglion impar.

the **ischiorectal fossa**, where it forms the medial wall of the *pudendal canal* (Figs. 3–13, 3–23, 3–26, and 3–56).

The fascia of the pelvic diaphragm covers both surfaces of the levator ani (Fig. 3–13). The fascia lining the superior (pelvic) surface of the levator ani is called the *superior fascia of the pelvic diaphragm.* This part of the pelvic fascia is attached to the posterior aspect of the body of pubis, the neck of the urinary bladder, the vagina, and the rectum in the female. *In the male* this fascia is attached to the prostate and the rectum. At the neck of the bladder the fascia is thickened to form two cord-like bands, called the **pubovesical ligaments** in the female and the **puboprostatic ligaments** in the male (Figs. 3–14, 3–21, and 3–22). *These ligaments, one on each side of the median plane, anchor the neck of the urinary bladder to the pubis.* The pubovesical ligaments in the female also attach to the wall of the vagina.

The inferior fascia of the pelvic diaphragm covers the inferior surface of the levator ani and forms the medial wall of the **ischiorectal fossa** (Figs. 3–2, 3–17, 3–20, 3–23, and 3–24). It is continuous with the fascia on the medial surface of the inferior half of the obturator internus muscle (Fig. 3–13) and on the inferior surface of the external anal sphincter (Figs. 3–4 and 3–5). The space between the pelvic fascia and the anterior surface of the bladder is called the **retropubic space** (Figs. 3–14, 3–17, 3–22, and 3–24). *It contains extraperitoneal* *fat, loose areolar tissue, blood vessels, and nerves.* The fat and areolar tissue accommodate the expansion of the urinary bladder.

THE OBTURATOR NERVE

The obturator nerve was briefly described before with the nerves of the lateral pelvic wall (Figs. 3-27, 3-56, 3-58 to 3-60, 3-63, 3-64, and 3-68). It *arises from the lumbar plexus and is formed in the substance of the psoas major* muscle from the anterior branches of the ventral rami of the *second, third, and fourth lumbar nerves* (principally L3). At the pelvic brim the obturator nerve emerges from the medial border of the psoas major on the lateral part of the sacrum (Fig. 3-58). It *runs behinds the common iliac vessels* and crosses the sacroiliac joint to enter the pelvis minor. It then *runs anteroinferiorly in the extraperitoneal fat medial to the fascia over the obturator internus muscle* (Figs. 3-27, 3-59, and 3-65). Here it lies lateral to the ureter, the internal iliac vessels, and the ductus deferens, or the round ligament of the uterus. It then passes along the **obturator groove** (Fig. 3-47) superior to the obturator artery and vein, where it divides into anterior and posterior divisions which leave the pelvis via the **obturator foramen** to supply the thigh (see Chap. 4).

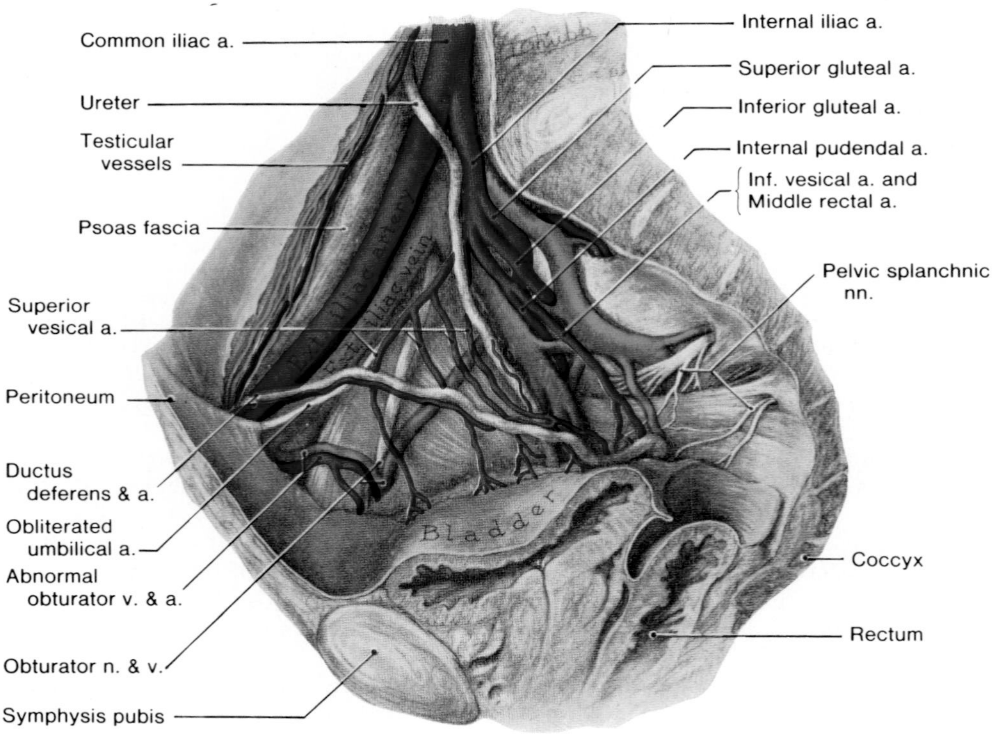

Figure 3-65. Drawing of a dissection of the side wall of the *male pelvis.* Observe the ureter and the ductus deferens running a strictly subperitoneal course across the external iliac vessels, umbilical artery, obturator nerve and vessels and each receiving a branch from a vesical artery. *Note that the ureter crosses the external iliac artery at its origin and the ductus deferens crosses it at its termination.* Observe that the umbilical artery, obliterated beyond the origin of the last superior vesical artery, creates a peritoneal fold. Note the obturator artery here springing from the inferior epigastric artery; *i.e.*, the artery is "abnormal." Observe the veins forming an open network through which the arteries are threaded.

CLINICAL ORIENTED COMMENTS

The obturator nerve is the only nerve supplying the lower limb which lies on the side wall of the pelvis in the extraperitoneal fat (Figs. 3-58 and 3-68). Here it is vulnerable to injury during removal of **cancerous lymph nodes** from the side wall of the pelvis (Fig. 3-65) in patients with **malignant pelvic disease**. Inadvertent removal of part of this nerve results in deficient adduction of the thigh on the affected side.

Because the obturator nerve lies posterolateral to the ovary in the pelvis minor, it may be involved in pathological changes in this reproductive gland.

BLOOD VESSELS OF THE PELVIS

Four different arteries enter the pelvis minor: (1) *internal iliac* (paired); (2) *median sacral*; (3) *superior rectal*; and (4) *ovarian* (paired).

The Internal Iliac Artery (Figs. 2-55, 3-65 to 3-68, and 3-74). The internal iliac (hypogastric) artery *supplies most of the blood to the pelvic viscera.* It is a terminal branch of the common iliac artery which arises from the bifurcation of this vessel, medial to the psoas major muscle and *anterior to the sacroiliac joint* (Fig. 2-142). Its origin is at the level of the intervertebral disc between L5 and S1 (**lumbosacral joint**), where it is crossed by the ureter (Figs. 3-67 and 3-68). It is separated from the sacroiliac joint by the internal iliac vein and the lumbosacral trunk (Figs. 3-58 and 3-68). It passes posteromedialy into the pelvis minor, medial to the external iliac vein and the obturator nerve (Figs. 3-65 and 3-68) and *lateral to the peritoneum.*

The branches of the internal iliac artery include both visceral branches and those supplying the body wall and the lower limb. *The arrangement of the visceral*

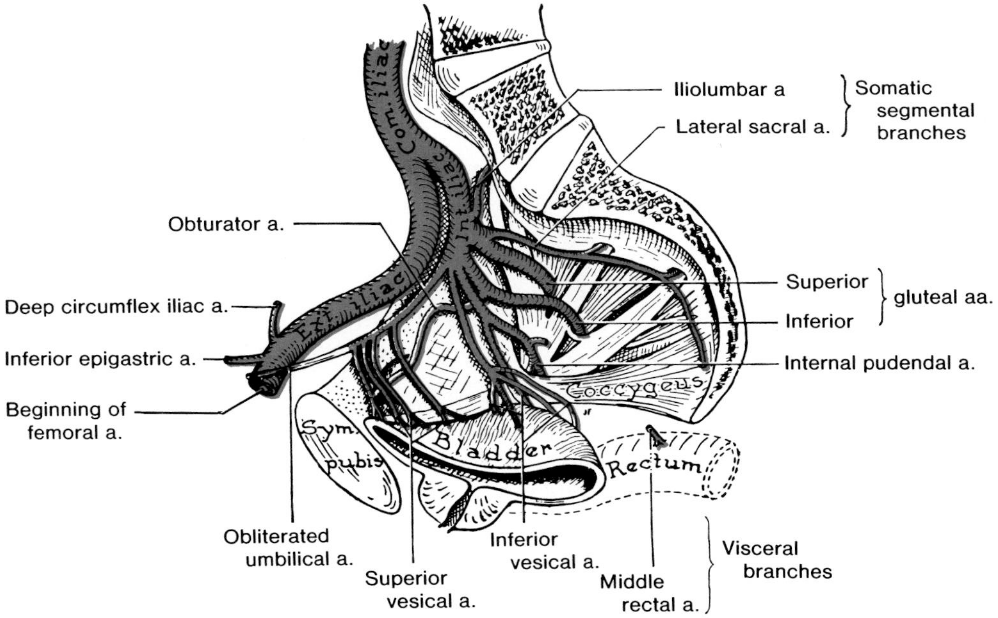

Figure 3-66. Drawing of a dissection of the *male pelvis* showing a lateral view of the right iliac arteries and their branches. Note that the internal iliac artery is smaller than the external iliac artery, which continues the direction of the common iliac artery. Observe that the common iliac artery has two terminal branches but no collateral branches. Note that the external iliac artery has two branches and ends as the femoral artery at the level of the inguinal ligament (Fig. 3-67). Examine the internal iliac artery, which forms the major blood supply to the pelvic viscera.

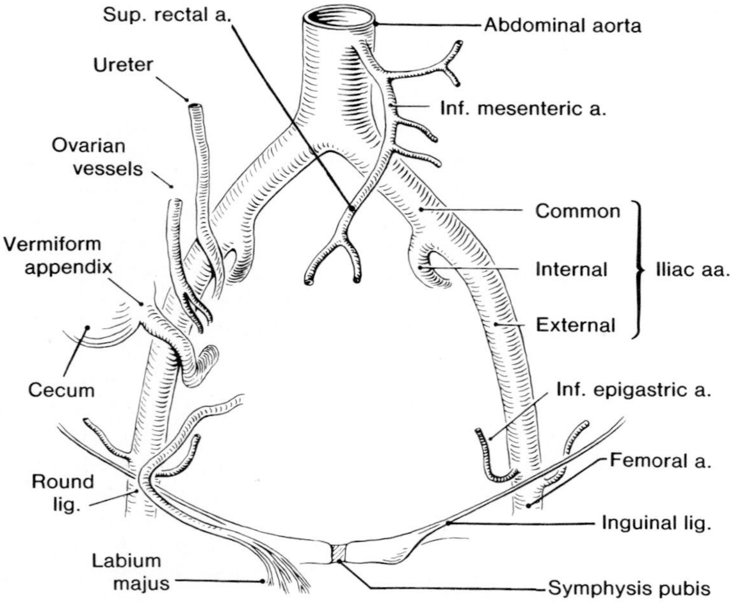

Figure 3-67. Drawing of the iliac arteries and certain structures crossing them to enter or leave the female pelvis minor. The sigmoid colon and mesocolon (left side only) are not shown. Observe the structures that cross the pelvic brim surrounding the superior pelvic aperture (ureter, ovarian vessels, round ligament of uterus, and sometimes the vermiform appendix).

branches is variable. As shown in Figure 3–66, the internal iliac artery often divides into two stems (sometimes called its anterior and posterior divisions) before giving off its named branches. The following branches of the internal iliac artery are listed in the order in which they commonly arise. **The anterior branches of the internal iliac artery** are the *umbilical*, the *obturator*, the *inferior vesical*, the *uterine*, the *middle rectal*, the *internal pudendal*, and the *inferior gluteal.*

The Umbilical Artery (Figs. 3–65, 3–66, 3–73, and 3–77*B*). This vessel runs anteroinferiorly between the urinary bladder and the side wall of the pelvis. It gives off the **superior vesical artery**, which supplies numerous branches to the superior part of the urinary bladder. *In the male* one of these gives rise to the **artery to the ductus deferens**, which passes into the spermatic cord (Fig. 2–27). *Prenatally the umbilical artery carries blood to the placenta for reoxygenation.* Postnatally its distal part atrophies and becomes a fibrous cord, called the **lateral umbilical ligament**, which runs on the deep surface of the anterior abdominal wall (Figs. 2–16, 3–17, 3–65, and 3–73).

The Obturator Artery (Figs. 3–65, 3–66, and 4–34*A*). The origin of this vessel is variable; usually it arises close to the umbilical artery and runs along the side wall of the pelvis, where it is crossed by the ureter near its origin. It passes anteroinferiorly on the obturator fascia *between the obturator nerve and vein* (Fig. 3–56) and passes through the obturator foramen to supply muscles of the thigh and the ligament of the head of the femur (see Chap. 4). Within the pelvis the obturator artery gives off some muscular branches, a *nutrient artery to the ilium*, and a pubic branch which ascends on the pelvic surface of the ilium to anastomose with the pubic branch of the inferior epigastric artery of the external iliac (Fig. 4–42*A*). This anastomosis may be quite large (*abnormal* or *accessory obturator artery*) and may replace part or all of the obturator artery (Fig. 4–42*B*). *A medially placed obturator artery is vulnerable to injury* during repair of a **femoral hernia** (see discussion in Chap. 4).

The Inferior Vesical Artery (Figs. 3–65

and 3–66). This vessel corresponds to the *vaginal artery in the female* (Figs. 3–69 and 3–72). It passes forward to the base of the bladder and *supplies the seminal vesicle, the prostate, and the posteroinferior part of the bladder.* It also gives rise to the artery of the ductus deferens (Figs. 2–27 and 3–65).

The Vaginal Artery (Figs. 3–69 and 3–72). This vessel passes forward and then along the side of the vagina, where it divides into numerous branches which supply the anterior and posterior surfaces of the vagina, posteroinferior parts of the bladder, and the pelvic part of the urethra.

The Uterine Artery (Figs. 3–69, 3–71, and 3–72). This vessel is homologus to the artery of the ductus deferens. The uterine artery usually arises separately from the internal iliac, but it may arise from the umbilical artery. It *descends on the side wall of the pelvis, anterior to the internal iliac artery* (Figs. 3–68) to enter the root of the broad ligament, where it passes superior to the lateral fornix of the vagina to reach the lateral margin of the uterus. It is im-

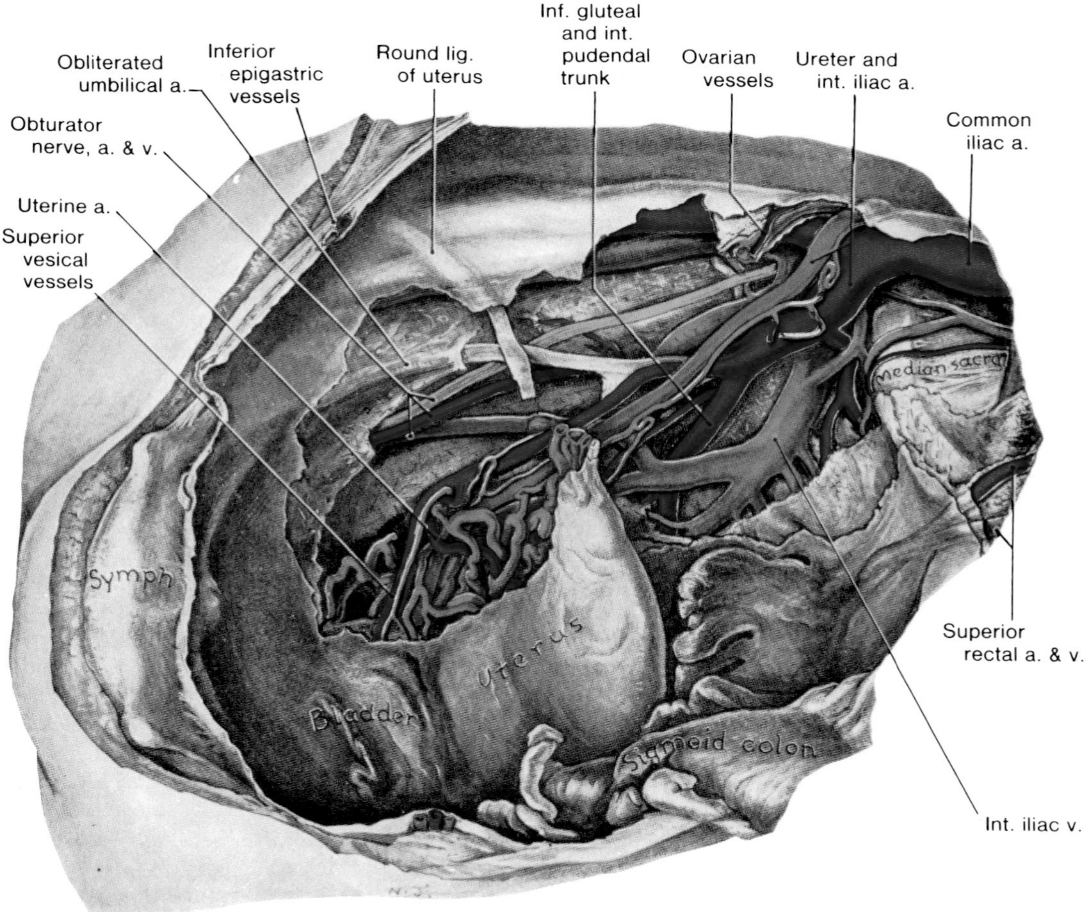

Figure 3-68. Drawing of a dissection of the blood vessels on the side wall of the *female pelvis*, viewed from the left side of a supine cadaver. In this older subject the uterus is retroverted (inclined backward). The inferior gluteal and internal pudendal arteries spring from a common trunk in this specimen (not separately as in Fig. 3-65). The uterine plexus of veins communicates with the superior rectal veins, thereby providing an additional area of portacaval anastomosis in the female (also see Fig. 2-112).

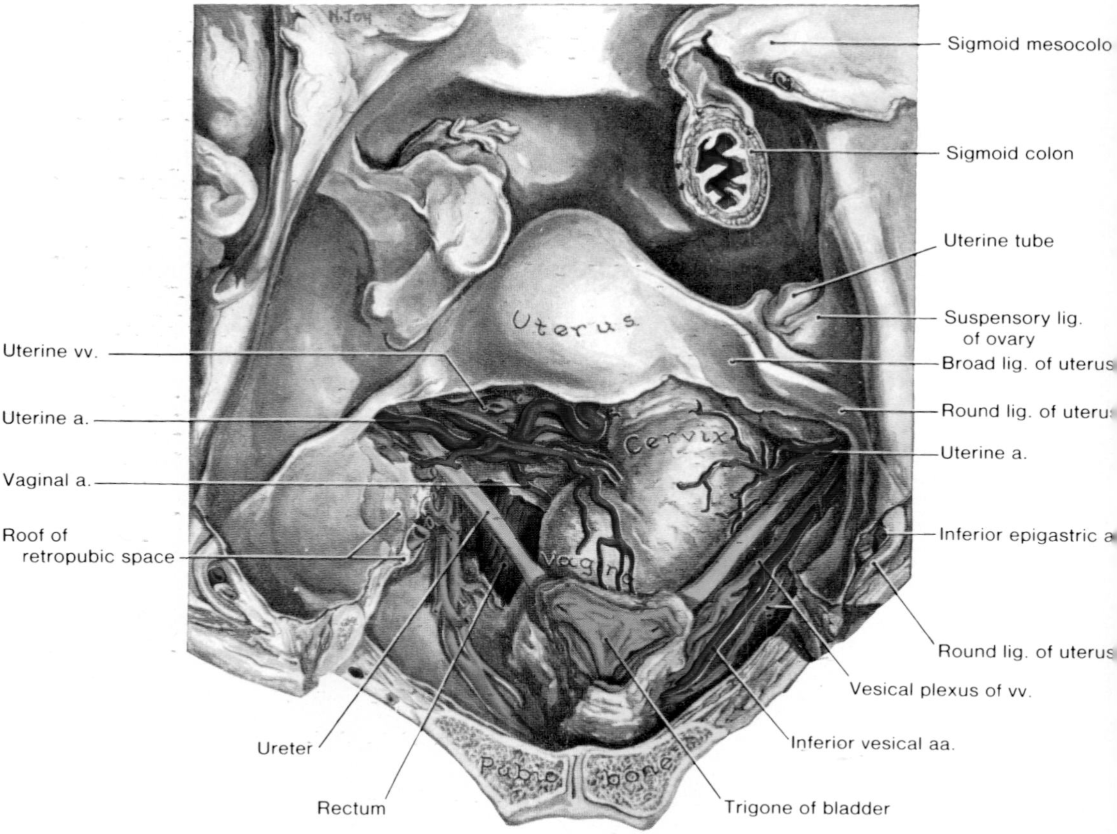

Figure 3-69. Drawing of an anterior view of the female internal genital organs. Part of the pubic bones and the entire bladder, except the trigone, are removed and with them parts of the broad ligaments. Observe that the uterus and vagina are asymmetrically placed, which is usual. As a result, one ureter, in this instance the left one, crosses the lateral fornix of the vagina and is close to the cervix of the uterus, whereas the other ureter is correspondingly far away. Note the uterine artery lying with its veins in the base of the broad ligament and running up the side of the uterus. Observe a large vaginal artery, a branch of the uterine artery, supplying the cervix and the anterior surface of the vagina. Note the vaginal artery arising from the internal iliac artery and supplying the posterior surface of the vagina. Examine the rectal fascia (not labeled) intervening between the foregoing arteries and the rectum. Observe the round ligament of the uterus curving round the inferior epigastric vessels at the deep inguinal ring and passing through the inguinal canal. Note the superior vesical vessels (not labeled) in the roof of the retropubic space.

portant to observe that *the uterine artery passes anterior to and above the ureter near the lateral fornix* of the vagina (Fig. 3–70). **This point of crossing lies about 2 cm superior to the ischial spine**. It may give a small branch to the ureter. The uterine artery becomes quite large during pregnancy.

On reaching the side of the cervix, the uterine artery divides into (1) a large *superior branch supplying the body and fundus of the uterus* and (2) a smaller *vaginal branch supplying the cervix and vagina.* The uterine artery pursues a tortuous course along the lateral margin of the uterus (Fig. 3–71) and ends when *its ovar-*

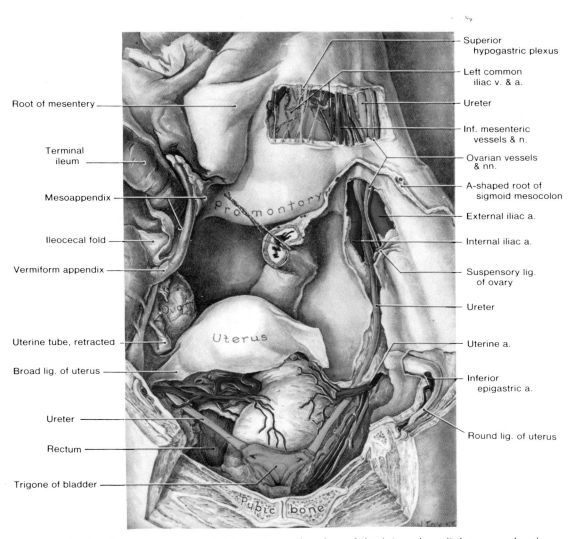

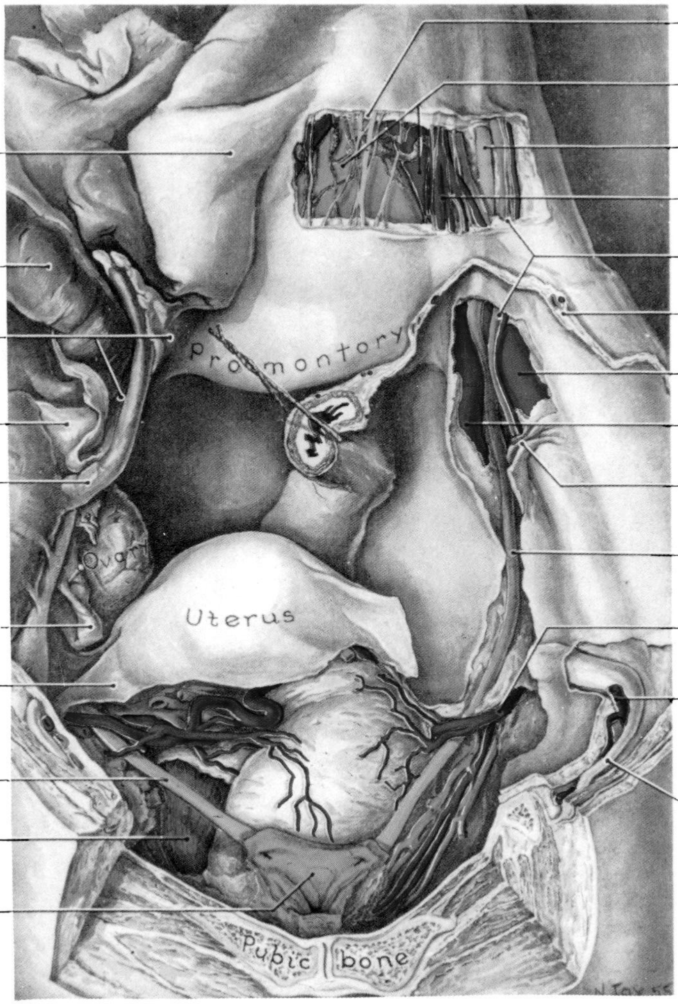

Figure 3-70. Drawing of a dissection of an anterior view of the internal genital organs showing the pelvic course of the ureter in the female. Observe the superior hypogastric plexus and some lymph vessels anterior to the left common iliac vein. Note that the left ureter, from above downward, is crossed by the sigmoid branches of the inferior mesenteric artery, the ovarian vessels, and the uterine artery. Examine the apex of the Λ-shaped root of the sigmoid mesocolon, which is situated in front of the left ureter and acts as a guide to it. Observe the ureter crossing the external iliac artery at the bifurcation of the common iliac artery and close behind the ovarian vessels and descending in front of the internal iliac artery. Note its subperitoneal course, from where it enters the pelvis to where it passes deep to the broad ligament and is crossed by the uterine artery. Observe that the vermiform appendix is in one of its unusual positions, *i.e.*, postileal. Note the ileocecal fold extending from the end of the ileum to the mesoappendix.

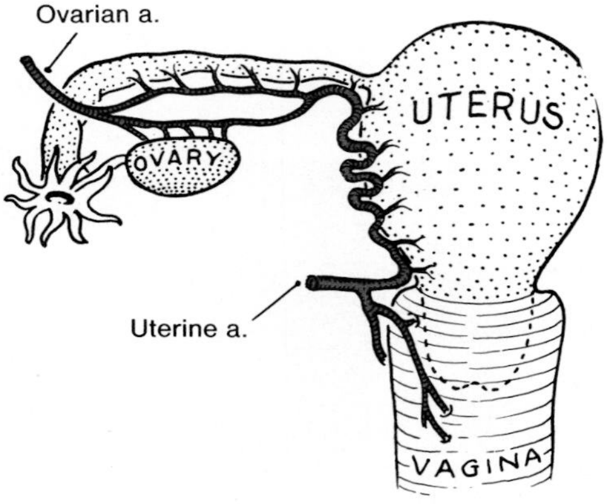

Figure 3-71. Drawing of an anterior view of the female internal genital organs illustrating the anastomosis of the ovarian and uterine arteries occurring in the broad ligament of the uterus. Each ovarian artery arises from the abdominal aorta inferior to the renal artery, whereas the uterine artery is a branch of the internal iliac artery (Fig. 3-70).

ian branch anastomoses with the ovarian artery between the layers of the broad ligament.

CLINICALLY ORIENTED COMMENTS

The fact that the uterine artery crosses anterior to and above the ureter near the lateral fornix of the vagina (Figs. 3-69 and 3-70) is clinically important. *The ureter is in danger of being inadvertently clamped* or severed during **hysterectomy** (G. *hystera*, uterus + *ektomē*, excision) when the uterine artery is tied off. The left ureter is particularly vulnerable because it is very close to the lateral aspect of the cervix (Fig. 3-70). The ureter is also vulnerable to injury when the ovarian vessels are being tied off during surgery (*e.g.*, **ovariectomy**) because these structures lie very close to each

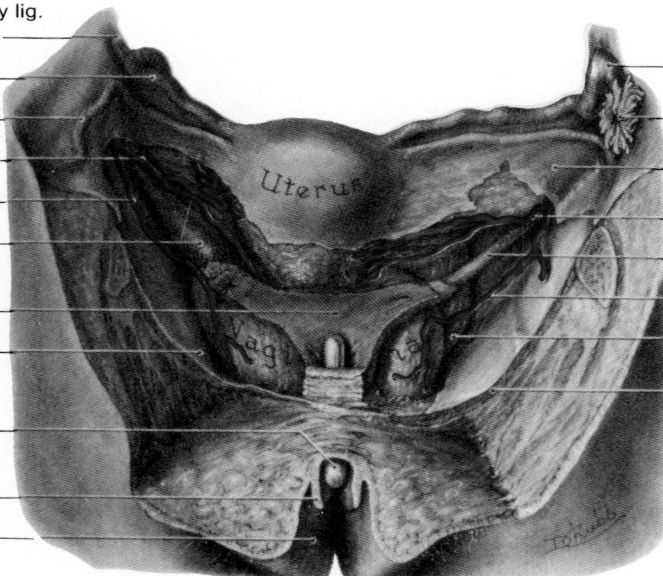

Figure 3-72. Drawing of an anterior view of the uterus and uterine tubes. The pubic bones and the bladder, except for the trigone, are removed. Examine the ureters, the trigone of bladder, and the urethra in relation to the asymmetrically placed uterus and vagina. Examine the ostium of the left uterine tube, which here happens to face forward. Note that the right ureter contains a calculus or stone (see Case 2-2 at the end of Chap. 2).

other where they cross the pelvic brim (Figs. 3–67 and 3–73). *Before clamping the uterine artery it is important to identify its relationship to the ureter.*

The Middle Rectal Artery (Figs. 3–65, 3–66, and 3–98). This small vessel runs medially to the rectum and also sends branches to the prostate and seminal vesicle in males and to the vagina in females. It anastomoses with the other rectal arteries.

The Internal Pudendal Artery (Figs. 3–17, 3–65, and 3–66). This vessel is larger in the male than the female. It passes inferolaterally, anterior to the piriformis muscle and the sacral plexus (Fig. 3–58) and *leaves the pelvis between the piriformis and coccygeus muscles* (Fig. 3–63) by passing through the lower part of the *greater sciatic foramen* (Fig. 3–66). It passes around the posterior aspect of the ischial spine or the sacrospinous ligament (Fig. 3–18) *to enter the ischiorectal fossa through the lesser sciatic foramen* (Fig. 3–43). It then passes with the internal pudendal veins and branches of the pudendal nerve through the **pudendal canal** in the lateral wall of the *ischiorectal fossa* (Figs. 3–23 and 3–56). Just before it reaches the sym-

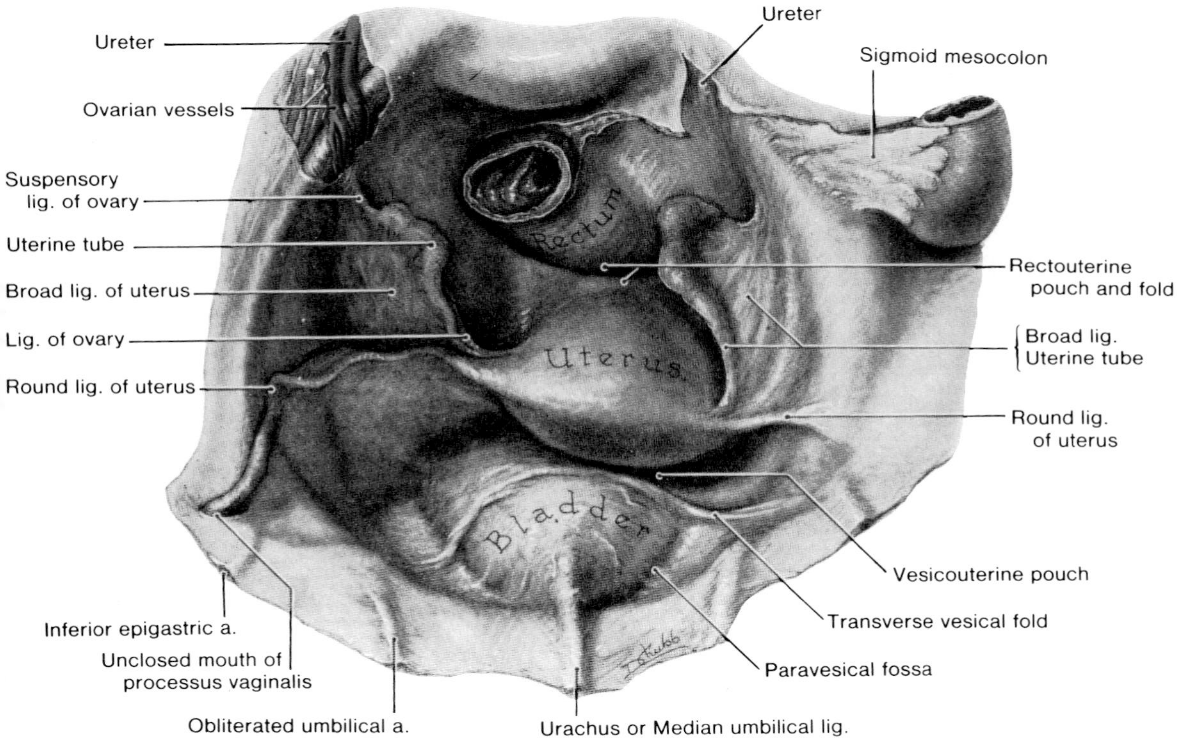

Figure 3-73. Drawing of a dissection of the female pelvis minor *from above.* Observe the pear-shaped uterus which is asymmetrically placed, as is usual, here leaning to the left. Note the right round ligament of the uterus, which here is longer than the left and has an acquired "mesentery." The round ligament of the uterus takes the same subperitoneal course as the ductus deferens in the male (Fig. 3-65). Examine the free edge of the medial four-fifths of the broad ligament which is one-fifth occupied by the ovarian vessels and is the suspensory ligament of the ovary. Observe the ovarian vessels crossing the external iliac vessels very close to the ureter. Note that the left ureter crosses at the apex of the Λ-shaped root of the sigmoid mesocolon. The obliterated umbilical artery raises a fold of peritoneum called the lateral umbilical ligament (also see Fig. 2-16).

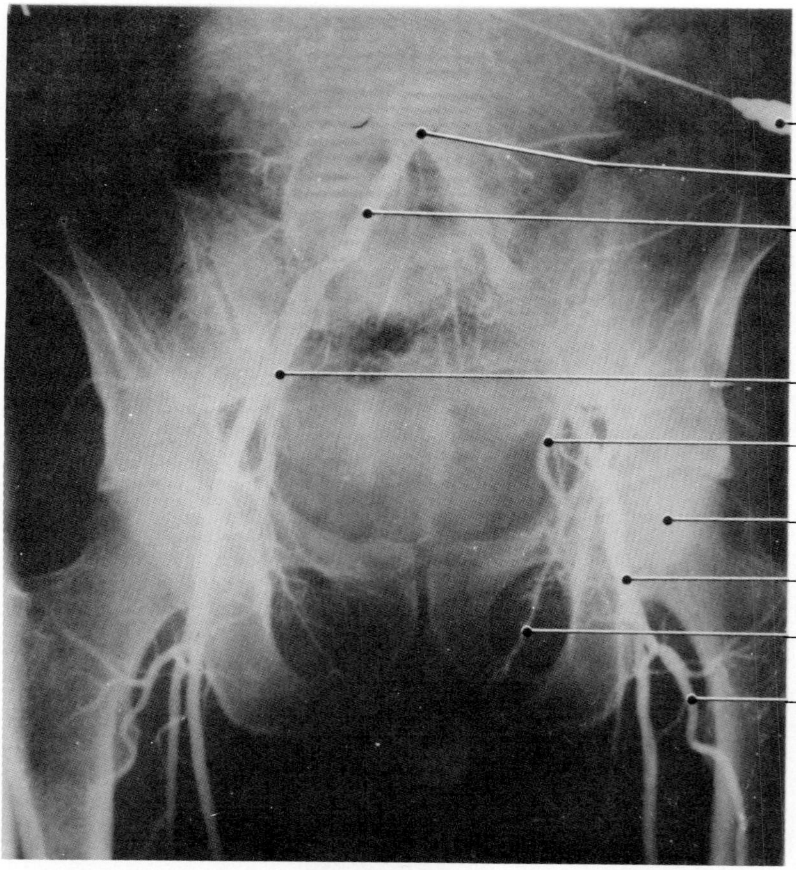

Figure 3-74. *Iliac arteriogram.* An injection of radiopaque material was made into the aorta in the lumbar region (note the needle). Observe the bifurcation of (1) the aorta into right and left common iliac arteries (anterior to L4 vertebra), and (2) the common iliacs into internal and external iliac arteries opposite the sacroiliac joint at the level of the lumbosacral disc (also see Fig. 4-34).

physis pubis, it divides into its terminal branches, the **deep** and **dorsal arteries of the penis** (Figs. 3–11 and 3–31) or **the clitoris** (Fig. 3–42).

The Inferior Gluteal Artery (Figs. 3–58, 3–63, 3–65, and 3–66). This vessel passes posteriorly between the sacral nerves (usually S2 and S3) and *leaves the pelvis through the inferior part of the greater sciatic foramen below the piriformis muscle* (Fig. 4–52) to supply the muscles and skin of the buttock and the posterior surface of the thigh (see Chap. 4).

The posterior branches of the internal iliac artery are the *superior gluteal*, the *iliolumbar*, and the *lateral sacral arteries*.

The Superior Gluteal Artery (Figs. 3–58, 3–63, 3–65, and 3–66). This large artery passes posteriorly through the pelvic fascia and **runs between the lumbosacral trunk and the ventral ramus of the first sacral nerve**. *It leaves the pelvis through the superior part of the greater sciatic foramen above the piriformis muscle* (Fig. 4–52) to supply muscles in the buttock (see Chap. 4).

The Iliolumbar Artery (Figs. 3–58 and 3–66). This vessel runs superolaterally to the iliac fossa, passing anterior to the sacroiliac joint and posterior to the psoas major muscle, where it **separates the obturator nerve from the lumbosacral trunk** (Fig. 3–58). In the iliac fossa it divides into (1) an *iliac branch* supplying the iliacus muscle and a nutrient artery to the ilium, and (2) a *lumbar branch* supplying the psoas major and the quadratus lumborum muscles.

The Lateral Sacral Arteries (Figs. 3–58 and 3–66). These vessels, usually a superior and an inferior one on each side, may arise from a common trunk. They pass medially and *descend anterior to the sacral ventral rami*, giving off spinal branches that pass through the pelvic sacral foramina and *supply the contents of the sacral canal* (**spinal meninges** and **roots of sacral nerves**; see Chap. 5). Some branches of the lateral sacral arteries pass from the sacral canal through the dorsal sacral foramina to supply muscles and skin overlying the sacrum.

The Median Sacral Artery (Fig. 2-55). This small unpaired artery arises from the posterior surface of the abdominal aorta just superior to its bifurcation and runs anterior to the body of the sacrum to end in a series of anastomoses that form the *coccygeal body*. The function of this structure is unknown.

The median sacral artery was originally the direct continuation of the abdominal aorta. It represents the caudal end of the dorsal aorta in the embryo and descends in the median plane anterior to L4 and L5 vertebrae and the promontary of the sacrum and passes into the hollow of the bone. It ends in the *coccygeal* body, a small cellular and vascular mass located anterior to the tip of the coccyx; its functional significance is unknown. Before the median sacral artery enters the pelvis, it often *gives rise to the fifth lumbar arteries* (Fig. 2-55) and sends small branches to the posterior part of the rectum. The median sacral artery anastomoses with the lateral sacral arteries.

The Superior Rectal Artery (Figs. 2-107, 3-67, and 3-98). This artery is the *direct continuation of the inferior mesenteric artery*. It crosses the left common iliac vessels and descends into the pelvis minor within the sigmoid mesocolon. At the level of S3 vertebra it divides into two branches which descend on each side of the rectum, supplying it as far down as the internal anal sphincter. The superior rectal artery anastomoses with branches of the middle rectal (Fig. 3-98), a branch of the internal iliac artery, and with the inferior rectal artery, a branch of the internal pudendal artery.

The Ovarian Artery (Figs. 3-66, 3-71, and 3-73). Each ovarian artery arises from the abdominal aorta inferior to the renal artery. It passes inferiorly *adherent to the parietal peritoneum and internal to the ureter* on the posterior abdominal wall. It crosses the proximal ends of the external iliac vessels and enters the pelvis minor and the superolateral part of the broad ligament to supply the ovary. It **anastomoses with the uterine artery** (Fig. 3-71).

Veins of the Pelvis (Figs. 2-85, 2-112, 3-65, 3-68, and 3-69). The pelvis is **mainly drained through the internal iliac veins** and their tributaries, but there is some drainage through the *superior rectal* (hemorrhoidal), the *median sacral*, and the *ovarian* veins. Some blood from the pelvis also passes to the *internal vertebral venous plexus* (Fig. 5-64). The internal iliac vein joins the external iliac vein to form the common iliac vein which unites with its partner to form the **inferior vena cava** at the level of L5 vertebra (Figs. 2-113 and 2-129). *The internal iliac vein lies posteroinferior to the internal iliac artery* (Fig. 3-68) and its tributaries are similar to the branches of this artery, except for the fetal **umbilical vein**, which drains into the left branch of the portal vein (Fig. 2-112), and the iliolumbar vein, which usually drains into the common iliac vein.

After birth the nonfunctional umbilical vein gradually becomes a fibrous cord called the **ligamentum teres** of the liver (Figs. 2-80 and 2-83). For a variable time after birth, the umbilical vein remains patent and may be used for exchange transfusions (see discussion in Chap. 2). *The superior gluteal veins*, *the vena comitantes of the superior gluteal arteries, are the largest tributaries of the internal iliac veins*, except during pregnancy when the uterine veins become larger.

Pelvic venous plexuses are formed by the veins in the pelvis (Figs. 3-24 and 3-75). *These intercommunicating networks of veins are clinically important.* The various plexuses (vesical, prostatic or uterine, and vaginal and rectal) unite and drain mainly into the internal iliac vein; some drain via

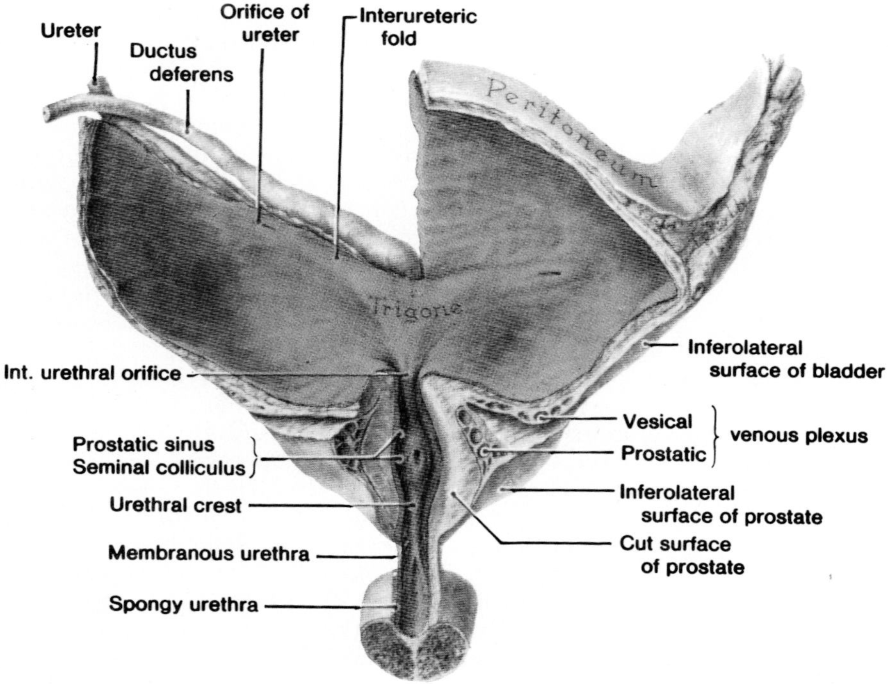

Figure 3-75. Drawing of the interior of the male urinary bladder and prostatic urethra. The anterior parts of the bladder, prostate, and urethra were cut away. The knife was then carried through the posterior wall of the bladder at the superior border of the right ureter and interureteric fold. This fold unites the two ureters along the upper limit of the smooth trigone. Observe that the right ureter does not join the bladder wall but traverses it obliquely, as far as its slitlike orifice, situated 2.5 to 3 cm from the left orifice. Note that the mucous membrane is smooth over the trigone and rugose elsewhere—especially when the bladder is empty. The embryological origin of the trigone differs from other parts of the bladder. Observe the slight fullness behind the internal urethral orifice which, when exaggerated, becomes the uvula vesicae. This small projection is caused by the median lobe of the prostate. Examine the orifice of the prostatic utricle at the summit of the seminal colliculus on the urethral crest. This orifice is homologous with the vaginal orifice in the female. Observe the tiny orifices of the ejaculatory ducts, one on each side of the prostatic utricle. Note that the urethral crest extends rather higher than usual and bifurcates rather lower than usual. Examine the prostatic fascia enclosing the important prostatic venous plexus.

the **superior rectal vein** into the inferior mesenteric vein (Fig. 2-112).

The rectal venous plexuses surround the rectum (Figs. 2-112, 3-24, and 3-100). The *external rectal plexus* is located on its surface outside the muscular coat and the *internal rectal plexus* in its submucosa. These plexuses drain into the superior, middle, and inferior rectal veins. *The superior rectal vein drains into the inferior mesenteric vein and forms one of the clinically important communications between the portal and systemic venous systems* (Fig. 2-112).

CLINICALLY ORIENTED COMMENTS

In some people the veins forming the internal rectal plexus become varicose (dilated and tortuous) and form **internal hemorrhoids** or piles (Case 3-3). *Internal hemorrhoids are covered by anal mucosa* and are located above the **pectinate line** (Fig. 3-100), the line along which the anal valves are located. The veins forming the internal rectal plexus are within loose areolar connective tissue which offers them little support. Hence, they are less able to resist rises in blood pressure. In addition, they are dragged down by hard feces during defecation, which tends to promote development of varicosities. **Portal obstruction** (*e.g.*, associated with *cirrhosis of the liver*) frequently results in the development of **rectal varicosities** (see discussion in Chap. 2, Fig. 2-112, and Case 2-8).

The prostatic venous plexus (Fig. 3-75) *lies on the front and sides of the prostate* within the lateral part of its fascial sheath. It is located posterior to the arcuate ligament and the symphysis pubis (Fig. 3-2) and *receives blood mainly from the deep dorsal veins of the penis* (Figs. 3-31 and 3-37), but it also receives blood from the anterior surface of the bladder and the prostate. *The prostatic venous plexus drains into the vesical venous plexus* and from it into the internal iliac veins. It may also drain via the sacral veins into the **vertebral venous plexus** (Fig. 5-64).

CLINICALLY ORIENTED COMMENTS

The connection between the prostatic venous plexus and the vertebral venous plexus is important clinically. Large valveless veins from the prostatic venous plexus drain into the valveless vertebral veins. Because *blood can flow in either direction*, it may be forced from the prostatic venous plexus into the vertebral veins during coughing, sneezing, and straining, which causes **compression of the inferior vena cava**. *Cancer cells from a prostatic tumor may metastasize via this route to the vertebral column*, invade the vertebrae, and establish **secondary cancerous growths**. Once blood reaches the vertebral venous plexus it may also pass into the segmental intervertebral veins and from there into the *azygos venous system* (Fig. 1-92). Hence, blood from the prostate and the bladder may reach the heart via the superior vena cava instead of via the inferior vena cava. *The internal vertebral venous plexus is large enough to carry the pelvic blood if the inferior vena cava is obstructed* (see Clinically Oriented Comments on this vein in Chap. 2).

The vesical venous plexus in the male (Fig. 3-75) *envelops the base of the bladder and the prostate, the seminal vesicles, the deferent ducts, and the inferior ends of the ureters* and is connected with the prostatic venous plexus. It mainly drains through the inferior vesical veins into the internal iliac veins, but it may drain via the sacral veins into the vertebral venous plexus (Fig. 5-64).

The vesical venous plexus in the female (Fig. 3-24) *envelops the pelvic part of the urethra and the neck of the bladder.* It receives blood from the dorsal vein of the clitoris and communicates with the vaginal plexus.

The vaginal venous plexuses (Fig. 3-24) *lie along the sides of the vagina and within its mucosa.* They communicate with the vesical, uterine, and rectal venous plexuses and drain chiefly through the vaginal veins.

The uterine venous plexuses (Fig. 3-69) *lie along the sides of the uterus between the layers of the broad ligament.* They communicate with the ovarian and vaginal venous plexuses and drain mainly through the uterine veins on each side.

The Pelvic Lymphatics (Figs. 2-14, 2-109, 2-134, and 3-85). There are many lymph nodes and lymph vessels in the pelvis; they are not easy to demonstrate in dissections of old cadavers. *In general the pelvic organs drain through the external and internal iliac lymph nodes and the sacral lymph nodes.* In addition there are small lymph nodes between the layers of the broad ligament and in the fascial sheaths of the bladder and the rectum. *From all these nodes, lymph drains to the common iliac and lumbar lymph nodes* (Fig. 2-134).

The external iliac lymph nodes (8 to 10) lie on the corresponding external iliac vessels and drain lymph from the lower limb, the abdominal wall, the *bladder*, and the *prostate* or the *uterus* and *vagina*.

The internal iliac lymph nodes surround the internal iliac vessels and their branches (Fig. 3-85). They *receive lymph* *from all the pelvic viscera*, deep parts of the perineum, and the gluteal and thigh regions.

The sacral lymph nodes lie on the median and lateral sacral arteries. They *receive lymph from the posterior pelvic wall, the rectum, the neck of the bladder, and the prostate or cervix* of the uterus (Fig. 3-22).

The common iliac lymph nodes form two groups: (1) a *lateral group* lies along the common iliac vessels, and (2) a *median group* in the angle between these vessels (Fig. 3-85). The lateral group receives lymph from the lower limb and the pelvis via the external and internal iliac lymph nodes, whereas the medial group receives lymph directly from the pelvic viscera and indirectly through the internal iliac and sacral lymph nodes.

The lumbar lymph nodes (Fig. 2-134) lie along the abdominal aorta and the inferior vena cava and receive lymph from the common iliac lymph nodes. The efferent vessels from these nodes form right and left **lumbar trunks** which drain into the **cisterna chyli** (Fig. 1-85). This long white *lymph sac* lying on the upper two lumbar vertebrae is discussed in Chapter 2.

THE PELVIC VISCERA

THE URINARY ORGANS

The urinary system (Fig. 2-114) consists of (1) the two excretory organs or **kidneys** (described in Chap. 2), (2) the **ureters**, which convey the urine to (3) the **urinary bladder**, a reservoir for temporarily hold-

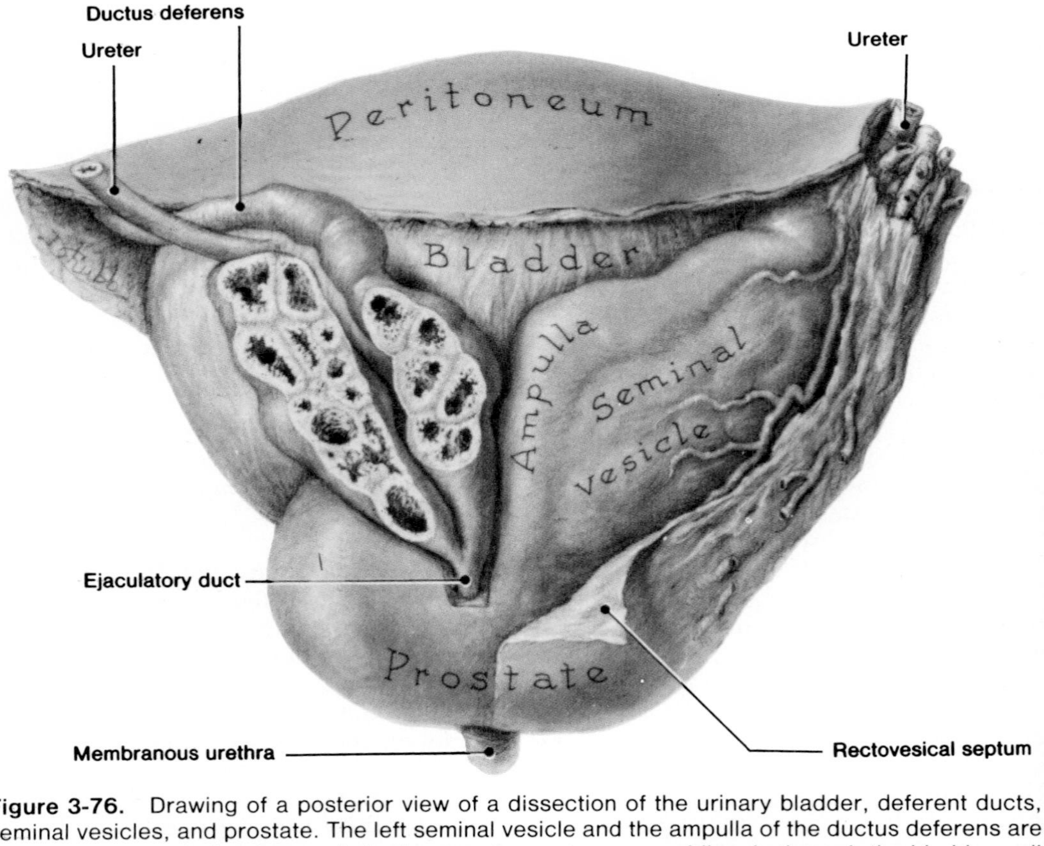

Figure 3-76. Drawing of a posterior view of a dissection of the urinary bladder, deferent ducts, seminal vesicles, and prostate. The left seminal vesicle and the ampulla of the ductus deferens are dissected free and sliced open. *In both sexes* the ureters pass obliquely through the bladder wall in an anteromedial direction to open into the corresponding superolateral angle of the trigone of the bladder (see Figs. 3-72 and 3-75).

ing urine which passes through (4) the **urethra** to reach the exterior.

The Ureters (Figs. 2-113, 2-115, 2-118, 2-124, 2-134, 3-69, 3-70, and 3-72). *The abdominal parts of the ureters*, about half of the 25 cm long muscular tubes, are described in Chapter 2. When leaving the abdomen to enter the pelvis minor *the ureters pass over the pelvic brim anterior to the origins of the external iliac arteries* (Figs. 3-67 and 3-68).

The pelvic part of the ureter courses posteroinferiorly, external to the parietal peritoneum on the side wall of the pelvis (Fig. 3-72) and *anterior to the internal iliac artery* (Fig. 3-70). It continues this course to a point about 1.5 cm superior to the **ischial spine** (Fig. 3-65) and then curves anteromedially, superior to the levator ani muscle.

In the male the ureter lies lateral to the ductus deferens and enters the posterosuperior angle of the bladder, just superior to the seminal vesicle (Figs. 3-75 and 3-76). *In the female* the ureter descends on the side wall of the pelvis minor (Fig. 3-68) where it forms the posterior boundary of the **ovarian fossa** (Figs. 3-69 and 3-86*B*). As it descends it *passes medial to the origin of the uterine artery* (Fig. 3-68) and continues to a point at the level of the ischial spine, where it *is crossed superiorly by the uterine artery* (Fig. 3-69). It then passes close to the lateral fornix of the vagina, especially on the left side, and enters the posterosuperior angle of the bladder (Fig. 3-70).

Vessels and Nerves of the Ureters (Figs. 2-113, 2-124, and 3-66). The vessels and nerves of the ureters are also discussed in Chapter 2. The **blood supply to the ureter** comes from *three main sources*: (1) the *renal artery* (superior end), (2) the *common iliac* or the *aorta*, and (3) the *vesical arteries*. In the pelvis the arteries supplying the ureter approach it from the lateral side. *In the female* the most constant arteries supplying the pelvic part of the ureter are branches of the **uterine artery** in the floor of the pelvis minor (Fig. 3-68). *In the male* similar branches are derived from the **inferior vesical artery** (Fig. 3-66). *Veins accompany all the above arteries and have corresponding names.*

The nerves of the ureter are derived from adjacent *autonomic plexuses* (renal, testicular or ovarian, and inferior hypogastric, Figs. 2-127 and 3-93) which contain pain fibers. The afferent fibers reach the spinal cord through the dorsal roots of T11, T12, and L1 nerves.

CLINICALLY ORIENTED COMMENTS

The ureters are expansile muscular tubes which become dilated if obstructed. An acute obstruction such as results from a **ureteric calculus** or stone (Fig. 3-72) causes colicky pain or colic, as discussed in Case 2-2 at the end of Chapter 2. *The colic results from hyperperistalsis in the ureter above the point of the obstruction.* Usually this **colicky pain** is accompanied or followed by a dull, more constant pain owing to distention of the ureter and renal pelvis.

Ureteric stones may cause complete or intermittent *obstruction of urinary flow.* The obstruction may occur anywhere along the ureter, but it occurs most often (1) where the ureter crosses the external iliac artery and the brim of the pelvis (Fig. 2-67) and (2) where it passes obliquely through the wall of the urinary bladder (Figs. 3-72 and 3-73).

The Urinary Bladder (Figs. 2-114, 3-14, 3-22, 3-32, 3-65, 3-72, 3-73, 3-75, and 3-77). The urinary bladder (L. *vesica*) is a muscular sac or **vesicle for urine storage**. *In the adult* the empty bladder lies in the pelvis minor posterior to the pubic bones from which it is separated by the connective tissue space, called the **retropubic space** (Figs. 3-14, 3-17, 3-22, and 3-24). *In infants and children the bladder is in the abdomen* even when empty; it begins to enter the pelvis major at about 6 years of age but is not entirely in the pelvis minor until after puberty (15 to 16 years).

The urinary bladder is a hollow viscus with strong muscular walls that is characterized by its distensibility. *Its shape, size, position, and relations vary with the*

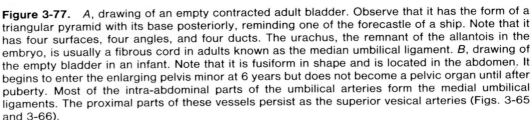

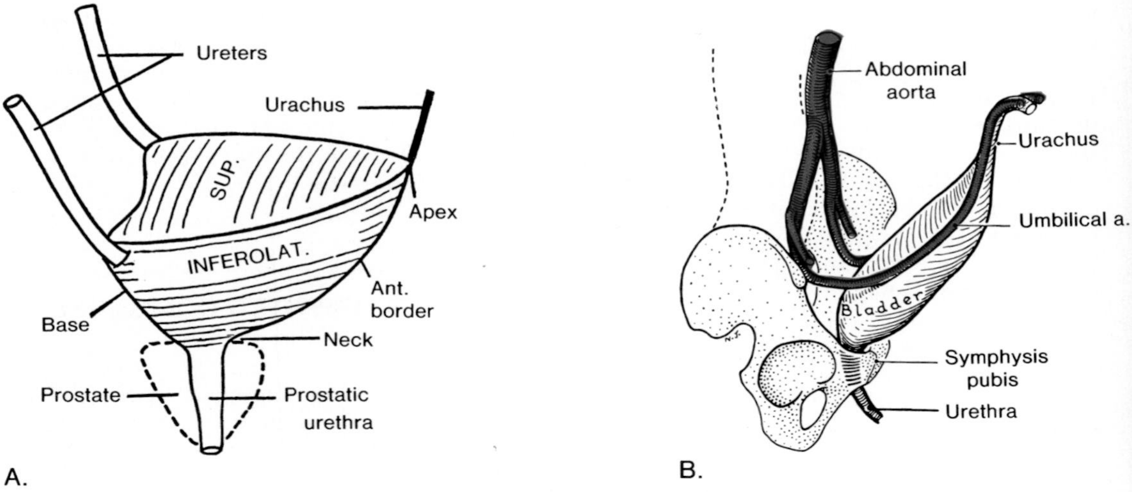

Figure 3-77. *A*, drawing of an empty contracted adult bladder. Observe that it has the form of a triangular pyramid with its base posteriorly, reminding one of the forecastle of a ship. Note that it has four surfaces, four angles, and four ducts. The urachus, the remnant of the allantois in the embryo, is usually a fibrous cord in adults known as the median umbilical ligament. *B*, drawing of the empty bladder in an infant. Note that it is fusiform in shape and is located in the abdomen. It begins to enter the enlarging pelvis minor at 6 years but does not become a pelvic organ until after puberty. Most of the intra-abdominal parts of the umbilical arteries form the medial umbilical ligaments. The proximal parts of these vessels persist as the superior vesical arteries (Figs. 3-65 and 3-66).

amount of urine it contains and with the age of the person. The mucous membrane lining the bladder is soft and only loosely connected to its muscular wall, except in a triangular area at its base called the **trigone of the bladder** (Figs. 3-69 and 3-72). The mucous membrane in the empty contracted bladder is thrown into numerous folds or rugae, except in the trigone where the mucous membrane is always smooth, because here it is firmly attached to the muscular wall.

When empty the bladder lies in the anteroinferior part of the pelvis minor, *inferior to the peritoneum* (Figs. 3-17, 3-65, and 3-77), on the pelvic floor posterior to the symphysis pubis. *In the female* the peritoneum is reflected from the superior surface of the bladder near its posterior border on to the anterior wall of the uterus at the junction of its body and cervix (Fig. 3-22). A **vesicouterine pouch** of peritoneum extends between the bladder and the uterus. This pouch is empty except when the uterus is retroverted (Fig. 3-68); in these cases a loop of bowel may lie in it. *In the male*, the peritoneum is reflected from the surface of the bladder over the superior surfaces of the deferent ducts and seminal vesicles (Figs. 3-14, 3-17, 3-65, and 3-77). The bladder is relatively free within the loose extraperitoneal fatty tissue (Fig. 3-56) except for its neck, which is held firmly by the **puboprostatic ligaments** in the male (Fig. 3-14) and the **pubovesical ligaments** in the female (Fig. 3-22). Hence, as the bladder fills it can expand superiorly into the extraperitoneal fatty tissue of the anterior abdominal wall (Figs. 3-14, 3-17, and 3-22). This lifts the peritoneum from the transversalis fascia of the anterior abdominal wall (Fig. 2-16).

In fixed cadaveric specimens, the empty bladder has the form of a triangular pyramid which is not unlike the forepart or forecastle of a ship (Fig. 3-78). *In living persons* the bladder always contains some urine; hence, it is usually more or less rounded (Fig. 2-118). The empty bladder is described as having *four aspects or sur-*

faces: a **superior surface** facing upward; **two inferolateral surfaces** facing downward, laterally, and forward; and a **posterior surface** facing backward and slightly downward. The inferolateral walls of the bladder are in contact with the fascia covering the levatores ani muscles (Figs. 3-23 and 3-56). The posterior surface is referred to as the **base of the bladder** and its anterior end is known as the **apex of the bladder** (Fig. 3-77). The inferior part of the organ where the base and the inferolateral surfaces converge is called the **neck of the bladder**. The lumen of the bladder opens into the urethra at the neck of the bladder (Fig. 3-75). *In the male* the neck rests on the prostate (Figs. 3-14 and 3-77).

The Bladder Bed (Figs. 3-17 and 3-56). The shape of the bladder is largely determined by the structures closely related to it. The entire organ is enveloped by areolar tissue, called the **vesical fascia**, in which is located the *vesical plexus of veins* (discussed previously). The bladder bed is formed on each side by the pubic bones and the **obturator internus** and **levator ani** muscles and posteriorly by the rectum (Fig. 3-14). *In the female* the base of the bladder is separated from the rectum by the cervix

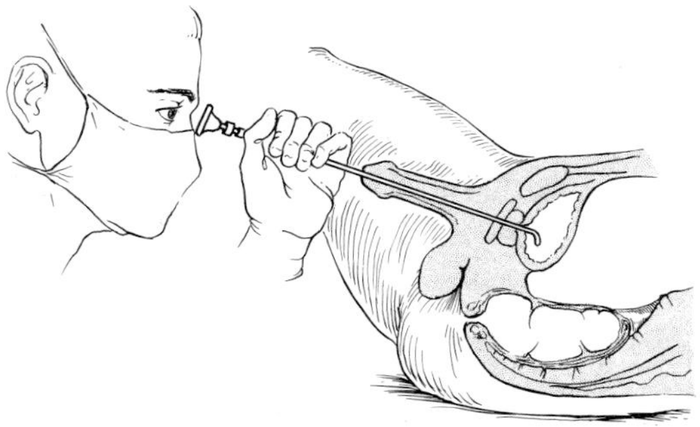

Figure 3-78. Drawing illustrating the use of a cystoscope to examine the interior of the urinary bladder. Various surgical procedures may also be performed through the cystoscope with the aid of carefully designed instruments that are inserted along the barrel of the instrument. A catheter may also be inserted into the ureter through the cystoscope to obtain a sample of urine from the pelvis of the kidney and to inject radiopaque contrast material for retrograde pyelography. This radiographic technique is discussed in Chapter 2. (Illustrated by Mrs. D. M. Hutchinson).

of the uterus and the superior part of the vagina (Fig. 3-22). The **base of the bladder** *in the male* is separated from the rectum by the ampullae of the deferent ducts and the seminal vesicles (Figs. 3-17 and 3-76).

Structure of the Bladder. The wall of the bladder is composed chiefly of smooth muscle called the **detrusor urinae muscle** (L. *detrudere*, to thrust out). It consists of three layers running in many directions. There are external and internal layers of longitudinal fibers and a middle layer of circular fibers. Toward the neck of the bladder these muscle fibers form the involuntary **internal sphincter** of the bladder. Some of these fibers run radially and assist in opening the *internal urethral orifice* (Fig. 3-75). *In the male* the muscle fibers in the neck region are continuous with the connective tissue stroma of the prostate, whereas *in the female* they are continuous with the muscle fibers in the wall of the urethra.

The **mucous membrane**, lined with transitional epithelium and pink in living persons, can undergo considerable stretching. The openings of the ureters (*ureteric orifices*) and the urethra (*internal urethral orifice*) are located at the base of the bladder and form the angles of the **trigone** (Fig. 3-72). *The ureters pass obliquely through the bladder wall in an inferomedial direction,* which helps to prevent urine from backing up into the ureters. An increase in bladder pressure presses the walls of the ureters together, thereby preventing the pressure in the bladder from forcing urine up the ureters and damaging the kidneys. The two orifices of the ureters are connected by a narrow **interureteric ridge** (Fig. 3-75) which forms the superior margin of the trigone.

Vessels and Nerves of the Bladder (Figs. 3-65, 3-66, 3-68, and 3-69). *The main arteries supplying the bladder are branches of the internal iliac arteries.* The **superior vesical arteries**, branches of the umbilical, supply anterosuperior parts of the bladder and the **inferior vesical arteries** supply the base of the bladder. The *obturator* and *inferior gluteal arteries* also supply small branches to the bladder. In the female the *uterine* and *vaginal* arteries also send small branches to this organ.

The veins correspond to the arteries and are *tributaries of the internal iliac veins*. They form the **vesical venous plexuses** described previously (Fig. 3-75).

The lymph vessels from superior parts of the bladder drain to the *external iliac lymph nodes* (Fig. 3-76), whereas those from inferior parts drain to the *internal iliac lymph nodes*. Some lymph vessels from the neck region of the bladder drain into the *sacral* or *common iliac lymph nodes*.

The nerve supply of the bladder is from the *pelvic splanchnic nerves* (**parasympathetic fibers**). They are *motor to the detrusor* muscle and *inhibitory to the internal sphincter*. Hence, when these fibers are stimulated by stretching, the bladder contracts, the internal sphincter relaxes, and urine flows from the bladder. The **sympathetic fibers** are derived from T11, T12, L1, and L2 nerves. These fibers are probably inhibitory to the bladder. *Sensory fibers* from the bladder are visceral and transmit pain sensations (*e.g.*, resulting from overdistention of the bladder). The nerves supplying the bladder form the **vesical nerve plexus**, consisting of both sympathetic and parasympathetic fibers. It is continuous with the *inferior hypogastric plexus* (Fig. 3-93).

CLINICALLY ORIENTED COMMENTS

As it expands, the bladder rises within the extraperitoneal fat and when excessively distended it rises to level of the umbilicus, or even higher in some cases. In so doing, it lifts several centimeters of parietal peritoneum from the suprapubic part of the anterior abdominal wall. The bladder then lies adjacent to this wall without the intervention of peritoneum. Thus, the distended bladder may be punctured (**suprapubic cystostomy**) or approached above the symphysis pubis surgically for the introduction of instruments into it without traversing the peritoneum and involving the peritoneal cavity. **Calculi**, foreign bodies, and small tumors may also be removed from the bladder by this suprapubic route.

Because of the high position of the distended bladder, it may be ruptured by injuries to the inferior part of the anterior abdominal wall or by fractures of the pelvis. The rupture may be extraperitoneal or intraperitoneal. *Rupture of the superior part of the bladder frequently tears the peritoneum, resulting in extravasation of urine into the peritoneal cavity* (Case 3-7 and Fig. 3-104). **Posterior rupture of the bladder** usually results in escape of urine extraperitoneally.

The interior of the bladder can be examined with a **cystoscope** (Fig. 3-78) inserted through the urethra. The bladder can also be examined radiographically after it has been filled with radiopaque material via a catheter.

The Male Urethra (Figs. 2-114, 3-11, 3-14, 3-31, 3-33, 3-35 to 3-37, and 3-75 to 3-78). The urethra in the male is a channel 15 to 20 cm long that *conveys urine from the urinary bladder to the external urethral orifice* (meatus) located at the tip of the glans penis (Figs. 3-30 and 3-36). The male urethra also *provides an exit for semen* or seminal fluid (sperms + glandular secretions). For descriptive purposes the male urethra is divided into three parts.

The Prostatic Part of the Urethra (Figs. 2-114, 3-14, and 3-75). This **first part**, about 3 cm long, *begins at the internal urethral orifice at the apex of the trigone* of the bladder and descends through the prostate, describing a gentle curve that is concave forward. It *ends at the superior layer of deep fascia of the sphincter urethrae muscle* (Fig. 3-14). Its lumen is narrower above and below than in the middle but is contracted except when fluid is passing through it.

The posterior wall of the prostatic part of the urethra has notable features. There is a distinct median, longitudinal ridge called the **urethral crest** (Fig. 3-75). The groove on each side of this crest is called the **prostatic sinus**. Most of the ducts of the prostate gland open into these sinuses (Fig. 3-80); the others open along the sides of the urethral crest. In the central part of the urethral crest there is an ovoid or rounded eminence called the **seminal colliculus** (2 to 4 mm long) on which there is a small slit-like opening. It leads backward and upward into a *blind cul-de-sac*, 0.5 to 1 cm in length, called the **prostatic utricle** (Fig. 3-14).

Explanatory Note. The seminal colliculus is often called the *verumontanum* by urologists. The term **utricle** is derived from a Latin word meaning a *small leather bag*, an appropriate description of the prostatic utricle, a vestigial structure that develops from the *uterovaginal canal* in the embryo. As it is homologous to the uterus and vagina in the female, you may hear it called by its old names, "vagina masculina" or "uterus masculinus," *i.e.*, male vagina and uterus, respectively.

On each side of the orifice of the prostatic utricle on the seminal colliculus is the minute *opening of an ejaculatory duct*. These openings are so small they are difficult to see in a cadaver; however, they can often be catheterized via the urethra in living persons.

CLINICALLY ORIENTED COMMENTS

Owing to the close relationship of the prostate to the prostatic part of the urethra (Figs. 3-14 and 3-75), enlargement of the prostate (**hypertrophy of the prostate**) may obstruct the urethra (see subsequent clinical comments on the prostate). Often such an obstruction can be relieved by an instrument called a *resectoscope* that is inserted into the urethra. This operation is called a **transurethral resection of the prostate**.

The Membranous Part of the Urethra (Figs. 3-10*B*, 3-13, 3-14, 3-16*C*, 3-32, 3-33, 3-56, 3-76, and 3-80). This **second part** is the shortest portion of the urethra (about 1 cm long) and is the **least dilatable.** Except for the *external urethral orifice* (Figs. 3-30 and 3-36), the membranous part is the narrowest portion of the urethra. It descends from the apex of the prostate to the bulb of the penis (Fig. 3-32) and *traverses the sphincter urethrae muscle and the perineal membrane* or inferior fascia of the urogenital diaphragm (Figs. 3-10, 3-11, and 3-16). It pierces the perineal membrane about 2.5 cm posterior to the symphysis pubis (Fig. 3-14). On each side of this part of the urethra is a small **bulbourethral gland** (Figs. 2-26, 3-16*C*, and 3-17).

CLINICALLY ORIENTED COMMENTS

The membranous urethra is the narrowest part of the urethra after the external urethral orifice has been entered. Its narrowness results from contraction of the sphincter urethrae (Figs. 3-14 and 3-16*C*). This circular investment of muscle also makes the membranous urethra the least distensible part of the channel.

The Spongy Part of the Urethra (Figs. 2-26, 2-114, 3-11, 3-14, 3-31, and 3-35 to 3-37). This **third part**, formerly called the cavernous portion, is the longest segment (about 15 cm) of the urethra. It begins where the urethra passes into the corpus spongiosum of the penis (Fig. 3-33) and ends at the external urethral orifice. Because it traverses the entire length of the penis, some people call the spongy part the *penile urethra*. Its lumen is about 5 mm in most places but is expanded in the bulb of the penis to form the **bulb of the urethra** (Fig. 3-14) and in the glans penis to form the **navicular fossa** (Figs. 3-14 and 3-36).

The ducts of the bulbourethral glands (Fig. 3-17) *open into the ventral wall of the proximal part of the spongy urethra* (Fig. 2-26). The orifices of these ducts are very small. There are also minute openings of the ducts of the mucous **urethral glands** (of Littré). These are most numerous on the dorsal surface of the spongy urethra (Fig. 3-36).

Blood Vessels Supplying the Urethra. The arteries are derived from the structures the urethra traverses. Hence, branches of prostatic vessels supply it as it passes through the prostate, and the artery of the bulb and the urethral artery supply its remaining parts. *Its nerves are branches of the pudendal nerve* (Fig. 3-82) and it receives autonomic fibers from the cavernous nerve plexuses.

CLINICALLY ORIENTED COMMENTS

The normal male urethra, about 5 mm in diameter, will expand enough to permit the passage of an instrument about 8 mm in diameter. However, the external urethral orifice is the narrowest and least distensible part of the urethra. Hence, an instrument that passes through this opening should pass through all other parts of the urethra. **Urethral stricture** may occur as the result of external trauma or infection; instruments called **sounds** are used to dilate the urethra.

Urethral catheterization is frequently done to remove urine from a patient who is unable to micturate (void). It is also performed to irrigate the bladder and to obtain an uncontaminated sample of urine. *When inserting catheters and sounds the curves in the urethra must be considered.* The membranous part runs downward and forward as it passes through the urogenital diaphragm (Fig. 3-10*B*) and the prostatic part takes a slight curve which is concave forward as it traverses the prostate (Figs. 2-26 and 3-14). Just below the perineal membrane (Figs. 3-10*B* and 3-14), the spongy urethra is well covered inferiorly and posteriorly by the erectile tissue of the bulb of the penis (Fig. 3-11), but a short segment of it is unprotected superiorly. Because the urethral wall is thin and distensible here, it is vulnerable to injury during rough instrumentation.

Rupture of the bulb of the spongy urethra is fairly common in **straddle injuries** (Case 3-2). The urethra is torn when it is caught between a hard object (*e.g.*, a steel beam, the horn of a saddle, or the bar of a bicycle) and the equally hard pubic arch. Thus, urine escapes into the superficial perineal space or pouch (Fig. 3-10) and from there downward into the scrotum and upward in the anterior abdominal wall, deep to the superficial fascia (see the discussion of Case 3-2 for details).

The most *common congenital abnormality* of the urethra is **hypospadias** (see Fig. 3-79 and Case 3-4). In these males there is a defect in the ventral wall of the spongy urethra so that it is open for a greater or lesser distance (Fig. 3-79). Hence, the urethral opening is in a more proximal position on the ventral surface of the penis or on the scrotum (Figs. 3-103 and 3-107). In the *glandular type of hypospadias* (Fig. 3-103), the prepuce is deformed and its frenulum may be absent.

The Female Urethra (Figs. 3-3, 3-22, 3-39, 3-42, and 3-72). *The female urethra is a short* (2 to 6 cm) *muscular tube* lined by mucous membrane. It corresponds to the prostatic and membranous parts of the male urethra. From the bladder *it passes anteroinferiorly*, posterior and then inferior to the symphysis pubis. *The external urethral orifice is located between the labia minora, just anterior to the vaginal orifice* (Figs. 3-22 and 3-39) *and inferoposterior to*

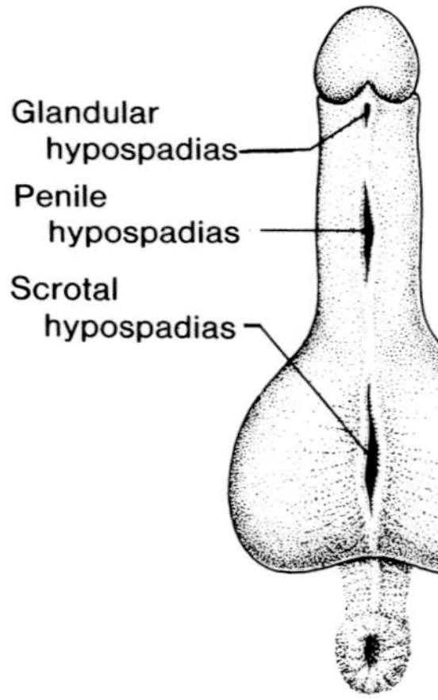

Figure 3-79. Drawing of the ventral or urethral surface of the penis, illustrating various abnormal locations of the urethral opening. From above downward are shown the glandular, penile, and scrotal types of hypospadias. The glandular and penile types result from failure of fusion of the urogenital folds and the scrotal type results from failure of fusion of the labioscrotal swellings (see Fig. 3-29).

the clitoris (Fig. 3-42). The urethra, 5 to 6 mm in diameter, is closed except during micturition; it lies anterior to the vagina and is separated from it superiorly by a **vesicovaginal space**. Inferiorly it is so intimately associated with the vagina that it appears to be embedded in it (Fig. 3-23). *It passes with the vagina through the pelvic and urogenital diaphragms and the perineal membrane* (Figs. 3-16, 3-57, and 3-60). The female urethra is surrounded by the **sphincter urethrae muscle** (Fig. 3-15) and some fibers of this voluntary sphincter enclose both the urethra and the vagina (Fig. 3-25). **Urethral glands** similar to those in the male urethra are present, particularly in its superior part.

The **blood supply to the female urethra** is from the *inferior vesical, internal pudendal,* and *vaginal arteries* (Fig. 3–69). **Lymph vessels** pass the *sacral* and *internal iliac lymph nodes* (Fig. 3-85); a few lymph vessels also pass to the *inguinal lymph nodes.*

CLINICALLY ORIENTED COMMENTS

The short female urethra is very distensible because it contains much elastic tissue as well as smooth muscle. Thus, it can easily be dilated to 1 cm without injuring it. Because of these anatomical features, *passage of catheters or cystoscopes is much easier than in the male.* Hence, **calculi**, foreign bodies, and small **tumors** may be removed from the bladder via the urethra. Urine may also be readily removed from a distended female bladder by passing a catheter through the urethra into the bladder. **Catheterization** is often performed before pelvic operations to decompress the bladder.

THE GENITAL ORGANS

The Male Genital Organs (Figs. 2-26, 3-14, 3-17, 3-30, 3-32, 3-35, 3-38, and 3-76). The male genital organs comprise the testes, the deferent ducts, the seminal vesicles, and the ejaculatory ducts. The **prostate** and **bulbourethral glands** are accessory or *auxiliary genital glands.*

The **testis** and **scrotum** are described in Chapter 2 (Figs. 2-19 and 2-24 to 2-27). The **penis** was described earlier in the present chapter.

The Ductus Deferens (Figs. 2-25 to 2-27, 3-17, 3-27, 3-65, 3-75, and 3-76). The ductus deferens (vas deferens) is a *thick-walled muscular tube* which begins in the tail of the epididymis and **ends in the ejaculatory duct** (Fig. 3-76), carrying sperms from one to the other. It ascends in the spermatic cord, passes through the inguinal canal (Fig. 2-26), and crosses over the external iliac vessels to enter the pelvis minor (Fig. 3-65). *The ductus deferens passes along the side wall of the pelvis where it lies external but adherent to the parietal peritoneum* and medial to the vessels and nerves. *It crosses the ureter near the posterolateral angle of the bladder, running between the ureter and the peritoneum* (Figs. 3-65 and 3-76) to reach the base of the bladder. At first it lies superior to the seminal vesicle and then it descends medial to the ureter and this vesicle. The ductus deferens enlarges to form the **ampulla** as it passes posterior to the bladder (Fig. 3-76). It then narrows and joins the duct of the seminal vesicle in the groove between the prostate and the bladder to form the **ejaculatory duct** (Figs. 3-77 and 3-80). The enlarged distal portion of the ductus deferens or ampulla (Figs. 3-76, 3-80, and 3-81) lies against the posterior wall of the bladder.

The tiny *artery to the ductus deferens* is closely applied to its surface (Fig. 2-27). It arises from the *umbilical artery* (Fig. 3-65) and terminates by anastomosing with the testicular artery posterior to the testis (Fig. 2-27). *The ductus deferens is richly innervated by autonomic nerve fibers,* thereby facilitating its rapid contraction for expulsion of sperms during ejaculation. For a discussion of **vasectomy** (excision of a segment of the ductus deferens or vas deferens), for sterilizing a male, see Chapter 2.

The Seminal Vesicles (Figs. 3-17, 3-32, 3-76, 3-80, and 3-81). The seminal vesicles (glands) consist of long tubes (15 cm) which are coiled to form vesicle-like masses on the

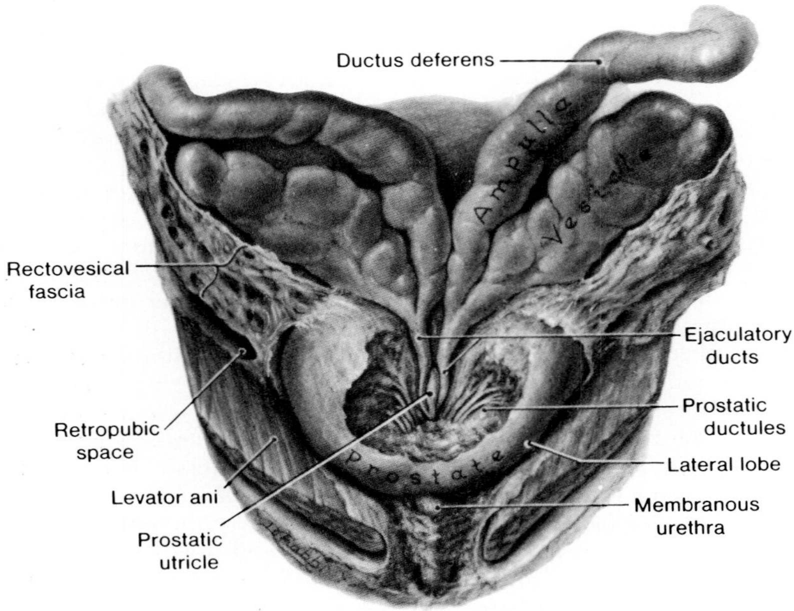

Figure 3-80. Drawing of a dissection of the prostate from behind. Observe the right and left ejaculatory ducts, each formed where the duct of a seminal vesicle joins the ampullary end of a ductus deferens. Note the vestigial prostatic utricle lying between the ends of the two ejaculatory ducts. All three open into the prostatic urethra (Fig. 3-75). The 20 to 30 prostatic ductules mostly open on to the prostatic sinus.

base of the bladder. For years it was thought that they stored seminal fluid because sperms have been observed in them in cadaveric specimens. It is now widely accepted that **they do not store sperms** in living persons. It would be more appropriate to call them *seminal glands* because they secrete a thick secretion which mixes with the sperms as they pass along the ejaculatory ducts (Figs. 3-80). This secretion is probably concerned with the activation of the sperms.

The seminal vesicles are situated at the base of the bladder, anterior to the rectum (Figs. 3-76 and 3-84). Their superior ends are covered with peritoneum and lie behind the ureters, where they are separated from the rectum by the peritoneum of the **rectovesical pouch** (Fig. 3-14). Their inferior ends are closely related to the rectum and are separated from it only by a layer of smooth muscle and fibers, called the **rectovesical septum** (Figs. 3-14, 3-21, and 3-77). *The duct of each seminal vesicle joins the ductus deferens to form the ejaculatory duct* (Figs. 3-77, 3-80, and 3-81), which opens into the posterior wall of the prostatic urethra (Fig. 3-75).

The artery to the ductus deferens also supplies the seminal vesicle. The muscular walls of the seminal vesicles contain a plexus of nerve fibers and also some sympathetic ganglia. The preganglionic sympathetic fibers emerge from the *upper lumbar nerves* and the parasympathetic fibers emerge from the *pelvic splanchnic nerves* (S2, S3, and S4, Fig. 3-82). All these fibers pass through the **inferior hypogastric plexus** (Figs. 2-127 and 3-93).

The Ejaculatory Duct (Figs. 2-26, 3-76, 3-80, and 3-81). Each of these ducts is a slender tube formed by the union of the duct of the seminal vesicle and the ductus deferens. The ejaculatory ducts are 2 to 2.5 cm long and are formed near the neck of the bladder (Figs. 3-76 and 3-77). The two ducts run close together as they pass anteroinferiorly through the prostate (Fig. 3-80) and along the sides of the minute prostatic utricle. *The ejaculatory ducts open by slit-*

like apertures into the prostatic urethra (Fig. 3-75), one on each side of the orifice of the prostatic utricle or just inside this vestigial organ.

The Prostate (Figs. 2-26, 3-14, 3-17, 3-20, 3-21, 3-32, 3-75, 3-76, and 3-80). *The prostate is the largest of the accessory glands of the male reproductive tract.* It is a partly glandular and partly fibromuscular organ about the size of a horse chestnut or a walnut and *surrounds the first part of the urethra, i.e.*, the **prostatic urethra**. It is situated low in the pelvis minor posterior to the symphysis pubis and is enclosed by a dense sheath of fascia, called the *fascial sheath of the prostate.* Posteriorly this fascia is part of the *rectovesical septum* (Figs. 3-14, 3-21, and 3-76), which separates the bladder, the seminal vesicles, and the prostate from the rectum. Inferiorly the fascial sheath of the prostate is continuous with the superior fascia of the urogenital diaphragm. The **prostatic venous plexus** (Fig. 3-75) lies between the capsule of the gland and its fascial sheath.

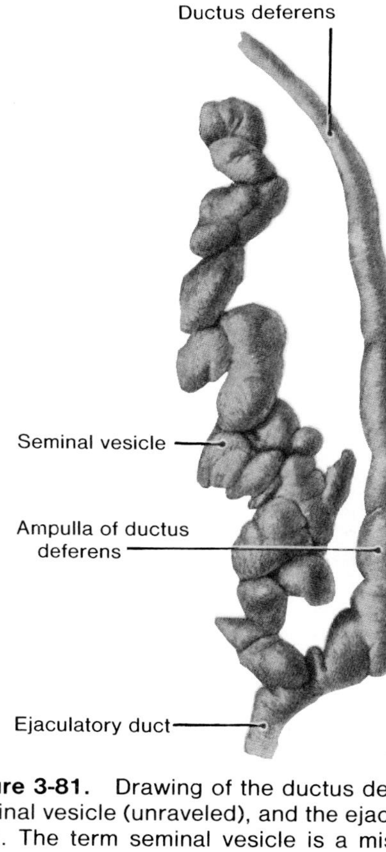

Figure 3-81. Drawing of the ductus deferens, seminal vesicle (unraveled), and the ejaculatory duct. The term seminal vesicle is a misnomer because it is a tortuous tube with numerous diverticula (outpouchings) and is coiled upon itself giving it the appearance of a vesicle (Fig. 3-80). *Understand the seminal vesicle does not store sperms or seminal fluid;* it secretes fluid which is added to the semen.

The prostate is somewhat conical in shape and has a base, an apex, and three surfaces (posterior and two inferolateral surfaces). The **base**, normally 3.5 to 4 cm in diameter, is *related to the neck of the bladder* (Fig. 3-77). The prostatic urethra enters the middle of the base of the prostate near its anterior border (Fig. 3-14). The **apex**, located about 3 cm distal to the base, is *related to the superior fascia of the urogenital diaphragm and rests on the sphincter urethrae muscle* (Figs. 3-13 and 3-14). The prostate is embraced by the medial margins of the levatores ani muscles (Figs. 3-13 and 3-17). The **posterior surface** of the prostate *is triangular and flattened transversely*, facing backward and slightly downward toward the urogenital diaphragm. The **inferolateral surfaces** meet anteriorly with the convex anterior surface and rest on the fascia covering the levatores ani (Fig. 3-56). *The prostatic urethra and the ejaculatory ducts pass through the substance of the prostate*, dividing it into median and lateral lobes.

Explanatory Note. Definitions of the divisions of the prostate are subject to much controversy. All divisions are arbitrary and not structurally distinct. In addition to the usual median and right and left lobes, some clinicians refer to a posterior lobe which is part of the lateral lobes that can be palpated through the rectum (Fig. 3-84).

The median lobe of the prostate lies anterosuperior to the prostatic utricle and the ejaculatory ducts (Figs. 3-75 and 3-80). In old men *the median lobe commonly produces a projection into the cavity of the bladder*, just posterior to the internal urethral orifice, called the uvula vesicae or **uvula of the bladder** (Fig. 3-75). Here the median lobe is in contact superiorly with

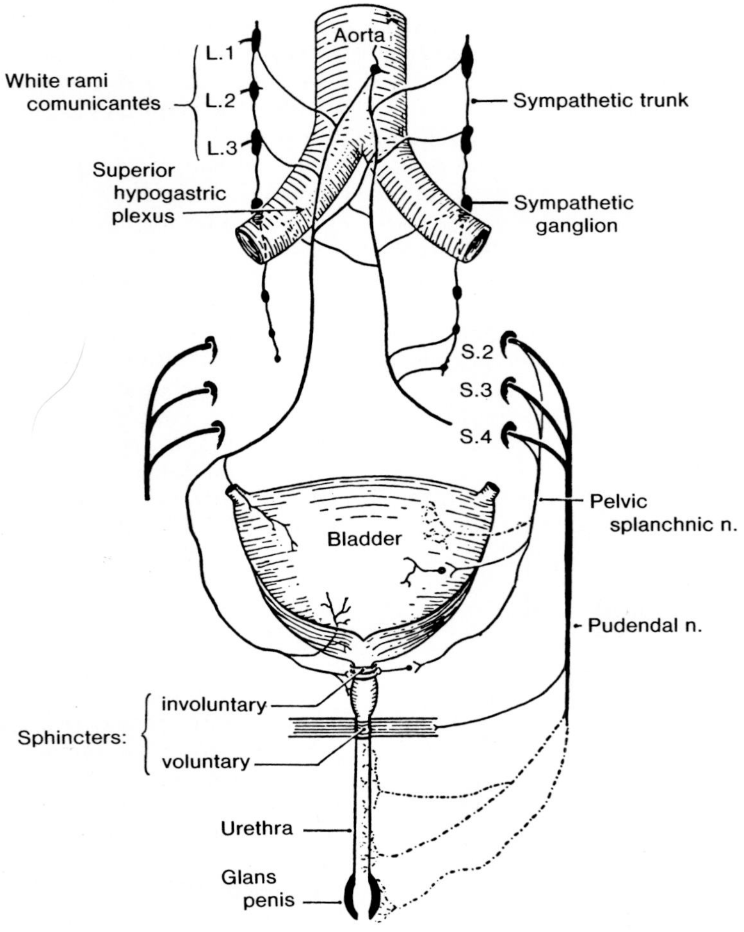

Figure 3-82. Diagram of the nerve supply to the urinary bladder and urethra. The *broken lines* indicate afferent fibers. The parasympathetic fibers are in the pelvic splanchnic nerves (nervi erigentes; S2, S3, and S4) and are the motor nerves to the bladder. When they are stimulated, the bladder empties, the blood vessels dilate, and the penis erects. They are also the sensory nerves of the bladder. The sympathetic fibers through the superior hypogastric plexus (presacral nerve; lower thoracic, L1, L2, and L3) are motor to a continuous muscle sheet comprising the ureteric musculature, the trigonal muscle, and the muscle of the urethral crest. They also supply the muscle of the epididymis, ductus deferens, seminal vesicle, and prostate. When the superior hypogastric plexus is stimulated, seminal fluid is ejaculated into the urethra but is hindered from entering the bladder, perhaps by the muscle sheet which is drawn toward the internal urethral orifice. The sympathetic fibers are also vasoconstrictor and to some slight extent are sensory to the trigone region. The pudendal nerve is motor to the sphincter urethrae and sensory to the glans penis and the urethra. It seems that the sympathetic supply to the bladder has a vasoconstrictor and a sexual effect, and that as regards micturition, it is not antagonistic to the parasympathetic supply.

the inferior part of the trigone of the bladder. The **right** and **left lobes** making up the remainder of the prostate cannot be clearly defined anatomically from the median lobe. They are separated by the prostatic urethra and are joined anteriorly by an isthmus. The **prostatic utricle** (Figs. 3-75 and 3-80), representing the *remains of the uterovaginal canal in the embryo* (fused paramesonephric ducts), is located in the substance of the median lobe of the prostate and appears as a blind tubule. It has no functional significance.

Most of the **prostatic ductules** (20 to 30) *open into the prostatic sinuses on each side of the urethral crest* on the posterior wall of the prostatic urethra (Fig. 3-75). This occurs because most of the glandular tissue is located posterior and lateral to the prostatic urethra. *The prostatic secretion is a thin, milky fluid* which is discharged into the urethra by contraction of its smooth muscle (Fig. 3-83).

The arteries of the prostate are derived from the *internal pudendal, inferior vesical,* and *middle rectal* arteries (Figs. 3-65 and 3-66). **The veins of the prostate** are wide and thin-walled and form the *prostatic venous plexus* around the sides and base of the prostate (Fig. 3-75). *This plexus drains into the internal iliac veins, but also communicates with the vesical plexus and the vertebral venous plexuses* (Fig. 5-64).

The lymph vessels of the prostate terminate chiefly in the *internal iliac* and *sacral lymph nodes* (Fig. 3-85); some vessels from the posterior surface pass with the lymph vessels of the bladder to the *external iliac lymph nodes,* and some from the anterior surface pass to the internal iliac group by joining those from the membranous urethra. **The nerves of the prostate** are derived from the *inferior hypogastric plexus* (Fig. 3-93). The prostate is well supplied with plexuses of nonmyelinated nerve fibers connected to small sympathetic ganglia. Various types of sensory nerve ending are located in the connective tissue of the gland.

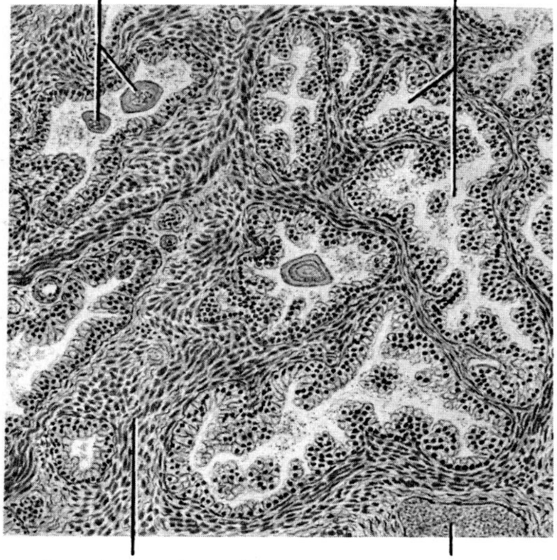

Figure 3-83. Drawing of a section of the prostate removed from a 54-year-old person killed in an accident. Observe the prostatic concretions in the alveoli of the gland. Hematoxylin-eosin, ×65.

CLINICALLY ORIENTED COMMENTS

The prostate is of great medical interest because *benign nodular hyperplasia of the prostate* is a common condition in older males. This disease begins in the mid 40s and results in varying degrees of *obstruction of the neck of the bladder.* The size and activity of the prostate are controlled by sex hormones. The prostate is small at birth but rapidly enlarges at puberty (13 to 16 years). In most males the prostate progressively enlarges (*i.e.,* undergoes **hypertrophy**) after the mid 40s, but in some males it becomes more fibrous and smaller (*i.e.,* undergoes **atrophy**). The etiology or cause of these changes is not known, but they are probably related to endocrine changes, primarily in the sex hormones occurring at this period of life.

Benign prostatic hypertrophy (Fig. 3-17) affects a high proportion of elderly men and is a common cause of urethral obstruction leading to **nocturia** (need to urinate during the night), **dysuria** (difficulty and/or pain during urination), and **urgency** (sudden desire to void). The enlarged prostate projects into the urinary bladder impeding the urinary flow by elevating the internal urethral orifice above the floor of the bladder and by lengthening and distorting the prostatic urethra. Sometimes the overgrowth of the prostate mainly involves the median lobe and forms a valve-like mechanism at the internal urethral orifice. Consequently, as the patient strains, the obstruction of the bladder outlet increases. The hypertrophied prostate gland may be removed surgically (*prostatectomy*).

Cancer (adenocarcinoma) of the prostate is one of the most common tumors of men, being found *microscopically* at autopsy within the gland in about 60% of men over 80 years of age. *Cancer of the prostate metastasizes via both blood* (**hematogenous spread**) *and lymph vessels* (**lymphogenous spread**). An anatomical basis for metastases to the vertebral column and pelvis is via the valveless *venous communications between the prostatic plexus of veins and the vertebral venous plexuses* (Fig. 5-64), especially the internal (extradural) vertebral plexus. The main connections are via the pelvic and common iliac veins to the **ascending lumbar vein**. It has been shown that straining to urinate, necessary because the prostatic cancer is impeding the flow of urine, causes the blood draining the **prostatic venous plexus** (Fig. 3-75) to reverse its flow and pass via the lumbar veins into the **vertebral venous plexuses.**

It is possible for cancer cells to spread via the pelvic lymphatics (**lymphogenous metastases**) to the lymph nodes around the internal iliac and common iliac arteries and the aorta (Fig. 3-85). *Tumor cells from the prostate may also pass via the pelvic veins to the inferior vena cava,* the right heart, the lungs, the left heart and then throughout the body. For some reason, prostatic cancer cells are more apt to produce **bone metastases** than organ metastases and are more likely to cause an *increase in bone density* than bone destruction.

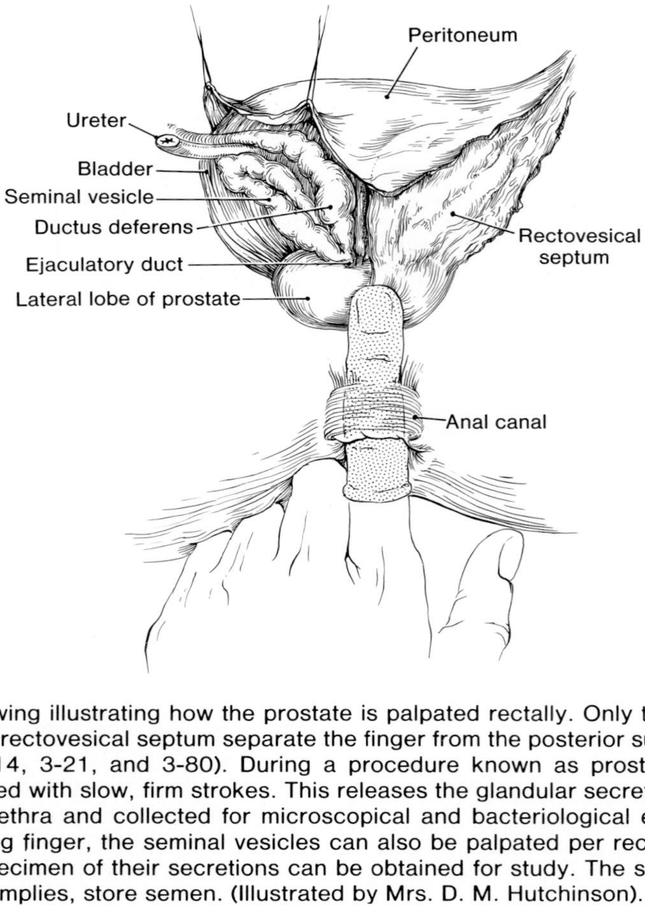

Figure 3-84. Drawing illustrating how the prostate is palpated rectally. Only the anterior wall of the rectum and the rectovesical septum separate the finger from the posterior surface of the gland (also see Figs. 3-14, 3-21, and 3-80). During a procedure known as prostatic massage, the prostate is massaged with slow, firm strokes. This releases the glandular secretions which can be milked from the urethra and collected for microscopical and bacteriological examination. If the examiner has a long finger, the seminal vesicles can also be palpated per rectum, particularly if enlarged, and a specimen of their secretions can be obtained for study. The seminal vesicles *do not*, as their name implies, store semen. (Illustrated by Mrs. D. M. Hutchinson).

The posterior surface of the prostate is palpable through the rectum (Fig. 3-84). Only the anterior wall of the rectum and the rectovesical septum (Fig. 3-14) separate the examiner's gloved finger from the prostate. Palpating the prostate rectally provides information about its size and consistency; *e.g.*, a **malignant prostate** feels hard and nodular and **prostatitis** (inflammation of the prostate) results in an enlarged, tender, *hot prostate.* In some cases **prostatic massage** is performed to obtain prostatic fluid for microscopical and bacteriological examination.

The position of the prostate depends on the fullness of the bladder. A full bladder displaces the gland inferiorly so that it is more readily palpable; hence, an unwary examiner may assume the gland is hypertrophied because it is so easily palpated when it is actually normal.

In histological sections of the prostate it is common to see spherical or ellipsoid lamellated bodies, called **prostatic concretions** (corpora amylacea), in the tubules or alveoli (Fig. 3-83). Their number increases with age. Small prostatic concretions pass out of the gland with its secretions and are added to the semen. Large concretions are unable to pass through the minute prostattic ductules (Fig. 3-80) and remain in the prostate. If the prostatic concretions become calcified they are known as **prostatic calculi** (stones). Some of these become very large and may be palpated during prostatic massage (Fig. 3-84) if they are near the surface. Because they are firmly embedded in the fibrous stroma of the prostate they *simulate the irregular hardness of a carcinoma.* In some cases the calculi are relatively free and give the palpating finger the impression of a bean bag.

The Bulbourethral Glands (Figs. 2-26, 3-16*C*, and 3-17). This pair of pea-sized yellowish glands, formerly called Cowper's glands, *lie posterolateral to the membranous urethra.* They are above the bulb of the penis and within the fibers of the sphincter urethrae muscle. Their relatively long ducts (2.5 to 3 cm) pass through the inferior fascia of the urogenital diaphragm or perineal membrane with the urethra and through the bulb of the penis, *to open by minute apertures into the proximal part of the spongy urethra* (Fig. 2-26). The bulbourethral glands receive their **blood supply** from the *arteries to the bulb of the penis* (Figs. 3-11 and 3-17).

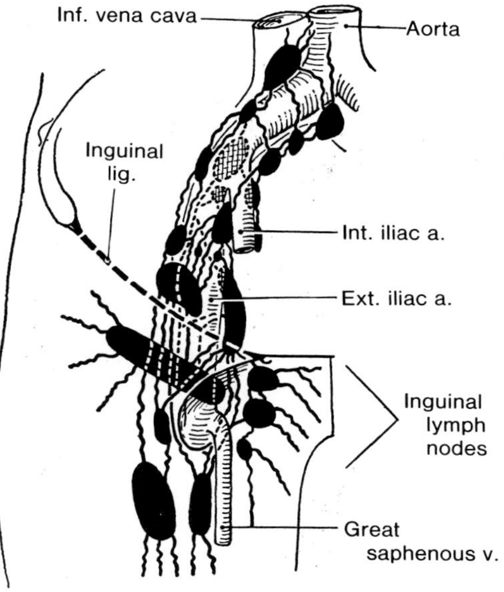

Figure 3-85. Drawing of a dissection of the inguinal and pelvic lymphatics. Observe that there are two groups of pelvic lymph nodes: (1) near the pelvic brim and (2) within the pelvic cavity. The lymph nodes near the pelvic brim (12 or more) are the external and common iliac lymph nodes which are arranged around the respective blood vessels and the nodes superior to the sacral promontory. The nodes within the pelvic cavity, not shown (internal iliac, lateral sacral, and median sacral) are arranged (1) on the respective blood vessels; (2) in the vesical fascia; (3) in the rectal fascia mainly behind the rectal (pararectal nodes); (4) on the course of the superior rectal artery in the broad ligament near the cervix; and (5) between the prostate and the rectum. The lymph nodes arranged along the external, internal, and common iliac vessels form a complex that is often referred to clinically as the *iliopelvic plexus of lymph nodes.*

The Female Genital Organs (Figs. 3-12, 3-15, 3-22 to 3-24, 3-68 to 3-73, 3-86, and 3-87). The *external female genitalia* (**vulva**, female pudendum) have been described and are illustrated in Figures 3-3 and 3-39 to 3-43. The *internal female gen-*

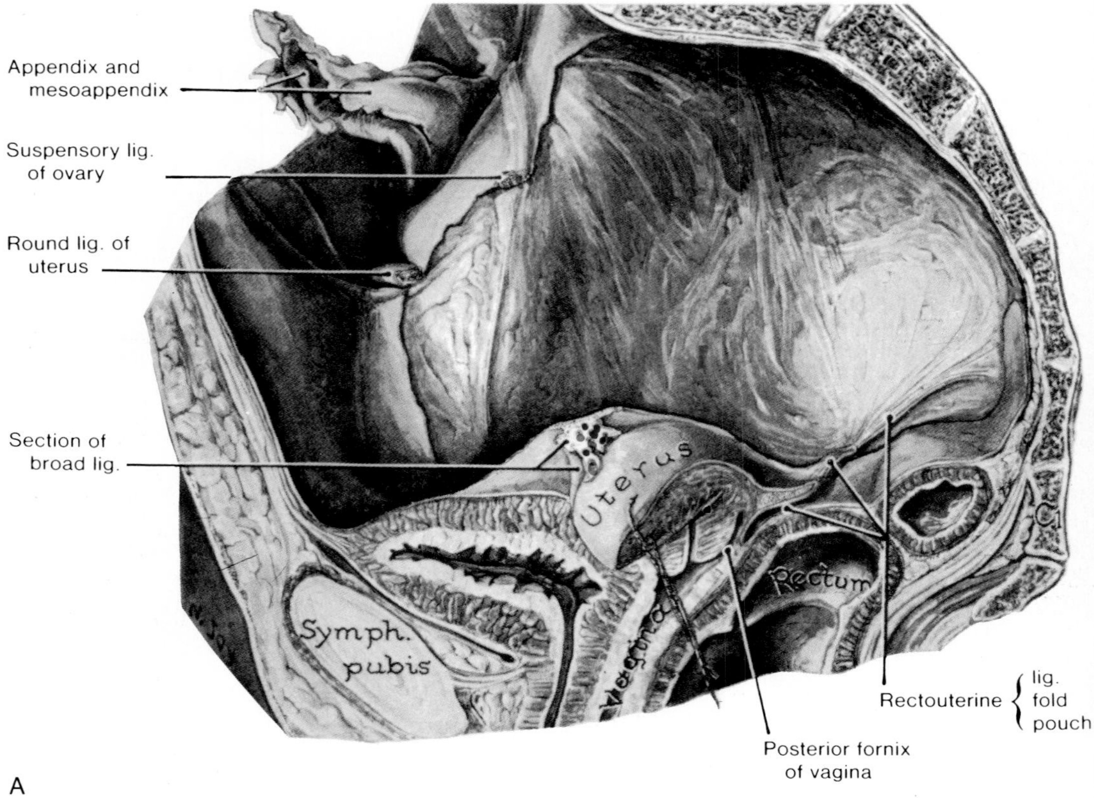

A

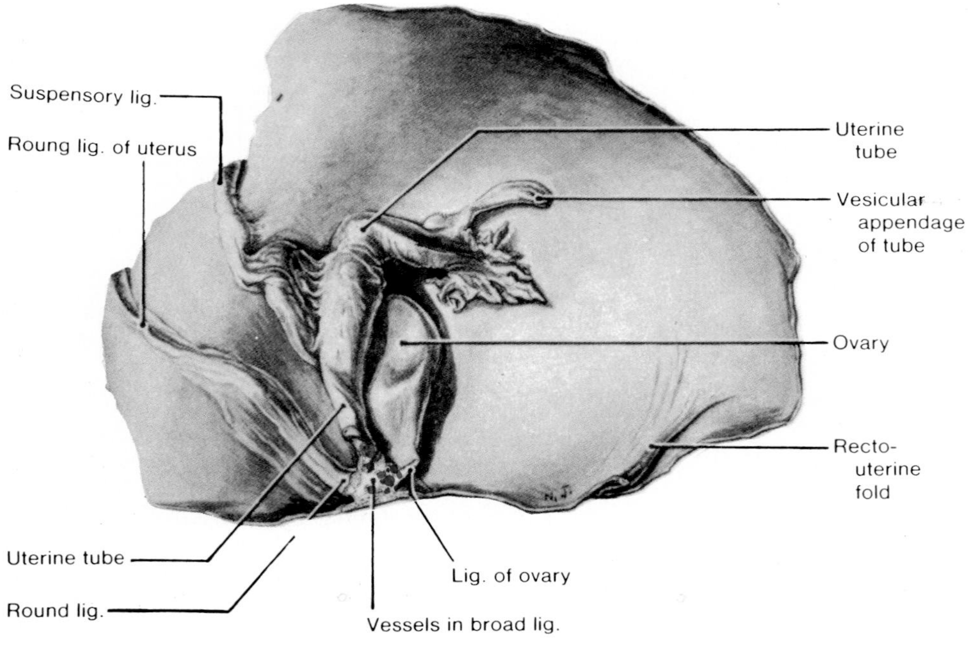

B.

Figure 3-86. *A*, drawing of a median section of the female pelvis. Note that the following structures have been divided at the pelvic brim: the round ligament and the suspensory ligament with the contained ovarian vessels and nerves. The following structures have been divided at the side of the uterus: the broad ligament with the uterine tube in its free margin, the round ligament anteriorly, the ligament of the ovary posteriorly, and several branches of the uterine vessels. *B*, drawing of the broad ligament and related structures which were peeled off the side wall of the pelvis shown in *A*, leaving the subperitoneal fatty-areolar tissue (tela subserosa) exposed.

italia consist primarily of the *vagina*, the uterus, the *uterine tubes*, and the *ovaries*.

The Vagina (Figs. 3-12, 3-22 to 3-24, 3-41, 3-69, and 3-72). The vagina (L. sheath), the **female organ of copulation**, is a *musculomembranous tube* lined with stratified epithelium. It forms the inferior portion of the female genital tract and *serves as the inferior end of the birth canal.* In the anatomical position the vagina descends anteroinferiorly from the **rectouterine pouch** (Fig. 3-22) and describes a slight curve that is convex anteriorly. Its anterior wall (6 to 8 cm long) and its posterior wall (7 to 10 cm) are normally in apposition (Fig. 3-23); hence, *the vagina is only a potential canal* except where it is held apart by the cervix of the uterus (Fig. 3-22). It opens inferiorly into the **vestibule of the vagina** between the labia minora (Figs. 3-12 and 3-41). It communicates superiorly with the cavity of the uterus (Fig. 3-87) and its posterior wall extends superior to the cervix of the uterus to the **posterior fornix** (discussed subsequently). A thin *fold of mucous membrane*, called the **hymen** (G. membrane), surrounds the entrance to the vagina or vaginal orifice (Fig. 3-15). After childbirth the hymen is much less visible and usually consists only of tabs (**hymenal caruncles**).

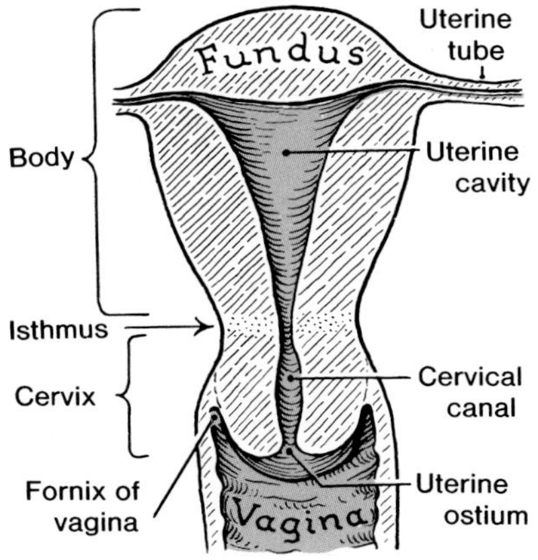

Figure 3-87. Diagram of the uterus and vagina illustrating the parts of the uterus and the relationship of its cervix (L. neck) to the superior end of the vagina (L. sheath). Observe that the superior end of the vagina surrounds the vaginal portion of the cervix. For brevity clinicians often call the uterine ostium (opening) the *external os* and the opening of the cervical canal into the uterine cavity the *internal os*.

The vagina lies posterior to the urinary bladder and anterior to the rectum (Figs. 3-22, 3-23, and 3-60) and *passes between the medial margins of the two levatores ani muscles.* It pierces the **urogenital diaphragm** with the sphincter urethrae muscle, the posterior fibers of which are attached to the vaginal wall (Figs. 3-15, 3-16*C*, and 3-25).

The cervix of the uterus projects into the uppermost part of the anterior wall of the vagina, slightly separating its walls (Fig. 3-22). As a result of the cervix projecting into the anterior wall of the vagina, *the uterus lies almost at a right angle to the axis of the vagina in its normal anteverted position* (Fig. 3-22). Because more of the posterior part of the cervix enters the vagina than does the anterior part, the recess or cul-de-sac between the vaginal wall and the cervix is deeper posteriorly than anteriorly. The recess anterior to the cervix is called the **anterior fornix** (L. arch, vault); the recess posterior to it is known as the **posterior fornix** (Fig. 3-86*A*); and the recesses at its sides are referred to as the **lateral fornices** (Fig. 3-87). Understand that these four fornices are parts of a continuous recess surrounding the cervix (Fig. 3-22).

The relations of the vagina are important. From above downward, *its anterior wall is in contact with the cervix, the base of the bladder, the terminal parts of the ureters, and the urethra* (Figs. 3-22, 3-69, and 3-70). *It is intimately connected to the neck of the bladder and to the urethra* and is joined to the pubis by the **pubovesical** and **pubourethral ligaments** (Fig. 3-22).

The superior limit of the vagina (i.e., the 1 to 2 cm of its posterior wall covering the posterior fornix) *is usually covered by peritoneum.* Thus, injuries to this part of the vagina may involve the peritoneal cavity (see subsequent clinical comments). Inferior to the posterior fornix, only the loose connective (areolar) tissue of the **rectovaginal septum** (Figs. 3-15 and 3-24) separates the posterior wall of the vagina from the rectum. The vagina is also related inferiorly to the **perineal body** (Fig. 3-12).

The narrow lateral walls of the vagina

in the region of the lateral fornices (Fig. 3-87) *are attached to the broad ligament* of the uterus (Fig. 3-70), where it contains the ureters and the uterine vessels (Figs. 3-69 and 3-86). Inferiorly, the lateral walls of the vagina *are in contact with the levatores ani muscles* (Fig. 3-60), *the greater vestibular glands, and the bulbs of the vestibule* (Figs. 3-12 and 3-46). Contraction of the levatores ani muscles decreases the size of the vaginal lumen by drawing the walls of the vagina together.

The arteries of the vagina (Figs. 3-69, 3-71, and 3-72) are the *vaginal*, the vaginal branch of the *uterine*, the *internal pudendal*, and the vaginal branches of the *middle rectal*. All these are branches of the internal iliac arteries.

The veins form *vaginal venous plexuses* along the sides of the vagina (Fig. 3-24) which are drained through the vaginal veins into the internal iliac veins.

The lymph vessels of the vagina are in three groups: (1) those from the superior part of the vagina accompany the uterine artery and drain into the **internal** and **external iliac lymph nodes** (Fig. 3-85); (2) those from the *middle part of the vagina* accompany the vaginal artery and drain into the **internal iliac lymph nodes**; and (3) those from the *vagina below the hymen (i.e.,* its vestibule) drain mainly into the superficial **inguinal lymph nodes** (Figs. 3-85 and 4-38). Some vessels from the vestibule drain into the sacral and common iliac lymph nodes.

The nerves of the vagina are derived from the *uterovaginal plexus* which lies in the base of the broad ligament *on each side of the supravaginal part of the cervix* (Figs. 3-92 and 3-93). Sympathetic, parasympathetic, and afferent fibers pass through this plexus. The lower nerve fibers from this plexus supply the cervix and the superior part of the vagina. The *vaginal nerves* follow the vaginal arteries and end in the wall of the vagina.

CLINICALLY ORIENTED COMMENTS

Usually the vagina is collapsed and its anterior and posterior walls are in contact (Figs. 3-23 and 3-24); however, the vagina serves as the inferior end of the **birth canal** and can be markedly distended by the fetal head, particularly in an anteroposterior direction. Distention of the vagina laterally is limited by the presence of the **ischial spines** and the sacrospinous ligaments (Figs. 3-9, 3-45, 3-46, and 3-52).

The interior of the vagina and the vaginal part of the cervix of the uterus can be examined through a **vaginal speculum** (Fig. 3-88) or by palpation with the fingers. Pulsations of the uterine arteries (Fig. 3-71) may be felt through the lateral fornices (Fig. 3-87).

Owing to the anatomical relationships of the vagina, an unsterilized instrument directed posteriorly into the vagina (*i.e.*, by an inexperienced person in an attempt to enter the uterus) may be pushed through the posterior wall of the vagina into the peritoneal cavity and may lead to **peritonitis** (Fig. 3-22). This has occurred when amateur attempts have been made to induce an **abortion** with a hatpin or some other sharp object.

Peritoneal abscesses in the rectouterine pouch (Fig. 3-22) may be drained by incising the posterior vaginal wall at the posterior fornix. Via this same route, a peritoneoscope or **culdoscope** may be inserted to examine the ovaries (*e.g.*, for cysts or tumors) or the uterine tubes (*e.g.*, for a tubal pregnancy). This procedure is used in the diagnosis of a number of pelvic diseases.

Surgical operations on the vagina are relatively common and they are usually performed via the *perineal approach.* These operations are commonly done to correct abnormal relaxation of the anterior and posterior vaginal walls when childbearing has resulted in weakening of the pelvic diaphragm. This may result in a bulging of the bladder into the anterior wall of the vagina, called a **cystocele**, or a bulging of the anterior wall of the rectum into the posterior wall of the vagina, called a **rectocele** (Fig. 3-62).

In some **virgins** the vaginal orifice may be only a few millimeters in diameter owing to failure of the hymen to rupture. More often the opening in the hymen will admit the tip of one finger. In these cases the initial coitus may result in tearing and slight bleeding of the hymen.

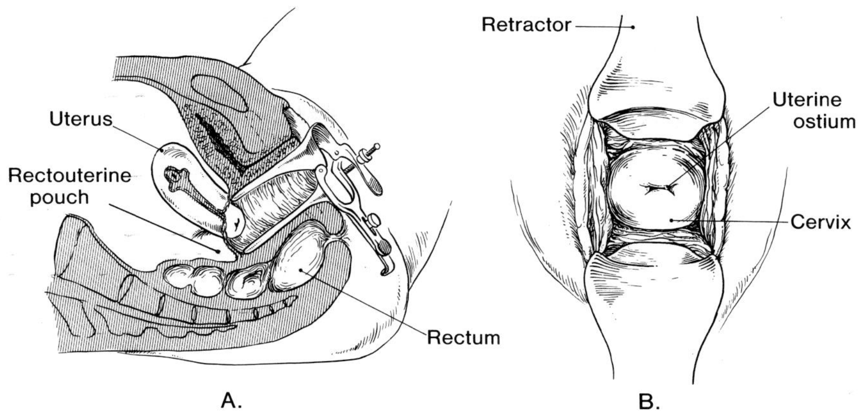

Figure 3-88. Drawings illustrating how the interior of the vagina and the vaginal aspect of the cervix of the uterus are examined. *A* shows the patient in the lithotomy position (Fig. 3-1) with a vaginal speculum separating the walls of the vagina. The uterine ostium (Fig. 3-87) is usually at the level of the ischial spines (Fig. 3-9), which can be felt from the vagina (Fig. 3-111). *B* shows a view of the cervix from the vagina with retractors in place. (Illustrated by Mrs. D. M. Hutchinson).

The Uterus (Figs. 3-22, 3-24, 3-69 to 3-73, and 3-86 to 3-90). The uterus (L. womb) of a nonpregnant woman is a hollow, thick-walled, pear-shaped **muscular organ** which is 7 to 8 cm long, 5 to 7 cm wide, and 2 to 3 cm thick. *During pregnancy the uterus enlarges greatly to accommodate the fetus.* The uterus normally projects anterosuperiorly over the bladder and the superior part of the vagina (Fig. 3-22). *The uterus consists of two major parts*: (1) the expanded upper two-thirds known as the **body**, and (2) the cylindrical lower third called the **cervix** (L. neck). Because the cervix projects into the vagina, it is divided into *vaginal* and *supravaginal parts* for descriptive purposes. The vaginal part communicates with the vagina via the **uterine ostium** (L. door, entrance, mouth) or *external os.* The **fundus** (L. bottom) of the uterus is the rounded *upper part of the body* superior to the line joining the points of *entrance of the two uterine tubes* (Fig. 3-89). The region of the body of the uterus on each side where the uterine tube enters (Fig. 3-87) is called the **cornu** (L. horn) of the uterus. The **isthmus of the uterus** is the narrow zone of transition between the body and cervix of the uterus (Fig. 3-87). This slight constriction is most obvious prior to the first pregnancy.

The uterus is normally bent anteriorly or **anteflexed** between the cervix and the body and the entire uterus is normally bent or inclined forward (**anteverted**, Fig. 3-22). Although anteflexion and and anteversion of the uterus are considered to be the normal anatomical position of the uterus, many women have **retroflexed** (L. *retro*, backward) and **retroverted** uteri which produce no symptoms. The uterus is frequently retroverted in older women (Fig. 3-68). Retroversion is a turning backward of the uterus without flexing the organ.

The wall of the uterus consists of three layers: (1) the outer serosa or **perimetrium**, consisting of a single layer of mesothelium supported by a thin layer of connective tissue; (2) the middle muscular layer or **myometrium**, consisting of 12 to 15 mm of smooth muscle; and (3) the inner mucosal layer or **endometrium**, which is firmly adherent to the underlying myometrium. *The blastocyst implants into the endometrium* (G. *endon*, within, + *mētra*, uterus) where it develops into an embryo and its fetal membranes.

The uterus has an anteroinferior surface or **vesical surface** related to the bladder and a posterosuperior or **intestinal surface** related to the intestines. These convex surfaces are separated by *right* and *left borders.* The uterine tubes extend laterally from the sides of the body of the uterus (Fig. 3-89). The **ligaments of the ovaries** are attached to the uterus posteroinferior

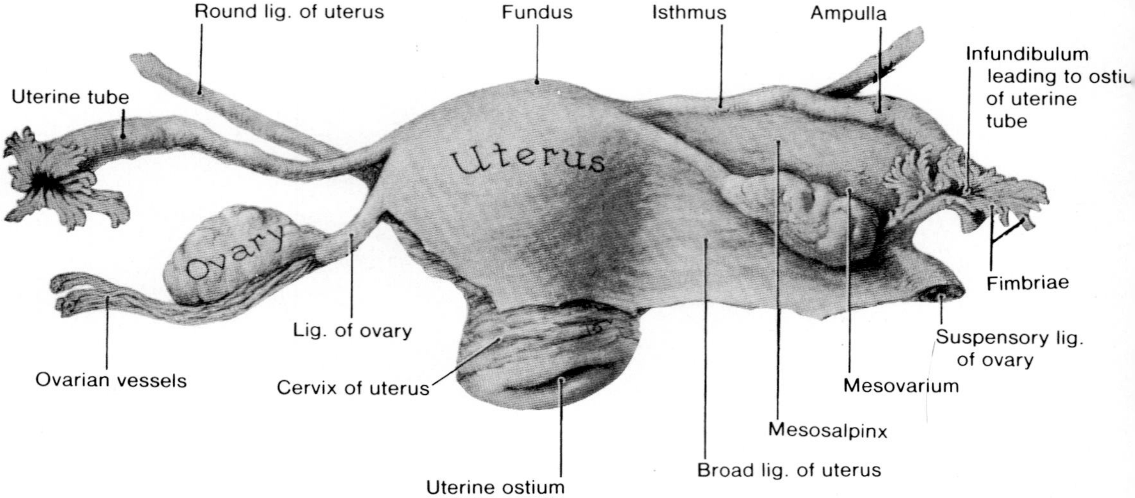

Figure 3-89. Drawing of a posterior view of the uterus, ovaries, uterine tubes, and related structures. *On the left side* the broad ligament of the uterus is removed, thereby setting free the uterine tube, the round ligament of the uterus, and the ligament of the ovary. These three structures are attached to the side of the uterus close together, at the junction of its fundus and body. *On the right side* is the "mesentery" of the uterus and uterine tube, called the broad ligament. Observe that the ovary is attached (1) to the broad ligament by a mesentery of its own called the mesovarium; (2) to the uterus by the ligament of the ovary; and (3) near the pelvic brim by the suspensory ligament of the ovary which transmits the ovarian vessels. The part of the broad ligament above the level of the mesovarium is called the mesosalpinx.

to the *uterotubal junction* and the **round ligaments of the uterus** are attached anteroinferior to this junction. *These ligaments are continuous within the wall of the uterus and are both derived from the gubernaculum* in the embryo. Each round ligament runs between the layers of the broad ligament and across the pelvic wall to the **deep inguinal ring**. After traversing the inguinal canal, the round ligament merges with subcutaneous tissues of the labium majus (Fig. 3-41).

The body of the uterus is enclosed between the layers of the broad ligament (Figs. 3-72, 3-89, and 3-90) and is freely movable. Hence, as the bladder fills the uterus rises, and when the bladder is fully distended, the uterus is inclined backward (*retroverted*) and lies in line with the vagina. As the bladder empties it moves back to its normal anteverted position. The cervix of the uterus is not so mobile because it is held in position by several structures. The **transverse cervical ligaments** (lateral cervical ligaments, cardinal ligaments, Fig. 3-24) extend from the cervix and the lateral fornices of the vagina (Fig. 3-87) to the side walls of the pelvis. The **uterosacral ligaments** pass from the sides of the cervix toward the sacrum; they are deep to the peritoneum and superior to the levatores ani muscles. These ligaments can be palpated through the rectum. *The uterosacral ligaments tend to hold the cervix in its normal relationship to the sacrum.*

The principal supports of the uterus are the *pelvic floor and the structures surrounding the uterus* (Figs. 3-24 and 3-60). The levatores ani and coccygei muscles and the muscles of the urogenital diaphragm (Fig. 3-16) are particularly important in supporting the uterus.

Peritoneum covers the uterus anteriorly and superiorly, except for the vaginal part of the cervix (Figs. 3-24, 3-68, 3-73, and 3-86). The peritoneum is reflected anteriorly from the uterus onto the bladder and posteriorly over the posterior fornix of the vagina onto the rectum (Fig. 3-22). Laterally the peritoneum forms the important folds called the broad ligaments.

The broad ligaments (Figs. 3-69, 3-72, 3-73, 3-89, and 3-90) *are folds of peritoneum with mesothelium on their anterior and posterior surfaces.* They extend from the sides of the uterus to the side walls and the floor of the pelvis. *They hold the uterus in relatively normal position.* The two layers of the broad ligament are continuous with each other at a free edge which is directed forward and upward to surround the uterine tube. *Enclosed in the free edge of each broad ligament is a uterine tube.* The **ligament of the ovary** lies *posterosuperiorly* and the **round ligment of the uterus** lies *anteroinferiorly* within the broad ligament (Figs. 3-72, 3-73, and 3-89).

The broad ligament has *a condensation of loose areolar tissue and smooth muscle,* called the **parametrium** (G. *para,* alongside, near + *mētra,* uterus), at its base and around the inferior end of the cervix. Here the connective tissue of the pelvic floor extends from the fibrous subserous coat of

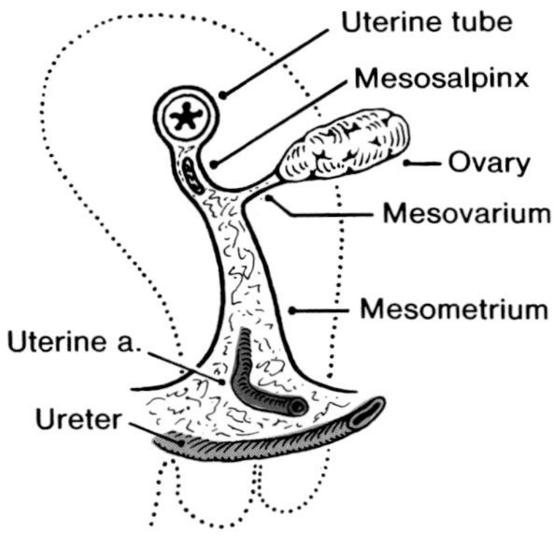

Figure 3-90. Diagram of a paramedian section of the broad ligament, the "mesentery" of the uterus and uterine tube. Observe that the ovary is attached to the broad ligament by a mesentery of its own called the mesovarium. The part of the broad ligament below the level of the mesovarium is called the mesometrium (mesentery of the uterus), whereas the part of the broad ligament above the level of the mesovarium is called the mesosalpinx. (In Fig. 3-89 observe the trumpet-like appearance of the uterine tube.)

the body of the uterus between the layers of the broad ligament.

The broad ligament gives attachment to the ovary through the **mesovarium** (Figs. 3-89 and 3-90); this short peritoneal fold connects the anterior border of the ovary (L. ovarium) with the posterior layer of the broad ligament.

The relations of the uterus are very important. *Anteriorly* the body of the uterus is separated from the bladder by the **vesicouterine pouch of peritoneum** (Fig. 3-22). Here the peritoneum is reflected from the uterus onto the posterior margin of the superior surface of the bladder. *The vesicouterine pouch is empty when the uterus is in its normal position* (Fig. 3-22), but it usually contains a loop of intestine when the uterus is retroverted (Fig. 3-68). *Posteriorly* the body of the uterus and the supravaginal part of the cervix are separated by a layer of peritoneum and the peritoneal cavity from the *sigmoid colon* (Fig. 3-70). The uterus is separated from the rectum by the **rectouterine pouch of peritoneum** (pouch of Douglas). The inferior part of this pouch is on the posterior fornix of the vagina (Figs. 3-22 and 3-73). The close relationship of the ureter to the uterine artery is very important. *The ureter is crossed superiorly by the uterine artery at the side of the cervix* (Fig. 3-69).

The blood supply of the uterus is derived mainly from the **uterine arteries** which are *branches of the internal iliac* (Figs. 3-69, 3-71, and 3-72). They enter the broad ligament beside the lateral fornices of the vagina (Fig. 3-87), *superior to the ureters.* At the isthmus of the uterus, the uterine artery divides into a larger **ascending branch** that *supplies the body of the uterus* and a smaller **descending branch** that *supplies the cervix and the vagina.* The uterus is also supplied by the **ovarian arteries** which are branches of the aorta. The uterine arteries pass along the sides of the uterus within the broad ligament and then turn laterally at the entrance to the uterine tubes, where they *anastomose with ovarian arteries* (Fig. 3-71).

The veins of the uterus are thin-walled and enter the broad ligament with the uterine arteries (Figs. 3-69 and 3-70). *The uter-*

ine veins form a plexus on each side of the cervix and their tributaries drain into the *internal iliac veins.*

The lymph vessels of the uterus follow three main routes. (1) Most lymph vessels from the **fundus of the uterus** pass with the ovarian vessels to the **lumbar lymph nodes** (Figs. 2-134), but some pass to the *external iliac lymph nodes* or run along the round ligament of the uterus to the *superficial inguinal lymph nodes* (Figs. 3-85 and 4-38). (2) Lymph vessels from the **body of the uterus** pass laterally through the broad ligament to the **external iliac lymph nodes**. On the way to these nodes, the lymph may pass through *parauterine lymph nodes* near the uterus. (3) Lymph vessels from the **cervix of the uterus** pass to the **internal iliac** and **sacral lymph nodes**. The lymph vessels of the uterus enlarge greatly during pregnancy.

The nerves of the uterus arise from the *inferior hypogastric plexus* (Fig. 3-93), largely from the **uterovaginal plexus** which lies in the base of the broad ligament on each side of the supravaginal part of the cervix. Sympathetic, parasympathetic, and afferent fibers pass through this plexus. Some nerves from this plexus run with the vaginal arteries; others pass directly to the cervix; and some run upward in the broad ligament with or near the uterine arteries to supply the body of the uterus and the uterine tubes. The **nerves to the cervix** form a plexus in which are located small *paracervical ganglia*, one of which is often large and is called the *uterine cervical ganglion.* The autonomic fibers of the uterovaginal plexus are mainly vasomotor. Most of the afferent fibers ascend through the hypogastric plexus and enter the spinal cord via T10 to T12 and L1 spinal nerves.

CLINICALLY ORIENTED COMMENTS

The uterus is mainly an abdominal organ in the newborn and its cervix is relatively large. During **puberty** (13 to 15 years) the uterus grows rapidly. During **menopause** (46 to 52 years) the uterus becomes inactive and thereafter shrinks. Most female cadavers have atrophic uteri; some have none, usually because they were removed surgically during an operation called a **hysterectomy** (G. *hystera*, uterus + *ektomē*, excision).

In rare cases the **paramesonephric ducts** degenerate in the embryo, as they normally do in the male; this results in *absence of the uterus and vagina.* More commonly fusion of these embryonic ducts is incomplete and a variety of congenital malformations results (Fig. 3-94). *If a vagina is present, some type of uterus usually exists, but when the vagina is absent, so is the uterus.* An **artificial vagina** can be created, *e.g.*, by inserting a skin graft from the buttocks into a space that is surgically dissected between the bladder and the rectum.

During pregnancy the uterus increases rapidly in size and weight and rises high into the abdomen. During the last weeks of pregnancy the uterus is about 20 cm in length and may weigh as much as 1 kg. After childbirth the uterus contracts but it is still large for several weeks and lies against the anterior abdominal wall almost as high as the umbilicus. By 8 weeks after childbirth the uterus is close to its normal size and weighs 40 g or less.

Prolapse of the uterus (Fig. 3-62) is rare. The uterus descends to an abnormally low level in the pelvis and in advanced cases the cervix protrudes through the vagina and the labia. Prolapse of the uterus usually results from stretching or tearing of the pelvic floor (Fig. 3-60) during childbirth (parturition).

The cervix and body of the uterus may be examined by **bimanual palpation.** Two fingers of the right hand are passed high into the vagina while the other hand is pressed downward and backward on the anterior abdominal wall, just above the symphysis pubis. The size and other characteristics of the uterus can be determined in this way (*e.g.*, whether the uterus is in its normal anteverted position as in Fig. 3-22 or retroverted as in Fig. 3-68). Owing to *softening of the isthmus of the uterus* (**Hegar's sign**) in early pregnancy, the cervix feels as though it were separate from the body of the uterus during bimanual examination. This softening of the uterine isthmus is an early probable **sign of pregnancy**.

The part of the mesonephric duct which forms the ductus deferens and ejaculatory duct in the male may persist in the female as the **duct of Gartner** and lie between the layers of the broad ligament alongside the lateral wall of the uterus or in the wall of the vagina. The vestigial remnants may also give rise to **Gartner's duct cysts.**

The degree of dilation of the cervix during labor can be determined by rectal examination. As the cervical canal dilates, a fingertip may be inserted into it (Case 3-8). The finger in the rectum can be passed across the fetal head as it presents in the uterine ostium (external os) and the degree of dilation can be estimated accurately without entering the vagina.

The Uterine Tubes (Figs. 3-22, 3-71 to 3-73, and 3-91). The uterine tubes (Fallopian tubes, oviducts) are a pair of ducts, 10 to 12 cm long and 1 cm in diameter, which extend laterally from the cornua or **horns of the uterus**. They are designed to *receive the oocytes discharged from ovarian follicles* and to convey the dividing **zygote** to the

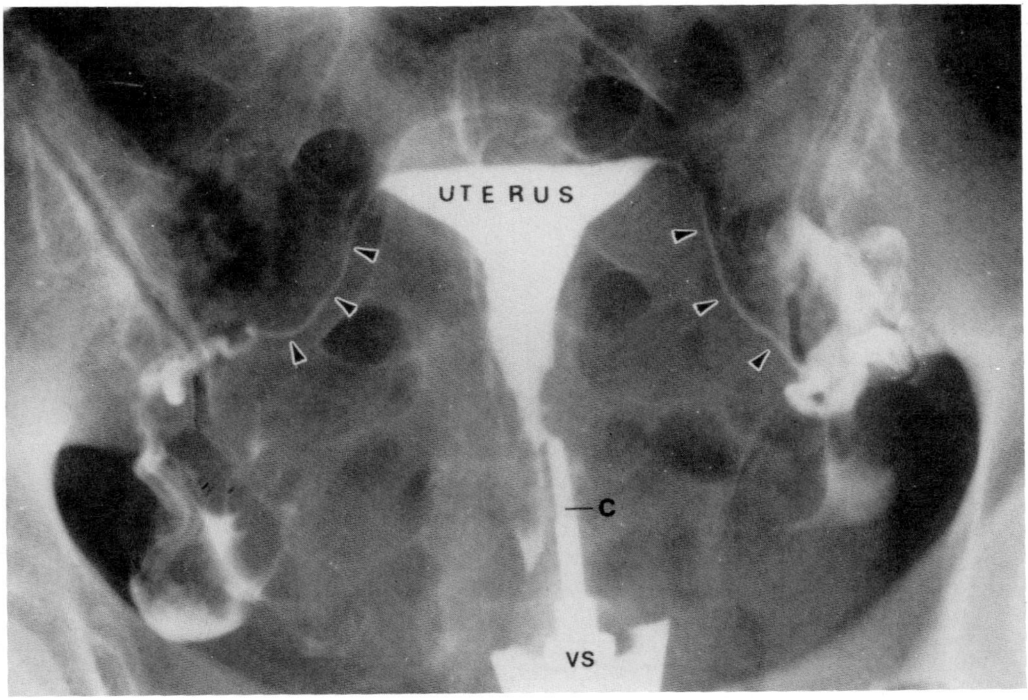

Figure 3-91. *Hysterosalpingogram* or radiograph of the uterus and uterine tubes taken after the injection of radiopaque material into the uterus through the uterine ostium. The triangular uterine cavity is clearly outlined (also see Fig. 3-87). The contrast medium has traveled through the uterine tubes, indicated by the *small arrows*, to the infundibulum (Fig. 3-89) and passed into the peritoneal cavity on both sides (lateral to the arrows). In comparison with the size of the uterus, the uterine cavity is small; this is related to the great thickness of the uterine wall (Fig. 3-22). The cavity of the body of the uterus when viewed from the side is a mere slit, whereas from behind the cavity is triangular with its base in the fundus and its apex continuous with the cervical canal. The lateral angles of the triangle indicate the entrance of the uterine tubes. *C*, catheter in cervical canal at internal uterine ostium (Fig. 3-87); *VS*, vaginal speculum in vagina (Fig. 3-88*A*). Understand that the female genital tract is the only direct communication into the peritoneal cavity from the exterior and is therefore a potential pathway for infection (*e.g.*, gonorrhea).

uterine cavity. The uterine tubes also convey the sperms to the ampulla of the tube (described subsequently), where the oocyte normally waits temporarily for **fertilization** to occur. Each tube opens at its proximal end into the horn (L. cornu) of the uterus and at its distal end into the **peritoneal cavity** near the ovary.

For descriptive purposes *the uterine tube is divided into four parts.* (1) **The infundibulum** (L. funnel) is the funnel-shaped distal end of the uterine tube. The **abdominal ostium** or opening of the tube, about 2 mm in diameter, lies at the bottom of the infundibulum and opens into the peritoneal cavity near the ovary. The margins of the infundibulum are drawn out into numerous fringed folds called **fimbriae** (L. fringes). These finger-like processes spread over most of the surface of the ovary and a large one, the **ovarian fimbria**, is attached to the superior pole of the ovary. During *ovulation* (expulsion of the oocyte from the ovary into the peritoneal cavity) the fimbriae trap the oocyte and the cilia of its mucosal lining sweep it through the abdominal ostium of the uterine tube. (2) **The ampulla** of the uterine tube receives the oocyte from the infundibulum and it is in this part that **fertilization of the oocyte** by a sperm usually occurs. *The ampulla is the widest and longest part of the uterine tube,* making up about two-thirds of its length. It is usually tortuous and thin-walled. (3) **The isthmus** (G. narrow passage) of the uterine tube is the short (2 to 5 cm), narow, thick-walled part which joins the *cornu* or *horn of the uterus.* (4) **The uterine part** of the uterine tube (*intramural portion,* interstitial part) is the short segment (about 2 cm) which pierces the wall of the uterus. The **uterine ostium** of the tube (1 mm) is smaller than its **abdominal ostium** (2 mm). The lumen of the uterine tube increases very gradually in width from the uterus toward the ovary (Fig. 3-91).

The uterine tubes lie in the free edges of the broad ligaments of the uterus (Figs. 3-72, 3-89, and 3-90). The part of the broad ligament between the uterine tube and the ligament of the ovary and the mesovarium is called the **mesosalpinx** or mesentery of the uterine tube (G. *salpinx,* trumpet). The uterine tubes extend posterolaterally to the side walls of the pelvis and then ascend and arch over the ovary. Except for the uterine parts, the uterine tubes are clothed in peritoneum (Figs. 3-72 and 3-90).

The arteries of the uterine tube are derived from the anastomosis between the *uterine* and *ovarian arteries.* These tubal branches pass along the tube (Fig. 3-71) between the layers of the mesosalpinx (Fig. 3-72). The ampullary and uterine parts of the tube are the most vascularized portions.

The veins of the uterine tube are arranged similarly to the arteries and drain into the *uterine* and *ovarian veins* (Fig. 3-69). **The lymph vessels of the uterine tubes** run with those of the fundus of the uterus and the ovary to the *lumbar lymph nodes* (Fig. 2-134).

CLINICALLY ORIENTED COMMENTS

Usually the oocyte is fertilized in the ampulla of the uterine tube and the dividing zygote passes into the uterus where it implants in the endometrium. Fertilization of an oocyte cannot occur when both tubes are blocked because the sperms cannot reach the oocyte in the ampulla. *One of the major causes of infertility in women is blockage of the uterine tubes resulting from infection (e.g.,* **gonorrhea**). The patency of a uterine tube may be determined by the **Rubin test**, a procedure in which CO_2 gas is introduced into the uterus to see if it enters the peritoneal cavity. Tubal patency can also be determined by injecting a radiopaque material into the uterus (**salpingography**, Fig. 3-91).

Ligation of the uterine tubes is one method of birth control. Oocytes discharged from the ovarian follicles in these patients die in the peritoneal cavity or in the infundibulum of the tube and soon disappear.

Because the female genital tract is in direct communication with the peritoneal cavity via the abdominal ostia of the uterine tubes, infections of the vagina, uterus, or tubes may involve the peritoneum of the abdomen and pelvis and result in **peritonitis** (inflammation of the peritoneum). Conversely, inflammation of the tube (**salpingitis**) may result from infections that spread from the peritoneal cavity. In some cases collections of pus may develop in the tube (**pyosalpinx**) and the tube may be partly occluded by *adhesions.* In these cases the zygote may not pass to the uterus and the blastocyst may implant in the wall of the uterine tube, producing an **ectopic tubal pregnancy.** Although implanation may occur in any part of the tube, the common site is somewhere along the ampulla. *Tubal pregnancy is the most common type of ectopic gestation* and occurs about once in every 250 pregnancies in North America. Ectopic tubal pregnancies usually result in **rupture of the uterine tube** and *hemorrhage into the abdominopelvic cavity* during the first 8 weeks of gestation. Tubal rupture and the associated severe hemorrhage constitute a threat to the mother's life.

The epoophoron lies in the mesosalpinx between the uterine tube and the ovary. *This vestigial structure* consists of a number of small rudimentary tubules which are *remnants of the cranial mesonephric tubules* associated with the mesonephric kidney in the embryo. They are homologous with the efferent ductules of the testis and they may develop into **paraovarian cysts.**

A vesicular appendage is sometimes observed near the infundibulum of the uterine tube (Fig. 3-86*B*). It represents the *remains of the cranial end of the mesonephric duct* which forms the ductus epididymis in the male but normally degenerates in females.

The Ovaries (Figs. 3-22, 3-70, 3-71, 3-86*B*, 3-89, and 3-90). The ovaries are oval or almond-shaped, pinkish-white bodies about 3 cm long, 1.5 cm wide, and 1 cm thick. They are located one on each side in a recess called the **ovarian fossa** on the side wall of the pelvis minor. *The ovarian fossa* (Fig. 3-86*B*) *is bounded anteriorly by the obliterated umbilical artery and posteriorly by the ureter and the internal iliac artery* (Fig. 3-68). The ampulla of the uterine tube curves over the lateral end of the ovary so that the infundibulum curls around the ovary (Fig. 3-71). The **ovarian fimbria** of the infundibulum attaches the tube to the ovary; hence, during ovulation the oocyte is picked up and carried into the ampulla of the uterine tube by the action of the cilia on the mucosa on the fimbriae.

Each ovary is attached to the posterosuperior aspect of the broad ligament and is suspended from the posterior layer of this ligament by a fold of peritoneum, called the **mesovarium** (Figs. 3-89 and 3-90), through which the ovarian vessels pass to and from the ovary. The ovary is also attached to the uterus by a band of fibrous tissue, the **ligament of the ovary** which runs in the broad ligament. Near the pelvic brim the ovary is attached by the **suspensory ligament of the ovary** (Figs. 3-73 and 3-89), a thickening of fibrous tissue which passes over the iliac vessels and the psoas major muscle. *The suspensory ligament of the ovary contains the ovarian vessels and nerves* (Figs. 3-72, 3-73 and 3-89) which pass to the lateral end of the ovary and into the mesovarium and the **hilum of the ovary.**

The surface of the ovary is not covered by peritoneum; hence, the oocyte is expelled into the peritoneal cavity. The surface of the ovary in young women is covered by a single layer of cuboidal epithelium ("germinal epithelium") which is continuous with the flattened mesothelium of the peritoneum at the mesovarium. *This epithelium does not give rise to the oocytes.* Oogonia develop before birth from **primordial germ cells.**

Before puberty the surface of the ovary is smooth, whereas after puberty the ovary becomes progressively scarred and distorted (Fig. 3-89) as successive **corpora lutea** degenerate. *The corpora lutea are endocrine structures* that develop from follicles that expel their oocytes. If the oocyte shed each month is not fertilized, the corpus luteum degenerates and is gradually replaced by a fibrous scar, the **corpus albicans.** As few oocytes are fertilized the ovarian surface becomes puckered by scars and irregular (Fig. 3-89).

The ovarian arteries arise from the abdominal aorta at about the level of L2 vertebra below the renal arteries and descend on the posterior abdominal wall. On reaching the pelvic brim, *the ovarian arteries cross over the external iliac vessels internal to the ureter* (Figs. 3-69, 3-70, and 3-73). The ovarian arteries then enter the pelvis minor and run medially in the **suspensory ligaments** of the ovaries to enter the broad ligament inferior to the uterine tubes. At the level of the ovary, the ovarian artery sends branches through the **mesovarium** to the ovary (Fig. 3-71) and then continues medially in the broad ligament to supply the uterine tube and to anastomose with the uterine artery.

The ovarian veins leave the hila of the ovaries and form a leash of vessels, called the **pampiniform plexus**, in the broad ligament near the ovary and the uterine tube. This plexus communicates with the uterine plexus of veins. The two veins leaving the **ovarian plexus of veins** form one ovarian vein at the pelvic brim. *The right ovarian vein ascends to the inferior vena cava, whereas the left ovarian vein drains into the left renal vein.*

The lymph vessels of the ovary join those from the uterine tube and the fundus of the uterus on the same side and ascend with the ovarian vein to the **lumbar lymph nodes.** These nodes are located between the bifurcation of the abdominal aorta and the renal vessels (Figs. 2-134).

The nerves of the ovary descend along the ovarian vessels from the **abdominal sympathetic plexus** (Fig. 2-127). The **ovarian plexus of nerves** lies on and follows the ovarian artery and supplies the ovary, the broad ligament, and the uterine tube and communicates with the **uterine plexus.** The parasympathetic fibers of the ovarian plexus are derived from the vagus (CN X).

CLINICALLY ORIENTED COMMENTS

The position of the ovaries varies considerably in women who have borne children. During pregnancy the broad ligaments and the ovaries are carried superiorly with the enlarging uterus. After childbirth the ovaries descend as the uterus contracts, but they may not return to their original locations. The ovaries are also very mobile and may be displaced by the intestines. *On the right side the vermiform appendix may lie very close to the ovary* (Fig. 3-86*A*). After **menopause** (cessation of menstrual cycles), the formation of ovarian follicles, corpora lutea, and corpora albicantia ceases and the ovaries gradually atrophy. The ovaries become small and shrivelled and those of older women contain no ovarian follicles.

In females with the **Turner syndrome** and *XO sex chromosome complex*, the ovaries are represented by slender streaks of connective tissue lacking oocytes. The common clinical features of these females are *short stature, a webbed neck, absence of sexual maturation*, and a broad *shield-like chest.*

THE RECTUM AND ANAL CANAL

The rectum and anal canal are **pelvic viscera** which are parts of the large intestine. They are briefly described with this part of the digestive system in Chapter 2 and are illustrated in Figures 2-33 and 2-42. The **sigmoid colon** is also in the pelvis; in fact it used to be called the *pelvic colon.* It usually lies in the pelvis minor with coils of small bowel on top of it (Fig. 2-33). The terminal portion of the **ileum** is almost always in the pelvis (Figs. 2-33 and 2-42), from which it ascends over the right iliac vessels to end in the cecum. Commonly the **vermiform appendix** hangs over the pelvic brim (Fig. 3-67) and in the female lies close to the right ovary. *Only those organs which cannot be removed from the pelvis minor without cutting are designated as pelvic viscera.* Thus, the terminal ileum and most of the sigmoid colon are not true pelvic contents.

The pelvic floor is formed by the *pelvic diaphragm* (Figs. 3-55, 3-57, and 3-60), which consists of muscles (levator ani and coccygeus) and their lining fascia. This muscle sheet, which *assists in supporting the pelvic viscera*, stretches somewhat like a hammock between the pubis anteriorly and the coccyx posteriorly. It is also attached along the side walls of the pelvis to the thickened band of obturator fascia known as the **tendinous arch** (Figs. 3-17 and 3-57). The fascia on the superior surface of the pelvic diaphragm, the **visceral pelvic fascia** (Fig. 3-56), forms investing sheaths and ligamentous thickenings which help to support and to fix the pelvic viscera (Figs. 3-17 and 3-24).

The Rectum (Figs. 3-14, 3-17, 3-21 to 3-24, 3-55, 3-57, 3-60, 3-61, 3-73, and 3-95). *The rectum is continuous superiorly with the sigmoid colon and begins on the pelvic surface of the third piece of the sacrum* (S3 vertebra, Fig. 3-14). About 12 cm long in both sexes, the rectum follows the curve of the sacrum and coccyx to about 3 cm beyond the tip of the coccyx. Here *the rectum ends by turning posteroinferiorly to become the anal canal* (Fig. 3-22). The **puborectalis muscle** forms a sling at the junction of the rectum and the anal canal, producing the anorectal angle (Fig. 3-61). Inferiorly *the rectum lies immediately posterior to the prostate in the male* (Fig. 3-57) *and the vagina in the female* (Fig. 3-60). The termination of the rectum lies posterior to the **central perineal tendon** or perineal body (Fig. 3-12) and also to the

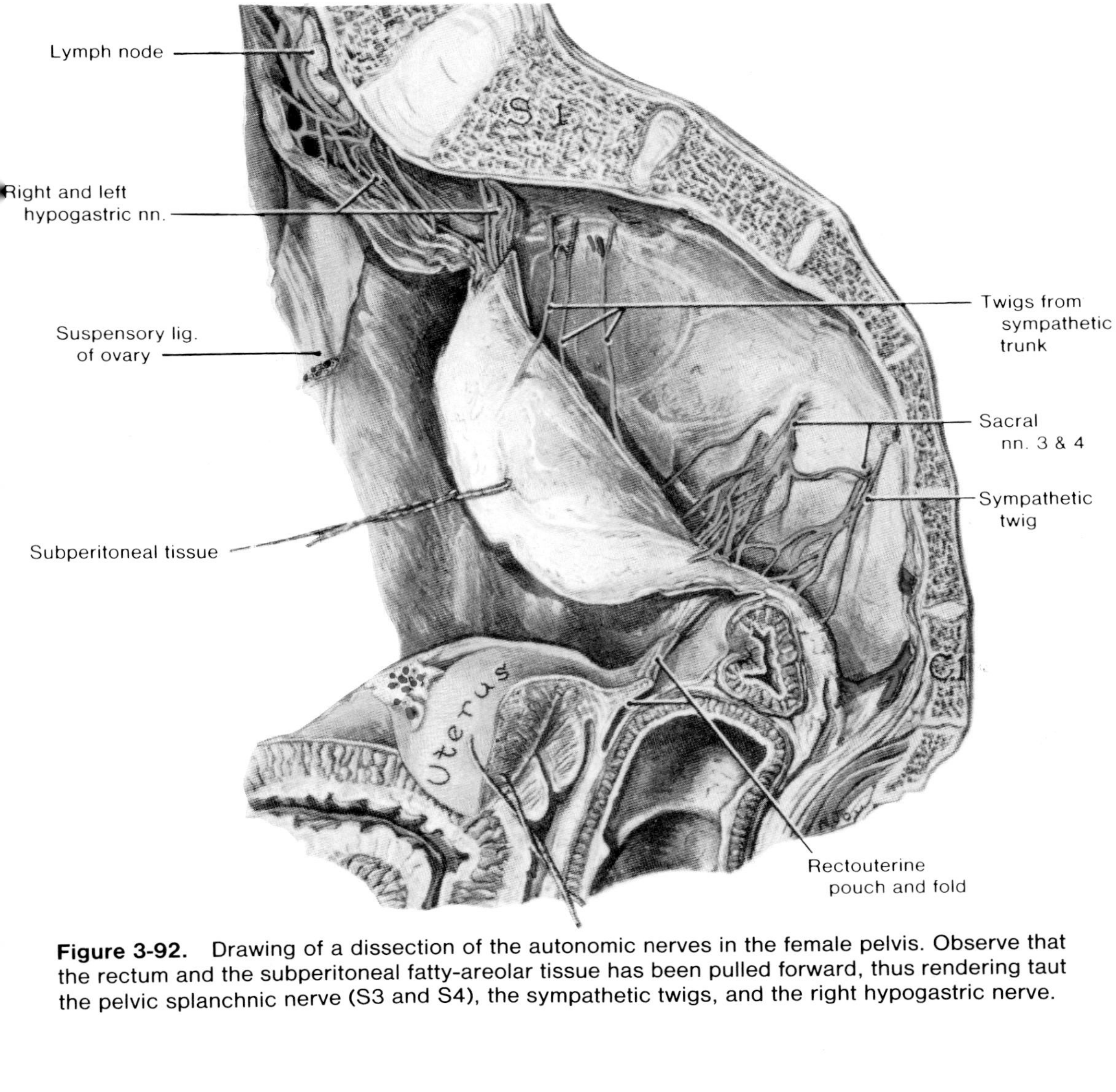

Figure 3-92. Drawing of a dissection of the autonomic nerves in the female pelvis. Observe that the rectum and the subperitoneal fatty-areolar tissue has been pulled forward, thus rendering taut the pelvic splanchnic nerve (S3 and S4), the sympathetic twigs, and the right hypogastric nerve.

apex of the prostate in the male (Figs. 3-14 and 3-17).

Peritoneal Covering of the Rectum (Figs. 3-14, 3-22, 3-65, 3-86*A*, 3-92 and 3-95). Peritoneum covers the superior third of the rectum on its front and sides; the middle third has peritoneum in front only; and *the inferior third has no peritoneal covering.* In the male the peritoneum is reflected from the anterior surface of the rectum to the posterior wall of the bladder (Fig. 3-14), where it forms the floor of the **rectovesical pouch.** In male infants and children in whom the bladder is in the abdomen (Fig. 3-77*B*), the peritoneum extends inferiorly as far as the base of the prostate. As the bladder moves into the pelvis minor, the adult peritoneal relationship is attained (Fig. 3-14).

In the female the peritoneum is reflected from the rectum to the **posterior fornix** of the vagina, where it forms the floor of the **rectouterine pouch** (Figs. 3-22, 3-73, and 3-88). The lateral reflections of perito-

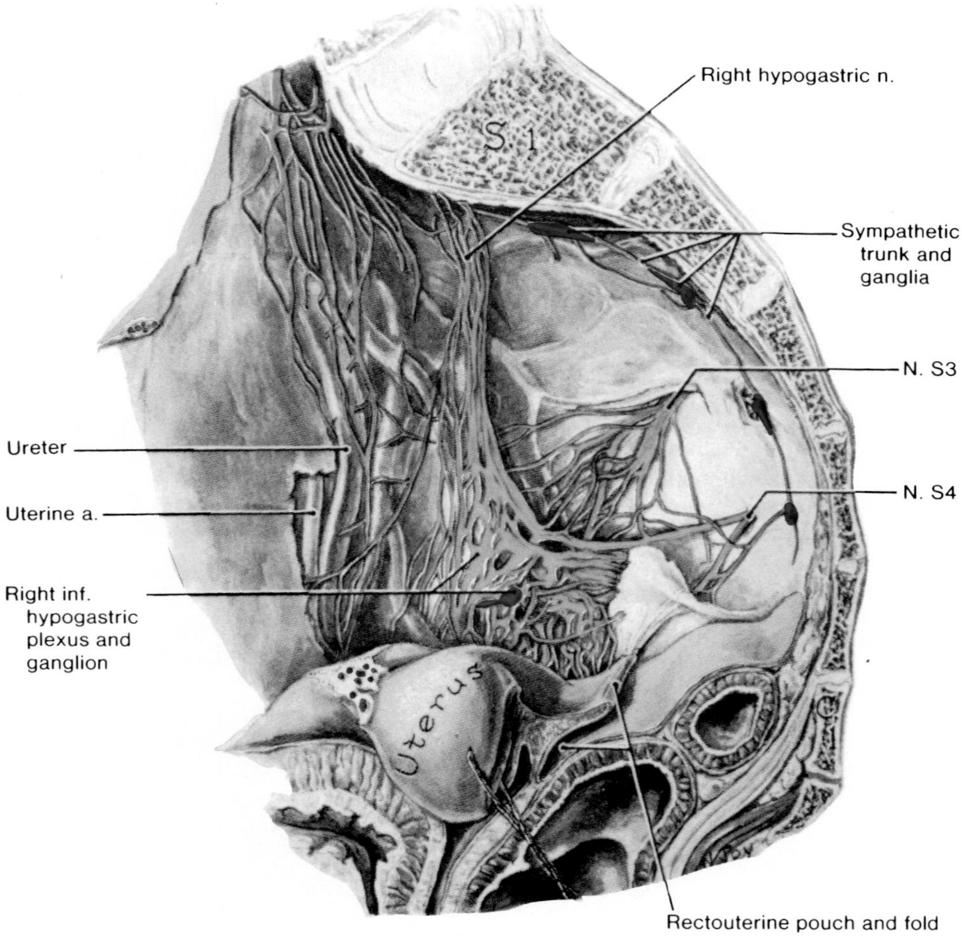

Figure 3-93. Drawing of a dissection of the autonomic nerves in the female pelvis. This is a later stage of the dissection shown in Figure 3-92. The inferior hypogastric (pelvic) plexus lies in the extraperitoneal connective tissue. *In the male* it is located on the side of the rectum, seminal vesicle, prostate, and posterior part of the bladder. *In the female,* as above, each plexus is situated on the side of the rectum, cervix, fornix of the vagina, and posterior part of the bladder and extends into the base of the broad ligament.

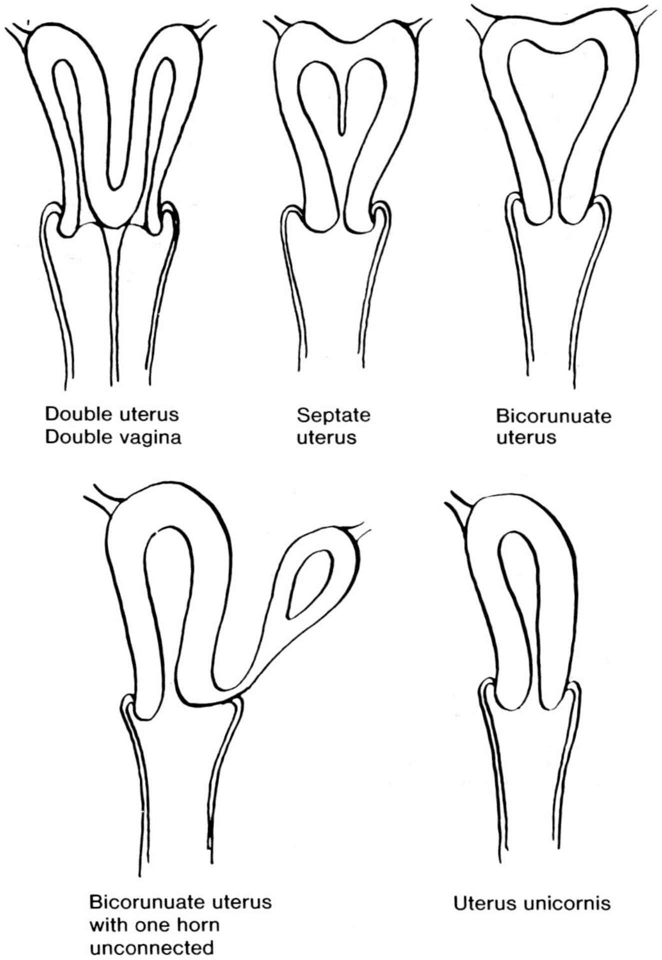

Figure 3-94. Sketches illustrating the common types of congenital malformation of the uterus and vagina which result from failure of fusion of the paramesonephric ducts during the early fetal period. The uterus with a single horn and uterine tube (uterus unicornis) results when only one paramesonephric duct develops.

neum from the rectum in both sexes form **pararectal fossae** which permit the rectum to distend (Figs. 3-95 and 3-97).

Shape and Flexures of the Rectum (Figs. 3-14, 3-19, 3-22, 3-61, and 3-95 to 3-98). Despite the origin of its name, the rectum (L. *rectus*, straight) is curved; it follows the curve of the sacrum and *its terminal part bends sharply backward to join the anal canal* (Fig. 3-61). Although generally smaller in caliber than the sigmoid colon (Fig. 3-95), its inferior part below the level of the peritoneal reflection is distended into the **rectal ampulla** just above the pelvic diaphragm (Figs. 3-22, 3-55, and 3-95). The rectum is S-shaped in the coronal plane (Fig. 3-95). At the three concavities in the rectum indicated by the flexures, there are internal folds (valves) of the mucous membrane called **transverse rectal folds** or *plicae transversales* (Fig. 3-97) which partly close the lumen of the rectum. These folds consist of mucous membrane and circular smooth muscle and their form is maintained by prolongations of the **teniae coli** (Fig. 3-95) in the anterior and posterior walls of the rectum.

Relations of the Rectum (Figs. 3-12, 3-22, 3-23, 3-57, 3-60, and 3-95). **Posteriorly** the rectum rests on the inferior three *sacral*

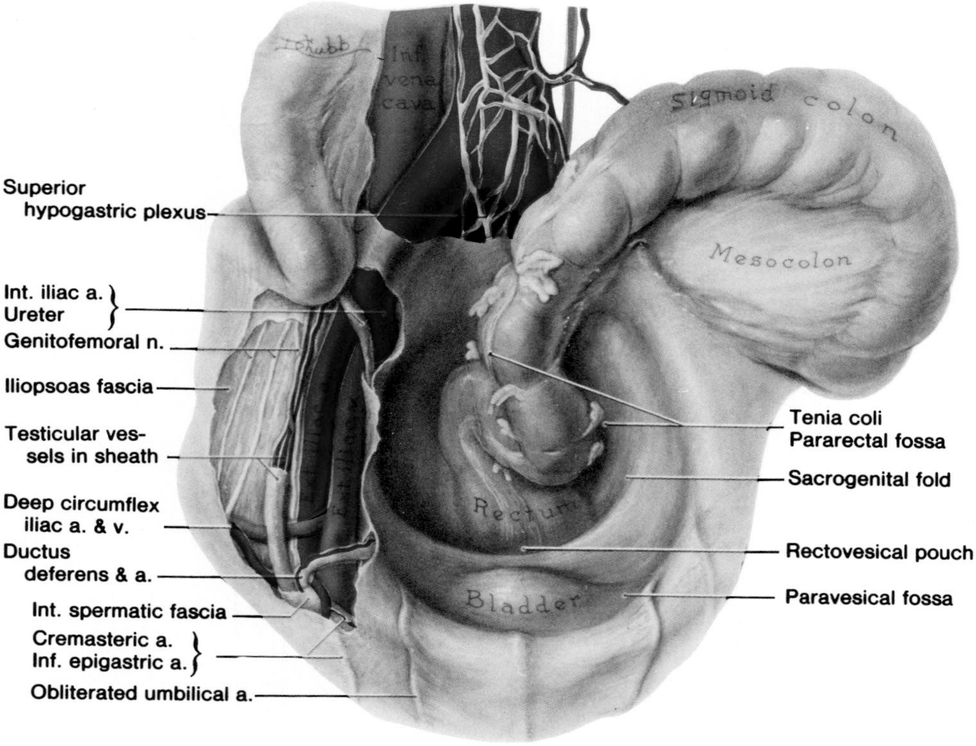

Figure 3-95. Drawing of an anterosuperior view of a dissection of the male pelvis and its surroundings. Observe the one limb of the Λ-shaped root of the sigmoid (pelvic) mesocolon ascending near the external iliac vessels and the other descending to the third piece of the sacrum. At the apex of this Λ-shaped root is the mouth of the intersigmoid recess, and behind the mouth lies the left ureter. Examine the teniae coli forming two wide bands, one in front of the rectum and the other behind. Note the crescentic fold of peritoneum called the sacrogenital fold. Observe the superior hypogastric plexus (presacral nerve) lying in the fork of the aorta and in front of the left common iliac vein (also see Fig. 2-127). Note the ureter adhering to the peritoneum, crossing the external iliac vessels, and descending in front of the internal iliac artery. Observe that the ductus deferens and its artery also adhere to the peritoneum, cross the external iliac vessels, and then hook around the inferior epigastric artery to join the other constituents of the spermatic cord. Observe the genitofemoral nerve on the psoas fascia; its two lateral (femoral) branches become cutaneous and its medial (genital) branch supplies the cremaster muscle before becoming cutaneous.

vertebrae, the *coccyx*, the *anococcygeal ligament* (Figs. 3-22 and 3-57), the *median sacral vessels*, the branches of the *superior rectal artery* (Fig. 3-96), and the inferior ends of the *sympathetic trunks* (Fig. 3-93). The rectum is surrounded by a fascial sheath and is loosely attached to the anterior surface of the sacrum. **Anteriorly**, in the male it is related to the base of the *bladder* (Fig. 3-95), the terminal parts of the *ureters*, the *deferent ducts*, the *seminal vesicles*, and the *prostate* (Figs. 3-77 and 3-84). The two layers of the **rectovesical septum** (Fig. 3-14) lie in the median plane between the bladder and the rectum and are closely associated with the seminal vesicles and the prostate. *The rectovesical septum represents a potential cleavage plane between the rectum and the prostate.* **In the female the anterior relation of the rectum is the vagina** (Figs. 3-22 and 3-60). The rectum is separated from the cervix of the uterus and the posterior fornix of the vagina by the **rectouterine pouch**

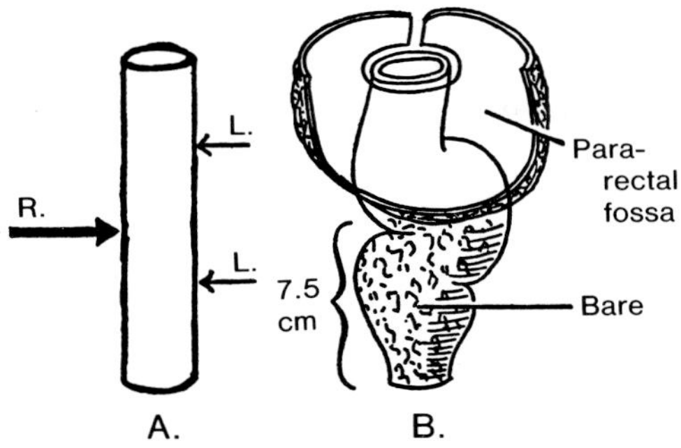

Figure 3-96. Sketches illustrating the peritoneal coverings and lateral flexures of the rectum, anterior view. The superior part of the rectum is covered with peritoneum in front and at the sides; the middle part is covered in front only; and the inferior part (ampulla) is not covered with peritoneum (*i.e.*, it is bare). As the rectum expands it fills the pararectal fossae (also see Fig. 3-95). The distance from the skin surface to the peritoneal cavity (*i.e.*, the rectovesical pouch, Fig. 3-14) measured anterior to the anal canal and rectum is 8 to 10 cm; measured behind (*i.e.*, to the pararectal fossa), it is 12 to 15 cm.

(Figs. 3-86*A* and 3-88). Inferior to this pouch the **rectovaginal septum** (Fig. 3-24) separates the vagina and the rectum.

The Rectal Vessels (Figs. 3-65, 3-66, and 3-98). There are *five rectal arteries* which anastomose freely with each other. The **superior rectal artery**, *the continuation of the inferior mesenteric* (Fig. 2-107), supplies the terminal part of the sigmoid colon and the superior part of the rectum (Fig. 3-98). It crosses the left common iliac vessels and descends into the pelvis minor within the sigmoid mesocolon. At the level of S3 vertebra, it divides into two branches which descend one on each side of the rectum (Fig. 3-98). The two **middle rectal arteries**, which are *branches of the internal iliacs* (Figs. 3-65 and 3-66), supply the middle and inferior parts of the rectum. The two **inferior rectal arteries**, *branches of the internal pudendal arteries* (Fig. 3-97), originate in the **ischiorectal fossae** (Figs. 3-4 and 3-27). They supply the inferior part of the rectum and the anal canal.

The **rectal veins form two plexuses** (Fig. 3-100): (1) an *internal rectal* (*submucous*) *plexus* located between the muscle layer and the mucous membrane, and (2) an *external rectal plexus* located superficial to the muscle layer below the level of the peritoneal reflection. Above the irregular **pectinate line** the veins of the internal plexus drain into the superior rectal vein. *The venous drainage of the rectum is via superior, middle, and inferior rectal veins.* There is a rich anastomosis between all three. Because *the superior rectal vein drains into the portal system* (Fig. 2-112), whereas the middle and inferior veins drain into the systemic system, this is an important area of portacaval anastomosis (see discussion in Chap. 2).

The lymph vessels from the *superior half* or more of the rectum *ascend along the superior rectal vessels* to the **pararectal lymph nodes** and then pass to the lymph nodes in the inferior part of the

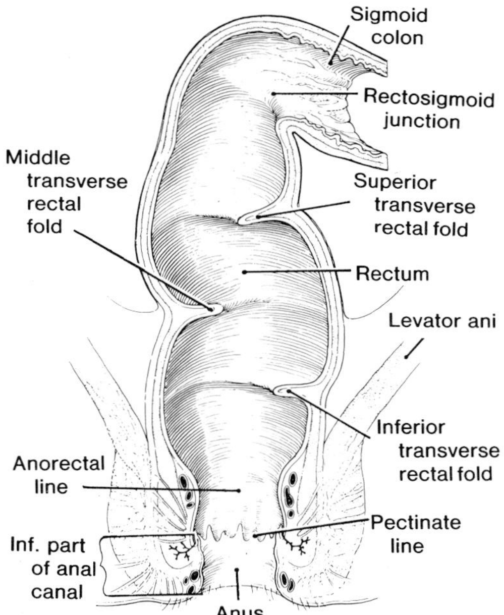

Figure 3-97. Drawing of the rectum and anal canal. The rectum in both sexes is about 12 cm long and the anal canal is about 3 cm (Fig. 3-19). Observe the curvature of the rectum and the acute flexion at the rectosigmoid junction. Note the three transverse rectal folds, two on the right and one on the left, which aid in the support of the feces (stool). The transverse rectal folds may also aid in the separation of the feces from gas (L. flatus, a blowing).

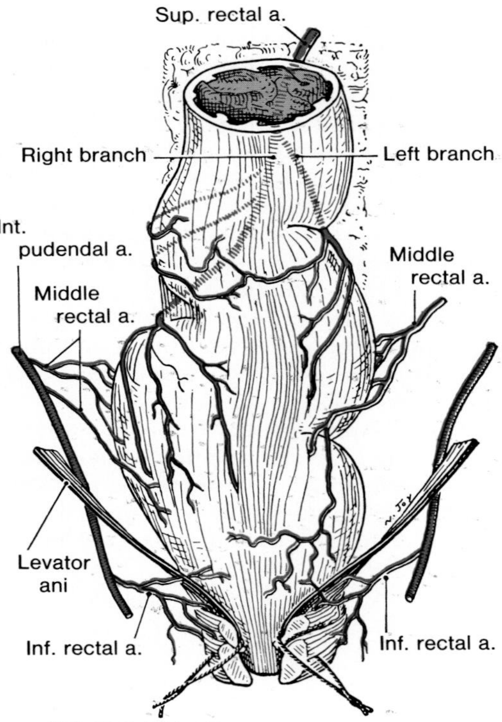

Figure 3-98. Drawing of an anterior view of the arteries of the rectum and anal canal. (The levatores ani muscles are semidiagrammatic.) Observe the branches of the right and left divisions of the superior rectal artery obliquely encircling the rectum, much as the branches of the dorsal arteries of the penis encircle the penis (Fig. 3-35). The middle rectal arteries (branches of the internal iliac arteries) are usually small; in this specimen the right artery is small but the left one is large and partly replaces the left division of the superior rectal artery. Note that the inferior rectal arteries (branches of the internal pudendal arteries) are largely expended on the anal canal. Observe the lateral flexures of the rectum (also see Fig. 3-97). These flexures and the transverse rectal folds help to support the weight of the feces. The anastomosis of arteries in the wall of the rectum is so extensive that the middle and inferior rectal arteries can supply the entire rectum if the inferior mesenteric artery (and thereby the superior rectal artery) is clamped.

mesentery of the sigmoid colon and around the **inferior mesenteric artery** (Fig. 2-109). From the *inferior half of the rectum,* most lymph vessels pass superiorly with the middle rectal arteries and drain into the **internal iliac lymph nodes** (Fig. 3-85); some vessels may pass into the *ischiorectal fossae* before going to the internal iliac nodes.

The Nerves of the Rectum (Figs. 3-38, 3-58, 3-65, 3-92, and 3-93). The nerve supply of the rectum is derived from the sympathetic and parasympathetic systems. The *sympathetic nerves* mainly run along the inferior mesenteric and superior rectal arteries and partly from the **inferior hypogastric plexuses** at the sides of the rectum (Fig. 3-93). The *parasympathetic nerves* are derived from the second, third, and fourth sacral nerves and run in the **pelvic splanchnic nerves** to join the *inferior hypogastric plexus.* The sensory nerves follow the path of the parasympathetic nerves and their fibers are stimulated by distention of the wall of the rectum. *The pelvic splanchnic nerves represent the sacral part of the parasympathetic portion of the autonomic nervous system.*

CLINICALLY ORIENTED COMMENTS

Many of the structures related to the inferior part of the rectum may be palpated through the walls of this part of the digestive tract, e.g., the prostate and seminal vesicles as discussed previously (Fig. 3-84). *In both sexes,* the pelvic surfaces of the sacrum and the coccyx may be felt posteriorly; also the **ischial spines** and **ischial tuberosities** (Figs. 3-45 and 3-46) may be palpated. *Enlarged internal iliac lymph nodes* (Fig. 3-85), pathological thickening of the ureters, swellings in the ischiorectal fossae (*e.g.*, an **ischiorectal abscess**, Case 3-3 and Fig. 3-99), and abnormal contents in the **rectovesical pouch** in the male (Fig. 3-14) or in the **rectouterine pouch** in the female (Figs. 3-22 and 3-88*A*) may be detected. Tenderness of an *inflamed vermiform appendix* can be detected rectally if this organ lies in the pelvis (Case 2-4 and Figs. 2-44 and Figs. 3-67).

The rectum can also be examined with a **proctoscope** (G. *prōktos*, anus + *skopēo*, to view) and biopsies of lesions may be taken through it. During insertion of a *sigmoidoscope* for **proctosigmoidoscopy** (inspection of the rectum and sigmoid colon through a sigmoidoscope), the curvatures of the rectum (Figs. 3-61 and 3-96) and the acute flexion at the **rectosigmoid junction** have to be kept in mind (Fig. 3-97) so that the patient will not undergo unnecessary discomfort. One must also know that the **transverse rectal folds** (valves) may temporarily impede passage of the instrument.

Herniation or prolapse of the rectum in females, called a **rectocele** (Fig. 3-62), occurs when there is a weakness of the fibromuscular layer of the posterior wall of the vagina. The vagina tends to bulge through the vaginal orifice with the attached wall of the rectum. In some cases defecation is difficult unless the patient presses on the rectocele with the fingers in the vagina. Repair of this type of hernia is called a **colporrhaphy** (G. *colpo*, vagina + raphē, suture).

The Anal Canal (Figs. 3-2, 3-14, 3-19, 3-20 to 3-22, 3-55, 3-97, and 3-98). The anal canal is 2.5 to 4 cm long in the adult and is *the terminal part of the large intestine* and the digestive tract (Fig. 2-33). The anal canal begins where the rectal ampulla narrows abruptly (Fig. 3-22) at the level of the U-shaped sling formed by the **puborectalis muscle** (Fig. 3-61). Hence, the *anorectal junction* is indicated by the sharp backward bend of the canal. The anal canal is contracted and forms an anteroposterior slit (Fig. 3-4), except during the passage of feces. *The anal canal is surrounded by internal and external anal sphincters* (Fig. 3-19*A*) and descends posteroinferiorly between the anococcygeal ligament (Figs 3-22 and 3-57) and the central perineal tendon or perineal body (Fig. 3-12). *The anal canal is surrounded by the levatores ani muscles which form the main part of the pelvic diaphragm* (Fig. 3-55) *within the anal region or triangle of the perineum* (Fig. 3-2). An **ischiorectal fossa** lies on each side of the anal canal (Figs. 3-3 and 3-20).

The internal anal sphincter (Figs. 3-19 to 3-21) consists of a thickening of the circular smooth muscle of the intestine. This *involuntary sphincter of the anal canal* (about 2.5 cm long) surrounds the upper two-thirds of the anal canal and has a *palpable inferior border*. The internal anal sphincter relaxes when it is stimulated by the parasympathetic nerves supplying it.

The external anal sphincter (Figs. 3-4, 3-14, 3-19 to 3-21, and 3-38) was described previously with the anal region of the perineum. Together with the **puborectalis muscle** (part of the levator ani), the external anal sphincter forms a muscular **anorectal ring** (Figs. 3-21 and 3-38). The external anal sphincter constitutes the large *voluntary sphincter of the anal canal and anus*. It surrounds the inferior two-thirds of the anal canal, forming a broad band on each side that overlaps the internal anal sphincter and the fibers of the levator ani (Fig. 3-19*A*). As described in detail previously, *the external anal sphincter has three* parts: subcutaneous, superficial, and deep. The **superficial part** is attached posteriorly to the coccyx and anteriorly to the central perineal tendon (Figs. 3-12 and 3-25). Hence, *the anorectal junction has an anorectal ring composed of voluntary and involuntary muscle fibers* which are responsible for maintaining rectal continence. *The innervation of the external anal sphincter* is primarily by S4 via the **inferior rectal nerve** (Fig. 3-4). *This nerve leaves the pudendal canal and runs anteromedially and superficially across the ischiorectal fossa* to supply the external anal sphincter. Hence, it is vulnerable during surgical treatment of an **ischiorectal abscess** (see Case 3-3 and Fig. 3-99).

The Interior of the Anal Canal (Figs. 3-14, 3-19, and 3-97). The superior half of the anal canal is characterized by a series of 5 to 10 longitudinal ridges, or folds of mucosa, called **anal columns** (rectal columns of Morgagni). These columns are clearly defined in infants and children but are often poorly marked in adults, particularly in older persons. The terminal "branches" of the superior rectal vessels are within the anal columns and it is here that *the superior rectal veins of the portal system anastomose with the middle and inferior rectal veins of the caval system* (Fig. 2-112). A clinically important plexus of veins is formed by these veins and its enlargement results in **internal hemorrhoids** (Fig. 3-100).

The superior ends of the anal columns indicate the **anorectal line** (Fig. 3-19*B*), where the rectum joins the anal canal. The rectum and the upper part of the anal canal are derived from the **hindgut** in the embryo.

The inferior ends of the anal columns are united to each other by small semilunar folds of mucosa called **anal valves** (Figs. 3-14 and 3-19*B*). These form a series of small recesses or pockets called the **anal sinuses** (crypts of Morgagni), one at the inferior end of a groove between two ridges. When compressed by feces, the mucous-containing anal sinuses exude mucous which aids in evacuation of the anal canal. The anal valves are at the level formerly occupied by the **anal membrane** in the embryo (Fig. 3-19*B*). The inferior comb-shaped limit of the anal valves is known as the **pectinate line** (Figs. 3-19*A* and 3-97). Inferior to the pectinate line is the **anal pecten** (L. comb). It is a *bluish-white zone in living persons* about 1 cm wide (Fig. 3-19*B*). About 2 cm superior to the anus there is an abrupt transition from simple columnar to stratified squamous epithelium. This transitional zone between the anal mucosa and the anal skin, known as the **anocutaneous line** (anal verge), can usually be identified in a living person as a bluish pink area; it is referred to clinically as the "white line" (of Hilton). The clinician is interested in this line because it *lies at the interval between the subcutaneous part of the external anal sphincter and the inferior border of the internal anal sphincter* (Fig. 3-19*A*). An **intersphincteric groove** can be felt at this site on digital examination of the

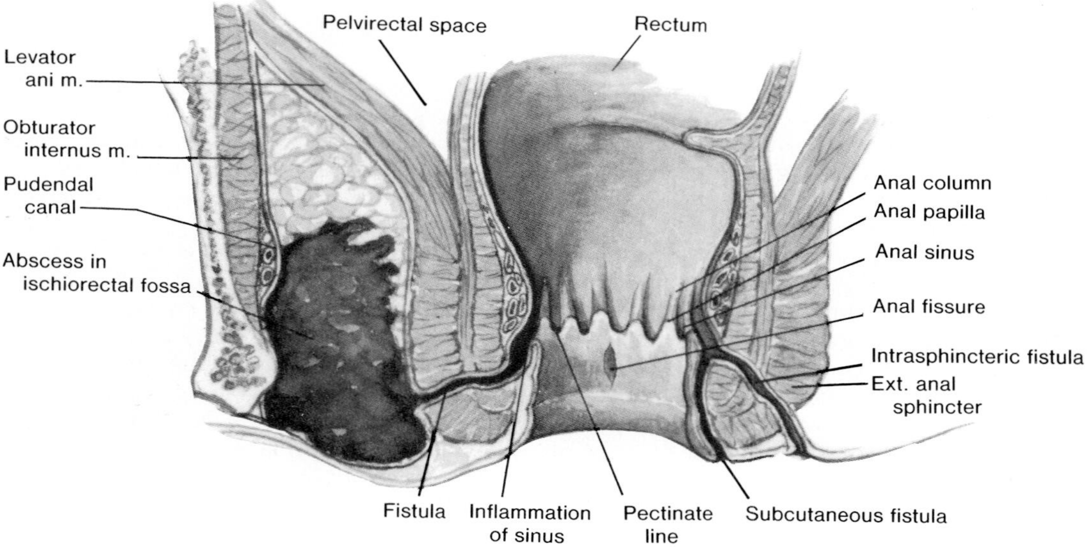

Figure 3-99. Drawing of a coronal section of the pelvis and perineum illustrating an ischiorectal abscess in the right ischiorectal fossa. Infection and inflammation of the anal sinuses or crypts (*cryptitis*) spread into the ischiorectal fossa and pus develops which aggregates to form an abscess (collection of pus). Anal fistulae are pathological channels that may develop following infection and carry the infection from the anal canal to one or more of the following sites: the ischiorectal fossa, the pelvirectal space, the perineum, and the buttock. Observe the tear of the anal mucosa called an anal fissure; over 90% of cases occur posteriorly in the midline. The anal mucosa appears to be vulnerable to injury here because the superficial part of the external anal sphincter (Fig. 3-19*A*) inserts posteriorly into the coccyx (Fig. 3-38), supporting the anal mucosa. As a result it is more easily torn by hard fecal material than elsewhere. The small epithelial projections on the anal valves, called anal papillae, are thought to be remnants of the *embryonic anal membrane.* Sometimes they become hypertrophied, as illustrated in Figure 3-100.

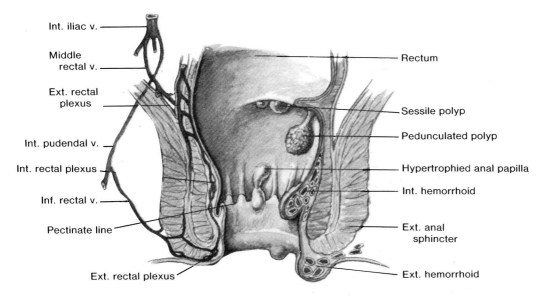

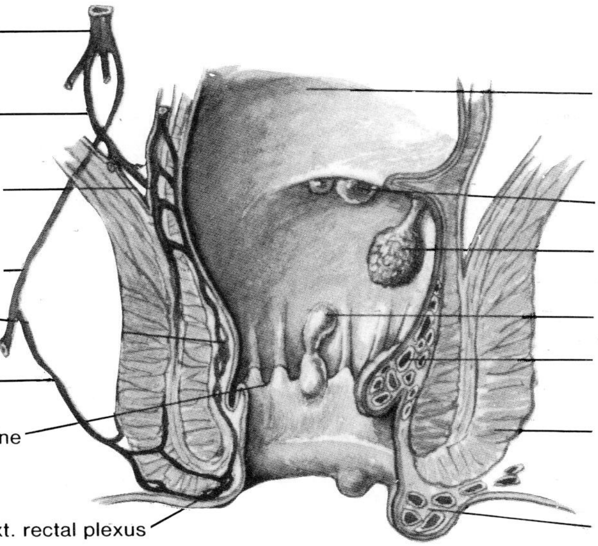

Figure 3-100. Drawing of a coronal section of the pelvis and perineum showing its venous drainage and illustrating various anorectal problems. Polyps are protruding growths from the mucous membrane. Internal hemorrhoids (piles) are covered with mucosa, whereas external hemorrhoids are covered with modified anal skin. *Internal hemorrhoids* are varicosities of tributaries of the superior rectal vein and *external hemorrhoids* are varicosities of the inferior rectal vein.

anal canal of living persons (Fig. 3-84). Distal to the anocutaneous or "white" line, the anal canal is lined with true skin which is often brownish in color. It contains sweat glands, sebaceous glands, and some hairs (Fig. 3-19*B*).

Blood Vessels of the Anal Canal (Figs. 2-55, 3-19*A*, 3-27, 3-65, 3-66, 3-98, and 3-99). The **superior rectal artery** supplies the *superior part of the anal canal*; its terminal branches run in the anal columns as far as the anal valves where they form anastomotic loops. The two **middle rectal arteries** help to supply the superior part of the anal canal by forming anastomoses with the superior rectal arteries. The two **inferior rectal arteries** supply the *inferior part of the anal canal* (*i.e.*, distal to the anal valves) as well as the surrounding muscles and the perianal skin. These arteries also have anastomoses with the middle rectal arteries. The **median sacral artery** (Fig. 2-55) gives off small branches that supply the posterior wall of the anorectal junction and of the anus.

The merging lamina propria and submucosa of the anal canal contain many convolutions of small veins called the **submucosal plexus of veins**. This plexus drains in opposite directions from the level of the pectinate line (Fig. 3-97). *Superior to the pectinate line the submucosal plexus of veins drains chiefly into the* **superior rectal veins** *and thereby into the portal system* (Fig. 2-112). The venous plexuses above the pelvic diaphragm anastomose to form left and right **middle rectal veins** which drain into the corresponding internal iliac veins. *Inferior to the pectinate line the submucosal plexus of veins drains into* **inferior rectal veins** *around the margin of the external anal sphincter*. These veins have communications with the middle and superior rectal veins.

The lymph vessels from the part of the anal canal *superior to the pectinate line* drain into the **internal iliac lymph nodes** and through them to the common iliac and aortic lymph nodes (Fig. 3-85), whereas the lymph vessels *inferior to the pectinate line* drain into the **superficial inguinal lymph nodes** (Figs. 3-85 and 4-38).

Nerves of the Anal Canal (Figs. 3-65, 3-92, and 3-93). The nerve supply of the anal canal superior to the pectinate line is the same as that for the rectum. The **sympathetic nerves** pass along the superior rectal vessels and partly form the *inferior hypogastric plexus.* The **parasympathetic nerves** are from S2 to S4 and run in the pelvic sphanchnic nerves to join the inferior hypogastric plexus. The *sensory nerves,* sensitive only to stretching, are derived from the inferior rectal branches of the **pudendal nerve** (Fig. 3-26). The fibers supplying the perianal skin are concerned with cutaneous sensations.

CLINICALLY ORIENTED COMMENTS

The anal canal superior to the pectinate line (Fig. 3-97) *develops from the hindgut* (endoderm) as does the rectum, whereas *the anal canal inferior to the pectinate line develops from the anal pit or proctodeum* (ectoderm). The pectinate line indicated by the anal valves indicates the approximate former site of the anal membrane. Because of its hindgut origin the superior part of the anal canal is supplied by branches of the **inferior mesenteric artery** (hindgut artery), whereas the inferior part of the canal derived from the anal pit is supplied by branches of the **internal pudendal artery**. The venous and lymphatic drainage and the nerve supply of these regions also differ (Figs. 3-19, 3-97, and 3-98) because of the different embryological origins of the superior and inferior parts of the anal canal.

The anal canal extends from the superior aspect of the pelvic diaphragm to the anus (Fig. 3-55) and is marked by the anorectal ring formed mainly by the puborectalis muscle (Fig. 3-61). In practice some surgeons regard only the part of the anal canal inferior to the pectinate line (Fig. 3-97) as the true anal canal because of the differences in blood and nerve supply and in venous and lymphatic drainage above and below this line. In the embryo the rectum is separated from the exterior by the **anal membrane**, but this normally breaks down at the end of the 8th week. If it persists, a condition known as **imperforate anus** exists. Some form of imperforate anus occurs once in about 5000 births and is more common in males. Most anorectal malformations result from abnormal development of the **urorectal septum** (Fig. 3-28*B*), resulting in incomplete separation of the cloaca into urogenital and anorectal portions.

Internal hemorrhoids (piles) are *varicosities of the tributaries of the superior rectal veins* and are covered by mucous membrane (Case 3-3 and Fig. 3-100). Some clinicans still refer to the superior rectal veins as the superior hemorrhoidal veins. **External hemorrhoids** are *varicosities of the tributaries of the inferior rectal veins* and are covered by skin (Fig. 3-100). As there are multiple anastomoses between the venous plexuses of the rectal veins, these communicating veins may also be dilated.

Mixed hemorrhoids are varicosities of the superior, communicating, and inferior rectal veins. Hemorrhoids prolapsing through the external anal sphincter are often compressed, impeding the blood supply. As a result they tend to ulcerate and strangulate. *Thrombus (clot) formation* is more common in external hemorrhoids than in internal hemorrhoids **Thrombosed hemorrhoids** are often painful. For a description of the etiology of hemorrhoids, see the discussion of Case 3-3. *The anastomosis between the superior and middle rectal veins forms a clinically important communication between the portal and systemic systems* (Fig. 2-112). Any abnormal increase in pressure in the valveless portal system may cause enlargement of the superior rectal veins contained in the anal columns, resulting in internal hemorrhoids. In **portal hypertension**, as in *hepatic cirrhosis* (Case 2-8), the tiny anastomotic veins in the anal canal and elsewhere (Fig. 2-112) become varicose and may rupture.

In chronically constipated persons, the anal valves may be torn by hard fecal material and the anal mucosa may also be torn. The slit-like lesion, known as an **anal fissure** (Fig. 3-99), is usually inferior to the anal valves and is very painful because this region is supplied by the inferior rectal nerve (Fig. 3-26). **Perianal abscesses** (collections of pus) may follow infection of anal fissures and the infection may spread to the

ischiorectal fossae (Case 3-3) or into the pelvis forming ischiorectal and pelvirectal abscesses, respectively (Fig. 3-99). An **anal fistula** may develop as a result of the spread of an infection; one end of the abnormal canal opens into the anal canal and the other opens into the perianal skin or buttock (Fig. 3-99).

As the anal canal superior to the pectinate line (Fig. 3-97) is supplied through the *autonomic plexuses*, an incision or a needle insertion in this region is painless. However, the anal canal inferior to the pectinate line is very sensitive (*e.g.*, to the prick of a hypodermic needle) because it is supplied by the *inferior rectal nerve*, which contains sensory fibers, including those carrying pain.

THE PELVIC AUTONOMIC NERVES

The Sympathetic Trunks (Figs. 3-58, 3-64, 3-82, 3-92, and 3-93). The *sacral sympathetic trunks* are directly continuous with the *lumbar sympathetic trunks* (Figs. 2-131 and 3-64) posterior to the common iliac vessels (Fig. 2-113). They are smaller than the lumbar trunks and each one has four ganglia (Fig. 3-64). The trunks descend on the pelvic surface of the sacrum just medial to the pelvic sacral foramina. The two trunks converge as they pass along the sacrum and unite in the small median ganglion impar (L. unequal, *i.e.*, unpaired) on the coccyx (Fig. 3-64). The sympathetic trunks run in the presacral fascia external to the peritoneum (Fig. 3-95).

Branches of the Sacral Sympathetic Trunks (Figs. 3-58, 3-82, 3-92, and 3-93). The sympathetic trunks send **gray rami communicantes** to each of the ventral rami of the *sacral* and *coccygeal nerves.* They also send small branches to the median sacral artery and to the inferior hypogastric plexus (Fig. 3-93). A few branches from the **ganglion impar** pass to the *coccygeal body* which lies anterior to the apex of the coccyx.

The Hypogastric Plexuses (Figs. 3-70, 3-82, 3-92, 3-93, and 3-95). The **superior hypogastric plexus** (presacral nerve, presacral plexus) descends into the pelvis and lies just below the bifurcation of the aorta (Fig. 3-95). It is the downward prolongation of the *intermesenteric plexus* (Fig. 2-127) which is joined by L3 and L4 splanchnic nerves (Fig. 3-82). Branches from the superior hypogastric plexus enter the pelvis and descend anterior to the sacrum as the **right** and **left hypogastric nerves** (Figs. 2-127, 3-92, and 3-93). These nerves descend on the lateral walls of the pelvis where they mingle with the **pelvic splanchnic nerves** (Figs. 3-38, 3-58, 3-65, and 3-82) to form the right and left pelvic or **inferior hypogastric plexuses** (Fig. 3-93). *The pelvic splanchnic nerves are parasympathetic and are derived from S2, S3, and S4* (Fig. 3-82). Hence, the inferior hypogastric plexuses contain both sympathetic and parasympathetic fibers. *Each plexus surrounds the corresponding internal iliac artery.* There are small ganglia scattered within these plexuses and each plexus receives small branches from the superior sacral ganglia of the sympathetic trunks. Branches from the hypogastric plexuses, containing sympathetic and parasympathetic fibers, are distributed to the pelvic viscera along the branches of the internal iliac artery (Fig. 3-65).

The visceral plexuses are *extensions of the inferior hypogastric plexuses on the walls of the pelvic viscera.* The **middle rectal plexus** arises from the superior part of the inferior hypogastric plexus and extends inferiorly as far as the internal anal sphincter. The branches from the rectal plexus pass directly to the rectum or along the middle rectal artery. It also sends parasympathetic fibers to the sigmoid and descending parts of the colon. The **vesical plexus** arises from the anterior part of the inferior hypogastric plexus and the branches from it pass to the bladder along the vesical arteries (Fig. 3-65). Branches from this plexus also pass to the seminal vesicles, the deferent ducts, and the prostate (Fig. 3-82). The **prostatic plexus** arises from the inferior part of the hypogastric plexus and is composed of rather large nerves which enter the base and sides of the prostate. These nerves are also distributed to the seminal vesicles, the ejaculatory ducts, the urethra, the bulbourethral glands, and the penis. The nerves supplying the corpora cavernosa of the penis are called the *cavernous nerves*. They arise from the anterior part of the prostatic plexus and join with branches from the **pudendal nerve** (Figs. 3-26 and 3-82). These nerves pass along the membranous urethra to the penis. The **uterovaginal plexus** arises mainly from the part of the inferior hypogastric plexus that lies in the base of the *broad ligament* (Fig. 3-93). Some nerves from the uterovaginal plexus pass inferiorly to the vagina and the cervix with the vaginal arteries; other nerves pass directly to the cervix with the vaginal arteries; some nerves pass directly to the cervix or superiorly with the uterine arteries to the body of the uterus. Some of these fibers also supply medial parts of the uterine tube. *The uterovaginal plexus is homologous with the prostatic plexus.* The **vaginal nerves** from the plexus also supply the urethra, the vestibular bulbs, the greater vestibular glands, and the clitoris. The nerves supplying the bulbs of the vestibule (Fig. 3-12) and the corpora cavernosa of the clitoris (Fig. 3-40) are called the *cavernous nerves*.

JOINTS OF THE PELVIS

THE LUMBROSACRAL JOINTS

The fifth lumbar vertebra (L5) and the first sacral vertebra (S1) articulate with one another by an *anterior fibrocartilaginous joint* between their bodies and by two *posterior synovial joints* between their articular processes. The articulations between L5 and S1 are similar to the joints between other typical vertebrae (Chap. 5); however, the **intervertebral disc** is wedge-shaped because it is thicker anteriorly (Figs. 3-22 and 5-27).

The right and left **zygapophyseal joints** (Figs. 5-33 and 5-34) are synovial joints between the inferior articular processes of L5 and the superior articular processes of the S1 part of the sacrum. The S1 facets face posteriorly and medially and thereby prevent L5 vertebra from sliding forward. These joints are similar to those in other parts of the vertebral column (see Chap. 5). Associated with them are the *ligamenta flava* and the *interspinous* and *supraspinous ligaments* (Figs. 5-31 to 5-34).

L5 vertebra is also attached to the ilium and the sacrum by the strong **iliolumbar ligaments** (Figs. 2-131 and 3-46*A*). *These ligaments unite each thick transverse process of L5 vertebra to the internal lip of the iliac crest posteriorly* (Fig. 3-8). The lower fibers of each iliolumbar ligament, often called the lumbosacral ligament, descend to the anterior part of the ala of the sacrum (Fig. 3-46*A*). *The iliolumbar ligaments help to stabilize the lumbosacral joint and are important because they limit axial rotation of L5 vertebra on the sacrum.*

CLINICALLY ORIENTED COMMENTS

There are numerous variations of the lumbosacral region. **Spina bifida occulta** (Fig. 5-30) of either L5 or S1 vertebra is present in about 10% of people with no back problems (*i.e.*, asymptomatic people). Partial or complete separation of S1 from the sacrum (**lumbarization of S1**, Fig. 5-26) or partial or complete fusion of L5 to the sacrum (**sacralization of L5**, Fig. 5-24) are somewhat less common and are seen in many asymptomatic persons. In sacralization of L5 there are fewer moving levels than normal in the lumbar region of the vertebral column and possibly this favors earlier or more severe disease at the moving lumbar joint levels. Large transverse processes on L5 are not uncommon and are more likely to strengthen the lumbosacral joint than to weaken it.

A curious condition called **spondylolysis** is found usually in the lower lumbar region in about 5% of white North American adults. It occurs more frequently in certain races, *e.g.*, Eskimos, Australian aborigines, and South African Bushmen. It is found about as often in people with low back pain as in those without. *In spondylolysis a defect is found in the vertebral arch between the superior and inferior facets*, the area called the **pars interarticularis**. When bilateral it results in the vertebra being in two pieces (Fig. 5-41): the posterior piece consists of the laminae, the inferior articular processes, and the spinous process; the anterior piece is the remainder of the vertebra.

If the two pieces separate, the condition is called **spondylolisthesis** (Fig. 3-101). The resulting anteroinferior displacement of the anterior piece of L5 reduces the AP diameter of the superior pelvic aperture (Fig. 3-52) and *may interfere with parturition*. Obstetricians test for spondylolisthesis by running their fingers down the lumbar spinous processes of the pregnant patient's back. If the spinous process of L5 is prominent, it indicates that the anterior part of L5 vertebra and the vertebral column above have moved forward (Fig. 3-101). Radiographs are then made to confirm the diagnosis and to measure the effective AP diameter of the superior pelvic aperture.

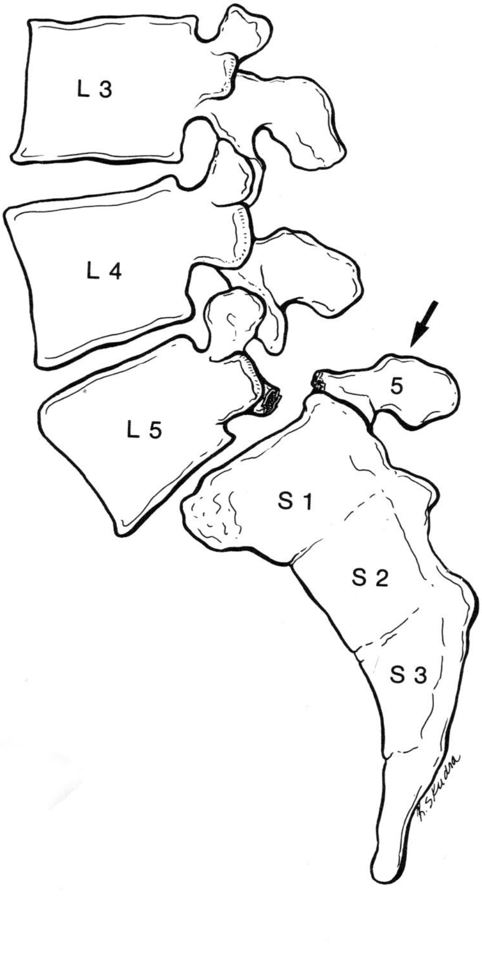

Figure 3-101. Drawing made from a lateral radiograph of a patient with spondylolisthesis of L5 vertebra. Observe that the anterior piece of L5 (body, pedicles, transverse processes, and superior articular processes) has moved forward taking the vertebrae above this level with it. Note that the posterior piece of L5 (laminae, inferior articular processes, and spinous process) stays with the sacrum. Often one or both pieces of the affected vertebra are hypoplastic (underdeveloped). The *arrow* points to the spinous process of L5, which is on a vertical plane posterior to the other lumbar spinous processes; thus it appears unduly prominent. *T*, transverse process shadow. Because spondylolithesis may interfere with parturition by reducing the AP diameter of the superior pelvic aperture (Fig. 3-52), obstetricians test their patients for this condition by running their fingers down the lumbar spinous processes to determine if the L5 spinous process is prominent. (For a radiograph of the normal lumbosacral region, see Fig. 5-27.)

THE SACROCOCCYGEAL JOINT

The sacrococcygeal joint is usually a symphysis (G. a growing together), a type of cartilaginous joint. The apex of the sacrum and the base of the coccyx are united by a thin fibrocartilaginous intervertebral disc (Figs. 3-14, 3-22, and 5-27) that is slightly thicker anteriorly. The **sacrococcygeal ligaments** correspond to the anterior and posterior longitudinal ligaments of the other intervertebral joints (Fig. 5-32). The *sacral* and *coccygeal cornua* are also united by **intercornual ligaments**. In persons up to middle age there is slight movement of the coccyx backward on defecation and during childbirth there is considerable posterior movement of the coccyx. In elderly persons the first coccygeal vertebra is frequently fused to the apex of the sacrum, thereby eliminating the sacrococcygeal joint (Fig. 5-1).

THE SACROILIAC JOINTS

These are very strong **synovial joints** between the articular surfaces of the sacrum and the ilium (Figs. 3-7*B*, 3-47, 3-48*A*, and 3-49). These articular surfaces have irregular elevations with depressions in the opposing surfaces, producing joints with little movement. The **articular capsule** is attached close to the articulating surfaces of the sacrum and the ilium. The sacrum is suspended between the iliac bones (Figs. 3-7 and 3-49) and the bones are firmly held together by very strong **interosseous** and **dorsal sacroiliac ligaments** (Figs. 3-46, 3-102, and 4-44).

The Interosseous Sacroiliac Ligaments (Fig. 3-102). These massive ligaments uniting the iliac and sacral tuberosities are *very strong*. They lie posterior to the synovial capsule and consist of short, strong bundles of fibers which blend with the dorsal sacroiliac ligament posteriorly. The bundles of fibers radiate from the iliac tuberosity to the lateral aspect of the ala of the sacrum, posterior to the auricular facets of the sacrum, and thus suspend the sacrum between the two ilia.

The Dorsal Sacroiliac Ligaments (Fig. 4-44). These ligaments are composed of (1) strong, short, transverse fibers joining the ilium and the first and second tubercles of the lateral crest of the sacrum; and (2) long vertical fibers that unite the third and fourth transverse tubercles of the sacrum to the posterior iliac spine. The dorsal sacroiliac ligament blends with the **sacrotuberous ligament** (Figs. 3-18 and 4-44).

The Ventral Sacroiliac Ligament (Fig. 3-18). This is a wide, thin sheet of transverse fibers located on the anterior and inferior aspects of the joint. It covers the abdominopelvic surface of this articulation.

The **sacrotuberous** and **sacrospinous ligaments** (Figs. 3-18, 3-46, and 4-44) discussed previously are accessory ligaments of the sacroiliac joints. The sacroiliac joints are covered posteriorly by the erector spinae and gluteus maximus muscles (Figs. 5-46 and 5-50). The **skin dimples**, indicating the posterior superior iliac spines (Figs. 5-11 and 5-48), lie at the level of the middle of the sacroiliac joints.

The sacroiliac joints are strong weight-bearing joints which are responsible for transmitting the weight of the body to the ossa coxae or hip bones (Fig. 5-2).

Movements of the Joints. Little movement occurs at the sacroiliac joints because they are designed primarily for weight bearing. *Movement of the sacroiliac joints is limited to a slight gliding and rotary movement*, except when a considerable force is applied to them such as occurs during a jump from a height. In this case the force is transmitted via the vertebral column to the superior end of the sacrum, which tends to rotate forward. This rotation is counterbalanced by the strong sacrotuberous and sacrospinous ligaments, allowing the force to be transmitted to each ilium and lower limb.

If the right lower limb is raised keeping

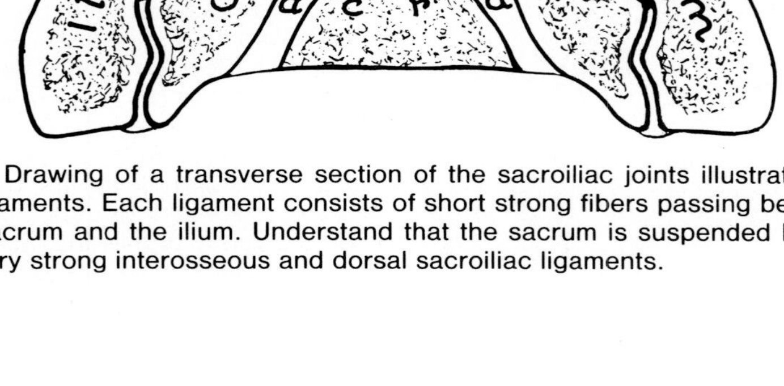

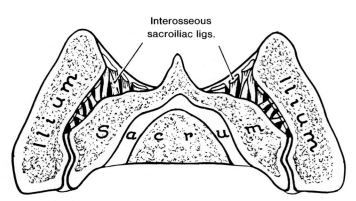

Figure 3-102. Drawing of a transverse section of the sacroiliac joints illustrating the powerful interosseous ligaments. Each ligament consists of short strong fibers passing between the tuberosities of the sacrum and the ilium. Understand that the sacrum is suspended between the iliac bones by the very strong interosseous and dorsal sacroiliac ligaments.

the left leg straight, the hamstring muscles (Fig. 4-45) and their extensions, the sacrotuberous ligaments, anchor the sacrum to the right hip bone and lower limb. If at the same time the left lower limb is extended, the iliofemoral and ischiofemoral ligaments anchor the left ilium to the left femur, and thus movement will take place at the left sacroiliac joint. By this maneuver, movements can be tested at each sacroiliac joint separately.

The above manipulation will also cause the L5 vertebra to rotate toward the side on which the lower limb is flexed owing to the pull of the iliolumbar ligament. In addition, the right pubic bone will be raised in relation to the left.

Arterial Supply of the Joints (Figs. 3-66 and 4-47). The articular branches to the sacroiliac joints are derived from the *superior gluteal, iliolumbar*, and *lateral sacral arteries*.

Nerve Supply of the Joints (Figs. 3-58 and 4-47). The articular branches are derived from (1) the *superior gluteal nerves*, (2) the *sacral plexus*, and (3) the dorsal rami of *S1* and *S2 nerves*.

CLINICALLY ORIENTED COMMENTS

When one falls from a height and lands on the feet, the sacroiliac joints transfer most of the body weight to the hip bones. Flexion of the legs also helps to prevent injury to the vertebral column. The resilience of the sacrotuberous and sacrospinous ligaments (Figs. 3-46 and 4-44) also cushions the shock to the back.

The sacroiliac ligaments (Fig. 3-102) *are thought to become softer and more yielding during the late stages of pregnancy.* Thus the range of movement of the joints is temporarily increased. Combined with similar changes in the pubic symphysis and in the associated ligaments (Fig. 3-46), the passage of the fetus through the birth canal is thus facilitated. The sacroiliac joints often become partially ossified during old age, especially in males. Calcification may occur in the anterior sacroiliac ligament making the joint space less visible on radiographs, even though still present.

THE SYMPHYSIS PUBIS

The symphysis pubis or pubic symphysis is a median **cartilaginous joint** between the bodies of the pubic bones (Figs. 3-8, 3-14, 3-22, 3-49, 3-57, and 3-60). Each articular surface is covered by a thin layer of hyaline cartilage which is connected to the cartilage of the other side by a thick fibrocartilaginous **interpubic disc** (Figs. 3-8 and 3-57). This disc is generally thicker in females than in males and often contains a cavity.

The **superior pubic ligament** connects the pubic bones superiorly and extends as far as the pubic tubercles (Fig. 3-46*A*). The **arcuate pubic ligament** (Figs. 3-2, 3-18, and 3-22) is a thick arch of fibers (1) connecting the inferior borders of the joint, (2) rounding off the subpubic angle (Fig. 3-46*B*), and (3) forming the superior border of the pubic arch (Fig. 3-7*A*). The arcuate pubic ligament is separated from the urogenital diaphragm by an interval through which the dorsal vein of the penis or clitoris enters the pelvis (Figs. 3-11 and 3-42).

PATIENT ORIENTED PROBLEMS

Case 3-1. A 23-year-old **primigravida** (L. *primus*, first + *gravida*, pregnancy) had been in labor for nearly 24 hr. The crown of the fetal head was now visible through the vaginal orifice. The obstetrician, fearing that her perineum might be torn, decided to perform a **mediolateral episiotomy** (Fig. 3-44*B*) to enlarge the inferior opening of the birth canal (vaginal orifice).

Problems. What structures would probably be cut during this surgical procedure? What perineal structures might have been injured if the perineum had been allowed to tear in an uncontrolled fashion? In severe **perineal lacerations**, what important muscles may be torn? *These problems are discussed on page 411.*

Case 3-2. A 31-year-old construction worker was walking along a steel beam when he fell, straddling it. He was in severe pain owing to *trauma to his testes and perineum.* Later he observed swelling and discoloration of his scrotum, and when he attempted to urinate, only a few drops of bloody urine appeared.

Urethrography (radiography of the urethra), performed by gently injecting a radiopaque contrast solution into his external urethral orifice with a syringe, revealed a **rupture of the spongy urethra** just below the inferior fascia of the urogenital diaphragm, or perineal membrane (Figs. 3-10 and 3-11). The **urethrograms** showed passage of contrast material out of the urethra into the surrounding tissues of the perineum, a process known as **extravasation of urine**.

Problems. When the patient tried to urinate, practically no urine came from his external urethral orifice. Where did it go? Explain why extravasated urine cannot pass posteriorly, laterally, or into the pelvis minor. During a discussion of this case, a clinician referred to Colle's fascia and Scarpa's fascia. What are these fascial layers now called? *These problems are discussed on page 412.*

Case 3-3. A 49-year-old family physician noted *tenderness and pain to the right of his anus.* The pain was aggravated by defecation and sitting. As he had a history of internal **hemorrhoids** (piles) and **pruritus** (L. an itching) **ani**, he suspected that he might be developing an *abscess in his ischiorectal fossa* and have an **anal fistula**.

After he had explained his symptoms and history to *his* doctor, his physician examined the rectum and anal canal. When he asked the patient to strain as if to defecate, **prolapsing internal hemmorrhoids** (Fig. 3-100) came into view. During digital examination of the rectum, the doctor detected some *swelling in the patient's right ischiorectal fossa.* The swelling produced severe pain when it was compressed. A diagnosis of an **ischiorectal abscess** was made (Fig. 3-99). The abscess was drained through an incision in the skin between the anus and the ischial tuberosity (see Figs. 3-23 and 3-44 for the site of the incision).

Problems. Differentiate between **internal** and **external hemorrhoids**. *What is an ischiorectal abscess*? What nerve is vulnerable to injury during surgical treatment of an ischiorectal abscess? If this nerve were severed, what structure would be partly denervated? *These problems are discussed on page 412.*

Case 3-4. During the physical examination of a male child, a congenital malformation of the penis known as **hypospadias** was detected. The urethra opened just proximal to the site where the frenulum (which was absent) usually attaches the **prepuce** (Fig. 3-35) to the penis on its ventral surface (Fig. 3-103). There was a slight indentation or blind urethra at the site of the normally located **external urethral orifice** at the tip of the glans penis. In addition, there was a slight ventral curvature of the penis (**chordee**) because its ventral surface was shorter than its dorsal parts. **Micturition** was esentially normal except that he dribbled downward if he urinated while standing up, wetting his clothing and his shoes.

Problems. What is the *embryological basis of hypospadias.* Discuss other types of hypospadias. Do you think this condition would subsequently interfere with reproductive function? *These problems are discussed on page 413.*

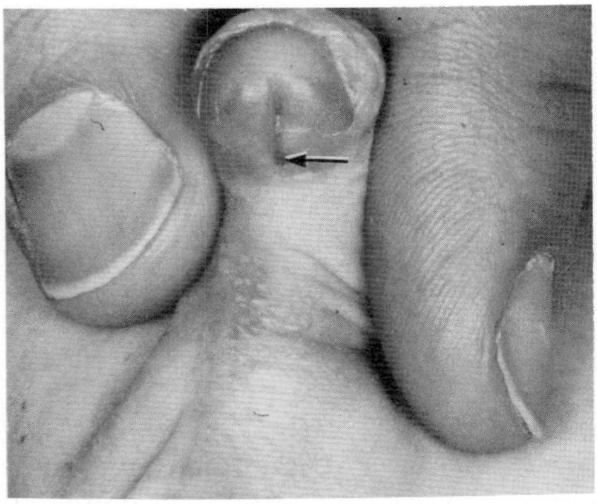

Figure 3-103. Photograph of a child's penis showing the external urethral orifice (*arrow*) on the ventral surface near the glans penis (glandular hypospadias). Observe that the glans is also abnormally formed, being bent toward the ventral surface of the penis (chordee).

Case 3-5. There was *uncertainty about the sex* of a full term infant whose birth weight was in the normal range. It was the mother's first pregnancy and there were no complications during the prenatal period or the delivery. The mother had been prescribed no medications except for a mineral and vitamin supplement. She stated emphatically that she had taken no drugs during her pregnancy. The intern thought that the baby was a boy with **hypospadias,** whereas the resident believed the infant was a **female pseudohermaphrodite** or intersex.

As careful examination revealed *ambiguous external genitalia* (Fig. 3-104), sex assignment was postponed. The small genital organ (**phallus**) measured 1.8 by 1.0 cm. *The labioscrotal folds were incompletely fused* but resembled a bifid scrotum. Between these folds there was a shallow, trough-like depression with a single opening through which the infant voided. **No gonads** (sex glands) were palpable. A rectal examination revealed a small midline structure which was thought to be a uterus.

The parents were informed that the infant's sex organs were poorly developed and that several tests would have to be done before the baby's sex could be determined. A buccal smear was taken for a **sex chromatin test** which was later reported to be *chromatin positive.* Other laboratory studies revealed that the infant's 17-ketosteroid output was elevated. A diagnosis of *female pseudohermaphroditism* resulting from **congenital adrenal hyperplasia** was made and the patient's sex was assigned as female.

Problems. Discuss the embryological basis of congenital adrenal hyperplasia? Is this baby an *intersex*? What kind of **teratogenic agents** can cause varying degrees of masculinization of female fetuses? State the basis of the sex chromatin test. What would the child's chromosome constitution be? *These problems are discussed on page 414.*

Case 3-6. A 40-year-old unconscious woman was rushed to the hospital because she had sustained *multiple injuries during an automobile accident.* Priority was given to securing a patent airway by inserting an **endotracheal tube**. Next, emergency care was directed toward controlling bleeding and treating the shock.

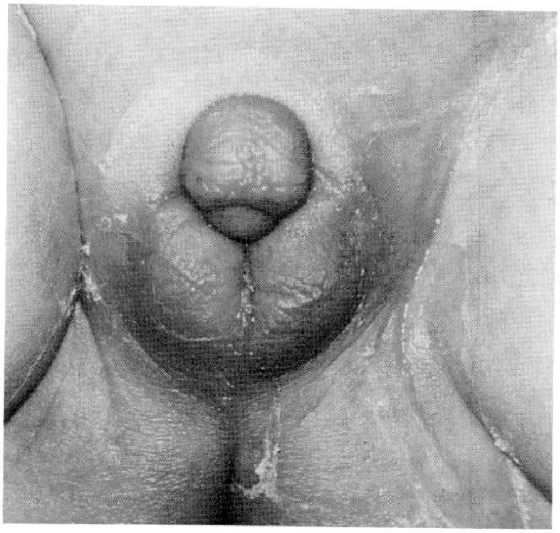

Figure 3-104. Photograph of the ambiguous external genitalia of a newborn infant.

When the patient's general condition had stabilized, radiographs were taken of the injured regions of her body. Because she had not urinated since being admitted, she was catheterized. The presence of blood in the bladder urine (**hematuria**) suggested rupture of the urinary bladder. Therefore, 100 ml of sterile dilute contrast solution were injected through a catheter and radiographs of the pelvis and abdomen were made. The radiologist reported that there were **fractures of the pubic rami** on both sides and that the *cystogram showed extravasation* (L. *extra*, out of + *vas*, vessel) of contrast material from the superior surface of the bladder (Fig. 3-105).

Problems. Where would the extravasated urine go? What covers the superior surface of the bladder? Thinking anatomically, what route do you think the surgeon would take in repairing the ruptured bladder? *These problems are discussed on page 415.*

Case 3-7. During the physical examination of a 15-year-old boy prior to summer camp, a doctor felt a firm *ovoid lump in his left inguinal region*, above the medial part of the inguinal ligament. On questioning,

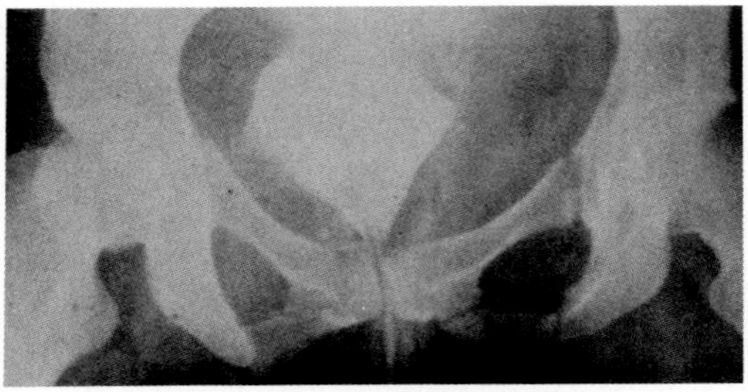

Figure 3-105. Radiograph of the pelvis showing fractures of the pubic rami on both sides. The contrast medium injected through the catheter in the urinary bladder may be seen passing out of the superior portion of the bladder.

the boy said that this swelling had always been in his groin and that it was very painful when it was hit. He also stated that the swelling had been increasing slightly in size for about 2 years.

During examination of the scrotum, the doctor noted that the left side was less rugose (wrinkled) than on the right side. Although he was able to palpate the right testis, he could not locate a left testis. Assuming it may have retracted into the **inguinal canal** and be the cause of the swelling there, he placed the tips of his index and middle fingers over the site of the deep inguinal ring and above the **inguinal lump**. Exerting moderate steady pressure he moved his fingers in the line of the inguinal canal. The mass moved slightly, far enough to emerge from the superficial inguinal ring, but could not be moved into the scrotum. A diagnosis of imperfect or *incomplete descent of the testis*, a condition known as **cryptorchidism** (G. *kryptos*, hidden + *orchis*, testis) was made.

Problems. This abnormality is often referred to as undescended testis, but this term is usually inappropriate. Explain why. What is the embryological basis of incomplete descent of the testis? Why did the mass enlarge between the 13 to 15 year period? Could such a mass ever be detected in a female? What kind of hernia would you expect to be associated with cryptorchidism? *These problems are discussed on page 415.*

Case 3-8. A 28-year-old **gravida** (pregnant woman) was experiencing pregnancy for the first time (*primigravida* or *gravida* I). Toward the end of the **gestational period** (L. *gestatio*, to bear) she suffered painful uterine contractions at night which subsided toward morning (**false pains**). When she called her doctor he told her that her **labor** (L. toil, suffering) was imminent. In a few days she observed a discharge of mucus and some blood, referred to as a *show*, which results from release of the **cervical plug** which had filled the cervical canal temporarily, forming a barrier between the uterus and the vagina.

When she reported that her "pains" (**uterine contractions**) were occuring every 10 minutes, her obstetrician asked her to go to the maternity hospital. Following admission the doctor examined her rectally and informed the intern that the **uterine ostium** (external os) was open about one fingertip (Fig. 3-87) and that she was still in the **first stage of labor** (the period of dilation of the uterine ostium). This stage usually lasts 8 to 10 hr in primigravidas. Later a large volume of fluid (*rupture of the fetal membranes* or "bag of waters") was expelled.

When the patient entered the **second stage of labor** (the period of expulsive effort beginning with complete dilation of the cervix and ending with delivery of the baby), she began to experience considerable pain. Although she had wanted to have a *natural birth* without the use of anesthetics, she was unable to bear the pain and asked for relief. Medication for pain relief was administered as ordered by her physician. When it was determined that her contractions were 2 minutes apart and lasting 40 to 60 sec, she was moved to the case room and placed on the delivery table. As the fetal head dilated the **birth canal** (cervix and vagina), it was obvious that the woman was suffering intense pain. The obstetrician decided to do a **mediolateral episiotomy** (Fig. 3-44*B*) when it appeared possible that a tear might occur in her perineum. He gave her an intradermal injection of an anesthetic agent into the region of the perineum concerned (for details about an episiotomy, see Case 3-1). Although the local anesthetic enabled the incision to be made without pain, it did not alleviate the severe pain of her labor.

Although **extradural (epidural) anes-**

thesia (Fig. 5-69*B*) is often used in obstetrics because it relieves the pelvic pains without interfering with uterine contractions, the obstetrician in this case decided to do **bilateral pudendal nerve blocks** (anesthetization of the pudendal nerves). Thereafter the patient completed the second stage and proceeded through the **third stage of labor** (beginning after delivery of the child and ending with expulsion of the placenta and fetal membranes) without complications (Fig. 3-106).

Problems. What membranes usually rupture during the first stage of labor or at the end of it? What fluid escapes? *Name the structures supplied by the pudendal nerve.* Based on your knowledge of the anatomy of this nerve, where would you inject the anesthetic agent to do a *pudendal nerve block*? What is the principal landmark in the perineal route. What other landmark is there when doing a perineal nerve block? When complete perineal anesthesia is required, branches of what other nerves would have to be blocked? *These problems are discussed on page 416.*

DISCUSSION OF PATIENT ORIENTED PROBLEMS

Case 3-1. During a **mediolateral episiotomy**, the following structures are usually cut (Figs. 3-3 and 3-42): (1) the posterior wall of the vagina, (2) the perineal skin, (3) the bulbospongiosus muscle, (4) the superficial transversus perinei muscle, and (5) the perineal membrane or inferior fascia of urogenital membrane (Fig. 3-11). Part of the deep transversus perinei muscle may be cut in some cases.

An episiotomy is performed to ease delivery of a fetus and/or when a tear of the perineum seems inevitable during **partu-**

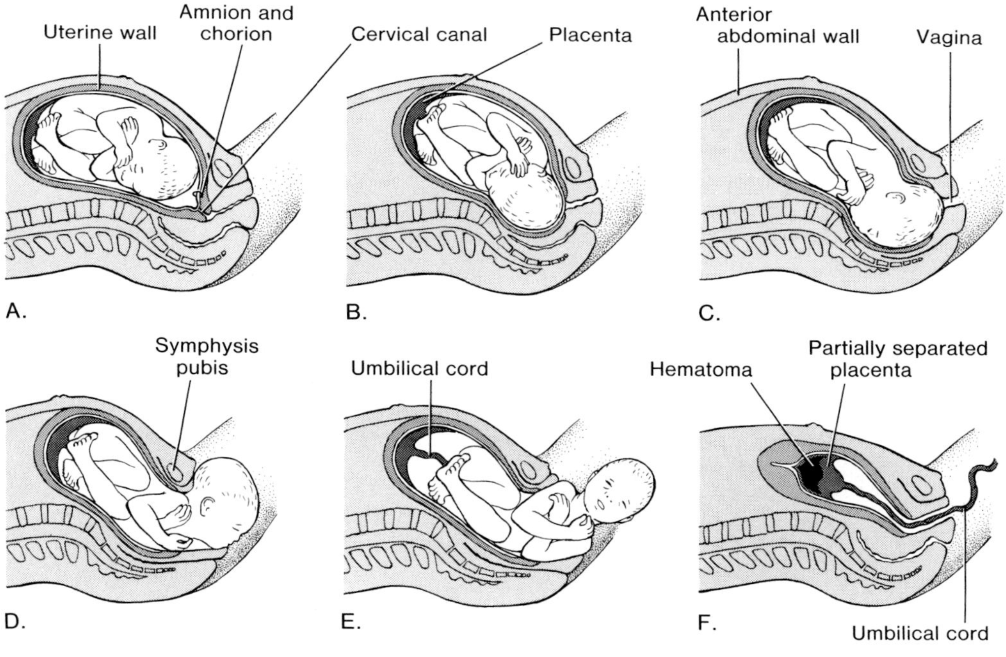

Figure 3-106. Drawings illustrating the process of birth (parturition or labor). *A* and *B*, the cervix is dilating during the *first stage of labor.* Note that the amnion and chorion are being forced into the cervical canal. *C* to *E*, the fetus passes through the cervical canal and vagina during the *second stage of labor. F*, as the uterus contracts during the *third stage of labor* the placenta folds up and pulls away from the uterine wall, resulting in bleeding and the formation of a hematoma between the uterus and the placenta. In 15 to 20 minutes the hematoma, the placenta, and the associated fetal membranes are expelled from the uterus (not shown) by further uterine contractions.

rition (birth of a baby). If a tear is allowed to occur spontaneously in whatever direction it may, the **central perineal tendon** (perineal body), the **external anal sphincter**, and the wall of the rectum may be torn. Episiotomy thus makes a clean cut away from important structures. Section of the levator ani muscle is avoided if possible during episiotomy.

Because the two **levatores ani** muscles and the two coccygeus muscles form the **pelvic diaphragm**, the chief function of which is to form the floor of the pelvis, it is important during repair of a lacerated perineum (**perineorrhaphy**) to repair the medial part of the levator ani muscle if it has been torn. Failure to do this results in poor perineal support for the pelvic organs, which may result in sagging of the pelvic floor in later life. This could lead to difficulty in bladder control, occasionally in control of the rectum, and could be the basis of a *prolapse of the uterus* in rare cases (Fig. 3-62).

Case 3-2. The traumatic rupture of the man's spongy urethra within the bulb of his penis (Fig. 3-31) resulted in superficial (subcutaneous) **extravasation of urine** when the patient attempted to urinate. Urine from the torn urethra passed into the perineum, *superficial to the inferior fascia of the urogenital diaphragm* or perineal membrane, but *deep to the superficial perineal fascia* (Colles' fascia). The urine in the superficial perineal space (pouch) passes *inferiorly* into the areolar tissue of the scrotum, *anteriorly* into the penis, and *superiorly* into the anterior wall of the abdomen.

The inferior fascia of the urogenital diaphragm or perineal membrane (Figs. 3-10 and 3-11) and the superficial fascia of the perineum are firmly attached to the ischiopubic rami. The urine cannot pass posteriorly because *the two layers are continuous with each other around the superficial transversus perinei muscles.* It does not extend laterally because these two layers are connected to the rami of the pubis and ischium and with the deep fascia of the thigh (**fascia lata**), where it is continuous with the membranous layer of the superficial fascia of the abdomen. It cannot extend into the pelvis minor because the opening into this cavity is closed by the inferior fascia of the urogenital diaphragm or perineal membrane (Fig. 3-10). Urine cannot pass into the thighs because the membranous layer of the superficial fascia of the anterior abdominal wall (Scarpa's fascia) blends with the fascia lata, just distal to the inguinal ligament. The fascia lata is the strong fascia enveloping the muscles of the thigh (Fig. 4-19).

Case 3-3. Hemorrhoids, or piles, are varicosities or dilations of one or more of the veins draining the anal canal. **Internal hemorrhoids** are varicosities of the tributaries of the *superior rectal vein.* This vein becomes the inferior mesenteric vein and belongs to the portal system of veins (Fig. 2-85). The tributaries of the superior rectal vein arise in the *internal rectal plexus*, which lies in the anal columns (Fig. 3-19*B*), where they frequently become varicose (dilated and tortuous). *Internal hemorrhoids are covered by mucous membrane.* At first they are contained in the anal canal (Fig. 3-100), but as they enlarge they may protrude through the anal canal on straining, as in the present case, and during defecation. Bleeding from these hemorrhoids is common. *Chronic constipation* with prolonged straining is a common predisposing factor in persons with internal hemorrhoids, but there are several other cases (*e.g.*, pregnancy and portal obstruction related to cirrhosis of the liver; see Case 2-8). *Most hemorrhoids do not result from portal obstruction.* They frequently occur in members of the same family, suggesting that the condition may be heritable (*i.e.*, there is an increased susceptibility to the development of hemorrhoids).

External hemorrhoids are varicosities of the tributaries of the *inferior rectal vein* arising in the *external* rectal plexus, which drains the inferior part of the anal canal. *External hemorrhoids are covered by modified anal skin* and are usually not painful unless they undergo thrombosis (G. clotting). This is referred to as a **thrombosed hemorrhoid**.

Perianal abscesses (collections of pus) often result from injury to the anal mucosa by hardened fecal material. Inflammation of the anal sinuses or crypts may result, producing a condition called **cryptitis**. The infection may spread through a small crack or lesion in the anal mucosa and pass through the anal wall into the *ischiorectal fossa*, producing an **ischiorectal abscess** (Fig. 3-99). Infections in the fat in the ischiorectal fossa (Fig. 3-23) are not uncommon. They can result from tears of the anal muscosa, disease of the perineal skin, and rarely from infection brought via the blood stream. The abscess may be connected medially, forming an **anorectal fistula** which joins the ischiorectal abscess to the anal canal and/or to the skin of the perineum and buttock. Untreated ischiorectal abscesses may extend upward into the **pelvirectal space** of the pelvis (Fig. 3-99), producing a supralevator or **pelvirectal abscess**.

The ischiorectal fossa is a wedge-shaped space lateral to the anus and the levator ani (Figs. 3-20 and 3-23). *The main component of the ischiorectal fossa is fat.* The branches of the nerves and vessels (pudendal nerve, internal pudendal vessels, and the nerve to the *obturator internus muscle*) enter the ischiorectal fossa through the **lesser sciatic foramen** (Figs. 3-17 and 3-18). The pudendal nerve and internal pudendal vessels pass in the *pudendal canal* lying in the lateral wall of the ischiorectal fossa (Figs. 3-23 and 3-56). The **inferior rectal nerve** leaves the pudendal canal and runs anteromedially and superficially across the ischiorectal fossa (Figs. 3-3, 3-6, 3-27). It passes to the **external anal sphincter** and supplies it (Fig. 3-4). Damage to this nerve results in impaired action of this voluntary sphincter.

Case 3-4. In 1 in 300 male infants, the external urethral orifice is on the ventral (under) surface of the penis. Most often the defect is of the glandular type, as in the present case (Fig. 3-103). In other patients the opening is on the body (shaft) of the penis (**penile hypospadias**, Fig. 3-107*A*), on the perineum (**penoscrotal hypospadias**, Fig. 3-107*B*), or on a bifid scrotum (scrotal or **perineal hypospadias**). In the latter case the external genitalia are usually ambiguous, which often results in the patients being classified as **male pseudohermaphrodites** (a type of intersexuality).

The embryological basis of hypospadias

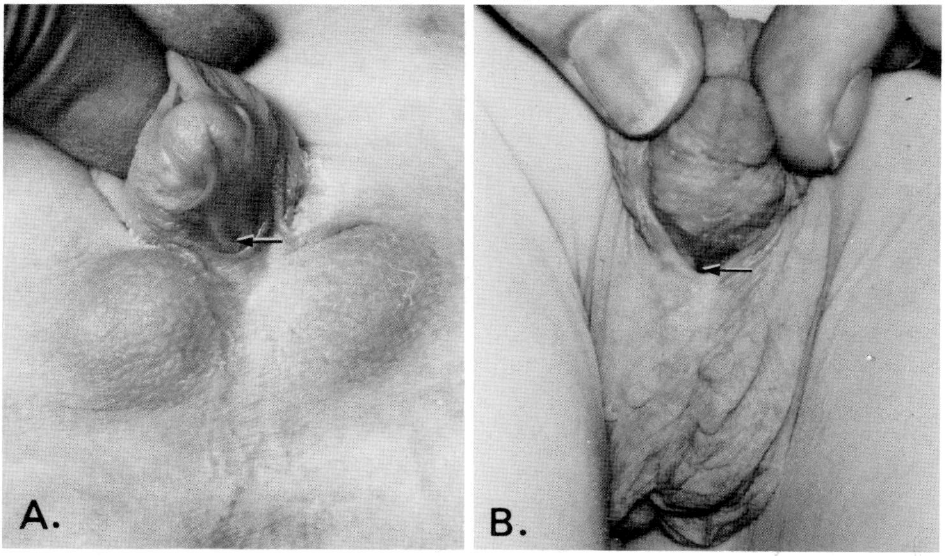

Figure 3-107. Photographs of the external genitalia of male infants with hypospadias. *A*, *penile hypospadias.* Note that the penis is short and curved (chordee) and that the external urethral orifice (*arrow*) is near the penoscrotal junction. *B*, *penoscrotal hypospadias.* Note that the external urethral orifice is at the penoscrotal junction; thus no part of the urethra is enclosed in the penis.

is failure of the **urogenital folds** to fuse on the ventral surface of the developing penis and form the spongy urethra (Fig. 3-29). It is usually combined with underdevelopment of the embryonic phallus, resulting in a short penis. The **glandular plate** of ectoderm in the glans penis usually develops and splits in the normal fashion, but it fails to join the urethral groove. Urine, therefore, is not discharged from the tip of the penis, but from an opening or openings somewhere along the ventral surface of the penis or, if the **labioscrotal swellings** have not fused, from the groove between them.

The **etiology** (cause) of hypospadias is not clearly understood, but it appears to have a multifactorial etiology (genetic and environmental factors). Close relatives of patients with hypospadias are more likely than the general population to have the abnormality. It is generally believed that hypospadias is associated with an *inadequate production of androgens by the fetal testes*. Differences in the timing and degree of **hormonal insufficiency** probably account for the gradations of hypospadias.

Because the urethral orifice is not located at the tip of the glans and there is ventral bowing of the penis (**chordee**), which is more marked when the penis is erect, reproduction by persons with this malformation is difficult. The degree of chordee is usually more pronounced when the urethral opening is located more proximally on the body of the penis. In some cases, the degree of curvature is so severe during erection that **intromission** (insertion of the penis into the vagina) and natural **insemination** (deposition of semen in the vagina) are impossible.

Surgical correction of the chordee to produce a straight body of the penis and repair of the urethra (**urethroplasty**) were recommended in the present case before the boy started school, so that it would be possible for him to urinate normally in the standing position and later be able to reproduce.

Case 3-5. The most common single cause of ambiguous external genitalia is the **adrenogenital syndrome**, resulting from *congenital virilizing adrenal hyperplasia*. Although classified as **intersexes**, *caution must be exercised in applying* this term. There is no ovarian abnormality and the ambiguous appearance of the external genitalia can be corrected so that no doubt as to sex exists.

Usually the fetal adrenal cortex disappears during the first postnatal year as the definitive cortex differentiates. In **adrenal hyperplasia**, *a genetically determined condition*, the fetal cortex becomes hyperplastic and produces excessive amounts of androgenic substances during the fetal period. These hormones cause masculinization of the genitalia of female fetuses (enlargement of the clitoris, fusion of the labia majora, and persistence of the urogenital sinus, Fig. 3-108).

Certain **progestogens** (ethisterone and norethisterone), administered during pregnancy (*e.g.*, to prevent a threatened abortion), may cause varying degrees of masculinization of female fetuses (usually **clitoral hypertrophy** and **labial fusion**). As every embryo has the potential to develop in a male or female direction, errors of sex development such as **intersexuality** can occur if there is a disturbance of sex determination, of differentiation of the genital ducts, or of development of the external genitalia.

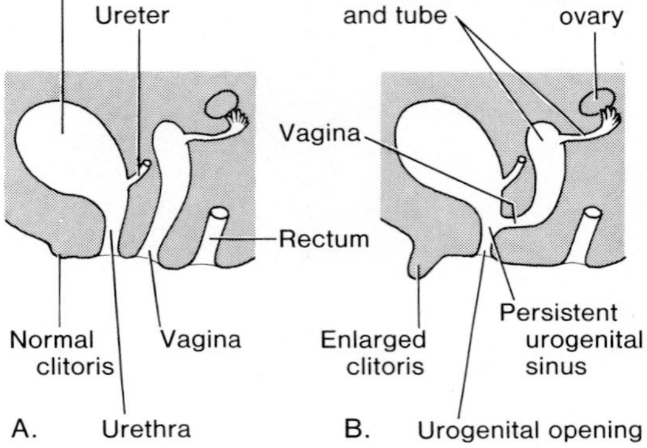

Figure 3-108. Schematic lateral views of the female urogenital system. *A*, normal. *B*, infant with congenital adrenal hyperplasia. Observe the enlarged clitoris and the persistent urogenital sinus and urogenital opening (i.e., the embryonic condition).

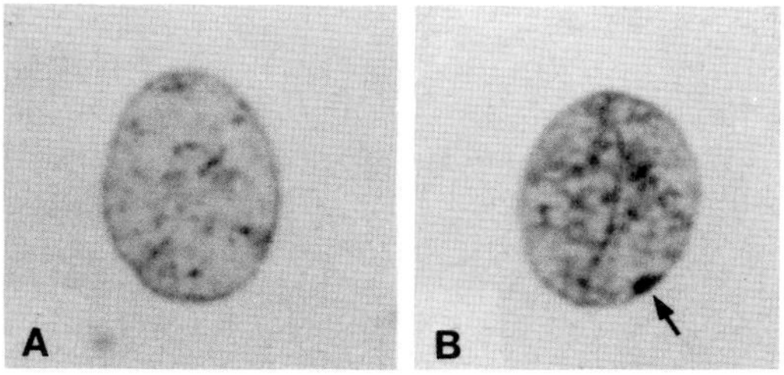

Figure 3-109. Photomicrograph of oral epithelial nuclei. *A*, chromatin negative nucleus from a normal male. No sex chromatin is visible. *B*, chromatin positive nucleus from a normal female. The *arrow* indicates a typical mass of sex chromatin. Cresyl echt violet stain, ×2000.

The sex chromatin test, developed by Moore and Barr in 1955, is based on the sex difference in the sex chromosome constitution in human cells. *In females* one of the two X chromosomes of the interphase nucleus is compact (**heterochromatic**) rather than elongated (**euchromatic**) like the other 45 chromosomes in the cell. The compact X chromosome appears as a mass of **sex chromatin** at the inner surface of the nuclear membrane in oral epithelial cells of females (Fig. 3-109*B*). *The sex chromatin test is an important laboratory aid in the clinical evaluation of intersexes.* With the exception of **true hermaphrodites** (persons with both ovarian and testicular tissue), the sex chromatin pattern and **karyotype** (characteristics of chromosomes) usually correspond to the **gonadal sex** (sex indicated by the type of sex glands present). The chromosome constitution of the present patient would be 46, XX (*i.e.*, a total of 46 chromosomes with an XX sex chromosome complex that is normal for a female).

Case 3-6. The urine which escaped from the patient's ruptured bladder would pass into the **peritoneal cavity** (Fig. 3-105). Although pelvic fractures are sometimes complicated by **bladder rupture**, the radiographs indicated that the rupture was not likely caused by a sharp bone fragment. Probably the bladder was ruptured by the same compressive blow to the region of the symphysis pubis that fractured the pelvis. A full bladder is especially liable to rupture at its dome or superior surface following a nonpenetrating blow.

The superior surface of the bladder is almost completely covered with peritoneum, but near its posterior border the peritoneum is reflected onto the uterus at the level of the internal ostium, forming the **uterovesical pouch** (Fig. 3-22). In the male the peritoneum is reflected from the surface of the bladder over the superior surfaces of the deferent ducts and seminal vesicles.

In a patient with *intraperitoneal bladder rupture*, signs and symptoms of peritoneal irritation are likely to develop. **Septic peritonitis** (G. *sepsis*, putrifaction) may develop if there are pathogenic organisms in the urine. As the urine accumulates in the peritoneal cavity, dullness will be detected over the **paracolic gutters** during percussion of the abdomen (Fig. 2-110). This dullness will disappear from the left side when the patient is rolled onto the right side and vice versa, indicating free fluid in the peritoneal cavity from a ruptured viscus (the bladder in this case).

Access to the bladder for surgical repair of its ruptured superior wall would most likely be via the **suprapubic route**, through the anterior abdominal wall and the peritoneum. The bladder is separated from the pubic bones by a thin layer of areolar tissue which may contain fat (Fig. 3-22). When the bladder is full, its anteroinferior surface is in contact with the anterior abdominal wall, without the interposition of peritoneum.

Case 3-7. The testis lies on the posterior abdominal wall of the embryo. If it remains

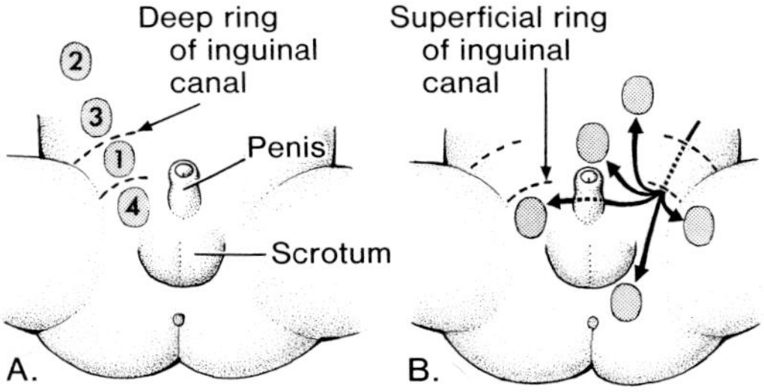

Figure 3-110. Diagrams illustrating cryptorchidism and ectopic testes. *A*, various positions of cryptorchid testes numbered in order of frequency. *B*, various sites of ectopic testes.

in this position, an extremely rare condition, it can be correctly referred to as an **undescended testis**. However in the present case, the testis began its descent but was arrested in the inguinal canal (Fig. 3-110*A*). Thus, it is better not to refer to this condition as undescended testis but as incomplete (imperfect) descent of the testis.

In boys, particularly infants, intermittent contraction of the **cremaster muscle** in response to cold pulls the testis into the inguinal canal. Thus, correct technique during the physical examination must be used to differentiate between a **retracted testis** and an imperfectly descended testis. The examination should be conducted in a warm room with warm hands. A retracted testis descends in response to heat, whereas an imperfectly descended one does not.

In some cases an **ectopic testis** may be located in the superficial fascia above the inguinal ligament, in front of the pubis, in the perineum, or in the thigh (Fig. 3-110*B*). A testis in the inguinal canal increases slightly in size during the 13 to 15 year period (**puberty**) because of the increased production of androgenic hormones at this time. It is generally assumed that a testis that does not enter the scrotum is sterile and that the incidence of malignancy is higher in a **cryptorchid testis** (G. *kryptos*, hidden + *orchis*, testis) than in one that has descended normally.

In females with **testicular feminization**, *a rare condition*, the testes may be located in the inguinal canals and the condition incorrectly diagnosed as **bilateral indirect inguinal hernias**. These females are not intersexes in the usual sense because their breast development and external genitalia are normal for a female. This abnormality results when the external genitalia do not become masculinized during the early fetal period probably because they were *insensitive to androgens*.

During normal development the **processus vaginalis** protrudes through the anterior abdominal wall (Fig. 2-18), forming the inguinal canal through which the testis usually descends before birth. If development of the processus is arrested, the patent processus vaginalis presents a hernial sac into which abdominal contents may herniate (Fig. 2-22). *Often indirect inguinal hernia is associated with incomplete descent of the testis.* The hernia may not be detected until surgical procedures are performed to move the testis into the scrotum.

Case 3-8. When the "bag of waters" break, the amniotic and chorionic sacs rupture (**amniochorionic membrane**), permitting the amniotic fluid to escape (up to 1000 ml in most cases). *The amniotic and chorionic sacs protrude into the cervical canal* during the first stage of labor and help to dilate the cervix (Fig. 3-106*A*). If only a small tear occurs in the amnion, the fluid escapes but the amnion may be pushed out and cover the head of the fetus. In these very rare cases, the fetus is said to be born with a **caul**, which must be removed to allow the infant to breathe. Many sailors consider this phenomenon good luck and assume when it occurs that they are unlikely to die from drowning.

The pudendal nerve, arising from the sacral plexus (S2, S3, and S4), is the *main nerve of the perineum*, which includes the **pudendum** (vulva). It is both motor and sensory to this region and also carries some of the postganglionic sympathetic fibers to the perineum. *In the female* the pudendal nerve divides into the perineal nerve and the dorsal nerve of the clitoris. The **perineal nerve** gives off two *posterior labial nerves* (Fig. 3-43) and divides into small terminal muscular branches which enter the superficial and deep perineal spaces to supply the muscles in them and the *bulb of the vestibule* (Fig. 3-42). The **dorsal nerve of the clitoris** supplies the prepuce and glans of the clitoris and the associated skin.

When the pudendal nerve is blocked via the perineal route, *the chief bony landmark is the ischial tuberosity* (Figs. 3-18, 3-43, and 3-46*B*). With the patient in the lithotomy position (Figs. 3-1 and 3-111), the **ischial tuberosity** is palpated and a **skin wheal** (lesion produced by an intradermal injection) is raised just medial to the tuberosity (Fig. 3-111), where the *pudendal nerve* emerges from the *pudendal canal* to distribute itself over the perineum (Fig. 3-43). The needle is inserted superomedially for about 2.5 cm before the injection is made. In some cases the needle is guided

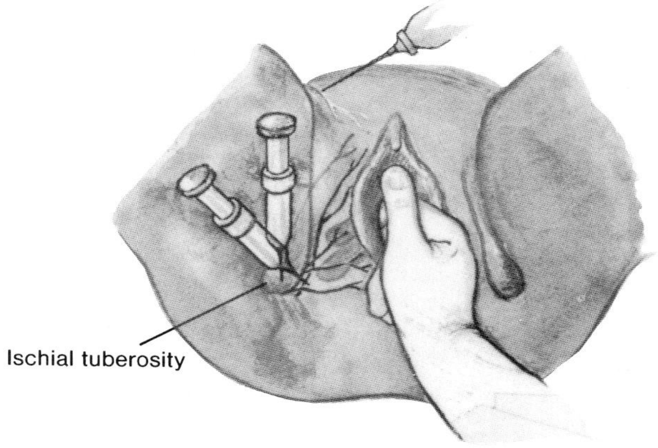

Figure 3-111. Drawing illustrating how a pudendal nerve block may be performed (refer to Fig. 3-39 for further orientation). In the perineal route the chief bony landmark is the ischial tuberosity. The needle is inserted toward and just medial to the tuberosity, where the pudendal nerve emerges from the pudendal canal (Fig. 3-43.) Some obstetricians guide the needle by the fingers placed in the vagina until its tip is posterior and inferior to the ischial spine where the pudendal nerve lies (Fig. 3-63). The injection at the top of the drawing blocks or anesthetizes the ilioinguinal nerve and the branches of the genitofemoral nerve supplying the vulva (Fig. 4-14).

by the fingers inserted in the vagina until it is about 1 cm posterior and inferior to the **ischial spine** where the pudendal nerve is located.

When complete perineal anesthesia is required the *genital branches of the genitofemoral nerve*, the *ilioinguinal nerve* (Figs. 3-110 and 4-14), and the *perineal branch of the posterior cutaneous nerve of the thigh* (Fig. 3-43) must also be anesthetized by making an injection along the outer margin of the labia majora. Pudendal nerve block and anesthetization of the above nerves is also performed when doing surgical operations on the urogenital and anal regions.

SUGGESTIONS FOR ADDITIONAL READING

1. Dilts, P. V., Jr., Greene, J. W., Jr., and Roddick, J. W., Jr. *Core Studies in Obstetrics and Gynecology*, Ed. 2, The Williams & Wilkins Company, Baltimore, 1978.

This relatively small book (262 pp.) presents the basic information all physicians should know about obstetrics and gynecology. It serves as an introduction to these specialities and clearly describes important basic material.

2. Doolas, A., Caldwell, R. G., Roseman, D. L., and de Peyster, F. A. Colon, appendix, rectum, and anus. In *Basic Surgery*, edited by J. A. McCredie, Macmillan Publishing Co., Inc., New York, 1977.

The important surgical diseases of the various organs are described. Principles of therapy rather than details of surgical technique are emphasized. First a summary of the essential anatomy is given and then the inflammatory diseases and neoplasms (malignant growths) are discussed. Physical examination of the rectum and anal canal is described and clearly illustrated.

3. Healey, J. E., Jr. *A Synopsis of Clinical Anatomy*. W. B. Saunders Co., Philadelphia, 1969.

This beautifully illustrated text makes it obvious why knowledge of the regional anatomy of the pelvic walls and pelvic viscera is of utmost importance to the physician in the diagnosis and treatment of intrapelvic and intra-abdominal pathology. You will find well illustrated accounts of digital rectal examinations, vaginal examinations, pelvic fractures, hemorrhoids, ischiorectal abscesses, developmental defects of the rectum and anal canal, and operations on the prostate.

4. Lowenfels, A. B. *Companion Guide to Surgical Diagnosis*. The Williams & Wilkins Company, Baltimore, 1975.

It is usually more difficult to make a differential diagnosis of abdominopelvic pain in women than in men because there are more genital organs in the female pelvis. Gynecological diseases such as acute salpingitis (inflammation of the uterine tube), hemorrhage into or torsion of an ovarian cyst, and ectopic pregnancy on the right side may produce symptoms similar to appendicitis. In addition certain diseases may mimic pregnancy and pregnancy does not protect a woman against the common surgical disorders. Enlargement of the uterus during pregnancy displaces the cecum and appendix into the upper part of the abdomen. If these patient oriented problems interest you, refer to this relatively small text (276 pp.). The approach is simple and informal.

5. Moore, K. L. *The Developing Human, Clinically Oriented Anatomy*, Ed. 2, W. B. Saunders Co., Philadelphia, 1977.

   Malformations of the genital organs are relatively common and frequently occur in association with abnormalities of the urinary system. To understand these conditions, including intersexuality, a good understanding of normal sex development is needed. If you are not clear about the role of the testes in sexual differentiation and hypospadias, or if you are unsure why congenital adrenal hyperplasia may cause masculization of a female fetus, you are urged to do additional reading.

CHAPTER 4

The Lower Limb

The lower limb (extremity or "leg" in lay language) is *the organ of locomotion* and is specialized for bearing the weight of the body and for maintaining equilibrium. For purposes of description, the lower limb is divided into the **hip** and **thigh,** the **knee** (genu), the **leg** (crus), the **ankle** (talus), and the **foot** (pes). The Latin word *pes* for the foot is the basis of the medical words *peduncle* and *pedicle* (Fig. 5-4). *Podos* (G. foot) appears in the term **podiatrist**, a specialist who, like an orthopaedic surgeon, treats foot disorders.

As the lower limb is involved in weight bearing, **some movement has been sacrificed to acquire stability** (*e.g.,* compare the mobility of your toes and your fingers). Although people use the term leg to refer to their lower limb, understand that the leg is only the distal part of the lower limb between the knee and the ankle.

Because *injuries and degenerative disorders* of the lower limbs are so common, it is essential for you to be familiar with the normal and abnormal functioning of these organs. To understand why a patient cannot walk or has an **abnormal gait,** you must know what structures are involved in normal walking.

The parts of the lower limb are comparable to those of the upper one (*e.g.,* the knee and the elbow). This is understandable when you know that they rotated through 90° in opposite directions during embryonic development. The upper limbs rotate laterally through 90° on their longitudinal axes bringing the thumb to the lateral side, whereas the lower limbs rotate medially through almost 90° bringing the great toe to the medial side. Hence the knee faces anteriorly when one stands in the anatomical position and the extensor muscles lie on the anterior aspect of the lower limb. Therefore, *extension occurs in opposite directions in the upper and lower limbs* (see Fig. I-10*B* and *C*).

As it is concerned with movement of the whole body and bearing its weight, the lower limb is stronger and heavier than the upper limb (*e.g.,* compare the size of the thigh and the arm and the weight of the femur and the humerus).

THE SKELETON OF THE LOWER LIMB

The bones of the lower limb form the inferior part of the **appendicular skeleton** (Figs. 4-1 and 4-2). The lower limb is connected to the vertebral column by the **pelvic girdle,** which is formed by the two **ossa coxae** (hip or innominate bones). The coxal bones articulate posteriorly with the **sacrum** (Fig. 5-25) and meet inferiorly and anteriorly at the **symphysis pubis** (Figs. 4-1 and 4-5). The ossa coxae, the sacrum, and the **coccyx** form the skeleton of the **bony pelvis** (Fig. 4-3), which surrounds the inferior part of the abdominal cavity. The anatomical term *pelvis* is a Latin word meaning basin; however, the pelvis in the anatomical position is tilted so that the anterior superior iliac spines and the symphysis pubis are in the same coronal plane (Fig. 3-48*B*). Verify this on a skeleton that is hanging in the anatomical position and observe that the opening into the pelvis (**pelvic inlet**) faces anterosuperiorly and not inferiorly as it does when you hold it as you would a washbowl or basin.

On the lateral aspect of the os coxae is the socket of the **hip joint,** where the head of the **femur** (thigh bone) articulates with the cup-shaped **acetabulum** (L. vinegar cup) of the os coxae (Figs. 4-3 and 4-8). The

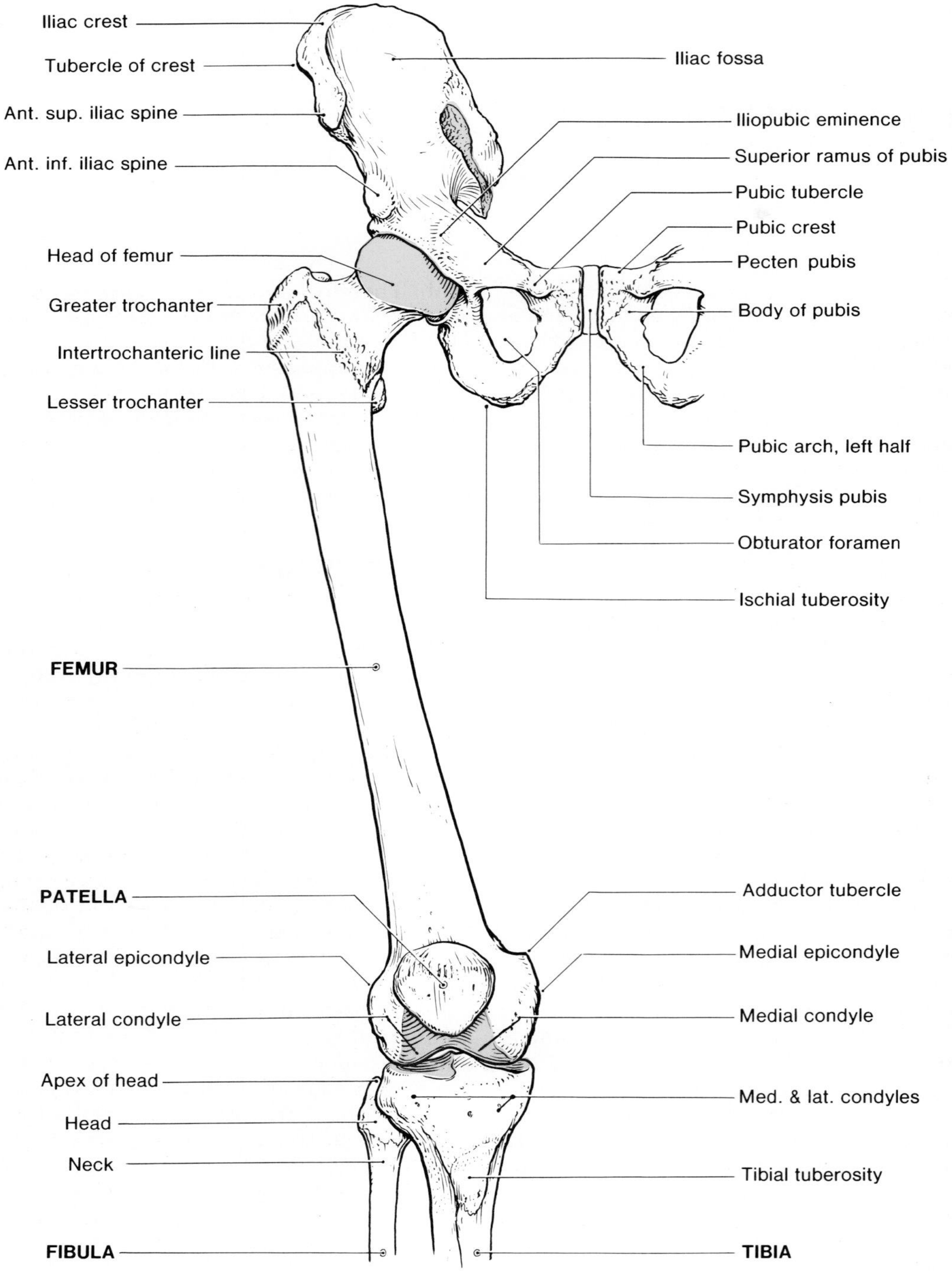

Figure 4-1. Drawing of an anterior view of the bones of the lower limb. The distal parts of the leg bones are not illustrated. The skeleton of the limb is connected to the vertebral column by the pelvic girdle which is formed by the os coxae (hip bone). Note that the ossa coxae meet at the symphysis pubis. For the surface anatomy of these bones, see Figures 4-5, 4-7, 4-25, and 4.27.

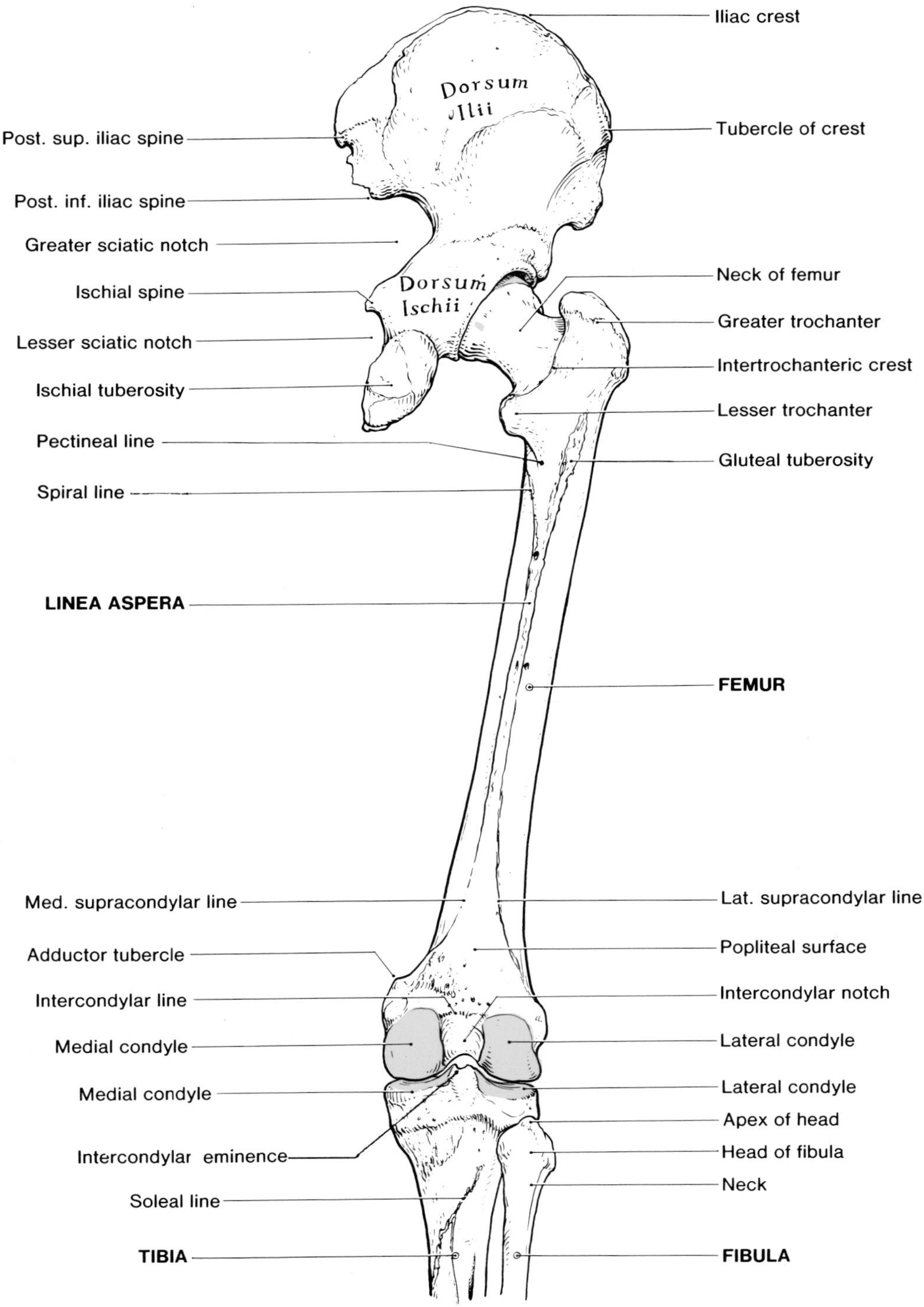

Figure 4-2. Drawing of a posterior view of the bones of the lower limb. The distal parts of tibia and fibula are not shown. With the sacrum and coccyx (not shown), the two ossa coxae form the skeleton of the bony pelvis (Fig. 4-3), which surrounds the lowest part of the abdominal cavity. The articular cartilages of the condyles of the femur and the tibia are colored *yellow*.

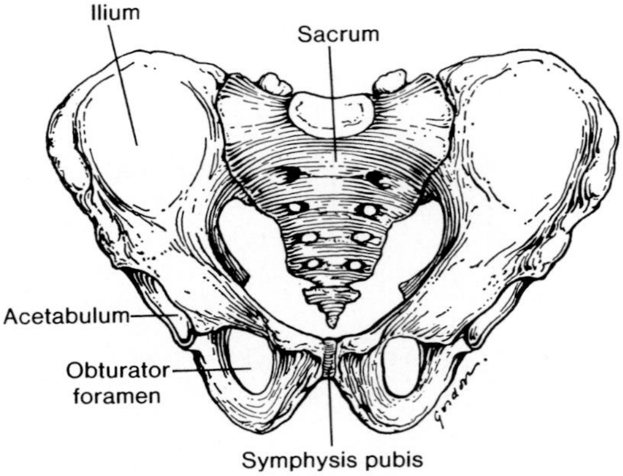

Figure 4-3. Drawing of an anterior view of the male pelvis. Note that the pelvis (L. basin) is inclined forward when it is in the anatomical position and that the ossa coxae articulate anteriorly with each other at the symphysis pubis and posteriorly with the sacrum.

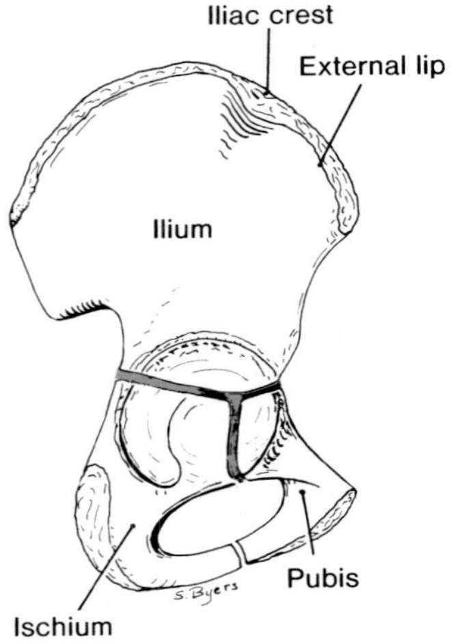

Figure 4-4. Drawing of an os coxae from a child. Observe that it is composed of three bones (ilium, ischium, and pubis) which meet at the cup-shaped acetabulum, the socket for the head of the femur (Fig. 4-1). Note that the bones have not fused at this stage and are united by cartilage (*blue*) along a Y-shaped line in the acetabulum. Fusion of these bones to form the os coxae occurs around the 16th year. The lines of fusion may be visible in the adult bone.

skeleton of the free limb consists of the **femur** in the thigh, the **tibia** and **fibula** in the **leg**, and the **tarsal bones**, **metatarsal bones**, and **phalanges** in the foot (Figs. 4-1, 4-68, and 4-72).

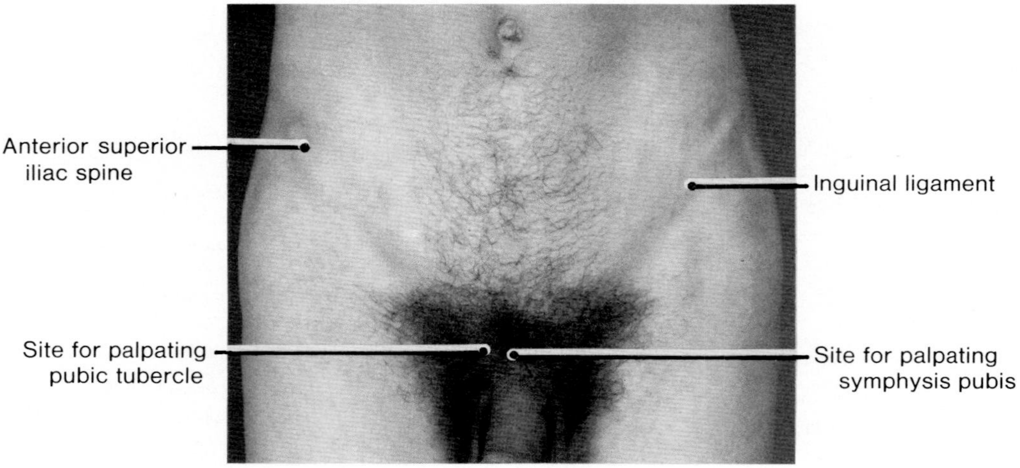

Figure 4-5. Photograph of the pelvic region of a 27-year-old man showing the principal surface landmarks. Observe the anterior end of the iliac crest, called the anterior superior iliac spine, at the lateral end of the groove of the groin. This important bony landmark indicates where the inguinal ligament attaches; its other end is attached to the pubic tubercle (Fig. 4-1). The entire symphysis pubis is readily felt in the midline at the inferior extremity of the anterior abdominal wall. The pubic tubercle can be palpated as a small protuberance on the superior border of the body of the pubis about 2.5 cm lateral to the symphysis pubis.

THE HIP AND THIGH

The region of the hip and thigh includes the whole *area from the iliac crest to the knee* (Fig. 4-1). The hip is the region between the iliac crest and the greater trochanter of the femur (Figs. 4-2 and 4-10), and the thigh is the part between the hip and the knee.

BONES AND SURFACE ANATOMY

The Os Coxae (Figs. 4-1 to 4-4). The coxal bone (L. *os*) is commonly called the **hip bone**. Large and irregularly shaped, it consists of three bones during childhood: the **ilium** (os ilium), the **ischium** (os ischium), and the **pubis** (os pubis). These bones fuse at 15 to 17 years and are indistinguishably joined in the adult.

The Ilium (Figs. 4-1 to 4-4 and 4-8). This bone forms the superior two-thirds of the os coxae and the superior two-fifths of the **acetabulum.** The ilium is the bone you can feel in your flank (latus), the fleshy part between your ribs and hip. When you put your hand on your hip, it rests on the superior margin (crest) of the ilium (Figs. 4-7, 4-8, and 4-10).

The ilium is roughly fan-shaped with the "handle of the fan" in the acetabulum. The margin of the ilium has internal and external lips and a curved superior margin or **iliac crest** between them. This crest is easily palpated as it extends through the inferior margin of the flank or side of the body (Fig. 4-7). Its highest point, as palpated from behind, is at the level of the spinous process of the fourth lumbar vertebra, an important landmark for the procedure of **lumbar puncture** (Fig. 5-69), used to obtain cerebrospinal fluid (CSF).

The iliac crest ends anteriorly in a rounded *anterior superior iliac spine* which is easily felt and may be visible (Figs. 4-1, 4-5, 4-7, and 4-8).

The iliac crest ends posteriorly in a sharp **posterior superior iliac spine** (Fig. 4-2). It is a little difficult to identify by palpation in most people, but its position can always be determined because it lies at the bottom of a dimple (skin depression) about 4 cm lateral to the median plane (Fig. 4-6). These dimples form because the skin and underlying fascia are attached to the bone in this area (Fig. 5-11).

Another palpable bony landmark, the **tubercle of the crest** (Figs. 4-1 and 4-2), is located about 6 cm superior and posterior

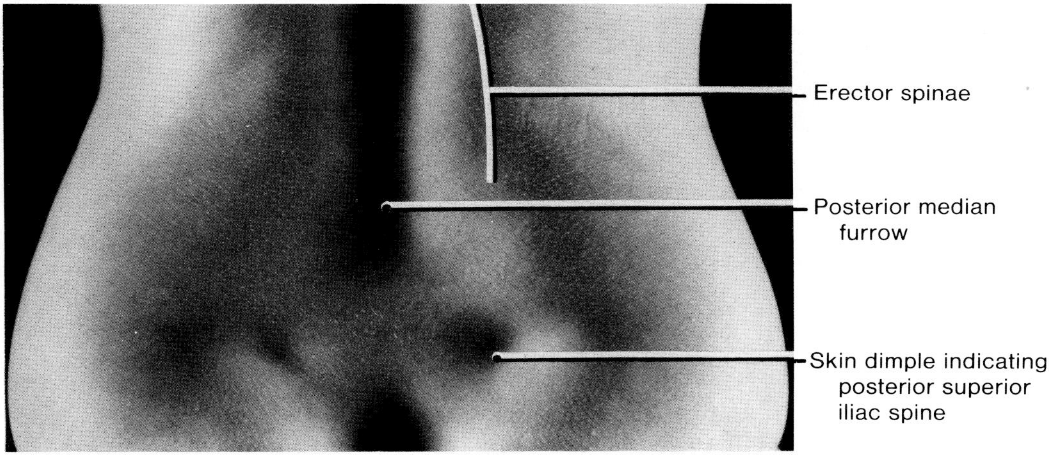

Figure 4-6. Photograph of the lower back region of a 21-year-old woman showing the principal surface features. The posterior superior iliac spines lie in the floor of the skin dimples, which are located about 4 cm from the posteromedian line (center of posterior median furrow). These dimples indicate where the deep fascia is attached to the posterior superior iliac spines. The line joining these dimples is at the level of the spinous process of the second sacral vertebra.

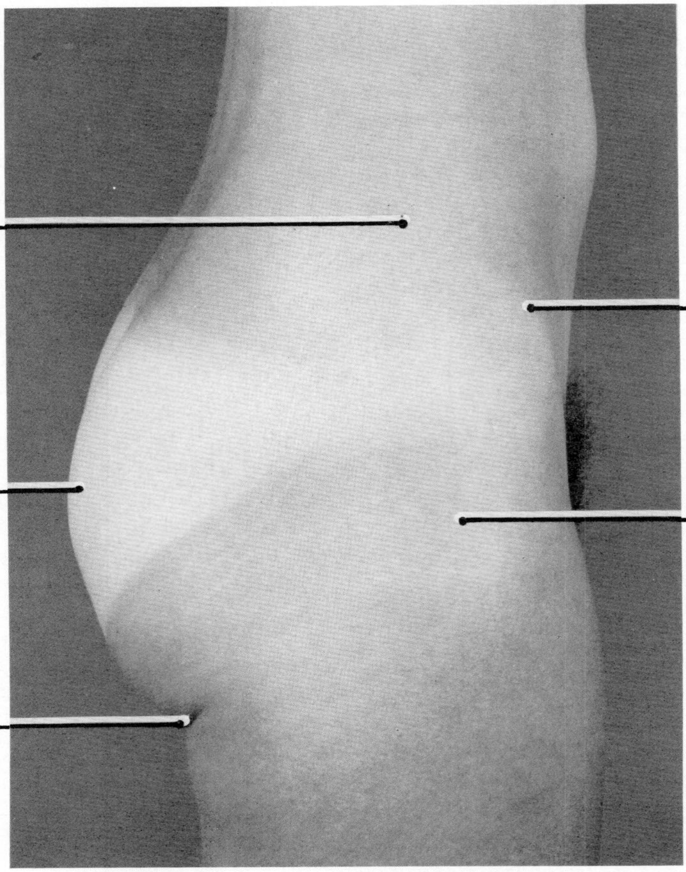

Figure 4-7. Photograph of a lateral view of the gluteal region of a 27-year-old woman showing the principal surface features. The iliac crest can be easily palpated by tracing posterosuperiorly from the anterior superior iliac spine. Note the prominence (buttock) formed mainly by the gluteus maximus muscle. When a person is standing, the gluteus maximus covers the ischial tuberosity (Fig. 4-45), but it can be felt by deep palpation through this large muscle just above the medial portion of the gluteal fold. This prominent fold coincides with the inferior border of the gluteus maximus. The groove or crease inferior to the gluteal fold is called the gluteal sulcus.

to the anterior superior iliac spine. The **anterior inferior iliac spines** (Fig. 4-1) and the **posterior inferior iliac spines** (Fig. 4-2) lie inferior to their respective superior spines.

The posterior part of the inner surface of the ilium articulates with the side of the sacrum at the **sacroiliac joint** (Fig. 5-2). Just inferior to this joint is the large **greater sciatic notch** (Fig. 4-2) through which pass the sciatic nerve and other structures (Fig. 4-44).

The Ischium (Figs. 4-1, 4-2, and 4-4). This bone forms the posteroinferior third of the os coxae and the posterior two-fifths of the acetabulum. The ischium (G. hip) is the roughly L-shaped part of the os coxae which passes inferiorly from the acetabulum and then turns anteriorly to join the pubis. It has three parts: a **body** adjoining the ilium, an **ischial tuberosity** projecting downward from the body (Fig. 4-2), and an **ischial ramus** passing upward from the tuberosity to join the corresponding part of the pubis.

The **ischial tuberosity** is covered by the gluteus maximus muscle when the hip is extended (Figs. 4-10 and 4-45), but it is uncovered when the hip is flexed. It bears the weight of the body when one sits up straight (Fig. 5-3) and can be felt upon deep palpation through the distal part of the gluteus maximus just above the medial portion of the **gluteal fold,** a prominent fold delimiting the buttock inferiorly (Figs. 4-7 and 4-10). Inferior to the gluteal fold is the **gluteal sulcus,** a groove or crease which separates the buttock from the posterior aspect of the thigh when the hip joint is extended. You can palpate the inferior surface and medial border of the ischial tuberosity during hip flexion; this is most easily done when you sit on your fingertips.

The triangular **ischial spine** separates the **greater sciatic notch** superiorly from the **lesser sciatic notch** inferiorly (Figs. 4-2 and 4-8). The lesser notch is located between the ischial spine and the ischial tuberosity.

The Pubis (Figs. 4-1, 4-4, and 4-8). This bone forms the anterior part of the os coxae and the anteromedial one-fifth of the acetabulum. It consists of three parts: a flattened **body** lying medially; a **superior ramus** passing superolaterally; and an **inferior ramus** passing posteriorly, inferiorly, and laterally to join the ramus of the ischium and form half of the pubic arch. The body of the pubis joins the body of the opposite pubis in the median plane at a cartilaginous joint called the **symphysis pubis** (Figs. 4-1, 4-3, and 4-5).

The anterior border of the body of the pubis is thickened to form a **pubic crest** (Fig. 4-1). At its lateral end there is a projection, known as the **pubic tubercle,** which provides the main pubic attachment for the **inguinal ligament** (Fig. 3-46). It can be palpated about 2.5 cm from the median plane (Fig. 4-5). This tubercle is a very important bony landmark in cases of **inguinal hernia** (Case 4-8).

Orientation of the Os Coxae (Fig. 4-8). To place the os coxae (hip bone) in the

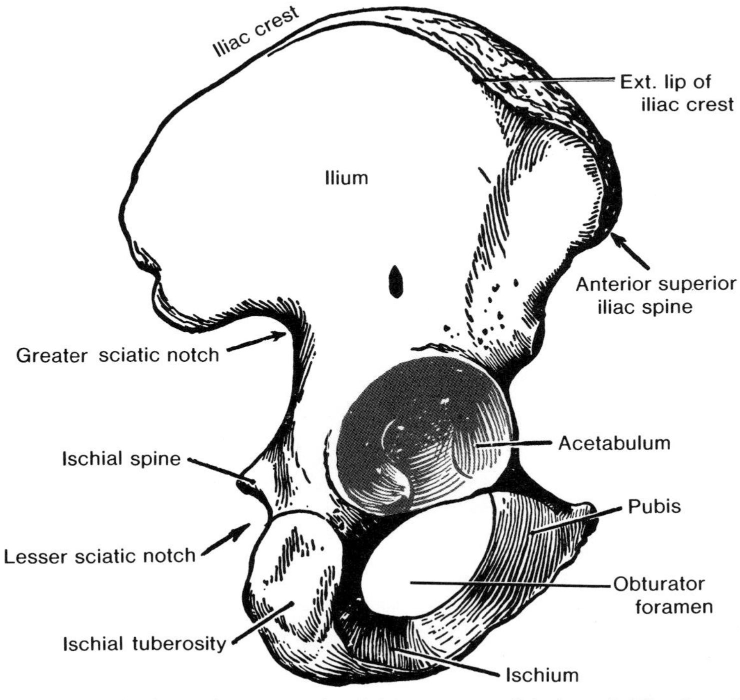

Figure 4-8. Drawing of the lateral aspect of a right os coxae (hip bone). The fan-shaped part of the ilium is sometimes called the wing of the ilium. Note that the acetabulum, the socket for the head of the femur, faces laterally, downward, and slightly forward. Most of the borders and surfaces of the hip bone are named according to this anatomical position.

anatomical position, move it until the anterior superior iliac spine and the symphysis pubis are in the same coronal plane. In this position the inner aspect of the body of the pubis faces almost directly upward. Verify this on a skeleton and on yourself. While standing erect, palpate one of your anterior superior iliac spines as you feel your symphysis pubis (also see Fig. 3-48*B*).

The Obturator Foramen (Figs. 4-1, 4-3, 4-4, and 4-8). This large oval aperture is surrounded by the bodies and the rami of the pubis and ischium. It lies inferior to the acetabulum and is nearly closed in the living body by the fibrous **obturator membrane** (Fig. 4-110).

The Acetabulum (Figs. 4-3, 4-4, and 4-8). This cup-shaped cavity in the os coxae articulates with the head of the femur. Until puberty the ilium, the ischium, and the pubis are united by a Y-shaped hyaline cartilage in the acetabulum (Fig. 4-4). At 15 to 17 years the three bones fuse to form a single bone, the os coxae, and the cartilage is replaced by bone.

The Femur (Figs. 4-1, 4-2, 4-9, and 4-10). The femur (thigh bone) is the longest, strongest, and heaviest bone in the body. *A person's height is roughly four times the length of the femur.* It extends from the hip joint, where its rounded head articulates with the acetabulum, to the knee joint,

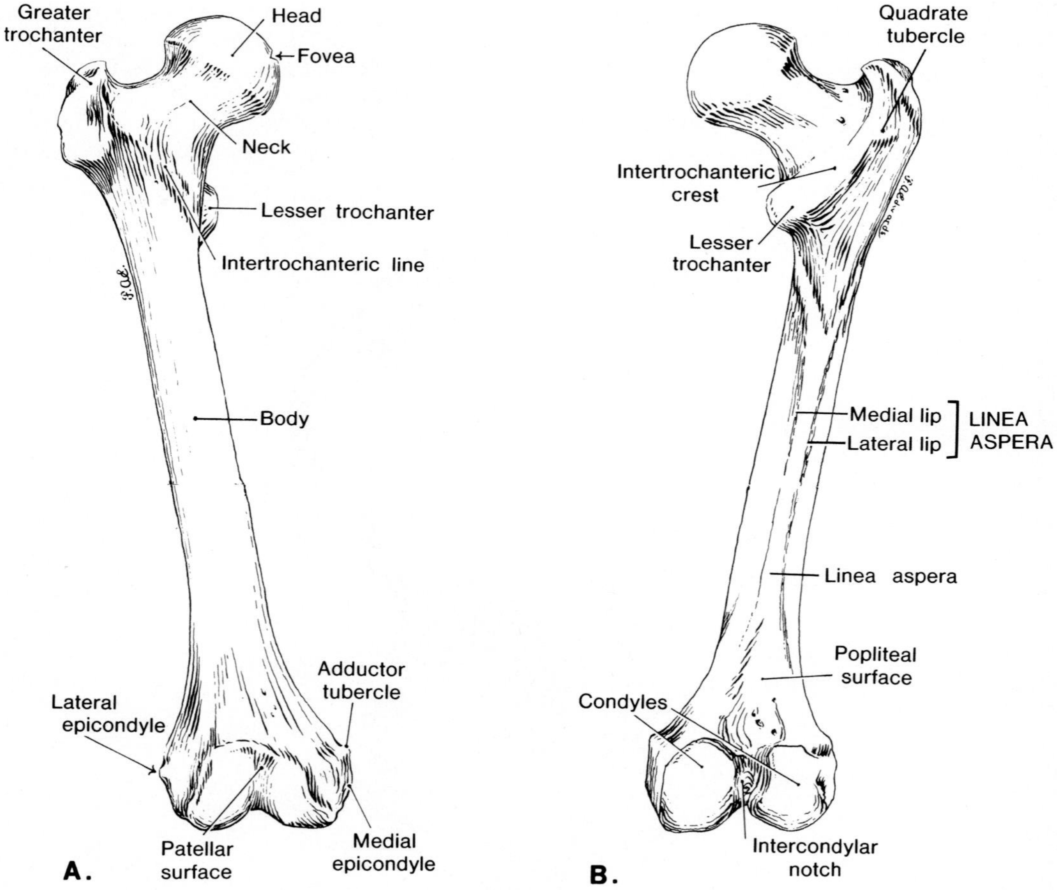

Figure 4-9. Drawings of the right femur in the anatomical position. *A*, anterior aspect. *B*, posterior aspect. The quadratus femoris muscle is attached to the quadrate tubercle and the bone below it. The linea aspera is a broad, rough ridge that usually forms a crest-like projection with distinct medial and lateral lips.

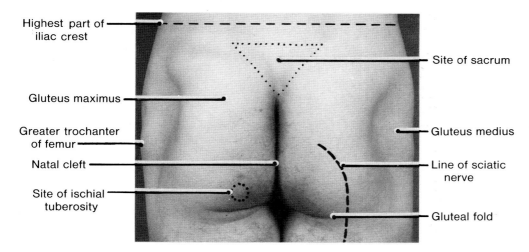

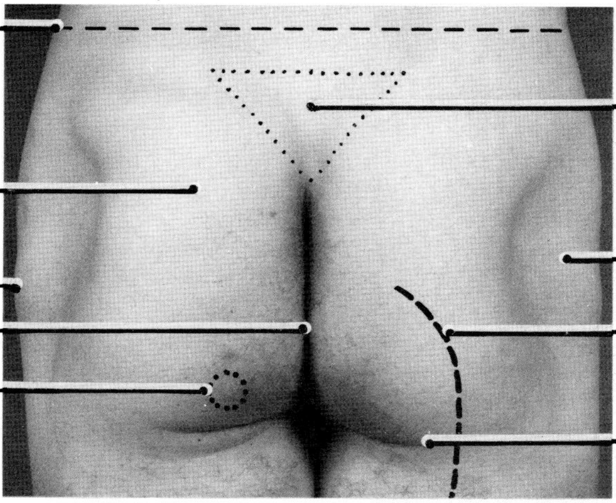

Figure 4-10. Photograph of the gluteal region of a 27-year-old man showing the principal surface landmarks. To produce these features the subject was asked to stand in the anatomical position and to press his heels together (*i.e.*, he was doing an isometric contraction of his lateral femoral rotators). Observe that the greater trochanter is the most lateral point of the hip region. The term buttock (L. *natis*) refers to the prominence produced by the underlying gluteal muscles. A line (– – –) joining the highest part of the iliac crests usually crosses the space between the spinous processes of the third and fourth lumbar vertebrae. Consequently, it serves as a useful guide for determining the site for inserting a lumbar puncture needle to obtain a sample of cerebrospinal fluid (Fig. 5-69). Observe the prominent gluteal fold that delimits the buttock inferiorly. The groove or crease inferior to the gluteal fold is called the gluteal sulcus; it separates the buttock from the posterior aspect of the thigh. To visualize its relationship to the gluteus maximus muscle, see Figure 4-45.

where its condyles articulate with the tibia. The femur consists of a **body** (shaft) and two **ends** (extremities), proximal and distal. The proximal end of the femur consists of a head, a neck, and greater and lesser trochanters.

The head of the femur forms about two-thirds of a sphere and is directed medially, upward, and slightly forward to fit deeply into the acetabulum of the os coxae. A little below and behind its center is a pit or **fovea** where the ligament of the head is attached (Figs. 4-113 and 4-114). The head of the femur can sometimes be palpated, particularly in thin males, when the thigh is rotated laterally.

The neck of the femur, about 5 cm long, connects the head to the shaft. It is an obliquely placed, thick bar of bone which is limited laterally by the **greater trochanter** and is narrowest in diameter at its middle. The neck, which is not palpable, is frequently fractured in older persons (Case 4-1 and Fig. 4-157).

A broad, rough **intertrochanteric line** runs obliquely downward between the two trochanters anteriorly (Fig. 4-9*A*). It is produced by the attachment of the strong, massive **iliofemoral ligament** (Fig. 4-116). A corresponding prominent rounded ridge, the **intertrochanteric crest** unites the two trochanters posteriorly (Fig. 4-9*B*).

The laterally placed **greater trochanter** is a large, somewhat rectangular projection from the junction of the neck with the shaft. It provides an insertion for several muscles of the gluteal region (Fig. 4-22). *The greater trochanter lies close to the skin* and can be easily palpated on the lateral side of the thigh about 10 cm (a handbreadth) inferior to the tubercle of the iliac crest (Figs. 4-1 and 4-10). To palpate your greater trochanter, abduct your right limb while supporting the weight of your body on your left foot. Palpate your right greater trochanter by pressing downward and medially 7 to 8 cm inferior to your iliac crest. If you lie on your back and abduct both limbs, you can feel both greater trochanters because the muscles are relaxed.

Because it is the most lateral point of the hip region, the greater trochanter makes you uncomfortable when you lie on your side on a hard surface. In the erect position, *a line joining the tips of the greater trochanters normally passes through the center of the heads of the femora and the pubic tubercles.* Verify this using Figures 4-1 and 4-9. The degree of prominence of the greater trochanter is increased if the gluteal muscles atrophy or waste away (*e.g.,* owing to injury to the gluteal nerves). It is, of course, displaced in dislocations of the hip (Case 4-6 and Figs. 4-118 and 4-154).

The rounded, conical **lesser trochanter** projects from the posteromedial surface of the femur at the inferior end of the intertrochanteric crest (Fig. 4-9). It is located in the angle between the neck and the shaft.

The body of the femur or shaft is slightly bowed anteriorly and is narrowest at the midshaft. Its middle two-quarters are approximately circular in cross-section. Below the neck the body is smooth and featureless except for a broad ridge of bone, the **linea aspera** (L. rough line), running down the middle of its posterior surface (Figs. 4-2 and 4-9*B*). This broad, rough line or ridge bifurcates proximally and distally into diverging lines that bound triangular areas. Many muscles and three intermuscular septa are attached to the linea aspera (Fig. 4-22).

The **pectineal line** of the femur runs from the lesser trochanter to the medial lip of the linea aspera (Fig. 4-2). The tendon of the pectineus muscle inserts into it (Fig. 4-22). The body of the femur is not usually palpable because it is so well covered with large muscles.

The distal end of the femur (Fig. 4-9) is divided into two large articular **condyles** (G. knuckles) which project posteriorly and are separated by a deep U-shaped **intercondylar notch.** The medial and lateral condyles blend with each other anteriorly and with the shaft superiorly. Although the two articular surfaces are confluent anteriorly (Figs. 4-1 and 4-9*A*), each one is separated from the **patellar surface** by a slight groove. This surface is where the patella (kneecap) slides during flexion and extension of the knee joint. The lateral and medial margins of the patellar surface can be palpated when the knee is flexed.

The **adductor tubercle,** a small prominence of bone (Fig. 4-9*A*), may be felt at the uppermost part of the medial femoral condyle. It should be palpated from above downward; stand beside a skeleton and observe its adductor tubercle as you feel yours.

The medial and lateral **condyles** of the femur are subcutaneous and easily palpable. Palpate them as you flex and extend your knee joint. At the center or "hub" of the nonopposed surface of each condyle is a prominent **epicondyle,** to which the tibial and fibular ligaments of the knee are attached (Fig. 4-125). The medial and lateral epicondyles are easily palpable.

CLINICALLY ORIENTED COMMENTS

The femur is large and strong, particularly its body, but a **violent direct injury** may fracture the femur and it may take up to 20 weeks for union of the fragments to occur.

Fractures of the neck of the femur or between the greater and lesser trochanters (**intertrochanteric fractures**), or through the trochanters (**pertrochanteric fractures**) are common in persons over 60 years of age. They are more common in older women than in men because their bones become markedly weakened owing to senile and **postmenopausal osteoporosis.** In this condition, resorption of bone is greater than bone formation. Generally when one hears that someone has "broken her hip," the usual injury involved is a **fracture of the femoral neck** (Case 4-1).

FASCIA OF THE THIGH

The Superficial Fascia. This comprises the subcutaneous connective tissue of the thigh, including that over certain bones and prominences (*e.g.,* the patella). The superficial fascia (tela subcutanea) of the thigh, as elsewhere, consists of loose areolar tissue containing a considerable amount of fat. Over the **ischial tuberosities** (Figs. 4-2 and 4-10) the fat is within much fibrous tissue. In the gluteal region the fat is deposited in a thick layer and is enormous in some people (*e.g.,* the bushmen of South Africa). This fat contributes to the contour of the buttocks (L. *nates*) and to the formation of the **gluteal folds** (Figs. 4-7 and 4-10).

In certain regions the superficial fascia splits into two layers, between which run the superficial vessels and nerves. The two layers are thick in the inguinal region where the superficial layer is continuous with the superficial fascia of the abdomen. In between these layers of fascia are the superficial **inguinal lymph nodes** (Fig. 4-38) and the great and small saphenous veins.

The superficial veins of the lower limb terminate in two trunks, the **saphenous veins** (Figs. 4-11 to 4-13), which drain most of the blood from the superficial fascia. There is only one saphenous vein in the thigh because the small saphenous vein passes from the foot to the back of the knee, where it ends in the **popliteal vein** (Fig. 4-12*A*).

The Great Saphenous Vein (Figs. 4-11 to

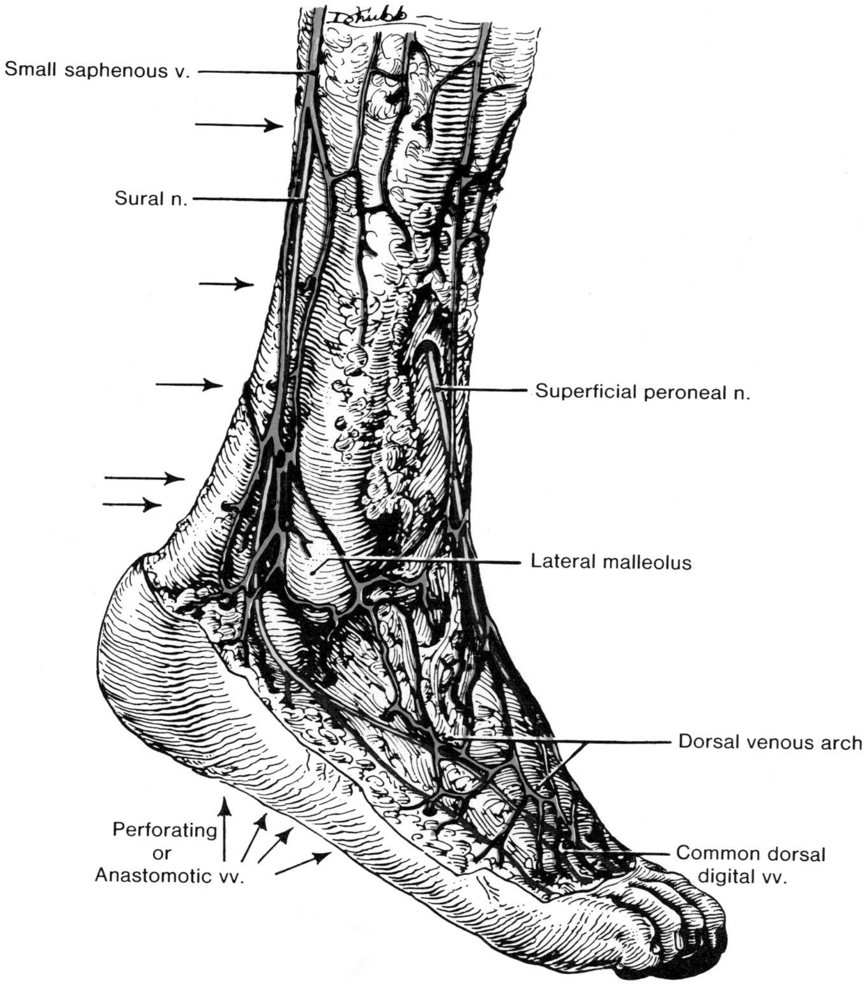

Figure 4-11. Drawing of an anterolateral view of the superficial veins of the ankle and the dorsum of the foot.

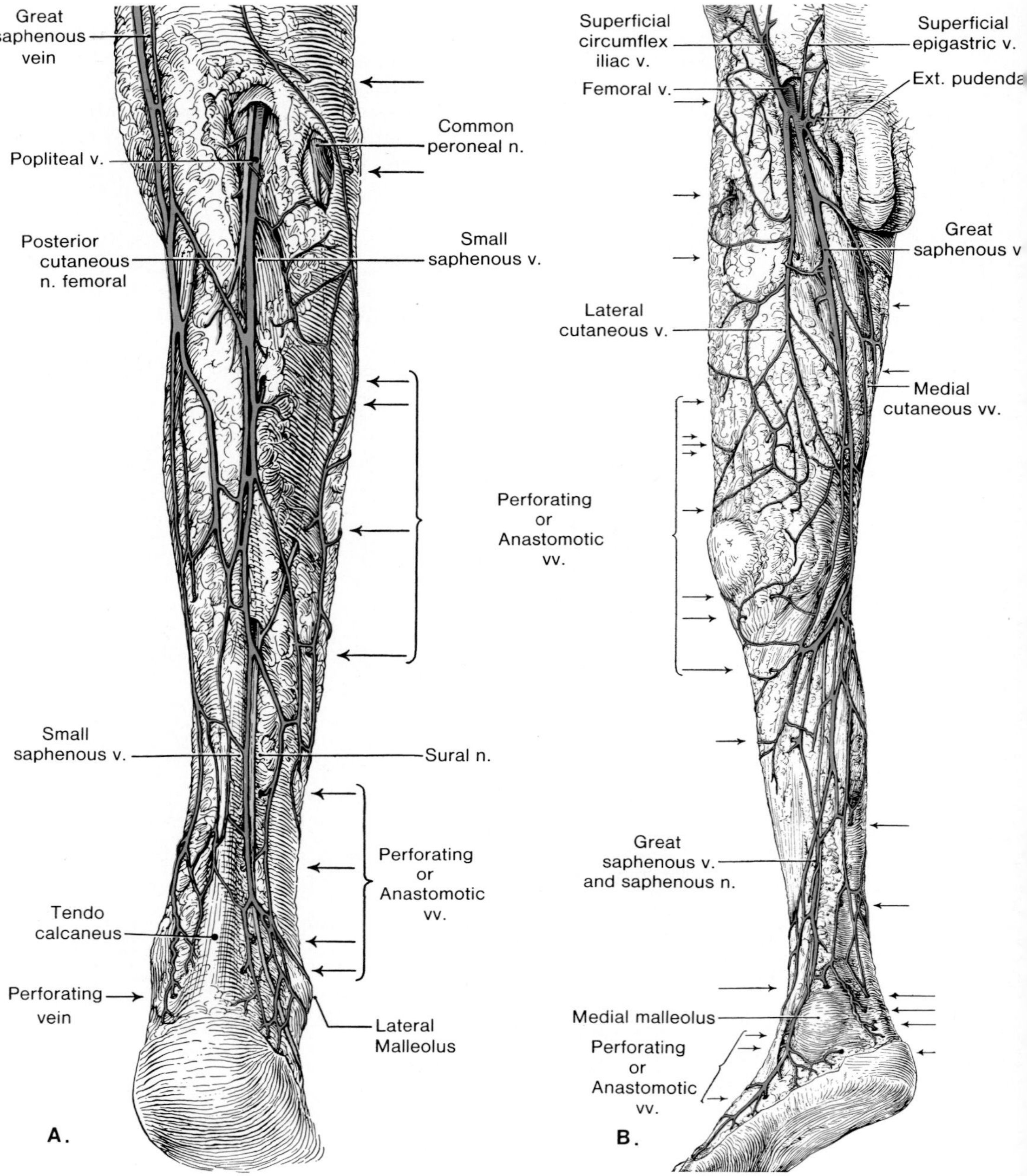

Figure 4-12. Drawings of the superficial veins of the lower limb; some of the nerves are also shown. *A*, posterior view. *B*, anteromedial view. Note the clinically important relationship of the great saphenous vein to the medial malleolus. The *arrows* indicate where anastomotic or perforating veins pierce the deep fascia and bring the superficial and deep veins into communication with each other. Note that the short saphenous vein accompanies the sural nerve and ends at the back of the knee. Often the saphenous veins become dilated and tortuous and their 8 to 20 bicuspid valves become incompetent (*i.e.*, their cusps do not meet and close the vein). The veins become dilated and tortuous and are then referred to as varicose veins.

4-16). This large vein is also called the long, large, or greater saphenous vein. It ascends from the foot to the groin in the subcutaneous fat, beginning at the medial end of the **dorsal venous arch** and passing anterior to the **medial malleolus** of the tibia (Fig. 4-12*B*). It then ascends obliquely across the lower third of the tibia to the knee. Here it lies superficial to the medial epicondyle about 10 cm posterior to the medial border of the patella (Fig. 4-13). From here it runs superolaterally to reach the anterior midline of the thigh and the **saphenous opening** (fossa ovalis) in the deep fascia (Figs. 4-13 and 4-16).

The great saphenous vein perforates the **cribriform fascia** and the **femoral sheath** (Fig. 4-19), two parts of the deep fascia, to end in the **femoral vein** (Fig. 4-13).The cribriform (L. *cribrum,* a sieve) fascia is a thin portion of the deep fascia that covers the saphenous opening (Fig. 4-16). It is perforated by the great saphenous vein, one or more superficial arteries, and some lymph vessels.

In Figure 4-12 observe that the great

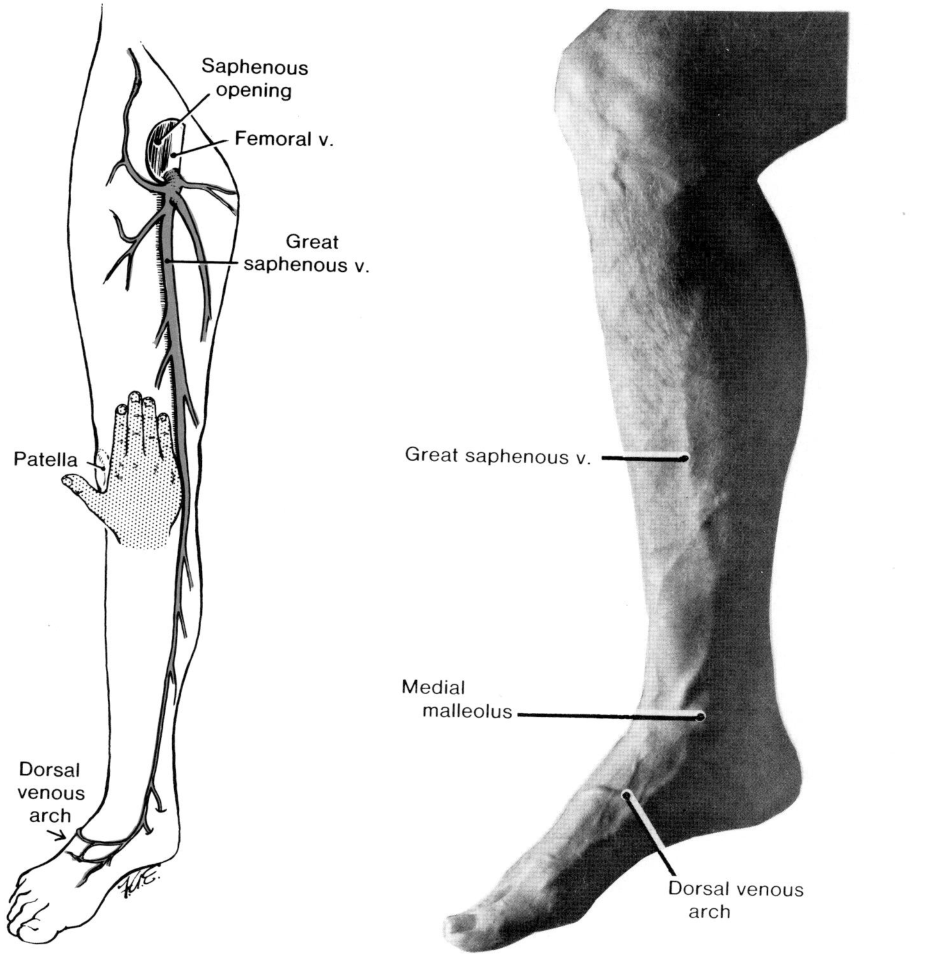

Figure 4-13. *A*, drawing of the right lower limb showing how to locate the site of the great saphenous vein at the knee. Observe that it is located about 10 cm (*i.e.*, a handbreadth) posterior to the medial border of the patella or kneecap. *B*, photograph of the right leg of a 75-year-old man. Note that the great saphenous vein begins at the medial end of the dorsal venous arch of the foot and passes anterior to the medial malleolus.

saphenous vein anastomoses freely with the small saphenous vein. Note also the clinically important **perforating veins** which connect the superficial veins with the deep veins (Figs. 4-12 and 4-35). The main perforating veins (often referred to as "perforators") from the great saphenous vein are arranged in three sets: one related to the adductor (subsartorial) canal, one related to the calf muscles, and one just proximal to the ankle joint.

CLINICALLY ORIENTED COMMENTS

When the valves of the distal set of perforating veins become **"incompetent"** (*i.e.*, dilated so that their cusps do not meet and close the vein), contractions of the calf muscles which normally propel the blood upward cause a **reverse flow** through the perforating veins (*i.e.*, deep to superficial), which makes the perforating and superficial veins become tortuous and dilated (*i.e.*, **varicose veins**).

Prior to therapy for varicose veins, **venography** is often done to locate all the perforating veins which are to be treated surgically (*e.g.*, ligated) or medically (injected with corrosive fluids) to prevent the passage of blood from the deep to the superficial veins.

Vein grafts using the great saphenous vein have been used to bypass obstructions (*e.g.*, atheromatous occlusion of the femoral and coronary arteries).

Coronary bypass surgery is becoming relatively common in some countries. When a portion of the great saphenous vein is removed and inserted as a bypass, the vein is reversed so that its valve cusps do not obstruct the blood flow. Following removal of the great saphenous vein, the blood from superficial parts of the leg reach the deep veins via the perforating or anastomotic veins (Fig. 4-12).

It is important to memorize the fact that *the great saphenous vein lies immediately anterior to the medial malleolus* (Figs. 4-12, 4-13 and 4-92). Even when it may not be visible in infants, in obese patients, or in those in shock whose veins are collapsed, this vein can always be located and punctured by making a skin incision at this site. This common clinical procedure, often referred to as a **"cutdown,"** is used to insert a cannula (L. reed) for prolonged administration of blood, plasma expanders, electrolytes, or drugs.

In Figure 4-12*B* observe that the **saphenous nerve** accompanies the great saphenous vein anterior to the medial malleolus. Should it be caught by a ligature during a saphenous "cutdown," the patient (if conscious) is likely to complain of pain along the medial border of the foot (Fig. 4-106).

The Small Saphenous Vein (Figs. 4-11 and 4-12*A*). This vein is also referred to as the short or lesser saphenous vein. It is formed by the union of vessels arising from the lateral part of the **dorsal venous arch.** It passes along the lateral side of the foot with the sural nerve, posterior to the **lateral malleolus** (Fig. 4-12*A*), and ascends along the lateral side of the **tendo calcaneus** (tendon of Achilles)* midway up the calf of the leg (Fig. 4-83). It passes to the **popliteal fossa** (space), the lozenge-shaped area posterior to the knee (Fig. 4-56), where it perforates the deep fascia and ends in the popliteal vein (Fig. 4-58). It has several communications with the great saphenous vein and the deep veins (Fig. 4-12*A*). Just before piercing the popliteal fascia, it frequently gives off a branch which unites with another vein to form the **accessory saphenous vein.** This becomes the main communication between the great and small saphenous veins.

CLINICALLY ORIENTED COMMENTS

Varicose veins are common in the posterior and medial parts of the lower limb,

* This common tendon for the gastrocnemius and soleus muscles (Fig. 4-83) is often referred to as Achilles tendon after the mythical Greek warrior who was vulnerable only in the heel. You will also hear about the Achilles reflex or ankle jerk, a contraction of the calf muscles that occurs when the tendo calcaneus is sharply struck.

particularly in older persons, and cause considerable discomfort and even pain. Varicose saphenous veins have a caliber greater than normal and their cusps do not meet (*i.e.,* they are incompetent); hence they allow blood to run from the deep into the superficial veins.

Varicose veins appear to have various causes, *e.g.,* where the normal venous return is impeded, such as in constipated persons, pregnant females, and persons with large abdominal tumors. They often develop in members of the same family, which may indicate a genetic weakness in the vein walls. Varicose veins and **hemorrhoids** (piles), a varicose condition of the rectal veins, are often associated.

Thrombophlebitis (inflammation of a vein with secondary thrombus or clot formation) of the deep veins of the leg destroys their valves, resulting in much of the blood from the leg being returned via the superficial veins. This causes them to become varicose (large and tortuous). Should such a **thrombus** (clot) break loose, it will be carried through the right side of the heart to the lung. Here it will be stopped as the branches of the pulmonary artery become progressively smaller. If the **pulmonary embolus** is small it may produce few or no symptoms, but if it is very large it may result in **sudden death.** (For a fuller discussion of **pulmonary embolism**, see Chap. 1)

The Cutaneous Nerves (Figs. 4-14 and 4-16 to 4-18). Several cutaneous nerves in the superficial fascia supply skin on the anterior, medial, and lateral aspects of the thigh.

The **ilioinguinal nerve** is distributed to the skin of the superomedial area of the thigh (Figs. 4-14 and 4-16). Femoral branches of the **genitofemoral nerve** supply the skin just below the middle part of the inguinal ligament.

The **lateral femoral cutaneous nerve** enters this region deep to the lateral end of the inguinal ligament, near the anterior superior iliac spine (Figs. 4-14 and 4-18), to supply the skin on the anterior and lateral aspects of the thigh.

The anterior cutaneous branches of the **femoral nerve** (intermediate and cutaneous nerves of the thigh) supply the skin on the anterior and medial aspects of the thigh, whereas the **saphenous nerve,** the longest branch of the femoral nerve, supplies skin on the medial side of the leg and foot (Figs. 4-14 and 4-106).

CLINICALLY ORIENTED COMMENTS

The anatomy of the lateral femoral cutaneous nerve (L2 and L3) is clinically important in a condition called **meralgia paresthetica,** a tingling and painful itching in the anterolateral region of the thigh in the area of distribution of this nerve (Fig. 4-14). It often occurs as people get older and fatter, especially when the abdomen bulges over the inguinal ligament and compresses this nerve.

The Deep Fascia (Figs. 4-15 to 4-19). The deep fascia of the thigh, known as the **fascia lata** (L. broad band) is an especially strong, dense, broad layer which invests the muscles of the thigh like a stocking. It is extremely strong laterally where it runs from the tubercle of the iliac crest to the tibia (Figs. 4-1, 4-2, and 4-43). This part of the fascia lata, known as the **iliotibial tract,** receives tendinous reinforcements from the tensor fasciae latae and gluteus maximus muscles. The distal end of the iliotibial tract of the fascia lata, which is about 2.5 cm wide, is attached to the lateral condyle of the tibia (Figs. 4-21 and 4-23*A*). To palpate it, raise your heel from the floor with your knee joint flexed (Figs. 4-27 and 4-55).

Just posterior and inferior to the anterior superior iliac spine, the fascia lata encases a muscle, the **tensor fasciae latae** (Fig. 4-20). It pulls on the strap-like iliotibial tract of the fascia lata, thereby steadying the trunk on the thigh and preventing posterior displacement of the iliotibial tract by the gluteus maximus, three-quarters of which inserts into the iliotibial tract (Fig. 4-45), which is a longitudinal thickening of the deep fascia or fascia lata.

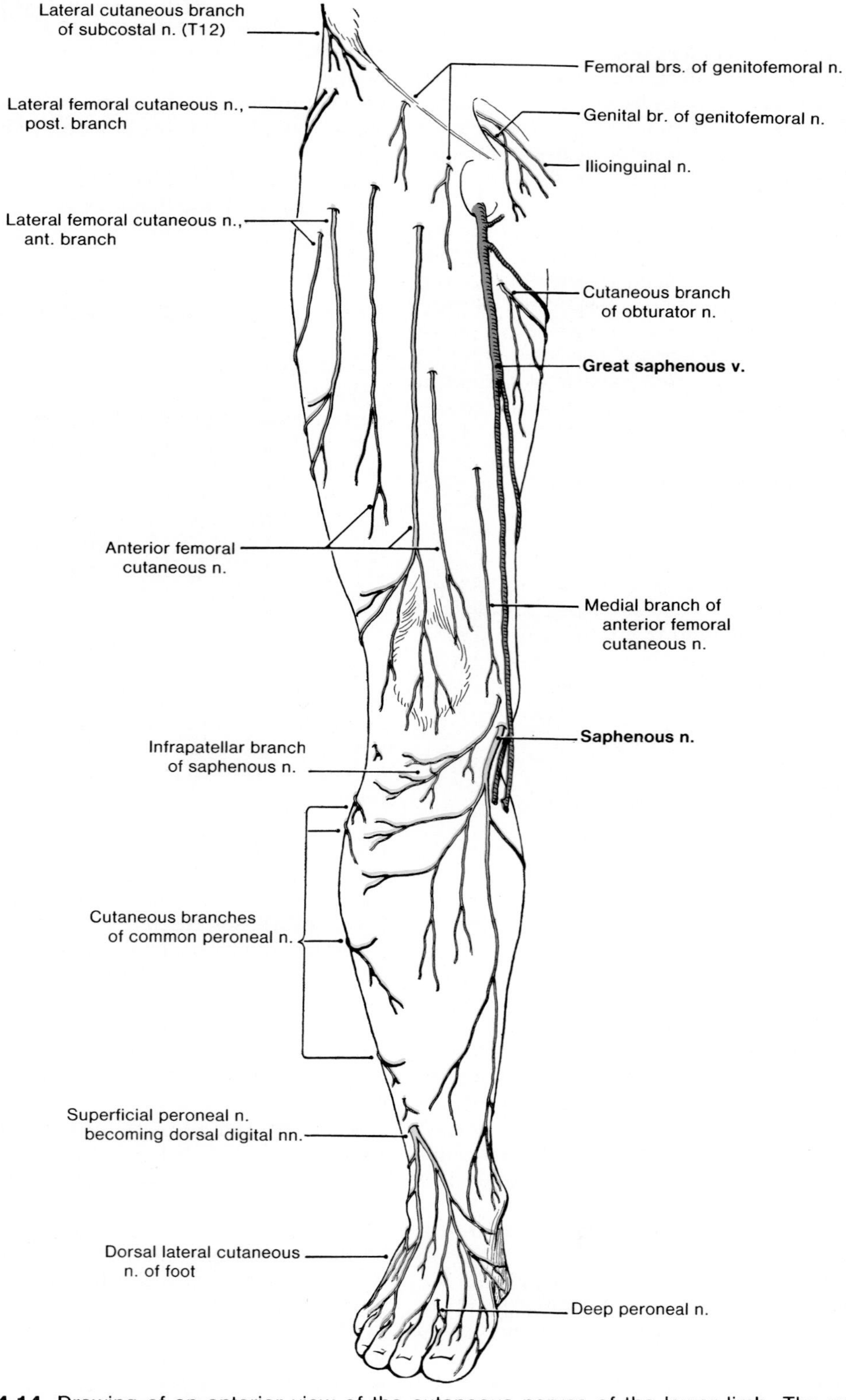

Figure 4-14. Drawing of an anterior view of the cutaneous nerves of the lower limb. The great saphenous vein is also shown.

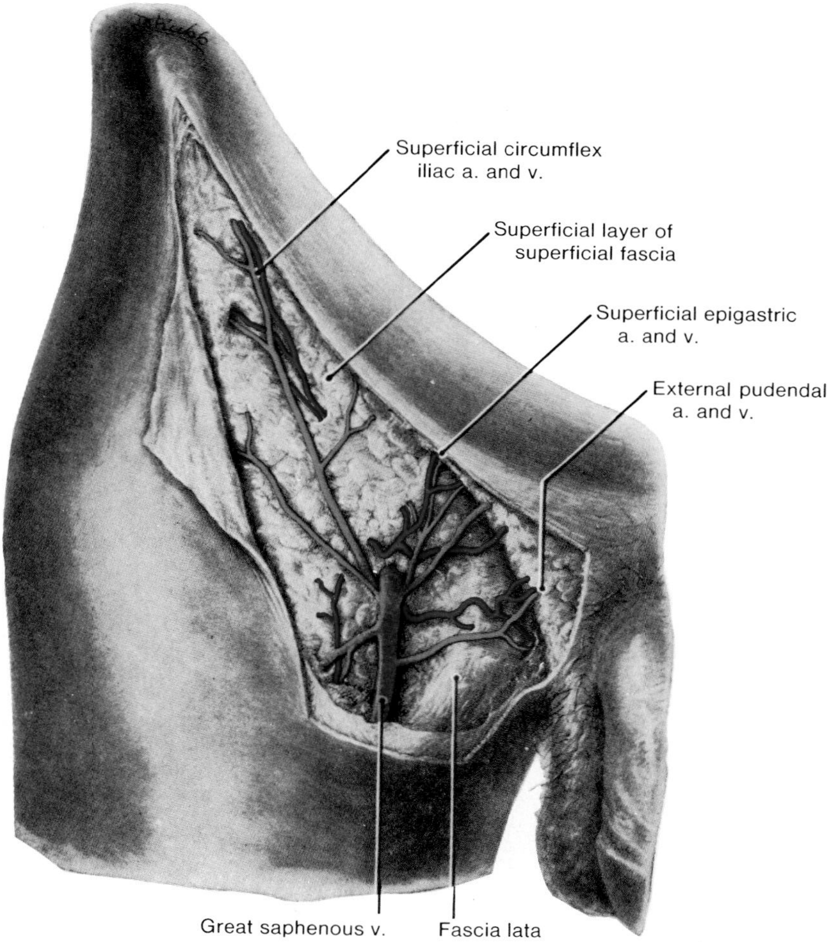

Figure 4-15. Drawing of a dissection of the superficial inguinal arteries and veins. The arteries are branches of the femoral artery and the veins are tributaries of the great saphenous vein. Observe that this vein passes through the cribriform fascia to enter the femoral vein. The cribriform fascia is a thin layer of deep fascia that fills the saphenous opening, an aperture through which pass the great saphenous vein and other smaller vessels (see Fig. 4-13 also).

The Saphenous Opening (Figs. 4-13 to 4-16). Just inferior to the inguinal ligament there is a deficiency in the fascia lata, known as the **saphenous opening,** through which the great saphenous vein passes to join the femoral vein. The center of this opening is about 6 cm (three finger-breadths) inferolateral to the pubic tubercle (Figs. 4-1 and 4-5). The saphenous opening is about 4 cm long and 1 to 2 cm wide (Fig. 4-16). Its medial margin is smooth but its superior, lateral, and inferior margins form a sharp crescentic edge, called the **falciform** (L. sickle form or shaped) **margin.** This margin of the saphenous opening is joined to the medial margin by fibrous and fatty tissue known as the **cribriform fascia** (Figs. 4-15 and 4-16). This thin part of the deep fascia spreads over the saphenous opening.

MUSCLES OF THE HIP AND THIGH

The large and powerful thigh muscles can be organized into **three main groups** on the basis of their location, action, and nerve supply. They are separated by three intermuscular septa (Fig. 4-17). The lateral

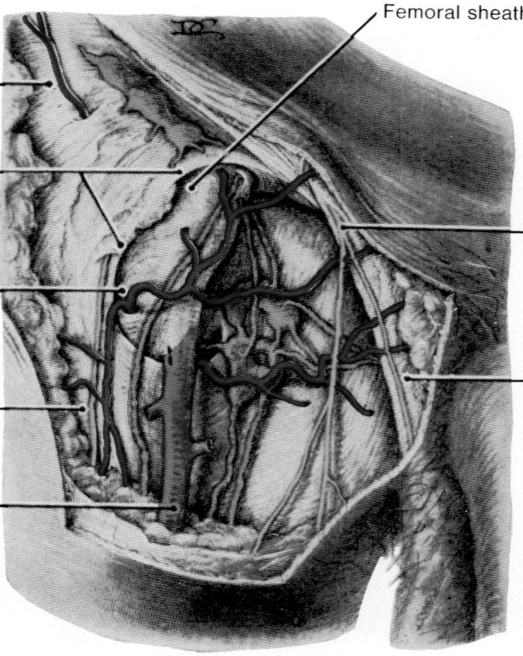

Figure 4-16. Drawing of a dissection of the superficial inguinal arteries and veins. Observe the saphenous opening in the fascia lata through which the great saphenous vein and other smaller vessels pass through the cribriform fascia to enter the femoral vein (Fig. 4-13*A*). Note that the superior, inferior, and lateral margins of this opening form a sharp crescentic edge of deep fascia, known as the falciform margin.

one is strong; the other two are relatively weak.

The anterior group of muscles (sartorius and quadriceps femoris) lies on the *anterior and lateral aspects of the thigh.* In general they are **extensors of the knee** joint and are supplied by the **femoral nerve.** The front of the thigh also contains the terminal parts of the **iliacus** and **psoas major** muscles (Fig. 4-20), which are the main flexors of the hip joint.

The adductor group of muscles (adductors magnus, brevis, and longus; gracilis; obturator externus; and pectineus) lies on the *medial side of the thigh* (Figs. 4-17 and 4-20). They are **adductors of the hip** joint and are supplied by the **obturator nerve,** except for the pectineus, which is supplied by the femoral nerve and occasionally by the obturator also.

The hamstring group of muscles (semitendinosus, semimembranosus, and biceps femoris) lies on the *back of the thigh* (Fig. 4-17) and is supplied by the **sciatic nerve** (Fig. 4-52). In general they are **flexors of the knee** joint and **extensors of the hip** joint. The hamstring group of muscles is described on page 478.

Muscles of Front of Thigh (Figs. 4-17, 4-18, 4-20, and 4-23). The anterior group of muscles in the thigh consists of the **sartorius** and the **quadriceps femoris** (composed of four parts). All these muscles are supplied by the **femoral nerve.**

The front of the thigh also contains the terminations of two muscles of the posterior abdominal wall (iliacus and psoas major) which are often described as a composite muscle, the **iliopsoas.** The abdominal parts of these muscles are described in Chapter 2.

The Psoas Major Muscle (Figs. 4-19, 4-20, 4-23, and 4-28). This long, thick, powerful muscle passes from the abdomen into the thigh by passing deep to the inguinal ligament.

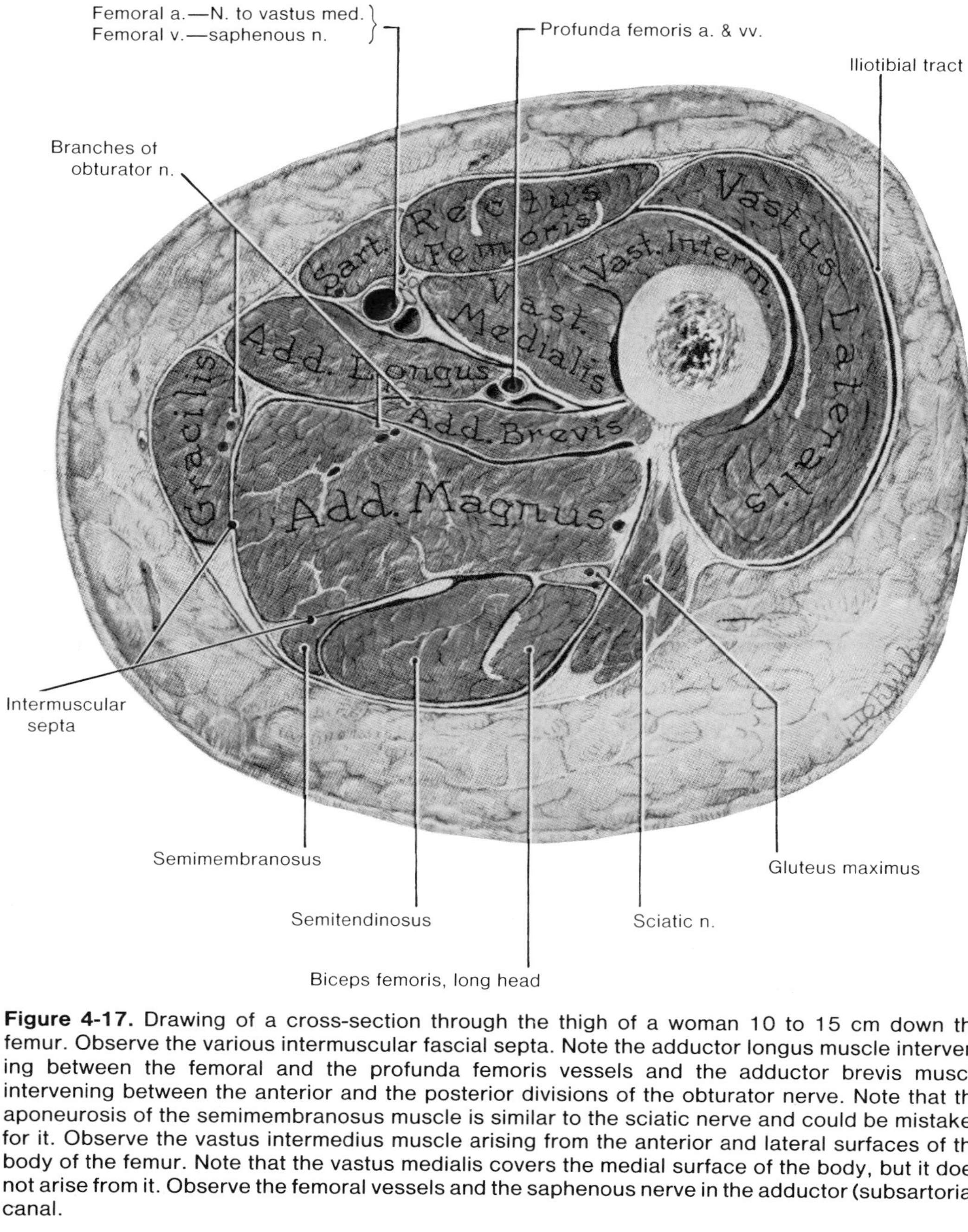

Figure 4-17. Drawing of a cross-section through the thigh of a woman 10 to 15 cm down the femur. Observe the various intermuscular fascial septa. Note the adductor longus muscle intervening between the femoral and the profunda femoris vessels and the adductor brevis muscle intervening between the anterior and the posterior divisions of the obturator nerve. Note that the aponeurosis of the semimembranosus muscle is similar to the sciatic nerve and could be mistaken for it. Observe the vastus intermedius muscle arising from the anterior and lateral surfaces of the body of the femur. Note that the vastus medialis covers the medial surface of the body, but it does not arise from it. Observe the femoral vessels and the saphenous nerve in the adductor (subsartorial) canal.

Origin. **Transverse processes,** sides of **vertebral bodies,** and **intervertebral discs** of **T12 to L5.**

Insertion (Fig. 4-21). **Lesser trochanter of femur** via iliopsoas tendon.

Nerve Supply. Ventral rami of upper three or four **lumbar nerves.**

Action. **Flexes hip joint** (assisted by iliacus).

The Iliacus Muscle (Figs. 4-18 to 4-20

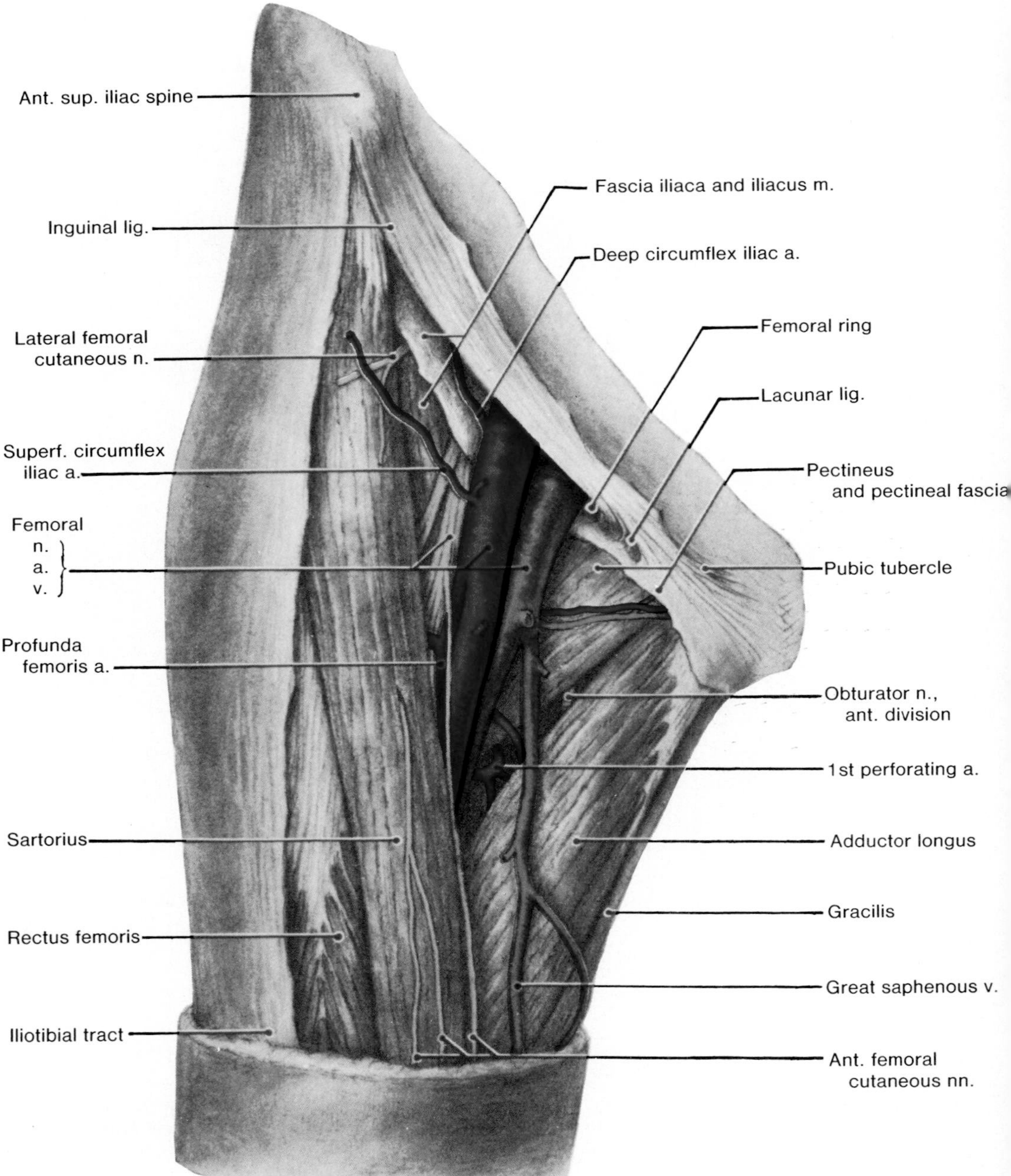

Figure 4-18. Drawing of a dissection of the femoral triangle. Observe the boundaries of this triangle: the inguinal ligament, superiorly; the medial border of the adductor longus, medially; and the medial border of the sartorius, laterally. The head of the femur lies posterior to the point where the inguinal ligament crosses the femoral artery (Fig. 4-32). Note that the femoral artery and vein lie anterior to fascia covering the iliopsoas and pectineus muscles, respectively, and that the femoral nerve lies posterior to it. Observe that the femoral artery is about midway between the anterior superior iliac spine and the pubic tubercle and disappears into the adductor canal where the medial border of the sartorius crosses the lateral border of the adductor longus.

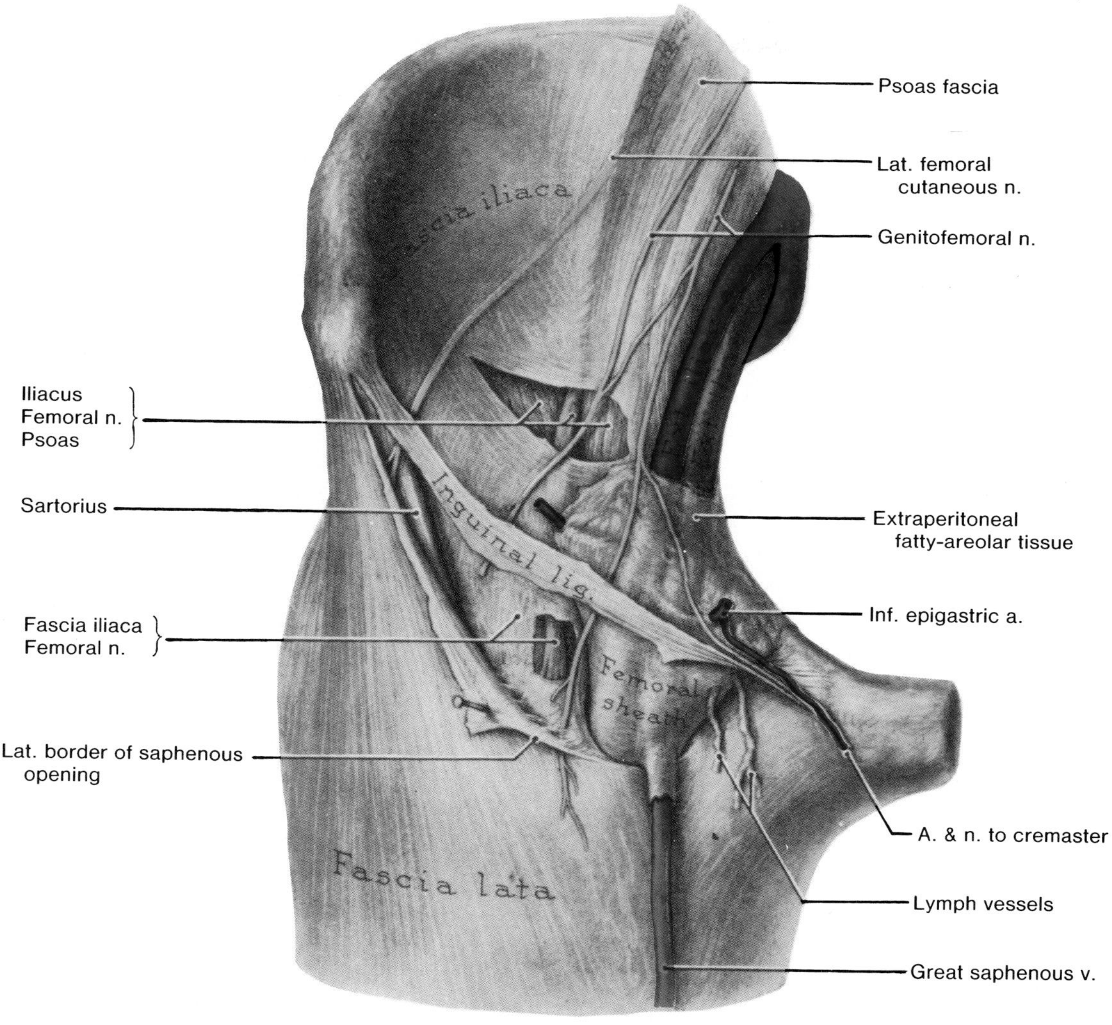

Figure 4-19. Drawing of a dissection of the femoral sheath. The three flat muscles of the abdominal wall are cut away from the superior border of the inguinal ligament and the fascia lata from the inferior border. The falciform margin of the saphenous opening in the fascia lata is cut and reflected. Observe the fascia iliaca, continuous medially with the psoas fascia and carried downward anterior to the iliacus muscle into the thigh. As it passes posterior to the inguinal ligament it adheres to it. Note that the extraperitoneal fatty-areolar tissue, which lines the abdominal cavity and in which the external iliac vessels run, is carried downward around these vessels into the thigh as a delicate funnel-shaped sac, called the femoral sheath. This is loosely adherent to the inguinal ligament anteriorly and to the pecten pubis posteriorly. Observe the femoral sheath containing the femoral artery, vein, and lymph vessels. Note that the femoral nerve, being posterior to the fascia iliaca, is external to the femoral sheath. The *contents of the femoral sheath* are clearly illustrated in Figures 4-36 and 4-39.

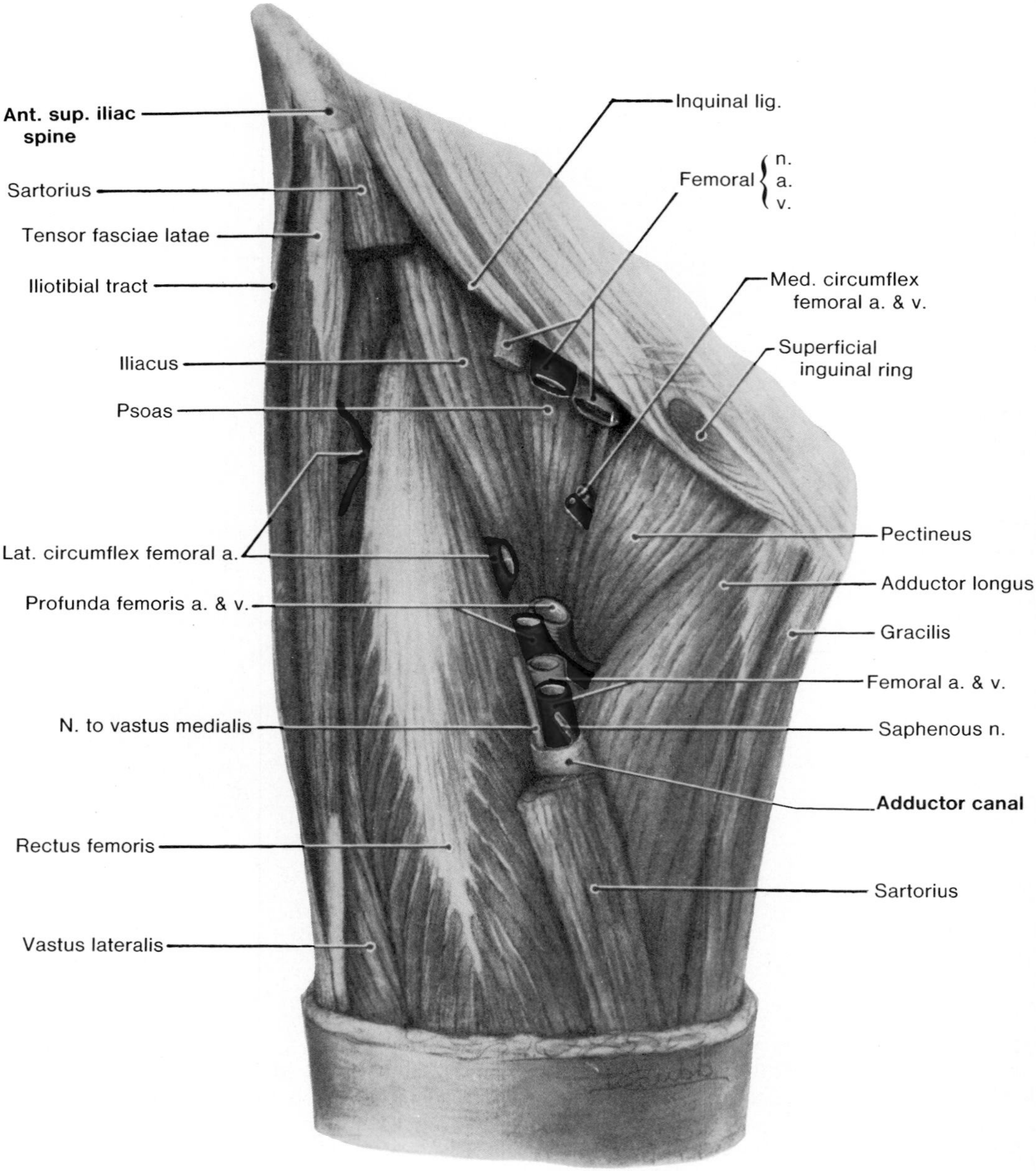

Figure 4-20. Drawing of a dissection of the femoral triangle. Sections are removed from the sartorius and the femoral vessels and nerve. Its lateral boundary is the medial border of the sartorius and its medial boundary is the medial border of the adductor longus. Observe that the floor of the triangle is composed of muscles (adductor longus, pectineus, psoas major, and iliacus). Note that the triangle is shallow at the base and deep at the apex. Observe that the femoral artery is entering the fascial tunnel called the adductor canal (subsartorial canal, Hunter's canal). It is accompanied in this canal by the femoral vein and the saphenous nerve.

and 4-23*A* and *B*). This large fan-shaped muscle lies along the lateral side of the psoas major in the pelvis.

Origin (Fig. 4-21). **Iliac crest,** floor of **iliac fossa,** and **ala of sacrum.**

Insertion (Figs. 4-21 and 4-30). **Lesser trochanter of femur** via iliopsoas tendon.

Nerve Supply. **Femoral** nerve (L2 and L3).

Action. **Flexes hip joint** (assisted by psoas major).

The Tensor Fasciae Latae Muscle (Figs. 4-20 and 4-22 to 4-24). This fusiform muscle lies on the lateral side of the front of the thigh, enclosed within the fascia lata.

Origin (Fig. 4-22). **Anterior part of outer lip of iliac crest,** lateral surface of **anterior superior iliac spine,** and notch below it.

Insertion (Figs. 4-17, 4-18, 4-27, 4-54, 4-55, and 4-57). **Iliotibial tract** (attached to lateral condyle of tibia).

Nerve Supply. **Superior gluteal** nerve (L4 and L5).

Actions. **Abducts** and **flexes hip joint** and helps to keep knee extended in erect posture by making iliotibial tract taut. It also **steadies the trunk on the thigh** and counteracts the backward pull of the gluteus maximus on the iliotibial tract (a longitudinal thickening of the fascia lata).

The Sartorius Muscle (Figs. 4-17, 4-20 to 4-24, and 4-28). This narrow, strap-like muscle is the longest in the body and is the most superficial muscle in the anterior group. It was given its name (L. *sartor*, a tailor) because it is used to cross the legs in the tailor's cross-legged sitting position. Throughout much of its course, the *sartorius covers the femoral artery* as it runs in the adductor (subsartorial) canal.

Origin (Figs. 4-20 to 4-22). **Anterior superior iliac spine** and upper part of notch below it.

Insertion (Fig. 4-26). **Upper quarter of medial surface of tibia**, anterior to gracilis and semitendinosus muscles.

Nerve Supply. **Femoral** nerve (L2 and L3).

Actions. **Flexes** and **laterally rotates hip joint**. It also aids in abducting this joint.

The Quadriceps Femoris Muscle (Figs. 4-17, 4-20 to 4-25, 4-28, and 4-30). The quadriceps consists of *four muscles* (**rectus femoris** and **vastus lateralis, medialis,** and **intermedius**) that *are collectively known as the quadriceps femoris.* This great extensor muscle of the leg covers the front and sides of the femur (Fig. 4-17). The names of its parts indicate their location: the **rectus femoris** (L. *rectus*, straight) has deep fibers that run straight down the thigh; the **vastus lateralis** lies on the lateral side of the thigh; the **vastus medialis** covers the medial aspect of the thigh; and the **vastus intermedius** is located between the vastus medialis and lateralis. To see the vastus intermedius, the rectus femoris must be sectioned and reflected upward (see Fig. 4-23*B*).

Origin (Figs. 4-21, 4-22, 4-30, and 4-48). **Rectus femoris**: *straight head,* **anterior inferior iliac spine**; *reflected head,* **groove above acetabulum. The three vasti muscles arise from the femur** (details below).

The **vastus lateralis** arises from the **intertrochanteric line,** the greater trochanter, the gluteal tuberosity (Fig. 4-2), the upper half of the lateral lip of the linea aspera, and the lateral intermuscular septum.

The **vastus medialis** arises from the intertrochanteric line, the **spiral line** (Fig. 4-2), the medial lip of **linea aspera,** and the medial intermuscular septum.

The **vastus intermedius** arises from the **upper two-thirds of the femur** and the distal half of the lateral intermuscular septum.

A small muscle, the **articularis genus** (Fig. 4-23*C*), is sometimes blended with the vastus intermedius. It arises from the inferior part of the femur and inserts into the synovial capsule of the knee joint and the walls of the **suprapatellar bursa** (Fig. 4-124). This small muscle pulls the synovial capsule upward during extension of the knee joint.

Insertion (Figs. 4-1, 4-21, 4-23, 4-26, and 4-54). **Base of patella** and **tibial tuberosity**. The tendons of all four muscles (heads of quadriceps) unite to form a strong quadriceps tendon which is inserted into the patella (kneecap). This *common tendon* continues inferiorly to the tibial tuberosity as the **patellar ligament (ligamentum patellae)**. In addition, expansions of the aponeuroses of the vasti, called the medial and lateral **retinacula of the patella**, insert into the condyles of the tibia.

Nerve Supply. All components of the quadriceps femoris muscle are supplied by

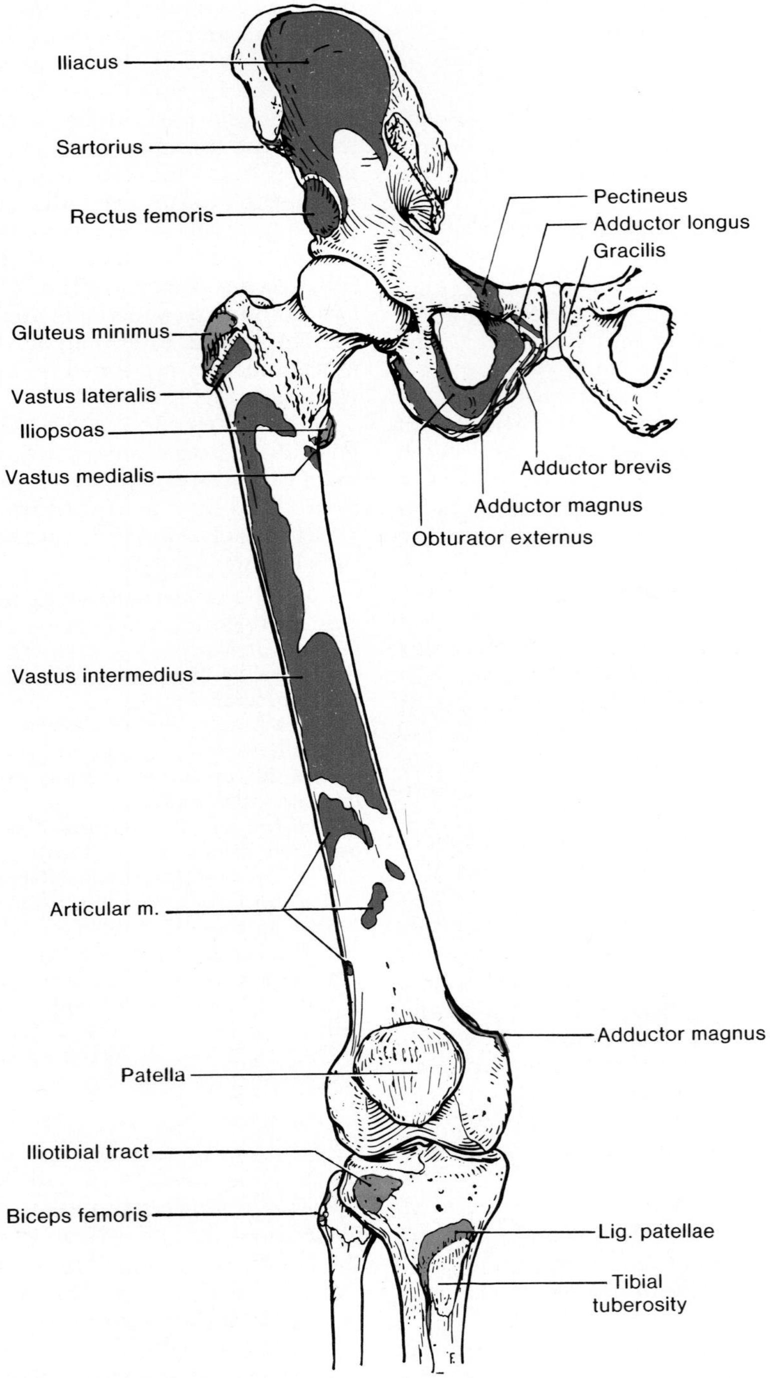

Figure 4-21. Drawing of an anterior view of the bones of the lower limb showing the attachments of muscles. Note that the rectus femoris arises from the ilium and that all the vasti muscles arise from the femur (see Fig. 4-22 also). *Red* indicates origins and *blue*, insertions of muscles.

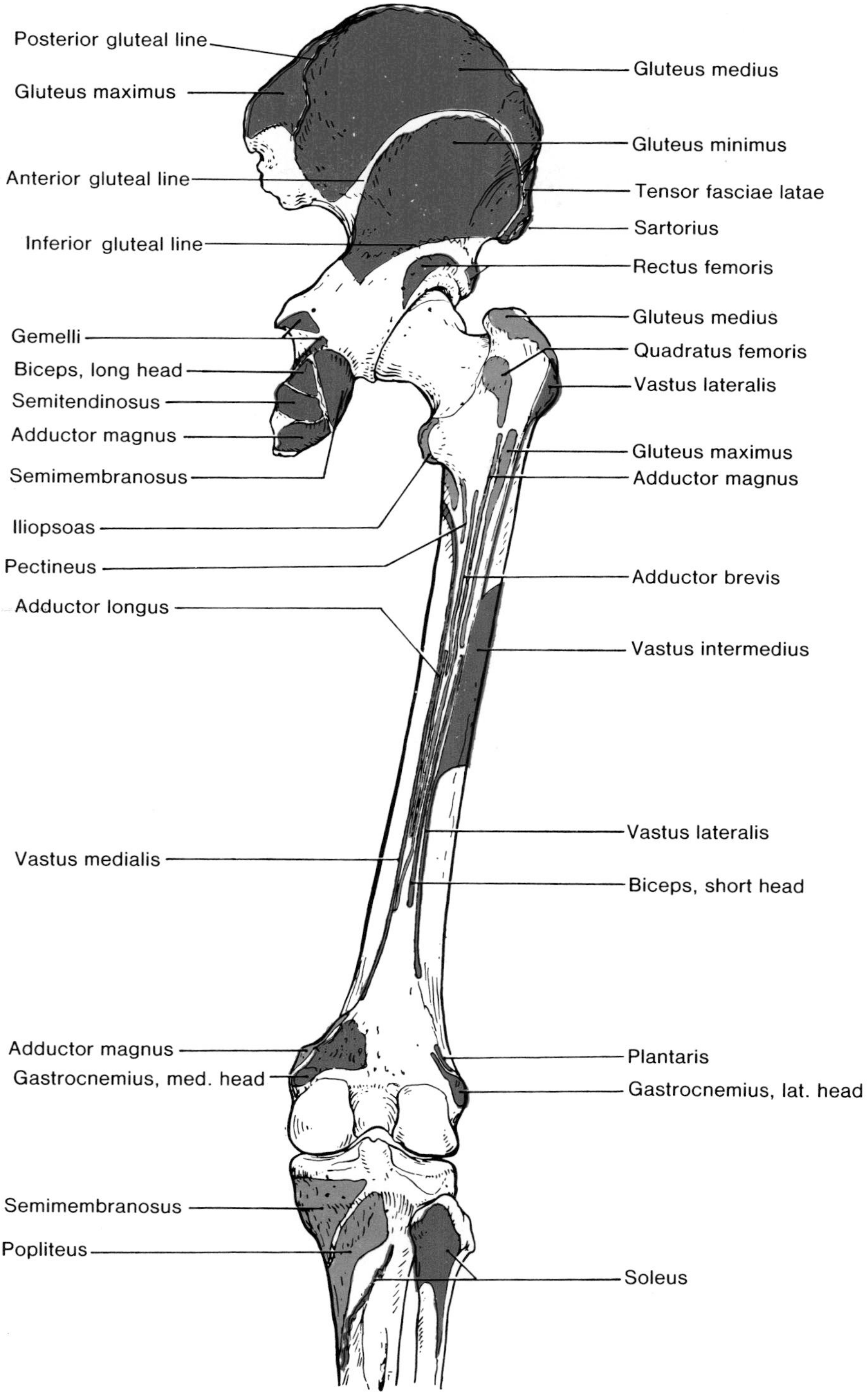

Figure 4-22. Drawing of a posterior view of the bones of the lower limb showing the attachments of muscles. Observe that several muscles are attached to the linea aspera (Figs. 4-2 and 4-9*B*). Note the extensive origin of the vastus lateralis, the largest of the four muscles making up the quadriceps femoris (also see Fig. 4-17).

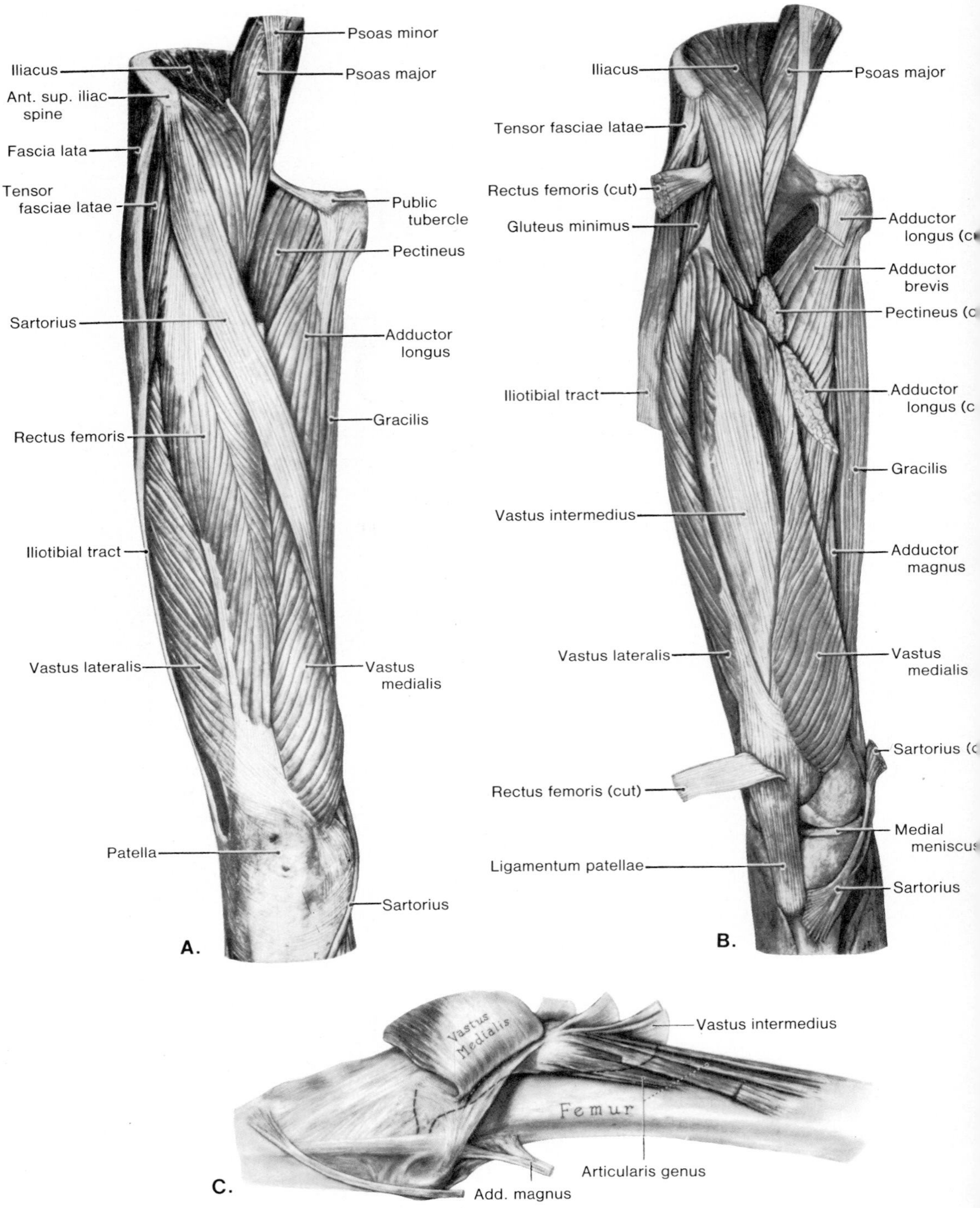

Figure 4-23. Drawings of the muscles of the front of thigh. *A*, superficial dissection. *B*, deep dissection with sections of the sartorius, rectus femoris, pectineus, and adductor longus excised. The pectineus, adductor longus, and gracilis originate from a curved line on the pubic bone (Fig. 4-21). *C*, deep dissection showing the articularis genus muscle which sometimes blends with the vastus intermedius muscle. The articularis genus retracts the synovial capsule during extension of the knee joint.

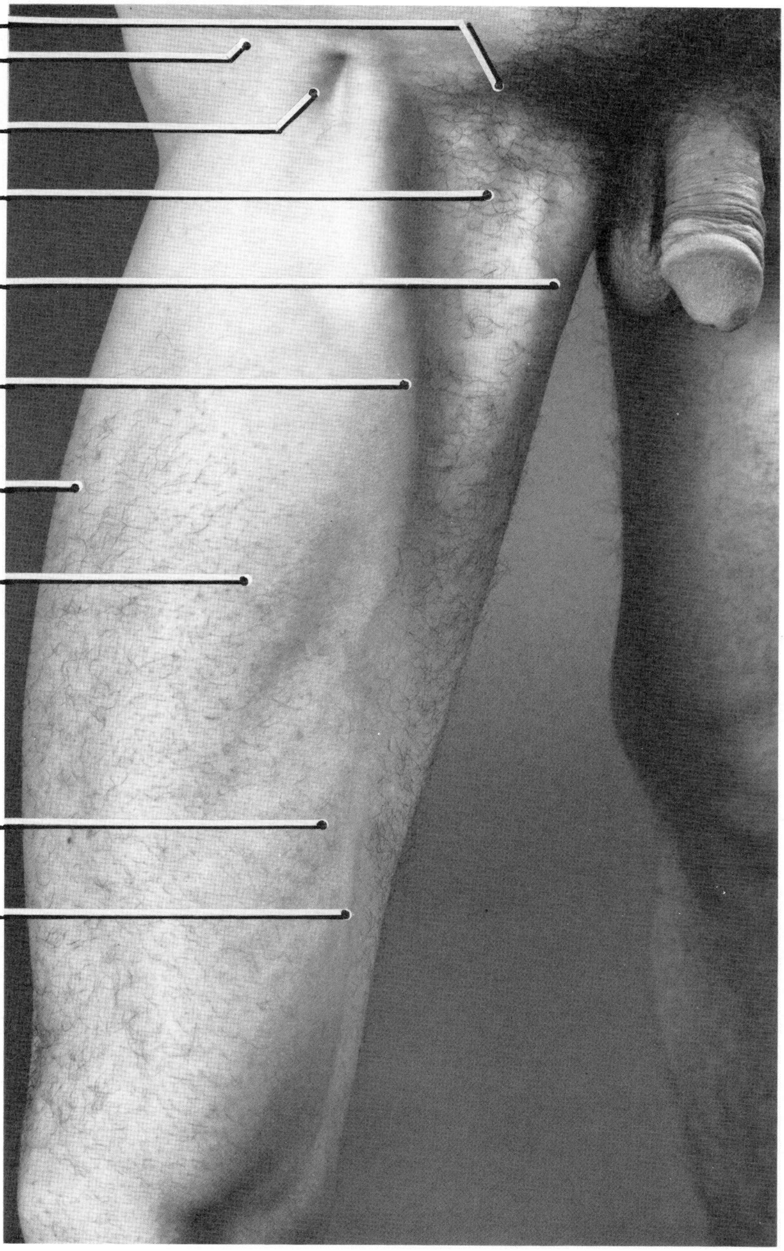

Figure 4-24. Photograph of the thigh of a 27-year-old man showing the sartorius in action. To display this muscle he was asked to flex, abduct, and laterally rotate his thigh. This photograph was taken with his pelvis somewhat rotated to the left, bringing the anterior superior iliac spine *apparently* near the midline of the thigh. The femoral triangle can be seen as a depression inferior to the inguinal ligament which forms its base. The lateral boundary of this area is the sartorius and its medial boundary is the adductor longus. Observe the great saphenous (G. clearly visible) vein.

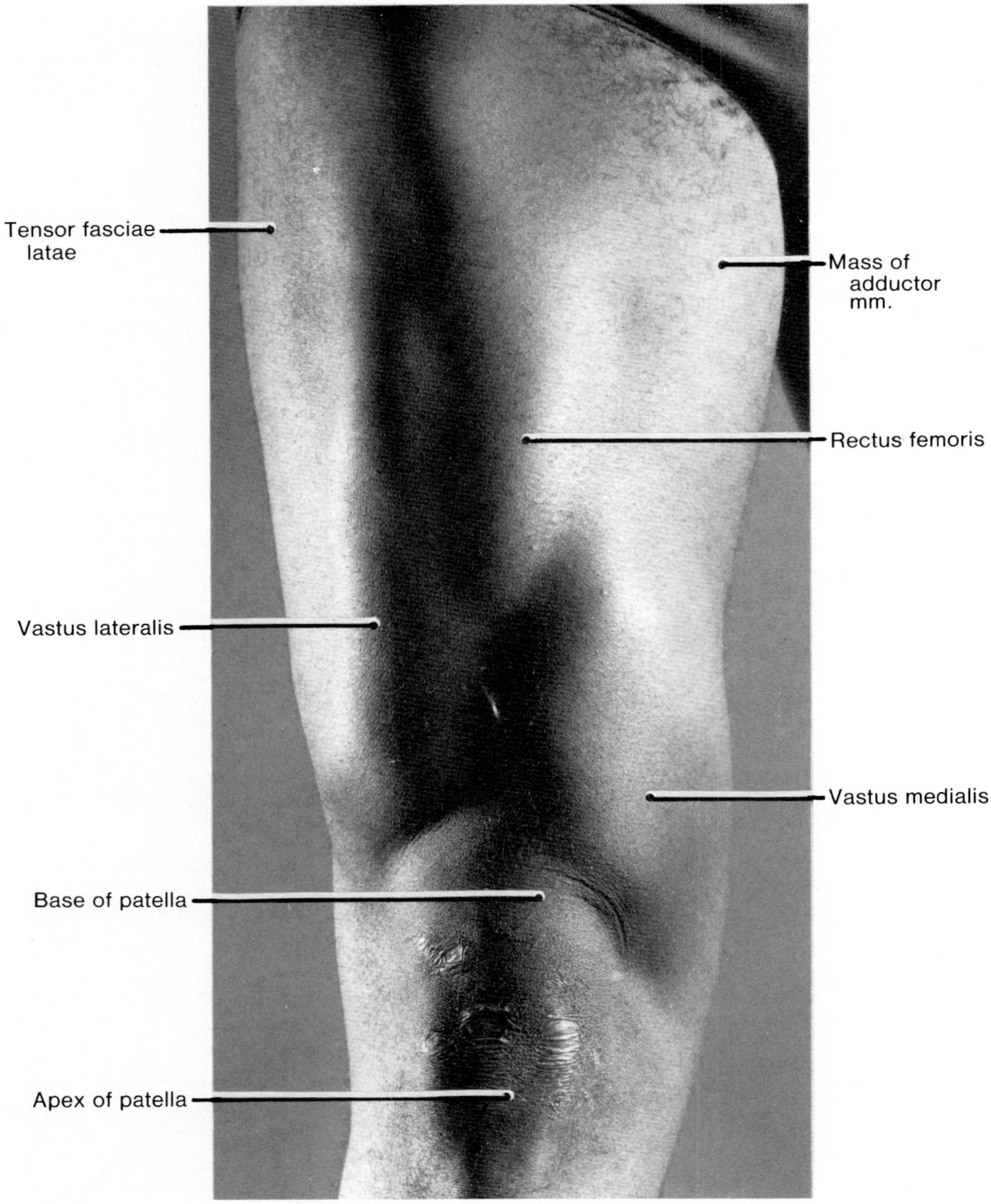

Figure 4-25. Photograph of the front of the thigh of a 35-year-old man showing the principal surface features. Compare with Figure 4-23*A*. The parts of the quadriceps femoris became visible when he extended his knee against resistance on his leg. Observe that the fleshy bulk of the vastus medialis extends more distally than does the vastus lateralis. This helps to counteract lateral displacement of the patella by the pull of the rectus femoris and vastus lateralis. When this muscle is relaxed the patella is freely movable from side to side. All four parts of the quadriceps converge on the base of the patella, a sesamoid bone in the quadriceps tendon. The deepest portion of the quadriceps (vastus intermedius) is not visible from the surface (view it in Fig. 4-23*B*).

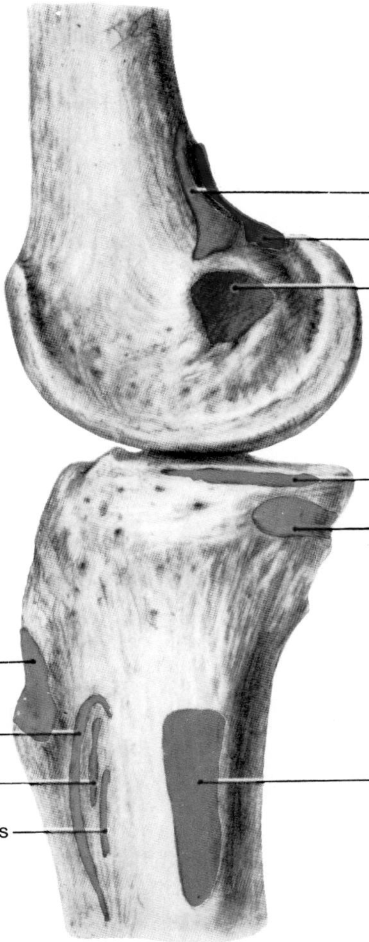

Figure 4-26. Drawing of a medial view of the bones of the right knee joint showing the attachment of muscles and ligaments.

branches of the **femoral** nerve (L2, L3, and L4).

Actions. **Extends leg at knee joint**. All four parts contribute to this action by pulling on the tibia via the patellar ligament. Verify this by extending your knee against resistance; three parts of the muscle can be palpated and observed (Figs. 4-24 and 4-25). Only one part of the quadriceps (rectus femoris) crosses the hip joint; thus, **rectus femorus flexes thigh at hip joint**.

All parts of the quadriceps are used in climbing, running, jumping, and rising from a chair. If you put your hands on your quadriceps as you get up from a chair, you can feel these large muscles contract.

CLINICALLY ORIENTED COMMENTS

If the quadriceps femoris is paralyzed the knee cannot be extended, but the patient can stand erect because body weight tends to overextend the knee. The patient can also walk with short steps if the pelvis is rotated to prevent extension of the hip so far as to flex the knee. Patients with **paralysis of the quadriceps** femoris often press on the distal end of their thigh during walking to prevent flexion of their knee from occurring.

In football broadcasts you often hear

about an injury known as a "**hip pointer**." This is a contusion or bruise over the bony prominence of the iliac crest, particularly the anterior superior iliac spine, from which the inguinal ligament and the sartorius muscle arise.

Another common term in sports language is "**Charley horse**." This is a contusion (L. a bruising) and a tearing of muscle fibers that result in the formation of a **hematoma** (a local mass of extravasated blood that escapes into the muscle from damaged vessels). The most common site of a Charley horse is the quadriceps muscle. It is associated with localized pain and/or muscle stiffness and commonly follows direct trauma (*e.g.*, a tackle in football).

The Patella (L. little plate). This is a triangular sesamoid bone with its apex pointing inferiorly (Fig. 4-1). It is located within the **quadriceps femoris tendon** (Fig. 4-23*A*) which continues inferiorly as the **ligamentum patellae** or patellar ligament (Fig. 4-23*B*) and attaches to the tibial tuberosity (Figs. 4-21 and 4-26). When a person is erect, the inferior margin or apex of the patella is about 1.5 cm proximal to the knee joint (Figs. 4-25 and 4-124).

The patella is subcutaneous and can be easily palpated. It lies anterior to the expanded distal end of the femur, hence its posterior surface is articular. The patella is thought to increase the power of the already strong quadriceps femoris muscle by increasing its leverage. Palpate your patella as you flex your knee, noting that it is pulled down. Kneel down and verify that it is the tibial tuberosity and the patellar ligament that receive most of the weight. Only the apex of the patella bears any weight in this position.

CLINICALLY ORIENTED COMMENTS

The patella is cartilaginous at birth and becomes ossified during the 3rd to 6th years, frequently from more than one center. Although these centers usually coalesce, they may remain separate on one or both sides, giving rise to a bipartite or tripartite patella. An unwary observer might interpret this condition on a radiograph as a **fracture of the patella**.

A direct blow on the patella may fracture it in two or more fragments. The patella may also be fractured transversely by sudden contraction of the quadriceps (*e.g.*, when one slips and attempts to prevent a backward fall). In these cases the proximal fragment is pulled superiorly with the quadriceps tendon and the distal fragment remains with the ligamentum patellae. This condition would have more tendency to occur in persons with unfused or poorly fused ossification centers in this bone.

Because of the tendency of the parts of a fractured patella to separate, the position of extension (in which the quadriceps femoris is relaxed) is used to reduce a fractured patella.

Tapping the patellar ligament with a percussion hammer normally leads to elicitation of the **quadriceps reflex** (patellar reflex, knee reflex, and **knee jerk**). This reflex is routinely tested as follows. The patient is seated on the edge of a table or bed with the legs hanging loosely, or the patient's knee is flexed over the supporting arm of the examiner with the heel resting lightly on the bed. The patellar ligament is tapped briskly until contraction of the quadriceps femoris is elicited; this results in extension of the knee joint.

Tapping the patellar ligament activates **muscle spindles** in the quadriceps femoris. Afferent impulses from these spindles travel in the femoral nerve to the spinal cord (L2, L3, and L4). From here, efferent impulses are transmitted via motor fibers in the femoral nerve to the quadriceps femoris, resulting in a jerk-like contraction of the muscle and extension of the leg at the knee joint. Diminution or **absence of the quadriceps reflex** may result from any lesion which interupts the reflex arc, *e.g.*, peripheral nerve disease.

Muscles of Medial Side of Thigh (Figs. 4-20, 4-23 to 4-25, and 4-28). The main action of the medial group of muscles is **adduction of the thigh** (*e.g.*, when holding oneself on a horse); hence, these muscles constitute the **adductor group**. It includes the pectineus, the gracilis, the adductors magnus, brevis, and longus, and the obturator externus. **All adductors are supplied by the obturator nerve** (L2, L3, and L4), *except the pectineus*, which is supplied by the femoral nerve (sometimes it receives a branch from the obturator), and the "hamstring" part of the adductor magnus (supplied by the sciatic nerve).

The Pectineus Muscle (Figs. 4-18, 4-20, 4-23, and 4-33). This short, flat quadrangular muscle is in the floor of the femoral triangle.

Origin (Figs. 4-1, 4-21, and 4-48). **Pecten pubis** (pectineal line) and pectineal surface of this bone. The pecten (L. comb) is a sharp ridge on the pubic bone.

Insertion (Figs. 4-2, 4-22, and 4-30). **Pectineal line** of femur.

Nerve Supply. **Femoral** nerve (L2 and L3); sometimes receives a branch from obturator nerve (L2 and L3).

Actions. **Adducts** and **flexes hip joint**.

The Gracilis Muscle (Figs. 4-17, 4-18, 4-20, 4-23, and 4-28). The gracilis (L. slender) is a long strap-like muscle that lies along the medial side of the thigh and the knee. It is the most superficial of the hip adductors and is the weakest member of the adductor group. It is the only one of this group to cross the knee joint.

Origin (Figs. 4-21 and 4-48). **Body** and **inferior ramus of pubis**.

Insertion (Fig. 4-26). **Upper quarter of medial surface of tibia,** posterior to sartorius.

Nerve Supply. Anterior division of **obturator** nerve (L2 and L3).

Actions. **Adducts hip joint**, **flexes knee joint**, and **medially rotates leg**.

The Adductor Longus Muscle (Figs. 4-17, 4-18, and 4-20 to 4-24). This triangular muscle is the most anterior of the adductor group. Its medial border forms the medial boundary of the femoral triangle.

Origin (Figs. 4-1, 4-21, and 4-48). Front of **body of pubis**, just below pubic crest.

Insertion (Figs. 4-2 and 4-22). **Middle third of linea aspera** of femur.

Nerve Supply. **Obturator** nerve (L2, L3, and L4).

Actions. **Adducts** and **flexes thigh at hip joint** and can **laterally rotate thigh** at this joint.

The Adductor Brevis Muscle (Figs. 4-17 and 4-23*B*). This short adductor lies deep to the pectineus and adductor longus (long adductor) and anterior to the adductor magnus (large adductor).

Origin (Figs. 4-21, 4-23*B*, and 4-48). **Body** and **inferior ramus of pubis**.

Insertion (Figs. 4-22 and 4-30). **Pectineal line** and **proximal part of linea aspera** of femur.

Nerve Supply. **Obturator** nerve (L2, L3, and L4).

Actions. **Adducts thigh at hip joint**, flexes it to some extent, and **laterally rotates thigh**.

The Adductor Magnus Muscle (Figs. 4-17, 4-23*B*, 4-28, and 4-46). This very large muscle is, as its name implies, the largest of the adductors. Actually it is a composite muscle (part adductor and part hamstring), as indicated by its nerve supply and actions.

Origin (Figs. 4-21, 4-22, and 4-48). **Inferior ramus of pubis**, **ramus of ischium**, and **ischial tuberosity.**

Insertion (Figs. 4-2, 4-21, 4-22, 4-26, and 4-30). Medial side of **gluteal tuberosity**, **linea aspera**, **medial supracondylar line**, and **adductor tubercle** of femur. There is a hiatus (L. an aperture) or opening in the aponeurotic insertion of the adductor magnus to the supracondylar line (Fig. 4-31), called the **tendinous hiatus (adductor hiatus)**, which allows the femoral vessels to pass into the **popliteal fossa**.

Nerve Supply. Posterior division of **obturator** nerve (L2, L3, and L4), except for the vertical "hamstring" part passing from the ischial tuberosity to the adductor tubercle, which is supplied by the tibial part of the **sciatic** nerve (L4).

Actions. Adductor part **adducts thigh at hip joint** and **laterally rotates it**, and *vertical hamstring part* **extends thigh at hip joint**.

The Obturator Externus Muscle (Figs. 4-29, 4-41, 4-47, and 4-116). This flat, fan-shaped muscle is deeply placed in the upper medial part of the thigh and overlies the external surface of the obturator membrane (Fig. 4-110).

Origin (Figs. 4-21 and 4-48). **Margins of**

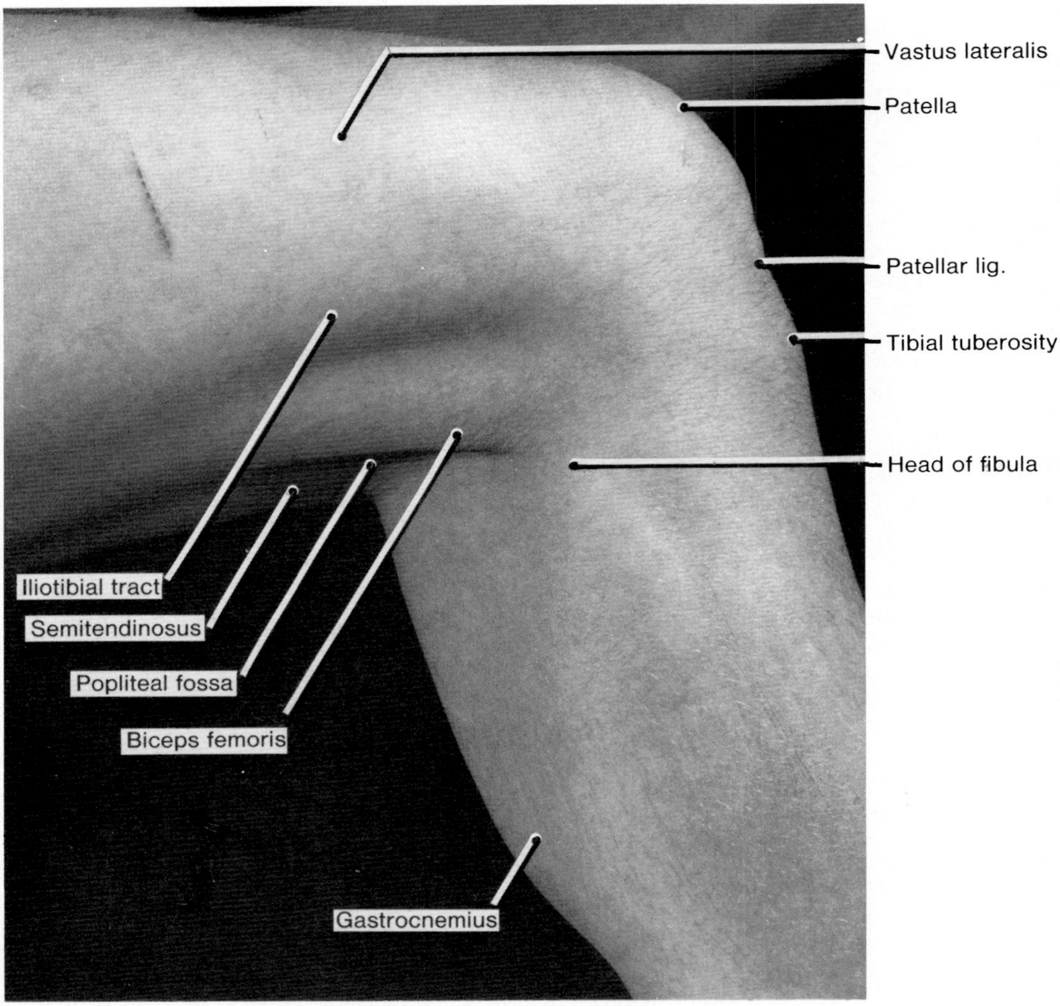

Figure 4-27. Photograph of the lateral aspect of the thigh and the proximal part of the right leg of a 12-year-old girl showing the principal surface features. The quadriceps femoris (rectus femoris and vastus lateralis showing) constitutes the major anterolateral mass of muscle that acts on the knee joint to extend the leg. All four of its parts insert into the base of the patella, which in turn attaches to the tibial tuberosity via the patellar ligament (Figs. 4-23 and 4-26). When this ligament is tapped with a reflex hammer, the quadriceps reflex (knee jerk) is elicited. The biceps femoris tendon may be traced distally and laterally by palpation to its insertion into the head of the fibula, which is on the same level as the tibial tuberosity.

obturator foramen and **obturator membrane**.

Insertion (Fig. 4-30). **Trochanteric fossa** of femur.

Nerve Supply. **Obturator** nerve (L3 and L4).

Action. **Laterally rotates thigh at hip joint**.

CLINICALLY ORIENTED COMMENTS

Occasionally you hear about an athlete with an injury called a "**pulled groin**." This means that there has been a strain, stretching, and probably some tearing away of the tendinous origins of the adductor

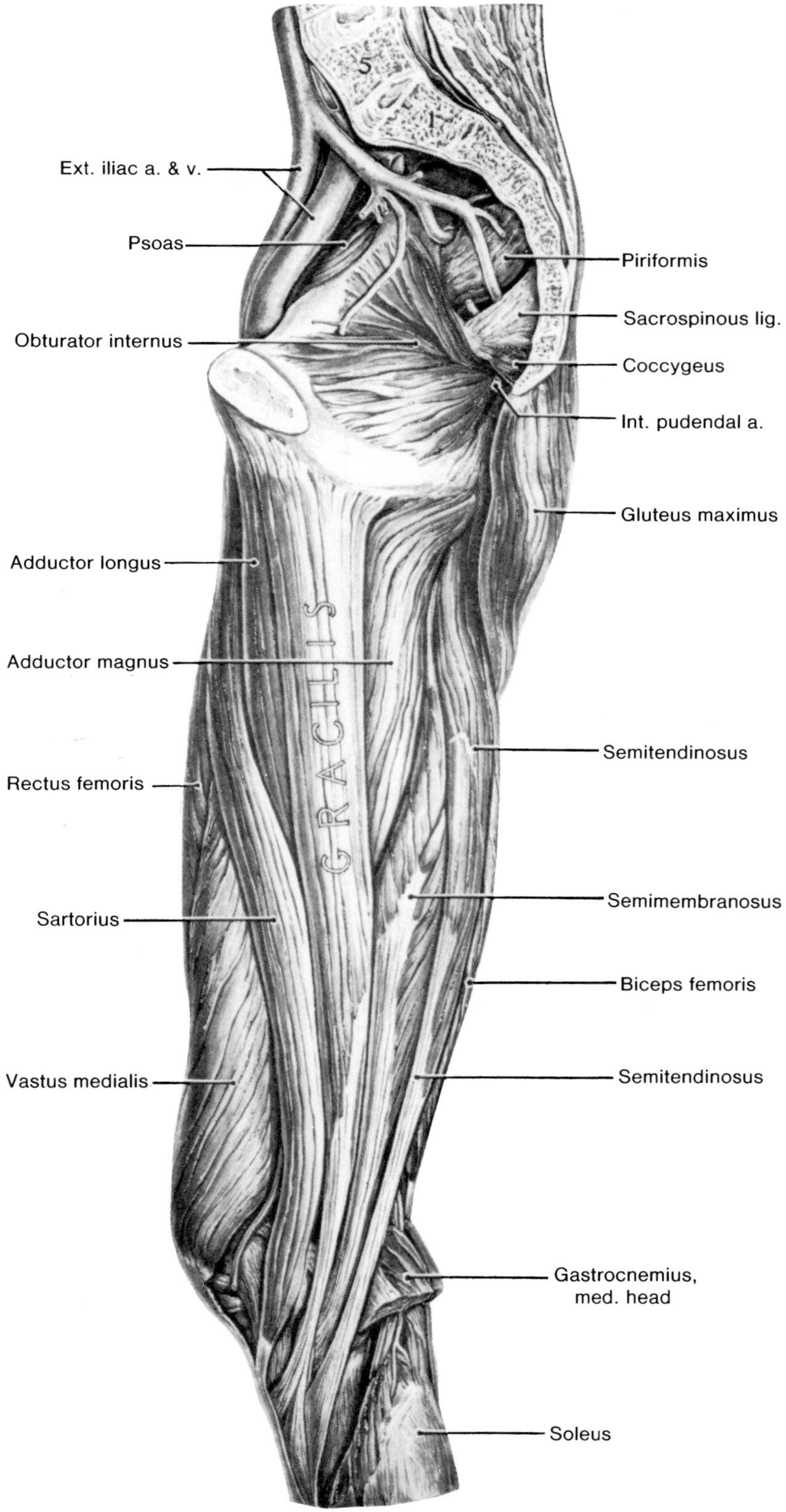

Figure 4-28. Drawing of a dissection of the muscles of the medial side of the right thigh. Observe that the adductor group of muscles forms a large mass that adducts the thigh at the hip joint.

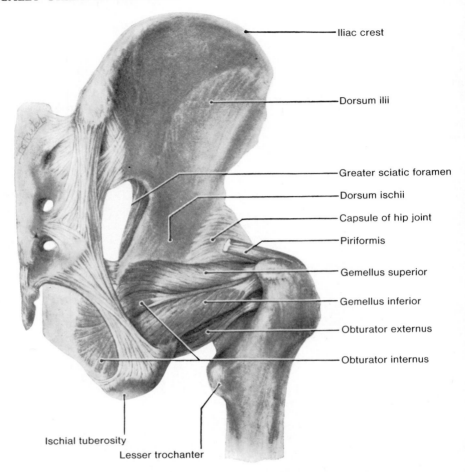

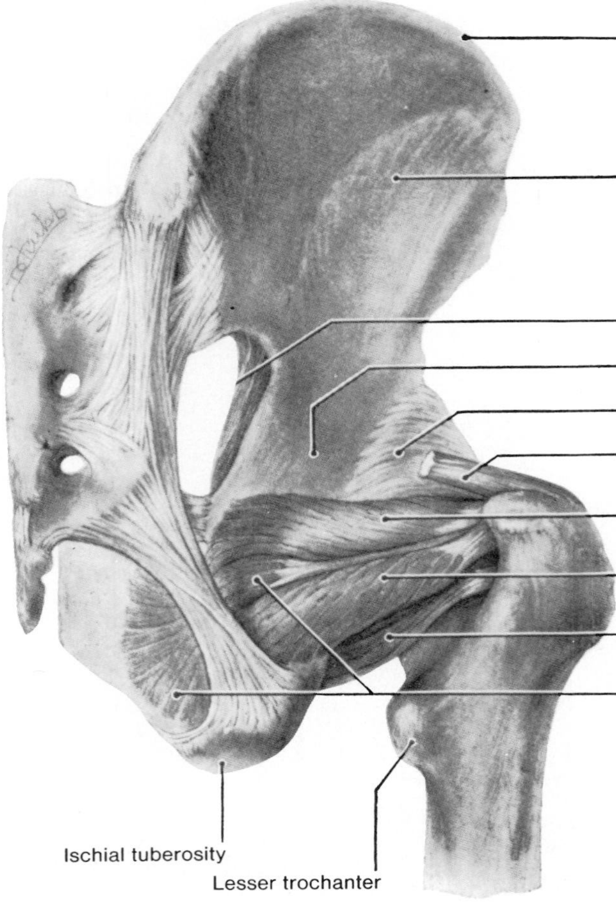

Figure 4-29. Drawing of a dissection of a posterior view of the obturator muscles. Note the inferior end of the ischial tuberosity is at the same level as the lesser trochanter.

group of muscles which arise from the external surfaces of the pubic rami and the ramus of the ischium (Fig. 4-48).

THE FEMORAL TRIANGLE

The femoral triangle is a *clinically important region* in the superomedial part of the thigh that appears as a depression (Fig. 4-24) inferior to the inguinal ligament.

Boundaries of the Femoral Triangle (Figs. 4-18, 4-20, 4-24, 4-32, and 4-33). The femoral triangle is bounded **superiorly** by the **inguinal ligament**, medially by the medial border of the **adductor longus** muscle, and **laterally** by the medial border of the **sartorius** muscle.

The apex of the femoral triangle is located where the medial borders of the sartorius and the adductor longus muscles meet. Note that the apex of this triangle is distal to the point where the femoral vessels pass under the sartorius muscle (Fig. 4-32).

The floor of the femoral triangle is gutter-shaped and is formed medially by the **adductor longus** and **pectineus muscles** and laterally by the iliopsoas muscle (the collective description for the iliacus and psoas muscles). Occasionally a small part of the adductor brevis lies in the floor

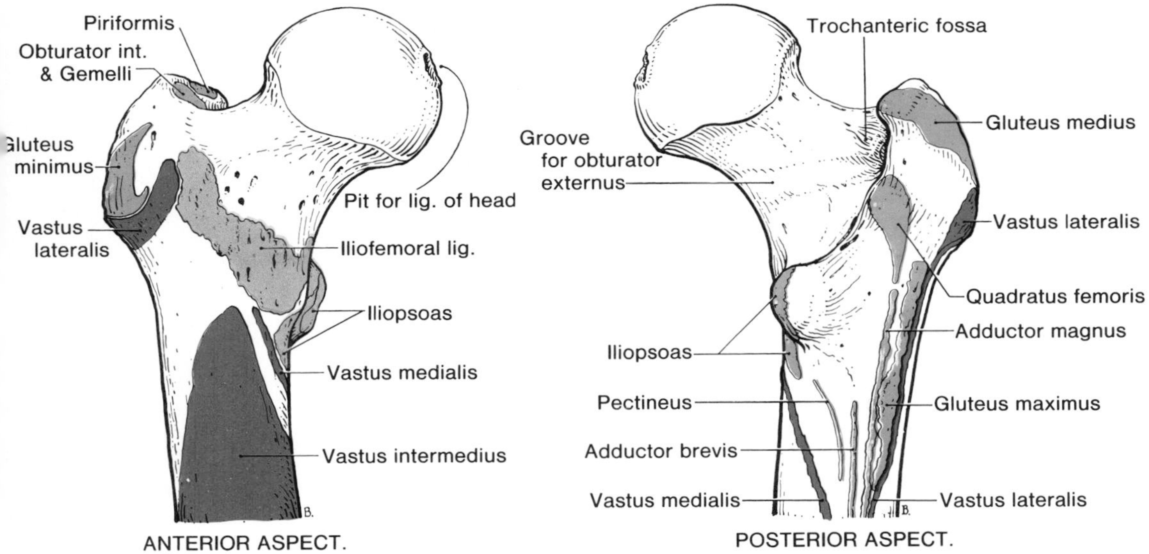

Figure 4-30. Drawing of the proximal end of the right femur showing the sites of attachment of muscles to it.

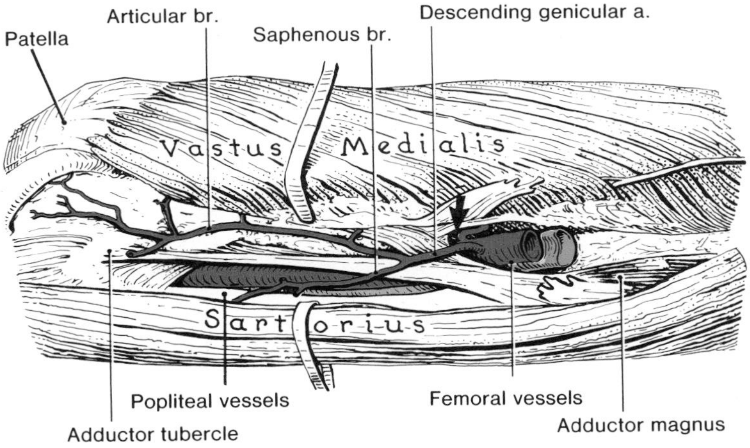

Figure 4-31. Drawing of a dissection of the distal end of the right thigh showing the adductor hiatus or hiatus tendineus (*arrow*) between the insertion of the adductor magnus muscle and the femur. This opening allows the femoral vessels to pass into the popliteal fossa, the diamond-shaped space posterior to the knee joint. Once in this fossa they are known as the popliteal vessels.

of the triangle. **The roof of the femoral triangle** is formed by skin and fasciae (superficial and deep).

Surface Anatomy of the Femoral Triangle (Fig. 4-24). When a person stands with the thigh somewhat flexed, abducted, and laterally rotated, the femoral triangle can be observed as a depression in the proximal third of the thigh. You can easily palpate and often observe its base, the inguinal ligament (Figs. 4-5, 4-24, and 4-32). Its lateral boundary, the medial edge of the

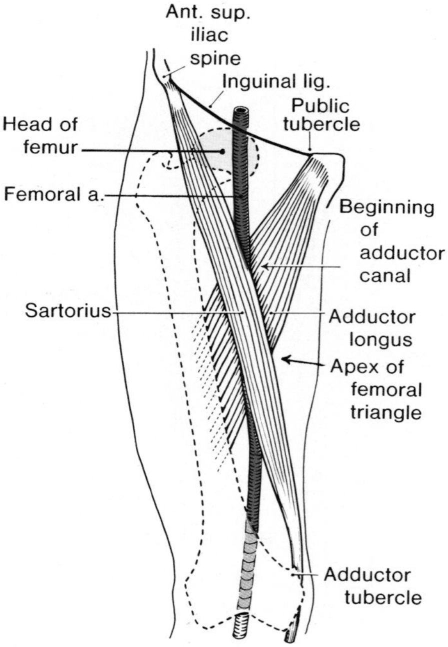

Figure 4-32. Drawing of the upper part of the right thigh showing the boundaries of the femoral triangle. Its base is formed by the inguinal ligament and its sides are formed by the medial border of the sartorius and the medial border of the adductor longus. These two muscles cross each other at the apex of the triangle. Observe the beginning of the adductor canal through which the femoral vessels pass to enter the popliteal fossa (Fig. 4-31). Note that the head of the femur (*yellow*) lies posterior to the femoral artery just inferior to the midpoint of the inguinal ligament; thus, compression of the femoral artery is easily effected at this site.

sartorius, is obvious, but its medial boundary (medial border of adductor longus) is not so easy to identify.

You can easily palpate the **femoral pulse** in the femoral triangle (Fig. 4-32), 2 to 3 cm inferior to the midpoint of the inguinal ligament. The floor of the femoral triangle (Figs. 4-20 and 4-33) becomes firm when the hip is in strong flexion.

Contents of the Femoral Triangle (Figs. 4-18, 4-36, and 4-39). This triangular area contains the **femoral vessels** and the **femoral canal** which are enclosed in the femoral sheath (Fig. 4-19). This triangle also contains the **profunda femoris vessels**, the **femoral nerve**, and some cutaneous nerves.

The Femoral Artery (Figs. 4-18, 4-20, 4-32, 4-34 to 4-37, and 4-40). This large vessel, providing the **chief arterial supply to the lower limb**, is the continuation of the **external iliac artery**. It enters the femoral triangle deep to the midpoint of the inguinal ligament and lateral to the femoral vein. In Figure 4-40 observe that the *femoral artery is under the deep fascia*, whereas the great saphenous vein is in the superficial fascia.

The femoral artery bisects the femoral triangle as it passes to its apex, running deep to the sartorius muscle within the adductor canal (Fig. 4-20). Toward the distal end of the femoral triangle, the femoral artery crosses the femoral vein so that at its apex it lies anterior to it.

The profunda femoris (deep femoral) artery is the largest branch of the femoral artery and is the *chief artery to the thigh.*

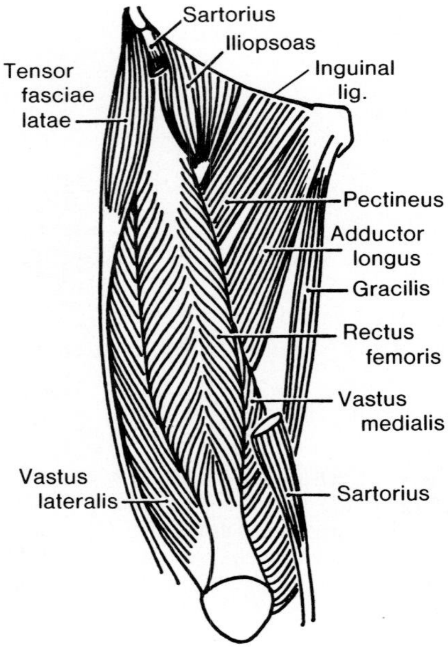

Figure 4-33. Drawing of the muscular floor of the right femoral triangle formed medially by the pectineus and adductor longus muscles and laterally by the ilipsoas muscle. The femoral vessels extend from near the center of the base of the triangle along its gutter-like floor to the apex of the triangle (see Figs. 4-20 and 4-32).

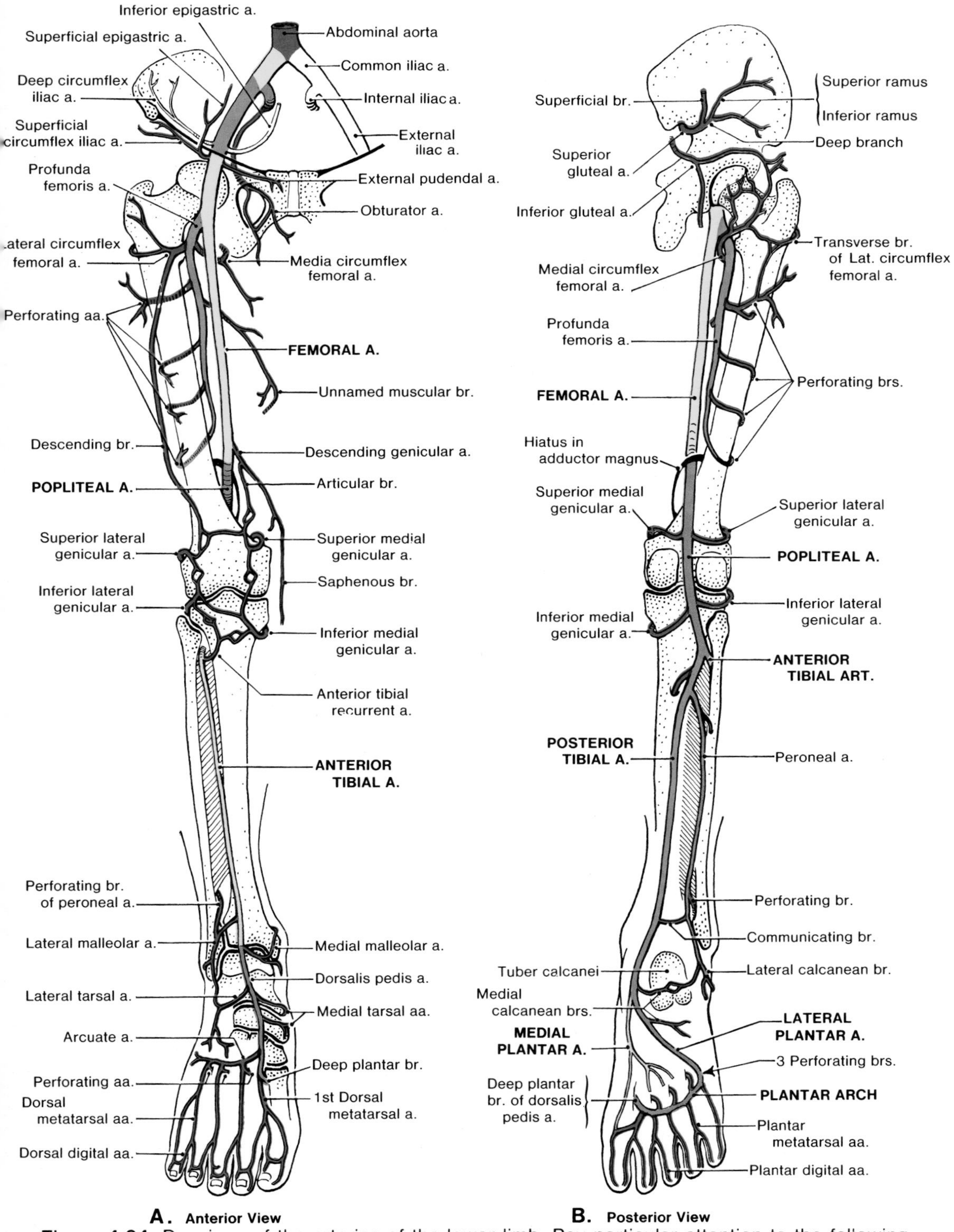

Figure 4-34. Drawings of the arteries of the lower limb. Pay particular attention to the following three substantial arteries: (1) profunda femoris artery; (2) lateral circumflex femoral artery; and (3) medial circumflex femoral artery. In *B*, observe the anastomoses between the internal iliac artery and the femoral artery via the superior and inferior gluteal branches of the internal iliac and the medial and lateral circumflex branches of the profunda femoris. These anastomoses are important in arteriosclerosis of the thigh arteries and in the blood supply of the head and neck of the femur.

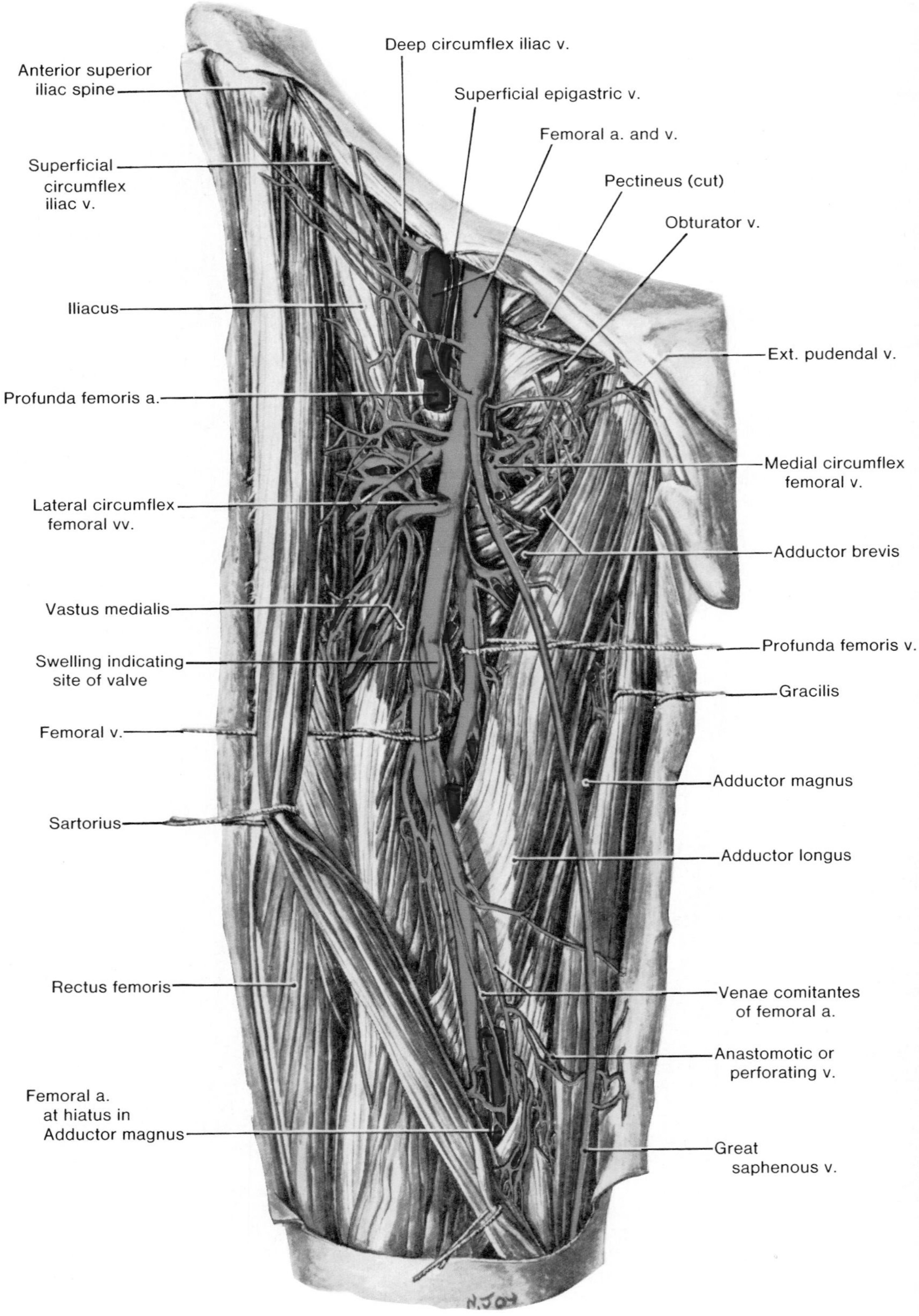

Anterior superior iliac spine
Superficial circumflex iliac v.
Iliacus
Profunda femoris a.
Lateral circumflex femoral vv.
Vastus medialis
Swelling indicating site of valve
Femoral v.
Sartorius
Rectus femoris
Femoral a. at hiatus in Adductor magnus
Deep circumflex iliac v.
Superficial epigastric v.
Femoral a. and v.
Pectineus (cut)
Obturator v.
Ext. pudendal v.
Medial circumflex femoral v.
Adductor brevis
Profunda femoris v.
Gracilis
Adductor magnus
Adductor longus
Venae comitantes of femoral a.
Anastomotic or perforating v.
Great saphenous v.

It arises from the lateral side of the femoral artery within the femoral triangle 3.5 to 4 cm inferior to the inguinal ligament. It runs medial to the femoral artery and then passes posterior to it and the femoral vein. It leaves the femoral triangle between the pectineus and adductor longus muscles (Fig. 4-20) and descends posterior to the latter muscle, giving off *perforating arteries* (Fig. 4-34) which perforate and supply the adductor magnus and hamstring muscles (Fig. 4-37).

The medial and lateral **circumflex femoral arteries** are branches of the profunda femoris that supply the thigh muscles (Fig. 4-34). The **medial circumflex femoral** artery passes deeply between the iliopsoas and pectineus muscles to reach the back of the thigh. This artery is clinically important because it *supplies most of the blood to the head and neck of the femur* (Figs. 4-34*B* and 4-114). The **lateral circumflex femoral** artery passes laterally, deep to the sartorius and rectus femoris muscles, and between the branches of the femoral nerve. Here it divides into branches that supply the muscles on the lateral side of the thigh (Figs. 4-34 and 4-37) and the head of the femur (Fig. 4-114).

CLINICALLY ORIENTED COMMENTS

For left heart or **renal angiography**, a long slender catheter is inserted into the femoral artery as it passes through the femoral triangle, similar to that subsequently described for **catheterization** of the femoral vein.

The superficial position of the femoral artery in the femoral triangle (Fig. 4-18) renders it liable to lacerations or puncture by gunshot wounds. Commonly both the femoral artery and vein are torn owing to their closeness within the femoral sheath. In these cases an **arteriovenous shunt** may occur as the result of communication between the injured vessels. If it is necessary to ligate the femoral artery, blood is supplied to the lower limb by the **cruciate anastomosis**, the union of the medial and lateral circumflex femoral arteries with the inferior gluteal arteries superiorly and the first perforating artery inferiorly (Fig. 4-34). At present, injured or obstructed segments of the femoral artery are commonly replaced by grafts rather than by ligating the proximal part of the vessel.

The Femoral Vein (Figs. 4-18, 4-20, 4-31, and 4-35 to 4-37). This large vessel ends posterior to the inguinal ligament, where it becomes the **external iliac vein**. It leaves the femoral triangle a little medial to the midinguinal point and the femoral artery. In the inferior part of the femoral triangle, the femoral vein lies deep to the femoral artery. While within the femoral triangle the femoral vein receives, as well as other tributaries, the profunda femoris and great saphenous veins (Fig. 4-13).

CLINICALLY ORIENTED COMMENTS

To secure blood samples and take pressure recordings from the right chambers of

Figure 4-35. Drawing of a dissection of the front of the thigh to illustrate the femoral vein. The thigh is rotated laterally at the hip joint. The veins are injected with latex; only stumps of the arteries remain. Note the profunda femoris vein joining the femoral vein inferior to the inguinal ligament. Observe the large size of the lateral circumflex femoral vein, here double and ending in the femoral vein. Note the many long, slender, paired venae comitantes that accompany the various arteries. Observe the superficial circumflex iliac vein, in this specimen receiving the superficial epigastric vein, communicating with the veins proximal and distal to it, and ending both in the great saphenous and femoral veins. Note the great saphenous vein communicating with a vena comitans of the femoral artery and the medial circumflex femoral vein communicating with the obturator vein. Observe the anastomotic or perforating vein (often called a "perforator") connecting the great saphenous and femoral veins via the venae comitantes. These "perforators" are important in the differentiation of the types and in the therapy of varicose veins. (See discussion in text.)

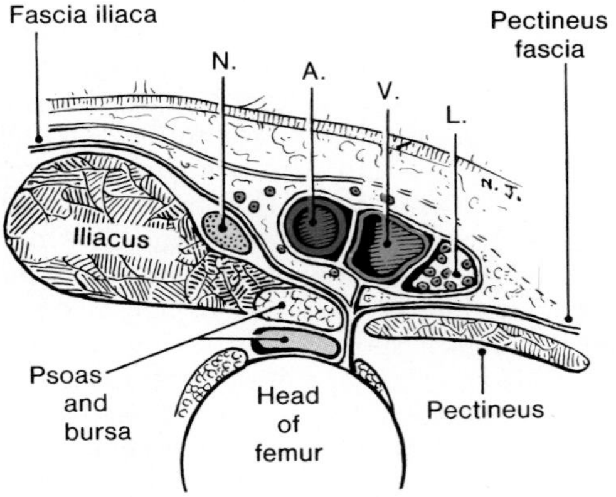

Figure 4-36. Diagram of a horizontal section of the thigh showing the femoral sheath and the relationship of the femoral vessels and the femoral nerve to each other and to the head of the femur. Note that the psoas tendon separates the femoral artery from the head of the femur. From medial to lateral the contents of the femoral sheath are (1) the *femoral canal* containing lymph vessels (*L*); (2) the *femoral vein* (*V*); and (3) the *femoral artery* (*A*). Note that the femoral nerve (*N*) lies under the deep fascia surrounding the iliacus muscle (fascia iliaca), lateral to the femoral sheath.

the heart and/or the pulmonary artery or for right **heart angiography** (serial radiographs of the heart), a long slender catheter is usually inserted into the femoral vein as it passes through the femoral triangle. The catheter is passed under fluoroscopic control through the external and common iliac veins and the inferior vena cava into the right atrium of the heart. A **series of radiographs** is made as a contrast medium is injected into the right atrium. These radiographs *record the passage of the opacified blood* from the right atrium to the right ventricle and to the pulmonary trunk and the right and left pulmonary arteries and their branches. Pressure records are made as the catheter is slowly withdrawn from a small pulmonary artery to a main pulmonary artery, to the right ventricle, and finally into the right atrium.

The Inguinal Lymph Nodes (Figs. 4-36, 4-38, and 4-40). A horizontal group of **superficial inguinal lymph nodes** lies about 2 cm inferior to the inguinal ligament and a vertical group lies along each side of the great saphenous vein. These nodes drain the lower limb, the abdomen (inferior to the umbilicus), the external genitalia, and the anus.

The **deep inguinal lymph** nodes, one to three in number, lie on the medial side of the femoral vein within as well as inferior to the **femoral canal.** In Figure 4-38 observe the free anastomosis between the lymph vessels in the inguinal region. About 24 efferent vessels leave these nodes, pass deep to the inguinal ligament, and enter the external iliac lymph nodes. Of these, less than half tranverse the femoral canal (Fig. 4-36); the others ascend alongside the femoral artery and vein, some inside and some outside the femoral sheath.

CLINICALLY ORIENTED COMMENTS

The superficial inguinal lymph nodes become enlarged in diseases of the parts which their lymph vessels drain. **Minor sepsis** and abrasions of the lower limb produce slight enlargement of these nodes in healthy people.

Malignancies of the external genital organs and perineal abscesses also result in enlargement of the superior group of superficial inguinal lymph nodes, whereas diseases affecting the lower limb produce enlargement of the inferior group of superficial inguinal lymph nodes.

The Femoral Nerve (Figs. 4-18 to 4-20, 4-36, and 4-37). The femoral nerve (L2, L3, and L4), the **largest branch of the lumbar plexus**, forms in the substance of the psoas major muscle. It descends posteriorly to the midpoint of the inguinal ligament, lateral to the femoral vessels and outside the **femoral sheath** (Figs. 4-36 and 4-117). After passing distally about 3 cm in the femoral triangle, the femoral nerve breaks up into several terminal branches to supply the muscles of the front of the thigh and articular branches to the hip and knee joints. It gives off several cutaneous branches which are distributed to skin on the anteromedial side of the lower limb (Figs. 4-14 and 4-18).

The saphenous nerve is regarded as the termination of the femoral nerve. It descends through the femoral triangle, lateral to the femoral sheath containing the femoral vessels. It *accompanies the femoral artery in the adductor canal* (Fig. 4-37) and then descends into the leg and the medial side of the foot to supply the overlying skin (Figs. 4-12*B*, 4-14, and 4-106).

THE FEMORAL SHEATH

The femoral sheath is an oval, funnel-shaped, **fascial tube** that encloses the femoral vessels and the femoral canal (Figs. 4-16, 4-19, 4-39, and 4-117). It is a diverticulum or downward prolongation of the fasciae lining the abdomen (transversalis fascia anteriorly and iliac fascia posteriorly). The femoral sheath is covered distally by the **fascia lata** (deep fascia of the thigh, Fig. 4-19).

The femoral sheath is bounded medially by the concave margin of the **lacunar ligament** (Fig. 4-40) and ends about 4 cm inferior to the inguinal ligament, where it is continuous with the adventitia of the femoral vessels.

Compartments of the Femoral Sheath (Figs. 4-36, 4-39, 4-40 and 4-117). The femoral sheath is subdivided by two vertical septa or partitions into **three compartments**: (1) a **lateral compartment** for the *femoral artery*; (2) an intermediate compartment for the *femoral vein*; and (3) a **medial compartment** (the **femoral canal**) for lymph vessels and a lymph node embedded in areolar tissue.

The Femoral Canal (Figs. 4-36, 4-39, and 4-40). This conical, **medial compartment of the femoral sheath** is short (about 1.25 cm.). Presumably it allows the femoral vein to expand. It contains lymph vessels, a lymph node, loose areolar tissue, and fat. It is widest at its abdominal end and extends distally to the level of the proximal end of the **saphenous opening** (Fig. 4-16).

The femoral ring (Fig. 4-40) is the small proximal end or *abdominal opening (mouth) of the femoral canal.* It is closed by extraperitoneal tissue called the **femoral septum**, which is pierced by the lymph vessels connecting the deep inguinal and the external iliac lymph nodes. There is also a lymph node (gland of Cloquet) at the femoral ring.

The boundaries of the femoral ring are: *laterally*, the **femoral vein**; *posteriorly*, the **superior ramus of the pubic bone** covered by the pectineus and its fascia; *medially*, the **lacunar ligament** and the conjoint tendon; and *anteriorly*, the **inguinal ligament** and the spermatic cord.

The **lacunar ligament** is composed of fibers from the posteromedial part of the inguinal ligament which pass posteriorly to the **pecten pubis** (pectineal line, Figs. 4-1 and 4-18). The continuation of these fibers laterally along the pecten pubis forms the **pectineal ligament** (Fig. 4-41).

CLINICALLY ORIENTED COMMENTS

The femoral ring is a weak point in the abdominal wall that normally admits the tip of the little finger. This is important in understanding the mechanism of femoral hernia, which is a protrusion of abdominal viscera (often small intestine) through the femoral ring into the femoral canal (Case 4-8). The normal contents of the femoral canal (lymph vessels, a small lymph node, and areolar tissue) are easily compressed to allow passage of the herniated material.

A femoral hernia can usually be palpated just inferior to the inguinal ligament. Initially it is relatively small because it is contained within the femoral canal, but it may enlarge by passing inferiorly through the saphenous opening (Fig. 4-16) into the loose areolar tissue of the thigh (Fig. 4-155).

Strangulation of a femoral hernia may occur owing to the sharpness and rigidness of the boundaries of the femoral ring, particularly the concave margin of the lacunar ligament. *Strangulation interferes with the blood supply* to the herniated bowel and this vascular impairment may result in death of the tissues concerned. Because the distal end of the femoral canal reaches the proximal part of the saphenous opening in the fascia lata (Fig. 4-40), a femoral hernia may herniate through the cribriform fascia and bulge anteriorly under the skin over the saphenous opening.

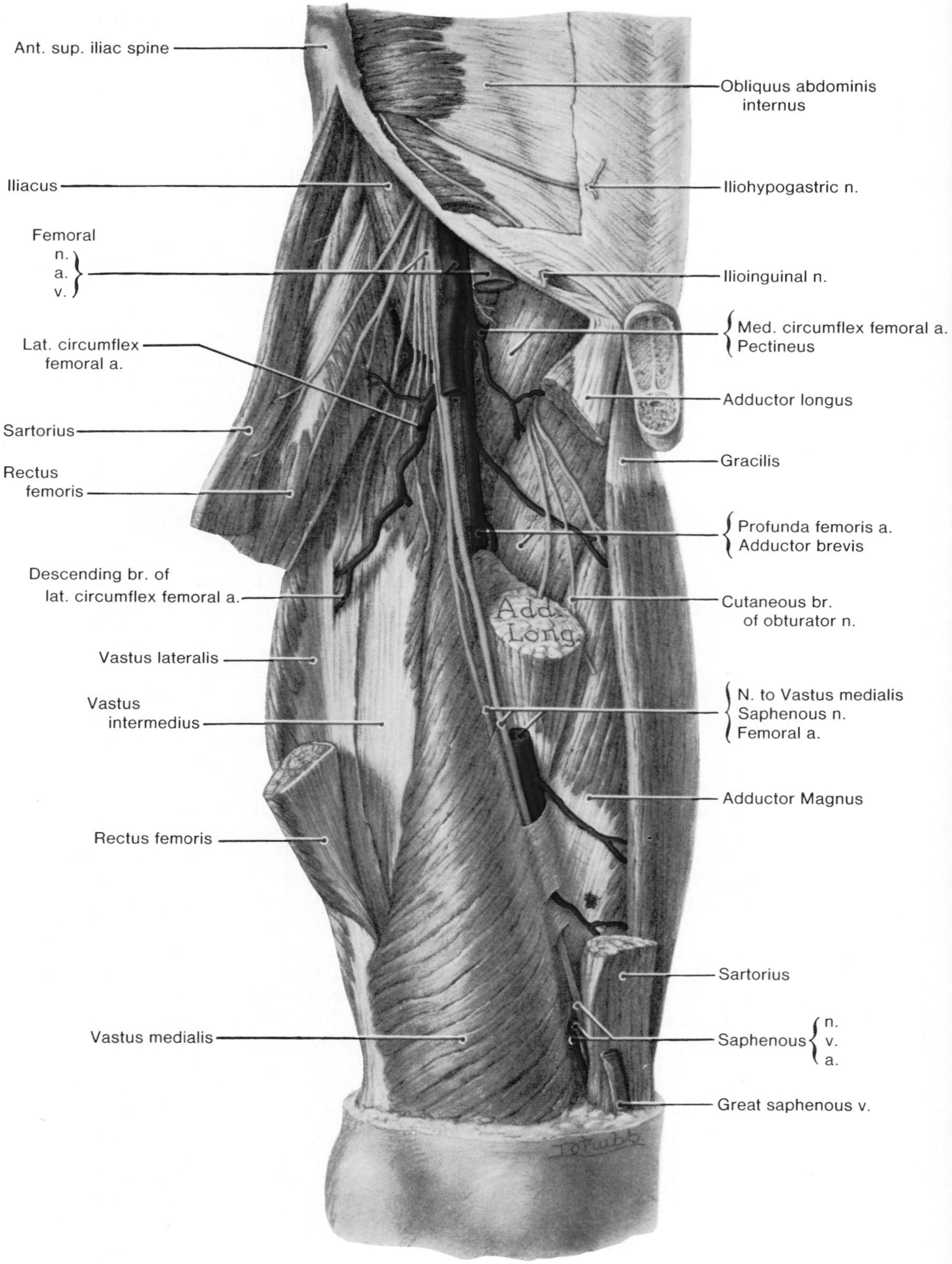

Ant. sup. iliac spine
Obliquus abdominis internus
Iliacus
Iliohypogastric n.
Femoral n. a. v.
Ilioinguinal n.
Med. circumflex femoral a.
Pectineus
Lat. circumflex femoral a.
Adductor longus
Sartorius
Gracilis
Rectus femoris
Profunda femoris a.
Adductor brevis
Descending br. of lat. circumflex femoral a.
Add. Long.
Cutaneous br. of obturator n.
Vastus lateralis
N. to Vastus medialis
Saphenous n.
Femoral a.
Vastus intermedius
Adductor Magnus
Rectus femoris
Sartorius
Saphenous n. v. a.
Vastus medialis
Great saphenous v.

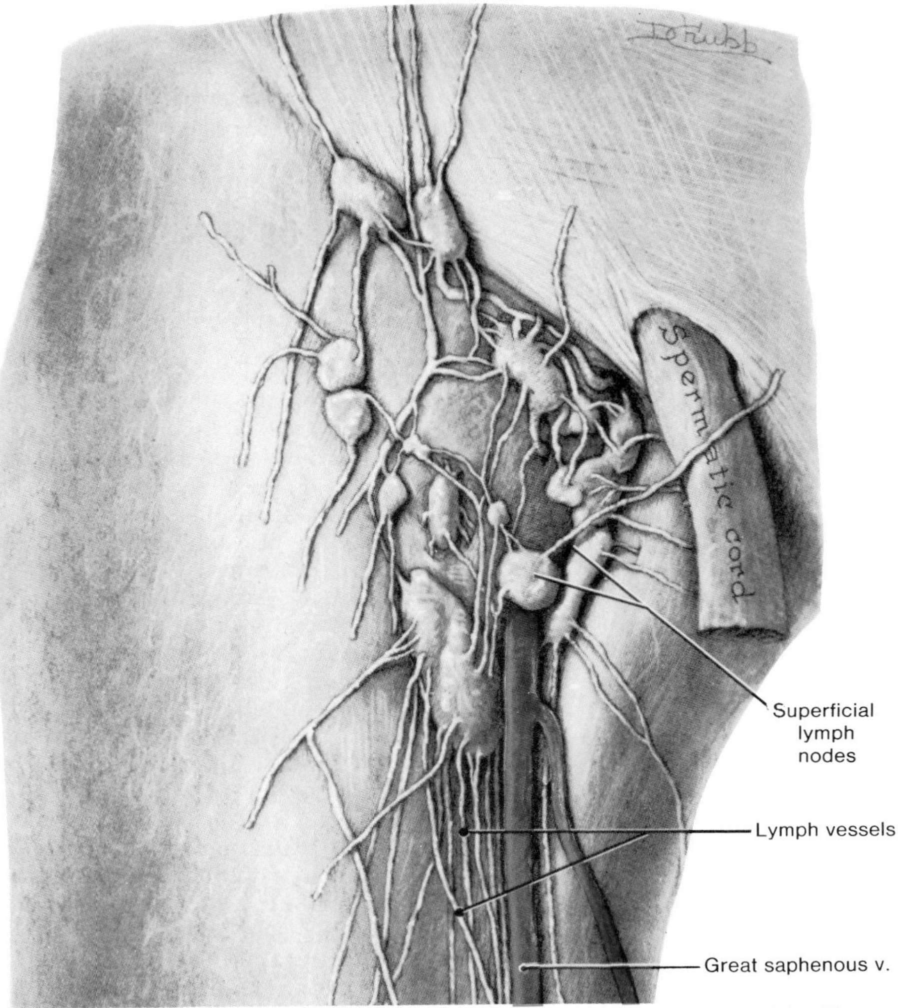

Figure 4-38. Drawing of a dissection of the inguinal lymph nodes on the right side. Observe (1) a proximal chain parallel to the inguinal ligament (*superficial inguinal nodes*); (2) a distal chain along the sides of the great saphenous vein (*superficial subinguinal nodes*); and (3) more deeply, a chain of two or three nodes on the medial side of the femoral vein (*deep inguinal nodes*), one being below the femoral canal and one or two within it. Minor sepsis (*e.g.*, presence of pus-forming organisms) and abrasions of the lower limb are so common that it is not unusual to find enlarged (*i.e.*, palpable) inguinal lymph nodes in healthy people.

Figure 4-37. Drawing of a dissection of the front of the right thigh and adductor region. The limb is rotated laterally. Observe the femoral nerve breaking up into a leash of nerves on entering the thigh. Note the femoral artery lying between two motor territories, namely, that of the obturator nerve which is medial and that of the femoral nerve which is lateral. Observe that no motor nerve crosses anterior to the femoral artery, but the twig to the pectineus is seen crossing posterior to it. Note that the nerve to vastus medialis and the saphenous nerve accompany the femoral artery into the adductor canal. Observe the saphenous nerve and artery and their companion anastomotic vein emerging from the lower end of this canal and becoming superficial between the sartorius and gracilis muscles. Note the profunda femoris artery arising about 4 cm below the inguinal ligament, lying behind the femoral artery, and disappearing behind the adductor longus muscle.

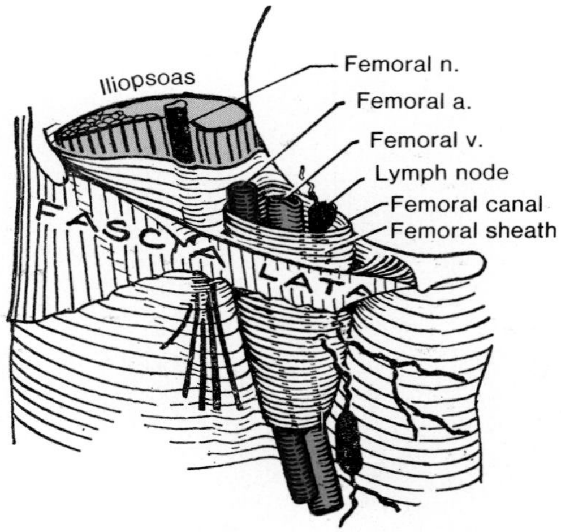

Figure 4-39. Drawing of the upper part of the thigh showing the femoral sheath. Note that this fascial wrapping for the femoral vessels and the femoral canal is funnel-shaped and has three compartments: a lateral one for the femoral artery, a middle one for the femoral vein, and a medial one (the femoral canal) for lymph vessels and a lymph node.

A femoral hernia presents as a mass inferolateral to the pubic tubercle and medial to the femoral vein. This type of hernia is more common in women than men largely because the femoral ring is larger owing to the greater breadth of the female pelvis.

The **obturator artery**, a branch of the internal iliac (Fig. 4-34*A*), passes through the obturator foramen to supply adjacent muscles. A posterior branch also supplies the hip joint and the ligament of the head of the femur (Fig. 4-113). In 20 to 30% of persons, an enlarged pubic branch of the **inferior epigastric artery** takes the place of the obturator artery or forms an abnormal **accessory obturator artery** (Fig. 4-42). This artery runs close to or across the femoral ring to reach the obturator foramen (canal) and is therefore closely related to the free margin of the lacunar ligament and the neck of a femoral hernia. This artery could be involved in strangulation of the hernia, but the important concern is its *vulnerability to damage during femoral hernial repair.*

THE ADDUCTOR CANAL

The adductor (subsartorial) canal is a narrow **fascial tunnel** (Fig. 4-20), deep to the sartorius muscle in the middle one-third of the medial part of the thigh, through which the **femoral vessels** pass into the popliteal fossa (Figs. 4-31 and 4-32) to become the popliteal vessels (Fig. 4-58).

The adductor canal *begins near the apex of the femoral triangle* inferior to the inguinal ligament, where the sartorius muscle crosses over the adductor longus muscle (Figs. 4-20 and 4-32) and *ends at the tendinous opening or adductor hiatus* in the tendon of the adductor magnus (Fig. 4-31).

Boundaries of the Adductor Canal (Figs. 4-18, 4-20, and 4-37). It is bounded laterally by the **vastus medialis,** posteromedially by the **adductor longus** and **adductor magnus,** and anteriorly by the **sartorius.** The sartorius and the subsartorial fascia form the roof of the adductor canal (Fig. 4-17); hence, this canal is *often called the subsartorial canal.* The adductor canal, about 15 cm in length, is an intermuscular tunnel that is triangular on cross-section with its apex posterior.

Contents of the Adductor Canal (Figs. 4-17, 4-20, 4-31, and 4-37). The **femoral vessels** enter the adductor canal near the apex of the femoral triangle, the vein lying posterior to the artery. The femoral artery and vein leave the adductor canal through the **adductor hiatus**, the tendinous opening in the adductor magnus. When the femoral artery enters the **popliteal fossa** it is called the **popliteal artery**; similarily, the femoral vein becomes the popliteal vein.

In Figure 4-20 observe that the profunda femoris artery and vein do not enter the adductor canal. The perforating branches of these deep vessels pierce the fibers of the adductor muscles to reach the posterior aspect of the thigh (Figs. 4-18 and 4-34).

The **saphenous nerve**, a cutaneous branch of the femoral nerve to the leg, accompanies the femoral vessels throughout the adductor canal (Fig. 4-20). It enters lateral to the vessels, crosses them anteriorly, and lies medial to them at the distal end of the canal (Fig. 4-37). The saphenous

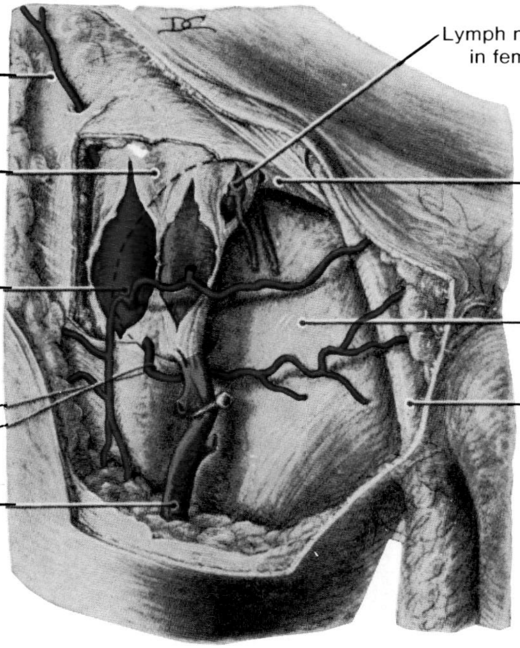

Figure 4-40. Drawing of a dissection of the upper part of the right thigh showing the femoral sheath, canal, and ring. The falciform edge of the saphenous opening or hiatus is cut away. Note the superior horn (cornu) of the opening passing toward the pubic tubercle and blending with the inguinal ligament and with the lacunar ligament. Observe the medial border of the opening formed by the fascia covering the pectineus muscle and as such passing laterally behind the femoral sheath. Note the three compartments of the sheath: (1) the lateral one for the artery; (2) the intermediate one for the vein; and (3) the medial one, called the femoral canal, for lymph vessels. Observe the proximal end of the femoral canal, called the femoral ring, bounded medially by the lacunar ligament, anteriorly by the inguinal ligament, posteriorly by the pectineal fascia, and laterally by the femoral vein. It is into the femoral canal that a hernia may bulge from above as in Case 4-8.

nerve does not leave the adductor canal by passing through the adductor hiatus; it emerges posterior to the sartorius muscle and anterior to the adductor magnus tendon. It pierces the deep fascia on the medial aspect of the knee and passes down the medial side of the leg with the saphenous vein (Fig. 4-14).

The **nerve to the vastus medialis** accompanies the femoral artery through the proximal part of the adductor canal (Figs. 4-20 and 4-37) and divides into branches that supply the muscle and the knee joint.

CLINICALLY ORIENTED COMMENTS

John Hunter, a Scottish anatomist and surgeon (1728 to 1793), was the first person to ligate the femoral artery in the adductor canal to reduce pressure in the vessel and its continuation when there was an **aneurysm** (circumscribed dilation) in the popliteal artery (Fig. 4-62). For this reason the adductor canal used to be referred to as Hunter's canal.

THE GLUTEAL REGION

The gluteal region of the thigh is bounded superiorly by the **iliac crest** and inferiorly by the inferior border of the **gluteus maximus** muscle, which forms the gluteal fold (Figs. 4-7 and 4-10). *The gluteal region is largely formed by the large gluteus maximus* muscle, which is superficially

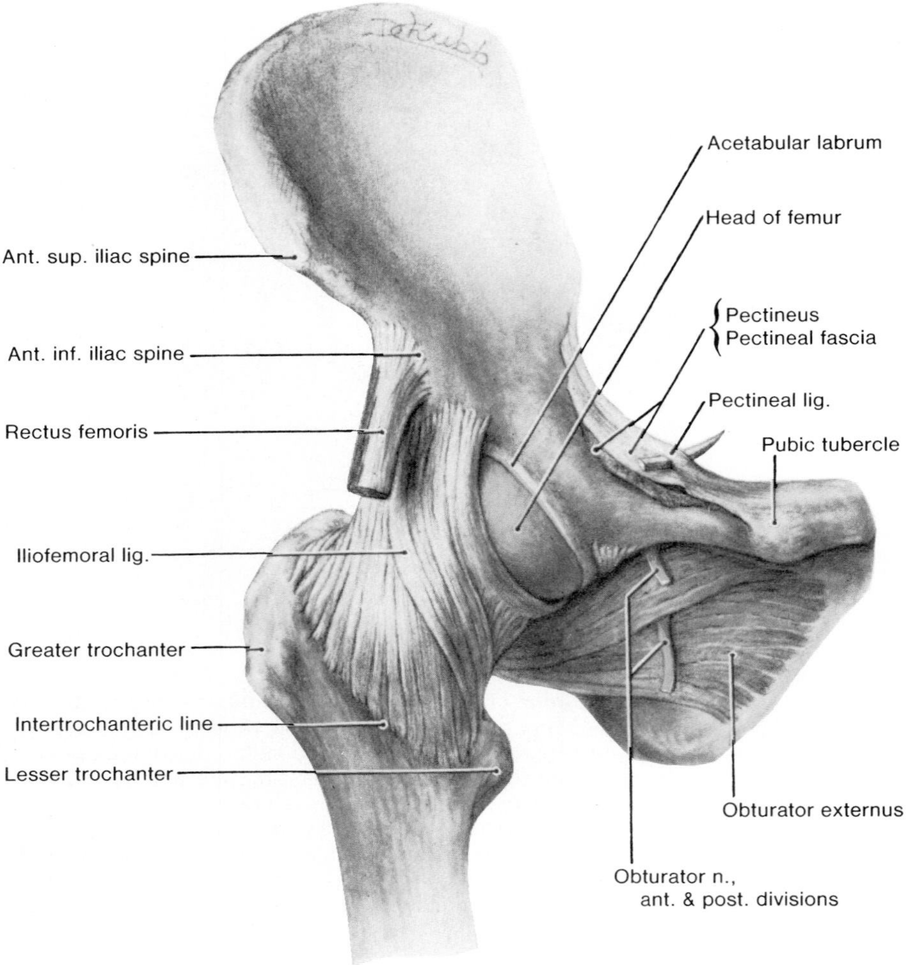

Figure 4-41. Drawing of a dissection of the right hip joint from the front. Observe the head of the femur exposed just medial to the iliofemoral ligament and facing not only upward and medially, but also forward. Note the obturator externus muscle crossing obliquely below the neck of the femur. Observe the thinness of the pectineus muscle and the blending of its fascia with the pectineal ligament along the pecten pubis (see this sharp ridge in Fig. 4-1).

located in the buttock (Fig. 4-45). The terms gluteal region, buttock ("butt"), nates, clunis, and "rump" all refer to the same area, although the term buttock is sometimes used wrongly to refer only to the prominence formed by the gluteus maximus muscle.

Bony Landmarks (Figs. 4-1, 4-2, 4-6, 4-7, 4-10, and 4-43). Refer to the various figures and to an articulated skeleton and revise your knowledge of the following: iliac crest, anterior superior iliac spine, greater sciatic notch, lesser sciatic notch, ischial spine, and posterior superior iliac spine.

Palpate your anterior and posterior **superior iliac spines** and your iliac crest. The posterior spines are somewhat difficult to feel but they always lie deep to the skin dimples in the lower back (Figs. 4-6 and 5-11).

Ligaments of the Gluteal Region (Fig. 4-44). The region between the sacrum and the bony pelvis is bridged by two important accessory ligaments of the sacroiliac joint

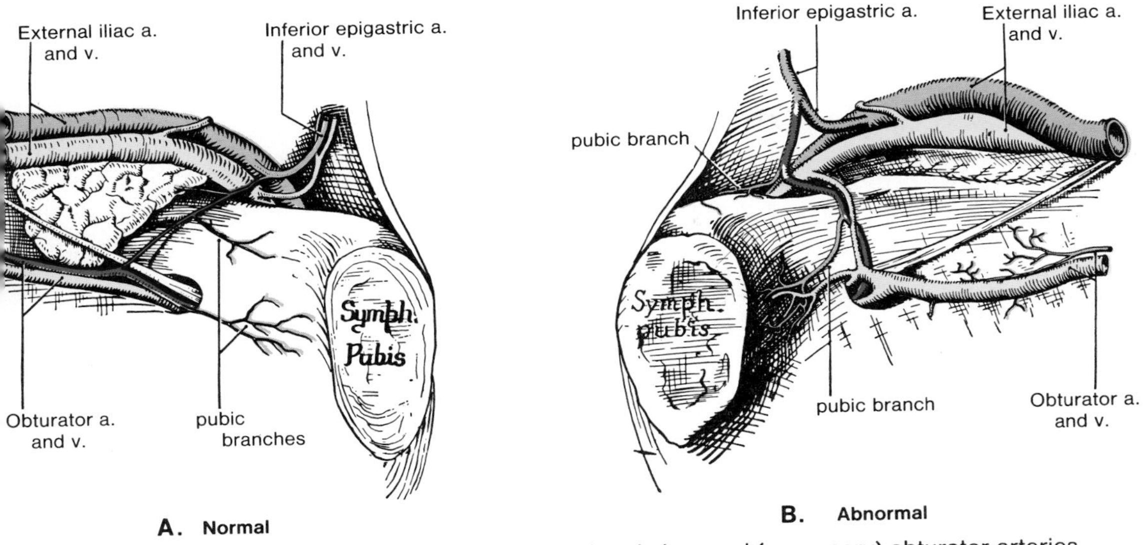

Figure 4-42. Drawing of dissections showing normal and abnormal (accessory) obturator arteries. In *B* the obturator artery arises from the inferior epigastric via the pubic anastomoses.

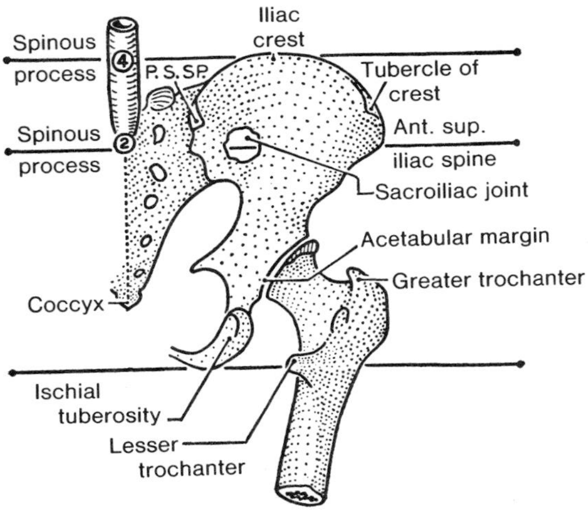

Figure 4-43. Drawing illustrating the bony landmarks of the gluteal region. The iliac crest is palpable because neither muscle nor tendon crosses it. The tubercle of the crest lies at the most lateral part of the crest and is the highest part visible from the front. A line joining the highest points on the iliac crests crosses the fourth lumbar spinous process and serves as a guide to it. A line joining the posterior superior iliac spines (*PSSp.*) crosses the second sacral spinous process and marks the bottom of the dural and arachnoid sacs containing cerebrospinal fluid. The top of the greater trochanter lies 9 to 10 cm below the tubercle of the iliac crest. Observe that a line drawn horizontally at the level of the ischial tuberosity crosses the lesser trochanter of the femur. Because you sit on your ischial tuberosities, it follows that the coccyx does not descend so far as the tuberosities. (See Figs. 4-7 and 4-10 also.)

called the **sacrotuberous** and **sacrospinous ligaments**. They close the sciatic notches of the os coxae (Fig. 4-2) producing the greater and lesser sciatic foramina (Fig. 4-44). The **greater sciatic foramen** is primarily a doorway for structures entering or leaving the pelvis (*e.g.*, the sciatic nerve), whereas the **lesser sciatic foramen** is a doorway for structures entering or leaving the perineum (*e.g.*, the pudendal nerve), the region between the thighs (Fig. 3-2).

The greater and lesser sciatic notches are separated by a beak-like process, the **ischial spine**, which gives attachment to the sacrospinous ligament (Fig. 4-44).

The Sacrotuberous Ligament (Figs. 4-44, 4-47, and 4-52). This long band extends from the posterior superior and posterior inferior iliac spines and the dorsum and sides of the sacrum and coccyx to the ischial tuberosity. Using Figures 4-44 to 4-46, verify that this ligament is in the same vertical line as the long head of the biceps femoris and semitendinosus muscles. The two *sac-*

rotuberous ligaments resist backward rotation of the inferior end of the sacrum and provide an origin for the gluteus maximus muscles.

The Sacrospinous Ligament (Fig. 4-44). This is a triangular connective tissue sheet that is sandwiched between the sacrotuberous ligament and the coccygeus muscle. Coextensive with the coccygeus, it extends from the ischial spine to the inferolateral border of the sacrum and coccyx (Fig. 3-18).

Muscles of the Gluteal Region (Figs. 4-7, 4-10, and 4-44 to 4-47). Most of the mass of the buttock is formed by the **gluteus maximus** muscle which overlies the

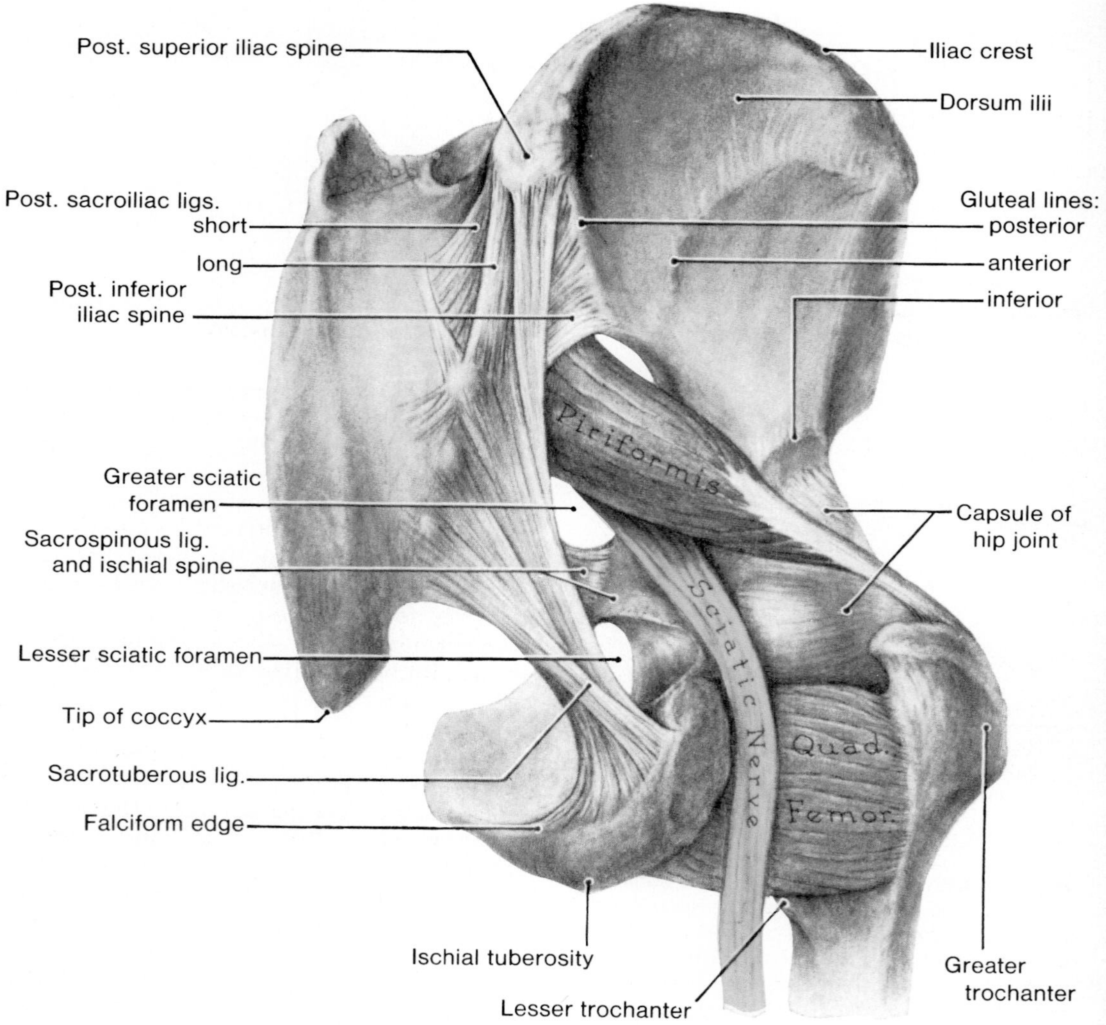

Figure 4-44. Drawing of a posterior view of the bony and ligamentous parts of the right gluteal region. Observe that the tip of the coccyx lies above the level of the ischial tuberosity and below that of the ischial spine. Note that the lower border of the piriformis muscle is defined by joining the midpoint between the tip of the coccyx and the posterior superior iliac spine to the top of the greater trochanter. Observe that the lower border of the quadratus femoris muscle is level with the inferior end of the ischial tuberosity and that it crosses the lesser trochanter of the femur. Note that the lateral border of the sciatic nerve lies midway between the lateral surface of the greater trochanter and the medial surface of the ischial tuberosity when the body is in the anatomical position (see Fig. 4-10 also).

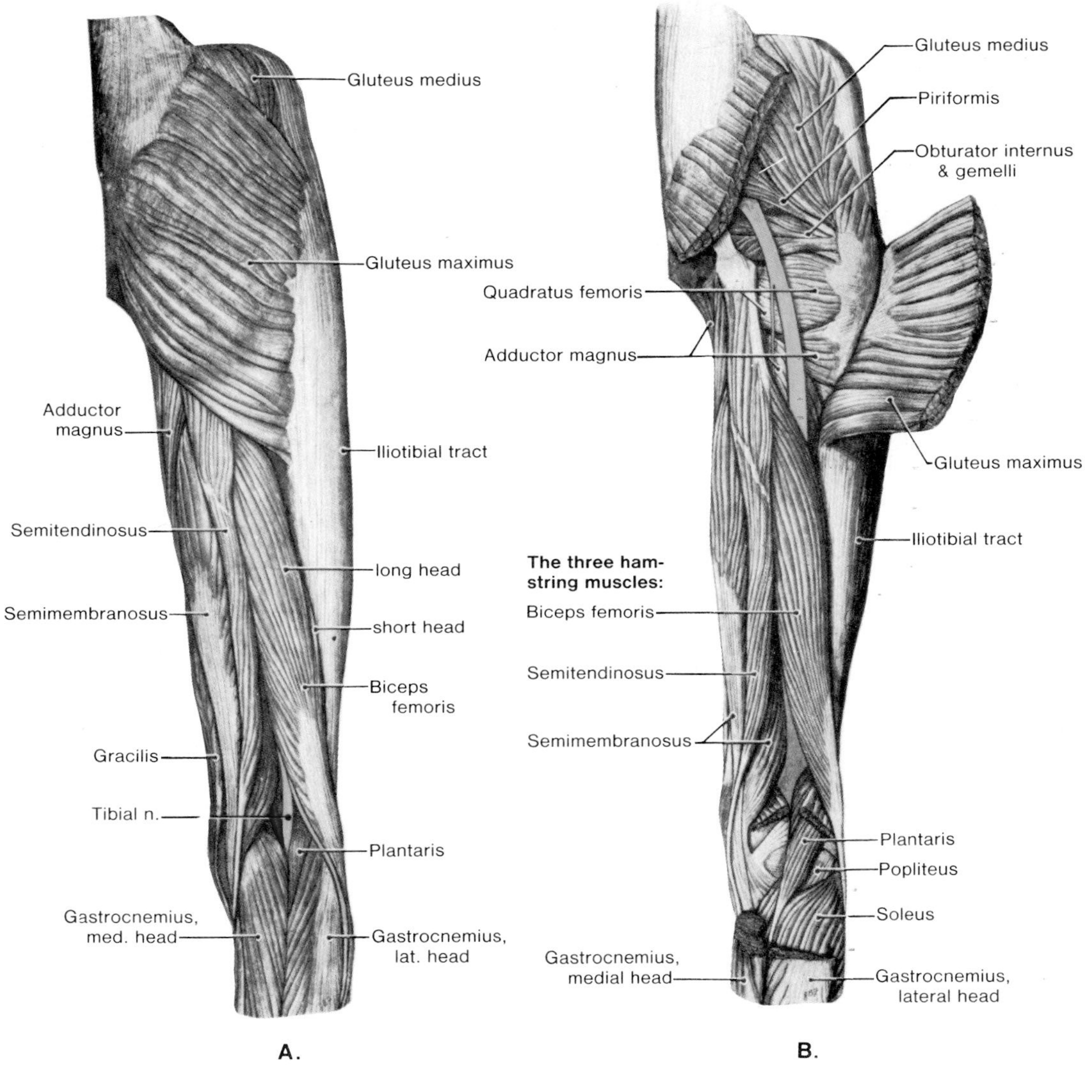

Figure 4-45. Drawings of dissections of the right gluteal region and the back of the thigh showing the muscles. In *B* observe that the large gluteus maximus muscle overlies the sciatic nerve and several other muscles.

sciatic nerve (Fig. 4-45*B*) and a number of muscles named from above downward as follows: gluteus medius, piriformis, superior gemellus, obturator internus, inferior gemellus, quadratus femoris, and adductor magnus. Deep to the gluteus medius is the gluteus minimus which fills in the gap between the greater trochanter of the femur and the wing of the ilium that is bridged by the gluteus medius.

The Gluteus Maximus Muscle (Figs. 4-10 and 4-45 to 4-47). The gluteus maximus is the largest, heaviest, and most coarsely fibered muscle in the body. It forms a thick, quadrilateral pad over the **ischial tuberosity** when the thigh is extended. This tuberosity can be felt on deep palpation through the distal portion of the gluteus maximus just superior to the medial portion of the gluteal fold (Fig. 4-10). When the thigh is flexed, the distal border of the gluteus maximus moves up off the ischial tuberosity leaving it subcutaneous.

Many people have the mistaken idea that

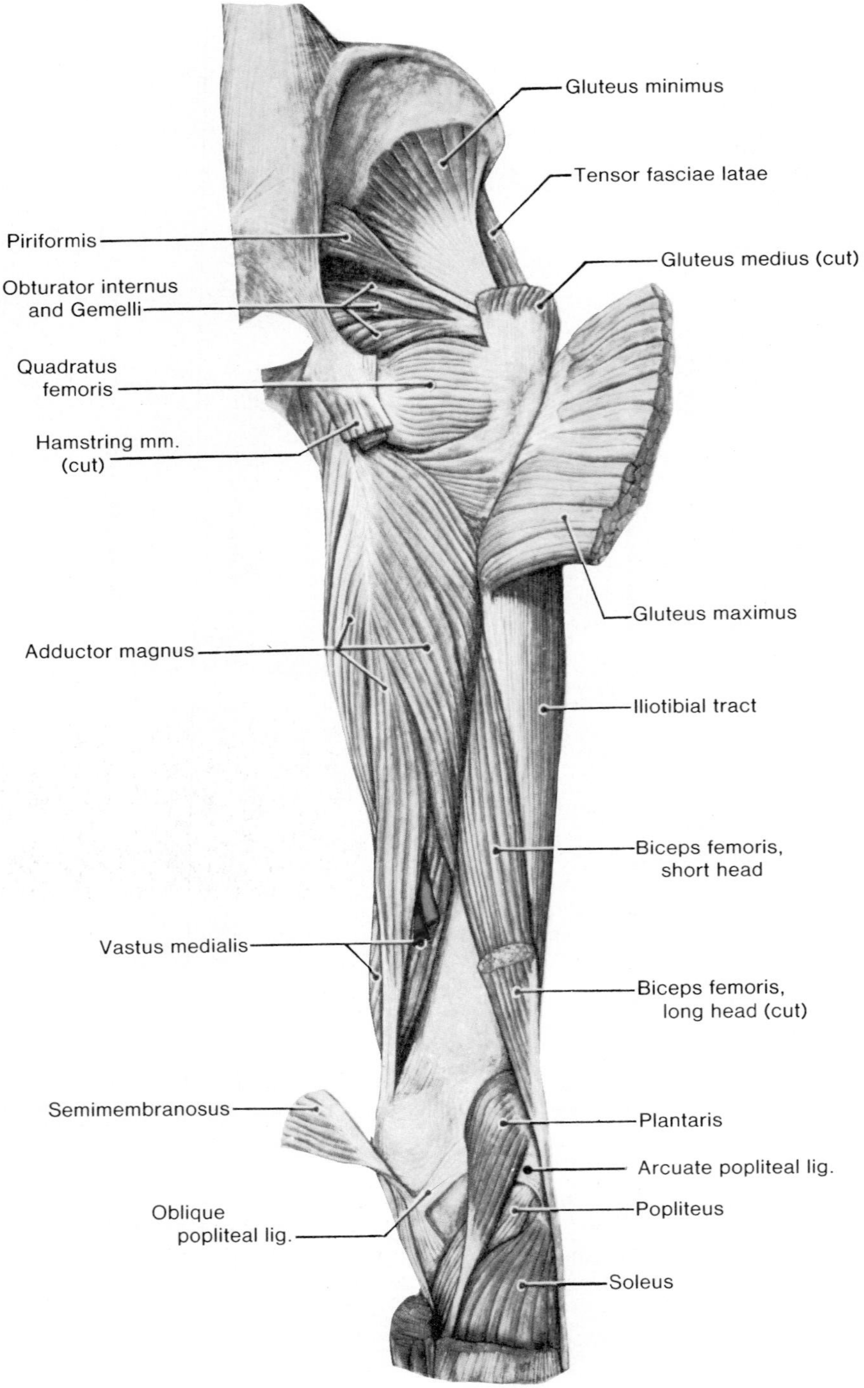

Figure 4-46. Drawing of a deep dissection of the muscles of the right gluteal region and the back of the thigh. Most of the hamstring muscles have been cut and reflected to show the adductor magnus muscle from behind.

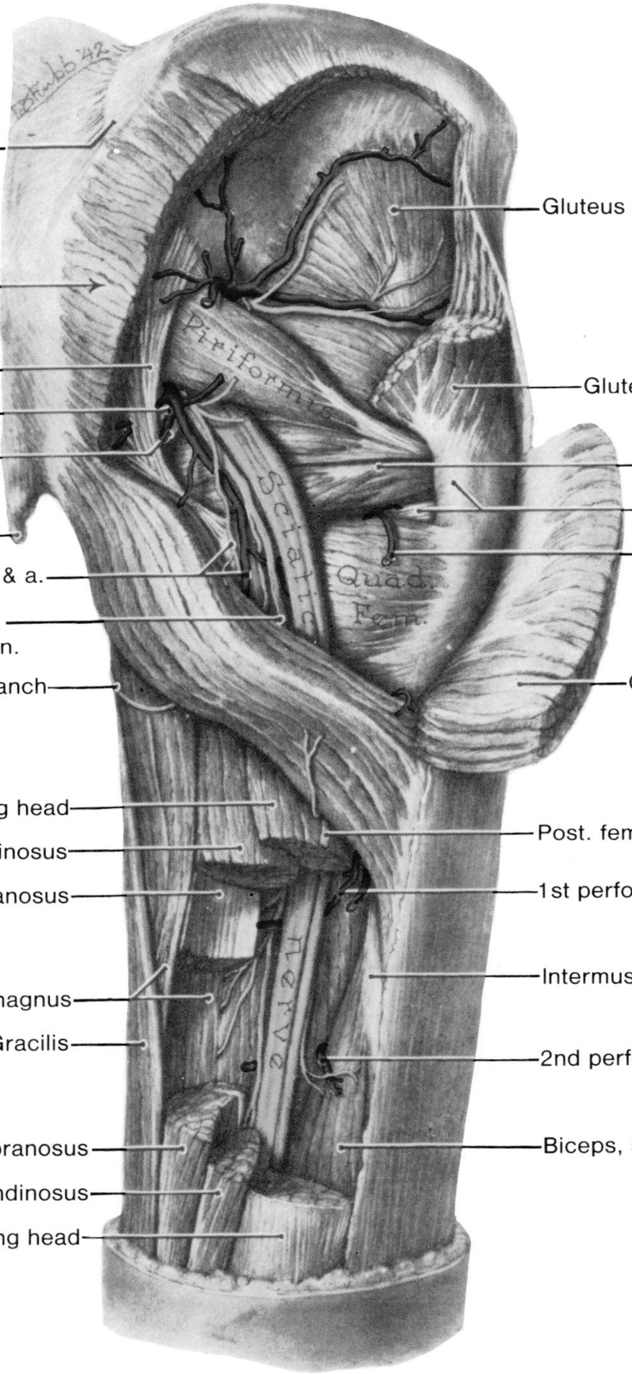

Figure 4-47. Drawing of a dissection of the right gluteal region and the back of the thigh. Most of the gluteus maximus is reflected and parts of the gluteus medius and the three hamstring muscles are excised. Observe that the superior gluteal vessels and nerve appear superior to the piriformis muscle and that all other vessels and nerves appear inferior to it. Note that there are no nerves and/or vessels of importance lateral to the sciatic nerve.

they sit on their gluteus maximus muscles. Hold your hand on your buttock as you sit down. Verify that the gluteus maximus moves up undercovering the ischial tuberosities (Figs. 4-10 and 5-3) on which you sit.

Origin. (Figs. 4-22 and 4-44). **Posterior gluteal line** and area superior and posterior to it, including **iliac crest**; dorsal surfaces of **sacrum** and **coccyx**; and **sacrotuberous ligament.**

Insertion (Figs. 4-22 and 4-30). **Iliotibial tract** of fascia lata (about three-fourths of its fibers), which inserts into lateral condyle of the tibia (Fig. 4-54) and **gluteal tuberosity** of femur (about one-fourth of its fibers).

Nerve Supply. **Inferior gluteal** nerve (L5, S1, and S2).

Actions. **Extends** and **rotates thigh laterally** at hip joint. The gluteus maximus is the **chief extensor of the thigh.** When acting with its insertion fixed, it is also a strong extensor of the pelvis (*e.g.*, when rising from the seated or stooped position).

Bursae Deep to Gluteus Maximus (Fig. 4-52). Usually there are three bursae separating this large muscle from underlying structures: (1) the **trochanteric bursa** separates it from the lateral side of the greater trochanter of the femur; (2) the **gluteofemoral bursa** separates it from the superior part of the origin of the vastus lateralis; and (3) the **ischial bursa** separates it from the ischial tuberosity.

CLINICALLY ORIENTED COMMENTS

The **ischial bursa** superficial to the **ischial tuberosity** may become inflamed as the result of repeated excessive friction. This produces a friction bursitis known as **ischial bursitis** (weaver's bottom). People who weave yarn to make cloth extend first one leg and then the other. This repeated friction on the ischial bursa may lead to inflammation of its walls, and the **inflammatory reaction** results in a painful swelling of the bursa.

As the ischial tuberosities bear the weight during sitting (Fig. 5-3), these pressure points may lead to **pressure sores** in debilitated patients, particularly paraplegic persons (*i.e.*, paralysis of both lower limbs and, generally, the trunk).

Trochanteric bursitis (inflammation of the trochanteric bursa) causes diffuse deep pain in the gluteal and lateral thigh regions. This type of **pelvic girdle pain** is characterized by tenderness over the greater trochanter of the femur (Figs. 4-10 and 4-52).

The Gluteus Medius Muscle (Figs. 4-10 and 4-45 to 4-47). Most of this thick, broad, fan-shaped muscle lies superior to the gluteus maximus on the superior half of the external surface of the ilium. This superficial portion is covered by the strong **fascia lata**; the inferior third of the muscle lies deep to the gluteus maximus.

Origin (Figs. 4-22 and 4-44). **External surface of ilium** between posterior and anterior gluteal lines.

Insertion (Figs. 4-22 and 4-30). **Lateral surface of greater trochanter of femur.** A bursa separates its tendon from the trochanter.

Nerve Supply **Superior gluteal** nerve (L4, L5, and S1).

Actions. **Abducts** and **medially rotates thigh.** It also **steadies the pelvis** so that it does not sag when the foot on the opposite side is raised (*e.g.*, during walking). Verify this action while standing by placing your right hand over your right gluteus medius as you raise your left foot. You should feel the gluteus medius contract and produce a depression in the thigh (Fig. 4-10). Note also that the pelvis does not sag (tilt down) on the left side.

The Gluteus Minimus Muscle (Figs. 4-46 and 4-47). This fan-shaped muscle, the smallest of the gluteal group, lies deep to the gluteus medius.

Origin (Figs. 4-22 and 4-44). **External surface of ilium** between anterior and inferior gluteal lines.

Insertion (Figs. 4-21 and 4-30). **Anterior surface of greater trochanter of femur.** A bursa separates its tendon from the trochanter.

Nerve Supply. **Superior gluteal** nerve (L4, L5, and S1).

Actions. **Abducts** and **medially rotates**

thigh and **steadies pelvis**; its actions are the same as the gluteus medius.

CLINICALLY ORIENTED COMMENTS

When the gluteus medius and minimus muscles are paralyzed (*e.g.*, owing to injury of the superior gluteal nerve or to a disease such as **poliomyelitis**), the suportive and steadying effect of these muscles on the pelvis is lost. Hence when the foot is raised on the normal side, the pelvis falls downward on that side (Case 4-2); similarly, when the person walks there is a **gluteus medius limp** (gluteal gait), characterized by listing or falling of the pelvis toward the unaffected side at each step.

A similar gait occurs in persons with unilateral posterior **dislocation of the hip** joint (Fig. 4-118). This condition prevents the normal functioning of the gluteus medius and minimus muscles.

The Piriformis Muscle (Figs. 4-28, 4-29, 4-44, and 4-44 to 4-47). Because of its position, this small muscle is used as the **landmark of the gluteal region** and is the key to understanding the relationships in this area because it determines the names of blood vessels and nerves to this region; *e.g.*, the superior gluteal vessels and nerve emerge above its superior border and the inferior gluteal vessels and nerve emerge below its inferior border (Fig. 4-47). Note that the sciatic nerve also emerges inferior to the piriformis, but its name is derived from the Greek word form ischium to indicate the nerve's relationship to this bone (Fig. 4-44).

Because the *piriformis occupies a key position in the gluteal region,* it is clinically important to be able to locate its position. **The surface marking of the inferior border of the piriformis** can be determined from the midpoint of the line joining the tip of the coccyx and the posterior superior iliac spine (Fig. 4-53). A line joining this point to the top of the greater trochanter of the femur indicates the inferior border of the piriformis.

Origin. (Figs. 3-27 and 3-57). **Anterior aspect of second, third,** and **fourth lateral masses of sacrum** (opposite greater sciatic notch) and from **sacrotuberous ligament.**

Insertion (Fig. 4-30). **Upper border of greater trochanter of femur.** It leaves the pelvis via the greater sciatic notch and passes posterior to the head of the femur to reach its insertion.

Nerve Supply. Branches of ventral rami of **first** and **second sacral nerves.**

Actions. **Laterally rotates thigh** when hip joint is extended and **abducts thigh** when hip joint is flexed. Helps to hold head of femur in acetabulum; *i.e.*, it stabilizes hip joint.

The Obturator Internus Muscle (Figs. 4-45 to 4-47). This muscle, like the piriformis, is one of the muscles of the pelvic wall. The two *gemelli* (L. twins) muscles (superior and inferior) are extrapelvic parts of the obturator internus.

Origin. **Internal surface of obturator membrane** and **margin of obturator foramen.** As it leaves the pelvis through the lesser sciatic foramen, it becomes tendinous and makes a sharp turn around the ischium just inferior to its spine. It is separated from the bone by a bursa. The **superior gemellus** and **inferior gemellus** arise from the **ischial spine** and **ischial tuberosity**, respectively.

Insertion (Fig. 4-30). **Medial surface of greater trochanter of femur.** The gemelli insert into the tendon of the obturator internus and often their bellies obscure it.

Nerve Supply. **Nerve to obturator internus** (L5 and S1), a branch of the sacral plexus. The superior gemellus is also supplied by this nerve, but the inferior gemellus is supplied by the **nerve to the quadratus femoris** (L5 and S1).

Actions. **Laterally rotates thigh** and **abducts thigh** when hip joint is flexed. **Helps to hold head of femur in acetabulum**; *i.e.*, it **stabilizes hip joint**. The gemelli assist the obturator internus in the performance of these actions.

The Quadratus Femoris Muscle (Figs. 4-44 to 4-47). This short, thick, flat, quadrilateral muscle is located inferior to the obturator internus and the gemelli.

Origin (Fig. 4-48). **Lateral border of ischial tuberosity**.

Insertion (Figs. 4-9, 4-22, and 4-30). **Quadrate tubercle** of femur and bone inferior to it. This tubercle is a rounded eminence on the intertrochanteric crest.

Nerve Supply. **Nerve to quadratus femoris** (L5 and S1) from sacral plexus.

Action. **Laterally rotates thigh.**

Nerves of the Gluteal Region. There are many nerves in the gluteal region; the deep ones are of most importance clinically.

The Superifical Nerves (Figs. 4-49 and 4-160). The skin of the gluteal region is richly innervated. It receives cutaneous branches from several lumbar and sacral segments. Although the correct terminology for these nerves is the **cluneal** (L. *clunis*, buttock) **nerves**, this designation is not commonly used at present.

The **superior cutaneous nerves (superior cluneal nerves)** are lateral branches of the *dorsal rami* of the upper three lumbar nerves (*i.e.*, L1, L2, and L3 of the lumbar plexus). They emerge from the deep fascia just above the iliac crest and descend over the buttock (Fig. 4-49).

The **middle cutaneous nerves (middle cluneal nerves)** are lateral branches of the *dorsal rami* of the first three sacral nerves (*i.e.*, S1, S2, and S3 of the sacral plexus). They become cutaneous along a line connecting the posterior superior iliac spine and the tip of the coccyx. They supply skin over the sacrum and the adjacent area of the buttock (Fig. 4-49).

The **inferior cutaneous nerves (inferior cluneal nerves)** are the gluteal branches of the **posterior femoral cutaneous nerves** which are larger than the

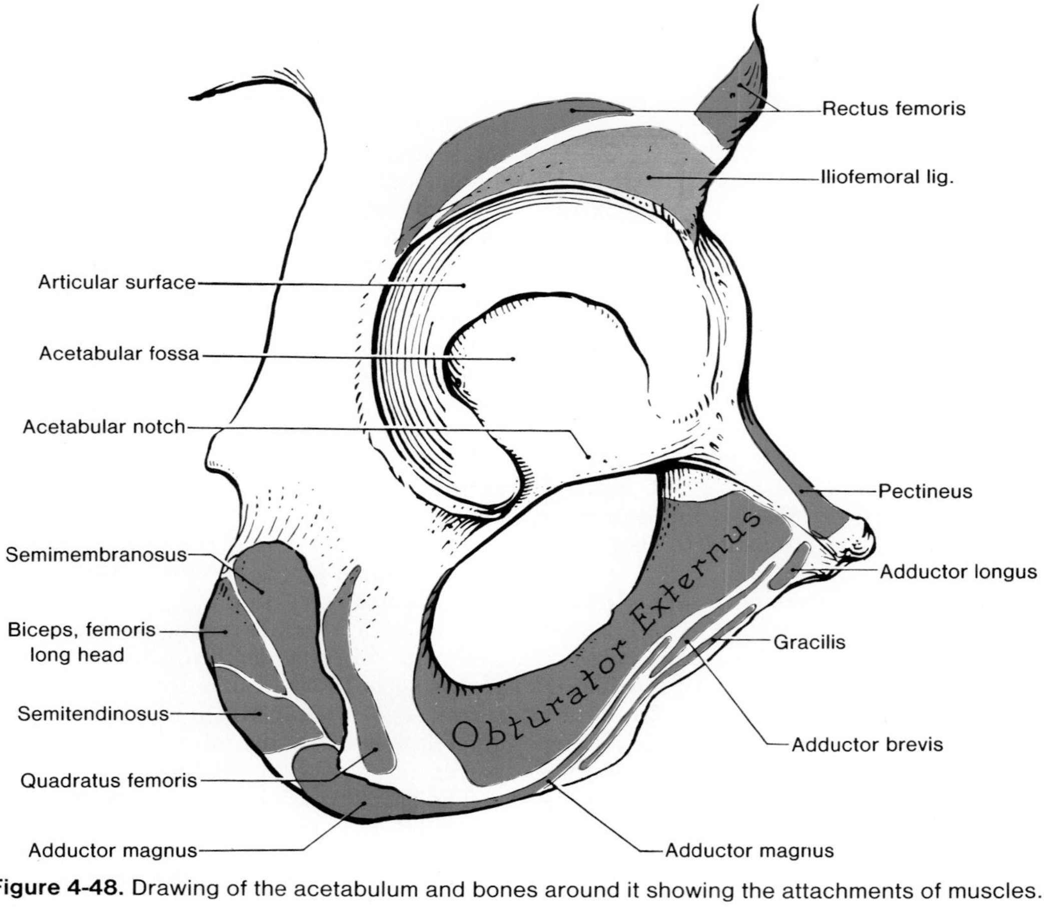

Figure 4-48. Drawing of the acetabulum and bones around it showing the attachments of muscles.

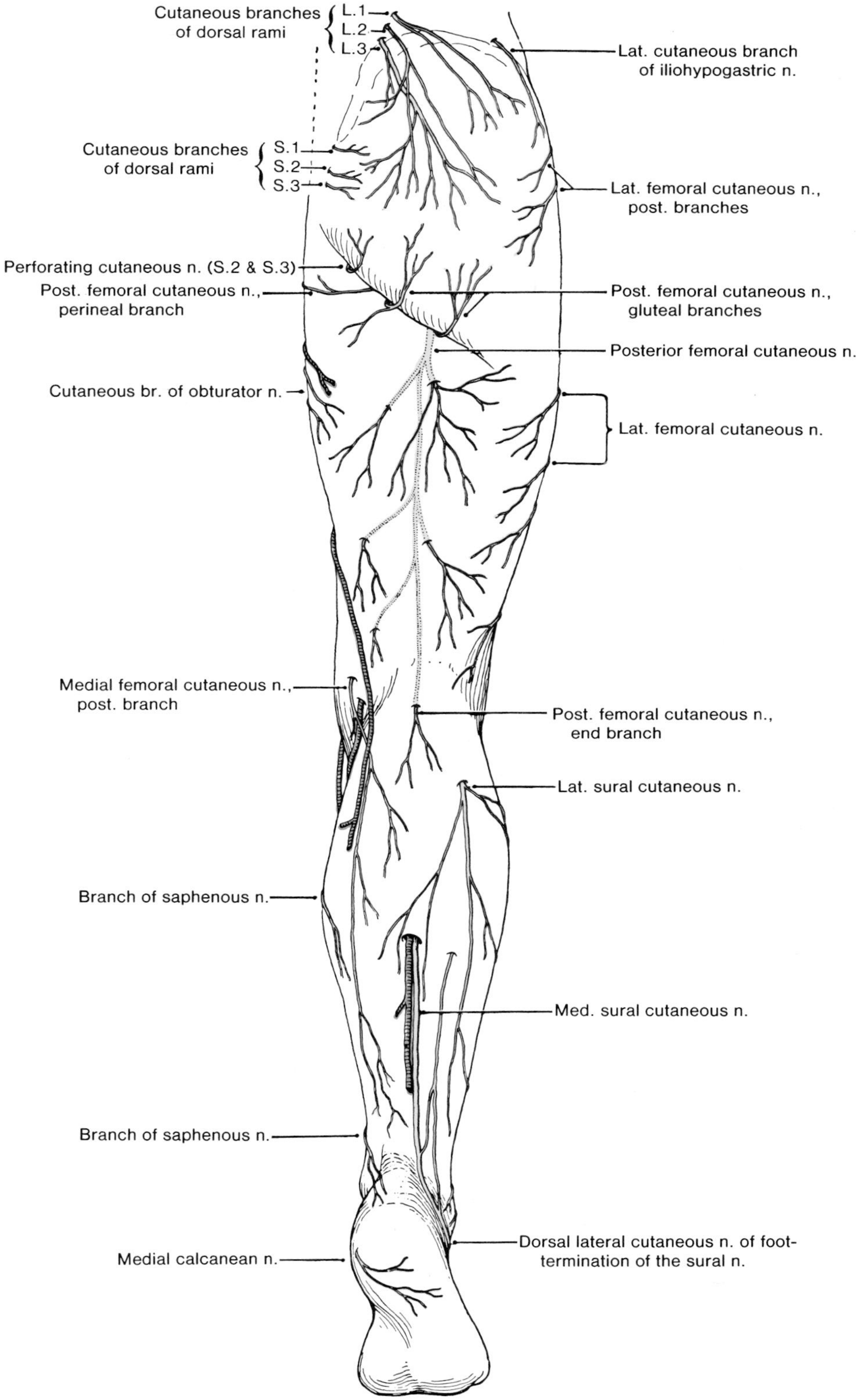

Figure 4-49. Drawing of a posterior view of the cutaneous nerves of the right lower limb. See Figure 4-14 for an anterior view. Observe that the chief supply to the buttock is from the dorsal primary rami of lumbar and sacral nerves and the sacral plexus. The cutaneous nerves to buttock are sometimes called cluneal nerves.

other cutaneous nerves. They are branches of the sacral plexus (S1, S2, and S3) and are derived from the *ventral rami* of these nerves. These nerves become cutaneous and curve around the inferior border of the gluteus maximus muscle to supply the lower part of the buttock (Fig. 4-49).

The **iliohypogastric nerve** arises from the first lumbar ventral ramus, with a small contribution from the 12th thoracic. It supplies cutaneous branches to the lateral area over the crest of the ilium and the greater trochanter of the femur (Figs. 4-37 and 4-49).

The Deep Nerves (Figs. 4-44, 4-45, and 4-47). These seven nerves are all branches of the **sacral plexus** within the pelvis. They all leave the pelvis via the **greater sciatic foramen** and, *except for the superior gluteal nerve*, **they emerge below the inferior border of the piriformis** muscle. The site of exit of these nerves can be detected by deep pressure (usually painful) just above the midpoint of a line joining the posterior superior iliac spine to the ischial tuberosity (Figs. 4-6, 4-10, and 4-53).

The Superior Gluteal Nerve (L4, L5, and S1). This nerve passes out of the greater sciatic foramen, *superior to the piriformis muscle* (Fig. 4-47), and runs laterally between the gluteus medius and minimus with the deep branch of the superior gluteal artery. It divides into a **superior branch** that supplies the gluteus medius and an **inferior branch** which supplies the gluteus minimus and the tensor fasciae latae muscles.

The Inferior Gluteal Nerve (L5, S1, and S2). This nerve passes out of the greater sciatic foramen, *inferior to the piriformis muscle* and superficial to the sciatic nerve (Fig. 4-47). It immediately breaks up into several branches that supply the overlying gluteus maximus muscle.

The Sciatic Nerve (L4, L5, S1, S2, and S3). This *very important nerve* is about 2 cm in diameter at its commencement and is the largest nerve in the body (Figs. 4-44, 4-47, 4-50, 4-52, and 4-94). **The sciatic nerve** leaves the pelvis through the greater sciatic foramen and *enters the gluteal region inferior to the piriformis muscle.* Once it passes from the piriformis, it runs inferolaterally deep to the gluteus maximus muscle, *midway between the greater trochanter of the femur and the ischial tuberosity.* It rests first on the ischium (hence its name) and then passes posterior to the obturator internus, quadratus femoris, and adductor magnus. The sciatic nerve is really two nerves, the **tibial** and **common peroneal**, bound together in the same connective tissue sheath (*epineurium*). The two nerves usually separate from each other in the lower third of the thigh, but occasionally they are separate when they leave the pelvis (Fig. 4-50*B* and *C*.) In these cases the tibial nerve passes inferior to the piriformis and the common peroneal pierces the muscle or passes superior to it.

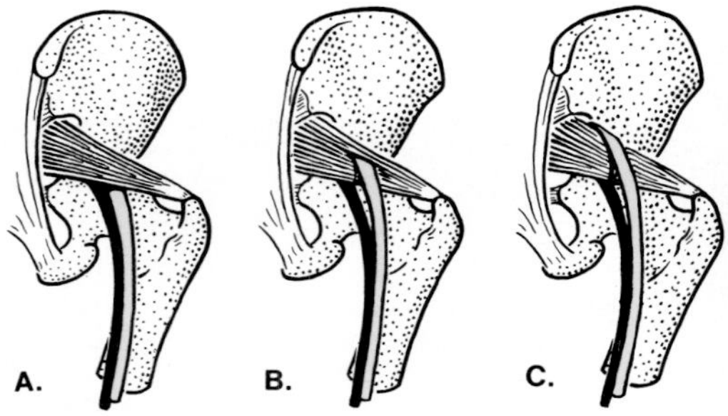

Figure 4-50. Diagrams illustrating the relationship of the sciatic nerve to the piriformis muscle. *A*, in most cases it passes inferior to the muscle. *B*, in 10 to 12% of cases the sciatic divides before entering the gluteal region and the common peroneal division (*yellow*) passes through the muscle. *C*, in 0.5% of cases the common peroneal division passes superior to the muscle, in which case it is vulnerable to injury during intragluteal injections.

CLINICALLY ORIENTED COMMENTS

Injury to the sciatic nerve may occur in wounds of the gluteal region (*e.g.*, gunshot or stab wounds); thus, knowledge of its course through the gluteal region midway between the ischial tuberosity and the greater trochanter of the femur is clinically important (Figs. 4-10 and 4-53). Because of the large sciatic nerve, the buttock has a **side of safety** (its lateral side) and a **side of danger** (its medial side). Wounds or

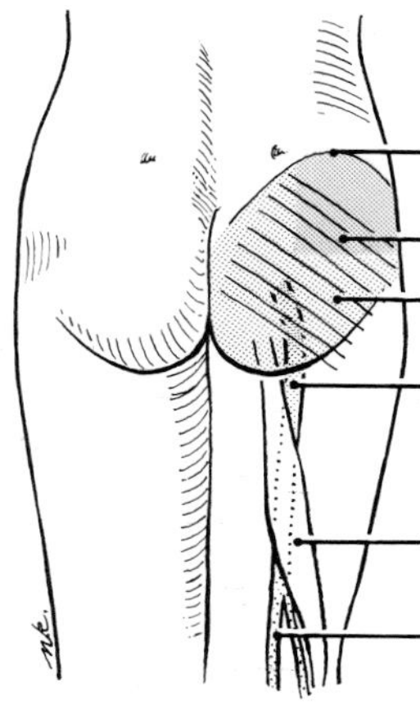

Figure 4-51. Diagram showing the extent of the buttock and the location of the sciatic nerve under the gluteus maximus muscle. The safe area (quadrant) for giving intramuscular injections is shown in *green*. The area to be avoided is shown in *red*. If injections are given into the rounded lower part (summit or prominence) of the buttock, just above the gluteal fold (Fig. 4-10), the sciatic or other nerves and vessels may be injured. Anatomically, injections are best given with the patient in the prone position (lying face down). If the injection is given when the patient is standing and leaning forward, a needle inserted into the apparent safe area may pierce the piriformis muscle and the stems of the posterior femoral cutaneous nerve (Fig. 4-49) or the common peroneal division of the sciatic nerve (Fig. 4-50*B* and *C*).

surgery on its medial side are liable to injure the sciatic nerve and its branches to the hamstring muscle on the back of the thigh (Fig. 4-47). Paralysis of these muscles results in impairment of extension of the hip joint and flexion of the knee joint.

Sciatica (sciatic pain) is a term commonly used for *pain in the area of distribution of the sciatic nerve.* The pain is generally over one or more of the following areas: the gluteal region, particularly in the region of the greater sciatic notch; the posterior aspect of the thigh; the posterior and lateral aspects of the lower leg; and the lateral part of the foot, particularly the area around the lateral malleolus.

Although sciatica may result from irritation of the sciatic nerve owing to inflammation, it is more often **caused by pressure on a dorsal root and/or a ventral root of** one of the nerves which form it. As the sciatic nerve is derived from the ventral rami of L4, L5, S1, S2, and S3 nerves, the location of the pain felt by a patient varies according to the nerve root(s) involved (Fig. 4-160). For example, if the intervertebral disc between L5 and S1 herniates posteriorly (Case 5-3), pressure would likely be exerted on the S1 roots or component of the sciatic nerve. As a result the patient would probably experience pain over the posterior region of the thigh and the posterolateral region of the leg.

Sciatica can also result from pressure on the sciatic nerve in the pelvis, in the gluteal region, or in the thigh.

The Posterior Femoral Cutaneous Nerve (S1, S2, and S3). This nerve leaves the pelvis with the inferior gluteal nerve and vessels and the sciatic nerve (Fig. 4-47) and passes deep to the gluteus maximus. It gives branches to the skin of the inferior part of the buttock (Fig. 4-49) and continues downward to supply *skin of the posterior thigh* and popliteal region.

The Nerve to the Quadratus Femoris Muscle (L4, L5, and S1). This nerve passes deep to the sciatic nerve and the obturator internus muscle and over the posterior surface of the hip joint. It supplies an articular branch to this joint and innervates the quadratus femoris and inferior gemellus muscles.

The Nerve to the Obturator Internus (L5, S1, and S2). This nerve passes through the greater sciatic foramen inferior to the piriformis muscle and across the base of the ischial spine (Fig. 4-52). It supplies the superior gemellus muscle and then passes posterior to the ischial spine, re-entering the pelvis via the lesser sciatic foramen to supply the obturator internus.

The Pudendal Nerve (S2, S3, and S4). This nerve is the most medial structure to pass through the greater sciatic foramen inferior to the piriformis muscle (Fig. 4-47). It passes lateral to the sacrospinous ligament, re-entering the pelvis via the lesser sciatic foramen to supply structures in the perineum (*e.g.*, voluntary anal sphincter and genitalia, see Chap. 3).

CLINICALLY ORIENTED COMMENTS

The gluteal region is a common site for intramuscular injection of drugs. Because of this, it is important to understand the extent of this area and the safe region for giving injections. Too many people restrict the area of the buttock to its summit ("cheek") or most prominent part. Its full extent is shown in Figure 4-51. As there are a number of important nerves and blood vessels in the gluteal region, **injections can only be made safely into the superolateral quadrant**. To locate the safe area, put the tip of your thumb on the anterior superior iliac spine and then place your closed hand posterior and inferior to the iliac crest. Your hand will cover the safe area for injection into the gluteal muscles.

Injections into either of the inferior two quadrants will endanger and possibly injure the sciatic or other nerves and vessels which emerge inferior to the piriformis muscle (Fig. 4-52). Similarly injections into the superomedial quadrant may injure the superior gluteal nerve and/or vessels (Fig. 4-47). In one in about 200 cases, injections into this quadrant could injure the common peroneal nerve (Fig. 4-50*C*) and produce **foot-drop** (paralysis of the dorsiflexor muscles of the foot and ankle, Case 4-3).

Improper intragluteal injection may also injure the gluteal branches of the **posterior cutaneous nerve femoral** (inferior cluneal nerves, S1, S2, and S3), resulting in **pain and dyesthesia** (some loss of sensation) in the area of skin supplied by them (Figs. 4-49, 4-52, and 4-160).

The safe area for giving intramuscular injections is into the superolateral quadrant (Fig. 4-51) just inferior to the iliac crest. The injection penetrates the belly of the gluteus medius and possibly the gluteus minimus.

The hazards of injecting drugs into the gluteal region of small infants are well recognized. Because of the danger of injuring the sciatic or other nerves, drugs are commonly injected into the muscles of the anterolateral region of the thigh. To avoid the femoral nerve (Fig. 4-37), injections are given inferolateral to the anterior superior iliac spine.

Vessels of the Gluteal Region (Figs. 4-34*B* and 4-47). The arteries supplying the gluteal region directly are branches of the **internal iliac artery** (Fig. 3-65).

The Superior Gluteal Artery (Figs. 4-47 and 4-52). This short large artery is the continuation of the posterior division of the **internal iliac artery** (Fig. 4-34*A*). It leaves the pelvis through the greater sciatic foramen *superior to the piriformis muscle* and divides immediately into superficial and deep branches (Fig. 4-34*B*). The superficial branch supplies the gluteus maximus and the deep branch supplies the gluteus medius and minimus and the tensor fasciae latae muscles. It anastomoses with the inferior gluteal and medial circumflex femoral arteries.

The Inferior Gluteal Artery (Figs. 4-34*B*, 4-47, and 4-52). This artery is the larger of the two terminal branches of the anterior division of the internal iliac artery. It leaves the pelvis through the greater sciatic foramen, *inferior to the piriformis muscle*, and supplies the gluteus maximus, obturator internus, quadratus femoris, and superior parts of the hamstring muscles. It anastomoses with the superior gluteal artery and participates in the **cruciate anastomosis** of the thigh, involving the first perforating arteries of the profunda femoris and the medial and lateral circumflex femoral arteries.

The Internal Pudendal Artery (Figs. 4-47 and 4-52). This is the smaller of the two terminal branches of the anterior division of the internal iliac artery. It descends anterior to the other terminal branch (inferior gluteal artery) and leaves the pelvis via the greater sciatic foramen *inferior to the piriformis muscle.* It then descends posterior to the ischial spine to enter the perineum via the lesser sciatic foramen with the puddendal nerve. It supplies the external genitalia and muscle in the pelvic and gluteal regions.

Veins of the Gluteal Region. The su-

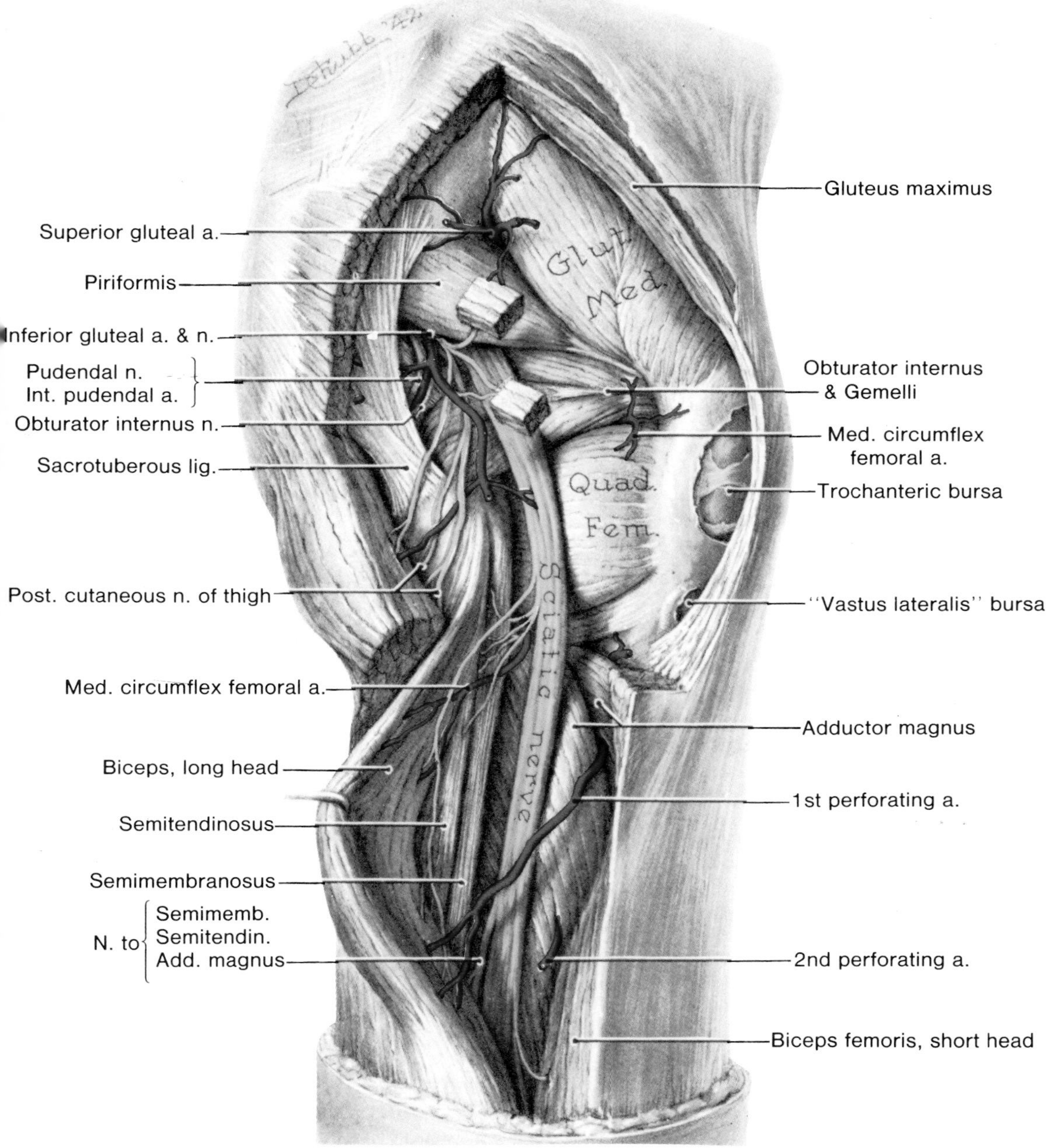

Figure 4-52. Drawing of a dissection of the gluteal region and the back of the right thigh. The gluteus maximus muscle is split (superiorly and inferiorly) in the direction of its fibers and the middle part is excised, but two cubes remain for identification of its nerve. Observe that the gluteus maximus is the only muscle to cover the greater trochanter and the aponeurosis of the vastus lateralis muscle. Note that the inferior gluteal nerve enters the gluteus maximus in two chief branches near its center. Observe that the sciatic nerve appears below the piriformis muscle and crosses, in turn, the dorsal aspect of the ischium, the obturator internus, the gemelli, the quadratus femoris, and the adductor magnus. Note, and this is clinically important, that its branches arise from its medial side at variable levels to supply the hamstring muscles and part of the adductor magnus. Only the branch to the biceps femoris (short head) arises from its lateral side. Obviously the lateral side ("safe side") is an effective surgical approach to the posterior aspect of the hip joint and to structures in the gluteal region.

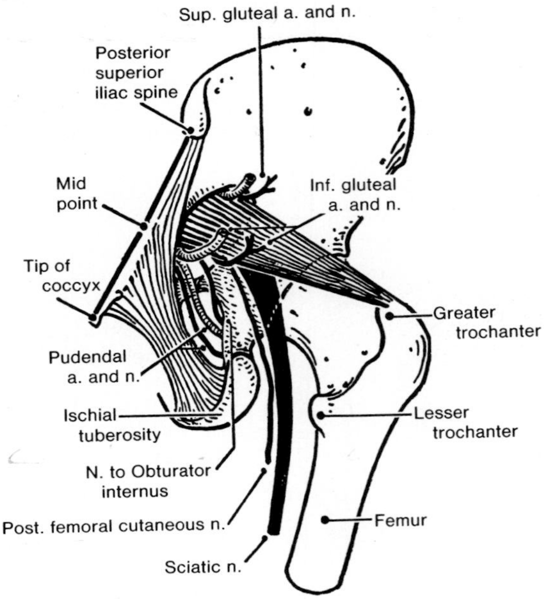

Figure 4-53. Drawing illustrating the structures passing through the right greater sciatic foramen, superior and inferior to the piriformis muscle. Obviously *the piriformis occupies a key position in the gluteal region*. The position of the inferior border of the piriformis can be determined on the surface of the buttock as indicated above and as follows: (1) find the midpoint of a line joining the tip of the coccyx to the posterior superior iliac spine; and (2) join this point to the top of the greater trochanter of the femur. The line so formed indicates the inferior border of the piriformis. Note the important nerves and vessels that enter the gluteal region below this muscle. Various surgical approaches through the gluteus maximus to the region of the hip joint and sciatic nerve depend on the location of the inferior border of the piriformis.

perior and inferior gluteal veins, tributaries of the internal iliac vein, accompany the corresponding arteries through the greater sciatic foramen. Usually each of these veins is double, *i.e.*, **venae comitantes** (L. accompanying veins). They communicate with the tributaries of the femoral vein and thus can provide an alternate route for blood return from the lower limb if the femoral vein is occluded or has to be ligated.

The internal pudendal veins also accompany the corresponding artery and join to form a single vein that enters the internal iliac vein. They drain blood from the external gentalia and the perineal region.

Muscles of Back of Thigh. The anterior and adductor groups of thigh muscles were discussed previously. Three large fusiform femoral muscles (Figs. 4-45 to 4-47, 4-52, 4-56, and 4-57) make up the **hamstring group** (*semitendinosus, semimembranosus*, and *long head of biceps femoris*) which can be made to stand out by flexing the knee joint against resistance. They have a *common site of origin* from the **ischial tuberosity** deep to the gluteus maximus, but one of them, biceps femoris, has an additional origin from the femur. They also have a *common nerve supply* from the **sciatic nerve.**

The hamstring muscles span two joints, the hip joint and the knee joint; hence, they are **extensors of the thigh** at the hip joint and **flexors of the leg** at the knee joint. Verify that you cannot perform both these actions fully at the same time. The hamstring muscles descend in the back of the thigh where their tendons form the "hamstrings" at the back of the knee (Fig. 4-56).

The posterior femoral muscles became known as the hamstrings ("hams") because their tendons behind the knee (Fig. 4-56) were used to hang up the hams (hip and thigh regions) of animals such as pigs. Furthermore, in ancient times it was common for foot soldiers to slash their opponent's horses behind the knees in order to cut their hamstrings, which would bring the horses and their riders down. Similarly, they cut the hamstrings of other soldiers so they could not run; this was called "hamstringing" your enemy.

The Semitendinosus Muscle (Figs. 4-17, 4-27, 4-28, and 4-45 to 4-47). As its name indicates, *it is half tendinous.* Its slender, cord-like tendon begins about two-thirds of the way down the thigh.

Origin (Figs. 4-22 and 4-48). **Ischial tuberosity** by common tendon with long head of biceps femoris.

Insertion (Fig. 4-26). **Medial surface of superior part of shaft of tibia,** posterior to insertions of sartorius and gracilis.

Nerve Supply. **Tibial division of sciatic** nerve (L5, S1, and S2).

Actions. **Extends thigh at hip joint, flexes leg at knee joint**, and with semimembranosus, **medially rotates tibia** on femur (particularly when the knee is flexed).

The Semimembranosus Muscle (Figs. 4-17, 4-28, 4-45 to 4-47, 4-52, 4-57, and 4-62). As its name indicates *it is half membranous.*

Origin (Figs. 4-22 and 4-48). **Ischial tuberosity.**

Insertion (Figs. 4-22, 4-26, 4-28, and 4-66). **Medial condyle of tibia** in horizontal groove on its posteromedial aspect.

Nerve Supply. **Tibial division of sciatic** nerve (L5, S1, and S2).

Actions. **Extends thigh at hip joint, flexes leg at knee joint** (common action of hamstrings), and with semitendinosus, **medially rotates tibia** on femur (particularly when the knee is flexed).

The Biceps Femoris Muscle (Figs. 4-17, 4-45 to 4-47, 4-52, and 4-55 to 4-60). As its name indicates, this muscle has *two heads of origin,* long and short. The long head is one of the three hamstring muscles.

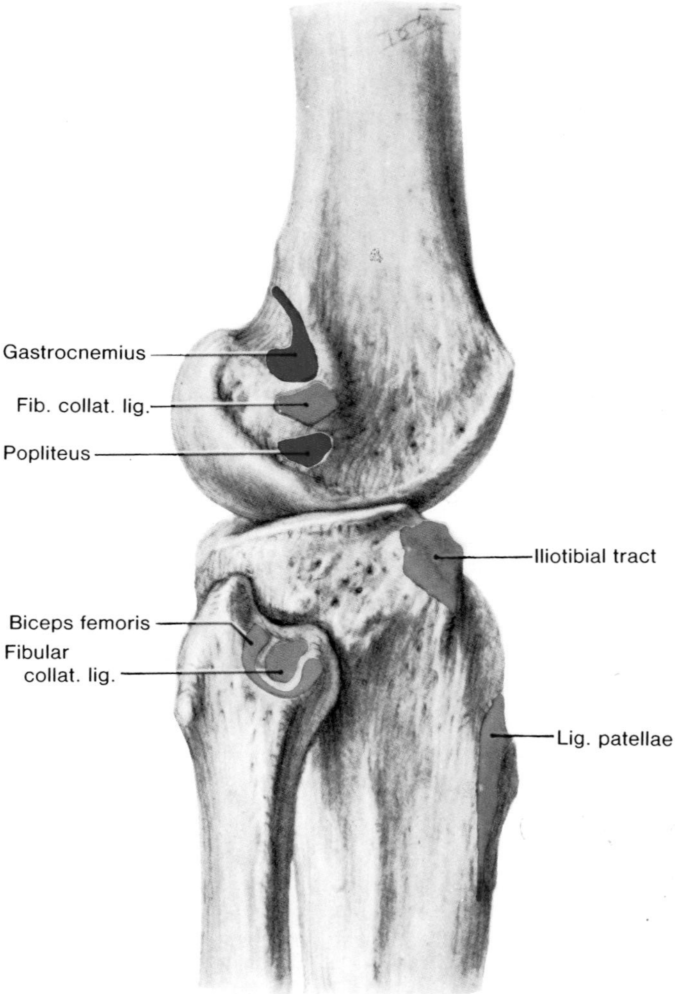

Figure 4-54. Drawing of a lateral view of the bones of the right knee joint showing the attachments of muscles and ligaments. Origins of muscles are shown in *red* and insertions in *blue.* The attachments of the fibular collateral ligament (Fig. 4-124) are shown in *green.*

Origin (Figs. 4-2, 4-22, and 4-48). *Long head,* **ischial tuberosity** by common tendon with semitendinosus muscle. *Short head,* **linea aspera** (lateral lip) and proximal part of **supracondylar line** of femur.

Insertion (Figs. 4-21, 4-54 to 4-56, and 4-124). **Head of fibula** by common tendon. The tendon is split by the **fibular collateral ligament** of the knee and sends some fibers to the lateral condyle of the tibia and the deep fascia of the leg (Fig. 4-125). The rounded tendon of the biceps femoris can easily be seen and felt where it passes the knee to insert into the head of the fibula, especially when the knee is flexed against resistance (Figs. 4-55 and 4-56).

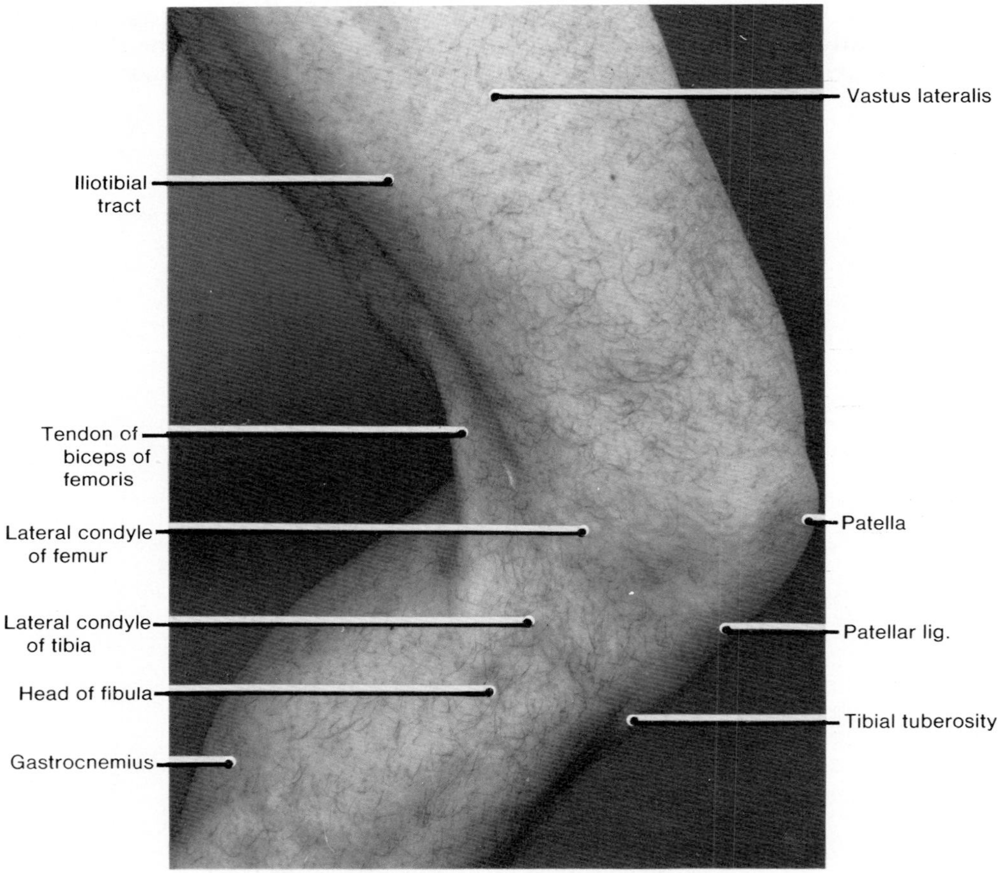

Figure 4-55. Photograph of the lateral surface of the right thigh and the proximal part of the leg of a 27-year-old man showing the principal surface features of the muscles and bones. The gluteus maximus and tensor fasciae latae muscles insert into the iliotibial tract posteriorly and anteriorly, respectively. This tract (band of deep fascia) inserts into the lateral condyle of the tibia (Fig. 4-54). The tendon of the biceps femoris may be traced by palpation from the posterior aspect of the distal extremity of the thigh inferolaterally to its insertion into the head of the fibula. Verify by palpation that the lateral condyles of the femur and the tibia, as well as the head of the fibula, are subcutaneous. The neck of the fibula can be felt just distal to the head of the bone. The tendon of the biceps femoris and the proximal extremity of the fibula are important guides to the common peroneal nerve. It is indicated by a line drawn along the tendon of the biceps femoris posterior to the head of the fibula and then around the lateral aspect of the neck of the fibula to its anterior aspect (see Fig. 4-67*A*). You should be able to feel this commonly injured nerve lateral to the neck of the fibula. It is particularly exposed to injury here because it is subcutaneous and is related deeply to bone (fibula).

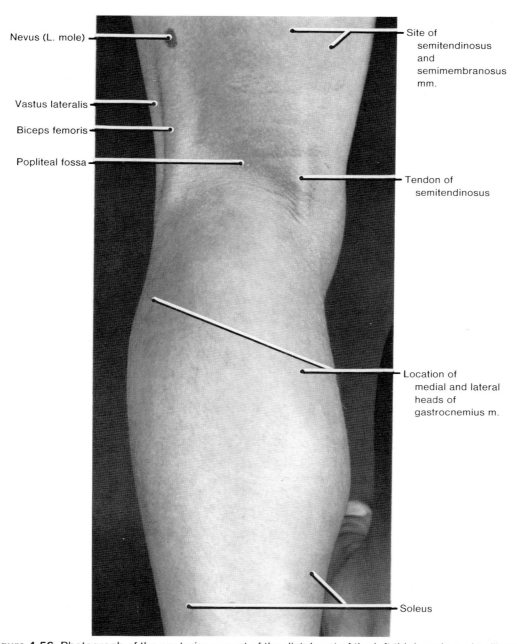

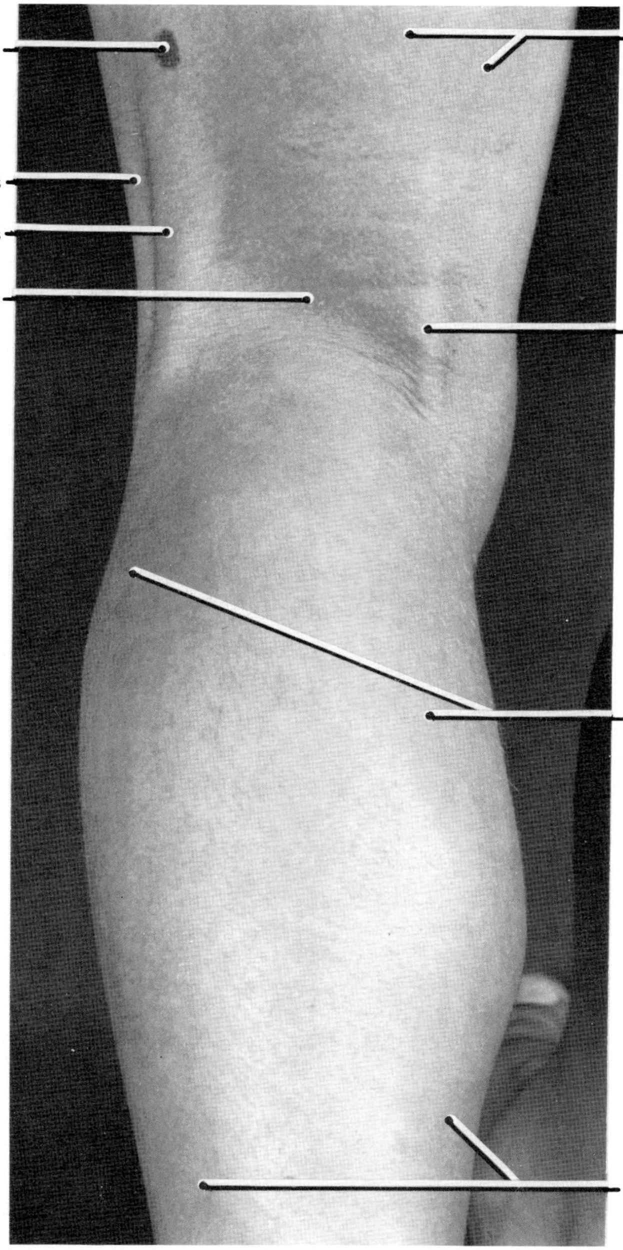

Figure 4-56. Photograph of the posterior aspect of the distal part of the left thigh and proximal part of the leg of a 12-year-old girl, showing the principal surface features of the muscles and the popliteal fossa. This fossa is visible only when the knee is flexed (as here). Note that the popliteal fossa is bounded above and laterally by the biceps femoris muscle and above and medially by the semitendinosus and semimembranosus muscles. To feel the tendons of your hamstrings as displayed here, sit on a chair and press your heel firmly against the chair leg. The common peroneal nerve passes on the medial side of the biceps femoris tendon and then passes posterior to the head of the fibula (Figs. 4-58 and 4-67*A*). The tendons of the semitendinosus and semimembranosus can be traced medially toward their insertion into the proximal part of the tibia (Fig. 4-26). Near its insertion the tendon of the semitendinosus is lateral to that of the semimembranosus and, as it is on a more superficial plane, is clearly visible. The gastrocnemius, forming the lower boundary of the popliteal fossa along with the soleus muscle, makes up the triceps surae which forms the prominence of the calf. The popliteal artery (Fig. 4-61) lies deeply in the popliteal fossa and the popliteal pulse may be palpated here; however, as it lies so deeply its pulsations are difficult to feel.

Nerve Supply. Long head, **tibial division of sciatic** nerve (L5, S1, and S2) like the other hamstrings. *Short head,* **common peroneal division of sciatic** nerve (L5, S1, and S2).

Actions. Long head, like the other hamstrings, **extends thigh at hip joint.** *Both heads,* **flex leg at knee joint** and **laterally rotate leg.**

CLINICALLY ORIENTED COMMENTS

Because the two *heads of the biceps femoris have a different nerve supply* (*i.e.,* from different divisions of the sciatic nerve), a wound in the thigh may paralyze one head and not the other.

The length of the hamstrings varies considerably in different persons. In some people they will not stretch enough to allow them to touch their toes when they flex their vertebral column and keep their knees straight; in other people the hamstrings are long and they can easily touch the floor with their palms or do a high kick with comparative ease. Some athletes are unable to excel in some sports (*e.g.,* gymnastics) despite rigorous exercises because of an anatomical insufficiency of their hamstrings.

"**Pulled hamstrings**" are common sports injuries in persons who run very hard (*e.g.,* half backs or pass receivers in football). Often the violent muscular exertion required to excel in sports tears off or **avulses part of the tendinous origin of the hamstrings** from the ischial tuberosity. Usually there is also contusion (bruising) and tearing of some of the muscle fibers, resulting in rupture of some of the blood vessels supplying these muscles. The resultant **hematoma** (collection of blood) is contained by the dense fascia lata of the thigh.

THE POPLITEAL FOSSA

Surface Anatomy of the Popliteal Fossa (Figs. 4-27, 4-56, and 4-57). The popliteal fossa (space) is the diamond or lozenge-shaped region at the **posterior aspect of the knee**. It lies opposite the distal third of the femur, the knee joint, and the proximal part of the tibia. The fossa appears as a hollow and is visible only when the knee joint is flexed. Popliteal is derived from the Latin word "*poples,*" meaning a ham, and this adjective was probably used to describe the fossa because the tendons of the hamstrings ("hams") form the proximal boundaries of the popliteal fossa.

Flex your knee and palpate the hollow (popliteal fossa) behind your knee and between the opposing borders of the semitendinosus and biceps femoris tendons (Fig. 4-56). Feel deeply in the fossa for the pulsations of the popliteal artery. You will probably find your "**popliteal pulse**" difficult to feel because the artery lies so deeply.

Extend your knee and feel the prominence formed partly by the fleshy semimembranosus muscle as it pushes laterally and bulges posteriorly. Fat in the fossa also contributes to this prominence or bulge.

Also palpate the deep popliteal fascia forming the roof of the fossa; it is best palpated when the knee joint is extended. Although this popliteal fascia is thin, it is very strong and is firmly attached to the muscles (Figs. 4-56 to 4-59) forming the boundaries of the fossa.

Roof of the Popliteal Fossa (Figs. 4-56 and 4-58). The roof or posterior wall of this fossa is formed by skin and superficial and deep popliteal fasciae. The **superficial popliteal fascia** contains some fat, the small saphenous vein, and three cutaneous nerves. The **deep popliteal fascia** forms a strong, dense sheet that affords a protective covering for the neurovascular structures passing from the thigh to the leg. When the knee is extended the semimembranosus muscle moves laterally offering further protection to these structures.

CLINICALLY ORIENTED COMMENTS

Because the deep popliteal fascia is tense and does not permit expansion, pain from an abscess or tumor in this region is usually severe. In addition, **popliteal abscesses** (collections of pus) tend to spread up the

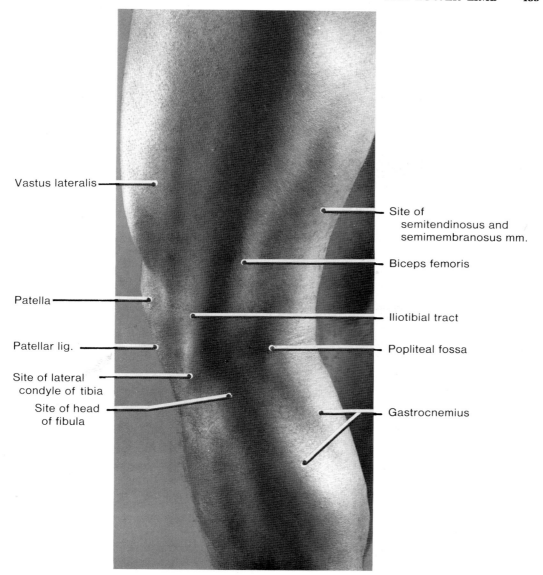

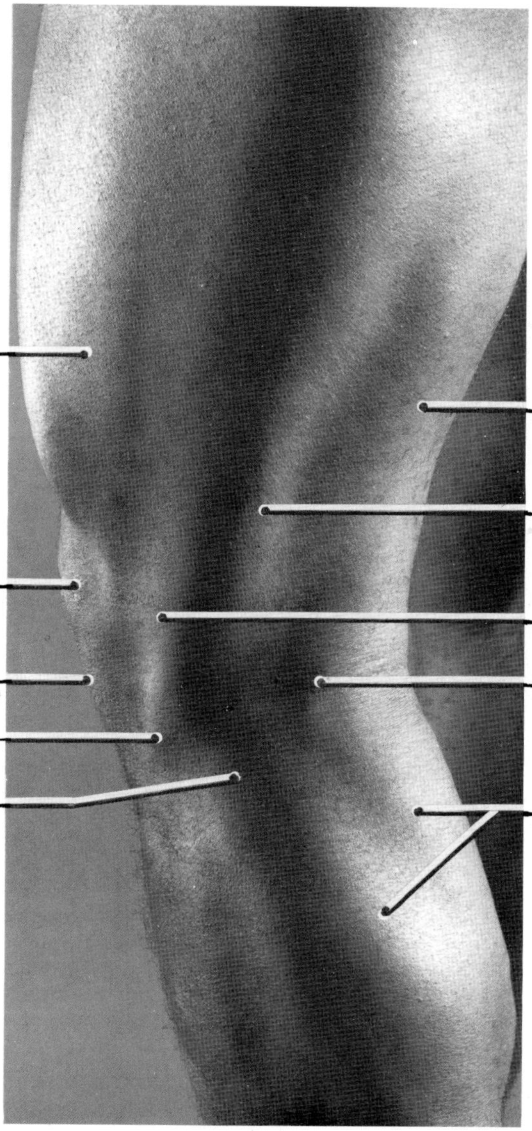

Figure 4-57. Photograph of the lateral aspect of the left thigh and the proximal half of the leg of a 35-year-old man showing the principal surface features of the muscles and bones when the knee is slightly flexed. Also observe the prominent posterior border of the iliotibial tract which inserts into the lateral condyle of the tibia (Fig. 4-54), the fibrous capsule of the knee joint, and the patella. About one fingerbreadth posterior to the iliotibial tract, observe the biceps femoris tendon that inserts on the head of the fibula (easily palpable but not visible in this photograph).

thigh or down the leg because the tough deep fascia enclosing them.

Boundaries of the Popliteal Fossa (Figs. 4-56 to 4-59). The muscles surrounding the popliteal fossa delineate a diamond-shaped space that is bounded *superolaterally* by the **biceps femoris** muscle, *superomedially* by the **semimembranosus** and **semitendinosus** muscles, and *inferolaterally* and *inferomedially* by the medial and lateral heads of the **gastrocnemius** muscle.

Contents of the Popliteal Fossa (Figs.

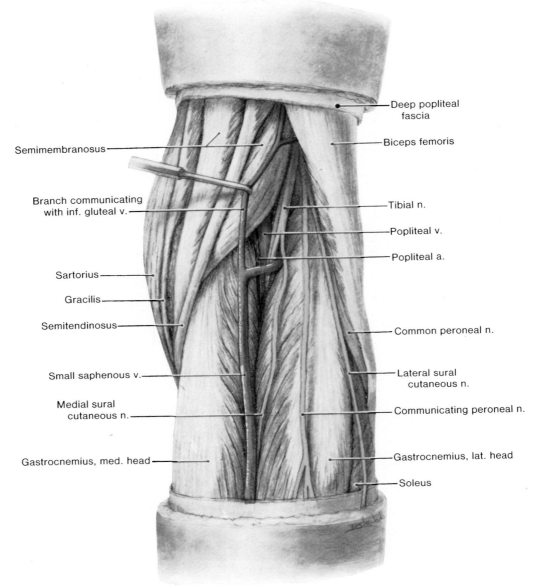

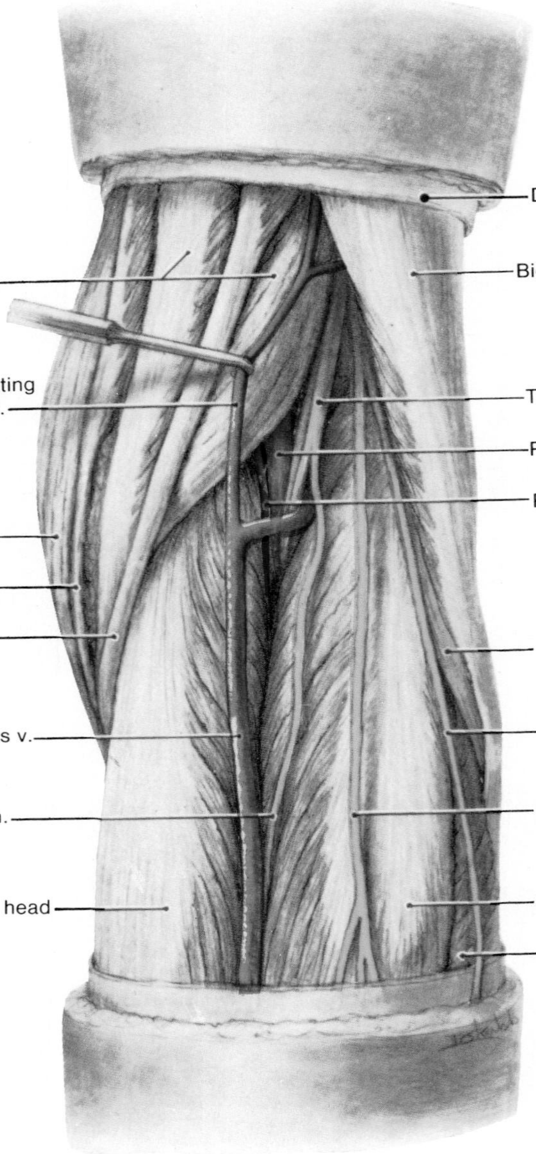

Figure 4-58. Drawing of a superficial dissection of the right popliteal fossa. Note that only a small part of the popliteal artery is not covered by muscles. Observe the two heads of the gastrocnemius, the semimembranosus, the semitendinosus, and the biceps femoris. These muscles form the boundaries of the diamond or lozenge-shaped popliteal fossa (see Fig. 4-59). To expose the contents of the fossa, the pad of fat which surrounds the various nerves and vessels was carefully removed. Note the small saphenous vein running between the two heads of the gastrocnemius. Deep to this vein is the medial sural cutaneous nerve which leads proximally to the tibial nerve. Observe that the tibial nerve is superficial to the popliteal vein, which in turn is superficial to the popliteal artery. Note the common peroneal nerve following the posterior border of the biceps femoris and here giving off two cutaneous branches. The common peroneal is the most commonly injured nerve in the lower limb (Case 4-3) mainly because of its exposed position as it winds around the neck of the fibula (Fig. 4-67*A*).

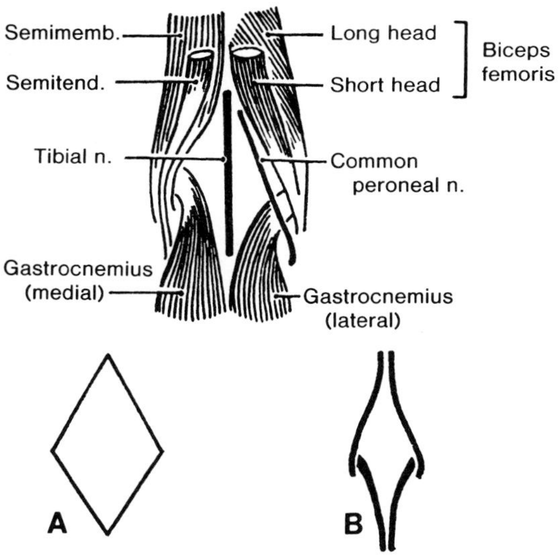

Figure 4-59. Drawings illustrating the boundaries of the right popliteal fossa and the two important nerves it contains. The muscular boundaries have been pulled apart to illustrate the diamond-shaped space. Understand that normally these muscles are closely packed together (Fig. 4-58) and that the fossa is only a small interval between the distal ends of the hamstring muscles. *A*, illustrates the lozenge or diamond shape of the fossa shown above and in *B*. Superolaterally the fossa is bounded by the biceps femoris muscle; superomedially it is bounded by the semitendinosus and semimembranosus muscles; and inferolaterally and inferomedially it is bounded by the medial and lateral heads of the gastrocnemius muscle. Note that the tibial nerve, the larger division of the sciatic nerve, passes through the middle of the fossa from its superior to its inferior angle.

4-58 to 4-61). When the muscles forming the boundaries of the fossa are pulled apart, especially the heads of the gastrocnemius, the popliteal fossa and its contents can be observed. Although the fossa appears large when this is done, understand that normally the muscles are packed closely together and the fossa is relatively small.

The principle contents of the popliteal fossa are fat, the **popliteal vessels** (artery, vein, and lymph) and their branches and tributaries, the **tibial** and **common peroneal nerves**, the **small saphenous vein**, the inferior part of the **posterior femoral cutaneous nerve** (Fig. 4-49), an articular branch of the **obturator nerve**, and four to six **popliteal lymph nodes**.

The Popliteal Artery (Figs. 4-58, 4-61, 4-62, and 4-88). The popliteal artery enters the popliteal fossa through the adductor hiatus in the tendon of the adductor magnus muscle (Fig. 4-31), which is located at the junction of the middle and distal thirds of the thigh (Fig. 4-34*B*). It begins here as the direct continuation of the **femoral artery**. From its origin it passes inferolaterally through the fat of the popliteal fossa, and it ends by dividing into two terminal branches, the **anterior** and **posterior tibial arteries**, at the inferior border of the popliteus muscle (Fig. 4-62).

The popliteal artery is located deeply throughout its course (Figs. 4-58 and 4-61). Anteriorly from proximal to distal, it lies against fat on the posterior surface of the femur, the fibrous capsule of the knee joint, and the fascia covering the popliteus muscle (Fig. 4-61). Posteriorly from proximal to distal, it lies deep to the semimembranosus muscle, the popliteal vein, the tibial nerve, and the gastrocnemius muscle.

Branches of the popliteal artery are numerous (Figs. 4-34*B*, 4-61, 4-62, and 4-127). They supply skin on the posterior aspect of the leg and muscles of the thigh and the leg. Five important **genicular branches** (L. *genu*, knee) supply the articular capsule and the ligaments of the knee joint. They are named as follows: **lateral superior** and **inferior**, **medial superior** and **inferior**, and **middle**. The small middle genicular artery, in addition to supplying ligaments (*e.g.*, the cruciate ligaments), supplies the synovial capsule of the knee joint (Fig. 4-123).

Muscular branches are given to the hamstrings and the calf muscles (gastrocnemius, soleus, and plantaris). The latter arteries (two in number and large) are called **sural arteries** (L. *sura*, the calf of the leg). The superior muscular branches of the popliteal artery have clinically important anastomoses with the terminal part of the profunda femoris and gluteal arteries.

Cutaneous branches arise from the popliteal artery and its branches. Usually one, the **superficial sural artery**, accompanies the small saphenous vein.

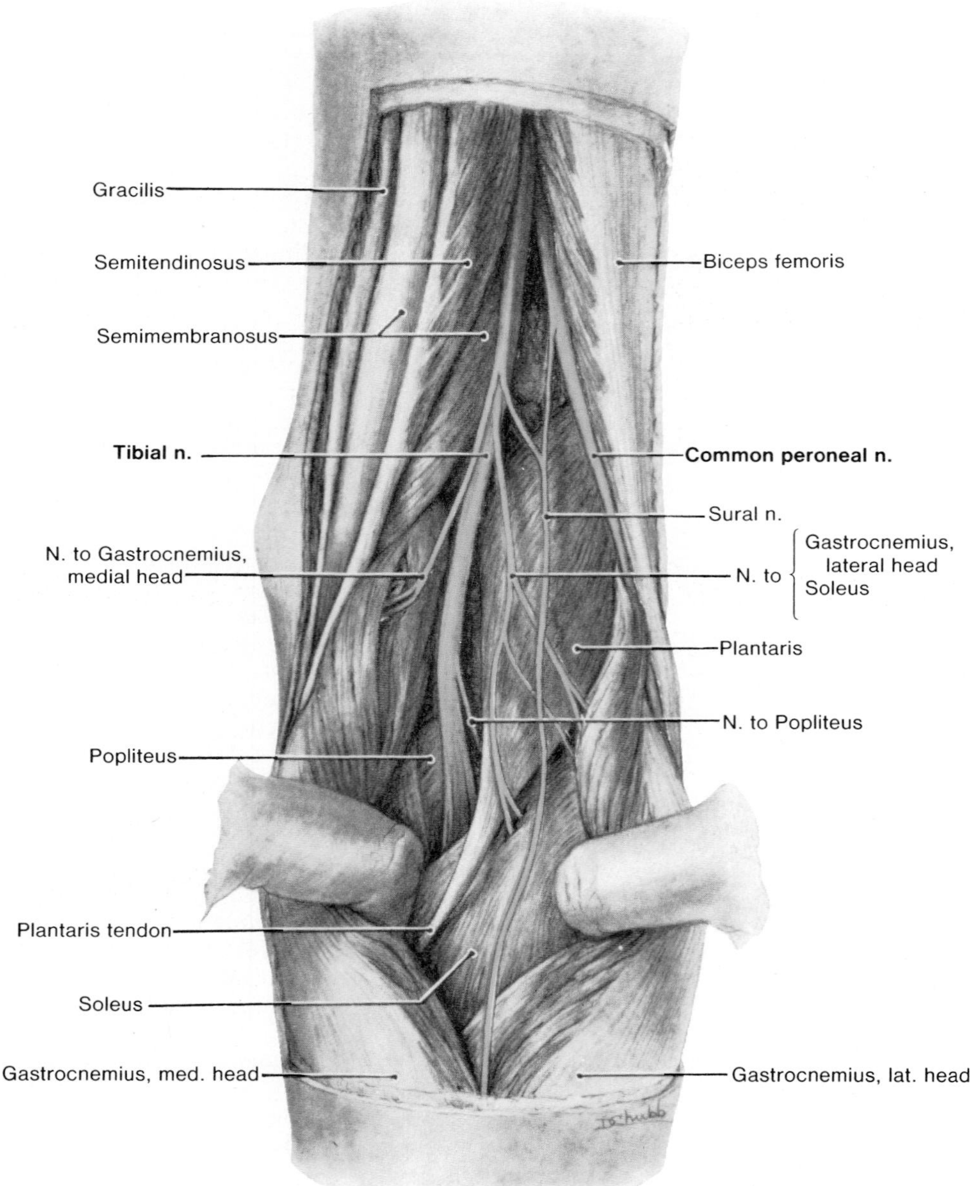

Figure 4-60. Drawing of a dissection of the nerves of the right popliteal fossa. The two most important nerves are the tibial and the common peroneal (terminal branches of the sciatic nerve). To expose them the medial and lateral heads of the gastrocnemius muscle are pulled forcibly apart. Observe a cutaneous branch of the tibial nerve joining a cutaneous branch of the common peroneal nerve to form the sural nerve. This junction is high; usually it is 5 to 8 cm above the ankle (Fig. 4-12*A*). Note that all motor branches in this region are springing from the tibial nerve, one branch coming from its medial side and the others from its lateral side.

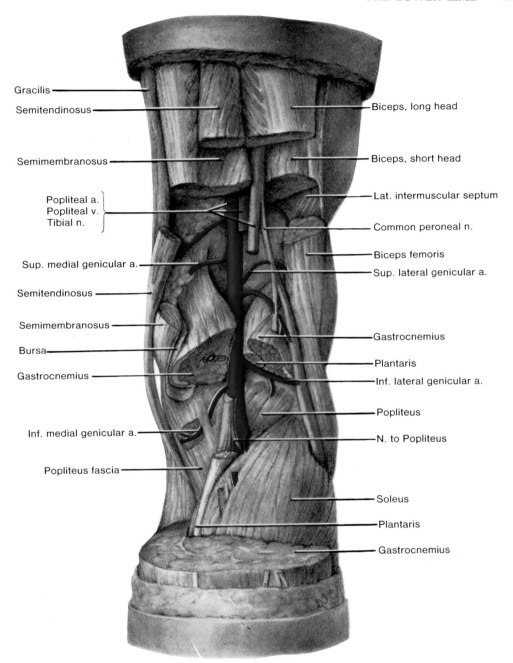

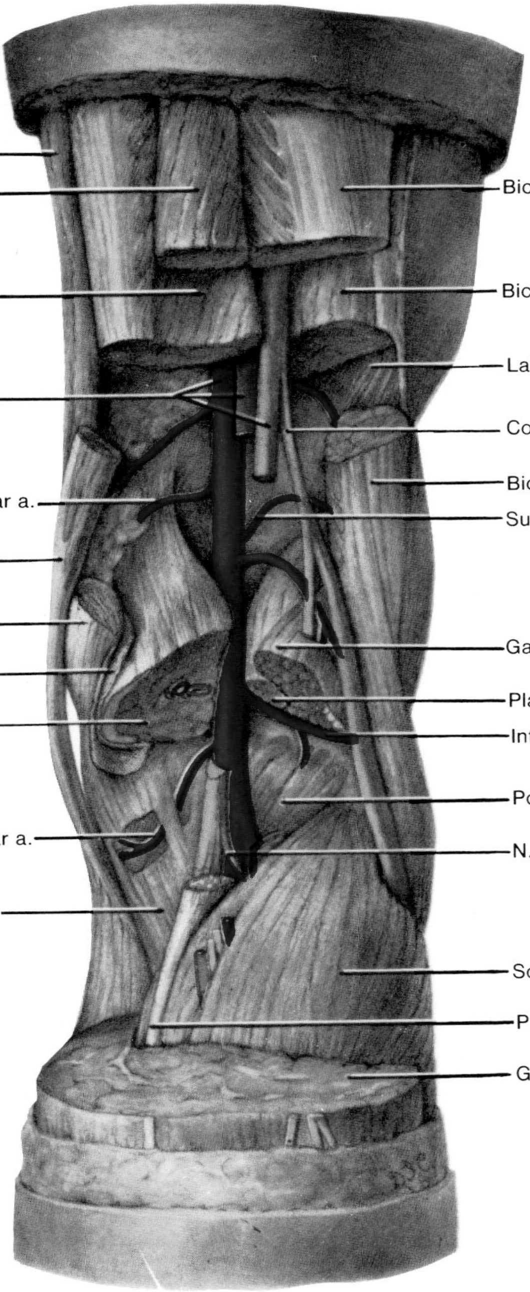

Figure 4-61. Drawing of a deep dissection of the right popliteal fossa. Observe the popliteal artery and its genicular branches lying deep on the floor of the fossa, which is composed of the popliteal surface of the femur, the capsule of the knee joint, and the popliteus fascia.

The Genicular Anastomosis (Figs. 4-34, 4-62, and 4-63). There is an intricate network of arterial vessels at the knee **involving 10 vessels**: the descending branch of the lateral circumflex femoral artery, a branch of the **profunda femoris**; the descending genicular branch of the **femoral artery**; the **five genicular branches of**

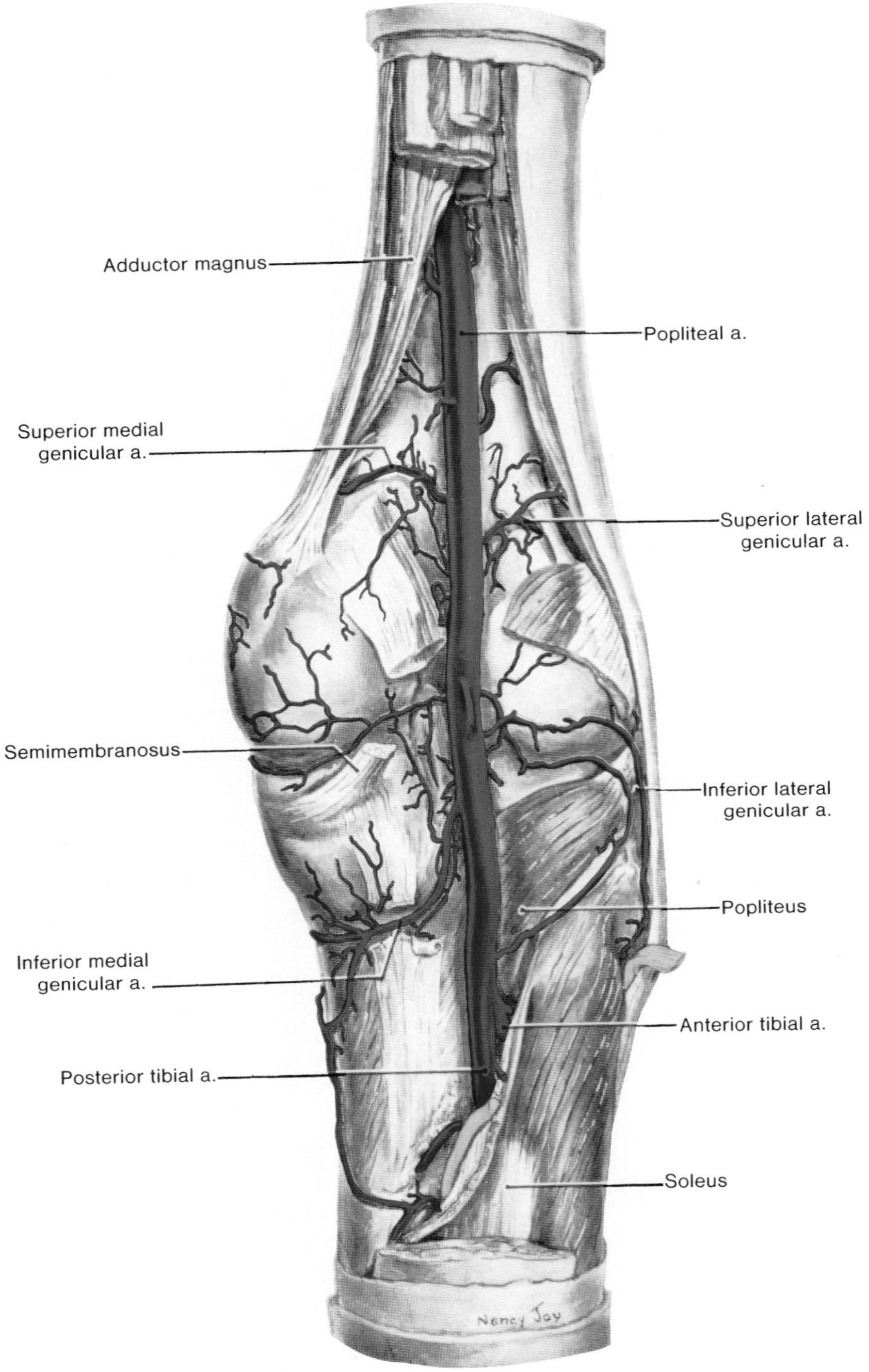

Figure 4-62. Drawing of the femoral artery showing a posterior view of the anastomoses around the right knee. Note that the popliteal artery begins at the hiatus in the adductor magnus proximally (not visible here, see Fig. 4-31) and ends at the inferior border of the popliteus muscle distally, where it bifurcates into the anterior and posterior tibial arteries. The three anterior relations of the popliteal artery are the femur (fat intervening), the fibrous capsule of the knee joint, and the popliteus muscle (covered with popliteus fascia, Fig. 4-61). Observe the four named genicular branches of the popliteal artery and one unnamed genicular artery on each side.

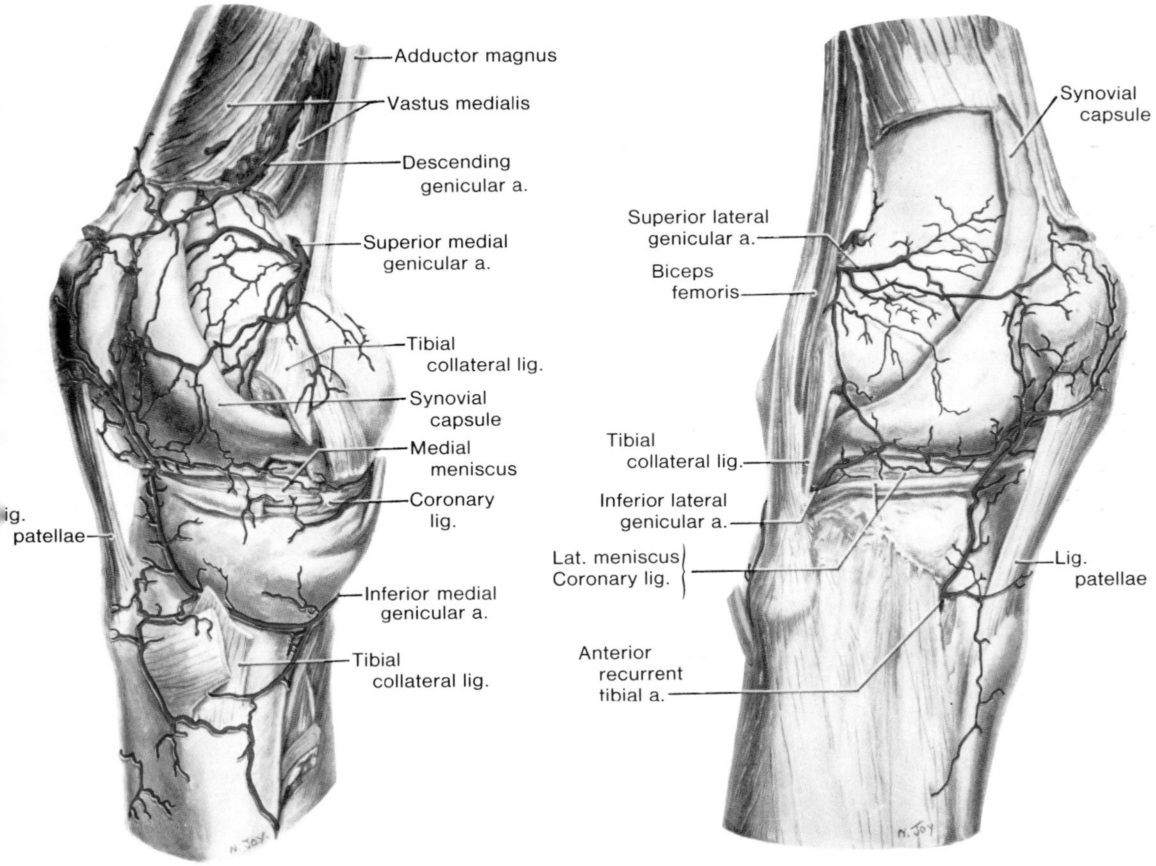

A. ANTEROMEDIAL VIEW B. ANTEROLATERAL VIEW

Figure 4-63. Illustrations of the clinically important anastomoses around the knee. Observe the two named genicular branches of the popliteal artery on each side, a superior and an inferior. Note also the descending genicular artery, a branch of the femoral artery superomedially, and the anterior recurrent branch of the anterior tibial artery, inferolaterally. Observe the inferior lateral genicular artery running along the lateral meniscus and an unnamed artery running similarly along the medial meniscus.

the popliteal artery; the **circumflex fibular artery**; and the anterior and posterior **tibial recurrent arteries**, branches of the posterior and anterior **tibial arteries**.

The genicular anastomosis is located around the patella and the proximal ends of the tibia and fibula. There is a **superficial network** between the deep fascia and the skin above and below the patella and in the fat posterior to the patella. There is also a **deep network** lying on the articular capsule of the knee joint and on the adjacent condyles of the femur and the tibia.

CLINICALLY ORIENTED COMMENTS

Sometimes there is little or no blood flow through the popliteal artery (*e.g.*, owing to obstructive disease resulting from **atherosclerosis**). Common sites for atheromatous occlusion are in the femoral artery at the adductor hiatus, *i.e.*, near the origin of the popliteal artery (Figs. 4-31 and 4-34).

When **obstructive disease** is suspected, an obvious sign would be loss of the popliteal pulse. Normally the pulsations of this artery can be felt on deep palpation when the knee is flexed. Palpation of this pulse is commonly done by placing the patient in the prone position (face down) on a table with the knee flexed to relax the popliteal fascia and the hamstring muscles.

Popliteal aneurysm (localized dilation of the popliteal artery owing to weakness of its wall) can cause swelling and pain in the popliteal fossa. To prevent rupture of the aneurysm, the femoral artery may be ligated in the **adductor canal** (formerly called Hunter's canal because Dr. Hunter devised this procedure many years ago).

When the femoral artery or the proximal part of the popliteal artery has been ligated or occluded owing to **obstructive disease**, blood can bypass the occlusion via the anastomoses around the knee and reach the artery again beyond the blockage. This is known as a **collateral circulation**. When an artery is blocked by an embolus or is ligated, the collateral anastomosing vessels become wider. Sudden blockage by an **embolus** (G. a plug) gives much less time for enlargement of the collateral vessels and the development of new ones than does gradual narrowing owing to obstructive disease.

The collateral circulation often provides an inadequate supply to the leg which, if very poor, can result in death of tissue (**necrosis**) owing to insufficiency of blood. Commonly the weakened region of the artery is replaced by a **prosthetic graft** or by a piece of the patient's great saphenous vein which is reversed so that its valves point in the direction of blood flow.

The Popliteal Vein (Figs. 4-58, 4-61, and 4-88). This vein is formed at the distal border of the popliteus muscle by the union of the venae comitantes of the anterior and posterior tibial veins. It ascends through the popliteal fossa, crossing from the medial to the lateral side of the popliteal artery. Throughout its course, it lies superficial to and in the same fibrous sheath as the popliteal artery.

The **small saphenous vein** (Fig. 4-58) pierces the popliteal fascia in the roof of the popliteal fossa and drains into the **popliteal vein**. The other tributaries of the popliteal vein correspond with the branches of the popliteal artery. The popliteal vein passes through the adductor hiatus in the tendon of the adductor magnus muscle and enters the **adductor canal** (Fig. 4-31), where it becomes the femoral vein (Fig. 4-35).

The Popliteal Nerves (Figs. 4-58 to 4-61 and 4-85). The sciatic nerve usually ends at the superior angle of the popliteal fossa by dividing into the tibial and common peroneal nerves, but this division may occur at a higher level (Fig. 4-50*B* and *C*).

The tibial nerve (medial popliteal nerve) is the *larger of the two terminal branches of the sciatic* nerve. It descends almost vertically through the popliteal fossa. In Figure 4-58 observe that the tibial nerve is the most superficial of the three main central components of the popliteal fossa (*i.e.*, nerve, vein, and artery). At first the tibial nerve is covered by the semimembranosus muscle and then it runs deep to the popliteal fascia. It then passes obliquely, posterior to the popliteal vessels and comes to lie medial to them, where it is covered by the converging heads of the gastrocnemius muscle (Figs. 4-58 to 4-61).

The tibial nerve gives rise to three articular branches to the knee joint. These **genicular branches** accompany the superior and inferior medial and middle genicular vessels to the joint. It also supplies muscular branches to the gastrocnemius, plantaris, popliteus, and soleus muscles.

Within the popliteal fossa, the tibial nerve gives off the **sural nerve**, which runs laterally within the fascia of the leg (Figs. 4-11, 4-12, 4-14, and 4-60). It is joined by the **sural communicating branch** of the common peroneal nerve and supplies the lateral aspect of the ankle and the foot. The tibial nerve also gives rise to the **medial sural cutaneous nerve** (Figs. 4-49 and 4-58), which supplies the skin of the calf.

The common peroneal nerve (lateral popliteal nerve) is the *smaller of the two terminal branches of the sciatic* nerve. It begins at the superior angle of the popliteal fossa and follows the medial border of the biceps femoris muscle and its tendon along the superolateral boundary of the fossa (Figs. 4-58, 4-60, and 4-61). It leaves the fossa by passing superficial to the lateral head of the gastrocnemius muscle. It then passes over the back of the head of the fibula before winding around the lateral surface of the neck of this bone. It then runs beneath the upper fibers of the peroneus longus muscle (Figs. 4-61, 4-67*A*, and 4-77).

The *common peroneal nerve is palpable* and can be rolled against the bone posterior to the head of the fibula and posterolateral to its neck. In this region the common peroneal nerve ends by dividing into **superficial** and **deep peroneal nerves** (Figs. 4-67*A* and 4-81). Within the popliteal fossa (*i.e.*, before dividing), the common peroneal nerve gives off articular branches to the knee and proximal tibiofibular joints. These **genicular branches** accompany the superior and inferior lateral genicular vessels to the knee joint.

Within the fossa it also gives off the **lateral sural cutaneous nerve** to the skin of the calf and a sural communicating branch which joins the **sural nerve** in supplying the lateral aspect of the ankle and foot (Figs. 4-49, 4-58, and 4-106).

CLINICALLY ORIENTED COMMENTS

The **common peroneal nerve** *is the most commonly injured nerve in the lower limb*, mainly because it is exposed where it winds superficially around the neck of the fibula (Fig. 4-81). Even when there is direct trauma to the sciatic nerve, the common peroneal division is usually more severely affected than the tibial division.

The common peroneal nerve may be lacerated at the side of the knee (*e.g.*, Case 4-3), severed during **fracture of the neck of the fibula** (Case 4-4), or severely stretched subsequent to fracture of the head of the fibula or rupture of the fibular collateral ligament (Fig. 4-125). In addition, it is susceptible to pressure exerted in the region of the head of the fibula by a tightly applied **plaster cast** or the buckle of a restraining strap on the operating table.

Severance of the common peroneal nerve results in paralysis of all the dorsiflexor and evertor muscles of the foot. Owing to the paralysis of the dorsiflexor muscles, this part of the lower limb hangs down, producing a condition known as "**foot-drop**" ("drop-foot"). As a result the patient shows a **high steppage gait** in which the foot is raised higher than is necessary so that the toes do not hit the ground, and the foot is brought down suddenly in a flapping manner that produces a distinctive "clop."

There is also a variable loss of sensation on the anterolateral aspect of the leg and the dorsum of the foot, including the web between the first and second toes, supplied by the superficial peroneal and deep peroneal nerves, respectively (Fig. 4-106).

The tibial nerve is not commonly injured because of its protected position in the popliteal fossa; however, it may be injured by gunshot or deep lacerations in this region (Case 4-10). **Severance of the tibial nerve** produces paralysis of the flexor muscles in the leg and the intrinsic muscles of the sole of the foot and loss of sensation on the sole of the foot. Persons with **tibial nerve injury** are unable to plantarflex their foot or toes (Fig. 4-75*B*).

THE LEG AND FOOT

The leg is the part of the lower limb between the knee and the ankle joint (Fig. 4-65); the foot is the part distal to the leg. For descriptive purposes, the foot is the part of the limb distal to a transverse line drawn through the malleoli.

BONES OF THE LEG

The bones of the leg (L. *crus*) are the **tibia** ("shin bone") and the **fibula** (Figs. 4-1, 4-2, and 4-65). The tibia supports most of the weight and articulates with the condyles of the femur superiorly and with the saddle-shaped superior surface of the talus inferiorly. The fibula is mainly for the attachment of muscles (Figs. 4-66 and 4-67), but it also provides stability to the ankle joint. Its lateral malleolus forms a **mortise**, or socket, with the inferior surface of the tibia and medial malleolus, into which the trochlea of the talus fits (Figs. 4-70 and 4-142). The bodies of the tibia and fibula are connected by an interosseous membrane

(Figs. 4-64 and 4-74) composed of strong oblique fibers (Fig. 4-81).

The Tibia (Figs. 4-1, 4-2, and 4-64 to 4-67). *The proximal end* of the tibia is large and has an almost flat superior surface bearing two **condyles** which articulate with the condyles of the femur. The superior surface of the tibia is so flat and horizontal that it is described as medial and lateral **tibial plateaus**. In Figures 4-2 and 4-65 note that the bifid **intercondylar eminence** fits into the intercondylar notch between the femoral condyles.

In Figure 4-67*B* observe that the lateral condyle has a facet inferiorly for the head of the fibula. Note the prominent **tibial tuberosity** anteriorly into which the ligamentum patellae (patellar ligament) inserts (Figs. 4-23*B*, 4-26, 4-27, 4-55, and 4-67*B*).

The distal end of the tibia is small and has facets for the fibula and the talus (Fig. 4-67*B*). It projects medially and inferiorly as the **medial malleolus**, which has a facet on its lateral surface for articulation with the talus (Fig. 4-65). On a dried talus, note that this facet is continuous with the facet on the inferior surface of the tibia. The body (shaft) of the tibia is approximately triangular in cross-section (Figs. 4-64 and 4-74) and has medial, lateral, and posterior surfaces.

In Figure 4-67*B* observe that muscles attach to the lateral surface of the tibia. The lateral border of the tibia is sharp where it gives attachment to the **interosseous membrane**, which unites the two leg bones (Figs. 4-64 and 4-74); hence, this border of the tibia is commonly referred to as the **interosseous border**.

On the posterior surface of the proximal part of the body of the tibia, observe a rough diagonal ridge known as the **soleal line** (Fig. 4-65). It runs inferomedially to the medial border, about a third of the way down the shaft. The popliteus muscle inserts into the tibia proximal to this line (Figs. 4-62 and 4-66). Note also the **vertical line** which runs inferiorly from the middle of the soleal line (Fig. 4-65). It separates the origin of the flexor digitorum longus medially from that of the tibialis posterior laterally (Fig. 4-66).

CLINICALLY ORIENTED COMMENTS

The body of the tibia is narrowest at the junction of the middle and lower thirds. This is the most frequent site of fracture and the region where *rickets* (a disease of growing bone) has its effect during infancy and childhood (Fig. I-35).

March fractures of the lower third of the tibia are common in persons who undertake long walks when they are not used to this activity (*e.g.*, march for millions). The strain of this strenuous activity may fracture the anterior cortex of the tibia.

Indirect violence may be applied to the tibia and fibula when the body turns during a fall with the foot fixed. Severe torsion during skiing may produce a **spiral fracture** of the tibia at the junction of the middle and lower thirds with a fracture of the neck of the fibula. A forward or backward fall may produce a "**boot-top fracture**" owing to the rigidity of the ski boot.

Fractures of the tibia and fibula may also result from a direct blow, *e.g.*, when the bumper of a car strikes the leg producing what are called "**bumper fractures**". The fractures usually occur at about the same level in both bones and are frequently compound, *i.e.*, a fracture in which there is an open wound of the soft parts leading to the bone fragments. As the tibia lies subcutaneously (Fig. 4-64), the blow often tears the skin, permitting the bone fragments to protrude.

As the body of the tibia is unprotected anteromedially throughout its course and is relatively slender at the junction of its lower and middle one-thirds, it is not surprising that it is the most common long bone to be fractured and to suffer compound injury. Its extensive subcutaneous surface, however, makes it an accessible site for obtaining pieces of bone for **grafting** (*e.g.*, insertion of a piece of bone into another one to replace a defect).

In fracture-dislocations of the ankle (*e.g.*, **Pott's fracture**, Case 4-5), the medial malleolus of the tibia may be avulsed (pulled off) by the strong deltoid ligament (Fig. 4-159).

A.

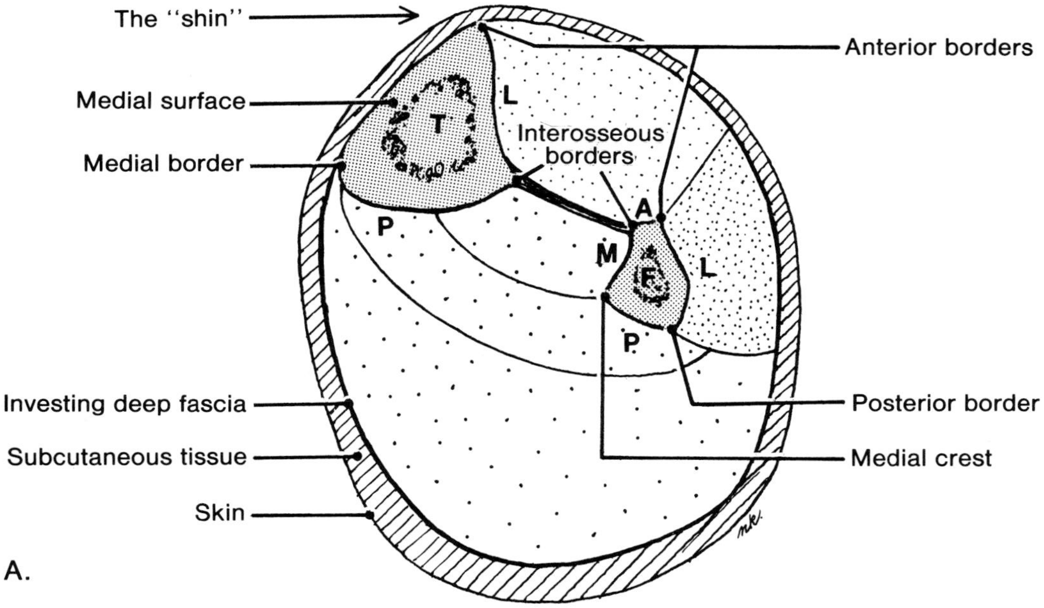

B.

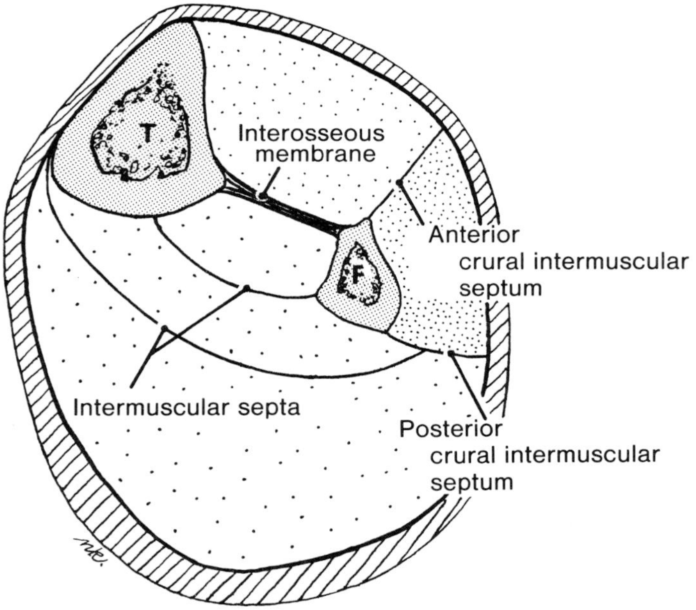

Figure 4-64. Drawings of the proximal aspect of cross-sections of the right leg, actual size, giving the terminology of the surfaces and borders of the tibia (*T*) and fibula (*F*). Observe the anterior (*A*), posterior (*P*), medial (*M*), and lateral (*L*) surfaces. Note that the medial surface of the tibia is subcutaneous, whereas the lateral surface of the smaller fibula is deeply placed. Observe that the tibia and fibula are connected by a strong interosseous membrane which is attached to their interosseous borders. Compare with the cross-section of the leg in Figure 4-74 containing the muscles. Note that the two bones, their interosseous membrane, and the anterior and posterior crural intermuscular septa divide the leg into three compartments: anterior, lateral, and posterior.

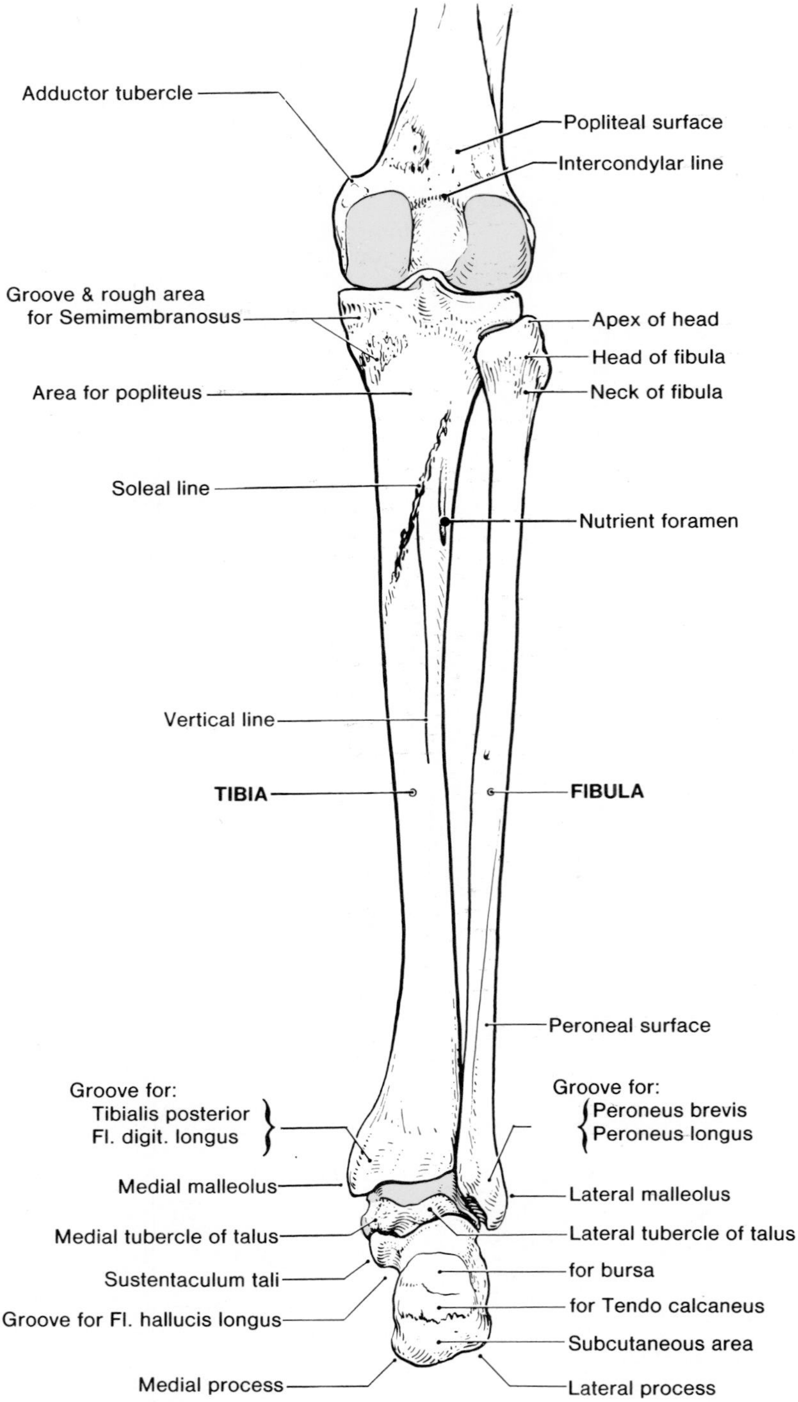

Figure 4-65. Drawing of a posterior view of the bones of the right lower limb. Observe that the two bones of the leg are unequal in size. The larger tibia lies medial and its medial surface is subcutaneous. The smaller fibula is deeply placed. In the body the tibia and the fibula are connected by an interosseous membrane. For more details of the proximal parts of these bones, see Figures 4-1 and 4-2. Observe that the lateral malleolus lies more inferior (1 to 2 cm) and posterior than does the medial malleolus. Note that the talus is held between the two sides of the mortise or cavity formed by the inferior surface of the tibia and the medial and lateral malleoli of the tibia and fibula, respectively (see Fig. 4-142 for a radiograph of this mortise).

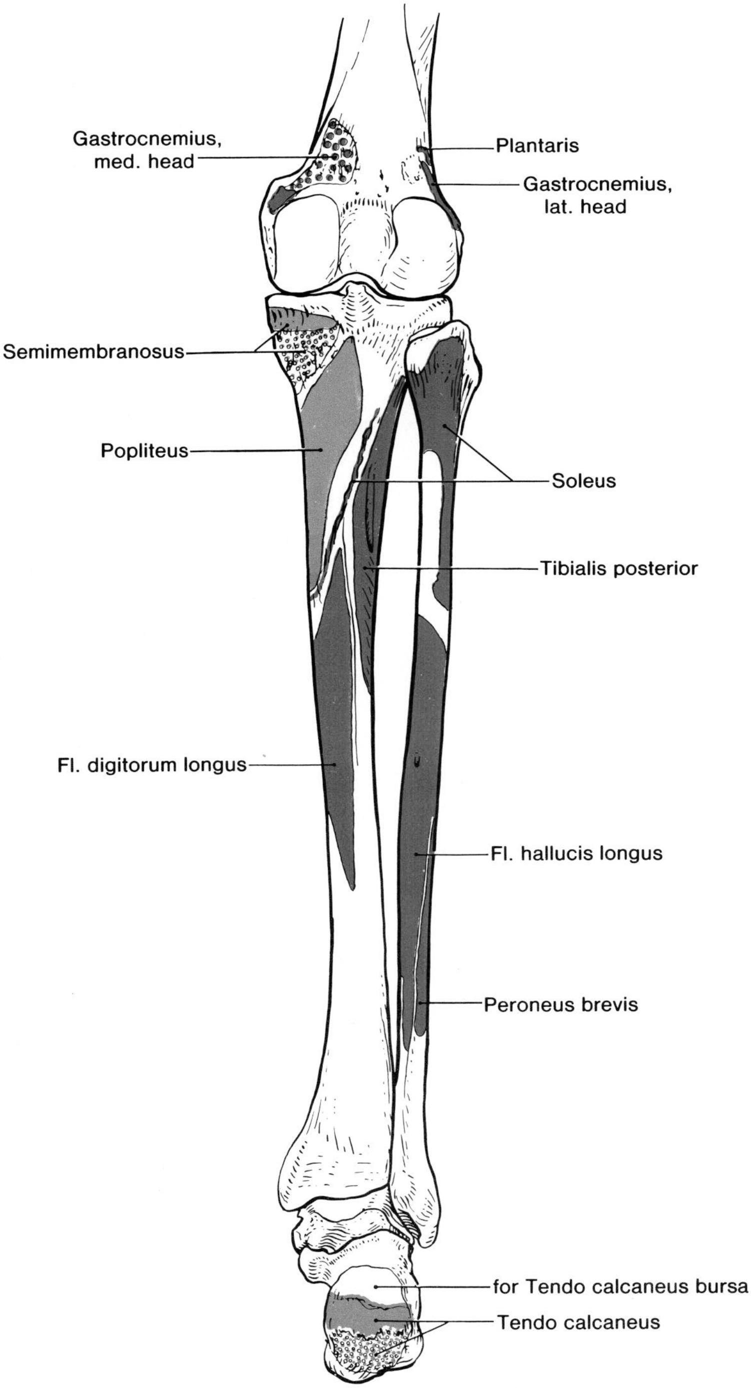

Figure 4-66. Drawing of the posterior aspect of the bones of the right lower limb showing the sites of attachment of muscles to it. Only the distal end of the bone of the thigh (femur) is shown. Although not indicated, the two leg bones are connected by a strong interosseous membrane (Figs. 4-64 and 4-74). The main attachment of the tendo calcaneus into the middle of the posterior surface of the calcaneus is shown in *blue*. The origins of muscles are shown in *red* and insertions in *blue*.

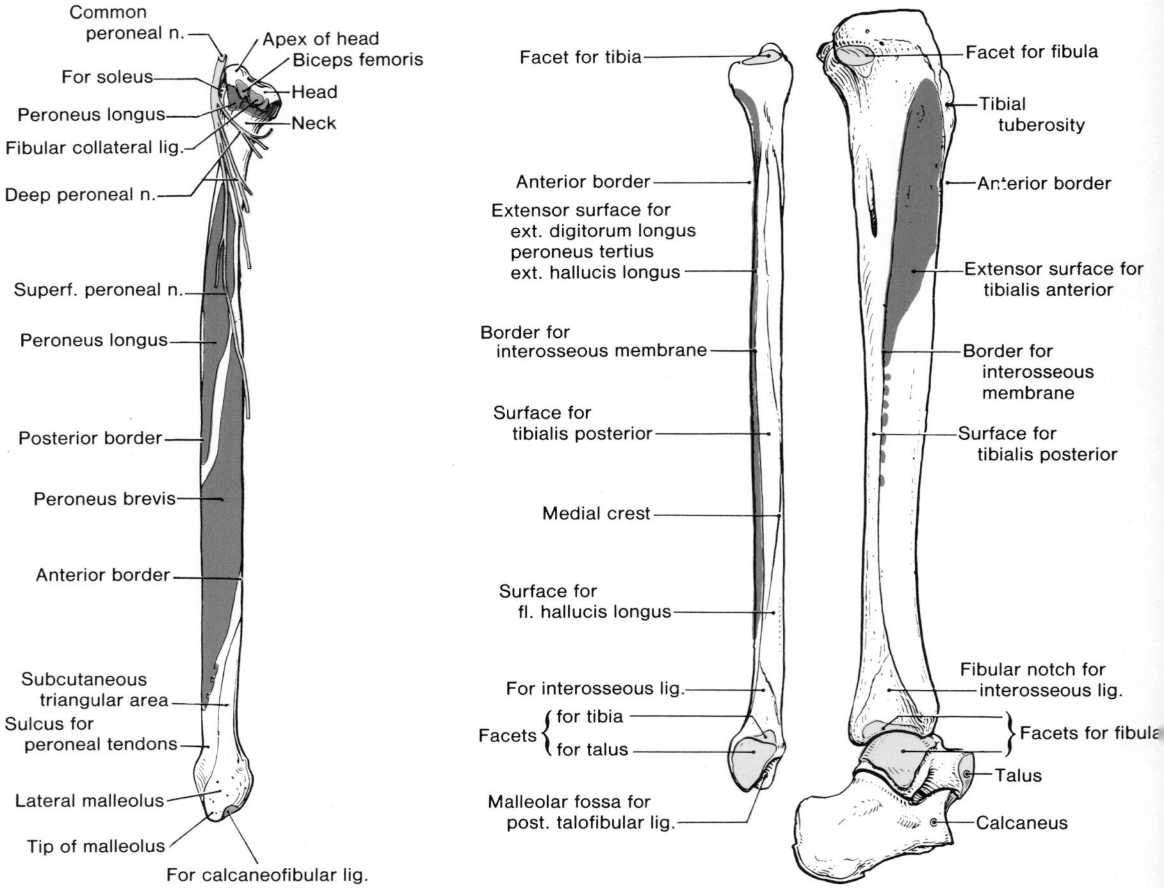

A. LATERAL SURFACE OF FIBULA

B. TIBIA AND FIBULA, OPPOSED ASPECTS

Figure 4-67. Drawings of the bones of the leg showing the attachments of muscles and ligaments. Some bones of the foot are shown in *B*. The tibia ("shin bone"), the weight bearer of the leg, has a proximal expanded end which articulates with the femoral condyles and the head of the fibula (Figs. 4-1 and 4-2). The fibula ("splint or brooch bone"), the lateral bone of the leg, bears little or no weight and plays no part in the knee joint, but its malleolus forms part of the mortise for the talus (Fig. 4-142). In *A*, note the *clinically important relationship of the common peroneal nerve* to the proximal end of the fibula. Observe that this nerve passes posterior to the head of the fibula and around the lateral aspect of the neck of this bone to its anterior aspect. The nerve is particularly exposed to injury here, being subcutaneous and related so closely to the fibula. In *B*, observe the rough triangular, opposed surfaces of the bones for attachment of the interosseous membrane; this ligament is the chief bond of the distal tibiofibular joint. It is also strengthened in front and behind by the anterior and posterior tibiofibular ligaments (Fig. 4-140).

The Fibula (Figs. 4-1, 4-2, and 4-64 to 4-67). The fibula (L. pin or skewer) is the *lateral bone of the leg*. Its slender body (shaft) has little or no function in weight bearing, but its malleolus helps to hold the talus in its socket (Fig. 4-142). It serves mainly for muscle attachments (nine of them) and probably acts as a brace in providing support for the tibia. The slightly constricted part of the shaft near the head is referred to as the **neck** of the fibula. Its sharp **interosseous border** is for the attachment of the **interosseous membrane** (Figs. 4-64 and 4-74).

Its knob-like **head** has a facet on its superior surface for articulation with the inferior surface of the lateral tibial condyle.

Its distal end, called the **lateral malleolus**, is also knob-like. The lateral surface of this bony prominence is subcutaneous (Figs. 4-79 and 4-86). The medial surface articulates with the lateral side of the tibia and the talus of the lower end of the body of the tibia. Posteroinferior to the facet for the talus is a depression, the **malleolar fossa**, into which you can insert the tip of your finger. The posterior talofibular ligament and part of the posterior tibiofibular ligament (Fig. 4-140) attach to this fossa (Fig. 4-67*B*). In Figure 4-65 observe that the lateral malleolus lies more inferior and posterior than does the medial malleolus. Verify this on yourself.

CLINICALLY ORIENTED COMMENTS

Fractures of the fibula commonly occur 2 to 5 cm proximal to the distal end of the lateral malleolus and are often associated with fracture-dislocations of the ankle (*e.g.*, a **Pott's fracture**, Case 4-5 and Fig. 4-159). The fibula breaks when the talus is forcibly tilted against the lateral malleolus, forcing it laterally. The **posterior tibiofibular ligament** (Fig. 4-140) acts as a fulcrum, translating the lateral force on the malleolus to a medial force on the body just proximal to the ankle joint, where it often breaks (Fig. 4-159); the medial malleolus is also often torn off.

Absence or deficiency of the fibula is not common and is often associated with other malformations (*e.g.*, absence of the peroneal and calf muscles and/or foot deformities).

The fibula is a common source of bone for grafting (*e.g.*, replacing the body of the humerus which has been removed because of a tumor). Removal of portions of the fibula does not affect leg or foot function. The missing piece of bone usually does not grow back (regenerate) because the periosteum and nutrient artery are generally removed so that the graft will remain alive.

Surface Anatomy of the Leg Bones. A thorough physical examination of the leg requires a good knowledge of the surface features of its bones.

Surface Anatomy of the Tibia. The surface features of the medial surface of the tibia (shin bone) are more or less familiar to most people. Palpate the medial surface of your tibia (Fig. 4-64), noting that it is subcutaneous, smooth, and flat; verify that the skin covering it is freely movable. As you run your hand distally, feel the prominence at the ankle known as the **medial malleolus**. Note that it is also subcutaneous and that its inferior end is blunt. You may be able to observe the **great saphenous vein** crossing the lowest third of the medial surface of your tibia obliquely (Figs. 4-12*B* and 4-92). The ankle joint is at the level of a point about 1.5 cm proximal to the tip of the medial malleolus.

Run your hand proximally along the medial surface of your tibia and palpate its medial condyle. Verify that it is also subcutaneous. Feel the anterior border of your tibia (Figs. 4-64 and 4-74), noting that it is sharp and subcutaneous. The skin here is very close to the periosteum of the bone; no wonder it hurts so much and bruises so easily when you hit the front of your leg (*i.e.*, shin, Fig. 4-64) on something hard. Run your hand proximally along the anterior aspect of the tibia until you feel the rounded elevation called the **tibial tuberosity** (Fig. 4-1). It is about 5 cm distal to the inferior border or apex of the patella (Figs. 4-25, 4-27, and 4-55).

Palpate the **patellar ligament (ligamentum patellae)**, which extends from the patella to the tuberosity of the tibia. It is most easily felt when the knee is extended. Flex your knee joint (*i.e.*, **genuflex**) and feel the depression on each side of the patellar ligament. Usually some indentation is visible at these sites when the leg is extended. The articular capsule of the knee joint is very superficial in these depressions (Fig. 4-122).

The **tibial tuberosity** is a useful bony landmark because it roughly indicates the level of the division of the popliteal artery into its terminal branches, the anterior and posterior tibial arteries, at the distal border of the popliteus muscle (Figs. 4-34*B* and 4-62). The smooth upper part of the tibial tuberosity (to which the **patellar ligament** is attached) is at the level of the head of the fibula. The subcutaneous, rough lower part of the tuberosity, which bears the weight during kneeling, is at the level of the neck of the fibula (Fig. 4-54).

Surface Anatomy of the Fibula. You can easily palpate the **head of the fibula** at the level of the upper part of the tibial tuberosity because this knob of bone is subcutaneous at the posterolateral aspect of the knee (Fig. 4-55). It is usually easiest to palpate from behind. A good guide to its location is the distal end of the tendon of the biceps femoris (Figs. 4-27 and 4-57).

The **neck of the fibula** (Fig. 4-67*A*) can be palpated just distal to the head. The **common peroneal nerve** may be rolled under your finger here, thereby causing a tingling sensation on the anterolateral aspect of your leg and the dorsal surfaces of your toes (Fig. 4-106).

Only the distal portion of the body of the fibula is subcutaneous. This portion of the fibula proximal to the lateral maleolus is commonly fractured (Case 4-5 and Fig. 4-159). Palpate the lateral prominence at the ankle or lateral malleolus (Fig. 4-79). Verify that it is subcutaneous and that its inferior end is sharp. Run your finger proximally and palpate the distal third of the fibula. You may be able to see it as you invert and evert your foot (Fig. 4-75*C* and *D*). Verify that the tip of your *lateral malleolus extends further distally* (1 to 2 cm) and posteriorly than does the tip of the medial malleolus. This relationship is important in the diagnosis and treatment of certain injuries in the ankle region (*e.g.*, **Pott's fracture-dislocation of the ankle**, Case 4-5).

BONES OF THE FOOT

The bones of the foot comprise the **tarsus**, the **metatarsus**, and the **phalanges**. Using an articulated foot, observe that its medial border is almost straight (Figs. 4-68 and 4-69). Note that the line joining the midpoints of the medial and lateral borders of the foot is oblique and that the metatarsal bones and the phalanges are located anterior to this line and the tarsal bones posterior to it.

There is relatively little free movement between the individual bones of the foot because of the way they fit together and are held in position by ligaments (Figs. 4-145 to 4-147). As a consequence, the foot is relatively stable.

The Tarsus (Figs. 4-65 and 4-68 to 4-72). The tarsus (G. *tarsos*, flat) consists of **seven tarsal bones**: talus, calcaneus, cuboid, navicular, and three cuneiforms. Only one of them, the talus, articulates with the two leg bones.

The Talus (Figs. 4-65 to 4-72 and 4-142). The talus (L. ankle bone) has a **body**, a **neck**, and a **head**. It looks somewhat like a turtle when it is viewed from above, resting on the anterior two-thirds of the calcaneus or heel bone. It also articulates with the tibia, the fibula, and the navicular bone. Its saddle-shaped superior surface bears the weight of the body transmitted via the tibia. **The body of the talus** is cuboidal in shape; its pulley-shaped superior articular surface, often called the **trochlea** (L. pulley), articulates with the inferior surface of the tibia as part of the ankle joint (Fig. 4-141). The body has three continuous facets for articulation (Fig. 4-68): one for the facet on the inferior surface of the tibia, one for the facet on the lateral surface of the medial malleolus, and one for the facet on the medial surface of the lateral malleolus (Fig. 4-142). The inferior surface of the body has an oval, deeply concave area for articulation with the calcaneus. There is a **posterior process** projecting posteriorly from the body which ends in medial and lateral tubercles, with a groove between them for the tendon of the flexor hallucis longus muscle (Figs. 4-65 and 4-68). Occasionally the **lateral tubercle** of the posterior process (Fig. 4-71) fails to unite with the body of the talus. This separate bone, known as the *os trigonum*, could be misinterpreted as a fracture by an inexperienced viewer of radiographs.

The head of the talus is its rounded anterior end, which is directed anteromedially (Figs. 4-69 to 4-71). It has a large facet for articulation with the navicular bone and one for articulation with the shelf-

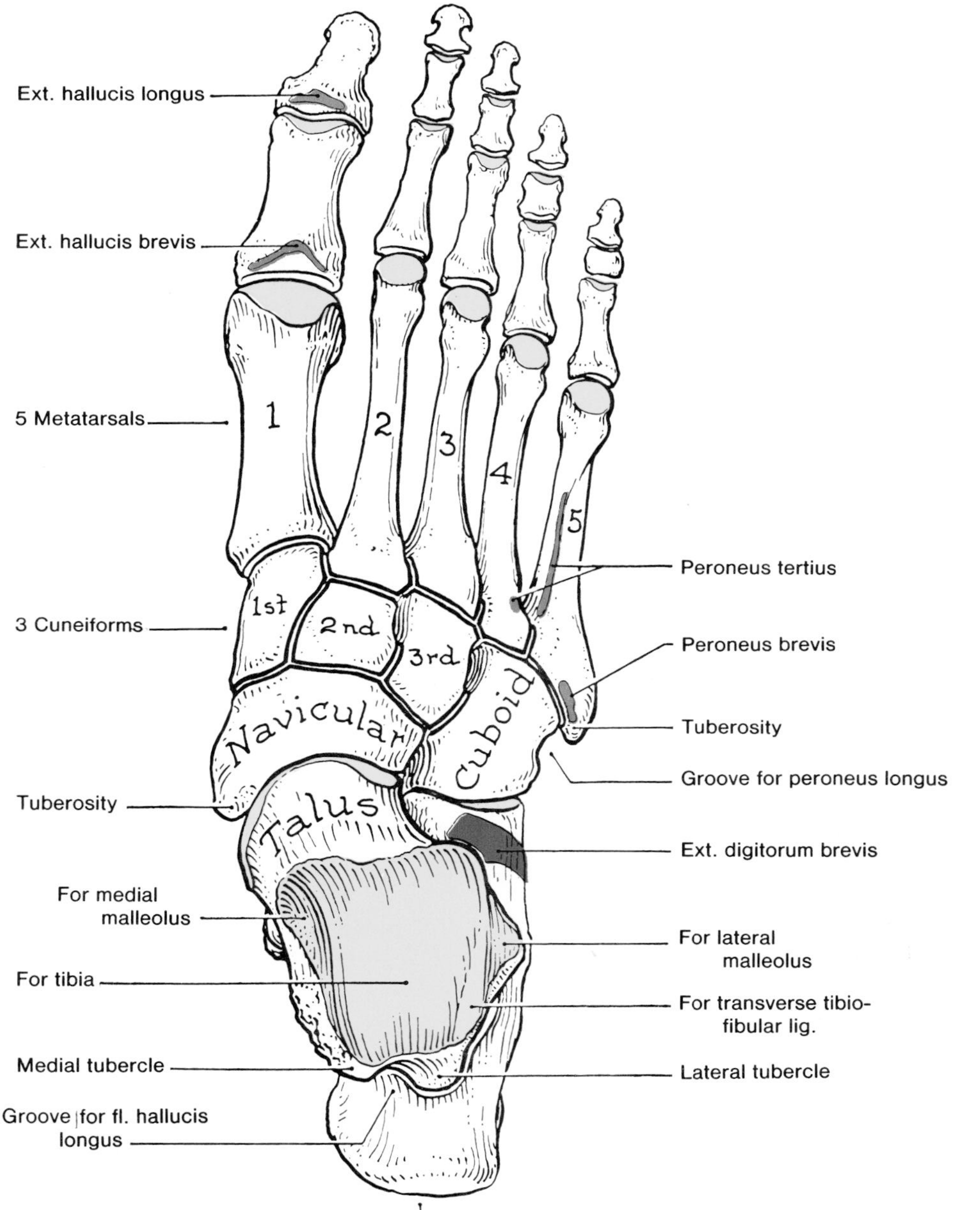

Figure 4-68. Drawing of the dorsal aspect of the bones of the right foot, showing the muscle attachments and articular cartilages (*yellow*). The arch or dorsum of the foot is sometimes referred to as the "instep." Observe the tuber calcanei (tuberosity) for attachment of the tendo calcaneus (see also Figs. 4-66 and 4-83). The origin of the extensor digitorum brevis is shown in *red*. Insertions of muscles are shown in *blue*.

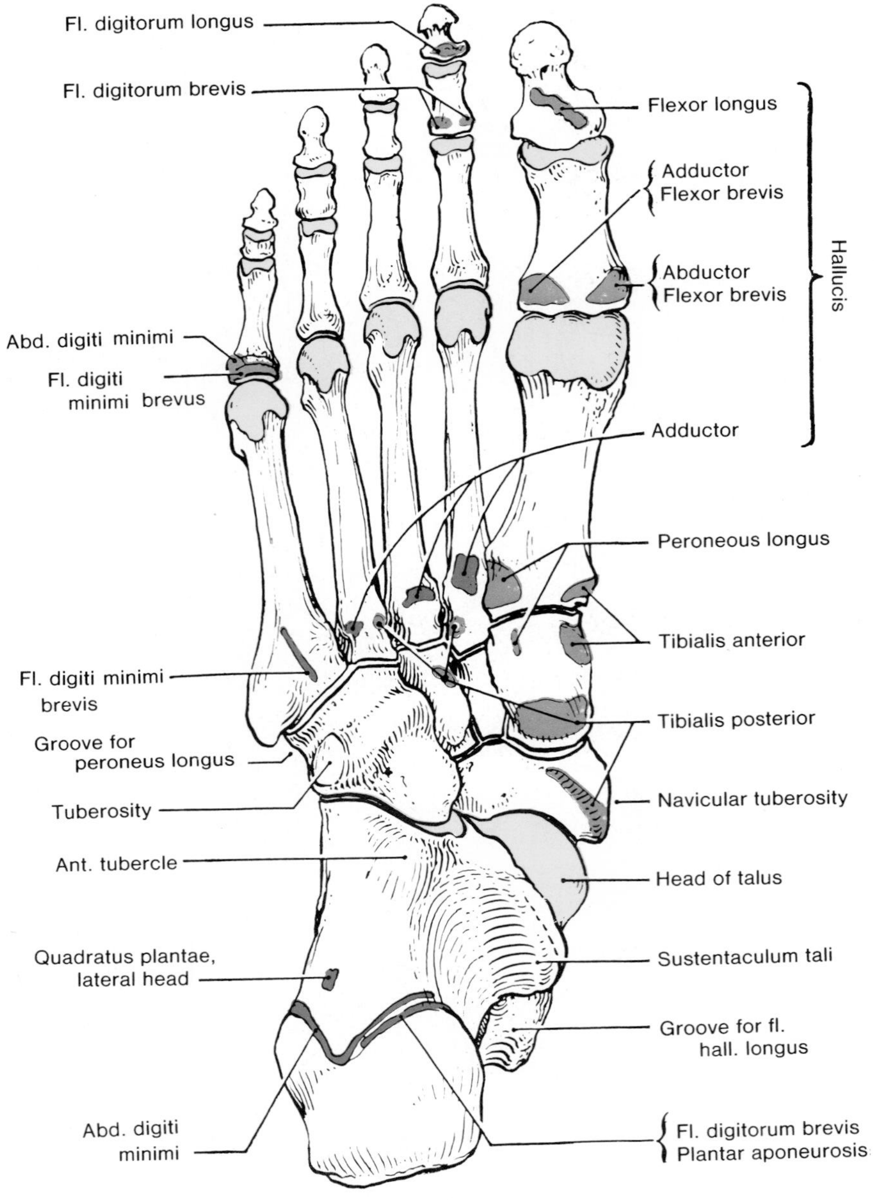

Figure 4-69. Drawing of the plantar aspect of the bones of the right foot showing the attachments of muscles and the features of the bones.

like projection of the calcaneus known as the **sustentaculum tali** (Figs. 4-65 and 4-69), as well as a small facet for articulation with the plantar calcaneonavicular ligament (Fig. 4-143).

The neck of the talus is the slightly constricted part between the head and the body (Fig. 4-71). Inferiorly there is a deep groove called the **sulcus tali** for the interosseous ligaments between the talus and the calcaneus (Fig. 4-145).

The Calcaneus (Figs. 4-65 to 4-72). The calcaneus (L. heel) is the largest and strongest bone of the foot. This heel bone is also

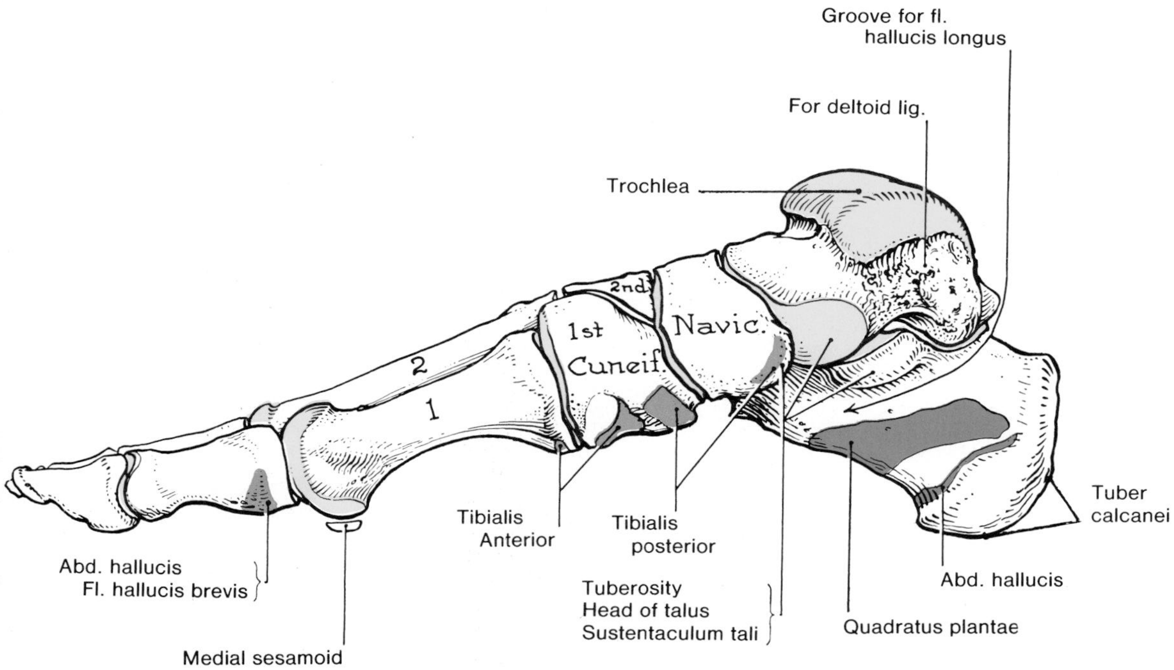

Figure 4-70. Drawing of the medial aspect of the bones of the right foot. The trochlea is the part of the body of the talus that articulates with the ankle socket or mortise (Fig. 4-142). The trochlea of the talus has a superior part (indicated here), a medial malleolar part (visible above), and a lateral malleolar part (shown below). In this and other drawings the colors indicate the articular cartilages (*yellow*), the origin of muscles (*red*), and the insertions of muscles (*blue*).

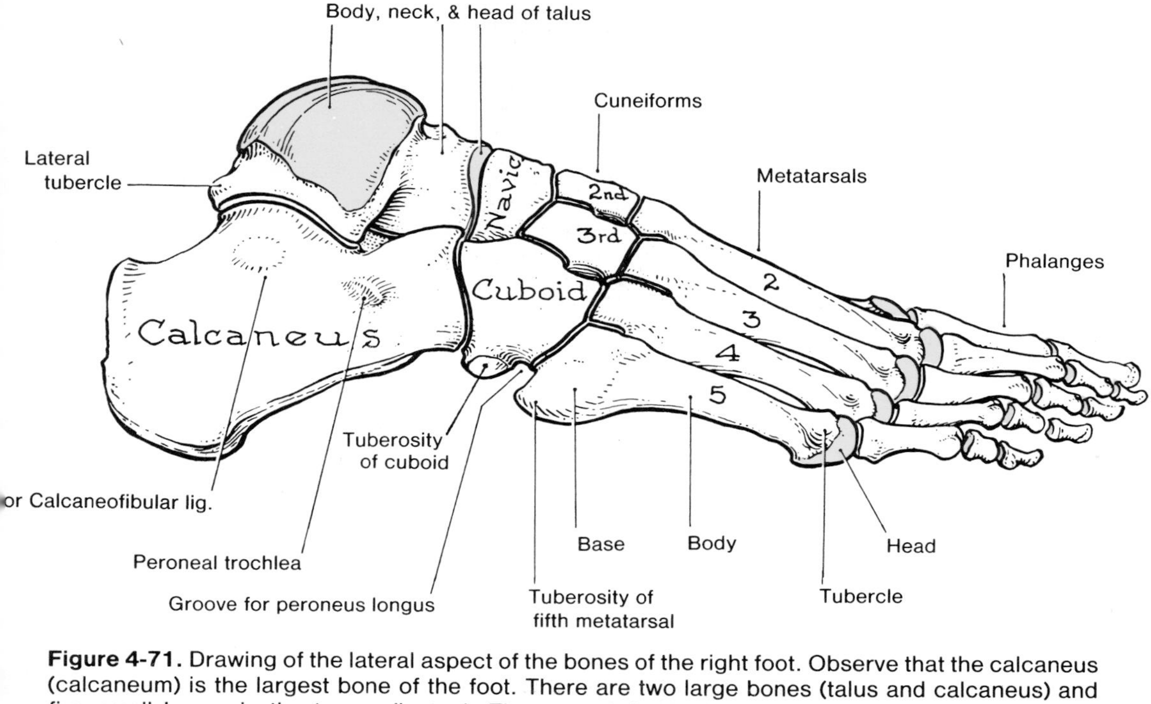

Figure 4-71. Drawing of the lateral aspect of the bones of the right foot. Observe that the calcaneus (calcaneum) is the largest bone of the foot. There are two large bones (talus and calcaneus) and five small bones in the tarsus (instep). The part of the body of the talus indicated here is the trochlea. It articulates with the tibia and the malleoli (Fig. 4-142).

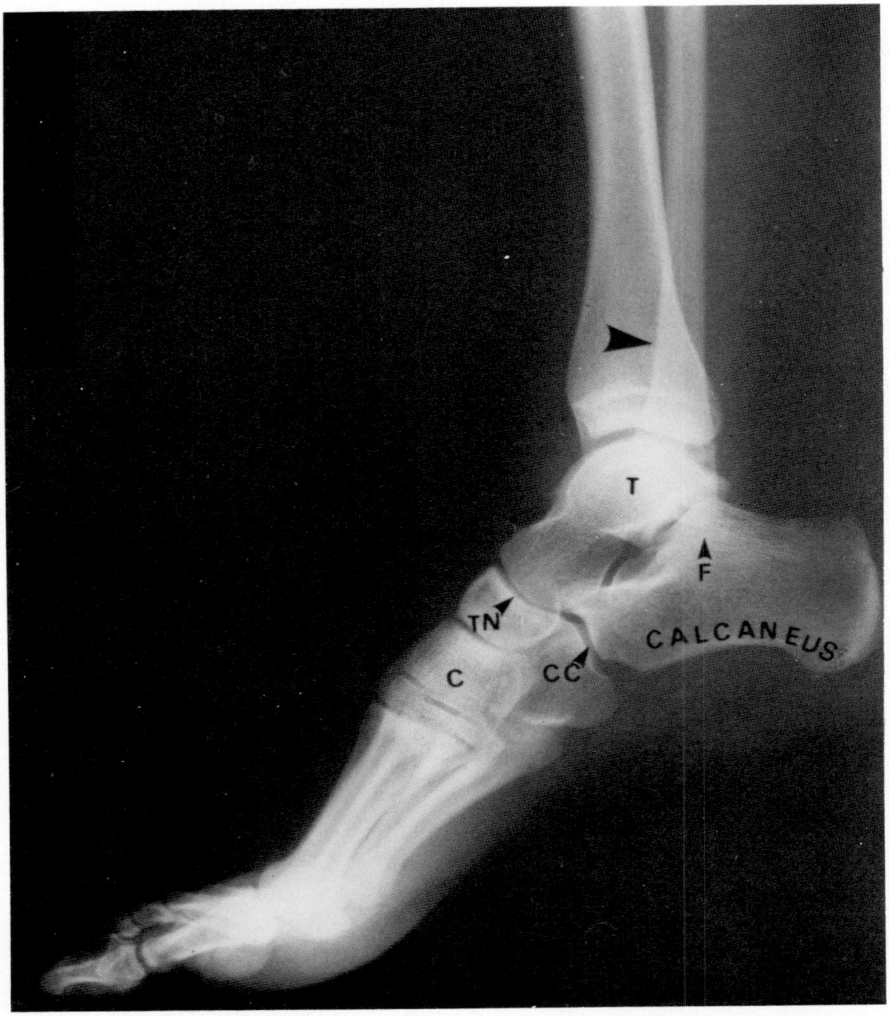

Figure 4-72. Lateral radiograph of the bones of the right leg and foot. This radiograph was taken with the foot raised as in walking. The *large arrow* points to the edge of the triangular area where the tibia and the fibula are superimposed on each other. The *small arrow* (*F*) indicates how far the fibula extends distally. The talus (*T*) participates in the talonavicular joint (*TN*) and the calcaneus in the calcaneocuboid (*CC*) joint. The cuneiforms (*C*) and the proximal ends of the metatarsals are superimposed upon each other.

referred to as the os calcis, or the calcaneum. The calcaneus lies inferior to the talus; thus its superior surface presents articular facets for it. The posterior one is demarcated anteriorly by a groove, the **sulcus calcanei**. Anterior to this sulcus is the **sustenaculum tali** (Figs. 4-65, 4-69, and 4-70), which helps to support the talus. The calcaneus projects posteriorly behind the bones of the leg and **forms the prominence of the heel** (Figs. 4-72 and 4-84). At the posterior end of the inferior surface there is a **tuber calcanei** projecting downward (Fig. 4-70). It is deep to the fibrous tissue and fat of the heel pad, and its inferior part transmits the weight of the body to the floor or ground.

On the medial surface of the calcaneus there is a groove on the inferior surface of the **sustentaculum tali** for the flexor hallucis longus tendon (Figs. 4-70 and 4-147), and on its lateral surface there is a tubercle, the **peroneal trochlea** (Fig. 4-71), with a slight groove posterior and inferior to it for the tendon of the peroneus longus muscle.

The Navicular (Figs. 4-68 to 4-72). The navicular (L. little ship) is a flattened oval bone that is shaped somewhat like a boat. It is located between the head of the talus and the three cuneiform bones and has facets for articulation with each of them. It also has an occasional facet for articulation with the cuboid bone. Medially and inferiorly there is a rough **tuberosity** to which the tendon of the tibialis posterior muscle attaches (Figs. 4-69 and 4-147).

The Cuboid (Figs. 4-68, 4-69, 4-71, and 4-72). This bone, as indicated by its name, is approximately cubical in shape. It is the most lateral bone of the distal row of the tarsus. Proximally it presents an articular surface for the calcaneus and distally two facets for the fourth and fifth metatarsals. On the medial surface there are facets for the lateral cuneiform and the navicular. Anterior to the **tuberosity** on the lateral and inferior surfaces of the bone (Fig. 4-71) there is a **groove for the peroneus longus** tendon (Fig. 4-147).

The Cuneiform Bones (Figs. 4-68 to 4-72, 4-144, and 4-148). These three bones are derived from a Latin word meaning "wedge-shaped." They are referred to as **medial** (first), **intermediate** (second), and **lateral** (third) cuneiform bones. Observe that the *medial cuneiform is the largest* and the intermediate cuneiform the smallest. Note also that each cuneiform articulates with the navicular bone posteriorly and with the base of its appropriate metatarsal anteriorly. In addition the lateral cuneiform articulates with the cuboid bone.

The Metatarsus (Figs. 4-68 to 4-72). The metatarsus consists of five metatarsals which are **miniature long bones**. In Figure 4-68 note that they are numbered from the medial side and that each bone consists of a base proximally, a body (shaft), and a head distally (Fig. 4-71). The bases articulate with the cuneiform and the cuboid bones and the heads articulate with the proximal phalanges.

In Figure 4-68 observe that the second metatarsal is wedged between the medial and lateral cuneiforms and between the first and third metatarsals and that it is the longest of the metatarsals. On the plantar surface of the head of the first metatarsal there are prominent medial and lateral **sesamoid bones** (Fig. 4-70). Examine Figures 4-70 to 4-72, noting that the heads of the metatarsals bear some of the weight of the body. Note that the base of the fifth metatarsal has a large **tuberosity** which projects over the lateral margin of the cuboid and provides attachment on its dorsal surface for the peroneus brevis tendon (Figs. 4-68 and 4-81).

CLINICALLY ORIENTED COMMENTS

Occasionally a supernumerary or accessory bone, called the *os vesalianum pedis* (Vesalius' bone), appears near the base of the fifth metatarsal. When examining radiographs, it is important to know of its possible presence so it will not be diagnosed as a fracture of this tuberosity. When this accessory bone is large, the tuberosity is small.

The Phalanges (Figs. 4-68 to 4-72). There are 14 phalanges: the great toe (L. *hallux*), or big toe, has two strong ones (proximal and distal) and the other four digits have three each (proximal, middle, and distal). Each phalanx consists of a base proximally, a body (shaft), and a head distally.

Surface Anatomy of Bones of the Foot. Because injuries and deformities of the foot are so common (*e.g.*, fractures, clubfoot, and flatfoot), familiarity with the surface anatomy of the bones of the feet is essential knowledge.

The Talus. Its head is often visible and is palpable in two places: anteromedial to the proximal part of the lateral malleolus on inversion of the foot (Fig. 4-75*D*) and anterior to the medial malleolus on eversion of the foot (Fig. 4-75*C*). The head occupies the space between the sustenaculum tali and the tuberosity of the navicular bone

(Fig. 4-70). When the foot is plantarflexed (Fig. 4-75*B*), the superior surface of the **body** of the talus can be palpated with difficulty on the anterior aspect of the ankle, distal to the inferior end of the tibia.

The Calcaneus. The posterior, medial, and lateral surfaces of this large bone can be easily palpated, but the inferior surface is not easily felt owing to the overlying plantar aponeurosis and plantar muscles (Figs. 4-97 and 4-100). The **sustentaculum tali** (Figs. 4-65 and 4-70) can be felt as a small prominence distal to the tip of the medial malleolus. To feel it, begin palpating well below this point and move proximally until you detect a medially projecting shelf-like process. The **peroneal trochlea** may be detectable as a small tubercle on the lateral aspect of the calcaneus (Fig. 4-71). It lies anteroinferior to the tip of the lateral malleolus. In some people it is too small to feel. Evert your foot (Fig. 4-75*C*) and palpate the **tendon of the peroneus longus** (Fig. 4-79) and peroneus brevis, which are separated by this small tubercle (Fig. 4-82). The anterior extremity of the calcaneus can be felt with difficulty on deep palpation anterior to the lateral malleolus.

The Navicular (Figs. 4-68, 4-90, and 4-92). The **tuberosity** of this bone is easily seen and palpated on the medial aspect of the foot, inferior and anterior to the tip of the medial malleolus. It is a prominent and *important bony landmark* in the foot. Actively invert your foot and palpate the tendon of the tibialis posterior muscle passing to and inserting into this tuberosity.

The Cuboid and Cuneiforms (Figs. 4-68 and 4-72). These bones are difficult to identify individually by palpation. The cuboid can be felt somewhat indistinctly on the lateral aspect of the foot posterior to the base of the fifth metatarsal. The medial cuneiform can be indistinctly palpated between the tuberosity of the navicular and the base of the first metatarsal bone.

The Metatarsus (Figs. 4-92 and 4-96). The head of the **first metatarsal** bone forms a prominence on the medial aspect of the foot. The medial and lateral sesamoids inferior to the head of this metatarsal (Fig. 4-70) can be felt to slide when the great toe is moved passively with the fingers.

The **base of the fifth metatarsal** forms a prominent landmark on the lateral aspect of the foot. The large tuberosity of the fifth metatarsal can easily be palpated at the midpoint of the lateral border of the foot (Fig. 4-79). In some people it even produces a prominence in their shoe.

The bodies of the metatarsals (Fig. 4-71) can be felt indistinctly on the dorsum of the foot between the extensor tendons (Figs. 4-79 and 4-81).

The Phalanges (Fig. 4-71). The dorsal surfaces of these bones can be felt indistinctly through the extensor tendons, and the interphalangeal joints can be identified.

CLINICALLY ORIENTED COMMENTS

In **flatfoot**, weakening of the supporting muscles and the plantar calcaneonavicular ligament (Fig. 4-146) removes the support for the head of the talus; as a result it descends, stretching the ligaments and flattening the longitudinal arch of the foot (Fig. 4-151). The depressed head of the talus can be palpated just anterior to the medial malleolus. For more information on the anatomical basis of flatfeet, see page 590.

Clubfoot (talipes equinovarus), in which the sole of the foot is turned medially and is inverted (Fig. 4-73), is quite common (1 in 1000 to 1500). The foot is bent so that the tuberosity of the navicular bone comes close to the sustenaculum tali (Fig. 4-69).

Fractures of the bones of the foot are common. Persons who jump or fall from a considerable height and land on their heels may fracture their calcanei. In falls on the heel the calcaneus often breaks into several fragments. A **calcaneal (calcanean) fracture** is very disabling because of disruption of the subtalar joint (Fig. 4-144).

Fractures of the neck of the talus occur during severe dorsiflexion of the ankle (*e.g.*, when a person is pressing hard on the brake of a car during a head-on collision). In some injuries the body of the talus is dislocated posteriorly.

Fractures of the metatarsals usually occur when a heavy object falls on the foot or the foot is run over by a metal wheel.

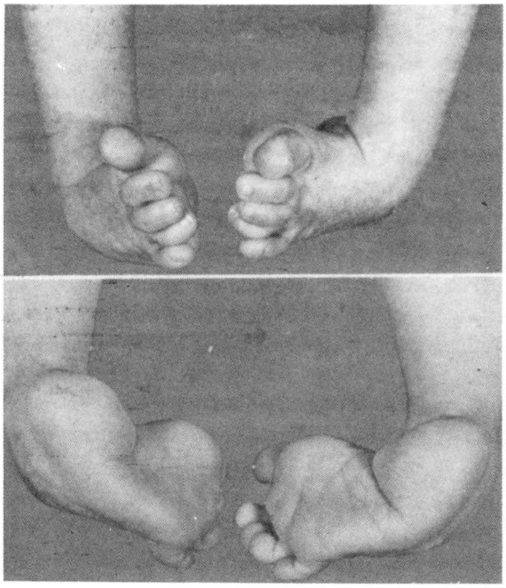

Figure 4-73. Photograph of the legs and feet of a newborn infant with the most common type of congenital clubfeet (*i.e.*, talipes equinovarus). Note that the feet are inverted and the ankles are plantarflexed.

When the foot is suddenly and violently inverted, the tuberosity of the fifth metatarsal may be avulsed (pulled off) by the tendon of the peroneus brevis muscle. **March fractures** of the second metatarsal bone are common in persons who go on long marches when they are unaccustomed to such prolonged strenuous activity.

Fractures of the phalanges most often result from heavy objects falling on them or from stubbing the bare toes (*e.g.*, on a doorstep).

THE CRURAL FASCIA

The deep fascia of the leg (**fascia cruris**) is continuous with the deep fascia of the thigh (**fascia lata**), but it does not completely invest the leg. The crural fascia is attached to the anterior and medial borders of the tibia (Figs. 4-74 and 4-77), where it is continuous with its periosteum. It is absent over the subcutaneous part of the medial surface of the tibia and over the triangular subcutaneous surface of the inferior one-quarter of the fibula (Fig. 4-81). In this region it is attached to the borders of the fibula.

The deep fascia is very thick in the proximal part of the anterior aspect of the leg where it forms part of the origin of the underlying muscles (*e.g.*, tibialis anterior, Fig. 4-80). Although thin in the distal part of the leg, it is thickened where it forms the superior and inferior retinacula.

The Superior Extensor Retinaculum (Figs. 4-76 to 4-78). This strong broad band of deep fascia passes from the fibula to the tibia, proximal to the malleoli. It binds down the tendons of the muscles in the anterior compartment of the leg, preventing them from bowstringing outward during dorsiflexion of the ankle joint (Fig. 4-75*A*).

The Inferior Extensor Retinaculum (Figs. 4-76 to 4-78). This is a Y-shaped band of deep fascia which is attached laterally to the anterosuperior surface of the calcaneus. It forms a very strong loop around the tendons of the peroneus tertius and the extensor digitorum longus. The band-like **proximal limb** of the Y-shaped band is attached to the medial malleolus. During its superomedial course it passes over the tendons of the tibialis anterior and extensor hallucis longus muscles, the dorsalis pedis vessels, and the deep peroneal nerve. The **distal limb** of the Y-shaped band is attached medially to the plantar aponeurosis (Fig. 4-97). During its inferomedial course, it also passes over the tendons of the tibialis anterior and extensor hallucis longus muscles, the dorsalis pedis vessels, and the deep peroneal nerve.

THE CRURAL COMPARTMENTS

The tibia and fibula, the interosseous membrane, and the crural intermuscular septa divide the leg into the **three crural compartments**: anterior, lateral, and posterior (Figs. 4-64 and 4-74). The anterior part of the leg contains the anterior and lateral compartments, which are separated by the **anterior crural intermuscular septum**. The peroneal muscles in the lateral crural compartment are separated from muscles in the posterior crural compartment by the **posterior crural intermuscular septum**.

The much larger posterior crural part of the leg is subdivided by a broad **transverse**

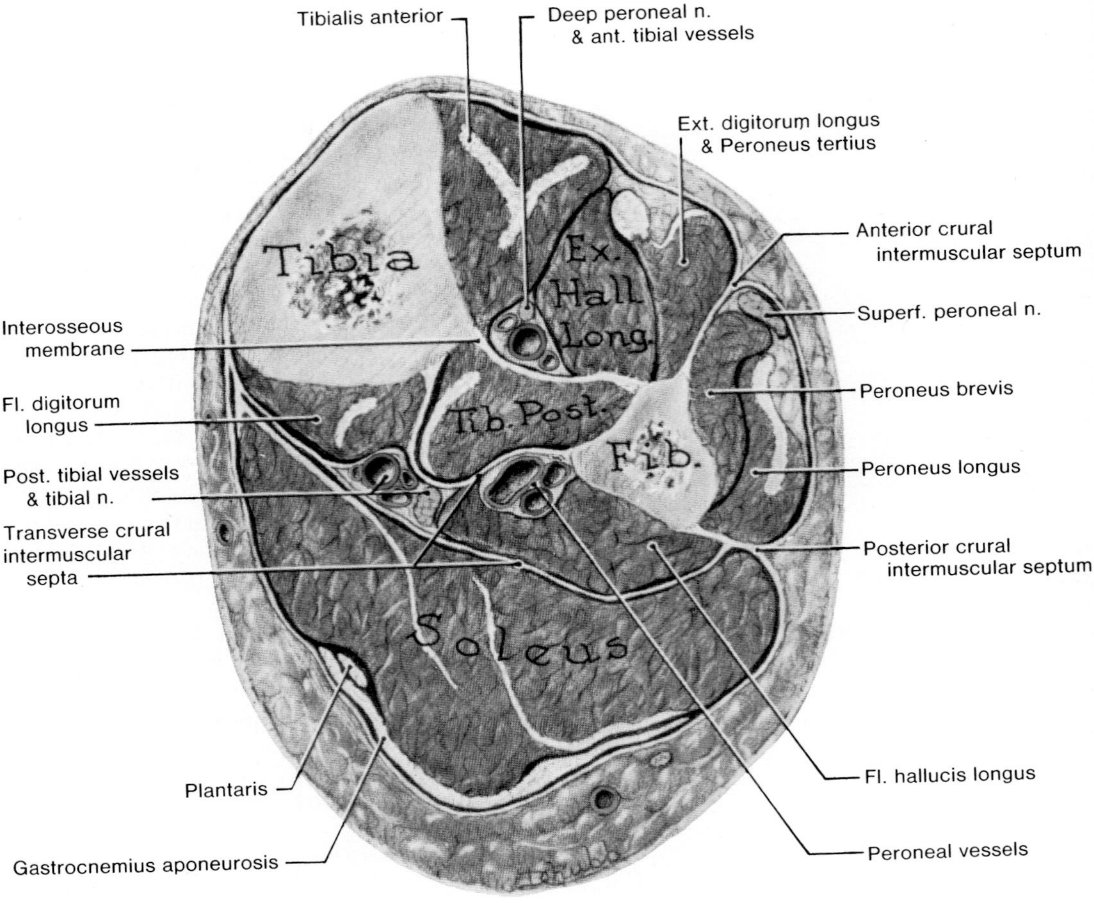

Figure 4-74. Drawing of a cross-section of the right leg of an adult male showing its three compartments and their contents. Observe the anterior crural compartment bounded by the tibia, the interosseous membrane, the fibula, the anterior crural intermuscular septum, and the deep fascia. It contains the anterior tibial vessels and the deep peroneal nerve. Note the lateral crural compartment bounded by the fibula, the anterior and posterior crural intermuscular septa, and the deep fascia. It contains the superficial peroneal nerve. Observe the posterior crural compartment bounded by the tibia, the interosseous membrane, the fibula, the posterior crural intermuscular septum, and the deep fascia. This compartment is subdivided by two coronal intermuscular septa into three subcompartments: (1) the deepest compartment contains the tibialis posterior muscle; (2) the intermediate compartment contains the flexor hallucis longus and flexor digitorum longus muscles, the posterior tibial vessels, and the tibial nerve; and (3) the superficial compartment contains the soleus, gastrocnemius, and plantaris muscles.

crural intermuscular septum (deep transverse fascia of the leg) into superficial and deep posterior crural compartments containing the superficial and deep muscles, respectively (Fig. 4-74).

The Anterior Crural Compartment (Fig. 4-74 and Table 4-1). The anterior compartment is located anterior to the interosseous membrane between the lateral surface of the tibia and the anterior crural intermuscular septum. It contains the **tibialis anterior**, **extensor hallucis longus**, **extensor digitorum longus**, and **peroneus tertius** muscles, which are mainly concerned with dorsiflexion of the ankle joint and extension of the toes (Fig.

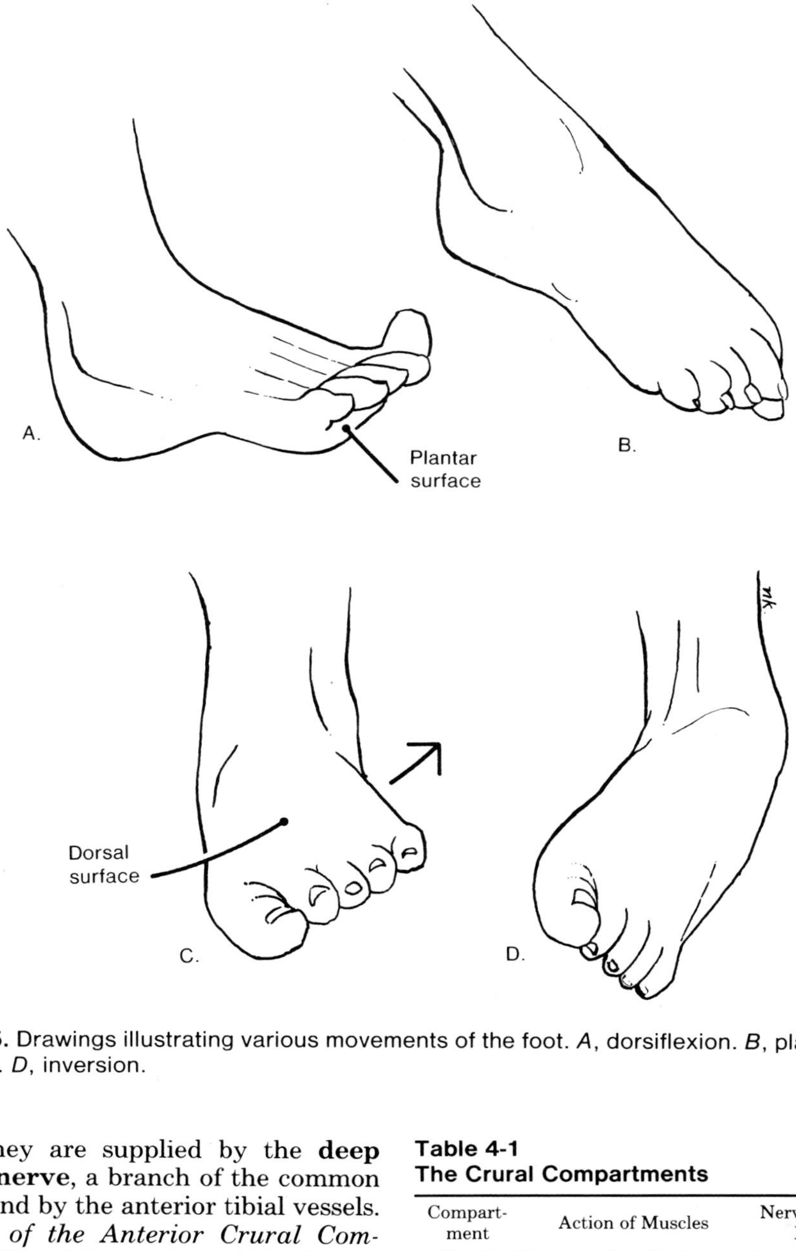

Figure 4-75. Drawings illustrating various movements of the foot. *A*, dorsiflexion. *B*, plantarflexion. *C*, eversion. *D*, inversion.

4-75*A*). They are supplied by the **deep peroneal nerve**, a branch of the common peroneal, and by the anterior tibial vessels.

Muscles of the Anterior Crural Compartment (Figs. 4-74 to 4-76 and Table 4-1). The four anterior crural muscles **dorsiflex the ankle joint** and are supplied by the **deep peroneal nerve**. As described subsequently, these muscles also have other actions.

The Tibialis Anterior Muscle (Figs. 4-74 and 4-76 to 4-78). This thick muscle lies against the lateral surface of the tibia, where its proximal muscular part is easy to palpate on the lateral side of the shin.

Table 4-1
The Crural Compartments

Compartment	Action of Muscles	Nerve Supply of Muscles
Anterior	Dorsiflexion	Deep peroneal
Posterior	Plantarflexion	Tibial
Lateral	Eversion	Superficial peroneal

Origin (Fig. 4-67*B*). **Lateral condyle**, proximal half or more of **lateral surface**

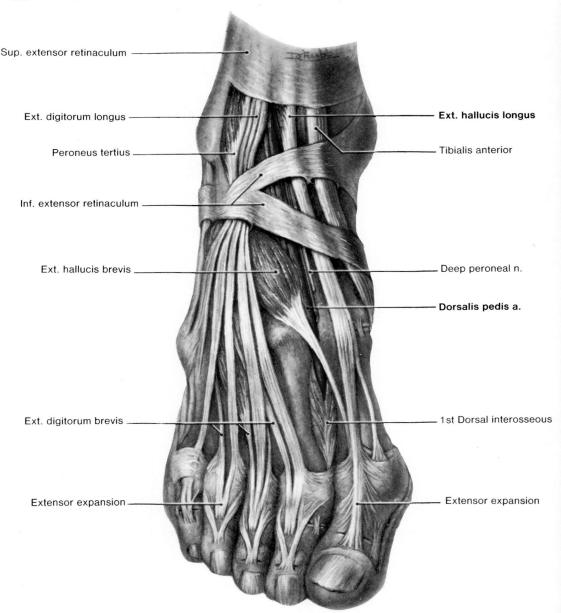

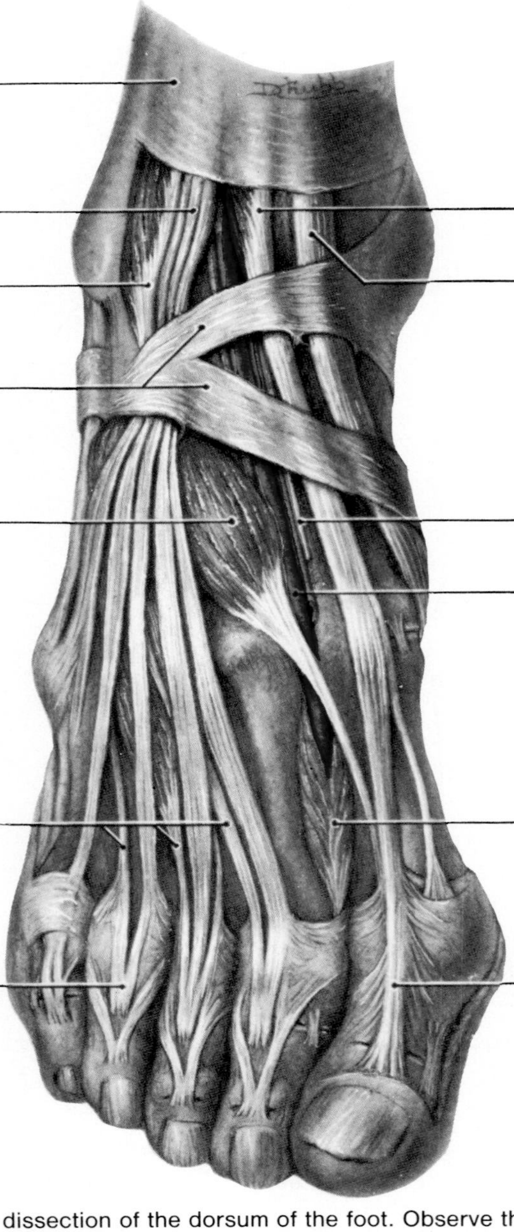

Figure 4-76. Drawing of a dissection of the dorsum of the foot. Observe the vessels and nerve at the ankle lying midway between the malleoli with two tendons on each side. Observe that the dorsalis pedis artery, the continuation of the anterior tibial, is crossed by the tendon of the extensor hallucis brevis muscle and then disappears between the two heads of the first dorsal interosseous muscle to end in the sole of the foot. The pulsations of this artery can easily be felt in most people just lateral to the tendon of the extensor hallucis longus muscle, where it passes over the navicular and cuneiform bones. A knowledge of how to feel the dorsalis pedis pulse is clinically important in cases of suspected arterial disease of the lower limb and of threatened or established gangrene of a toe or toes (necrosis or death owing to obstruction of blood supply). Observe the inferior extensor retinaculum restraining the tendons from bowstringing forward and/or medially.

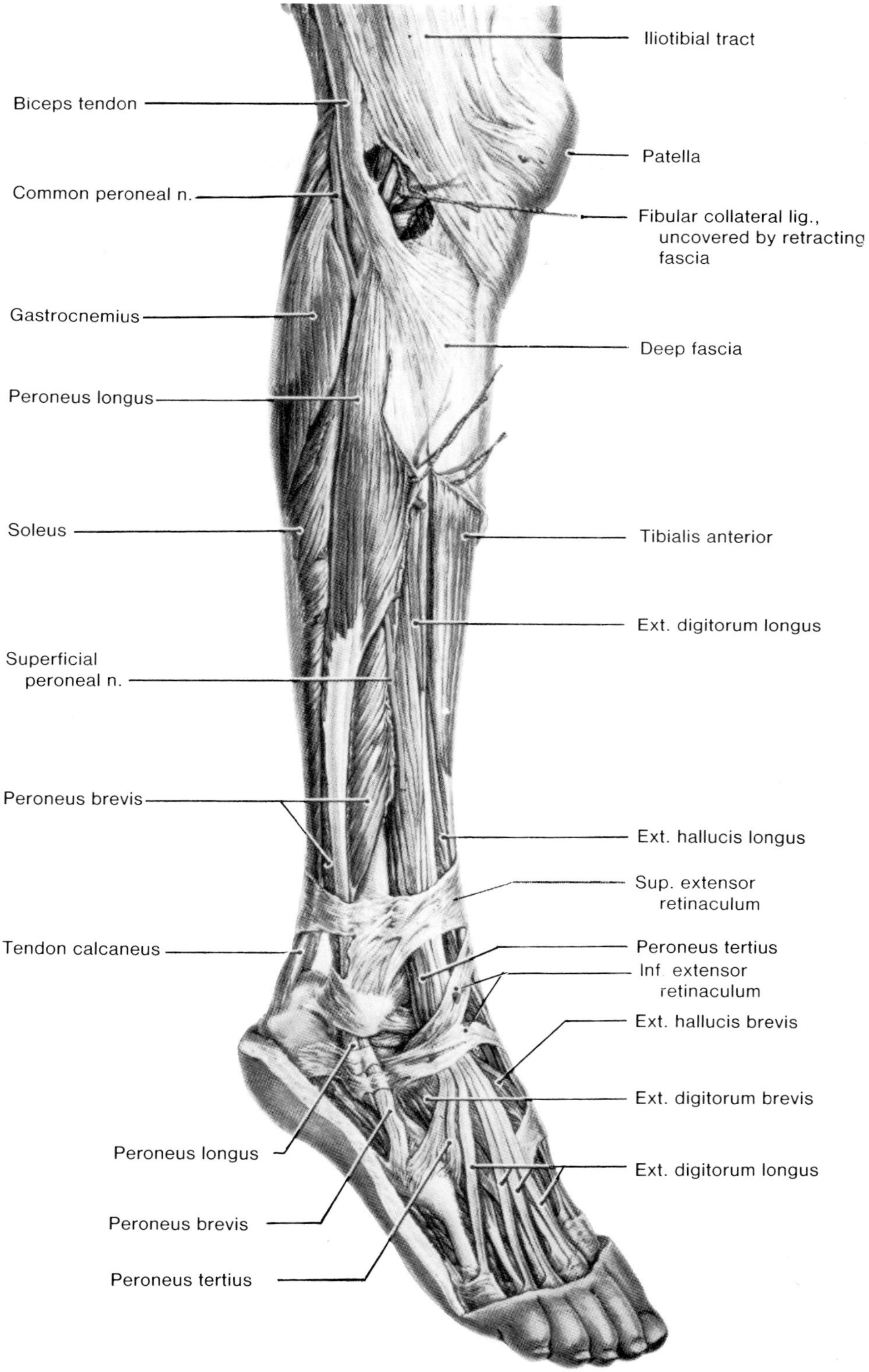

Figure 4-77. Drawing of a dissection of the muscles of the right leg and foot, anterolateral view. Observe the superficial position of the common peroneal nerve (L4, L5, S1, and S2), a terminal branch of the sciatic nerve. Because the common peroneal nerve is subcutaneous in the knee region, it is commonly injured when the neck of the fibula is fractured or when there is a deep laceration on the lateral side of the knee.

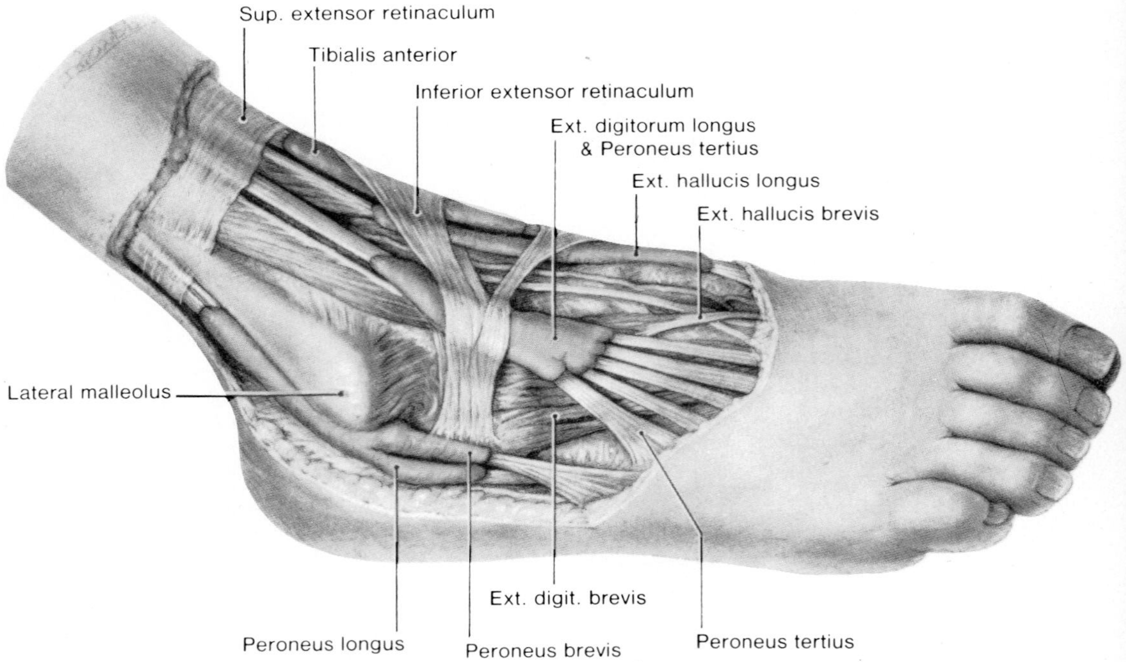

Figure 4-78. Drawing of a dissection of the right foot showing the synovial sheaths of the tendons at the ankle, anterolateral view. Observe that the tendons of the peroneus longus and peroneus brevis muscles are enclosed in a common synovial sheath posterior to the lateral malleolus. Distal to this it splits into two, one for each tendon. Note that the tendon of the small peroneus tertius muscle runs with the tendons of the extensor digitorum longus within a common synovial sheath. The peroneus tertius muscle is a partially separated portion of the extensor digitorum longus.

of tibia, **deep fascia** of leg, and **interosseous membrane**.

Insertion (Figs. 4-69, 4-70, and 4-78). Medial and inferior surfaces of **medial cuneiform** bone and base of **first metatarsal** bone. The tendon, which becomes free in the distal third of the leg, passes deep to the extensor retinacula.

Nerve Supply. **Deep peroneal** nerve (L4 and L5).

Actions (Fig. 4-75*A* and *D*). **Dorsiflexes ankle joint** and **inverts foot**.

CLINICALLY ORIENTED COMMENTS

When the tibialis anterior is paralyzed owing to **injury of the common peroneal nerve** (Case 4-3) or to its deep peroneal branch supplying this muscle, the foot drops (*i.e.*, it falls into plantarflexion when it is raised from the ground). In this condition, known as **foot-drop**, the foot makes a slapping noise during walking because the foot is raised higher than normal to keep the toes from dragging on the ground and tripping the patient. As the foot is lowered it makes a characteristic "clop" or flapping noise.

"**Shin splints**" is a lay term for a painful condition of the anterior compartment of the leg that follows vigorous and/or lengthy exercise. Often persons who lead sedentary lives (*e.g.*, office workers) develop pains in the anterior part of their legs when they undertake long walks (*e.g.*, miles for millions). As a result their anterior tibial muscles swell from overuse. The swollen muscles in their tight osseofibrous anterior compartment reduce the blood flow to the muscles, which may develop cramps if they continue to be used. Even at rest the swollen muscles are painful and tender to pressure. The condition may also occur in trained athletes who do not warm up adequately or warm down sufficiently after excessive exercise (*e.g.*, figure skaters and marathon runners).

People living in Alaska and Northern Canada commonly get shin splints after the first heavy snow fall that requires them to use snowshoes; their anterior tibial muscles, and probably their peroneal muscles, are used in **snowshoeing** to raise the toes of the snowshoes and to keep them straight. Because they have not been used strongly during the summer, the first severe demand on these muscles causes severe shin splints, referred to as **snowshoe leg**. Trappers sometimes treat their swollen and painful muscles by cauterizing the overlying skin with a hot iron; this is an example of the therapeutic use of **counterirritation** (irritation or inflammation of the skin with the object of relieving a deep inflammatory process).

The Extensor Hallucis Longus Muscle (Figs. 4-74 and 4-76 to 4-78). This thin muscle lies between and partly deep to the tibialis anterior and the extensor digitorum longus muscles.

Origin (Fig. 4-67*B*). **Middle half of anterior surface of fibula** and **interosseous membrane**.

Insertion (Fig. 4-68). **Dorsal aspect of base of distal phalanx of great toe**. Its tendon passes deep to the superior and inferior extensor retinacula where it is easy to observe and to palpate when the great toe is dorsiflexed, particularly when performed against resistance.

Nerve Supply. **Deep peroneal** nerve (L5 and S1).

Actions (Fig. 4-75*A*) **Dorsiflexes ankle joint** and **extends great toe**.

The Extensor Digitorum Longus Muscle (Figs. 4-74 and 4-76 to 4-80). This muscle lies lateral to the tibialis anterior and can be easily palpated. Its tendons may be seen and felt when the toes are dorsiflexed.

Origin. (Fig. 4-67*B*). **Lateral condyle of tibia**, **proximal two-thirds of anterior surface of fibula**, and **interosseous membrane**.

Insertion (Figs. 4-69 and 4-76). **Middle and distal phalanges of lateral four toes**. Its tendon passes deep to the superior extensor retinaculum and divides into four tendons anterior to the ankle which pass through a loop formed by the stem of the

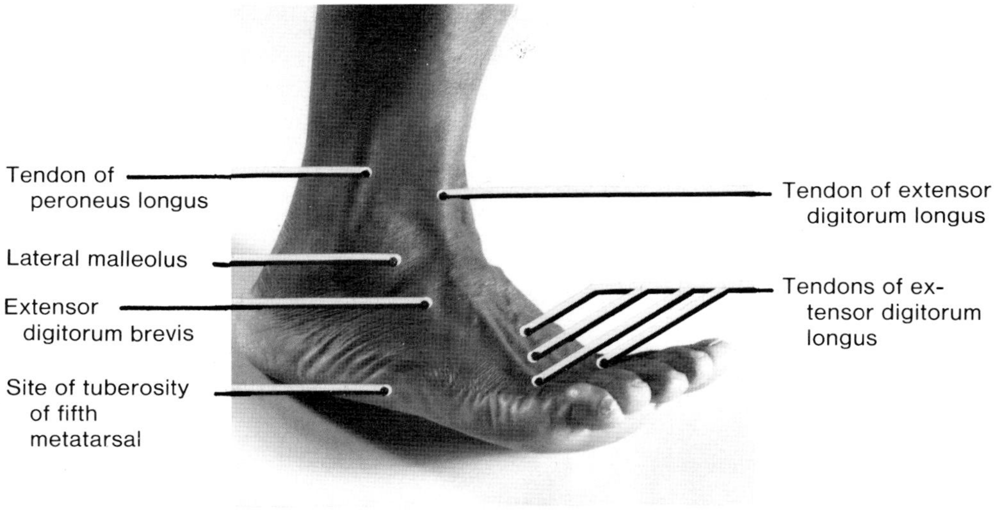

Figure 4-79. Photograph of the right lower leg and foot of a 35-year-old man with the toes dorsiflexed and the foot everted. Observe the tendons of the extensor digitorum longus which run to the lateral four toes. A common synovial sheath surrounds the four tendons (Fig. 4-78). The tuberosity of the fifth metatarsal bone (Fig. 4-71) can be felt half-way along the lateral border of the foot. This tuberosity may be avulsed in acute inversion of the foot.

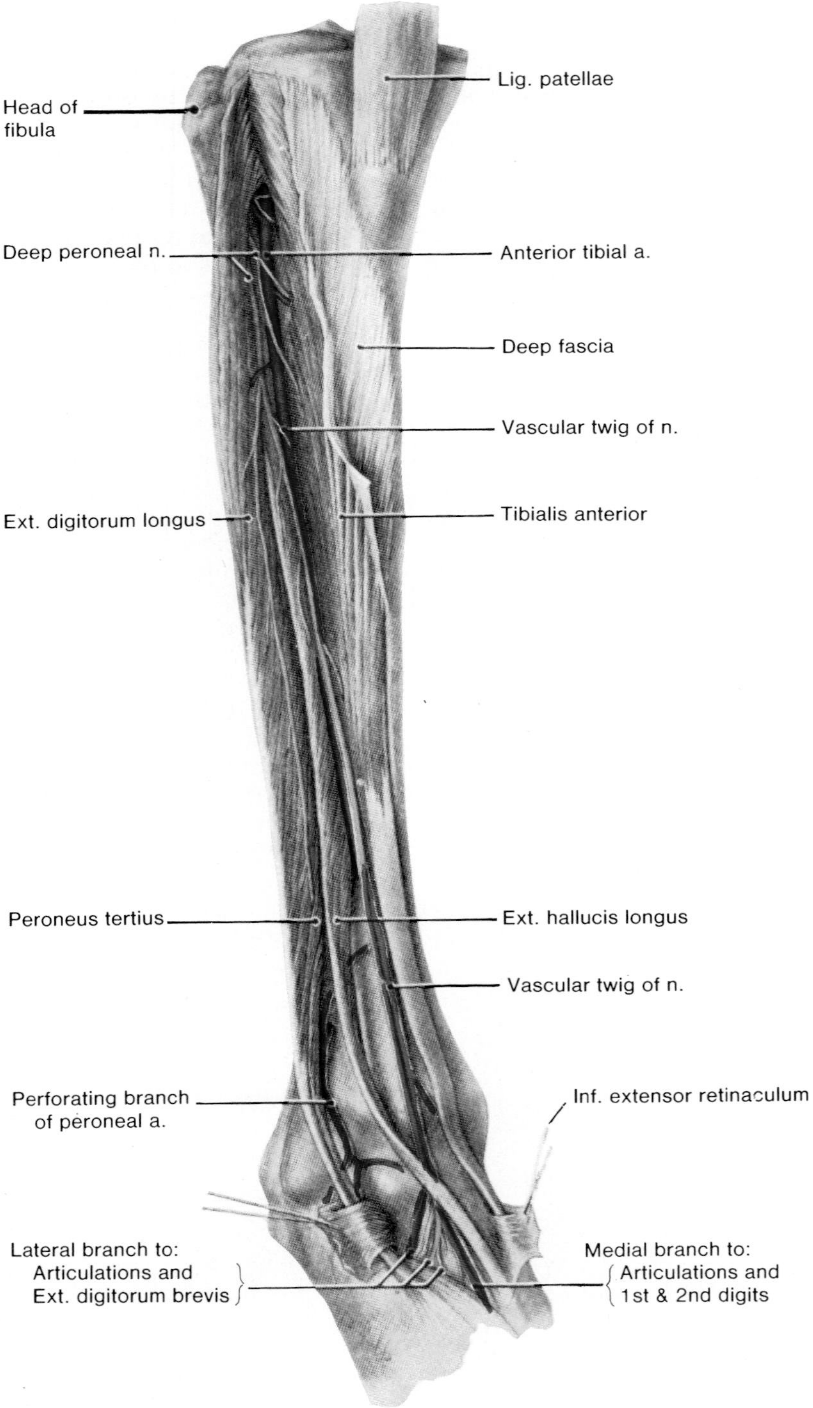

Figure 4-80. Drawing of a dissection of the anterolateral aspect of the right leg. The muscles are separated in order to display the artery and the nerve. Observe the tibialis anterior muscle arising in part from the deep fascia. Note the peroneus tertius muscle, which is really the lower part of the extensor digitorum longus muscle. The origins of these muscles are illustrated in Figure 4-67. Observe the vascular and articular branches of the deep peroneal nerve. Note that at the ankle the deep peroneal nerve is covered by only one tendon, that of the extensor hallucis longus muscle.

inferior extensor retinaculum (Figs. 4-76 to 4-78). A **common synovial sheath** surrounds the four tendons, which diverge on the dorsum of the foot as they pass to their insertions into the phalanges of the lateral four toes. Each tendon forms a membranous **extensor expansion** over the dorsum of the proximal phalanx, which divides into two lateral slips and one central slip. The central slip inserts into the base of the middle phalanx and the lateral slips converge to insert into the base of the distal phalanx.

Nerve Supply. **Deep peroneal** nerve (L5 and S1).

Actions (Figs. 4-75 and 4-79). **Dorsiflexes ankle joint**, **everts foot**, and **extends lateral four toes** at the metatarsophalangeal and interphalangeal joints.

The Peroneus Tertius Muscle (Figs. 4-74 and 4-76 to 4-78). This small muscle (not always present) is a partially separated inferior part of the extensor digitorum longus muscle.

Origin (Fig. 4-67*B*). **Distal one-third of anterior surface of fibula** and **interosseous membrane**.

Insertion (Fig. 4-68). **Dorsum of base of fifth metatarsal** bone or nearby deep fascia. Its tendon runs with those of the extensor digitorum longus through the strong loop formed by the stem of the inferior extensor retinaculum.

Nerve Supply. **Deep peroneal** nerve (L5 and S1).

Actions (Fig. 4-75*A* and *C*). **Dorsiflexes ankle joint** and **everts foot**.

Nerve of the Anterior Crural Compartment (Figs. 4-74, 4-77, 4-80, and 4-81). The nerve of the anterior compartment is the deep peroneal; it is one of the two terminal branches of the common peroneal nerve (L4, L5, S1, and S2).

The deep peroneal nerve begins between the neck of the fibula and the peroneus longus muscle (Fig. 4-81) and then runs inferomedially on the fibula, deep to the extensor digitorum longus (Fig. 4-80). After piercing the anterior crural intermuscular septum and the extensor digitorum longus, it descends anterior to the interosseous membrane in the anterior crural compartment, where it joins the anterior tibial artery between the extensor hallucis longus and tibialis anterior muscles (Fig. 4-74). It passes deep to the extensor retinacula with the anterior tibial artery, where it ends by dividing into medial and lateral branches which supply structures on the dorsum of the foot (Figs. 4-14 and 4-80).

In addition to supplying muscles in the anterior crural compartment, the deep peroneal nerve gives twigs to the peroneus longus muscle in the lateral compartment and to the posterior tibial and peroneal arteries. It also sends articular branches to the ankle joint and other joints it crosses and supplies the skin between the great and second toes (Figs. 4-14 and 4-106).

Arteries of the Anterior Crural Compartment. Structures in the anterior compartment are supplied by the anterior tibial artery and its branches.

The Anterior Tibial Artery (Figs. 4-34*A*, 4-62, 4-74, 4-76, 4-80, and 4-81). The smaller of the terminal branches of the popliteal artery, the anterior tibial begins opposite the distal border of the popliteus muscle and ends at the level of the ankle joint midway between the malleoli, where it becomes the **dorsalis pedis artery** Fig. 4-76).

In Figures 4-80 and 4-81, observe that the proximal part of the anterior tibial artery is deeply located but readily accessible distally. From its origin in the back of the leg, the anterior tibial artery passes anteriorly through the interosseous membrane via an opening in its proximal part. It then descends on the anterior surface of this membrane between the extensor hallucis longus and the tibialis anterior muscles with the deep peroneal nerve and two veins. In the distal part of the leg the artery lies directly on the tibia where it is crossed by the tendon of the extensor hallucis longus muscle (Fig. 4-76).

In addition to supplying muscles in the anterior crural compartment, the anterior tibial artery has several other named branches. The anterior and posterior **tibial recurrent arteries** join the anastomoses around the knee (Fig. 4-62), and the medial and lateral anterior **malleolar arteries** ramify over the medial and lateral malleoli, respectively (Fig. 4-34*A*), contributing to the networks around the ankle.

The Lateral Crural Compartment

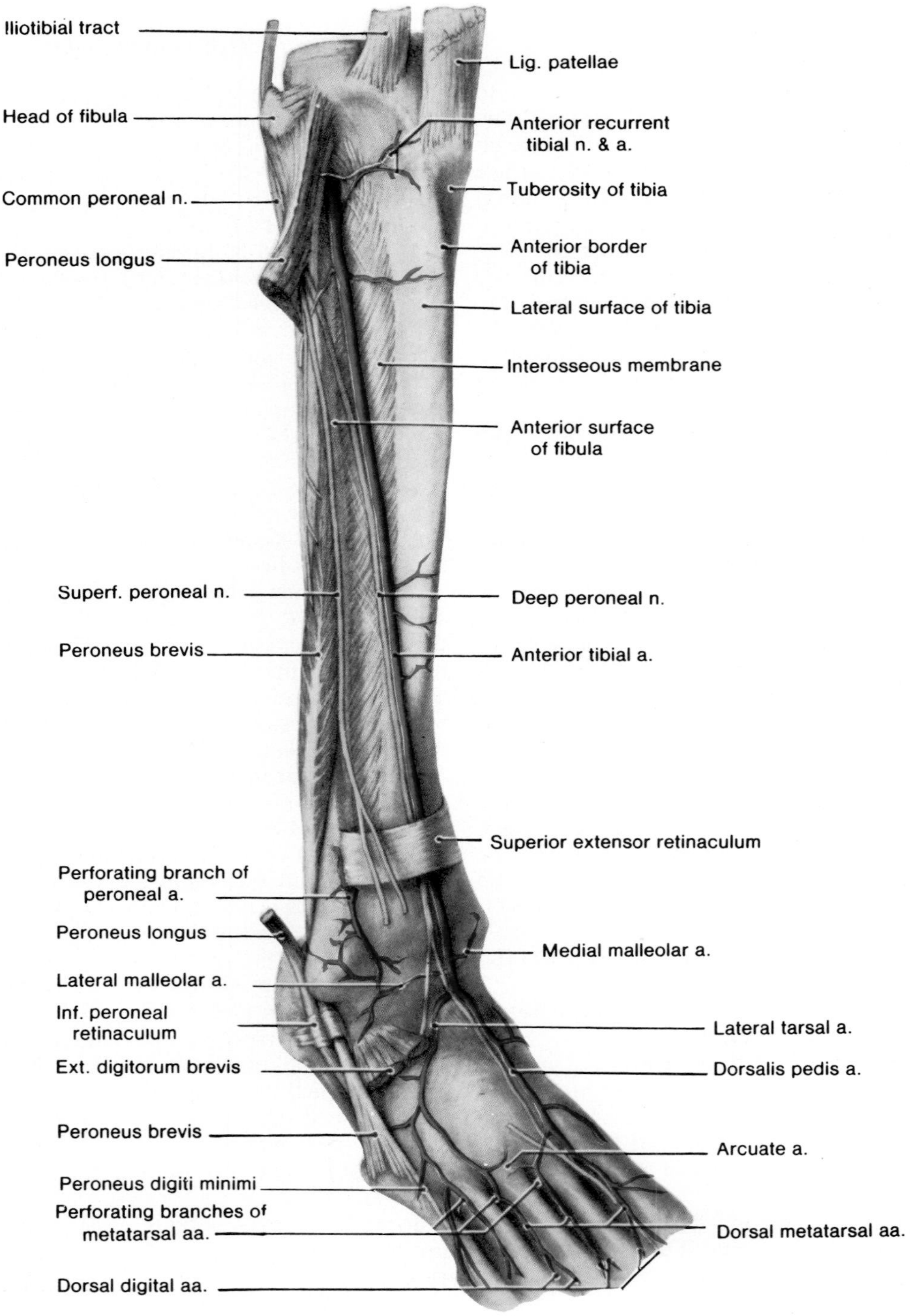

Figure 4-81. Drawing of a dissection of the front of the leg and the dorsum of the right foot displaying the arteries and nerves. The anterior crural muscles are removed and the peroneus longus is excised. Observe the anterior tibial artery entering the region in contact with the medial side of the neck of the fibula and the nerve in contact with its lateral side. Hence, the nerve approaches the artery from the lateral side. Note that the artery and nerve and their named branches lie on the skeletal plane and are undisturbed by the removal of the muscles. Observe the superficial peroneal nerve following the anterior border of the peroneus brevis muscle which guides it to the surface, a variable distance above the triangular subcutaneous area of the fibula. Note that the fibers of the interosseous membrane are so directed to allow the fibula to be forced upward but not pulled downward.

(Figs. 4-64, 4-74, and Table 4-1). The lateral compartment is bounded by the lateral surface of the fibula, the anterior and posterior crural intermuscular septa, and the crural fascia. It contains the **peroneus longus** and **peroneus brevis** muscles, which are concerned with plantarflexion of the ankle joint and eversion of the foot (Fig. 4-75*B* and *C*). They are supplied by the **superficial peroneal nerve**, a branch of the common peroneal (Fig. 4-74). Because the adjective *peroneal* is the Greek equivalent of the Latin *fibular*, the lateral compartment is occasionally called the peroneal or fibular compartment.

Muscles of the Lateral Crural Compartment (Figs. 4-74, 4-76 to 4-79, 4-82, and 4-83). The two peroneal muscles in this compartment arise mainly from the fibula (G. *peronē*). **The two peroneal muscles evert the foot** (Fig. 4-75*C*) and are both supplied by the superficial peroneal nerve. The tendons of these muscles are held in position by thickened bands of the deep fascia known as the **peroneal retinacula**, which prevent displacement of the peroneal tendons (Fig. 4-82).

The Peroneus Longus Muscle (Figs. 4-74, 4-76 to 4-79, 4-82, and 4-83). This is the more superficial of the two peroneal muscles and it arises higher on the fibula (Fig. 4-67*A*). Its tendon can easily be palpated

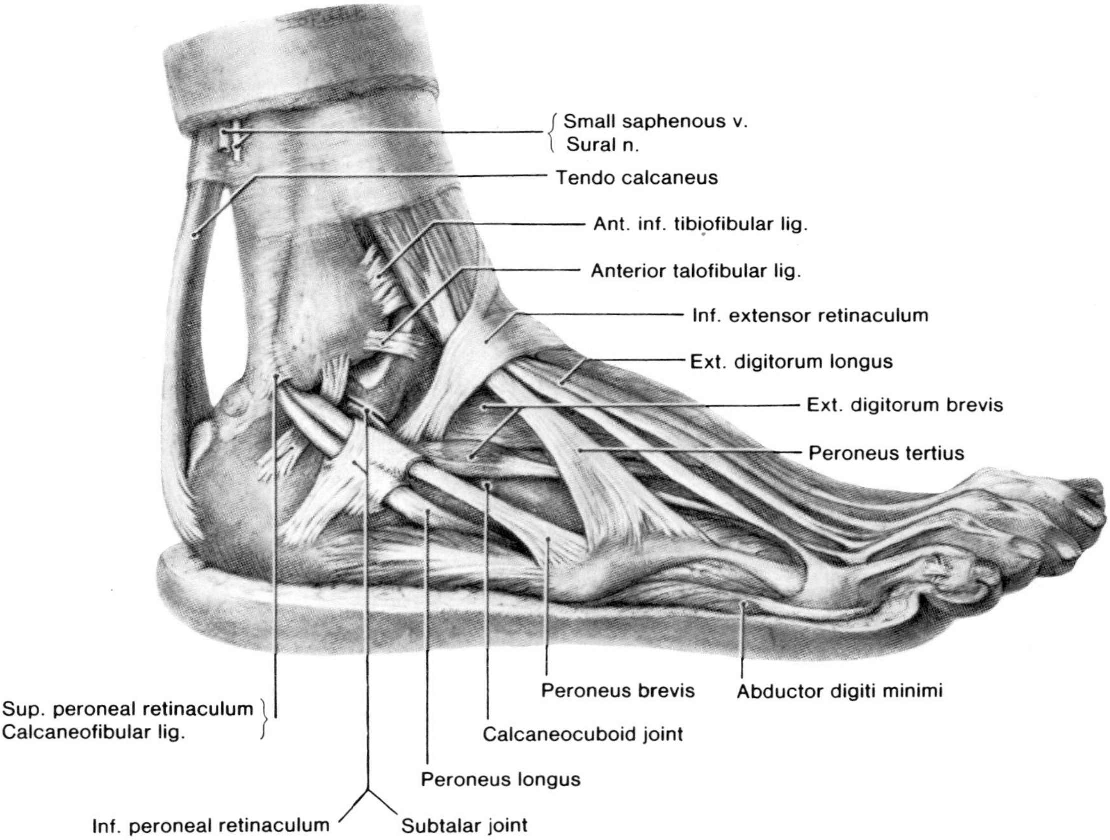

Figure 4-82. Drawing of a lateral view of a dissection of the dorsum of the right foot showing the ankle, subtalar, and calcaneocuboid joints. Observe the round calcaneofibular ligament attached anteriorly to the lateral malleolus and that its tip overlaps the peroneal tendons, preventing them from slipping forward. Note that the inferior peroneal retinaculum is attached to the lateral surface of the calcaneus and is in line with the inferior extensor retinaculum which is attached to its superolateral surface.

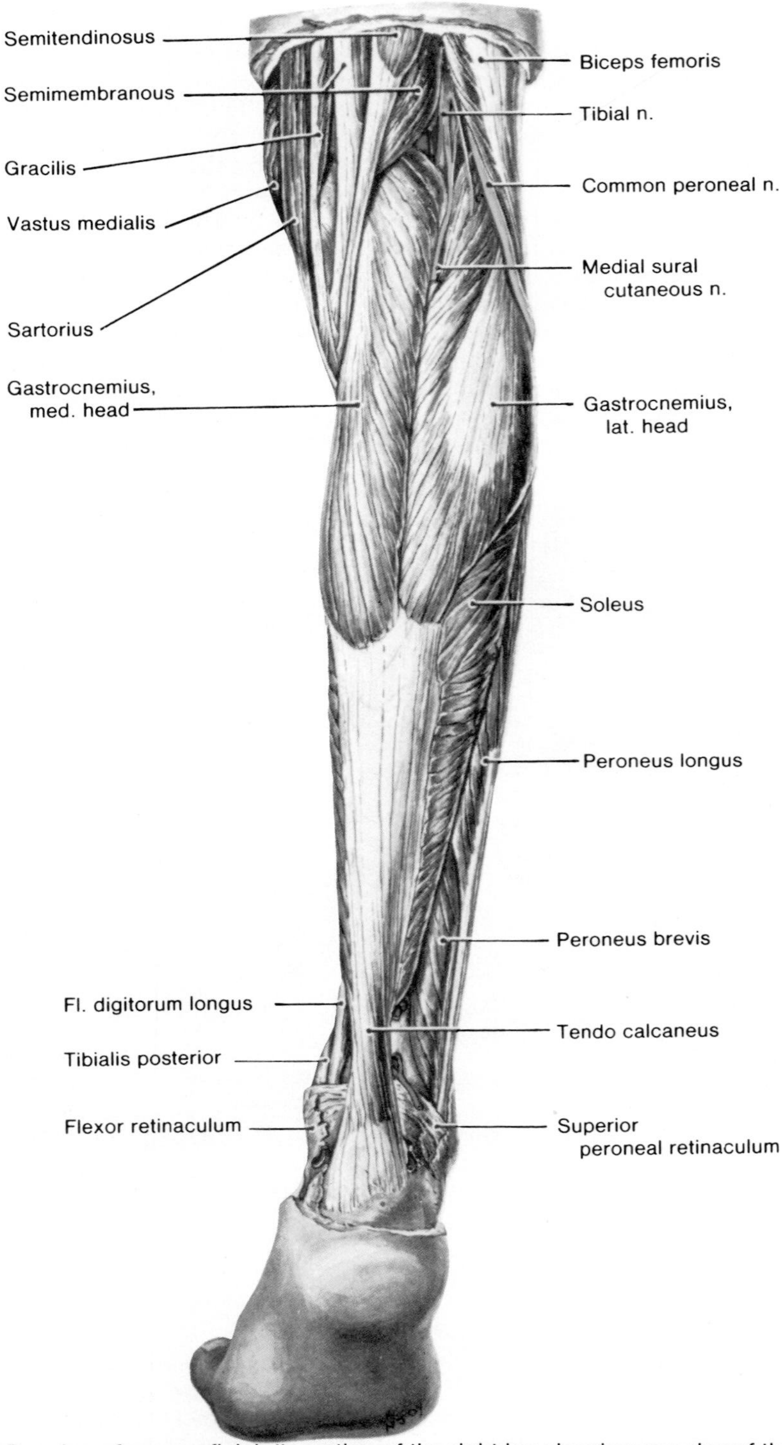

Figure 4-83. Drawing of a superficial dissection of the right leg showing muscles of the superficial posterior crural compartment. The triceps surae muscle, consisting of the gastrocnemius and the soleus, forms the prominence of the calf (Fig. 4-84). Note that the tendon of the gastrocnemius joins the tendon of the soleus to form the tendo calcaneus or calcaneal tendon.

and usually observed proximal and posterior to the lateral malleolus (Fig. 4-79).

Origin (Fig. 4-67*A*). **Head** and **proximal two-thirds of lateral surface of fibula**.

Insertion (Figs. 4-69, 4-90, and 4-147). **Base of first metatarsal** bone and **medial cuneiform** bone. Its long tendon runs deep to the superior peroneal retinaculum and curves posterior to the lateral malleolus, which it uses as a pulley (Fig. 4-82). It runs in a common synovial sheath with the peroneus brevis muscle (Fig. 4-78), passing inferior to the **peroneal trochlea** or tubercle (Fig. 4-71) to enter a groove on the anteroinferior aspect of the cuboid bone. It then crosses the sole of the foot, running obliquely and distally to reach its insertion.

Nerve Supply. **Superficial peroneal** nerve (L5 and S1).

Actions (Fig. 4-75*B* and *C*). **Plantarflexes ankle joint** and **everts foot**. Its tendon crosses obliquely in the sole of the foot (Fig. 4-147) and helps to maintain the transverse and lateral longitudinal arches of the foot (Fig. 4-151). To make the tendon of your peroneus longus muscle stand out (Fig. 4-79), evert your foot against resistance.

The Peroneus Brevis Muscle (Figs. 4-74, 4-77, 4-78, 4-82, and 4-139). This muscle lies deep to the peroneus longus and, as its name indicates, is shorter and smaller than its partner in the lateral crural compartment.

Origin (Figs. 4-66 and 4-67*A*). **Distal third of lateral surface of fibula** and **intermuscular septa**.

Insertion (Figs. 4-68, 4-77, and 4-82). **Tuberosity and dorsal surface of base of fifth metatarsal** bone. Its tendon can be felt inferior to the lateral malleolus where it lies anterior to the tendon of the peroneus longus (Fig. 4-82). The tendon of the peroneus brevis can be easily traced to its insertion into the base of the fifth metatarsal bone (Fig. 4-139). A slip from the muscle often inserts into the long extensor tendon of the little toe and is known as the *peroneus digiti minimi* (Fig. 4-81).

Nerve Supply. **Superficial peroneal** nerve (L5 and S1).

Actions (Fig. 4-75*B* and *C*). **Plantarflexes ankle joint** and **everts foot**. Its actions are the same as the peroneus longus, except that it appears to be less important in supporting the arches of the foot (Fig. 4-151) because its tendon does not pass inferior to them.

CLINICALLY ORIENTED COMMENTS

The tuberosity of the fifth metatarsal bone (Fig. 4-71) may be avulsed (pulled off) by the peroneus brevis tendon during violent eversion of the foot. This kind of fracture may be associated with a sprained ankle (Case 4-5).

An accessory bone (*os vesalianum pedis*) is sometimes present near the base of the fifth metatarsal bone. An awareness of its possible presence is necessary so that it will not be interpreted in a radiograph as a fracture of the tuberosity of the fifth metatarsal.

In children and adolescents there is often a **secondary ossification center** for the lateral surface of the tuberosity of the fifth metatarsal bone. This **chip-like piece of bone** should not be mistaken in a radiograph for a **flake fracture** of the tuberosity. The presence of similar secondary centers in both feet would usually indicate that a fracture is not present. These centers are not observed in adults because they have fused.

Nerves of the Lateral Crural Compartment (Figs. 4-74, 4-77, 4-81, and 4-106). The nerve of the lateral crural compartment is the superficial peroneal nerve, one of the two terminal branches of the common peroneal nerve.

The superficial peroneal nerve begins between the peroneus longus muscle and the neck of the fibula and descends posterolateral to or in the anterior crural intermuscular septum. It lies anterolateral to the fibula between the peroneal muscles and the extensor digitorum longus (Fig. 4-74). It supplies the peroneal muscles and then pierces the deep fascia to become superficial in the distal third of the leg (Fig. 4-77). It passes in the superficial fascia to supply the skin on the lower part of the anterior surface of the leg, nearly all the dorsum of the foot, and most of the toes (Figs. 4-14 and 4-106).

Arteries of the Lateral Crural Compartment (Fig. 4-74). There are no arteries in the lateral compartment, except for muscular branches to the peroneal muscles which arise from the peroneal branch of the posterior tibial artery.

The Posterior Crural Compartment (Figs. 4-64, 4-74, and Table 4-1). From medial to lateral the posterior compartment lies posterior to the tibia, the interosseous membrane, the fibula, and the **posterior crural intermuscular septum**. The muscles in it are concerned with plantarflexion of the ankle joint (Fig. 4-75*B*) and are divided into superficial and deep groups by the **transverse crural intermuscular septum**. The superficial group of muscles consists of the gastrocnemius, plantaris, and soleus, and the deep group of muscles consists of the tibialis posterior, flexor digitorum longus, and flexor hallucis longus.

In Figures 4-74 and 4-88 observe that the tibial nerve and the posterior tibial vessels supply both divisions of the posterior crural compartment and run between the superficial and deep groups of muscle.

Muscles of the Posterior Crural Compartment (Figs. 4-64, 4-74, and 4-83 to 4-90). All posterior crural muscles are supplied by the tibial nerve. In Figure 4-74 observe that this nerve and the posterior tibial vessels are deep to the **transverse crural intermuscular septum** and that the muscles of the posterior compartment are much larger than those of the anterior compartment. They are also more powerful because they are sometimes required to sustain the whole weight of the body (*e.g.*, when rising on the toes).

1. Muscles in the Superficial Posterior Compartment (Figs. 4-74 and 4-83 to 4-86). These muscles are separated from muscles in the deep posterior compartment by the transverse crural intermuscular septum. *Understand that this septum lies in the coronal plane of the body* (Fig. I-5).

Three muscles comprise the superficial group: the **gastrocnemius**, the **soleus**, and the **plantaris** (when present). The gastrocnemius and the soleus together are sometimes referred to as the **triceps surae** muscle. Note that it forms the prominence of the calf (Figs. 4-84 and 4-86).

The muscles of the superficial compartment *act together in plantarflexing the ankle joint*; they raise the heel against the weight of the body, *e.g.*, in walking, dancing, and standing on the tiptoes.

The Gastrocnemius Muscle (Figs. 4-55 to 4-60 and 4-83 to 4-86). The gastrocnemius, the most superficial of the posterior crural muscles, forms most of the prominence of the calf. It has *two heads of origin*; its medial head is slightly larger and extends a little more distally than does the lateral head. The two heads of the muscle come together at the inferior margin of the **popliteal fossa** where the converging heads form the inferolateral and inferomedial boundaries of the popliteal fossa.

Origin (Figs. 4-22, 4-26, and 4-54). **Posterior aspects of femoral condyles** just proximal to articular surfaces. To be more specific, the smaller *lateral head* arises from the proximal and posterior part of the *lateral surface* of the **lateral condyle** and the distal part of the supracondylar line, and the larger *medial head* arises from the *popliteal surface of the femur* just proximal to the **medial condyle**. The lateral head often contains a sesamoid bone, called the **fabella** (L. bean), close to its origin (Fig. 4-121*C*), which is usually visible on lateral radiographs of the knee.

Insertion (Figs. 4-66 and 4-84 to 4-88). Middle part of **posterior surface of calcaneus** via tendo calcaneus. It shares this stout, very strong tendon with the soleus muscle. The calcaneal tendon is the *thickest and strongest tendon in the body.*

Nerve Supply. **Tibial** nerve (S1 and S2).

Actions (Figs. 4-75*B*, 4-84, and 4-86). **Plantarflexes ankle joint** and **flexes knee joint**. It acts with the soleus muscle in plantarflexing the ankle (*e.g.*, in walking) and contracts to produce this movement when this action is resisted (*e.g.*, when standing on the toes, as illustrated in Figs. 4-84 and 4-86). Although the gastrocnemius acts on the knee and ankle joints, it is unable to exert its full power on both joints at the same time.

CLINICALLY ORIENTED COMMENTS

Rupture of the tendo calcaneus is not uncommon, especially in older males. Although it may occur during games such as squash, it often happens during a stumble or when the person is startled, causing him to jump or start to run (*e.g.*, when crossing a street). Complete rupture of the tendo calcaneus usually results in *abrupt pain in the posterior aspect of the lower leg*, an inability to walk, and a lump or increase in the prominence of the calf owing to shortening of the triceps surae muscle.

The tendon may also rupture in young persons, frequently at the start of a 100-m dash when the tendon is severely stressed during the take-off. Ruptures of the tendon may also occur when it becomes weaker than normal as a result of **ischemia** (lack of a good blood supply). The rupture usually occurs about 3 cm proximal to the insertion of the tendon into the calcaneus and a distinct gap can easily be felt in it. Following rupture of the tendon, the *foot can be dorsiflexed to a greater extent than is normal* and the patient is unable to plantarflex his/her ankle joint against resistance.

Persons who continually wear high heels may develop shortening of the triceps surae because the origin of this muscle is continually brought closer to its insertion. If this occurs, transitory **calf pain** may be experienced when walking without shoes or in flat shoes owing to tightness of the muscle.

Tennis leg is a painful calf injury resulting from partial *tearing of the medial belly of the gastrocnemius* at or near the musculotendinous junction. It is caused by overstretching the muscle by concomitant full extension of the knee and dorsiflexion of

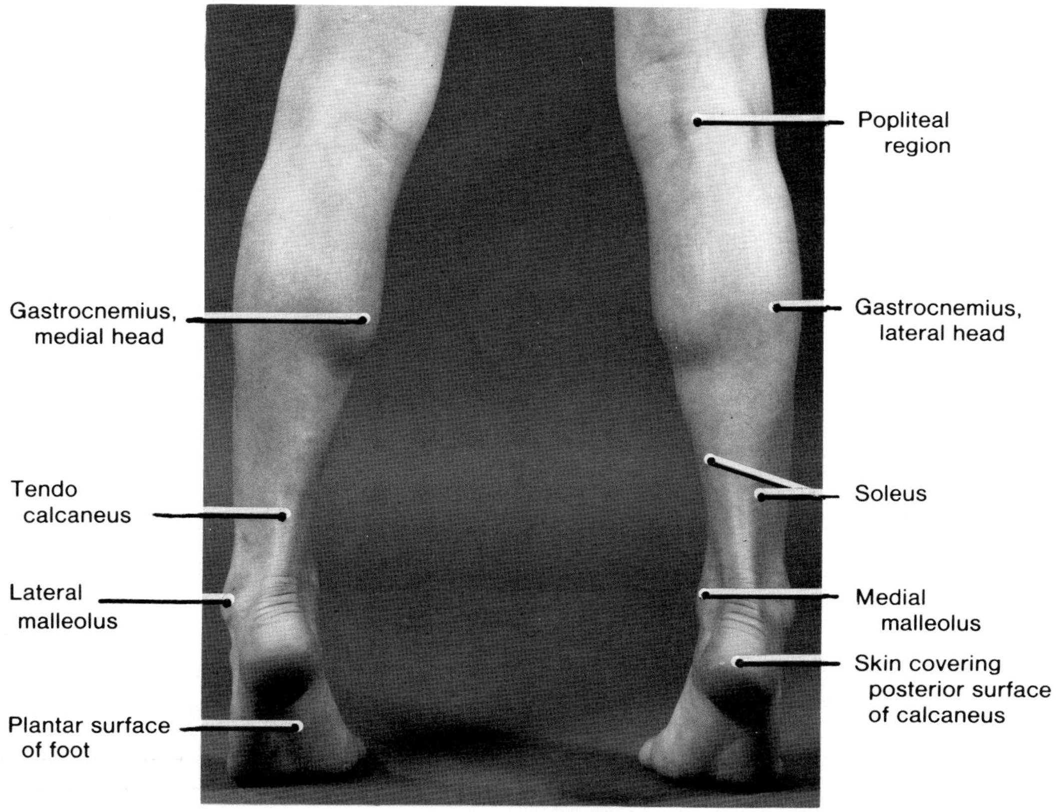

Figure 4-84. Photograph of the posterior aspect of the legs of a 12-year-old girl who is standing on her tiptoes to show the principal surface features. The fleshy posterior part of the leg, formed by the gastrocnemius and soleus muscles (collectively known as the triceps surae), is often referred to as the "calf of the leg." The triceps surae is the principal plantarflexor of the ankle joint; hence, when it is paralyzed, the patient cannot stand on the tiptoes as demonstrated.

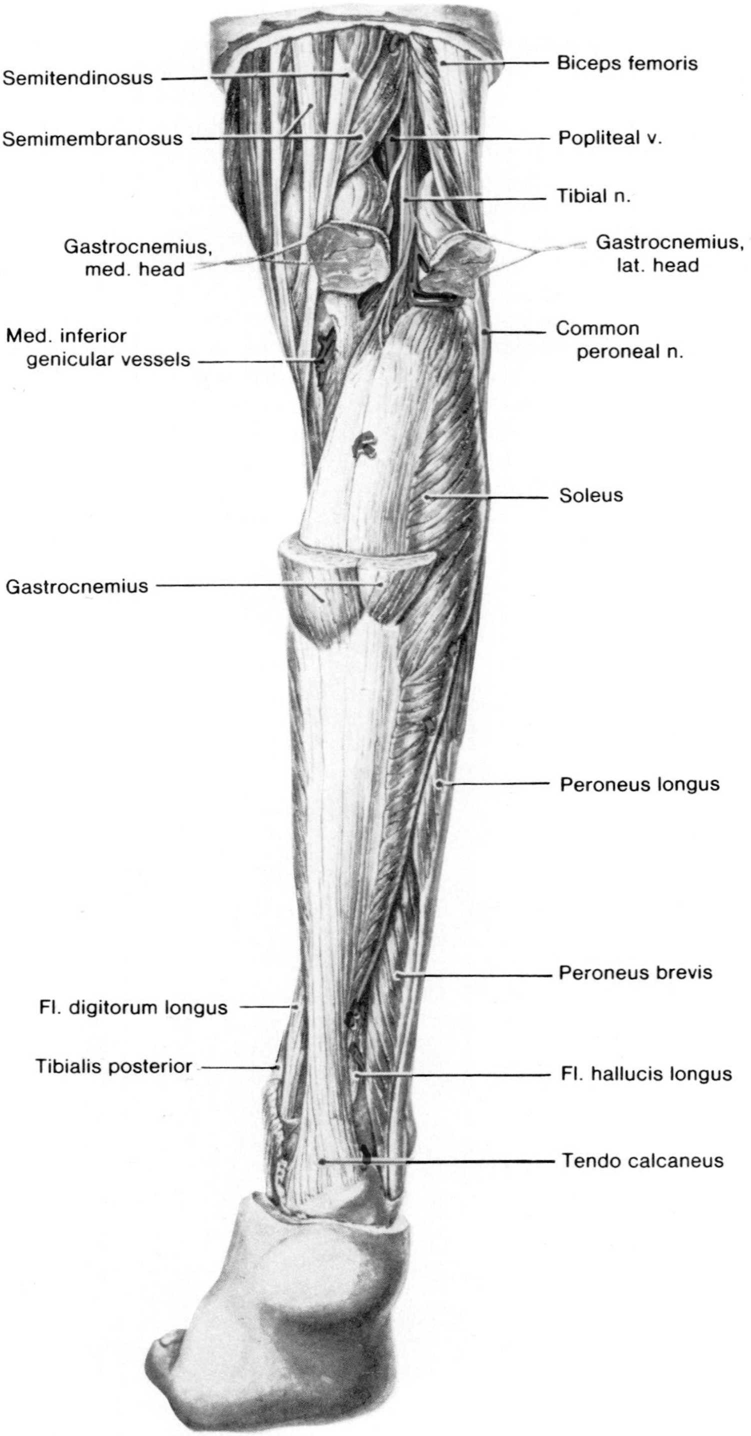

Figure 4-85. Drawing of a deep dissection of the muscles of the superficial posterior crural compartment. The fleshy bellies of the gastrocnemius muscle are largely excised, exposing the origin of the soleus muscle.

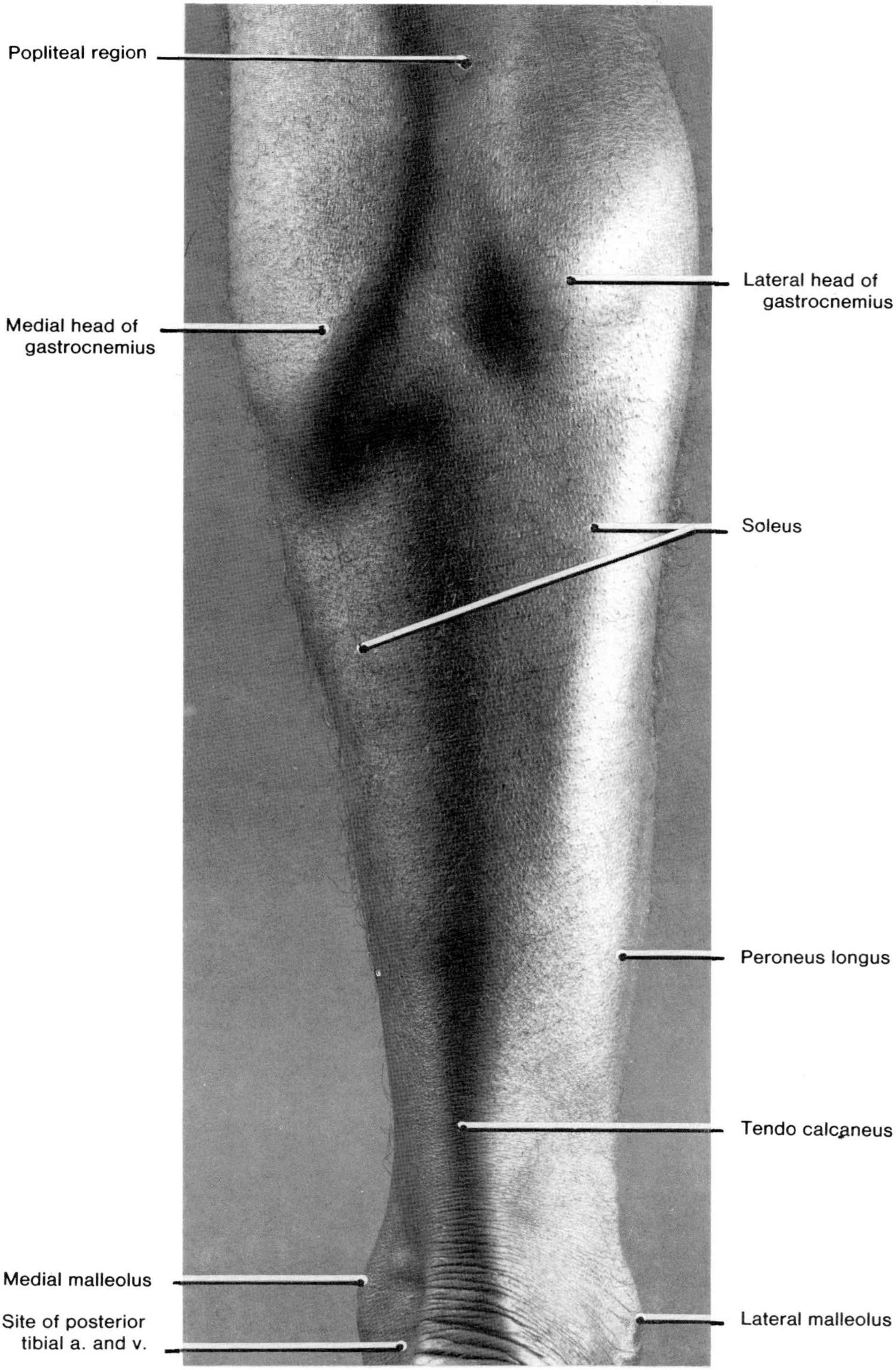

Figure 4-86. Photograph of the posterior aspect of the right leg of a 35-year-old man standing on his tiptoes to show the principal surface features. Observe that the medial and lateral malleoli are subcutaneous and prominent. Note that the tip of the lateral malleolus is more distal than that of the medial malleolus and is farther posteriorly. Observe that the two heads of the gastrocnemius come together to form a single muscle (also see Fig. 4-83), the tendon of which joins the tendon of the soleus muscle to make up the tendo calcaneus that inserts into the posterior surface of the calcaneus. The two-headed gastrocnemius, together with the soleus, forms the triceps surae muscle, which produces the prominence of the calf. Compare with Figure 4-83.

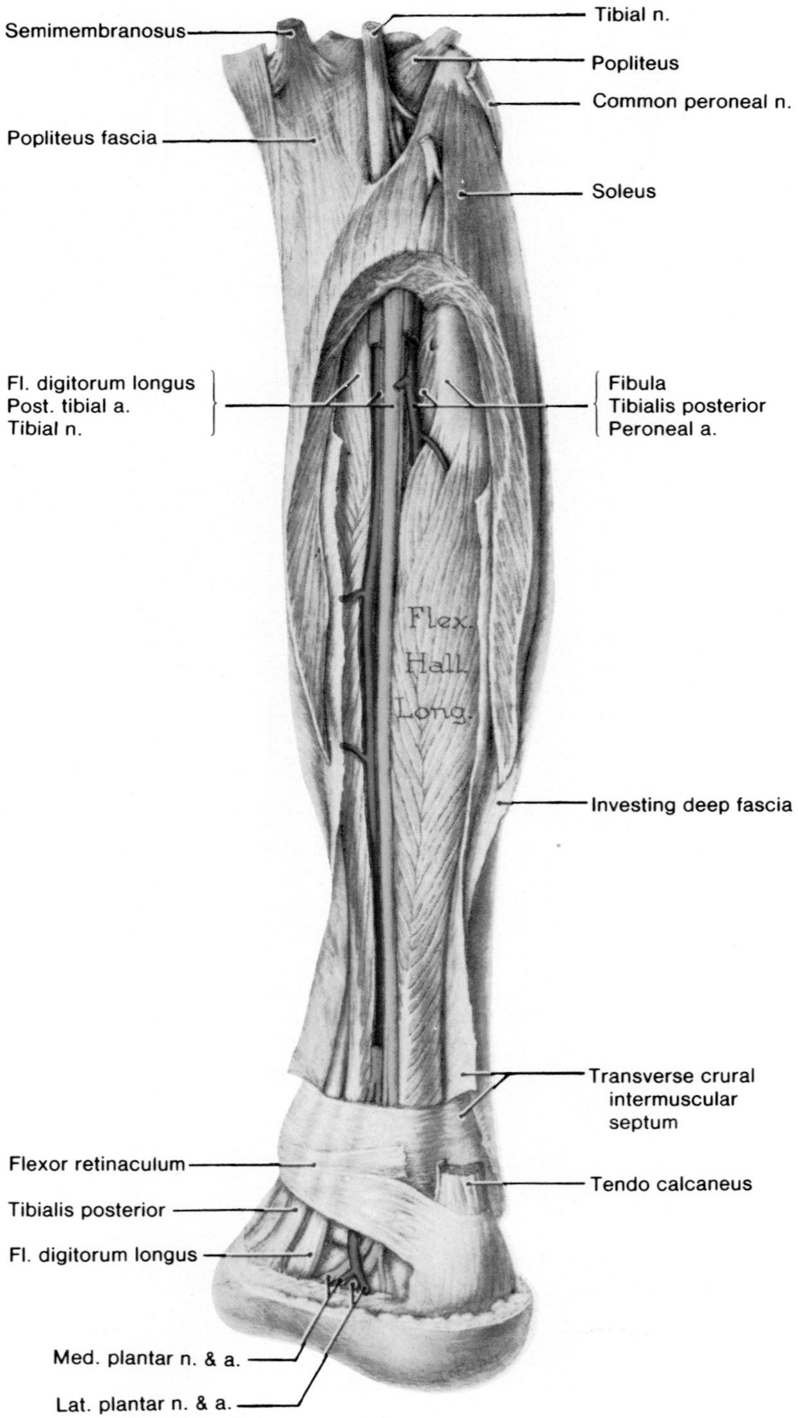

Figure 4-87. Drawing of a dissection of the posterior compartment of the right leg showing the deep structures. The tendo calcaneus is divided and the gastrocnemius muscle and a horseshoe-shaped section of the soleus muscle are removed. Observe the posterior tibial artery and the tibial nerve descending between the large flexor hallucis longus and the smaller flexor digitorum longus muscles. Note the transverse crural intermuscular septum deep to soleus (Fig. 4-74) and the tendo calcaneous that acts as a restraining ''anklet'' at the ankle; here it blends medially with the weaker investing deep fascia to form the flexor retinaculum.

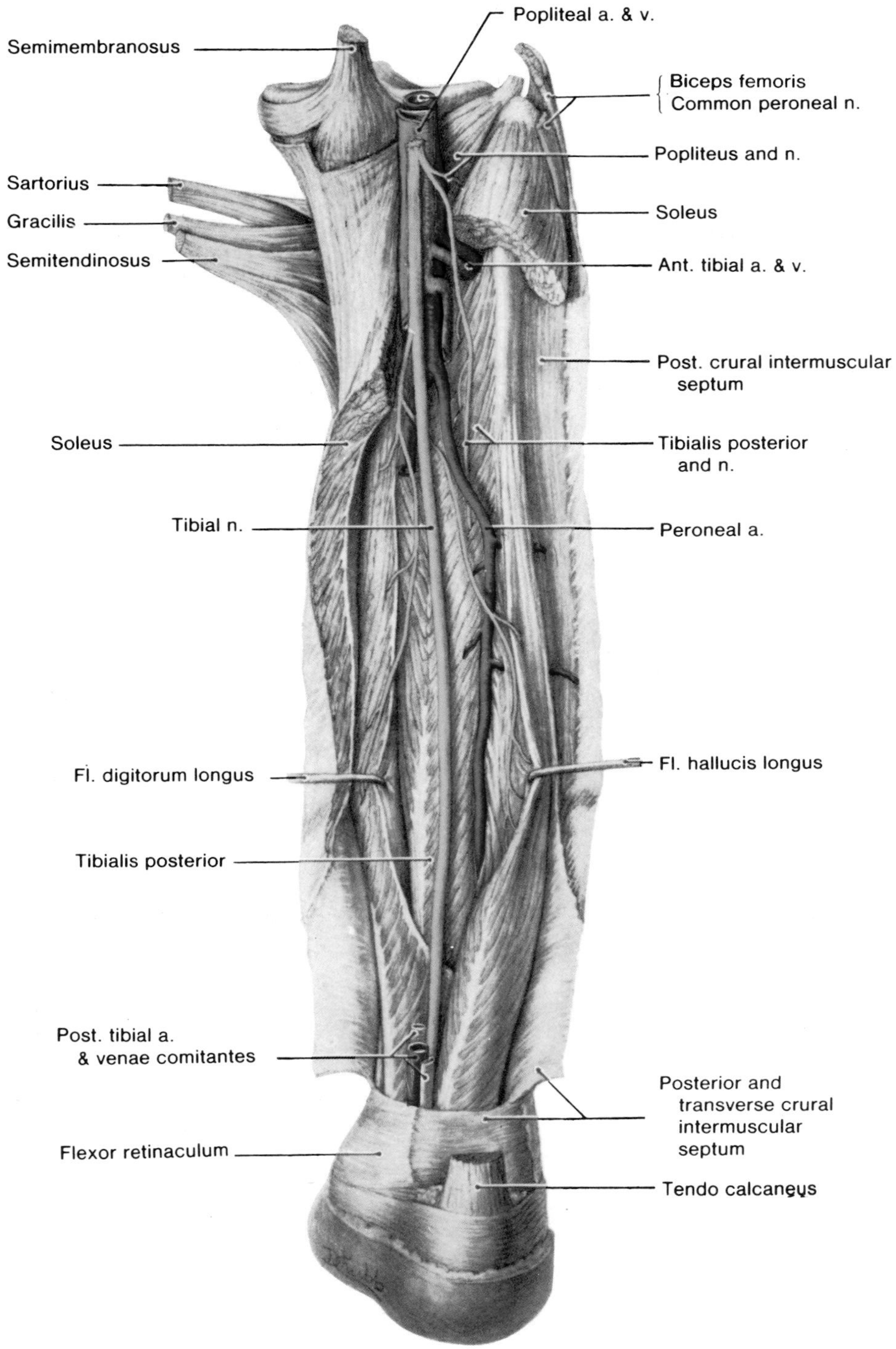

Figure 4-88. Drawing of a dissection of the posterior compartment of the right leg displaying the deep structures. The soleus muscle is largely cut away, the two long digital flexors are pulled apart, and the posterior tibial artery is excised. Observe the bipennate tibialis posterior muscle lying deep to the long digital flexors (see Fig. 4-74 also) and that the peroneal artery is overlapped by the flexor hallucis longus muscle. Note that the nerve to the tibialis posterior here arises in conjunction with the nerve to the popliteus, and the nerve to the flexor digitorum longus arises in conjunction with the nerve to the flexor hallucis longus. Observe that in the popliteal fossa the tibial nerve is superficial to the popliteal artery, whereas at the ankle the posterior tibial artery is superficial to the tibial nerve.

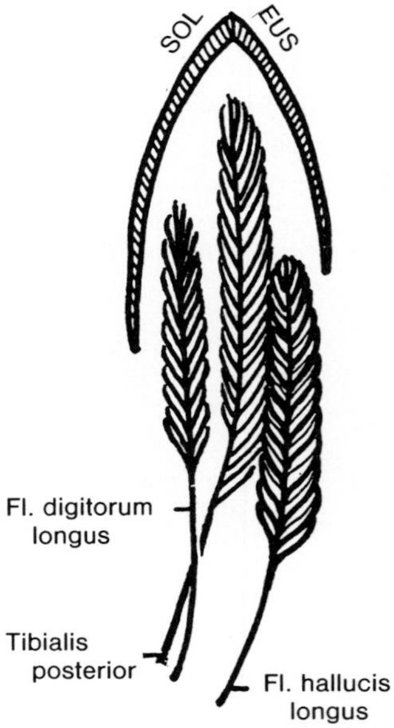

Figure 4-89. Diagram illustrating the three bipennate (feather-like) muscles of the deep posterior compartment of the right leg that lie deep to the soleus muscle (Fig. 4-87). The quill-like tendons pass inferomedially to enter the sole of the foot (Fig. 4-90). The tibialis posterior is in the deepest subcompartment of the posterior crural compartment (see Fig. 4-74) and is separated from the other two muscles by a strong transverse intermuscular septum.

the ankle joint. Contributory factors appear to be muscle fatigue and degenerative changes in the muscle. It usually occurs when a middle-aged tennis player is serving the ball or stretches for a difficult shot.

The gastrocnemius is one of a few muscles with only one source of blood supply, [*i.e.*, the sural (L. *sura*, calf) arteries from the popliteal]. They are virtually end arteries, *i.e.*, with no anastomoses except by capillaries. If one branch is blocked, the part supplied by it dies. The term "**football calf**" is sometimes used to describe the doughy sensation that is felt on palpation of the calf of a person whose gastrocnemius has undergone necrosis owing to an infarct in the muscle, resulting from **acute ischemia** caused by an **embolus** (G. plug) in the popliteal artery.

The Soleus Muscle (Figs. 4-74 and 4-83 to 4-86). This broad, flat, fleshy muscle was named because of its resemblance to the sole, a flatfish. The soleus lies immediately deep to the gastrocnemius and can be palpated on each side of this muscle and below the midcalf when the person is standing on his/her tiptoes.

Origin (Figs. 4-2, 4-22, and 4-66). **Posterior aspect of head** and **upper fourth of fibula**, **soleal line of tibia**, **tendinous arch** over tibial vessels, and middle third of **medial border of tibia**. Observe that the soleus has a *horseshoe-shaped origin from the tibia and the fibula just below the knee.*

Insertion (Figs. 4-66 and 4-84 to 4-87). Middle part of **posterior surface of calcaneus** via tendo calcaneus. It shares this strong tendon with the gastrocnemius muscle.

Nerve Supply. **Tibial** nerve (S1 and S2).

Actions. **Plantarflexes ankle joint** and **steadies leg on foot** during standing. It acts with the gastrocnemius in plantarflexing the ankle (*e.g.*, in walking and dancing).

CLINICALLY ORIENTED COMMENTS

Swelling of the bursa between the tendo calcaneus and the superior part of the tuberosity of the calcaneus, called **calcaneal bursitis**, is fairly common in long distance runners and Scottish dancers owing to excessive friction on the bursa as the tendon slides over it.

When standing the venous return of the leg depends largely on muscular activity, especially of the calf muscles. The efficiency of this "**calf pump**" is improved by the tight sleeve of deep fascia covering these muscles (Fig. 4-74). When the calf muscles contract the blood is pumped upward in the **deep veins** (the anterior and posterior tibial veins unite to form the popliteal vein, which becomes the femoral vein). Normally blood is prevented from flowing into the **superficial veins** by the valves in the communicating veins. If these valves become incompetent, blood is forced into the superficial veins (Fig. 4-12) during contraction of the leg muscles and by hydrostatic pressure when straining or stand-

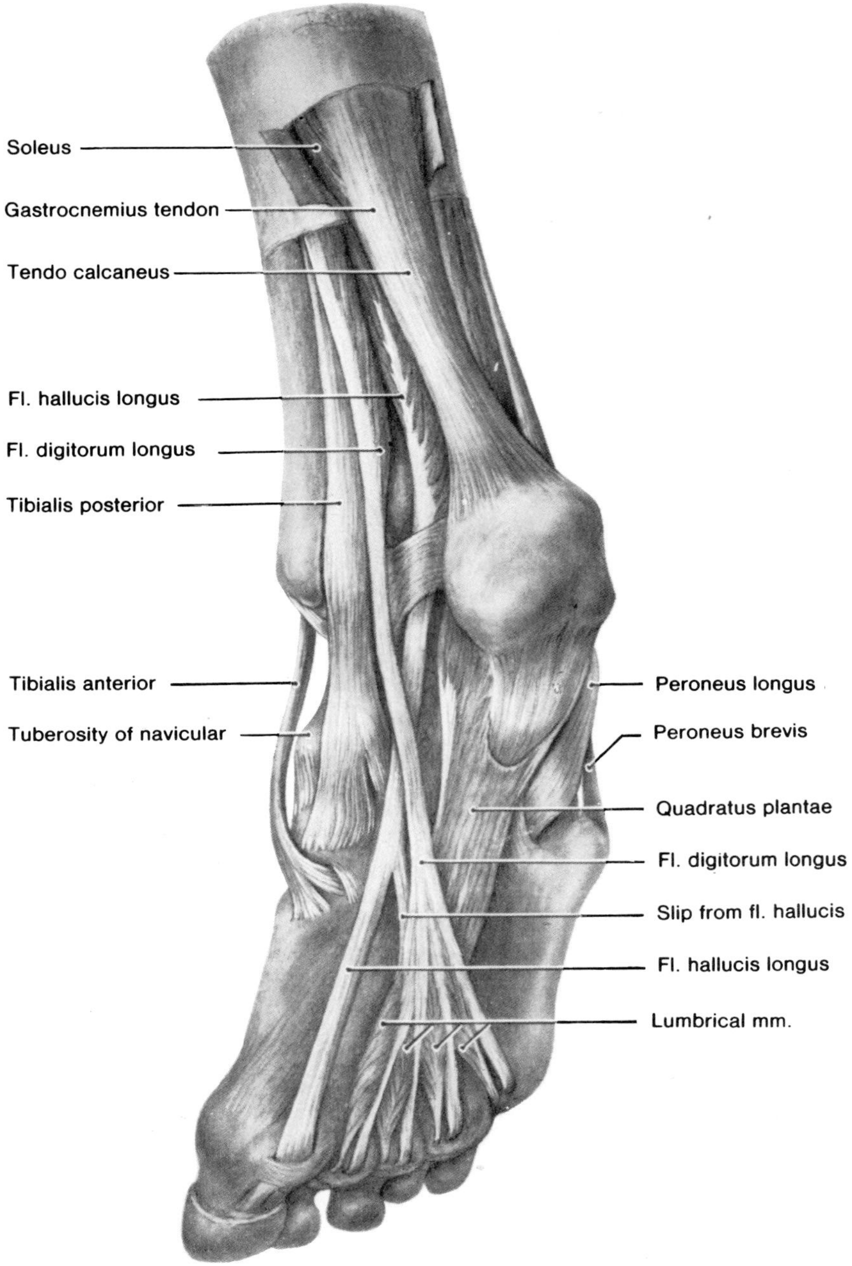

Figure 4–90. Drawing of a dissection of the distal part of the right leg and the foot displaying the second layer of plantar muscles, consisting of the flexor hallucis longus, the flexor digitorum longus, the four lumbricals, and the quadratus plantae. Observe that the flexor digitorum longus crosses superficial to the tibialis posterior muscle, posterior to the medial malleolus, and superficial to the flexor hallucis longus in the foot. Note the four lumbrical muscles passing to the medial sides of the toes. Observe that the flexor hallucis longus sends a strong tendinous slip to the flexor digitorum longus muscle.

ing. The distented perforating and superficial veins are called **varicose veins**.

The Plantaris Muscle (Figs. 4-45, 4-46, 4-60, 4-61, and 4-74). This small muscle is variable in size and extent; it may be absent. When present it has a fleshy belly and a long, slender tendon which runs obliquely between the gastrocnemius and soleus muscles. *It is of no practical importance.*

Origin (Figs. 4-22 and 4-66). Inferior end of **lateral supracondylar line** and **popliteal surface of femur** above lateral head of gastrocnemius muscle.

Insertion (Fig. 4-66). Middle part of **posterior surface of calcaneus** as part of tendo calcaneus or separately on the medial side of it.

Nerve Supply. **Tibial** nerve (S1 and S2).

Actions. **Flexes knee joint** and **plantarflexes ankle joint**. It acts with the gastrocnemius and soleus muscles, but its role is minor.

CLINICALLY ORIENTED COMMENTS

The clinical importance of the plantaris lies in the possibility of its rupture during violent movements. Sudden dorsiflexion of the ankle joint may rupture its slender tendon. In most cases of apparent **rupture of the plantaris tendon**, muscle fibers of the triceps surae are also torn (see tennis leg, p. 519).

This injury is common in basketball players, sprinters, and ballet dancers. Surprisingly the pain following rupture may be so severe that the person is unable to bear weight on the foot. Usually some fibers of the gastrocnemius are also torn, resulting in internal bleeding and **pain in the calf**. This is called a "**Charley horse**" by athletes, as is pain in the front of the thigh, following injury to the quadriceps femoris muscle. The pain of a Charley horse is more severe and prolonged than an **athletic cramp** (painful muscle spasm).

2. Muscles in the Deep Posterior Compartment (Figs. 4-60, 4-61, 4-74, 4-87, and 4-88). Four muscles comprise the deep group of the posterior crural compartment: the **popliteus**, the **flexor digitorum longus**, the **flexor hallucis longus**, and the **tibialis posterior**. The popliteus acts on the knee (rotator), whereas the others act on the ankle and the joints of the foot.

The Popliteus Muscle (Figs. 4-60 to 4-62, 4-88, and 4-124). This thin, flat, triangular muscle forms the floor of the inferior part of the **popliteal fossa**; thus it lies in the proximal part of the leg.

Origin (Figs. 4-54 and 4-66). **Lateral surface of lateral condyle of femur**, just inferior to the attachment of the fibular collateral ligament of the knee. Its stout cord-like tendon arises from a rough pit on the condyle known as the **popliteal groove** of the femur. *The origin of the popliteus is inside the fibrous capsule of the knee joint* and deep to the fibular collateral ligament; thus, the deep surface of its tendon is covered by synovial membrane (Figs. 4-124 and 4-126). Some fibers of the popliteus arise from the posterior surface of the lateral meniscus of the knee joint.

Insertion (Figs. 4-22 and 4-66). **Posterior surface of tibia**, **proximal to soleal line**; hence, the inferior border of the popliteus is adjacent to the superior border of the soleus.

Nerve Supply. **Tibial** nerve (L5).

Actions. **Flexes** and **rotates knee joint**. It **unlocks the knee** joint at the beginning of flexion of the fully extended knee by rotating the tibia medially on the femur. It is a lateral rotator of the femur on the tibia when the foot is fixed (*e.g.*, on the ground).

Three muscles in the deep posterior crural compartment (Figs. 4-87 to 4-89) lie deep to the three superficial plantarflexors of the ankle joint (*i.e.*, the calf muscles in the superficial posterior compartment). These deep muscles assist the muscles of the superficial compartment in plantarflexion of the ankle joint, with inversion of the foot, and in steadying the leg on the foot when standing.

In Figures 4-87 to 4-90 note that the tendons of these deep muscles pass posterior to the medial malleolus and deep to the **flexor retinaculum** as they enter the foot. The flexor retinaculum is a thickening of deep fascia that passes from the medial process of the calcaneus (Fig. 4-65) to the tip of the medial malleolus (Figs. 4-88 and 4-93). Distally the flexor retinaculum is continuous with the deep fascia on the dorsum of the foot. It holds the tendons of the deep posterior muscles and the posterior tibial vessels and nerve close to the bones of the ankle, preventing displacement of the tendons during movements of the foot.

The Flexor Hallucis Longus Muscle (Figs. 4-74 and 4-87 to 4-89). This powerful bipennate muscle, the largest of the three deep muscles, *lies lateral* and is closely *attached to the fibula.*

Origin (Figs. 4-66 and 4-67*B*). **Inferior two-thirds of posterior surface of fibula, interosseous membrane**, and **intermuscular septa**. Its tendon passes posterior to the distal end of the tibia and deep to the flexor retinaculum (Fig. 4-87), where it occupies a broad shallow groove on the posterior surface of the talus which is continuous with the groove on the plantar surface of the sustenaculum tali (Fig. 4-70). The tendon then crosses deep to the tendon of the flexor digitorum longus in the sole of the foot, giving a tendinous slip to its tendon (Fig. 4-90). As it passes to the great toe, the flexor hallucis longus tendon runs between two sesamoid bones in the tendons of the flexor hallucis brevis (Figs. 4-101 and 4-104); thus, its tendon is protected from the pressure of the head of the first metatarsal bone.

Insertion (Figs. 4-69 and 4-90). **Base of distal phalanx of great toe**.

Nerve Supply. **Tibial** nerve (S1 and S2).

Actions. **Flexes great toe** at all joints, **plantarflexes ankle joint**, and helps to maintain the medial longitudinal arch of foot (Fig. 4-151). It is *the "push-off" muscle during walking* and running and provides much of the spring to the step. It is also important in holding the leg in the normal position on the foot.

The Flexor Digitorum Longus Muscle (Figs. 4-74, 4-85, and 4-87 to 4-90). This long narrow muscle (long flexor of the toes) *lies medial* and is closely *attached to the tibia.* It is smaller than the flexor hallucis longus, even though it moves four toes.

Origin (Fig. 4-66). **Posterior surface of tibia** (inferior to the popliteus and soleal line) and **intermuscular septum**.

Insertion (Figs. 4-69 and 4-90). **Distal phalanges of lateral four digits**. Its tendon runs inferiorly passing posterior to the tibialis posterior tendon and the medial malleolus. It then passes diagonally in the sole of the foot superficial to the tendon of the flexor hallucis longus. As the tendon reaches the middle of the sole, it divides into four tendons which pass to the bases of the lateral four phalanges.

Nerve Supply. **Tibial** nerve (S1 and S2).

Actions. **Flexes all joints of lateral four toes, plantarflexes ankle joint**, and *helps to maintain medial longitudinal arch of foot* (Fig. 4-151). Flexion of the toes is important in walking and running because it gives the foot a grip on the ground.

The Tibialis Posterior Muscle (Figs. 4-74 and 4-87 to 4-91). This large important muscle, the deepest one in the posterior compartment, lies between the flexor digitorum longus and the flexor hallucis longus in the same plane as the tibia and fibula.

Origin (Figs. 4-66, 4-67*B*, and 4-91). **Interosseous membrane**, lateral part of **posterior aspect of tibia** (inferior to soleal line), and upper two-thirds of **medial surface of fibula**.

Insertion (Figs. 4-70, 4-91, 4-143, and 4-147). **Tuberosity of navicular** bone with slips to cuneiforms, cuboid, and **bases of second, third, and fourth metatarsals**.

Nerve Supply. **Tibial** nerve (L4 and L5).

Actions (Fig. 4-75*B* and *D*). **Plantarflexes ankle joint, inverts foot**, and *helps to maintain medial longitudinal arch of foot* (Fig. 4-151), owing to its muscle insertions into the plantar surfaces of several tarsal bones and the direction of its pull.

Nerves of the Posterior Crural Compartment (Figs. 4-60, 4-61, 4-74, 4-87, and 4-88). The **tibial nerve** (medial popliteal) supplies all muscles in the posterior compartment. The *larger terminal branch of the sciatic nerve*, the tibial, arises from the ventral branches of the ventral rami of L4, L5, S1, S2, and S3. It descends along the posterior aspect of the thigh, through the middle of the popliteal fossa posterior to the popliteal vein and artery. At the distal border of the popliteus muscle, it passes with the posterior tibial vessels deep to the tendinous arch of the soleus muscle. It then descends deep to the soleus muscle and

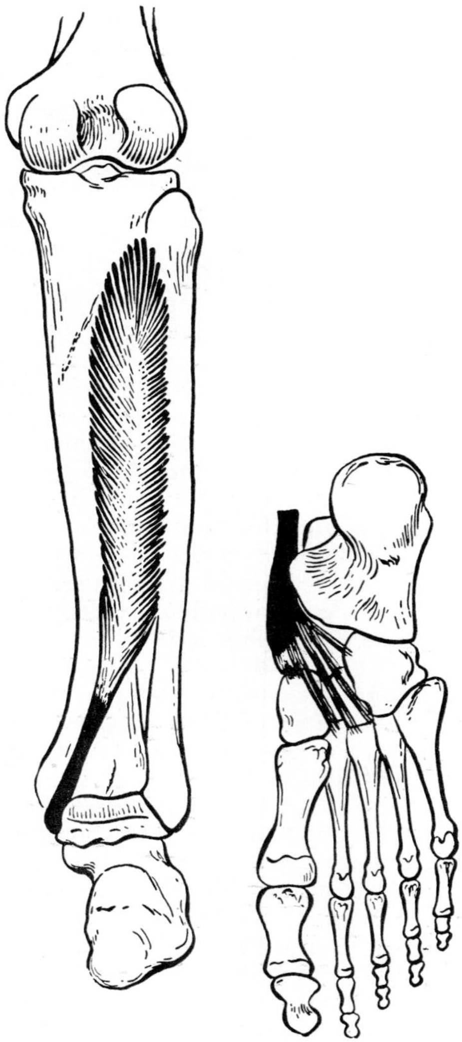

Figure 4–91. Drawings to illustrate the origin and insertion of the right tibialis posterior muscle. It arises from the interosseous membrane and the adjoining tibia and fibula (Fig. 4–74) and inserts into the tuberosity of the navicular bone (Figs. 4–69 and 4–92). Note that it also sends slips to adjacent bones and to the bases of the second, third, and fourth metatarsal bones.

runs inferiorly on the tibialis posterior muscle in company with the above vessels (Fig. 4-74). It leaves the posterior crural compartment by passing deep to the flexor retinaculum in the interval between the medial malleolus and the calcaneus (Figs. 4-87 and 4-88). Here it lies between the posterior tibial vessels and the tendon of the flexor hallucis longus muscle (Fig. 4-93). Posteroinferior to the medial malleolus, the tibial nerve divides into the **medial** and **lateral plantar nerves** (Figs. 4-87 and 4-93).

The tibial nerve gives branches to all muscles in the posterior crural compartment (Fig. 4-94) and to the **sural nerve** (Fig. 4-60), which supplies skin of the lateral and posterior part of the lower third of the leg and the lateral side of the foot (Figs. 4-12 and 4-106). Articular branches of the tibial nerve supply the knee joint and medial calcaneal branches supply the skin of the heel.

CLINICALLY ORIENTED COMMENTS

Because the tibial nerve is deep and fairly well protected, it is not commonly injured. Lacerations in the popliteal fossa (Case 4-10) or posterior **dislocations of the knee joint** may damage this nerve, producing paralysis of the muscles in the posterior compartment of the leg and the intrinsic muscles in the sole of the foot. When the plantarflexors of the foot are paralyzed, the patient is unable to curl the toes or stand on the tiptoes. In addition, there is loss of sensation in the sole of the foot (Fig. 4-106), making it vulnerable to the development of pressure sores.

Arteries of the Posterior Crural Compartment. Structures in the posterior compartment are supplied by the posterior tibial artery and its branches.

The Posterior Tibial Artery (Figs. 4-34*B*, 4-62, 4-74, 4-87, 4-88, 4-93, and 4-95). This artery **begins at the distal border of the popliteus** muscle, between the tibia and the fibula, as the larger terminal branch of the popliteal artery. As the direct continuation of the popliteal, the posterior tibial artery passes deep to the origin of the soleus muscle and, after giving off the **peroneal artery** (its largest branch), it passes inferomedially on the posterior surface of the tibialis posterior muscle (Fig. 4-95). In its descent it is accompanied by the tibial nerve and two venae comitantes, deep to the transverse crural intermuscular septum (Fig. 4-74). At the ankle the posterior tibial artery runs posterior to the medial malleolus, from which it is separated by the tendons of the tibialis posterior and flexor digitorum longus muscles (Fig. 4-93). Inferior to the medial malleolus, it runs between the tendons of the flexor hallucis longus and flexor digitorum longus muscles. Deep to flexor retinaculum and the origin of the abductor hallucis muscle, the posterior tibial artery divides into **medial** and **lateral plantar arteries** (Figs. 4-87 and 4-93).

Branches of the Posterior Tibial Artery (Figs. 4-87, 4-88, and 4-95).

The peroneal artery is the largest and *most important collateral branch of the posterior tibial* artery. It begins 2 to 3 cm inferior to the distal border of the popliteus muscle and the tendinous arch of the soleus and descends obliquely toward the fibula and along its medial side within the flexor hallucis longus muscle or between it and the intermuscular septum and the tibialis posterior. The peroneal artery gives off muscular branches to the popliteus and to other muscles in the posterior and lateral compartments of the leg. It also supplies a **nutrient artery to the fibula** and a communicating branch which joins that of the posterior tibial artery (Fig. 4-95). The peroneal artery usually pierces the interosseous membrane and passes to the dorsum of the foot, where it anastomoses with the **arcuate artery** (Figs. 4-81 and 4-95).

The posterior tibial artery also gives branches to the muscles of the posterior compartment and to the skin on the medial aspect of the leg.

A **circumflex fibular branch** is given off at the knee, which passes laterally over the neck of the fibula to the anastomoses around the knee (Fig. 4-62).

The **nutrient artery of the tibia** arises from the posterior tibial artery near its origin (Figs. 4-34*B* and 4-95). It is the *largest of the nutrient arteries to long bones* in the body and the nutrient foramen through which it passes is obvious, just distal to the soleal line on the posterior surface of the tibia (Fig. 4-65).

Other branches of the posterior tibial artery are a **communicating branch** that unites it to the peroneal artery (Fig. 4-95); **calcanean branches** to the tissues of the heel which pass medial and posterior to the tendo calcaneus (Fig. 4-93) and anastomose with branches of the peroneal artery; and a **malleolar branch** which joins the network of vessels on the medial malleolus (Fig. 4-34).

CLINICALLY ORIENTED COMMENTS

The **pulse of the posterior tibial artery** can usually be palpated about half way between the posterior surface of the medial malleolus and the medial border of the tendo calcaneus (Figs. 4-93 and 4-96). The pulse of this artery is usually easy to feel in children and in some cases its pulsations are visible. In older persons in whom the pulse may be difficult to palpate with the foot relaxed, it is usually easier to feel with the patient's foot dorsiflexed and inverted.

A knowledge of how to palpate the pulse of the posterior tibial artery is essential for examining patients with **intermittent claudication**, a condition caused by ischemia (insufficient blood supply) to the leg muscles owing to **arteriosclerotic stenosis** (narrowing) or occlusion (complete blockage) of the leg arteries. It is characterized by leg cramps which develop during walking and disappear soon after. When a few more steps are taken, the cramps reappear.

When a patient complains of **leg cramps**, often the peripheral *pulses in the leg are absent or markedly diminished.* These cramps develop during exercise because the narrowed arteries and the collateral circulation to the leg muscles (Fig. 4-34) are unable to supply the extra blood that is required by the actively contracting leg muscles. When examining a patient with leg cramps, it is important to determine whether the circulatory failure in the leg results from narrowing (**arteriosclerosis**) or spasm of the arteries supplying the leg muscles.

THE FOOT

The foot is the part of the lower limb distal to the leg. It is concerned mainly with support and locomotion of the body. The bones of the foot are illustrated in Figures 4-68 to 4-72. The clinical importance of the foot is indicated by the estimate that the average orthopaedic surgeon devotes about 20% of his practice to foot problems and foot surgery. The entire practice of podiatry is devoted to the foot.

Skin of the Foot. The skin on the dorsum of the foot is thin and mobile; hair is sparse and there is relatively little subcutaneous fat. Generally there is a well marked tuft of hair on the skin over the proximal phalanges of men. Because of the thinness of the skin and superficial fascia on the dorsum of the foot, the tendons of the foot are usually clearly visible on this surface, especially during dorsiflexion (Figs. 4-79 and 4-92).

The skin on the plantar surface or sole of the foot is thick, particularly over the heel and the ball of the foot (base of great toe). This skin contains many sweat glands and much fat in the subcutaneous tissue which is firmly bound down to underlying structures by cords and septa of fibrous connective tissue (Fig. 4-97). The structure of the sole of the foot is designed for weight bearing and for protection of the underlying nerves and vessels.

Fascia of the Foot. The deep fascia of the foot is continuous with that of the leg. It is thin on the dorsum of the foot and here is continuous with the **extensor retinacula** (Fig. 4-76). Over the lateral and posterior aspects of the foot it is continuous with the **plantar fascia**.

The Plantar Aponeurosis (Fig. 4-97). This is a fibrous membranous *expansion of the plantar fascia* that covers the entire sole; its central part is the thickest. It consists of longitudinally arranged bands of dense fibrous connective tissue which *help support the longitudinal arches* of the foot (Fig. 4-151) and hold the parts of the foot together. It stretches from the calcaneus posteriorly and widens as it extends anteriorly before dividing into slips for the five digits. These slips split to enclose the digital tendons and are attached to the margins of the fibrous digital sheaths and to the sesamoid bones of the great toe (Fig. 4-104). At

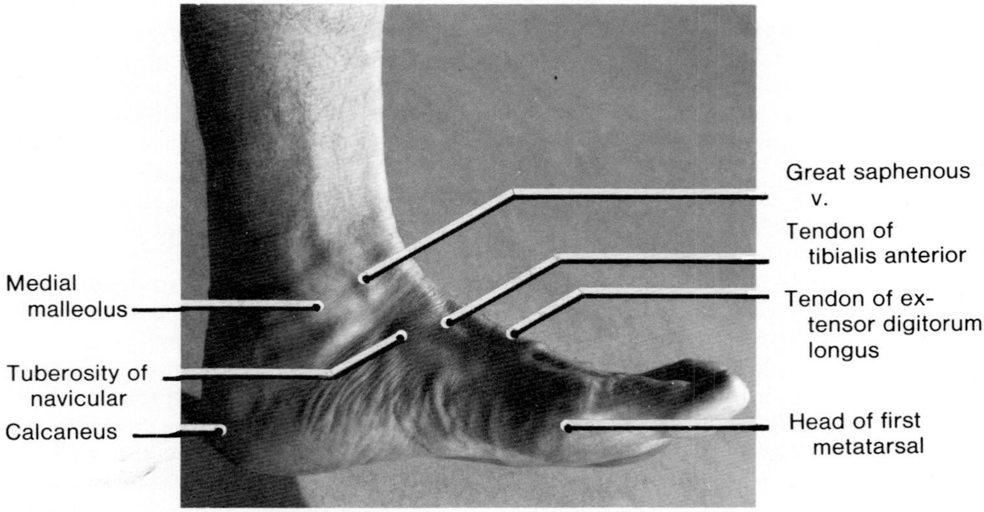

Figure 4–92. Photograph of the medial aspect of the left ankle of a 45-year-old man showing the principal surface features visible when the ankle joint is dorsiflexed. The medial malleolus does not form a very prominent bony landmark in this person. The great saphenous vein is very constant in position, as here, anterior to the medial malleolus. During a "cutdown" (venostomy) this vein is dissected in order to insert a cannula for prolonged administration of intravenous fluids or medication. Observe this vein in Figures 4–13 and 4–93.

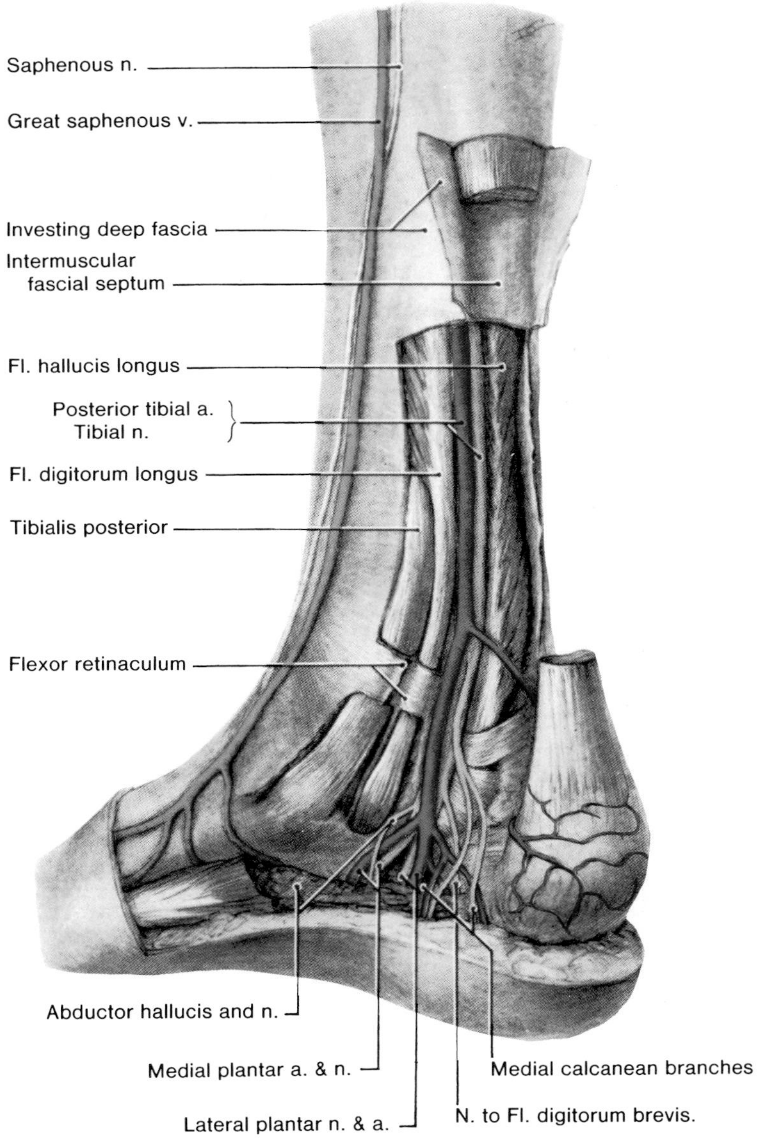

Figure 4–93. Drawing of a medial view of a dissection of the right ankle and heel. The posterior part of the abductor hallucis muscle is excised. Observe the posterior tibial artery and the tibial nerve lying between the flexor digitorum longus and the flexor hallucis longus muscles. They divide into medial and lateral plantar branches on the surface of the osseofibrous tunnel of the flexor hallucis longus. Note that the tibialis posterior and the flexor digitorum longus occupy separate and individual osseofibrous tunnels behind the medial malleolus, which acts as their pulley. Observe the medial and lateral plantar nerves lying within the fork formed by the medial and lateral plantar arteries. Note the deep veins of the foot emerging to join the great saphenous vein.

the margins of the plantar aponeurosis, vertical septa extend deeply to form **three compartments of the sole** of the foot: the medial (great toe) compartment, the lateral (small toe) compartment, and the central compartment. The muscles, nerves, and vessels in the sole may be described according to these compartments, but the muscles

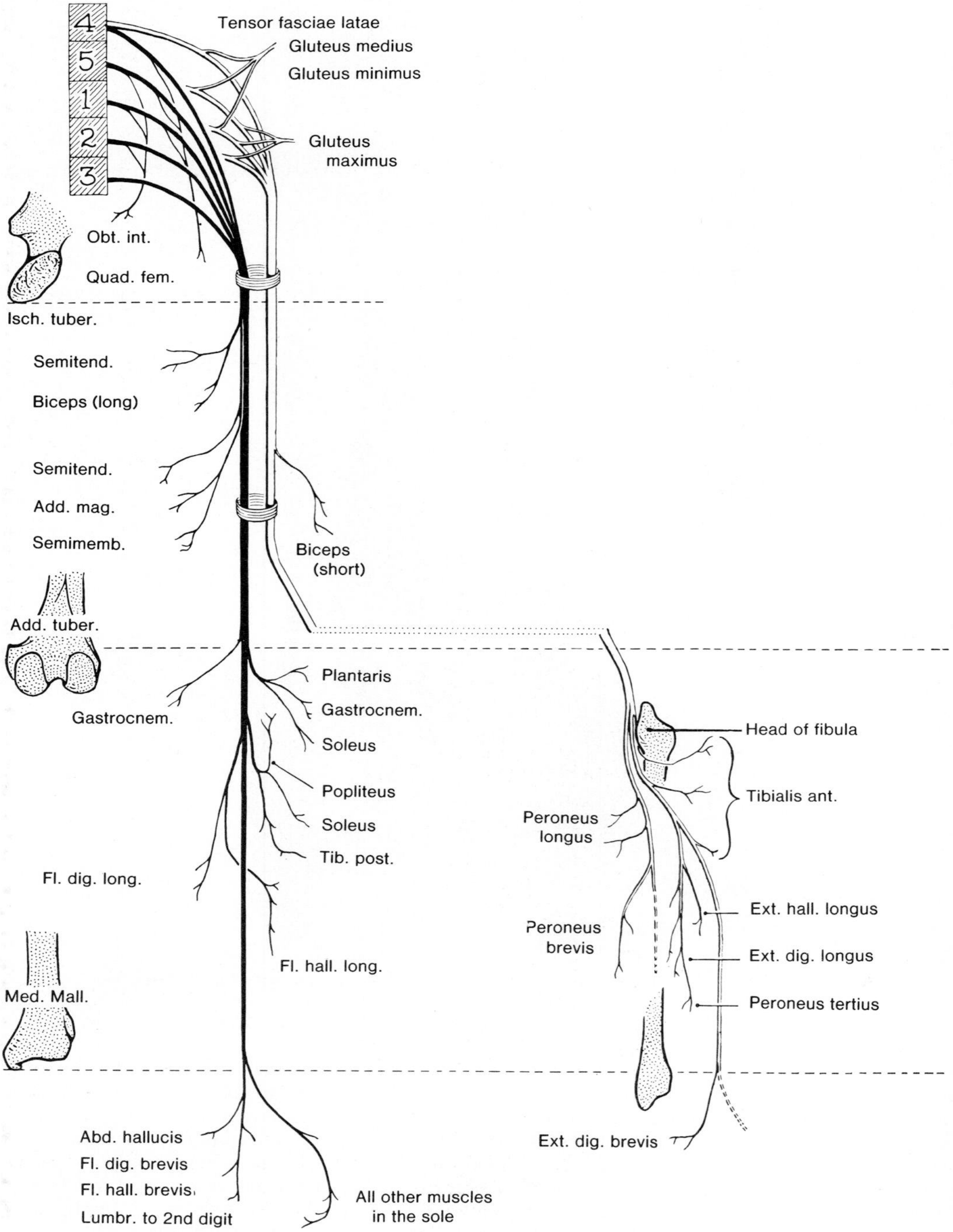

Figure 4–94. Scheme of the motor distribution of the sciatic nerve and its branches and the tibial (*black*) and common peroneal nerves. The tibial nerve, the larger of the two terminal branches of the sciatic nerve, arises from the ventral branches of the ventral rami of L4, L5, S1, S2, and S3. The common peroneal nerve, about half the size of the tibial nerve, is derived from the dorsal branches of the ventral rami of L4, L5, S1, and S2. The sciatic is really two nerves enclosed in a sheath of fascia.

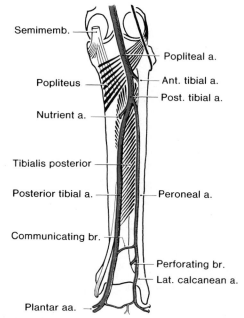

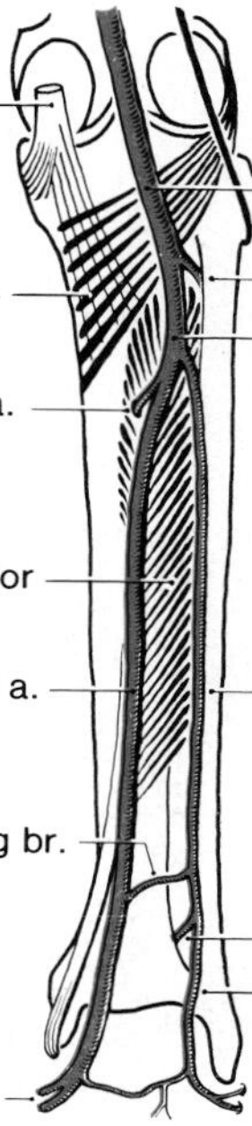

Figure 4–95. Drawing of the arteries in the posterior crural compartment. Note that the posterior tibial artery, the larger of the two terminal branches of the popliteal, begins at the inferior border of the popliteal muscle as the direct continuation of the popliteal artery. Observe the peroneal artery, its largest branch, and the nutrient artery to the tibia. Note the important anastomoses at the back of the heel between the posterior tibial and peroneal arteries.

of the sole are usually dissected and described by layers (Fig. 4-98).

Muscles of the Dorsum of the Foot. There is only one small muscle on the dorsum of the foot and it is relatively unimportant.

The Extensor Digitorum Brevis Muscle (Figs. 4-76 to 4-82). This broad thin muscle forms a fleshy mass on the lateral part of the dorsum of the foot.

Origin (Fig. 4-68). **Dorsal surface of calcaneus.**

Insertion (Fig. 4-76). **Base of proximal phalanx of great toe** and **tendons of extensor digitorum longus of toes 2 to 4.**

Nerve Supply (Fig. 4-80). **Deep peroneal** nerve (S1 and S2).

Action. **Extends toes** 1 to 4 at interphalangeal and metatarsophalangeal joints.

CLINICALLY ORIENTED COMMENTS

Probably the only clinical reason for knowing about the presence of the extensor digitorum brevis muscle is that contusion and/or tearing of its fibers resulting in a **hematoma** often produces a swelling anterior to the lateral malleolus. A person who has injured his/her ankle commonly thinks the swollen muscle, which has not been seen before, indicates a sprained ankle. It might also be interpreted as a possible fracture of the cuboid bone or a sprained transverse tarsal joint.

Muscles of the Sole of the Foot (Figs. 4-98 to 4-105). There are **four layers of intrinsic muscles** in the sole of the foot which are specialized to help maintain the longitudinal and transverse arches of the foot (Fig. 4-151) and to enable one to stand on uneven ground. The specialization of these **plantar muscles** has resulted in the loss of many of their functions; as a result, several muscles in the foot have names implying functions that they are rarely called upon to perform or are unable to perform. The muscles of the sole of the foot are of little importance individually because the fine control of the individual toes is not important to most people.

The First Layer of Plantar Muscles (Figs. 4-98 to 4-100). The **three muscles** of this superficial layer *all extend from the posterior part of the calcaneus to the phalanges* of the toes. They consist of the abductors of the great (big) and small (little) toes and the short flexor of the toes. They comprise a functional group that acts as an elastic spring or tie for the arches of the foot that is capable of assisting in the maintenance of its concavity.

The Abductor Hallucis Muscle (Figs. 4-98 to 4-100). This abductor of the great toe lies superficially along the medial border of the foot.

Origin (Figs. 4-70, 4-93, and 4-99). Medial process of **tuber calcanei**, flexor retinaculum, and plantar aponeurosis.

Insertion (Fig. 4-69). Medial side of **base of proximal phalanx of great toe**.

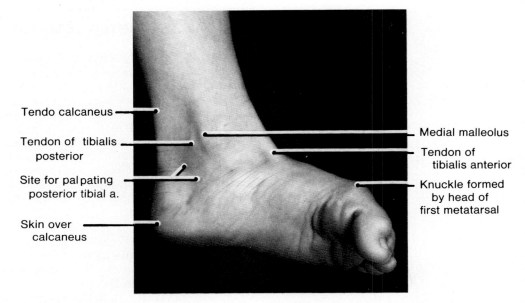

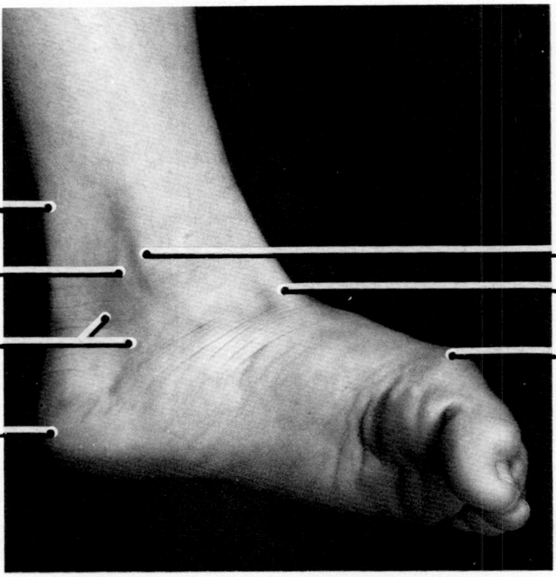

Figure 4–96. Photograph of the medial aspect of the left ankle of a 12-year-old girl whose foot is inverted. During this action, the tendon of the tibialis posterior (an invertor of the foot) may be observed and palpated as it passes posterior and distal to the medial malleolus. The tendon can be easily traced to its insertion into the navicular bone (Fig. 4–91). The pulse of the posterior tibial artery may be palpable where it passes posteroinferior to the medial malleolus. It can often be felt about a fingerbreadth posterior to the medial malleolus. An examination of the pulse here may yield valuable information in cases of suspected arteriosclerotic stenosis of the posterior tibial artery.

Nerve Supply. **Medial plantar** nerve (S2 and S3).

Actions. **Abducts** and **flexes great toe.**

The Flexor Digitorum Brevis Muscle (Figs. 4-69, 4-100, and 4-102). This short flexor of the toes lies between the abductor hallucis and the abductor digiti minimi.

Origin (Fig. 4-69). Medial process of **tuber calcanei**, plantar aponeurosis, and **intermuscular septa.**

Insertion (Fig. 4-69). By four tendons into **middle phalanges of lateral four toes.**

Nerve Supply. **Medial plantar** nerve (S2 and S3).

Action. **Flexes lateral four toes** at proximal interphalangeal joints.

The Abductor Digiti Minimi Muscle (Figs. 4-100 to 4-102). You may hear this abductor of the small toe called the abductor digiti quinti (V). It is the most lateral of the three muscles in the first layer.

Origin (Fig. 4-68). Medial and lateral processes of **tuber calcanei**, plantar aponeurosis, and intermuscular septum.

Insertion (Fig. 4-69). Lateral side of base of **proximal phalanx of small toe.**

Nerve Supply. **Lateral plantar** nerve (S2 and S3).

Actions. **Abducts** and **flexes small toe.**

The Second Layer of Plantar Muscles (Figs. 4-90, 4-98, and 4-101). This layer of muscles and tendons, located deep to the first layer, consists of **quadratus plantae** and **lumbrical muscles** and the **tendons of two leg muscles** (flexor hallucis longus and flexor digitorum longus). The tendon of the flexor hallucis longus crosses deep to the tendon of the flexor digitorum longus as it passes from the lateral to the medial side of this tendon to reach the great toe.

The Quadratus Plantae Muscle (Figs. 4-90, 4-101 and 4-102). This small, flat, accessory muscle (sometimes called the flexor digitorum accessorius) joins the tendon of the flexor digitorum longus to the calcaneus and forms a fleshy sheet of muscle in the posterior half of the foot. Its *two heads of origin* embrace the calcaneus.

Origin (Figs. 4-69 and 4-70). *Medial*

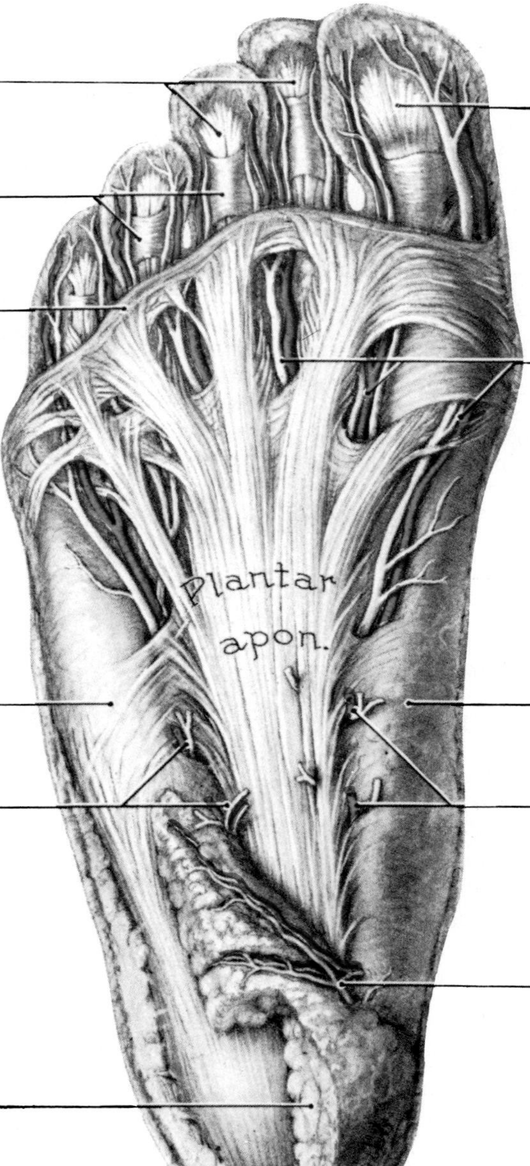

Figure 4–97. Drawing of a superficial dissection of the plantar aspect or sole (L. *planta*) of the right foot. The strong plantar aponeurosis acts as a strong tie for the maintenance of the longitudinal arches of the foot (Fig. 4–151); to fill this role it has to be extremely sturdy. It stretches from the calcaneus posteriorly to the five digits anteriorly.

head, **body of calcaneus** and **plantar fascia**; *lateral head,* lateral margin of **plantar surface of calcaneus.**

Insertion (Figs. 4-90 and 4-101). **Tendon of flexor digitorum longus.**

Nerve Supply (Fig. 4-102). **Lateral plantar** nerve (S2 and S3).

Action. **Assists flexor digitorum longus** in flexing lateral four toes by adjusting pull of flexor digitorum longus (*i.e.,* it brings

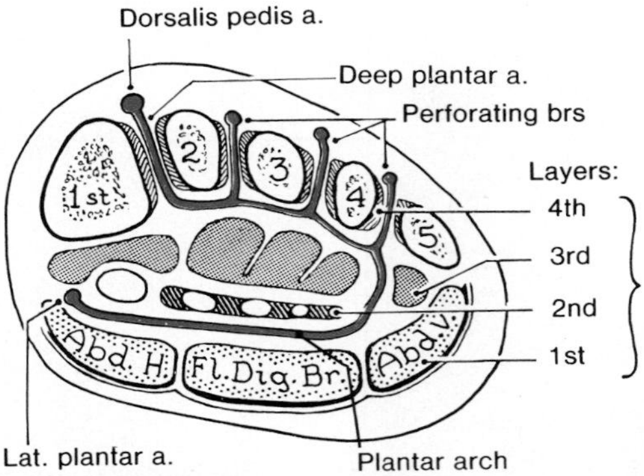

Figure 4–98. Drawing of a cross-section of the right foot near the bases of the metatarsals showing the four layers of intrinsic muscles in the sole of the foot and the plantar arteries. See Figure 4–107 for a drawing of the arteries of the dorsum of the foot.

its tendon more directly in line with the long axes of the digits).

The Lumbrical Muscles (Figs. 4-90 and 4-100). There are four of these slender muscles.

Origin (Fig. 4-90). **Tendons of flexor digitorum longus**.

Insertion (Fig. 4-90). **Base of proximal phalanx of lateral four toes** and medial aspect of **extensor expansions** of tendons of extensor digitorum longus.

Nerve Supply. Medial one, **medial plantar** nerve (S1 and S2); *lateral three,* **lateral plantar** nerve (S1 and S2).

Actions. **Flex metatarsophalangeal joints** and **extend interphalangeal joints of lateral four toes**.

The Third Layer of Plantar Muscles (Figs. 4-102 to 4-104). These short muscles of the great and small toes lie in the anterior half of the sole of the foot.

The Flexor Hallucis Brevis Muscle (Figs. 4-102 to 4-104). This fleshy muscle with two bellies covers the first metatarsal bone on its plantar surface.

Origin (Fig. 4-103). **Cuboid** and **lateral cuneiform bones**.

Insertion (Fig. 4-69). **Base of proximal phalanx of great toe** by two tendons, the medial one inserting with the abductor hallucis and the lateral one with the adductor hallucis. Two **sesamoid bones** are usually present in these tendons (Figs. 4-101, 4-103, and 4-104). The sesamoids protect the tendon of the flexor hallucis longus from pressure from the head of the first metatarsal bone during standing and walking.

Nerve Supply. **Medial plantar** nerve (S1 and S2).

Action. **Flexes great toe** at metatarsophalangeal joint.

The Adductor Hallucis Muscle (Figs. 4-102 and 4-103). This adductor of the great toe has *two heads of origin.*

Origin (Figs. 4-69 and 4-103). *Oblique head,* **bases of second, third**, and **fourth metatarsal bones**, and fibrous sheath of peroneus longus tendon; *transverse head,* **plantar ligaments of lateral four metatarsophalangeal joints**.

Insertion (Figs. 4-69 and 4-103). Lateral side of **base of proximal phalanx of great toe**.

Nerve Supply. **Lateral plantar** nerve (S2 and S3).

Actions. Oblique head, **adducts great toe** (*i.e.*, toward second toe) and **flexes metatarsophalangeal joint**; transverse head **draws heads of metatarsal bones together**, **adducts great toe**, and **helps to maintain curvature of transverse arch** of foot.

The Flexor Digiti Minimi Brevis Muscle (Figs. 4-102 and 4-103). This relatively insignificant muscle, also called the flexor digiti quinti (V), is only a fleshy slip.

Origin (Fig. 4-69). **Base of fifth metatarsal** bone and sheath of peroneus longus tendon.

Insertion (Fig. 4-69). **Base of proximal phalanx of small toe.**

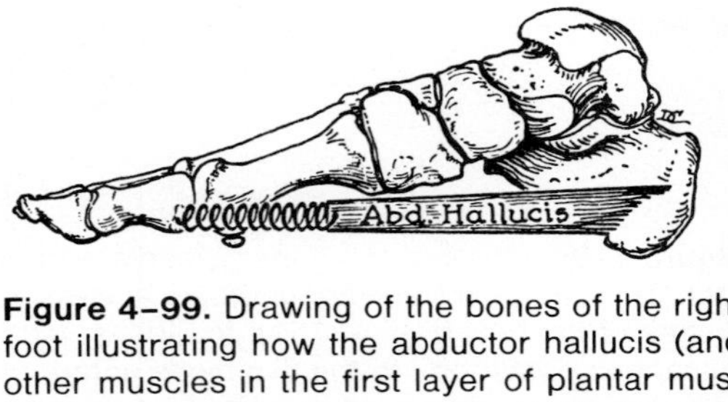

Figure 4–99. Drawing of the bones of the right foot illustrating how the abductor hallucis (and other muscles in the first layer of plantar muscles) acts as an elastic spring or tie beam in helping to maintain the arches of the foot (Fig. 4–151). The shape of the interlocking bones and the strength of the ligaments are more important however in maintaining these arches.

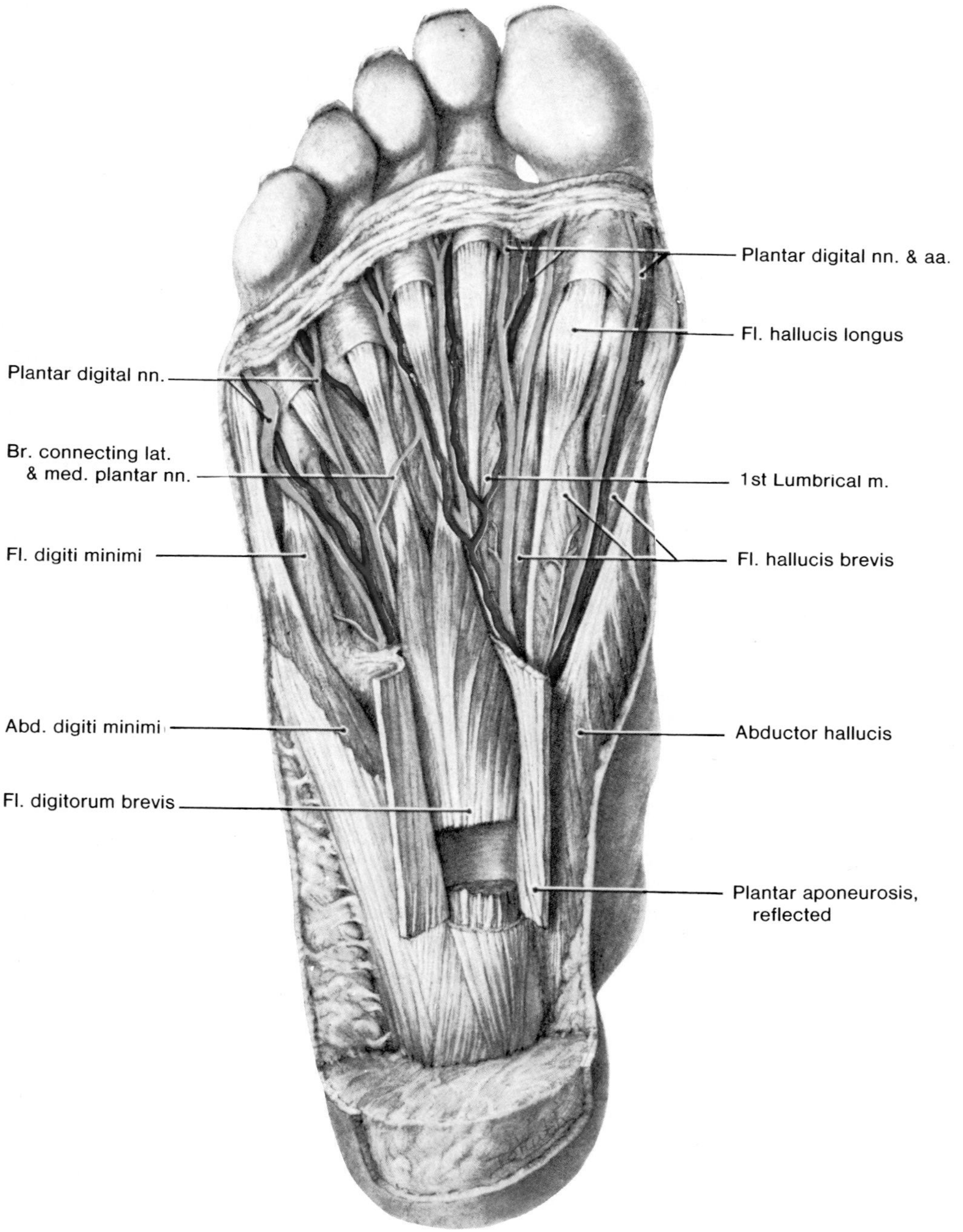

Figure 4–100. Drawing of a dissection of the plantar aspect of the right foot demonstrating the *first layer of plantar muscles*, the digital nerves, and the arteries. The plantar aponeurosis and fascia are reflected or removed and a section is taken from the flexor digitorum brevis to show the "fibrous box" encasing it. Observe the muscles of the first layer: abductor digiti minimi, flexor digitorum brevis, and abductor hallucis. Note that the lateral and medial plantar digital nerves supply one and one-half and three and one-half digits respectively and are united by a connecting (communicating) branch. The lateral nerve to the small toe is thickened in this specimen and the flexor digitorum brevis fails to send a tendon to the small toe.

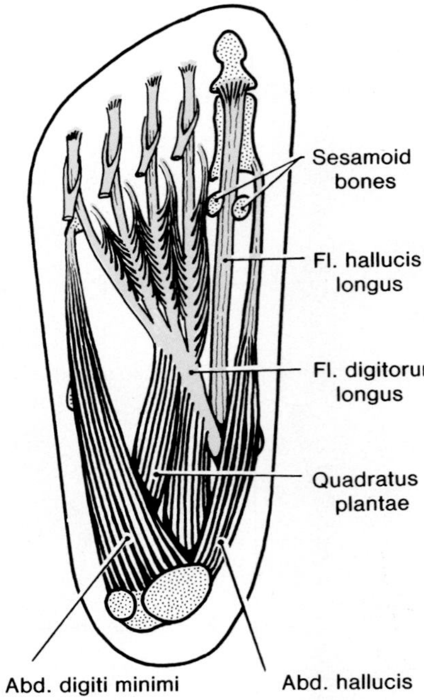

Figure 4–101. Drawing of some of the muscles of the sole of the right foot. The *second layer of muscles*, displayed by removal of the flexor digitorum brevis (Fig. 4–100), is framed by the abductor muscles of the great and small toes.

Action. **Flexes small toe** at metatarsophalangeal joint.

The Fourth Layer of Muscles (Figs. 4-104 and 4-105). This layer consists of the interosseous muscles and the tendons of the peroneus longus and tibialis posterior muscles which cross the sole of the foot.

The Interosseous Muscles (Figs. 4-104 and 4-105). There are three plantar and four dorsal interossei and, as their name indicates, they are between bones (metatarsals).

Origin (Figs. 4-104 and 4-105). *Plantar interossei:* medial sides of **third**, **fourth**, and **fifth metatarsal bones**. *Dorsal interossei:* adjacent **sides of two metatarsal bones** (between which they lie).

Insertion (Figs. 4-104 and 4-105). *Plantar interossei:* medial sides of **bases of proximal phalanges of third**, **fourth**, and **fifth toes**. *Dorsal interossei: first,* **medial side** and **second, lateral side** of **proximal phalanx of second toe**; *third* and *fourth,* **lateral sides** of **proximal phalanges of third** and **fourth toes**. *All interossei* are also attached to the **extensor expansions** (dorsal expansions) of the corresponding toes (Fig. 4-76).

Nerve Supply. **Lateral plantar** nerve (S2 and S3).

Actions. The plantar interossei adduct (*key*: **PAD**, Plantar **AD**duct) and the dorsal interossei adduct (*key*: **DAB**, **D**orsal **AB**-duct) to and from the line of the second toe, respectively. These actions are not important to most people. They are important, however, in **maintaining the integrity of the forefoot** by approximating the bones during weight bearing. The interossei also flex the toes at the metatarsophalangeal joints and extend them at the interphalangeal joints via their insertion into the extensor expansions.

Nerves of the Foot (Figs. 4-93, 4-94, 4-97, 4-100, 4-102, and 4-106). The plantar nerves are branches of the **tibial nerve**, which divides posterior to the medial malleolus into medial and lateral **plantar nerves**. They supply the intrinsic muscles of the foot, except for the extensor digitorum brevis, which is supplied by the deep peroneal nerve. These nerves also supply the skin of the foot.

The Medial Plantar Nerve (Figs. 4-87, 4-93, 4-94, 4-97, 4-100, 4-102, and 4-106). This is the larger of the two terminal branches of the **tibial nerve**. It passes deep to the abductor hallucis muscle and runs anteriorly between this muscle and the flexor digitorum brevis on the lateral side of the medial plantar artery. It terminates near the bases of the metatarsal bones by dividing into **three digital nerves** which supply cutaneous branches to three and one-half digits and motor branches to the abductor hallucis, flexor digitorum brevis, flexor hallucis brevis muscles, and the most medial lumbrical muscle.

The Lateral Plantar Nerve (Figs. 4-87, 4-93, 4-97, 4-100, 4-102, and 4-106). This is the smaller of the two terminal branches of the **tibial nerve**. It begins deep to the flexor retinaculum and the abductor hallucis muscle and runs anterolaterally, medial to the lateral plantar artery and between the first and second layers of muscles. It

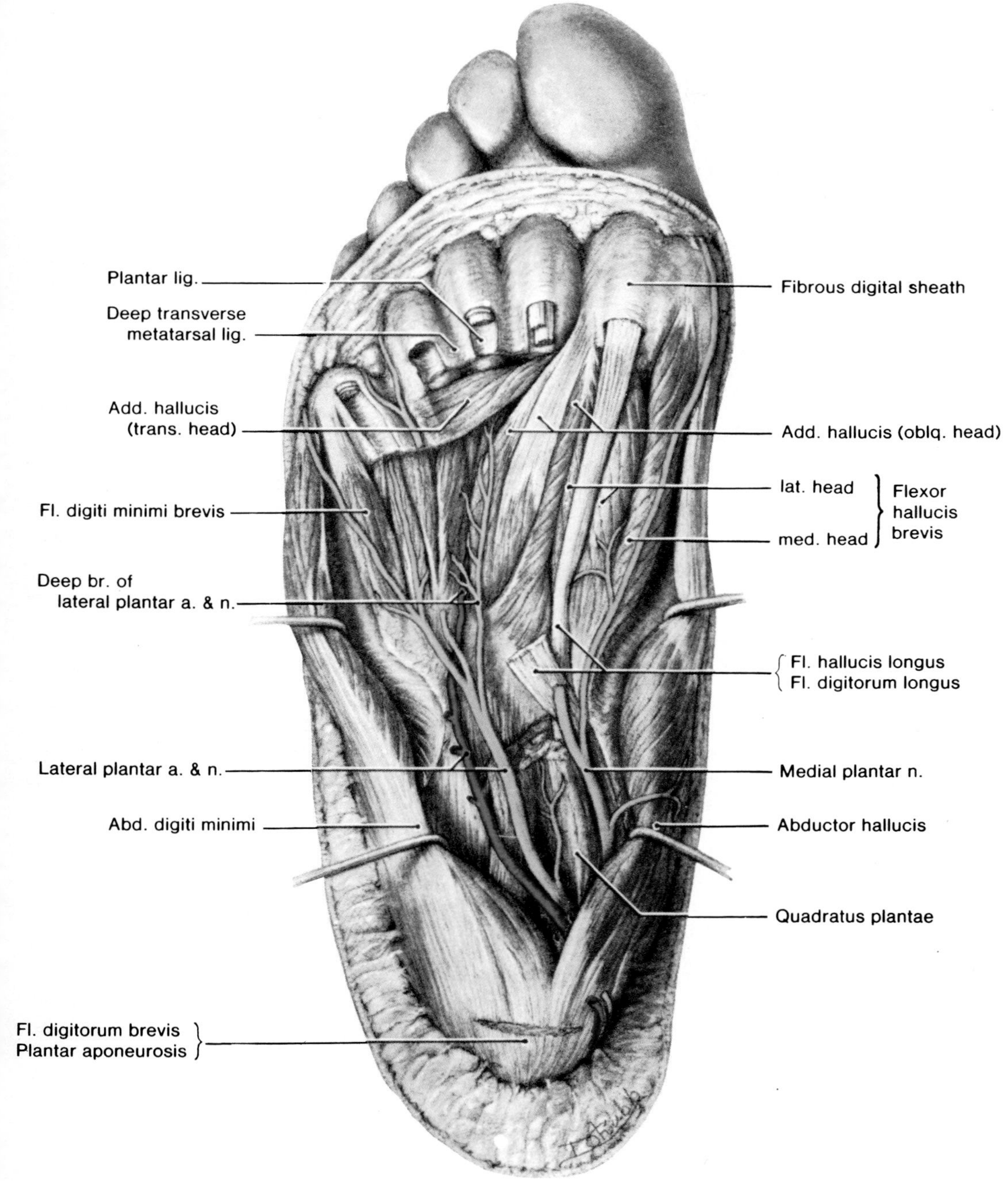

Figure 4–102. Drawing of a dissection of the *third layer of plantar muscles* in the right foot. The abductor digiti minimi and the abductor hallucis muscles of the first layer are pulled aside and the flexor digitorum brevis is cut short. The flexor digitorum longus and the lumbricals of the second layer are excised and the quadratus plantae is cut. Observe the muscles in the third layer: flexor digiti minimi, adductor hallucis, and flexor hallucis brevis. Note the lateral interossei and that the lateral plantar nerve and artery course laterally between the muscles of the first and second layers.

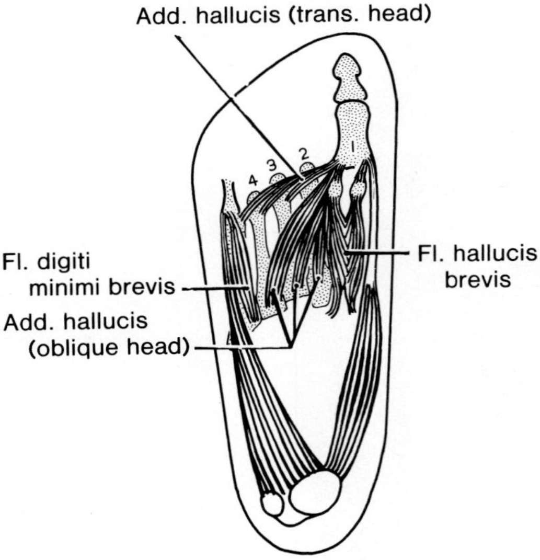

Figure 4–103. Diagramatic illustration of the *third layer of plantar muscles* in the right foot. The three muscles of this layer are the adductor and short flexor of the great toe and the short flexor of the small toe. Note that these muscles form three sides of a square in the anterior half of the sole which is largely filled by the oblique head of the abductor hallucis muscle.

sends cutaneous branches to one and one-half digits and motor branches to all muscles of the sole that are not supplied by the medial plantar nerve.

The Sural Nerve and the Sural Communicating Branch (Figs. 4-14, 4-49, and 4-106). These nerves are cutaneous branches of the tibial and common peroneal nerves, respectively. They supply the posterior aspect of the leg and the lateral margin of the foot.

The Saphenous Nerve (Figs. 4-14 and 4-106). This is the *largest cutaneous branch of the femoral* nerve. In addition to supplying skin and fascia on the anterior and medial side of the leg, it supplies the proximal half of the medial side and adjacent dorsum of the foot.

Arteries of the Foot (Figs. 4-81, 4-87, 4-93, 4-95, 4-97, 4-98, 4-100, 4-102, 4-107, and 4-108). The arteries of the foot are the terminal branches of the anterior and posterior tibial arteries.

The Dorsalis Pedis Artery (Figs. 4-34*A*, 4-76, 4-81, and 4-107). This vessel is the direct continuation of the **anterior tibial artery**. It begins anterior to the ankle joint midway between the two malleoli and passes forward, deep to the inferior extensor retinaculum, to the proximal end of the first interosseous space. Here it divides into a **deep plantar artery**, which passes to the sole of the foot, and an **arcuate artery**.

The **arcuate artery**, a branch of the dorsalis pedis, runs laterally across the bases of the metatarsal bones, deep to the extensor tendons. It gives off the second, third, and fourth **dorsal metatarsal arteries** (Fig. 4-107). These vessels run to the clefts of the toes where each divides into two **dorsal digital arteries** to the sides of the toes.

The **deep plantar artery**, a terminal branch of the dorsalis pedis, passes deeply through the first interosseous space to join the lateral plantar artery and form the **deep plantar arch** (Figs. 4-107 and 4-108).

CLINICALLY ORIENTED COMMENTS

The ability to palpate the **pulse of the dorsalis pedis** artery is essential for clinical practice, particularly in cases of **intermittent claudication** (leg cramps in the calf brought on by exercise and relieved by rest).

The **dorsalis pedis pulse** can usually be felt where it passes over the navicular and cuneiform bones lateral to the extensor hallucis longus tendon (Fig. 4-76). It may also be felt distal to this at the proximal end of the first interosseous space (between first and second metatarsals). In some people (10 to 12%) the dorsalis pedis artery may be too small to palpate or it may be absent from its usual position; thus, *failure to detect a dorsalis pedis pulse* does not always indicate the presence of **arteriosclerotic disease**.

The **arteries of the sole of the foot** (medial and lateral plantar arteries) are derived from the posterior tibial artery which divides deep to the flexor retinacu-

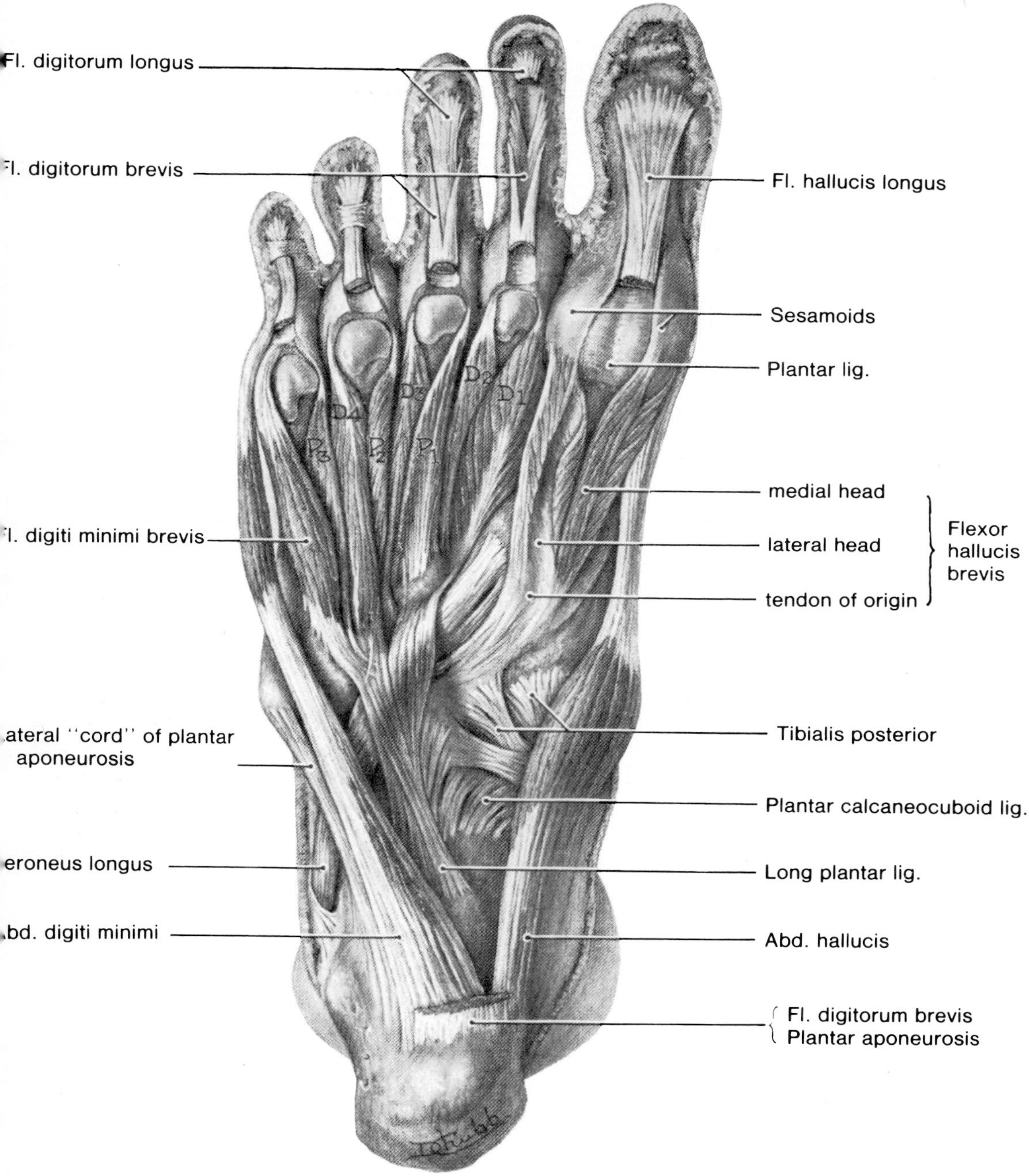

Figure 4–104. Drawing of a dissection of the *fourth layer of the plantar muscles* in the right foot. The abductor and flexor brevis of the small toe and the abductor and flexor brevis of the great toe of the first and third layers of muscles remain for purposes of orientation. Observe the muscles of the fourth layer: three plantar and four dorsal interossei in the anterior half of the foot and the tendons of peroneus longus and tibialis posterior in the posterior half. The plantar interossei adduct the three lateral toes toward an axial line that passes through the second metatarsal bone and second toe, whereas the dorsal interossei abduct from this line.

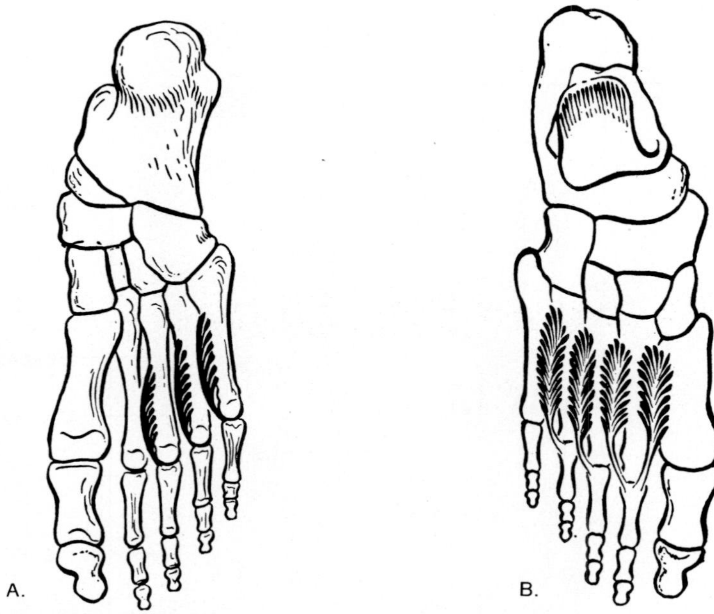

Figure 4–105. Drawings illustrating the interossei of the fourth layer of muscles in the sole of the right foot. *A*, plantar interossei from below. *B*, dorsal interossei from above. Note that the axis of abduction and adduction in the toes is the second digit rather than the third digit as in the hand. All interosseous muscles are supplied by the lateral plantar nerve (S2 and S3).

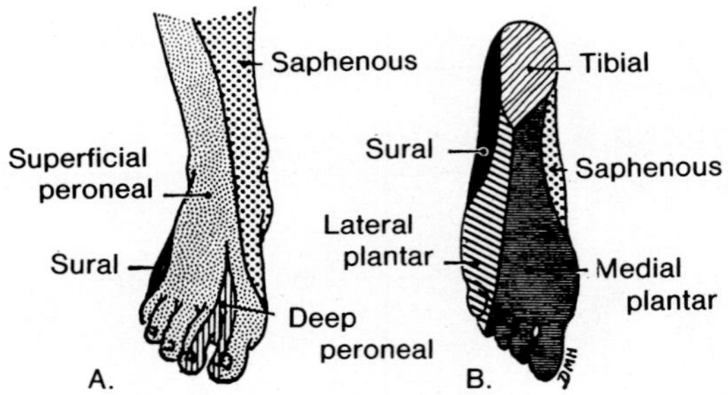

Figure 4–106. Diagrams illustrating the cutaneous distribution of the nerves of the distal part of the leg and foot. The superficial and deep peroneal nerves are branches of the common peroneal nerve, the most commonly injured nerve in the lower limb. *A*, dorsum of right leg and foot. *B*, plantar surface of left foot.

lum (Fig. 4-87). These arteries supply the plantar muscles and anastomose with arteries on the dorsum of the foot (Figs. 4-98 and 4-108).

The Medial Plantar Artery (Figs. 4-34*B*, 4-87, 4-93, 4-97, 4-100, and 4-108). This vessel is the smaller of the two terminal branches of the **posterior tibial artery**. It arises deep to the flexor retinaculum and passes distally on the medial side of the foot between the abductor hallucis and flexor digitorum brevis muscles. It supplies branches to the medial side of the great toe, giving off muscular, cutaneous, and articular branches during its course.

The Lateral Plantar Artery (Figs. 4-34*B*, 4-87, 4-93, 4-97, 4-100, 4-102, and 4-108). This vessel is the larger of the two terminal branches of the **posterior tibial artery**. It arises deep to the flexor retinaculum and runs obliquely across the sole of the foot on the lateral side of the lateral plantar nerve. It *passes laterally* between the flexor digitorum brevis and quadratus plantae muscles (*i.e., between the first and second layers of muscles*), giving off calcaneal, cutaneous, muscular, and articular branches as it passes to the base of the fifth metatarsal bone. Here it curves medially between the third and fourth muscular layers and terminates at the base of the first metatarsal bone, where it joins the deep plantar branch of the dorsalis pedis artery to form the **plantar arch** (Figs. 4-98 and 4-108).

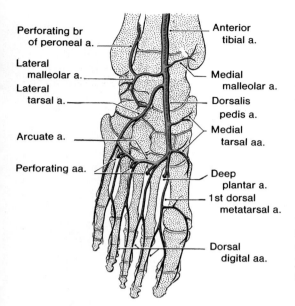

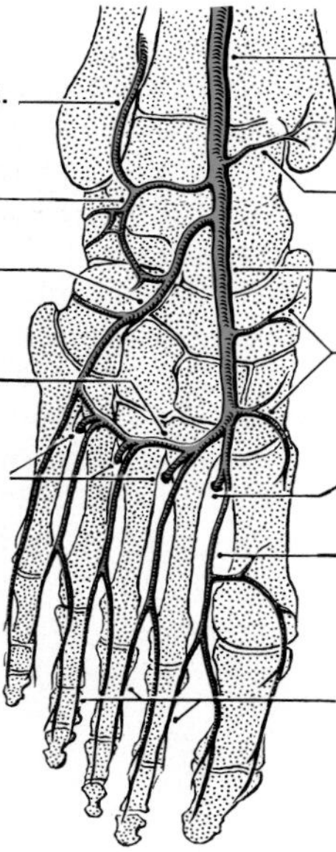

Figure 4–107. Drawing of the arteries of the dorsum of the right foot. Observe that the anterior tibial artery takes a straight course anterior to the ankle joint and ends midway between the malleoli as the *dorsalis pedis artery*. This clinically important artery can be palpated where it passes over the navicular and cuneiform bones. As the artery can be easily compressed against bone here, this is the common site for taking the pedal pulse.

As the plantar arch crosses the foot it gives off four **plantar metatarsal arteries** and branches to the tarsal joints and muscles. These arteries join with the superficial branches of the medial and lateral plantar arteries to form common **digital arteries.** Each of these arteries divides into two plantar digital arteries (Figs. 4-34*B* and 4-108) that supply adjacent sides of the toes.

Veins of the Foot (Figs. 4-11 to 4-13, 4-92, and 4-93). The dorsal digital veins run along the dorsal margins of each toe and unite at their webs to form dorsal metatarsal veins. These join to form a **dorsal venous arch**. From here efferents pass medially to the **great saphenous vein** and laterally to the **small saphenous vein.**

The superficial veins of the sole unite to form a **plantar venous arch**, from which efferents pass to medial and lateral marginal veins that join the great and small saphenous veins.

The deep veins begin as **plantar digital veins** on the plantar aspects of the toes. Most blood returns via the deep veins which are connected with the superficial veins by many **perforating veins** (Figs. 4-11 and 4-12). These anastomotic veins are important in the differentiation of the types and in the therapy of varicose veins (p. 432).

JOINTS OF THE LOWER LIMB

As the **pelvic girdle**, consisting of the two ossa coxae, connects the lower limb to the trunk, its articulations are included with those of the lower limb. The sacroiliac joints and the symphysis pubis are described with the pelvis in Chapter 3.

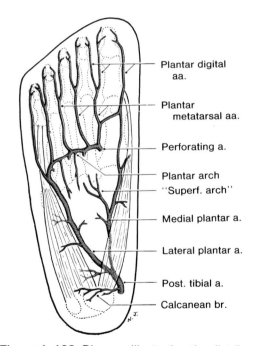

Figure 4–108. Diagram illustrating the distribution of the plantar arteries in the sole of the right foot, derived from the posterior tibial artery. Observe that the medial plantar artery is the smaller of the two terminal branches and that the lateral plantar artery runs across the sole of the foot to the fifth metatarsal bone near its base. It then runs medially, crossing the sole again and forming the plantar arch.

THE HIP JOINT

This articulation is a multiaxial **ball and socket type of synovial joint** and is the best example of this kind of joint in the body.

Articular Surfaces (Figs. 4-41, 4-48, 4-109, 4-110, and 4-117). The globular head of the femur articulates with the cup-like acetabulum of the os coxae (hip bone). The head of the femur forms about two-thirds of a sphere and is completely covered with hyaline cartilage, except over the roughened **fovea** (pit), to which the **ligament of the head** is attached. Observe the extensive articular area of the head of the femur.

The articular or **lunate surface of the acetabulum** is horseshoe-shaped. The acetabulum has a centrally located, nonarticular **acetabular fossa** (*i.e.*, within the horseshoe) which is occupied by a fatpad covered with synovial membrane (Fig. 4-110). The cartilage is absent inferiorly opposite the acetabular notch (Fig. 4-48). The acetabular fossa is closed inferiorly by the **transverse acetabular ligament**.

The Acetabular Labrum (Figs. 4-110 and 4-113). The depth of the acetabulum is in-

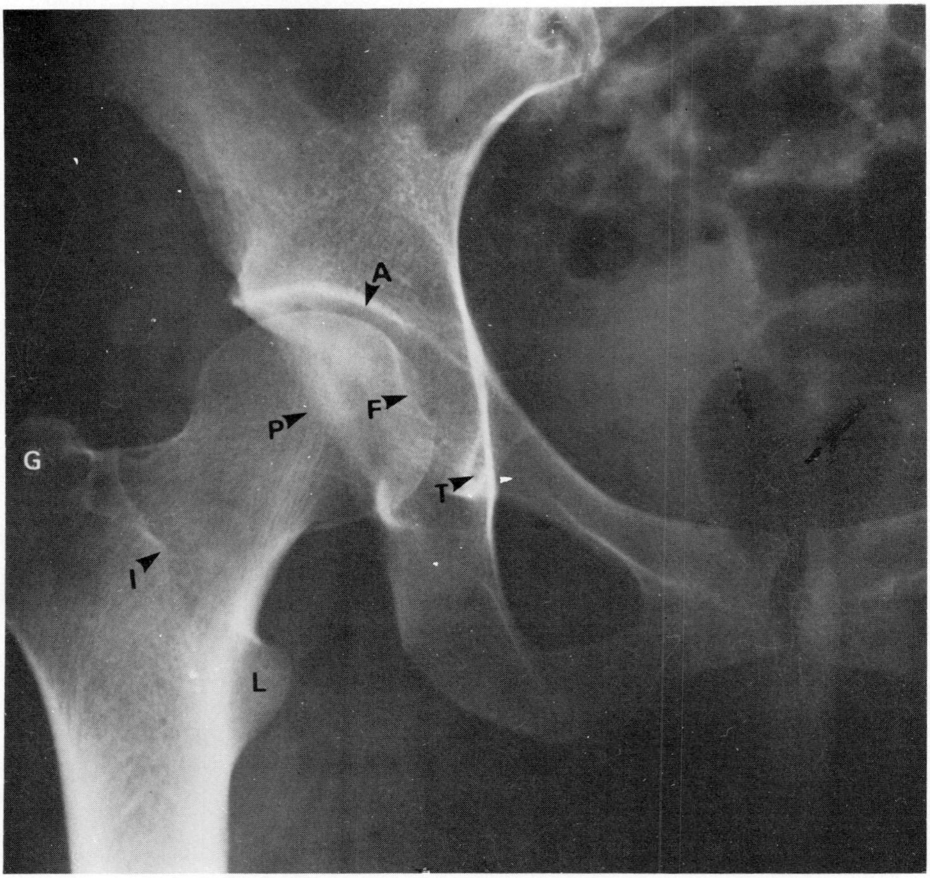

Figure 4–109. Radiograph of the hip joint (anteroposterior projection). *On the femur* observe the greater (*G*) and lesser (*L*) trochanters, the intertrochanteric crest (*I*), and the pit or fovea (*F*) for the ligament of the head. *On the pelvis* observe the roof (*A*) and posterior rim (*P*) of the acetabulum and the "teardrop" appearance (*T*) caused by the superimposition of structures at the lower margin of the acetabulum. The hip joint is the best example in the body of a ball-and-socket joint. Its strength depends largely upon the depth of the acetabulum and the strength of the surrounding ligaments and muscles.

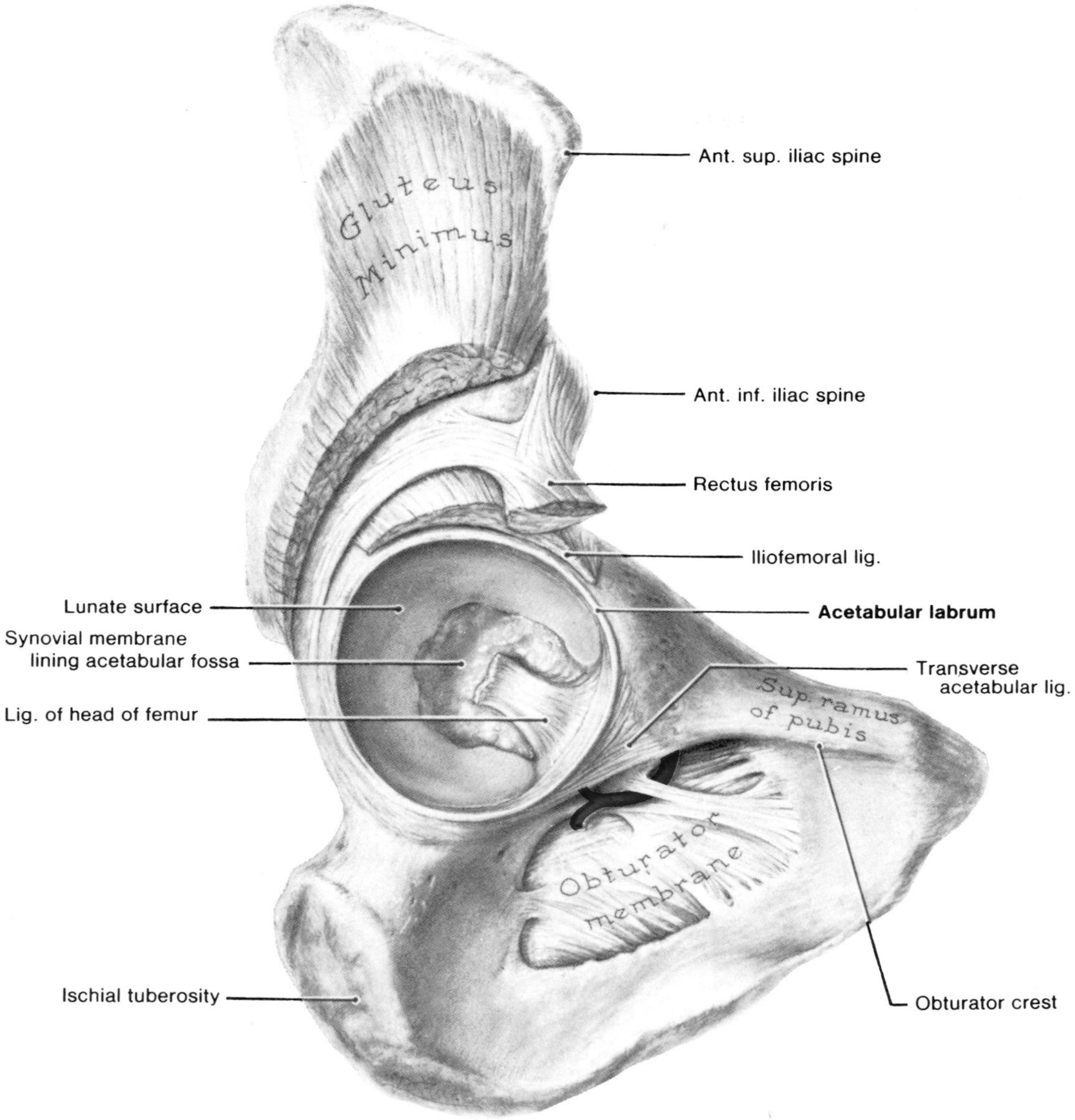

Figure 4–110. Drawing of a dissection of the socket for the head of the right femur. Observe the transverse acetabular ligament, the fibers of which convert the acetabular notch into the acetabular foramen. Note the acetabular labrum attached to the acetabular rim and to the transverse ligament. It forms a complete ring around the head of the femur beyond its equator. Observe the articular or lunate surface and the synovial membrane attached to the margin of the articular cartilage and covering the pad of fat and the vessels in the acetabular fossa. Note the ligament of the head of the femur, which is a hollow cone of synovial membrane compressed between the head of the femur and its socket. It resembles a collapsed bell-tent which envelops ligamentous fibers that are attached above to the pit on the head of the femur and below to the transverse ligament and the margins of the acetabular notch, which faces directly inferiorly in the anatomical position (Fig. 4–48). Through it passes the artery to the head of the femur. Note that only the lunate surface of the acetabulum is covered with articular cartilage (*yellow*). Also see Figure 4–113.

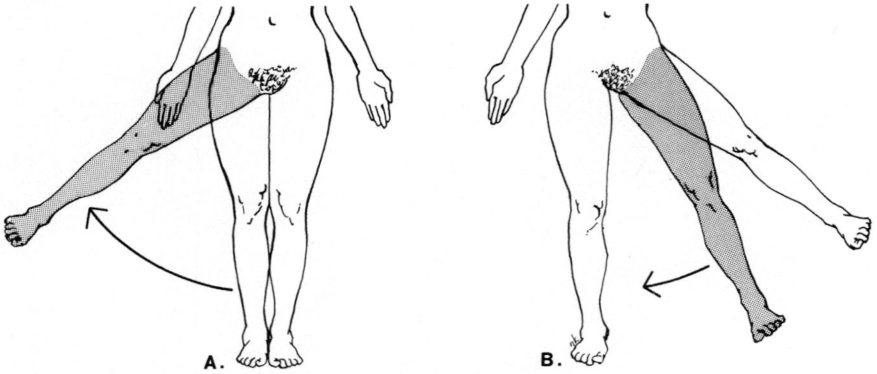

Figure 4–111. Drawings illustrating abduction (*A*) and adduction (*B*) of the lower limb at the hip joint. Note that abduction takes the limb away from the median plane of the body and adduction brings it back toward the median plane.

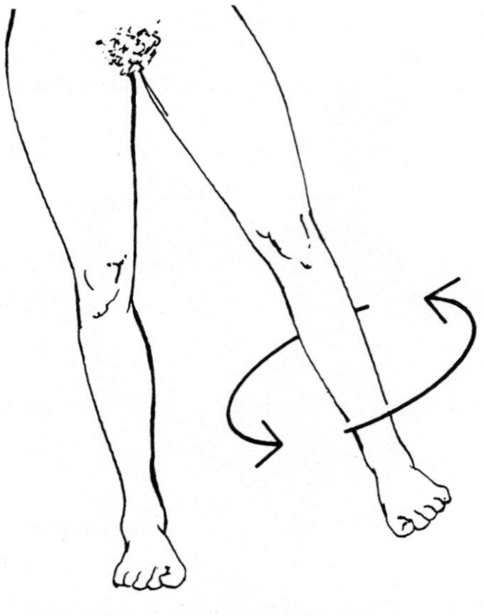

Figure 4–112. Drawing illustrating circumduction of the lower limb at the hip joint. Note that the cone of movement results from a combination of flexion-extension and abduction-adduction. Verify that rotation is not a component of circumduction.

creased by the *fibrocartilaginous* acetabular labrum (L. lip). It is attached to the bony rim of the acetabulum and to the transverse acetabular ligament which spans the acetabular notch; thus, the labrum forms a circle and completes the socket for the femoral head. It narrows the acetabular outlet and its free thin edge cups around the head and helps to hold it firmly in its socket.

Movements of the Joint (Figs. 4-111 and 4-112). The range of movement is not so great as at the shoulder joint because some movement has been sacrificed in order to provide stability and strength.

The movements occurring at the hip joint are flexion-extension, abduction-adduction, medial and lateral rotation, and circumduction.

The Articular Capsule (Figs. 4-41, 4-113, and 4-115 to 4-117). The fibrous capsule is strong and dense. **Proximally** it is attached to the edge of the acetabulum just beyond the acetabular labrum and to the transverse acetabular ligament. **Distally** the capsule is attached to the neck of the femur as follows: *anteriorly* to the intertrochanteric line and the root of the greater trochanter; *posteriorly* it is loosely attached to the neck about a fingerbreadth proximal to the intertrochanteric crest. Thus, *the fibrous capsule forms a cylindrical sleeve that encloses the hip joint* and most of the femoral neck.

Most fibers of the articular capsule take a spiral course from the os coxae to the lateral portion of the intertrochanteric line of the femur, but some deep fibers (the **orbicular zone** or **zona orbicularis**) pass

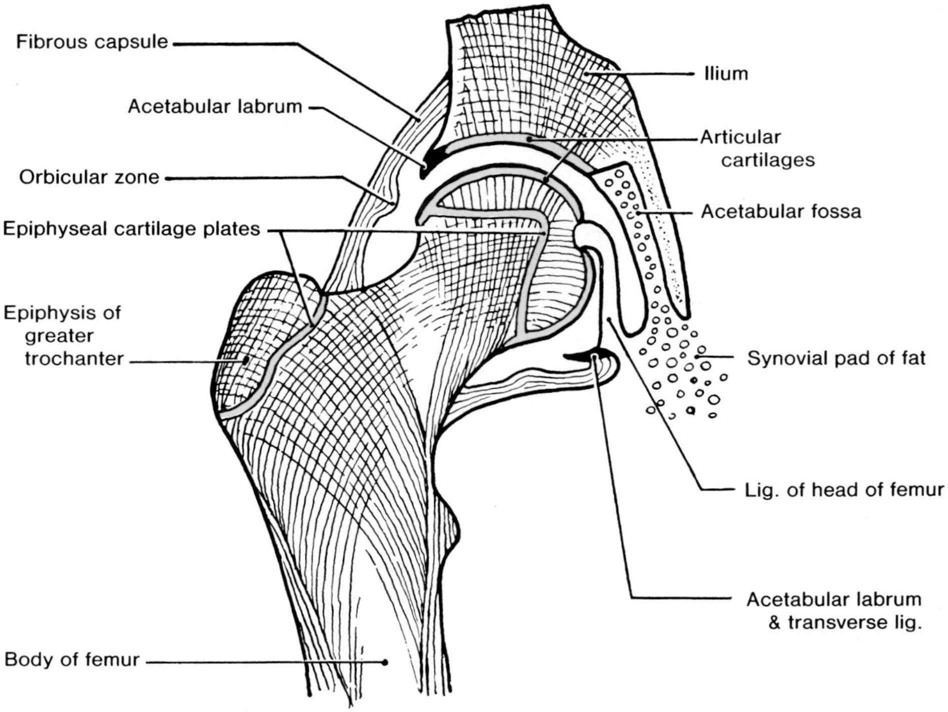

Figure 4–113. Drawing of a coronal section of the right hip joint. Observe that the bony trabeculae of the ilium are projected into the head of the femur as lines of pressure and that the trabeculae of the femur cross these as lines of tension. Note that the epiphysis of the head of the femur is entirely within the fibrous capsule of the joint. Observe that the ligament of the head of the femur is a synovial tube that is fixed above at the fovea on the head of the femur (Fig. 4–109) and is open below at the acetabular foramen. Here it is continuous with the synovial membrane covering the fat in the acetabular fossa and also with the synovial membrane covering the transverse acetabular ligament (Fig. 4–110). Understand that the ligament of the head becomes taut during adduction of the hip joint (*e.g.*, when crossing the legs).

circularly around the neck of the femur (Figs. 4-113 and 4-116). These capsular fibers form a collar around the neck of the femur which constrict the capsule and help to hold the femoral head in the acetabulum.

Some deep longitudinal fibers, called **retinacula**, are reflected upward along the neck of the femur as longitudinal bands. The **retinacula of the neck of the femur** contain blood vessels that supply the head and neck of the femur (Fig. 4-114).

Four main groups of longitudinal capsular fibers (intrinsic ligaments) are given names according to the region of the acetabulum that is attached to the femur (*e.g.*, iliofemoral ligament, Fig. 4-115).

The Intrinsic Ligaments of the Capsule (Figs. 4-41 and 4-115 to 4-117). These **thickened parts of the fibrous capsule** strengthen the hip joint.

The iliofemoral ligament (Figs. 4-41, 4-115, and 4-116) is a *very strong, thick band that covers the anterior aspect of the joint.* It is shaped like an inverted Y, the stem or apex of which is attached proximally to the anterior inferior iliac spine and the acetabular rim. Its base is attached distally to the intertrochanteric line of the femur. This ligament is *tense in full extension of the hip joint* and has an important role in preventing overextension of the hip joint during standing (*i.e.*, it helps to maintain the erect posture). It is *one of the strongest ligaments in the body.*

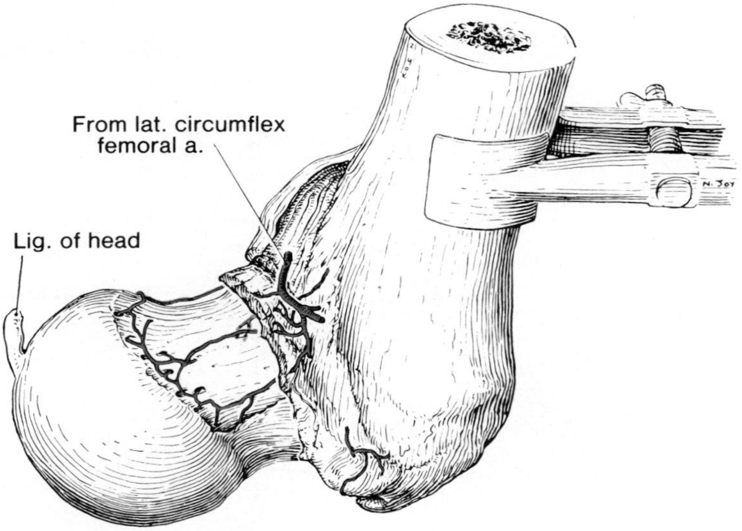

ANTERIOR VIEW

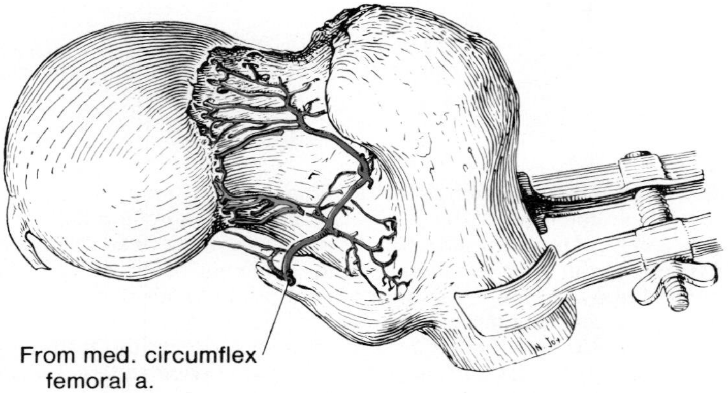

POSTEROSUPERIOR VIEW

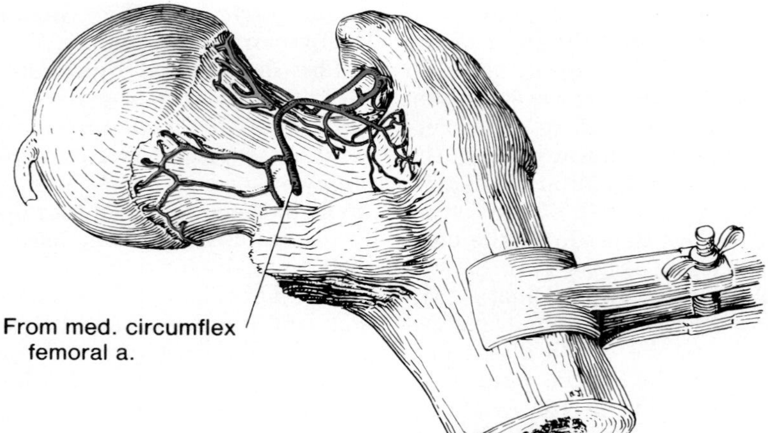

POSTEROINFERIOR VIEW

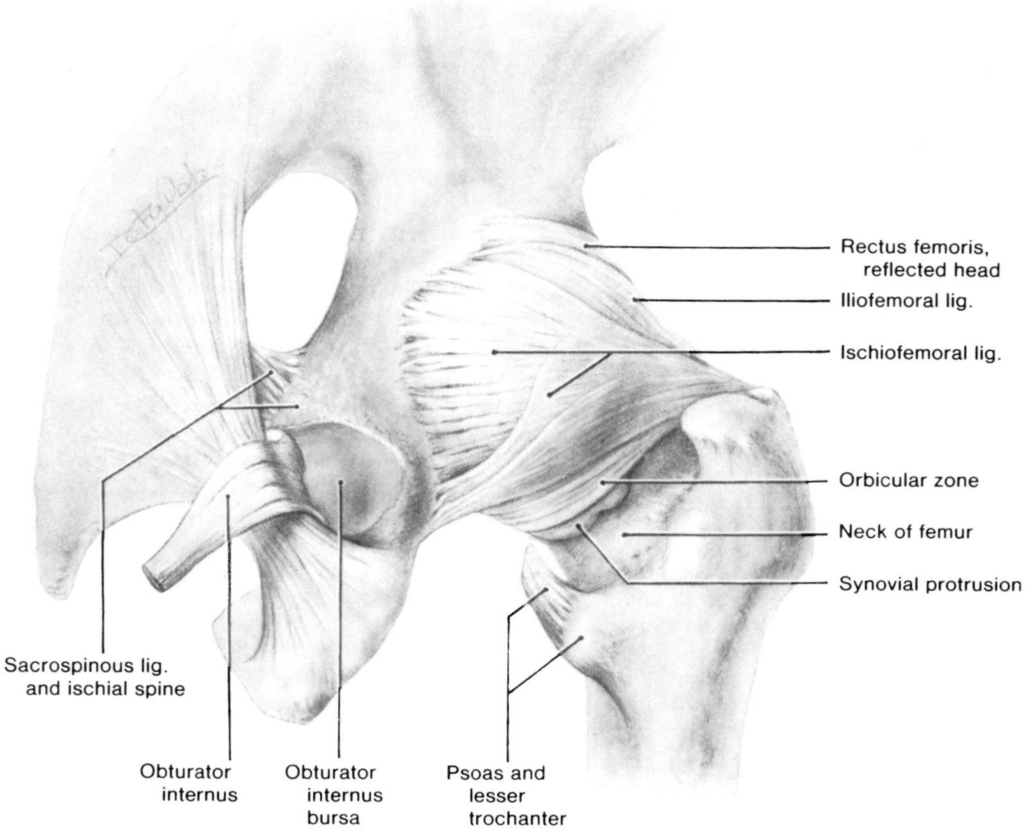

Figure 4-115. Drawing of a dissection of the right hip joint from behind. Observe that the fibrous capsule is directed spirally so it becomes taut during extension and medial rotation of the femur. Note that the fibers cross the neck posteriorly about a fingerbreadth above the intertrochanteric crest and at this point are closely blended with the tendon of the obturator externus. Observe that the synovial membrane (*blue*) protrudes below the fibrous capsule and there forms a bursa for the tendon of the obturator externus muscle. The intrinsic ligaments of the articular capsule, particularly the very strong iliofemoral ligament, reinforce the capsule of the hip joint.

Figure 4-114. Drawings illustrating the blood supply to the head of the femur. Observe that the femoral head receives *three sets of arteries*: (1) the main set ends in the synovial retinacula on the posterosuperior and posteroinferior parts of the neck; it perforates just distal to the head, bends at 45° toward its center, and anastomoses freely with (2) terminal branches of the medullary artery of the body and in most cases with (3) the artery of the ligament of the head. This artery enters the head only when the ossification of the center for the epiphysis of the head has extended to the fovea of the femoral head (12 to 14 years). This anastomosis persists even in advanced age, but in 20% of people it is never established. It is obvious that the blood supply to the head of the femur is endangered in fractures of the neck of the femur (Case 4-1).

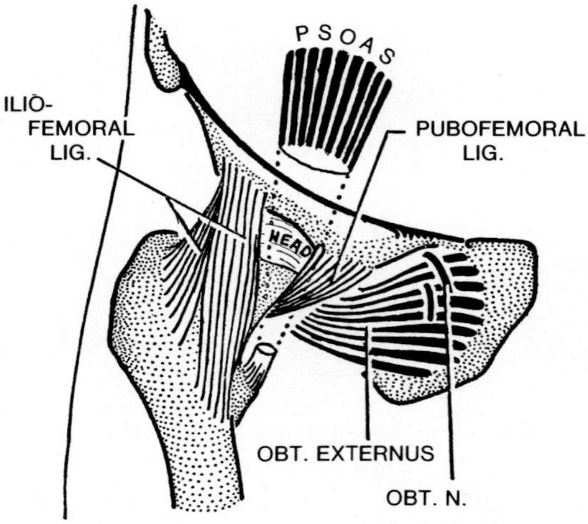

Figure 4–116. Drawing of an anterior view of the fibrous capsule of the right hip joint. Observe that the psoas muscle guards the weak point of the capsule between the iliofemoral and pubofemoral ligaments. Note the iliofemoral ligament, which is very strong and shaped like an inverted Y. Examine the flat, fan-shaped obturator externus muscle crossing backward and laterally below the neck of the femur and the fibrous capsule of the hip joint.

CLINICALLY ORIENTED COMMENTS

When one stands at ease, there is a tendency to thrust the pelvis anteriorly, thereby hyperextending the hip joints. In this position, much of the weight of the body is borne by the exceedingly strong iliofemoral ligaments. Because no muscles need to contract to maintain the stand easy or slouching position, it is a relaxing way to stand.

The iliofemoral ligament is rarely torn in dislocations of the hip joint. In fact it is used as the fulcrum to a lever during reduction of a dislocation of the hip joint.

The pubofemoral ligament (Fig. 4-116) arises from the pubic part of the acetabular rim and the iliopubic eminence (Fig. 4-1). Distally its fibers blend with the medial part of the iliofemoral ligament. It *strengthens the inferior and anterior part of the fibrous capsule.* The pubofemoral ligament tightens during extension of the hip joint and becomes tense during abduction; thus, it checks overabduction of the hip joint. It is a *relatively weak ligament,* however.

The ischiofemoral ligament (Fig. 4-115) *reinforces the fibrous capsule posteriorly.* It arises from the ischial portion of the acetabular rim and spirals superolaterally to the neck of the femur, medial to the base of the greater trochanter. It is a relatively strong ligament.

Observe the spiral arrangement of the three ligaments of the fibrous capsule in Figures 4-115 and 4-116. This anatomical construction tends to screw the femoral head medially into the acetabulum during extension of the hip joint, thereby resisting hyperextension of it.

The ligament of the head of femur (ligamentum capitis femoris) is a weak flattened ligament that you may hear referred to clinically as the ligamentum teres (L. round) ligament, Figs. 4-113, 4-114, and 4-117). It appears to be of little importance in strengthening the hip joint. Its wide end is attached to the margins of the acetabular notch and to the transverse ligament and its narrow end is attached to the fovea of the femur. In about 80% of cases it carries a **small artery to the head,** which is a branch of the obturator artery. The ligament of the head is stretched when the flexed thigh is adducted or laterally rotated. Understand that this flat ligament is **within the hip joint** and is surrounded by synovial membrane; thus, *it is intracapsular but extrasynovial* (*i.e.,* outside the synovial capsule but inside the fibrous capsule).

CLINICALLY ORIENTED COMMENTS

The ligament of the head of the femur varies in size and in strength in different people; sometimes it is absent. Its function, other than as a pathway for the artery to the femoral head, is unclear. It appears to be of limited value in strengthening the hip joint because no appreciable disability occurs when it ruptures or does not develop.

In **fractures of the femoral neck** close to the head (Case 4-1), there is often disruption of the blood supply to the head of the femur (Fig. 4-114). In some cases the

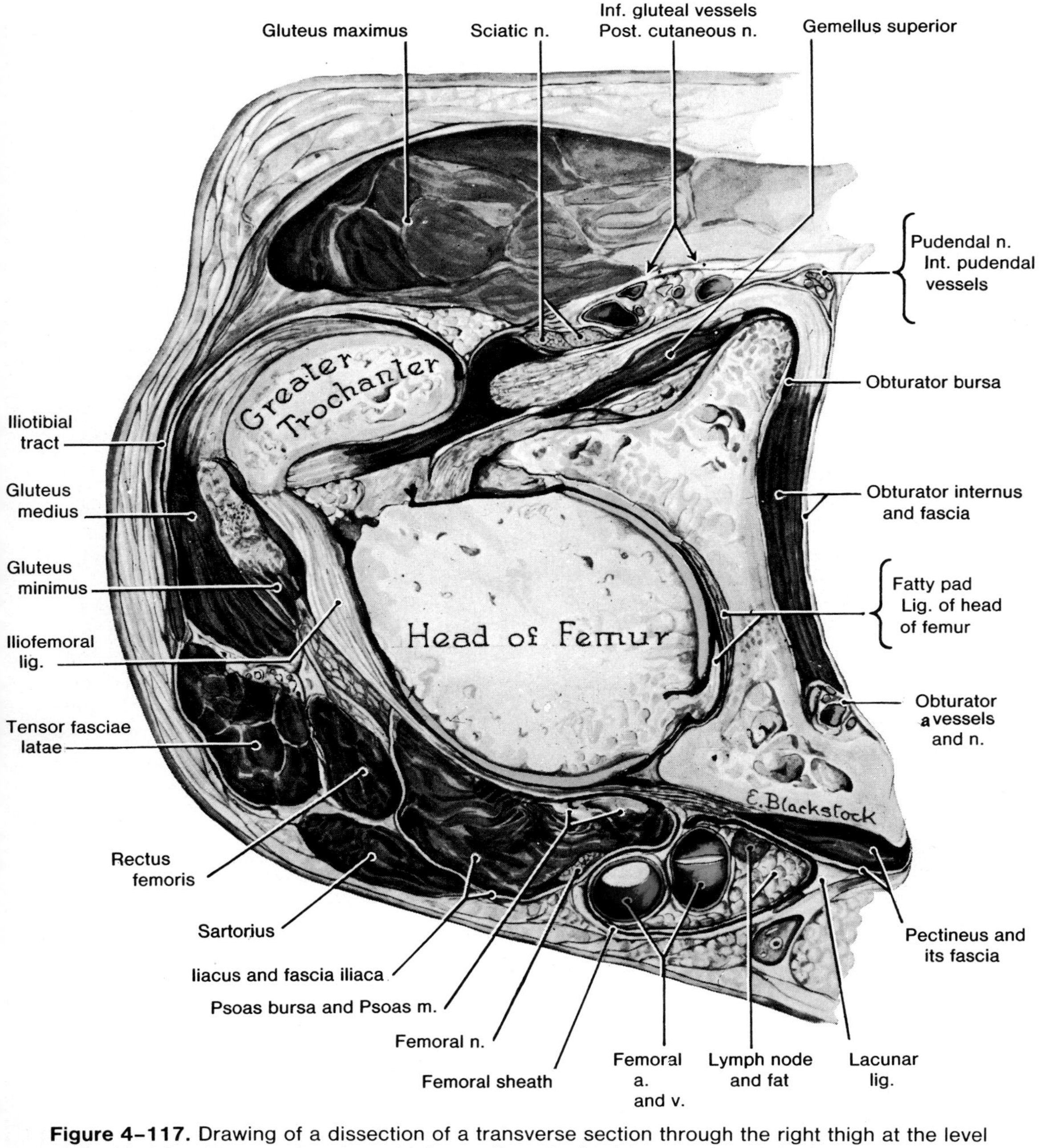

Figure 4-117. Drawing of a dissection of a transverse section through the right thigh at the level of the hip joint. Observe that the articular cartilage (*yellow*) is spread over the head of the femur. Note that the fibrous capsule of this joint is very thick where it forms the iliofemoral ligament (Fig. 4-116) and is thin dorsal to the psoas tendon, where the psoas bursa intervenes. Observe the femoral sheath enclosing the femoral artery and vein, a lymph node, lymph vessels, and fat, is free except posteriorly, where, between the psoas and pectineus muscles, it is attached to the capsule of the hip joint. Note that the femoral artery is separated from the hip joint by the tough psoas tendon (also see Fig. 4-36). Note the femoral nerve lying between the iliacus muscle and its fascia.

blood supplied via the artery in the ligamentum capitis femoris may be the only blood received by the proximal fragment of the head. If the ligament has been ruptured or is absent (20% of cases), the fragment of bone may receive no blood and, as a result, undergo **aseptic necrosis** (death in the absence of infection).

The synovial capsule (Figs. 4-110, 4-113, 4-115, and 4-117) lines the inner surface of the fibrous capsule and is reflected from it on to the neck of the femur and covers the bone as far as the margin of the articular cartilage of the head.

It forms a sleeve for the ligament of the head of the femur which is attached around the margins of the fovea of the femoral head. The synovial capsule also lines the acetabular fossa (Fig. 4-110) and covers the fatty pad in the acetabular notch. It is attached around the edge of the acetabular fossa and to the transverse acetabular ligament. *The synovial capsule protrudes below the fibrous capsule posteriorly* (Fig. 4-115), where it acts like a **bursa** for the tendon of the obturator externus muscle.

Stability of the Joint (Figs. 4-109 and 4-115 to 4-117). The hip joint is a very strong and *stable articulation*. It is surrounded by powerful muscles and the articulating bones are united by a dense fibrous capsule that is strengthened by strong intrinsic ligaments, particularly the iliofemoral ligament.

Blood Supply (Figs. 4-34 and 4-114). The articular arteries are derived from the **obturator, medial circumflex femoral**, and the superior and inferior **gluteal arteries**.

Nerve Supply (Figs. 4-37, 4-41, and 4-47). The articular nerves are derived from (1) the **femoral** via the nerve to the rectus femoris muscle; (2) the **obturator** (anterior division); (3) the **sciatic** via the nerve to the quadratus femoris muscle; and (4) the **superior gluteal.**

CLINICALLY ORIENTED COMMENTS

Congenital dislocation of the hip joint is common, occurring in about 1.5 per 1000 live births, and is bilateral in about half the cases.

Traumatic (acquired) dislocation of the hip joint is not common because the head of the femur has a deep socket and the joint is strongly supported by its articular capsule, intrinsic ligaments, and related muscles.

Congenital Dislocation of the Hip Joint. Despite its name, this abnormality is not usually obvious at birth and may not become so for several months. In some cases the diagnosis is not made until late infancy (1 to 2 years). *Females are affected much more often than males* (8:1). Some studies have shown that the articular capsule of the hip joint is loose at birth and that there is often underdevelopment (hypoplasia) of the acetabulum and the femoral head.

A **characteristic clinical sign** of this condition is an inability to abduct the lower limb; in addition, the affected leg *seems* to be shorter because the dislocated femoral head is higher than on the normal side.

Traumatic (Acquired) Dislocation of the Hip Joint. Dislocation of the hip joint may occur during an **automobile accident** when the hip joint is flexed, adducted, and medially rotated (Case 4-6). When the person's *knee strikes the dashboard* with the limb in this position, the force transmitted up the femur drives the head out of its socket (*i.e.*, the acetabulum, Fig. 4-154). In this position the femoral head is covered posteriorly by capsule rather than bone; as a result, the capsule ruptures inferiorly and posteriorly allowing the femoral head to pass through the tear in the capsule and over the posterior margin of the acetabulum. *Often the acetabular margin fractures*, producing a fracture-dislocation of the hip joint. When the femoral head dislocates, it usually carries the acetabular bone fragment and the acetabular labrum with it. Dislocation of the hip joint can occur in other directions, *e.g.*, anteriorly if the thigh is abducted when the knee is struck.

Owing to the close relationship of the **sciatic nerve** (L4, L5, S1, S2, and S3) to the hip joint (Fig. 4-117), it may be injured (stretched and/or compressed) during posterior dislocations or fracture-dislocations of the hip joint. This may result in **paralysis of the hamstrings** and the muscles distal to the knee supplied by it (Fig. 4-94), as well as sensory changes in the skin over the posterior and lateral aspects of the lower leg and over much of the foot (Fig. 4-160).

THE KNEE JOINT

This articulation, the largest and most complicated in the body, is a modified **hinge type of synovial joint** that also permits some rotation. Its structure is complicated because it consists of three joints merged into one: an intermediate one between the patella and the femur, and lateral and medial ones between the femoral and tibial condyles (Figs. 4-1 and 4-122).

Articular Surfaces (Figs. 4-26, 4-54, and 4-119 to 4-122). The bones involved in the knee joint are the **femur**, the **tibia**, and the **patella**. The fibula is only indirectly associated. The articular surfaces are the large curved condyles of the femur, the flattened condyles of the tibia, and the patella (the largest sesamoid bone in the body).

Verify that when you stand in the anatomical position your knees are almost in contact, unless you have bow legs. Understand that your tibiae are parallel, or almost so, in the anatomical position, but your femora are not. They are set obliquely because their heads are separated by the width of the pelvis (Fig. 4-21). This produces an open angle at the lateral side of the knee, toward which the patella tends to be displaced when the quadriceps femoris muscle contracts.

CLINICALLY ORIENTED COMMENTS

The long axis of the body of the femur lies at an angle of 80° to the vertical in males and 76° in females. This angular difference in females results from their wider pelves designed for child bearing. This *sex difference in the femora* has medicolegal significance for the sexing of skeletal remains (*e.g.,* in suspected homicide).

Although **dislocation of the patella** is uncommon, it tends to occur more often in females because of the previously mentioned angle of the femur. The vastus medialis tends to prevent lateral dislocation of the patella because its muscle fibers are attached to the medial border of the patella and blend with the quadriceps femoris tendon (Figs. 4-25 and 4-127). Consequently, weakness or **paralysis of the vastus medialis** will predispose to patellar dislocation.

On the superior surface of each tibial condyle there is an articular area for the corresponding femoral condyle. These articular areas, commonly referred to as the medial and lateral **tibial plateaus** (Figs. 4-120 and 4-132*A*), are separated from each other by a narrow nonarticular area which widens anteriorly and posteriorly into anterior and posterior **intercondylar areas**, respectively.

Surface and Radiographic Anatomy (Figs. 4-55 and 4-121). The knee joint may be felt as a slight gap on each side of the knee between the corresponding femoral and tibial condyles. When the knee is flexed or extended, a depression appears on each side of the ligamentum patellae; the articular capsule of the knee joint is very superficial in these depressions.

The knee joint lies deep to the apex of the patella (Fig. 4-25) or just distal to it, but it may be located as low as the midpoint of the ligamentum patellae (Fig. 4-124).

Movements of the Joint. The principal movements occurring at the knee joint are **flexion** and **extension**, but a variable amount of medial and lateral **rotation** also occurs. Owing to the shapes of the articular surfaces and to the fact that the center of the femoral condyle is posterior to the midpoint of the distal end of the femur (Fig. 4-119), the chief knee movements of flexion and extension are combined with gliding and rotation about the vertical axis.

Sit on a table with your legs dangling over the edge and rotate one leg as far medially as you can and then as far laterally

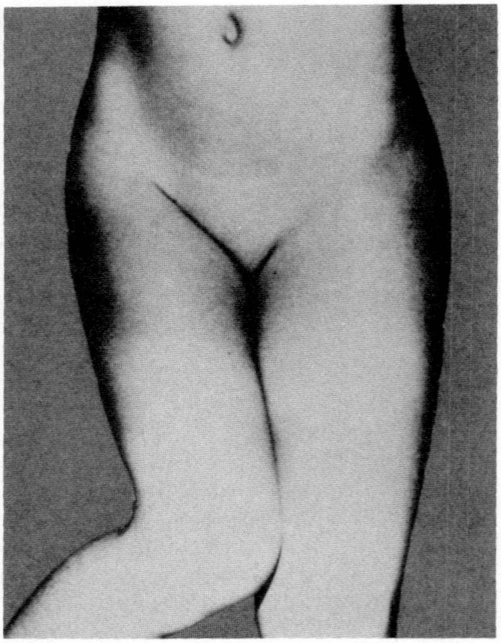

A.

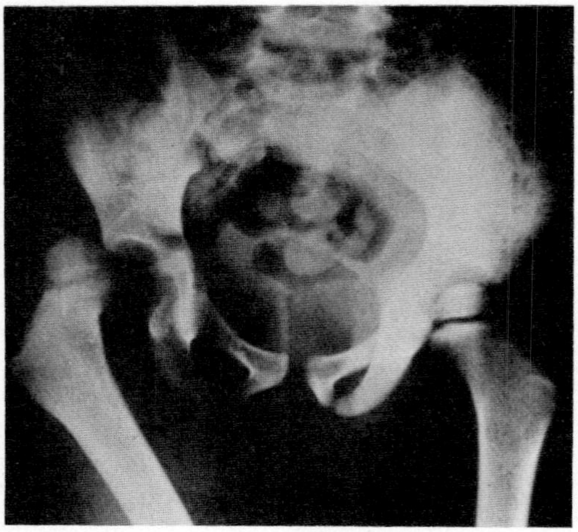

B.

Figure 4–118. *A*, photograph of a female child showing the typical clinical deformity associated with a traumatic *posterior dislocation of the right hip* joint. Observe that her hip is medially rotated, adducted, and slightly flexed. *B*, radiograph of the pelvis of this child (anteroposterior projection) showing the right femoral head out of the acetabulum and displaced posteriorly. On the *left side*, the epiphysis of the femoral head is clearly visible and the head is in its socket (acetabulum).

as it will go. While doing this, put the fingers of both your hands on the sides of the joint and you will feel the tibia rotate medially and laterally on the femur. Thus rotation is permitted while the knee is flexed or semiflexed. A slight degree of medial rotation of the femur is also necessary to achieve complete extension of the knee joint. When the knee is fully extended, as when sitting on a chair with the heel resting

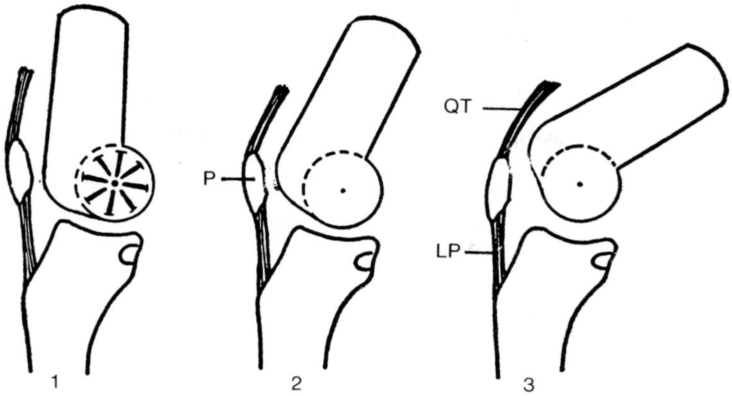

Figure 4–119. Diagrams illustrating the right knee joint during extension, slight flexion, and flexion. At the hub of the wheel-like condyle (center of circle) lies the epicondyle. Note that the condyle of the femur moves on the condyle of the tibia and that the center of the wheel-like condyle is posterior to the midpoint of the distal end of the femur. *P*, patella. *LP*, ligamentum patellae, *QT*, quadriceps tendon.

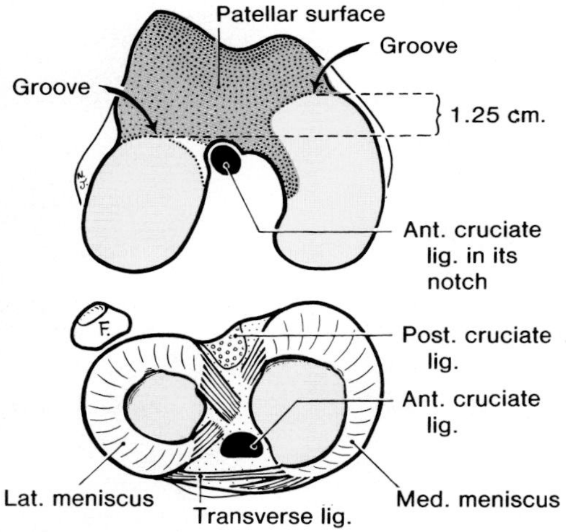

Figure 4–120. Diagrams illustrating the menisci and the articular surfaces of the right knee joint (*yellow*). These surfaces of the knee joint are characterized by their large size and their complicated and incongruent shapes, which are related to the movements at this joint.

on another chair, the skin anterior to the patella is loose and can easily be picked up between the fingers and the thumb. This laxity of the skin helps flexion to occur. Verify this by noting that the slackness disappears as the knee is flexed.

When some people fully extend their knee, it "locks" owing to medial rotation of the femur on the tibia. This makes the lower limb a solid column and more adapted for weight bearing. To "unlock" the knee the popliteus muscle contracts, thereby rotating the femur laterally so that flexion of the knee can occur.

The Articular Capsule (Figs. 4-122 to 4-124). *The fibrous capsule* surrounding the knee joint is mostly loose and thin, except in a few places where local thickenings occur; these are called **intrinsic ligaments.** A few **extrinsic ligaments** and several tendons, located outside the fibrous capsule, also strengthen the joint.

In some places the fibrous capsule has disappeared and has been replaced by bone, cartilage, or tendon; for example, the expansion of the tendon of the quadriceps femoris replaces the anterior part of the fibrous capsule. This arrangement allows the knee the full range of flexion.

Fibrous Capsular Attachments (Figs. 4-54, 4-65, 4-122, and 4-124). **Superiorly** the fibrous capsule is attached to the femur just proximal to the articular margins of the condyles and to the intercondylar line posteriorly. It is deficient on the lateral condyle to allow the tendon of the popliteus muscle, the origin of which is intracapsular, to pass out of the joint and insert into the tibia.

Inferiorly the capsule is attached to the articular margin of the tibia, except where

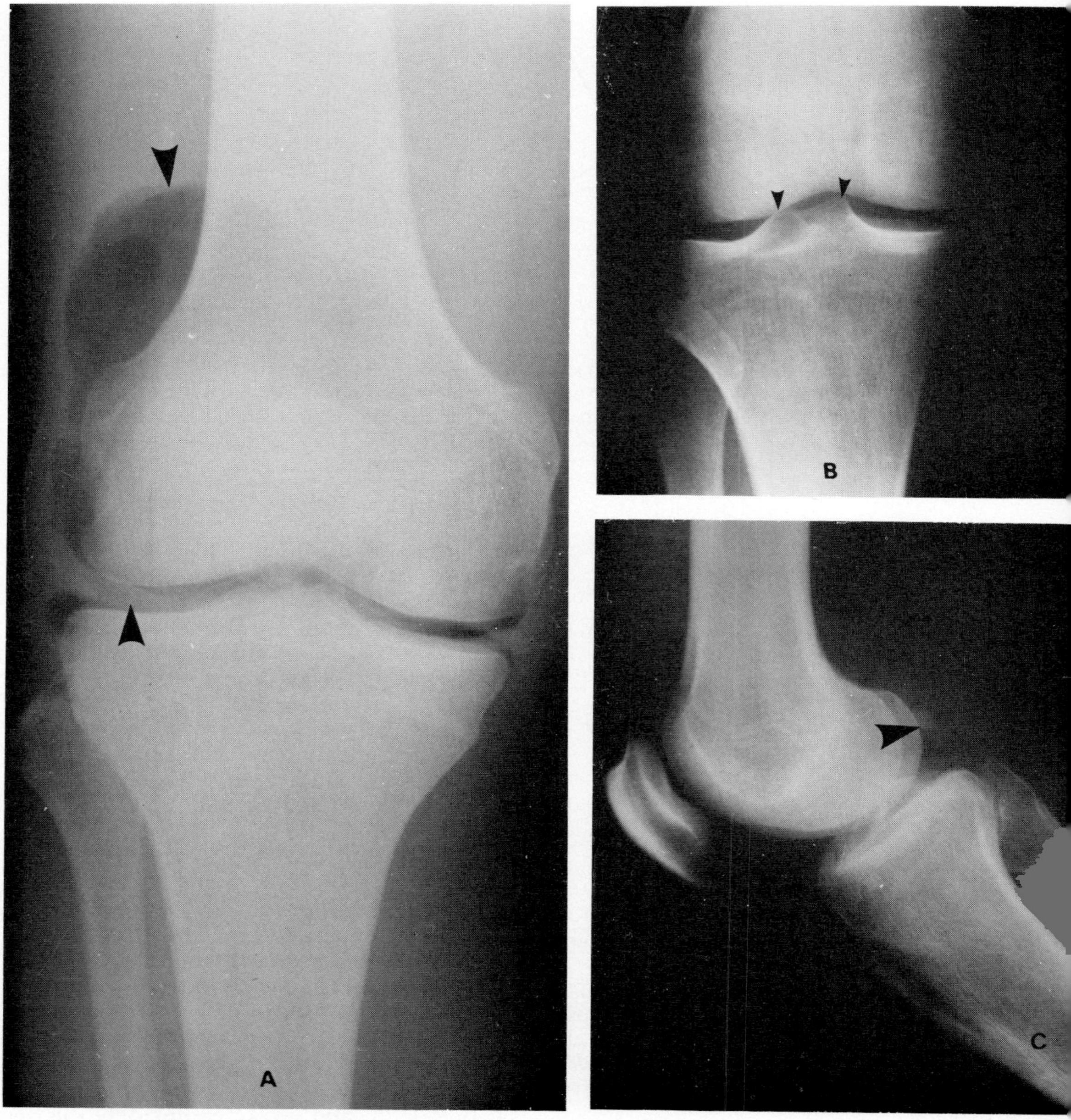

Figure 4–121. Radiographs of the knee. Before taking the film in *A*, air was injected into the joint cavity. Being less opaque than bone and other tissues, it appears black. The *upper arrow* points to the highest margin of the suprapatellar (quadriceps) bursa (see Fig. 4–124). The *lower arrow* indicates the lateral meniscus that is outlined with air. *B*, *arrows* point to the lateral and medial intercondylar tubercles in this AP view. *C*, lateral view of the flexed knee joint. The *arrow* points to a fabella which is a sesamoid bone in the tendon of the lateral head of the gastrocnemius muscle. Athletic injuries, particularly those occurring during football and hockey, are the most frequent cause of trauma to the menisci (cartilages) and the ligaments of the knee joint.

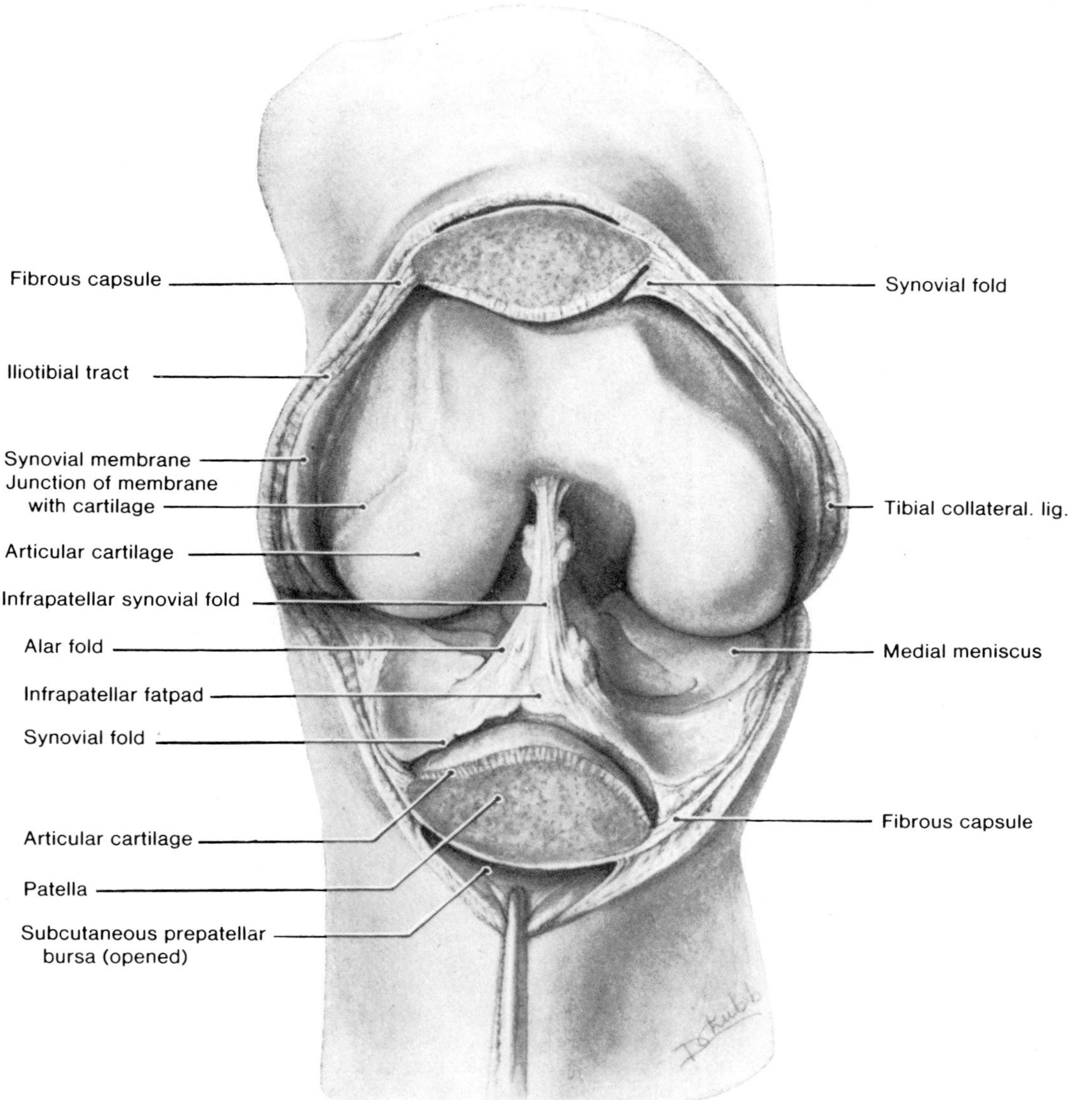

Figure 4–122. Drawing of a dissection of a right knee joint which has been opened from the front. The patella is sawn through, the skin and the fibrous capsule are cut through, and the joint is flexed. Observe that peripherally the articular cartilage of the patella becomes thin. Note the infrapatellar synovial fold resembling a partially collapsed bell-tent whose apex is attached to the intercondylar notch and whose base is below the patella. Observe that the infrapatellar fatpad is continued into the "tent." Understand that a fracture of the patella would bring the prepatellar bursa into communication with the joint cavity. Note that the articular cartilage and the synovial membrane are continuous with each other on the side of the condyle, as in other joints. The tibial collateral ligament is simply a thickening of the fibrous capsule of the knee joint but is unique in that it is attached to the medial meniscus. The fibular collateral ligament is not visible in this dissection because it is located more posteriorly than the tibial collateral ligament (Fig. 4–125).

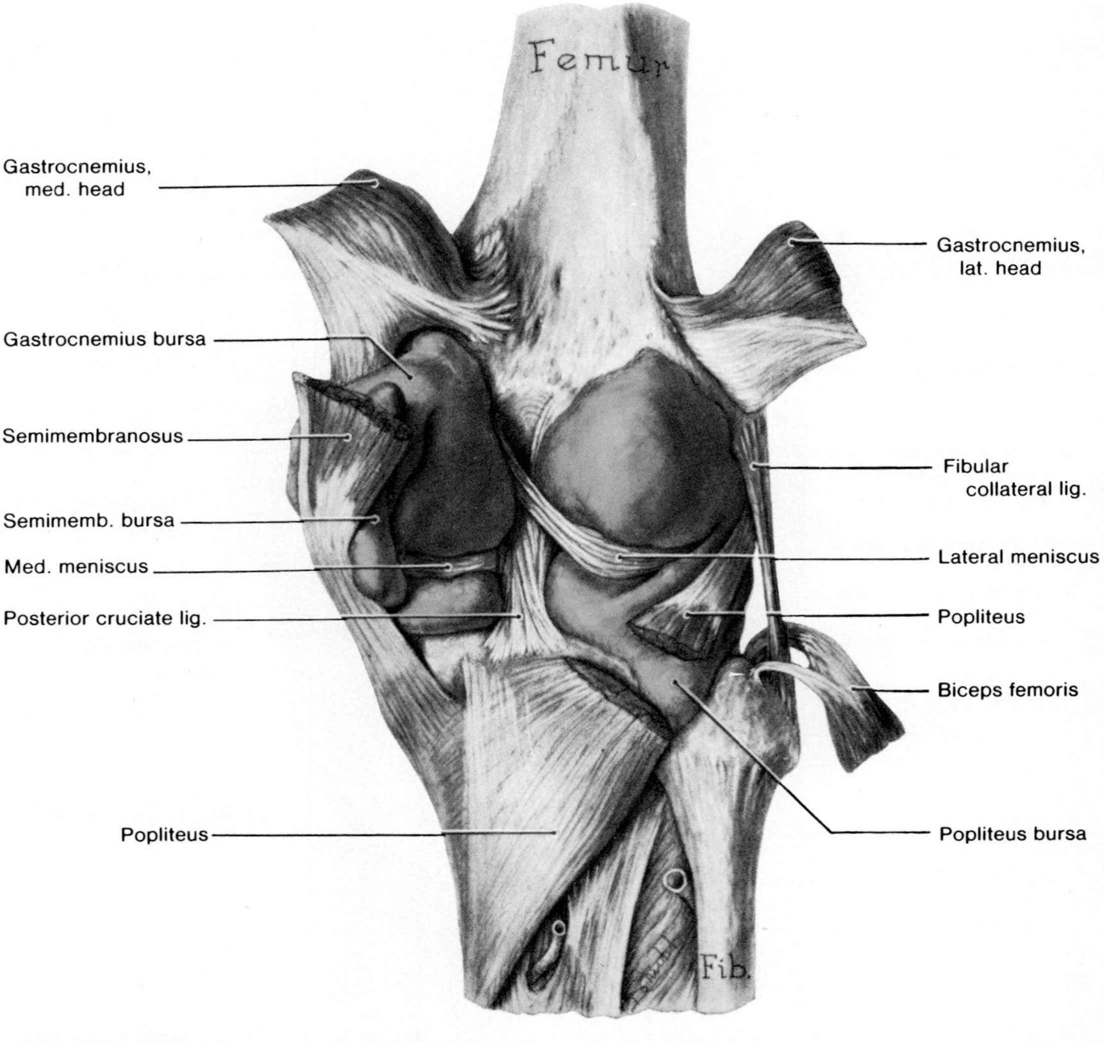

Figure 4–123. Drawing of a posterior view of a dissection of a distended right knee joint. The heads of the gastrocnemius are turned upward, the biceps is turned downward, and a section is removed from the popliteus muscle. Observe the posterior cruciate ligament which is exposed from behind without opening the synovial capsule or joint cavity. Note the origins of the gastrocnemius muscle limiting the extent to which the synovial membrane can rise. Observe the semimembranosus bursa here communicating with the gastrocnemius bursa, which in turn communicates with the joint cavity. Note that the popliteus tendon is separated from the lateral meniscus, the upper end of the tibia, and the proximal tibiofibular joint by an elongated bursa. This bursa communicates with the cavity of the knee joint both above and below the meniscus, and in this specimen it also communicates with the proximal tibiofibular joint cavity as shown in Figure 4–124.

the tendon of the popliteus muscle crosses the bone (Figs. 4-60 and 4-125). Here the capsule is prolonged inferolaterally over the popliteus to the head of the fibula, forming the **arcuate popliteal ligament** (Fig. 4-46).

Ligaments of the Fibrous Capsule. The fibrous capsule is supplemented and strengthened by five ligaments: **ligamentum patellae, fibular collateral ligament** (proximal part), **tibial collateral ligament, oblique popliteal ligament,**

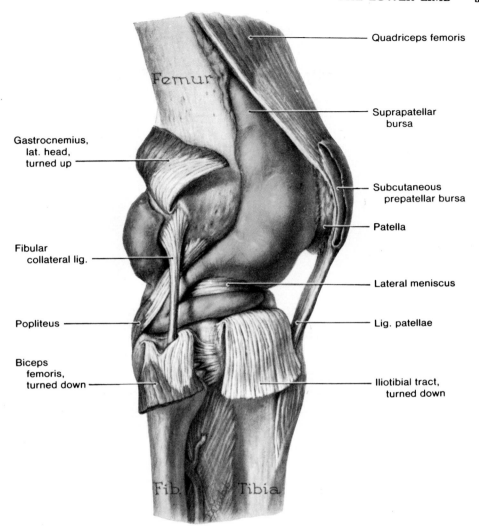

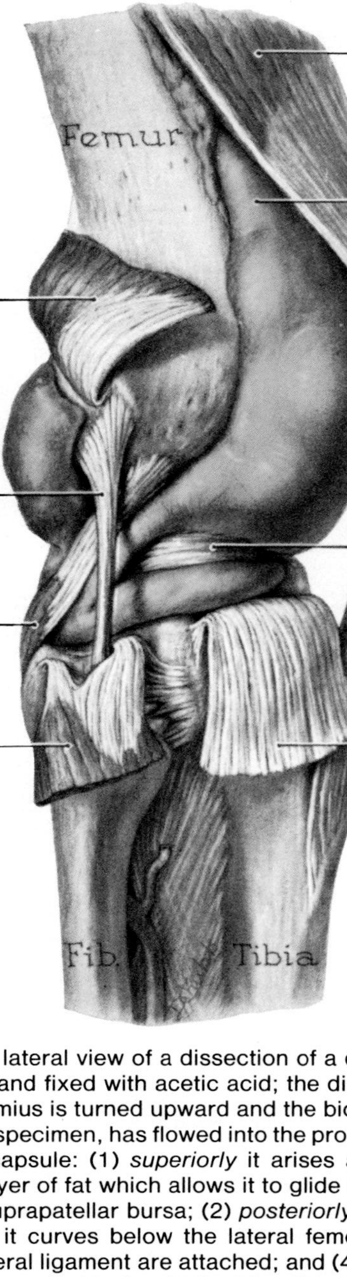

Figure 4–124. Drawing of a lateral view of a dissection of a distended right knee joint. Latex was injected into the joint cavity and fixed with acetic acid; the distended synovial capsule is exposed and cleaned. The gastrocnemius is turned upward and the biceps and the iliotibial tract are turned downward. The latex, in this specimen, has flowed into the proximal tibiofibular joint cavity. Observe the extent of the synovial capsule: (1) *superiorly* it arises about two fingerbreadths above the patella where it rests on a layer of fat which allows it to glide freely in movements of the joint. This superior part is called the suprapatellar bursa; (2) *posteriorly* it arises as high as the origin of the gastrocnemius; (3) *laterally* it curves below the lateral femoral epicondyle where the popliteus tendon and the fibular collateral ligament are attached; and (4) *inferiorly* it bulges below the lateral meniscus overlapping about one-thrid of an inch of the tibia. The coronary ligament is removed to show this. Note that the biceps femoris muscle and the iliotibial tract protect the joint laterally. Observe the subcutaneous prepatellar bursa, which is slightly more extensive here than is usual (Fig. 4–126).

and **arcuate popliteal ligament**. They are often called external ligaments to differentiate them from the internal ligaments (*e.g.,* the cruciate ligaments) which are internal to the fibrous capsule (*i.e.,* intra-articular).

The Ligamentum Patellae (Figs. 4-23*B*, 4-27, and 4-124 to 4-126). The **patellar**

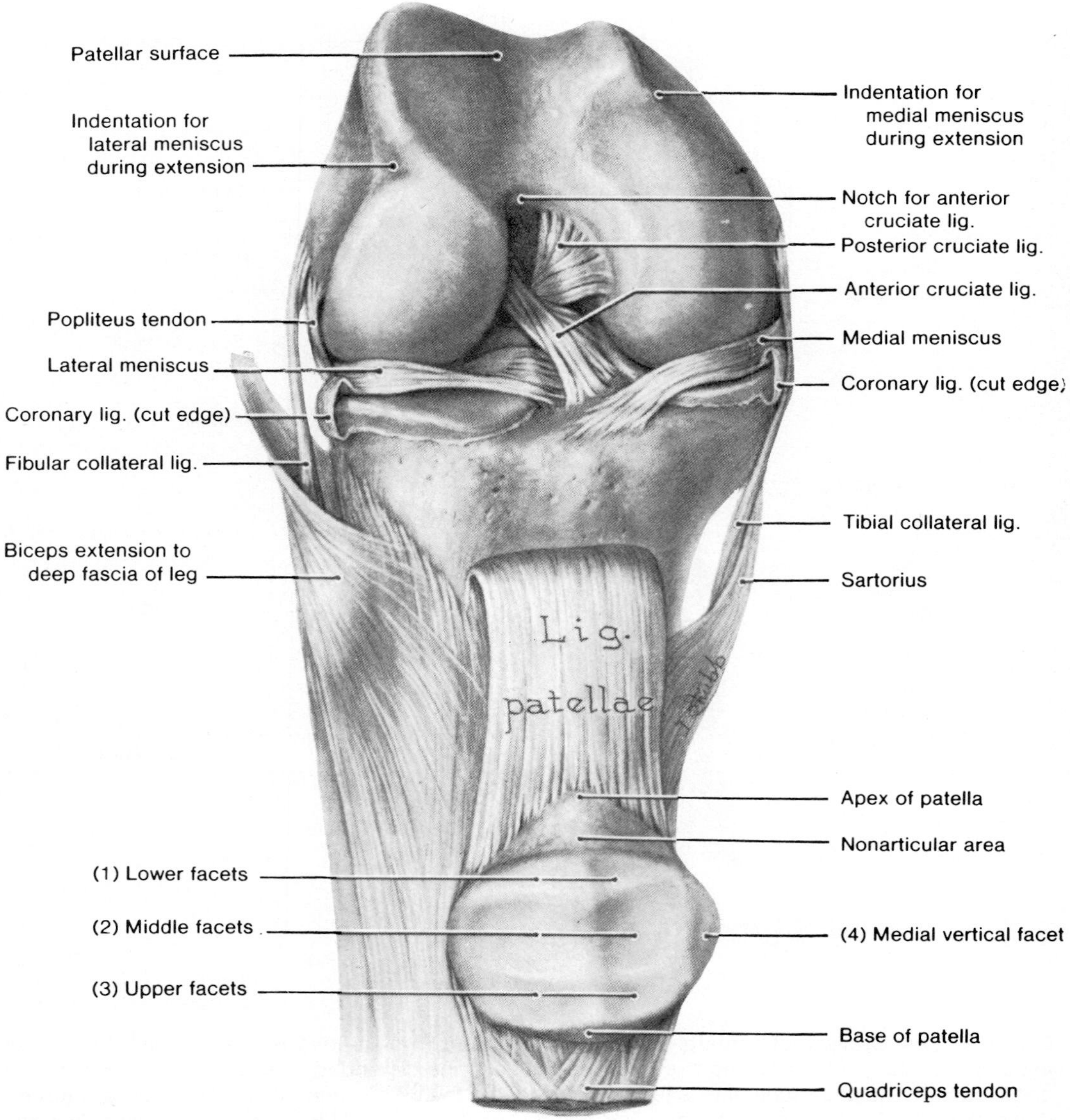

Figure 4-125. Drawing of an anterior view of a dissection of the ligaments of the right knee joint. The patella is turned downward and the joint is flexed. Observe the indentations on the sides of the femoral condyles at the junction of the patellar and tibial articular areas. Note that the lateral tibial articular area is shorter than the medial one. Observe the subsidiary notch at the anterolateral part of the intercondylar notch for the reception of the anterior cruciate ligament on full extension. Note the three paired facets on the posterior surface of the patella for articulation with the patellar surface of the femur successively during (1) extension, (2) slight flexion, (3) flexion; and the most medial facet on the patella (4) for articulation during full flexion with the crescentic facet that skirts the medial margin of the intercondylar notch of the femur.

ligament is a very strong, thick band, 3 to 5 cm long, which is in fact the *continuation of the tendon of the quadriceps femoris* muscle and is continuous with the fibrous capsule of the knee joint. Verify by palpation that it extends from the inferior border or apex of the patella to the tuberosity of the tibia (Figs. 4-25, 4-27, and 4-55).

The patellar ligament is most easily felt when the knee is extended. The superior part of its deep surface is separated from the synovial membrane of the knee joint by a mass of loose fatty tissue called the **infrapatellar fatpad** (Fig. 4-122). The inferior part of the patellar ligament is separated from the anterior surface of the tibia by the **deep infrapatellar bursa** (Fig. 4-126). For clinically oriented comments on the patellar ligament and the quadriceps reflex (knee jerk), see page 448.

The Fibular Collateral Ligament (Figs. 4-54, 4-77, and 4-123 to 4-126). This round cord (formerly called the lateral ligament) is about 5 cm long and extends inferiorly from the **lateral epicondyle of the femur** to the lateral surface of the **head of the fibula**, anterior to its apex. In Figure 4-126 observe that the tendon of the popliteus muscle passes deep to the fibular collateral ligament, separating it from the lateral meniscus. Also observe that the tendon of the biceps femoris muscle is split in two by this ligament (Fig. 4-123). As the rounded tendon of the biceps femoris can be easily observed and felt (Fig. 4-27), it serves as a guide to the attachment of the inferior end of the fibular collateral ligament.

Superiorly the fibular collateral ligament fuses with the underlying fibrous capsule of the knee joint; hence, this part is an intrinsic ligament. Inferiorly the fibular collateral ligament is separated from the fibrous capsule by fatty tissue; hence, this part is an extrinsic ligament. In Figure 4-125 observe that *the fibular collateral ligament is not attached to the lateral meniscus.*

CLINICALLY ORIENTED COMMENTS

The fibular collateral ligament is not commonly torn because it is very strong, and severe blows to the medial side of the knee that might force it outward (**genu varum**) and open the knee joint on the lateral side are uncommon. However, lesions (*e.g.,* sprains or tears) of the fibular

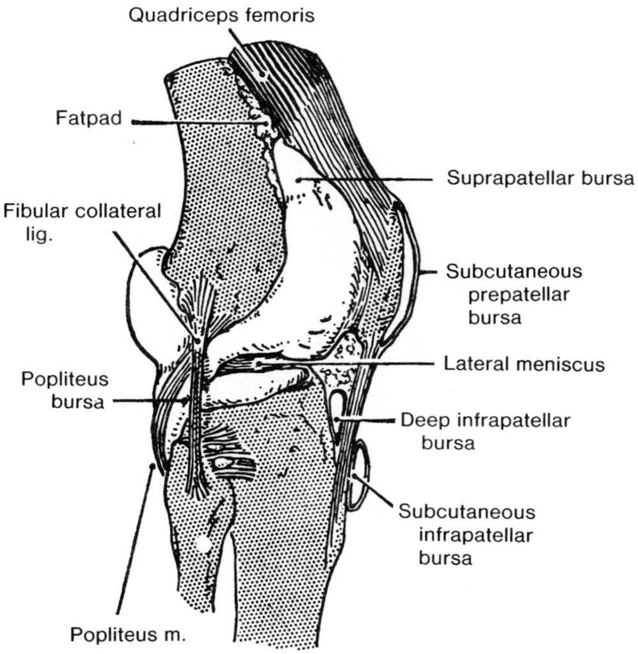

Figure 4–126. Drawing of a lateral view of a right knee joint filled with latex to show the extent of the synovial capsule. The fibular collateral ligament prevents disruption of the joint at the side. Observe that it extends from the lateral epicondyle of the femur to the head of the fibula.

collateral ligament can have serious consequences. Usually it is the distal end of the ligament that tears, and sometimes the head of the fibula is avulsed (pulled off) before the ligament ruptures. Complete tears of the fibular collateral ligament are often associated with *stretching of the common peroneal nerve* (Fig. 4-77). This affects the muscles of the anterior and lateral compartments of the leg and may produce **foot-drop** owing to paralysis of the dorsiflexor and evertor muscles of the ankle and foot.

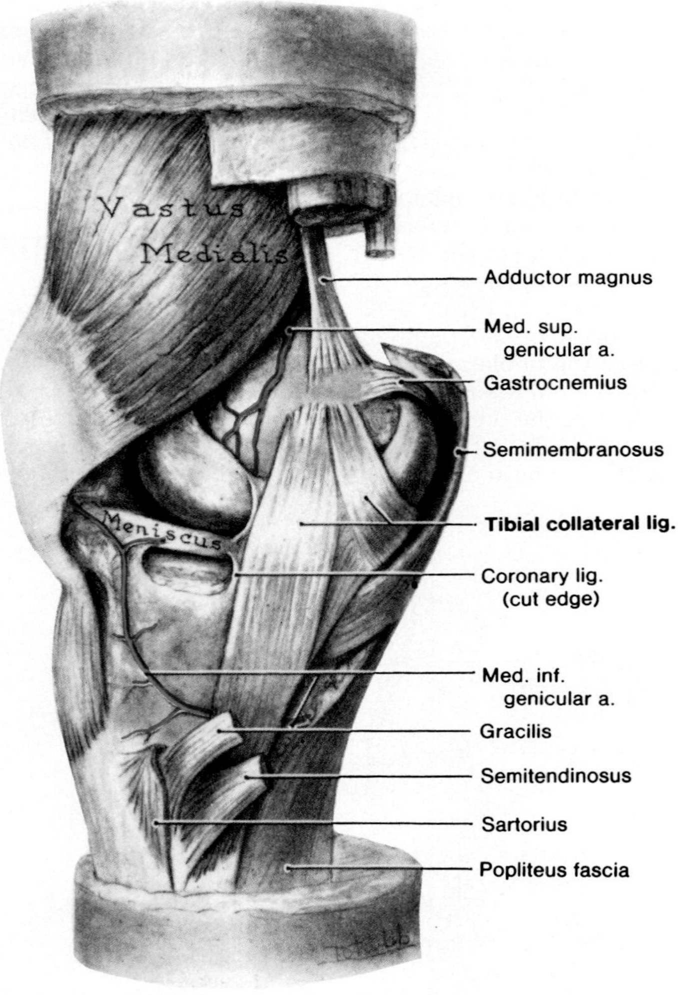

Figure 4–127. Drawing of a dissection of the medial aspect of the right knee joint. Observe the band-like part of the tibial collateral ligament which is attached to the medial epicondyle, almost in line with the adductor magnus tendon and crossing the insertion of the semimembranosus. Note that it crosses the medial inferior genicular artery and is crossed by the tendons of the three medial rotators (sartorius, gracilis, and semitendinosus), each of which is supplied by a different nerve (femoral, obturator, sciatic). The tibial collateral ligament prevents disruption of the joint at the side. *Observe that the medial meniscus is firmly attached to the tibial collateral ligament*; this relationship is more obvious in Figure 4–136. Because of this attachment, injury to this ligament commonly results in a concomitant injury to the medial meniscus (*e.g.*, a cartilage tear). Note that the posterior part of the tibial collateral ligament fans out, giving it a triangular shape.

This causes the foot to fall and become inverted. As a result, the toes drag on the ground when walking (Case 4-3).

The Tibial Collateral Ligament (Figs. 4-26, 4-122, 4-125, and 4-127). This strong, broad, flat band (formerly called the medial ligament) is about 9 cm long and extends from the medial epicondyle of the femur to the medial condyle and upper part of the medial surface of the tibia. Figure 4-122 illustrates that this ligament is a thickening of the fibrous capsule of the knee joint and that the tendon of the adductor magnus is partly continuous with the tibial collateral ligament. Figure 4-127 shows that they have a similar direction of fibers. Its inferior end is separated from the tibia by the medial inferior genicular vessels and nerve. The deep fibers of the straight band-like part of the ligament are firmly **attached to the medial meniscus** and to the fibrous capsule of the knee joint. Some fibers of this ligament also pass posteriorly to attach to the medial meniscus and the tibia.

CLINICALLY ORIENTED COMMENTS

As the collateral ligaments are slack during flexion, they permit rotation of the tibia and the femur in this position (Fig. 4-137). The firm attachment of the tibial collateral ligament to the medial meniscus is of considerable clinical significance because injury to the ligament frequently results in concomitant injury to the medial meniscus (Case 4-9).

Rupture of the tibial collateral ligament, often associated with tearing of the medial meniscus and the anterior cruciate ligament (Fig. 4-131*B*), is the *most common type of football injury.* It is caused by a blow to the lateral side of the knee (Fig. 4-156). Consequently, when examining soft tissue injuries of the knee, always think of **the three C's** that may be damaged: **C**ollateral ligaments, **C**ruciate ligaments, and **C**artilages (menisci).

The Oblique Popliteal Ligament (Fig. 4-46). This broad band is an expansion of the tendon of the semimembranosus muscle; *it supports the fibrous capsule posteriorly.* This ligament can be demonstrated by pulling on the tendon of this muscle, because it arises from it posterior to the medial condyle of the tibia. It then passes superolaterally to attach to the central part of the posterior aspect of the fibrous capsule of the knee joint.

The Arcuate Popliteal Ligament (Fig. 4-46). This Y-shaped band of capsular fibers also *strengthens the fibrous capsule posteriorly.* The stem of the ligament arises from the posterior aspect of the head of the fibula. As it passes superomedially over the tendon of the popliteus muscle, it spreads out over the posterior surface of the joint and inserts into the intercondylar area of the tibia and the posterior aspect of the lateral epicondyle of the femur.

The synovial capsule (Figs. 4-122 to 4-124, 4-126, 4-128, and 4-129) lines the inner aspect of the fibrous capsule and reflects onto the articulating bones as far as the edges of their cartilages. *The synovial capsule of the knee joint is more extensive than that of any other joint*; thus, the synovial cavity of the knee joint is the largest in the body.

In the embryo the knee joint possesses three synovial cavities, a patellar and two condylar ones. The partition separating the patellar from the condylar cavities disappears during development, leaving the vestigial **alar folds** and the infrapatellar synovial fold (Fig. 4-122).

During prenatal development, the medial and lateral halves of the knee joint were originally two independent joint cavities, which were separated by the membranes of the intercondylar septum. This septum partially broke down anterior to the anterior cruciate ligament (Fig. 4-128); the perforation is generally large and extends back to the anterior cruciate ligament. It divides the septum into an anterior part, the **infrapatellar synovial fold** (Fig. 4-122), and a posterior part in which the anterior and posterior **cruciate ligaments** develop; here the synovial membrane is reflected across the sides of both cruciate ligaments, excluding them from the synovial capsule of the joint. Therefore, *the cruciate ligaments are situated outside the synovial cavity, but within the articular capsule.*

Fluid can pass from one condylar cavity to the other, by way of the patellar cavity (*i.e.*, over the infrapatellar synovial fold) or through the perforation that appears in the intercondylar septum between the infrapatellar fold (Fig. 4-128) and the anterior cruciate ligament. Each condylar cavity is divided into a superior and inferior part by one inwardly projecting meniscus. The two parts communicate around the free concave margin of the meniscus (Fig. 4-162).

The synovial capsule is attached around the periphery of the patella. With the knee flexed to a right angle, you can palpate and often observe a depression on each side of the ligamentum patellae. Study Figures 4-123 to 4-125, verifying that the synovial cavity is very superficial at each side of this ligament.

From the synovial surface of the **infrapatellar fatpad** (Fig. 4-122), the infrapatellar synovial fold extends as a cresentic fold that runs posterosuperiorly to attach to the femur at the anterior border of the intercondylar notch (Figs. 4-122 and 4-128). Inferiorly the edges of the infrapatellar synovial fold are attached to the intercondylar eminence of the tibia. In Figure 4-128 observe that the synovial capsule is separated from the ligamentum patellae by the infrapatellar fatpad.

CLINICALLY ORIENTED COMMENTS

Injections are made into the synovial cavity of the knee joint for diagnostic or therapeutic purposes. When a joint is inflamed (*e.g.*, owing to infection or arthritis), the amount of synovial fluid may increase. Aspiration of this fluid may be necessary to relieve pressure or to obtain a sample for diagnostic studies. In other cases it may be necessary to evacuate blood that has entered the joint (*e.g.*, after a fracture in which the fracture line extends into the joint).

In **pneumoarthrography** (air contrast study of a joint) air is injected into the joint cavity to facilitate study of the structures in it (Fig. 4-121*A*). Being less opaque than

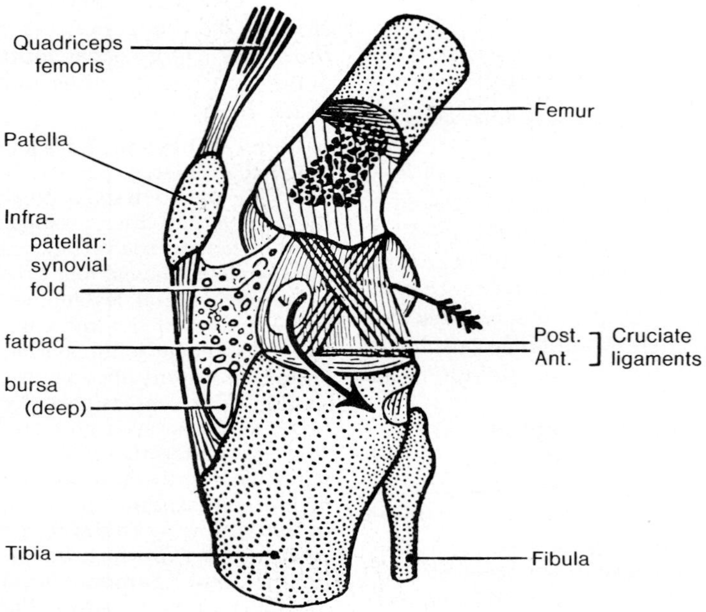

Figure 4–128. Drawing of a medial view of the right knee joint showing the intercondylar septum. The *arrow* passes through the perforation that formed in the septum before birth. This perforation divides the septum into an anterior part, the infrapatellar synovial fold, and a posterior part in which the cruciate ligaments develop. These ligaments are named according to their tibial attachments (*e.g.*, anterior cruciate to anterior part of intercondylar area, Fig. 4-131).

these structures (*e.g.*, the menisci), it appears black on radiographs and outlines the soft tissues which appear as gray images.

Sometimes the cavity of the knee joint is examined for injury or disease using an **arthroscope** (an instrument for examining the interior of a joint). The knee joint cavity can also be irrigated or washed out using saline. Steroids are sometimes injected into the knee joint cavity for treatment of **non-infectious joint diseases**.

Injections are generally given into the lateral side of the knee joint, with the patient sitting on the side of a table with the knee flexed and the leg hanging. *To determine the site of injection,* three bony points are located: the apex of the patella, the lateral plateau of the lateral tibial condyle, and the anterior prominence of the lateral femoral condyle. Joining these three points forms a triangle, the center of which indicates the proper injection site. To enter the joint cavity, the needle must pass posteromedially. Draw this triangle on your knee and insert your fingernail into the center of it. You should be able to feel the gap between the corresponding tibial and femoral condyles.

Any procedure involving entry into the knee joint cavity is performed under sterile conditions (*e.g.*, injections for diagnostic or therapeutic purposes). Should the joint become infected, toxins (G. poisons) or bacteria may readily pass into the circulation, resulting in **toxemia** and **bacteremia**, respectively.

Bursae About The Knee (Figs. 4-122 to 4-126, 4-128, and 4-129). There are several bursae about the knee because most tendons around the knee run parallel to the bones and pull lengthwise across the knee joint. Some bursae have been mentioned in the foregoing account. Almost invariably, *three bursae communicate with the synovial cavity of the knee joint*; these lie deep to the tendons of the quadriceps femoris, the popliteus, and the medial head of the gastrocnemius muscle.

The Suprapatellar Bursa (Figs. 4-121*A*, 4-124, and 4-129). This large saccular extension (flat pouch) of the synovial capsule passes superiorly between the femur and the tendon of the quadriceps femoris muscle. It extends about four fingerbreadths superior to the base of the patella (Fig. 4-129). This bursa *permits free movement of the quadriceps tendon over the distal end of the femur* and facilitates the full range of extension and flexion of the knee joint. The bursa is held in position by part of the vastus intermedius muscle, called the articularis genus muscle (Fig. 4-23*C*).

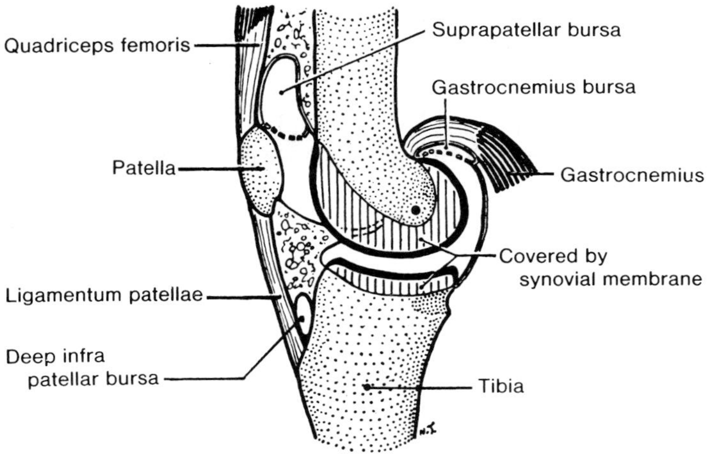

Figure 4–129. Drawing of a medial view of the right knee joint showing the suprapatellar and gastrocnemius bursae communicating with the synovial cavity.

CLINICALLY ORIENTED COMMENTS

Because the suprapatellar bursa almost invariably communicates freely with the synovial cavity of the knee joint, it is regarded as a part of it; hence, stab or puncture wounds proximal to the knee in the anterior aspect of the distal part of the thigh may infect the knee joint via the suprapatellar bursa. It may also be involved in fractures of the distal end of the femur, resulting in **hemarthrosis** (blood in the joint).

The Popliteus Bursa (Figs. 4-123 and 4-135). This **subpopliteal recess** or extension of the synovial cavity lies between the tendon of the popliteus muscle and the lateral condyle of the tibia. It opens into the lateral condylar part of the synovial cavity of the knee joint inferior to the lateral meniscus. Sometimes this bursa is also continuous with the synovial cavity of the **proximal tibiofibular joint** (Fig. 4-123) owing to perforation of the partition between the popliteus and that joint cavity.

The Gastrocnemius Bursa (Fig. 4-123). This is an extension of the synovial cavity of the knee joint which lies deep to the tendon of origin of the medial head of the gastrocnemius muscle. As it separates the tendon from the femur, it is often called the **subtendinous bursa** (of the medial head) of the gastrocnemius.

The following bursae around the knee do not communicate with the synovial cavity of the knee joint; they are all related to the patella.

The Subcutaneous Prepatellar Bursa (Figs. 4-122, 4-124, and 4-126). This large bursa lies between the skin and the anterior surface of the patella and allows free movement of the skin over the underlying patella, *e.g.*, during flexion of the knee joint.

CLINICALLY ORIENTED COMMENTS

Because of its superficial and exposed position, the subcutaneous prepatellar bursa may become inflamed (*e.g.*, after prolonged working on the hands and knees when scrubbing a hard floor). **Prepatellar bursitis** is an example of friction bursitis caused by friction between the skin and the patella. If the inflammation is chronic, the bursa becomes distended with fluid and forms a soft fluctuant swelling anterior to the knee (Fig. 4-130). This condition is commonly called "*housemaid's knee.*" Miners and other people who work on "all fours" also develop prepatellar bursitis. It may be called "beat knee" (*i.e.*, worn out).

The Subcutaneous (Superficial) Infrapatellar Bursa (Fig. 4-126). This bursa lies between the skin and the fascia anterior to the tuberosity of the tibia. It allows the skin to glide over the tibial tuberosity and to withstand pressure when kneeling with the trunk upright (*e.g.*, during praying).

CLINICALLY ORIENTED COMMENTS

Subcutaneous infrapatellar bursitis involving the subcutaneous infrapatellar bursa (Fig. 4-126) may result from excessive friction between the skin and the tibial tuberosity; thus, the swelling occurs over

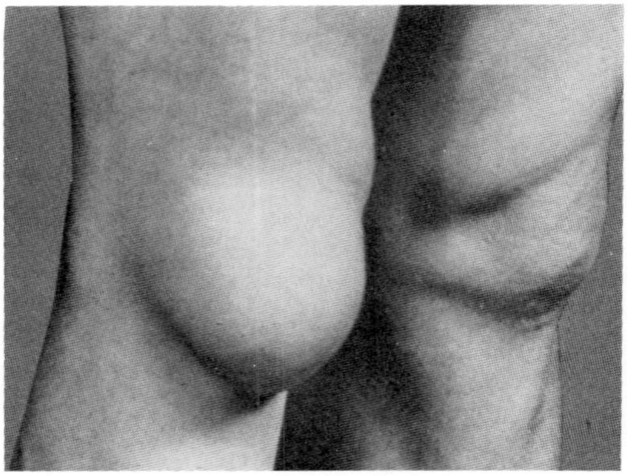

Figure 4–130. Photograph of the knees of a patient with prepatellar bursitis ("housemaid's knee"), resulting from inflammation of the subcutaneous prepatellar bursae (Fig. 4–126). The amount of fluid in the bursa over her right patella is greater than is usually seen in this type of friction bursitis.

the proximal end of the tibia and not over the knee. This condition has been called "*clergyman's knee,*" but it occurs more often now in roofers and carpet layers.

The Deep Infrapatellar Bursa (Figs. 4-126, 4-128, and 4-129). This small bursa lies between the ligamentum patellae and the tibial tuberosity. It is separated from the knee joint by the infrapatellar fatpad.

CLINICALLY ORIENTED COMMENTS

Deep infrapatellar bursitis results in a swelling between the patellar ligament and the tibial tuberosity. The swelling is usually less pronounced than that associated with superficial prepatellar bursitis. Enlargement of this bursa obliterates the dimples on each side of the patellar ligament, as does an **effusion** (L. a pouring out) of the knee joint (*i.e.,* escape of fluid from the vessels in the joint cavity).

The Intra-articular Ligaments (Figs. 4-120, 4-123, 4-125, and 4-131). Within the articular capsule of the knee joint, there are two ligaments that attach the femur to the tibia. It is important that you understand that the **cruciate ligaments** are *within the articular capsule, but outside the synovial cavity* of the knee joint. They are located between the medial and lateral condylar joints and are separated from the joint cavity by synovial membrane. Recall that the synovial capsule lines the fibrous capsule, except posteriorly where it is reflected anteriorly around the cruciate ligaments.

The cruciate (L. shaped like a cross) ligaments are strong, rounded bands that cross each other obliquely like the limbs of a St. Andrew's cross (*i.e.,* an X, Fig. 4-128). They are named anterior and posterior according to their site of attachment to the tibia; *i.e.,* the **anterior cruciate ligament** attaches to the tibia *anteriorly* and the **posterior cruciate ligament** attaches to the tibia *posteriorly.*

The Anterior Cruciate Ligament (Figs. 4-120, 4-125, and 4-131 to 4-133). This is the

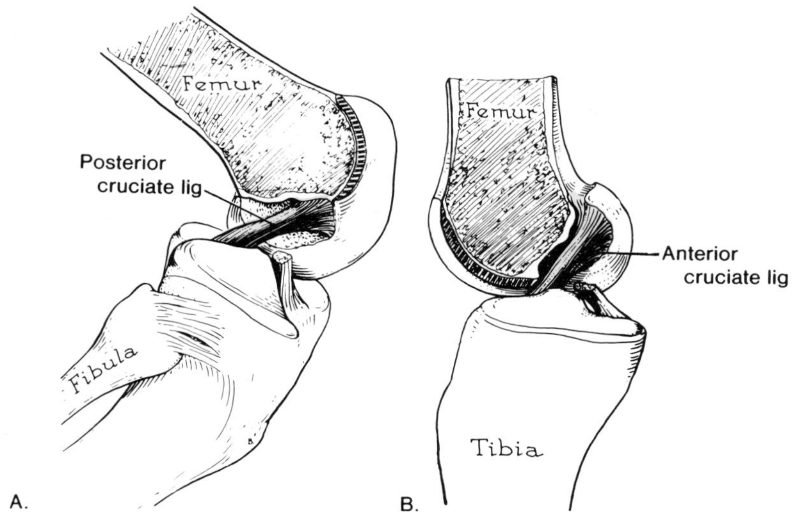

Figure 4–131. Drawings illustrating the cruciate ligaments. In each illustration one-half of the right femur is removed with the proximal part of the corresponding cruciate ligament. *A*, lateral view showing that the posterior cruciate attaches the femur to the tibia posteriorly and prevents forward sliding of the femur, particularly when the knee is flexed. *B*, medial view showing that the anterior cruciate ligament attaches the femur to the tibia anteriorly and prevents backward sliding of the femur and hyperextension of the knee. It also limits medial rotation of the extended knee when the foot is on the ground (*i.e.*, when the leg is fixed).

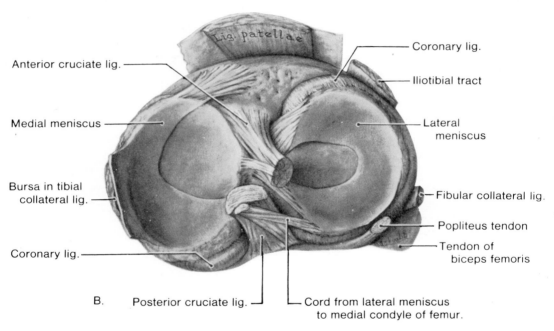

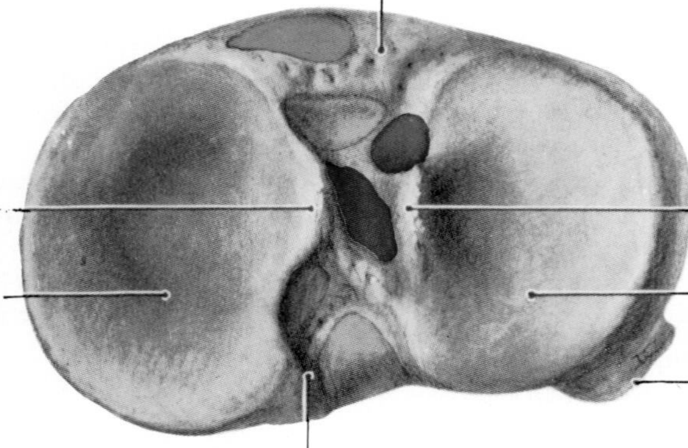

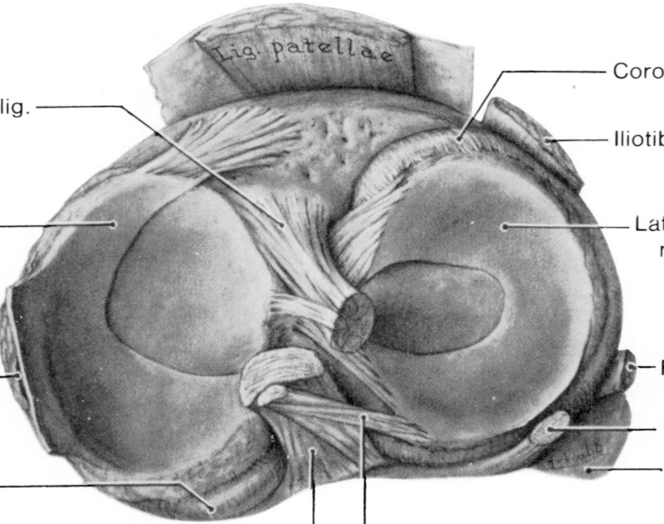

Figure 4–132. Drawings of dissections of the right knee joint demonstrating the cruciate ligaments and the menisci. *A*, the superior aspect of the proximal end of the tibia showing the medial and lateral plateaus (articular surfaces). Sites of attachment of the cruciate ligaments are colored *yellow*; those of the medial meniscus, *blue*; and those of the lateral meniscus, *red*. *B*, this view shows the menisci and their attachment to the intercondylar area of the tibia. The tibial attachments of the cruciate ligaments are also shown. The menisci are cartilaginous and tough where they are compressed between the femur and the tibia, but they are ligamentous and pliable at their attachments. The menisci conform to the shapes of the surfaces on which they rest. As the horns of the lateral meniscus are attached close together and its coronary ligament is slack, this meniscus can slide forward and backward on the condyle. Because the horns of the medial meniscus are attached far apart, its movements on the condyle are restricted. Movement of the medial meniscus is also restricted because of its attachment to the tibial collateral ligament; hence, it is commonly torn.

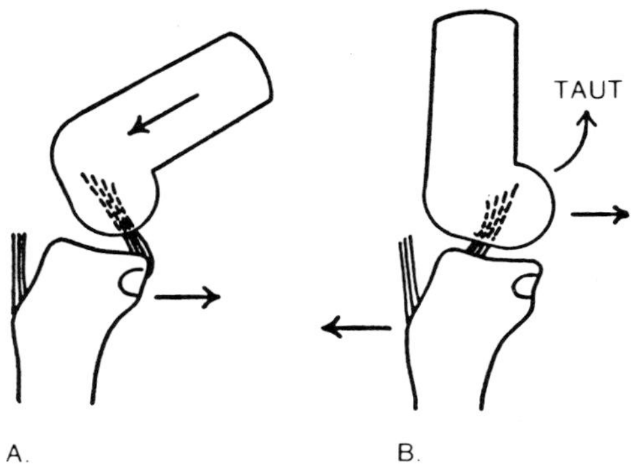

Figure 4–133. Diagrams illustrating the functions of the cruciate ligaments. *A*, the posterior cruciate ligament prevents forward displacement of the femur or backward displacement of the tibia. *B*, the anterior cruciate ligament prevents backward displacement of the femur and hyperextension of the knee joint.

weaker of the two cruciate ligaments. It arises from the anterior rough part of the intercondylar area of the tibia just posterior to the attachment of the medial meniscus. It extends upward, backward, and laterally to attach to the posterior part of the medial side of the lateral condyle of the femur. It is slack when the knee is flexed and **taut when the knee is fully extended** (Fig. 4-133*B*).

The anterior cruciate ligament prevents backward displacement of the femur on the tibia and hyperextension of the knee joint. When the knee joint is flexed to a right angle, the tibia cannot be pulled forward because it is held by the anterior cruciate ligament.

CLINICALLY ORIENTED COMMENTS

The relatively weak anterior cruciate ligament is *sometimes torn concomitantly with the tibial collateral ligament* when the knee is hit hard from the lateral side while the foot is on the ground (Case 4-9). First the tibial collateral ligament ruptures which opens the knee joint on the medial side and forces the knee inward (**genu valgum**). This may tear the medial meniscus and the anterior cruciate ligament.

The anterior cruciate ligament may also be torn when (1) the tibia is driven anteriorly on the femur, (2) the femur is driven posteriorly on the tibia, and (3) the knee joint is severely hyperextended. The knee joint becomes very unstable when the anterior cruciate ligament is torn (Fig. 4-134). To test its stability, the tibia is pulled in an anterior direction, and if there is forward movement (the "*anterior drawer sign*"), a tear of the anterior cruciate ligament is indicated.

The Posterior Cruciate Ligament (Figs. 4-120, 4-123, 4-131, 4-132, and 4-136). This is the *stronger of the two* cruciate ligaments. It arises from the posterior part of the intercondylar area of the tibia and passes upward and forward on the medial side of the anterior cruciate ligament to attach to the anterior part of the lateral surface of the medial condyle of the femur. The posterior cruciate ligament **tightens during flexion of the knee** joint, preventing forward displacement of the femur

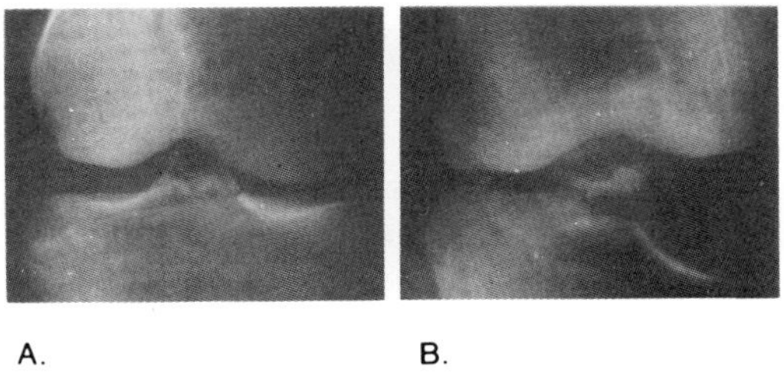

Figure 4–134. Radiographs of the right knee (frontal projections) of a 21-year-old football player after he was hit hard from the lateral side (Fig. 4–156). *A*, shows a normal relationship between the femur and the tibia. Note the undisplaced fracture of one of the tubercles of the intercondylar eminence of the tibia (also called the medial tibial spine). *B*, shows the same knee radiographed while it was being stressed in abduction with the patient under anesthesia. Note that the knee joint has opened up on the medial side, which indicates a complete tear of the tibial collateral ligament. Note also the displacement of the fracture, which indicates that the anterior cruciate ligament and the bone which attaches it to the tibia have been torn away (avulsed), rendering the ligament incompetent (unable to perform its function).

or backward displacement of the tibia, *i.e., it prevents hyperflexion and the femur from sliding forward off the tibial plateaus* (Figs. 4-132 and 4-133*A*).

CLINICALLY ORIENTED COMMENTS

The posterior cruciate ligament may be injured when the anterior aspect of the tibia is struck with the knee flexed. Although this kind of injury may occur when a passenger's leg is driven against the dashboard, dislocation of the hip (Case 4-6) is more likely to occur.

If the tibia is driven forcefully backward on the femur, or the femur is driven forward on the tibia, or the knee joint is severely hyperflexed, the posterior cruciate ligament may be torn. When this occurs, the flexed knee is unstable. To test its stability, the tibia is forced in a posterior direction. If there is backward movement (the "*posterior drawer sign*"), a tear of the posterior cruciate ligament is indicated.

The Menisci of the Knee Joint (Figs. 4-120 to 4-127, 4-132, and 4-136). The two menisci (G. crescents) are *crescentic plates of fibrocartilage* within the knee joint that are interposed between the femoral and tibial condyles. Because of their shape, they are sometimes called the *semilunar cartilages.* Wedge-shaped in cross-section, they are firmly attached at their ends to the **intercondylar areas** of the tibia.

The menisci deepen the articular surfaces of the proximal end of the tibia which articulate with the femoral condyles. Their superior surfaces are slightly concave for reception of the femoral condyles, whereas their inferior surfaces that rest on and fit the tibial condyles are flatter. They are thick at their peripheral attached margins and thin at their internal unattached edges. Being smooth and slightly movable, the menisci fill the gaps between the femur and the tibia that would otherwise be present during movements of the joint. Their external margins are attached to the capsule of the joint and through it to the edges of the articular surface of the tibia. The capsular fibers which attach the menisci to the tibial condyles are called medial and lateral **coronary ligaments** (Figs. 4-125, 4-127, and 4-135). As they are attached to the condylar surfaces of the tibia, they move with it; however, the looseness of their attachments allows them to move slightly on the tibia.

The transverse ligament of the knee joins the anterior parts of the two menisci; this connection allows them to move together during movements of the femur on the tibia. The thickness of this ligament varies in different people and sometimes it is absent.

The thick *peripheral margins of the menisci are vascularized* by genicular branches of the popliteal artery (Fig. 4-127), but their thin unattached edges in the interior of the joint are avascular.

The Medial Meniscus (Figs. 4-23*B,* 4-120, 4-122, 4-123, 4-125, 4-127, 4-132, and 4-136). The longer medial meniscus is a rather oval or *C-shaped cartilage* and is broader posteriorly than anteriorly. Its anterior horn (L. *cornu,* end) is attached to the

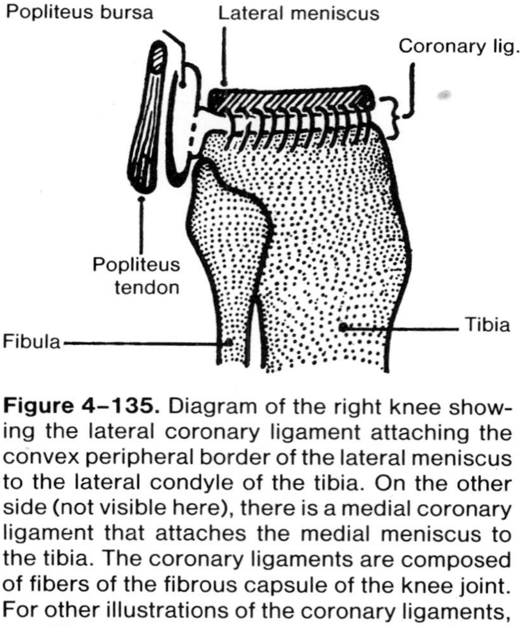

Figure 4–135. Diagram of the right knee showing the lateral coronary ligament attaching the convex peripheral border of the lateral meniscus to the lateral condyle of the tibia. On the other side (not visible here), there is a medial coronary ligament that attaches the medial meniscus to the tibia. The coronary ligaments are composed of fibers of the fibrous capsule of the knee joint. For other illustrations of the coronary ligaments, see Figures 4–125 and 4–127. This diagram also illustrates the communication of the popliteus bursa with the synovial cavity of the knee joint.

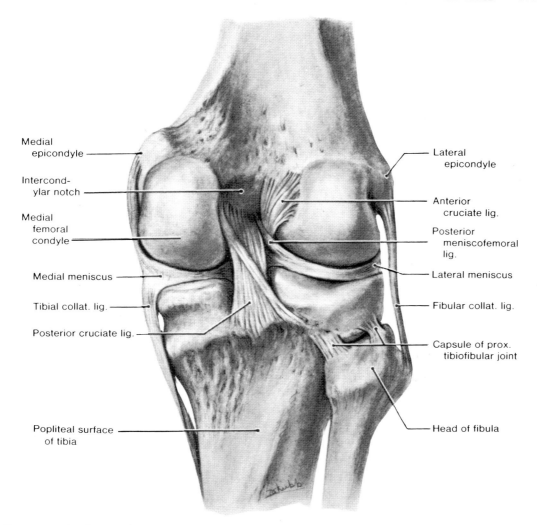

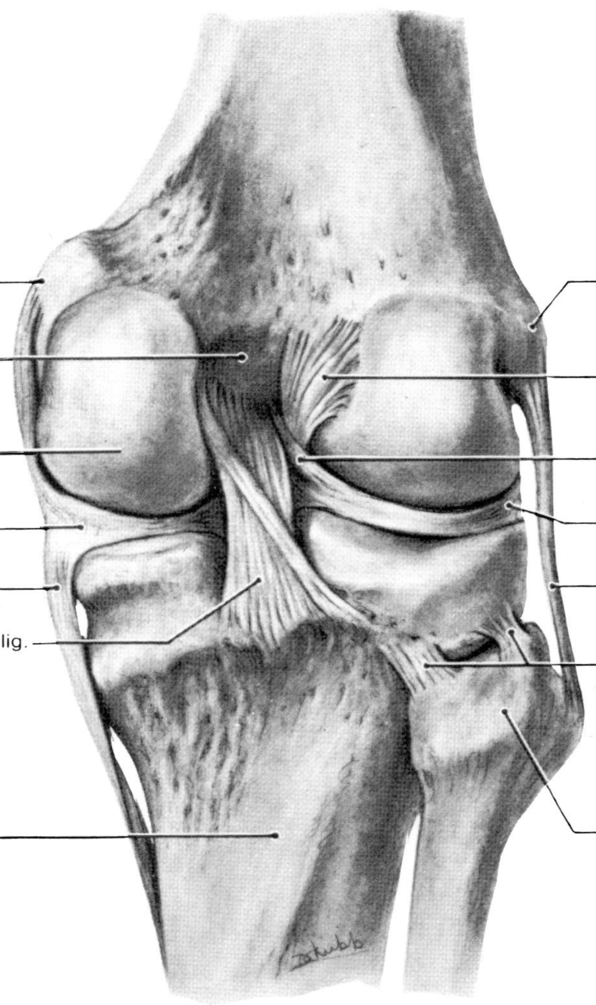

Figure 4–136. Drawing of a dissection of the ligaments of the right knee joint from behind. Observe the band-like tibial collateral ligament attached to the medial meniscus. Note that the cord-like fibular collateral ligament is separated from the lateral meniscus by the width of the popliteus tendon (removed here; see Figs. 4–123 and 4–126). Thus, *undue stress on the tibial collateral ligament may tear the medial meniscus*, whereas the lateral meniscus is usually not torn by stress on the fibular collateral ligament. Note that the posterior cruciate ligament is joined by the posterior meniscofemoral ligament that runs from the lateral meniscus to the lateral surface of the medial femoral condyle. Observe the attachment of the anterior cruciate ligament to the lateral femoral condyle. Athletic injuries are the most frequent cause of trauma to the collateral and cruciate ligaments. Because the medial meniscus is firmly attached to the tibial collateral ligament, it is often torn also (see Fig. 4-163).

intercondylar area of the tibia, anterior to the attachment of the anterior cruciate ligament (Fig. 4-132). Moreover, it is the most anterior of the structures attached to the intercondylar area. Its posterior horn is attached to the posterior intercondylar area, anterior to that of the posterior cruciate ligament and between the attachments of the lateral meniscus and the posterior cruciate ligament (Figs. 4-120 and 4-132).

The peripheral border of the medial meniscus is firmly adherent to the deep surface of the tibial collateral ligament.

CLINICALLY ORIENTED COMMENTS

Injuries to the knee joint are common because it is a major weight-bearing joint and its stability depends almost entirely upon its associated ligaments and muscles. **Ligamentous injuries** may result from any blow that forces the knee to move in an abnormal plane.

A blow on the lateral side of the knee when a person is bearing weight on the leg stresses the tibial collateral ligament. If the blow is relatively minor, most fibers are stretched and some may be torn; this is called a **sprained ligament.** When the blow is severe all the fibers may be torn, either partially or completely. This is called a **torn ligament**; the tear usually occurs near its femoral attachment (Case 4-9 and Fig. 4-163).

Localized tenderness and pain in the flexed knee on the medial side of the patellar ligament just proximal to the medial tibial plateau may indicate **injury to the medial meniscus.** Injury to this meniscus is a common occurrence (about 20 times more common than injury to the lateral meniscus). It results from a **twisting strain** that is applied to the knee when it is flexed (Fig. 4-137). Because it is firmly attached to the tibial collateral ligament (Fig. 4-136), sprains of this ligament may tear the cartilage or detach it from the fibrous capsule. Part of the torn cartilage may become displaced toward the center of the joint and become lodged between the tibial and femoral condyles. This "locks the knee" in the flexed position and prevents the patient from fully extending the knee.

Because the menisci are poorly supplied with blood, tears in them heal poorly unless they are near the peripheral margins, which are vascularized by genicular branches of the popliteal artery (Fig. 4-127).

When weight is borne by the flexed knee joint, a sudden twist of the knee may cause **rupture of the medial meniscus**, usually splitting it longitudinally. This injury is common in athletes (*e.g.,* football players) who twist their flexed knees while running. It also occurs in coal miners and other persons who topple over when they are working in a crouched or squatting position.

Usually a torn medial meniscus is surgically excised (**medial meniscectomy**) because repeated displacements of the torn part of the meniscus are temporarily disabling and may lead to degenerative disease of the joint. Regeneration occurs from the vascular fibroareolar tissue around the periphery of the joint cavity.

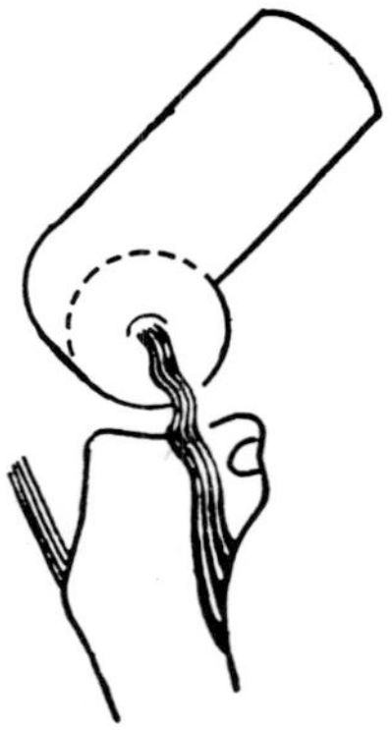

Figure 4–137. Diagram showing that the collateral ligaments are slack during flexion and permit rotation. Thus, the menisci usually tear when the knee is flexed and able to rotate.

The Lateral Meniscus (Figs. 4-120, 4-121, 4-123 to 4-126, and 4-132). The shorter lateral meniscus is *nearly circular* in shape, conforming to the more circular lateral tibial condyle. In Figure 4-132*B* note that it covers a larger area of articular surface than does the medial meniscus. In Figures 4-123 and 4-125 note that the tendon of the popliteus muscle separates the lateral meniscus from the fibular collateral ligament.

The anterior and posterior horns of the lateral meniscus are attached close together in the anterior and posterior intercondylar areas, respectively. A strong tendinous slip called the *posterior meniscofemoral ligament* joins the lateral meniscus to the posterior cruciate ligament and to the medial femoral condyle (Fig. 4-136).

CLINICALLY ORIENTED COMMENTS

The lateral meniscus, smaller and more freely movable than the medial meniscus, is less likely to be injured, mainly because it is not attached to the fibular collateral ligament. The popliteus tendon and the popliteus bursa intervene between the lateral meniscus and this ligament (Figs. 4-123 to 4-126).

When air and/or dense contrast material are injected into the synovial cavity of the knee joint before radiographs are taken, the menisci can be observed (Fig. 4-121). **Pneumoarthrograms** (radiographs taken after air injection) or **double contrast arthrograms** are helpful in demonstrating soft tissue lesions of the knee joint. Because air is less opaque than the menisci, it appears black in the radiograph and outlines the soft tissues (*e.g.,* the lateral meniscus in Fig. 4-121*A*). When dense contrast materials are used, the articular cartilages and menisci appear as radiolucent images within the dense contrast medium.

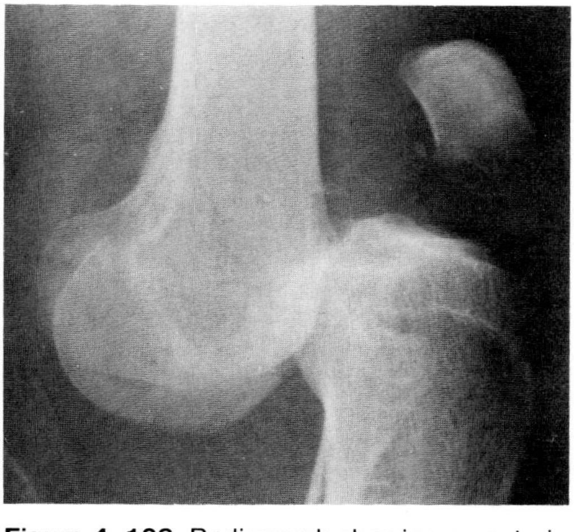

Figure 4–138. Radiograph showing an anterior dislocation of the knee joint in a 28-year-old man who sustained multiple injuries in an automobile accident. The amount of dislocation indicates that all the collateral and cruciate ligaments are torn. In addition the menisci are probably torn and displaced. There was also severe injury to the popliteal artery, which required surgical reconstruction with an arterial prosthesis.

Stability of the Joint. Although the knee joint is one of the strongest joints in the body, particularly when extended, it is the one whose function is commonly deranged (*e.g.,* in body contact sports such as hockey and football).

The stability of the knee joint *depends upon the strength of the surrounding muscles and ligaments.* Of these supports, the muscles are the most important. Thus, many sports injuries are preventable through appropriate conditioning and training.

The most important muscle in stabilizing the knee joint is the quadriceps femoris, particularly the lower fibers of the vastus medialis and the vastus lateralis (Fig. 4-23). Evidence for this is that the knee joint will function surprisingly well following damage to the ligaments if the quadriceps femoris is well developed.

CLINICALLY ORIENTED COMMENTS

The quadriceps femoris muscle undergoes considerable atrophy during periods of disuse (*e.g.,* while the lower limb is in a cast). Thus, it must be exercised to prevent disuse atrophy and resulting instability of the knee. Without good muscular support, repaired knee ligaments may be more easily sprained or retorn, either partially or completely. **Residual instability of the knee joint** is one of the most troublesome complications of ligamentous injuries of the knee.

Because the knee joint possesses great stability in most people, **traumatic dislocation of the knee joint** is not common; however, this severe injury may occur during automobile accidents (Fig. 4-138). In addition to disruption of the ligaments of the knee, the popliteal artery and the tibial nerve (Fig. 4-61) may be injured.

Blood Supply (Figs. 4-34, 4-62, 4-63, and 4-127). The articular arteries to the knee joint are branches of the vessels that enter into the **genicular anastomosis** around the knee. The middle genicular artery penetrates the fibrous capsule posteriorly and supplies structures in the intercondylar region.

Nerve Supply. The articular nerves are branches of the obturator, femoral, tibial, and common peroneal nerves (Fig. 4-60).

THE TIBIOFIBULAR JOINTS

The fibula articulates with the tibia at the proximal and distal tibiofibular joints. In addition, the bodies of the two bones are connected by a strong **interosseous membrane** (Figs. 4-64, 4-74, and 4-81) which plays an important role in the articulations between the tibia and the fibula.

The Proximal (Superior) Tibiofibular Joint (Figs. 4-67*B,* 4-124, and 4-136). This articulation is a **plane type of synovial joint** between the head of the fibula and the inferior edge of the lateral condyle of the tibia.

Articular Surfaces (Figs. 4-54, 4-66, and 4-136). The flat, oval-to-circular facet on the head of the fibula articulates with a similar facet located posterolaterally on the inferior aspect of the lateral condyle of the tibia. These facets are covered with hyaline cartilage.

Movements of the Joint. Slight movement occurs at the proximal tibiofibular joint during dorsiflexion of the ankle joint which presses the lateral malleolus laterally and causes movement of the body and the head of the fibula. Some movement of the joint also occurs during plantarflexion of the ankle joint.

The Articular Capsule (Figs. 4-124, 4-126, and 4-136). The **fibrous capsule** surrounds the joint and is attached to the margins of the articular facets on the fibula and the tibia. It is much thicker anteriorly than posteriorly where it is strengthened by the anterior and posterior **ligaments of the head of the fibula** (Figs. 4-124 and 4-136). The fibers of these ligaments run superomedially from the fibula to the tibia. In Figure 4-123 observe that the tendon of the popliteus muscle is intimately related to the posterosuperior aspect of the proximal tibiofibular joint.

The **synovial capsule** (Figs. 4-123 and 4-124) lines the fibrous capsule. The pouch of synovial membrane prolonged under the tendon of the popliteus muscle, known as the **popliteus bursa**, sometimes communicates with the synovial cavity of the proximal tibiofibular joint through an opening in the superior part of the capsule. Consequently, the proximal tibiofibular joint may be indirectly in communication with the synovial cavity of the knee joint.

Blood Supply (Figs. 4-34 and 4-62). The articular arteries to this joint are derived from the inferior lateral **genicular** and anterior **tibial recurrent arteries.**

Nerve Supply (Figs. 4-60, 4-80, and 4-81). The articular nerves are derived from the **common peroneal** nerve, the **nerve to the popliteus,** and the **anterior tibial recurrent** nerve.

The Distal (Inferior) Tibiofibular Joint (Figs. 4-65, 4-67*B,* 4-139, 4-140, and 4-142). This articulation is a **fibrous type of joint** of the syndesmosis type (*i.e.,* the bony surfaces are held together by fibrous tissue). It is located between the inferior end of the body of the fibula and the inferior end of the tibia.

Articular Surfaces (Fig. 4-67*B*). The rough, convex, triangular articular area on the medial surface of the distal end of the shaft of the fibula just above the facet for the talus articulates with a triangular concave area at the inferolateral lower end of the tibia, called the **fibular notch**. There is a small upward projection of the synovial capsule of the ankle joint into the inferior part of the distal tibiofibular joint.

A strong **interosseous ligament** which is continuous superiorly with the interosseous membrane (Fig. 4-81) forms the principal connection between the tibia and fibula. It consists of strong bands which extend from the fibular notch of the tibia to the medial surface of the distal end of the body of the fibula (Fig. 4-67*B*).

The joint is also strengthened anteriorly and posteriorly by the anterior and posterior **tibiofibular ligaments** (Figs. 4-139 and 4-140). They extend from the borders of the fibular notch of the tibia to the anterior and posterior surfaces of the lateral malleolus, respectively. The inferior and deep part of the posterior tibiofibular ligament is called the **transverse tibiofibular**

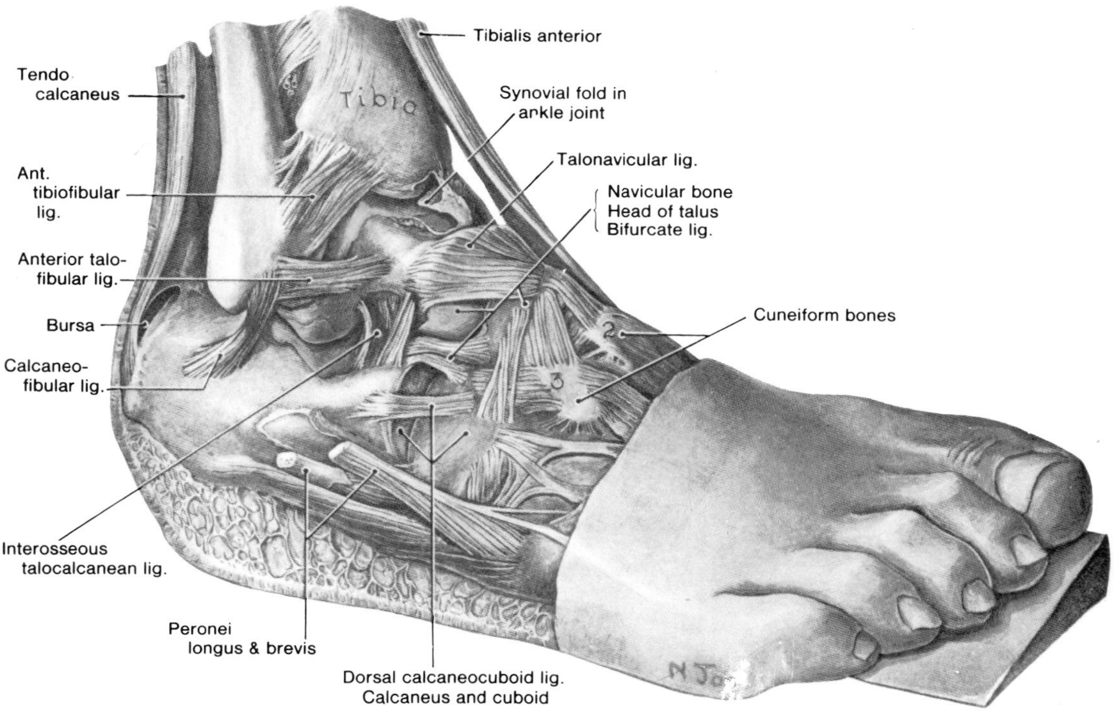

Figure 4–139. Drawing of a dissection of a lateral view of the right ankle joint and the joints of inverson and eversion. The foot has been inverted in order to demonstrate the articular areas (*yellow*) and the ligaments that become taut during inversion of the foot. The joints of inversion and eversion are (1) the subtalar (posterior talocalcanean) joint, (2) the talocalcaneonavicular (combined anterior talocalcanean and talonavicular) joint, and (3) the transverse tarsal (combined calcaneo-cuboid and talonavicular) joint. Note that the talonavicular joint is involved twice. The articular areas colored *yellow* are (1) the posterior talar facet of the calcaneus, (2) the anterior surface of the calcaneus, (3) the head of the talus, and (4) the upper and lateral parts of the trochlea of the talus. The anterior talofibular and the dorsal calcaneocuboid ligaments are weak and easily torn.

ligament. This strong band closes the posterior angle between the tibia and the fibula.

CLINICALLY ORIENTED COMMENTS

The posterior tibiofibular ligament is much stronger than the anterior tibiofibular ligament, and in severe ankle injuries it may avulse the posteroinferior part of the tibia. In these cases the fracture enters the ankle joint. If, in addition to this fracture, the medial and lateral malleoli are fractured, the injury is sometimes referred to as a **trimalleolar fracture** (*i.e.,* a fracture both malleoli and the posterior part of the inferior border of the tibia).

Stability of the Joint. This articulation forms a **strong union** between the distal extremities of the tibia and the fibula and much of the strength of the ankle joint is dependent on it.

Movement of the Joint. Slight movement of the distal tibiofibular joint occurs to accommodate the talus during dorsiflexion of the ankle joint.

Blood Supply (Figs. 4-80 and 4-81). The articular arteries are derived from the perforating branch of the **peroneal artery**

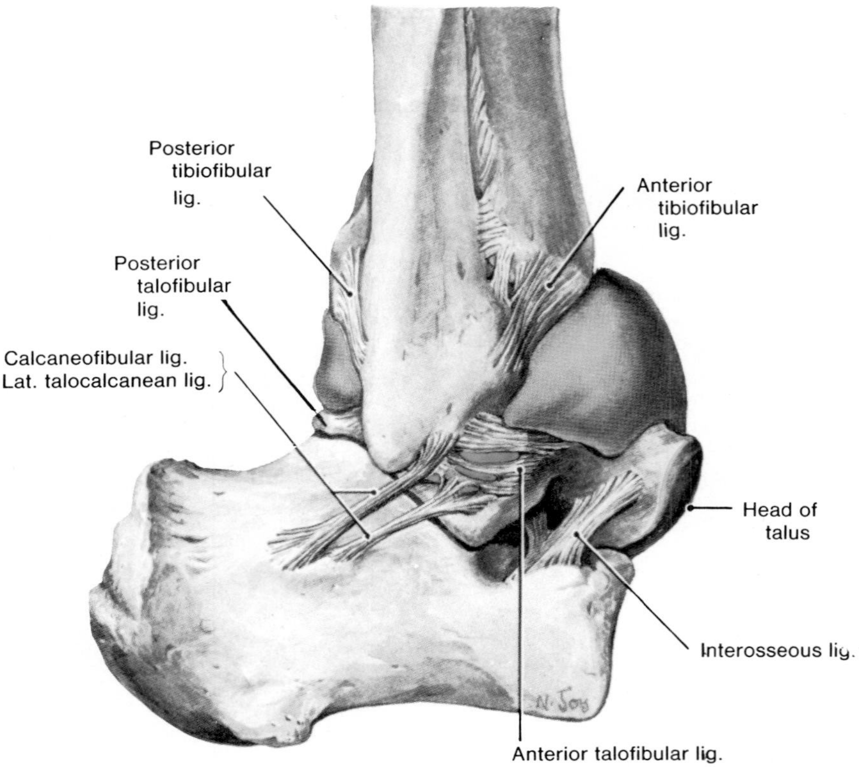

Figure 4–140. Drawing of a dissection of a lateral view of a distended right ankle joint. Observe the forward extension of the synovial cavity over the neck of the talus. Posteriorly and laterally, note the closeness of the synovial cavity of the ankle joint to the subtalar (posterior talocalcanean) joint.

and the medial malleolar branches of the anterior and posterior **tibial arteries**.

Nerve Supply (Figs. 4-81 and 4-93). The articular nerves are derived from the **deep peroneal**, the **tibial**, and the **saphenous** nerves.

THE ANKLE JOINT

This talocrural articulation is a **hinge type of synovial joint** between the distal ends of the tibia and fibula and the upper part of the talus. This joint can be felt between the tendons on the front of the ankle as a slight depression about 1 cm proximal to the tip of the medial malleolus.

Articular Surfaces (Figs. 4-67*B*, 4-68, 4-71, 4-72, and 4-139 to 4-143). The inferior extremities of the tibia and the fibula form a deep socket or box-like **mortise** into which the superior part or pulley-shaped trochlea (L. pulley) of the talus fits (Fig. 4-142). The articular surfaces are covered with hyaline cartilage.

The **fibula** has an articular facet on its lateral malleolus which faces medially and articulates with the facet on the lateral surface of the talus (Figs. 4-67*B* and 4-141).

The **tibia** articulates with the talus in two places (Figs. 4-141 and 4-142). Its distal surface forms the roof of the mortise which is wider anteriorly than posteriorly and slightly concave from front to back. The lateral surface of its medial malleolus also articulates with the talus (Fig. 4-142).

The **talus** has three articular facets which articulate with the inferior surface of the tibia and the malleoli (Figs. 4-67*B* and 4-141). The superior articular surface of the talus is wider anteriorly than posteriorly, convex from front to back, and slightly concave from side to side.

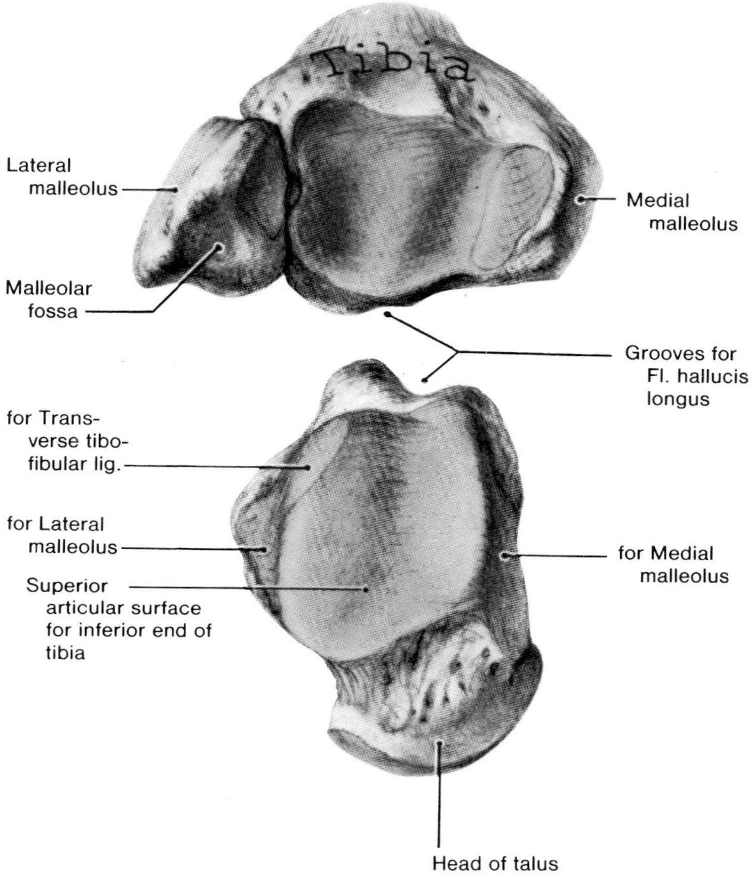

Figure 4–141. Drawings illustrating the articular surfaces of the right ankle joint. Note that the superior or trochlear articular surface of the talus is broader in front than behind; hence, the tibial and fibular malleoli which form a mortise for the talus (Fig. 4–142) are forced apart in dorsiflexion. The distal tibiofibular joint, on which the brunt of the strain then falls, gives resilence to the ankle joint. The superior articular surface of the talus is also called the trochlea of the talus (also see Fig. 4-142).

Movements of the Joint (Fig. 4-75*A* and *B*). The active movements of the ankle joint are **dorsiflexion** and **plantarflexion**. During dorsiflexion the trochlea tali rocks backward in its mortise (Fig. 4-141) and the malleoli tend to be forced apart because the superior articular surface of the talus is wider anteriorly than posteriorly. The lateral malleolus moves laterally during dorsiflexion as the tibia and fibula are forced slightly apart. This separation of the bones requires some movement of the proximal tibiofibular joint (Fig. 4-136). When the ankle joint is plantarflexed, some rotation, abduction, and adduction are possible.

The ankle joint is unstable during plantarflexion. Verify this by standing on your tiptoes and walking on them.

CLINICALLY ORIENTED COMMENTS

The range of plantarflexion (about 55°) is greater than that of dorsiflexion (about 35°), but there is considerable variation in these movements in different people. Some cannot dorsiflex beyond a right angle, especially women who wear high heels much of the time. These persons feel muscle

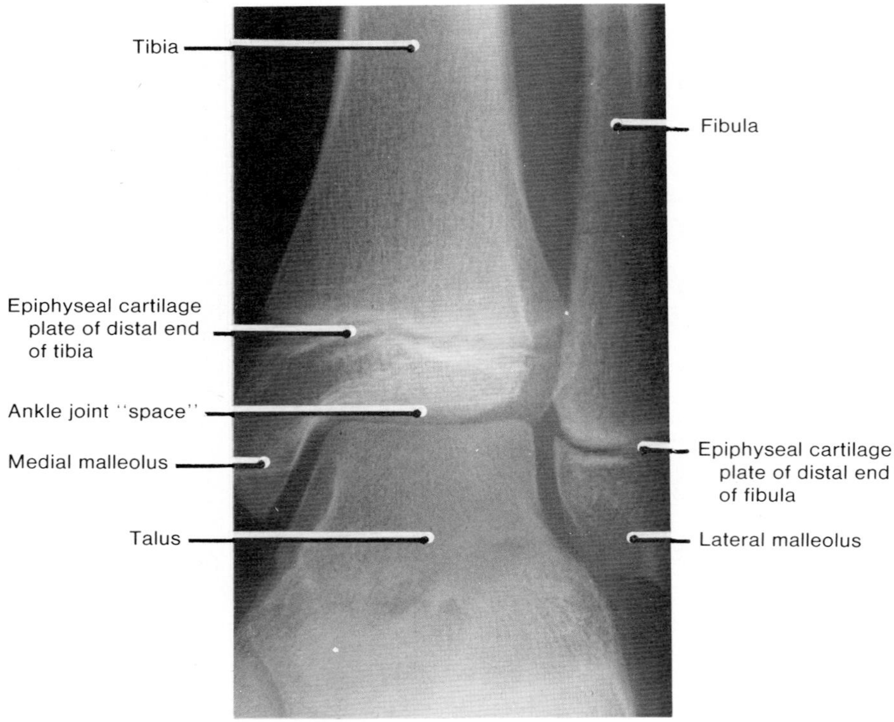

Figure 4–142. A slightly oblique frontal radiograph of the ankle joint of a 14-year-old boy showing how the talus fits into the mortise formed by the medial and lateral malleoli. After fracture and/or dislocation, it is essential to reduce the displaced fragments so that the normal mortise is regained; failure to do so will result in a painful ankle. The radiolucent lines crossing the tibia and fibula near their ends are the epiphyseal cartilage plates separating the primary ossification centers (diaphyses) from the secondary ossification centers (epiphyses). The "spaces" between the talus and the malleoli represent the radiolucent articular cartilages.

strain (calf pain) when they switch from high-heeled to low-heeled shoes.

A bony outgrowth commonly develops on the anterior aspect of the distal end of the tibia and the superior surface of the neck of the talus in persons who repeatedly kick a football or soccer ball. The plantarflexion, associated with kicking a ball, pulls the attachments of the anterior tibiotalar ligament, inducing such a characteristic bony outgrowth on these bones that the condition is commonly called a **footballer's (soccer player's) ankle**.

The Articular Capsule (Figs. 4-139 and 4-140). The *fibrous capsule* surrounding the ankle joint is thin anteriorly and posteriorly but is supported on each side by strong collateral ligaments. It is attached superiorly to the borders of the articular surfaces of the tibia and the malleoli and inferiorly to the talus close to the trochlear articular surface (Fig. 4-141), except anteroinferiorly, where it is attached to the dorsum of the neck of the talus (Fig. 4-143). The fibrous capsule is strengthened medially and laterally by two strong **collateral ligaments** (deltoid and lateral ligaments). The attachments and functions of these ligaments are clinically important.

The Deltoid Ligament (Fig. 4-143). This **strong medial ligament** *attaches the medial malleolus to the tarsus.* Its apex is attached to the margins and the tip of the **medial malleolus** and its broad base fans out to attach to **three tarsal bones**: the talus, the navicular, and the calcaneus.

The deltoid ligament is composed of four parts which are named according to their bony attachments: **tibionavicular, tibiotalar** (anterior and posterior), and **tibiocalcaneal ligaments**. Part of the deltoid ligament also attaches to the **calcaneonavicular (spring) ligament** (Fig. 4-143).

The deltoid ligament strengthens the ankle joint and holds the calcaneus and navicular bones against the talus. In addition, by supporting the spring ligament, it helps to maintain the medial side of the foot and the medial longitudinal arch (Fig. 4-151).

CLINICALLY ORIENTED COMMENTS

Medial dislocations of the ankle joint are not very common owing to the strength of the deltoid ligament (Fig. 4-143). In **fracture-dislocations of the ankle joint**, the distal end of the tibia and/or the fibula is usually fractured. The common **Pott's fracture** occurs when the foot is forceably everted (Fig. 4-159); this pulls on the extremely strong **deltoid ligament**, often tearing off the medial malleolus, allowing the talus to move laterally, and shearing off the lateral malleolus or, more commonly, breaking the fibula above the distal tibiofibular joint. If the tibia is carried forward, the posterior margin of the distal end of the tibia is sheared off by the talus.

The Lateral Ligament (Figs. 4-139 and 4-140). This ligament *attaches the lateral malleolus to the tarsus*; it is not nearly so strong as the deltoid ligament. It consists of three parts (*anterior and posterior talofibular and calcaneofibular ligaments*); sometimes these components are referred to as the lateral ligaments.

The **anterior talofibular ligament**

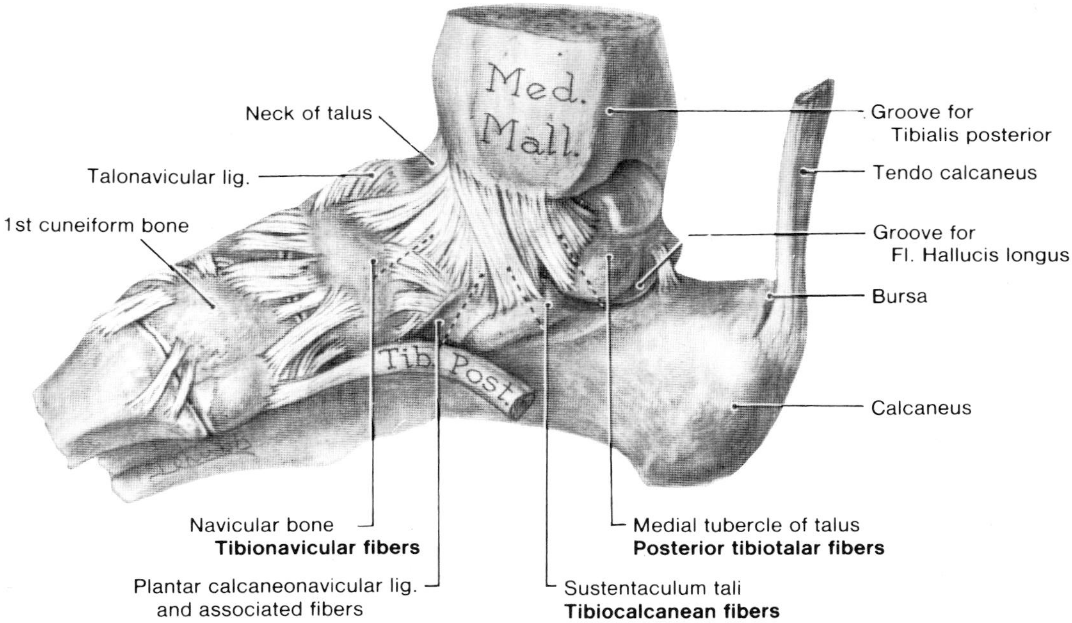

Figure 4–143. Drawing of a dissection of the right ankle joint and the tarsal joints from the medial side showing the ligaments. Observe the parts of the extremely strong deltoid ligament (*bold-face type*); another part (the anterior tibiotalar ligament) is not visible here. Note that the deltoid ligament radiates from the lower border of the medial malleolus and inserts into three foot bones. Observe that the deltoid ligament is also attached to the medial side of the plantar calcaneonavicular ligament. The deltoid ligament is so strong that instead of rupturing when the foot is strongly everted, it often avulses the tip of the medial malleolus (Fig. 4–159).

(Figs. 4-82, 4-139, and 4-140) extends medially from the lateral malleolus to the neck of the talus. It is not very strong.

The **posterior talofibular ligament** (Fig. 4-140) is thick and fairly strong. It runs horizontally medially and slightly backward from the fossa of the lateral malleolus to the lateral tubercle of the posterior process of the talus.

The **calcaneofibular ligament** (Figs. 4-139 and 4-140) is a round cord that passes posteroinferiorly from the tip of the lateral malleolus to the lateral surface of the calcaneus. This ligament is separated from the articular capsule of the ankle joint by fatty tissue and is crossed superficially by the tendons of the peroneus longus and brevis muscles (Fig. 4-82).

CLINICALLY ORIENTED COMMENTS

In adults the ankle is the most frequently injured major joint in the body. The lateral ligament of the ankle joint is the one most frequently injured in traumatic injuries of the ankle joint; one or more of its three parts may be torn (Fig. 4-158).

The usual **sprained ankle** results from twisting of the weight-bearing foot and is nearly always an **inversion injury**. The typical history is as follows:

1. The person steps on an uneven surface and falls.
2. This causes stretching of most and tearing of some fibers of the lateral ligament.
3. The ankle is soon painful and localized swelling and tenderness appear anteroinferior to the tip of the lateral malleolus.

In **severe sprains** some fibers are torn, either partially or completely, resulting in instability of the ankle joint. Unless the foot is held in the everted position until the torn ligaments heal, a fracture-dislocation of the ankle may occur if the ankle is severely inverted again (Case 4-5).

The synovial capsule (Fig. 4-140) lines the fibrous capsule of the joint and projects superiorly between the tibia and the fibula for a short distance.

CLINICALLY ORIENTED COMMENTS

The synovial cavity of the ankle joint is somewhat superficial on each side of the tendo calcaneus (Fig. 4-140); hence, when the ankle joint is inflamed (*e.g.,* owing to **arthritis**) the synovial fluid may increase, causing swelling in these locations.

Stability of the Joint (Figs. 4-77 and 4-139). The ankle joint is **very strong**, particularly in dorsiflexion, because it is supported by powerful ligaments and is crossed by several tendons that are tightly bound down by thickenings of the deep fascia (retinacula). Its stability is greatest in dorsiflexion, because in this position the trochlea of the talus fills the **mortise** formed by the malleoli (Fig. 4-142). The malleoli grip the talus tightly as it rocks backward and forward during movements of the ankle joint. *The grip of the malleoli is strongest during dorsiflexion* because this movement forces the anterior part of the trochlea of the talus posteriorly, spreading the tibia and fibula slightly apart. This spreading is limited by the strong interosseous ligament and the anterior and posterior tibiofibular ligaments that unite the leg bones (Figs. 4-67*B* and 4-140).

In plantarflexion the trochlea of the talus moves forward in the mortise and the malleoli come together. However, their grip on the trochlea is not so strong as during dorsiflexion and some side movement can be demonstrated in full plantarflexion. The wedge-shaped form of the trochlea in the mortise assists the ligaments in preventing posterior displacement of the foot when jumping and stopping suddenly.

In most people the joint is very unstable in plantarflexion. Appropriate training and conditioning may strengthen the joint in this position (e.g., as occurs in ballet dancers and persons who wear shoes with high heels).

CLINICALLY ORIENTED COMMENTS

As inversion of the foot tends to occur with active plantarflexion, **inversion injuries** of the ankle tend to occur more often than do eversion injuries when the foot is in this position. When one or more of the three components of the lateral ligament are stretched or torn, the ankle becomes very unstable. In severe injuries, a **fracture-dislocation** occurs in which the tip of the lateral malleolus is avulsed (Fig. 4-158). This injury often occurs when the foot is fixed against some object (*e.g.,* a large stone) and is thrown into an inverted position. Consequently, the body weight is violently transferred to the lateral ligament of the ankle. Usually the **calcaneofibular ligament** tears, partially or completely, often along with the anterior talofibular ligament. As the latter ligament is fused with the fibrous capsule of the ankle joint, this membrane may also be torn.

As the peroneus brevis muscle tends to prevent overinversion of the foot (Fig. 4-77), thereby aiding the lateral ligament, violent eversion of the foot may also result in **avulsion of the tuberosity of the fifth metatarsal bone,** into which the tendon of this muscle inserts. For this reason, radiologists routinely ensure that this bone is visible in radiographs of persons referred to them because of ankle injuries.

Blood supply (Figs. 4-34, 4-81, and 4-107). The articular arteries are derived from the four malleolar branches of the **peroneal** and anterior and posterior **tibial** arteries.

Nerve Supply (Figs. 4-80 and 4-93). The articular nerves are derived from the **tibial** nerve and the lateral branch of the **deep peroneal** nerve.

JOINTS OF THE FOOT

There are many joints in the foot involving the tarsal and metatarsal bones and the phalanges.

The Intertarsal Joints (Figs. 4-139 and 4-144 to 4-146). Only the large and clinically important intertarsal joints are described. The other joints are relatively small and are so tightly joined by ligaments that only slight movement occurs between them. All the bones are united by **dorsal** and **plantar ligaments** (Figs. 4-139 and 4-146). These small joints are named according to the bones involved (*e.g.,* cuneocuboid and cuneonavicular joints).

The Subtalar Joint (Figs. 4-139, 4-144, and 4-145). This joint, sometimes called the *talocalcanean joint,* is distal to the ankle joint. It is located where the talus rests on

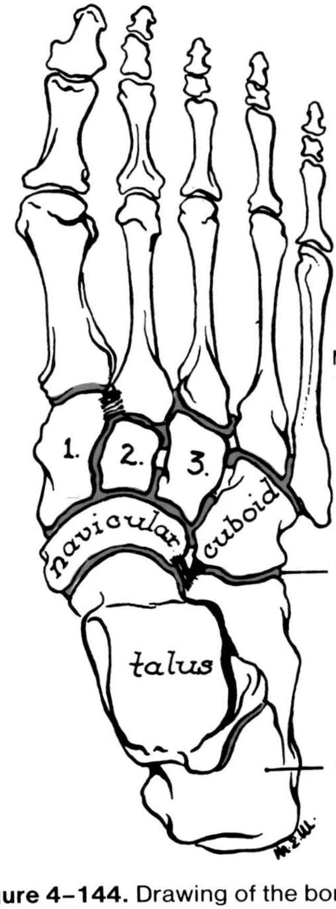

Figure 4–144. Drawing of the bones of the right foot showing the six separate joint cavities (*red*). The transverse tarsal joint is the articular plane that extends from side to side across the foot; it is composed of the talonavicular joint medially and the calcaneocuboid joint laterally. Although anatomically separate, these joints act together during movements of the foot.

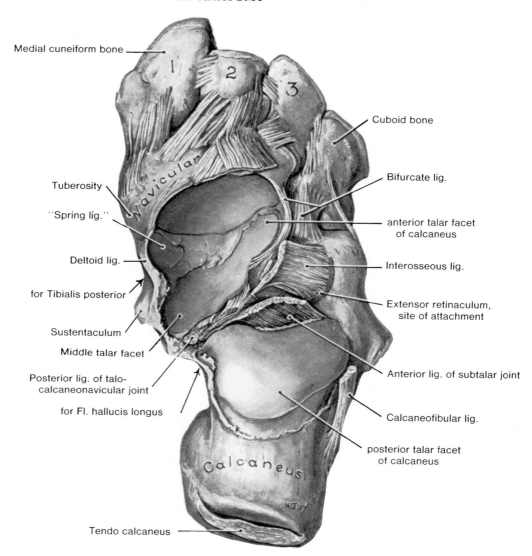

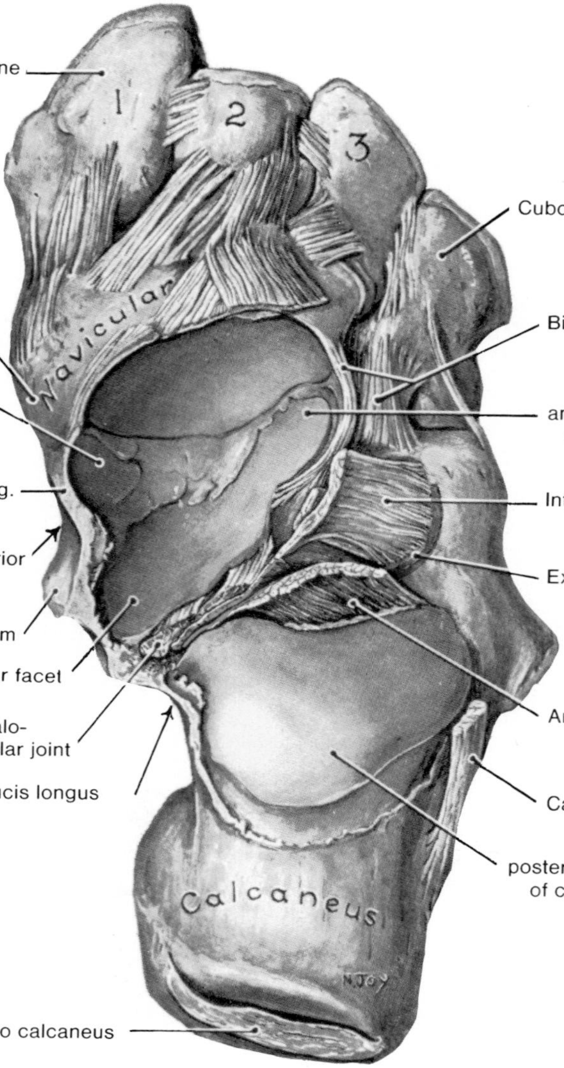

Figure 4–145. Drawing of a dissection of the right foot showing the joints of inversion and eversion. This specimen was prepared by sawing through the body of the talus and, after discarding it, nibbling away the neck and head of the talus. Observe the convex posterior talar facet separated from the concave middle and anterior facets by the ligamentous structures within the tarsal sinus. At the wide lateral end of this sinus note the strong interosseous talocalcanean ligament and the extensor retinaculum (*in blue*) which extends medially between the posterior ligament of the anterior talocalcanean joint and the anterior ligament of the posterior talocalcanean or subtalar joint. Observe that the subtalar joint has a synovial cavity to itself, whereas the talonavicular joint and the anterior talocalcanean joint share a common synovial cavity; hence, the collective name, talocalcaneonavicular joint. Note that the angular space between the navicular bone and the middle talar facet on the sustenaculum tali is bridged by the plantar calcaneonavicular (spring) ligament, the central part of which is fibrocartilaginous. Observe that the socket for the head of the talus is deepened medially by the part of the deltoid ligament that is attached to the spring ligament (Fig. 4–143) and laterally by the calcaneonavicular part of the bifurcate ligament.

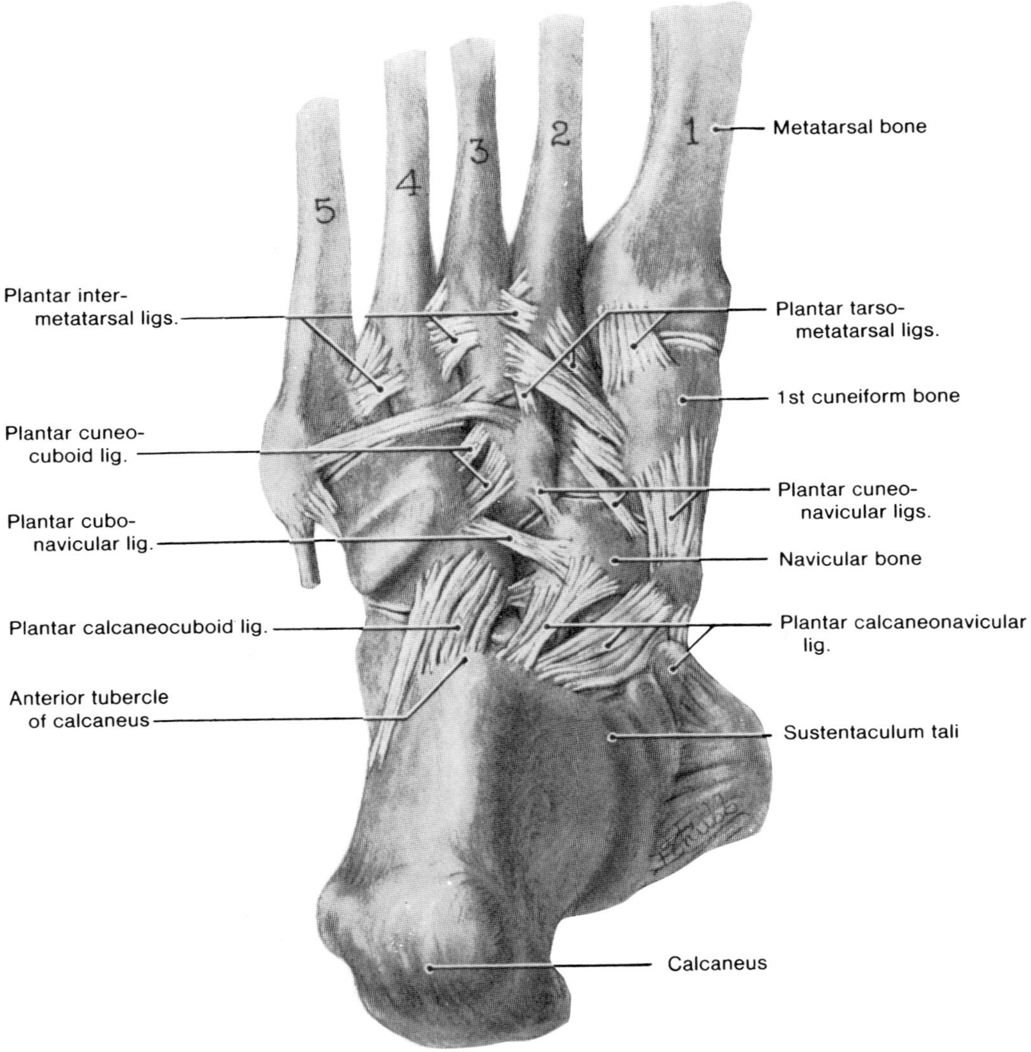

Figure 4–146. Drawing of a dissection of the plantar ligaments of the right foot. Observe that the plantar calcaneocuboid (short plantar) ligament and the plantar calcaneonavicular (spring) ligament are the inferior ligaments of the transverse tarsal joint. Having a common purpose, they have a common direction. Note that the ligaments in the forepart of the foot diverge backward from each side of the long axis of the third metatarsal and third cuneiform bones. Hence, a backward thrust to the first metatarsal (*e.g.*, when rising on the great toe in walking) is transmitted directly to the navicular and the talus by the first cuneiform and indirectly by the second metatarsal and second cuneiform and also by the third metatarsal and third cuneiform. A backward thrust to the fourth and fifth metatarsals is transmitted directly to the cuboid and calcaneus. These four bones (*i.e.*, the bones of the lateral longitudinal arch of the foot) are not displaced backward because of the adjoining ligaments.

and articulates with the calcaneus. It is a **gliding type of synovial joint** between the inferior surface of the body of the talus and the superior surface of the calcaneus. It is surrounded by an articular capsule which is attached near the margins of the articular facets. The fibrous capsule is supported by medial, lateral, and posterior **ta-**

localcaneal ligaments; in addition, the joint is supported anteriorly by the **interosseous talocalcanean ligament**.

Movements of the subtalar joint result in **inversion** (Fig. 4-75*D*) and **eversion** (Fig. 4-75*C*) of the foot. These movements are closely associated with those at the talocalcaneonavicular and calcaneocuboid joints.

The Talocalcaneonavicular Joint (Figs. 4-68, 4-72, 4-139, and 4-143 to 4-145). This joint is located where the head of the talus articulates with the head of the posterior surface of the navicular bone, the superior surface of the plantar calcaneonavicular ligament, the sustentaculum tali, and the articular surface of the calcaneus. The head of the talus has three facets, one for the navicular and two for articulation with the calcaneus. These articular surfaces are surrounded by a single articular capsule which blends with the interosseous talocalcaneal ligament posteriorly. It is reinforced dorsally by the dorsal talonavicular ligament, a broad band connecting the neck of the talus and the dorsal surface of the navicular bone.

The thick, fibroelastic **plantar calcaneonavicular (spring) ligament** is a triangular sheet that extends from the *sustentaculum tali* to the posteroinferior surface of the *navicular bone* and blends with the deltoid ligament medially. It forms part of the socket for the head of the talus and plays an important role in maintaining the longitudinal arch of the foot (Fig. 4-151).

The Calcaneocuboid Joint (Figs. 4-68, 4-72, 4-139, 4-144, and 4-145). This joint is between the anterior surface of the **calcaneus** and the posterior surface of the **cuboid**. The articular capsule of the joint is strengthened by the calcaneocuboid (lateral part of *bifurcate ligament,* Fig. 4-145) and plantar calcaneocuboid ligaments and is supported by the long plantar ligament. Its joint cavity does not communicate with that of any other joint.

The strong, **long plantar ligament** passes from the plantar surface of the calcaneus, including the anterior tubercle, to both lips of the groove on the cuboid bone (Fig. 4-147). Some of its fibers extend to the bases of the second, third, and fourth metatarsal bones, thereby forming a tunnel for the tendon of the peroneus longus muscle that passes through the groove in the cuboid bone to insert into the base of the first metatarsal and the adjoining part of the medial cuneiform bone (Fig. 4-69). The long plantar ligament is *important in maintaining the arches of the foot* (Fig. 4-151).

The wide **plantar calcaneocuboid (short plantar) ligament** is deep to the long plantar ligament (Figs. 4-146 and 4-147). It extends between the anterior aspect of the inferior surface of the calcaneus and the inferior surface of the cuboid just posterior to its ridge.

The Transverse Tarsal Joint (Figs. 4-70, 4-139, and 4-144). Although the talonavicular and calcaneocuboid joints are separate from each other, they extend right across the tarsus and lie in almost the same transverse plane. As they are **important in inversion and eversion** of the foot, the two joints are often referred to collectively as the transverse tarsal (midtarsal) joint. Understand that anatomically these joints are separate, but functionally they act together.

Movements of the Joints. During dorsiflexion and plantarflexion of the ankle joint, the body of the talus glides on a transverse axis in the mortise formed by the malleoli. In addition, the tarsus and metatarsus move as a unit. Movements occurring at the tarsal joints produce inversion and eversion of the foot (Fig. 4-75*C* and *D*).

The joints of inversion and eversion (Figs. 4-139 and 4-145) are (1) the subtalar (posterior talocalcanean) joint; (2) the talocalcaneonavicular (*i.e.,* combined anterior talocalcanean and talonavicular) joint; and (3) the transverse tarsal (*i.e.,* combined calcaneocuboid and talonavicular) joint. Hence, the talonavicular joint is involved twice.

In inversion the foot is adducted and directed so that the medial border is raised and the lateral border is depressed; thus, the sole is turned toward the median plane (Figs. 4-75*D* and 4-96).

In eversion the foot is abducted and directed so that the lateral border is raised and the medial border lowered; thus, the sole is turned away from the median plane (Fig. 4-75*C*).

Inversion and eversion occur during

walking on rough ground in adjusting the foot to stones or depressions. The strong **deltoid ligament** tends to prevent overeversion of the foot and the weaker **lateral ligament** (with the assistance of the peroneus longus and brevis muscles) tends to prevent overinversion of the foot. Consequently, inversion injuries of the foot are much more common than eversion injuries.

The Tarsometatarsal Joints (Figs. 4-68, 4-139, and 4-144 to 4-148). These articulations are the **plane type of synovial joint** which permit only gliding or sliding movements. In Figure 4-148 note that the four anterior tarsal bones articulate with the bases of the metatarsal bones. The metatarsal bones are very firmly attached to the tarsal bones by dorsal, plantar, and interosseous ligaments. *There are three separate tarsometatarsal joint cavities.*

The first or **medial tarsometatarsal joint** occurs between the medial cuneiform bone and the base of the first metatarsal bone. It has more range of movement than the other two joints.

The second or **intermediate tarsometatarsal joint** is between all three cuneiform bones and the second and third metatarsal bones. In Figure 4-144 observe that the base of the second metatarsal bone fits into a socket or mortise formed by the cuneiform bones; thus, it is the *strongest of the three tarsometatarsal joints.* As the second metatarsal is also firmly attached to the cuneiform bones, it has little independent movement. The cavity of this joint is continuous with that between the two medial cuneiform bones and through it with the synovial cavity of the cuneonavicular joint.

The third or **lateral tarsometatarsal joint** occurs between the cuboid bone and the fourth and fifth metatarsal bones. There is more movement permitted at this joint than at the second joint but not so much as at the first joint.

CLINICALLY ORIENTED COMMENTS

Because the second metatarsal bone has little movement at the second tarsometatarsal joint, it is particularly liable to fracture when sudden, unaccustomed stresses are applied to the distal part of the foot. When a person who is "out of condition" begins to participate in exercise programs, long walks, track and field activities, or ballet dancing a **stress fracture** (fatigue fracture) may occur in one of the weight-bearing bones. Stress fractures in the metatarsals are usually referred to as "**march fractures.**"

Resections of part of the foot (**amputations**) may be necessary following trauma (*e.g.,* crush injuries) or in cases of cancer, arteriosclerosis, or peripheral vascular diseases of the foot. In one type, the *Lisfranc amputation,* the foot is resected through the tarsometatarsal joints. In another, the *Syme amputation,* the foot is resected through the midtarsal joint.

The Intermetatarsal Joints (Figs. 4-68, 4-144, 4-146, and 4-147). These articulations between the bases of the metatarsal bones are the **plane type of synovial joint** which permit a slight gliding movement. Their joint cavities are extensions from the tarsometatarsal joints.

The bases of the second to fifth metatarsal bones are very firmly bound together by dorsal, plantar, and interosseous ligaments. A **deep transverse metatarsal ligament** connects indirectly the heads of the metatarsal bones (Fig. 4-102) and, with the interosseous ligaments, helps to maintain the transverse arch of the foot. Owing to the tight binding of the bases of the metatarsal bones, little individual movement of the metatarsals is possible.

The Metatarsophalangeal Joints (Figs. 4-68 to 4-72 and 4-144). These articulations are between the heads of the metatarsal bones and the bases of the proximal phalanges. They are the **condyloid (knuckle-like) type of synovial joint** which permit flexion, extension, and some abduction, adduction, and circumduction.

The **first metatarsophalangeal joint** is by far the largest owing to the size of the head of the first metatarsal bone and the presence of the sesamoid bones in the two tendons of the flexor hallucis brevis muscle (Fig. 4-104).

An **articular capsule** surrounds each joint and is attached near the margins of the articular surfaces. In Figure 4-68 note that the articular surfaces pass well onto the dorsal surfaces of the metatarsal bones. This part of the articular surface of the first metatarsophalangeal joint is particularly large and is related to its dorsiflexion during walking.

The **fibrous capsules** of these joints are

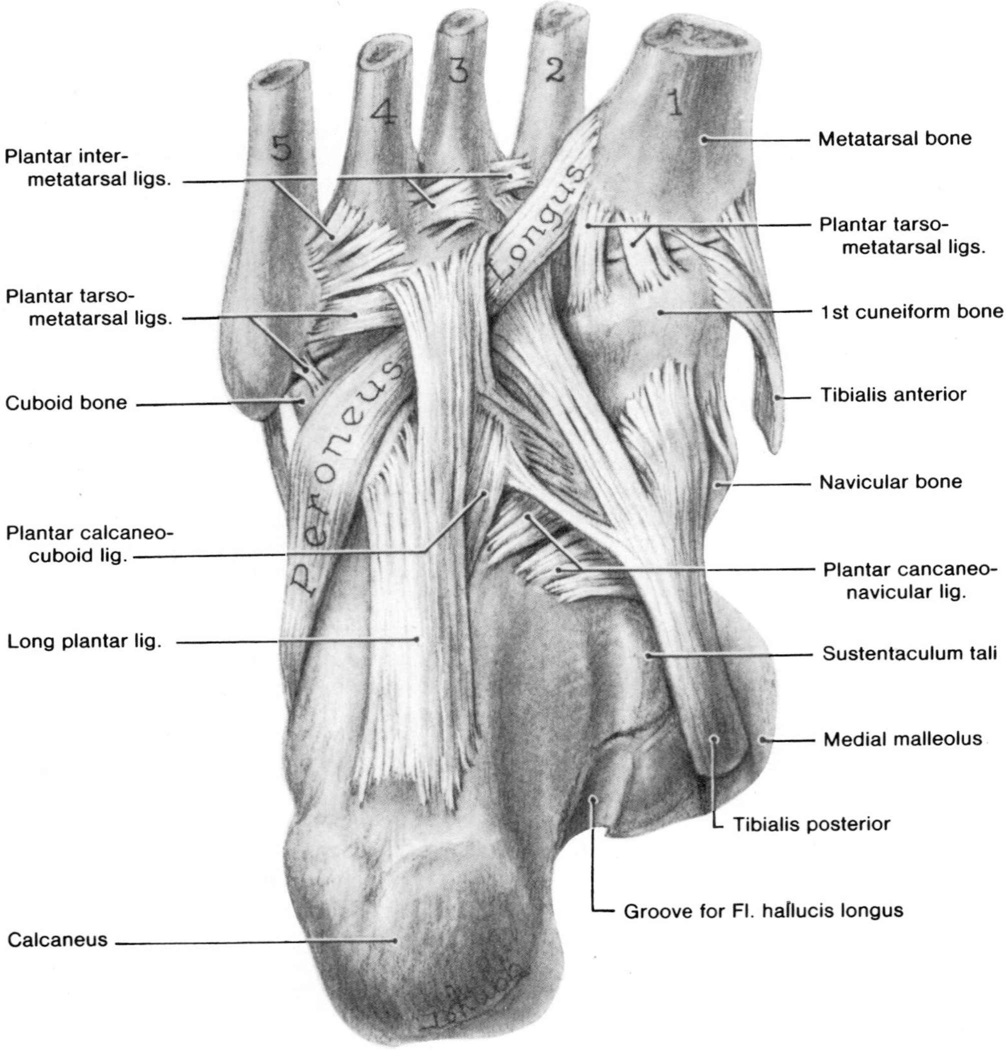

Figure 4–147. Drawing of a dissection of the sole of the right foot showing the plantar ligaments and the insertion of three long tendons (peroneus longus, tibialis anterior, and tibialis posterior). Observe the tendon of the peroneus longus crossing the sole of the foot in the groove anterior to the ridge of the cuboid which is bridged by some fibers of the long plantar ligament. Note that the tendon of the peroneus longus is inserted into the base of the first metatarsal bone. Recall that it also inserts into the adjoining part of the medial cuneiform bone (Fig. 4–69) and that it is an evertor of the foot. Observe that slips of the tendon of the tibialis posterior muscle extend like the fingers of an open hand to grasp the bones anterior to the transverse tarsal joint (*i.e.*, the five small tarsal bones and several metatarsal bones). The tibialis posterior is an evertor of the foot.

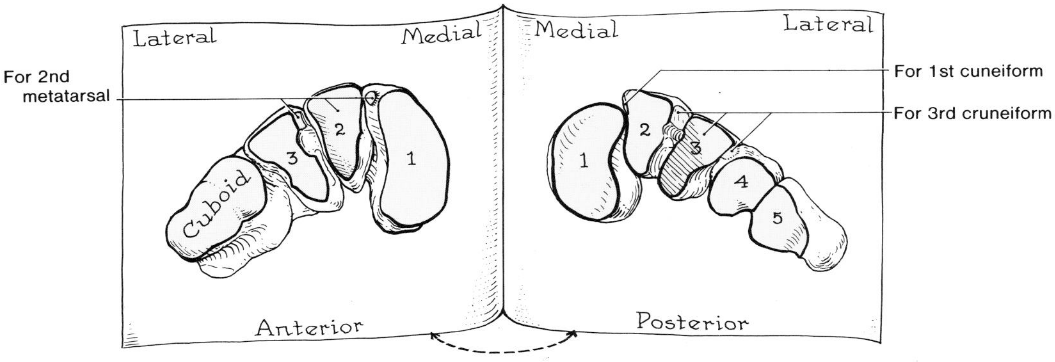

Figure 4–148. Drawing of the bony surfaces of the tarsometatarsal joints of the right foot. The anterior surfaces of the cuboid, the three cuneiform bones, and the posterior surfaces of the bases of the five metatarsal bones are displayed like the pages of a book. Note that the bases of the first three metatarsal bones articulate with the three cuneiform bones and that the bases of the fourth and fifth metacarpals articulate with the cuboid bone. Observe that the bones generally are wedge-shaped; this bony shape helps to maintain the transverse arch of the foot.

strengthened on each side by thick, triangular, collateral ligaments. The plantar part of the capsule is greatly thickened to form the **plantar ligament** (Fig. 4-102). This is a fibrocartilaginous plate that is firmly attached to the proximal plantar border of the phalanx and forms part of the socket for the head of the first metatarsal. The margins of the plantar ligament give attachment to the fibrous flexor sheath, slips of the plantar aponeurosis, and the deep transverse metatarsal ligaments.

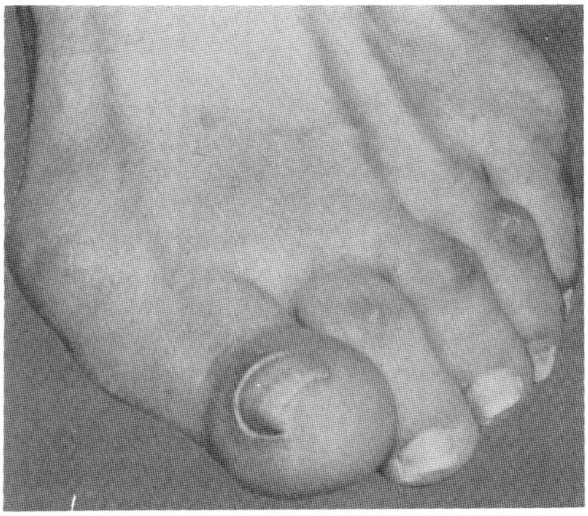

Figure 4–149. Photograph of the left foot of a woman showing the hallux valgus deformity and a localized swelling (bunion) on the medial aspect of her first metatarsophalangeal joint. A bunion is a type of friction bursitis. Note also the corns caused by pressure on the skin by the patient's shoe over the underlying proximal interphalangeal joints of toes 2 to 4. Observe the tendons of the extensor hallucis longus and the extensor digitorum longus. The "clawing" position of the lateral four toes and the resulting corns are caused by shortening of their extensor tendons.

CLINICALLY ORIENTED COMMENTS

The first metatarsophalangeal joint is often enlarged and deformed with permanent lateral displacement of the great toe (L. *hallux*). This adduction condition, known as **hallux valgus** (Fig. 4-149), is common in persons who wear pointed shoes. They are unable to move their great toe away from the second toe because the sesamoids under the head of the first metatarsal bone are usually displaced and lie in the space between the heads of the first and second metatarsal bones.

Gout, a metabolic disorder, is characterized by *urate deposits* in connective tissue, including cartilage and bone. This condition commonly affects the first metatarsophalangeal joint, which becomes swollen and painful, a condition referred to as *gouty arthritis.*

Degenerative joint disease (osteoar-

thritis) is also common in the metatarsophalangeal joint of the great toe. When this painful condition is present without deformity, it is known as **hallux rigidus**.

The Interphalangeal Joints (Figs. 4-68 and 4-69). The interphalangeal joints are between the head of one phalanx and the base of the more distal one. They are the **hinge type of synovial joint** permitting only flexion and extension. In most people the lateral four toes are, to a varying degree, partially flexed at the interphalangeal joints.

CLINICALLY ORIENTED COMMENTS

Hammer toe is a common deformity in which the proximal phalanx is permanently dorsiflexed at the metatarsophalangeal joint and the middle phalanx is plantarflexed at the interphalangeal joint. The distal phalanx is also flexed or extended, giving the toe (usually the second) a **hammer-like appearance**. This deformity may result from weakness of the lumbrical and interosseus muscles (Fig. 4-90), which flex the metatarsophalangeal joints and extend the interphalangeal joints.

The Arches of the Foot (Figs. 4-150 and 4-151). The bones of the foot are arranged in longitudinal and transverse arches that are designed as **shock absorbers** for supporting the weight of the body in the erect posture and for propelling it during movement (*e.g.,* walking). Consequently, *the design of the foot makes it adaptable to changes in surface and weight.* The resilient arches of the foot provide it with this adaptability. The weight of the body is first transmitted to the talus from the tibia and the fibula (Fig. 4-142). It is then transmitted posteroinferiorly to the calcaneus or anteroinferiorly to the heads of the metatarsal bones (Figs. 4-72 and 4-150).

Body weight is divided about equally be-

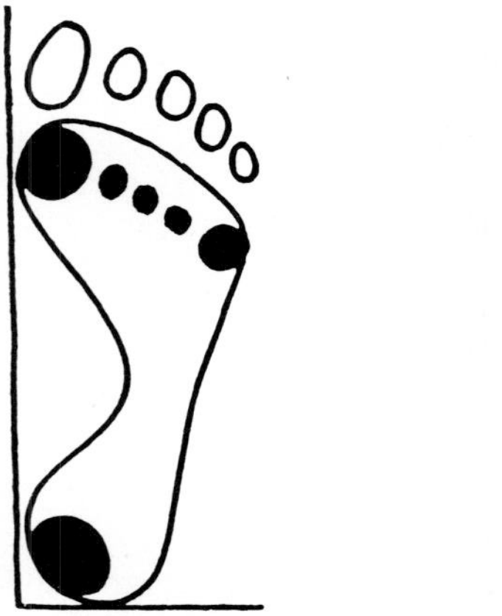

Figure 4–150. Diagram illustrating the weight-bearing points of the right foot. Body weight is divided about equally between the calcaneus and the heads of the metatarsals. The forepart of the foot has six points of contact with the ground: two with the sesamoid bones under the head of the first metatarsal and four with the heads of the lateral four metatarsals. Hence the first metatarsal supports a double load.

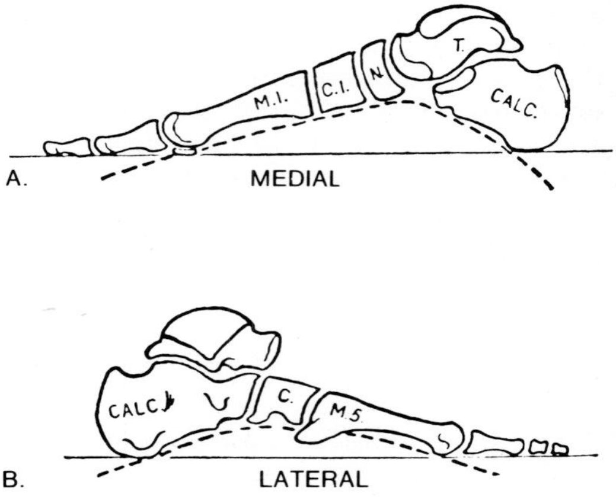

Figure 4–151. Drawings of the medial and lateral longitudinal arches of the right foot. Observe that the foot is arched longitudinally and that the posterior pillar of both arches is the calcaneus. Note that from the medial side the longitudinal arch is high, whereas from the lateral side it is low. This explains the appearance of the footprints of persons with normal feet (Fig. 4–150) and flatfeet (*i.e.,* flattened medial longitudinal arch). The arches act somewhat like springs (*i.e.,* normally they give a little but not completely). The bearing points illustrated in Figure 4–150 indicate the ends of the longitudinal arches.

tween the calcaneus and the heads of the metatarsal bones. Between these weight-bearing points are the arches of the foot, which are formed by the tarsal and metatarsal bones. The relatively elastic arches, convex superiorly and disposed both longitudinally and transversely, become slightly flattened by the body weight (*e.g.,* during standing), but they normally resume their curvature when the pressure is removed. There are two arches, longitudinal and transverse.

The Longitudinal Arch (Fig. 4-151). For purposes of description, the longitudinal arch is often regarded as being composed of two parts, medial and lateral. The medial longitudinal arch is higher and more important. Functionally, both parts of the longitudinal arch act as a unit with the transverse arch, through which the weight is spread out in all directions.

The **medial longitudinal arch** is composed of the calcaneus, the talus, the navicular, the three cuneiforms, and the three medial metatarsal bones (Figs. 4-70, 4-72, and 4-151*A*). The two sesamoid bones in the tendons of the flexor hallucis brevis muscle act as a "footstool" for the first metatarsal bone, giving it increased height (Fig. 4-104). The **head of the talus**, located at the summit of the arch and therefore the "*keystone,*" receives the weight of the body. At the articular surfaces between the talus and the navicular and also between the navicular and the three cuneiforms, the medial arch yields slightly when weight is put on it and recoils when it is removed.

The **lateral longitudinal arch** rests on the ground during standing; hence, the usual footprint (Fig. 4-150). It is composed of the calcaneus, the cuboid, and the lateral two metatarsal bones (Figs. 4-71 and 4-151*B*). It yields slightly at the hinge surfaces between the cuboid and the lateral two metatarsal bones when weight is put on it and recoils when weight is removed.

The Transverse Arch (Fig. 4-148). This arch runs from side to side of the foot. It is formed by the cuboid, the three cuneiforms, and the bases of the metatarsal bones. The medial and lateral longitudinal arches serve as pillars for the transverse arch. The peroneus longus muscle (Fig. 4-147) helps to maintain the transverse curvature of the transverse arch.

Maintenance of the Arches (Figs. 4-146 to 4-151). The integrity of the bony arches of the foot is maintained by (1) the **shape of the interlocking bones** (i.e., at the joints); (2) the **strength of the ligaments** and the **plantar aponeurosis** (Fig. 4-97); and (3) by the **action of muscles** (intrinsic and extrinsic) through the bracing action of their tendons.

Of these three factors the plantar ligaments and the plantar aponeurosis bear the greatest stress and are most important in maintaining the arches while standing quietly. **Electromyographic studies** indicate that the muscles are relatively inactive until walking begins. The invertor and evertor muscles of the foot appear to control the weight distribution of the foot (*e.g.,* when walking on rough ground).

The maintenance of the arches is also dependent on the intertarsal, tarsometatarsal, and intermetatarsal joints, because at these articulations the bones are bound together as parts of the arches of the foot. The plantar ligaments of these joints are the strongest and they are supported by robust interosseous ligaments.

The following fibrous structures, *listed in order of importance,* are essential for maintaining the arches of the foot.

1. **The plantar calcaneonavicular ligament** (Figs. 4-143, 4-146, and 4-147) is the **most important ligament in the foot** because it is the *main supporter of the medial longitudinal arch*; its principal attachments are the sustentaculum tali and the tuberosity of the navicular bone. This strong fibrocartilaginous band, acting as a tie between the calcaneus and navicular bones, prevents collapse of the arch formed by the three bones (*i.e.,* calcaneus, talus, and navicular, Fig. 4-70). Because of the resilience this medial ligament gives to the medial longitudinal arch when it is stressed, it is commonly called "**the spring ligament.**" It is supported by the tendon of the tibialis posterior muscle and by the deltoid ligament.
2. **The long plantar ligament** (Fig. 4-

147) is the next most important ligament in the foot; its principal attachments are the tubercle of the calcaneus and the plantar surface of the cuboid bone. It is longer and more superficial than the spring ligament and stretches like a tie beam under nearly the whole length of the lateral longitudinal arch; thus, it *provides the main support for the lateral longitudinal arch.*

3. **The plantar aponeurosis**, part of the plantar fascia (Fig. 4-97), is very strong and also acts as a *strong tie beam for the maintenance of the longitudinal arches.* One part of it, a dense fibrous band known as the **calcaneometatarsal ligament**, extends from the lateral process of the tuberosity of the calcaneus to the tuberosity of the fifth metatarsal bone. It is particularly important in helping the long plantar ligament to maintain the lateral longitudinal arch. The medial part of the plantar aponeurosis, through its attachment to the sesamoid bones ofthe flexor hallucis brevis (Figs. 4-97 and 4-100), is important in strengthening the medial longitudinal arch during standing on the toes.
4. **The plantar calcaneocuboid ligament** (short plantar ligament) is broader than the long plantar ligament (Figs. 4-146 and 4-147); its main attachments are the anterior end of the calcaneus and the proximal edge of the cuboid bone. This ligament aids the plantar calcaneonavicular and long plantar ligaments in supporting the longitudinal arches. In Figure 4-147 note that the peroneus longus tendon forms a sling beneath the lateral part of the longitudinal arch and acts as a tie beam for the transverse arch.

CLINICALLY ORIENTED COMMENTS

Flatfoot (pes planus) is a common condition that sometimes causes pain. In infants the flat appearance of the feet is normal and results from the subcutaneous fat pads in the soles of their feet. The condition persists for a variable time after the infant begins to walk, sometimes as long as 2 years.

Flatfeet in adolescents and adults are caused by "**fallen arches**," usually the medial longitudinal arches. During standing the plantar ligaments and the plantar aponeurosis are important in maintaining the arches of the foot, and they stretch somewhat under the body weight. If these *ligaments become abnormally stretched during long periods of standing,* the plantar calcaneonavicular (spring) ligament can no longer adequately support the head of the talus and, as a result, some flattening of the medial longitudinal arch occurs. There is concomitant lateral deviation of the forefoot.

In the **common type of flatfoot**, the foot resumes its arched form when the weight is removed from it. Flatfeet are common in older persons, particularly if they undertake much unaccustomed standing or if they gain weight rapidly, because of the added stress on the muscles and the increased strain on the ligaments.

Flattening of the transverse arch of the foot may also occur. Frequently callus formation occurs under the heads of the lateral four metatarsal bones. This thickening of the skin is a protective measure where abnormal pressure is exerted.

PATIENT ORIENTED PROBLEMS

Case 4-1. While visiting your home, your elderly grandmother slipped on the polished floor in the front hall. As you approached her, she was lying on her back in severe pain. Her right lower limb immediately attracted your attention because it was laterally rotated and noticeably shorter than her other limb. She was unable to get up or to lift her leg off the floor, and when she attempted to do so, experienced considerable pain.

Fortunately you had spent a summer in the emergency department of the local hospital and realized the probable seriousness of your grandmother's injury. You asked your mother to call the doctor indicating that your grandmother may have a "fractured hip." In the meantime you made her comfortable on the floor, resisting your sister's demands that she be moved to her bed.

Problems. What bone was probably fractured? Name the common fracture site of this bone in elderly people, particularly women. Why is this bone so fragile in older persons? Explain anatomically why her injured limb was shorter than the other one. What are the anatomical reasons for the complications commonly associated with these fractures? *These problems are discussed on page 595.*

Case 4-2. A construction worker fell from a ladder and landed on a piece of wood that had a 4-inch spike protruding from it. The large nail deeply penetrated the superomedial quadrant of his left buttock (Fig. 4-152).

He was taken to the hospital, where the board with the spike in it was removed, the bleeding stopped, and the wound treated.

As he walked out of the examining room

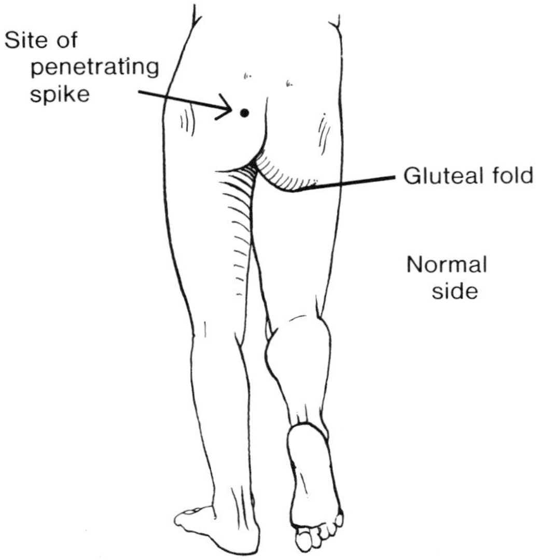

Figure 4–152. Drawing of the patient showing the place where the spike penetrated the left buttock. Observe the tilting of the pelvis to the right when the patient stands on the affected side. Also note the fallen gluteal fold on the right side.

in obvious pain, the doctor observed that he had a **distinct limp**. Each time he raised his right foot, his pelvis dropped to that side. During a subsequent examination, the doctor asked him to stand on his left leg with his other leg raised off the floor (Fig. 4-152). He observed that his gluteal fold and pelvis fell on the right side and concluded that there was a **severe nerve injury**. Sensation was normal in both lower limbs.

Problems. What peripheral nerve appears to have been injured when the man fell on the spike? What muscles were paralyzed? What is the anatomical basis for the patient's limp? What was the probable source of the bleeding? *These problems are discussed on page 596.*

Case 4-3. While playing in an old-timer's hockey game, a 45-year-old man was accidentally kicked with the point of a skate on the lateral surface of his right leg just below the knee. The **superficial wound** was treated by the trainer, but the man was unable to continue playing because of pain in the region of the laceration and some loss of power in his leg and foot. He also had numbness and tingling on the lateral surface of his leg and the dorsum of his foot. When he removed his skates, he found that he was unable to turn his right foot or toes upward (*i.e.,* dorsiflex them). He was advised to see his doctor forthwith.

As he walked into the examining room, the doctor observed that he had an **abnormal gait**, in that he raised his right foot higher than usual and brought it down suddenly, making a flapping noise. During the physical examination, the doctor detected tenderness over the neck region of the patient's fibula and a sensory deficit on the lateral side of the lower part of his leg, including the dorsum of his foot. Radiographs revealed a **fracture of the neck of the fibula**.

Problems. What is the anatomical basis of the loss of sensation and impaired function in the patient's foot? What nerve appears to have been severed? What is its relationship to the neck of the fibula? If the skate blade had not severed the nerve, what probably would have injured it if he had continued to play? What is the name given to the foot condition exhibited by the patient when he walked? *These problems are discussed on page 597.*

Case 4-4. While a 26-year-old worker was loading a heavy crate, it fell on his knee. He suffered severe pain and was unable to get up. The first aid team carried him to the doctor's office on a stretcher.

Following a physical examination, the doctor requested x-rays of the man's knee. The radiographs showed **comminuted fractures** of the proximal end of the shaft of the tibia and the neck of the fibula (Fig. 4-153).

Problems. What artery (arteries) might have been torn by the bone fragments? Using your anatomical knowledge, where would you check the patient's pulse to determine whether there has been damage to these arteries? What nerve may have been injured during fracture of the fibula? *These problems are discussed on page 597.*

Case 4-5. A 32-year-old man slipped on a patch of ice and fell. After he was helped up, he was unable to bear weight on his right foot and noticed that his ankle was beginning to swell. He hailed a cab and went to the hospital for treatment of what he thought was a badly "**sprained ankle**."

On examination it was found that the patient could barely move his ankle because of pain. Maximum tenderness was located over the lateral malleolus, about 2 cm proximal to its tip. Radiographs of the ankle revealed a transverse **fracture of the lateral malleolus** at the level of the superior articular surface of the talus.

Problems. What abnormal movement usually results in a sprained ankle? Discuss what is meant by the term "sprain." Explain anatomically how this fracture probably occurred. What structures were probably torn or ruptured? Is this what is usually referred to as a Pott's fracture? *These problems are discussed on page 598.*

Case 4-6. A 22-year-old woman was a front seat passenger in a car that was involved in a **head-on collision**. Although she sustained head injuries, her chief complaint was a **sore right hip** which prevented her from standing up. Believing that she might have broken her hip, she was rushed to the nearest hospital.

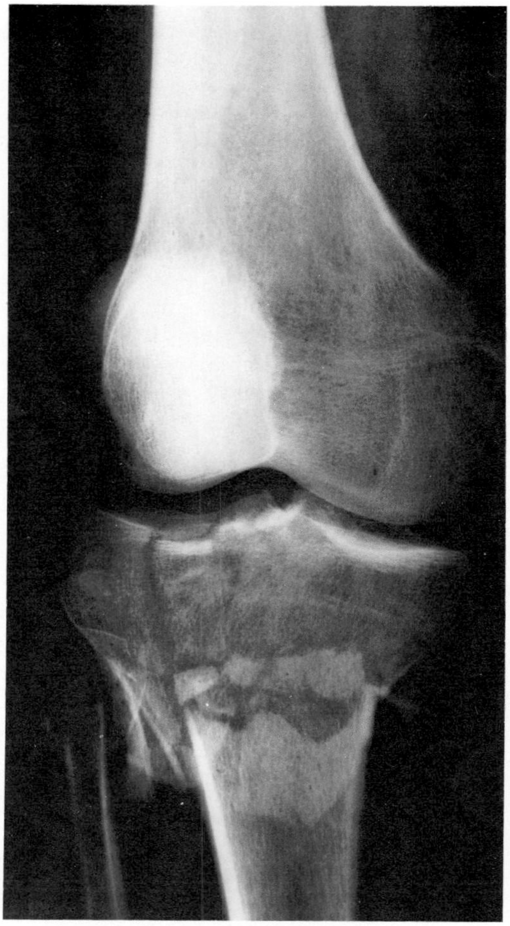

Figure 4–153. Radiograph of the patient's right knee region showing comminuted fractures of the proximal ends of the tibia and the fibula. Note the increased width of the upper end of the tibia caused by the comminution (breaking into fragments) and spreading of the pieces of bone.

A physical examination revealed that her lower limb was slightly flexed, adducted, medially rotated, and appeared shorter than the other limb (Fig. 4-154). Radiographs showed that there was a posterior **dislocation of her right hip** joint with a fracture of the posterior margin of her acetabulum.

Problems. Explain anatomically how this injury probably occurred. What nerve may have been injured? When paralysis of this nerve is complete, which is rare, what muscles would be paralyzed and where may cutaneous sensation be lost? *These problems are discussed on page 598.*

Case 4-7. A 62-year-old man presented with an **aching pain in his left buttock** which extended down the posterior aspect of his left thigh. During the examination the patient pointed to the area where he felt most pain, which was in the region of the greater sciatic notch. Tenderness was also elicited by pressure along a line beginning from a point midway between the top of the greater trochanter of his femur and the ischial tuberosity to a point in the midline of the thigh about half-way to the knee. When seated the patient was unable to extend his left knee fully because of severe pain.

With the patient in the supine position, the doctor grasped the patient's left ankle and placed his other hand on the front of the knee in order to keep the leg straight. He then slowly raised the left lower limb; when it reached about 75°, the man grimaced with pain. Even more pain was elicited when the patient's ankle joint was dorsiflexed.

Problems. What nerve or nerve root is involved in this case? From which segments of the spinal cord does it arise? Why does the *straight leg-raising test* elicit pain? Why did the pain increase when his ankle joint was dorsiflexed? Can you name the kind of pain experienced by this patient? What **back lesion** probably produced the pain in the buttock and thigh region? Thinking anatomically, what other lesions (*e.g.,* resulting from disease or injury) do you think might cause the patient's symptoms? *These problems are discussed on page 599.*

Case 4-8. A 55-year-old woman complained of a globular **swelling in her right groin** (Fig. 4-155*A*). She stated that the swelling became smaller when she lay down, but never completely disappeared. She also said that the mass occasionally got quite large and bulged under the skin on the front of her thigh. When this occurred, she stated that she got a pain down the medial side of her thigh.

On examination the doctor noted that the swelling was inferior to the medial third of the inguinal ligament and **lateral to the pubic tubercle**. When he inserted his index finger into her **inguinal canal** and asked her to cough, he felt no mass or protruding gut but observed a slight increase in the size of the swelling. When the

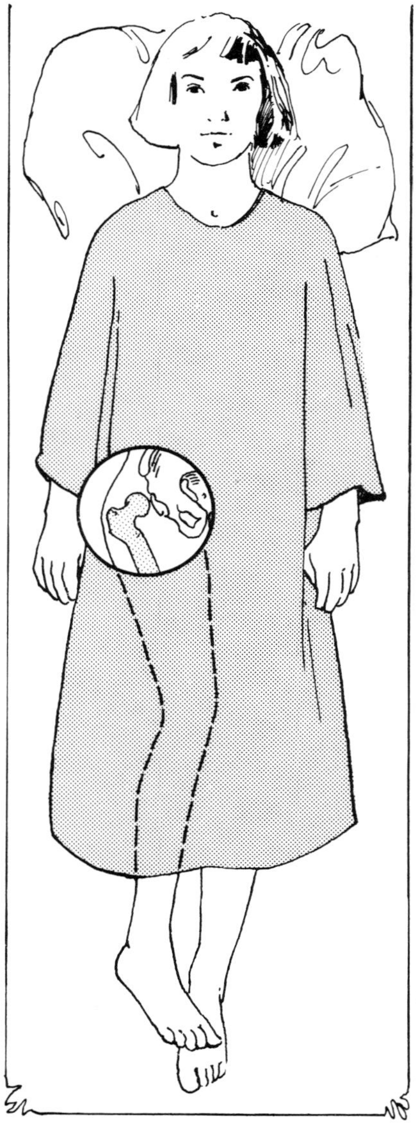

Figure 4–154. Drawing illustrating a traumatic posterior dislocation of the right hip. Observe that the woman's leg is flexed, adducted, medially rotated, and *appears* shorter than her left limb.

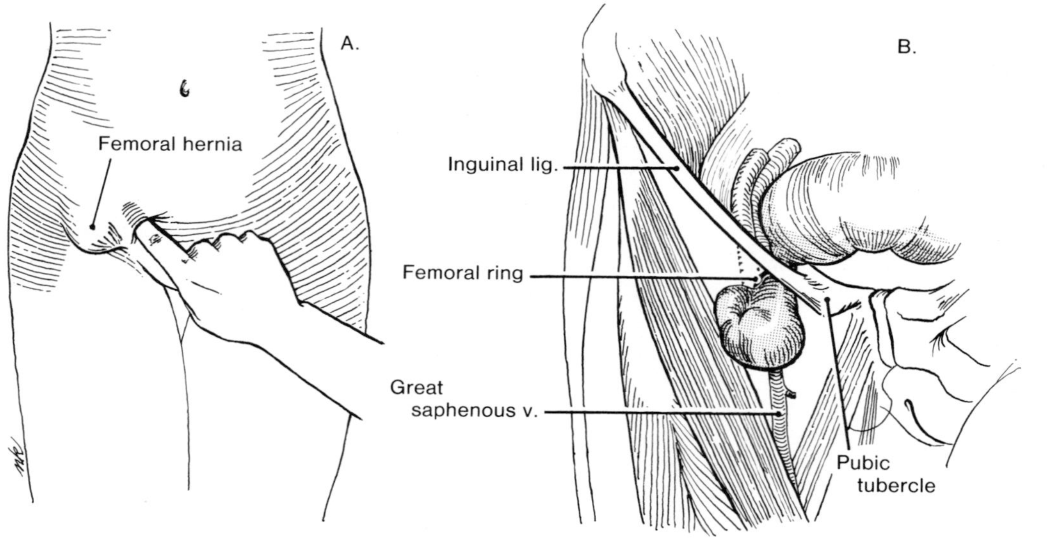

Figure 4–155. *A*, drawing of the external appearance of the femoral hernia. Note that it lies inferolateral to the pubic tubercle and the external ring of the inguinal canal. No mass was palpable in this canal during the invagination test illustrated. *B*, dissection of the thigh and pelvic regions showing the loop of bowel passing deep to the inguinal ligament and into the femoral canal. When it reaches the distal end of this canal it turns superiorly.

patient was asked to point to the site where the swelling first appeared, she placed her finger over the site of the femoral ring (Fig. 4-40). When asked in which direction the swelling came down when she felt pain, she ran her finger along her thigh to the region of the **saphenous opening** (Fig. 4-16).

The doctor applied extremely gentle manual pressure (taxis) to the swelling with the thigh flexed and medially rotated but was unable to reduce the protrusion. A diagnosis of irreducible, complete **femoral hernia** was made.

Problems. Define the terms femoral ring, femoral canal, and femoral hernia. What are the usual contents of the femoral canal? Use your anatomical knowledge to explain why a femoral hernia curves upward (Fig. 4-155*B*). Can you think of any anatomical reasons why femoral hernia is more common in females than in males? Explain anatomically why strangulation of this type of hernia is common. Enlargement of what structure in the femoral canal might be mistaken for a femoral hernia? *These problems are discussed on page 599.*

Case 4-9. A football player was clipped (blocked from the rear) as he was about to tackle the ball carrier (Fig. 4-156). The lineman's hip hit the runner's knee from the side. It was obvious on the slow motion videotape replay that the tackler's knee was slightly flexed and his foot firmly implanted in the frozen turf when he was hit. As he lay on the ground clutching his knee, it was obvious from his face that he was in severe pain.

While he was being helped to the sidelines, you said to your friend, "I'm afraid he has **torn knee ligaments**." Not knowing much about the functioning of the knee joint, your friend said, "Which knee ligaments are probably torn?"

Problems. How would you explain this injury to your friend, assuming he has little knowledge of the anatomy of the knee joint? What ligament was probably ruptured? What ligament may have been torn? Would the menisci be injured? *These problems are discussed on page 601.*

Case 4-10. A 48-year-old inebriated man fell through a glass door and was **slashed behind the right knee** by several deeply penetrating pieces of broken glass. Small

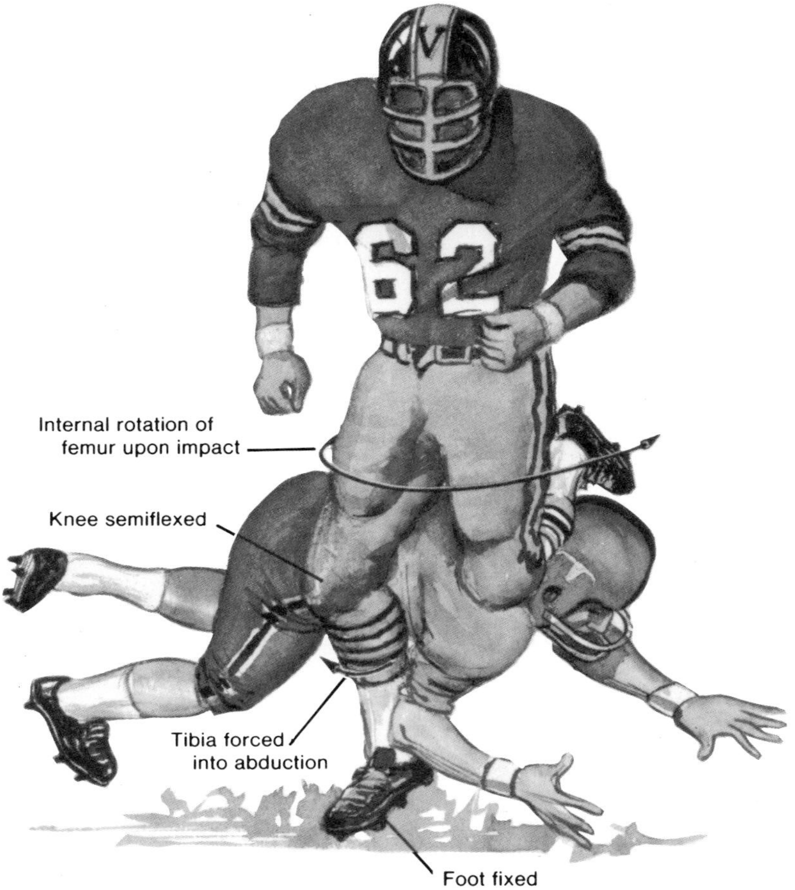

Figure 4–156. Drawing illustrating the way the patient's knee injury probably occurred. This infraction of football rules is called "clipping."

spurts of bright red blood were coming from several parts of the wound until a passing boy scout applied a tourniquet around the man's thigh. Closer examination revealed that one of the deep lacerations extended around the side of his knee, at about the level of the neck of the fibula.

Problems. What tendons might have been lacerated? What vessels were most likely severed? Where would you apply pressure to the main artery to stop blood flowing to the lacerated arteries? What nerve(s) may have been injured? Describe the relationship of the vessels and nerves to each other in this region. What would be the probable effects of nerve injuries in this region? *These problems are discussed on page 602.*

DISCUSSION OF PATIENT ORIENTED PROBLEMS

Case 4-1. It is very likely that your grandmother has a **fractured neck of her femur**, one of the common fractures in elderly women (Fig. 4-157). This injury is often wrongly referred to as a "fractured hip," implying that the hip bone (os coxae) is fractured.

As your grandmother tried to "catch herself," she probably exerted a torsional force on one hip, producing a fracture of the femoral neck, which is the most fragile part of the femur in elderly persons. She fell when the bone fractured; hence, the frac-

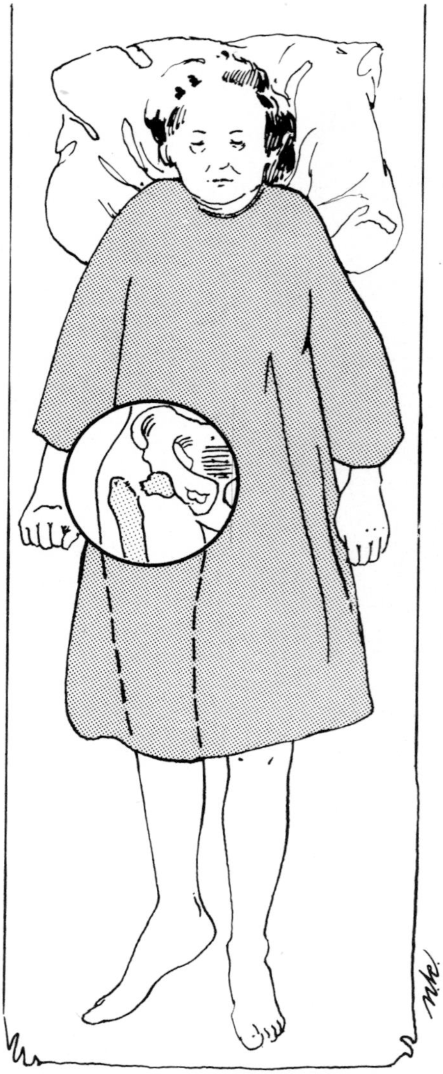

Figure 4–157. Drawing showing the fracture of the neck of the right femur and the shortening and lateral rotation of the lower limb of the elderly patient.

ture was probably the cause of her fall rather than the result of it.

The lateral rotation and shortening of her limb are characteristic clinical features following fractures of the proximal part of the femur. The rotation results from the change in the axis of the limb owing to separation of the shaft and head of the femur. The **shortening of the lower limb** results from the upward pull of the muscles connecting the femur to the os coxae. **Spasm** (sudden involuntary muscular contraction) of these muscles causes this pull. The bones lose mineral with advancing age, a disorder called **osteoporosis**; as a result, the neck of the femur becomes weaker. Consequently, fractures of the proximal part of the femur can result from slight or little trauma. In this bone disorder of post-menopausal women and elderly men, *absorption of bone is greater than bone formation.*

The blood vessels to the proximal part of the femur are derived mostly from the medial and lateral circumflex femoral arteries (Fig. 4-114). Branches of these arteries run in the retinacula or reflections of the fibrous capsule of the hip joint. A variable amount of blood may reach the femoral head through a branch of the obturator artery that runs in the ligamentum capitis femoris, called the **artery of the ligament of the head**. This ligament may be absent or may be ruptured during fractures of the femoral neck or head. Furthermore, this vessel is often not patent (open) in elderly patients who commonly have **arteriosclerosis** (hardening and narrowing of the arteries).

Sometimes other blood vessels supplying the femoral head (Fig. 4-114) are torn when the femoral neck fractures. Generally, the more proximal the fracture, the greater are the chances of interrupting the vascular supply. A poor blood supply may result in nonunion and **avascular necrosis** of the femoral head (death and collapse of the proximal bone fragment owing to poor blood supply). **Intracapsular fractures** (*e.g.,* a fracture high in the neck) almost always present healing problems because they usually interfere with the blood supply to the proximal fragment. The importance of preserving the blood supply to the proximal part of the femur is one reason why patients with this type of injury are handled with extreme care; another is that this injury is very painful.

Case 4-2. The spike obviously penetrated the skin, the gluteus maximus, the gluteus medius, and the superior gluteal nerve (Fig. 4-47). Injury to this nerve resulted in **paralysis of the gluteus medius**, the **gluteus minimus**, and the **tensor fasciae latae**. Normally the gluteus medius, assisted by the gluteus minimus and the tensor fasciae latae, steadies the pelvis so that the opposite side does not drop when the other limb is lifted. Owing to paralysis of these abductors of the thigh, the weight of the body forces the pelvis to tilt downward on the normal side when the person stands on the affected limb (Fig. 4-152). This **Trendelenburg sign** also occurs when other conditions exist, *e.g.*, an old unreduced or congenital dislocation of the hip joint.

Penetrating wounds or **intramuscular injections of drugs** into the superomedial quadrant of the gluteal region may also injure the superior gluteal vessels (Fig. 4-51). Had the spike penetrated the superolateral quadrant, it is unlikely there would have been damage to any nerves or blood vessels. This is the reason why this area is the common site for giving intramuscular injections (Fig. 4-51).

The characteristic dipping gait observed in this patient following **superior gluteal nerve injury** is often referred to as the **gluteus medius limp**. This gait may also be observed in some persons who have had **poliomyelitis**; in these cases the poliovirus destroys the nerve cells of origin of the superior gluteal nerve in the spinal cord (L4, L5, and S1, Fig. 4-160).

Case 4-3. The close relationship of the **common peroneal nerve** to the head and neck of the fibula (Fig. 4-67*A*) makes it vulnerable to injury when this region of the bone is fractured. As the nerve lies on the lateral aspect of the neck of the fibula, it can be easily injured by superficial lacerations (Fig. 4-77).

This patient's signs and symptoms make it obvious that the common peroneal nerve was injured. Superficial wounds, prolonged pressure by hard objects (*e.g.*, the sharp edge of a bed during sleep), or compression by a tight plaster cast may present similar clinical features.

Injury to the common peroneal nerve affects the muscles in the lateral compartment of the leg (peroneus longus and brevis supplied by the superficial peroneal nerve) and in the anterior compartment (muscles on the front of the leg and the extensor digitorum brevis supplied by the deep peroneal nerve). Consequently, eversion of the foot, dorsiflexion of the ankle joint, and extension of the toes are impaired.

This patient showed the characteristic **foot-drop** (plantarflexion and slight inversion of the foot) and the resulting **steppage gait**. As the patient walked, his toes dragged and his foot slapped the floor. In attempting to prevent this from happening, he raised his foot higher than usual.

The **dysesthesia** of the skin (impairment of sensation short of anesthesia) on the patient's leg and foot resulted from injury to sensory fibers in the cutaneous branches of the common peroneal nerve. The injury to the nerve resulted from the skate grazing the nerve or the nerve being compressed by bone fragments or a hematoma (collection of extravasated blood).

Although the fibula is not a weight-bearing bone, fractures of its shaft or proximal end cause pain on walking because the pull of muscles attached to it causes the fragments to move, which is painful.

Case 4-4. As the **popliteal artery** lies deep in the popliteal fossa against the fibrous capsule of the knee joint, it could have been torn by fragments from the comminuted fractures of the proximal ends of the tibia and fibula (Fig. 4-153). As this artery divides into its terminal branches (the anterior and posterior tibial arteries) at the lowest extremity of the **popliteal fossa** (Fig. 4-62), they may also have been torn when these bones fractured. Undoubtedly one or more of the five **genicular arteries**, branches of the popliteal artery, would have also been torn. They supply the capsule and ligaments of the knee joint (Fig. 4-34).

Pulsations of the posterior tibial artery may be felt halfway between the medial malleolus and the heel (Figs. 4-93 and 4-96). The **dorsalis pedis artery** can also be palpated where it passes over the navicular and cuneiform bones in the foot (Figs. 4-34*A* and 4-76). These are good places to take the pulse of the arteries because they are superficial here and can be compressed against the bones. Loss of a pulse in these arteries in the present case would suggest a torn popliteal and/or tibial arteries.

There is also a chance that the **tibial nerve** would be injured in this patient, as it is the most superficial of the three main central structures in the popliteal fossa (Fig. 4-58). Severence of this nerve would result in **paralysis of the popliteus** and the **muscles of the calf** (gastrocnemius, soleus, flexor hallucis longus, and tibialis posterior), together with those in the sole of the foot. Probably some of the genicular branches (articular nerves) to the knee joint would also be served.

The close relationship of the **common peroneal nerve** to the neck of the fibula (Fig. 4-67*A*) makes it vulnerable to injury when this region of the bone is fractured. For the signs and symptoms resulting from severance of this nerve, see Case 4-3.

Case 4-5. The usual sprained ankle results from **abnormal inversion of the weight-bearing foot**, which causes rupture of the anterolateral portion of the capsule of the ankle (talocrural) joint and of the calcaneofibular and talofibular ligaments. The term "*sprain*" is used to indicate some degree of tearing of the ligaments without fracture or dislocation. In severe sprains many fibers of the ligaments are completely ruptured and often considerable instability of the ankle joint results.

In the present case, the sprain and fracture occurred when the patient slipped in such a way that his foot was forced into an excessively inverted position. His body weight then caused a forceful inversion of the ankle joint. The calcaneofibular and anterior talofibular ligaments were torn partly or completely. Normally the deep mortise formed by the distal end of the tibia and the malleoli holds the talus firmly in position (Fig. 4-142). When the ankle ligaments tear, the talus is forcibly tilted against the lateral malleolus of the fibula, shearing it off (Fig. 4-158).

Had the man's ankle been forced in the opposite direction (*i.e.,* in an extremely everted position), the strong deltoid ligament could have avulsed (pulled off) the medial malleolus (Fig. 4-159). As the force continued it would have tilted the talus, moving it and the lateral malleolus laterally. Because the interosseous tibiofibular ligament (Fig. 4-67*B*) acts as a pivot, the fibula breaks above the distal tibiofibular joint. This injury is really a **fracture-dislocation of the ankle joint** caused by forceful eversion of the foot, and it is what is usually called a **Pott's fracture** because it is the kind of fracture-dislocation sustained and described by Dr. Percival Pott, an English surgeon. However, the term Pott's fracture is often used loosely to describe most fractures and fracture-dislocation of the malleoli.

Case 4-6. *Dislocation of the hip joint* is uncommon owing to its stability. The head of the femur is deeply seated in the acetabulum and is held there by an exceedingly strong articular capsule. *Traumatic dislocations commonly occur during automobile accidents* when the hip is flexed, adducted, and *medially rotated.* Very likely

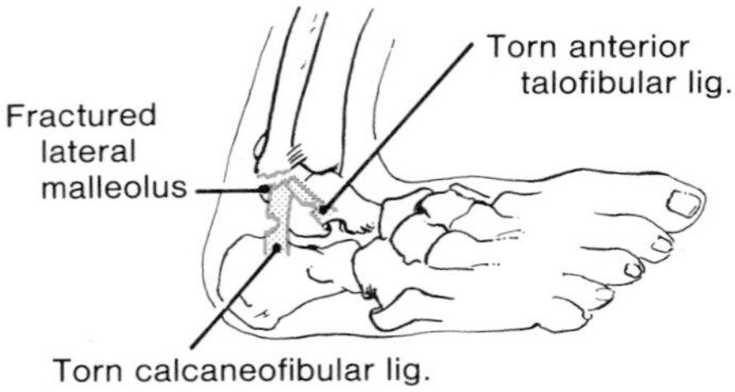

Figure 4–158. Drawing illustrating incomplete rupture of the calcaneofibular and talofibular ligaments and a fracture of the lateral malleolus, following forced inversion of the right foot.

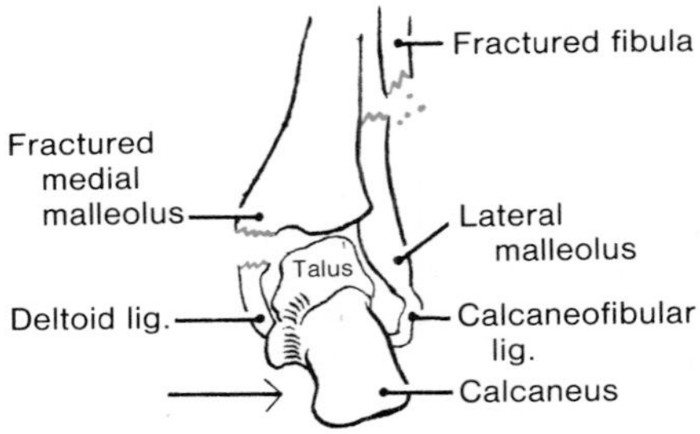

Figure 4–159. Drawing illustrating a fracture-dislocation (Pott's fracture) of the ankle caused by forced eversion of the right foot. Note that the strong deltoid ligament has not ruptured but has avulsed the medial malleolus. Observe the associated fracture of the fibula.

the patient's knee struck the dashboard when her right lower limb was in the position just described. Consequently the force was transmitted up the femur, driving its head and the posterior margin (lip) of the acetabulum posteriorly. As the head in this position is covered posteriorly by capsule rather than bone, the articular capsule probably ruptured inferiorly and posteriorly; this permitted the head to dislocate posteriorly and carry the fractured posterior margin of the acetabulum and the acetabular labrum with it. As a result, the head of the femur comes to lie on the gluteal surface of the ilium.

The close relationship of the **sciatic nerve** (L4 to S3) to the posterior surface of the hip joint makes it vulnerable to injury in posterior dislocations. If the paralysis is complete, which is rarely the case, the hamstring muscles and those distal to the knee would all be paralyzed. In addition there would probably be anesthesia in the lower leg and foot, except for the skin on the medial side which is supplied by the saphenous nerve (L3 and L4), a terminal branch of the femoral nerve (Figs. 4-106 and 4-160).

Case 4-7. The site of the patient's pain and its course down the posterior aspect of the thigh clearly implicates the **sciatic nerve**, the largest branch of the sacral plexus, which arises from spinal cord segments L4 to S3 (Fig. 4-160). It leaves the pelvis through the inferior part of the greater sciatic notch and extends from the inferior border of the piriformis muscle to the distal third of the thigh, along the course clearly indicated by the patient's pain (Figs. 4-47 and 4-52).

The straight leg-raising test (hip flexed and knee extended) elicits pain because the sciatic nerve is stretched when the leg is raised. Dorsiflexion of the ankle further increases the pull on the sciatic nerve and its roots (nerve fibers from ventral primary rami of L4 to S3).

Sciatica is the name given to *pain in the area of distribution of the sciatic nerve.* Variation occurs in the location of the pain in different patients owing to involvement of different nerve roots. A posterior **protrusion of an intervertebral disc** is a common cause of sciatica, most often affecting the first sacral nerve roots. A protruding L5/S1 disc exerts pressure on these dorsal and ventral roots, producing sciatica, which may be accompanied by "*lumbago*" (low back pain).

Sciatic pain can also result from pressure (*e.g.,* a tumor) on the sciatic nerve or its components in the pelvis, in the gluteal region, or in the thigh. Pain could also be produced by irritation of the sciatic nerve resulting from inflammation of the nerve (**neuritis**) or its sheath. Pain in the area of distribution of the sciatic nerve can also be caused by disease in an adjacent structure (*e.g.,* the sacroiliac joint, Fig. 5-2).

Case 4-8. A *femoral hernia* is a protrusion of fat, peritoneum, omentum, and usually a loop of intestine through the femoral ring into the femoral canal (Fig. 4-155*B*). **Bowel sounds** may be heard with a stethoscope when intestine is in the hernial sac.

The conical **femoral canal** is a short, blind, potential space in the medial compartment of the **femoral sheath** (Fig. 4-161), which is a prolongation of the fascial lining of the interior of the abdomen (fascia transversalis anteriorly and fascia iliaca posteriorly). Normally this space contains lymph vessels and at least one lymph node embedded in connective tissue.

The *femoral canal is a source of weakness in the abdominal wall*; thus, when intra-abdominal pressure rises very high (as may occur when a chronically constipated person attempts to defecate), abdominal contents (*e.g.,* a loop of intestine) may be forced through the femoral ring into the femoral canal. The intestine carries a pouch of parietal peritoneum before it as it descends along the femoral canal and through the saphenous opening. Being prevented from extending further down by the deep fascia of the thigh, the hernial sac is directed anteriorly and then superiorly, forming a swelling inferior to the inguinal ligament.

While the hernia is in the femoral canal (**incomplete femoral hernia**) it is usually small, but after it passes anteriorly through the saphenous opening into the loose areolar tissue of the thigh, it becomes much larger (**complete femoral hernia**). The differential diagnosis between indirect in-

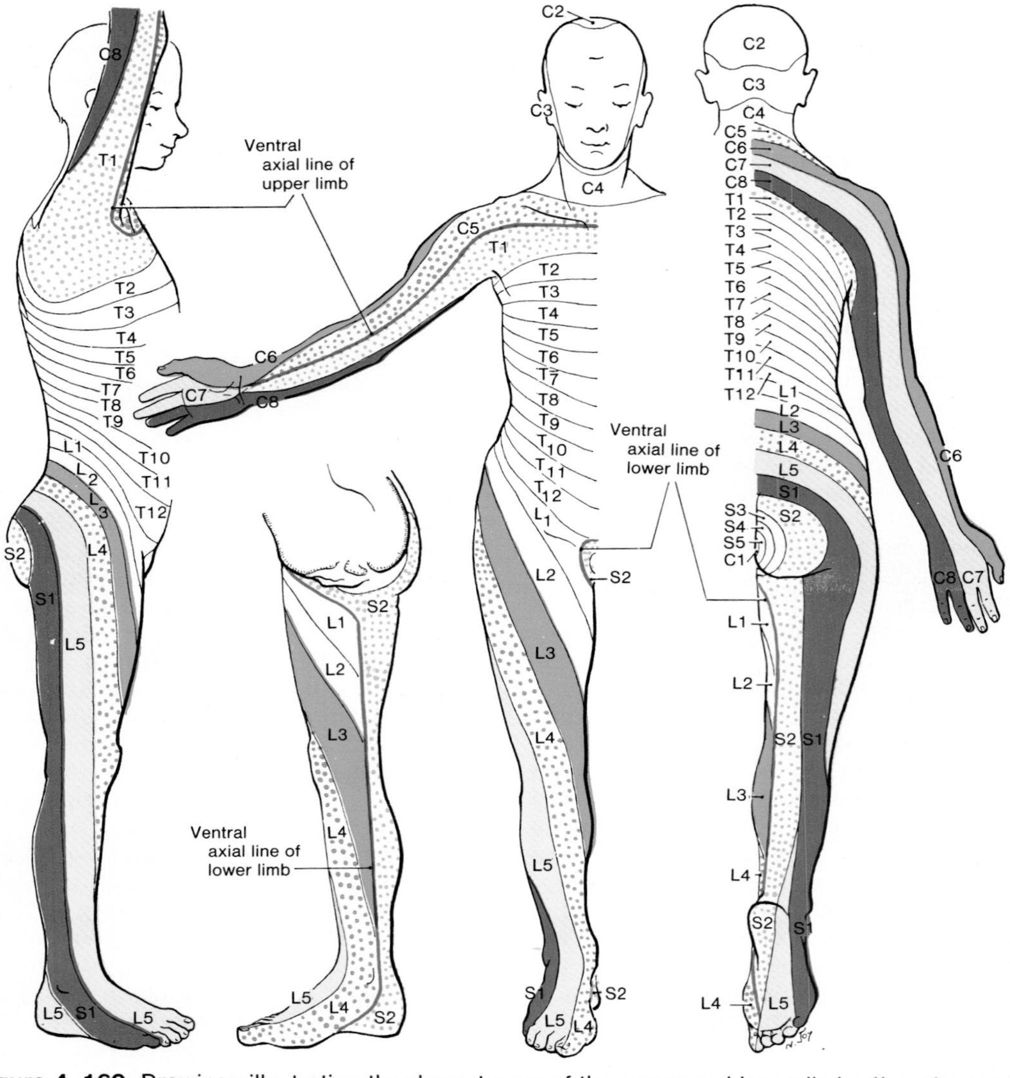

Figure 4–160. Drawings illustrating the dermatomes of the upper and lower limbs (*i.e.*, the areas of skin supplied by the spinal nerves and therefore the segments of the spinal cord). When the function of even a single dorsal nerve root is interrupted, faint but definite diminution of sensitivity can be demonstrated in the dermatome. The usual method for detecting the area of diminished sensitivity is by the use of a light pin scratch for pain sensation, although it can be found for temperature and tactile sensation also. In Case 4-7 pain was detected in the area of distribution of the sciatic nerve which comes from spinal cord segments L4 to S3. In Case 4-3 the patient had numbness and tingling on the lateral surface of his leg and the dorsum of his foot which implicated the common peroneal nerve (L4 to S2). Understand that the area of total anesthesia is less than might be anticipated owing to overlapping of the areas of distribution of nerve fibers.

guinal hernia and complete femoral hernia is at times difficult, because advanced types of femoral hernia sometimes produce a swelling above the inguinal ligament. The swelling produced by femoral hernia is more lateral, however, than one caused by indirect inguinal hernia. The **pubic tubercle** is an important bony landmark in differentiating an inguinal from a femoral hernia. The neck of an **inguinal hernial sac**

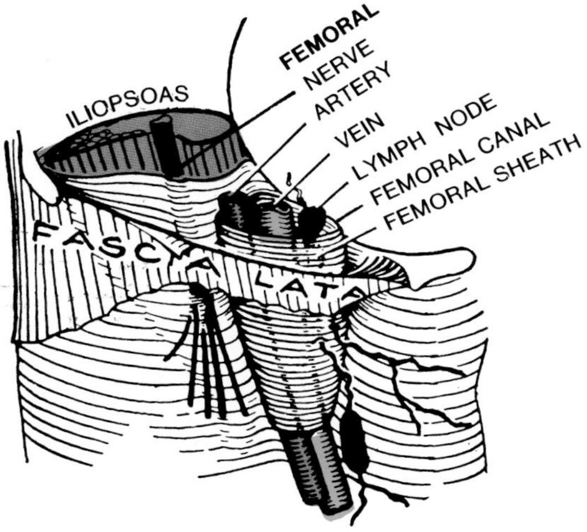

Figure 4–161. Drawing showing the upper part of the right thigh and femoral sheath. Note that the femoral sheath surrounds (from medial to lateral) the femoral canal, the femoral vein, and the femoral artery, but not the femoral nerve. The femoral canal contains lymph vessels, one or more lymph nodes, and areolar tissue. The conical femoral canal is a potential space in femoral sheath and the femoral ring is the mouth of the femoral canal. In femoral hernia the hernial sac enters the femoral canal via the femoral ring.

is *superomedial to the tubercle* at the superficial inguinal ring, whereas the neck of a **femoral hernial sac** is *inferolateral to the tubercle* at this site. In addition, if a hernia does not present in the inguinal canal during the **invagination test**, as in the present case, the hernia cannot be an indirect inguinal hernia.

If the hand is placed gently over the hernia and eased downward, the fold of the groin produced by the inguinal ligament will be seen passing superior to a femoral hernia, whereas if the hand is eased upward, the fold of the groin will be seen passing inferior to an inguinal hernia.

Femoral hernia is more common in females than in males (about 3:1) because the femoral ring is larger in women than in men owing to the greater breadth of the female pelvis, the smaller size of their femoral vessels, and the changes that occur in the associated tissues if pregnancy occurs.

Strangulation of a complete femoral hernia is common. The tendency for this type of hernia to strangulate (*i.e.,* compress the vessels of the hernia) results from the sharp boundaries of the femoral ring (*e.g.,* the inguinal ligament anteriorly and the lacunar ligament medially). Stricture of the hernia may also be produced by the sharp edges of the saphenous opening (Fig. 4-16).

Because of the relatively small size of the femoral ring and the saphenous opening and the rigidity of the surrounding structures, blockage of the venous return from the protruded loop of intestine often occurs. As arterial blood continues to pass into the loop, it becomes engorged with blood and circulation through it soon stops. Early surgical intervention is required to prevent **necrosis** (death) of the strangulated loop of intestine.

A soft enlarged lymph node in the femoral canal (Fig. 4-40) could be mistaken for a femoral hernia, although it would likely be more firm. Recall that the femoral canal or medial compartment of the femoral sheath normally contains one or more deep **inguinal lymph nodes** (Fig. 4-40). Cancer or infections in the areas drained by these nodes could cause them to enlarge.

Case 4-9. The knee joint, located between the two longest bones in the body (the femur and the tibia), is one of the most secure joints in the body. Although these bones are bounded together by strong ligaments (Fig. 4-162), the knee is subject to a wide range of injuries because of the severe strain that is placed on its attachments, especially in contact sports like hockey and football.

The blow on the lateral side of the tackler's knee by the lineman's hip occurred while he was running and his foot was fixed in the ground (Fig. 4-156). As he was bearing weight on his leg, the hard blow bent the runner's knee inward relative to the fixed tibia. This severely stressed the ligament on the inside of the knee, known as the **tibial collateral ligament**. Some fibers of this ligament may have ruptured and he may only have a sprain; however, because of the severity of the blow, probably the entire ligament ruptured near its attachment to the medial femoral epicondyle (Fig. 4-163). Because the **medial meniscus** of the knee, a fibrocartilaginous articular disc, is attached to this ligament, the

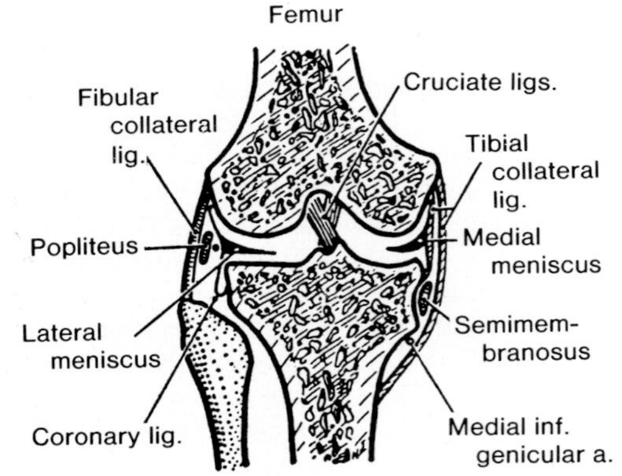

Figure 4–162. Drawing of a coronal section of the right knee joint. Note that the cruciate (cross-like) ligaments attach the femur to the tibia. Because the medial meniscus is attached to the tibial collateral ligament, it is usually torn when there is undue stress on it as the result of a hard blow to the lateral side of the knee.

meniscus may tear or become detached from it.

This may have been the full extent of the athlete's injury, but he may also have ruptured his **anterior cruciate ligament** (Figs. 4-125 and 4-133). This ligament, which prevents backward displacement of the femur and hyperextension of the knee joint, is sometimes torn when the knee is hit hard from the lateral side.

In summary, the forced abduction and lateral rotation of the runner's leg by the block probably resulted in the simultaneous rupture of three structures: the tibial collateral ligament, the medial meniscus, and the anterior cruciate ligament. If this **common triad of injuries** has occurred, the player will most likely be out of the lineup for the rest of the season.

Case 4-10. The two tendons likely to be lacerated by deep cuts behind the knee are those of the semitendinosus and the biceps femoris muscles (Figs. 4-56 and 4-58). In ancient times warriors used to slash these tendons at the back of their opponents' knees so they would be unable to run, or they would slash the horses' "hamstrings" to bring the riders to the ground.

The **small saphenous vein** and the **tibial nerve** would certainly be cut and probably the popliteal vein would also be severed. Because the popliteal artery is so deeply located, it is unlikely that it would be lacerated (Figs. 4-61 and 4-62). Probably the small amounts of spurting blood were coming from lacerated genicular and/or muscular branches of the popliteal artery.

Clamping the popliteal artery as it emerges from the adductor hiatus in the tendon of the adductor magnus muscle would cut all blood flow to the popliteal artery and its branches. The vessel would be occluded only long enough for the lacerated vessels to be repaired. The popliteal artery would not be ligated because the ligature would be above the origin of the important genicular branches to the **anastomoses around the knee** (Figs. 4-61 and 4-62). Ligation might lead to **gangrene** of the leg and foot, but in some people the descending branch of the lateral circumflex femoral artery and the descending genicular branch of the femoral artery (Fig. 4-34*A*) are large enough to compensate for the lack of blood flow through the tibial artery.

Throughout its course the popliteal artery lies deep in the popliteal fossa against the femur or the articular capsule of the knee joint. The anterior and posterior tibial veins unite in the distal part of the popliteal fossa to form the popliteal vein. This vessel lies superficial to the popliteal artery, me-

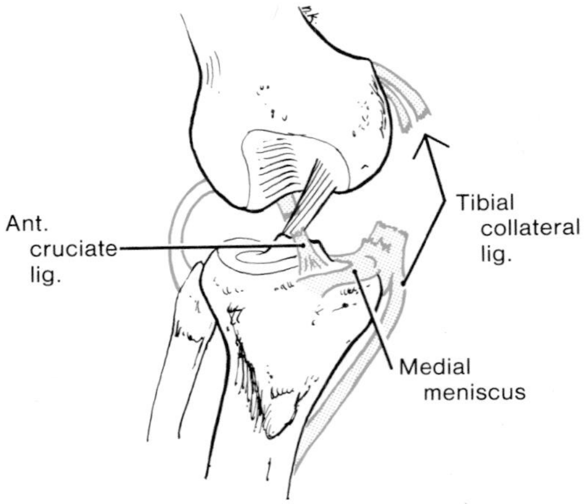

Figure 4–163. Diagrammatic illustration showing how the force from the hard blow (*arrow*) on the lateral side of the right knee had the effect of abducting the tibia on the femur. This probably ruptured the tibial collateral ligament, the medial meniscus, and the anterior cruciate ligament.

dial to it distally, and lateral to it proximally. As the artery and vein are bound wall-to-wall in a dense vascular sheath, an **arteriovenous shunt** may develop when they are lacerated simultaneously in the same region.

As the **tibial nerve** is the most superficial of the three central structures in the popliteal fossa (Fig. 4-58), it was probably severed. Because the laceration extended over the neck of the fibula, probably the other division of the sciatic nerve, the **common peroneal nerve**, was also cut. It is the most commonly injured nerve in the lower limb mainly because of its exposed position near the neck of the fibula. A deep laceration in the popliteal fossa probably would also cut the nerves to the lateral head of the gastrocnemius, the soleus, and the popliteus muscles (Fig. 4-60).

The tibial and common peroneal nerves are the terminal branches of the sciatic nerve. The tibial nerve passes vertically through the popliteal fossa superficial to the popliteal vessels, just beneath the deep popliteal fascia (Fig. 4-58). **Injury to the tibial nerve** produces paralysis of the flexor muscles in the leg and the intrinsic muscles in the sole of the foot. In addition, there would be a loss of sensation in the sole of the foot (Fig. 4-106).

Injury to the common peroneal nerve results in paralysis of all the dorsiflexor and evertor muscles of the foot, producing a condition known as **foot-drop**. There would also be a variable loss of cutaneous sensation on the anterolateral aspect of the leg and the dorsum of the foot. The nerve injuries probably sustained by this patient would result in a severe disability of his right leg and foot for many months until the nerves that would be rejoined at surgery regenerated (about 2.5 cm/mo).

SUGGESTIONS FOR ADDITIONAL READING

1. Haymaker, W., and Woodhall, B. *Peripheral Nerve Injuries. Principles of Diagnosis,* Ed. 2, W. B. Saunders Co., Philadelphia, 1953.

   This is a very good source of information concerning injuries to nerves derived from the lumbar and sacral plexuses. It includes a good analysis of the segmental and peripheral nerve supply of the skin, muscles, and skeleton, which provides a background for the diagnosis of peripheral nerve injuries.

2. Hollinshead, W. H. The lower limb. In *Functional Anatomy of the Limbs and Back.* Ed. 3, W. B. Saunders Co., Philadelphia, 1969.

   The chief emphasis is on the muscles of the lower limb and their actions, including discussions of the skeletal, nervous, and vascular systems. This book was written for the beginning student in physical therapy and, as the title indicates, takes a functional approach.

3. Nerve Injuries Committee, Medical Research Council. *Aids To The Investigation of Peripheral Nerve Injuries.* M.R.C. War Memorandum No. 7, Ed. 2, His Majesty's Stationery Office, 1943.

   This short booklet or atlas (48 pp.) is a gold mine of practical information about the examination of patients with lesions of peripheral nerves. It gives instructions with photographs and drawings for testing the actions of muscles and for determining areas of sensory deficit. This atlas is recommended for beginning students and persons less experienced in examining patients with lesions of peripheral nerves.

4. Romanes, G. J. (Ed.). *Cunningham's Textbook of Anatomy,* Ed. 11, Oxford University Press, London, 1972.

   This book of reference is sufficiently comprehensive to allow you to expand your knowledge of anatomy considerably. It contains a good coverage of surface and surgical anatomy and many practical discussions of peripheral nerve injuries. Many good radiographs are included which clearly demonstrate important features of radiographic anatomy.

5. Salter, R. B. *Textbook of Disorders and Injuries of the Musculoskeletal System,* The Williams & Wilkins Company, Baltimore, 1970.

   You will find this an excellent introduction to orthopaedics, rheumatology, metabolic bone disease, rehabilitation, and fractures. Although written for medical students, it will be of interest to all who are involved in the care of patients with disabilities of the musculoskeletal system. The author is recognized internationally for fundamental scientific investigations of disorders and injuries of the musculoskeletal system.

6. Trueta, J. The growth and development of bones and joints: Orthopedic aspects. In *Scientific Foundations of Pediatrics,* edited by J. A. Davies and J. Dobbing, W. B. Saunders Co., Philadelphia, 1974.

   This is an excellent account of the development and blood supply of the epiphyseal growth cartilage. Changes in this cartilage resulting from interruption of the blood supply to the body of the long bone and the action of hormones and vitamins on skeletal development are discussed. Disturbances of growth and development of bones and joints (*e.g.,* slipping of the proximal femoral epiphysis) are described.

7. Williams, J. G. P. *Sports Medicine,* The Williams & Wilkins Company, Baltimore, 1962.

   This book discusses the etiology, diagnosis, treatment, and prevention of disorders and injuries of athletes and describes methods of athletic training. It also gives an insight into the specialty of sports medicine.

CHAPTER 5

The Back

Low back pain ("lumbago") is a commonly encountered complaint in medical practice. To understand the anatomical basis of back problems (diseases of the vertebral column and/or of the soft tissues associated with it) that cause disabling pain, a good understanding of the structure and function of the back is required.

THE VERTEBRAL COLUMN

The vertebral column, commonly called **the spine** or the spinal column, forms the skeleton of the back and is part of the axial skeleton (Fig. 5-1). It consists of a number of bones called **vertebrae** which are united by a series of intervertebral articulations or joints to form a strong but flexible shaft that supports the trunk and its appendages (the limbs). It extends from the base of the skull through the whole length of the neck and trunk (Figs. 5-9 and 5-10).

The vertebral column is stabilized by ligaments which limit somewhat the movements produced by the muscles of the back. The **spinal cord**, the nerve roots, and their coverings, or meninges, are located within a canal, the **vertebral canal**, in this long column of bones.

The **spinal nerves** and their branches are located outside the vertebral canal, except for the meningeal nerves, which return through the intervertebral foramina to innervate the **spinal meninges** (G. membranes).

The vertebral column provides a partly rigid and partly flexible axis for the body and a pivot for the head. Thus, it has an important role in posture, in support of body weight, in locomotion, and in protection of the spinal cord and the nerve roots.

During sitting the vertebral column transmits the weight of the body across the **sacroiliac joints** to the ilia and then to the ischial tuberosities (Figs. 5-2 and 5-3). When standing the weight is transferred from the sacroiliac joints to the acetabula and then to the femora.

THE VERTEBRAL COLUMN AS A WHOLE

Although the adult vertebral column consists of **33 vertebrae**, observe that only 24 of them (7 cervical, 12 thoracic, and 5 lumbar) are movable (Fig. 5-1). The five sacral vertebrae are fused to form the **sacrum** (Fig. 5-25), which can be felt or palpated in the low back region (Fig. 5-11). Usually the four rudimentary coccygeal vertebrae (also called pieces or elements) are fused to form a slender tapering bone called the **coccyx** (Figs. 5-1 and 5-3), but the first coccygeal vertebra may be separate from the rest.

The presacral vertebrae are connected by resilient **intervertebral discs** (Figs. 5-4 and 5-8) which play an important role in movements between the vertebrae and in absorbing shocks transmitted up or down the vertebral column. The presacral vertebrae are also connected to each other by paired, posterior, synovial zygapophyseal joints between the articular processes (Figs. 5-4 and 5-33) and by anterior and posterior longitudinal ligaments (Figs. 5-31 and 5-32). These ligaments extend the length of the vertebral column and are attached to the intervertebral joints and the vertebral bodies. *The intervertebral ligaments and intervertebral joints prevent excessive flexion and extension of the vertebral column.*

The bodies of the vertebrae contribute about three-fourths of the length of the presacral part of the vertebral column and

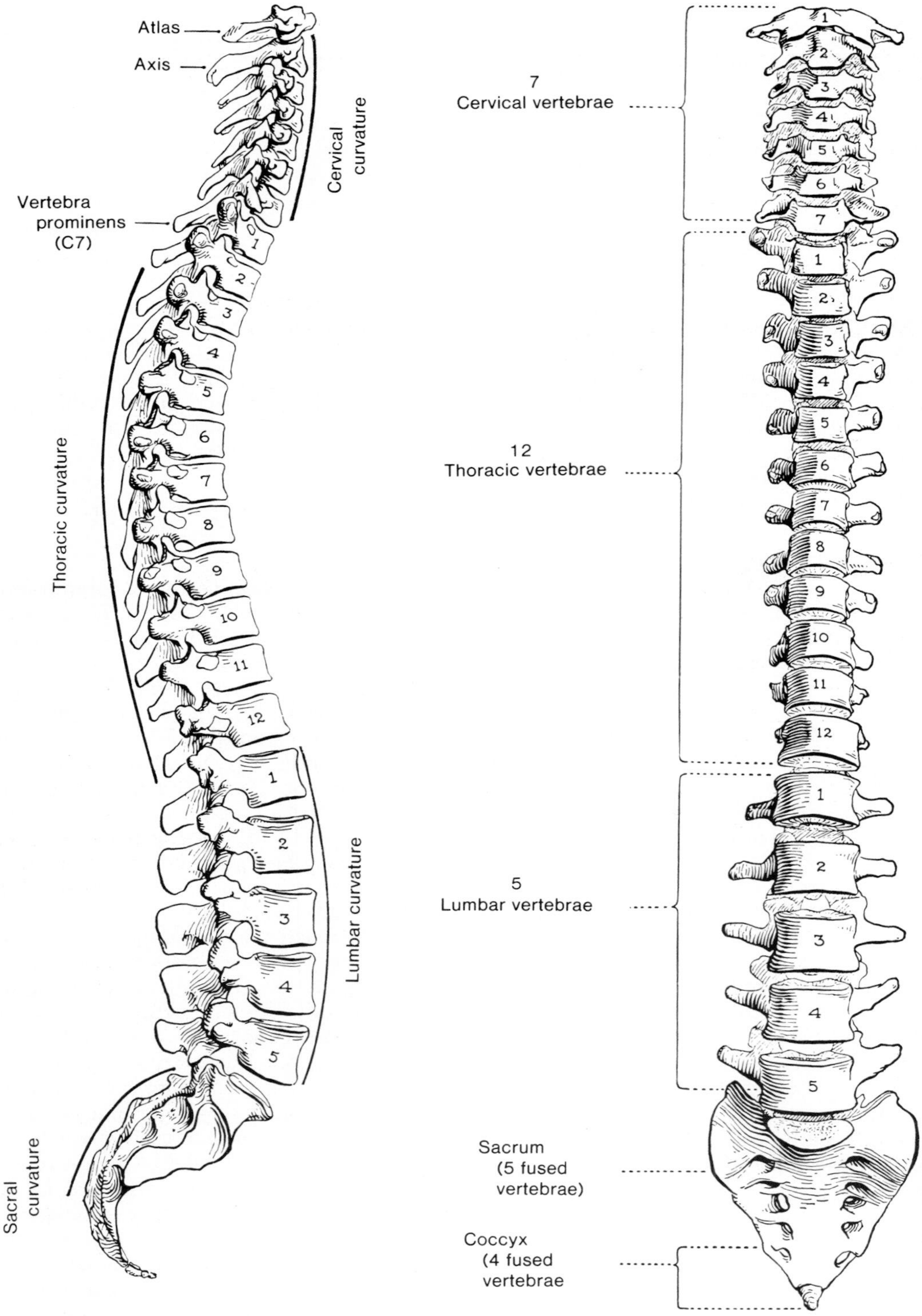

Figure 5-1. Drawings of the vertebral column showing the 24 presacral vertebrae, the sacrum, the coccyx, and the curvatures of the vertebral column. Note that the first coccygeal vertebra has fused with the sacrum. Most vertebral columns range between 72 and 75 cm in length, of which about one-fourth is contributed by the fibrocartilaginous intervertebral discs (Figs. 5-4 and 5-33).

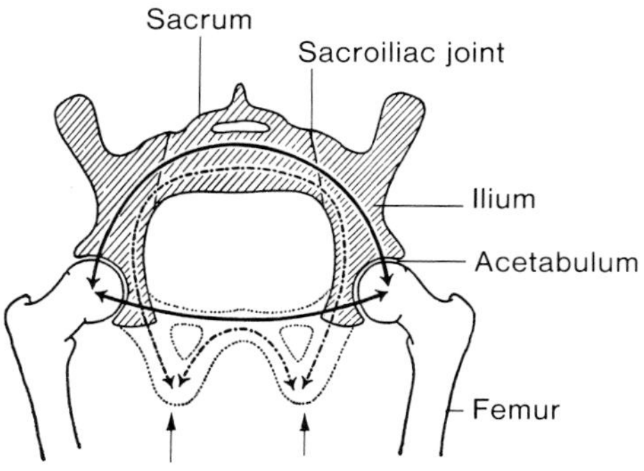

Figure 5-2. Diagram illustrating the weight-bearing mechanism of the pelvis: ——, the standing arch; – – –, the sitting arch.

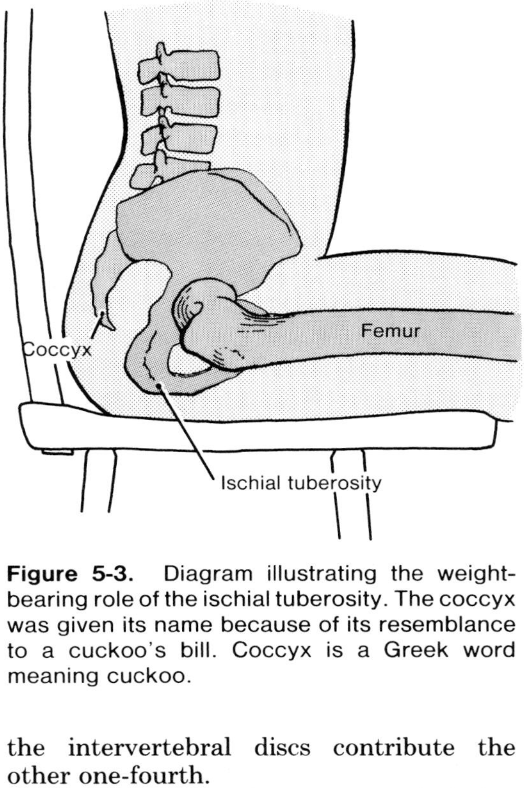

Figure 5-3. Diagram illustrating the weight-bearing role of the ischial tuberosity. The coccyx was given its name because of its resemblance to a cuckoo's bill. Coccyx is a Greek word meaning cuckoo.

the intervertebral discs contribute the other one-fourth.

When counting the vertebrae, it is important to begin at the base of the neck (Fig. 5-10), because what may appear to be an extra lumbar vertebra in a radiograph may be an extra thoracic or sacral vertebra. In Figure 5-1 observe that the vertebral bodies gradually become larger as the sacrum is approached and then become progressively smaller toward the coccyx. These

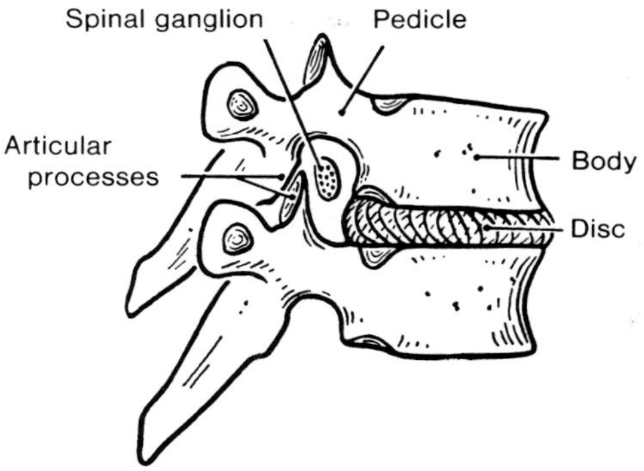

Figure 5-4. Lateral view of two thoracic vertebrae illustrating the intervertebral disc between them and the intervertebral foramen containing a spinal (dorsal root) ganglion. Note the articular processes which form small synovial zygapophyseal joints on each side at each level.

structural differences are related to the fact that the lumbosacral region of the vertebral column carries more weight than the cervical and thoracic regions.

CLINICALLY ORIENTED COMMENTS

Not everyone has 33 vertebrae, but the number of cervical vertebrae (7) is very constant in mammals, including man. Even the giraffe has only 7, but they are long! However, variations occur in the number of thoracic, lumbar, and sacral vertebrae in about 5% of otherwise normal people. Differences in number can be either a change in one region (+ or −) without change in other regions or a change in one region at the expense of another. Although numerical variations may be clinically important, many have been detected at autopsy or in radiographs of persons with no history of back problems. Caution, therefore, is required in ascribing symptoms to numerical variations of vertebrae.

In some people the fifth lumbar vertebra is partly or completely incorporated into the sacrum (**sacralization of the fifth lumbar vertebra**, Fig. 5-24); in others, the first sacral vertebra is separated from the sacrum (**lumbarization of the first sacral vertebra**, Fig. 5-26). The relationship between sacralization or lumbarization and back symptoms is unclear.

Curvatures of the Vertebral Column (Figs. 5-1 and 5-5). In the articulated vertebral column and in lateral radiographs, four sagittal curvatures are visible in the adult.

The thoracic and sacral curvatures develop during the fetal period (Fig. 5-5); thus, they are **primary curvatures.** *Secondary curvatures* begin to appear in the cervical and lumbar regions during the fetal period, but they are not noticeable until infancy. The *cervical curvature* develops as the infant begins to hold its head erect (about 3 months), and the *lumbar curvature* appears as the child begins to walk (about 13 months).

CLINICALLY ORIENTED COMMENTS

The vertebral column in some people does not have normal curvatures because abnormal development and pathological processes, *e.g.*, **osteoporosis** (L. *os*, bone + *porosis*, porous), affect the bodies of one or more vertebrae in such a way that abnormal curvatures develop.

Kyphosis (G. humpback), characterized by an abnormal curve that is convex posteriorly (*i.e.*, a **dorsal curvature** of the vertebral column), usually occurs in the thoracic region. Some increase in thoracic kyphosis usually develops in elderly people which is generally more marked in women (*e.g.*, the "*dowager's hump*").

Scoliosis (G. crookedness) indicates that the curve is convex to the side (*i.e.*, a **lateral curvature** of the vertebral column (Fig. 5-6). In some cases there is only one curve, *e.g.*, *coxitic scoliosis* in the lumbar region, which results from tilting of the pelvis to the side owing to hip disease.

Scoliosis may also result from an asymmetric weakness of the vertebral muscles (*myopathic scoliosis*) or from failure of one half of the body and the arch to develop (**hemivertebra**, Fig. 5-7). Many cases of scoliosis are of unknown origin (*i.e.*, *idiopathic scoliosis*).

Lordosis (G. backward bending) is characterized by an increased curve of the vertebral column that is **convex anteriorly**. Excessive lordosis, often referred to as swayback or saddleback, generally occurs in the lumbar region. Pregnant women often develop lordosis during the later stages of pregnancy in attempting to restore their line of gravity to the normal position.

Movements of the Vertebral Column (Figs. 5-8 to 5-10). Movements between adjacent vertebrae take place on the resilient nuclei pulposi of the intervertebral discs (Figs. 5-4 and 5-8) and at the zygapophyseal joints (Figs. 5-4 and 5-33). Although move-

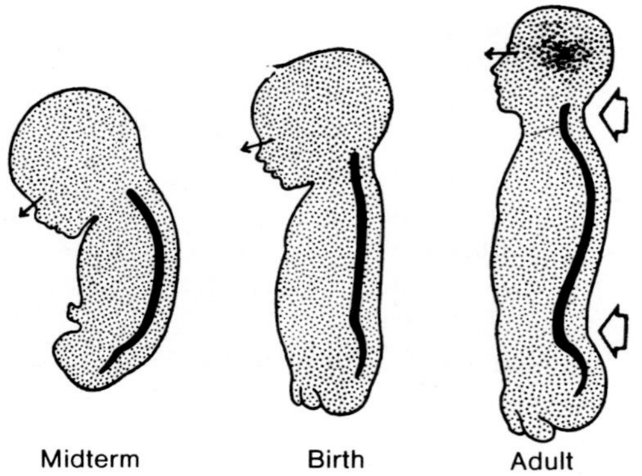

Figure 5-5. Drawings illustrating the development of curvatures of the vertebral column. In the adult the cervical and lumbar curvatures are indicated by *open arrows*.

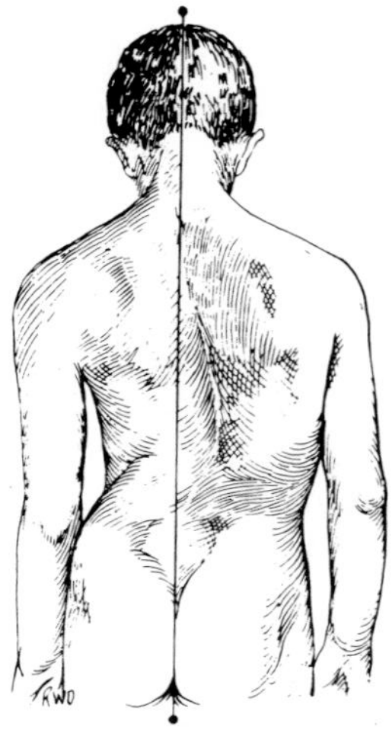

Figure 5-6. Drawing illustrating scoliosis or lateral curvature of the vertebral column.

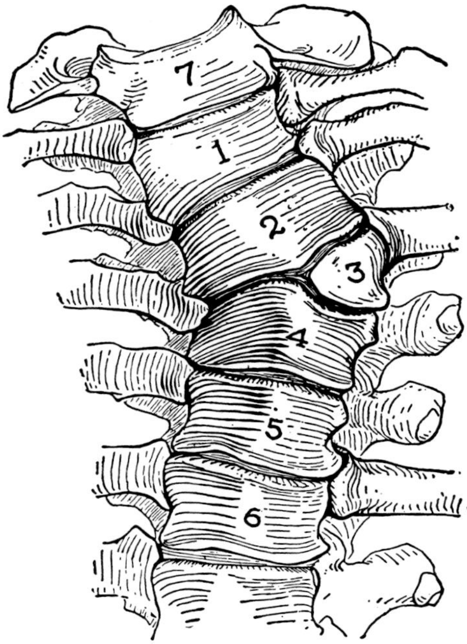

Figure 5-7. Drawing of a half vertebra (hemivertebra) that has produced a scoliosis (lateral curvature of the vertebral column). Half of the third thoracic vertebra and the corresponding rib are absent. In some cases hemivertebrae are in addition to the normal vertebrae.

ments between adjacent vertebrae are relatively small, especially in the thoracic region, the result of all the small movements is a considerable range of movement of the vertebral column as a whole (Figs. 5-9 and 5-10). Movements are freer in the cervical and lumbar regions than elsewhere.

The main movements of the vertebral column are **flexion** (forward bending), **extension** (backward bending), **lateral bending** (lateral flexion), and **rotation** (twisting of the vertebrae relative to each other). Some **circumduction**, a combination of flexion-extension and lateral bending, also occurs.

The thoracic region is relatively stable owing to its connection to the sternum via the ribs and the costal cartilages. In addition, its intervertebral discs are slightly thinner and its spinous processes overlap (Fig. 5-1).

Palpation of the Vertebral Column. In the adult there is often a slight hollow posterior to the first cervical vertebra (**C1** or **atlas**), just inferior to the external occipital protuberance (Fig. 5-55), but the atlas is not palpable posteriorly because it has no spinous process (Fig. 5-18). However, the transverse processes of the atlas can be felt on deep palpation about 1.5 cm inferior to the tips of the mastoid processes (Figs. 5-18 and 5-55).

The spinous process of the second cervical vertebra (**C2** or **axis**) can be palpated about 10 cm inferior to the external occipital protuberance (Fig. 5-55); it is the first bony point that can be felt inferior to this prominence.

The spinous processes of the third to fifth cervical vertebrae are difficult to palpate because they are short, but the spinous process of the sixth cervical vertebra is palpable in some people. In most people the distinct posterior bony projection at the base of the neck is the spinous process of the seventh cervical vertebra (Fig. 5-10). Because of the prominence of its spinous process, **C7 is called the vertebra prominens** (Figs. 5-10, 5-18, and 5-20). Its spinous process can be palpated and observed most easily when the neck is flexed.

Thoracic and lumbar spinous processes can be palpated, particularly in thin persons. In some people the spinous process of T1 may be almost as prominent as that of C7 (Fig. 5-10). **To count the vertebrae,** *begin below the vertebra prominens* be-

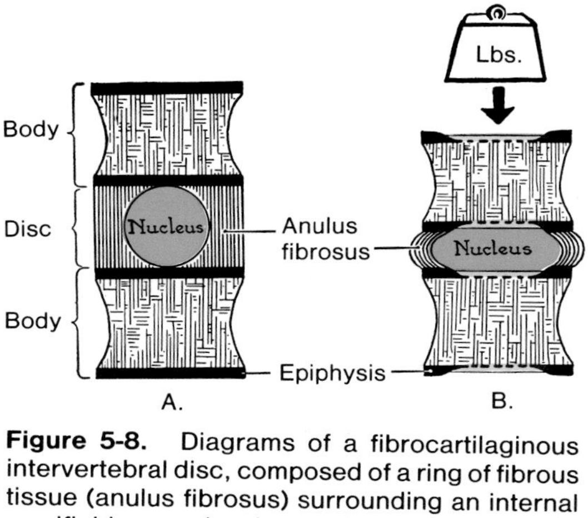

Figure 5-8. Diagrams of a fibrocartilaginous intervertebral disc, composed of a ring of fibrous tissue (anulus fibrosus) surrounding an internal semifluid mass (nucleus pulposus), illustrating the cushioning value of the nucleus pulposus during weight bearing.

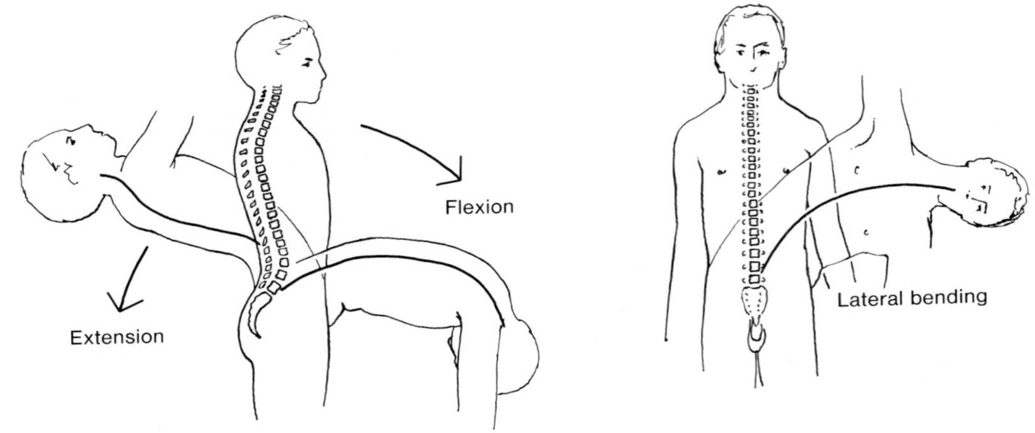

Figure 5-9. Drawings illustrating movements of the vertebral column: flexion (forward bending), extension (backward bending), and lateral bending (lateral flexion). Rotation and circumduction are also possible.

cause the number of cervical vertebrae (7) is very constant.

The median crest of the sacrum (Fig. 5-25*B*), formed by the reduced spinous processes (tubercles) of three or four of its vertebrae, can be palpated, but it is difficult to count them with certainty. *A line joining the skin dimples formed by the posterior superior iliac spines crosses the spinous process of the second sacral vertebra* (Figs. 5-11 and 5-48). The superior end of the natal cleft between the buttocks usually lies over the spinous process of S4.

THE VERTEBRAE

A clear understanding of the general characteristics of vertebrae in the different regions of the vertebral column described here is essential knowledge. Should you specialize later (*e.g.*, in radiology, or orthopaedics, or neurosurgery), you will need to learn the distinctive features of all vertebrae.

A Typical Vertebra (Fig. 5-12). The idealized or "typical" vertebra (*e.g.*, a midlumbar vertebra) is composed of two parts, each of which has a specific function. Typical vertebrae vary in size and in other characteristics from one region to another and to a lesser degree within each region (*e.g.*, examine the thoracic vertebrae in Figure 5-1 noting that their bodies gradually become larger, particularly from T4 inferiorly).

Parts of a Typical Vertebra (Fig. 5-12). A typical vertebra consists of a body anteriorly and a vertebral arch posteriorly. Seven processes arise from the vertebral arch.

The Body (Figs. 5-12 to 5-15). The heavy anterior part of a vertebra or body resembles a *short, long bone.* Its function, like long bones (*e.g.*, the femur), is to support weight. The bodies of the vertebrae from C3 to S1 become progressively larger in order to bear progressively greater weight (Fig. 5-1).

The Vertebral Arch (Figs. 5-12 to 5-14). The posterior part of a vertebra, the vertebral (neural) arch, is attached to the body. It *protects the neural tissues* (*e.g.*, the spinal cord) from injury. The vertebral arch is formed by two **pedicles** (L. little feet) and two **laminae** (L. thin plates). Four articular processes, two transverse processes, and one spinous process arise from the vertebral arch.

The vertebral arch encloses an aperture known as the **vertebral foramen.** Successive vertebral foramina form the **vertebral canal** (spinal canal), which contains the spinal cord and its meninges, nerve roots, and blood vessels (Figs. 5-56 to 5-60).

The pedicles are attached anteriorly to the body and are continuous posteriorly

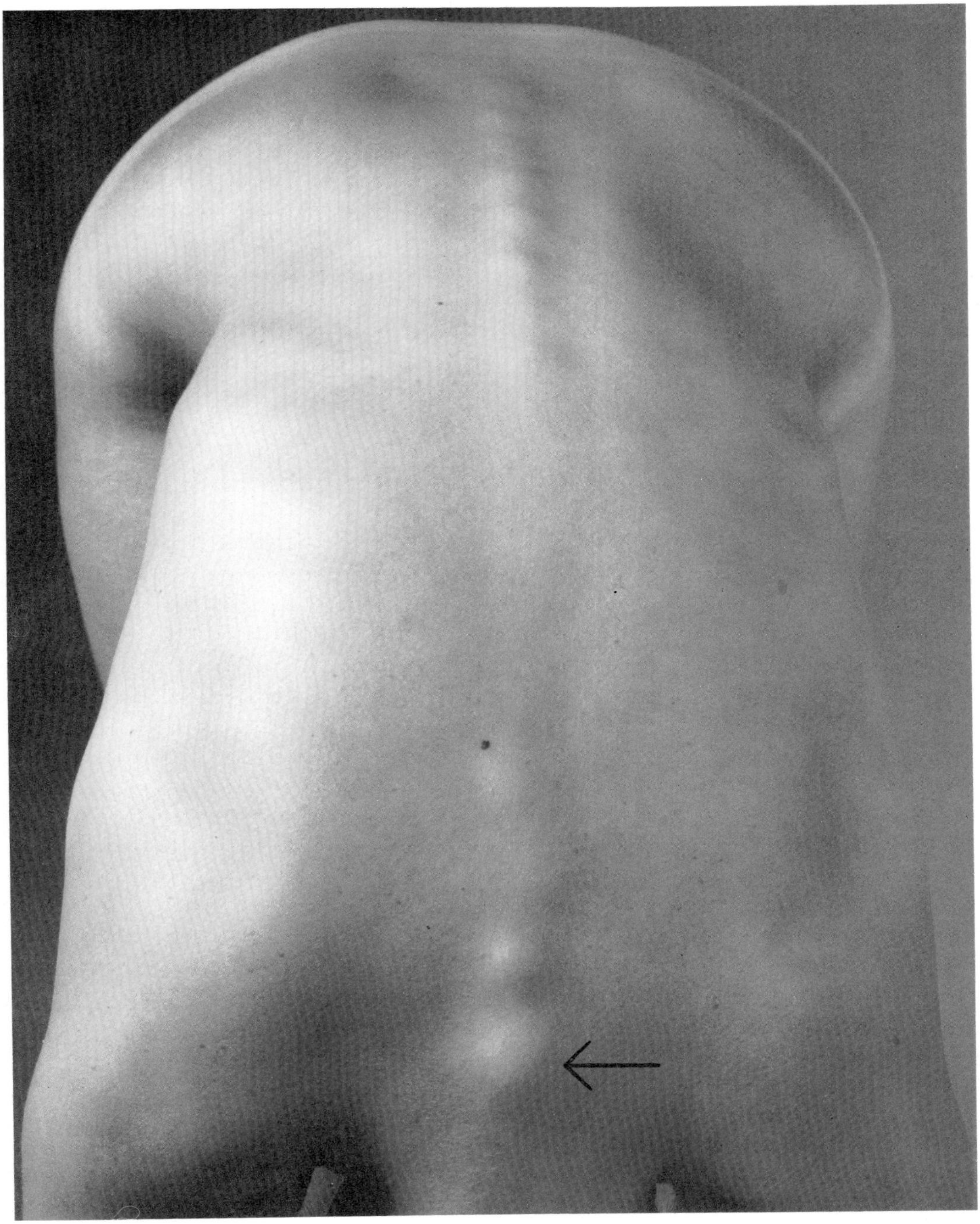

Figure 5-10. Photograph of the back of a 27-year-old woman illustrating flexion of the vertebral column and showing the vertebra prominens (*arrow*). Note that the spinous process of T1 is also prominent and that those of the lumbar vertebrae are visible in the "small of her back." (Also see Fig. 5-53.)

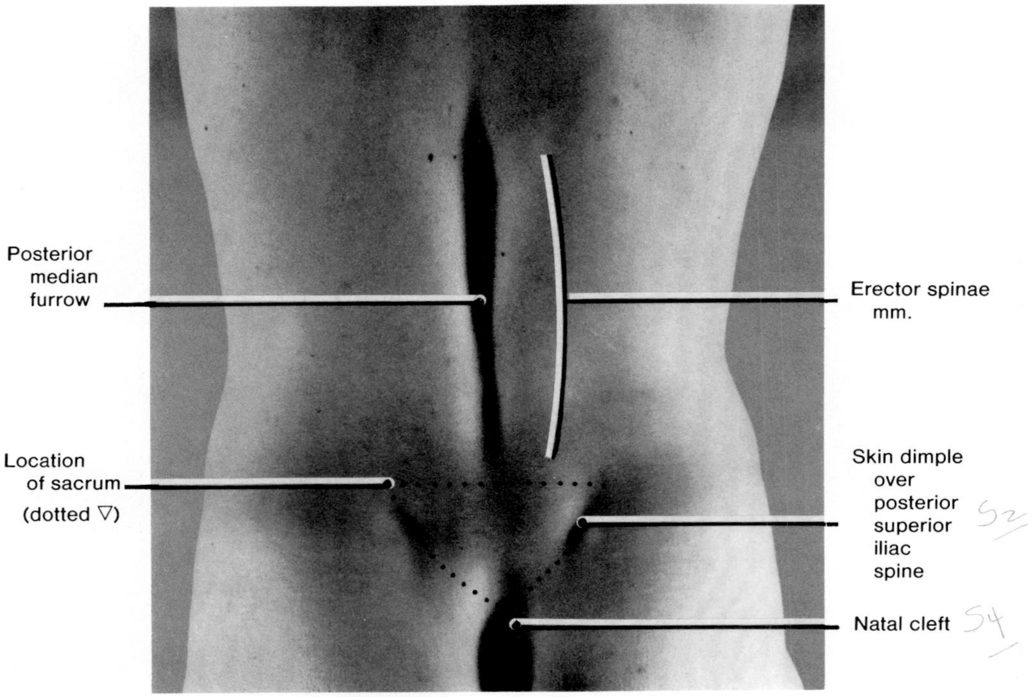

Figure 5-11. Photograph of the back of a 28-year-old man showing the principal surface landmarks. The dimples indicating the posterior superior iliac spines are very pronounced in this person. Compare with the back of the woman shown in Figure 5-48. For a dissection showing the erector spinae muscles, see Figure 5-46.

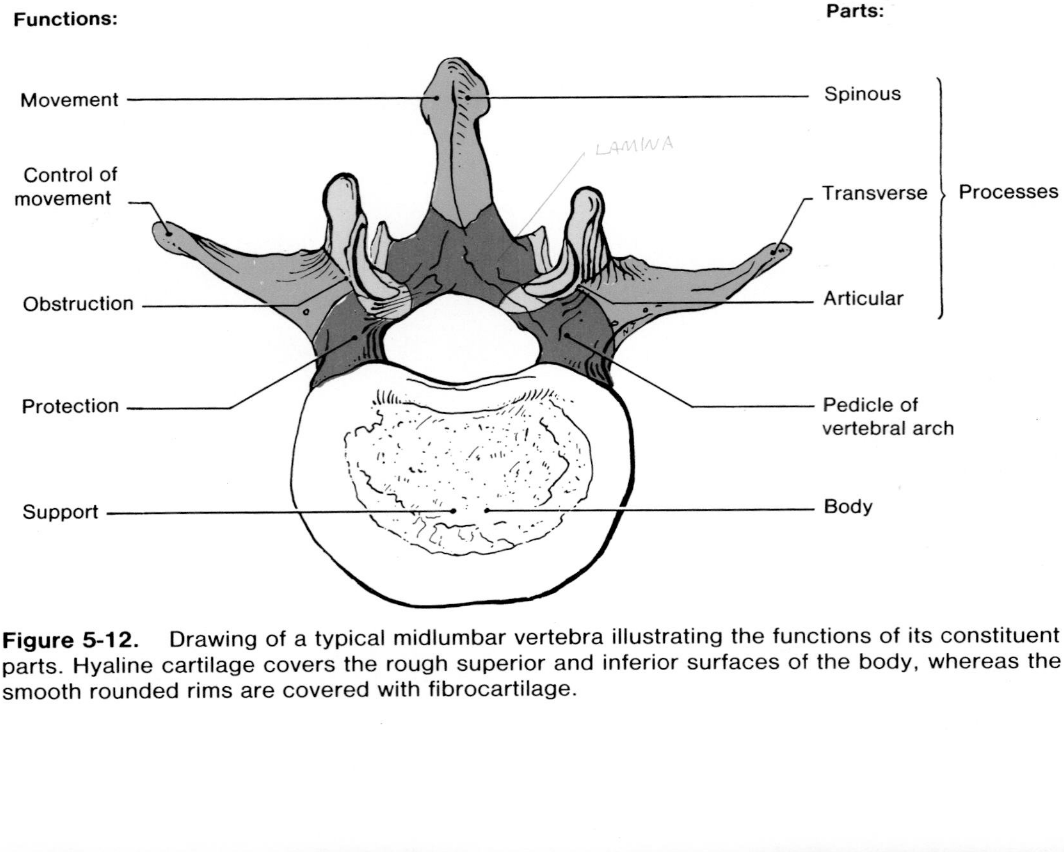

Figure 5-12. Drawing of a typical midlumbar vertebra illustrating the functions of its constituent parts. Hyaline cartilage covers the rough superior and inferior surfaces of the body, whereas the smooth rounded rims are covered with fibrocartilage.

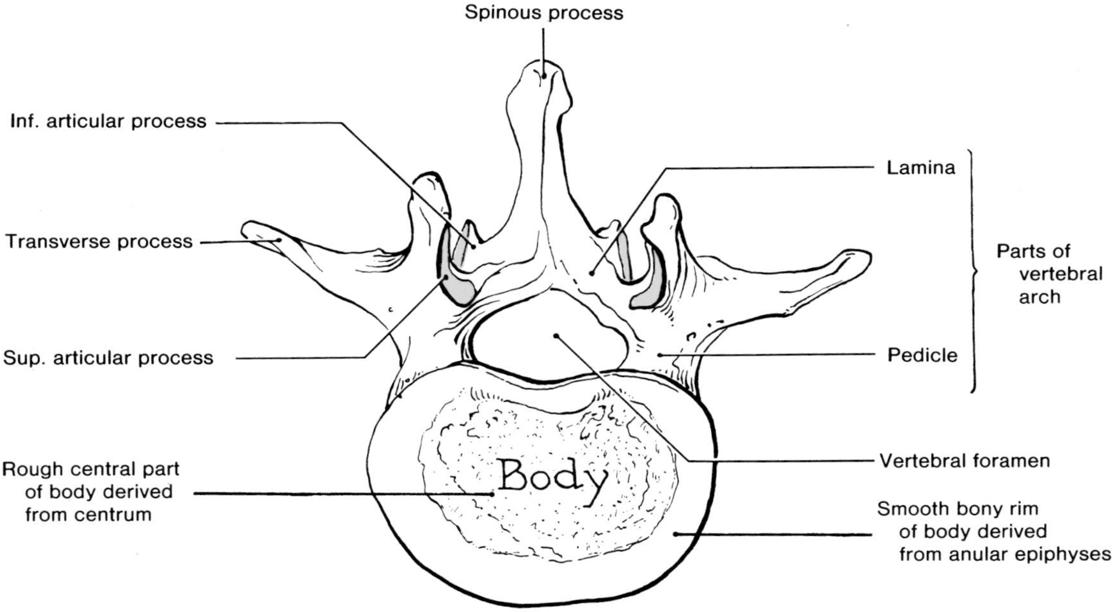

Figure 5-13. Drawing showing the parts of the second lumbar vertebra, viewed from above. For an explanation of the terms centrum and anular epiphyses, see Figures 5-28 and 5-29.

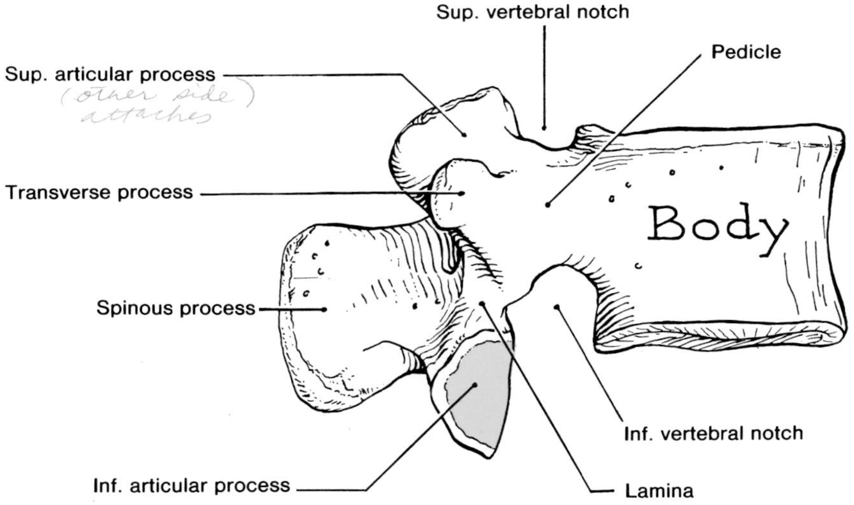

Figure 5-14. Drawing of a lateral view of a second lumbar vertebra. Each articular process has an articular facet (*yellow*).

with the flat laminae. There is a small notch above each pedicle, the **superior vertebral notch** (Fig. 5-14), which varies in size at different levels of the vertebral column. The notch below each pedicle, the **inferior vertebral notch**, is usually larger. When two vertebrae are in articulation (Fig. 5-4), these notches are adjacent to each other and form an almost complete bony ring, the **intervertebral foramen**.

The dorsal and ventral nerve roots are in the vertebral canal and the **spinal (dorsal**

root) ganglia are in the intervertebral foramina (Figs. 5-4 and 5-59). These roots join each other at the outer edge of the intervertebral foramen to form a **spinal nerve**.

The Vertebral Processes (Figs. 5-12 to 5-15). Typical vertebrae have seven processes projecting from the vertebral arch; three are lever-like (the spinous process and the transverse processes) and four are articular. Muscles and ligaments attach to the lever-like processes which act as levers for helping to move the vertebrae.

The **spinous process** (spine) projects posteriorly, usually in the median plane, from the place of union of the laminae (Figs. 5-12 to 5-15). The **transverse processes** project laterally on each side from the junction of the pedicle and the lamina. The **articular processes** (zygapophyses) arise near the junction of the pedicles and the laminae (Figs. 5-12 to 5-15). Each one bears an articular facet (Fig. 5-14). The contact between the upper and lower **articular facets** of an articulated vertebral column helps to prevent forward movement of an upper vertebra on a lower one, especially in the thoracic and lumbar regions. The articular facets allow some flexion and extension as well as varying degrees of lateral bending and rotation.

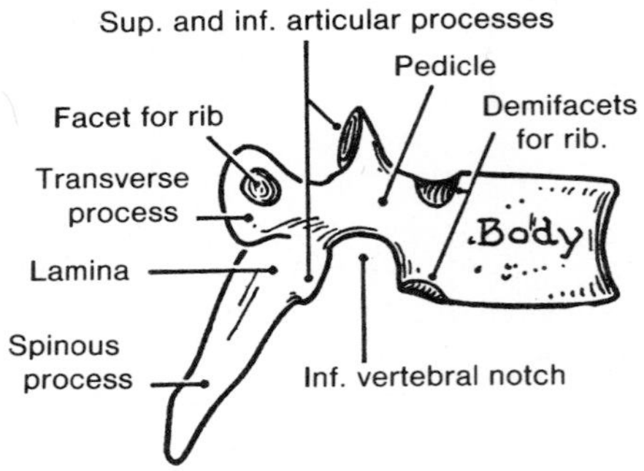

Figure 5-15. Drawing of a lateral view of a typical midthoracic vertebra.

Regional Characteristics. The vertebrae in the various regions of the vertebral column have distinctive characteristics which enable them to be identified with relative ease. In addition, there are obvious differences in the size of the vertebral foramen in the same regions of different persons (Fig. 5-16). There are also differences in the size of the foramina in the various regions. Verify this by inserting your finger into the vertebral foramen of a midthoracic vertebra, as shown in Figure 5-17, and then

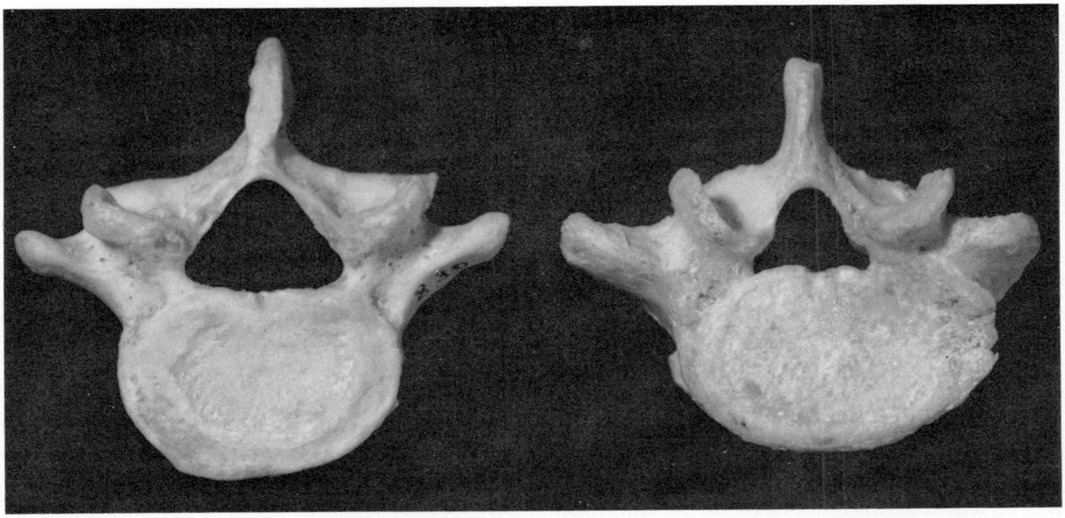

Figure 5-16. Photographs of superior views of fifth lumbar vertebrae illustrating the varying sizes and shapes of the vertebral canal in different persons. The common oval-triangular form is shown on the left, whereas the uncommon trifoliate (trefoil) pattern is illustrated on the right. A small trefoil-shaped canal is a contributory factor in cases of sciatica and/or cauda equina claudication (lower limb pain resulting from pressure on spinal nerve roots).

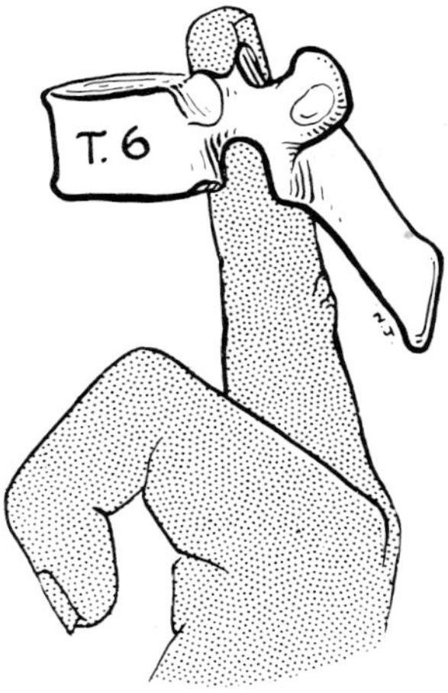

Figure 5-17. Diagram demonstrating the small size of the vertebral foramen of a midthoracic vertebra.

into the foramen of a first and a twelfth thoracic vertebra. Note that the vertebral foramina are larger in these regions because the spinal cord is enlarged in these locations for innervation of the limbs (Fig. 5-62).

Although there are characteristic regional differences in the vertebrae, only an expert can differentiate a fifth from a sixth thoracic vertebra or a second from a third lumbar vertebra. However, everyone who takes an anatomy course should be able to distinguish a cervical vertebra from a thoracic vertebra and a thoracic vertebra from a lumbar vertebra.

Cervical Vertebrae (Figs. 5-18 to 5-20). The cervical vertebrae form the *bony axis of the neck*. Their distinctive feature is the large oval **foramen transversarium** (transverse foramen) in each transverse process. The foramina transversaria in C7 are smaller than those of the other cervical vertebrae; occasionally they are absent. The vertebral arteries pass through these foramina (Fig. 5-59), except in C7, which transmit only small accessory vertebral veins.

The spinous processes of the third to sixth cervical vertebrae are short and bifid, with two knobs on their tips. Another characteristic is the almost equal sizes of their superior and inferior vertebral notches.

The first, second, and seventh cervical vertebrae are atypical.

The first cervical vertebra, a ring-shaped bone, is called the **atlas** (Figs. 5-18 to 5-20). Because it supports the skull, it was named after Atlas, who, according to Greek mythology, supported the heavens. Its kidney-shaped, concave, superior articular facets receive the **occipital condyles** (Figs. 5-19 and 5-55). *The atlas has no spinous process or body*; it consists of anterior and posterior arches, each of which bears a tubercle and a lateral mass (Figs. 5-18 and 5-19).

The second cervical vertebra, known as the **axis** (Fig. 5-18), has two flat bearing surfaces, the superior articular facets, upon which the atlas rotates. Its distinguishing feature is the blunt tooth-like **dens** (odontoid process). The strong dens (G. tooth) is held in position by the transverse ligament of the atlas (Fig. 5-19), and it prevents horizontal displacement of the atlas.

The seventh cervical vertebra is usually called the *vertebra prominens* because its long spinous process is visible through the skin (Fig. 5-10). C7 also has large transverse processes (Fig. 5-18).

Thoracic Vertebrae (Figs. 5-21 and 5-22). All 12 thoracic vertebrae **articulate with ribs**; thus, they are characterized by articular facets for them. There is one or more on each side of the body for articulation with the head of a rib and one on each transverse process of the upper 10 for the tubercle of a rib. The spinous processes tend to be long and slender, and those of the middle ones are directed downward over the vertebral arch of the vertebra below (Fig. 5-21*B*).

The middle four thoracic vertebrae are typical. The outline of their bodies, viewed from above, is heart-shaped, and their vertebral foramina are circular (Fig. 5-21*A*). Sometimes an impression is visible on the left sides of the bodies of the middle thoracic vertebrae; it is produced by the descending thoracic aorta (Fig. 1-19).

The first four thoracic vertebra have some cervical features. The first thoracic vertebra differs from typical thoracic vertebrae in that it has an almost horizontal spinous process and long transverse processes. It has a complete costal facet on the superior edge of the body for the first rib and a demifacet on the inferior edge which

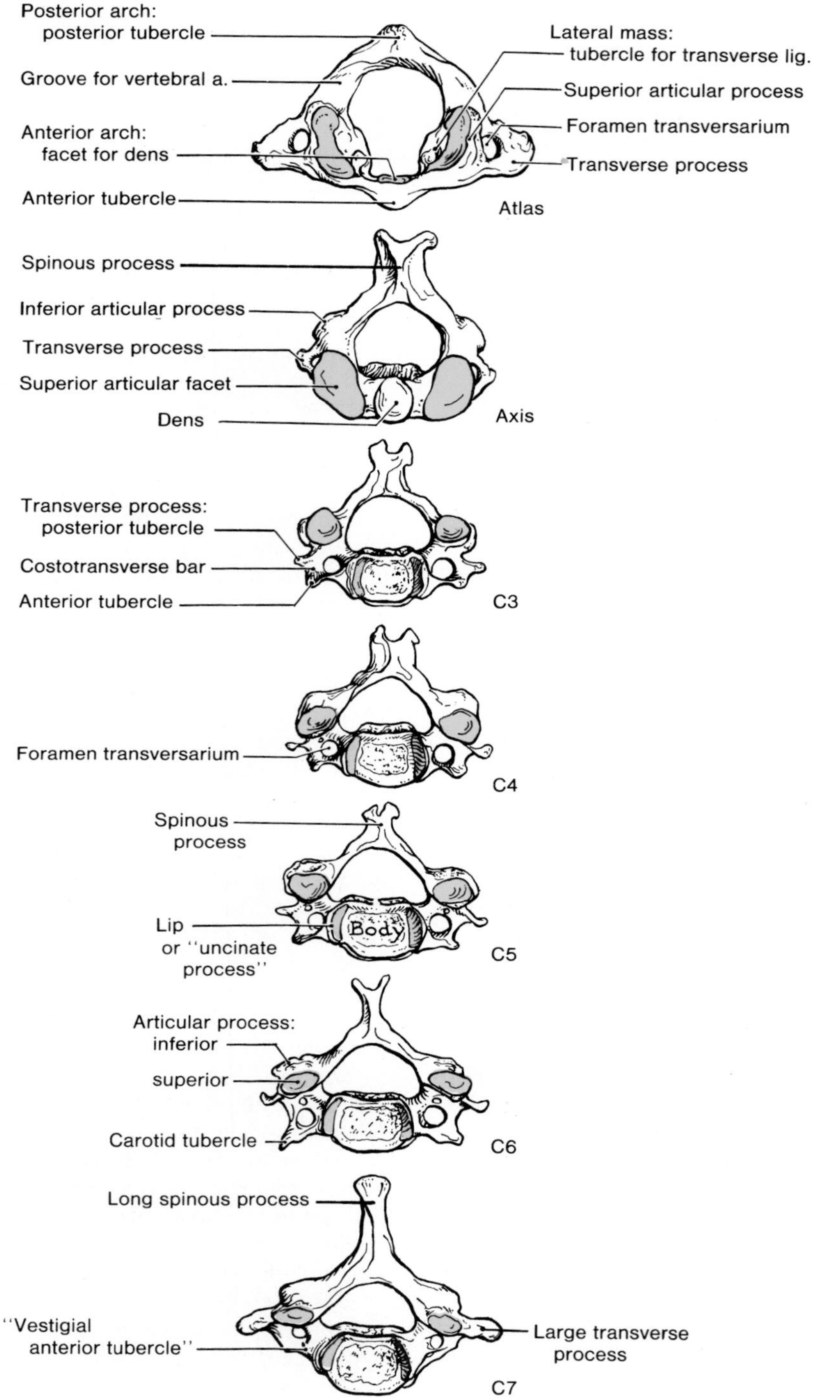

Figure 5-18. Drawings of the cervical vertebrae from above. Note that the foramina transversaria in C7 are smaller than those of the other cervical vertebrae; occasionally they are absent. Observe that the seventh cervical vertebra has a long spinous process and large transverse processes. It is often called the vertebra prominens (Figs. 5-10 and 5-20).

contributes to the articular surface for the second rib.

The lower four thoracic vertebrae are atypical (Fig. 5-22). They often have features of lumbar vertebrae and possess mammillary, accessory, and lateral tubercles.

Lumbar Vertebrae (Figs. 5-12 to 5-14, 5-16, and 5-23). These vertebrae are in the "small of the back," and their spinous processes are prominent when the vertebral column is flexed (Fig. 5-10). Lumbar vertebrae may be distinguished by their relatively *large bodies*, as compared with cervical and thoracic vertebrae, and by the *absence of costal facets*. Their vertebral bodies, seen from above, are kidney-shaped, and their vertebral foramina are oval to triangular (Figs. 5-12, 5-13, and 5-23). It is not difficult to identify lumbar vertebrae and it is easy to arrange them in their proper order (Fig. 5-23).

The fifth lumbar vertebra, the largest of all movable vertebrae, is characterized by *stout transverse processes* which arise

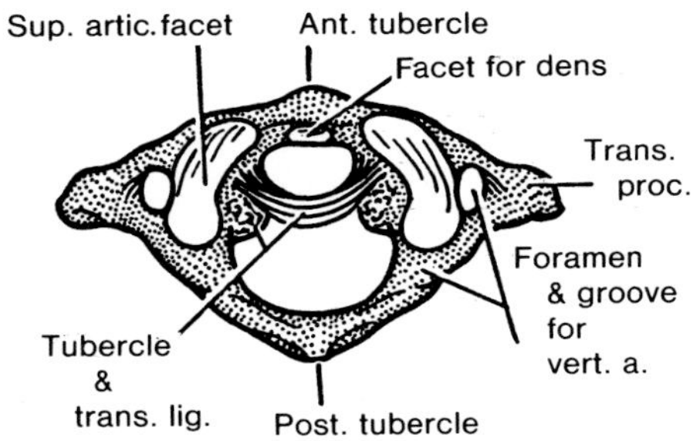

Figure 5-19. Drawing of a superior view of the atlas showing the transverse ligament.

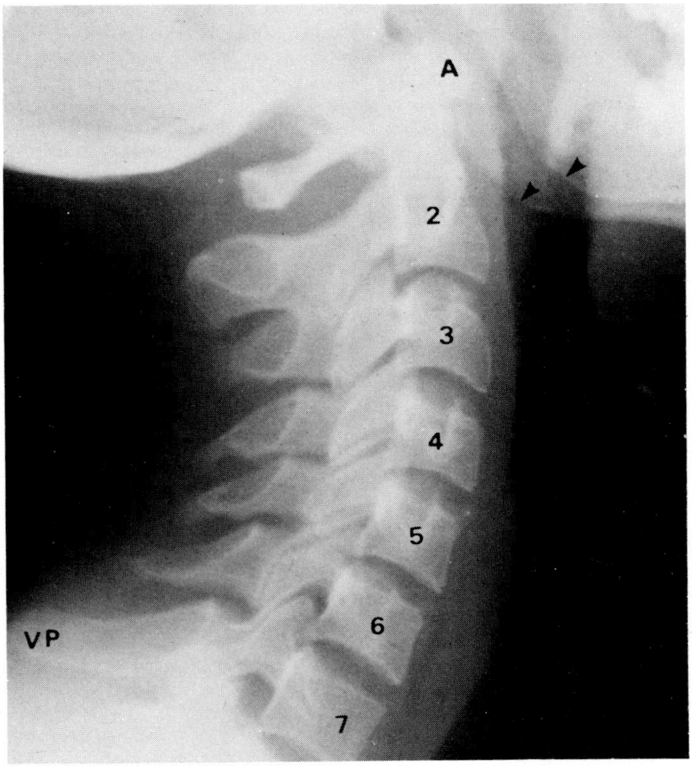

Figure 5-20. Lateral radiograph of the cervical region of the vertebral column in which the bodies of cervical vertebrae 2 to 7 have been numbered. Note that the anterior arch of the atlas (*A*) is in a plane anterior to the curved line joining the front of the bodies of the vertebrae. Note also the vertebra prominens (C7), characterized by its long spinous process, labeled *VP*. The *arrows* point to the angles of the mandible which are not perfectly superimposed upon each other.

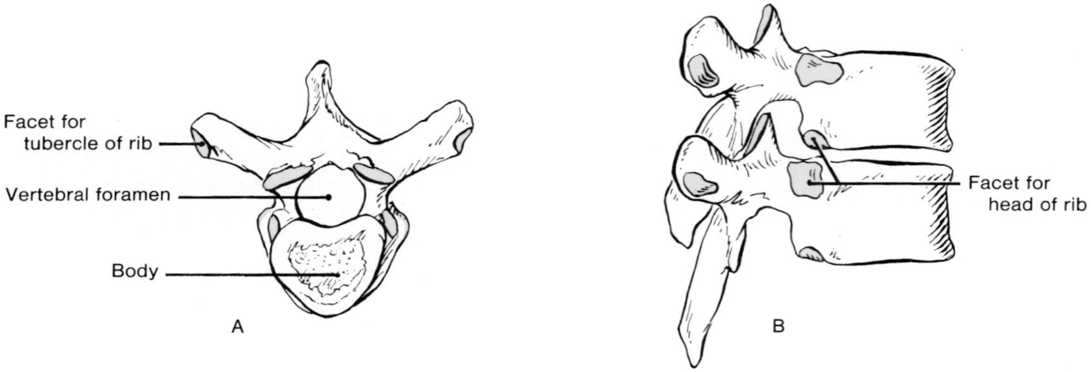

Figure 5-21. Drawings of middle or typical thoracic vertebrae showing their distinctive features. *A*, superior view. *B*, lateral view.

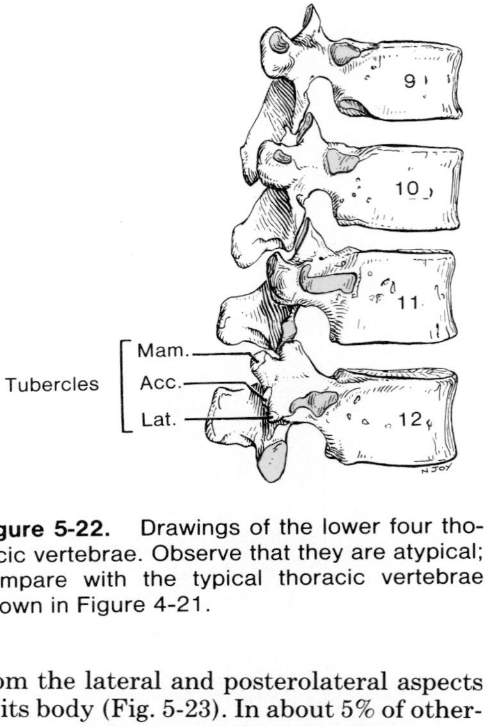

Figure 5-22. Drawings of the lower four thoracic vertebrae. Observe that they are atypical; compare with the typical thoracic vertebrae shown in Figure 4-21.

from the lateral and posterolateral aspects of its body (Fig. 5-23). In about 5% of otherwise normal persons, L5 is partly or completely incorporated into the sacrum, a condition known as hemisacralization or **sacralization of the fifth lumbar vertebra** (Fig. 5-24).

The Sacrum (Fig. 5-25). This large triangular, **wedge-shaped bone** is usually composed of five fused sacral vertebrae in the adult. The sacrum, derived from a Latin word meaning sacred, *provides strength and stability to the pelvis.*

On the pelvic (ventral, Fig. 5-25*A*) and dorsal surfaces (Fig. 5-25*B*) there are typically four pairs of foramina for the exit of the anterior and posterior primary divisions of the sacral nerves. In Figure 5-25*A* observe that the pelvic foramina are larger than the dorsal ones (Fig. 5-25*B*). Also notice that there are four transverse lines on the pelvic surface which indicate where fusion of the vertebrae occurred after the 20th year.

The base of the sacrum is formed by the superior surface of the first sacral vertebra. The superior articular processes that articulate with the inferior articular processes of L5 project upward from the base (Fig. 5-25*A*). The projecting anterior edge of the body of the first sacral vertebra is called the **sacral promontory** (L. *promontorium*, mountain ridge).

The sacrum supports the vertebral column and forms the posterior part of the pelvis (Fig. 5-2). It is tilted so that it articulates with L5 at an angle, the **lumbosacral angle** (Fig. 5-1). The sacrum is often wider in proportion to length in the female than in the male, but the body of the first sacral vertebra is usually larger in males.

The posterior aspect of the sacrum is rough, convex, and marked by five prominent longitudinal ridges. The central one, or **median sacral crest**, represents the fused spinous processes of the upper sacral vertebrae (Fig. 5-25*B*). The intermediate crest represents the fused articular processes, and the lateral crest represents portions of the transverse processes.

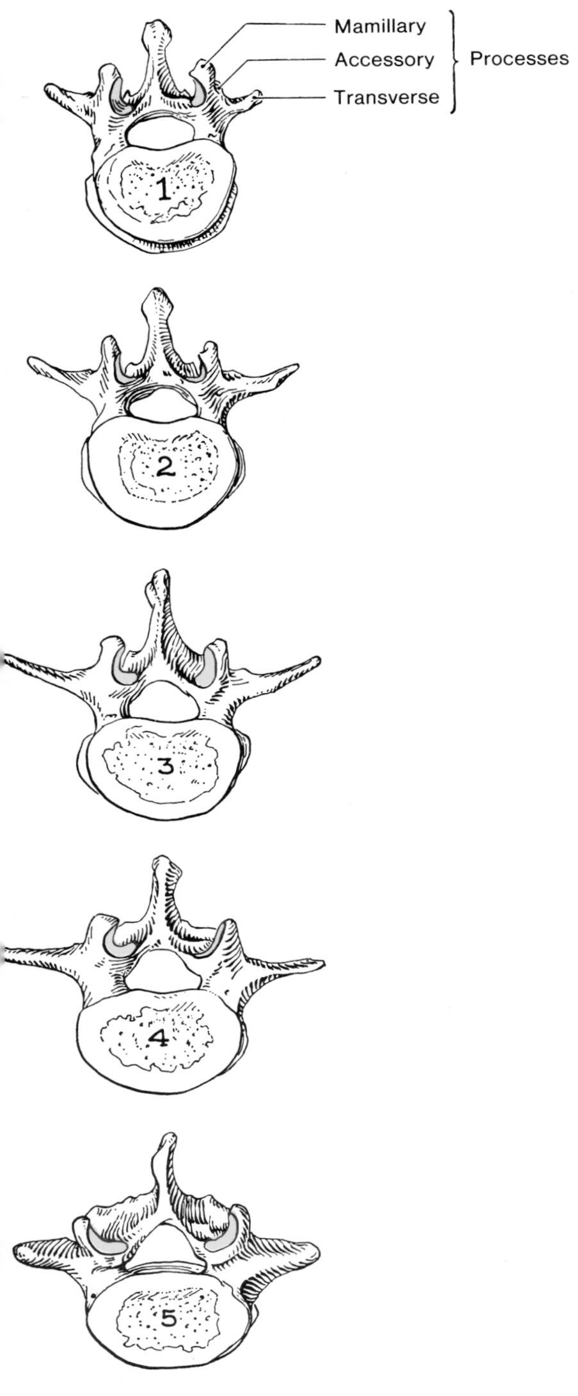

Figure 5-23. Drawings of the lumbar vertebrae from above. Note their kidney-shaped bodies and their oval and triangular vertebral foramina. Observe the stout transverse processes of L5 that are connected to the whole of the lateral surface of the pedicle and to the posterolateral part of the body.

Because the articular surface of the lateral aspect of the sacrum is like an auricle (L. external ear), it is called the **auricular surface** (Fig. 5-25*B*). This is where a synovial joint, the sacroiliac joint (Fig. 5-2), is located between the sacrum and the ilium. Note the $\wedge$-shaped **sacral hiatus** (L. opening) on the dorsal surface and the **sacral cornua** (L. horns) which project down on each side of the hiatus (Fig. 5-25*B*). Palpate the hiatus and cornua in your natal cleft (Fig. 5-11).

CLINICALLY ORIENTED COMMENTS

Anesthetic agents are sometimes injected through the sacral hiatus (**caudal anesthesia**, Fig. 5-69*B*). The anesthetic acts on the sacral and coccygeal nerves (Fig. 5-60). As the sacral hiatus is between the sacral cornua, they are important bony landmarks for locating the hiatus. Anesthetic agents can also be injected through the dorsal sacral foramina (Fig. 5-25*B*).

In some people the first sacral vertebra is more or less separated from the sacrum (**lumbarization of the first sacral vertebra**). In some cases of lumbarization of S1 (Fig. 5-26) or sacralization of L5 (Fig. 5-24), it is the first "normal articulation" (intervertebral disc plus two zygapophyseal joints) that takes the strain and that may degenerate prematurely or extensively. For example, when L5 is sacralized (Fig. 5-24) the L5/S1 level is strong and the L4/L5 level degenerates, often producing symptoms (*e.g.*, backache).

You are encouraged to become familar with the main radiographic features of the lumbosacral region of the vertebral column because low back pain is such a common complaint (Fig. 5-27). The planes of the lumbar **zygapophyseal joints** are variable, but this variation is of debatable clinical significance. In perfect lateral views of the lumbosacral region, the images of the

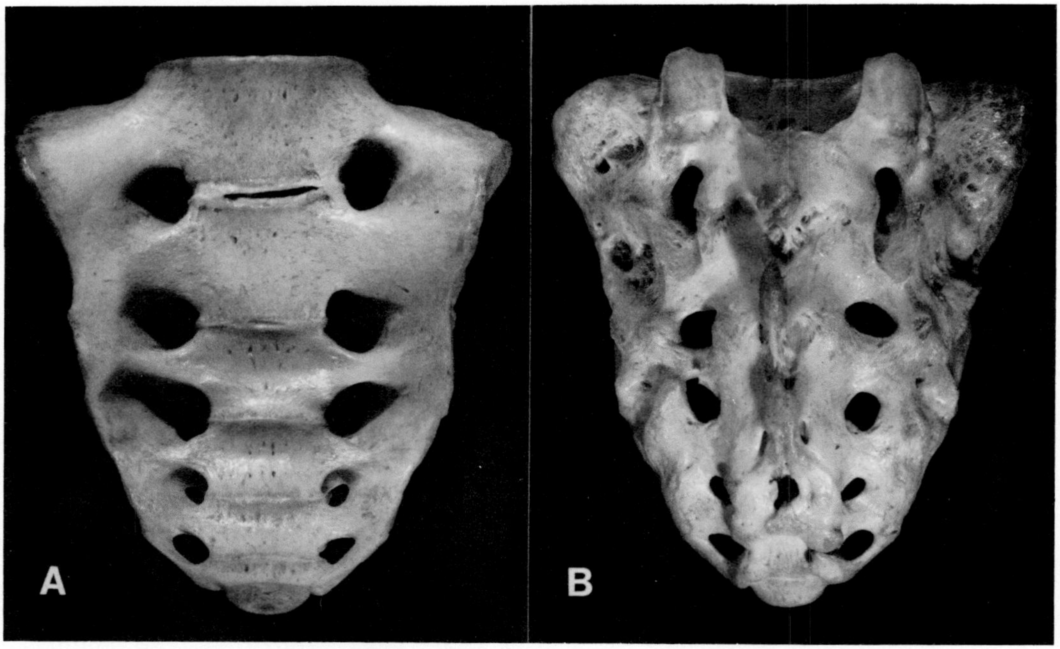

Figure 5-24. Photographs of a sacrum showing sacralization of the fifth lumbar vertebra. *A*, pelvic (ventral) surface. *B*, dorsal surface. As fusion of the fifth lumbar vertebra with the sacrum is almost complete in this case, only four lumbar type vertebrae would probably be recognized in a radiograph.

right and left articular processes and the intervertebral foramina are projected on each other so they appear as single rather than double images (Fig. 5-27*B*).

The Coccyx (Fig. 5-25). The coccyx (tailbone) is the vestigial remnant of the tail which embryos have until the 8th week. Usually four rudimentary vertebrae (segments or pieces) are present, but there may be one less or one more. The vertebrae consist of bodies only, except for the first coccygeal vertebra, which has **cornua** that represent remnants of the pedicles and transverse processes (Fig. 5-25*B*).

The three inferior coccygeal vertebrae often fuse during middle life, forming a beak-like bone; this accounts for the name coccyx, the Greek word for a cuckoo. During old age the first coccygeal vertebra often fuses with the sacrum, as illustrated in Figure 5-1.

The coccyx gives no support to the vertebral column, but it gives origin to part of the gluteus maximus and coccygeus muscles and to the anococcygeal ligament (Fig. 3-22). The coccyx can be palpated with the forefinger in the rectum and the thumb in the natal cleft (Fig. 5-11).

CLINICALLY ORIENTED COMMENTS

The coccyx is joined to the sacrum by cartilage (a synchondrosis or cartilaginous joint); therefore, it can bend to some extent during childbirth. In unusual cases the coccyx may separate from the sacrum, producing **coccydynia** (pain in the coccygeal region, usually marked during sitting). This condition more commonly results from a fall directly on the coccyx.

Development of Vertebrae (Fig. 5-28). The vertebrae begin to develop during the embryonic period as condensations of mesenchyme around the notochord (Fig. 5-28*A*). Chondrification centers soon appear

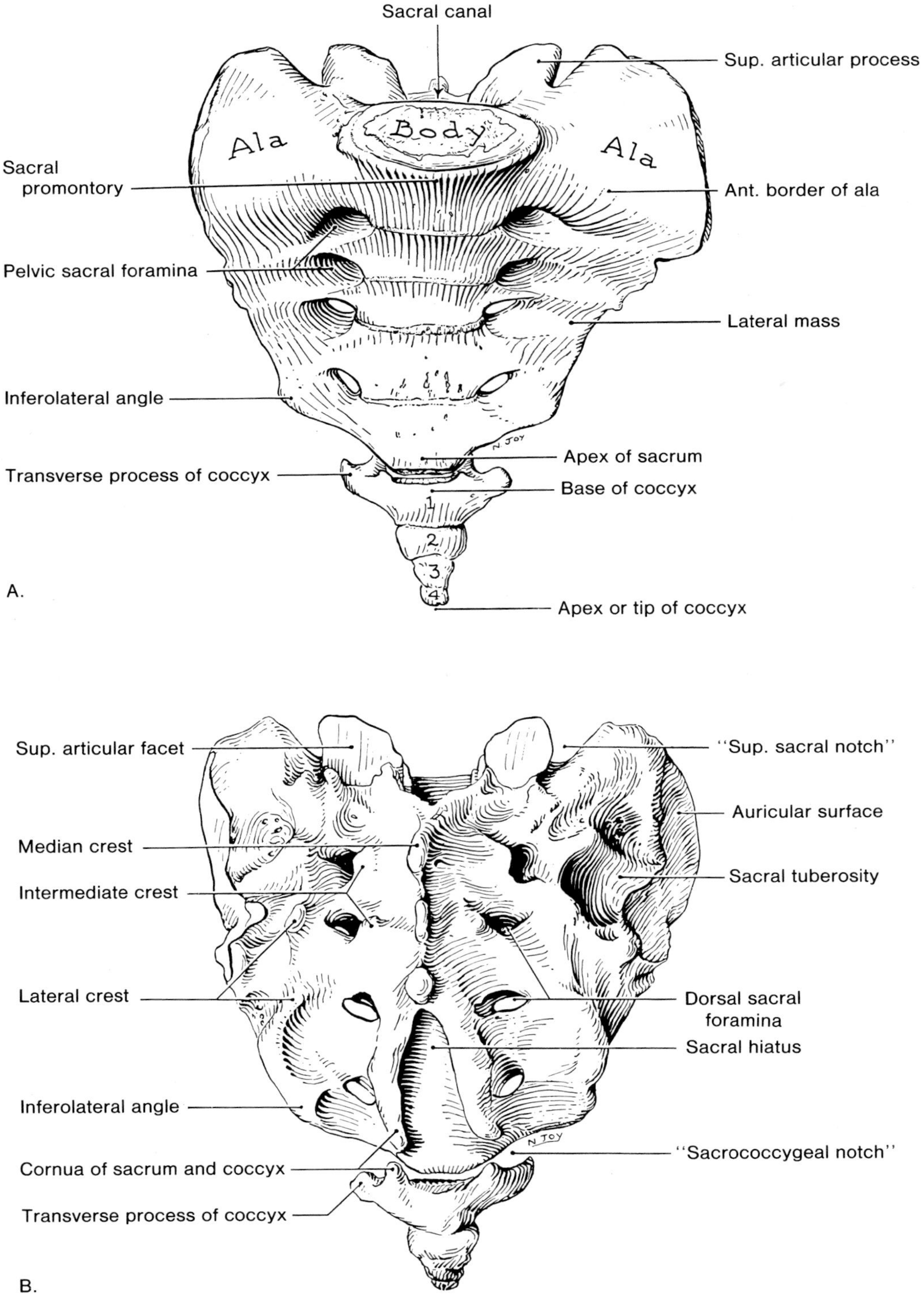

Figure 5-25. Drawings of the sacrum and coccyx. *A*, the pelvic (ventral) surface faces downward and forward and is concave from above down and from side to side (Fig. 5-1). *B*, the dorsal surface is rough and has a series of longitudinal ridges formed by the fused posterior parts of the five fused vertebrae.

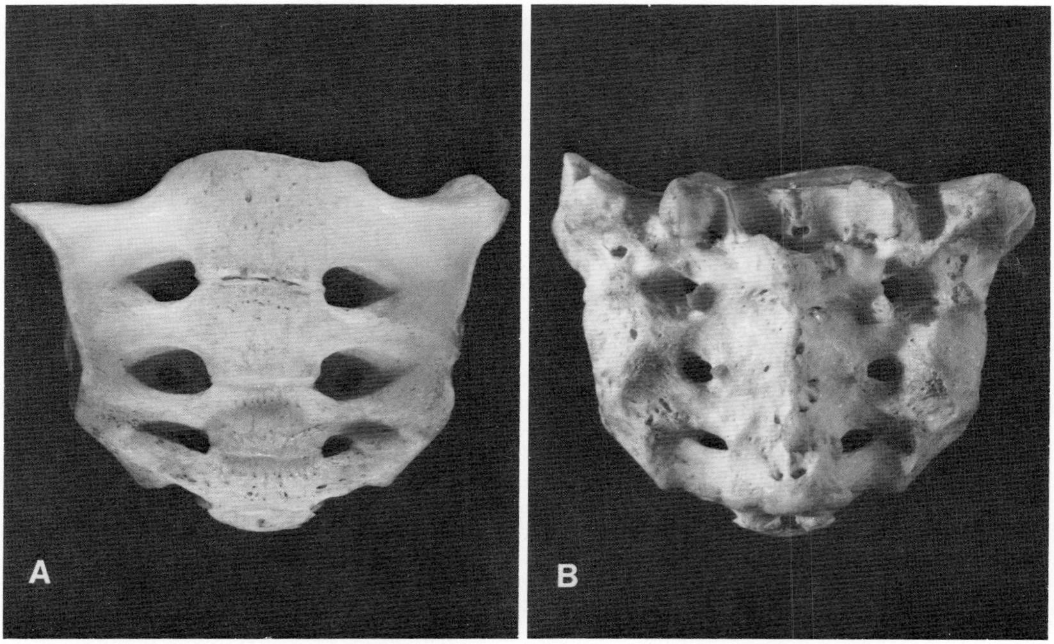

Figure 5-26. Photographs of a sacrum showing only four fused vertebrae, probably as a result of lumbarization of the first sacral vertebra. *A,* pelvic surface; *B,* dorsal surface. Compare with normal sacrum (Fig. 5-25).

and form a cartilaginous vertebra (Fig. 5-28*B*).

Typical vertebrae begin to ossify toward the end of the embryonic period. **Three primary ossification centers** begin in each cartilaginous vertebra, *one in the centrum and one in each half of the vertebral arch* (Fig. 5-28*C*). At birth the lower sacral and the coccygeal vertebrae are cartilaginous; they begin to ossify during infancy.

At birth each typical vertebra consists of three bony parts united by hyaline cartilage (Figs. 5-28*D* and 5-29*A*). The halves of the vertebral arch begin to fuse in the cervical region during the 1st year and fusion is usually complete in the lumbar region by the 6th year (Fig. 5-29*B*). In children the vertebral arch is joined to the centrum at **neurocentral joints** or synchondroses (*i.e.,* joints where the surfaces are connected by plates of cartilage). The vertebral arch fuses with the centrum during childhood (usually 5 to 8 years).

Shortly after puberty (12 to 16 years), **five secondary ossification centers** develop in each typical vertebra—*one at the tip of the spinous process, one at the tip of each transverse process,* and *two ring or* **anular epiphyses**, one on the superior and one on the inferior edge of the centrum (Fig. 5-28*E* and *F*). The body of the vertebra forms mainly from growth of the centrum with the addition of the anular epiphyses, more appropriately called **rim apophyses** (G. offshoots) because they add only raised rims to the edges of the vertebral bodies (Fig. 5-13).

All secondary ossification centers are usually united with the vertebra by the 25th year, but the times of their union are variable. Caution must be exercised so that a persistent epiphysis is not mistaken for a fracture in a radiograph.

Exceptions to the typical ossification of vertebrae occur in the atlas, the axis, the seventh cervical vertebra, the lumbar vertebrae, the sacrum, and the coccyx. For details of their ossification, consult the anatomy reference book listed at the end of this Chapter.

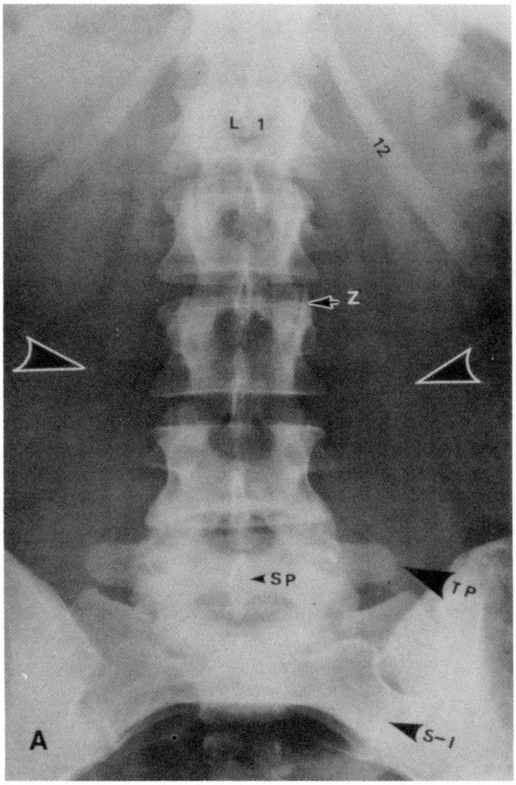

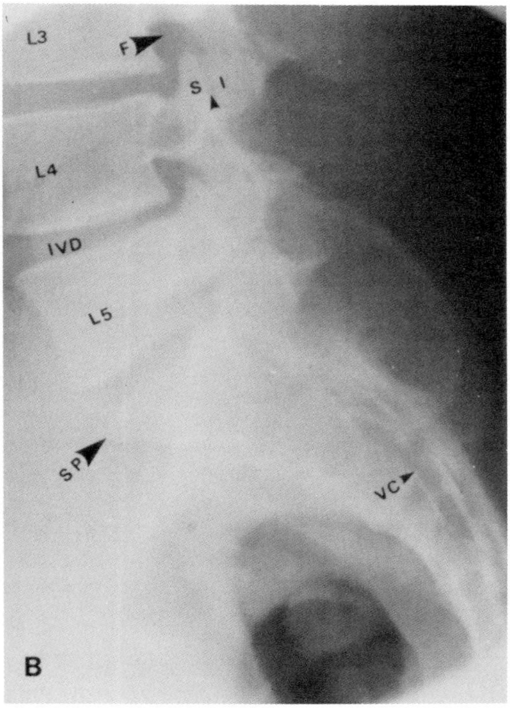

Figure 5-27. Radiographs of the lumbosacral region. *A,* anteroposterior (*AP*) view. Observe the articulation of the last (12th) "floating" rib with the last thoracic vertebra and the bodies and processes of the five lumbar vertebrae. The spinous process (*SP*) and a transverse process (*TP*) of L5 are labeled. The left zygapophyseal joint (*Z*) between L2/L3 is indicated. The *large arrows* indicate the margins of the psoas muscles. *B,* lateral view. Observe particularly the last three lumbar vertebrae and the spaces for the intervertebral discs. The space between L4/L5 is marked *IVD*. Note the angulation at the lumbosacral junction, producing the sacral promontory (*SP*). An *arrow* points to the joint between the superior articular process of L4 (*S*) and the inferior articular process of L3 (*I*). A *small arrow* points to the anterior margin of the vertebral canal (*VC*) and a large arrow points to the intervertebral foramina (*F*).

CLINICALLY ORIENTED COMMENTS

The most common developmental abnormality of vertebrae is **spina bifida occulta** (Fig. 5-30). The defect is in L5 and/or S1 in about *10% of people*, but this abnormality may occur anywhere along the vertebral axis. This defect results from failure of the halves of the vertebral arch to grow enough to meet each other and undergo **synostosis** (osseous union).

Often there is a tuft of hair over the vertebral defect, which varies from a slight deficiency to almost complete absence of the vertebral arch (Fig. 5-30). If several vertebrae are involved, the condition is called posterior **rachischisis** (G. *rachis*, spine + *schisis*, split).

Although most persons with spina bifida occulta have no specific complaints, some present with low back pain. Nearly all persons with rachischisis have a varying degree of nerve involvement, the distribution and amount depending mainly on the position and extent of the lesion.

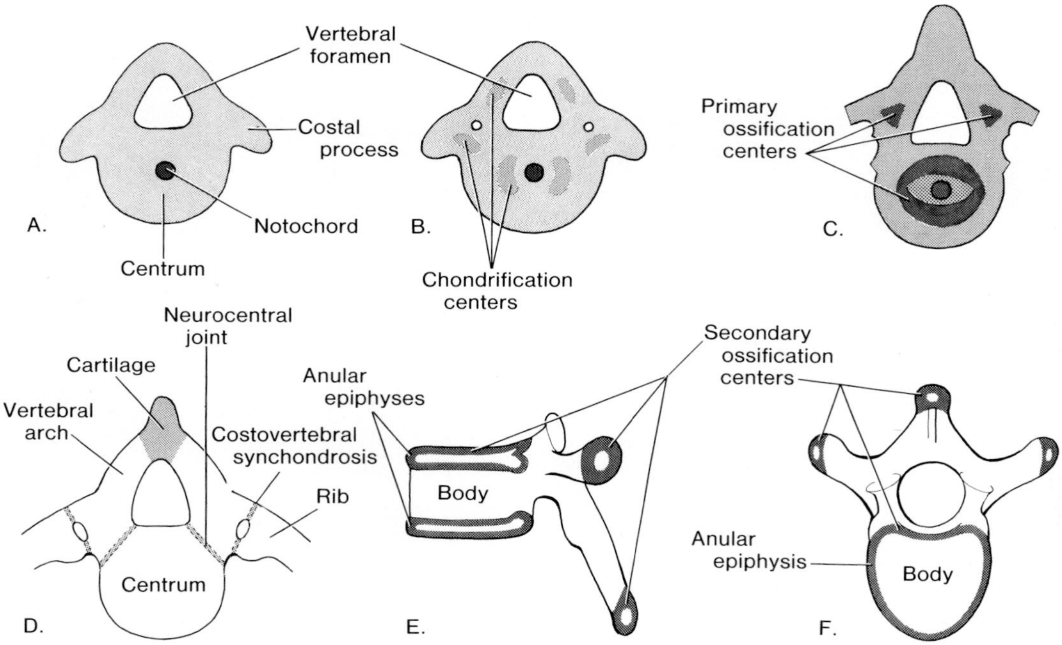

Figure 5-28. Drawings illustrating the stages of vertebral development. *A,* precartilaginous (mesenchymal) stage (7 weeks). *B,* chondrification centers appear. *C,* primary ossification centers appear at 7 weeks. *D,* a midthoracic vertebra at birth consisting of three bony parts. Note the cartilage between the halves of the vertebral arch and between the centrum and the vertebral arch. *E* and *F,* lateral and superior views of a midthoracic vertebra showing the location of the secondary centers of ossification.

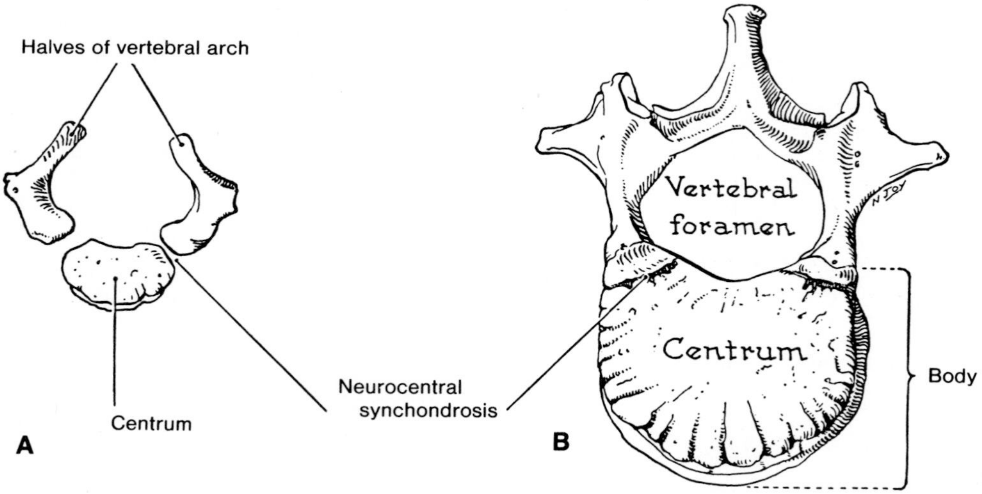

Figure 5-29. Drawings of dried vertebrae. *A,* at birth. The hyaline cartilage separating the halves of the vertebral (neural) arch from each other and from the centrum is not shown. *B,* early childhood. The halves of the vertebral arch have fused, but the neurocentral synchondroses are present; they begin to undergo synostosis during the 5th to 8th years.

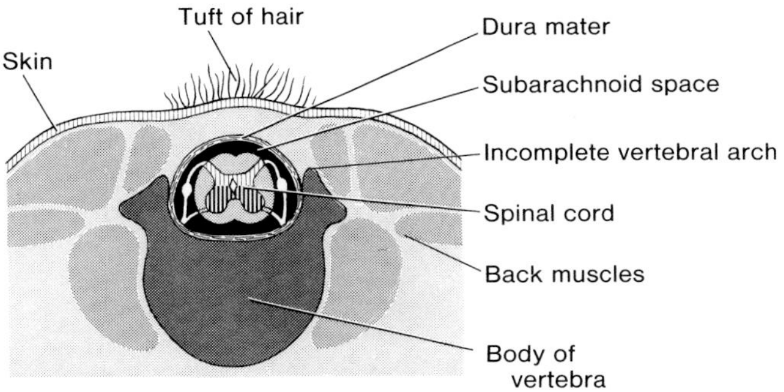

Figure 5-30. Diagrammatic sketch illustrating spina bifida occulta. Note that the halves of the vertebral arch have failed to develop and fuse with each other.

JOINTS OF THE VERTEBRAL COLUMN

The vertebrae from C2 to S1 articulate with each other at **three joints**: one anterior intervertebral nonsynovial joint, the **intervertebral disc**; and two posterior intervertebral synovial joints, the **zygapophyseal joints** (apophyseal or facet joints). Various ligaments and muscles also join the vertebrae together.

Joints of the Vertebral Bodies (Figs. 5-31 to 5-34). The anterior intervertebral joints, or intervertebral discs, are classified as **symphyses**, which are *fibrocartilaginous articulations of a nonsynovial type* that are designed for strength.

The Longitudinal Ligaments (Figs. 5-31, 5-32, and 5-36). In addition to the anuli fibrosi of the intervertebral discs (Figs. 5-8 and 5-34), the bodies of the vertebrae are united by anterior and posterior longitudinal ligaments.

The anterior longitudinal ligament is a strong, broad, fibrous band that runs longitudinally along the anterior surfaces of the intervertebral discs and the bodies of the vertebrae (Figs. 5-32 and 5-36). It extends from the pelvic surface of the sacrum to the anterior tubercle of the atlas and the base of the skull. *Its fibers are firmly fixed to the intervertebral discs and to the periosteum* of the vertebral bodies. The broad anterior longitudinal ligament **tends to prevent hyperextension** of the vertebral column.

CLINICALLY ORIENTED COMMENTS

The anterior longitudinal ligament is severely stretched and is sometimes torn during severe **hyperextension of the neck**. The association of rear end automobile collision and this injury is well known, especially to litigation lawyers (Case 5-2).

The posterior longitudinal ligament (Figs. 5-31, 5-32, 5-36, and 5-51 is a narrow and somewhat weaker band than the anterior longitudinal ligament. *It extends inside the vertebral canal* from the atlas to the sacrum and is attached to the intervertebral discs and to the edges of the vertebral bodies. The posterior longitudinal ligament **tends to prevent hyperflexion** of the vertebral column.

The Intervertebral Discs (Figs. 5-31 to 5-34 and 5-52). These fibrocartilaginous discs are formed of somewhat circular anuli fibrosi enclosing gelatinous nuclei pulposi. The anuli fibrosi insert into the smooth, compact bony rims on the articular surfaces of the vertebral bodies (Figs. 5-8, 5-13, and 5-34). The nuclei pulposi contact the articular cartilages (hyaline plates), which are attached to the rough parts (endplates) of the vertebral bodies (*i.e.*, inside the smooth, bony rims). Poorly developed intervertebral discs are present between the bodies of the sacral vertebrae in young persons, but they usually ossify with advancing age.

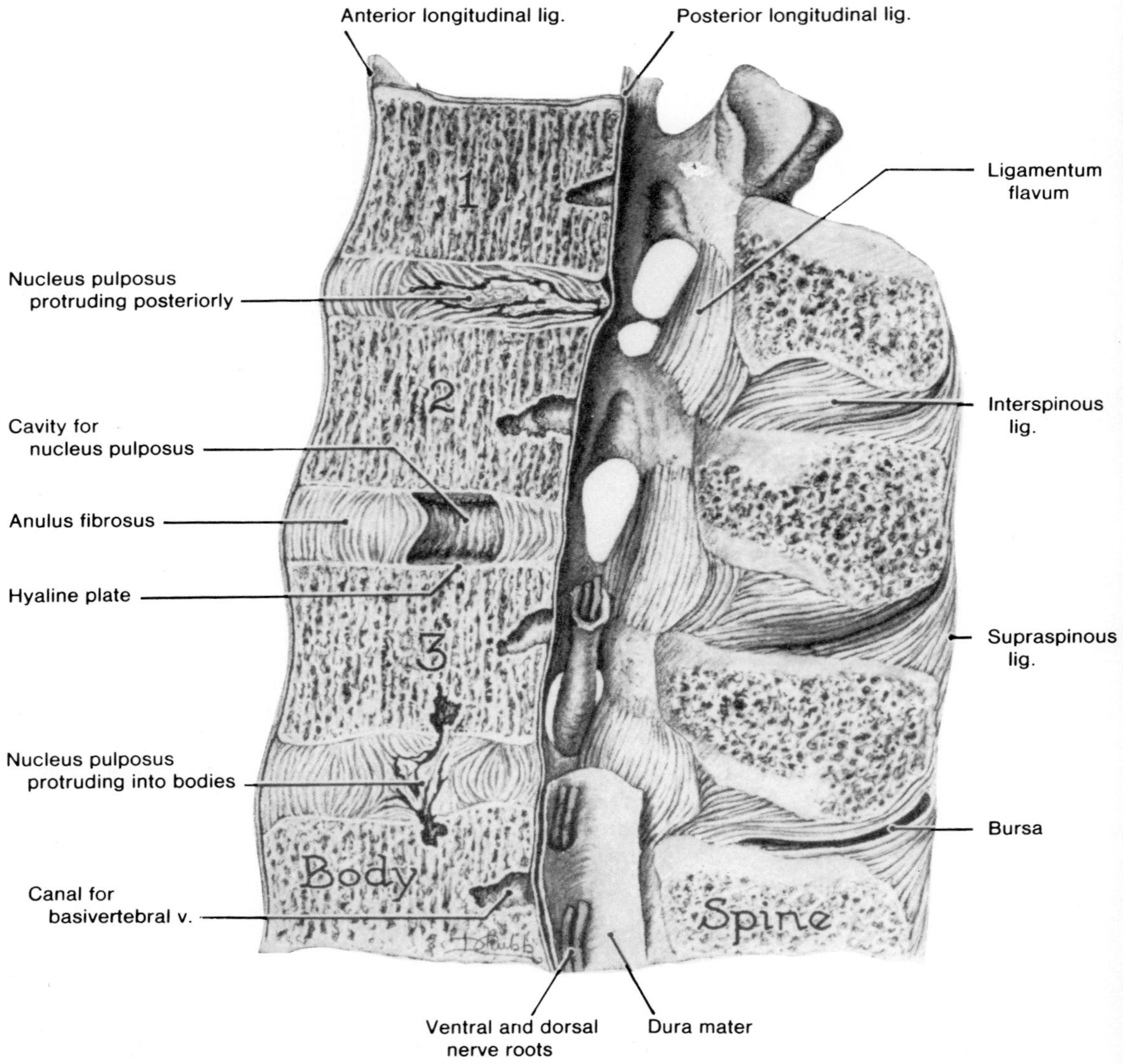

Figure 5-31. Drawing of a median section of the lumbar region of the vertebral column showing the ligaments and anuli fibrosi of the intervertebral discs that connect the vertebrae. Note the protrusions of the nuclei pulposi (called "slipped discs" by laymen) between L1/L2 and L3/L4; these are degenerative changes.

The anulus fibrosus (Figs. 5-33 and 5-52) is composed of concentric lamellae of collagenous fibers which run obliquely from one vertebra to another. Some fibers in one lamella are at right angles to those in adjacent ones; this arrangement, while allowing some movement between adjacent vertebrae, provides a strong bond between them. The lamellae are thinner and less numerous posteriorly than they are anteriorly or laterally.

The nucleus pulposus (L. fleshy) acts like a shock absorber for axial forces and like a semifluid ball bearing during flexion, extension, and lateral bending of the vertebral column (Figs. 5-8 and 5-9). It is a

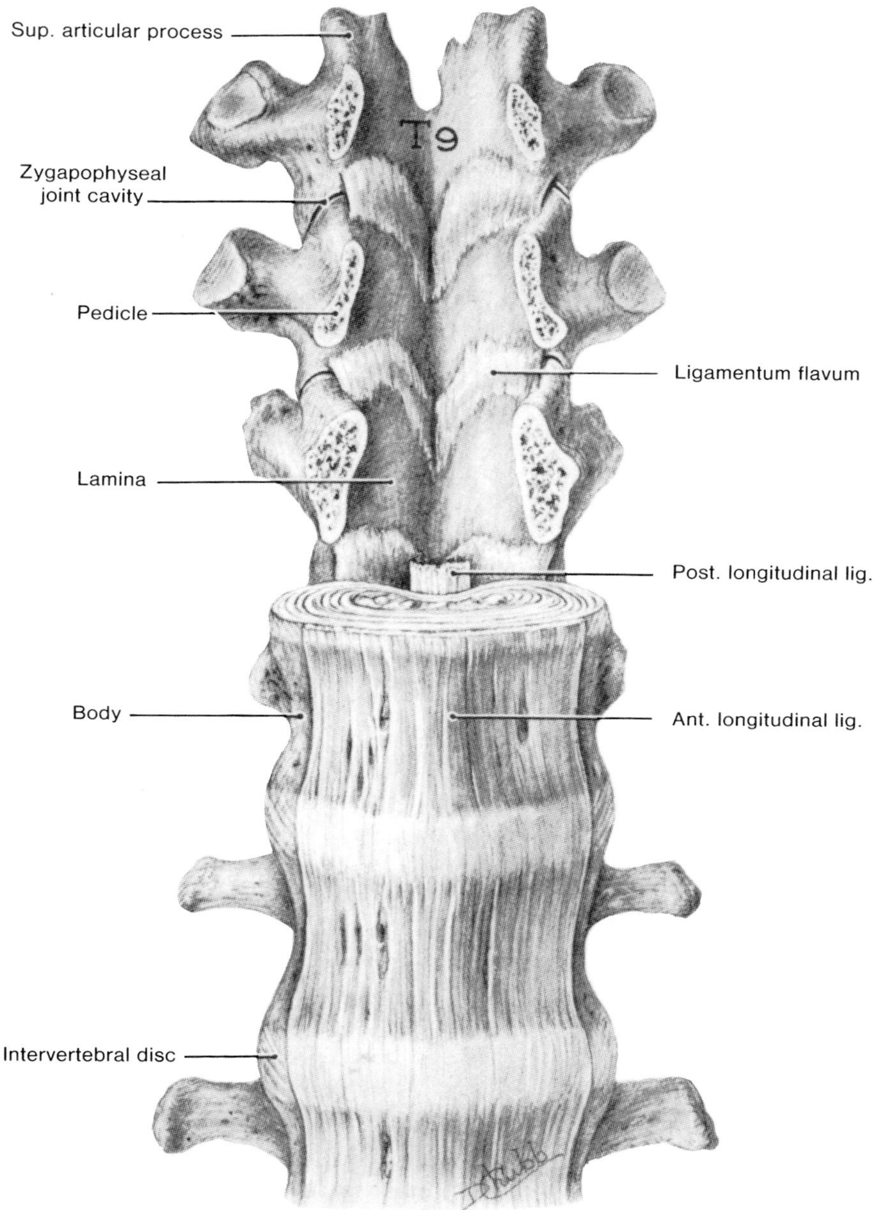

Figure 5-32. Drawing of the thoracic and lumbar regions of the vertebral column showing its ligaments. The pedicles of T9 to T11 vertebrae have been sawn through and their bodies have been discarded.

derivative of the notochord in the embryo and consists of reticular and collagenous fibers embedded in mucoid material. In young adults the water content of the nuclei pulposi is about 88%, and their fullness, or turgor (L. to swell), is great.

CLINICALLY ORIENTED COMMENTS

As people get older, their nuclei pulposi lose their turgor and become thinner owing

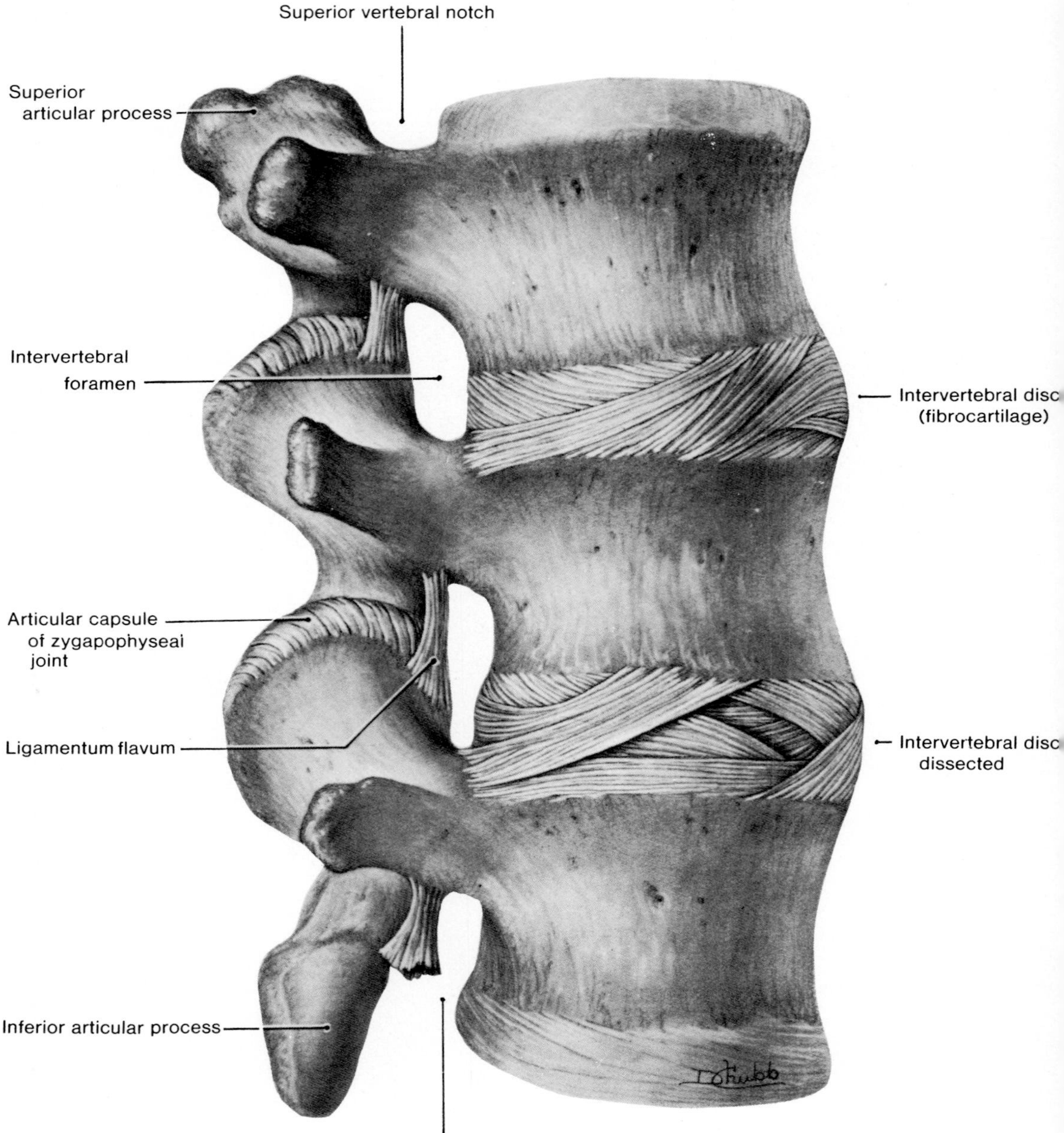

Figure 5-33. Drawing of a portion of the upper lumbar region of the vertebral column, lateral view, primarily to show the structure of the anuli fibrosi of the intervertebral discs (Fig. 5-34).

to dehydration and degeneration. These age changes account in part for the slight loss in height that occurs during old age.

The intervertebral discs are also subject to pathological changes that may result in protrusion of the nucleus pulposus through the anulus fibrosus, a condition known as a **herniated** or **prolapsed disc** (often incor-

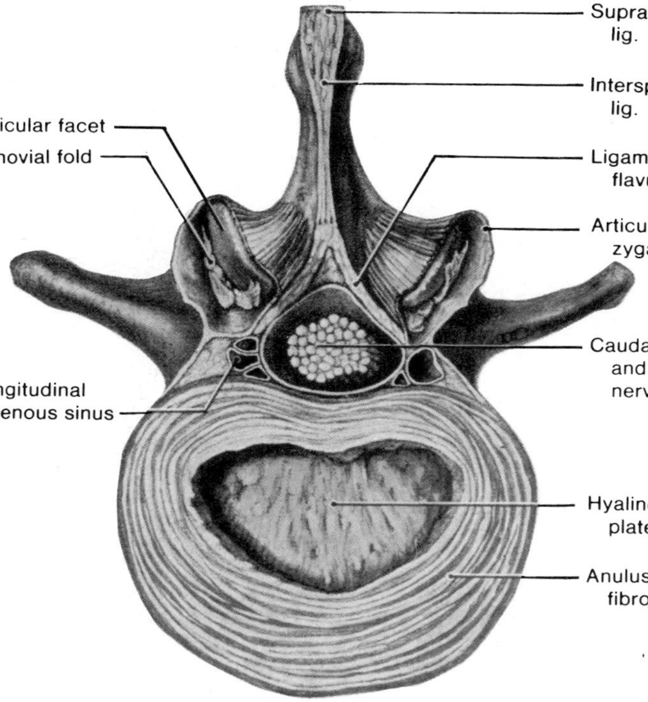

Figure 5-34. Diagram of a cross-section of an intervertebral disc and the vertebral ligaments. The nucleus pulposus has been scooped out to show the hyaline cartilage plate of the upper surface of the vertebral body. The nucleus pulposus contacts the hyaline plate, which is attached to the rough part of the vertebral body (Fig. 5-13). The anulus fibrosus inserts into the smooth bony rim of the body which is derived from the anular epiphysis.

rectly called a "slipped disc"). These nuclear protrusions usually occur posterolaterally, where the anulus fibrosus is weakest and poorly supported by the posterior longitudinal ligament (Figs. 5-31 and 5-34). The protruding part of the nucleus pulposus may compress an adjacent spinal nerve root, causing leg pain (*sciatica*) and/or low back pain (Case 5-3 and Fig. 5-80).

Acute low back pain (*lumbago*) and sciatica are often caused by a posterolateral protrusion of a lumbar intervertebral disc. The clinical picture varies considerably from patient to patient, but pain of acute onset in the mid and low back is a common presenting symptom. The terms lumbar and lumbago are derived from the Latin word *lumbus*, meaning the loin (the part of the side and back between the ribs and the pelvis). Because of the muscle spasm associated with low back pain, the lumbar region of the vertebral column is rigid and movement is painful. With treatment this type of pain usually begins to fade after a few days but may be gradually replaced by sciatica. In other cases both sciatica and low back pain may be present from the beginning.

Sciatica is an ache or pain in the area of the sciatic notch (lateral to ischial tuberosity) and the posterior aspect of the thigh, often spreading distal to the knee to the calf, ankle, and foot. *Sciatica often results from a posterolateral herniation of the nucleus pulposus through a rupture in the anulus fibrosus of the intervertebral disc.* In about 20% of patients with sciatica there is no back pain.

Lumbar intervertebral discs that herniate posterolaterally exert pressure on the spinal nerve roots (Fig. 5-80). In young persons the discs are so strong that when longitudinal force is applied to the vertebral column, the vertebrae usually break first, provided the discs are in a healthy condition. Discs are more often damaged by twisting or flexing the vertebral column. Posterior herniations of the nucleus pulposus may be also in the midline and may exert pressure on the spinal cord at cervical or thoracic levels and on the cauda equina at lower levels (Figs. 5-31 and 5-34).

Symptom-producing disc protrusions occur in the cervical region almost as often as in the lumbar region. A forcible flexion in the cervical region may rupture the disc posteriorly without fracturing the vertebral body. The cervical discs most commonly ruptured are those between C5/C6 and C6/C7, compressing spinal nerve roots C6 and C7, respectively. This results in pain in the neck, shoulder, arm, and often the hand (Fig. 4-160).

In older people degenerative changes may occur in the discs, resulting in *desication of the nucleus pulposus* and weakening of the anulus fibrosus. Consequently, a relatively minor stress (*e.g.*, as occurs during lifting a heavy object or pushing a stalled car) may tear the anulus fibrosus and allow the nucleus pulposus (if still in a semifluid condition) to protrude through the torn anulus fibrosus, usually in a posterolateral direction (Fig. 5-80 and Case 5-3).

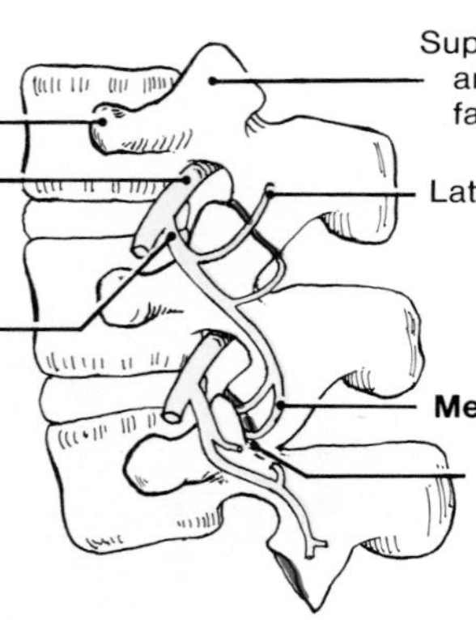

Figure 5-35. Drawing of part of the lumbar region of the vertebral column showing the innervation of the zygapophyseal joints. Observe that the dorsal primary ramus arises from the spinal nerve outside the intervertebral foramen and then divides into medial and lateral branches (Fig. 5-59). The medial branch descends in a groove posterior to the transverse process beside the superior articular process. It sends small articular branches to the capsule of the posterior or zygapophyseal joint beside it and to the subjacent joint as well.

Joints of the Vertebral Arches (Figs. 5-33 to 5-35). True synovial joints of the plane variety, known as **zygapophyseal joints**, are formed by the opposing articular processes (zygapophyses) of adjacent vertebral arches. Because the contact surfaces of these articular processes are called articular facets, clinicians often refer to zygapophyseal joints as "*facet joints*." The articular surfaces consist of smooth, shiny compact bone covered with hyaline cartilage. Each joint is surrounded by a thin loose **articular capsule** which is attached just peripheral to the articular margins of the adjacent articular processes (Figs. 5-33 and 5-34). These capsules are longer and looser in the cervical region than in the thoracic and lumbar regions. The fibrous capsule is lined by a synovial membrane.

In the cervical and lumbar regions, the zygapophyseal joints bear some weight, sharing this function with the intervertebral discs. These joints help to control flexion, extension, and rotation of adjacent cervical and lumbar vertebrae, where most of the motion of the vertebral column takes place.

The laminae of adjacent vertebral arches are joined by broad, yellow elastic bands called **ligamenta flava** (Figs. 5-32 and 5-34). Their fibers extend to the capsules of the zygapophyseal joints between the articular processes and contribute to the posterior boundary of the vertebral foramen (Fig. 5-33).

The adjacent edges of the spinous processes are joined by weak **interspinous ligaments** (Fig. 5-31), and their tips are joined by strong **supraspinous ligaments** (Figs. 5-31 and 5-69*B*). These ligaments expand to form the **ligamentum nuchae**, a triangular, median septum between the muscles on each side of the back of the neck. (Fig. 5-44). It extends from the spinous process of C7 to the posterior border of the foramen magnum, the external occipital crest, and the external occipital protuberance.

The **intertransverse ligaments** connect adjacent transverse processes and are insignificant, except in the lumbar region, where they are thin and membranous.

Innervation of the Zygapophyseal Joints (Fig. 5-35). These joints are innervated by nerves that arise from the *medial branches of the dorsal primary rami of spinal nerves.* As these nerves pass posteriorly and caudally, they lie in grooves on the posterior surfaces of the medial parts of the transverse processes. Each of these articular branches supplies the zygapophyseal joint beside it and possibly sends twigs to the subjacent joint as well.

CLINICALLY ORIENTED COMMENTS

Low back pain may result from disease of the zygapophyseal joints in the lumbar region (*e.g.*, owing to **osteoarthritis**). *Denervation of lumbar zygapophyseal joints* is a procedure currently being evaluated for treatment of low back pain thought to be caused by disease of these joints. In some cases the nerves are sectioned in the region near these joints; in other cases the nerves are destroyed by radiofrequency percutaneous **rhizolysis** (G. *rhiza*, root + *lysis*, dissolution). In each procedure the destructive process is directed at the medial branches of the dorsal primary rami of the spinal nerves (Fig. 5-35), usually at the L1 to L4 level. The value of these techniques in relieving low back pain has not been proven at this time.

Joints of the Suboccipital Region (Figs. 5-36 and 5-37). These joints are between the skull and the atlas and between the atlas and the axis.

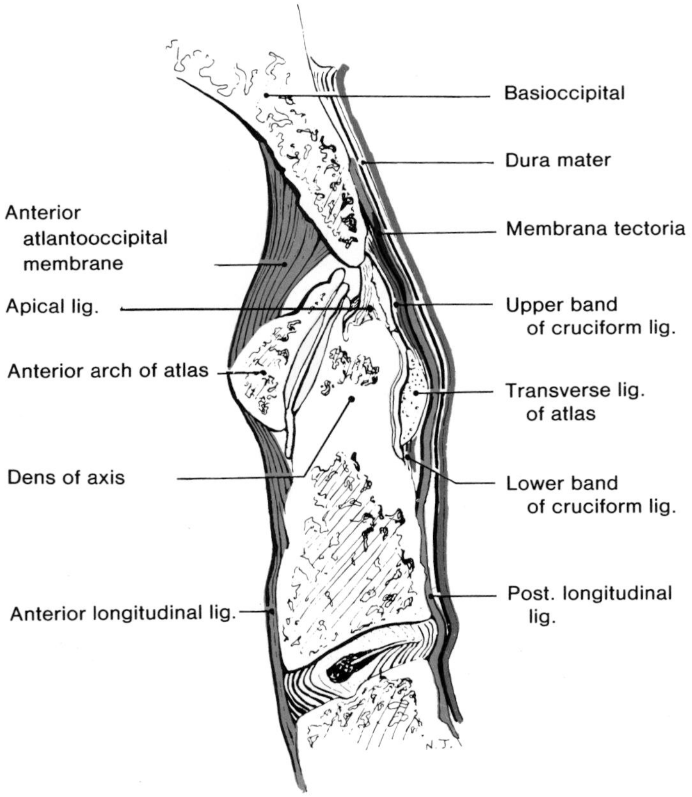

Figure 5-36. Drawing of the ligaments of the atlantoaxial and atlantooccipital joints on median section.

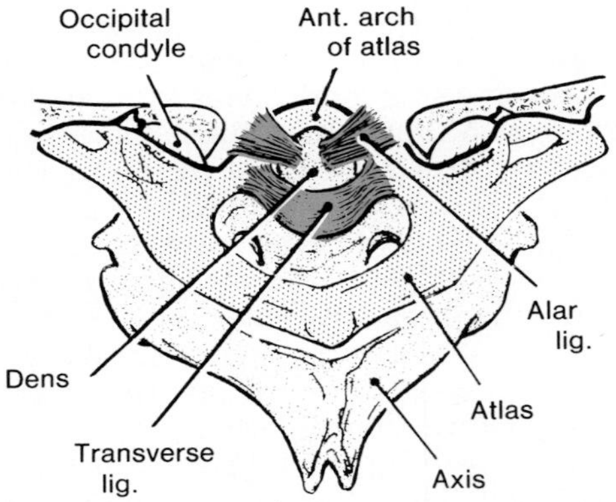

Figure 5-37. Drawing of the craniovertebral joints showing the transverse and alar ligaments. Note that the transverse ligament embraces the dens of the axis.

The atlantooccipital joints, between the atlas and the occipital bone, enable us to nod our heads (*e.g.*, the flexion and extension of the neck that occurs when indicating approval). The atlantooccipital joints, one on each side, are between the superior articular facets on the lateral masses of the atlas and the **occipital condyles** (Fig. 5-55). They are synovial joints with thin loose articular capsules.

The skull and atlas are also connected by anterior and posterior **atlantooccipital membranes** which extend from the anterior and posterior arches of the atlas to the anterior and posterior margins of the foramen magnum (Fig. 5-36).

The transverse ligament of the atlas is a strong band extending between the tubercles on the medial sides of the lateral masses of the atlas (Figs. 5-19, 5-36, and 5-37). It holds the dens of the axis against the anterior arch of the atlas, with a synovial joint between them. Vertically oriented upper and lower bands pass from the transverse ligament to the occipital bone superiorly and to the body of the axis inferiorly, forming the **cruciform ligament** (L. *crux*, cross). It was given this name because of its resemblance to a cross (Fig. 5-38).

The alar ligaments extend from the dens to the lateral margins of the foramen magnum (Figs. 5-37 and 5-38). These strong, short, rounded cords, which are almost as thick as pencils, *check lateral rotation and side-to-side movements of the head* and attach the skull to the axis.

The membrana tectoria is the upward continuation of the posterior longitudinal ligament (Fig. 5-36). It runs from the body of the axis to the internal surface of the occipital bone and covers the alar ligaments and the transverse ligament (Fig. 5-38).

The atlantoaxial joints (two lateral and one medial) *allow the head to be turned from side to side* (*e.g.*, when rotating the head to indicate disapproval). During this movement, the skull and the atlas rotate as a unit on the axis.

The apical ligament, an adult derivative of the notochord in the embryo, extends from the tip of the dens to the internal surface of the occipital bone (Fig. 5-36).

Movements between the skull and the atlas and between the atlas and the axis, occurring at the craniovertebral joints (antlantooccipital and atlantoaxial), are augmented by the flexibility of the neck owing to movements of the vertebral joints in the middle and lower cervical regions.

CLINICALLY ORIENTED COMMENTS

During rotation of the head, the dens of the axis is held in a collar formed by the anterior arch of the atlas and the transverse ligament and acts as a pivot (Fig. 5-37). If the transverse ligament ruptures, the dens may be driven into the cervical region of the spinal cord, causing **quadriplegia** (paralysis of the upper and lower limbs), or into the lower end of the medulla, causing sudden death. This injury often occurs when persons are hung or hang themselves. There is some controversy about the "*hangman's fracture*," but it is generally agreed that it is a complex fracture of the axis.

Fractures of the Vertebral Column. *All back and neck injuries are potentially serious* because of the possibility of fracturing vertebrae and injuring the spinal cord and/or the cauda equina (Figs. 5-34 and 5-58).

Some regions of the vertebral column tend to have greater numbers of certain

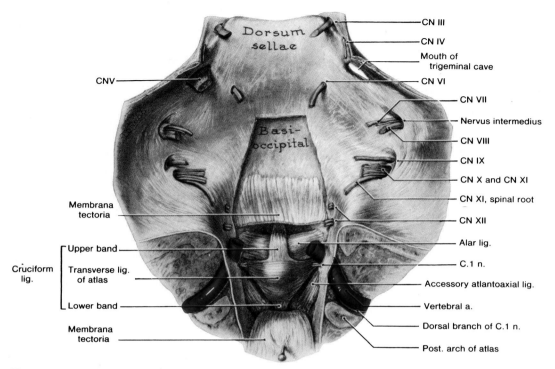

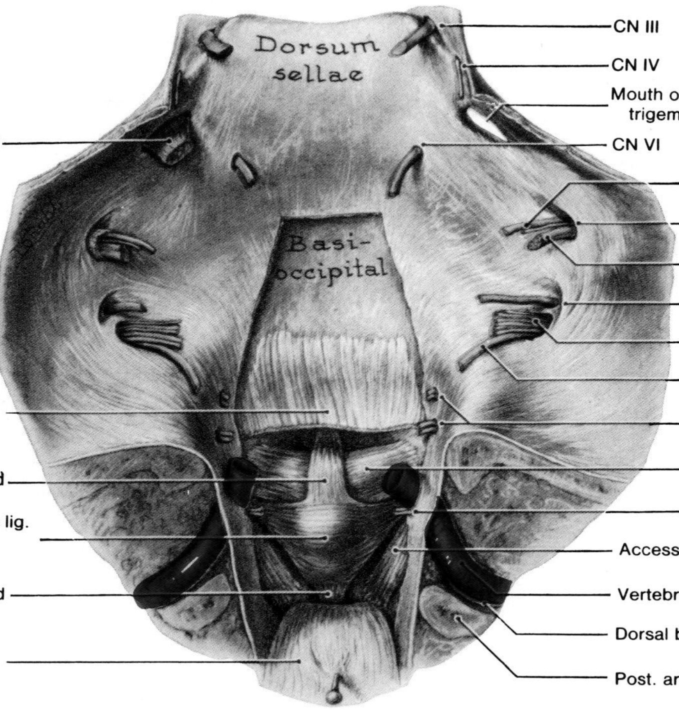

Figure 5-38. Drawing of the craniovertebral region from above showing the ligaments of the atlantoaxial and atlantooccipital joints. Observe the cross-shaped cruciform ligament.

types of fracture owing to their mobility and curvatures. *The cervical region is especially vulnerable to injury.* Injuries to the spinal cord in the cervical region, with compression or **transection of the cord**, may result in loss of all sensation and voluntary movement below the lesion or in sudden death, depending on the level of injury. Compression of any part of the central nervous system (brain and spinal cord), rendering it ischemic (G. ischo, to hold back + *haima*, blood), for 3 to 5 minutes results in death of nervous tissue, particularly nerve cells.

Fractures, dislocations, and fracture-dislocations of the vertebral column often result from a sudden forceful flexion, as may occur in a car accident (Case 5-9) or from a violent strike on the back of the head. The common fracture is a **crush (compression) fracture** of the body of one or more vertebrae, often in the middle or lower cervical regions of the vertebral column or near the junction of the thoracic and lumbar regions.

In severe **flexion injuries**, the posterior longitudinal and interspinous ligaments may be torn, and the vertebral arches may be dislocated and/or fractured along with crush fractures of the vertebral bodies. *In these cases there are injuries to the spinal cord.* The anterior longitudinal ligament is usually not torn in flexion injuries; thus, patients with injuries to the thoracolumbar vertebral bodies, without fracture or dislocation of the vertebral arches, are commonly placed in a position of extension so that this ligament will be tightened and the degree of compression of the vertebral bodies will be reduced.

When a person falls from a height and lands on the top of the head, the violence is transmitted along the axis of the vertebral column. Falling on the feet or the buttocks from a height or hitting the head while diving produces a similar axial force.

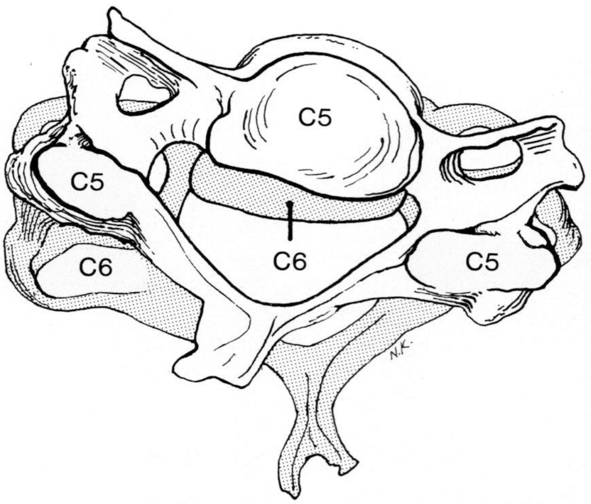

Figure 5-39. Rotary dislocation of C5 on C6 as seen from above. The right articular processes and transverse processes of C5 and C6 are projected over each other. The left articular and transverse processes of C5 are projected anterior to the similar processes of C6, exposing the left superior facet of C6. The hidden inferior facet of C5 is resting in the superior vertebral notch of C6 (locked facets). The spinous process of C5 is to the left of the midline.

A fall on the head may force the occipital condyles into the ring-shaped atlas, splitting it into two or more fragments. In other cases, the thin bone around the occipital condyles fractures, with the result that they pass upward with the atlas and axis into the posterior cranial cavity.

Injuries can also be caused by extension forces to the vertebral column. The details of **extension fractures** and/or dislocations vary from one vertebral region to another, but in general the posterior portions of the vertebral column are most likely to be injured.

In the cervical region, severe **hyperextension of the neck** may pinch the posterior arch of the atlas between the occiput and the axis. The atlas usually breaks at one or both grooves for the vertebral arteries, at the junctions of the lateral masses and the posterior arches (Fig. 5-18). If the force is continued, the arch of the axis also may be pinched off and may break at the isthmus, between the lateral mass and the posterior articular processes, unilaterally or bilaterally. If the force is even greater, the anterior longitudinal ligament and adjacent anulus fibrosus of the C2/C3 intervertebral disc are ruptured. At the moment of impact, the skull, atlas, and axis are separated from the rest of the vertebral column, and the spinal cord is usually severed. Such patients seldom survive more than 5 minutes, as the injury to the spinal cord is above the **phrenic outflow**, the origin of the phrenic nerves (C3, C4, and C5) which innervate the diaphragm (Fig. 1-86); thus respiration is severely affected. If the patient, who would be quadriplegic, lives long enough to reach a hospital, radiographs show the vertebrae and their fragments in surprisingly normal position. This results from the patient being in the **supine position** (on the back) during radiography, which reduces displacements of the bones and their fragments. However, often a tiny flake of bone is avulsed from the anteroinferior corner of the body of C2, where the anterior longitudinal ligament and the adjacent anulus fibrosus are attached, enabling one to deduce what has happened.

Hyperextension injuries of the vertebral column are rarely seen in the thoracic re-

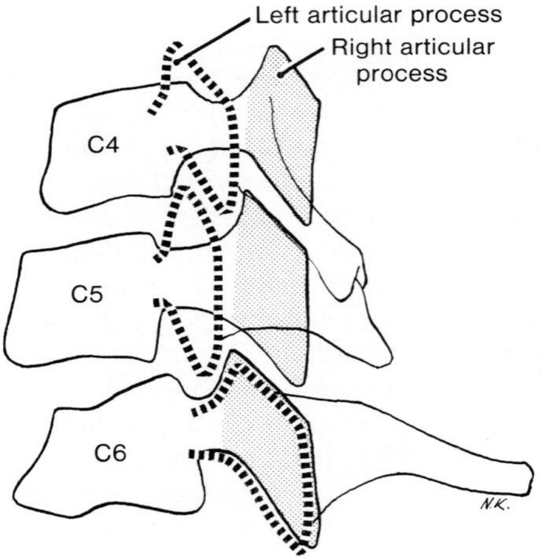

Figure 5-40. Diagram of a lateral radiograph of a patient with a rotatory dislocation of C5 on C6. The images of the two articular processes (pillars) of C6 are projected on each other; those at C5 are not. The left articular pillar of C5 is projected anterior to its mate on the right side. The lower edge of the left inferior facet of C5 rests in the left superior vertebral notch of C6 (locked facets).

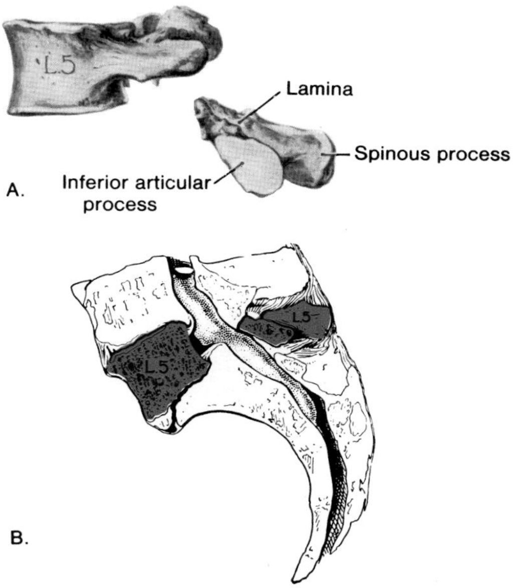

Figure 5-41. *A*, bipartite fifth lumbar vertebra. Note that one piece, consisting of the spinous process, laminae, and inferior articular processes, is separated from the body, pedicles, and superior articular processes. *B*, the body and superimposed vertebrae tend to slide forward, a condition known as spondylolisthesis.

gion owing to support provided by the ribs and because extension forces to the vertebral axis expend themselves on the moveable portions of the vertebral column, *i.e.*, the cervical and lumbar regions. However, the last two thoracic vertebrae, being freer to move than the others, may sustain injuries similar to lumbar vertebrae.

Extension injuries of the lumbar vertebral column also tend to injure the posterior elements. In addition to fractures of the laminae and articular processes, there are sometimes small crush fractures of posterior parts of the vertebral bodies. In marked hyperextension, the forces on the anterior longitudinal ligament and adjacent anulus may tear off the anterosuperior or anteroinferior corner of a lumbar vertebral body. In these cases, one can deduce that there was a great displacement of the vertebrae and their fragments at the moment of impact and the spinal cord and/or cauda equina was probably damaged.

Longitudinal forces up to 1200 psi on excised lumbar regions of the vertebral columns of young adults have shown that the body of the vertebra will fracture before the anulus fibrosus ruptures. The bone breaks inferior or superior to the nucleus pulposus (Fig. 5-8).

The patient's head or body is sometimes rotated to some extent when an injury takes place. At other times, the head or trunk receives the force on the anterolateral or posterolateral surface. In these cases a rotary element affects the injury, sometimes alone and sometimes combined with flexion or extension injuries.

The **rotatory dislocation** or fracture-dislocation of the cervical region is the best example of a rotatory injury of the vertebral column (Figs. 5-39 and 5-40). The zygapophyseal joint at one level on one side only is dislocated. The inferior facet of the superior vertebra slips forward and off the superior facet of the inferior vertebra; the displaced facets lock because of their shape (Fig. 5-40). Often there is minor fracturing of the tips of the facets which is not always obvious on radiographs. One side of the body of the superior vertebra is slightly forward and, if undue attention is paid to this, the dislocation of the zygapophyseal joint may be missed. Strong traction along the long axis of the body is needed to unlock the facets; this is usually controlled radiologically. When the facets have been un-

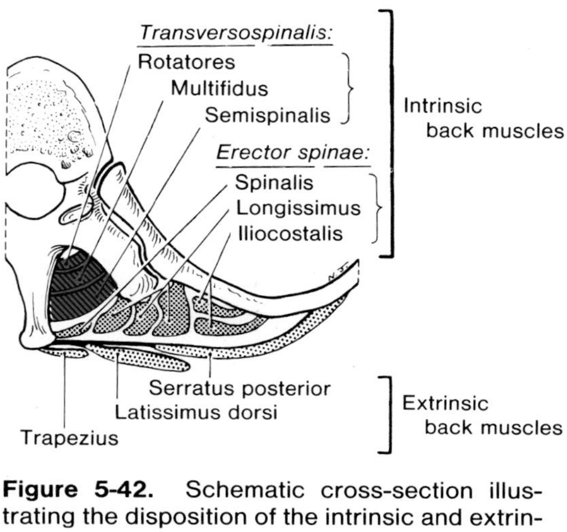

Figure 5-42. Schematic cross-section illustrating the disposition of the intrinsic and extrinsic muscles of the back.

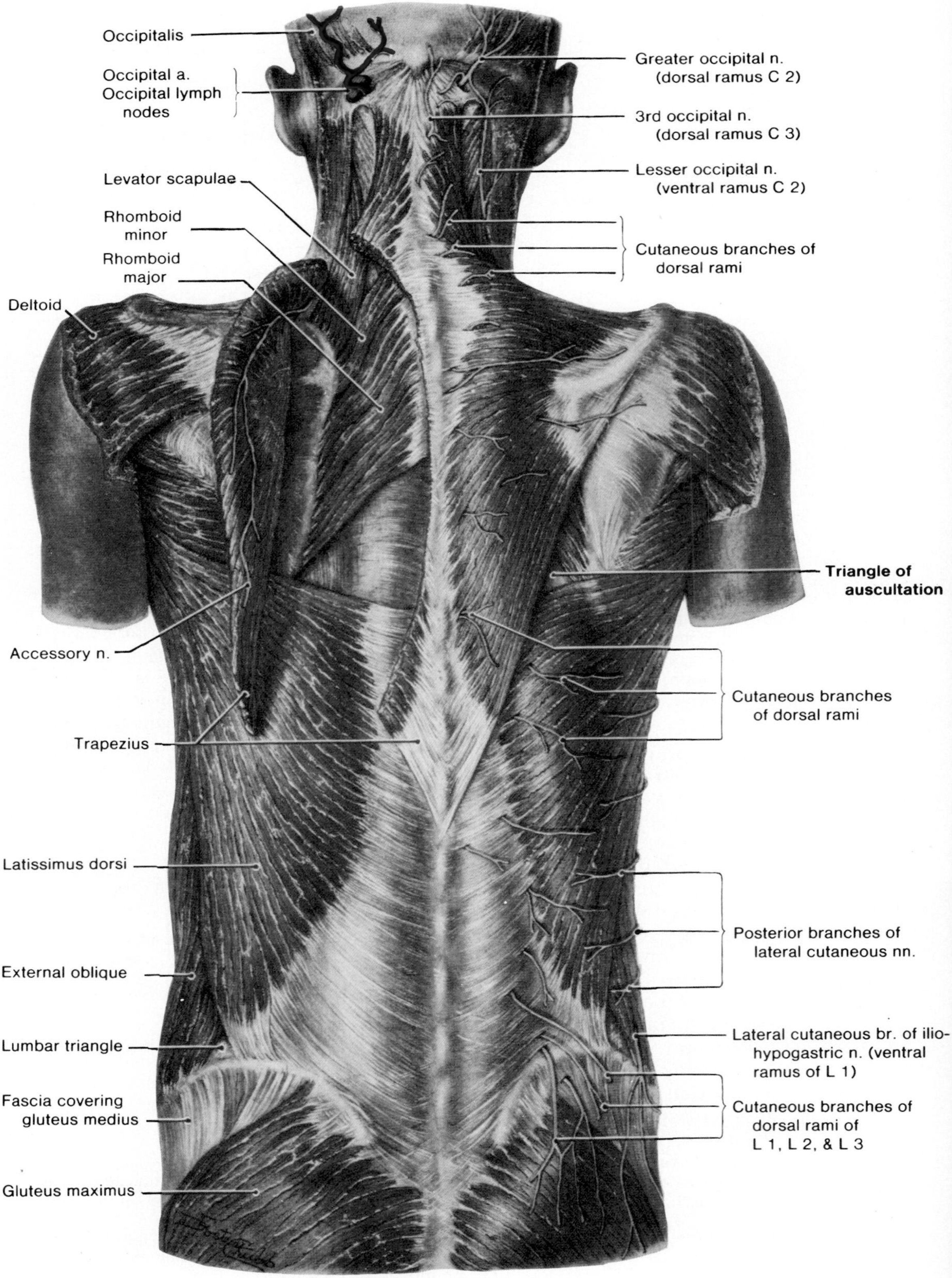

Figure 5-43. Drawing of a dissection of the back showing the superficial muscles. The trapezius has been reflected on the left side to show the underlying muscles. The superficial group acts on the upper limb.

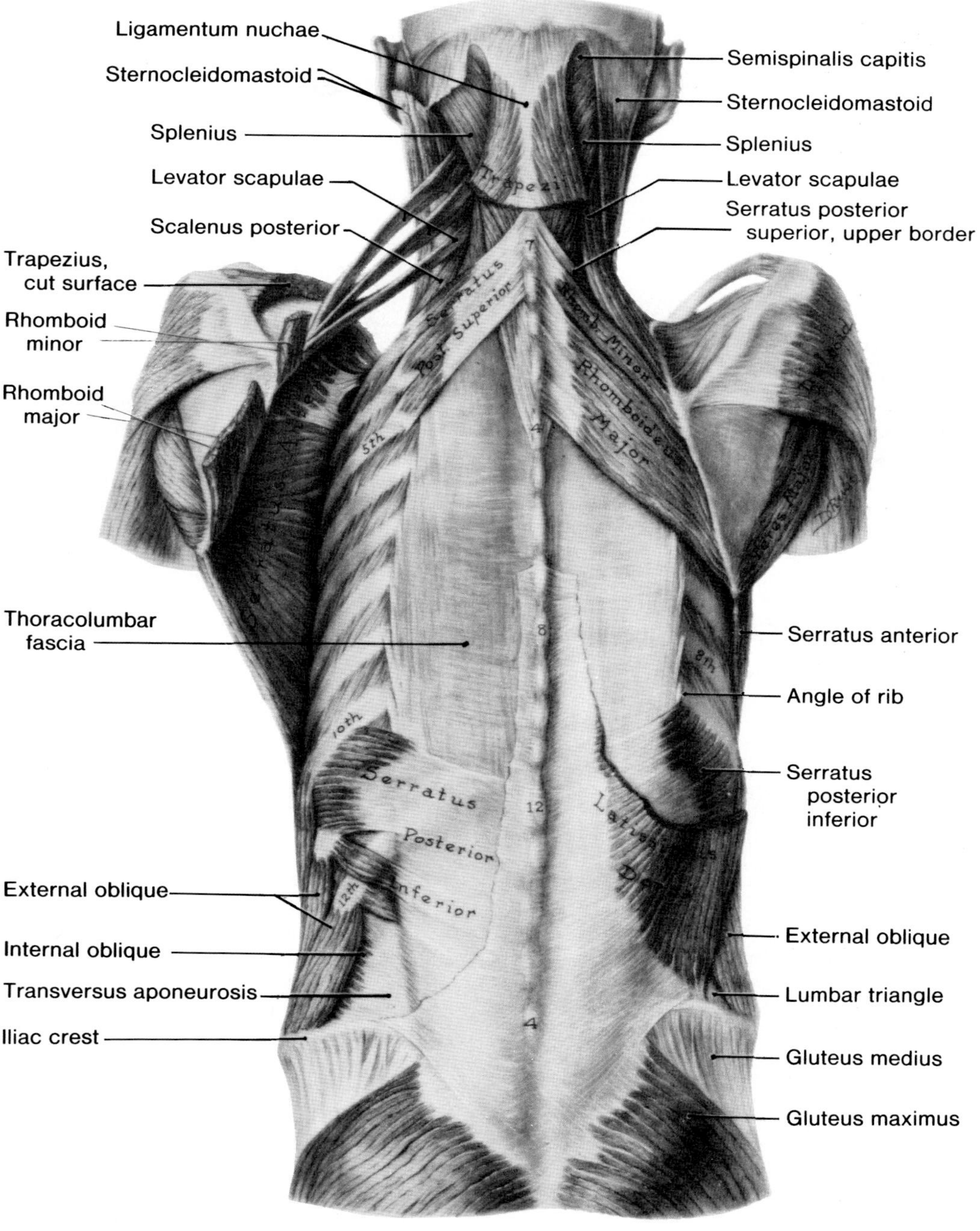

Figure 5-44. Drawing of a dissection of the back showing the intermediate muscles. The superficial muscles (trapezius and latissimus dorsi) have been largely cut away on both sides. The ligamentum nuchae, representing the cervical part of the supraspinous ligament, is a thin fibroelastic partition attached to the spinous processes of the cervical vertebrae, the external occipital crest, and the external occipital protuberance (Fig. 5-55). It gives origin to certain neck muscles, *e.g.*, splenius capitis and cervicis. The intermediate group of muscles functions in respiration.

locked, they usually come into alignment, and when traction is lessened, the dislocation has been reduced.

Rotatory forces often cause fractures of the articular processes, particularly in the lower thoracic and lumbar regions. These fractures are usually unstable, and an operation is necessary to produce stability (posterior **spinal fusion**) and to remove any bone, disc, or blood clot that may be pressing on nervous tissues.

Dislocation of vertebrae without fracture is rare, except in the cervical region, because of the interlocking of the thoracic and lumbar articular processes. Fortunately *the vertebral canal in the cervical region is usually somewhat larger than the spinal cord*; thus, there can be some displacement of the vertebrae without causing serious damage to the spinal cord (Fig. 5-59).

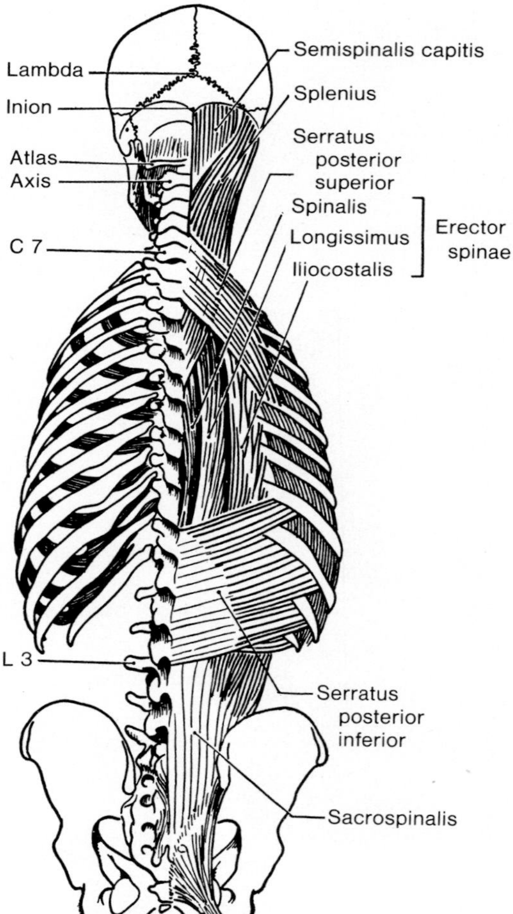

Figure 5-45. Drawing showing the intermediate and deep muscles of the back. The serratus posterior superior and inferior are muscles of the thorax.

Displacement of the Vertebral Column. In a few people, particularly Australian aborigines, South African bushmen, and Eskimos above the Yukon River, the fifth lumbar vertebra consists of two parts (Fig. 5-41). The posterior fragment, consisting of the spinous process, the laminae, and the inferior articular processes, remains in normal relation to the arch of the sacrum. The anterior fragment of this divided vertebra and the superimposed vertebra may occasionally move forward. This anterior displacement of most of the vertebral column is called **spondylolisthesis** (G. *spondylos*, vertebra + *olisthesis*, a slipping and falling). If the anterior part of the bone does not move forward, the condition is called **spondylolysis**.

Spondylolisthesis at L5 may result in pressure on the spinal nerves as they pass into the upper part of the sacrum. The cause of this condition, which develops postnatally and may cause acute low back pain (lumbago), is unknown. Most people believe it is a strain or "**march fracture**" of L5.

MUSCLES OF THE BACK

For descriptive purposes, the muscles of the back are divided into three groups: *superficial*, *intermediate*, and *deep*. The superficial and intermediate groups are **extrinsic back muscles** that are concerned with movements of the limbs and respiration, whereas the deep or **intrinsic back muscles** are concerned with movements of the vertebral column (Fig. 5-9).

THE EXTRINSIC MUSCLES OF THE BACK

Superficial Muscles of the Back (Figs. 5-42 and 5-43). The trapezius, latissimus dorsi, levator scapulae, and rhomboid muscles connect the upper limb to the axial skeleton and are related to movements of the upper limbs (see Chap. 6).

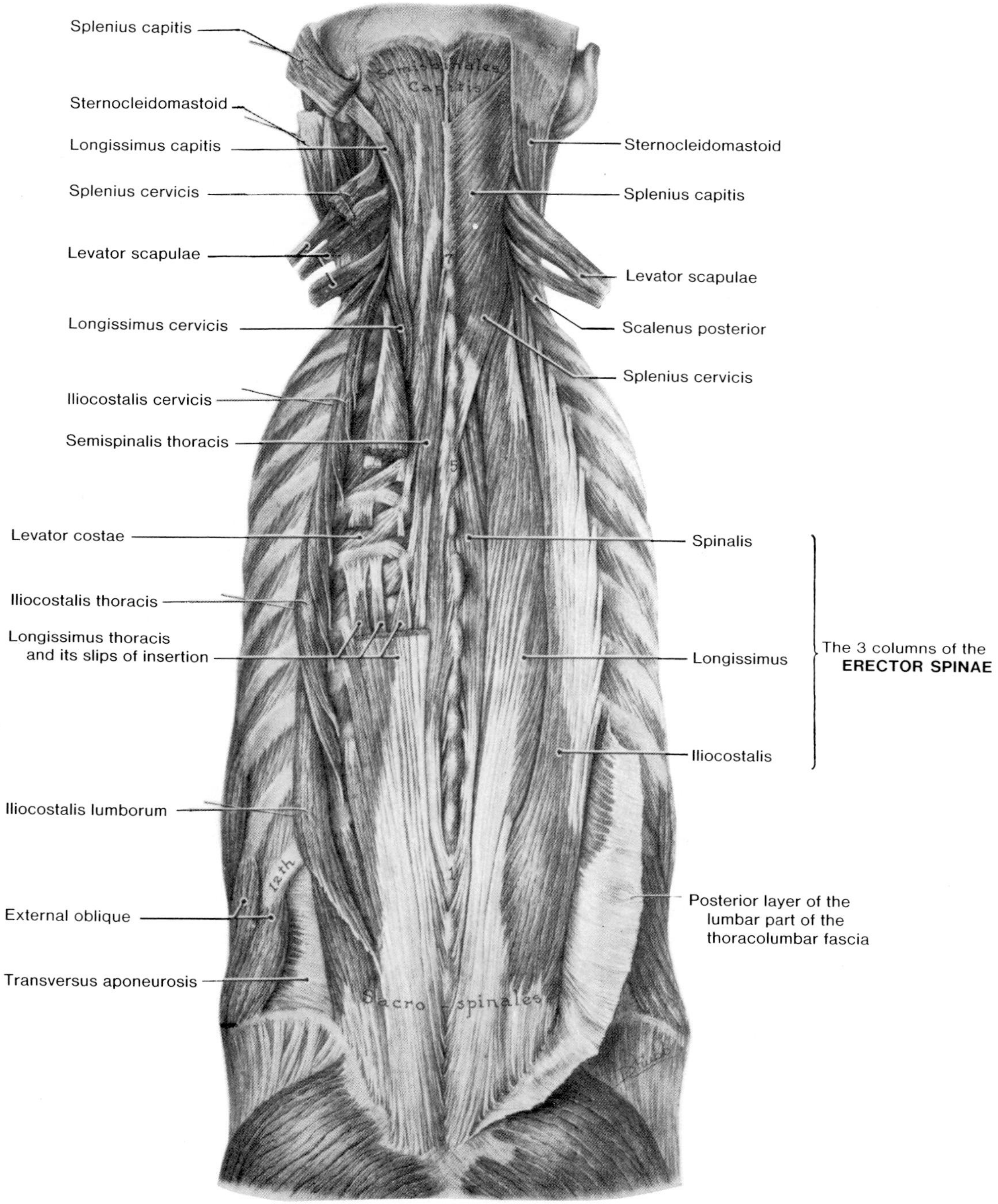

Figure 5-46. Drawing of a dissection illustrating the deep muscles of the back. The superficial layer of deep muscles (splenius capitis and cervicis) is reflected on the left side. The intermediate layer of deep muscles (erector spinae) is intact on the right side, lying between the spinous processes of the vertebrae medially and the angles of the ribs laterally. *The deep group are the intrinsic or true muscles of the back.*

Intermediate Muscles of the Back (Figs. 5-44 and 5-45). The serratus posterior, superior, and inferior are respiratory muscles and are described with the thorax in Chapter 1.

The superficial and intermediate groups of muscles concerned with *limb and forced respiratory movements* largely cover the deep or intrinsic muscles of the back (Figs. 5-43 to 5-45). Consequently, to expose the underlying intrinsic muscles, the extrinsic muscles must be reflected.

THE INTRINSIC MUSCLES OF THE BACK

The muscles of the deep or intrinsic group, **the true back muscles**, are concerned with the *maintenance of posture and movements of the vertebral column* (flexion, extension, lateral bending, rotation, and circumduction). The deep back muscles are covered posteriorly by a tough sheet of fascia which fuses with the aponeuroses of several extrinsic muscles (*e.g.*, the latissimus dorsi) in the lower thoracic and lumbar regions to form the **thoracolumbar (lumbar) fascia** (Fig. 5-44). When this fascia is removed, paired muscular columns are exposed which lie in longitudinal bands on each side of the spinous processes (Fig. 5-42). They are supplied by branches of the **dorsal primary rami** of spinal nerves that pass through them to supply the overlying skin (Fig. 5-43).

There are three layers of intrinsic back muscles, which are named according to their relationship to the surface and to the direction of their fibers (Fig. 5-42): (1) *a superficial layer*, the fibers of which pass superiorly and laterally; (2) *an intermediate layer*, with fibers that run longitudinally, parallel to the long axis of the vertebral column; and (3) *a deep layer*, in which the fibers extend superiorly and medially.

Superficial Layer of Intrinsic Muscles (Figs. 5-44 and 5-45). The splenii (G. *splenion*, bandage) consist of two large muscles in the back of the neck, which somewhat resemble bandages as they ascend from the midline of the neck to the base of the skull, and the transverse processes of the upper cervical vertebrae.

The Splenius Capitis and Cervicis Muscle (Fig. 5-46). This broad thin muscle, composed of two parts (capitis and cervicis), runs upward and laterally over the deeper muscles of the neck.

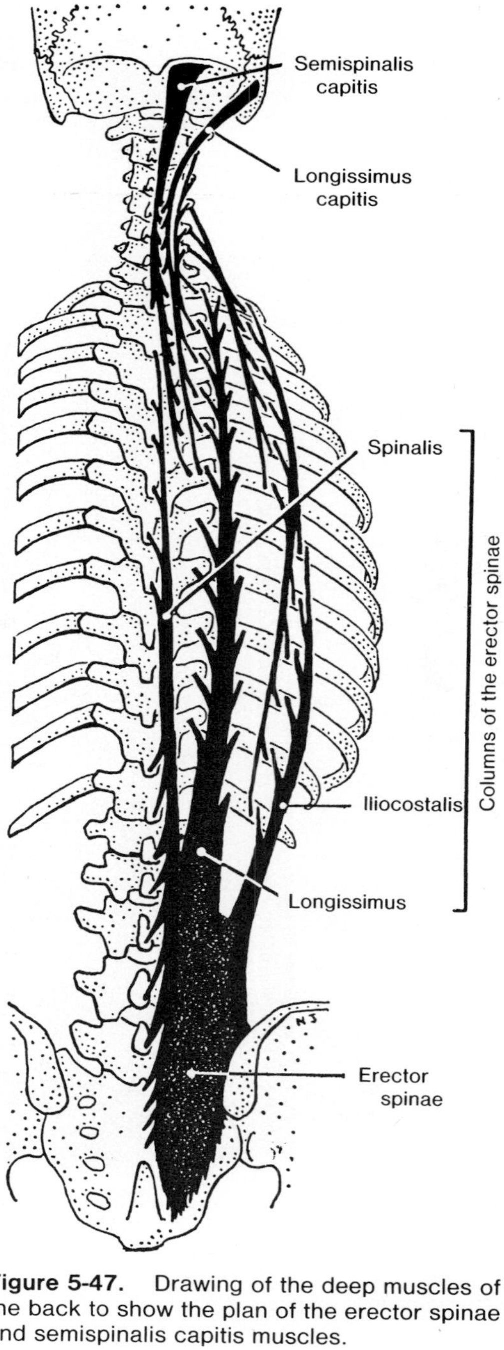

Figure 5-47. Drawing of the deep muscles of the back to show the plan of the erector spinae and semispinalis capitis muscles.

Origin. **Lower half of ligamentum nuchae** and **spinous processes of C7 to T6**.

Insertion. The capitis (L. *caput*, head) part inserts into the **mastoid process** of the temporal bone and the adjacent **occipital bone**, whereas the cervicis part inserts into the **transverse processes of the upper two to four cervical vertebrae**.

Actions. Acting alone, the splenius **laterally bends and rotates the neck**, turning the face to the same side. *Acting together*, the splenii **pull the head backward**.

Nerve Supply. Lateral branches of the dorsal rami of the middle (capitis part) and lower (cervicis part) **cervical spinal nerves**.

Intermediate Layer of Intrinsic Muscles (Figs. 5-45 to 5-48). This layer is formed by a large **erector spinae muscle** (sacrospinalis) lying on each side of the vertebral column. It is characterized by long muscle bundles running vertically (Fig. 5-47). This massive muscle, extending from the pelvis to the skull, can be readily palpated, and its lateral border is obvious in most people (Figs. 5-11 and 5-48). Inferior to the ribs, it divides into **three columns**: *iliocostalis, longissimus*, and *spinalis.*

The Iliocostalis Muscle (Figs. 5-45 to 5-47). As its name indicates, this lateral column of muscle arises from the iliac crest and inserts into the ribs (L. *costae*). It consists of *three parts*: (1) the iliocostalis **lumborum**, inserting into the angles of the lower six or seven ribs; (2) the iliocostalis **thoracis**, arising from the lower six ribs and inserting into the angles of the upper

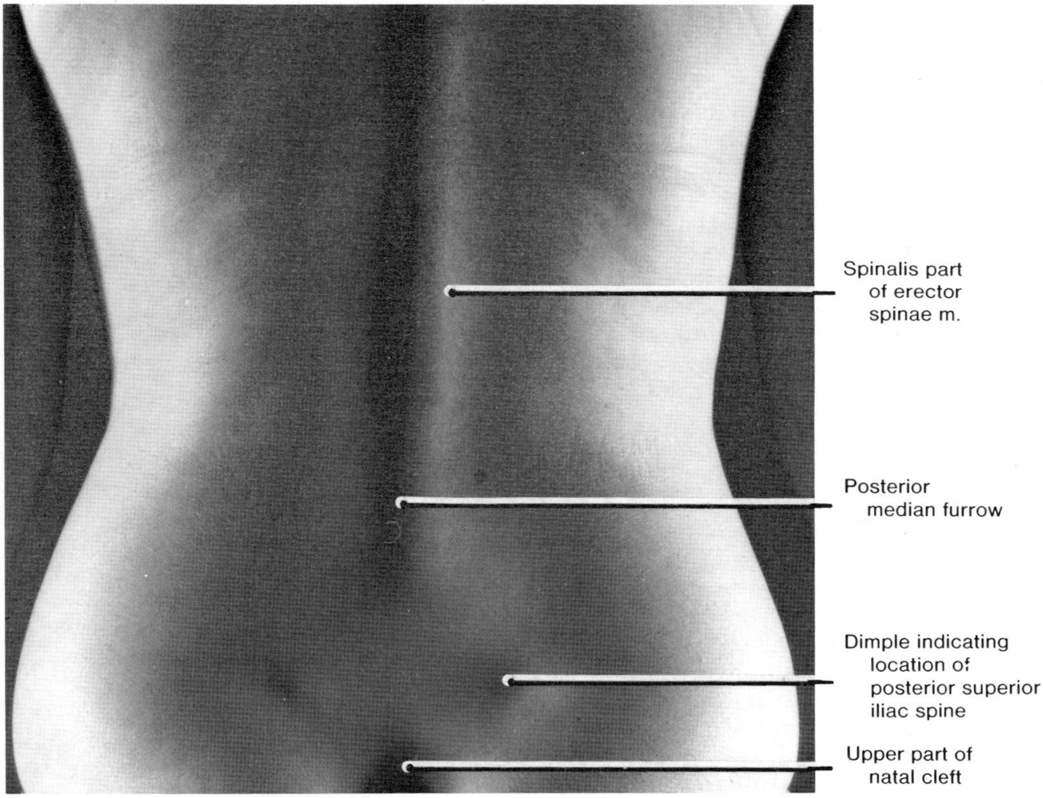

Figure 5-48. Photograph of the back of a 21-year-old woman showing the principal surface landmarks and the external appearance of the erector spinae muscles. The dimples indicating the posterior superior iliac spines are obvious because the skin and underlying fascia are attached to bone in this area (Fig. 5-50). A line joining these dimples crosses the spinous process of the second sacral vertebra. The spinalis part of the erector spinae is only 2 cm wide and is attached to the spinous processes (Fig. 5-47).

six ribs and the transverse process of C7; and (3) the iliocostalis **cervicis**, arising from the third to sixth ribs and inserting into the transverse processes of C6 to C4. The iliocosotalis muscles **extend the vertebral column** and, acting on one side, **bend it laterally** (Fig. 5-9).

The Longissimus Muscle (Figs. 5-42 and 5-45 to 47). The longissimus (L. longest), an intermediate column of muscle running mainly between the vertebral transverse processes, may be divided into *three parts*: longissimus **thoracis**, longissimus **cervicis**, and longissimus **capitis**, to indicate the sites of the insertion of its fibers. Distal fibers of the longissimus arise from the sacrum, and proximal fibers originate from successively higher transverse processes.

The longissimus thoracis (G. *thorax*, chest) inserts into the tips of the transverse processes of all thoracic vertebrae and into the inferior 9 to 10 ribs between their tubercles and angles.

The longissimus cervicis (L. *cervix*, neck) inserts into the posterior tubercles of the transverse processes of the cervical vertebrae (C2 to C6).

The longissimus capitis (L. caput, head) inserts into the mastoid process of the temporal bone.

The longissimus *thoracis and cervicis* **extend the vertebral column** and, acting on one side, **bend it laterally**, whereas the longissimus *capitis* **extends the head** and **turns the face toward the same side**.

The Spinalis Muscle (Figs. 5-42 and 5-45 to 5-48). This medial column of the erector spinae muscle *arises from spinous processes and inserts into spinous processes*, mainly in the thoracic region. It may also be divided into three parts (thoracis, cervicis, and capitis). *The spinalis muscle is an extensor of the vertebral column.*

Deep Layer of Intrinsic Muscles (Figs. 5-49 to 5-52). When the massive erector spinae muscle is removed, several short muscles (semispinalis, multifidus, and rotatores) are visible in the groove between the processes of the vertebrae (Fig. 5-42). Collectively these muscles are known as the **transversospinalis** because they are obliquely disposed and run from the *transverse processes to the spinous processes* of most vertebrae.

The Semispinalis Muscle (Figs. 5-42 and 5-49 to 5-53). As its name indicates, this muscle *originates from about half the length of the vertebral column or spine* (*i.e.*, T10 upward). It can be divided into *three parts* according to its insertions: semispinalis **thoracis**, into the cervical (C7) and thoracic (T1 to T4) spinous processes; semispinalis **cervicis**, into the spinous processes of C2 to C5; and semispinalis **capitis**, into the occipital bone.

The semispinalis thoracis and cervicis *extend the thoracic and cervical regions* of the vertebral column and *rotate them toward the opposite side*. The semis-

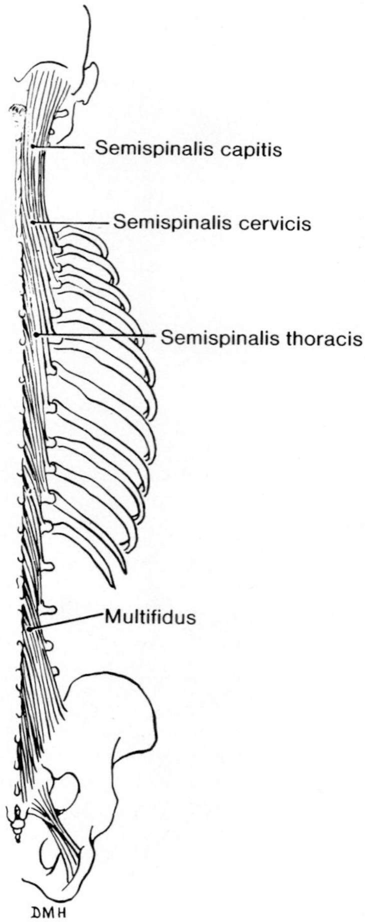

Figure 5-49. Drawing showing two of the deep oblique layers of muscle (transversospinalis). The rotatores muscles, forming the deepest layer, are not shown (see Figs. 5-42 and 5-51).

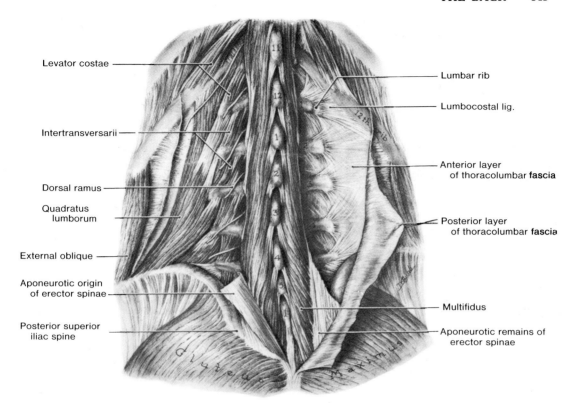

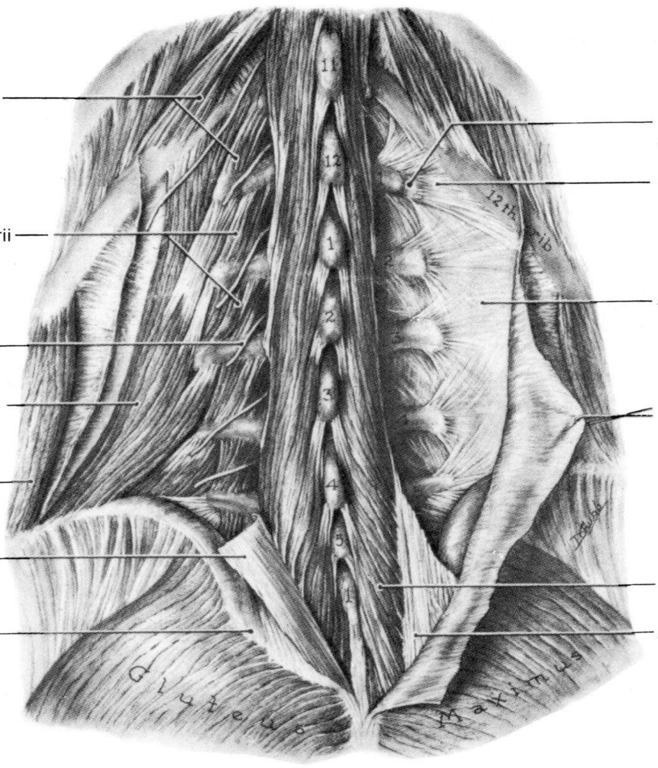

Figure 5-50. Drawing of a deep dissection of the back showing the multifidus and other intrinsic muscles.

pinalis **capitis** *extends the head and turns the face toward the opposite side.*

The Multifidus Muscle (Figs. 5-42, 5-49, and 5-50). The name (L. *multus*, many + *findo*, to cleave) indicates that this muscle is divided into several bundles. They occupy the groove on each side of the spinous processes of the vertebrae from the sacrum to the axis. Each bundle of muscle (heaviest in the lumbar region) ascends obliquely from its origin and inserts two to five vertebrae superiorly.

The multifidus muscle extends the vertebral column and rotates it toward the opposite side. *It is also a stabilizer.*

The Rotatores Muscles (Figs. 5-42 and 5-51). These short muscles form the deepest group in the groove between the spinous and transverse processes. They run the entire length of the vertebral column, but they can be demonstrated best in the thoracic region.

The rotatores *arise from the transverse process* of one vertebra and *insert into the base of the spinous process* of the vertebra above.

The action of the rotatores muscles is the same as the multifidus (*i.e.*, they **extend the vertebral column and rotate it** toward the opposite side. It also stabilizes the vertebral column).

The Interspinales and Intertransversarii Muscles (Figs. 5-50 and 5-52). These small insignificant muscles unite the spinous and transverse processes, respectively; they are well developed only in the cervical region. The interspinales are capable of producing extension of the vertebral column and the intertransversarii can produce lateral bending of the vertebral column.

General Comments. Try to gain an overview of the intrinsic back muscles and their actions because they are so important clinically and because backache is such a common complaint. It may help you to understand the arrangement of these muscles if you *visualize the erector spinae muscles as fanning out from the vertebral column* (Fig . 5-47). These deep muscles span the vertebral column as they extend superolaterally. Still deeper muscles (transversospinalis) span shorter distances and are directed superomedially (Fig. 5-49). The deepest muscles (rotatores) span the shortest distance, running from a transverse process below and lateral to the spinous process above and medial (Fig. 5-51).

When you step out with the left foot, the muscles on that side contract, whereas those on your right side may or may not contract. *The vertebral column is controlled by the intrinsic muscles* of the back (*i.e.*, they regulate its posture). When you are standing at attention, many of your back muscles are active, whereas when you stand at ease, many of them are inactive much of the time. They relax completely during standing when you flex your back as far as possible (Figs. 5-9 and 5-10), because in this position the ligaments of the vertebral column support the back.

SUBOCCIPITAL REGION

Suboccipital Muscles (Figs. 5-53 and 5-54). These four small muscles, lying deep to the semispinalis capitis, *extend and rotate the head*.

The rectus capitis posterior major (*rectus major*) originates from the spinous process of the axis, whereas the **rectus capitis posterior minor** (*rectus minor*) arises from the posterior tubercle of the atlas (Fig. 5-18). These muscles insert, side

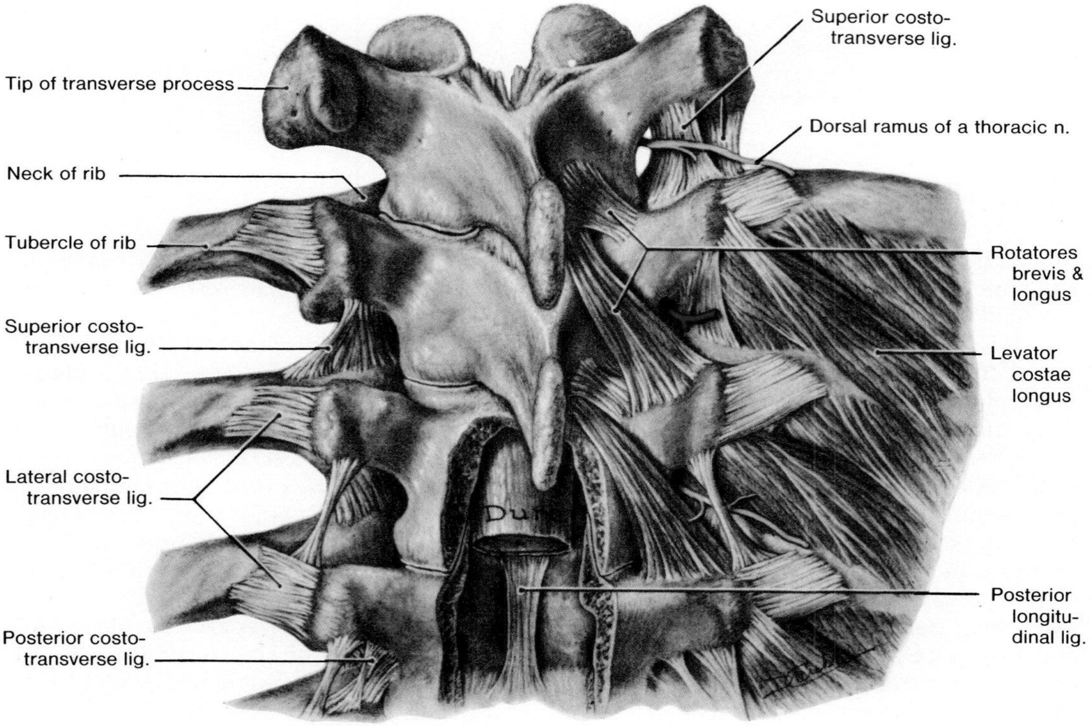

Figure 5-51. Drawing of a dissection showing the rotatores muscles of the back and the costotransverse ligaments. Of the three layers of transversospinalis or oblique muscles of the back (semispinales, multifidus, rotatores), the rotatores are the deepest and the shortest. They pass from the root of the transverse process to the junction of the transverse process and the lamina of the vertebra above.

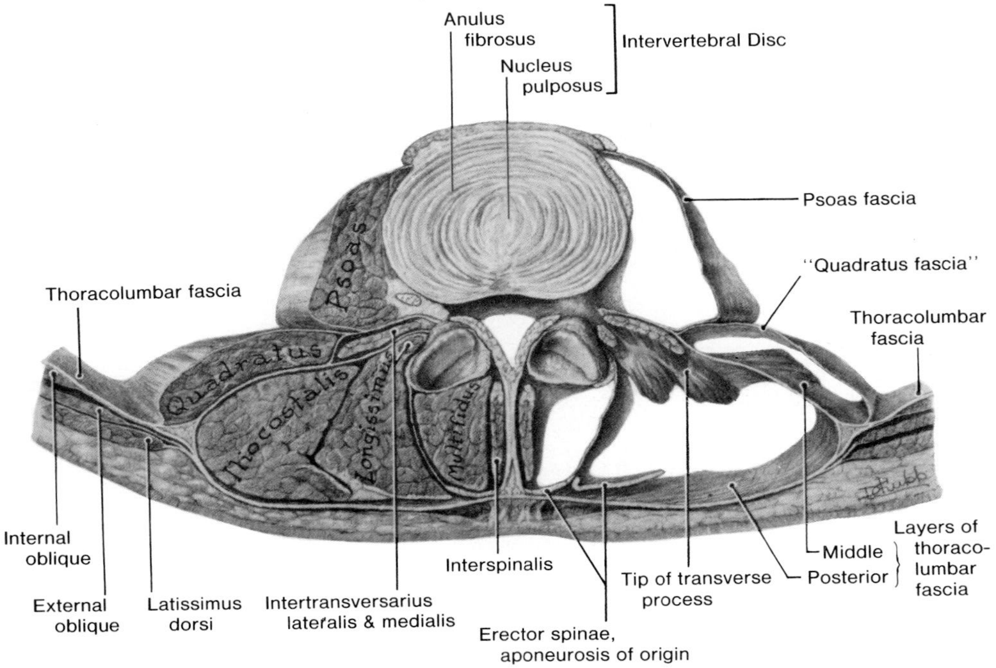

Figure 5-52. Drawing of a dissection of the deep muscles of the back. The muscles have been removed from their sheaths on the right side. Observe the laminated form of the anulus fibrosus of the intervertebral disc. No such organization is present in the nucleus pulposus, which consists mainly of fibrocartilage in older persons. Note that the anulus fibrosus is strongest anteriorly and laterally.

by side, into the occipital bone inferior to the inferior nuchal line (Figs. 5-53 and 5-55).

The obliquus capitis inferior (*inferior oblique*) is a thick round muscle that arises from the spinous process of the axis and runs obliquely upward and forward to insert into the tip of the transverse process of the atlas (Figs. 5-53 and 5-54). Although this muscle is not attached to the skull, it *rotates the head by pulling on the atlas* and it turns the face to the same side. The inferior oblique bounds the suboccipital triangle inferiorly (Fig. 5-53).

The obliquus capitis superior (*superior oblique*) is a flat triangular muscle that arises from the tip of the transverse process of the atlas and runs obliquely upward and backward to insert into the occipital bone (Figs. 5-53 and 5-54). The superior oblique bounds the suboccipital triangle laterally. *It bends the head backward and to the same side.*

The Suboccipital Triangle (Figs. 5-53 and 5-54). The boundaries of the suboccipital triangle are formed by three muscles: the rectus capitis posterior major, above and medially; the obliquus capitus superior, above and laterally; and the obliquus capitis inferior, below and laterally.

The **floor** of the suboccipital triangle is formed by the posterior atlantooccipital membrane and the posterior arch of the atlas; its **roof** is formed by the semispinalis capitis muscle.

CLINICALLY ORIENTED COMMENTS

The suboccipital triangle is important clinically because it contains the **vertebral artery** and the **suboccipital nerve** (dorsal ramus of the first cervical nerve). These structures lie in a groove on the superior

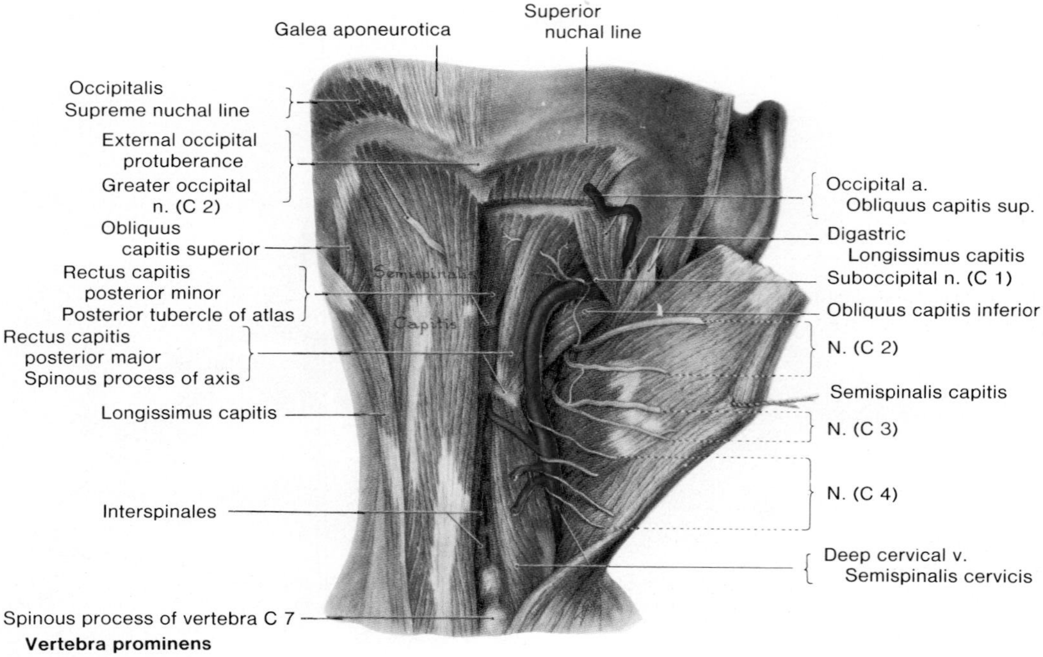

Figure 5-53. Drawing of a dissection of the suboccipital region. The trapezius, sternocleidomastoid, and splenius muscles have been removed.

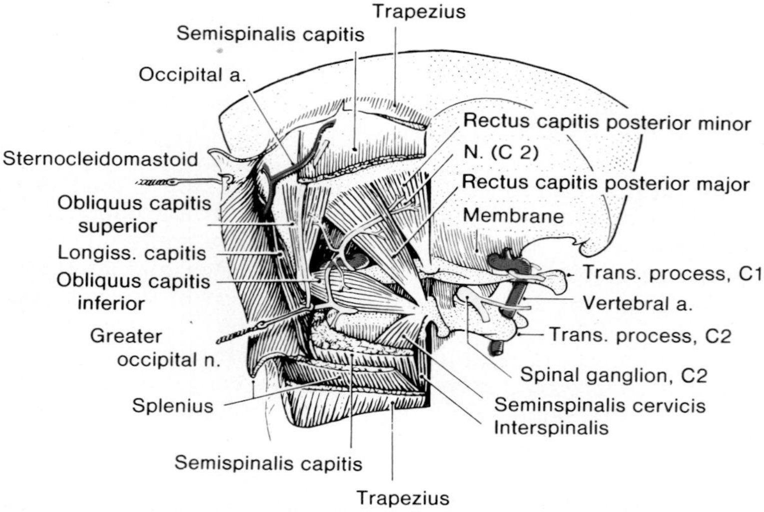

Figure 5-54. Diagram of the suboccipital region. The suboccipital triangle is bounded by three muscles: obliquus capitis inferior, obliquus capitis superior, and rectus capitis posterior major. Observe the vertebral artery winding behind the superior articular process of the atlas to enter the foramen magnum of the skull.

surface of the posterior arch of the atlas (Figs. 5-18, 5-53, and 5-54).

The curves in the vertebral arteries as they wind their way from the vertebral column, behind the superior articular process of the atlas (Fig. 9-34), to enter the foramen magnum of the skull (Fig. 5-54), may be clinically significant when blood

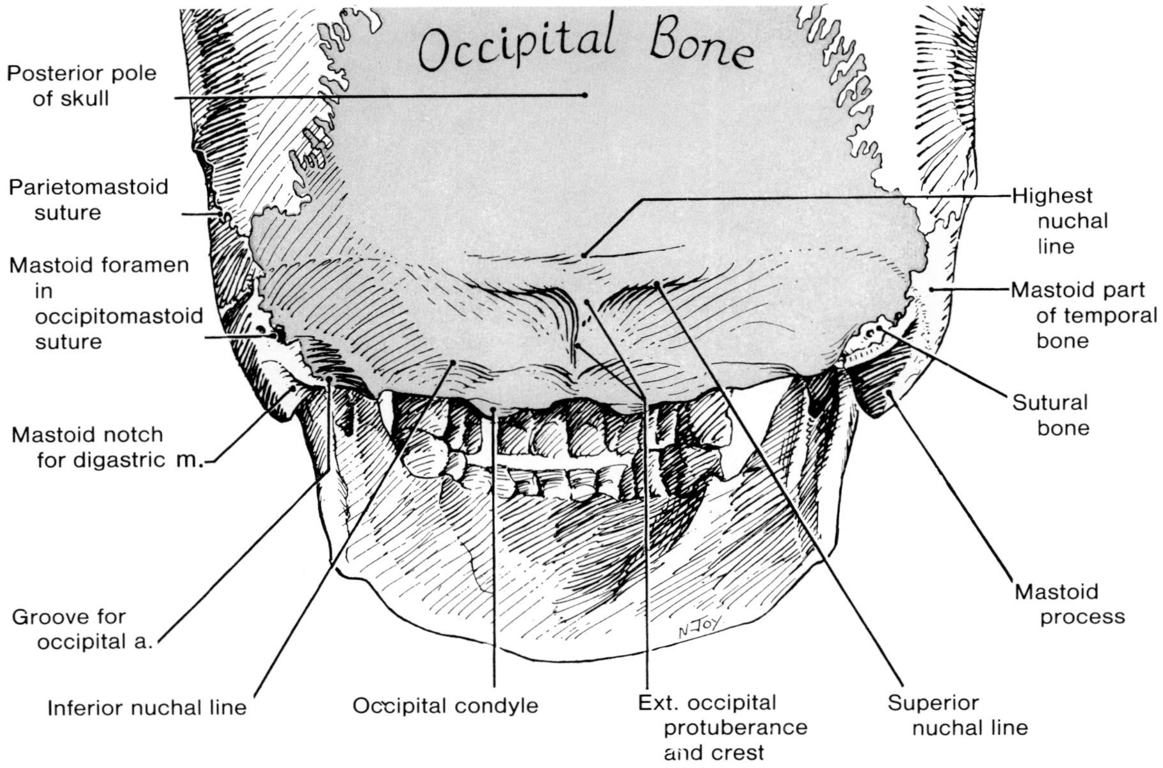

Figure 5-55. Drawing of part of the skull, from behind, to show the occipital bone.

flow through them is reduced (*e.g.*, owing to **arteriosclerosis** or hardening of the arteries). Under these conditions, prolonged turning of the head, as may occur during the backing up of a car, may cause dizziness and other symptoms because of interference with the blood supply to the brain stem.

A puncture needle can be inserted in the midline above the arch of C1 into the subarachnoid space **(cerebellomedullary cistern**, Fig. 7-82) for the collection of cerebrospinal fluid (CSF). This method of obtaining CSF is called **cisternal puncture**. This subarachnoid cistern, occupying the interval between the cerebellum and the medulla of the brain, receives CSF from the fourth ventricle of the brain through its median aperture (Figs. 7-80 and 7-82).

CSF is collected for determination of the alterations and variations in cells or in the concentration of chemicals in it. Cisternal puncture and injection of a contrast material is also performed by radiologists to outline the superior end of a tumor in the vertebral column (intraspinal tumor) after a **myelogram** (p. 000) has shown that the inferior end of the tumor completely blocks the vertebral canal.

CSF is usually obtained by lumbar puncture (Fig. 5-69), a procedure during which a needle is inserted between the spinous processes of L3 and L4 (or L4 and L5) into the subarachnoid space caudal to the spinal cord.

THE SPINAL CORD

The spinal cord is a cylindrical structure that is slightly flattened dorsoventrally and lies within the vertebral canal (Figs. 5-56, 5-57, 5-59, and 5-66). It is protected by the vertebrae, their ligaments, the spinal meninges (membranes), and the CSF.

The spinal cord averages about 45 cm in length in adult males and 42 cm in adult females. It extends from the foramen mag-

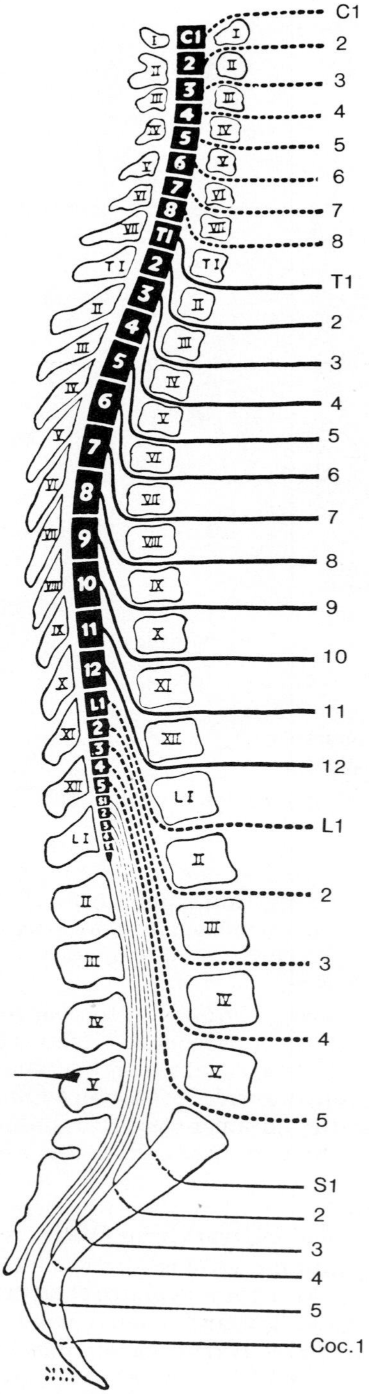

Figure 5-56. Diagram illustrating the relation of segments of the spinal cord and the spinal nerves to the vertebral column. Note that there are 31 pairs of spinal nerves (8 cervical, 12 thoracic, 5 lumbar, 5 sacral, and 1 coccygeal). Take special note that the spinal cord begins at the superior border of C1 (*i.e.*, at the foramen magnum) and ends opposite the intervertebral disc between L1 and L2. It does not extend into the inferior part of the vertebral canal.

num of the skull, where it is continuous with the medulla of the brain, to the superior part of the lumbar region of the vertebral column (Figs. 2-139 and 5-56). *The spinal cord in adults often ends opposite the intervertebral disc between L1 and L2,* but it may terminate as high as T12 or as low as L3 (Fig. 5-69*B*). Thus, **the spinal cord occupies only the upper two-thirds of the vertebral canal.**

The spinal cord is enlarged in two regions (Fig. 5-62) for innervation of the limbs. The **cervical enlargement** extends from C4 to T1 segments of the spinal cord, and most of the corresponding spinal nerves form the brachial plexus for innervation of the upper limb (Fig. 6-25). The **lumbosacral enlargement** extends from L2 to S3 segments of the spinal cord, and the corresponding nerves make up the lumbar and sacral plexuses for innervation of the lower limb (Fig. 4-52).

It is clinically important for you to understand that the spinal cord segments do not correspond with the vertebral levels, e.g., the lumbosacral enlargement (L2 to S3 segments of the spinal cord) extends from about the body of T11 to the level of the body L1. In Figure 5-56 note that the thoracic region of the spinal cord is the longest and that *the sacral region is well above the sacrum* and is the shortest region of the spinal cord.

Internal Structure of the Spinal Cord (Fig. 5-57). The gray matter of the spinal cord has an H-shaped or butterfly outline and is surrounded by white matter. The ventral and dorsal limbs of the H, called gray horns or columns, divide the white matter on each side into three columns (funiculi): ventral, lateral, and dorsal. A groove anteriorly, called the anterior or **ventral median fissure**, and a septum posteriorly, the posterior or **dorsal median septum**, partially separate the right and left sides of white matter. The central

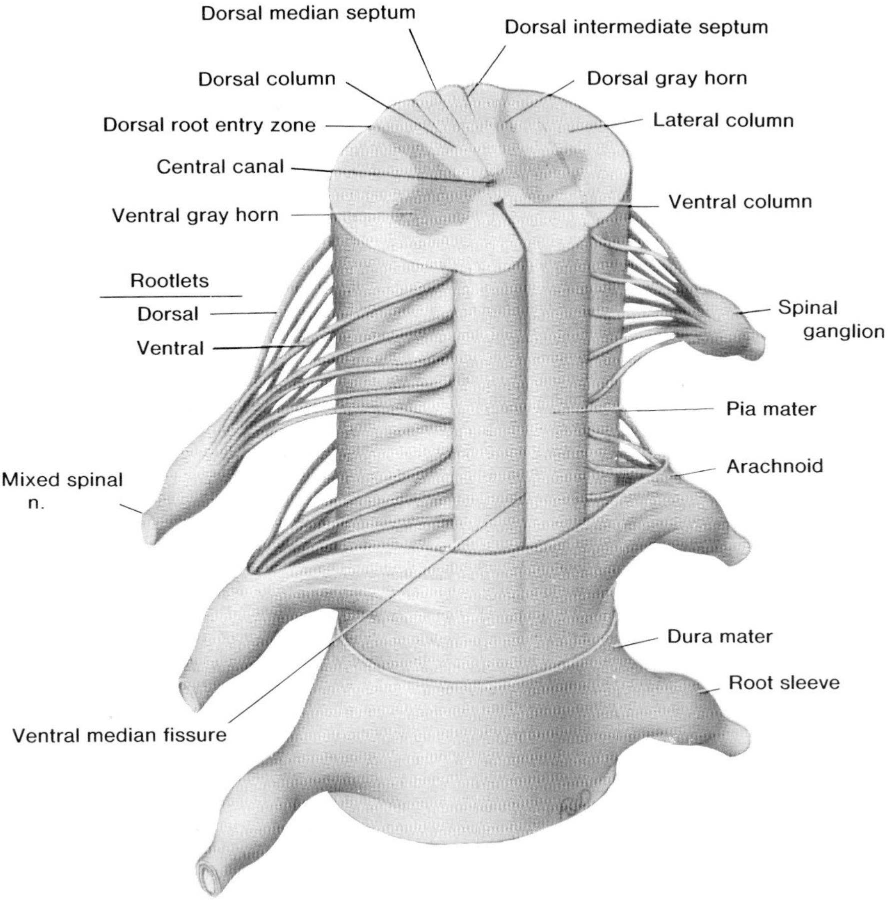

Figure 5-57. Drawing of the spinal cord, nerve roots, and meninges illustrating their general structure. Observe that each root emerges as a series of rootlets and that each spinal nerve is formed by the union of dorsal and ventral spinal nerve roots.

canal of the spinal cord is narrow and is usually not patent in older people (Fig. 5-57).

Structure of the Spinal Nerves (Figs. 5-56 to 5-60). There are 31 pairs of spinal nerves attached to the spinal cord by dorsal and ventral roots. The **ventral roots** leaving the cord contain efferent (motor) fibers, whereas the **dorsal roots** entering the cord contain afferent (sensory) fibers.

The cell bodies whose axons make up the ventral roots are in the ventral gray horn of the spinal cord (Figs. 5-57 and 5-59), whereas the nerve cells whose axons make up the dorsal roots are outside the spinal cord in the **spinal (dorsal root) ganglia**. Thus, the dorsal root of each spinal nerve has a spinal ganglion which is located in the intervertebral foramen and rests on the pedicle of the vertebral arch (Figs. 5-58 to 5-60).

Just outside the intervertebral foramen, the dorsal and ventral nerve roots unite to form a **spinal nerve** (Figs. 5-58 to 5-60). It divides at once into a ventral (anterior) **ramus** (L. branch) and a dorsal (posterior) ramus, each of which contains many afferent and efferent nerve fibers.

Positional Changes of the Spinal Cord (Fig. 5-61). In the embryo the spinal cord extends the entire length of the vertebral canal, and the spinal nerves form just

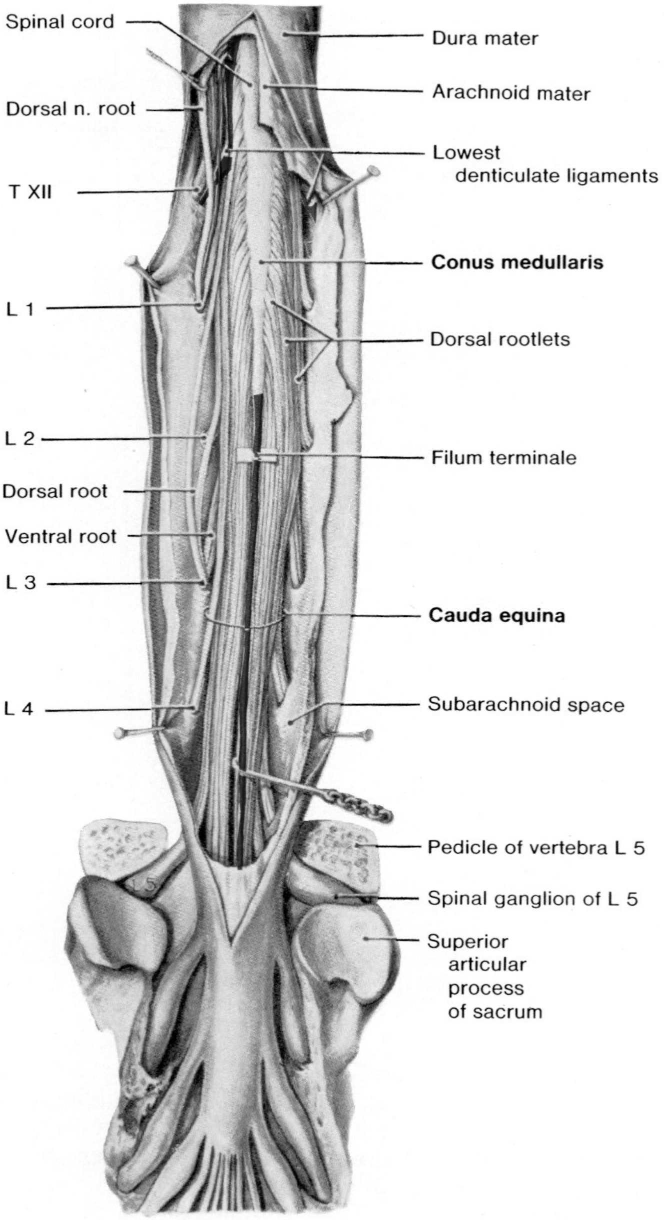

Figure 5-58. Drawing of a dissection of the lower end of the spinal cord. The dura mater and arachnoid have been incised to expose the lower end of the spinal cord and the cauda equina (bundle of spinal nerve roots).

outside the intervertebral foramina at their levels of origin (Fig. 5-61*A*). Because the vertebral column grows more rapidly than the spinal cord in the embryo and fetus, this relationship does not persist. The caudal end of the spinal cord comes to lie at relatively higher levels. At 24 weeks it ends at the level of S1 (Fig. 5-61*B*); **in the newborn it terminates at L2 or L3** (Fig. 5-61*C*); and *in the adult it usually ends at the lower border of L1* (Fig. 5-61*D*).

The position of the spinal cord during

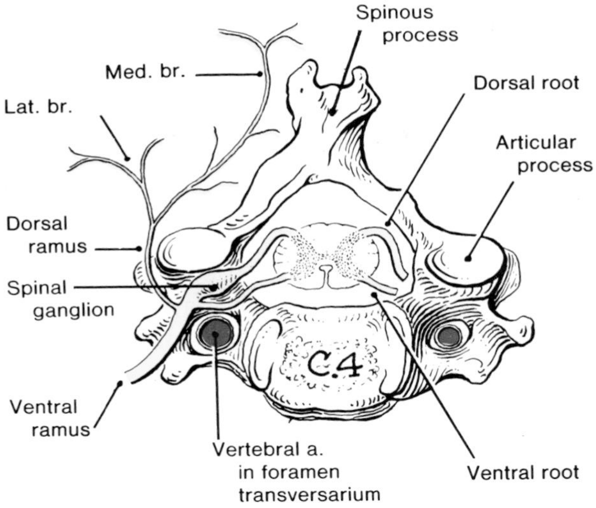

Figure 5-59. Drawing of the superior surface of the fourth cervical vertebra showing the spinal cord in its vertebral foramen. The meninges are not illustrated. Note that a typical spinal nerve arises from the spinal cord by dorsal and ventral roots. The spinal ganglion is located on the dorsal root and is within the intervertebral foramen. Note also that the dorsal and ventral roots join at about the level of the outer edge of the intervertebral foramen to form a spinal nerve. Observe that the fourth cervical nerve leaves the intervertebral foramen above the pedicle of C4. Just outside the foramen the nerve divides into two parts called dorsal (posterior) and ventral (anterior) primary rami.

development determines the direction of the spinal nerve roots in the subarachnoid space. The dorsal and ventral roots of the spinal nerves from C1 to C7 leave the vertebral canal through the intervertebral foramina above the corresponding pedicles of the vertebrae (Figs. 5-56 and 5-59). The spinal nerves from C1 and C2 lie on the vertebral arches of the atlas and the axis, respectively. The dorsal and ventral roots of the eighth cervical nerve pass through the intervertebral foramen between C7 and T1 because there are eight cervical nerves and only seven cervical vertebrae.

The length and obliquity of the nerve roots increase progressively as the inferior end of the vertebral column is approached because of the increasing distance between the spinal cord segments and the corresponding vertebrae (Figs. 5-56, 5-60, and 5-61). Thus, the lumbosacral and coccygeal nerve roots are the longest, and they form a collection of dorsal and ventral nerve roots in the subarachnoid space caudal to the termination of the spinal cord called the **cauda equina** (L. horse's tail). This *bundle of spinal nerve roots* extends into the inferior part of the vertebral canal (Figs. 5-56 and 5-58).

The spinal cord tapers rather abruptly into the **conus medullaris** (Figs. 5-58 and 5-61). From its inferior end, a long slender filament called the **filum terminale** (L. *filum*, a thread) arises; it lies within the cauda equina (Figs. 5-58, 5-61, and 5-62). Its subarachnoid part ends at S2, where it is attached to the end of the **dural sac** (Fig. 5-61), and its extradural prolongation inserts into the dorsum of the coccyx (Figs. 5-60 and 5-61). The filum terminale, which has no functional significance, consists of connective tissue, pia mater, and neuroglial elements.

Blood Supply and Venous Drainage of the Spinal Cord and its Meninges. *The Spinal Arteries* (Figs. 5-62 and 5-63). The spinal cord is supplied by three longitudinal vessels (an anterior spinal artery and two posterior spinal arteries) and anterior and posterior radicular arteries.

The anterior spinal artery, formed by the union of two small branches of the vertebral arteries (Fig. 5-62*A*), runs the length of the spinal cord in the ventral

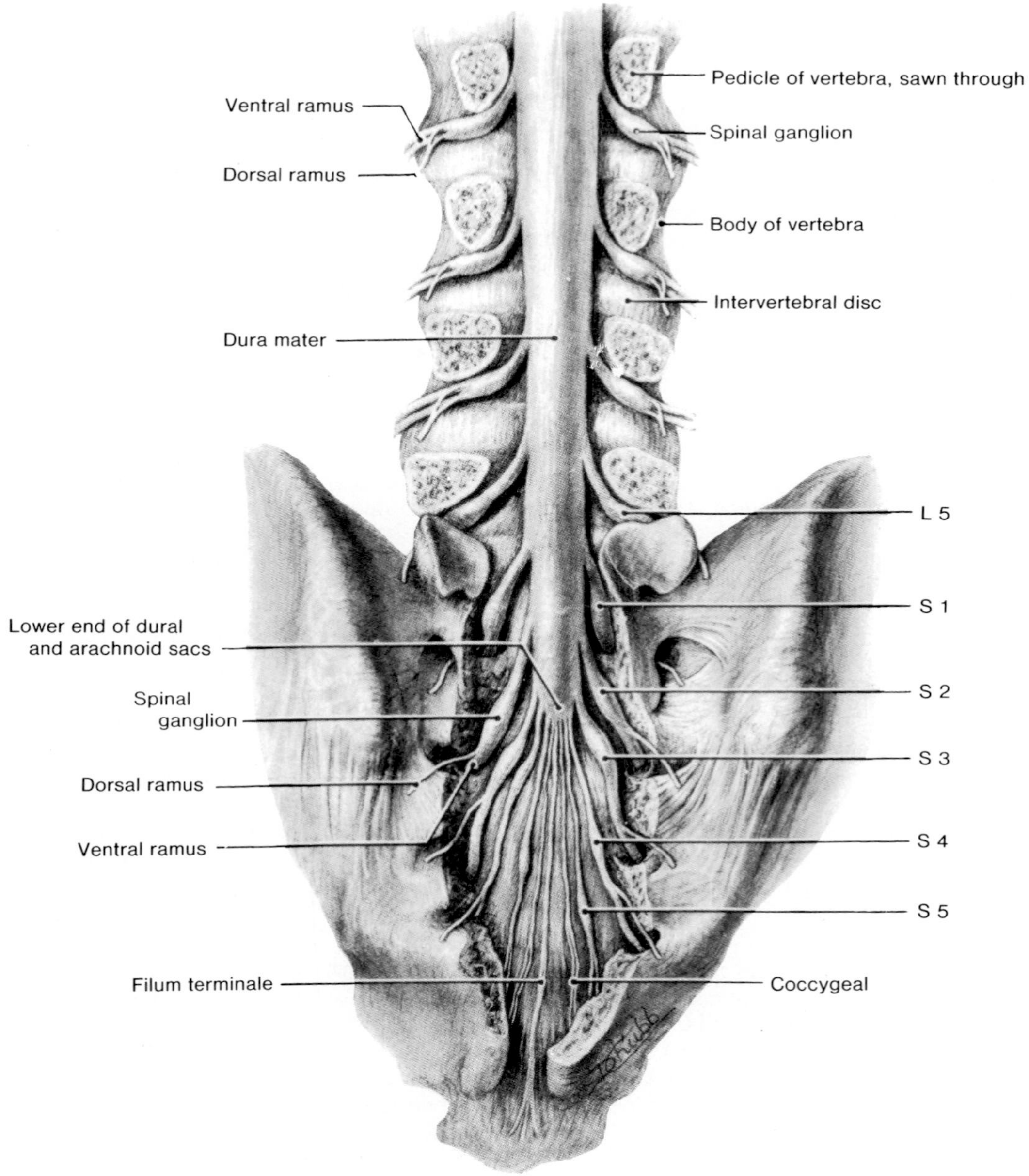

Figure 5-60. Drawing of a dissection of back to show the inferior end of the dural sac from behind. The posterior parts of the lumbar and sacral vertebrae have been removed. Understand that a posterolateral protrusion of the nucleus pulposus of a lumbar disc usually compresses the nerve root in its dural sleeve close to its point of exit from the spinal dural tube or sac. The nerve root passes downward, laterally to emerge from the vertebral column one foramen below the protruding disc, *e.g.*, a L5/S1 posterior disc protrusion usually compresses the S1 component of the sciatic nerve as in Case 5-3.

median fissure (Fig. 5-57). It *supplies the anterior two-thirds of the spinal cord.* The caliber of the anterior spinal artery varies according to its proximity to a major radicular artery. It is usually smallest in the T4 to T8 regions of the spinal cord.

Each posterior spinal artery arises as a small branch of either the vertebral or the posterior inferior cerebellar artery (Fig. 5-62*B*). These arteries form two descending vessels that anastomose frequently with each other and with the anterior spinal artery (Fig. 5-63) as they *supply the posterior one-third of the spinal cord.*

The blood supplied by the anterior and posterior spinal arteries is sufficient only for the upper cervical segments of the spinal cord. The remaining segments of the cord receive most of their blood from the many radicular arteries which join either the anterior or posterior spinal arteries (Figs. 5-62 and 5-63).

The radicular arteries arise from the spinal branches of the vertebral, deep cervical, ascending cervical, posterior intercostal, lumbar, and lateral sacral arteries. They enter the vertebral canal through the intervertebral foramina and divide into anterior and posterior radicular arteries that supply the vertebrae, the meninges, and the spinal arteries (Fig. 5-63). Usually one of the anterior radicular arteries supplying the lumbosacral enlargement of the cord is much larger than the others; it is called the **arteria radicularis magna** (artery of Adamkiewicz). It arises more frequently on the left from a lower intercostal or an upper lumbar artery (T6 to L3). *The large radicular artery or arteria radicularis magna is clinically important because it usually provides the main blood supply to the lower two-thirds of the spinal cord.*

The radicular arteries supplying the midthoracic region of the spinal cord are few and small. This **watershed area of the spinal cord** is a junctional zone between

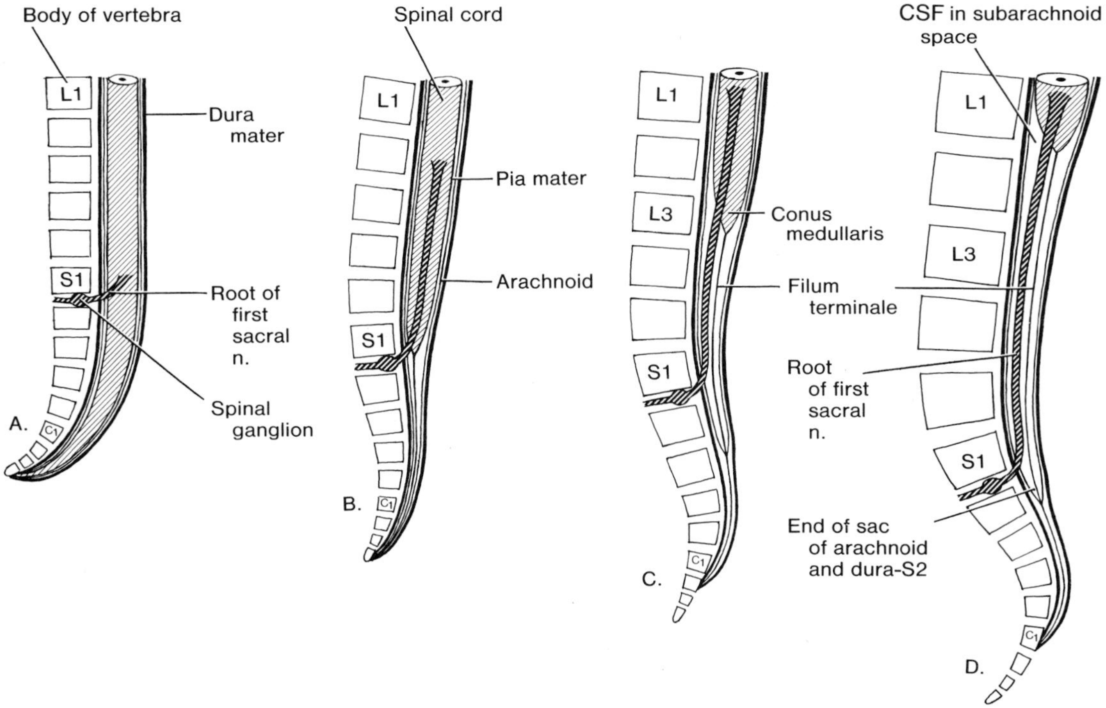

Figure 5-61. Drawings showing the position of the inferior end of the spinal cord in relation to the vertebral column and the meninges at various stages of development. The increasing length and obliquity of the nerve roots is also shown. *A,* 8 weeks; *B,* 24 weeks; *C,* newborn; *D,* adult.

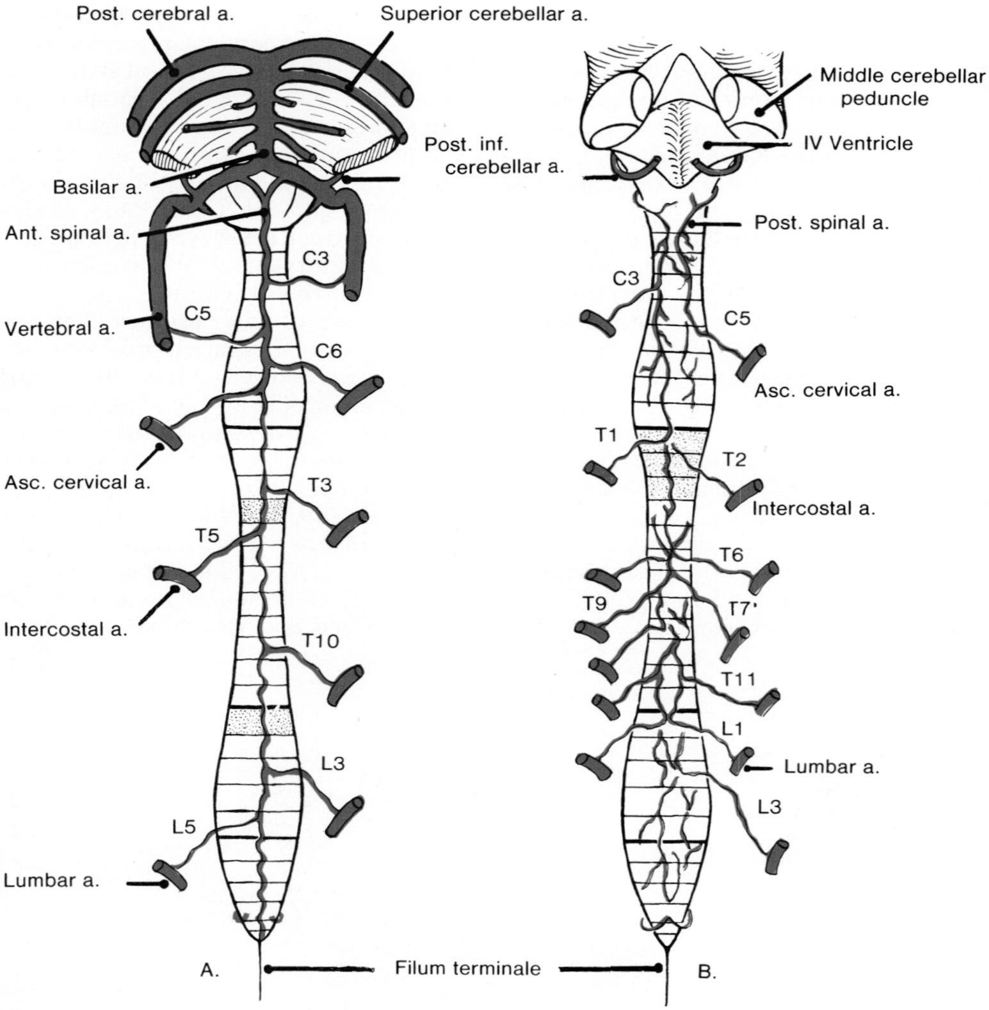

Figure 5-62. Drawings illustrating the arteries of the spinal cord. *A*, ventral aspect; *B*, dorsal aspect. The stippled areas of the cord indicate the regions most vulnerable to vascular deprivation when contributing arteries are injured. The levels of entry of the common radicular branches are shown (*e.g.*, C5 and T5). Note that the spinal cord is enlarged in two regions for innervation of the limbs.

the segments superior and inferior to it that are well supplied with blood.

CLINICALLY ORIENTED COMMENTS

The spinal cord may suffer circulatory impairment if the radicular arteries, particularly the **arteria radicularis magna**, are compromised by obstructive arterial disease or by ligation of their parent posterior intercostal or lumbar arteries during surgery. These patients may lose all sensation and voluntary movement below the level of impaired blood supply to the spinal cord (*i.e.*, **paraplegia**, paralysis of both lower limbs and generally the lower trunk).

When there is a *severe drop in systemic blood pressure* for 3 to 5 minutes, blood flow through the small radicular arteries supplying the watershed area of the spinal cord may be reduced or stopped, resulting in necrosis of neurons in the midthoracic region of the cord. These patients may also lose sensation and voluntary movement below the affected level of the spinal cord.

The Spinal Veins (Figs. 5-63 and 5-64). The spinal veins have a distribution somewhat similar to that of the spinal arteries. There are several anterior and posterior longitudinal veins on the spinal cord which communicate freely with each other and which are drained by numerous radicular veins.

The vertebral canal contains a profuse plexus of thin-walled, valveless veins which surround the spinal dura mater (Fig. 5-67). This plexus communicates via the anterior and posterior longitudinal sinuses with the venous sinuses of the dura mater (Figs. 5-82 and 7-69).

The spinal veins and vertebral venous plexuses drain into intervertebral veins, and from there into the **vertebral veins,** or the **ascending lumbar veins,** or the **azygos venous system** (Fig. 5-64).

CLINICALLY ORIENTED COMMENTS

The vertebral venous plexus is important clinically because blood may return from the pelvis or the abdomen by way of it and reach the heart through the superior venal cavae. When the prostate gland is cancerous, blood may pass from it to the vertebral venous plexus and the superior vena cava instead of by its usual route via the inferior vena cava. Tumor cells from a prostatic cancer may be deposited via these veins in the vertebrae and may develop as a secondary cancer (**metastasis**).

The vertebral canal varies considerably in size and shape from level to level, particularly in the cervical and lumbar regions

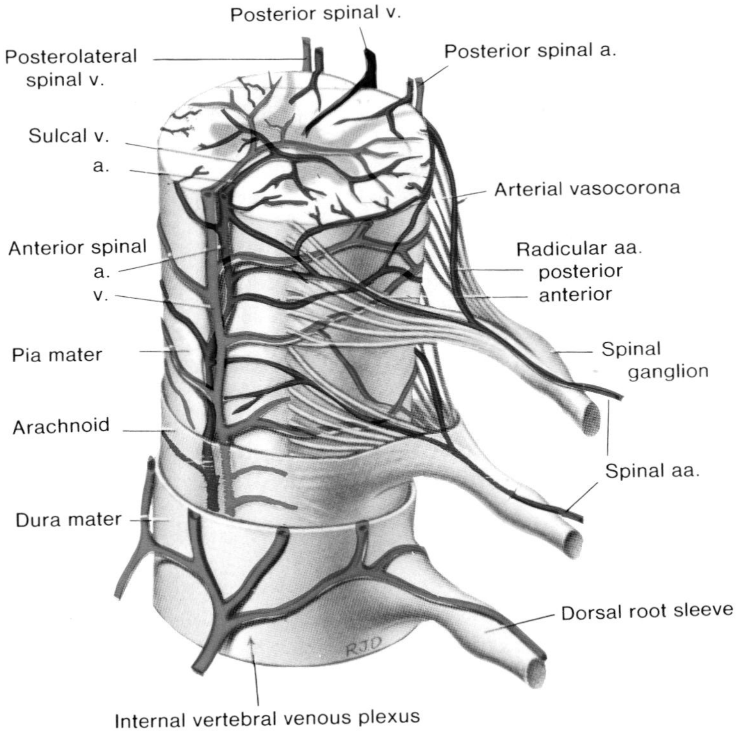

Figure 5-63. Drawing showing the blood supply and venous drainage of the spinal cord.

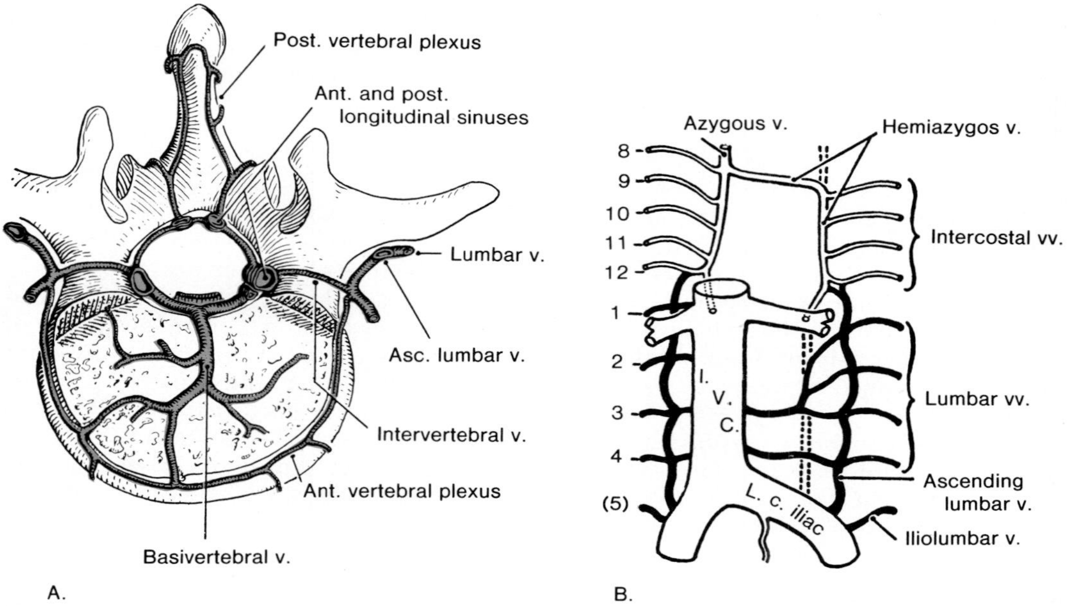

Figure 5-64. Drawings illustrating the vertebral venous plexuses and the azygos venous system. *A*, the vertebral venous plexuses. Note that the vertebral canal contains an internal plexus of veins which surrounds the spinal dura mater. This plexus communicates above with the occipital and basilar sinuses. Observe also the communications of the external plexus. *B*, the ascending lumbar vein and the azygos venous system. Note how the vertebral venous plexuses connect with this system (also see Fig. 5-34).

(Figs. 5-18 and 5-23). A small vertebral canal in the cervical region, into which the spinal cord fits as tightly as a finger in a glove, is potentially dangerous because a minor fracture and/or dislocation of the cervical vertebrae may damage the spinal cord. In addition, the transitory protrusion of a cervical intervertebral disc following an injury may cause "spinal cord shock," associated with paralysis below the site of the lesion. In these cases no fracture or dislocation of cervical vertebrae can be found, but if the patient dies, a **softening of the spinal cord** at one level may be found.

A small, trefoil-shaped vertebral canal is sometimes found at L5 (Fig. 5-16*B*), but rarely at L4. Such a three-lobed canal may be a contributory factor in cases of **sciatica** (pain along the distribution of the sciatic nerve) and/or **cauda equina claudication** (L. *claudicatio*, to limp). Encroachment on part or all of such a canal by a protruding intervertebral disc, by swollen ligamenta flava, or as a result of **osteoarthritis** of the zygapophyseal joints may exert pressure on one or more of the spinal nerve roots of the cauda equina and may produce sensory and motor symptoms. This group of bone and joint abnormalities is often called **lumbar spondylosis.**

In older people the nuclei pulposi of the intervertebral discs degenerate, the vertebrae come together, and the anuli fibrosi bulge anteriorly, posteriorly, and laterally; this leads to bony outgrowths called **osteophytes.** In the neck this condition is called **cervical spondylosis** and often is accompanied by swollen ligamenta flava and osteoarthritis of the zygapophyseal joints. In these conditions there is often encroachment on the intervertebral foramina and/or vertebral canal that may cause pressure on the cervical nerve roots and/or spinal cord, resulting in various neurological symptoms and signs.

Complete transection of the spinal cord results in loss of all sensation and voluntary movement below the lesion.

The patient is **quadriplegic** (upper and lower limbs paralyzed) if the cervical cord above C3 and/or C4 is transected, and the patient may die owing to respiratory failure. The patient is **paraplegic** (lower limbs paralyzed) if the transection is between the cervical and lumbosacral enlargements. The abdominal and back muscles are also affected, causing additional problems for the patient.

THE SPINAL MENINGES AND CSF

The dura mater, the arachnoid mater, and the pia mater are known collectively as the meninges (G. membranes). *The spinal meninges surround and support the spinal cord* (Figs. 5-65 to 5-68).

Between the dura mater and the arachnoid there is a *potential space*, the **subdural space**, containing only a capillary layer of fluid, but between the arachnoid and the pia mater there is an *actual space*, the **subarachnoid space**, containing CSF and the vessels of the spinal cord (Fig. 5-66).

The Dura Mater (L. *dura*, hard + *mater*, mother). The dura mater is a tough fibrous membrane composed mostly of collagen fibers and some elastic tissue. The **spinal dura mater** (dural sac) is free within the vertebral canal (Figs. 5-51 and 5-60) but is adherent to the margin of the foramen magnum of the skull and is continuous with the cranial dura mater. The **dura mater** hangs down from the skull like a tube, with a closed lower end that usually ends at the level of the lower border of S2 in adults (Figs. 5-61*D* and 5-66).

The spinal cord is suspended in the dura mater by a saw-toothed **denticulate ligament** (L. *dentatus*, toothed) on each side (Figs. 5-67 and 5-68). This ribbon-like ligament, composed of pia mater, is attached along the lateral surface of the spinal cord, midway between the dorsal and ventral nerve roots. The lateral edge of the denticulate ligament is notched, or serrated (L. *serratus*, a saw). There are 21 tooth-like processes attached to the dura mater between the foramen magnum and the level at which the dura is pierced by the nerve roots of S1.

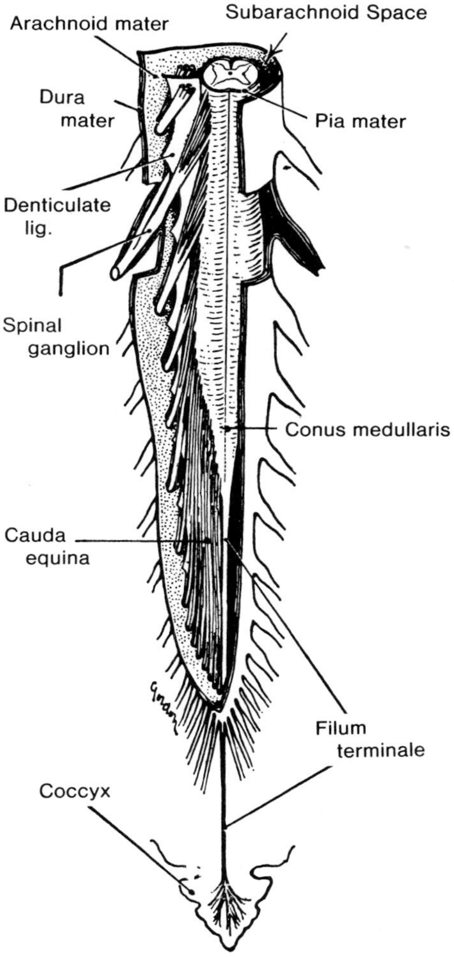

Figure 5-65. Drawing of the spinal cord and cauda equina exposed from behind. The structures in the subarachnoid space on the *right* have been removed for illustrative purposes.

The dura mater is evaginated along the dorsal and ventral nerve roots of the spinal nerves, forming **dural sleeves** for them which continue into the intervertebral foramina (Figs. 5-57, 5-63, and 5-67). Beyond the spinal ganglia, these dural sleeves fuse where the spinal nerve roots unite to form a spinal nerve just outside the intervertebral foramen (Fig. 5-59). Here the dura mater becomes continuous with the **epineurium** (G. *epi*, upon + *neuron*, nerve), the connective tissue sheath surrounding a peripheral nerve (Fig. I-58).

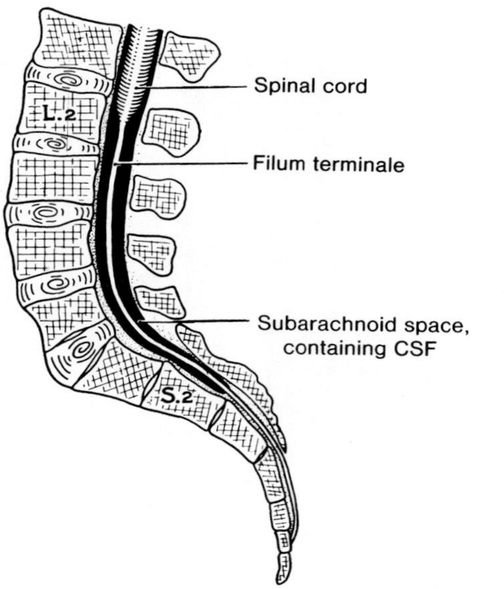

Figure 5-66. Diagram of the lower part of the spinal cord within the vertebral canal. In this case the spinal cord ends just caudal to the disc between L1 and L2 and the subarachnoid space ends just above the disc between S2 and S3.

CLINICALLY ORIENTED COMMENTS

Sometimes it is necessary to expose a patient's spinal dura, spinal cord, and/or nerve roots. **Laminectomy**, the surgical procedure used to make this exposure, was the name given because the spinous processes and the laminae of the vertebral arch are removed.

Using this procedure, pressure on neural structures from bony fragments, protruding nuclei pulposi of intervertebral discs, tumors, or hematomas (local masses of extravasated blood) may be relieved.

Sometimes operations are performed on the spinal cord to relieve **intractable pain** (*e.g.*, in the late stages of malignant disease of a pelvic viscus). In surgical section of the spinal cord (**open chordotomy**), the cut is made in the ventrolateral portion of the cord in order to interrupt the pain pathway (**lateral spinothalamic tract**). When the operation is completed, the edges of the dura are carefully joined and the muscles are replaced before the skin is sutured.

Percutaneous chordotomy, the use of high frequency electricity, has almost completely replaced open chordotomy. Because it can be performed on a conscious patient, the position and size of the lesion in the cord may be controlled by asking the patient what she/he feels (or does not feel) while the electrode is in place. The electrode is usually inserted between C1 and C2 (the atlas and the axis) to destroy all ascending pain fibers in the spinal cord on one side.

The Arachnoid Mater (G. spider-like). The spinal arachnoid is the delicate, filamentous, avascular covering of the spinal cord (Figs. 5-63 and 5-65). It is composed mostly of collagen fibers and some elastic tissue and is coextensive in length with the dura mater; however, it is separated from this layer by a potential **subdural space** (Figs. 5-67 and 5-68). The arachnoid is separated from the pia mater by an actual space, the **subarachnoid space**, but the two meningeal layers are connected by delicate strands of connective tissue called **arachnoid trabeculae** (Figs. 5-67 and 5-82). The arachnoid and pia mater developed as one layer in the embryo and then separated, but numerous connections (trabeculae) remained. Together, the pia mater and the arachnoid are called the **leptomeninges** (G. slender membranes) or the **pia-arachnoid**.

The Pia Mater (L. *pius*, tender). The spinal pia mater, composed of two fused layers of loose connective tissue (Fig. 5-67), encloses a fine network of blood vessels and adheres to the surface of the spinal cord. It also covers the roots of the spinal nerves and blood vessels (Figs. 5-63, 5-65, and 5-67). The **denticulate ligament** (discussed previously) is continuous with the pia mater at each side of the spinal cord (Fig. 5-68) and its lateral border is fixed at intervals to the spinal dura mater (Figs. 5-68 and 5-69).

The subarachnoid space (Figs. 5-61 and 5-66) is between the arachnoid and the pia. It contains CSF, a clear slightly alkaline fluid. The subarachnoid space extending from L2 to S2 is known as the **lumbar cistern** (L. *cisterna*, an under-

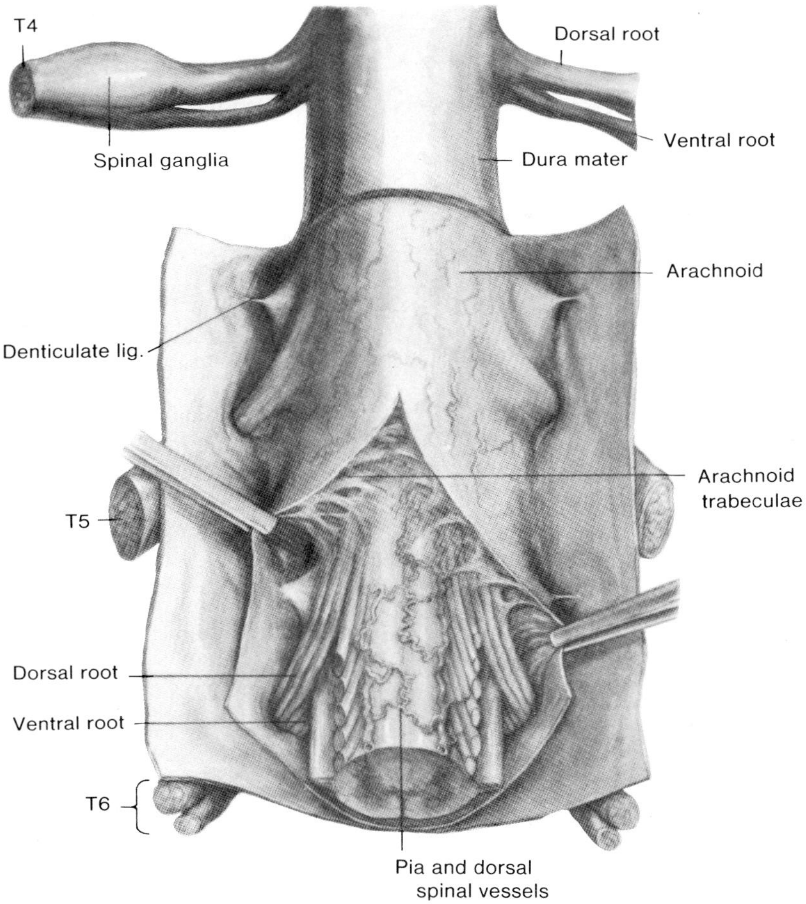

Figure 5-67. Drawing of a posterior view of the superior part of the thoracic spinal cord. *Below,* the dura mater and arachnoid have been split in the midline to expose the spinal cord and the pial and dorsal vessels. *Above,* the intact dura covers the spinal cord and the spinal nerve roots.

ground reservoir). In addition to CSF, it contains the cauda equina, and the filum terminale (Figs. 5-58 and 5-66).

CLINICALLY ORIENTED COMMENTS

CSF can be obtained from the lumbar cistern located in the lower part of the vertebral canal (Fig. 5-69*B*). As the spinal cord usually ends between L1 and L2, there is little danger of injuring the spinal cord when a **lumbar puncture needle** is inserted between the spinous processes of L3/L4 or L4/L5 into the lumbar cistern to obtain a sample of CSF (Fig. 5-69). The needle may touch a spinal nerve root in the cauda equina if it is not inserted exactly in the midline (Fig. 5-60). Touching a nerve root results in sharp pain in the **dermatome** or area of skin supplied by the nerve root concerned (Fig. 4-160). If this occurs, the needle is withdrawn about 1 cm and rotated 90° to move the bevel of the needle so that the nerve root is not injured when the needle is reinserted. Precautions are taken to avoid introducing infection into the subarachnoid space during lumbar puncture.

Lumbar puncture is performed to obtain CSF for diagnostic procedures such as

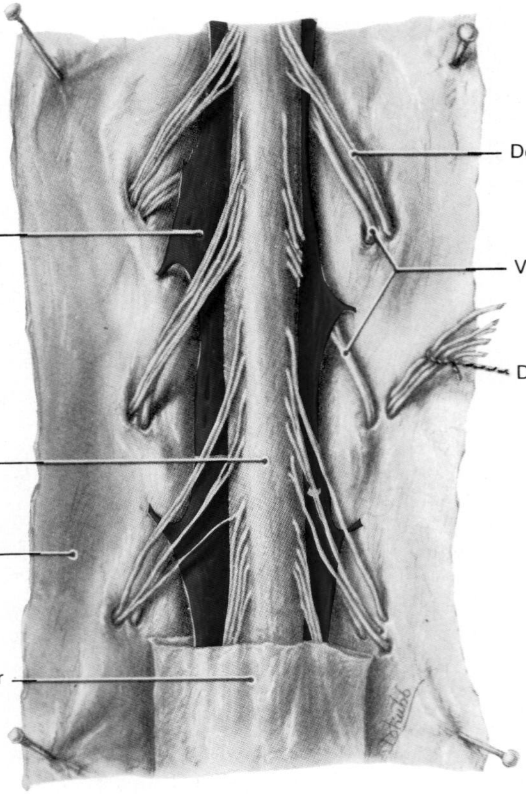

Figure 5-68. Drawing of a dissection of the spinal cord within the spinal meninges, posterior view. The dura mater and arachnoid have been split and pinned to expose the spinal cord and the nerve roots.

pneumoencephalography or myelography. During **pneumoencephalography** (G. *pneuma*, air + *enkephalos*, brain + *graphē*, a drawing), some CSF is replaced by air, and then skull radiographs are taken in various positions. These radiographs, called **pneumoencephalograms**, permit visualization of the ventricles and the subarachnoid space (Fig. 7-85).

During **myelography** a radiopaque substance is injected into the lumbar cistern, and then a fluoroscopic examination is performed on a tilting table. For these examinations an apparatus known as **fluoroscope** is used which makes the shadows of organs visible on a fluorescent screen. These radiographs, called **myelograms**, permit visualization of the spinal cord and the spinal subarachnoid space. The term myelogram is derived from the Greek words *myelos*, meaning medulla and *graphē*, a drawing. The spinal cord is sometimes called the spinal medulla, which explains the use of the prefix "myelo" in this term.

Spina bifida (L. *bifidus*, cleft in two parts) is used to describe a wide range of developmental defects. In its most simple form, **spina bifida occulta**, the halves of the vertebral arch fail to develop fully (Fig. 5-30); **spina bifida cystica** is a more serious abnormality in which there is herniation of the meninges and/or the spinal cord through the bony defect (Figs. 5-70 and 5-71). When the meninges alone are herniated, the condition is known as **spina bifida with meningocele** (Fig. 5-70*A*), whereas when the meninges and the spinal cord are herniated, the condition is known as **spina bifida with meningomyelocele** (Fig. 5-70*B*). In these cases the patients may exhibit evidence of spinal cord or nerve root malfunction, *e.g.*, paralysis of the limbs and incontinence of urine and feces. (Fig. 5-71*B*). *Spina bifida cystica involving the meninges and/or the spinal cord occurs about once in every 1000 births.*

Although the term spina bifida refers only to the vertebral defect, it is used clinically to refer to conditions involving both vertebral and neural defects (*e.g.*, spina bifida with meningocele or spina bifida with meningomyelocele). Most clinically significant cases of spina bifida probably result from a local overgrowth of the developing neural tube, commonly referred to as a **neural tube defect**. The excessive development of the neural tube (primordium or source of the brain and spinal cord) results in nonfusion of the halves of the vertebral arch (Fig. 5-70). Usually several vertebrae in the thoracic, lumbar, or sacral regions are involved (Fig. 5-71).

PATIENT ORIENTED PROBLEMS

Case 5-1. During a fight, a 16-year-old boy was stabbed in the back of the neck with a knife. As he ducked attempting to avoid his attacker, he flexed his neck. Much to the surprise of his assailant, the boy fell to the ground completely immobilized from the neck down.

Problems. How did this serious injury probably occur? Use your anatomical knowledge of the vertebral column and its contents to explain the basis of the injury. How might this knowledge be utilized in the diagnosis and treatment of diseases of the nervous system and in the administration of anesthetic agents? *These problems are discussed on page 666.*

Case 5-2. A 51-year-old man was relaxing while waiting for the traffic light to turn green when his car was "rear ended" (rammed very hard from behind). His body was pushed forward and his head was thrown violently backward (Fig. 5-78). He

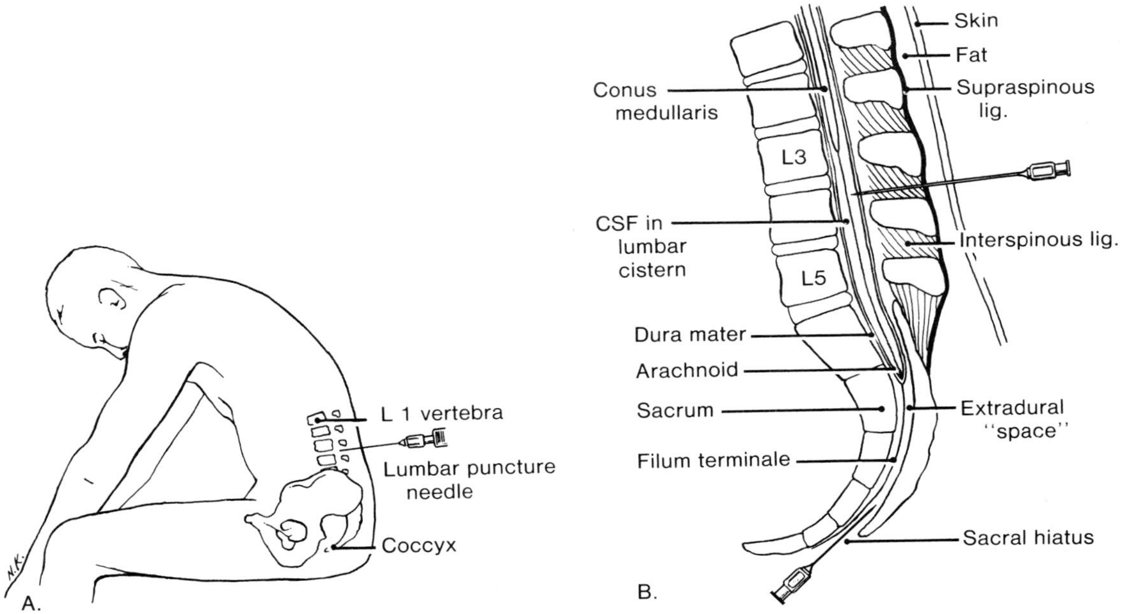

Figure 5-69. *A,* drawing illustrating the technique of lumbar puncture (spinal tap). Note that the person's back is flexed; this is done to open the spaces between the spinous processes and laminae of the vertebrae. *B,* median section of the inferior end of the vertebral column containing the spinal cord and its membranes. A lumbar puncture needle has been inserted at L3/L4 for withdrawal of CSF. A needle is also shown in the sacral hiatus, the site sometimes used for extradural (epidural) anesthesia. Note that the spinal cord in this person ends at the body of L3 vertebra, which is unusual.

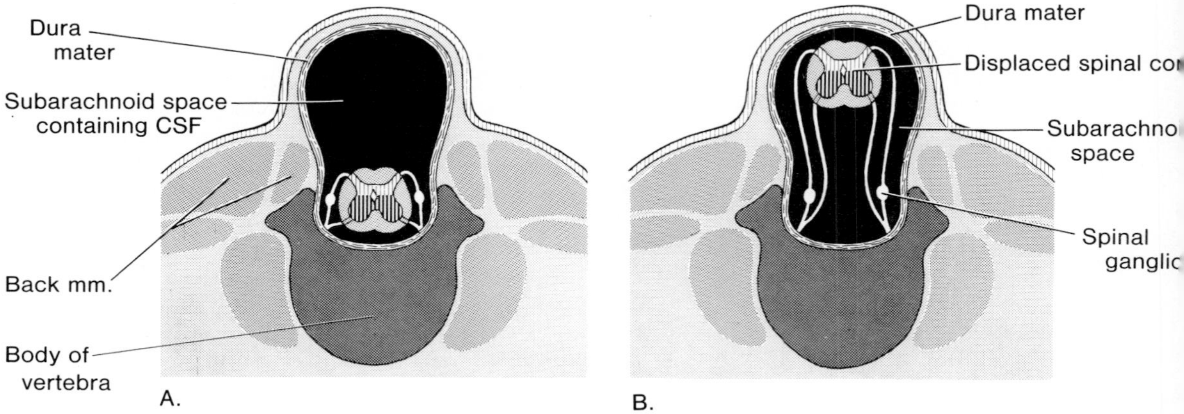

Figure 5-70. Diagrammatic sketches illustrating two types of spina bifida. *A,* with meningocele; *B,* with meningomyelocele.

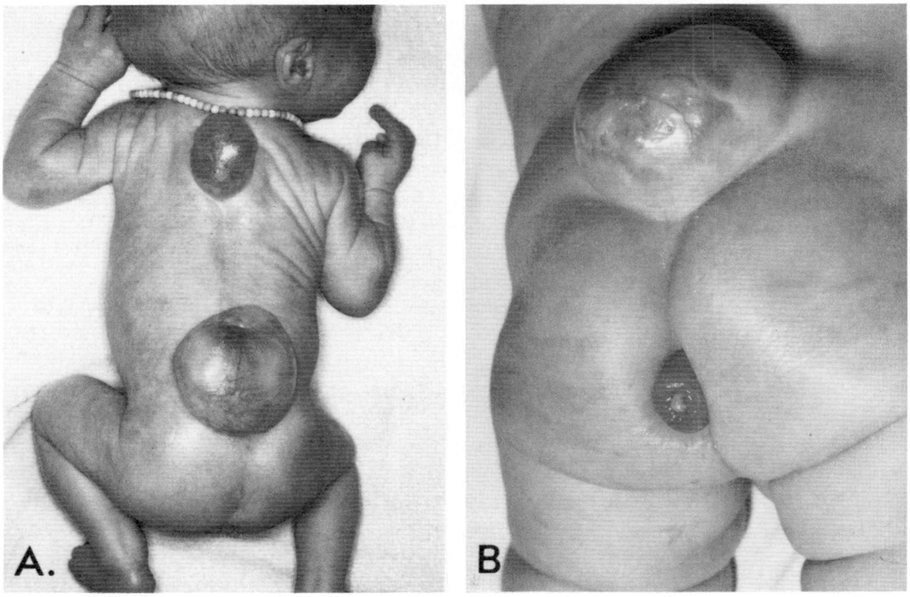

Figure 5-71. Photographs of infants with spina bifida with meningomyelocele, the common type of spina bifida cystica. In *B,* note the prolapsed rectum due to a relaxed external anal sphincter secondary to nerve involvement.

suffered a slight **concussion** (momentary loss of consciousness) and felt shaky. When he talked to the man who had hit his car and to the traffic officer, he informed them that he was not badly hurt. The officer noted that the headrest in his car was below the level of his head (Fig. 5-78).

The next morning his neck was stiff and painful and there was pain in his left trapezius region and left arm. The neck pain was aggravated by movement of his head. Gradually he developed a "crick in his neck" (Fig. 5-72).

On examination the doctor noted that he held his head rigidly and tilted to the right. He also observed that his chin was pointed to the left and that his neck was slightly flexed. Palpation revealed some tenderness

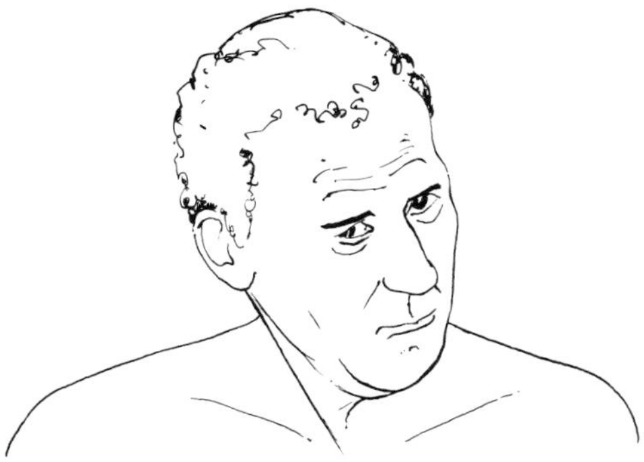

Figure 5-72. An illustration of the posture of the patient's head and neck, indicating that his neck muscles were probably injured during the accident.

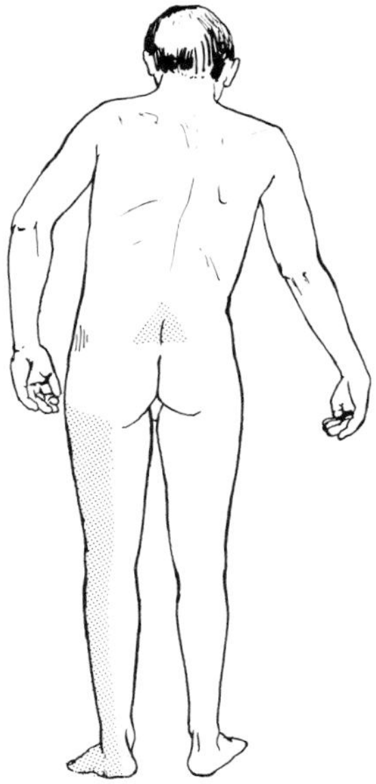

Figure 5-73. Drawing showing the patient's lumbar deviation and the regions where he felt pain (*stippled*).

over the spinous processes of his lower cervical vertebrae. **Percussion** (tapping with the finger) of the ligamentum nuchae and the spinous processes of his cervical vertebrae was not painful. The **biceps reflex** was weak on his left side.

Radiographs showed thin intervertebral discs at C5/C6 and C6/C7 with small fringes of bone on the opposing edges of the bodies of C5, C6, and C7. A diagnosis of **hyperextension injury of the neck** was made.

Problems. What is the anatomical basis of the patient's concussion, stiff neck, and pain in the neck and arm? What spinal nerve root was probably compressed? What muscles were likely injured? What probably caused the thinning of the patient's intervertebral discs and the formation of the bony fringes on the edges of the vertebral bodies of C5, C6, and C7. *These problems are discussed on page 667.*

Case 5-3. You decided to move into an apartment on the third floor of an old house. While helping you carry a heavy box of books, your father suddenly experienced an acute severe pain in his lower back. Later he developed a dull ache in the posterior and lateral aspects of his left thigh and leg (Fig. 5-73). A lateral deviation or tilt of the lumbar region of his vertebral column was also observed. He limped when he walked because he did not fully extend his hip joint.

On examination the orthopaedist told you that your father's back muscles were in spasm. When asked to indicate the site of most severe pain, your father pointed to his lower lumbar region.

During the examination you noted that he had **no ankle (Achilles tendon) reflex** on the left side and that he experienced increased pain when the doctor raised his lower limb on that side. The radiographs showed slight narrowing of the space between the vertebral bodies of L5 and S1.

The orthopaedist explained that the nucleus pulposus of one of your father's intervertebral discs was protruding and that he would be confined to bed for several weeks. The doctor urged you not to refer to a **protruding disc** as a "*slipped disc*" because this expression gives an erroneous concept of the condition. He emphasized that part of your father's intervertebral disc (torn anulus fibrosus and ruptured nucleus pulposus) had protruded, not slipped.

Problems. What is the anatomical basis of protrusion of an intervertebral disc and the resulting low back pain? What produced the lumbar deviation? Why did the patient experience pain in his thigh and leg? Why did the pain increase when the doctor raised the patient's lower limb?

These problems are discussed on page 668.

Case 5-4. A 6-year-old boy was taken to the doctor because of deformities that his mother described as a limp and a crooked back (Fig. 5-74).

On examination the doctor observed that his pelvis and shoulders were tilted and that his thorax was deformed. The deformity of his back disappeared when he bent toward the convex (left) side of the curve in his back. The curvature in his vertebral column also disappeared when a 3-cm block was placed under his left foot and when he sat down.

By measuring the distance between the anterior superior iliac spines of his ossa coxae (hip bones) and the tips of his lateral malleoli, the doctor determined that the boy's left lower limb was 3 cm shorter than his right one. Radiographs of the thoracic and lumbosacral regions of his vertebral column revealed a very slight curvature, convex to the left.

Problems. What is the medical term for a **lateral curvature of the vertebral column**? What caused the tilting of his pelvis? Would you describe his deformity as a structural or a functional abnormality of the vertebral column? What developmental malformation of the vertebral column can cause a lateral curvature? How do you think the boy's back might be straightened? *These problems are discussed on page 669.*

Case 5-5. A 1-month-old female infant was brought to the emergency room with a short history of weakness, reluctance to feed, occasional vomiting, and diarrhea.

During the physical examination the doctor noted that the infant was limp ("flat") until handled; she then became irritable. He detected tenseness of her **anterior fontanelle** (Fig. 5-75) and questionable resistance to flexion of the neck.

The doctor informed you that **bacterial meningitis** (inflammation of the meninges caused by a bacterial infection) was foremost on his list of **differential diagnoses** (possible causes or diseases that could give rise to the patient's symptoms). When he said that he was going to perform a **lumbar puncture** to obtain a sample of CSF for microscopic and bacteriological examination, you asked if you could observe the procedure. Before agreeing to this, he decided to test your anatomical knowledge of CSF and the spinal cord by asking you several questions.

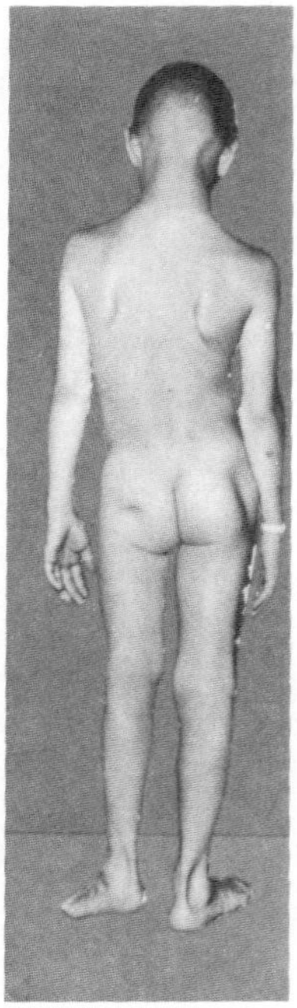

Figure 5-74. Photograph of a 6-year-old boy showing the tilt of his pelvis and shoulders and the deformity of his vertebral column.

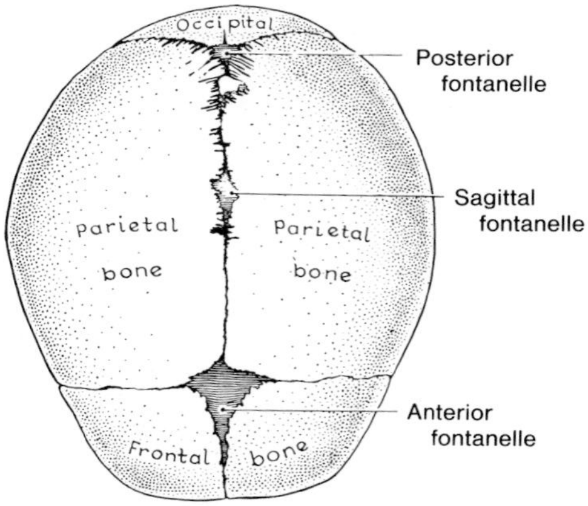

Figure 5-75. Drawing of an infant's skull from above illustrating the fontanelles (membranous intervals at the angles of the cranial bones).

Problems. Where is CSF produced? Where does it circulate? What is the main site of absorption of CSF into the venous system? Where do you think the puncture needle should be inserted into the subarachnoid space to avoid damaging the spinal cord? How would you locate the proper site for inserting the puncture needle? *These problems are discussed on page 669.*

Case 5-6. One day you were walking down the street with two other medical students when you noticed a woman with a "*dowager's hump.*" In attempting to impress your friends you said, "Hey look, there's a lady with thoracic **scoliosis**." Immediately your friends disagreed. One said she had a thoracic **kyphosis** and the other said she had a swayback or **lordosis**. You then said, "I'll bet each of you a buck you're wrong."

Problems. Who was right? What causes this deformity of the vertebral column that is commonly observed in older people? *These problems are discussed on page 671.*

Case 5-7. An 18-year-old man was thrown from a horse and sustained a spinal cord injury as the result of severe hyperextension of his neck. He died in about 5 minutes.

Problems. What vertebrae were most likely fractured and dislocated? What associated structures of the vertebral column were probably also ruptured? Although one would expect the patient to be quadriplegic following an upper **cervical cord transection**, what probably caused his death? *These problems are discussed on page 671.*

Case 5-8. During surgery for resection of an abdominal **aortic aneurysm** (Fig. 5-76), there was extensive mobilization of the aorta and several arteries were ligated. Although the aneurysm was successfully removed and replaced by a prosthesis, the patient was **paraplegic** (unable to move his lower limbs) and his bladder and bowel functions were no longer under voluntary control.

Problems. What is the anatomical basis of the patient's paraplegia? What arteries were probably ligated? Name the artery supplying the spinal cord that was likely deprived of blood. Why is its supply to the spinal cord so important? *These problems are discussed on page 671.*

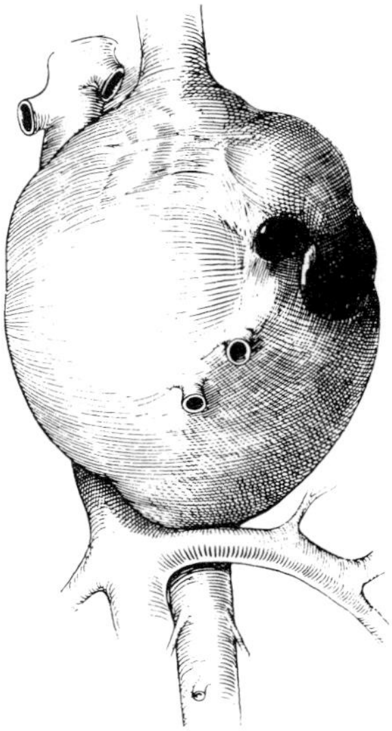

Figure 5-76. Large aortic aneurysm or circumscribed dilation of the abdominal aorta.

Case 5-9. A 28-year-old man was involved in a head-on collision. When removed from the car he complained of a sore neck and loss of sensation and voluntary movement in his lower limbs. There was also impaired ability of upper limb movements, particularly in the hand.

Radiographs showed **dislocation of C6 on C7** and a chip fracture of the anterosuperior corner of the body of C7 (Fig. 5-77*A*). Open reduction was carried out and the spinous processes of C6 and C7 were wired together to hold the vertebrae in normal relation to each other (Fig. 5-77*B*). The reduction was maintained by immobilization of the neck in a plastic collar, thereby allowing the patient to exercise his upper limbs and to sit up within a day or so after the injury.

Problems. What name is applied to the condition of patients with paralysis of both lower limbs? What joints of the vertebral column were dislocated? What ligaments binding the vertebrae together were probably torn? What was the most likely cause of the patient's paralysis? What other func-

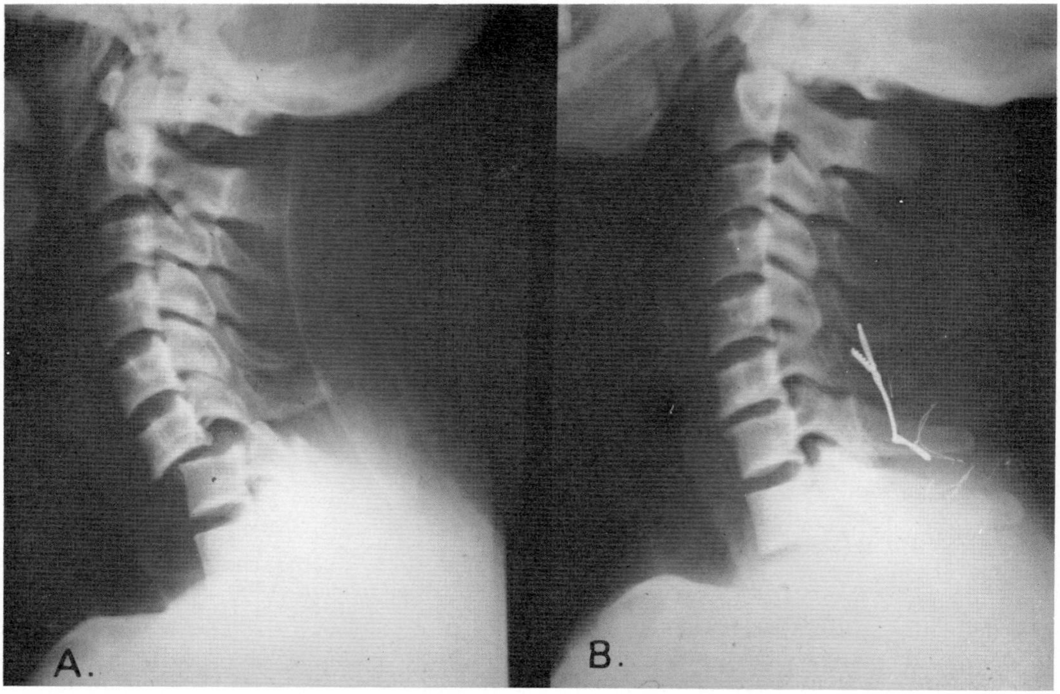

Figure 5-77. Radiographs of the cervical region of the vertebral column, lateral views. *A,* dislocation of C6 on C7. Note the small fragment of bone that has been broken off the superior corner of the body of C7. *B,* the spinous processes of C6 and C7 have been wired to hold the vertebrae in their normal position.

tions would no longer be under voluntary control? Discuss the difference in the method of numbering cervical and lumbar spinal nerves. *These problems are discussed on page 672.*

DISCUSSION OF PATIENT ORIENTED PROBLEMS

Case 5-1. The spinous processes and laminae of the vertebrae usually protect the spinal cord from injury; however, when the neck is flexed, the spaces between them increase. This would permit a knife to pass between two adjacent vertebral arches and to enter the vertebral canal. A knife entering the cervical vertebral canal would partly or completely sever the spinal cord. You can verify this movement of the cervical vertebrae by placing your hand on the back of your neck and then flexing it. Note that the space between the external occipital protuberance and the spinous process of C2 widens, as do the spaces between the spinous processes of C2 to C7. Had the knife severed the spinal cord above C3, the lesion would have stopped the patient's breathing because it would be above the **phrenic outflow** (C3, C4, and C5), the nerve supply to the diaphragm. As a result, the patient would have died in a few minutes.

Complete transection of the spinal cord results in loss of all sensation and voluntary movement inferior to the lesion. The patient is **quadriplegic** (upper and lower limbs paralyzed) when the lesion is superior to C5 because the brachial plexus of nerves supplying the upper limb is derived from C5 to T1 segments of the spinal cord. Had the boy been stabbed in the same place when his head was erect, he might not have been so severely injured. Very likely the knife would have struck the spinous processes or the laminae of the cervical vertebrae and perhaps glanced off without damaging the spinal cord.

Similar gaps exist between the lumbar spinous processes, enabling a clinician to insert a **lumbar puncture needle.** In adults the needle is usually inserted between the spinous processes of L3 and L4 into the **subarachnoid space**, caudal to the termination of the spinal cord, to obtain a sample of CSF. This procedure, known as **lumbar puncture**, is illustrated in Figure 5-69. Lumbar punctures are performed during the investigation of some diseases of the nervous system (*e.g.*, **meningitis**, Case 5-5).

Local anesthetic solutions may be injected into the **extradural (epidural) space** for several reasons. Of course, the extradural space is not a real "space" because it is filled with areolar tissue, fat, and veins. **Extradural (epidural) anesthesia** is often used in obstetrics because it relieves the pelvic pains without interfering with uterine contractions. The needle may be inserted through the **sacral hiatus** at the caudal end of the sacrum which is inferior to the level of the dural sac in most patients (Fig. 5-69*B*). In some people the dura mater and the subarachnoid space extend into the lower sacrum, and if the injection is made through the sacral hiatus in such a person, the anesthetic solution could be injected into the subarachnoid space and could mix with the CSF. If the anesthetic should reach the cervical part of the spinal cord, death would probably occur owing to interruption of the motor innervation of the diaphragm (*i.e.*, the phrenic outflow).

Extradural anesthesia is sometimes performed in the lumbar region. The needle is passed into the supraspinous and interspinous ligaments, as for lumbar puncture, but when the needle is part way in, the stylet is removed and a drop of saline solution put into the hub of the needle. The needle is slowly advanced, and as its tip leaves the interspinous ligament and enters the epidural space, the drop of saline disappears because of the relatively low pressure in the epidural space. The anesthetic solution is then slowly injected to infiltrate the extradural soft tissues and the **perineurium**, the connective tissue sheath that surrounds the lumbar nerves and is continuous with the dura mater (Fig. I-58).

Sometimes an anesthetic solution of greater density than CSF is injected into the subarachnoid space (Fig. 5-69), and produces a temporary blockage of sensory, motor, and autonomic nerve impulses. The subarachnoid administration of anesthetic solutions is referred to as **spinal anesthesia** and is occasionally used for abdominal or pelvic surgery. The head end of the operating table is kept slightly elevated to keep the anesthetic solution in the caudal part of the subarachnoid space. Should the anesthetic agent reach the cervical region of the spinal cord, death might occur owing to interruption of the nerve supply to the diaphragm (C3, C4, and C5, *i.e.*, the phrenic outflow).

Case 5-2. The association of rear end collisions and hyperextension injuries of the soft tissues of the cervical region is well-known. Headrests and bucket seats have been designed to minimize these injuries; however, a headrest is useless, as in the present case, if it is not raised so that the occipital region of the head will hit it if there is a rear end collision (Fig. 5-78).

The mechanism of injury is primarily one of severe hyperextension of the neck. Because the headrest was not in the correct

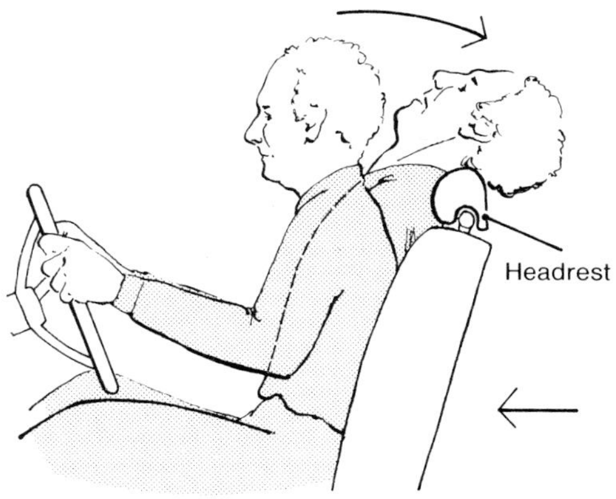

Figure 5-78. Illustration showing how the patient's head was thrown violently backward, producing a hyperextension injury of the neck. Note that the headrest was not raised to a position where it would have prevented severe hyperextension of the neck.

position, there was nothing to restrict the backward movement of the head. In addition, the muscles of the neck, the chief stabilizers of the cervical region of the vertebral column, were relatively relaxed because the patient was caught off guard when his car was hit from behind. As a result, his **anterior longitudinal ligament** and neck muscles (strap, scalene, sternocleidomastoid, and longus colli) were severely stretched and some fibers were probably torn, leading to small hemorrhages in these muscles. The resulting muscle spasm would give him a stiff and painful neck.

The concussion experienced by the patient probably resulted from the sudden impact of the frontal and sphenoid bones against the frontal and temporal poles of his brain (Fig. 5-79).

The pain in his left shoulder and the weakness of the biceps reflex on the left very likely resulted from *compression of the left sixth cervical nerve root*, probably by a posterolateral protrusion of the disc (tearing of the anulus fibrosus and herniation of the nucleus pulposus) between the fifth and sixth cervical vertebrae.

The musculocutaneous nerve (C5 and C6) supplies the biceps brachii muscle and the **biceps reflex** is mediated through C5

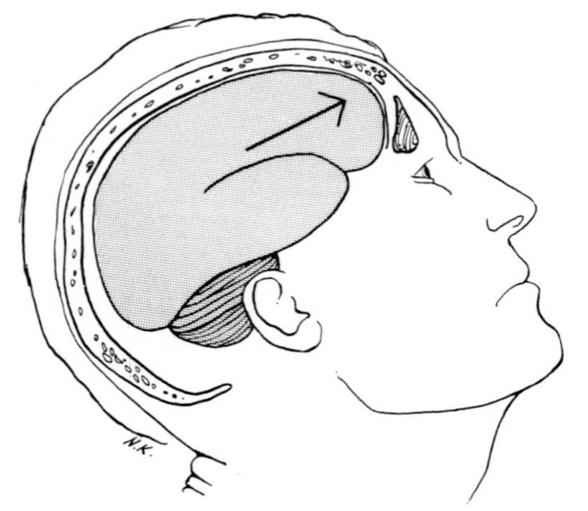

Figure 5-79. Illustration of the way contusion of the brain occurs as the result of sudden pressure on the frontal and temporal lobes when they are compressed against the front of the skull during hyperextension of the neck.

and C6. It should be pointed out that in most people in this patient's age group, some degree of degeneration of the lower intervertebral discs would already be present.

Although a **hyperextension injury of the neck** is popularly called a "*whiplash injury*," especially by litigation lawyers, many doctors consider the term an unacceptable medical designation because there is no well defined clinical syndrome or fixed pathology associated with the injury.

The thinning of the intervertebral discs in the cervical region probably resulted from desiccation (drying) of the nuclei pulposi of the intervertebral discs, which occurs with advancing age. This produces bulging of the anuli fibrosi of the discs, which results in fringes of subperiosteal new bone on the edges of the vertebral bodies.

Case 5-3. The **low back pain**, commonly called "*lumbago*" by laymen, was probably caused by rupture (tearing) of the posterolateral part of the anulus fibrosus and protrusion of the nucleus pulposus of the intervertebral disc between L5 and S1. The lumbar deviation or tilt of the vertebral column was produced by spasm of the deep back (intrinsic) muscles, resulting in a **protective splinting** effect on the vertebral column. As your father lifted, the strain on his intervertebral disc was so severe that the anulus fibrosus tore, resulting in **herniation of the nucleus pulposus** (Fig. 5-80). This protrusion exerted pressure on the S1 component of the sciatic nerve.

Disc protrusions most commonly occur posterolaterally where the anulus fibrosus

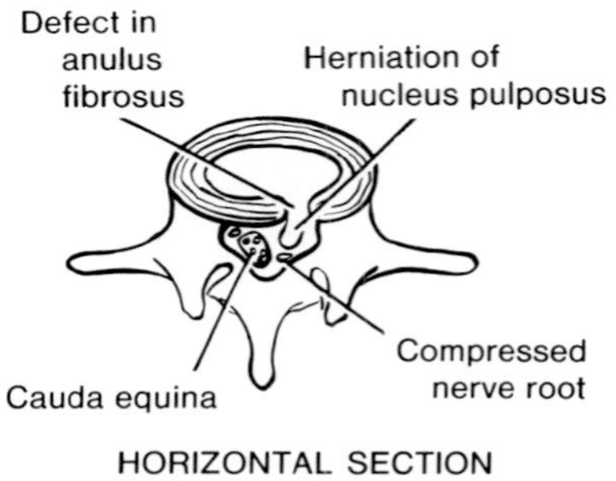

Figure 5-80. Drawing to illustrate how a posterolateral herniation of the nucleus pulposus of an intervertebral disc compresses a nerve root.

is thin. The posterior longitudinal ligament strengthens the middle portion of the posterior part of the anulus fibrosus (Fig. 5-32); consequently, midline posterior protrusions of lumbar discs are unusual. As the dorsal and ventral nerve roots cross this region, the protruding nucleus pulposus often affects one or more spinal nerve roots. Some hemorrhage, muscle spasm, and edema (swelling owing to fluid) would be present at the site of the rupture and would probably cause some of the initial back pain.

In the present case, pressure appears to have been placed on the S1 component of the sciatic nerve as it passes inferiorly behind the L5/S1 intervertebral disc (Fig. 5-60). As a result, the patient experienced pain over the posterolateral region of his thigh and leg (Fig. 4-160). When the doctor raised the patient's lower limb, the sciatic nerve was stretched. As its S1 component is compressed by the protruding disc (Fig. 5-80), the lower limb pain increased because of the stretching of the compressed fibers in that root.

Sciatica is the name given to pain in the area of distribution of the sciatic nerve (L4 to S3, Fig. 4-94). Pain is felt in one or more of the following areas: the buttock, especially the region of the greater sciatic notch, the posterior aspect of the thigh, the posterior and lateral aspects of the leg, and usually parts of the lateral aspect of the ankle and foot. The variation in the location of the pain is caused by the fact that a laterally situated posterior protrusion of a single lumbar disc presses on only one nerve root. However, the sciatic nerve is composed of several lower lumbar and upper sacral roots. The paravertebral muscle spasm and pain is caused by the muscles being in continuous tonic contraction to prevent the vertebrae from moving.

The narrowing or thinning of the space between the vertebral bodies noted in the radiographs is caused by the reduction of disc material between the adjacent vertebral bodies which normally occurs with advancing age.

Case 5-4. The medical term for a lateral curvature of the vertebral column is **scoliosis**, a Greek word meaning crookedness. The tilting of his pelvis was caused by his short leg, which also caused his scoliosis. To compensate for the tilt of the pelvis, a lumbar scoliosis occurred in order to keep the line of gravity running through the center of the body. The fact that the curvature could be corrected by placing a block under the foot of the short leg or by bending toward the convex side of the curve indicates that the curvature is a functional or **nonstructural scoliosis**. This condition may also be caused by muscle spasm secondary to trauma or a protrusion of the nucleus pulposus of a lumbar intervertebral disc (Fig. 5-80).

A fixed scoliosis that cannot be corrected by bending the vertebral column is called a **structural scoliosis**. This may result from a developmental abnormality known as **hemivertebra** (Fig. 5-7) or from destruction of vertebrae by an infection or a tumor. Structural scoliosis of unknown cause (**idiopathic scoliosis**) occurs most often in adolescent girls.

In the present case, the boy's deformity of the vertebral column could be corrected by putting a lift under the short left leg (*e.g.*, by putting a 3-cm sole on his shoe) or by placing staples across the epiphyses at the knee on the opposite side to stop growth of the femur and tibia. The staples would be removed when the legs were of equal length.

Case 5-5. CSF is produced by the **choroid plexuses** of the lateral, third, and fourth ventricles of the brain (Fig. 5-81). The plexuses in the lateral ventricles are the largest and most important producers of CSF.

The flow of CSF is from the lateral ventricles through the **interventricular foramina** into the third ventricle and from there via the **cerebral aqueduct** into the fourth ventricle. CSF leaves the fourth ventricle through the median and **lateral apertures** and enters the **cerebellomedullary cistern** (cisterna magna) and the **pontine cistern** (cisterna pontis), respectively. There is a sluggish movement of CSF from these cisterns through the spinal subarachnoid space. Movement of CSF in the subarachnoid space around the spinal cord is effected by movements of the vertebral column. The CSF from the cisterns

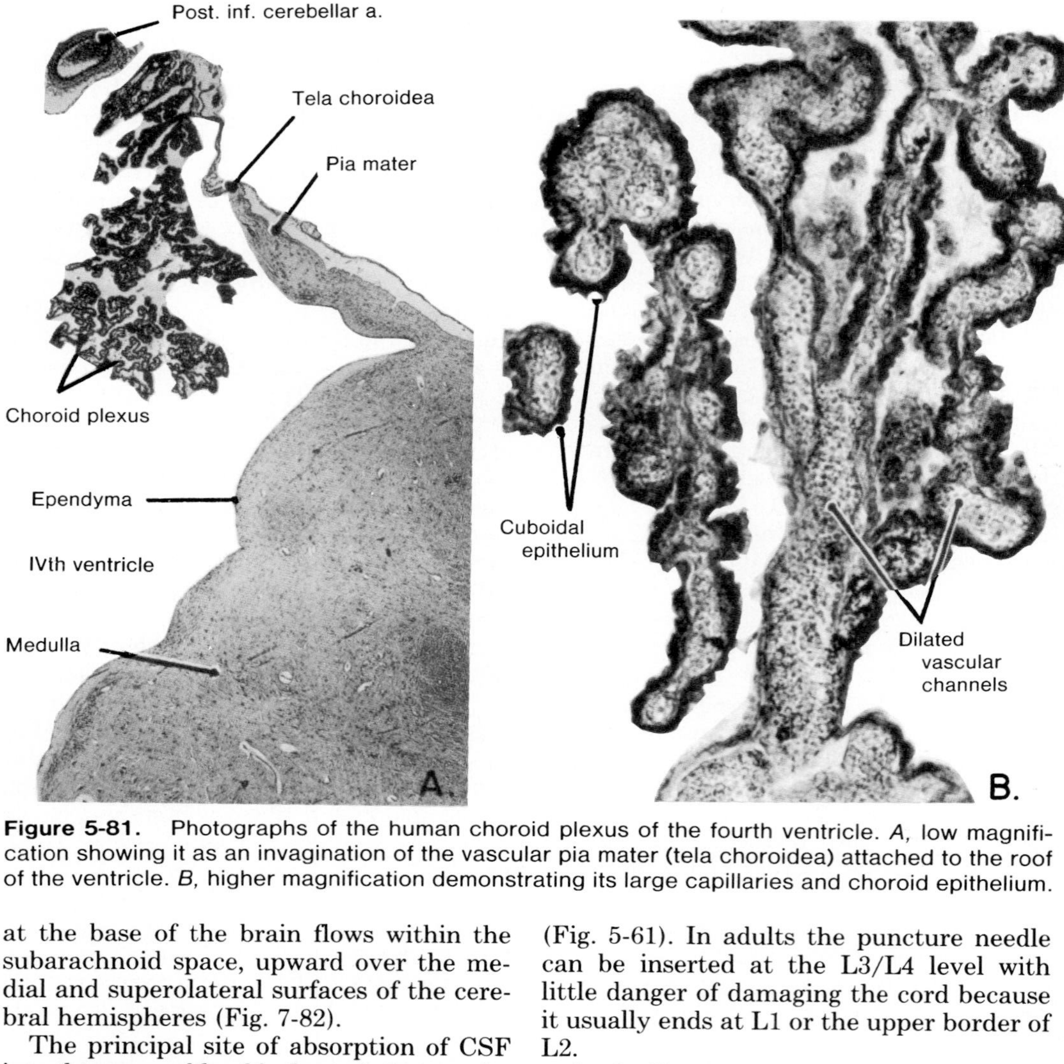

Figure 5-81. Photographs of the human choroid plexus of the fourth ventricle. *A*, low magnification showing it as an invagination of the vascular pia mater (tela choroidea) attached to the roof of the ventricle. *B*, higher magnification demonstrating its large capillaries and choroid epithelium.

at the base of the brain flows within the subarachnoid space, upward over the medial and superolateral surfaces of the cerebral hemispheres (Fig. 7-82).

The principal site of absorption of CSF into the venous blood is through the **arachnoid villi** projecting into the **dural venous sinuses** (Fig. 5-82), particularly the superior sagittal sinus. Many arachnoid villi become hypertrophied (overgrown) in older persons and are called **arachnoid granulations** (Pacchionian bodies). They may be sufficiently enlarged to cause pitting of the skull cap (Fig. 7-71).

There is little danger that a lumbar puncture needle will damage the spinal cord if it is inserted between the spinous processes of L4 and L5 into the subarachnoid space because the spinal cord in an infant usually terminates at L2 or the upper border of L3 (Fig. 5-61). In adults the puncture needle can be inserted at the L3/L4 level with little danger of damaging the cord because it usually ends at L1 or the upper border of L2.

As the line joining the posterior superior iliac spines usually crosses the spinous process of S2, one can move cranially from this bony landmark to locate the desired intervertebral interspace (*e.g.*, between the spinous processes of L4 and L5).

The doctor was so pleased with your answers that he asked you to assist him. You were asked to hold the infant upright with the neck and back in a flexed position to widen the spaces between the vertebral spinous processes and laminae. You observed while the doctor anesthetized the skin in the lumbar region and then slowly inserted a short, small needle (*e.g.*, no. 23).

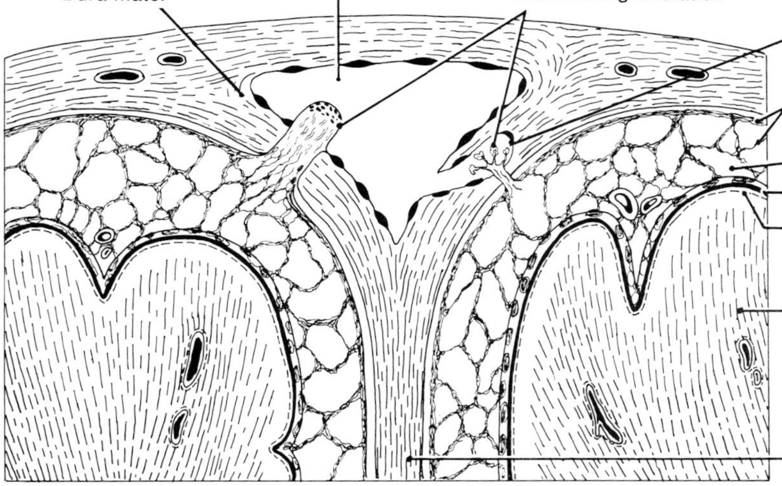

Figure 5-82. Diagram showing the meningeal-cortical relationships. Observe the superior saggital sinus, a venous sinus of the dura mater. It is one of the venous channels which drain blood from the brain and the bones of the skull. Note that the sinus is between the two layers of the dura mater and that the arachnoid granulations penetrate the sinus or a lateral lacunus of the sinus. The subarachnoid space between the arachnoid and the pia mater contains CSF.

He soon obtained a few milliliters of turbid CSF, some of which he smeared on a glass slide; he sent the remainder to the laboratory for culturing.

Case 5-6. You lost a dollar because you were wrong and so was one of your friends. The one who said the lady had a **thoracic kyphosis** made the correct diagnosis. Kyphosis (humpback) is characterized by a curve that is convex posteriorly (*i.e.*, a dorsal curvature of the vertebral column). Kyphosis often develops in elderly persons and is usually more marked in women; thus, the expression "dowager's hump."

The curvature occurs partly because the intervertebral discs lose their turgor owing to dehydration and degeneration and they become thinner in elderly persons. The bodies of thoracic vertebrae sometimes collapse in elderly women owing to **postmenopausal osteoporosis** (deossification with an absolute decrease in bone tissue). These degenerative changes also account for the loss in height that commonly occurs during old age.

Scoliosis is a lateral curvature of the vertebral column, whereas **lordosis** is characterized by a curve of the vertebral column that is convex anteriorly.

Case 5-7. Severe **hyperextension of the neck** usually causes fractures of the atlas at one or both grooves for the vertebral arteries, at the junction of the lateral masses and the posterior arch. The arch of the axis may break at the isthmus between the lateral mass and the inferior articular process. Probably his anterior longitudinal ligament and the anterior part of the C2/C3 intervertebral disc were also ruptured. As the patient hit the ground, hyperextending his neck, his skull, atlas, and axis were probably separated from the rest of his vertebral column. As a result his *spinal cord was probably torn* in the upper cervical region. Such patients rarely survive more than a few minutes because the injury to the spinal cord is above the phrenic outflow (the origin of the phrenic nerves, C3, C4, and C5). As these nerves are the sole motor supply to the diaphragm, respiration is severely affected; in addition, the action of the intercostal muscles is lost.

Case 5-8. During certain surgical procedures in the thorax and the abdomen, it is necessary to ligate aortic segmental branches (intercostal or lumbar). If the **arteria radicularis magna** arises from one of the intercostal or lumbar arteries that have been ligated, the blood supply to the lumbar enlargement of the spinal cord may be severely impaired. As a result **spinal cord infarction** (necrosis or death of nervous tissue), **paraplegia** (paralysis of the lower limbs), and loss of all sensation inferior to the lesion may follow.

Arising more frequently on the left from a lower intercostal (T6 to T12) or lumbar (L1 to L3) artery, the arteria radicularis magna enters the vertebral canal through an intervertebral foramen. It supplies blood mainly to the lower two-thirds of the spinal cord; thus, it is understandable why function is lost in the lower limbs, bladder, and bowels when this artery and part of the spinal cord are deprived of blood. This may occur during a **lumbar sympathectomy** (excision of one or more sympathetic ganglia) if the intercostal or lumbar artery giving rise to the arteria radicularis magna is ligated because it happens to pass anterior to the sympathetic trunk.

Case 5-9. The patient is paraplegic (lower limbs paralyzed) and the condition is known as **paraplegia**. Both the anterior (intervertebral disc) and posterior (**zygapophyseal) joints** between the bodies and vertebral arches of C6 and C7 respectively were dislocated in this case. Probably the posterior longitudinal and interspinous ligaments, as well as the anulus fibrosus, ligamenta flava, and articular capsules of the zygapophyseal joints were torn.

The cervical region of the vertebral column, being the most mobile part, is the most vulnerable to injuries such as dislocations and fracture-dislocations. Most of these injuries occur when a person's head moves forward suddenly and violently, as in the present case, or when struck by a hard blow.

In flexion injuries of the neck, the anterior longitudinal ligament is usually not torn, and when the patient's neck is placed in a position of extension, this ligament tightens and tends to hold the vertebrae together. Open operation was carried out in order to visualize the contents of the vertebral canal and to reduce the dislocation. The spinous processes of C6 and C7 were wired together to help stabilize the vertebral column during the initial part of the rehabilitation program and to promote healing of the torn ligaments and the intervertebral disc.

The vertebral bodies are bound together by the longitudinal ligaments and the anuli fibrosi of the intervertebral discs. The **posterior longitudinal ligament**, a narrower and weaker band than the anterior longitudinal ligament, is attached to the intervertebral discs and the edges of the vertebral bodies. It lies inside the vertebral canal and tends to prevent excessive flexion of the vertebral column. As dislocation occurred in this case, the posterior longitudinal ligament and the ligamenta flava were severely stretched and probably torn.

As the anulus fibrosus of the intervertebral disc attaches to the compact bony rims on the articular surfaces of the vertebral bodies, its posterior part would also have been stretched and probably torn at the C6/C7 level. It is possible that **protrusion of the nucleus pulposus** of the disc between these vertebra also occurred, because these nuclei are semifluid in young adults.

Because the vertebral canal in the cervical region is usually larger than the spinal cord, there can be some displacement of the vertebrae without causing damage to the spinal cord. In view of the patient's **paraplegia**, it is likely that the spinal cord was severely stretched or torn. At the moment of impact the displacement of C6 on C7 was undoubtedly greater than shown in the radiograph. There is an initial period of **spinal shock**, lasting from a few days to several weeks, during which all somatic and visceral activity is abolished. On return of reflex activity, there is spasticity of muscles and exaggerated tendon reflexes inferior to the level of the lesion. In addition bladder and bowel functions are no longer under voluntary control.

In patients with incomplete lesions, some tracts in the spinal cord escape damage at the level of injury. Consequently, there is a chance that damage to other tracts is not so severe as to be permanent and that some recovery may be expected.

Cervical nerves are numbered according to the vertebrae below them, except for the eighth cervical nerve, because the spinal nerves from C1 to C7 segments of the spinal cord leave the intervertebral foramina above the pedicles of the corresponding vertebrae (Figs. 5-56 and 5-59). The eighth cervical nerve leaves the foramen between C7 and T1 vertebrae because there are eight cervical nerves and only seven cervical vertebrae. However thoracic, lumbar, and sacral nerves are numbered according to the vertebrae above them because these spinal nerves leave the intervertebral foramina below the pedicles of their corresponding vertebrae (Fig. 5-59).

SUGGESTIONS FOR ADDITIONAL READING

1. Armstrong, J. R. *Lumbar Disc Lesions. Pathogenesis and Treatment of Low Back Pain and Sciatica*, Ed. 3, E. & S. Livingstone, Ltd., Edinburgh, 1965.
   An authoritative and comprehensive account of lesions of the lower lumbar intervertebral discs and of disturbances of the vertebral column.
2. Brain, W. R., and Wilkinson, M. *Cervical Spondylosis*, William Heinemann Medical Books, Ltd., London, 1967.
   A classical book on the neck dealing with disorders of the cervical region of the vertebral column. Anatomy, radiology, pathology, and treatment are discussed.
3. Epstein, B. S. *The Spine. A Radiological Text and Atlas*, Ed. 4, Lea & Febiger, Philadelphia, 1976.
   A standard textbook for radiology students presenting a clinical approach to radiological manifestations of diseases of the vertebral column. Common conditions are stressed.
4. Helfet, A. J., and Grubel Lee, D. M. *Disorders of the Lumbar Spine*, J. B. Lippincott Co., Philadelphia, 1978.
   This book discusses a number of clinical syndromes that cause pain in the back and describes the anatomical features of mechanical breakdown of the vertebral column in the lumbar region.
5. McRae, D. L. Protrusions of intervertebral discs and painful syndromes of the extremities. In *Clinical Neuroradiology*, edited by K. Decker, the Blakiston Division, McGraw-Hill Book Co., New York, 1966.
   A well illustrated account of the development of discs and vertebrae, types of disc lesion, bone changes secondary to disc lesions, myelography, and the relation of disc lesions to symptoms and signs.
6. Rothman, R. H., and Simeone, F. A. (Eds.) *The Spine*, Vol. 1, W. B. Saunders Co., Philadelphia, 1975.
   A comprehensive textbook on the vertebral column, with chapters on its development and applied anatomy and the diagnosis and treatment of spinal disease. The chapters are written by specialists in orthopaedic surgery, neurosurgery, psychiatry, and physical medicine.
7. Warwick, R., and Williams, P. L. (Eds.). *Gray's Anatomy*, Ed. 35 (British), W. B. Saunders Co., Philadelphia, 1973.
   This is an ideal reference book if you wish details that are not included in the present book. In the chapter on osteology there is a good illustrated account of the bones of the vertebral column, including details of their ossification.
8. Weinstein, P. R., Ehi, G., and Wilson, L. B. *Lumbar Spondylosis*, Year Book Medical Publishers, Chicago, 1977.
   A good reference for the pathology of the lumbar region of the vertebral column. There is also a good discussion of the surgical treatment of lumbar spinal stenosis and spondylosis.

CHAPTER 6

The Upper Limb

The upper limb (extremity) or "arm" in lay language is the **organ of manual activity** and is freely movable, especially the hand, which is adapted for grasping and manipulating.

For purposes of description, the upper limb is divided into the **shoulder** (junction of arm and trunk), the **arm** (brachium), the **elbow** (cubitus), the **forearm** (antebrachium), the **wrist** (carpus), and the **hand** (manus). *Note that the arm is only one part of the upper limb.*

As the upper limb is not usually involved in weight bearing, stability has been sacrificed to gain mobility. The digits (thumb and fingers) are the most mobile, but other parts are still more mobile than comparable parts of the lower limb.

Because the disabling effect of an injury to the upper limb, particularly the hand, is far out of proportion to the extent of the injury, it is important to obtain a sound understanding of the essential anatomy of this organ. However, knowledge of its structure without an understanding of its functions is almost useless clinically, because the aim of treating injured limbs is to preserve or restore their functions.

The bones of the upper limb form the *superior part of the appendicular skeleton* (Fig. 6-1). They are the **clavicle** (collar bone) and the **scapula** (shoulder blade) in the pectoral girdle; the **humerus** in the arm; the **radius** and the **ulna** in the forearm; the **carpal bones** in the carpus (wrist); the **metacarpal bones** in the hand; and the **phalanges** in the digits (thumb and fingers).

THE PECTORAL REGION AND AXILLA

The pectoral region (L. *pectus*, chest) is located anteriorly on the thoracic (chest) wall, extending from the root of the neck to the **axilla** (armpit) laterally and nearly to the costal (L. *costa*, rib) margin inferiorly. The right and left pectoral regions meet at the *anteromedian line.*

The pectoral region includes the breast and the pectoral muscles (pectoralis major, pectoralis minor, subclavius, and serratus anterior). These anteriorly located muscles act on the upper limb and connect it to the **thoracic skeleton** (thoracic vertebrae, ribs, and sternum). All these muscles insert into the pectoral girdle, except the pectoralis major, which inserts into the humerus (Fig. 6-3). The **pectoral girdle** consists of the clavicle and the scapula and articulates with the humerus.

SURFACE ANATOMY

The Clavicle (Figs. 6-1 to 6-3). The clavicle (L. little key) is located at the thoracocervical junction (root of neck) and can be palpated throughout its entire length. The medial (sternal) extremity (end) of the clavicle can be easily palpated because it projects above the superior margin of the **manubrium sterni.** Between these two medial elevations is the deep **jugular notch** (suprasternal notch).

As the clavicle passes laterally in the horizontal plane, its medial part can be felt to be convex anteriorly. The large vessels and nerves to the upper limb pass posterior to this convexity (Fig. 6-23).

The lateral (acromial) end of the clavicle does not reach the *"point of the shoulder"* formed by the **acromion** (acromion process) of the scapula (Figs. 6-1 to 6-3). The small **acromioclavicular joint** where the clavicle and the acromion articulate can be palpated 2 to 3 cm medial to the lateral border of the acromion, particularly when the upper limb is swung backward and forward.

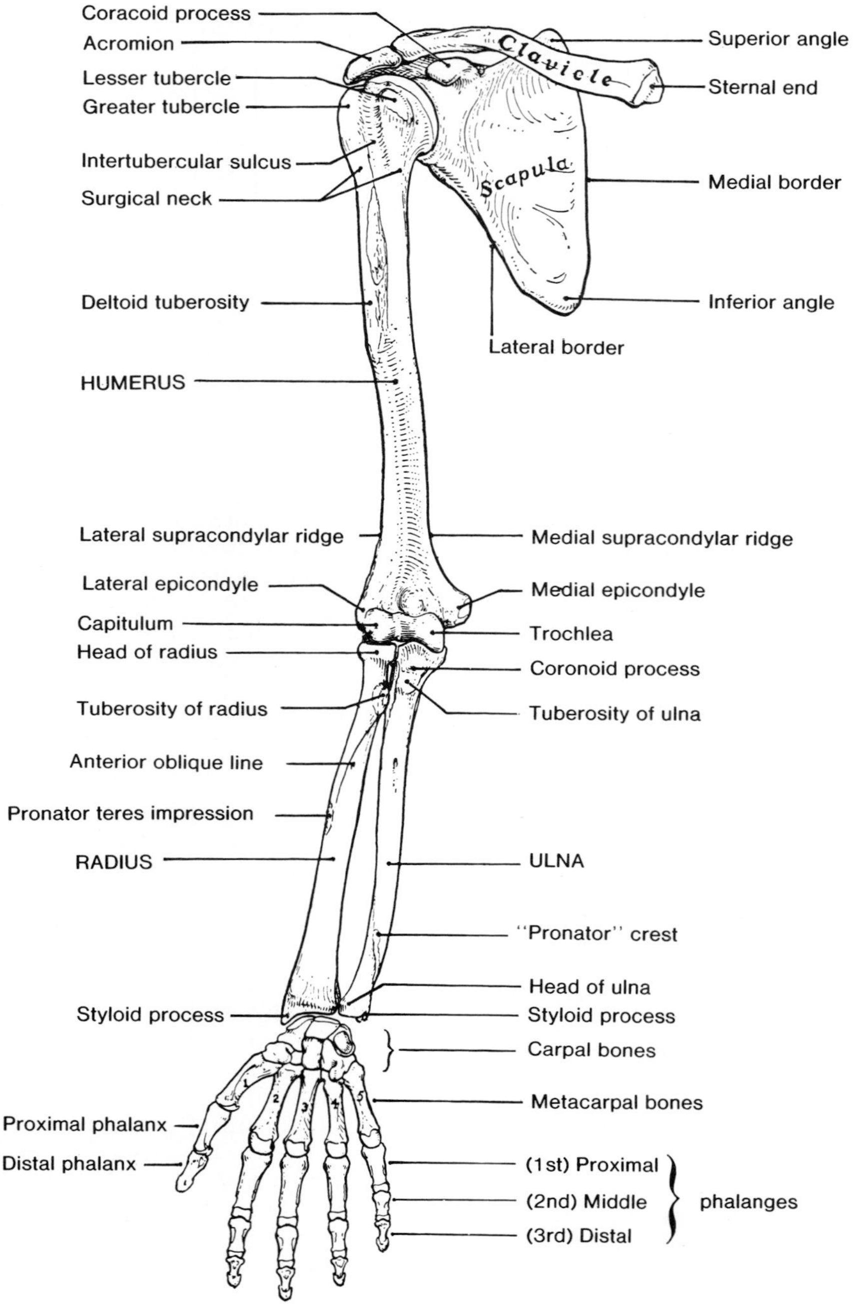

Figure 6-1. Drawing of an anterior view of the bones of the upper limb. Note that the shoulder region is supported by the bones of the pectoral girdle (scapula and clavicle). Observe the beak-like coracoid process of the scapula; coracoid is derived from a Greek word meaning "a crow"; actually it looks more like a bent finger (Fig. 6-42).

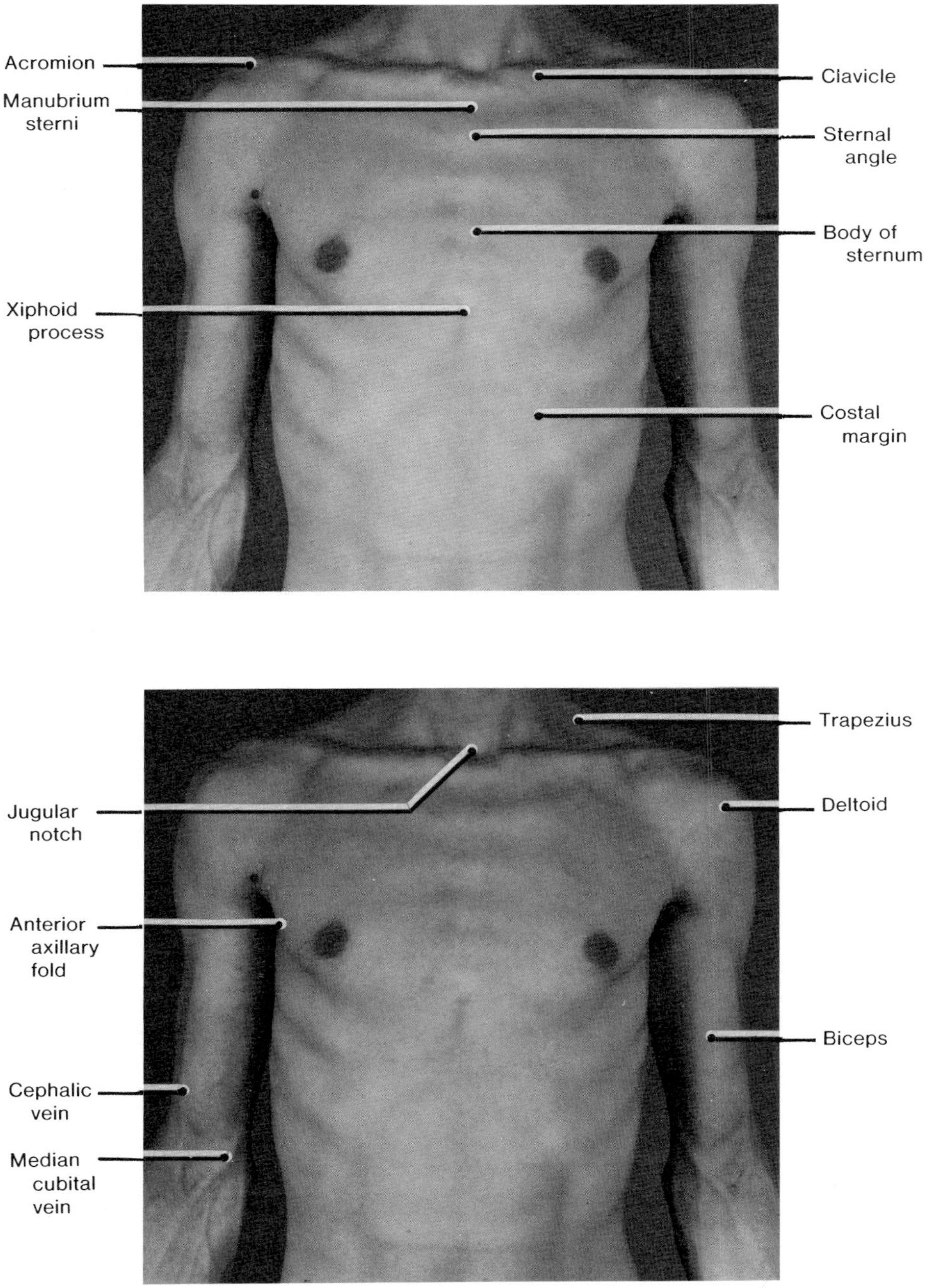

Figure 6-2. Photograph of a 27-year-old man illustrating the surface anatomy of the pectoral region and arm. The term acromion is derived from Greek words meaning "tip of the shoulder." Laymen refer to it as the "point of the shoulder" because of its prominence. Understand that it is part of the scapula, not the clavicle (Fig. 6-1). The costal (L. *costa*, rib) margin, extending inferolaterally from the sternum, is palpable with ease.

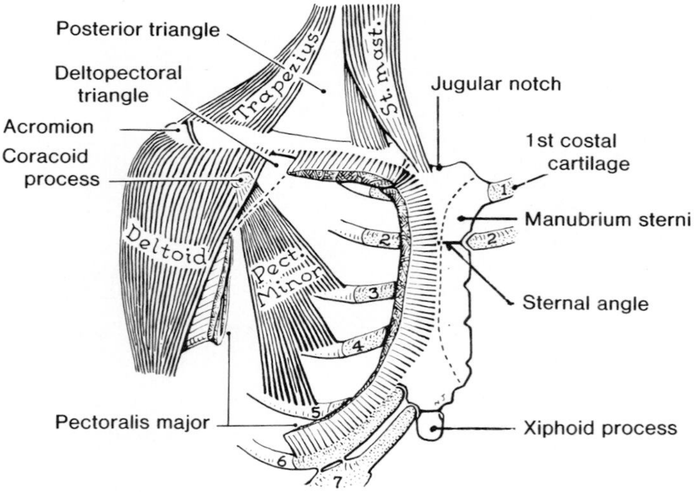

Figure 6-3. Drawing showing the muscles of the pectoral region and axilla. Most of the pectoralis major muscle is excised. See Figure 6-19 for an illustration of this muscle.

Either or both extremities of the clavicle may be prominent in some people (Fig. 6-2). When this condition is present it is usually bilateral; this point may be of significance in deciding when such prominence on one side is normal (to the patient concerned) or abnormal. Bilaterality, as in Figure 6-2, indicates normality.

The Sternum (Figs. 6-2 and 6-3). This elongated, nearly flat "*breast bone*" lies in the anterior midline of the chest. The sternum is subcutaneous throughout and, as there is usually no fat anterior to it, is almost always easily palpable. Vaguely resembling a dagger, the sternum consists of a **manubrium** (L. handle), a **body**, and a **xiphoid process** (G. *xiphoid,* sword-like).

The manubrium is united to the body of the sternum at the **manubriosternal joint**, which acts like a hinge, allowing the sternal body to swing anteriorly during inspiration. Viewed from the side, the sternum is slightly angled at this joint, which you can easily feel as a transverse ridge across the front of the joint. This **sternal angle** (of Louis) is a *clinically important bony landmark* (Figs. 6-2, 6-3, and 6-21), because if you run your finger laterally, the costal cartilage of the second rib can be palpated. Starting with it, you can easily count the ribs. Count them in the person shown in Figure 6-2, noting that his nipple lies at the level of the fourth intercostal space (*i.e.,* between ribs 4 and 5) in the **midclavicular line.** *The nipple in adult females is not a useful surface landmark* because its position varies with the size and pendulousness of the breast. Thus, the sternal angle is the only reliable clinical landmark for identifying the ribs and the intercostal spaces. As the accurate identification of ribs is of considerable importance, you should practice counting your ribs and those of your colleagues. Verify that the upper seven ribs articulate through their costal cartilages with the sternum; these are referred to as **true ribs.** The lower five ribs (*i.e.,* 8 to 12) are called **false ribs** because they do not articulate directly with the sternum. The lower two false ribs are known as "**floating ribs**" because they are not attached to the sternum at all, but they are not really floating because they are attached posteriorly to vertebrae.

The flat, sword-like **xiphoid process** is cartilaginous until about the 3rd year; thereafter, it slowly begins to ossify. It can be palpated between the seventh costal cartilages (Figs. 6-2 and 6-3) and is slightly movable until middle age; thereafter it becomes fused to the body of the sternum. Unossified areas may be present in the xiphoid process owing to incomplete fusion of the halves of the sternum during development. These perforations, which appear as holes in the dried sternum, are of no clinical significance.

The anterior axillary fold (Figs. 6-2, 6-3, and 6-7) is formed by the lateral border of the pectoralis major muscle. This fold can easily be felt between your forefinger and thumb. Make the fold more prominent by putting your hand on your hip and pressing hard against it. You can feel the pectoralis major muscle contracting within this fold.

The posterior axillary fold (Figs. 6-5, 6-15, and 6-16) contains the latissimus dorsi and teres major muscles. It can also be easily palpated. The head of the humerus (Fig. 6-4) can sometimes be palpated through the floor of the axilla with the arm elevated, particularly in thin persons, because the head faces inferiorly in this position (Fig. 6-143). You should also be able to feel the pulsations of the axillary artery in the axilla (Fig. 6-23).

The Scapula (Figs. 6-1 and 6-4 to 6-6). The scapula (L. shoulder blade) is a thin, flat, triangular bone located in the superior part of the back of the thorax. The **spine of the scapula** is on the superior part of the dorsal surface of the bone (Fig. 6-4). Its posterior border (crest) is subcutaneous throughout and is easily felt (Fig. 6-6). Note that its medial end (root) is opposite the spinous process of the third thoracic vertebra when the arm is by the side (Fig. 6-4).

The **acromion** projects forward from the lateral end of the spine and is clearly visible in some people (Fig. 6-2). In Figure 6-4, observe that the clavicle and the scapular spine form the arms of a "V" and that the acromion is located where these arms join. The **angle of the acromion** can be palpated with the thumb and the index finger (Fig. 6-6). It is formed by the junction of the lateral border of the acromion and the inferior border of the crest of the scapular spine (Figs. 6-4 and 6-6). *The acromial angle is important because it is the proximal point from which clinicians measure the length of the upper limb.* The acromion, often called the "point of the shoulder," is subcutaneous and can be easily observed and palpated (Figs. 6-2 and 6-6). Just inferior to the lateral border of the acromion is the smooth rounded curve of the shoulder formed by the deltoid muscle (Figs. 6-2 and 6-5).

The **superior angle** of the scapula lies at about the level of the spinous process of T2, and the **inferior angle** of the scapula lies on a level with the spinous process of T7 (Fig. 6-4). The inferior angle usually lies at the level of the seventh intercostal space when the arm is by the side.

The **medial (vertebral) border** of the

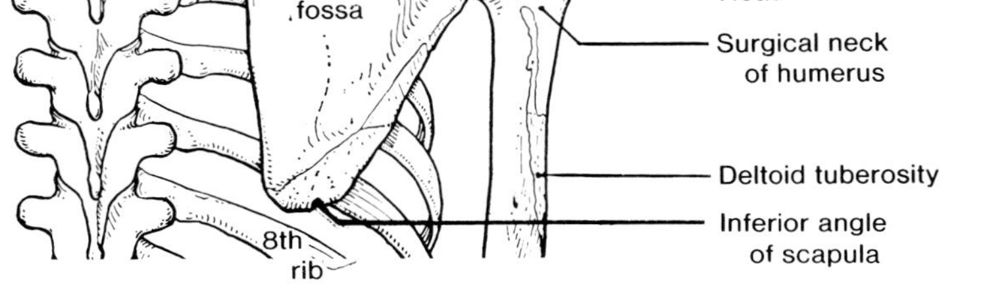

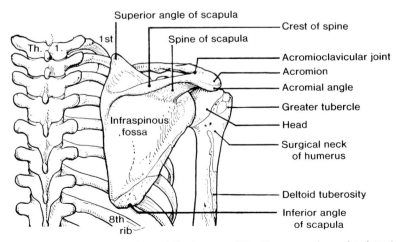

Figure 6-4. Drawing of a posterior view of the bones of the thorax and proximal part of the upper limb. The posterior border or crest of the spine is often referred to as "the spine" for the sake of brevity, but note that this is only the subcutaneous part of the spine.

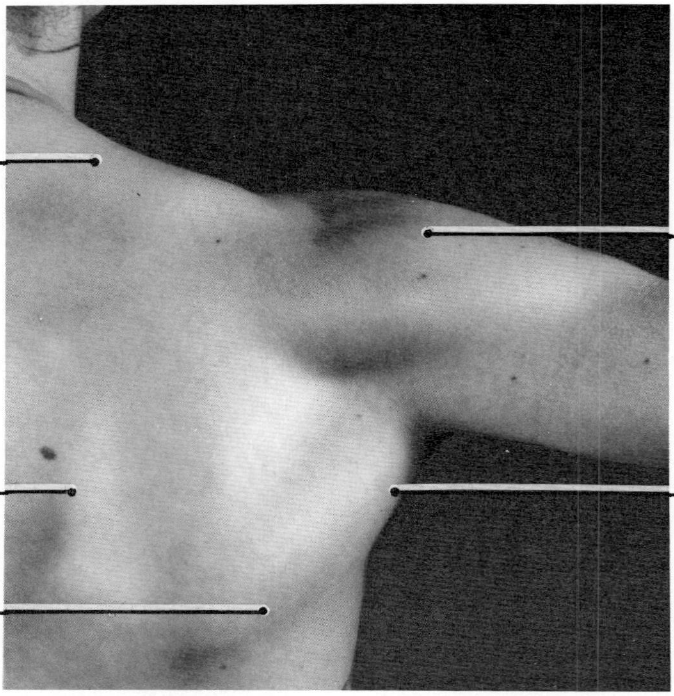

Figure 6-5. Photograph of the shoulder and scapular regions of a 12-year-old girl. To make her deltoid muscle stand out she abducted her arm against resistance. For an illustration of this muscle in an adult male, see Figure 6-57. Figure 6-4 demonstrates the bones of these regions.

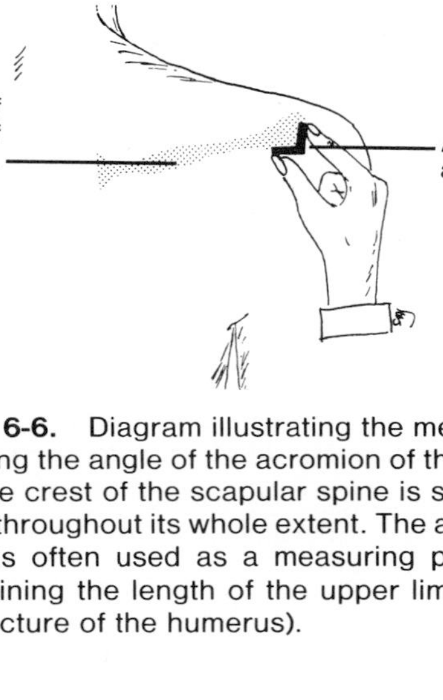

Figure 6-6. Diagram illustrating the method of palpating the angle of the acromion of the scapula. The crest of the scapular spine is subcutaneous throughout its whole extent. The acromial angle is often used as a measuring point for determining the length of the upper limb (*e.g.*, in a fracture of the humerus).

scapula is covered in its upper half by the trapezius muscle (Figs. 6-2, 6-3, and 6-5), but it can be easily palpated and observed from the superior to the inferior angle of the scapula. Note that the medial border of the scapula crosses ribs 2 to 7 (Fig. 6-4). The **lateral (axillary) border** is not easily palpated, except for its inferior part.

The tip of the **coracoid process** of the scapula can be palpated by pressing deeply about 2.5 cm inferior to the lateral part of the clavicle, *i.e.,* in the **deltopectoral triangle** (Figs. 6-19 and 6-20).

THE MAMMARY GLANDS

The mammary glands are accessory organs of the female reproductive system. They are located in the **breasts** (mammae) which overlie two of the muscles in the pectoral region, *i.e.,* the pectoralis major and, laterally, the serratus anterior (Figs. 6-7, 6-8, and 6-19). Although the breasts lie mainly anterior to the thorax, they are usually described with the upper limb because they must be removed during dissection to study the pectoral muscles.

Although both males and females have

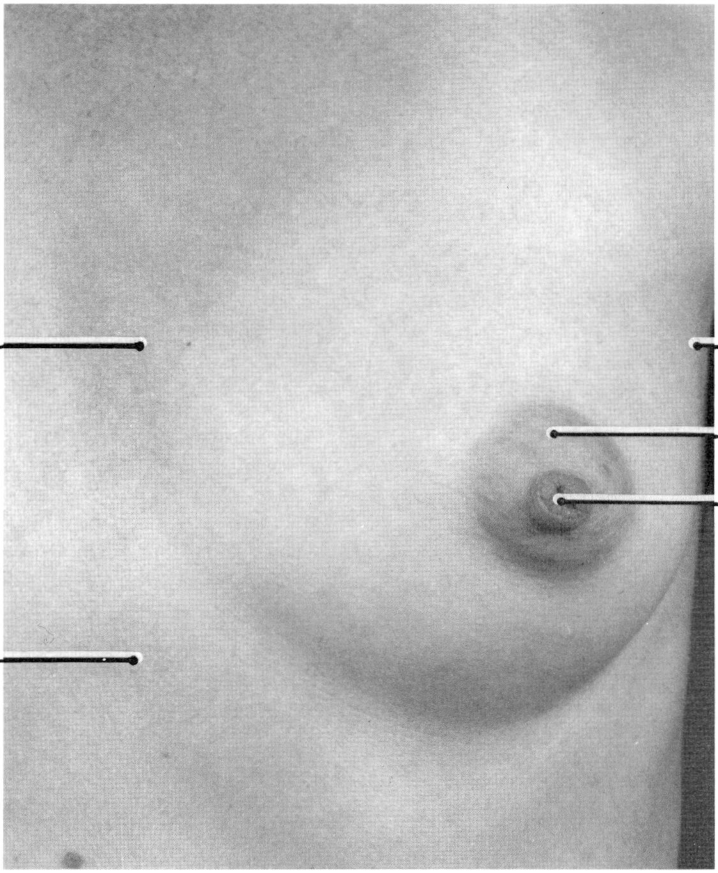

Figure 6-7. Photograph of the smooth conical breast (mamma) of a 27-year-old nulliparous woman. Note that the skin of the nipple is thrown into numerous wrinkles and, on the areola, exhibits many minute, rounded projections or tubercles owing to the underlying areolar glands. The median area or cleavage between the breasts is known as the sinus mammarum. An extension of the mammary gland into the anterior axillary fold is obvious in some women but not in the photograph of the breast shown above.

breasts, usually only females have well developed mammary glands. These glands in males are normally rudimentary throughout life and consist of only a few small ducts with some fat and fibrous tissue.

The Female Breast (Figs. 6-7 to 6-12). At puberty (12 to 15 years) the breasts normally grow and the circular areas of skin around the **nipples** (mammillary papillae), called **areolae**, enlarge and become more pigmented. The lactiferous ducts bud and form 15 to 20 lobules of glandular tissue (mammary glands), but true secretory alveoli do not form until pregnancy occurs. Each lobule is drained by a **lactiferous duct** (Figs. 6-8 and 6-9), each of which opens on the nipple. The ducts extend out from the nipple like the spokes of a wheel. Under the areola each duct has a dilated portion, called the **lactiferous sinus,** in which milk accumulates during lactation (milk production).

The areolae contain numerous sebaceous **areolar glands** which enlarge during pregnancy and secrete an oily substance that provides a protective lubricant for the areola and nipple. The areolae are pink in **nulliparous women** (ones who have not

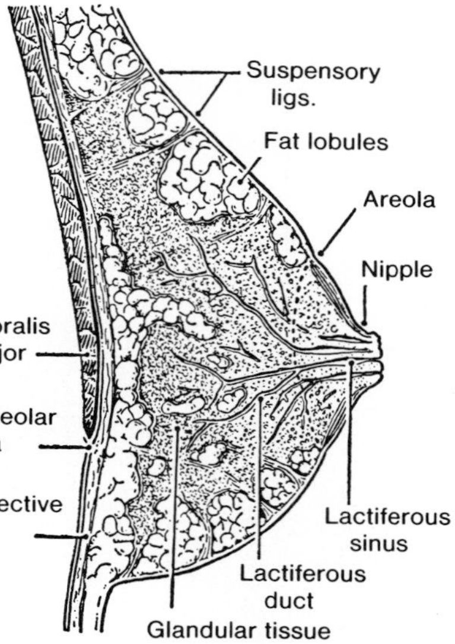

Figure 6-8. Drawing of a vertical section of the female breast. Observe that it consists of glandular, fibrous, and adipose tissues. Note that the breast is separated from the pectoralis major muscle by deep fascia. The loose areolar tissue between the breast and the deep fascia allows the breast some degree of movement.

borne children). During pregnancy the areolae enlarge and become deep brown, the depth of color depending upon the woman's complexion. The color diminishes after pregnancy, but the areolae never return to their original rosy-pink color.

As the mammary gland is a modified skin gland, it has no special capsule or sheath and it lies in the **superficial fascia**, chiefly anterior to the thorax but partly on its lateral aspect (Figs. 6-7 and 6-8). Although easily separated from the fascia covering the pectoralis major and serratus anterior muscles, the mammary gland is firmly attached to the skin of the breast by fibrous suspensory ligaments (of Cooper). These fibrous bands, which support the breast, run from the deep fascia between the lobes of breast tissue to the dermis of the skin (Figs. 6-8 and 6-9). The **suspensory ligaments** of the breast are often particularly well developed over the upper part of the breast.

The superolateral part of the mammary gland frequently projects upward and laterally toward the axilla, forming an **axillary tail** (Fig. 6-7). It extends along the inferior border of the pectoralis major in close relationship to the pectoral group of axillary lymph nodes (Fig. 6-10).

The rounded contour and most of the bulk of the breast are produced by fat lobules (Figs. 6-7 to 6-9), except during pregnancy and lactation. The shape of the breast varies considerably in different persons and races and in the same person at different ages. In **multiparous women** (ones who have borne several children), the breasts may be very large and pendulous. In elderly women the breasts are usually small and wrinkled owing to a decrease in adipose and glandular tissue.

Although breasts vary markedly in size, their roughly circular bases are fairly constant and have the following limits in a well developed female: *superior,* **second rib;** *inferior,* **sixth costal cartilage;** *medial,* edge of **sternum;** and *lateral,* **midaxillary line.**

Arterial Supply of the Breast (Figs. 6-23 and 6-31). There is an abundant blood supply to the breast. The arteries are derived from (1) perforating branches of the **internal thoracic artery** (intercostal spaces 2 to 4); (2) lateral mammary branches of the **lateral thoracic artery,** a branch of the axillary; and (3) lateral and anterior cutaneous branches of the **intercostal arteries** (intercostal spaces 3, 4, and 5).

Venous Drainage of the Breast (Figs. 6-16 and 6-44). Veins from the breast drain into the **axillary**, the **internal thoracic,** the lateral thoracic, and the upper intercostal veins.

Nerve Supply of the Breast. The breast is supplied by lateral and anterior cutaneous branches of the **second to sixth intercostal nerves.**

Lymphatic Drainage of the Breast (Fig. 6-10). The lymph vessels of the breast are numerous and originate from an extensive perilobular plexus. Most lymph vessels follow the lactiferous ducts to the areola, where they form a *subareolar lymphatic plexus.* From here, the lymph vessels pass to the **pectoral group of axillary lymph nodes.**

Some lymph vessels pass to (1) the *supraclavicular lymph nodes,* (2) the *opposite breast,* (3) the *parasternal lymph*

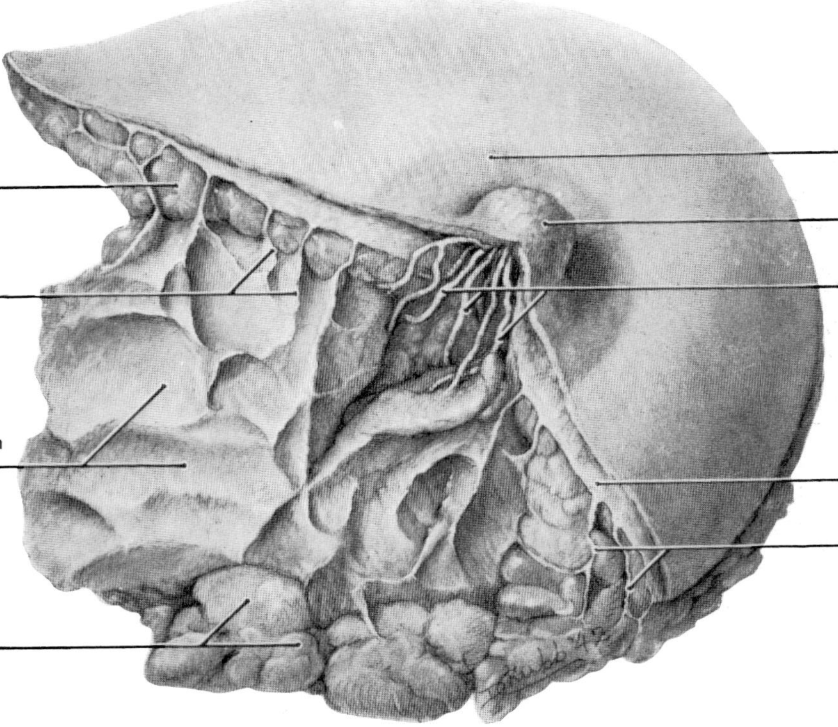

Figure 6-9. Drawing of a dissection of the mammary gland of an adult woman. The superficial fat has been scooped out of the compartments on the surface of the glandular tissue, which has been incised in order to trace the lactiferous ducts. Understand that the breast (mamma) consists of (1) the mammary gland; (2) the superficial fascia in which the gland is located; and (3) the overlying skin, including the nipple and the areola.

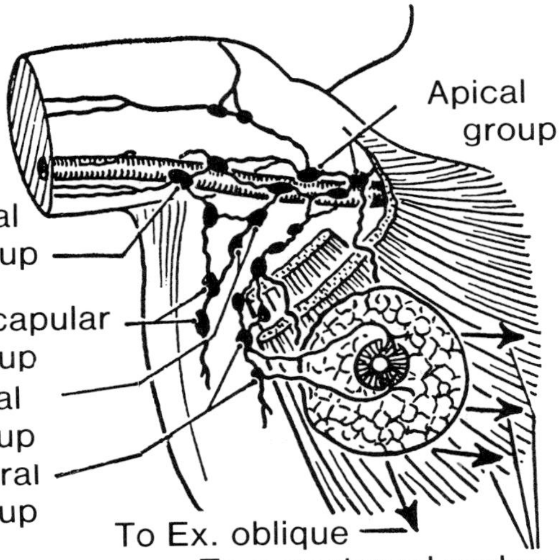

Figure 6-10. Drawing illustrating the lymphatics of the breast and the axilla. The main drainage of the breast is into the axillary lymph nodes, chiefly into the anterior or pectoral group. See Figure 6-47 for a drawing of a dissection of the axillary lymph nodes.

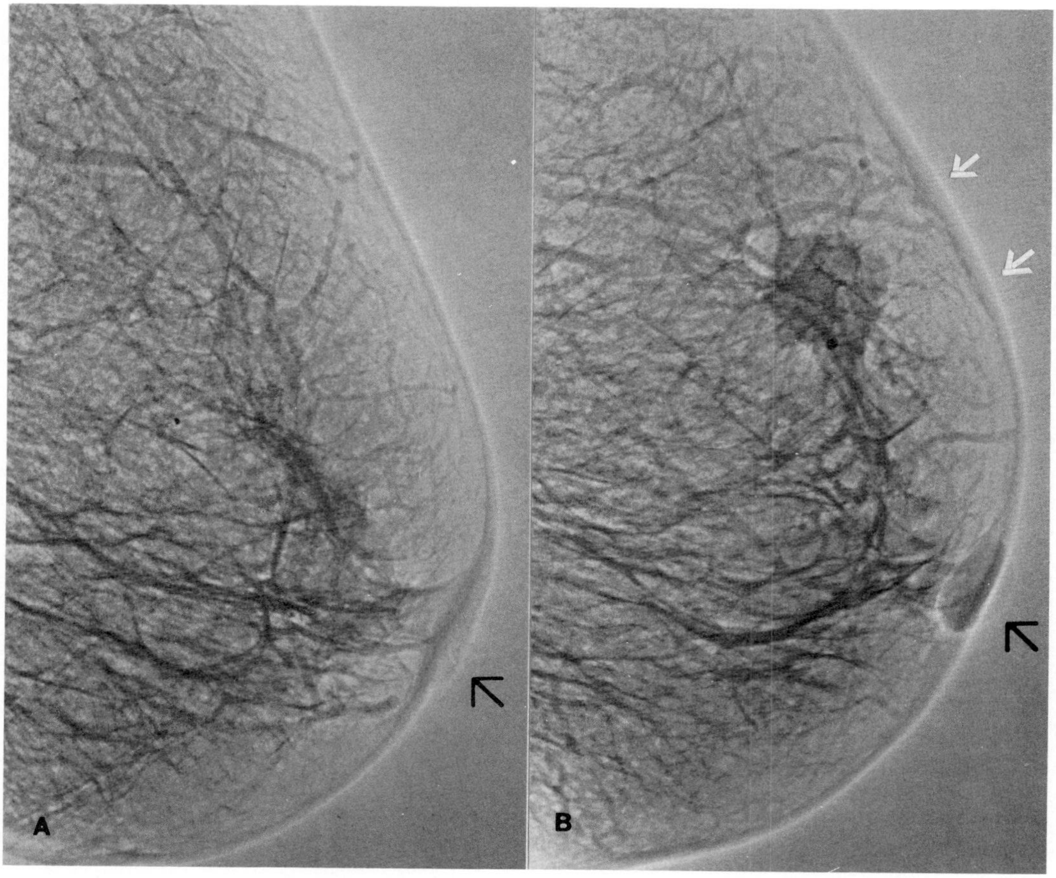

Figure 6-11. Xeromammograms, mediolateral projection. *A*, normal breast showing the suspensory ligaments between the lobules of fat. Veins may also be seen. The skin thickness is uniform except at the nipple (*arrow*). *B*, the carcinoma (cancer) appears as a jagged, rounded density. Note the overlying skin thickening (*white arrows*) secondary to impaired lymph drainage. The jagged appearance of the tumor results from the infiltration of cancer cells along the suspensory ligaments and the lymphatics. The *black arrow* indicates the nipple.

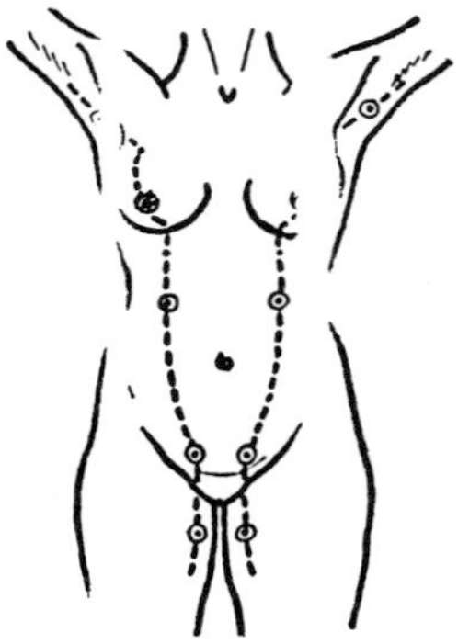

Figure 6-12. Diagram showing where accessory "breasts" (nipples) may appear along the former mammary ridges or "milk lines."

nodes into the thorax, and (4) the *abdominal lymph nodes*.

CLINICALLY ORIENTED COMMENTS

A clear understanding of the lymphatic drainage of the breast must be obtained because of its importance in the spread of **carcinoma of the breast** (breast cancer), *one of the two most common types of female cancer* (Fig. 6-11*B*). Cancer cells are carried by the lymph vessels to lymph nodes where they lodge, producing nests of tumor cells called **metastases** (G. *meta,* beyond + *stasis,* a placing). Consequently, metastases may develop in the supraclavicular lymph nodes, the axillary lymph nodes, the opposite breast, or in the abdomen.

The axillary lymph nodes are the most common site of metastases from carcinoma of the breast (Case 6-12); thus, enlargement of the axillary lymph nodes in a female suggests the possibility of breast cancer. Cancerous nodes tend to be hard and are usually not tender.

It must be stressed that enlargement of the axillary lymph nodes does not necessarily indicate cancerous involvement. Infection of lymphatic vessels (**lymphangitis**), *e.g.,* resulting from a thumb infection, spreads to the axillary lymph nodes causing them to enlarge and become tender (**lymphadenitis**). It is also important to know that the absence of enlarged axillary lymph nodes is no guarantee that metastasis from a breast cancer has not occurred.

Often there is dimpling and a leathery thickening of the skin over the site of a carcinoma of the breast (Fig. 6-11*B*), giving the skin the appearance of an orange peel; this skin change is called *peau d'orange.* Interference with the lymphatic drainage of the breast produces the leathery thickening, whereas the dimpling of the skin is mainly caused by infiltration of the cancer cells along the suspensory ligaments of the breast. This shortens the ligaments and causes the skin to invaginate (dimple). **Subareolar cancers** may cause inversion of the nipple by the same mechanism; however, one must be certain that the inversion was not a congenital abnormality.

Mastectomy is not an uncommon operation in females. In *simple mastectomy* the breast (nipple, areola, and glandular, fibrous, and fatty tissues) is removed down to the pectoralis fascia (Figs. 6-8 and 6-9). *Radical mastectomy* is a more extensive operation during which the breast, pectoral muscles, fat, fascia, and all the lymph nodes in the axilla and pectoral region are removed. Sometimes the fascia covering the superior part of the rectus sheath, the serratus anterior, the subscapularis, and the latissimus dorsi muscles is also removed.

During mastectomy, care must be taken to preserve the **long thoracic nerve** (Fig. 6-31). Cutting this nerve results in paralysis of the serratus anterior and inability to rotate the scapula upward during abduction of the shoulder; as a result, there is difficulty in elevating the arm above the head. In addition the vertebral border and inferior angle of the scapula protrude posteriorly, producing a "**winged scapula**" (Fig. 6-39), because normally the serratus anterior holds the scapula against the chest wall.

The foregoing information is intended to exphasize the importance of knowing the structure and lymphatic drainage of the breast and the anatomy of the pectoral region and axilla. It is not intended to give you sufficient knowledge to determine the significance of a palpable lesion in the breast. You will acquire this knowledge in your course in clinical diagnosis.

The breasts of some males enlarge at puberty when the rudimentary ducts give rise to glandular tissue; this is usually a transient occurrence in normal adolescence. In a few males this **gynecomastia** (G. *gyné,* woman + *mastos,* breast) is a characteristic of the **Klinefelter syndrome** resulting from an abnormal sex chromosome complement, usually XXY. Other characteristics of this condition are small testes, hyalinization of the seminiferous tubules, and aspermatogenesis.

Accessory breasts (**polymastia**) or nipples (**polythelia**) may occur above or below the normal breasts (Fig. 6-12). Usually supernumerary "breasts" consist only of a small nipple and areola that may be mistaken for a mole (nevus). They may appear anywhere along a line extending from the axilla to the groin, which is the location of the embryonic **mammary ridge.** Accessory mammary tissue may appear elsewhere (*e.g.,* on the neck or genital organs) owing to displacement of parts of the embryonic mammary ridges.

THE PECTORAL MUSCLES

The pectoral or chest region contains three muscles, all of which are associated with the upper limb.

The Pectoralis Major Muscle (Figs. 6-13, 6-14, 6-16, and 6-18 to 6-24). This large,

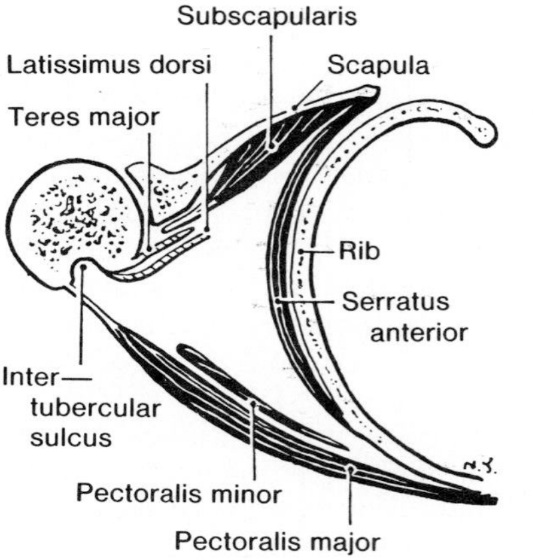

Figure 6-13. Diagram of a cross-section through the axilla showing its walls. Note the pectoral muscles in the *anterior wall*, the scapula and subscapularis in the *posterior wall*, the rib and serratus anterior in the *medial wall*, and the intertubercular sulcus in the *lateral wall*.

thick, triangular muscle covers the upper part of the chest, and its lateral border forms the **anterior axillary fold** (Fig. 6-16) and most of the anterior wall of the axilla.

The pectoral fascia enclosing this muscle is attached at its origin to the clavicle and the sternum (Figs. 6-14 and 6-19). It leaves the lateral border of the muscle to form the **axillary fascia** in the floor of the axilla.

In Figure 6-19, observe that the pectoralis major and deltoid muscles diverge slightly from each other superiorly and, along with the clavicle, they form the **deltopectoral triangle** (Figs. 6-19 and 6-20). It allows passage of the cephalic vein, its accompanying arterial twig to the deltoid, and lymph vessels. Note that the **cephalic vein**, one of the two major superficial veins draining the upper limb, occupies the furrow between the deltoid and the pectoralis major muscles before it enters the deltopectoral triangle on its way to the **axillary vein** (Figs. 6-19 and 6-44). The deltopectoral triangle, obvious in Figure 6-20, is a useful landmark when visible; in some people it is very small or absent. *The pectoralis major has two heads of origin.*

Origin (Figs. 6-19 and 6-21). **Medial half of clavicle** (*clavicular head*); **sternum, upper six ribs,** and aponeurosis of external oblique muscle of the abdomen (*sternal head*). The two heads of this muscle meet at the sternoclavicular joint.

Insertion (Figs. 6-13 and 6-21). **Lateral lip of intertubercular sulcus** of humerus (crest of greater tubercle of humerus).

Nerve Supply (Figs. 6-18, 6-22, and 6-23). **Lateral pectoral** nerve from lateral cord of brachial plexus and **medial pectoral** nerve from medial cord of this plexus.

Actions. **Adducts** and **medially rotates humerus** at the shoulder joint. Acting alone, the *clavicular head* **flexes the shoulder joint** (*i.e.,* raises arm forward) and from this position the sternocostal head **extends shoulder joint** (*i.e.,* carries arm backward). Place your hand on your pectoralis major and perform these movements against resistance. Verify that it can act as a whole and that its parts can act separately.

The Pectoralis Minor Muscle (Figs. 6-3, 6-13, 6-14, 6-18, and 6-21 to 6-26). This flat, triangular muscle lies in the anterior wall of the axilla, deep to the much larger pectoralis major (Fig. 6-14). The pectoralis minor, **the landmark of the axilla,** and

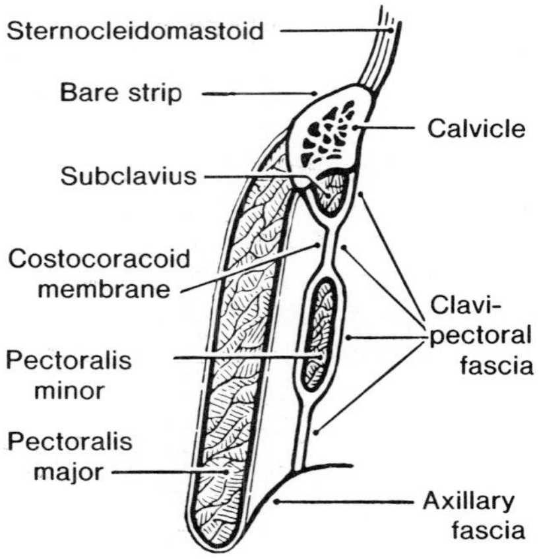

Figure 6-14. Drawing of a sagittal section of the axilla illustrating its anterior wall. The clavipectoral fascia is a strong sheet of connective tissue attached to the clavicle and enclosing the subclavius above and the pectoralis minor below. It then joins the floor of the axilla formed by axillary fascia. The clavipectoral fascia protects the contents of the axilla by filling in the interval between the clavicle and the pectoralis minor muscle.

the subclavius are surrounded by the clavipectoral fascia (Figs. 6-14 and 6-22). This thin sheet of fibrous tissue runs from the clavicle to the fascial floor of the axilla. This connection of the **clavipectoral fascia** with the clavicle supports and suspends the floor of the axilla, composed of axillary fascia and skin.

Origin (Figs. 6-21 and 6-23). Upper margins and outer surfaces of **ribs 3, 4,** and **5** and fascia of associated intercostal spaces.

Insertion (Fig. 6-21). Medial border of **coracoid process** of scapula.

Nerve Supply (Figs. 6-18 and 6-23). **Medial pectoral** nerve.

Actions. **Stabilizes scapula** by drawing it forward and downward. The chief importance of this muscle is that it is a useful landmark for many structures in the axilla because, with the coracoid process, it forms an arch deep to which pass the vessels and nerves to the arm (Figs. 6-26 and 6-41).

The Subclavius Muscle (Fig. 6-23). As its name indicates, this small **relatively unimportant muscle** lies below the clavicle. Because of its location it may serve as a protective cushion between a fractured clavicle and the subclavian vessels (Fig. 6-24) when this bone is fractured (Fig. 6-65).

Origin (Fig. 6-23). Junction of **first rib** and its costal cartilage.

Insertion (Fig. 6-23). **Inferior surface of clavicle.**

Nerve Supply (Fig. 6-24). **Nerve to subclavius.**

Actions. **Depresses lateral end of clavicle,** draws it toward sternum, and **steadies clavicle** during shoulder movements. Paralysis of this muscle produces no demonstrable effect.

THE AXILLA

The axilla (armpit) is a roughly pyramidal space (fossa) between the arm and the upper part of the thorax; it has four sides, an apex, and a base. The axilla provides continuity between the thoracocervical region and the upper limb and a passageway for the nerves and vessels of the upper limb (Fig. 6-31).

The truncated **apex of the axilla** is directed toward the root of the neck and is located at the medial side of the root of the coracoid process (Fig. 6-1). It is formed by the convergence of the bones in its three major walls: the **clavicle** in the anterior wall, the **scapula** in the posterior wall, and the **first rib** in the medial wall. The interval between these bones is the entrance to the axillary space through which all nerves and vessels pass to the upper limb.

The **base of the axilla,** facing inferiorly, is formed by the fascia and skin of the concave axilla. The skin of the axillary base is usually covered with hair in postpubertal persons.

Boundaries of the Axilla (Figs. 6-13 and 6-14). These boundaries can be visualized best in a cross-section through the axilla.

The Anterior Wall (Figs. 6-2, 6-7, 6-14, 6-16, and 6-19). The clavicle and the pectoral muscles form the anterior wall. The lateral border of the pectoralis major forms the **anterior axillary fold.** Place your hand on your hip and press medially as you palpate your anterior axillary fold with the thumb and forefinger of your other hand.

Posterior to the pectoralis major, the pectoralis minor and subclavius muscles form the deep layer of the anterior wall (Fig.6-14). These muscles are unimportant except that *the pectoralis minor is a useful landmark* for the vessels and nerves passing deep to it on their way to the upper limb (Fig. 6-26).

The Posterior Wall (Figs. 6-5, 6-13, 6-15, and 6-16). This wall is formed chiefly by the scapula and the subscapularis muscle. Inferior to the subscapularis is the teres major which combines with the latissimus dorsi to form the **posterior axillary fold.**

The Medial Wall (Figs. 6-13, 6-17, and 6-19). This wall is formed by the ribs and the intercostal muscles, covered by the serratus anterior muscle. To palpate your serratus anterior, put your hand on a shelf and press downward as you feel the side of your chest with the fingers of your other hand.

The Lateral Wall (Figs. 6-1, 6-13, and 6-18). This narrow wall is formed by the floor of the **intertubercular sulcus** (groove) in the humerus which lodges the tendon of the long head of the biceps muscle. This muscle and the coracobrachialis can be felt in the lateral wall of the axilla.

Contents of the Axilla (Figs. 6-18 and

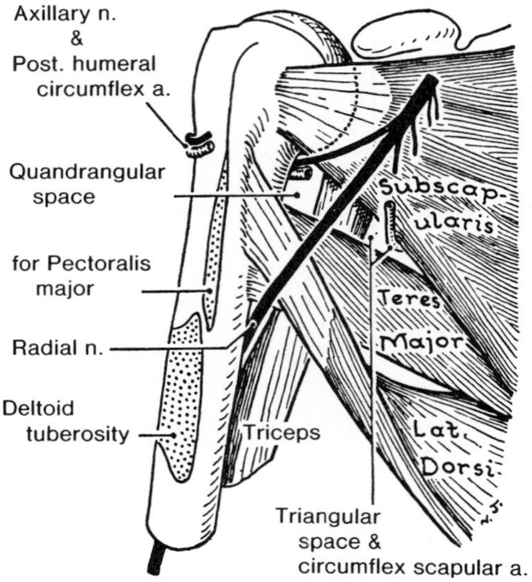

Figure 6-15. Drawing of a dissection of the axilla showing its posterior wall formed by the scapula and the subscapularis, teres major, and latissimus dorsi muscles.

6-23). The axilla contains large important nerves which are branches of the **brachial plexus** passing from the neck to supply almost all the upper limb. It also contains the **axillary vessels** (the axillary artery and its branches, the axillary vein and its tributaries, and the axillary lymph vessels) and several groups of important **axillary lymph nodes** (Fig. 6-10).

The Brachial Plexus (Figs. 6-23 to 6-27). This network of nerves extends from the neck to the axilla and supplies motor, sensory, and sympathetic nerve fibers to the upper limb. Its supraclavicular part is deep to the floor of the posterior triangle (Fig 6-24) and its infraclavicular part is in the axilla (Figs. 6-23 and 6-25).

The brachial plexus is usually formed by the union of the ventral primary rami of nerves C5 to C8 and T1. The ventral (anterior) rami that form the brachial plexus are sometimes referred to as the **roots of the brachial plexus.** Be careful not to confuse these with the dorsal and ventral roots which unite to form a spinal nerve (Fig. 6-25). The roots of the brachial plexus lie between the scalenus anterior and medius muscles (Fig. 6-24).

The plan of the brachial plexus is usually as follows (Figs. 6-24 to 6-27):

1. As the ventral primary rami enter the posterior triangle of the neck, those from C5 and C6 unite to form an **upper (superior) trunk**. The ventral ramus of C7 continues as a **middle trunk** and the ventral rami of C8 and T1 unite at the neck of the first rib to form a **lower (inferior) trunk**. The lower trunk lies on the first rib behind the subclavian artery (Figs. 6-25 and 6-26).
2. Each of the three trunks divides into an **anterior** and a **posterior division** behind the clavicle. These divisions are of fundamental significance because the anterior divisions supply the anterior (flexor) and the posterior divisions supply the posterior (extensor) parts of the upper limb.
3. The three *posterior divisions* unite to form the **posterior cord.** The anterior divisions of the upper and middle trunks unite to form the **lateral cord** and the anterior division of the lower trunk continues as the **medial cord** (Fig. 6-25). In Figure 6-26, observe that the cords of the plexus bear the relationship to the second part of the axillary artery that is indicated by their names (*e.g., the lateral cord is lateral to the axillary artery*).
4. Each cord of the brachial plexus divides into **two terminal branches** (Figs. 6-25 to 6-27): (1) the *lateral cord* divides into the **musculocutaneous nerve** and the **lateral root of the median nerve**; (2) the *medial cord* divides into the **ulnar nerve** and the **medial root of the median nerve**; and (3) the *posterior cord* divides into the **axillary nerve** and the **radial nerve.** Note that three nerves (musculocutaneous, median, and ulnar) form the letter **M** (Figs. 6-25 and 6-26), which serves as the **key to the brachial plexus.** Always locate it during dissections of the axilla and use it to identify the parts of the brachial plexus.

Variations of the brachial plexus from the usual pattern are not uncommon.

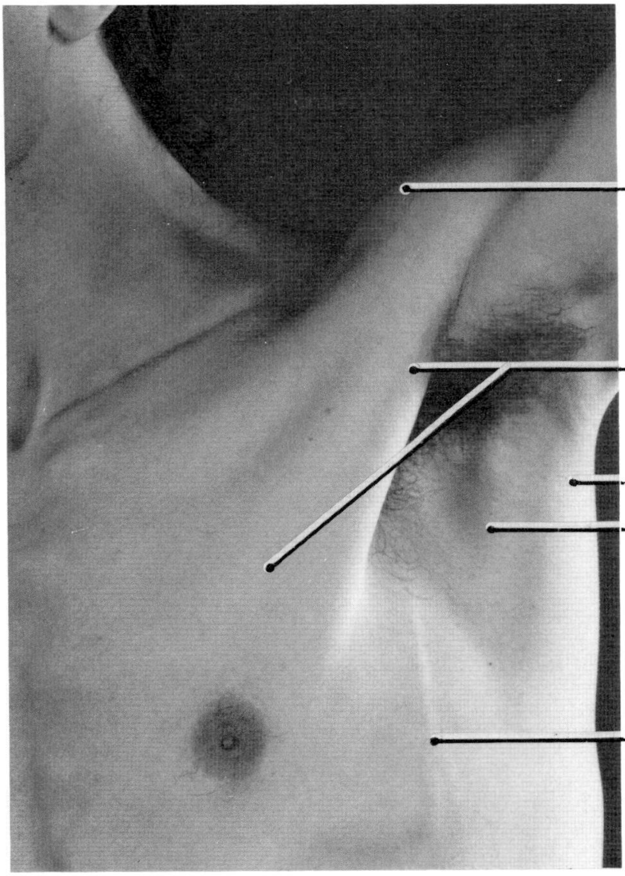

Figure 6-16. Photograph of the left axilla of a 27-year-old man exposed by abducting the upper limb. It is uncommon to see the teres major as illustrated here. Observe that the breast is rudimentary, the nipple is small, and the areola is surrounded by sparse hairs. The mammary gland (not visible here because it is within the breast) is also rudimentary in males.

In many cases part of the ventral ramus of C4 joins the plexus; this is called a **prefixed type of brachial plexus** (*i.e.,* C4 to C8). In some cases part of the ventral ramus of T2 joins the plexus; this is called a **postfixed type of brachial plexus** (*i.e.,* C6 to T2).

In some persons trunk division or cord formation may be absent in one or other parts of the plexus; however, the make-up of the ultimate terminal branches is unchanged. In addition the lateral or medial cords may receive fibers from ventral rami below or above the usual levels, respectively. In some people the median nerve has two medial roots instead of one, but the **M** is still recognizable.

The branches of the brachial plexus may be divided into supraclavicular branches (of the roots and trunks) and infraclavicular branches (of the cords). Only the infraclavicular branches are approachable through the axilla.

The supraclavicular branches of the roots and trunks of the brachial plexus are as follows (Fig. 6-27):

1. The **dorsal scapular nerve** (Figs. 6-27 and 9-14) arises from the ventral ramus of **C5** and pierces the scalenus medius muscle (Fig. 6-24) to supply

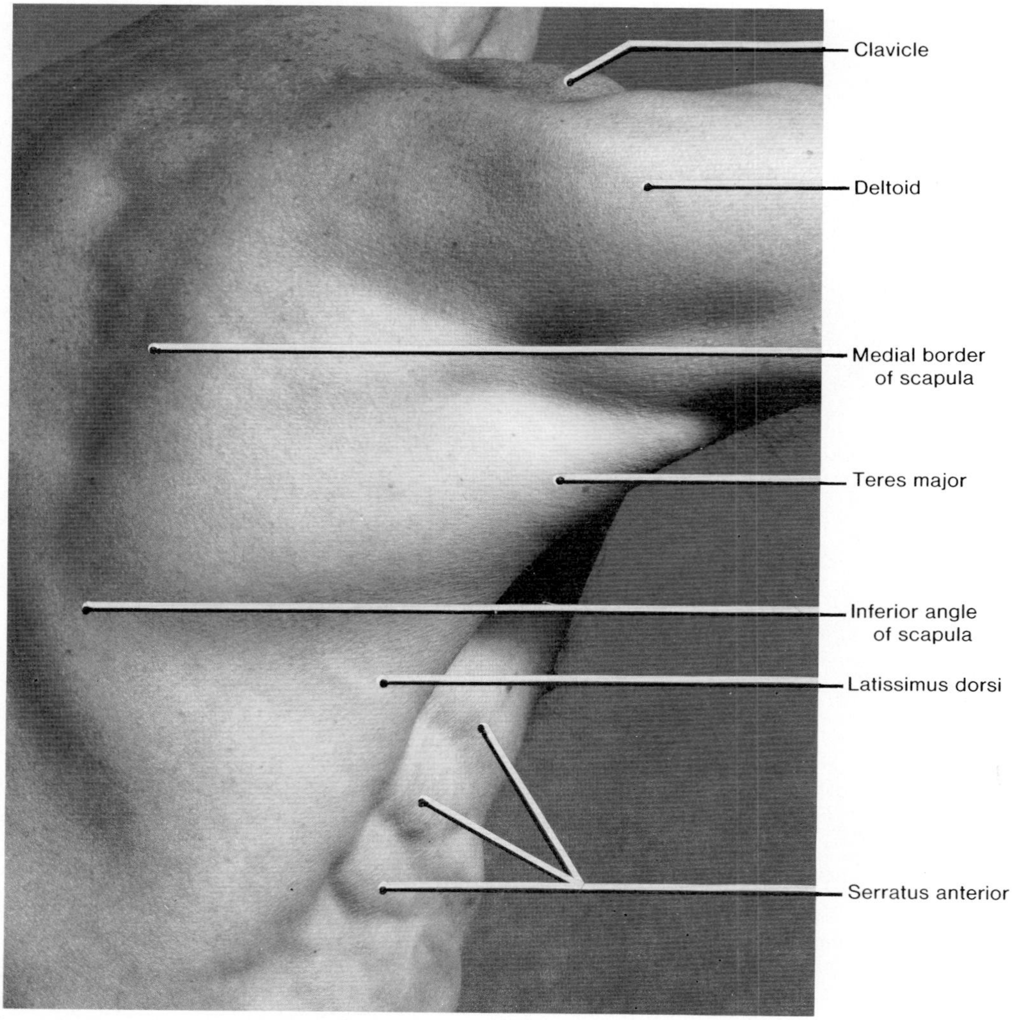

Figure 6-17. Photograph of the posterior aspect of the shoulder and axilla of a 46-year-old man. The teres major and the latissimus dorsi form the posterior axillary fold.

both rhomboid muscles and the levator scapulae.

2. The **long thoracic nerve** (Figs. 6-27, 6-31, and 6-32) arises from the ventral rami of C5 to C7 and passes through the apex of the axilla posterior to the other components of the brachial plexus to supply the serratus anterior.
3. The **nerve to the subclavius** (Figs. 6-24 and 6-27) arises from the ventral rami of C5 and C6 and descends in front of the brachial plexus to supply the subclavius muscle.
4. The **suprascapular nerve** (Figs. 6-27 and 6-58) arises from the upper trunk, receiving fibers from C5 and C6, and passes laterally across the posterior triangle superior to the brachial plexus. After passing through the **suprascapular notch** in the scapula, it supplies the supraspinatus and infraspinatus muscles and the shoulder joint.

The infraclavicular branches of the cords of the brachial plexus are as follows (Fig. 6-27).

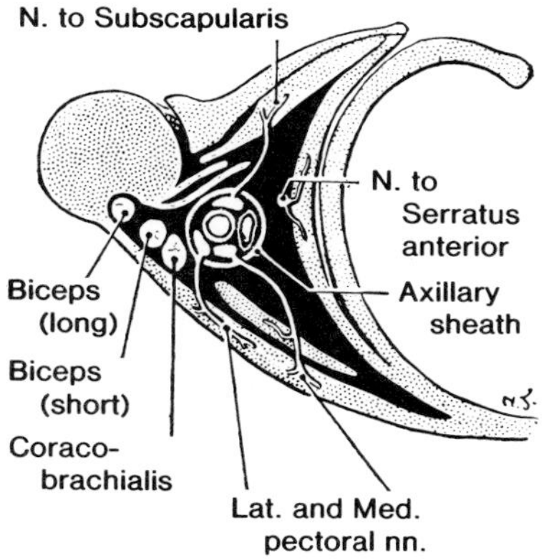

Figure 6-18. Drawing of a cross-section of the axilla showing some of its contents, *e.g.*, the principal vessels and nerves to the upper limb.

The lateral cord of the brachial plexus has three branches (Fig. 6-27).

1. The **lateral pectoral nerve** (C5 to C7) pierces the clavipectoral fascia to supply the **pectoralis major** (Figs. 6-18 and 6-23). *This nerve is called lateral because it arises from the lateral cord.* Remember this, otherwise you will be confused when you observe that it lies more medial on the chest wall than does the medial pectoral nerve.
2. The **musculocutaneous nerve** (C5 to C7), supplying the muscles of the front of the arm, is one of the two terminal branches of the lateral cord (Figs. 6-23, 6-26 to 6-28, and 6-32). It

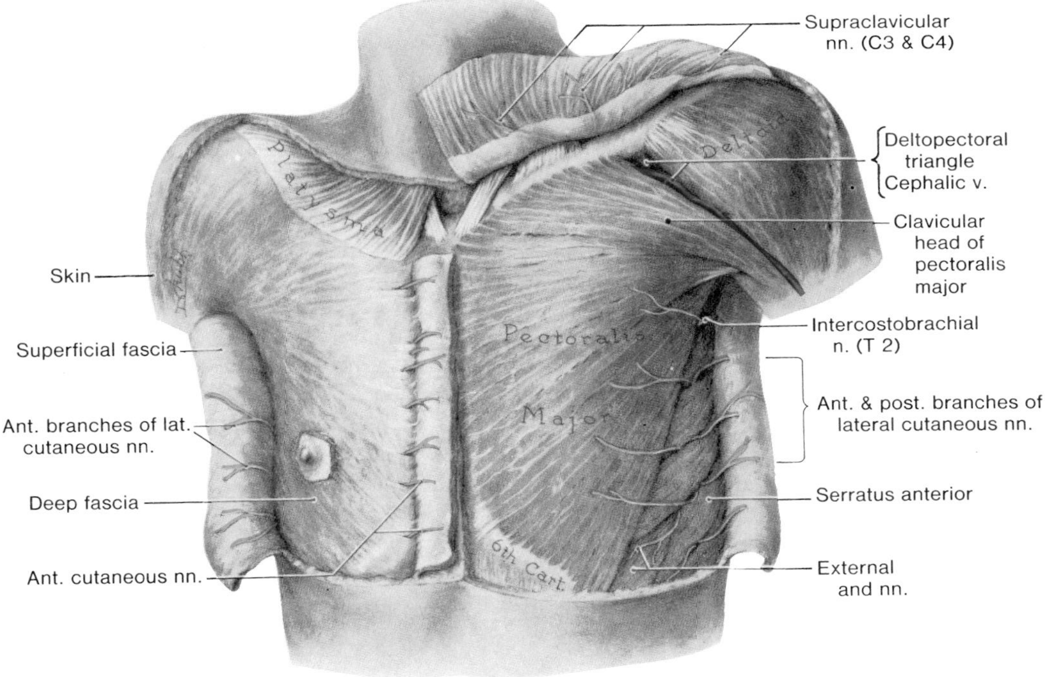

Figure 6-19. Drawing of a superficial dissection of the pectoral region. The platysma, a muscle of facial expression which descends to the second or third rib, is cut short on the right side and, together with the supraclavicular nerves, is turned up on the left side. Observe that the deep fascia covering the pectoralis major is filmy and the intermuscular bony strip running along the clavicle is both subcutaneous and subplatysmal. Note that the two heads of the pectoralis major meet at the sternoclavicular joint. Also observe the cephalic vein traversing the deltopectoral triangle (see Fig. 6-22 also).

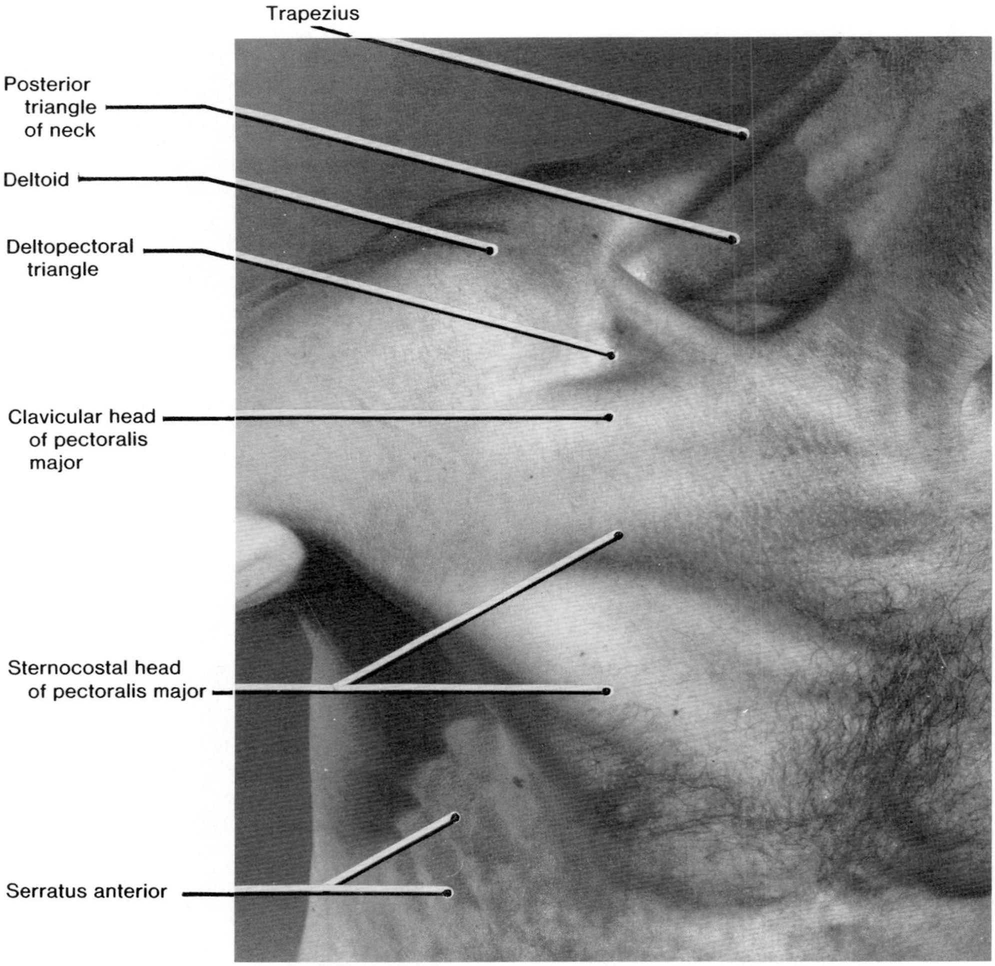

Figure 6-20. Photograph of the cervical, pectoral, and axillary regions of a 46-year-old man showing the principal surface markings. Compare with the dissection of the pectoral region shown in Figure 6-22. The brachial plexus (Fig. 6-24) is located in the posterior cervical triangle. The depression in the deltopectoral triangle is called the infraclavicular fossa.

enters the deep surface of the **coracobrachialis** muscle and supplies it, and then it continues on into the arm to supply the **biceps brachii** and the **brachialis** muscles. Just proximal to the elbow joint, it pierces the deep fascia and becomes superficial. From here it is called the **lateral cutaneous nerve of the forearm** and supplies skin on the lateral aspect of the forearm (Figs. 6-76, 6-102, and 6-103).

3. The **lateral root of the median nerve** is the continuation of the lateral cord; *i.e.,* it is the other terminal branch. It is joined by the medial root of the median nerve, lateral to the axillary artery, to form the **median nerve** (Figs. 6-23 and 6-25 to 6-29). This nerve passes inferiorly to supply primarily flexor muscles in the forearm, five muscles in the hand, and the skin of the hand.

The medial cord of the brachial plexus has five branches (Fig. 6-27).

1. The **medial pectoral nerve** (C8 and T1) enters the deep surface of the

pectoralis minor muscle (Fig. 6-18), supplying it and part of the **pectoralis major.** *This nerve is called medial because it arises from the medial cord.* In Figure 6-23, note that it lies lateral to the lateral pectoral nerve.

2. The **medial brachial cutaneous nerve,** or medial cutaneous nerve of the arm (C8 and T1), is a slender nerve that supplies skin over the medial surface of the arm and the upper part of the forearm (Fig. 6-102). It usually

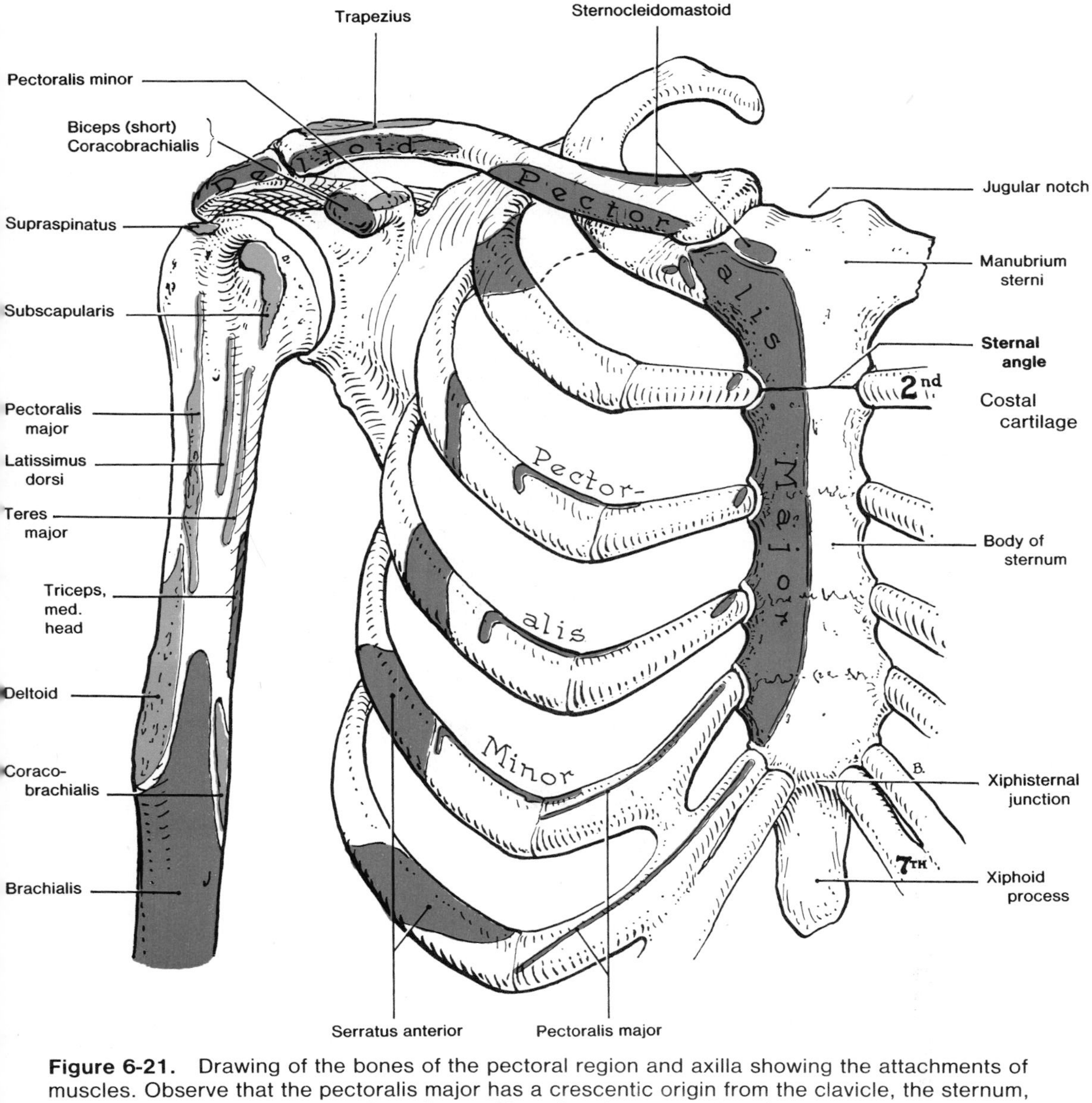

Figure 6-21. Drawing of the bones of the pectoral region and axilla showing the attachments of muscles. Observe that the pectoralis major has a crescentic origin from the clavicle, the sternum, and the upper five or six costal cartilages. Note that the pectoralis minor arises from the third, fourth, and fifth ribs. Observe the clinically important sternal angle. It may be felt as a horizontal ridge at the junction of the manubrium and the body of the sternum. The sternal angle is an important bony landmark for the identification of ribs.

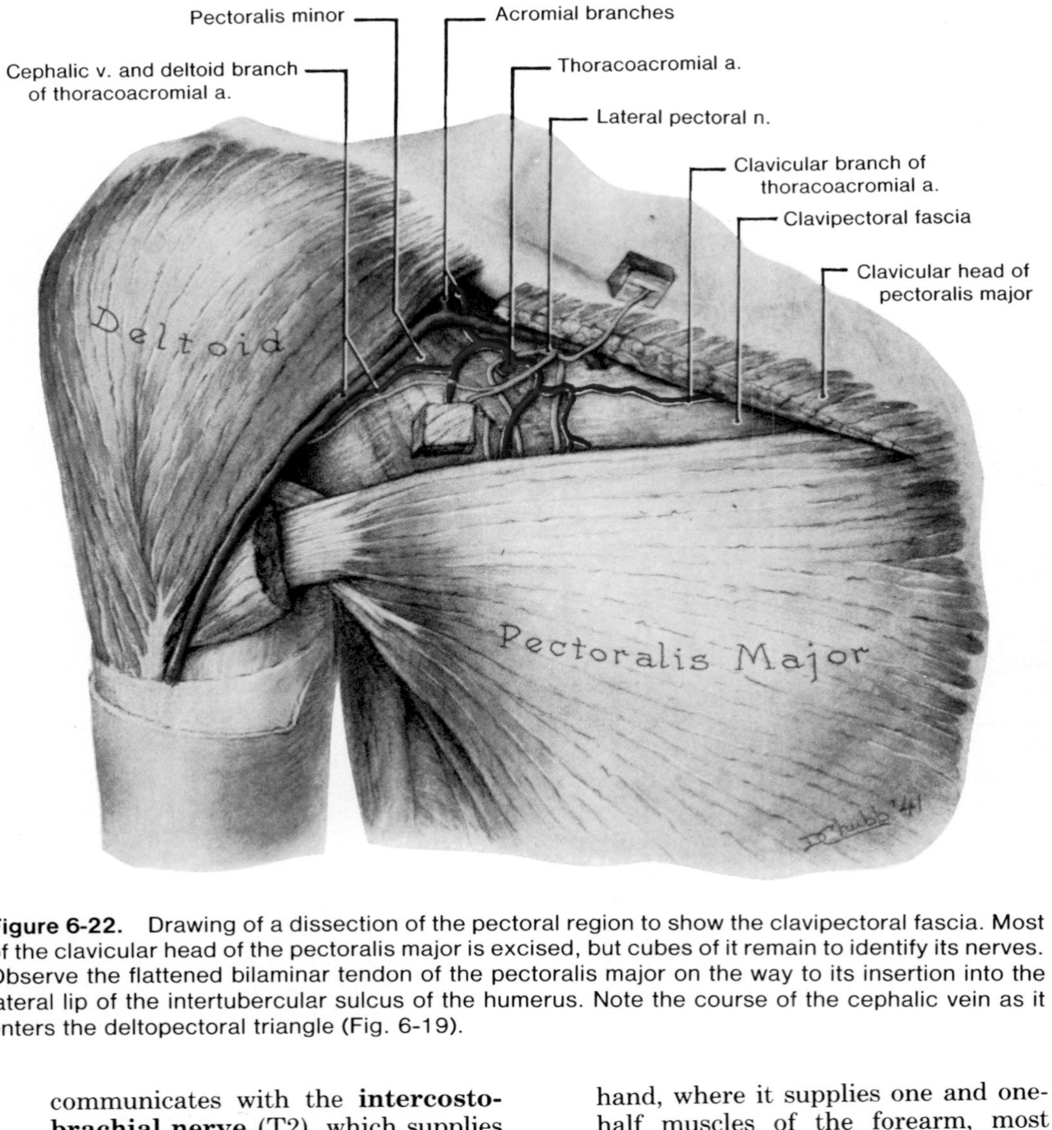

Figure 6-22. Drawing of a dissection of the pectoral region to show the clavipectoral fascia. Most of the clavicular head of the pectoralis major is excised, but cubes of it remain to identify its nerves. Observe the flattened bilaminar tendon of the pectoralis major on the way to its insertion into the lateral lip of the intertubercular sulcus of the humerus. Note the course of the cephalic vein as it enters the deltopectoral triangle (Fig. 6-19).

communicates with the **intercostobrachial nerve** (T2), which supplies skin of the floor of the axilla and adjacent regions of the arm.

3. The **medial antebrachial cutaneous nerve,** or medial cutaneous nerve of the forearm (C8 and T1), runs down between the axillary artery and vein to supply skin over the medial surface of the forearm (Fig. 6-102).
4. The **ulnar nerve** (C8, T1, and often C7) is a terminal branch of the medial cord of the brachial plexus (Fig. 6-27). **This important nerve** passes through the arm into the forearm and hand, where it supplies one and one-half muscles of the forearm, most small muscles of the hand, and some skin (Figs. 6-28 and 6-29).
5. The **medial root of the median nerve** is the other terminal branch of the medial cord. As stated previously, it joins with the lateral root to form the median nerve.

The posterior cord of the brachial plexus has five branches (Figs. 6-27 to 6-30). In general, they supply muscles that extend the joints of the upper limb. These branches also supply cutaneous nerves to the extensor surface of the upper limb.

1. The **upper subscapular nerve** (C5 and C6) is a small nerve that supplies the **subscapularis muscle** (Figs. 6-30 and 6-31).
2. The **thoracodorsal nerve** (C6, C7, and C8) arises between the upper and lower subscapular nerves and runs inferolaterally to supply the **latissimus dorsi muscle** (Figs. 6-30 and 6-31).
3. The **lower subscapular nerve** (C5 and C6) passes downward and laterally, deep to the subscapular artery and vein, giving a branch to the **subscapularis muscle** and ending by supplying the **teres major muscle** (Figs. 6-30 and 6-31).
4. The **axillary nerve** (circumflex nerve), from C5 and C6, is a large important *terminal branch* of the posterior cord of the brachial plexus (Figs. 6-27 and 6-32). It passes to the back of the arm through the quadrangular

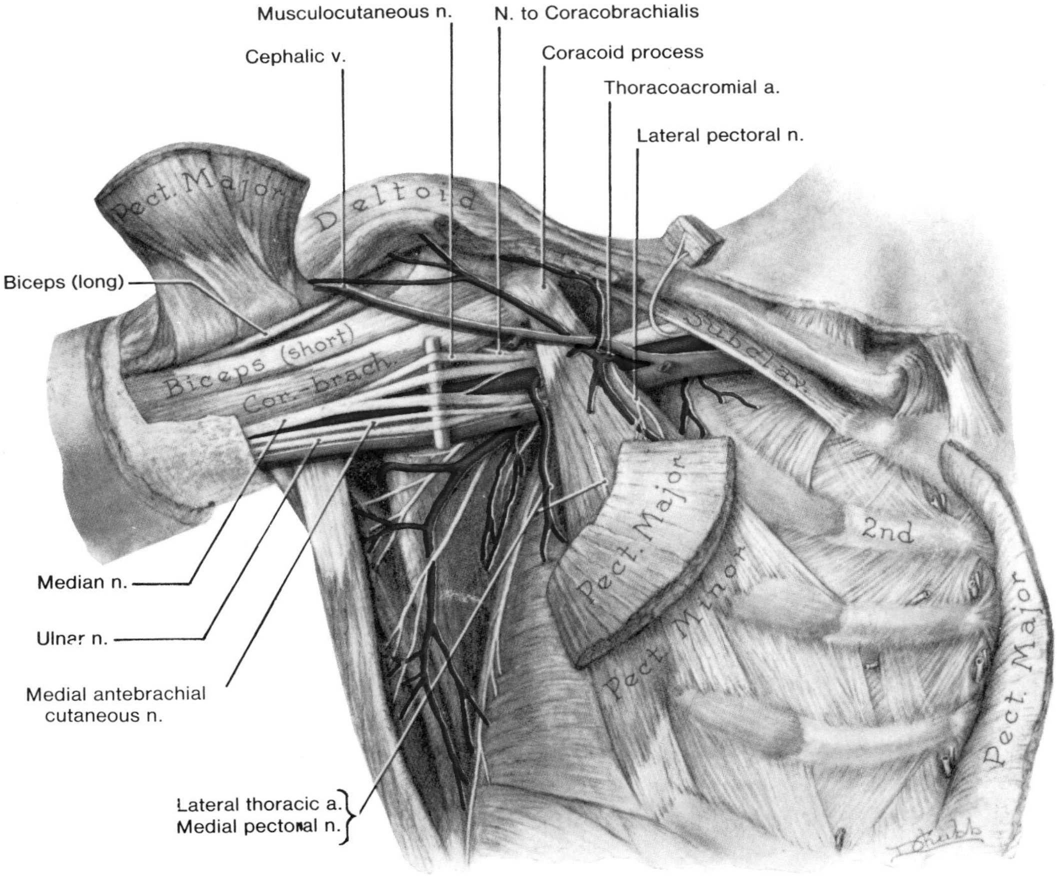

Figure 6-23. Drawing of a dissection of the pectoral region and axilla illustrating the anterior structures of the axilla. The pectoralis major is reflected and the clavipectoral fascia is removed. Observe the subclavius and pectoralis minor, the two deep muscles of the anterior wall. Note the axillary artery lying behind the pectoralis minor, a fingerbreadth from the tip of the coracoid process of the scapula with the lateral cord lateral to it and the medial cord medial to it. Observe that the axillary vein lies medial to the axillary artery. Note the median nerve, followed proximally, leading by its lateral root to the lateral cord and the musculocutaneous nerve and by its medial root to the medial cord and the ulnar nerve. These and the medial antebrachial cutaneous nerve are raised on a stick.

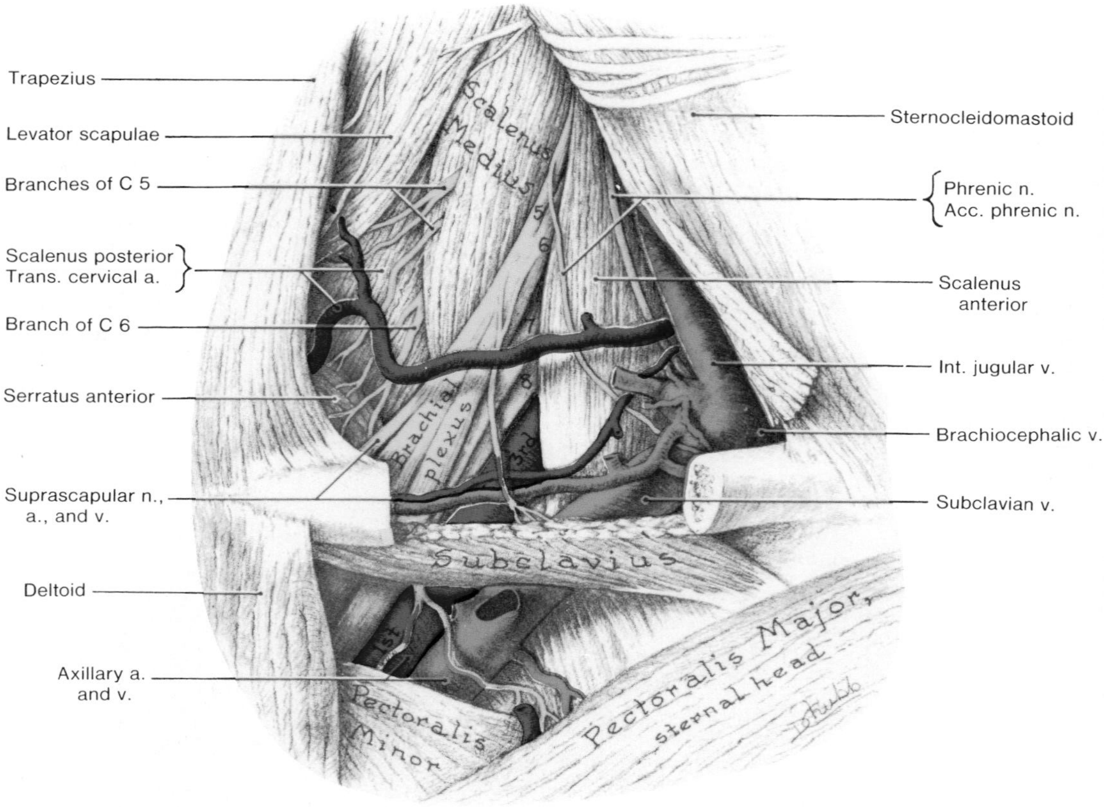

Figure 6-24. Drawing of the posterior triangle of the neck, the pectoral region, and the axilla, *right side*. Observe the third part of the subclavian artery and the first part of the axillary artery. Note the muscles forming the floor of the lower part of the posterior triangle (scaleni posterior, medius, and anterior and serratus anterior). Note the brachial plexus and the subclavian artery appearing between the scalenus medius and scalenus anterior. The lowest root of the plexus (T1) is concealed by the third part of the artery. The suprascapular nerve may be found by following the lateral border of the brachial plexus caudally. Note the subclavius, a relatively unimportant muscle, that may serve as a buffer between a fractured clavicle and the subclavian vessels.

(quadrilateral) space in company with the posterior circumflex humeral vessels (Figs. 6-31 and 6-32) and supplies articular branches to the shoulder joint. On emerging from the **quadrangular space** posteriorly, it winds around the surgical neck of the humerus and *supplies the teres minor and deltoid muscles.* It ends as the **upper lateral brachial cutaneous nerve** (Fig. 6-102) and supplies skin over the lower half of the deltoid and adjacent areas of the arm.

5. The **radial nerve** (C5 to C8 and T1) is the other terminal branch of the posterior cord (Figs. 6-27 and 6-31). *This large important nerve* provides the **major nerve supply to the extensor muscles** of the upper limb (Fig. 6-30) and supplies cutaneous sensation to **the skin of the extensor region,** including the hand (Figs. 6-29 and 6-103). As it leaves the axilla it runs backward, downward, and laterally between the long and medial heads of the **triceps** muscle to enter the **radial groove** of the humerus (Fig. 6-32). The radial nerve gives

branches to the triceps, anconeus, brachioradialis, and extensor muscles of the forearm (Figs. 6-30 to 6-32).

CLINICALLY ORIENTED COMMENTS

Injuries to the brachial plexus are of great importance. Because the plexus is located in the neck and the axilla, it can be injured by disease, stretching, and wounds in both these regions. The injury may involve the dorsal and ventral roots of the spinal nerves, the ventral rami (roots of plexus), the trunks, the divisions, the cords, or the branches of the cords (Figs. 6-25 to 6-27). The signs and symptoms depend on which part of the brachial plexus is involved.

Injuries to the brachial plexus result in loss of muscular movement (**paralysis**) and usually in loss of cutaneous sensation (**anesthesia**). The degree of paralysis may be assessed by testing the patient's ability to perform movements. In **complete paralysis** no movement can be detected, whereas in **incomplete paralysis** a movement can be performed but it is weak compared with that on the normal side. The explanation for this is that not all muscles concerned with the movement are para-

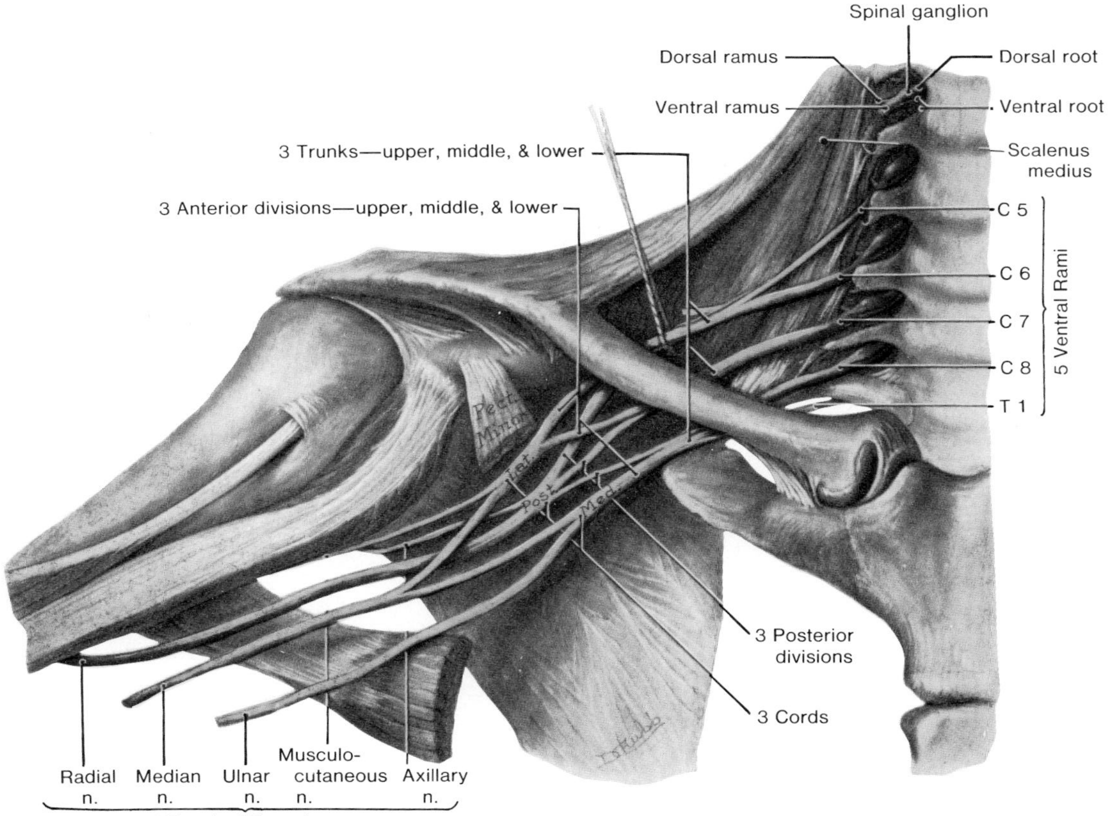

Figure 6-25. Drawing of the brachial plexus extending from the neck to the axilla. Observe the five ventral rami forming the brachial plexus. As there are only seven cervical vertebra, the T1 ramus arises below the pedicle of the first thoracic vertebra. The rami unite to form the three trunks of the plexus and each trunk divides into two divisions, an anterior and a posterior. From the divisions, observe that three cords lie behind the pectoralis minor muscle. Note that the large brachial plexus allows the mingling of nerve fibers from several segments of the spinal cord.

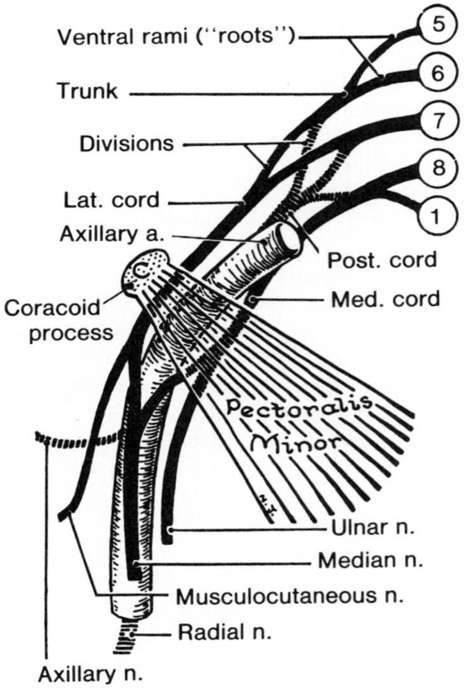

Figure 6-26. Diagram illustrating the plan of the brachial plexus. Note that the axillary artery is surrounded by the three cords of the plexus and that they bear the relation indicated by their names to the second part of the axillary artery, *i.e.*, the part behind the pectoralis minor. For descriptive purposes it is usual and useful to designate the parts of the brachial plexus as ventral rami ("roots"), trunks, divisions, and cords.

lyzed. The degree of anesthesia (G. absence of feeling) may be tested by determining the ability of the person to feel pain (*e.g.*, a pin-prick).

Recovery from first degree injuries (*e.g.*, caused by pressure on a nerve) usually occurs in a few weeks, but when a nerve is cut or crushed, **anterograde (Wallerian) degeneration** occurs distal to the lesion involving the axons, their terminals, and the myelin sheaths. However, if the cut ends of the nerve are brought together and sutured soon after injury, partial function may be restored to the part within a few months.

Upper Brachial Plexus Injuries (*e.g., Erb's Palsy and Erb-Duchenne Palsy*). Injuries to the upper part of the brachial plexus usually result from excessive separation of the neck and shoulder; this may occur in football when one tackler is pulling a person's arm as another one hits or pulls the person's head (*e.g.,* pulling the face mask). These injuries can also occur when a person is thrown from a horse and lands on the shoulder in a way that widely separates the neck and the shoulder (Fig. 6-33). Most often these injuries result from **motorcycle accidents.** When thrown, the shoulder often hits something (*e.g.,* a tree); as a result, the person's shoulder stops but the head and trunk continue forward. Similar damage to the brachial plexus can result from stretching an infant's neck during delivery (Fig. 6-34).

In an upper brachial plexus injury, the dorsal and ventral roots of the spinal nerves from C5 and C6 may be pulled out of the spinal cord (Fig. 6-25); thus, there is usually paralysis of the dorsal axial musculature and loss of sensation over the region of the back supplied by the dorsal primary rami, in addition to **paralysis of muscles and loss of sensation in the upper limb.**

If the lesion is confined to C5, usually no sensory changes can be detected because this nerve is not responsible for the exclusive supply of any definite area of skin; however, when both C5 and C6 are involved, there is usually some loss of sensation on the lateral aspect of the upper limb (Case 6-1).

In stab and bullet wounds of the neck, the upper trunk of the brachial plexus is often torn or severed where it emerges between the scalenus anterior and scalenus medius muscles (Fig. 6-24). These injuries result in loss of flexion, abduction, and lateral rotation of the shoulder joint, as well as loss of flexion of the elbow joint. Injury to the upper trunk of the brachial plexus may be recognized by the characteristic position of the limb (Fig. 6-35). It hangs by the side in medial rotation, a position referred to as the "tip-taking" or "**waiter's tip" position** because it is the way some waiters indicate their desire for a tip.

The following muscles that receive nerve fibers from C5 and C6 are most severely affected (*i.e.,* paralyzed): deltoid, biceps brachii, brachialis, brachioradialis, supraspinatus, infraspinatus, and teres minor (Figs. 6-28 and 6-30).

Incorrect use of crutches (*e.g.*, ones that are too long) may cause **injury to the posterior cord** of the brachial plexus. Often only the radial nerve is affected; as a result, the triceps, anconeous, and extensors of the wrist are paralyzed (Fig. 6-30). The person is unable to extend the elbow, the wrist, or the fingers. This type of paralysis, often called "**crutch palsy**," produces a **wrist-drop** and an inability to extend the wrist joint and the digits (Case 6-6 and Fig. 6-181*A*).

Lower Brachial Plexus Injuries (*e.g., Klumpke's Palsy*). These injuries are not so common as upper brachial plexus injuries. They may occur when the upper limb is suddenly pulled upward, *e.g.*, a forceful upward pull of the shoulder during birth (Fig. 6-36). It may also occur in adults when grasping something to break a fall (Fig. 6-37).

These accidents injure the lower trunk of the brachial plexus (C8 and T1), often pulling the dorsal and ventral roots of the spinal nerves out of the spinal cord. Generally the paralysis and anesthesia affect the muscles and skin supplied by the **ulnar nerve** (C8 and T1). Typically, the chief disabilities are in wrist and finger movements, *e.g.*, impairment of wrist flexion and of movements of the intrinsic muscles of the hand (Fig. 6-28). There is likely to be reduced sensation along the ulnar side of the arm, forearm, and hand (Figs. 6-29 and 6-102).

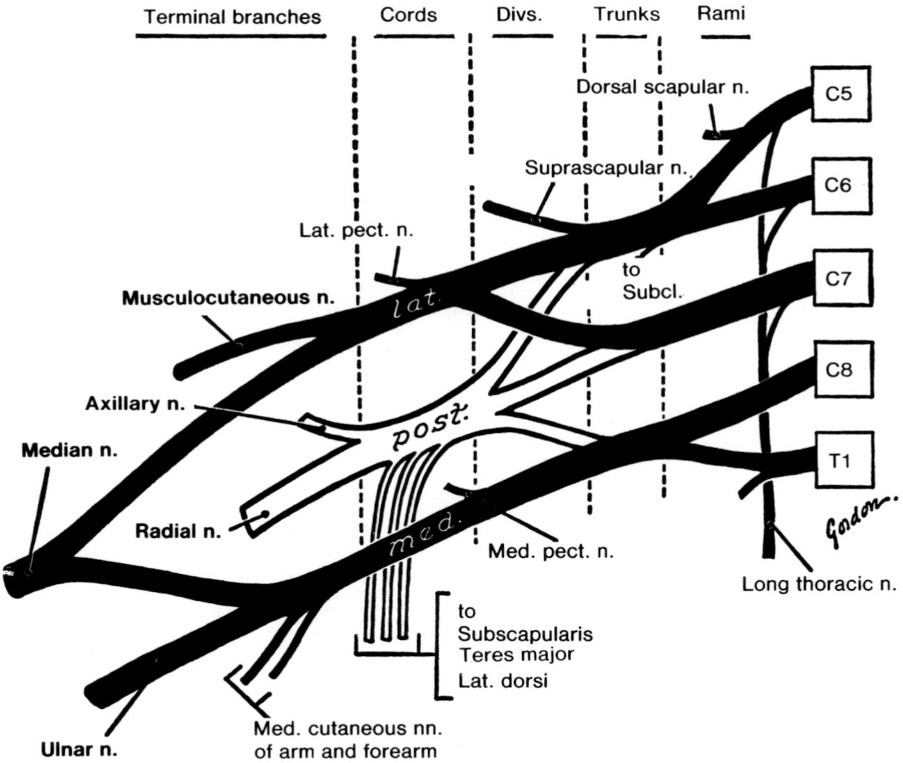

Figure 6-27. Schematic diagram of an anterior view of the right brachial plexus. Note the parts of the brachial plexus as follows: five ventral primary rami (C5 to C8, and T1) three trunks (upper, middle, and lower); six divisions (three anterior and three posterior); three cords (medial, lateral, and posterior); and five terminal nerves (radial, axillary, ulnar, median, and musculocutaneous). The most important branches of the brachial plexus (printed in **bold type**) are the median, ulnar, radial, musculocutaneous, and axillary nerves.

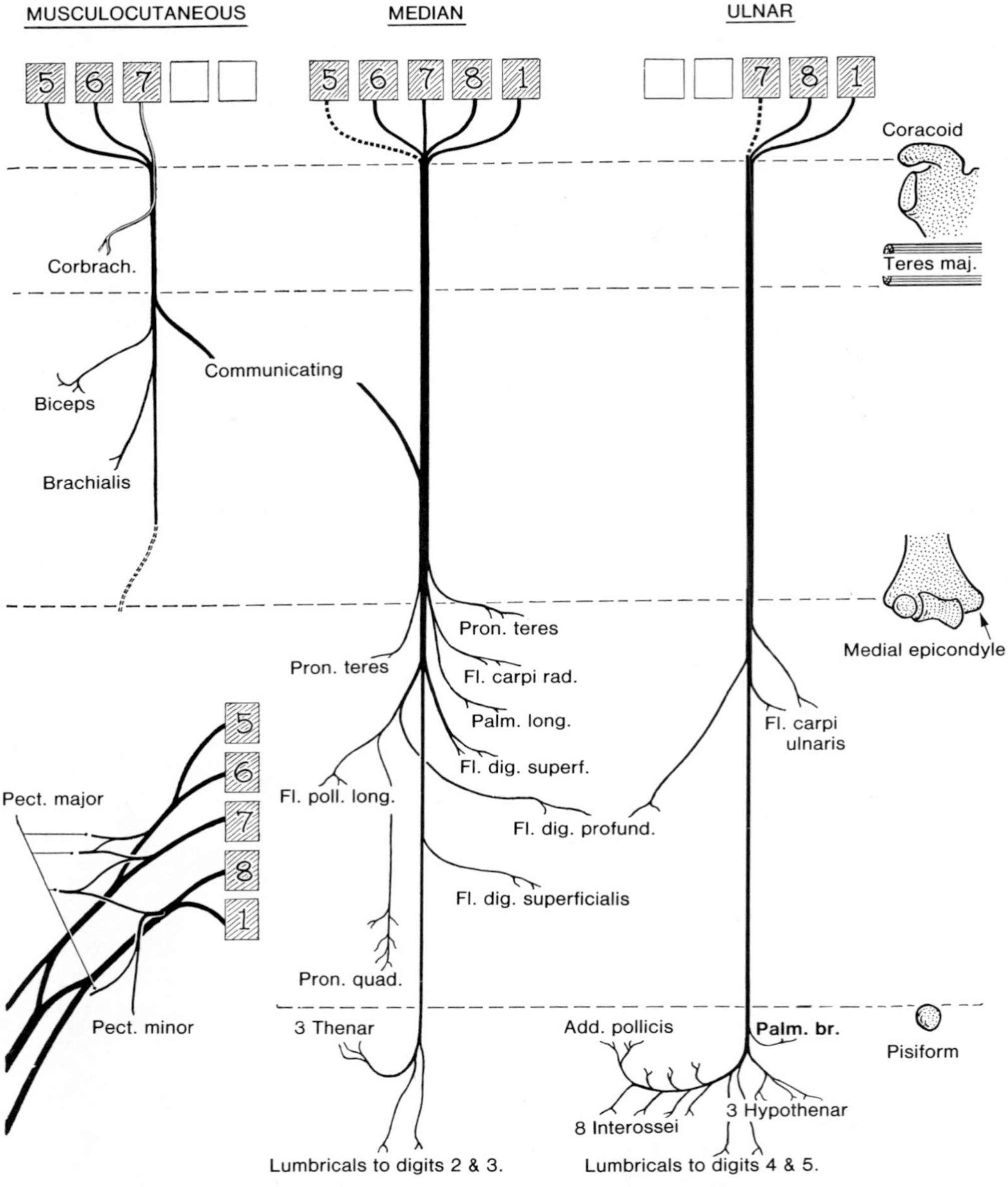

Figure 6-28. Diagrams illustrating the segmental origin and the motor distribution of the ventral nerves of the upper limb. The average levels at which the motor branches leave the stems of the main nerves are shown with reference to the lower border of the axilla (teres major), the elbow joint (medial epicondyle), and the wrist (pisiform bone).

Cervical Rib Syndrome. A rib in the neck or a **cervical rib** (Fig. 6-38) can exert pressure on the lower trunk of the brachial plexus, producing symptoms of nerve compression. The accessory rib on the seventh cervical vertebra exerts pressure on the lower trunk of the brachial plexus, particularly when the upper limb is pulled down (*e.g.,* when carrying a heavy suitcase). This probably affects the nerves by compressing the blood vessels supplying them and causing **anoxia** (lack of oxygen) of the axons sufficient to interfere with their function. Sensory fibers are more readily affected by pressure than motor fibers (*e.g.,* producing tingling and numbness). When the pressure is released (*e.g.,* when the suitcase is dropped), recovery of sensation and motor function often occurs in a few minutes.

The cervical rib syndrome has an embryological basis. Early in development each vertebra has two costal elements which form ribs in the thoracic region, but usually become parts of the vertebrae in other regions. In 0.5 to 1% of persons, the costal elements of the seventh cervical vertebra form projections called **cervical ribs** (Fig. 6-38). The cervical rib may be free anteriorly or attached to the first rib and/or the sternum. Usually these ribs produce no symptoms, but in some cases the **subclavian artery** and the lower trunk of the **brachial plexus** are kinked where they pass over the cervical rib. Compression of these structures between this extra rib and the anterior scalene muscle may produce symptoms of nerve and arterial compression, producing the **neurovascular compression syndrome.** Often the tingling, numbness, and impaired circulation to the upper limb do not appear until the age of puberty when the neck elongates and the shoulders tend to droop slightly.

The symptoms do not develop until middle life in some persons. These symptoms of a cervical rib probably result from the fact that posture becomes more stooped as the tone of muscles of the pectoral girdle relaxes. This allows the shoulder to fall forward and downward, making it easier for the cervical rib to compress the subclavian artery and the lower trunk of the brachial plexus.

Paralysis of Branches of the Brachial Plexus. When a nerve arising from the brachial plexus is injured, the effects de-

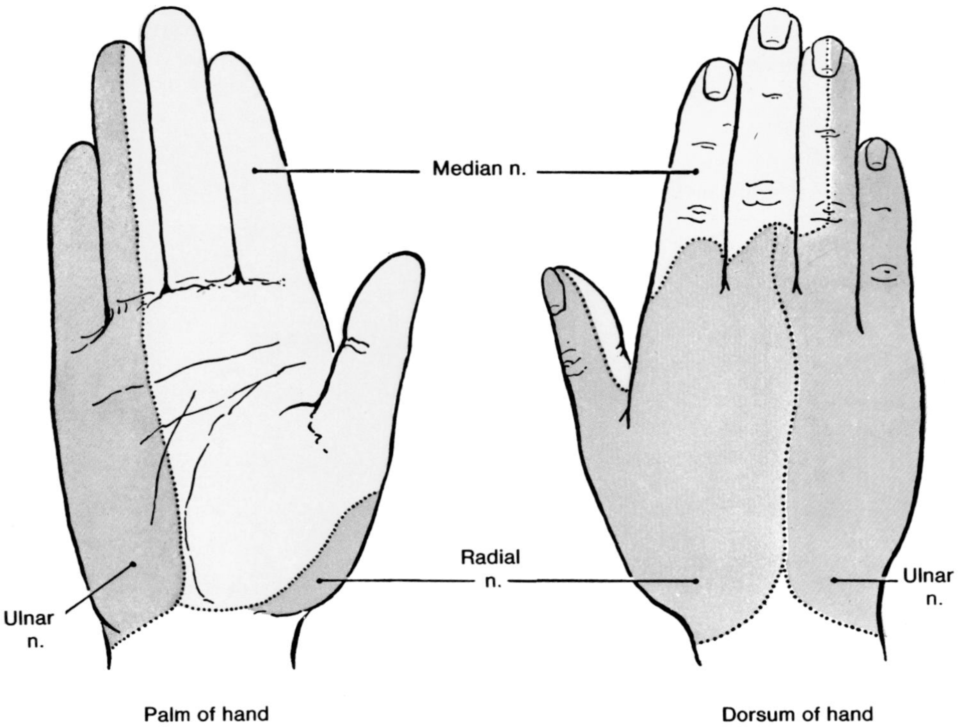

Figure 6-29. Diagrams illustrating the distribution of the cutaneous nerves to hand. Note that they are derived from three major nerves.

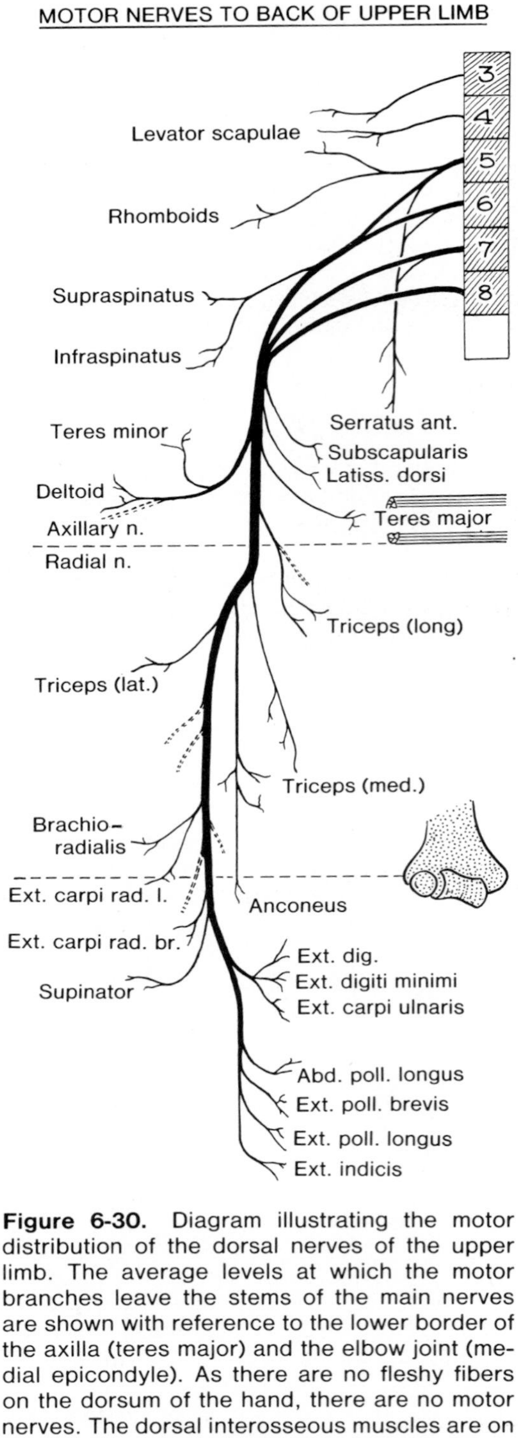

Figure 6-30. Diagram illustrating the motor distribution of the dorsal nerves of the upper limb. The average levels at which the motor branches leave the stems of the main nerves are shown with reference to the lower border of the axilla (teres major) and the elbow joint (medial epicondyle). As there are no fleshy fibers on the dorsum of the hand, there are no motor nerves. The dorsal interosseous muscles are on the dorsum of the hand (Fig. 6-114), but they are innervated anteriorly by the deep branch of the ulnar nerve.

pend upon the level at which the injury occurs; *e.g.,* if the radial nerve is severed above the origin of the branches to the triceps muscle (Figs. 6-30 to 6-32), extension of the elbow joint is impossible (Case 6-2). If the radial is cut below the origin of these nerves (*e.g.,* at the midshaft of the humerus), extension of the elbow joint is not affected, but there is paralysis of the extensor muscles of the forearm and the digits (Case 6-6).

As the **long thoracic nerve** (C5 to C7) to the serratus anterior muscle lies on the medial wall of the axilla (Figs. 6-31 and 6-32), it may be injured by a stab wound or during thoracic surgery (*e.g.,* for removal of a lung). Carrying a heavy object on the shoulder (*e.g.,* a steel beam) may also compress this nerve between the clavicle and the lateral part of the first rib (Fig. 6-31).

Crushing or cutting the long thoracic nerve results in paralysis of the serratus anterior muscle and in "**winging of the scapula.**" As a result, the vertebral border and inferior angle of the scapula become unusually prominent (Fig. 6-39). This "winging" is accentuated when the person pushes against a wall with both hands. Instead of keeping the scapula applied to the chest wall, as is normal, the paralyzed muscle allows the scapula to be pushed out like a wing. Difficulty is also experienced in flexing or abducting the arm above 45° from the side of the body because the serratus anterior muscle normally protracts and rotates the scapula so the glenoid cavity of the scapula faces upward when carrying out such a movement.

The **axillary nerve** (C5 and C6) passes through the quadrangular space (Figs. 6-31 and 6-32) and its anterior branch winds around the surgical neck of the humerus; thus, it may be injured during fracture of this part of the bone or during dislocation of the shoulder joint (Case 6-4). Following *severance of the axillary nerve,* the deltoid muscle is paralyzed and undergoes atrophy (**wasting**), and a loss of sensation (**anesthesia**) occurs over the lateral side of the proximal part of the arm (Fig. 6-40).

Injuries of other nerves arising from the brachial plexus (*e.g.,* the median and ulnar nerves) are discussed in subsequent sections and in Cases 6-5 and 6-10.

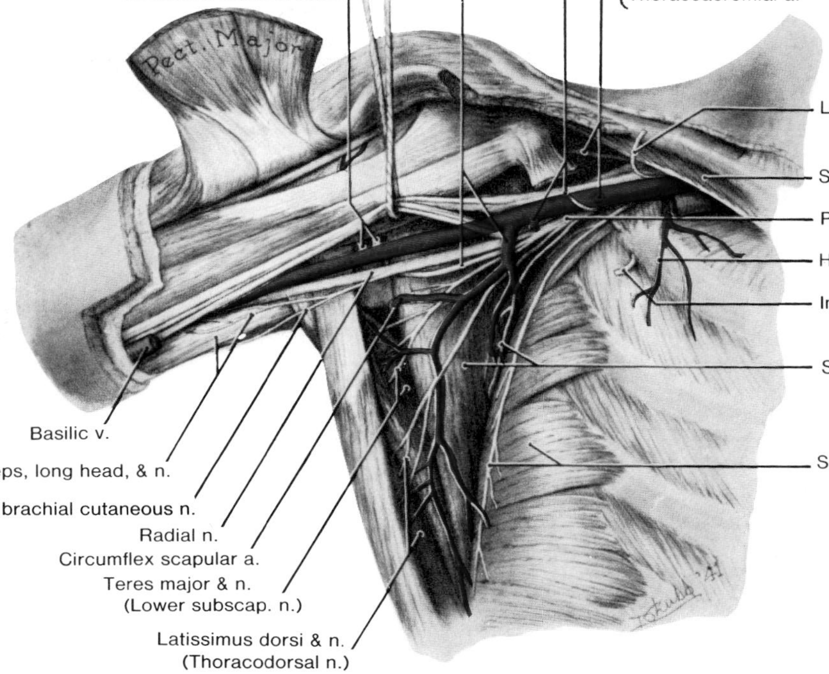

Figure 6-31. Drawing of a dissection of the posterior and medial walls of the axilla. The pectoralis minor is excised, the lateral and medial cords are retracted, and the axillary vein is removed. Observe the posterior cord and its two terminal branches (the radial and axillary nerves) lying behind the axillary artery. Note the nerves to the three posterior muscles: (1) the thoracodorsal nerve or nerve to the latissimus dorsi enters the deep surface of the muscle, 2.5 cm from its free border at a point midway between the chest and the abducted arm; (2) the upper subscapular nerve to the subscapularis lies parallel to (1) but above it; and (3) the lower subscapular nerve to the subscapularis and the teres major lies parallel to (1) but below it. The nerve to the serratus anterior is clinging to its muscle throughout. Observe the suprascapular nerve passing toward the root of the coracoid process and the subscapular artery, the largest branch of the axillary artery. Observe the posterior circumflex humeral artery accompanying the axillary nerve through the quadrangular space.

The Axillary Artery (Figs. 6-23, 6-26, and 6-41). This large vessel *begins at the outer border of the first rib* as a continuation of the **subclavian artery** and *ends at the lower border of the teres major muscle,* where it passes into the arm as the **brachial artery.** During its course through the axilla, the axillary artery passes posterior to the pectoralis minor muscle. For purposes of description the axillary artery is divided into three parts by this muscle (Fig. 6-41).

The first part of the axillary artery is located between the first rib and the superior border of the pectoralis minor. It has one branch, the **highest thoracic artery** (supreme or superior thoracic artery), which helps to supply the first and second intercostal spaces and the superior part of the serratus anterior muscle (Figs. 6-31 and 6-41). It anastomoses with the intercostal arteries.

The second part of the axillary artery lies deep to the pectoralis minor (Fig. 6-41). The lateral cord of the brachial plexus is lateral to the artery (Fig. 6-26),

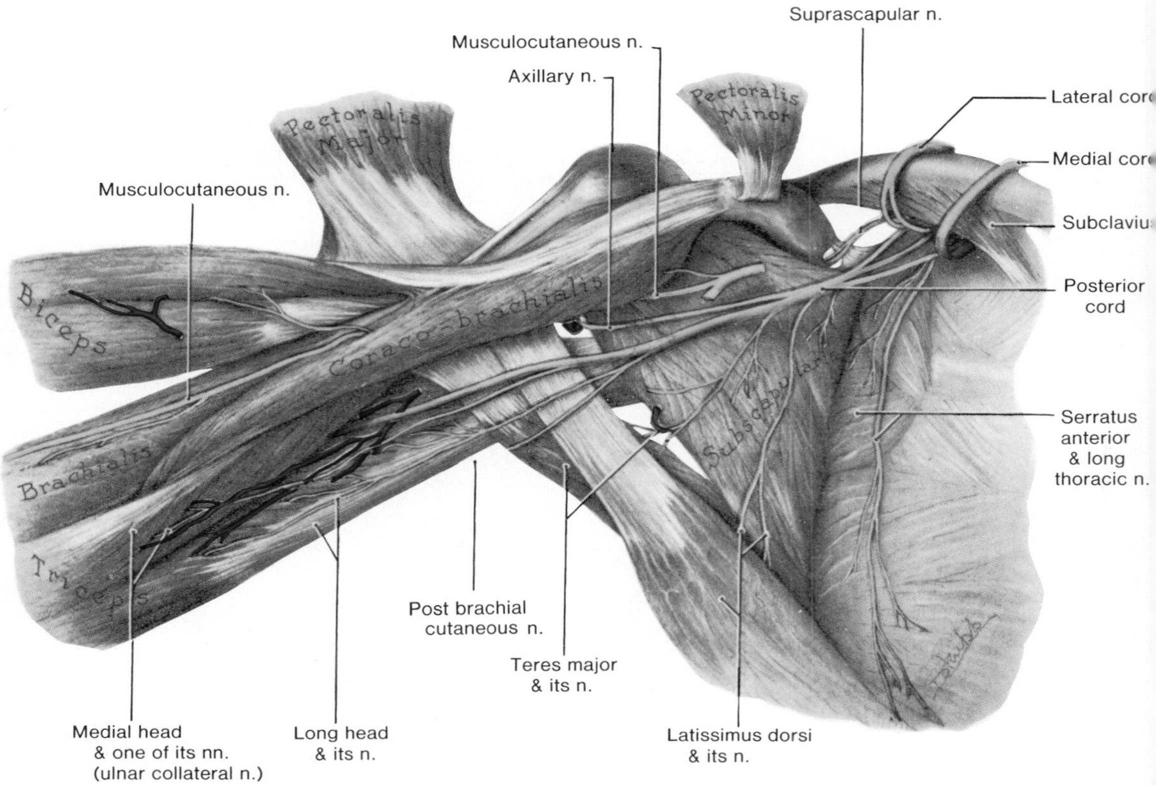

Figure 6-32. Drawing of a dissection of the posterior wall of the axilla demonstrating the posterior cord of the brachial plexus and its branches. The pectoralis major and pectoralis minor muscles are turned laterally; the lateral and medial cords of the brachial plexus are turned upward; the arteries, veins, and median and ulnar nerves are removed. Observe the coracobrachialis muscle arising with the short head of the biceps from the tip of the coracoid process and inserting half way down the humerus. Note the musculocutaneous nerve piercing the coracobrachialis and supplying it, the biceps, and the brachialis before becoming cutaneous. Observe the posterior cord of the plexus, formed by the union of the three posterior divisions, supplying the three muscles of the posterior wall of the axilla and soon ending as the radial and axillary nerves. Note that the radial nerve gives off, in the axilla, the nerve to the long head of the triceps and a cutaneous branch and, in this specimen, the ulnar collateral branch to the medial head of the triceps. It then enters the radial groove of the humerus with the profunda brachii artery. Note the axillary nerve passing through the quadrangular space with the posterior circumflex humeral artery.

the medial cord is medial to it, and the posterior cord is posterior to it. The second part of the axillary artery has two branches, the thoracoacromial and the lateral thoracic arteries (Fig. 6-31).

The **thoracoacromial artery,** a short wide trunk, arises from the axillary under the pectoralis minor and pierces the **costocoracoid membrane,** a part of the clavipectoral fascia (Fig. 6-14). It then divides into four branches (acromial, deltoid, pectoral, and clavicular) deep to the clavicular head of the pectoralis major muscle (Fig. 6-22).

The **lateral thoracic artery** descends along the axillary border of the pectoralis minor (Figs. 6-23 and 6-41) and supplies the serratus anterior, the pectoral muscles, and the axillary lymph nodes. In the female, it is *an important source of blood to the lateral part of the mammary gland.*

The third part of the axillary artery

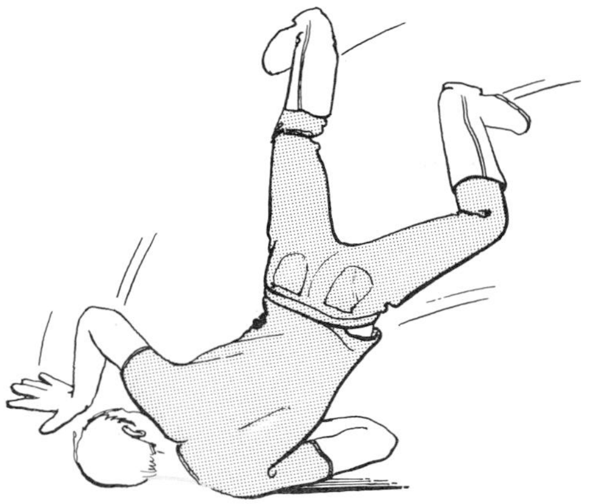

Figure 6-33. Drawing illustrating how the neck and shoulder are violently separated during a fall on the acromion of the scapula, producing an upper brachial plexus injury (Case 6-1).

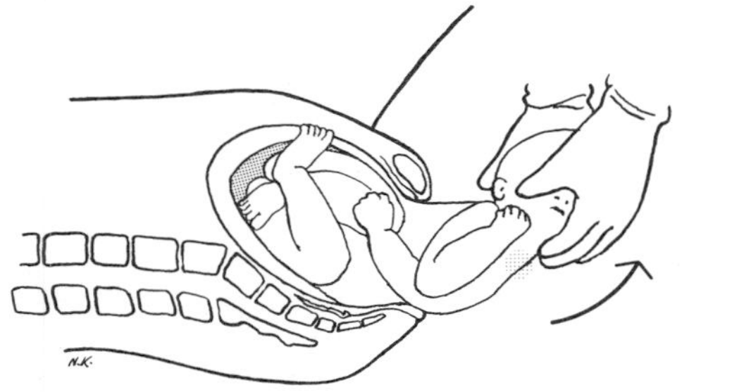

Figure 6-34. Drawing illustrating how the upper part of the brachial plexus may be injured by stretching the neck of the baby during delivery.

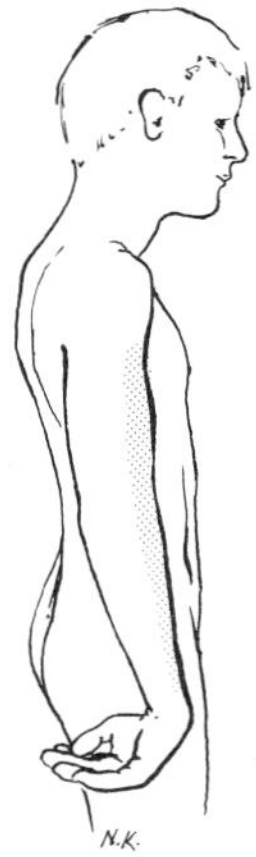

Figure 6-35. Illustration of the ''tip-taking'' position of the upper limb of a young man with an upper brachial plexus injury. Note the characteristic waiter's tip position of his hand. The area of skin that is usually anesthetic is shown in red.

extends from the lower border of the pectoralis minor to the lower border of the teres major (Fig. 6-41). It has three branches (subscapular, anterior circumflex humeral, and posterior circumflex humeral). In Figures 6-31 and 6-41, observe that the caliber of the axillary artery diminishes just beyond the origin of the subscapular and posterior circumflex humeral arteries.

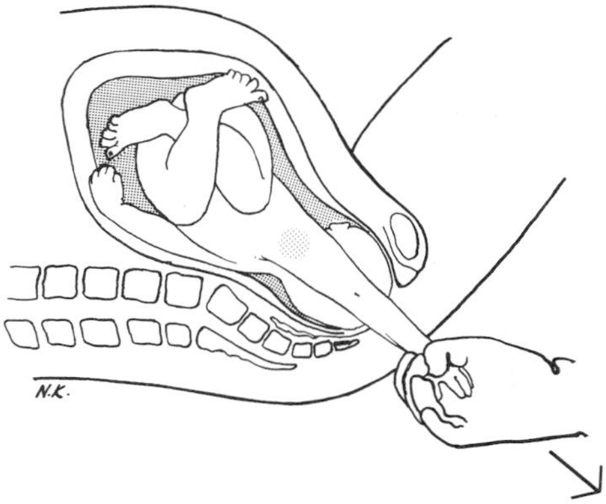

Figure 6-36. Illustration of the most common way lower type brachial plexus injuries occur, as the result of a forceful upward pull of the shoulder during birth.

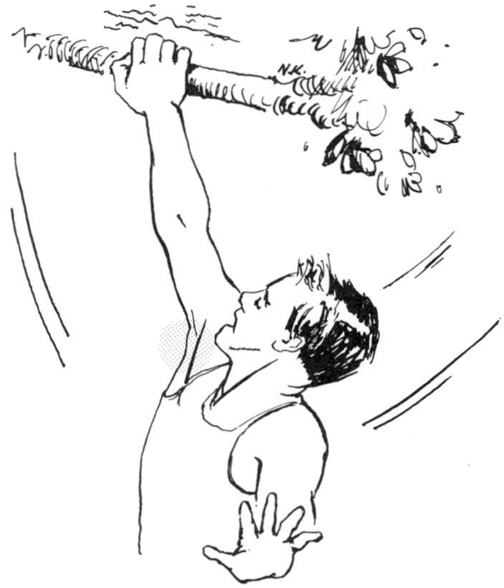

Figure 6-37. Drawing illustrating how a person may stretch and possibly tear the lower part of the brachial plexus by grasping for a limb during a fall.

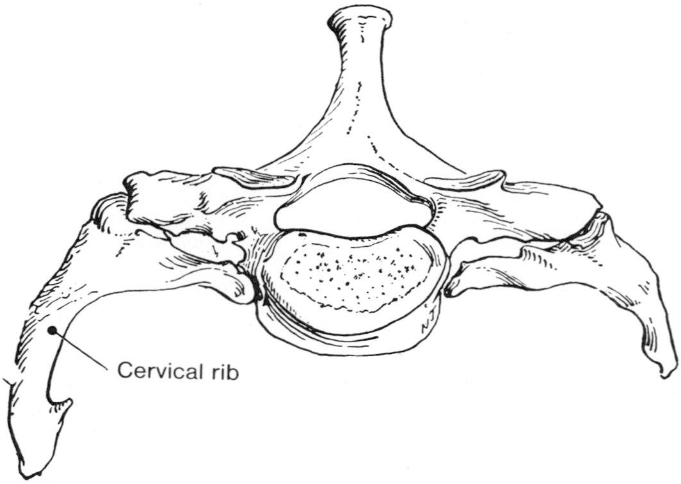

A.

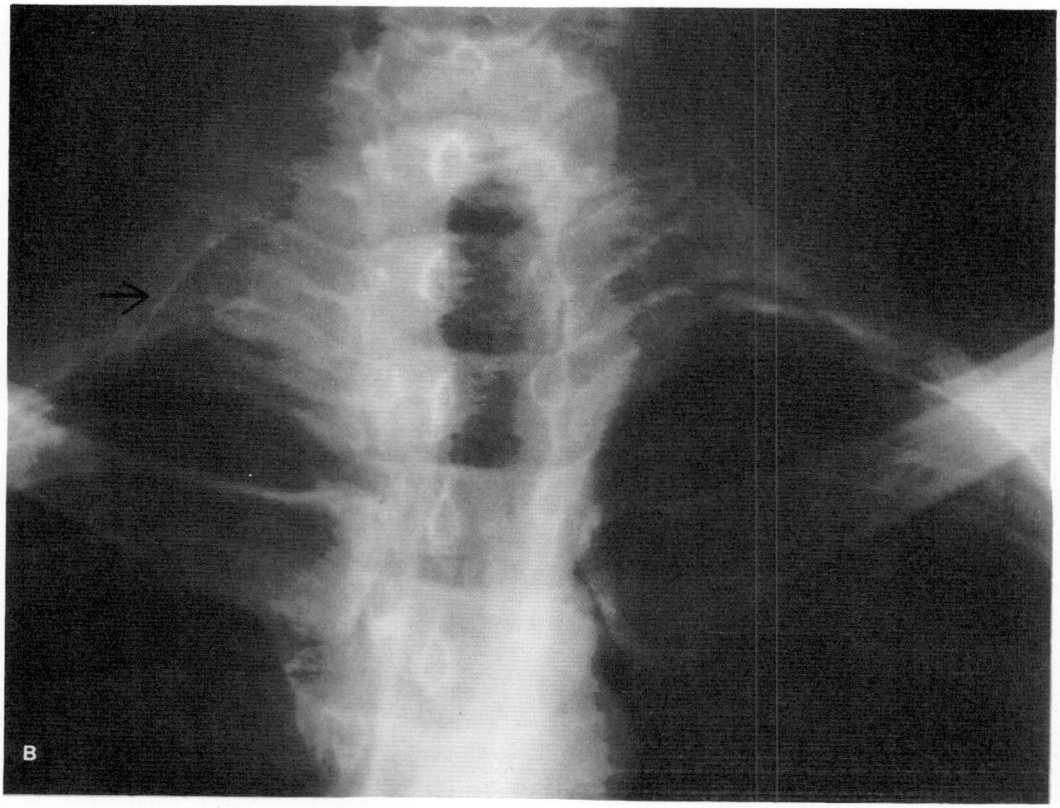

Figure 6-38. *A*, drawing of a seventh cervical vertebra and cervical ribs. Instead of becoming parts of the vertebra, the costal elements developed as rudimentary ribs. The subclavian artery and usually the lower trunk of the brachial plexus pass over the rib. *B*, anteroposterior radiograph of the thorax and the cervical vertebral column. Observe the long cervical rib (*arrow*) passing superior to the first (thoracic) rib.

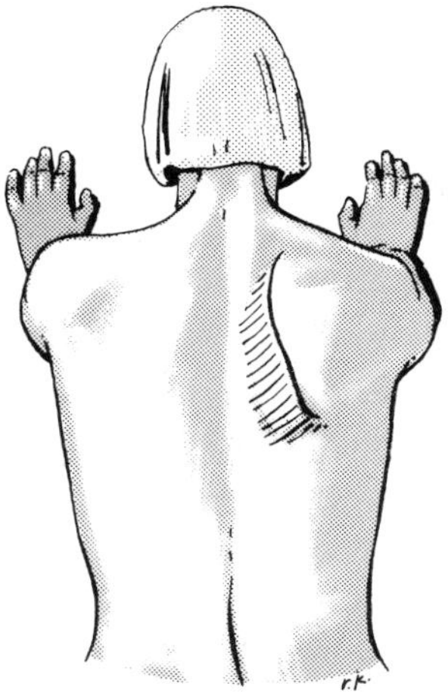

Figure 6-39. Drawing of a woman showing winging of the right scapula that resulted from a lesion of the long thoracic nerve. When the patient pushes against a wall with both hands, the vertebral or medial border of her right scapula stands out like a small wing. The patient is unable to raise her right arm fully.

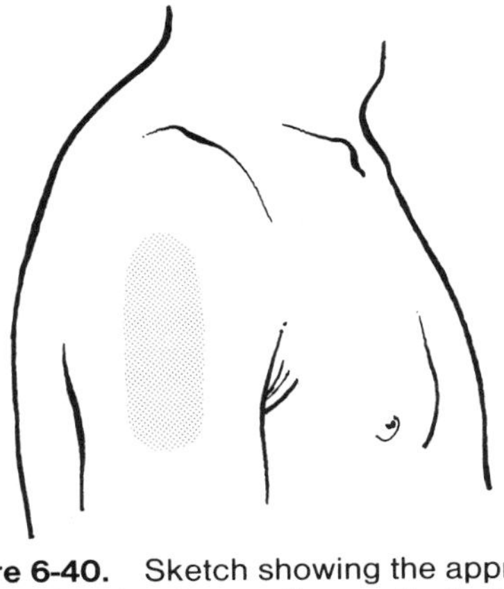

Figure 6-40. Sketch showing the approximate area of skin that is usually anesthetic in lesions of the axillary nerve.

The **subscapular artery** (Figs. 6-31 and 6-41), the largest branch of the axillary, descends along the axillary border of the scapula and ends as the circumflex scapular and thoracodorsal arteries. The **circumflex scapular artery** passes around the lateral border of the scapula to supply muscles on the dorsum of the scapula. The **thoracodorsal artery** continues the general course of the subscapular artery and supplies adjacent muscles, principally the **latissimus dorsi.**

The **anterior and posterior circumflex humeral arteries** pass around the surgical neck of the humerus and anastomose with each other (Fig. 6-41). The larger posterior circumflex humeral artery passes through the posterior axillary wall via the quadrangular space (Figs. 6-31 and 6-58) to supply the surrounding muscles (*e.g.,* the deltoid and triceps brachii).

CLINICALLY ORIENTED COMMENTS

There is much variation in the branching pattern of the axillary artery; hence, it is important to realize that *the branches of the axillary artery are named according to their distribution rather than their point of origin.*

There is extensive **arterial anastomosis around the scapula** (Fig. 6-42). Various vessels join to form extensive networks on both the costal and dorsal surfaces of the scapula. The surgical importance of this **collateral circulation** becomes apparent during ligation of an injured axillary or subclavian artery. Using Figure 6-43, verify that the axillary artery may be ligated between the thyrocervical trunk and the subscapular artery. In this case, the direction of blood flow in the subscapular artery becomes reversed and blood reaches the distal portion of the axillary artery first. Note that the subscapular artery receives its blood via several anastomoses with the suprascapular artery, transverse cervical artery, and some intercostal arteries. Understand that *ligation of the axillary artery distal to the subscapular artery would cut off the blood supply to the arm* (Figs. 6-41 and 6-43).

Axillary aneurysm (circumscribed dilation of the axillary artery) produces a fluctuant and pulsatile swelling in the axilla. If the first part of the artery is involved, the swelling projects forward, below the lateral part of the clavicle. When the aneurysm involves the third part of the artery, the

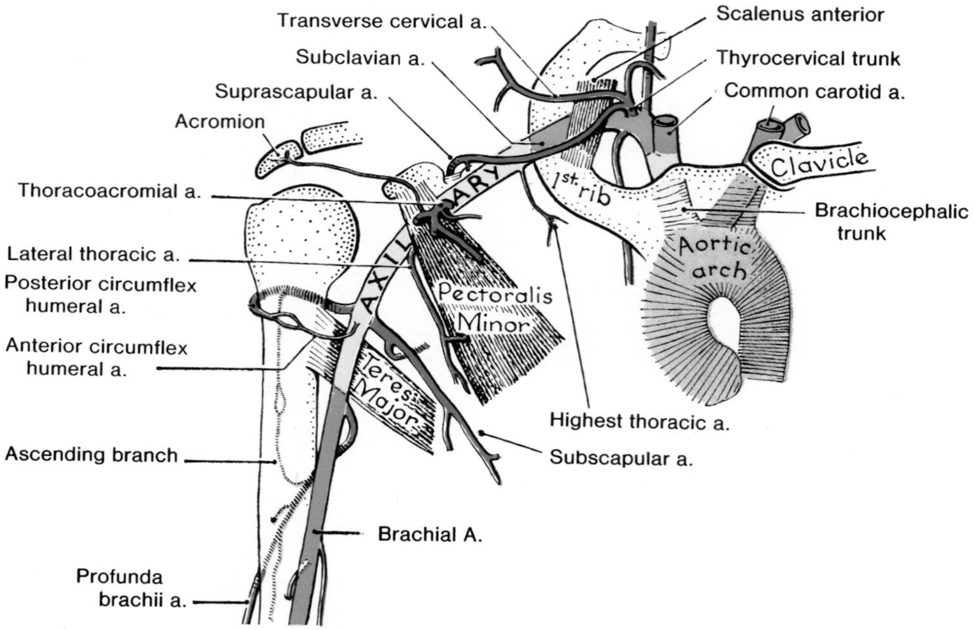

Figure 6-41. Diagram showing the named arteries of the axilla and arm. Note that the subclavian becomes the axillary artery at the lateral border of the first rib and that the axillary becomes the brachial artery at the lower border of the teres major.

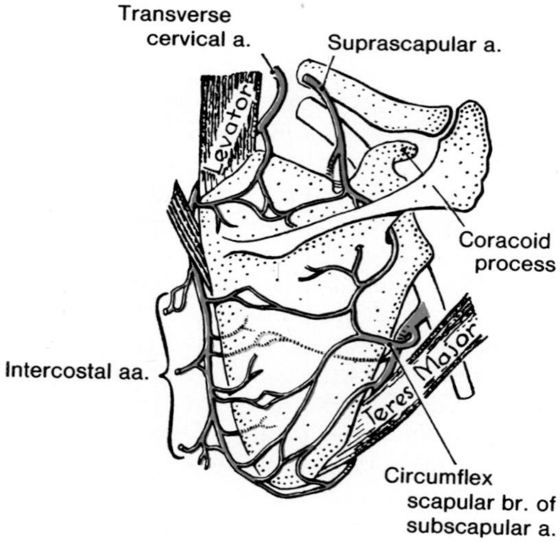

Figure 6-42. Drawing of a posterior view of the scapular region showing the extensive arterial anastomoses. Note that the various branches of the axillary artery take part in many anastomotic junctions with other branches of the axillary and with the branches of other arteries. See Figure 6-43 also.

anterior axillary fold is raised and the hollow of the axilla disappears owing to the presence of the soft pulsating mass. Because of the thinness of the **axillary sheath** (Figs. 6-45 and 6-46), the aneurysm commonly enlarges rapidly and compresses the nerves of the brachial plexus. This causes pain and subsequently loss of cutaneous sensibility (anesthesia) in the areas of the arm and forearm supplied by the nerves concerned. Weakness of the arm may result from pressure on the motor nerves, and edema of the forearm and the hand may result from compression of the axillary vein.

The Axillary Vein (Figs. 6-44 to 6-46). The large axillary vein lies on the medial side of the axillary artery and partly overlaps it. It completely overlaps the artery anteriorly when the arm is abducted.

The axillary vein *begins at the inferior border of the teres major* muscle as the continuation of the basilic vein (Fig. 6-44), which drains the medial surface of the fore-

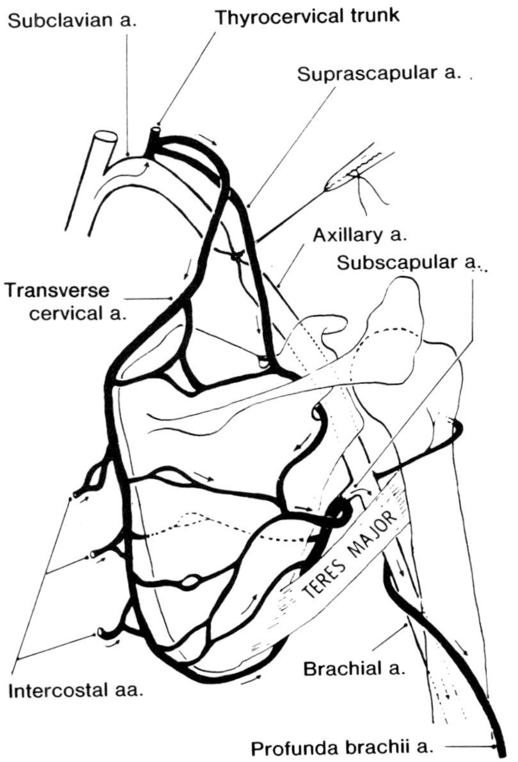

Figure 6-43. Drawing of a posterior view of the scapula and humerus showing the collateral circulation to the arm after ligation of the axillary artery. The *arrows* indicate the direction of blood flow.

arm and arm (Fig. 6-44). The axillary vein *ends at the outer border of the first rib,* where it becomes the **subclavian vein.** It receives tributaries that correspond to the six branches of the axillary artery, and at the lower margin of the subscapularis muscle, it receives the two **venae comitantes of the brachial artery** (Fig. 6-44). The venae comitantes are paired veins that are united by short branches to form a network around an artery. Above the level of the pectoralis minor, the axillary vein is joined by the **cephalic vein** (Figs. 6-23 and 6-44).

CLINICALLY ORIENTED COMMENTS

Wounds in the axilla often involve the axillary vein owing to its large size and exposed position (Fig. 6-44). A wound in the superior part of the vein, where it is largest, is particularly dangerous not only because of profuse hemorrhage, but also because of the risk of air entering the vessel. The walls of the axillary vein tend to be held apart by fibrous expansions from the clavipectoral fascia (Fig. 6-14). For this reason the axillary vein is isolated and cleared in axillary operations to avoid injuring it during subsequent dissection (*e.g.*, during removal of lymph nodes in radical mastectomy).

The cephalic vein can be punctured near the elbow (Fig. 6-77) for passing a fine pliable tube through it, the axillary vein, the subclavian vein, and onward into the heart. This is one technique used for doing **angiographic studies** of these vessels and the heart (*e.g.*, a radiograph of the heart after injection of radiopaque material).

The Axillary Sheath (Figs. 6-45 and 6-46). The axillary artery and vein and the cords of the brachial plexus are enveloped in a thin fascial (fibroareolar) sheath or tube which is continuous with the prevertebral layer of **cervical fascia.**

The Axillary Lymph Nodes (Figs. 6-10 and 6-47). There are 20 to 30 lymph nodes scattered in the fibrofatty connective tissue of the axilla; they are the main lymph nodes of the upper limb. The axillary lymph nodes are arranged in *five principal groups,* four of which lie below the pectoralis minor tendon and one (the apical group) above it.

The pectoral group (anterior group) consists of three to five lymph nodes that lie along the medial wall of the axilla in relation to the lateral thoracic artery and the lower border of the pectoralis major (Fig. 6-23). *The pectoral nodes receive lymph mainly from the anterior thoracic wall including* **the breast.** The efferent lymph vessels from these nodes pass to the central and apical groups of lymph nodes (Fig. 6-10).

The lateral group (brachial group) consists of four to six lymph nodes that lie along the lateral wall of the axilla, medial and posterior to the axillary vein. *The lateral nodes receive lymph from most of* **the**

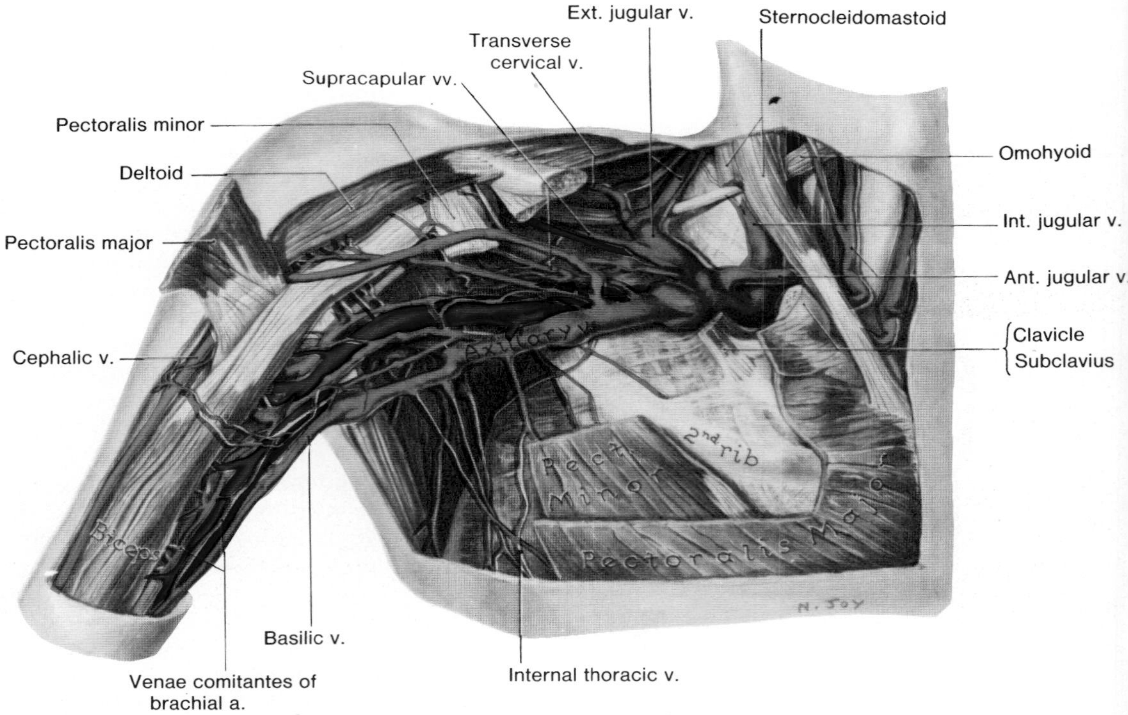

Figure 6-44. Drawing of a dissection of the axilla primarily to show its veins. Observe the basilic vein becoming the axillary at the lower border of the teres major; the axillary vein becoming the subclavian at the first rib; and the subclavian vein joining the internal jugular to become the brachiocephalic vein behind the sternal end of the clavicle. Many venous valves are visible (*e.g.*, one in the basilic, three in the axillary, and one in the subclavian). Note the venae comitantes (L. accompanying veins) of the brachial artery uniting and joining the axillary vein. Observe the cephalic vein here bifurcating to end both in the axillary and in the external jugular vein; usually it drains to the axillary vein.

upper limb; a few vessels accompany the cephalic vein and drain into the infraclavicular lymph nodes.

CLINICALLY ORIENTED COMMENTS

The lateral group of axillary lymph nodes is the first one to be involved in **lymphangitis** (inflammation of the lymphatic vessels) of the upper limb (*e.g.,* resulting from a hand infection).

The subscapular group (posterior group) consists of six or seven lymph nodes situated along the posterior axillary fold and the **subscapular blood vessels** (Fig. 6-31). *The subscapular nodes receive lymph from the posterior aspect of the thoracic wall and the* **scapular region.** Efferent vessels pass from them to the central group of axillary lymph nodes (Fig. 6-10).

The central group consists of three or four *large lymph nodes* situated near the base of the axilla in association with the second part of the axillary artery (*i.e.,* in the fat deep to the pectoralis minor). As its name indicates, *the central group receives lymph from* **three other groups of nodes** (pectoral, lateral, and subscapular). Efferent vessels from the central group pass to the apical group of axillary lymph nodes (Fig. 6-10).

The apical group consists of 6 to 12 lymph nodes situated in the **apex of the axilla,** along the medial side of the axillary vein and the first part of the axillary artery (Figs. 6-10 and 6-47). *The apical nodes* *receive lymph from* **all other axillary lymph nodes** and the efferent vessels from them unite to form the subclavian lymphatic trunk, which joins the jugular and bronchomediastinal trunks to form the **right lymphatic duct** on the right side; on the left side, it joins the **thoracic duct** (Figs. 1-48 and 9-40).

CLINICALLY ORIENTED COMMENTS

The axillary lymph nodes frequently become enlarged in **infections of the hand**, arm, shoulder, and axilla. Infections of adjacent parts (*e.g.*, the pectoral region and the breast) and the upper part of the front and side of the abdomen can also produce enlargement of the axillary nodes.

The axillary lymph nodes are frequently enlarged in later stages of cancers of the skin of the upper limb. In **breast cancer** they may be involved in any stage of the disease.

In carcinoma of the apical group (*e.g.*, owing to metastases from the mammary gland), the lymph nodes often adhere to the axillary vein, thereby necessitating excision of a part of this vessel. Enlargement of the apical nodes sometimes obstructs the cephalic vein where it pierces the coracoclav-

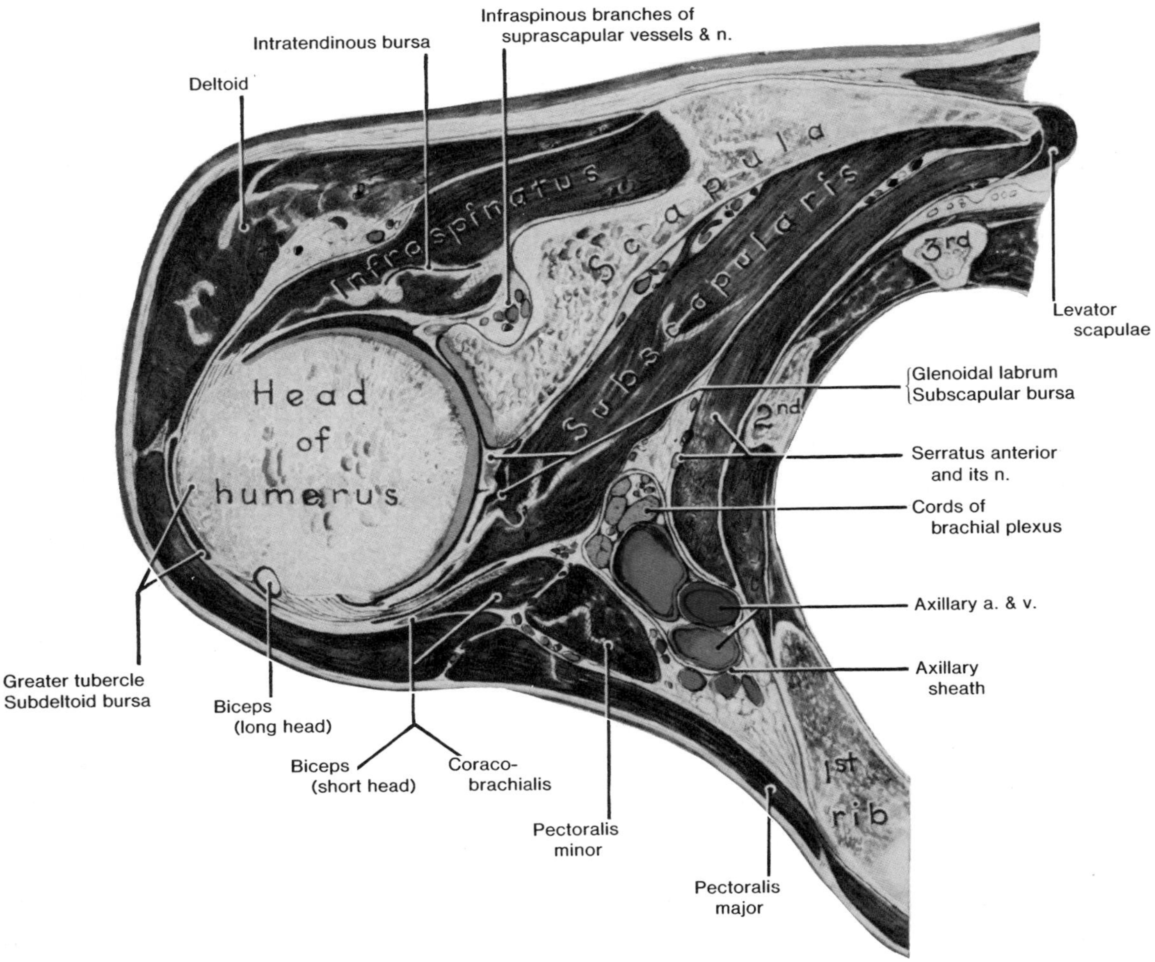

Figure 6-45. Drawing of a cross-section through the shoulder joint and the axilla near its apex. Observe the delicate axillary sheath of areolar tissue enclosing the axillary artery and vein and the three cords of the brachial plexus (and here an extra vein) to form a neurovascular bundle.

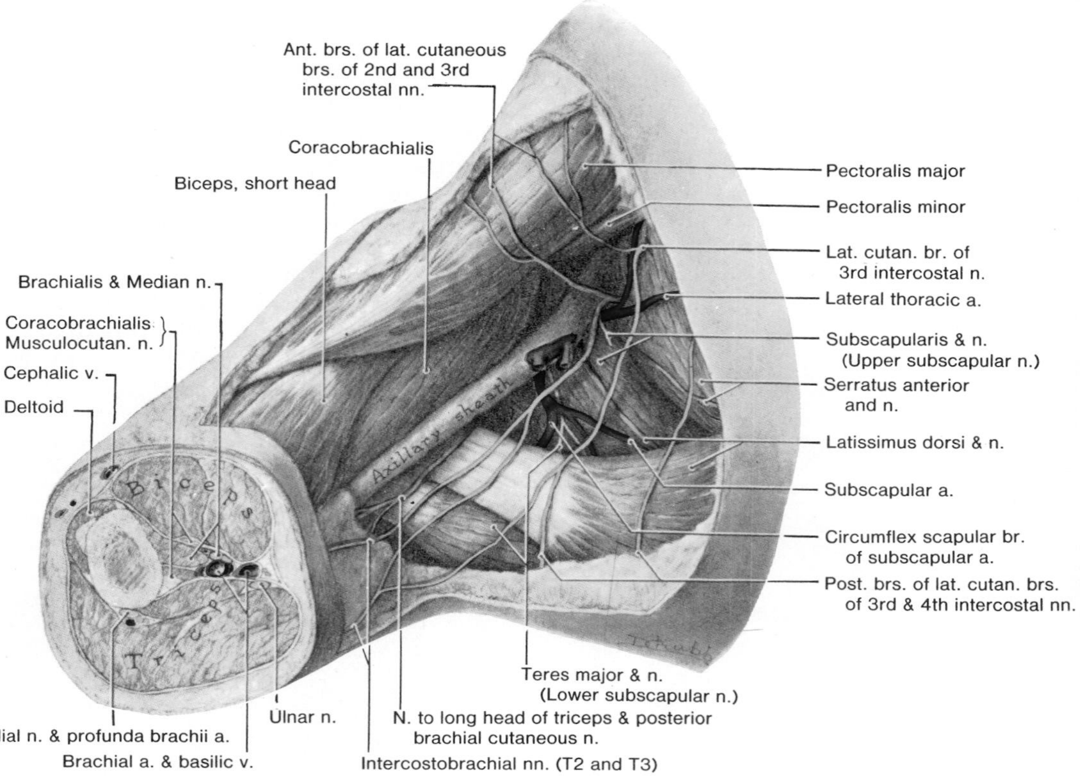

Figure 6-46. Drawing of a dissection of the axilla from below and of a cross-section of the arm. Observe the axillary sheath and the cutaneous nerves crossing the latissimus dorsi muscle. The most lateral of these nerves is also the sole nerve supply to the long head of the triceps muscle. Note that the axillary sheath transmits the great nerves and vessels of the upper limb; thus it is a neurovascular bundle.

icular membrane, superior to the pectoralis minor muscle (Figs. 6-14 and 6-23). *The axillary nodes are the most common site for metastases from a* **carcinoma of the breast** (Case 6-12).

THE BACK AND SHOULDER REGION

Although the back is described in Chapter 5, the superficial and intermediate groups (the extrinsic back muscles) that attach the upper limb to the vertebral column are described in this chapter.

The musculature of the shoulder may be divided into three groups: (1) **superficial extrinsic muscles** (trapezius and latissimus dorsi); (2) **deep extrinsic muscles** (levator scapulae, rhomboids, and serratus anterior); and (3) **intrinsic muscles** (deltoid, supraspinatus, infraspinatus, teres minor, teres major, and subscapularis). The muscles in the third group are described as intrinsic muscles because they arise and insert on the skeleton of the upper limb, running from the pectoral girdle (scapula and clavicle) to the humerus.

MUSCLES CONNECTING UPPER LIMB TO VERTEBRAL COLUMN

These muscles (trapezius, latissimus dorsi, levator scapulae, and rhomboidei minor and major) are extrinsic muscles of the back. In Figure 6-48, observe the dorsal rami of the spinal nerves supplying the skin of the back. Although these nerves supply

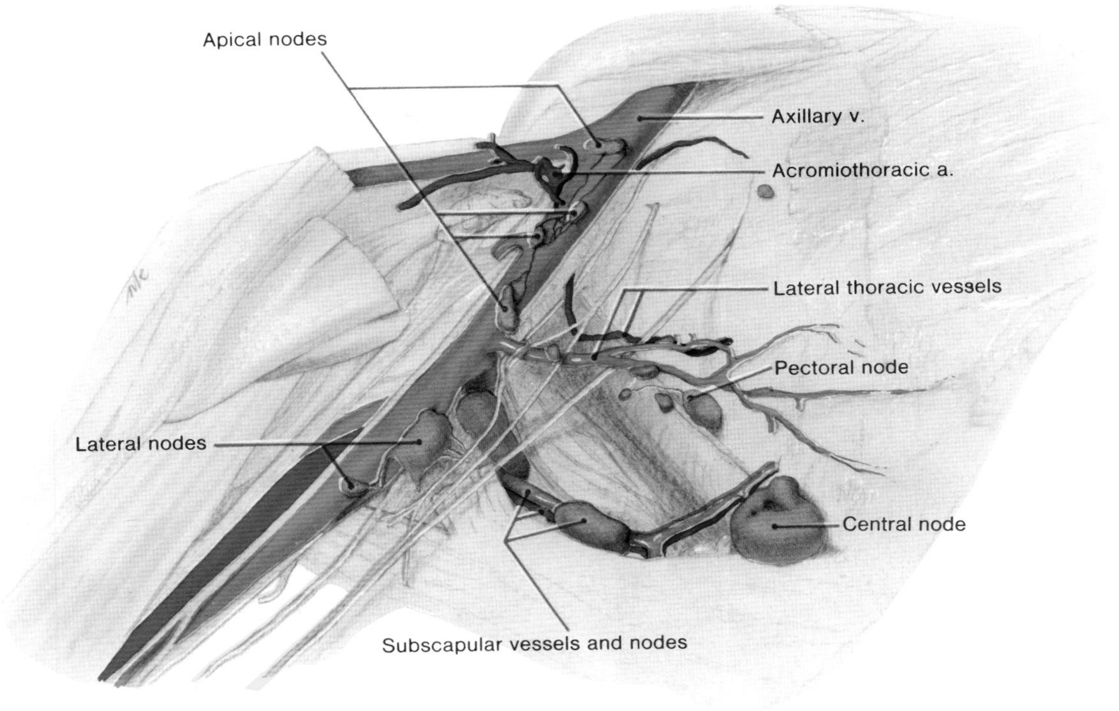

Figure 6-47. Drawing of a dissection of the axillary lymph nodes. These nodes, particularly the pectoral and subscapular groups, commonly receive over 75% of the lymph from the breast (dissected by Dr. Ross Mackenzie, Department of Anatomy, University of Toronto).

deep muscles of the back, they pass through the superficial layers of musculature of the shoulder without innervating them. These **extrinsic back muscles** are supplied by the ventral primary rami of cervical nerves. The explanation for this situation is that the superficial muscles develop as a ventrolateral sheet which migrates posteriorly in order to gain attachment to the vertebral column.

The Trapezius Muscle (Figs. 6-48 to 6-51). This large, flat, triangular muscle covers the back of the neck and upper half of the trunk. It was given its name because the muscles of the two sides form a *trapezion* (G. an irregular four-sided figure). The trapezius attaches the pectoral girdle to the skull and the vertebral column and assists in suspending pectoral girdle.

Origin (Fig. 6-48). Medial third of **superior nuchal line** of occipital bone, **external occipital protuberance, ligamentum nuchae, spinous processes of C7 to T12,** and supraspinous ligament.

Insertion (Figs. 6-3 and 6-50). **Lateral third of clavicle** (superior fibers), **acromion** and **spine of scapula** (middle fibers), and **base of scapular spine** (inferior fibers).

Nerve Supply (Fig. 6-48). Motor supply, **accessory** nerve (CN XI) and sensory branches from **third** and **fourth cervical** nerves.

Actions (Fig. 6-49). **Steadies, raises, retracts,** and **rotates scapula** so that the glenoid cavity faces upward and forward. *The superior fibers elevate the shoulder (e.g.,* when squaring the shoulders), *the middle fibers retract the scapula* (*i.e.,* pull it backward toward the midline), and *the inferior fibers depress the scapula and lower the shoulder,* assisting the superior fibers in rotating the scapula so that the glenoid cavity faces upward and forward.

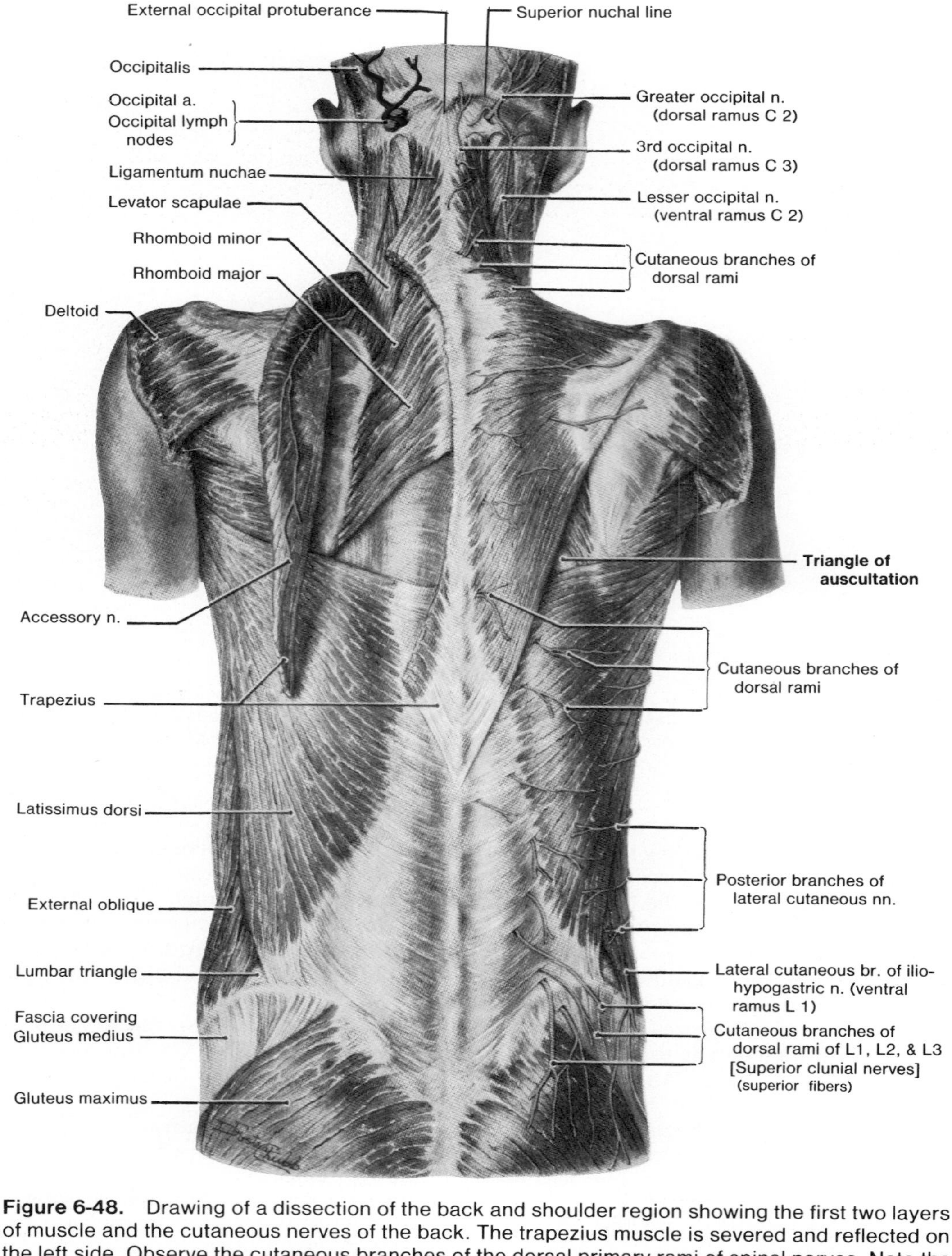

Figure 6-48. Drawing of a dissection of the back and shoulder region showing the first two layers of muscle and the cutaneous nerves of the back. The trapezius muscle is severed and reflected on the left side. Observe the cutaneous branches of the dorsal primary rami of spinal nerves. Note the trapezius and latissimus dorsi of the first layer and the levator scapulae and rhomboids of the second layer. These muscles help to attach the upper limb to the trunk. Observe the *triangle of auscultation* and the lumbar triangle. The ligamentum nuchae is a sheet of fibrous and elastic tissue interposed between the muscles of the two sides. It extends from the external occipital protuberance to the spinous processes of C1 to C7.

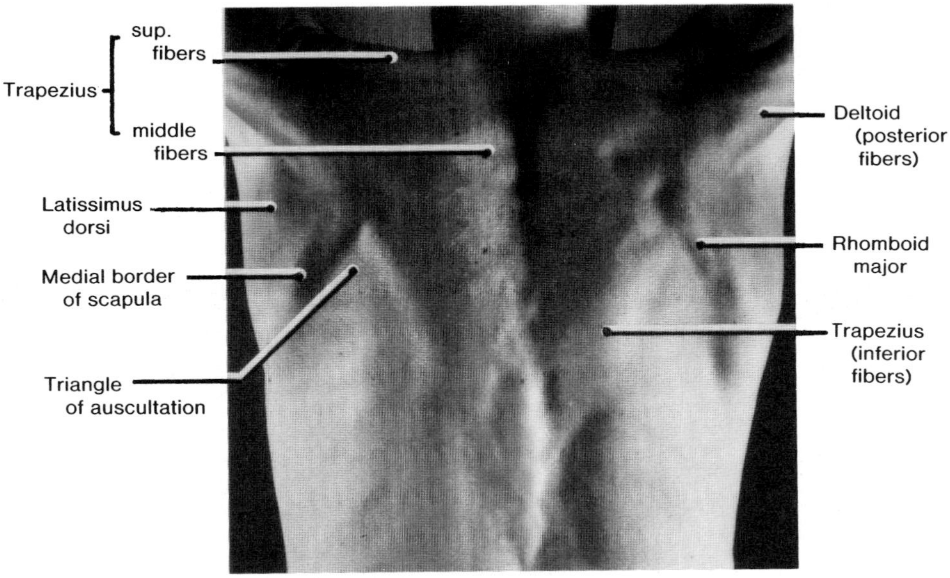

Figure 6-49. Photograph of the upper back region of a 46-year-old man with his arms elevated above his head. Observe the location of the medial (vertebral) border of the scapula. Compare with Figure 6-17. Because the superior fibers of the trapezius are attached to the lateral end of the spine of the scapula and the inferior fibers to its medial end, the scapula rotates when both groups of fibers contract. As a result the glenoid cavity faces upward and forward. This rotary action of the scapula which has occurred in the person photographed is essential for elevating the arms above the head.

The Latissimus Dorsi Muscle (Figs. 6-17, 6-48, 6-49, and 6-51). The Latin name of this muscle, meaning "widest of the back," is a good one because it covers the lower half of the back (T6 to iliac crest). This wide, thin, fan-shaped muscle passes between the trunk and the humerus and acts on the shoulder joint and indirectly on the pectoral girdle.

Origin (Fig. 6-48). **Spinous processes of lower six thoracic vertebrae** and, through the **thoracolumbar fascia** covering the extensor muscles of the vertebral column, to the **lumbar and sacral spinous processes.** Its lower lateral portion arises from the **iliac crest** and the **lower three** or **four ribs.**

Insertion (Figs. 6-1 and 6-54). Floor of **intertubercular sulcus** of humerus. In Figure 6-32, observe that its ribbon-like tendon winds around the inferior border of the teres major muscle. Also observe that this muscle approaches the axilla from behind (Fig. 6-48) and runs in the posterior wall of the axilla before inserting into the humerus (Fig. 6-15).

Nerve Supply. **Thoracodorsal** nerve (C6 to C8) from posterior cord of brachial plexus.

Actions. **Extends, adducts,** and **medially rotates humerus at shoulder** joint. Its most powerful action is in drawing the arm down from above the head (*e.g.,* when climbing). It is also very active when paddling a canoe and in swimming, particularly during the crawl stroke.

CLINICALLY ORIENTED COMMENTS

In Figure 6-48, observe that the superior border of the latissimus dorsi and a part of the rhomboideus major are overlapped by the trapezius. The triangle formed by the borders of these three muscles is called the **triangle of auscultation** (L. to listen). If

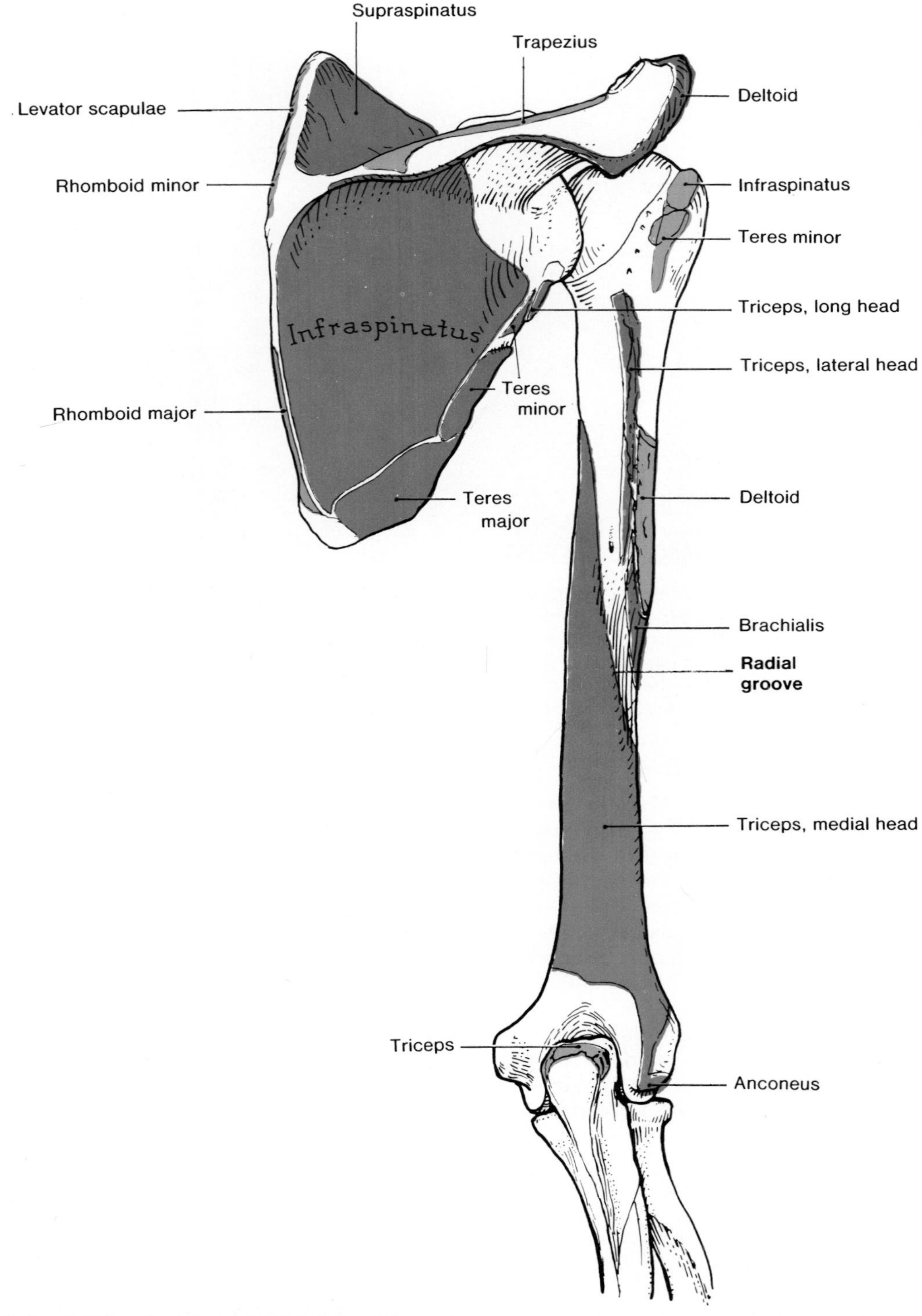

Figure 6-50. Drawing of a posterior view of the scapula and the bones of the arm and forearm, *right side*, showing the attachment of muscles to them. Observe that the lateral head of the triceps arises above and lateral to the groove for the radial nerve and that the medial head arises below and medial to this radial groove.

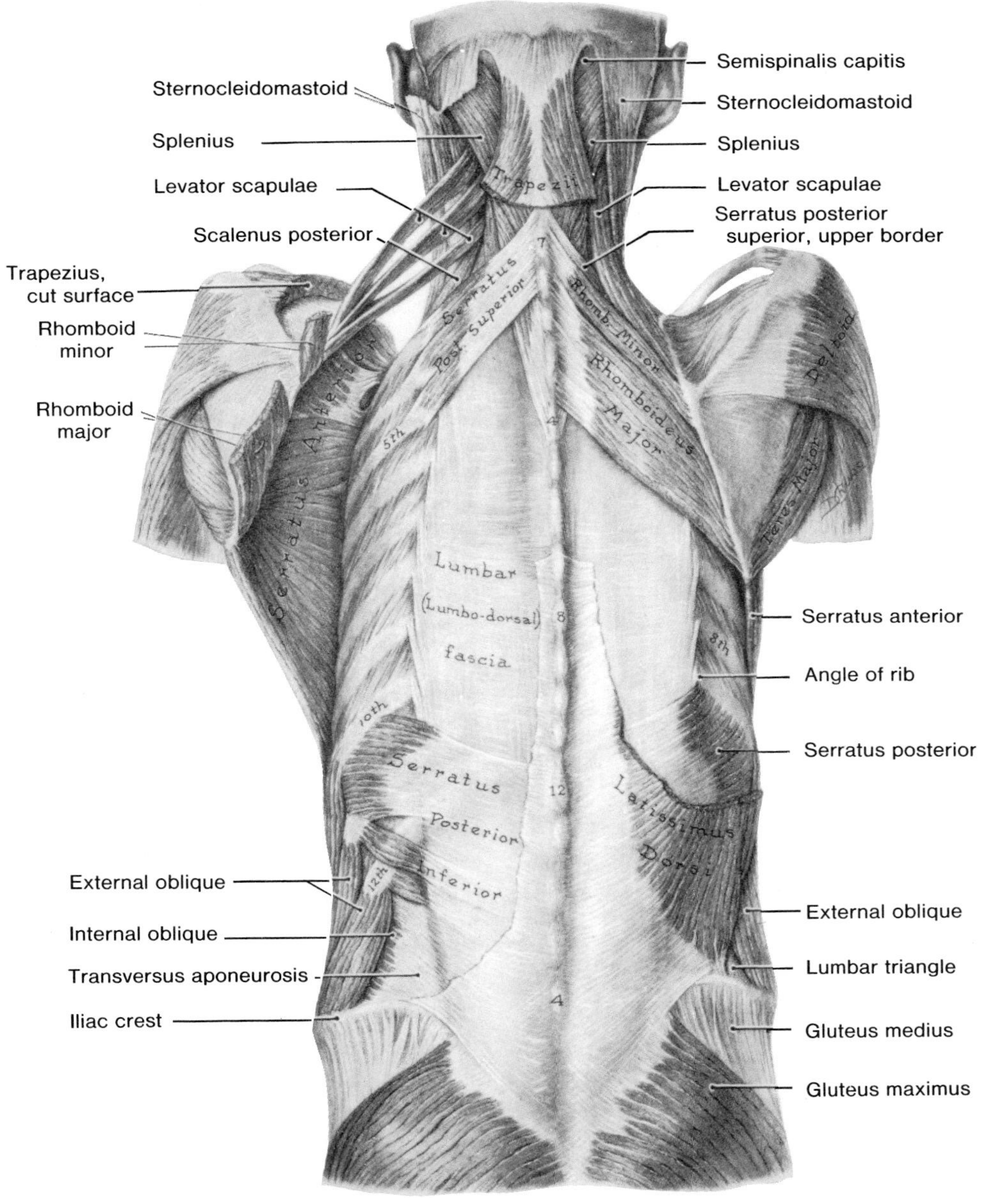

Figure 6-51. Drawing of a dissection of the back showing the intermediate muscles. The trapezius and latissimus dorsi are largely cut away on both sides. On the *right side*, observe the levator scapulae and rhomboidei. Note the serratus superior rising above the rhomboid minor. On the *left side*, observe the rhomboidei severed and allowing the vertebral border of the scapula to part from the thoracic wall. Note the three digitations (slips) of the levator scapulae. Observe the thoracolumbar (lumbar) fascia, extending laterally to the angles of the ribs, becoming thin superiorly, passing deep to serratus superior, and reinforced inferiorly by the latissimus dorsi and serratus inferior.

the scapula is drawn forward by folding the arms across the chest and the trunk is flexed, the triangle enlarges and its lateral side is formed by the medial border of the scapula. Parts of the sixth and seventh ribs and the sixth intercostal space between them become subcutaneous; consequently, *respiratory sounds may be heard with a stethoscope in the auscultatory triangle* (Fig. 6-69).

The Levator Scapulae Muscle (Figs. 6-48 and 6-51). The superior third of this thick, strap-like muscle lies deep to the sternocleidomastoid and the inferior third lies deep to the trapezius.

Origin (Fig. 6-51). **Transverse processes of first three** or **four cervical vertebrae.**

Insertion (Figs. 6-48 and 6-50). **Upper part of medial border of scapula** from superior angle to spine.

Nerve Supply. **Dorsal scapular** nerve (C5) and **third** and **fourth cervical** nerves.

Actions. **Elevates scapula** and **helps to tilt the glenoid cavity downward** by rotating the scapula. It also *helps to retract the scapula and fix it against the trunk.*

MUSCLES CONNECTING UPPER LIMB TO THORACIC WALL

This group includes the serratus anterior, the pectoralis minor, the pectoralis major, and the subclavius. All these muscles, except the serratus anterior, have been previously described with the pectoral muscles.

The Serratus Anterior Muscle (Figs. 6-51 to 6-54). This large, thin, foliate, powerful muscle overlies the lateral portion of the thorax and the intercostal muscles. It was given its name (L. *serratus*, a saw) because of the saw-toothed appearance of the fleshy digitations at its origin.

Origin (Figs. 6-51 to 6-53). **Outer surfaces of first eight ribs**, about midway between their angles and costal cartilages. Its lower three digitations interdigitate with the origin of the external oblique muscle of the abdomen.

Insertion (Fig. 6-54). **Entire anterior surface of medial border of scapula.**

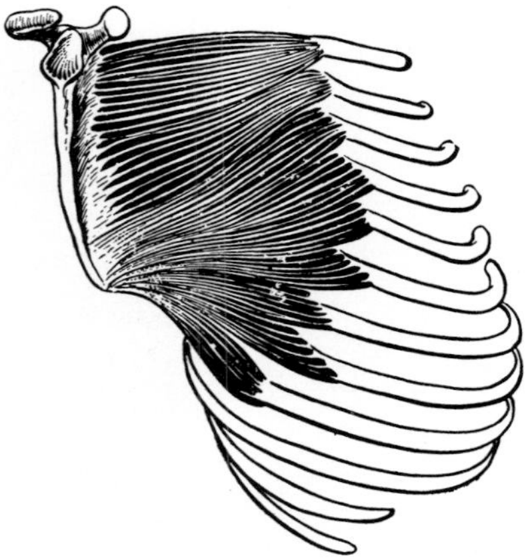

Figure 6-52. Drawing of the right serratus anterior arising *in this specimen* from the outer surfaces of the upper nine ribs. The scapula has been swung away from the chest wall to expose the entire muscle.

Nerve Supply (Fig. 6-32). **Long thoracic** nerve (C5 to C7).

Actions. **Protracts scapula** and **holds it against chest** wall. Because it acts when pushing or punching, it is often called "*the boxer's muscle.*" By fixing the scapula to the chest, it acts as an anchor for this bone allowing other muscles to use it as a fixed bone for producing movements of the humerus. *Its lower fibers* help to **rotate glenoid cavity of scapula upward** (*e.g.*, when arm is raised above the head as in Figures 6-49 and 6-53).

CLINICALLY ORIENTED COMMENTS

When the serratus anterior is paralyzed owing to **injury of the long thoracic nerve**, the scapula stands out like a wing when the person presses forward with the outstretched limb, *e.g.*, when pressing against a wall (Fig. 6-39). This condition is called a "**winged scapula.**" When the arm is raised, the scapula is pulled away from the chest wall in an uncontrollable fashion and the arm cannot be abducted farther than the horizontal position because the serratus anterior is unable to rotate the glenoid cavity upward.

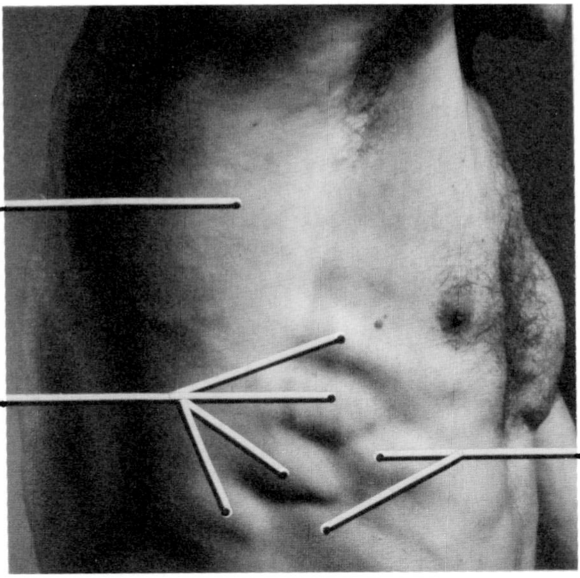

Figure 6-53. Photograph of a lateral view of the thorax of a 46-year-old man. Observe that the lower three digitations of the serratus anterior muscle interdigitate with the external oblique muscle of the abdomen. As it is inserted into the entire length of the medial margin of the scapula (Fig. 6-54), the serratus anterior is a powerful protractor of the scapula. It also holds the scapula against the chest wall.

The Rhomboid Muscles (Figs. 6-48 to 6-51). These two muscles lie deep to the trapezius. The **rhomboideus major** is about two times wider than the **rhomboideus minor**. The muscles appear as parallel bands that pass obliquely downward and laterally from the vertebrae to the scapula. They have a rhomboid appearance, *i.e.*, they form an oblique parallelogram.

Origin (Fig. 6-48). **Ligamentum nuchae** and **spinous processes of C7 to T5 vertebrae** (rhomboideus minor C7 and T1; rhomboideus major T2 to T5).

Insertion (Fig. 6-50). **Medial border of scapula** from base of spine to inferior angle.

Nerve Supply (Fig. 6-27). **Dorsal scapular** nerve (C5).

Actions. **Retract** and **elevate scapula** and help serratus anterior to fix it against trunk. Acting with the latissimus dorsi, they **rotate glenoid cavity downward** when the arm is lowered against resistance (*e.g.*, when paddling a canoe).

THE SCAPULAR MUSCLES

Six short muscles (deltoid, supraspinatus, infraspinatus, subscapularis, and teres major and minor) pass from the scapula to the humerus and act on the shoulder joint.

The Deltoid Muscle (Figs. 6-5, 6-17, 6-19 to 6-24, 6-48 to 5-51, and 6-55 to 6-58). This thick, powerful, triangular muscle covers the shoulder joint and, along with the underlying skeleton, forms the rounded contour of the shoulder. As its name indicates, it is triangular in outline, *i.e.*, shaped like the Greek letter *delta* (Δ) inverted.

Origin (Figs. 6-50 and 6-55). Anterior border of **lateral third of clavicle**, lateral border of **acromion**, and **crest of spine** of scapula. In Figures 6-55 and 6-56, observe the V-shaped origin from the pectoral girdle.

Insertion (Figs. 6-21, 6-54, 6-55, and 6-67). **Deltoid tuberosity of humerus.**

Nerve Supply (Figs. 6-32 and 6-58). **Axillary** nerve (C5 and C6) from posterior cord of brachial plexus.

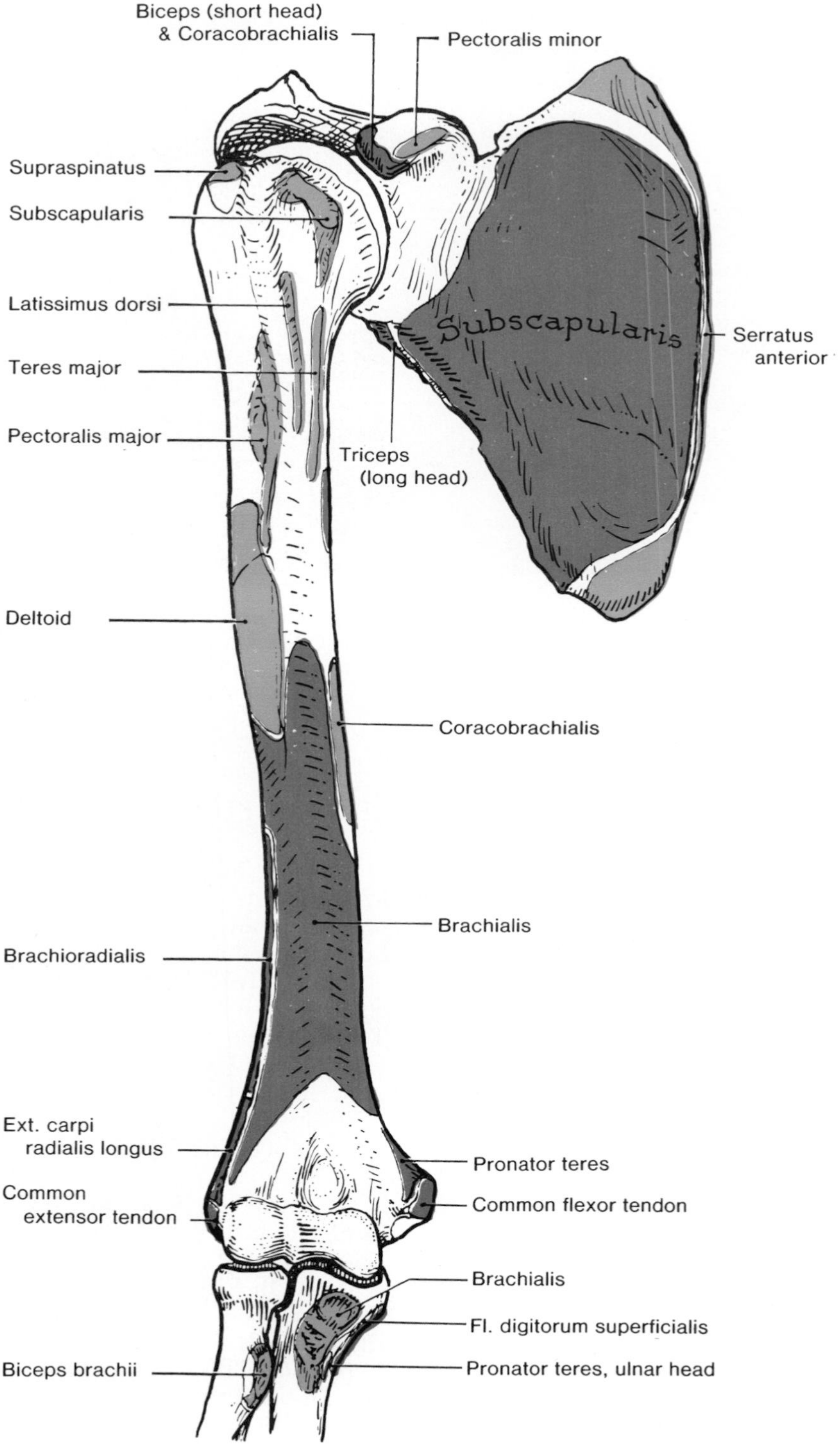

Figure 6-54. Drawing of an anterior view of the scapula and the bones of the arm and forearm, *right side*, showing the attachment of muscles to them.

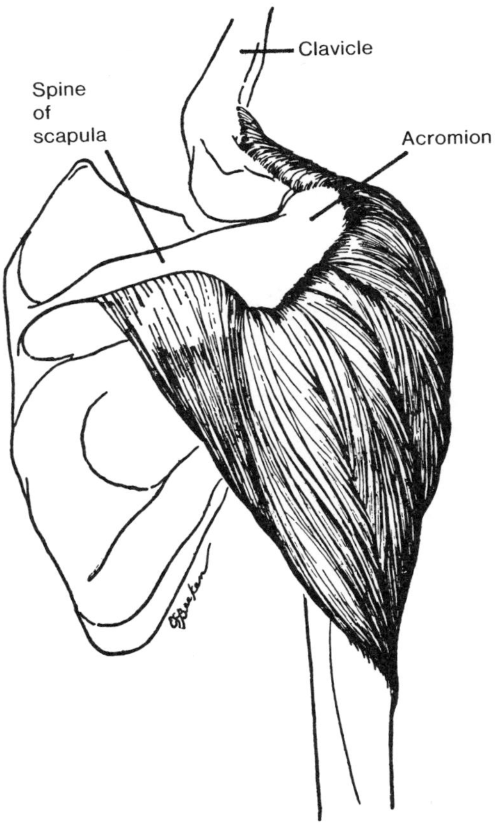

Figure 6-55. Drawing of the posterior aspect of the right deltoid muscle showing its extensive origin from the lateral third of the clavicle, the acromion and spine of the scapula. Note that the triangular-shaped deltoid caps the shoulder and gives it a rounded contour (Figs. 6-5, 6-56, and 6-71).

Actions. Functionally, the fibers of the deltoid may be divided into three parts: anterior, middle, and posterior, but the *muscle is capable of acting in part or as a whole.*The actions of its three parts are as follows: (1) the *anterior part* is a strong **flexor** and **medial rotator of humerus**; (2) the *middle (acromial) part* is the **chief abductor of humerus**; and (3) the *posterior part* is a strong **extensor** and **lateral rotator of humerus**. In performing the above movements, the deltoid works with other muscles, *e.g.*, the anterior part acts with the pectoralis major in flexing the arm, and the middle part acts with the supraspinatus in abducting the arm. The deltoid is active during arm swinging (*e.g.*, during walking).

CLINICALLY ORIENTED COMMENTS

Although the deltoid is a powerful abductor of the humerus, particularly the middle fibers, it cannot initiate this movement because when the arm is by the side the line of pull of the intermediate part of the muscle is parallel to the shaft of the humerus. The supraspinatus muscle (Figs. 6-60 and 6-63) is very important during the early phases of abduction but both muscles act together throughout abduction of the arm.

Each of these muscles is supplied by the fifth and sixth cervical nerve segments via the axillary (deltoid) and suprascapular (supraspinatus) nerves. Hence injury to these nerves or to the fifth and sixth cervical segments will affect abduction of the arm. The deltoid atrophies in cases of paralysis of the axillary nerve; thus, the rounded shape of the shoulder is lost, giving it a flattened appearance similar to that present with dislocation of the shoulder (Fig. 6-155).

To test the deltoid clinically, the patient's arm is abducted in the plane of the scapula to about 45°, and then the patient is asked to hold it there against resistance. Inability to do this indicates injury to the axillary nerve supplying the deltoid, *e.g.*, associated with fracture of the surgical neck of the humerus.

The Teres Major Muscle (Figs. 6-46, 6-51, 6-57, and 6-58). The teres (L. round) major forms a raised oval area on the dorsum of the scapula, beginning at the inferior angle. The lower border of this thick, rounded muscle forms the lower border of the posterior wall of the axilla (Fig. 6-13). The teres major and the tendon of the latissimus dorsi form the posterior axillary fold (Figs. 6-16 and 6-57).

Origin (Figs. 6-50 and 6-51). Oval area on **dorsal surface of scapula close to inferior angle.**

Insertion (Fig. 6-54). **Medial lip of intertubercular sulcus** (crest of lesser tubercle) of humerus.

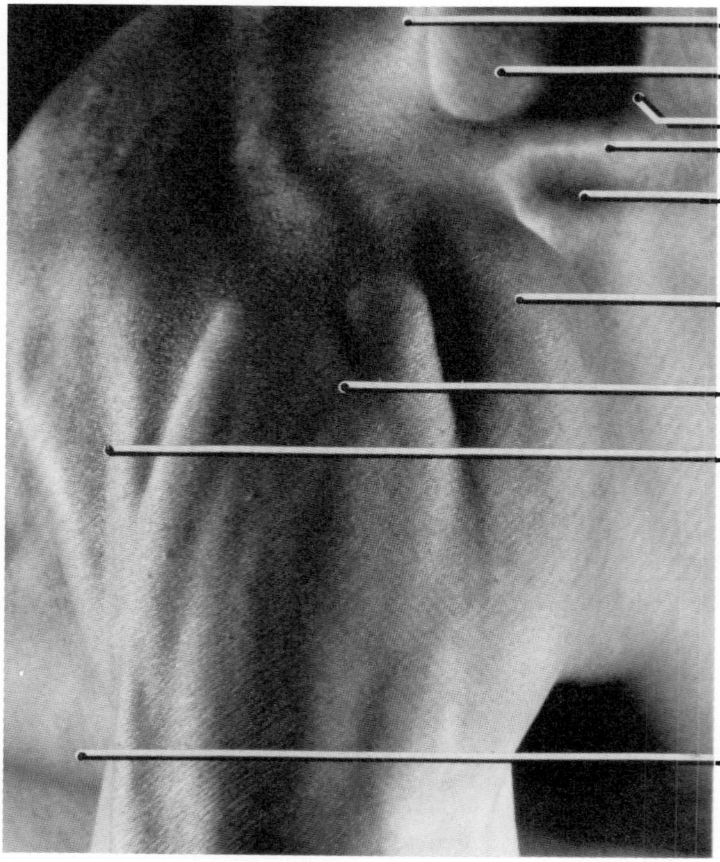

Figure 6-56. Photograph of a lateral view of the neck and shoulder regions of a 46-year-old man. To make parts of his deltoid muscle stand out, the subject abducted his arm against resistance. For a good illustration of this muscle in a child, see Figure 6-5. The appearance of the deltoid and the way its parts attach to the pectoral girdle (Fig. 6-55) give clues to the muscle's actions. The anterior fibers flex the arm at the shoulder joint and medially rotate it; the posterior fibers reverse these movements; and the middle fibers, acting with the supraspinatus, abduct the arm at the shoulder joint.

Nerve Supply (Fig. 6-31). **Lower subscapular** nerve (C6 and C7) from posterior cord of brachial plexus.

Actions. **Adducts** and **medially rotates humerus.** It can help to extend it from the flexed position and is an **important stabilizer** of the proximal end of the humerus during abduction.

The Rotator Cuff Muscles (Figs. 6-58 and 6-60). Four muscles joining the scapula to the humerus (**supraspinatus, infraspinatus, teres minor**, and **subscapularis**) are referred to as the rotator cuff or guardian muscles of the shoulder joint because **their main function is to hold the head of the humerus in the glenoid cavity** of the scapula. They are also concerned with rotation of the humerus about its longitudinal axis.

The tendons of the rotator cuff muscles blend to form a musculotendinous sheath, called **the rotator cuff**, which is attached to the underlying fibrous capsule of the shoulder joint. This rotator cuff protects the shoulder joint and gives it stability by holding the head of the humerus in the glenoid cavity.

Bursae of various sizes (Figs. 6-59 and 6-

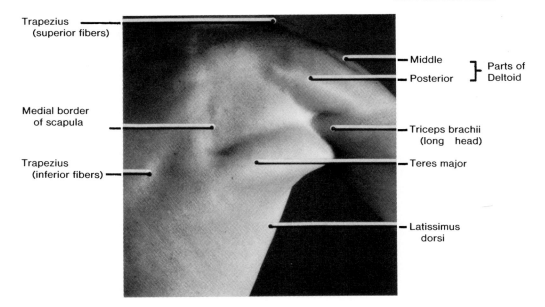

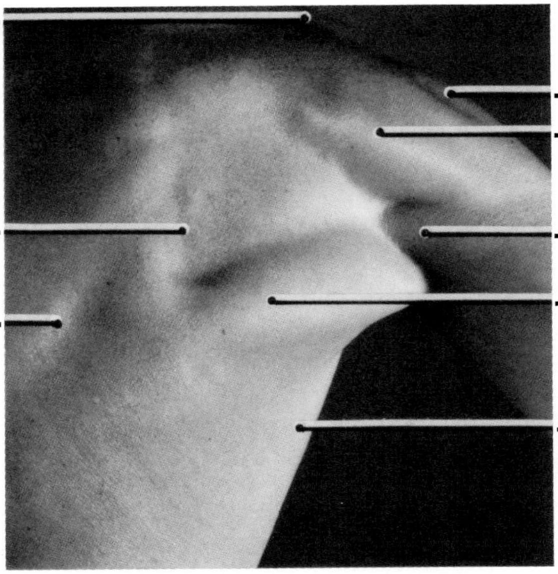

Figure 6-57. Photograph of the back and scapular region of a 46-year-old man showing the scapular and arm muscles. The teres major muscle was made to stand out by asking him to adduct his arm against resistance.

61) are located between the tendons making up the rotator cuff and the fibrous capsule of the shoulder joint. They reduce the friction on tendons passing over bones or other areas of resistance.

The Supraspinatus Muscle (Figs. 6-60 and 6-63). This rounded muscle lies in the supraspinatus fossa of the scapula, deep to the trapezius and the **coracoacromial arch** (Fig. 6-60). Its tendon is covered by the deltoid.

Origin (Fig. 6-50). Medial two-thirds of **floor of supraspinous fossa** of scapula.

Insertion (Figs. 6-21, 6-54, and 6-60). **Top of greater tubercle** of humerus.

Nerve Supply (Fig. 6-31). **Suprascapular** nerve (C5 and C6) from upper trunk of brachial plexus.

Actions. **Stabilizes shoulder joint** and **abducts humerus.**

The supraspinatus and the deltoid act together and progressively in elevating the humerus at the shoulder joint. The supraspinatus alone is unable to initiate abduction. It also acts strongly when the shoulder is adducted, preventing downward dislocation of the humerus in the glenoid cavity (*e.g.*, when carrying a heavy suitcase).

CLINICALLY ORIENTED COMMENTS

When the supraspinatus muscle is paralyzed, some patients produce initial abduction of the humerus by leaning slightly to the side, thereby using gravity to replace the action of the supraspinatus. Other patients initiate abduction of the humerus by knocking their elbow out with a jerk of the hip, which allows the deltoid to take over abduction.

The subacromial bursa (Fig. 6-61) is always large. It separates the acromion and the superior part of the deltoid muscle from the muscles that lie on the superior surface of the capsule of the shoulder joint. It contains a small amount of synovial fluid that makes its inner surface slippery; thus, it is able to reduce friction during movements of the shoulder when the supraspinatous tendon passes inferior to the coracoacromial arch (Fig. 6-60). It also facilitates movement of the deltoid over the fibrous capsule of the shoulder joint and the musculotendinous rotator cuff.

The Subscapularis Muscle (Figs. 6-45,

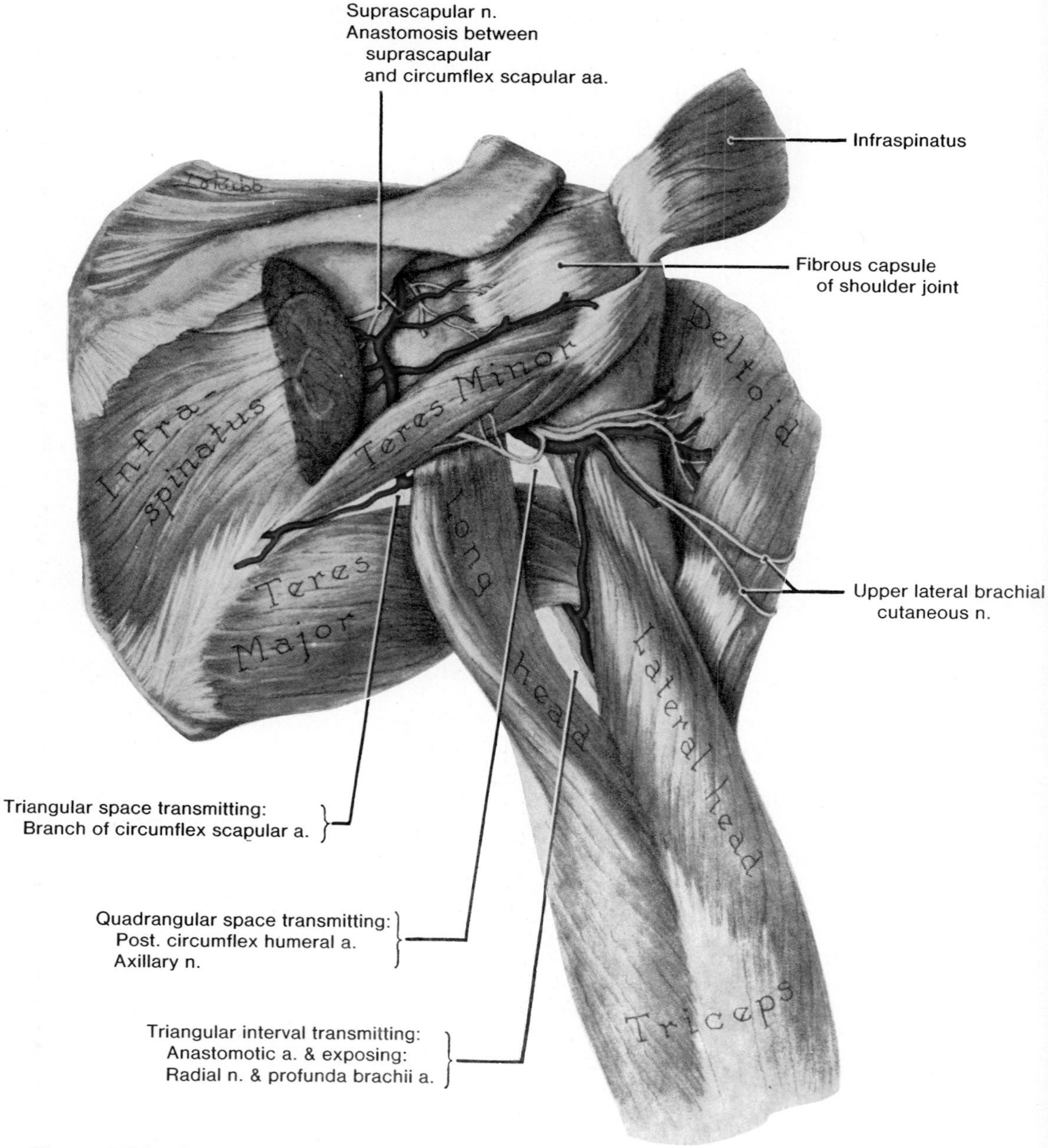

Figure 6-58. Drawing of a dissection of the posterior scapular and subdeltoid regions. Observe the thickness of the infraspinatus muscle which, aided by the teres minor and posterior fibers of the deltoid, rotates the humerus laterally. Note the long head of the triceps muscle passing between the teres minor, a lateral rotator, and the teres major, a medial rotator. Observe the long head of the triceps separating the quadrangular space from the triangular space and the teres major separating the quadrangular space from another triangular space. Note that the axillary nerve passes through the quadrangular space and winds around the surgical neck of the humerus. Consequently this nerve may be injured in a fracture of the humerus in this region. Note the arterial anastomoses on and around the scapula and the distribution of the suprascapular and axillary nerves. Each comes from C5 and C6; each supplies two muscles (supraspinatus and infraspinatus, teres minor and deltoid, respectively); each supplies the shoulder joint; only one (the axillary nerve) has cutaneous branches.

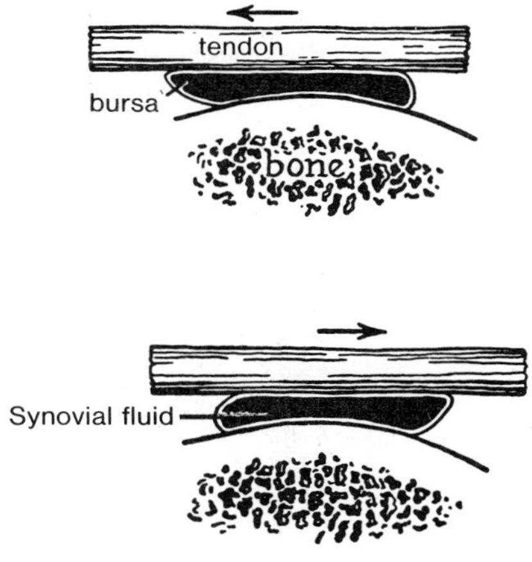

Figure 6-59. Drawings illustrating that a bursa (L. purse) is a device for eliminating friction wherever a muscle or tendon is liable to rub on another muscle, tendon, or bone. Understand that a bursa is a flattened sac and that its walls are separated merely by a *capillary film of synovial fluid* which acts as a lubricant that enables its walls to slide freely over each other.

6-60, and 6-62). This large, thick triangular muscle lies on the costal surface of the scapula and forms much of the posterior wall of the axilla.

Origin (Fig. 6-54). **Medial two-thirds of subscapular fossa** on costal surface of scapula.

Insertion (Fig. 6-54). **Lesser tubercle of humerus.** Its stout tendon is attached to the fibrous capsule of the shoulder joint and is separated from the neck of the scapula by the large **subscapularis bursa** (Fig. 6-45).

Nerve Supply (Fig. 6-31). **Upper** and **lower subscapular** nerves (C5 to C7) from posterior cord of brachial plexus.

Actions. **Medially rotates humerus** and **holds humeral head in glenoid cavity** (*i.e.*, stabilizes shoulder joint).

The Teres Minor Muscle (Figs. 6-58 and 6-63). This narrow, elongated muscle is often inseparable from the infraspinatus muscle and lies along its inferior border.

Origin (Figs. 6-50 and 6-63). Upper two-thirds of **lateral border of scapula** on dorsal surface, superior to origin of teres major.

Insertion (Figs. 6-50 and 6-63). Lowest facet on **greater tubercle of humerus.** The long head of the triceps muscle separates its tendon from the teres major, thereby producing a triangular space and a larger quadrangular space (Fig. 6-58).

Nerve Supply (Figs. 6-31 and 6-32). **Axillary** nerve (C5 and C6) from posterior cord of brachial plexus.

Actions. **Laterally rotates** and **adducts humerus** and **holds humeral head in glenoid cavity** (*i.e.*, stabilizes shoulder joint).

The Infraspinatus Muscle (Figs. 6-58, 6-60, and 6-63). This thick, triangular muscle occupies most of the infraspinous fossa.

Origin (Figs. 6-50 and 6-63). **Medial two-thirds of infraspinous fossa.**

Insertion (Figs. 6-50 and 6-63). Middle facet on **greater tubercle of humerus.** Its tendon is adherent to the fibrous capsule of the shoulder joint.

Nerve Supply (Fig. 6-31). **Suprascapular** nerve (C5 and C6) from upper trunk of brachial plexus.

Actions. **Laterally rotates humerus** and **holds humeral head in glenoid cavity** (*i.e.*, stabilizes shoulder joint).

CLINICALLY ORIENTED COMMENTS

The musculotendinous **rotator cuff** that holds the head of the humerus in the glenoid cavity of the scapula may be damaged by injury or disease. Trauma may tear or rupture the tendons of the rotator cuff muscles. **Degenerative tendonitis** is the most common disease, especially in older people, and calcium deposits may be demonstrated on radiographs in the supraspinatus tendon or in other tendons of the cuff. Tendonitis often leads to adherence of the supraspinatus tendon to the floor of the subacromial bursa and predisposes the tendon to rupture (Fig. 6-64). The calcium deposit often ruptures into the bursa producing a very painful **chemical bursitis**.

The supraspinatus tendon does not rupture very often in young people because their tendons are usually so strong that they tear away (avulse) the top of the greater tubercle of the humerus rather than rupture.

Tendonitis and inflammation of the subacromial bursa (**bursitis**) *result in shoul-*

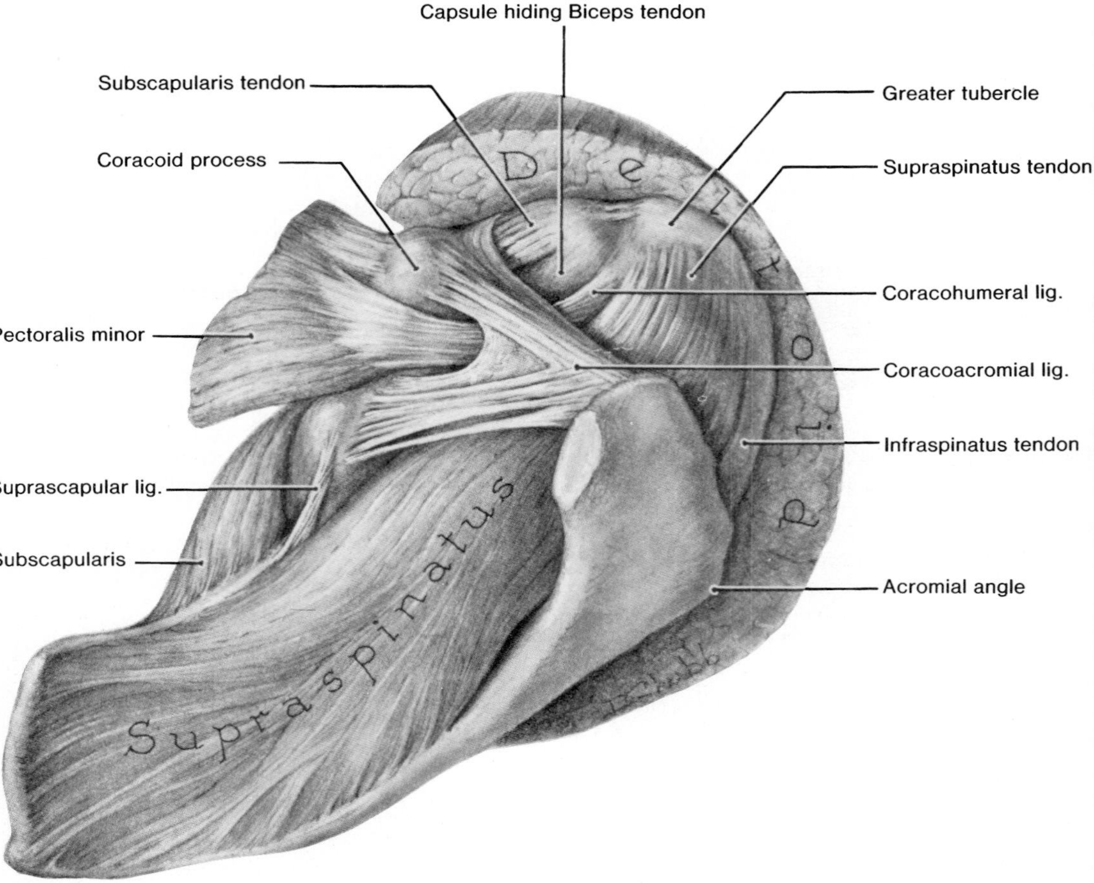

Figure 6-60. Drawing of a dissection of the supraspinous and subdeltoid regions. Observe the supraspinatus muscle passing inferior to the *coracoacromial arch* formed by the coracoid process, the coracoacromial ligament, and the acromion. Understand that this muscle lies between the deltoid above and the articular capsule of the shoulder joint below. The supraspinatus and the middle fibers of the deltoid are abductors of the arm at this joint. In this action the powerful middle part of the deltoid (Fig. 6-56) is the main abductor, but it requires help from the supraspinatus in the early phases of abduction in particular.

der pain which is intensified by attempts to abduct or laterally rotate the arm. Curiously when both shoulders are radiographed, there may be no calcium in the tendon or bursa on the side giving symptoms, but calcium may be observed in the asymptomatic shoulder region.

The main stability of the shoulder joint is provided by the tendons of the rotator cuff muscles that fuse with the capsule of the joint and insert into the greater and lesser tubercles of the humerus. This musculotendinous cuff strengthens the shoulder joint, except inferiorly; consequently, if a person falls when the humerus is abducted, the head of this bone may be levered out of the glenoid cavity of the scapula, producing a condition known as **dislocation of the shoulder** joint (Case 6-4). During dislocation, the acromion acts as the fulcrum of the lever.

Fractures of the clavicle are relatively common. *The weakest part of the clavicle is at the junction of the middle and lateral thirds.* One function of the clavicle is to transmit forces from the upper limb to the

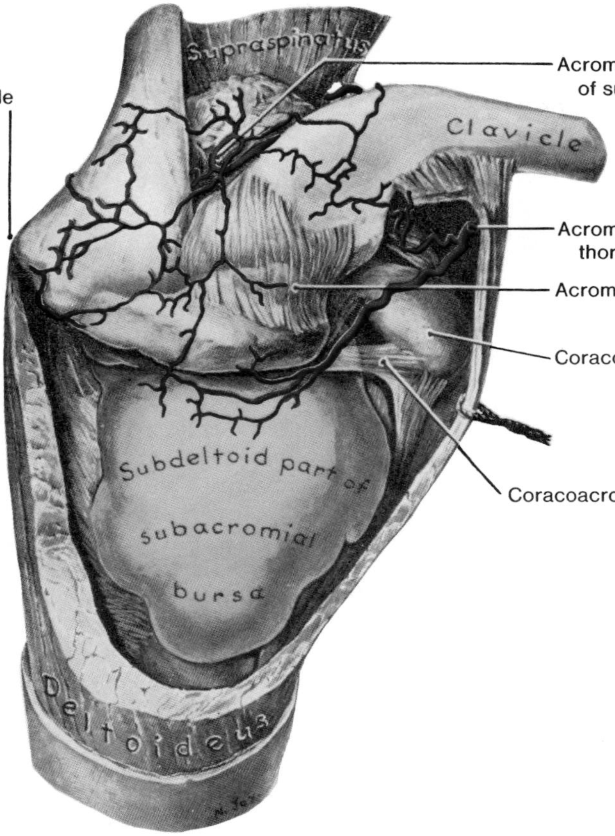

Figure 6-61. Drawing of a superolateral view of the shoulder region showing the subacromial bursa that has been injected with latex. The term "subacromial bursa" is usually understood to include the subdeltoid bursa because the two bursae are generally combined. Note that *superficial to the bursa* are parts of the deltoid, the acromion, the coracoacromial ligament, and the acromioclavicular joint and that *deep to the bursa* are the greater tubercle of the humerus and the supraspinatus tendon (not shown here). This bursa may, as the result of attrition, communicate with the shoulder and acromioclavicular joints (Fig. 6-64).

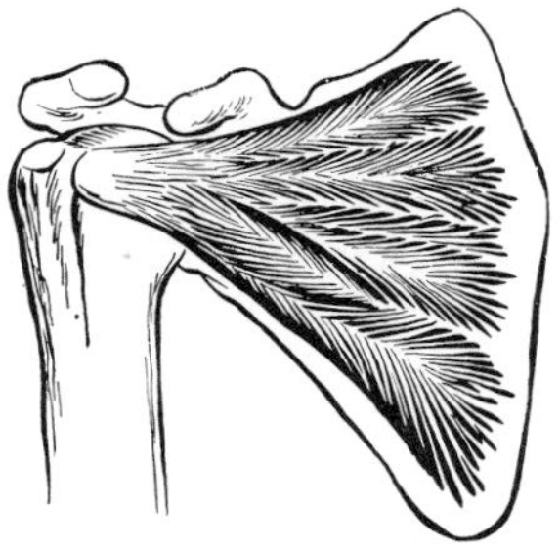

Figure 6-62. Drawing of the anterior aspect of the right scapula and humerus showing how the subscapularis muscle, which is *part of the rotator cuff*, guards the front of the shoulder joint and holds the humeral head in the glenoid cavity of the scapula.

axial skeleton; hence, in falls on the shoulder or hand, the force may be greater than the strength of the bone and fracture of the clavicle results. Fractures of the shaft of the clavicle medial to the point of attachment of the coracoclavicular ligament are common, especially in children and young adults (Fig. 6-65). In children the fracture is often incomplete, *i.e.*, a **green-stick fracture** in which one cortex of the bone breaks and the opposite one bends.

After fracture of the clavicle, the clavicular head of the sternocleidomastoid muscle elevates the medial fragment. As the trapezius is unable to hold up the lateral fragment owing to the weight of the upper

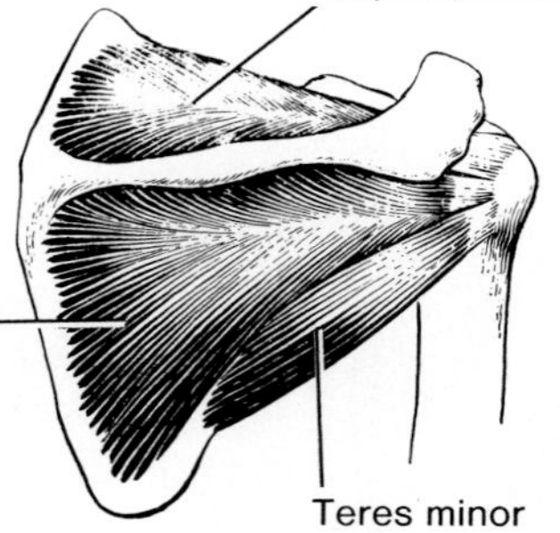

Figure 6-63. Drawing of the posterior aspect of the right scapula and humerus showing how the supraspinatus muscle guards the shoulder joint above and the infraspinatous and teres minor guard it behind. The fourth rotator cuff or stabilizer muscle, the subscapularis, passes anterior to this joint (Fig. 6-62). These four *rotator cuff muscles* have a steadying effect on the head of the humerus, maintaining it in correct apposition to the glenoid cavity of the scapula.

limb, it drops. Hence, a patient with a fractured clavicle frequently presents with his/her arm in a sling or supporting the sagging limb with the other arm.

In addition to being depressed, the lateral fragment of the clavicle is pulled medially by the adductors of the arm, principally the latissimus dorsi and pectoralis major muscles. This overriding of the bone fragments shortens the clavicle (Fig. 6-65).

Occasionally a communicating vein from the cephalic vein in the deltopectoral triangle (Fig. 6-19) passes anterior to the clavicle to join the external jugular vein (Fig. 6-44). This may be torn during fracture of a clavicle and give rise to a subcutaneous extravasation of blood (**hematoma**).

THE ARM OR BRACHIUM

The arm or brachium extends from the shoulder to the elbow. The rounded eminence on the anterior surface of the arm when the elbow is flexed is the **biceps brachii** muscle (Fig. 6-70). The body (shaft) of the **humerus** (the arm bone) is easy to palpate, as are its medial and lateral epicondyles (Figs. 6-1, 6-66, and 6-67). The **triceps brachii** muscle occupies the posterior part of the arm (Figs. 6-66 and 6-70 to 6-73).

THE HUMERUS

This is the largest bone of the upper limb (Figs. 6-1 and 6-67). Its smooth, ball-like head articulates with the glenoid cavity of the humerus. Close to the head are the **greater** and **lesser tubercles** for the insertion of certain muscles that surround and move the shoulder joint. The lesser tubercle is separated from the greater tubercle by the **intertubercular sulcus** (groove) in which lies the tendon of the long head of the biceps muscle. At the circumferential margin of the head lies the **anatomical neck**, separating the head and the tubercles. Distal to the head and tubercles, where the body narrows, is the **surgical neck**. *This is the site of most frequent fracture of the proximal end of the body.*

The upper half of the body is cylindrical. Anterolaterally at the midshaft, note the roughness known as the **deltoid tuberosity**. Observe the shallow, oblique **radial groove** or *sulcus of the radial nerve* that extends inferiorly from the medial to the lateral sides on the posterior aspect of the body (Fig. 6-67*B*). The distal end of the body is expanded from side to side and flattened from front to back. Observe a dry bone, noting that the distal end of the humerus curves forward slightly. The **trochlea** (L. pulley) fits into the **trochlear notch** of the ulna (Fig. 6-80), which swings on this pulley (trochlea) when the elbow is flexed. Just proximal to the trochlea are the **coronoid fossa** and the **olecranon fossa** for accommodating corresponding parts of the ulna. Adjoining the lateral part of the trochlea is a rounded ball of bone called the **capitulum** (L. little head). A prominent process, the **medial epicondyle**, projects from the trochlea and the **lateral epicondyle** projects from the capitulum. From each epicondyle a ridge runs proximally, known as the **medial** and **lateral supracondylar ridges** (Fig. 6-67*A*). The epicondyles, being subcutaneous, are easily felt. The medial epicondyle is the more prominent (Fig. 6-70).

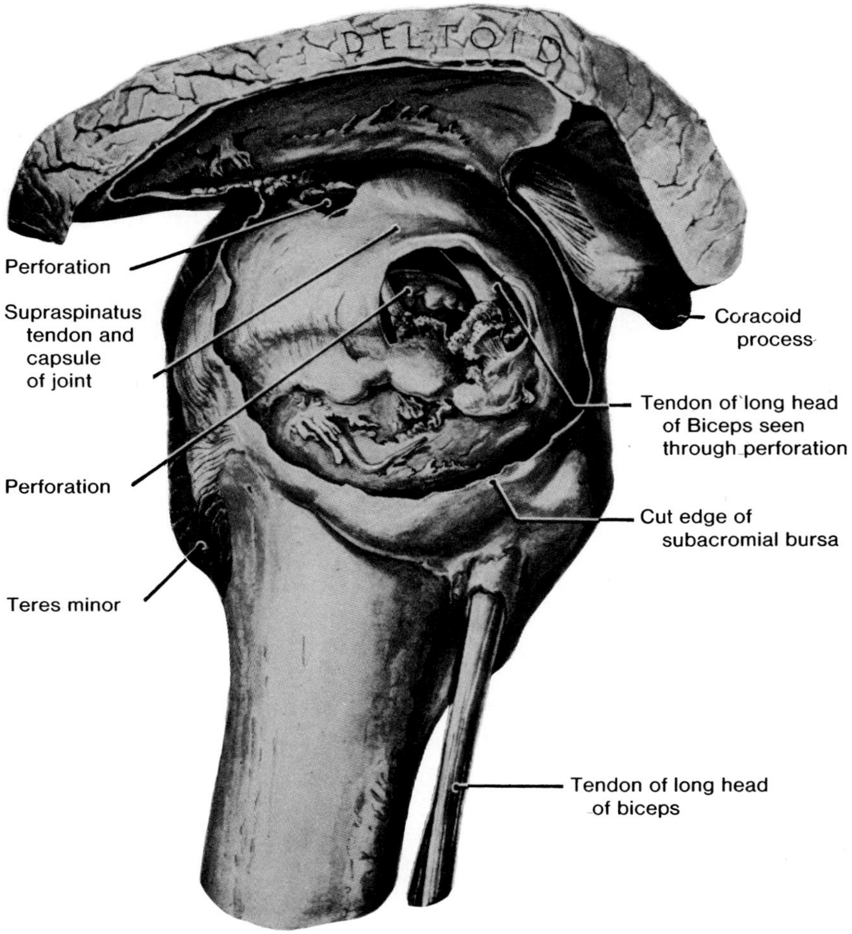

Figure 6-64. Illustration of a shoulder joint showing attrition (wearing away) of the supraspinatus tendon. As a result, the joint capsule and the wall of the subacromial bursa have perforated, and the shoulder joint cavity communicates with the bursa.

CLINICALLY ORIENTED COMMENTS

Fractures of the upper end of the humerus may be through the anatomical or the surgical neck of the humerus (Fig. 6-67). *Fractures of the surgical neck are common in elderly persons* and usually result from falls on the elbow when the arm is abducted. The fracture line occurs above the insertion of the pectoralis major, teres major, and latissimus dorsi muscles (Fig. 6-54).

Traumatic separation of the proximal epiphysis of the humerus (Fig. 6-68) can occur in persons under age 20 because this epiphysis does not fuse with the body until about the 20th year in males and about 2 years earlier in females. The displacement of the head which occurs is similar to that which occurs in fractures through the surgical neck of the humerus in elderly persons.

THE INTERMUSCULAR SEPTA

The muscles of the arm are contained in two fascial compartments (Figs. 6-66 and 6-69). These condensations of connective tissue extend from the medial and lateral **su-**

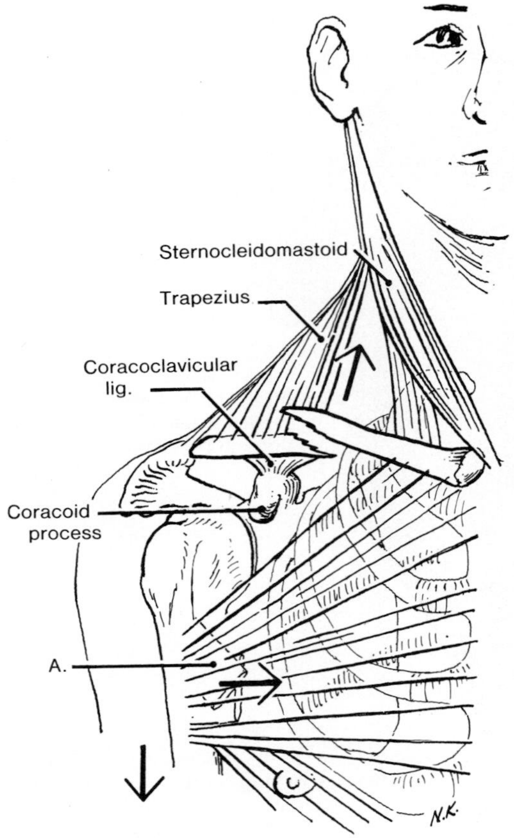

Figure 6-65. Sketch showing a fracture of the clavicle near the junction of the middle and lateral thirds (its weakest part). Note that the patient's shoulder has sagged slightly owing to the weight of the limb. *A*, pectoralis major, an adductor and medial rotator of the upper limb.

pracondylar ridges of the humerus to the brachial fascia, the strong tubular investment of deep fascia that ensheaths the arm. The **brachial fascia** is continuous proximally with the pectoral and axillary fasciae and distally with the fascia of the forearm.

The **anterior (flexor) compartment** contains three muscles (biceps, brachialis, and coracobrachialis), their nerves, and their vessels. The **posterior (extensor) compartment** contains one muscle (triceps), its nerve, and its vessels. The positions of these intermuscular septa are indicated by medial and lateral supracondylar ridges between the biceps, which bulge anteriorly, and the triceps, which bulge posteriorly (Fig. 6-67*A*).

THE BRACHIAL MUSCLES

There are five muscles in the arm, three flexors (supplied by the musculocutaneous nerve) and two extensors (supplied by the radial nerve).

The important brachial muscles are the **biceps brachii**, the **brachialis**, and the **triceps brachii**.

The Biceps Brachii Muscle (Figs. 6-66, 6-70, 6-71, 6-73, and 6-75). As its name indicates, this long fusiform muscle has *two heads of origin*. The two bellies of the muscle unite just distal to the middle of the arm.

Origin (Fig. 6-54). *Short head*, tip of **coracoid process**; *long head*, **supraglenoid tubercle** of scapula. The tendon of the long head crosses the humeral head within the capsule of the shoulder joint (Fig. 6-45) and descends into the intertubercular sulcus of the humerus (Figs. 6-18 and 6-67*A*).

Insertion (Figs. 6-54, 6-67, and 6-80). **Tuberosity of radius**. The *bicipitoradial bursa* separates its tendon from the anterior part of the tuberosity (Fig. 6-101). The biceps also inserts by the **bicipital aponeurosis** (Figs. 6-70 and 6-75), a broad, strong, triangular, membranous band which runs from the biceps tendon at the level of the elbow across the **cubital fossa** into the deep fascia over the flexor muscles in the medial side of the forearm.

The proximal part of the bicipital aponeurosis can be easily felt where it passes obliquely over the brachial artery and the medial nerve (Figs. 6-70, 6-73, and 6-75). This aponeurosis affords some protection for these and other structures in the cubital fossa. It also helps to lessen the pressure of the biceps tendon on the radial tuberosity during pronation and supination (Fig. 6-79).

Nerve Supply. **Musculocutaneous** nerve (C6 and C7).

Actions. **Flexes elbow** joint and **supinates forearm**; usually these actions occur together. It is also a weak flexor of the shoulder joint. You can easily feel your biceps contract as you supinate your forearm against resistance with the elbow flexed to 90°. It may help you recall the actions of this muscle if you know that it is an important muscle used when inserting a

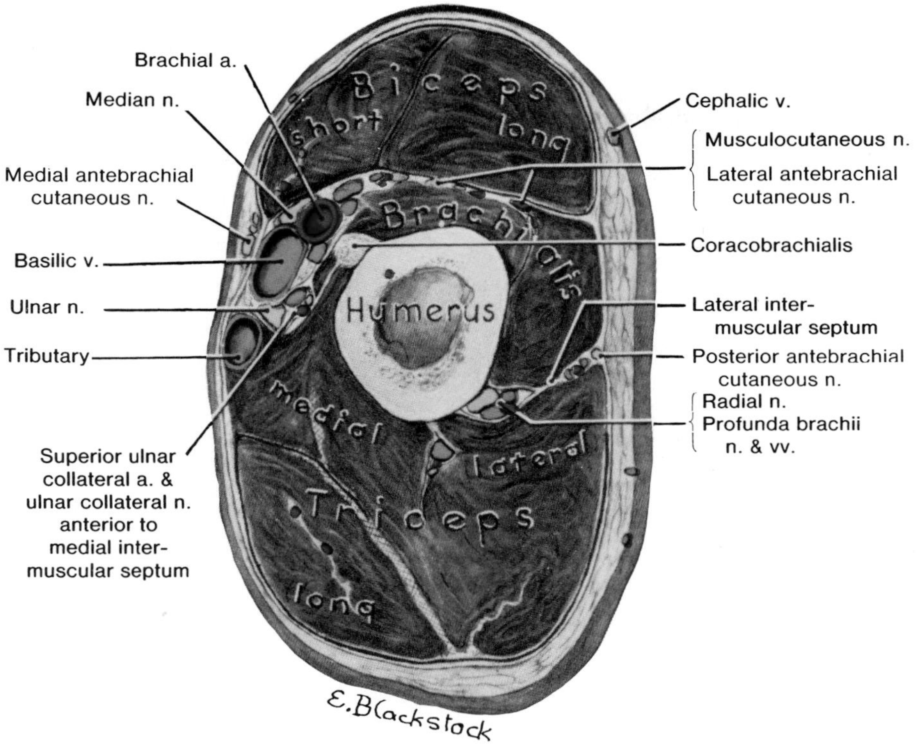

Figure 6-66. Drawing of a cross-section through the arm distal to its midpoint. Observe that the body (shaft) of the humerus is nearly circular; its cortex is thickest here. Note the three heads of the triceps in the posterior compartment of the arm, *i.e.*, behind the medial and lateral intermuscular septa. Observe that the radial nerve and its companion vessels are in contact with the bone. Note the two heads of the biceps, the brachialis, and the insertion of the coracobrachialis in the anterior compartment of the arm, *i.e.*, in front of the medial and lateral intermuscular septa. Observe the musculocutaneous nerve and its companion vessels in the septum between the biceps and the brachialis. Note the median nerve crossing to the medial side of the brachial artery and its venae comitantes. Observe the ulnar nerve moving posteriorly on to the side of the triceps and that the basilic vein (here as two vessels) has pierced the deep fascia. Note that the skin and subcutaneous tissues are thicker posterolaterally, where they are more exposed to injury, than anteromedially, where they are protected.

corkscrew and pulling out the cork of a wine bottle.

The Brachialis Muscle (Figs. 6-66, 6-71, 6-73, and 6-75). This strong muscle lies posterior to the biceps brachii. *It is the main flexor of the elbow joint.*

Origin (Fig. 6-54). **Distal half of anterior surface of humerus** and intermuscular septum.

Insertion (Figs. 6-54 and 6-80). **Coronoid process** and **tuberosity of ulna**.

Nerve Supply. **Musculocutaneous** nerve (C6 and C7). Its lateral part also receives a sensory branch from the **radial** nerve (C5 and C6).

Actions. **Flexes elbow** joint. Flex your forearm against resistance and feel the brachialis alongside the tendon of the biceps and on each side of the belly of this muscle.

The Triceps Brachii Muscle (Figs. 6-58, 6-66, and 6-70 to 6-73). This large muscle is the only one in the posterior compartment of the arm (Fig. 6-66), and it makes up the bulk of its posterior portion (Fig. 6-70). As its name indicates it has *three heads of origin.*

Origin (Figs. 6-50 and 6-54). *Long head,* **infraglenoid tubercle of scapula**; *lateral head,* **posterior surface** and **lateral border of humerus** proximal to radial groove;

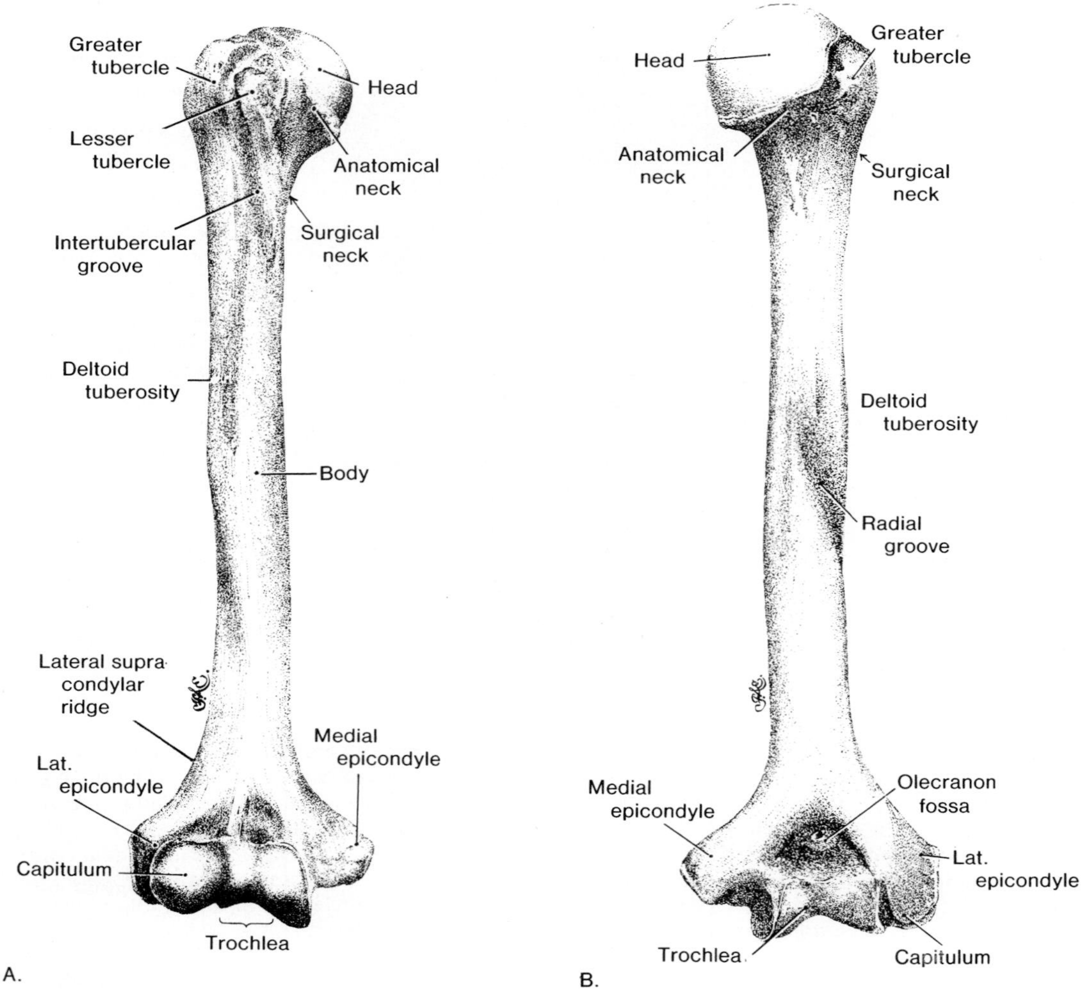

Figure 6-67. Drawings of the right humerus. *A*, anterior view. *B*, posterior view. Note the roughened area on the anterolateral surface of the body, termed the deltoid tuberosity, into which the tendon of the deltoid muscle inserts (Fig. 6-55). Posterior to it is the groove for the radial nerve and the profunda brachii artery (Fig. 6-74).

and *medial head*, **posterior surface of humerus** (inferior to radial groove) and **medial intermuscular septum.**

Insertion (Figs. 6-50 and 6-72). Upper surface of **posterior part of olecranon** of ulna and deep fascia of forearm. Just proximal to its insertion, there is a subtendinous olecranon bursa between the triceps tendon and the olecranon (Fig. 6-157*B*).

Nerve Supply. **Radial** nerve (C6 to C8).

Actions. **Extends elbow** joint. The medial head acts in all forms of extension; the other heads act when extra power is required (*e.g.*, when the forearm is acting against resistance, as occurs during pushing).

The Coracobrachialis Muscle (Fig. 6-73). This short, fairly slender, rounded muscle in the upper medial part of the arm is important mainly as a landmark (*e.g.*, the musculocutaneous nerve pierces it).

Origin (Figs. 6-54 and 6-73). **Tip of coracoid process** of scapula in common with short head of biceps.

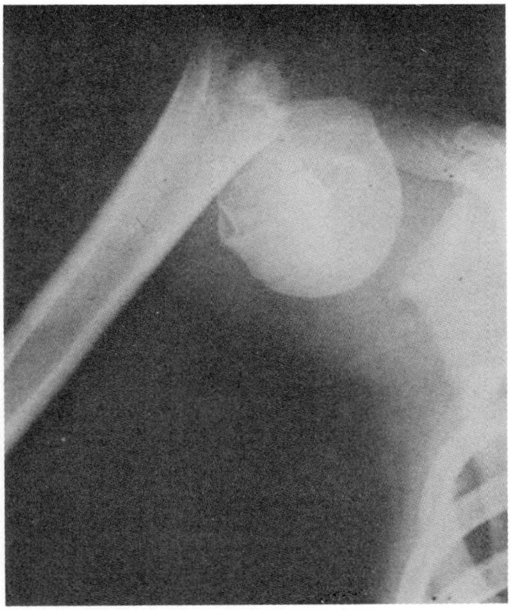

Figure 6-68. Radiograph of the right shoulder of a 14-year-old boy showing separation of the proximal epiphysis of the humerus. Although the humeral head has rotated, it has otherwise retained a fairly normal relationship with the glenoid cavity of the scapula.

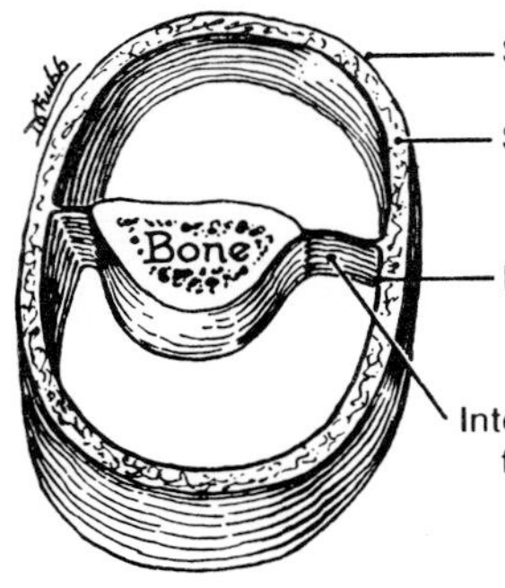

Figure 6-69. Drawing of the two fascial compartments of the arm which contain muscles (Fig. 6-66). Observe the medial and lateral intermuscular fascial septa which pass from the enveloping deep fascia to the supracondylar ridges of the humerus (Fig. 6-67*A*).

Insertion (Fig. 6-54). **Middle third of medial surface of humerus.**

Nerve Supply. **Musculocutaneous** nerve (C6 and C7).

Actions. **Flexes** and **adducts arm** at shoulder joint and stabilizes this joint.

The Anconeus Muscle (Figs. 6-72 and 6-163). This small, short, triangular muscle is on the lateral part of the posterior aspect of the elbow. It is usually partially blended with the triceps.

Origin (Figs. 6-50 and 6-67). **Lateral epicondyle of humerus.**

Insertion (Figs. 6-50 and 6-81). **Lateral border of olecranon** and upper part of **posterior surface of ulna**.

Nerve Supply. **Radial** nerve (C7, C8, and T1).

Actions. **Abducts ulna during pronation** of forearm through an axis that passes through the middle finger. It can also act as an extensor of the elbow joint.

THE CUBITAL FOSSA

This triangular space or hollow is in front of the elbow (Fig. 6-82) distal to the skin crease. It is bounded **superiorly** by an imaginary line connecting the epicondyles of the humerus (Figs. 6-67), **medially** by the pronator teres muscle (Fig. 6-70), and **laterally** by the brachioradialis muscle (Figs. 6-75 and 6-84).

The floor of the fossa is formed by the brachialis and supinator muscles of the arm and forearm, respectively (Fig. 6-84). **The roof** is formed by deep fascia that is strengthened by the bicipital aponeurosis (Fig. 6-75) and is covered by superficial fascia and skin.

Contents of the Cubital Fossa (Figs. 6-75 to 6-77 and 6-84). The cubital fossa is an important area because it contains the **biceps tendon**, the **brachial artery** and its terminal branches (**radial** and **ulnar arteries**), and parts of the **median** and **radial nerves**. The cubital fossa will be understood better when its contents and all the muscles forming its boundaries have been studied.

THE BRACHIAL ARTERIES

The Brachial Artery (Figs. 6-41, 6-66, 6-73 to 6-75, and 6-84). This artery provides the main arterial supply to the arm. It **begins at the lower border of the teres major** as the continuation of the axillary artery (Fig. 6-74). It runs downward and slightly laterally to the cubital fossa, where

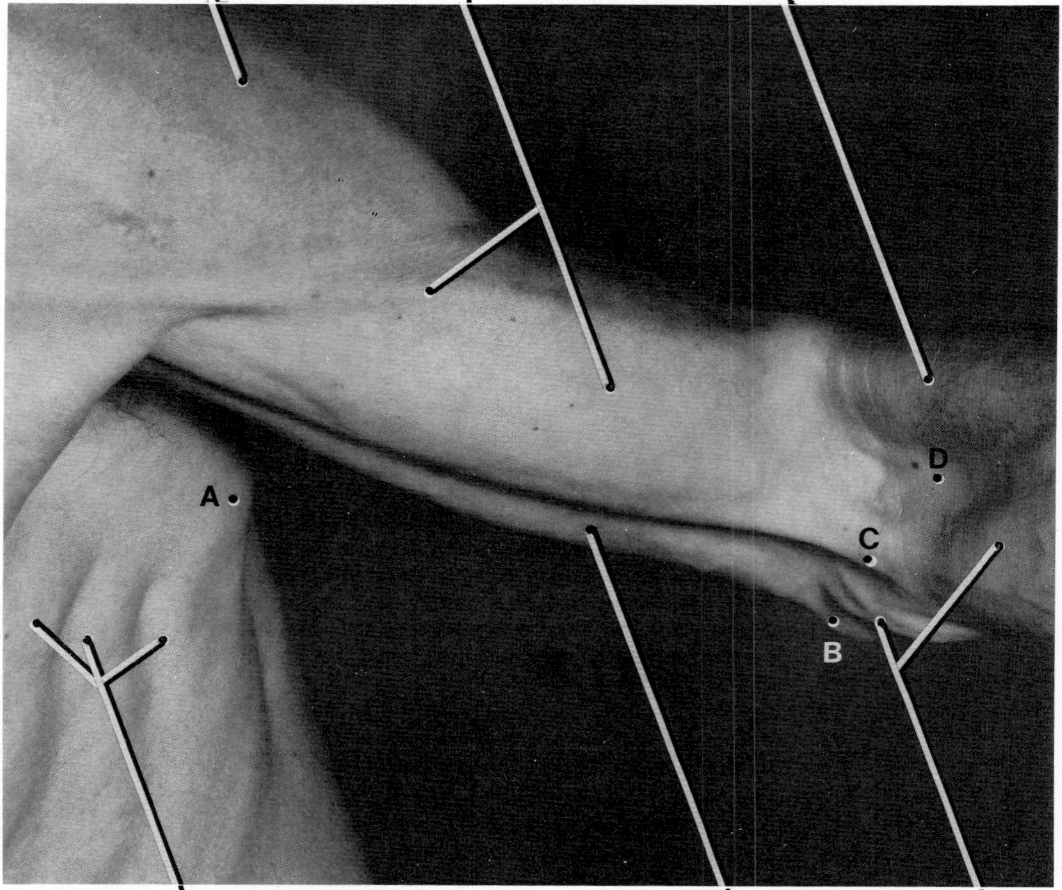

Figure 6-70. Photograph of the anterior surface of the shoulder, arm, elbow, and lateral chest region of a 46-year-old man. *A*, inferior angle of scapula. *B*, medial epicondyle of humerus. *C*, bicipital aponeurosis. *D*, cubital fossa.

it **ends opposite the neck of the radius** by dividing into the **radial** and **ulnar arteries** (Fig. 6-74). Its course through the arm is represented by a line connecting the midpoint of the clavicle with the midpoint of the cubital fossa.

In Figure 6-84, note that the brachial artery bifurcates medial to the tendon of the biceps, about 2.5 cm distal to the middle of a line joining the medial and lateral epicondyles of the humerus.

The brachial artery, *superficial and palpable throughout its course*, at first lies medial to the humerus and then anterior to it. It lies anterior to the triceps and brachialis muscles and is overlapped by the coracobrachialis and biceps muscles (Fig. 6-73). As the brachial artery passes downward and slightly laterally, it **accompanies the median nerve**, which crosses anterior to the artery in the middle of the arm (Fig. 6-73). In the cubital fossa the **bicipital**

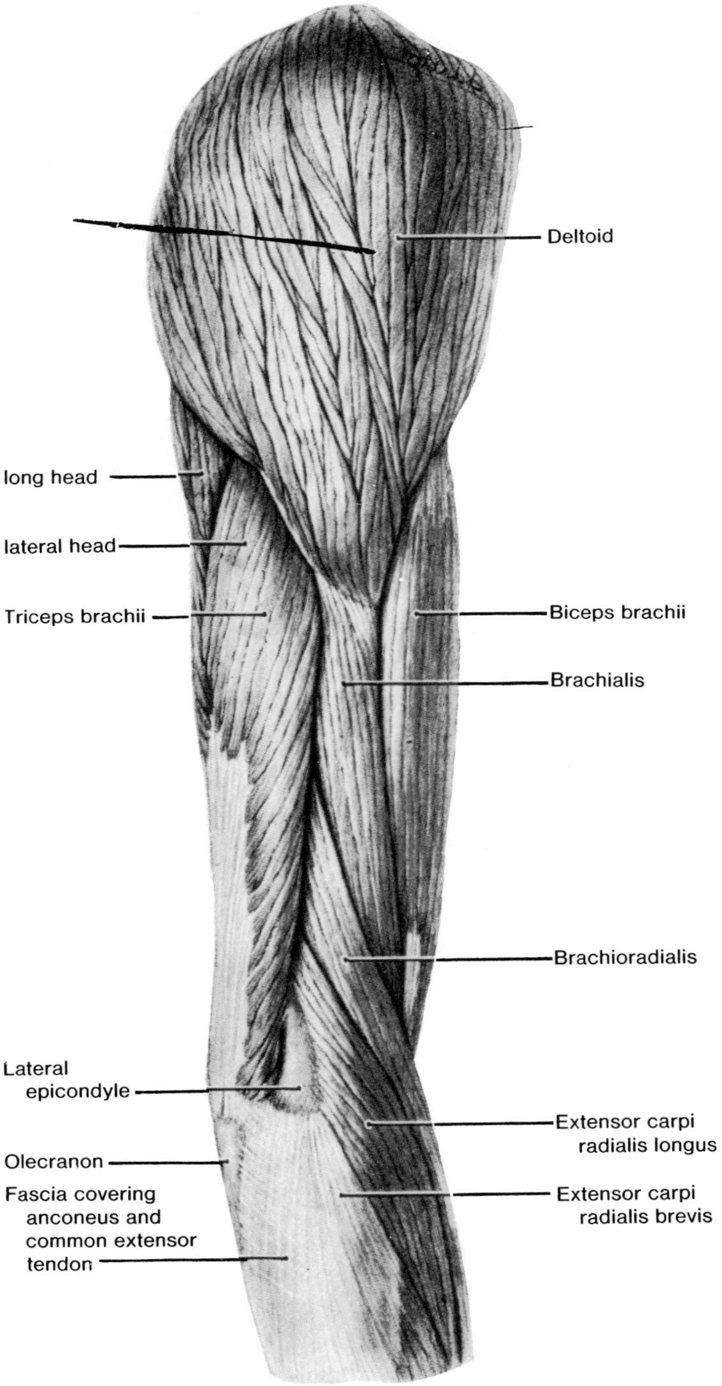

Figure 6-71. Drawing of a lateral view of a dissection of the arm and the proximal part of the forearm showing the muscles. Note particularly the thick triangular deltoid muscle which was given its name because its form is like the Greek letter delta (Δ) inverted (Fig. 6-55). The tendon of this muscle inserts into the deltoid tuberosity of the humerus (Fig. 6-67).

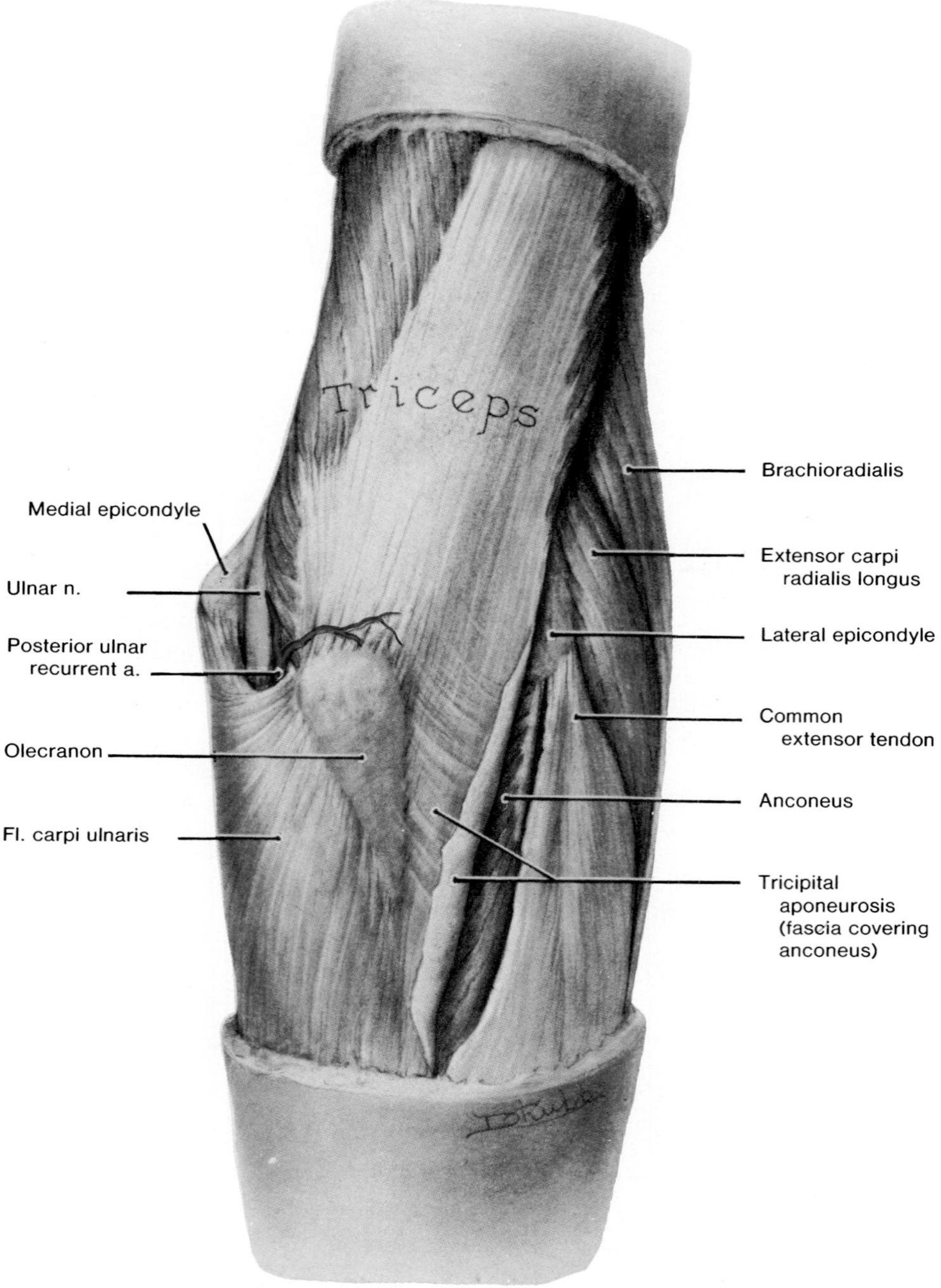

Figure 6-72. Drawing of a dissection of the elbow region from behind. The fascia covering the anconeus muscle is cut and lifted up. Observe that the triceps is inserted not only into the upper surface of the olecranon but also via the "tricipital aponeurosis" (deep fascia covering the anconeus) into the lateral border of the olecranon. Observe the subcutaneous and palpable posterior surfaces of the medial epicondyle, the lateral epicondyle, and the olecranon. Note the ulnar nerve, easily palpable, running subfascially behind the medial epicondyle and that distal to this point it disappears deep to the two heads of origin of the flexor carpi ulnaris. Observe these heads: one arising from the common flexor tendon, the other from the medial border of the olecranon and posterior border of the shaft of the ulna. Note the continuous linear origin from the humerus of the superficial extensor muscles. These are the brachioradialis, the extensor carpi radialis longus, the common extensor tendon, and the anconeus (see Figs. 6-85 and 6-86 also).

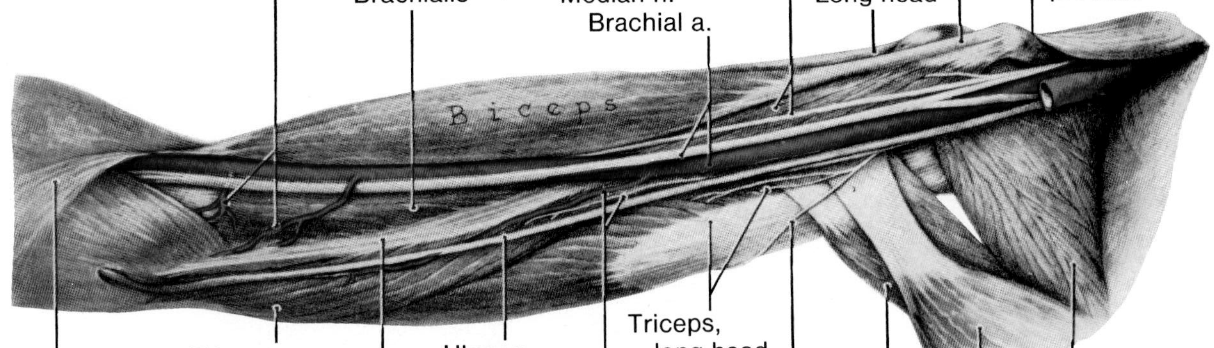

Figure 6-73. Drawing of a dissection of a medial view of the arm and the proximal part of the forearm. Observe the biceps brachii, the coracobrachialis, and the brachialis occupying the front of the arm and the triceps brachii occupying the back (see Fig. 6-66 also). Note the medial intermuscular septum separating these two muscle groups in the distal two-thirds of the arm. Observe the brachial artery (the great artery of the limb) lying a fingerbreadth from the tip of the coracoid process and applied to the medial side of the coracobrachialis superiorly and to the front of the brachialis inferiorly.

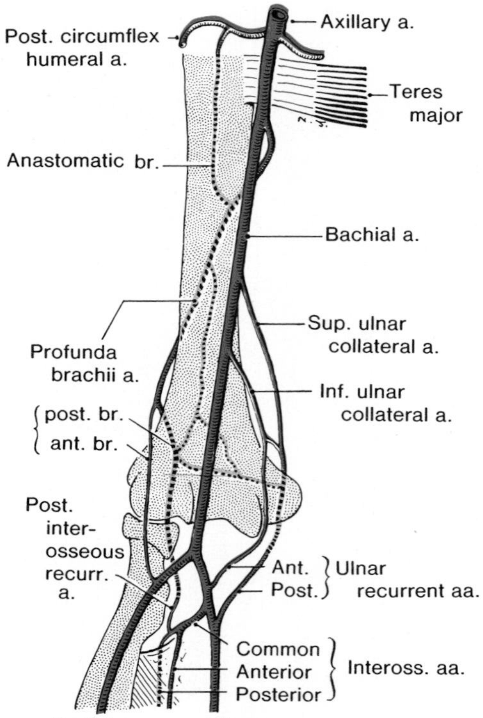

Figure 6-74. Drawing of an anterior view of the arterial supply of the arm and the proximal part of the forearm, showing the clinically important *anastomoses of the elbow region.* Note that the brachial artery divides opposite the neck of the radius into the ulnar and radial arteries. This bifurcation occurs about 2.5 cm distal to the crease of the elbow. Observe the anastomoses in front of and behind the elbow. The profunda brachii artery accompanies the radial nerve through the radial groove of the humerus (Figs. 6-32 and 6-67).

aponeurosis bridges and protects the median nerve and the brachial artery (Fig. 6-75) and separates them from the medial cubital vein (Fig. 6-76).

During its course through the arm, the brachial artery gives rise to many unnamed muscular branches, mainly from its lateral side. *Its named branches* are the **profunda brachii** artery (deep brachial artery, arteria profunda brachii), the **nutrient humeral** artery, and the **superior** and **inferior ulnar collateral** arteries (Fig. 6-74).

The **profunda brachii** artery is the *largest branch of the brachial* and has the highest origin (Fig. 6-74). It follows the radial nerve closely, accompanying it along the **radial groove** for this nerve in the posterior surface of the humerus (Figs. 6-67*B* and 6-74). Posterior to the humerus the profunda brachii artery divides into anterior and posterior descending branches, both of which help to form the arterial anastomoses of the elbow region (Fig. 6-74).

The **nutrient humeral artery** arises from the brachial around the middle of the arm and enters the nutrient canal on the anteromedial surface of the humerus.

The **superior ulnar collateral artery** (Figs. 6-73 and 6-74) arises from the brachial near the middle of the arm and accompanies the ulnar nerve posterior to the medial epicondyle of the humerus; here it anastomoses with the posterior ulnar recurrent branch of the ulnar artery and the inferior ulnar collateral artery.

The **inferior ulnar collateral artery** (Figs. 6-73 and 6-74) arises about 5 cm proximal to the elbow crease, passes anterior to the medial epicondyle of the humerus, and joins the anastomoses of the elbow region.

CLINICALLY ORIENTED COMMENTS

The anastomoses of the elbow region provide a functionally and surgically important **collateral circulation.** The brachial artery may be clamped or even ligated distal to the inferior ulnar collateral artery without producing tissue damage owing to inadequate circulation (ischemia). The anatomical basis for this is that the ulnar and radial arteries still receive sufficient blood through the anastomoses of the elbow region (Fig. 6-74).

Arterial blood pressure is routinely taken using a **sphygmometer** (sphygmomanometer), consisting of an inflatable (pneumatic) cuff and a mercury manometer. The cuff is placed around the arm and inflated with air; this compresses the brachial artery against the humerus and eventually occludes it. A **stethoscope** is placed over the artery in the cubital fossa, medial to the

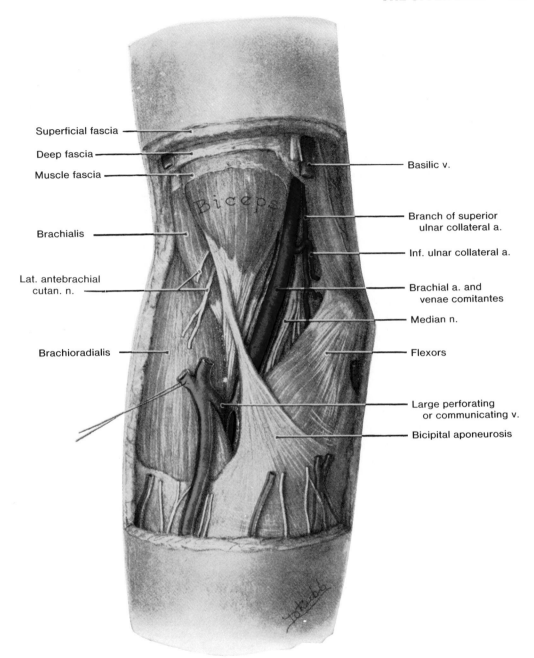

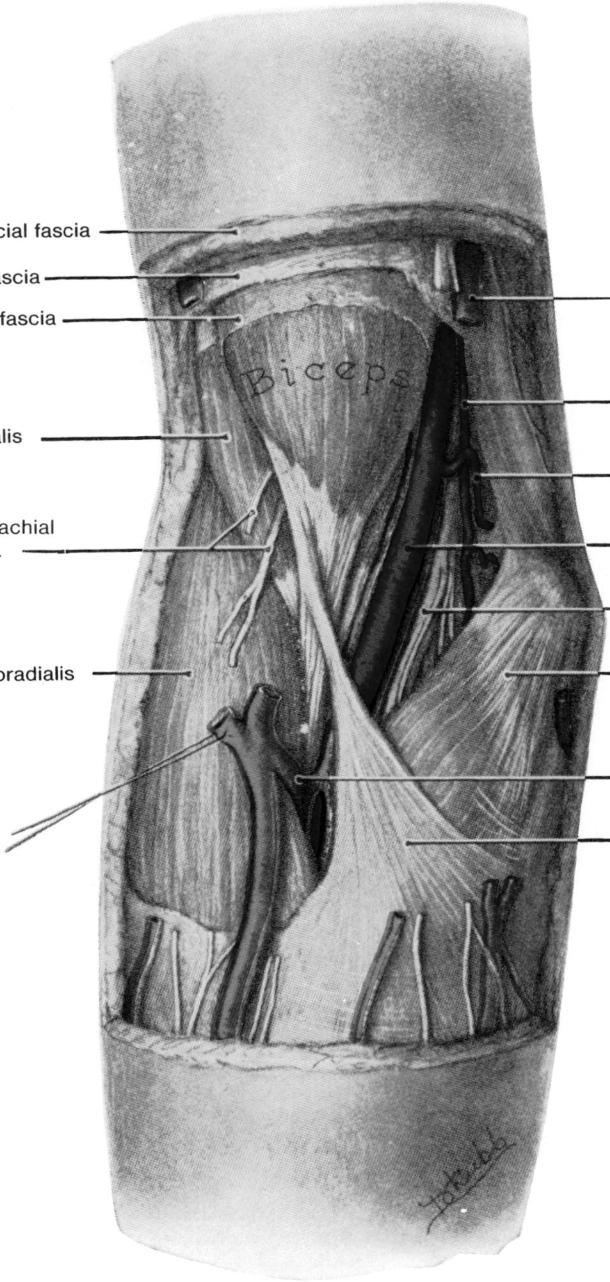

Figure 6-75. Drawing of a dissection of the right *cubital fossa*, the triangular space distal to the elbow crease. It is bounded laterally by the extensor muscles (represented by the brachioradialis) and medially by the flexor muscles (represented by the pronator teres). The apex of the fossa is where these two muscles meet distally. Observe the three chief contents of the cubital fossa: the biceps tendon, the brachial artery, and the median nerve. Note the biceps tendon rotating through a right angle and the bicipital aponeurosis springing from the tendon. Observe that the brachial artery lies medial to the biceps muscle and its tendon; this is where the stethoscope is placed for listening to pulsations of the brachial artery while measuring the blood pressure.

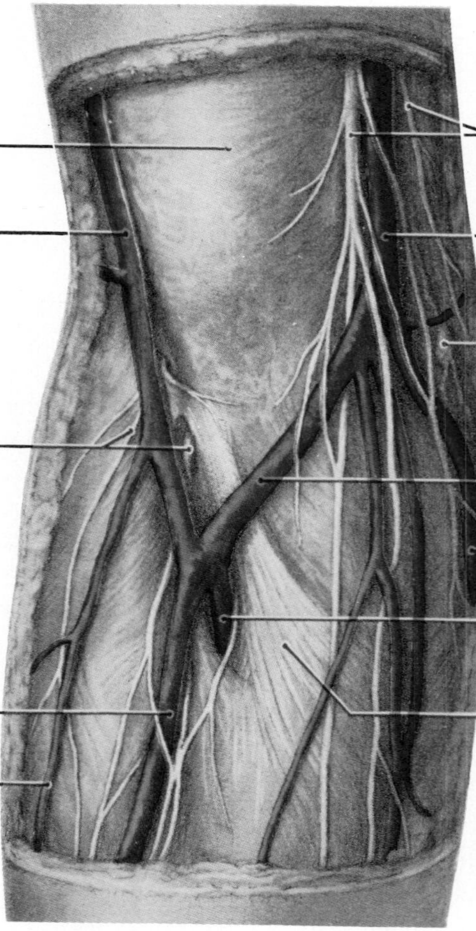

Figure 6-76. Drawing of a dissection of the superficial structures at the front of the right elbow. Observe the superficial veins—cephalic, median, basilic, and their connecting channels—making a variable M-shaped pattern. Note that the median cubital vein is separated from the brachial artery only by the bicipital aponeurosis. Observe the perforating vein, lateral to the bicipital aponeurosis, connecting the deep veins to the median cubital vein. Blood is commonly taken from the cubital veins, usually the median cubital vein (Fig. 6-77). Note that the cephalic and basilic veins occupying the bicipital furrows in the arm, one on each side of the biceps brachii muscle.

biceps brachii and its tendon. As the pressure in the cuff is reduced, blood begins to spurt through the artery. The first audible spurt indicates the *systolic blood pressure.*

Compression of the brachial artery may be produced in almost its entire course (*e.g.*, to control hemorrhage owing to injuries of the forearm or hand). The best place to compress the brachial artery is near the middle of the arm, where it lies on the tendon of the coracobrachialis muscle medial to the humerus (Figs. 6-73 to 6-75). In old people it is often tortuous and subcutaneous here, and its pulsations may be visible. To compress the brachial artery in the lower arm, pressure has to be directed posteriorly because the artery lies anterior to the humerus in this region (Fig. 6-74).

THE BRACHIAL VEINS

The deep brachial veins are arranged in pairs which accompany the brachial artery

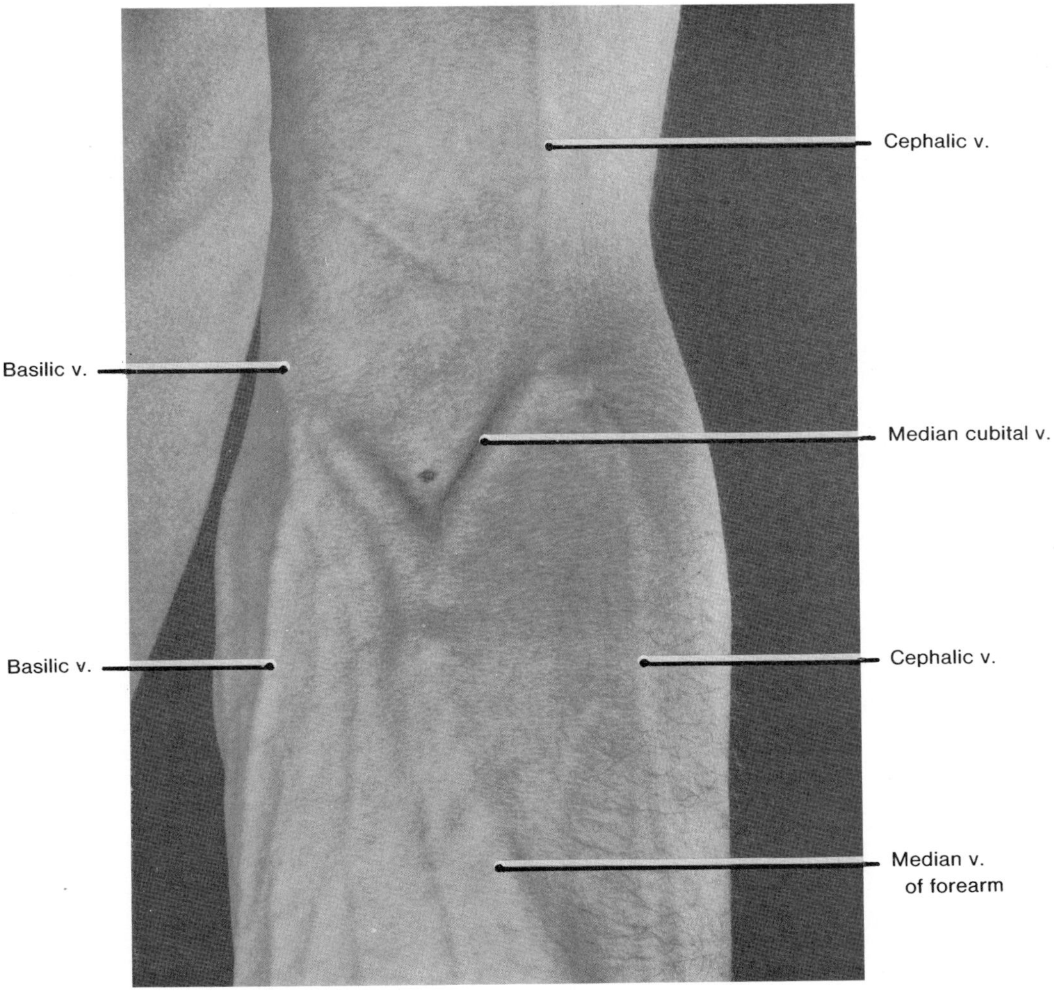

Figure 6-77. Photograph of the superficial veins at the front of the left elbow region of a 27-year-old man. The pattern is similar to that illustrated at the right elbow in Figure 7-76. Note that the basilic and cephalic veins are small and that a median vein of the forearm is present which ends in the basilic. The superficial veins of the forearm are extremely variable. The cubital veins are the common site for blood sampling, transfusion, and intravenous injections. The largest vein, usually the median cubital, is commonly selected.

(Fig. 6-44). They begin at the elbow by union of the **venae comitantes** (companions) of the ulnar and radial arteries and end in the axillary vein. The brachial veins contain valves and are connected at intervals by short transverse branches.

The superficial veins of the arm are the **cephalic** and **basilic veins** (Figs. 6-75 to 6-77). The **median cubital vein** is commonly used for **venipuncture** (taking blood). It links the cephalic and basilic veins anterior to the bicipital aponeurosis (Figs. 6-76 and 6-77). Considerable variation occurs in the connection of these venous channels.

THE BRACHIAL NERVES

The *four nerves of the arm* (median, ulnar, musculocutaneous, and radial) are terminal branches of the brachial plexus (Fig. 6-27), as is the axillary nerve which supplies the skin of the arm over the lower half of the deltoid and adjacent regions of the arm (Fig. 6-58). Two brachial nerves (median and ulnar) supply no brachial muscles, but they do supply the elbow joint and muscles in the front of the forearm (Fig. 6-28).

The Median Nerve (Figs. 6-25 to 6-29, 6-73, and 6-75). This major nerve is formed in the axilla by the union of a lateral root from the lateral cord and a medial root from the medial cord of the brachial plexus. The nerve runs distally in the arm on the lateral side of the brachial artery (Fig. 6-66) until it reaches the middle of the arm, where it crosses to its medial side (Fig. 6-73) in contact with the brachialis. It descends to the cubital fossa where it lies deep to the bicipital aponeurosis and the median cubital vein (Figs. 6-75 and 6-76). *The median nerve has no branches in the axilla or the arm* but passes deeply into the forearm to supply all but one and one-half of the muscles in the anterior part of the forearm (Fig. 6-28). It supplies articular branches to the elbow joint.

CLINICALLY ORIENTED COMMENTS

Injury to the median nerve proximal to the elbow results in a loss of sensation on the lateral portion of the palm, the palmar surface of the thumb, and the lateral two and one-half fingers, including their nailbeds (Fig. 6-29).

As the median nerve supplies no muscles in the arm, they are not affected; however, pronation, flexion of the wrist and fingers, and important movements of the thumb are lost or are severely affected because the muscles producing these movements are supplied by the median nerve after it enters the forearm [*e.g.*, pronator teres, flexor carpi radialis, and the three thenar (thumb) muscles] (Fig. 6-28).

The Ulnar Nerve (Figs. 6-27 to 6-29, 6-72, 6-73, and 6-78). This is the larger of the two terminal branches of the medial cord of the brachial plexus. It passes distally anterior to the triceps muscle on the medial side of the brachial artery. Around the middle of the arm, it pierces the medial intermuscular septum and descends between it and the medial head of the triceps (Fig. 6-73). *It enters the forearm by passing between the medial epicondyle of the humerus and the olecranon* (Figs. 6-72 and 6-78); here the ulnar nerve is superficial and easily palpable. The ulnar nerve has *no branches in the arm*, but it supplies one and one-half muscles in the forearm (Fig. 6-28). It also supplies articular branches to the elbow joint.

CLINICALLY ORIENTED COMMENTS

Injury to the ulnar nerve in the arm results in impaired flexion and adduction of the wrist and impaired movement of the thumb, ring, and little fingers (*e.g.*, poor grasp). *The characteristic clinical sign of ulnar nerve damage is inability to adduct or abduct the medial four digits* owing to loss of power of the interosseous muscles (Case 6-5). The way to test for weakness of the interossei is by trying to remove a piece of paper from between the adducted fingers when they are fully extended, as shown in Figure 6-186.

A later sign of ulnar nerve damage is **clawhand** (Fig. 6-104), in which the ring and middle fingers are hyperextended at the metacarpophalangeal joints and flexed at the interphalangeal joints. After several months there is usually considerable wasting (atrophy) of the interosseous muscles, producing depressions between the metacarpal bones. Usually the hypothenar muscles, or short muscles of the little finger (Figs. 6-127 and 6-130), also undergo atrophy because they are supplied by the deep branch of the ulnar nerve.

The Musculocutaneous Nerve (Figs. 6-23, 6-25 to 6-28, 6-32, and 6-73). This nerve arises as one of the terminal branches of the lateral cord of the brachial plexus, opposite the lower border of the pectoralis

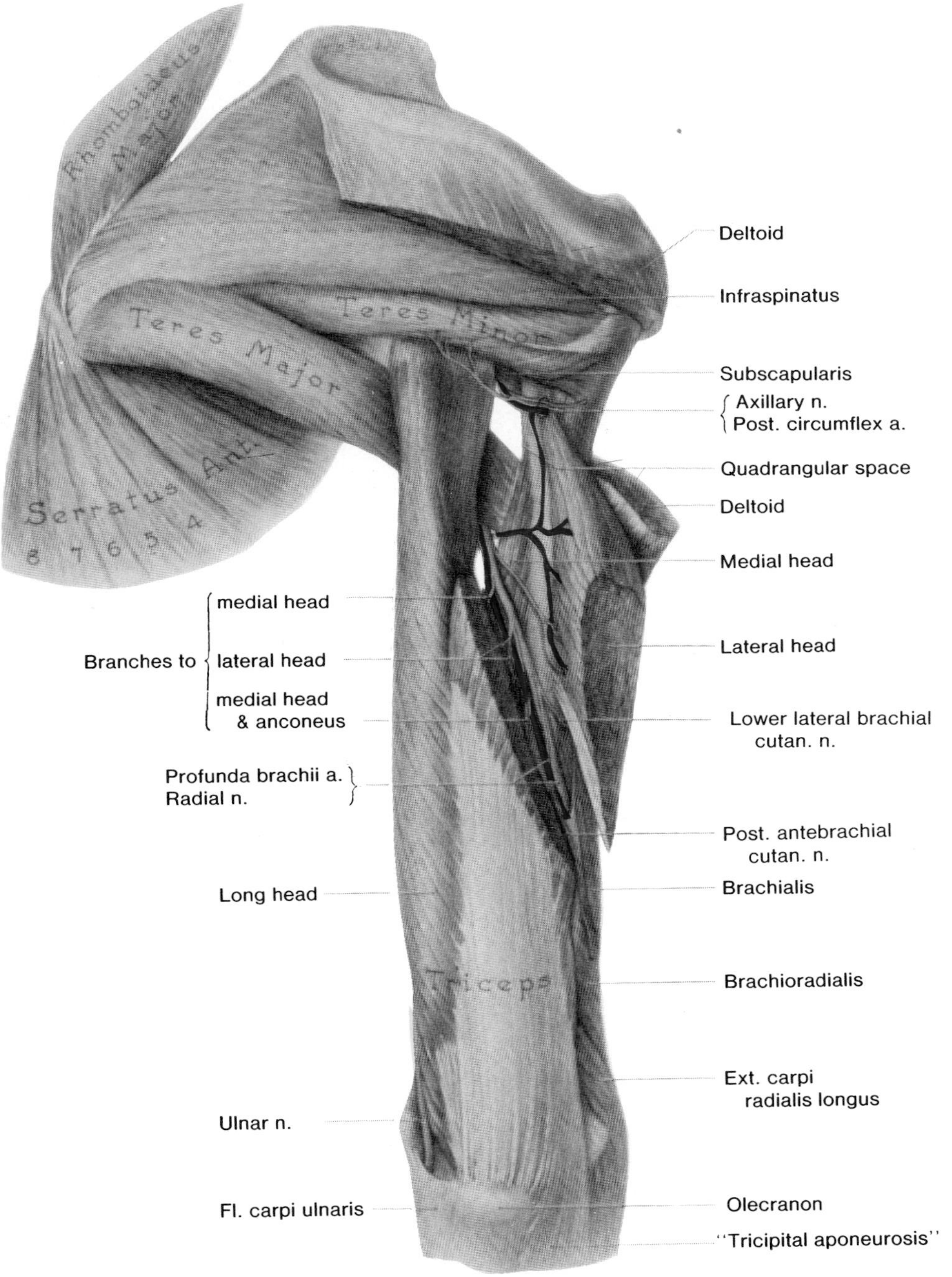

Figure 6-78. Drawing of a posterior view of a dissection of the triceps and its three related nerves (axillary, radial, and ulnar). Observe the radial nerve supplying the lateral and medial heads of the triceps and the anconeus. Note that the triceps is inserted into the upper aspect of the olecranon and also into the deep fascia of the forearm. Observe that the teres major, rhomboideus major, and serratus anterior muscles are mainly inserted into the inferior angle of the scapula.

minor muscle (Fig. 6-26). It pierces the coracobrachialis muscle near its midlength and then continues distally between the biceps and brachialis muscles (Fig. 6-73). It supplies all three of these muscles (Fig. 6-28) and pierces the deep fascia as it emerges between the biceps and the brachioradialis (Fig. 6-90), just proximal to the crease of the elbow. At the lateral border of the tendon of the biceps, it becomes the **lateral antebrachial cutaneous nerve** (Figs. 6-75, 6-76, and 6-102).

CLINICALLY ORIENTED COMMENTS

Injury to the musculocutaneous nerve in the arm (*e.g.*, resulting from a laceration) before it innervates any muscles (Fig. 6-28) results in paralysis of the coracobrachialis, the biceps, and the brachialis. As a result, flexion at the elbow joint and supination are greatly weakened. There may also be loss of sensation on the lateral surface of the forearm supplied by the lateral antebrachial cutaneous nerve. The area of sensory loss varies, depending on the extent to which the supply to this area is overlapped by adjacent nerves (Fig. 6-102).

The Radial Nerve (Figs. 6-25 to 6-27, 6-29 to 6-31, and 6-78). This nerve is the *direct continuation of the posterior cord of the brachial plexus.* The largest branch of the brachial plexus, it usually contains nerve fibers from all five nerves contributing to the plexus (*i.e.*, C5 to T1). It enters the arm posterior to the brachial artery, medial to the humerus, and anterior to the long head of the triceps (Fig. 6-78). It then passes inferiorly with the profunda brachii artery around the body of the humerus in the **radial groove** or *spiral sulcus for the radial nerve* (Figs. 6-67*B*, 6-74, and 6-78) to reach the lateral border of the humerus, where it pierces the lateral intermuscular septum. It then continues inferiorly between the brachialis and brachioradialis muscles to the level of the lateral humeral epicondyle, where it divides into deep and superficial branches (Fig. 6-84). The deep branch is entirely muscular and articular in its distribution (Fig. 6-30). The superficial branch supplies sensory fibers to the back of the hand and the fingers (Figs. 6-29 and 6-103).

CLINICALLY ORIENTED COMMENTS

Injury to the radial nerve proximal to the origin of the triceps (Fig. 6-30) results in paralysis of the triceps, the brachioradialis, the supinator, and the extensors of the wrist, thumb, and fingers. There would also be loss of sensation in the areas of skin supplied by this nerve (Case 6-2 and Figs. 6-29 and 6-181*A*).

When the radial nerve is injured where it lies in the radial groove, the triceps is not completely paralyzed, but paralysis of the other muscles supplied by it occurs. (Case 6-6). *The characteristic clinical sign of radial nerve injury is wrist-drop,* (*i.e.*, inability to extend or straighten the wrist, Fig. 6-181*A*).

THE FOREARM OR ANTEBRACHIUM

The forearm or antebrachium extends from the elbow to the wrist and contains two bones, the **radius** and the **ulna**, which lie parallel in the anatomical position (*i.e.*, in supination, Fig. 6-79). During pronation the radius lies across the ulna.

The interosseous membrane, joining these bones, fills the gap between the lateral border of the ulna and the medial border of the radius (Figs. 6-80 and 6-167). It consists of connective tissue fibers and, although thin, is a **very strong fibrous sheet**. In addition to tying the forearm bones together, the interosseous membrane provides attachment for some deep forearm muscles (*e.g.*, flexor digitorum profundus, Fig. 6-97).

THE ANTEBRACHIAL BONES

The Radius (Figs. 6-1, 6-79 to 6-81, and 6-157). The radius (L. spoke of a wheel) is the shorter and the lateral of the two fore-

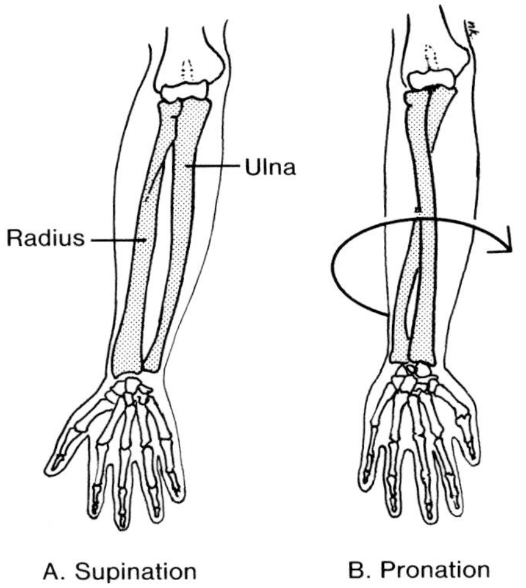

Figure 6-79. Drawing of the bones of the forearm and hand showing how the positions of the radius and ulna change during supination (*A*) and pronation (*B*) and that the axis of rotation passes throught the middle finger. The strong supinators are the biceps brachii and supinator muscles. The chief pronators are the pronator teres and pronator quadratus muscles. Both supination and pronation are most powerful when the elbow is flexed to a right angle.

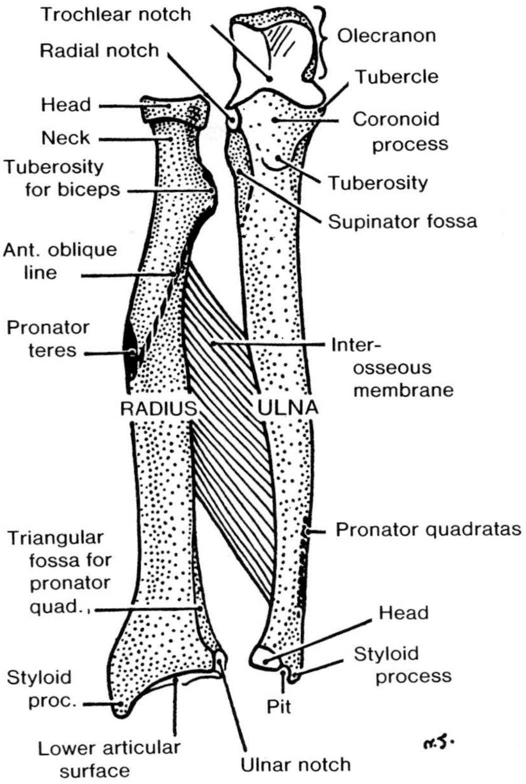

Figure 6-80. Drawing of the anterior aspect of the radius and ulna in the anatomical position. Observe that the radius is shorter than the ulna, but its distal end (styloid process) projects further inferiorly (about 1.2 cm) than does the distal end (styloid process) of the ulna. This relationship is important in the diagnosis of certain injuries in the wrist region (*e.g.*, Colles' fracture, Case 6-11).

arm bones. Its proximal end has a disc-shaped **head**, a smooth cylindrical **neck**, and an oval **radial tuberosity** (Fig. 6-80).

The **body** (shaft) of the radius increases in size from the proximal to the distal end and it has an obvious lateral convexity or bowing. It is concave anteriorly in its upper three-fourths and flattened in its distal one-fourth. The **anterior oblique line** of the radius runs obliquely across the front of the body from the region of the radial tuberosity to the area of greatest bowing (Fig. 6-80). The medial aspect of the body has a sharp **interosseous border** for attachment of the interosseous membrane; its lateral border is rounded.

The distal end bears an **ulnar notch** medially into which the head of the ulna fits (Fig. 6-80). Laterally the distal end of the radius tapers abruptly into the prominent pyramidal **styloid process**. Of the two forearm bones, only the radius articulates with the carpal bones of the wrist (Fig. 6-1). It carries the wrist about the ulna during pronation and supination (Fig. 6-79). The inferior surface of the distal end of the radius is smooth and concave where it articulates with the carpal bones. Posteriorly there is a prominent **dorsal tubercle** (Fig. 6-81).

The Ulna (Figs. 6-1, 6-79 to 6-81, and 6-157). The ulna (L. elbow) is the longer and the medial of the two forearm bones. This prismatic bone looks somewhat like a wrench, with the **olecranon** resembling the upper jaw, the **coronoid process** (G. crown-like) the lower jaw, and the **trochlear notch** the mouth. The pulley-shaped trochlea of the humerus articulates with the trochlear notch (Figs. 6-1 and 6-161).

Observe that the proximal "wrench-like" end of the ulna is larger than the rounded

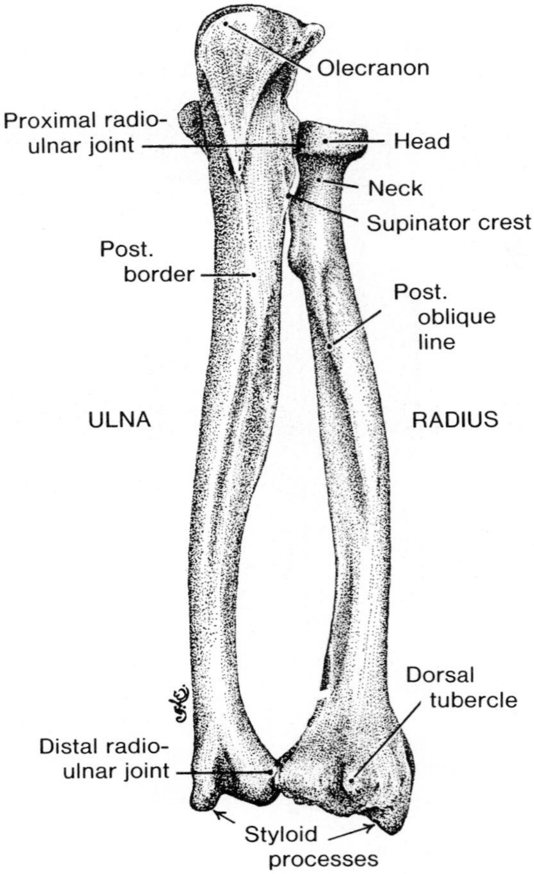

Figure 6-81. Drawing of the posterior aspect of the radius and the ulna. Note the disc-shaped head of the radius. Its posterior surface can be felt through the skin in the depression that is visible on the lateral side of the posterior surface of the extended elbow (Fig. 6-83).

head or distal end. The lateral side of the coronoid process has a small, shallow **radial notch** for the head of the radius (Fig. 6-80). Below the radial notch and extending on to the body is a triangular **supinator fossa** which gives origin to the supinator muscle (Fig. 6-80). It is bounded posteriorly by a distinct **supinator crest** (Figs. 6-81 and 6-157*B*). The anterior surface of the coronoid process is rough and ends distally in the **tuberosity of the ulna** (Fig. 6-80).

The **body** (shaft) of the ulna is thick proximally. The small slender distal end is composed of a rounded **head** and a small, conical **styloid process** (Fig. 6-81). The lateral aspect of the body of the ulna has a sharp interosseous border for attachment of the interosseous membrane (Fig. 6-80).

SURFACE ANATOMY OF THE FOREARM

The head of the radius can be palpated and felt to rotate in the depression on the posterolateral aspect of the extended elbow, just distal to the lateral epicondyle of the humerus (Fig. 6-83). Feel the head of your radius rotate during pronation and supination of your forearm (Fig. 6-79).

The body of the radius is partly palpable and the radial styloid process is easily palpated on the lateral side of the wrist (Fig. 6-82). It is located about 2 cm more distal than the ulnar styloid (Fig. 6-81). *This relationship is important* in the diagnosis of certain injuries in the wrist region (*e.g.*, **Colles' fracture**, Case 6-11). Just above the radial styloid the anterior, lateral, and posterior surfaces of the radius are palpable for a few centimeters. Note that the anterior and posterior surfaces are deep to the tendons. The lateral surface of the radius is easier to palpate and can often be palpated to the middle of the forearm. The entire posterioinferior margin of the radius is palpable medially from the styloid process to the distal radioulnar joint (Fig. 6-171). Insert your fingernail a short distance into the groove in the posterior part of the distal radioulnar joint. Grasp the distal end of the radius between your forefinger and thumb; it is located about 2 cm proximal to the distal skin crease at the wrist (Figs. 6-82 and 6-122).

The olecranon can be easily palpated and the skin covering it is often rough (Fig. 6-83) because the elbow frequently rests on it. The subcutaneous posterior border of the ulna can be palpated along its entire length.

The ulnar nerve can be palpated as a rounded cord where it lies posterior to the medial epicondyle of the humerus (Figs. 6-72, 6-73, and 6-83). Roll it against the bone and tap it with your finger. You may feel a tingling along the ulnar side of your hand, the area of skin supplied by the ulnar nerve (Figs. 6-29, 6-102, and 6-103).

The head of the ulna forms a rounded

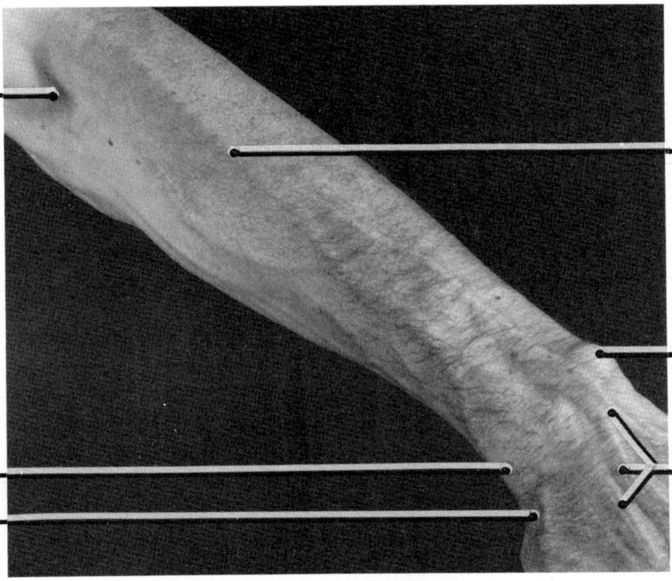

Figure 6-82. Photograph of the left forearm and hand in pronation of a 46-year-old man showing the principal surface landmarks. Compare with Figure 6-80. The head of the ulna is a rounded subcutaneous prominence that is easily seen and felt on the medial part of the dorsal aspect of the wrist region when the hand is pronated. The styloid process of the ulna is also subcutaneous and can be felt slightly distal and considerably ventral to the head of the ulna. The styloid process of the radius is not subcutaneous; it is overlaid by the tendons of the abductor pollicis longus and extensor pollicis brevis in the proximal part of the anatomical snuff box. For a close-up of this man's snuff box, see Figure 6-113.

subcutaneous prominence that can be easily seen and felt on the medial part of the dorsal aspect of the wrist when the hand is pronated (Figs. 6-82 and 6-83). The **styloid process**, also subcutaneous, may be felt slightly distal and posterior to the head.

MUSCLES OF CUBITAL REGION

The **brachialis muscle**, forming part of the floor of the cubital fossa (Figs. 6-75 and 6-84), was described previously.

The Supinator Muscle (Figs. 6-84, 6-97, and 6-101). This muscle lies deeply with the brachialis and forms part of the floor of the cubital fossa. Its *humeral and ulnar heads of origin* envelop the neck and proximal part of the shaft of the radius.

Origin (Figs. 6-86, 6-157*B*, and 6-160). *Humeral head*, **lateral epicondyle** of humerus, **radial collateral ligament** of elbow joint, and **anular ligament** of radius; *ulnar head*, **supinator fossa** and **supinator crest** of ulna.

Insertion (Figs. 6-85 and 6-86). **Lateral surface of proximal third of shaft of radius** (*i.e.*, distal to neck).

Nerve Supply (Fig. 6-84). **Deep branch of radial** nerve (C5 and C6).

Action (Fig. 6-79*A*). **Supinates forearm** (*i.e.*, rotates palm of hand anteriorly). *The biceps brachii assists the supinator in forceful supination*, particularly when the forearm is flexed (*e.g.*, when driving a screw).

The Brachioradialis Muscle (Figs. 6-70, 6-71, 6-84, 6-89, and 6-90). This *important muscle* forms the lateral boundary of the cubital fossa and is the most superficial muscle on the radial side of the forearm.

Origin (Figs. 6-67*A* and 6-85). Proximal two-thirds of **lateral supracondylar ridge** of humerus and **lateral intermuscular septum**.

Insertion (Figs. 6-85 and 6-86). **Lateral side of distal end of radius**, near base of styloid process.

Nerve Supply. **Radial** nerve (C5 and C6).

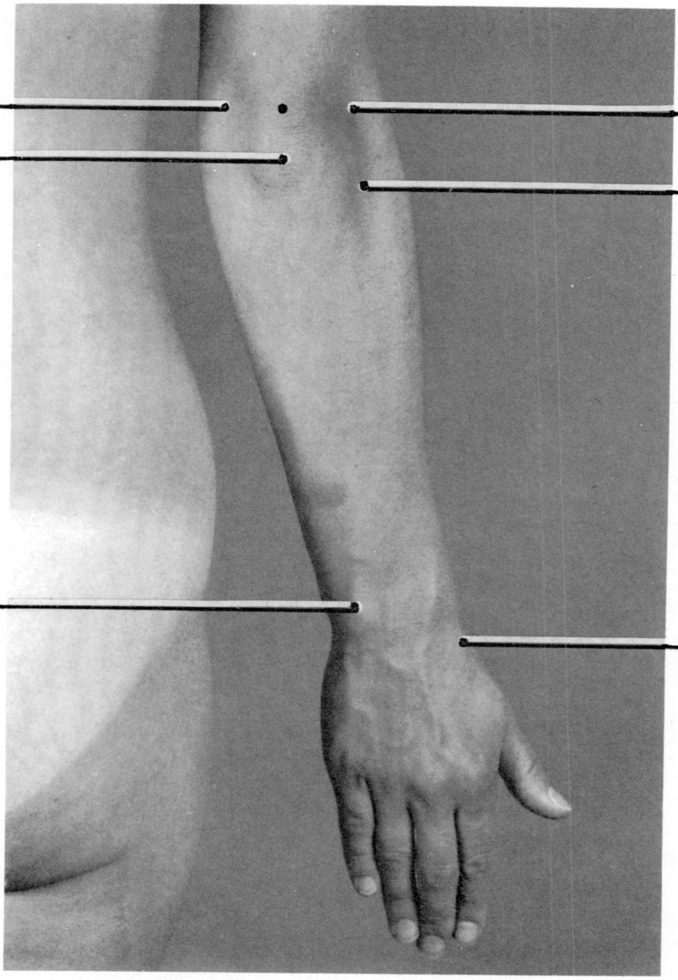

Figure 6-83. Photograph of the posterior aspect of the forearm and hand of a 27-year-old woman showing the principal surface landmarks of the bones (Figs. 6-81 and 6-86). In full extension of the elbow joint, as here, the tip of the olecranon (*black dot*) and the two humeral epicondyles are practically in a straight line. This relationship is important in the diagnosis of certain injuries of the elbow region, *e.g.*, dislocation of the elbow (Fig. 6-166). The head of the radius may be palpated in the depression on the lateral side of the elbow. The styloid process of the radius can be felt just distal to the lateral aspect of the distal end of the radius.

This is an important exception; usually the radial supplies extensors.

Action. **Flexes elbow** joint. It acts to best advantage when the forearm is in the midprone position (*i.e.*, midway between pronation and supination). Put your forearm in this position and flex it against resistance; observe and feel your brachioradialis as shown in Figure 6-70.

The Pronator Teres Muscle (Figs. 6-70, 6-84, and 6-90). This fusiform muscle forms the medial boundary of the cubital fossa as it crosses the front of the proximal half of the forearm obliquely. It has **two heads of origin.**

Origin (Figs. 6-54 and 6-85). *Humeral head,* **medial epicondyle** of humerus by common flexor tendon; *ulnar head,* **coronoid process** of ulna.

Insertion (Fig. 6-86). **Middle of lateral**

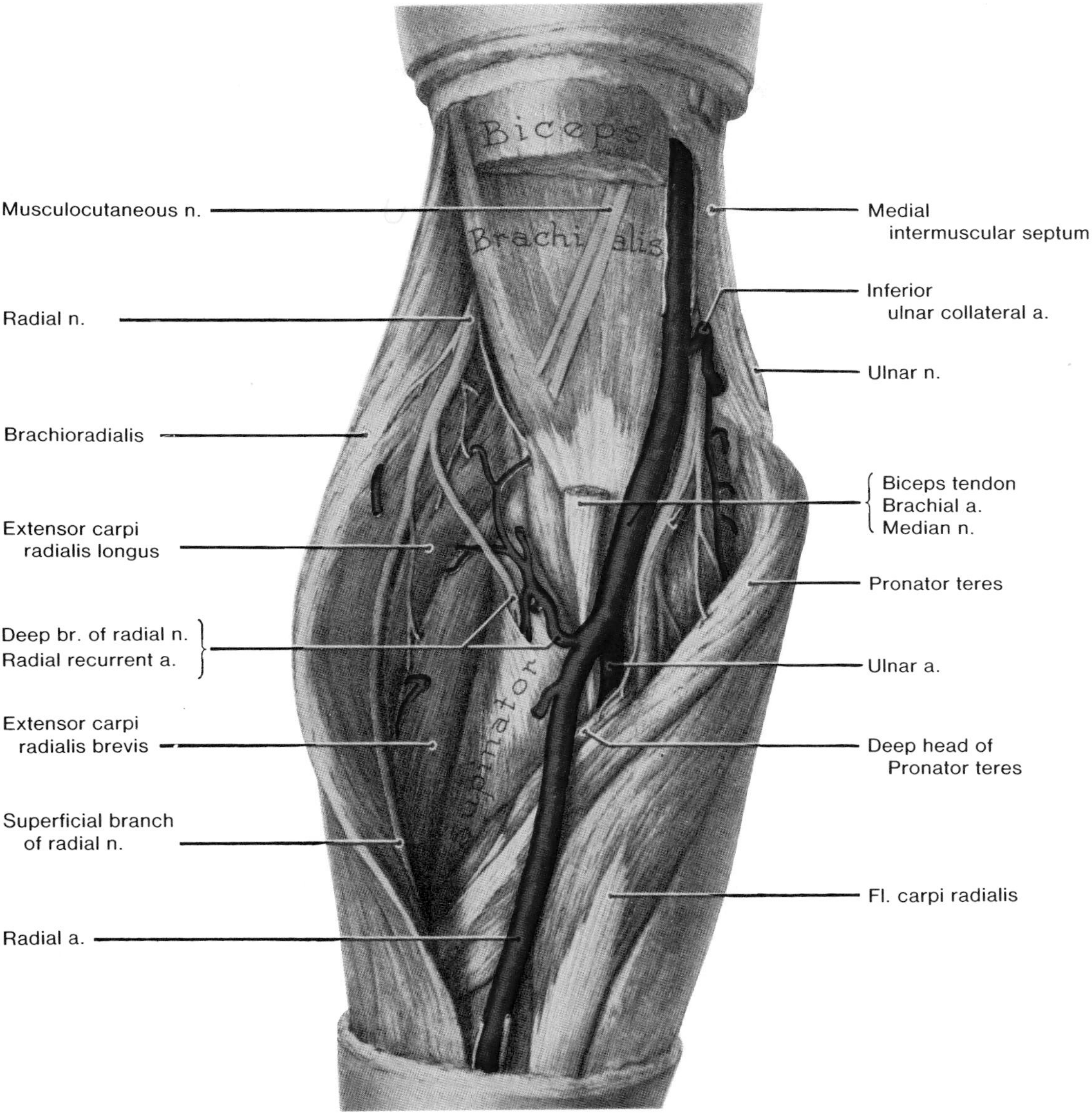

Figure 6-84. Drawing of a dissection of the front of the right elbow. Part of the biceps is excised and the cubital fossa is opened widely. Note the brachialis and supinator muscles which form the floor of the cubital fossa. Observe the brachial artery lying between the biceps tendon and the median nerve and dividing into two nearly equal branches, the ulnar and radial arteries. Observe the median nerve supplying flexor muscles; its motor branches arise from its medial side, except for the twig to the deep head of the pronator teres. Note the radial nerve supplying extensor muscles; its motor branches arise from its lateral side, except for the twig to brachialis. The radial nerve has been displaced laterally so its lateral branches appear to run medially in the drawing. Observe the deep branch of the radial nerve piercing the supinator muscle. It appears in the posterior compartment of the forearm as the posterior interosseous nerve (Fig. 6-109).

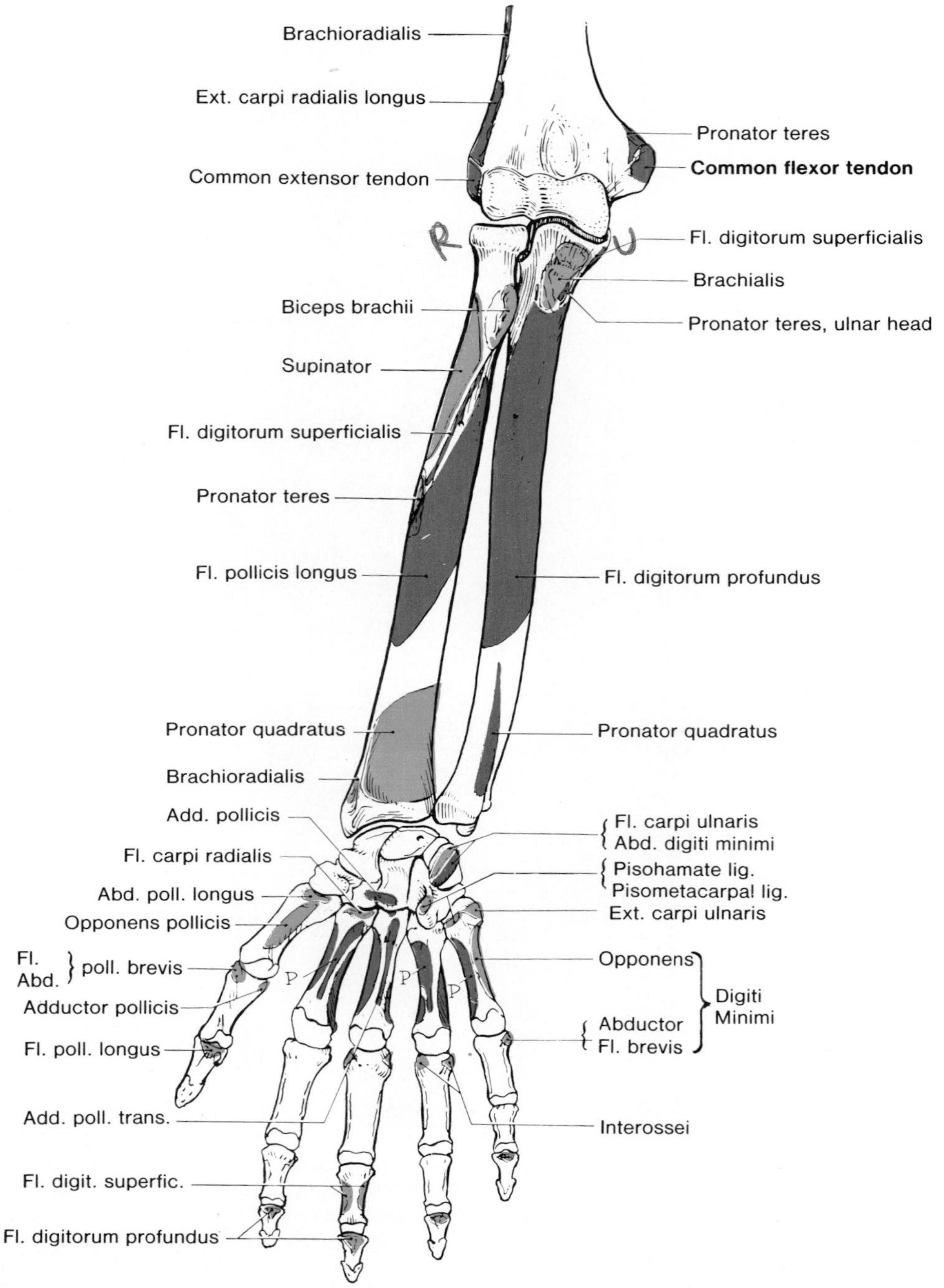

Figure 6-85. Drawing of an anterior view of the bones of the arm, forearm, and hand showing the attachment of muscles. Note particularly the origin of the *common flexor tendon* from the front of the medial epicondyle, from which the superficial flexor muscles arise and diverge like a narrow fan (Figs. 6-90 and 6-94). In general they pass to the anterior surface of the forearm and hand.

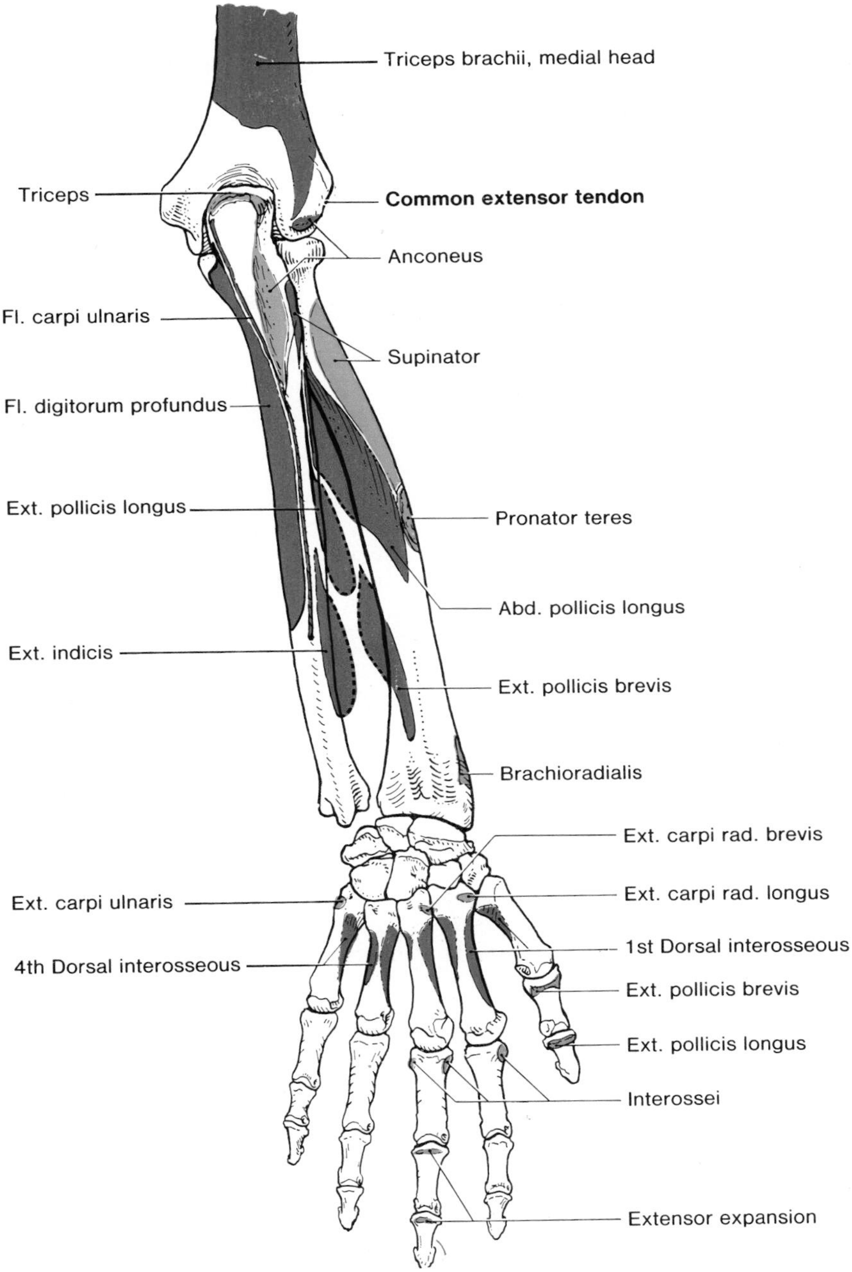

Figure 6-86. Drawing of a posterior view of the bones of the arm, forearm, and hand showing the attachments of muscles. Note particularly the origin of the *common extensor tendon* from the lateral epicondyle of the humerus; however, observe that the main origin of this tendon is from the lower anterior part of the epicondyle (Fig. 6-85). Four superficial extensor muscles arise by this common tendon and in general pass to the dorsum of the forearm and hand.

surface of radius on the summit of its main curve.

Nerve Supply. **Median** nerve (C6 and C7).

Actions (Fig. 6-79*B*). **Pronates forearm** and **flexes elbow** joint.

BONES OF HAND

To understand the insertions of antebrachial muscles, it is necessary to consider the skeleton of the hand with the forearm.

The Carpus or Wrist Bones (Figs. 6-85 to 6-88). The eight small bones of the wrist are referred to collectively as the carpus (L. wrist) and individually as the carpal bones. They are arranged in proximal and distal rows, each containing four bones.

The proximal row of carpal bones (lateral to medial) consists of the **scaphoid** (navicular), the **lunate**, the **triquetrum** (triangular), and the **pisiform** (Fig. 6-87*A*). The pea-shaped pisiform is included in the proximal row even though it is a sesamoid bone in the tendon of the flexor carpi ulnaris (Figs. 6-92, 6-93, and 6-97). *The pisiform bone is a clinically important landmark that is easily palpable* (Fig. 6-92).

The distal row of carpal bones (lateral to medial) consists of the **trapezium**, the **trapezoid**, the **capitate**, and the **hamate** bones. The hamate can be identified by its prominent process, the hamulus or **hook of hamate**, which can be palpated inferolateral to the pisiform bone (Fig. 6-87*A*). You should also be able to identify the **tubercle of the scaphoid** and a distinct ridge, the **tubercle of the trapezium** (Figs. 6-87*A* and 6-88). You can palpate the tubercle of the scaphoid on the anterior aspect of the wrist, just proximal to the thenar eminence (thickening of palm at base of thumb). If you have trouble feeling it, extend your wrist and then palpate at the junction of the middle and lateral thirds of the transverse distal wrist crease (Figs. 6-92 and 6-121).

The carpal bones articulate with each other by synovial joints and are bound together with ligaments to form a compact mass which has a posterior convexity and anterior concavity. This **carpal sulcus** is converted into an osseofibrous **carpal tunnel** (canal) by the flexor retinaculum which is attached to the scaphoid and trapezium laterally and to the pisiform and lunate medially (Fig. 6-88). This tunnel is completely filled in our bodies by tendons and the median nerve (Fig. 6-97).

CLINICALLY ORIENTED COMMENTS

The scaphoid and trapezium lie in the floor of the anatomical snuff box (Fig. 6-109). *The scaphoid is the most frequently fractured of the carpal bones.* Injury to this bone results in localized tenderness in this depression at the base of the thumb (Case 6-9).

Although fracture of the lunate is rare, anterior dislocation is not uncommon. A displaced lunate may compress the median nerve against the flexor retinaculum (Fig. 6-97). For the effects of this nerve injury, see Case 6-10.

The Metacarpus (Fig. 6-87). The five bones of the hand (**metacarpal bones**) are miniature long bones. They extend from the carpus to the digits (thumb and fingers) and are numbered from the lateral side; thus, the thumb contains the first metacarpal. In Figures 6-87 and 6-122, note that the first metacarpal is shorter than the others. Although covered with tendons, the metacarpals can be easily palpated throughout their whole length on the dorsum of the hand (Fig. 6-120).

The **heads** of the metacarpals are at their distal ends where they articulate with the phalanges (bones of digits). These heads form the proximal row of knuckles, which become visible when the fist is clenched. On the dorsal surface of each head there is a small **tubercle** on each side for attachment of collateral ligaments and joint capsules (Figs. 6-87*A*).

The **bodies** (shafts) of the metacarpals are slightly concave on their medial and lateral sides, where the dorsal interosseous muscles attach (Fig. 6-132). The **bases** of the metacarpals, which are arranged fanwise around the distal row of carpal bones, differ considerably from each other (Fig. 6-78*B*).

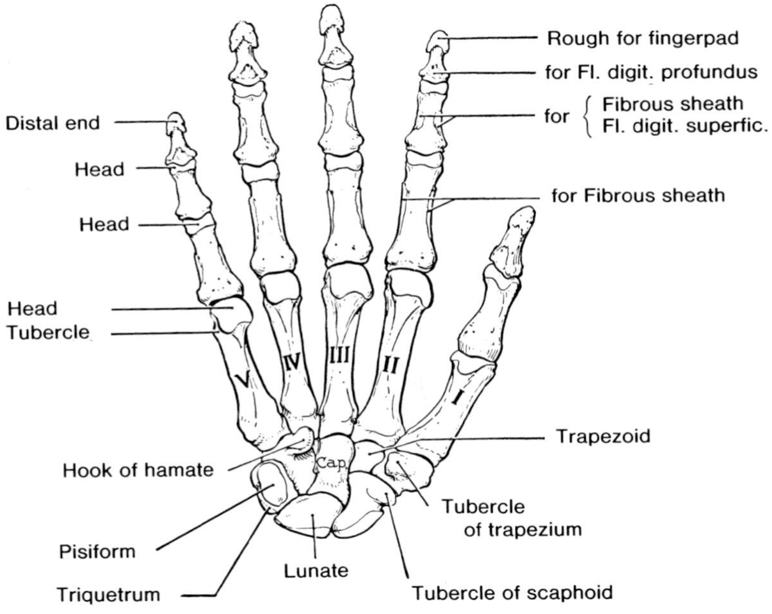

A. PALMAR ASPECT

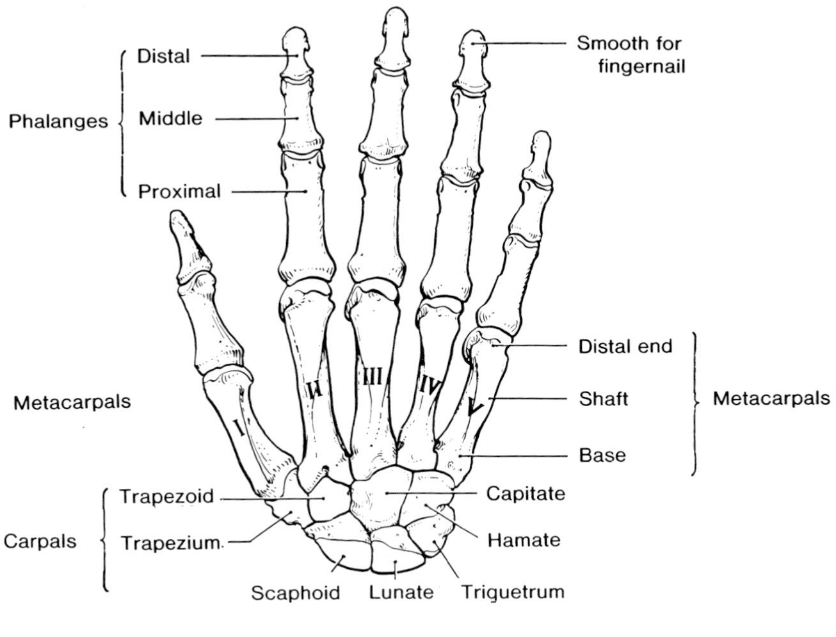

B. DORSAL ASPECT

Figure 6-87. Drawings of the bones of the hand. The skeleton consists of three segments: (1) the carpal bones of the wrist, (2) the metacarpal bones of the palm, and (3) the phalanges of the digits. The heads of the metacarpals form the distinctive knuckles of the hand. The phalanges may be felt easily; their heads form the knuckles of the fingers.

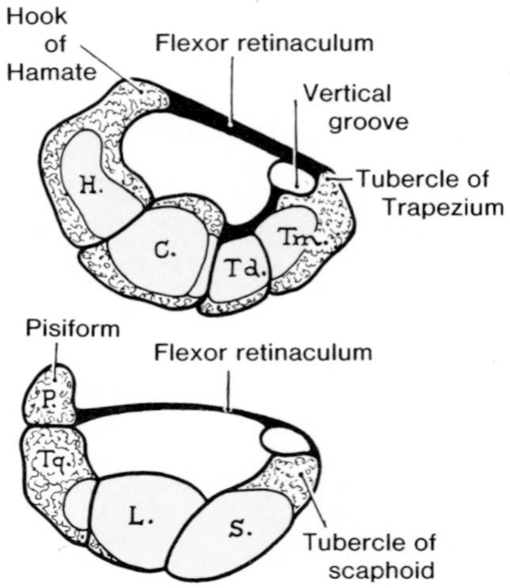

Figure 6-88. Drawings of the carpal bones (Fig. 6-87) showing how the flexor retinaculum stretches between the ends of the concavity of the carpal bones and forms a 2- to 3-cm osseofibrous carpal tunnel through which pass several tendons and the median nerve to the hand. The flexor carpi radialis runs through a small tunnel called the vertical groove.

The Phalanges (Fig. 6-87). Each phalanx is also a miniature long bone consisting of a **body** (shaft), a larger proximal end or **base**, and a smaller distal end or **head**. The thumb (digit 1) has two phalanges (proximal and distal) and each finger (digits 2 to 5) has three phalanges (proximal, middle, and distal). The phalanges of the thumb are shorter and broader than those of the fingers. The proximal phalanges of the digits are the longest and the distal ones the shortest.

THE ANTERIOR ANTEBRACHIAL MUSCLES

Disposition of the Antebrachial Muscles (Figs. 6-75 and 6-84 to 6-86). The elbow joint is covered anteriorly by the biceps and brachialis muscles, and the bicipital aponeurosis forms the deep part of the roof of the cubital fossa (Fig. 6-75). The elbow joint is covered posteriorly by the triceps muscle; as a consequence, the flexor and extensor muscles of the forearm originating from the humerus must arise from the medial and lateral epicondyles, respectively. Thus, the flexor-pronator group arises by a *common flexor tendon* from the medial epicondyle, referred to as the **common flexor origin** (Fig. 6-85), and the extensor-supinator group arises by a *common extensor tendon* from the lateral epicondyle, referred to as the **common extensor origin** (Figs. 6-85 and 6-86).

Distal to the elbow joint, the other and deeper flexor and extensor muscles originate from the anterior and posterior aspects of the shafts of the ulna and radius, respectively. The dividing line on the posterior aspect of the forearm between the extensor and flexor groups is the posterior border of the ulna, which is palpable from the olecranon to the wrist (Fig. 6-89).

All the flexor tendons are located on the anterior surface of the wrist and most of them are held in place by the **flexor retinaculum**, a thickening of deep fascia (Fig. 6-97).

The eight muscles in the front of the forearm are classified as **flexors** (Fig. 6-89), and they can be organized into *three functional groups* as follows: (1) **muscles that rotate the radius on the ulna** (pronator teres and pronator quadratus—the supinator also performs this activity but it is grouped with the extensor muscles); (2) **muscles that flex the hand at the wrist** (flexor carpi radialis, flexor carpi ulnaris, and palmaris longus); and (3) **muscles that flex the digits** (flexor digitorum superficialis, flexor digitorum profundus, and flexor pollicis longus).

The anterior antebrachial muscles can be divided into *three layers*: (1) **superficial** (pronator teres, flexor carpi radialis, palmaris longus, and flexor carpi ulnaris); (2) **intermediate** (flexor digitorum superficialis); and (3) **deep** (flexor digitorum profundus, flexor pollicis longus, and pronator quadratus). A septum separates the deep flexors from the superficial and intermediate flexors (Fig. 6-89). Observe that *within the septum are located the ulnar artery and the ulnar nerve.*

Flex and extend your fingers (*i.e.*, make a fist and open it) and feel the contraction of the superficial and deep flexors. Verify by palpation that this flexor group of muscles originates by a common flexor tendon

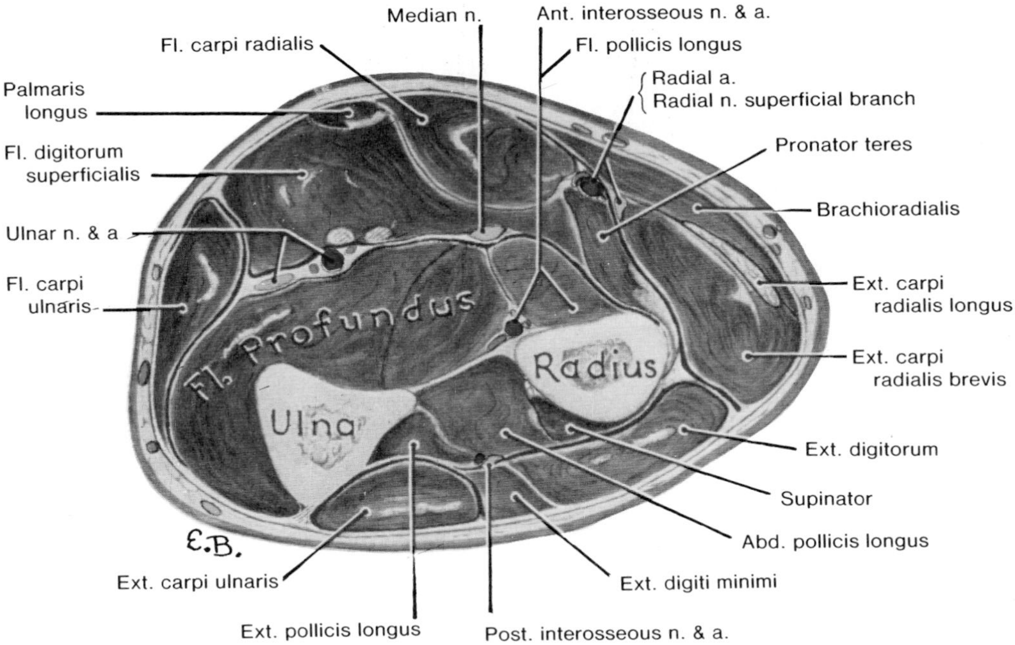

Figure 6-89. Drawing of a cross-section through the middle of the forearm at the level of insertion of the pronator teres (Fig. 6-86). Observe the interosseous membrane stretching from the interosseous (lateral) border of the ulna to the interosseous (medial) border of the radius and spreading far on to the anterior surface and not so far on to the posterior surface of the radius. Note the ulnar nerve and artery and the median nerve lying in the areolar septum between the superficial and the deep digital flexors. Observe the flexor digitorum profundus and flexor pollicis longus around the medial and anterior surfaces of the ulna and the anterior surface of the radius; this is flexor territory. Note the pronator teres inserted into the lateral surface of the radius (see Fig. 6-86). Because it invades the extensor territory, it has the ability to pronate the forearm and hand (Figs. 6-79*B* and 6-173).

from the medial humeral epicondyle (Figs. 6-85, 6-90, and 6-94).

The Superficial Flexor Muscle Layer (Figs. 6-89 and 6-90). This group of four muscles arises by the **common flexor tendon** from the medial epicondyle and its supracondylar ridge (Fig. 6-85). This **common flexor origin** also includes the antebrachial fascia (deep fascia of the forearm) and the intermuscular septa (Fig. 6-89). The superficial muscles are mainly pronators of the forearm and/or flexors of the hand at the wrist joint.

The Pronator Teres Muscle (Figs. 6-84, 6-89, and 6-90). This muscle, a pronator of the forearm and weak flexor of the elbow joint, has been described with the muscles of the cubital region.

The Flexor Carpi Radialis Muscle (Figs. 6-89 to 6-94). This muscle lies immediately medial to the pronator teres. In the middle of the forearm its fleshy belly is replaced by a long, flattened tendon that becomes cordlike as it passes to the wrist.

Origin (Fig. 6-85). **Medial epicondyle** of humerus by *common flexor tendon.*

Insertion (Fig. 6-85). **Base of second metacarpal** bone. To reach its insertion, its long tendon passes through a canal in the lateral part of the flexor retinaculum (Fig. 6-91) and the vertical groove in the trapezium (Fig. 6-88). The stout tendon of the flexor carpi radialis can be easily palpated and observed a little lateral to the midline of the wrist (Fig. 6-92); thus, its tendon may be used as a **guide to the radial artery** (Fig. 6-90) which lies just lateral to it.

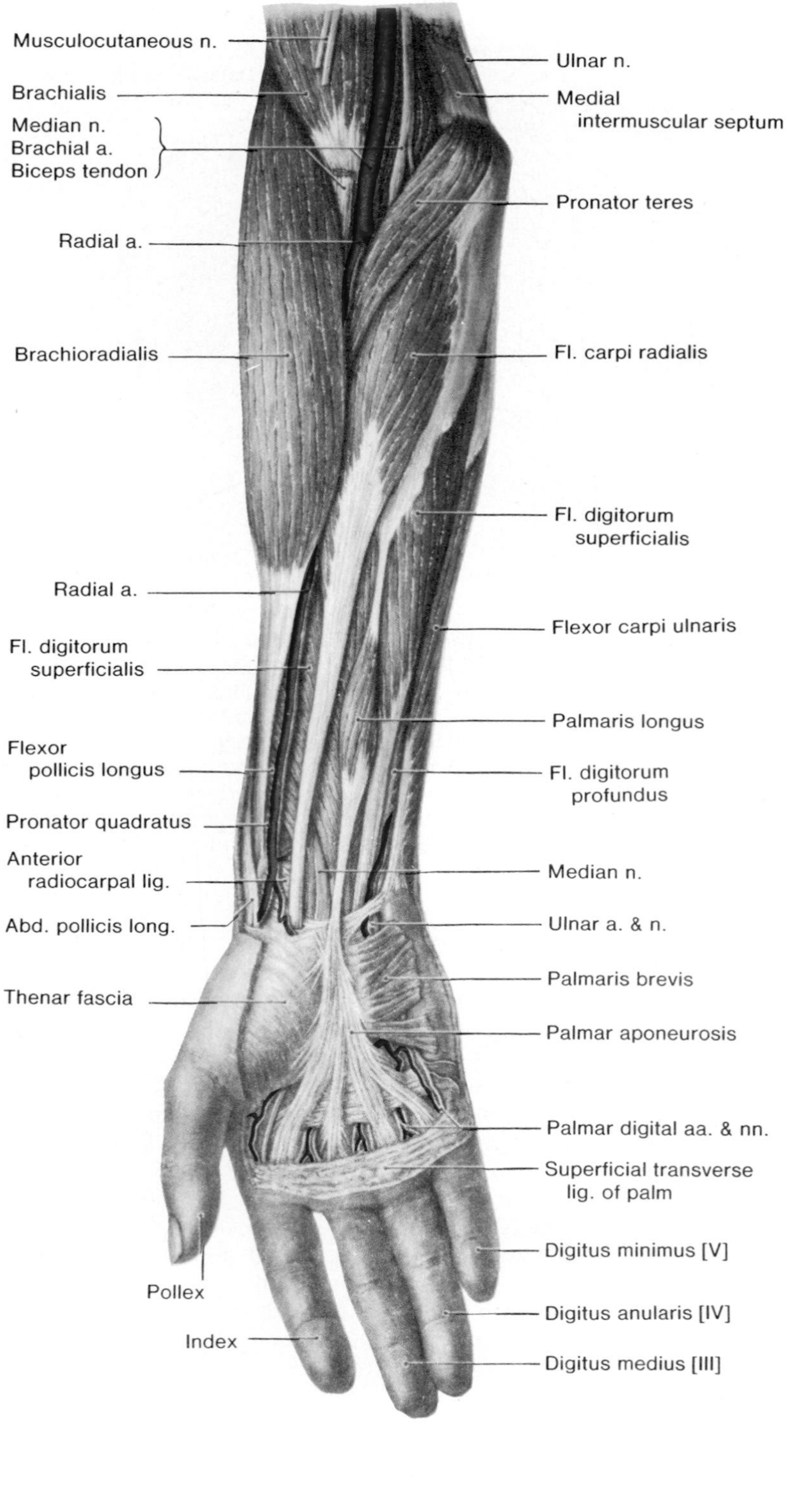
Musculocutaneous n.
Brachialis
Median n.
Brachial a.
Biceps tendon
Radial a.
Brachioradialis
Radial a.
Fl. digitorum superficialis
Flexor pollicis longus
Pronator quadratus
Anterior radiocarpal lig.
Abd. pollicis long.
Thenar fascia
Pollex
Index
Ulnar n.
Medial intermuscular septum
Pronator teres
Fl. carpi radialis
Fl. digitorum superficialis
Flexor carpi ulnaris
Palmaris longus
Fl. digitorum profundus
Median n.
Ulnar a. & n.
Palmaris brevis
Palmar aponeurosis
Palmar digital aa. & nn.
Superficial transverse lig. of palm
Digitus minimus [V]
Digitus anularis [IV]
Digitus medius [III]

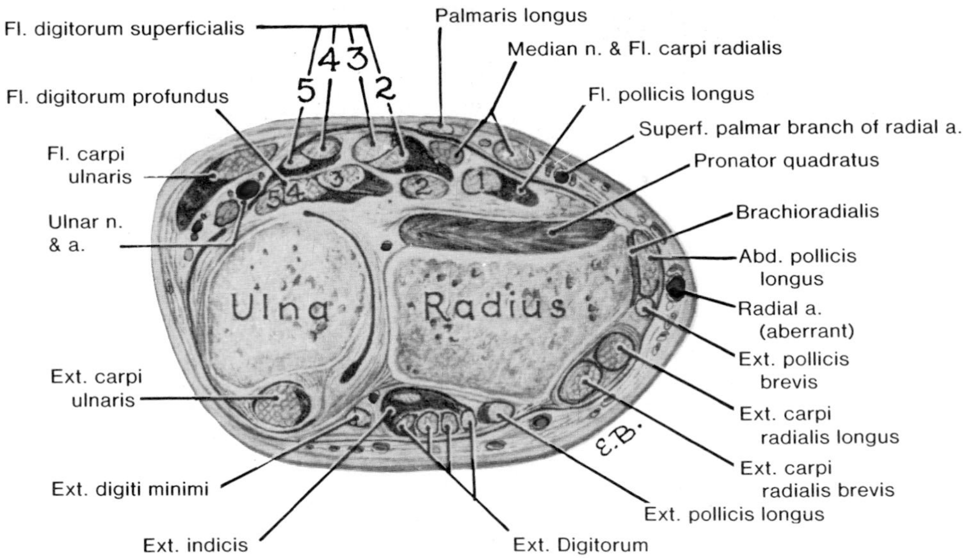

Figure 6-91. Drawing of a cross-section through the forearm above the wrist. Observe the flexor carpi radialis, palmaris longus, and flexor carpi ulnaris constituting a surface layer of flexors of the wrist. Deep to these, the long flexors of the digits: (1) the four tendons of the flexor digitorum superficialis, those to the middle and ring fingers being anterior to those to the index and little fingers; and (2) the five tendons of the deep digital flexors, lying side by side, those to the thumb (flexor pollicis longus) and index being free. Note that the ulnar nerve and artery are under the flexor carpi ulnaris; hence, the pulse of the artery cannot be felt here. Note the median nerve at the midpoint on the front of the wrist, deep to the palmaris longus, and at the lateral border of the flexor digitorum superficialis. Note the three large extensor tendons on the dorsum of the wrist; they are inserted into the metacarpal bones and work as synergists with the powerful flexors of the digits, whereas the remaining tendons, being extensors of the digits, are slender.

Nerve Supply. **Median** nerve (C6 and C7).

Actions. **Flexes** and **abducts wrist**. It also flexes the elbow joint to some extent.

The Palmaris Longus Muscle (Figs. 6-89 to 6-94). Although this small fusiform muscle is absent on one or both sides in about 13% of people, its actions are not missed.

Origin (Fig. 6-85). **Medial epicondyle** of humerus by *common flexor tendon.*

Insertion (Fig. 6-90). **Palmar aponeurosis.** Its long thin tendon passes superfi-

---

Figure 6-90. Drawing of a dissection of the superficial muscles in the front of the forearm. *At the elbow* observe the brachial artery lying between the biceps tendon and the median nerve and bifurcating into the radial and ulnar arteries. *In the forearm* observe the radial artery lying between two muscle groups. The muscles lateral to this artery are supplied by the radial nerve, whereas those medial to it are supplied by the median and ulnar nerves; thus, *no motor nerve crosses the radial artery*. Note the lateral group of muscles, represented by the brachioradialis, slightly overlapping the radial artery which is otherwise superficial. Note that the four superficial muscles (pronator teres, flexor carpi radialis, palmaris longus, and flexor carpi ulnaris) radiate from the medial epicondyle by a *common flexor tendon* (Fig. 6-85). Note that the palmaris longus is continued into the palm as the palmar aponeurosis which receives an accession of fibers from the flexor retinaculum and divides into four longitudinal bands, one for each finger. *At the wrist* note the radial artery lateral to the flexor carpi radialis tendon and the ulnar artery lateral to the flexor carpi ulnaris tendon. Compare the wrist with the photograph of this region (Fig. 6-92).

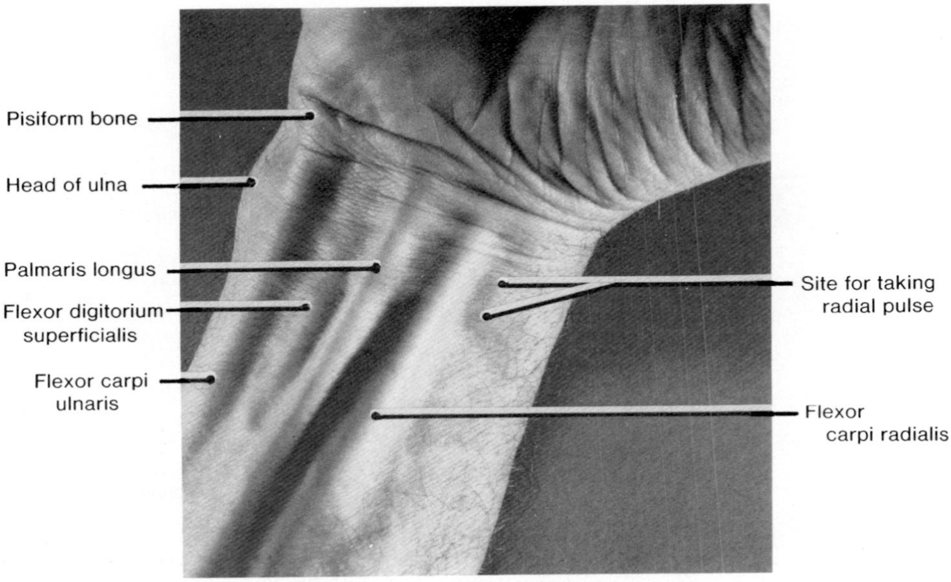

Figure 6-92. Photograph of the anterior aspect of the wrist of a 46-year-old man showing the principal surface markings and the favorite site for taking the pulse of the radial artery. The cord-like tendon of the flexor carpi radialis serves as a guide to the radial artery which lies lateral to it (Figs. 6-90 and 6-93). The long slender tendon of the palmaris longus (absent in about 13% of people) serves as a guide to the median nerve which is deep and lateral to it (Figs. 6-90, 6-91, and 6-93). The flexor carpi ulnaris muscle overlies the ulnar nerve throughout its length (Fig. 6-91), but at the wrist its tendon may be used as a guide to the ulnar nerve and artery which are just lateral to it (Fig. 6-93).

cial to the flexor retinaculum (Fig. 6-91) and, when present, it is easily felt and observed (Fig. 6-92). It may be used as a **guide to the median nerve** which is just lateral to it at the wrist (Fig. 6-93).

Nerve Supply. **Median** nerve (C7 and C8).

Action. **Flexes wrist** and may act as tensor of palmar fascia.

The Flexor Carpi Ulnaris Muscle (Figs. 6-89 to 6-95 and 6-97). This is the most medial of the superficial flexor muscles. It has *two heads of origin* between which the ulnar nerve passes distally.

Origin (Figs. 6-85 and 6-86). *Humeral head,* **medial epicondyle** of humerus by common flexor tendon; *ulnar head,* **medial border of olecranon** and **posterior border of ulna.**

Insertion (Figs. 6-85 and 6-93). **Pisiform bone** and through two strong ligaments (pisohamate and pisometacarpal) into **hook of hamate** and **base of fifth metacarpal bone**, respectively. The tendon of the flexor carpi ulnaris is easily felt and observed in front of the ulnar border of the wrist, where it is inserted into the pisiform bone (Figs. 6-90, 6-92, and 6-93). Its tendon is a good **guide to the ulnar nerve and artery** (Fig. 6-93) which are on its lateral side at the wrist.

Nerve Supply. **Ulnar** nerve (C7 and C8).

Actions. **Flexes** and **adducts wrist**.

The Intermediate Flexor Muscle Layer (Fig. 6-89). Deep to the four flexor muscles, comprising the superficial layer just described, lies the flexor digitorum superficialis. Although it forms an intermediate layer, it is part of the superficial group of muscles.

The Flexor Digitorum Superficialis Muscle (Figs. 6-89 to 6-93 and 6-95). This is the largest superficial muscle in the forearm; it has **two heads of origin.**

Origin (Fig. 6-85). *Humeroulnar head,* **medial epicondyle** of humerus by common flexor tendon, **ulnar collateral ligament** of elbow joint, and **coronoid pro-**

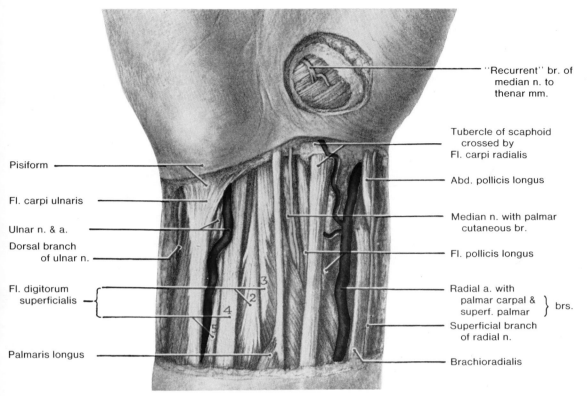

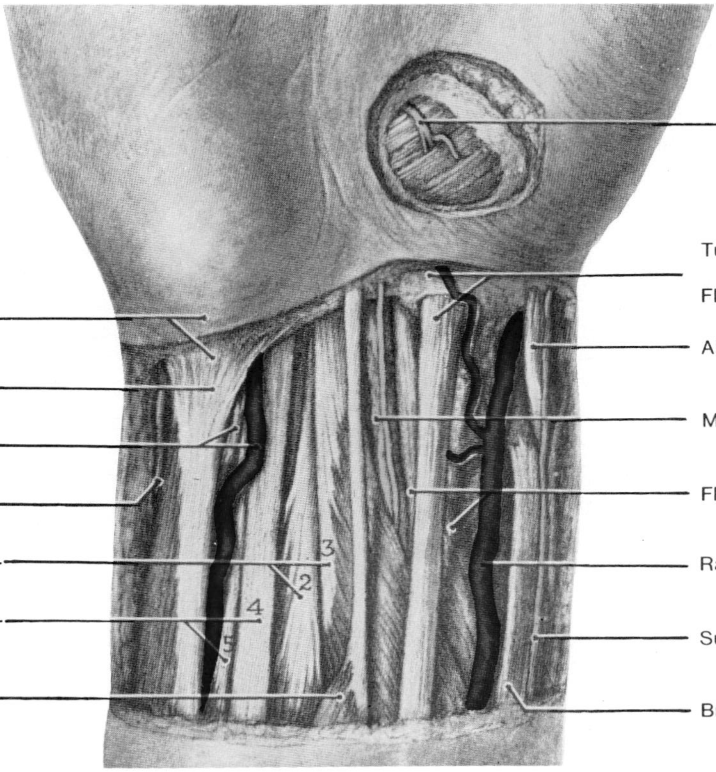

Figure 6-93. Drawing of a dissection of the structures at the front of the wrist. The distal transverse skin incision was made along the distal wrist crease (Fig. 6-94). This crease crosses the pisiform bone to which the flexor carpi ulnaris is attached. Observe the palmaris longus tendon bisecting the distal skin crease, exactly at the middle of the wrist. Note that the median nerve is deep to the lateral margin of the palmaris longus tendon. Observe also that the ulnar nerve and artery are sheltered by the flexor carpi ulnaris tendon and by the expansion this tendon gives to the flexor retinaculum (see Figure 6-90). Note the flexor digitorum superficialis tendons to digits 3 and 4 are somewhat anterior to those to digits 2 and 5. Observe the "recurrent" branch of the median nerve to the thenar muscles lying within a circle, the center of which is 2 to 4 cm distal to the tubercle of the scaphoid (Fig. 6-87*A*). This nerve may be severed by lacerations in this region, resulting in impairment of movements of the thumb (Fig. 6-129).

cess of ulna. *Radial head*, upper half of **anterior border of radius.**

Insertion (Fig. 6-85). Palmar aspect of **shafts of middle phalanges of medial four digits.** As the wrist is approached, the flexor digitorum superficialis gives rise to four tendons which pass deep to the flexor retinaculum (Figs. 6-91 and 6-95). The superficial pair of tendons passes to the middle and ring fingers (Figs. 6-93 and 6-95) within **synovial sheaths** in osseofibrous tunnels in the fingers (Figs. 6-96 and 6-98).

Nerve Supply. **Median** nerve (C7, C8, and T1).

Actions. **Flexes middle phalanges of medial four digits** (*i.e.*, flexes proximal interphalangeal joints). In continued action, it **flexes metacarpophalangeal** and **wrist joints.**

The Deep Flexor Muscle Layer (Figs. 6-89 and 6-97). This comprises the third layer of muscles in the forearm and consists of the flexor digitorum profundus, the flexor pollicis longus, and the pronator quadratus. None of these muscles arises from the humerus; they arise from the radius or the ulna.

The Flexor Digitorum Profundus (Figs.

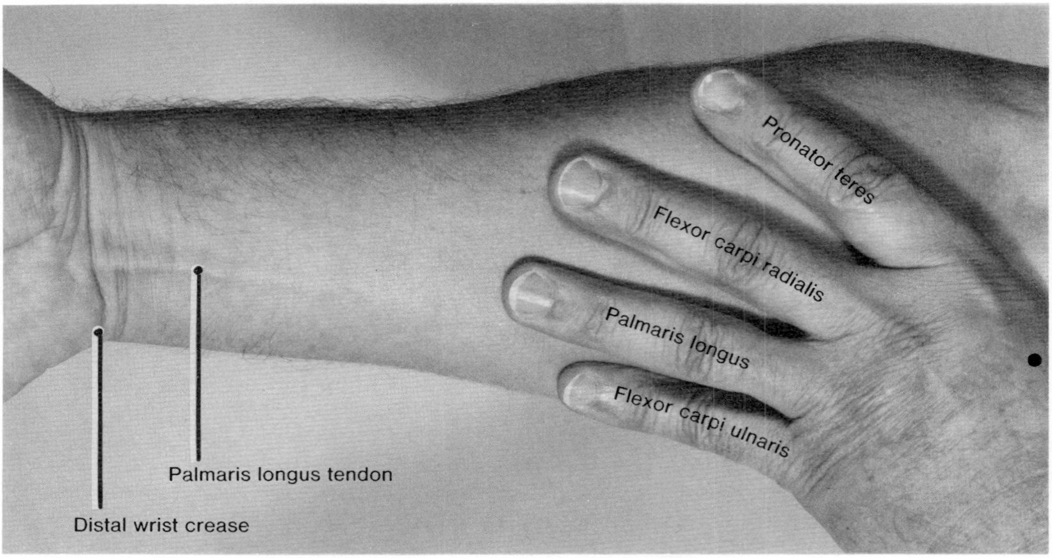

Figure 6-94. Photograph of the anterior surface of the right forearm and wrist region of a 53-year-old man who is showing how to locate the position of the four superficial flexor muscles. The thumb of the person's left hand is placed posterior to the elbow around the medial epicondyle of the humerus (deep to *black dot*), from which arises the common flexor tendon of these superficial muscles (Fig. 6-85).

6-89 to 6-91, 6-97, and 6-101). This long, thick, deep (L. profundus) muscle is the only one which can flex the distal interphalangeal joints of the fingers (*i.e.*, it flexes all joints of the fingers).

Origin (Fig. 6-85). Proximal three-fourths of **medial** and **anterior surfaces of ulna** and medial half of **interosseous membrane**. The muscle divides into four parts which end in four tendons that pass posterior to the tendons of the flexor digitorum superficialis and the flexor retinaculum (Figs. 6-90, 6-91, and 6-97). Each tendon enters the fibrous sheath of its digit posterior to the tendon of the flexor digitorum superficialis (Fig. 6-98).

Insertion (Fig. 6-85). Palmar surfaces of **bases of distal phalanges of medial four digits**.

Nerve Supply. The *medial part* associated with the little and ring fingers is supplied by the **ulnar** nerve (C8 and T1), and the *lateral part* associated with the index and middle fingers is supplied by the **median** nerve (C8 and T1) via its anterior interosseous branch.

Actions. **Flexes distal phalanges**. It is the only muscle that can flex the distal interphalangeal joints of the medial four digits. Clench your extended fist tightly and feel this muscle contract on the medial side of the sharp posterior border of the ulna. Although its action is to flex the distal interphalangeal joints of these fingers, it helps to flex all joints crossed by its tendons (*i.e.*, the wrist joint, the metacarpophalangeal joints, and the two interphalangeal joints).

The Flexor Pollicis Longus Muscle (Figs. 6-89 to 6-93, 6-97, and 6-98). This flexor of the thumb (L. *pollex*), the first digit of hand, lies lateral to the flexor digitorum profundus.

Origin (Figs. 6-80 and 6-85). **Anterior surface of radius, distal to oblique line** and lateral half of **interosseous membrane**. Its flat tendon passes deep to the flexor retinaculum (Fig. 6-97), enveloped in its own synovial sheath (Fig. 6-98).

Insertion (Fig. 6-85). Palmar surface of **base of distal phalanx of thumb.**

Nerve Supply. Anterior interosseous branch of **median** nerve (C8 and T1).

Actions. **Flexes phalanges of thumb**

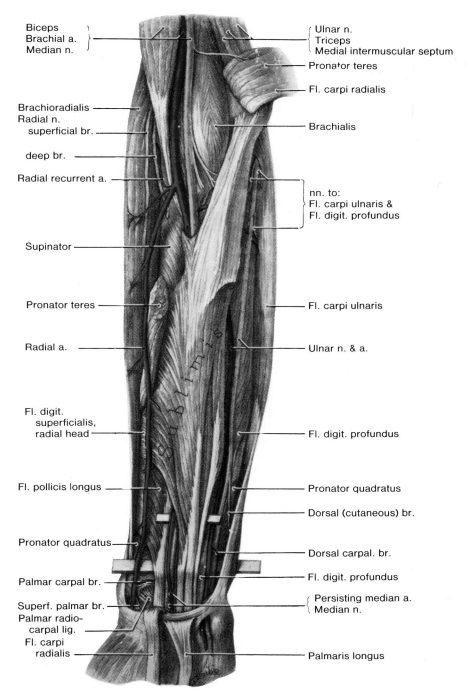

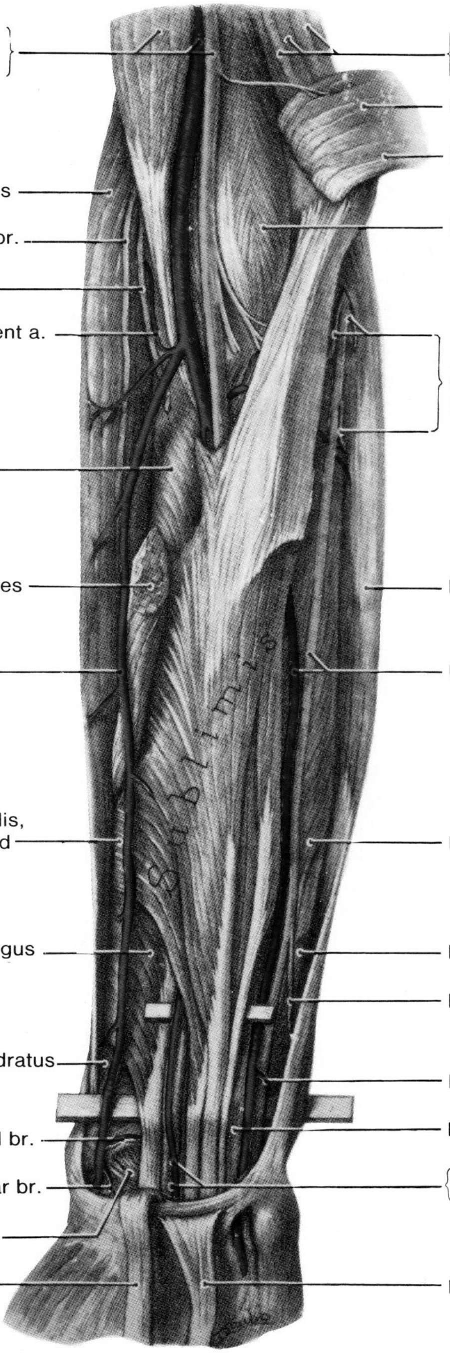

Figure 6-95. Drawing of a dissection showing the flexor digitorum superficials (sublimis) and related structures. Observe the oblique origin of the superficialis from (1) the medical epicondyle of the humerus, (2) the ulnar collateral ligament of the elbow, (3) the tubercle of the coronoid process, and (4) the upper two-thirds of the radius. The superficialis, like the three muscles anterior to it and the two and one-half muscles posterior to it, is supplied by the median nerve. Observe the ulnar artery descending obliquely behind the superficialis to join the ulnar nerve. Note the median nerve descending vertically behind the superficialis, clinging to it, and appearing at its lateral border. Observe the digital tendons of this muscle at the wrist (for a better view of them, see Fig. 6-93).

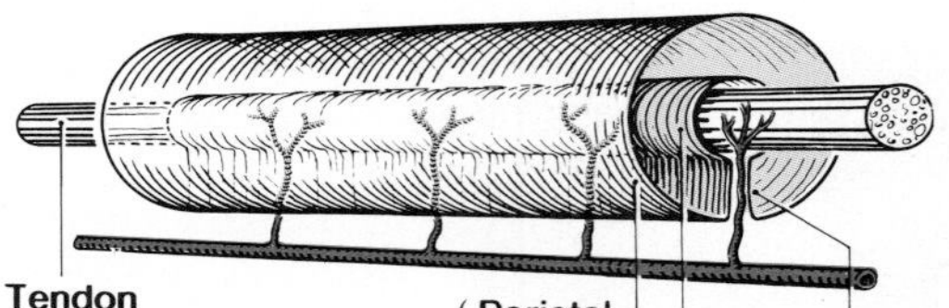

Figure 6-96. Illustration showing the structure of a synovial sheath. This tubular bursa is a lubricating device that envelopes the long digital tendons where they pass through the osseofibrous tunnels in the fingers (Fig. 6-98). The layers of the synovial sheath are separated by a capillary film of synovial fluid. Note that the mesotendons convey small blood vessels to the tendons. In the fingers these mesotendons are represented by fibrous cords called vinculae (Fig. 6-132*A*).

and is the only muscle that flexes the interphalangeal joint of the thumb. It also flexes the metacarpophalangeal and carpometacarpal joints of the thumb and assists in flexion of the wrist joint.

The Pronator Quadratus Muscle (Figs. 6-90, 6-91, 6-95, and 6-97). As its name indicates, this small, fleshy muscle is quadrangular (*i.e.*, four angles and four sides). It cannot be palpated or observed, except in dissections, because it is the deepest muscle in the front of the forearm and comprises the fourth layer. Located just proximal to the wrist, *the pronator quadratus is the only muscle that arises only from the ulna and inserts only into the radius.*

Origin (Figs. 6-85 and 6-99). **Distal fourth of anterior surface of ulna**.

Insertion (Figs. 6-85 and 6-99). **Anterior surface of distal fourth of radius**.

Nerve Supply. Anterior interosseous branch of **median** nerve (C8 and T1).

Actions (Figs. 6-79 and 6-99). **Pronates forearm**. It also **holds the radius and ulna together**, particularly when upward thrusts are transmitted through the wrist.

Summary. All muscles on the anterior surface of the forearm are supplied by the median and ulnar nerves, except the brachioradialis. This muscle, which belongs to the extensor group, lies in the lateral part of the anterior aspect of the forearm. Although functionally a flexor of the elbow joint, it is supplied by the radial nerve.

The median nerve supplies all but one and one-half muscles on the anterior surface of the forearm (Fig. 6-28). The flexor carpi ulnaris and the medial half of the flexor digitorum profundus are supplied by the ulnar nerve.

The long flexors of the fingers (flexor digitorum superficialis and flexor digitorum profundus) also flex the metacarpophalangeal and wrist joints. The flexor digitorum profundus flexes the fingers in slow action, but this activity is reinforced by the flexor digitorum superficialis when speed and flexion against resistance are required.

When the wrist, metacarpophalangeal, and interphalangeal joints are flexed, the flexor muscles are shortened and their action is consequently weakened. In addition, some weakening results from the ligamentous action of the extensor muscles. Verify this by flexing your wrist and gripping a pencil and then extending your wrist and gripping it again. Note that your grip is firmer in the first position.

THE ANTERIOR ANTEBRACHIAL NERVES

The nerves of the forearm are the **median**, the **ulnar**, and the **radial**. The median nerve is the principal nerve of the anterior compartment. The radial nerve appears in the cubital region and soon enters the posterior compartment.

The Median Nerve (Figs. 6-84, 6-89 to 6-93, 6-95, 6-97, 6-102, and 6-137). The median nerve enters the forearm from the cubital fossa by passing between the two heads of the pronator teres muscle (Fig. 6-84). It descends deep to the flexor digitorum superficialis, to which it is closely attached by the muscle's fascial sheath. It continues distally between this muscle and the flexor digitorum profundus.

Near the wrist the median nerve becomes superficial by passing between the tendons of the flexor digitorum superficialis and the flexor carpi radialis, deep to the tendon of the palmaris longus (if this muscle is present, Figs. 6-90 and 6-100). *The median nerve can be easily palpated at this site* (Fig. 6-92), just before it passes deep to the flexor retinaculum (Fig. 6-97). Verify this

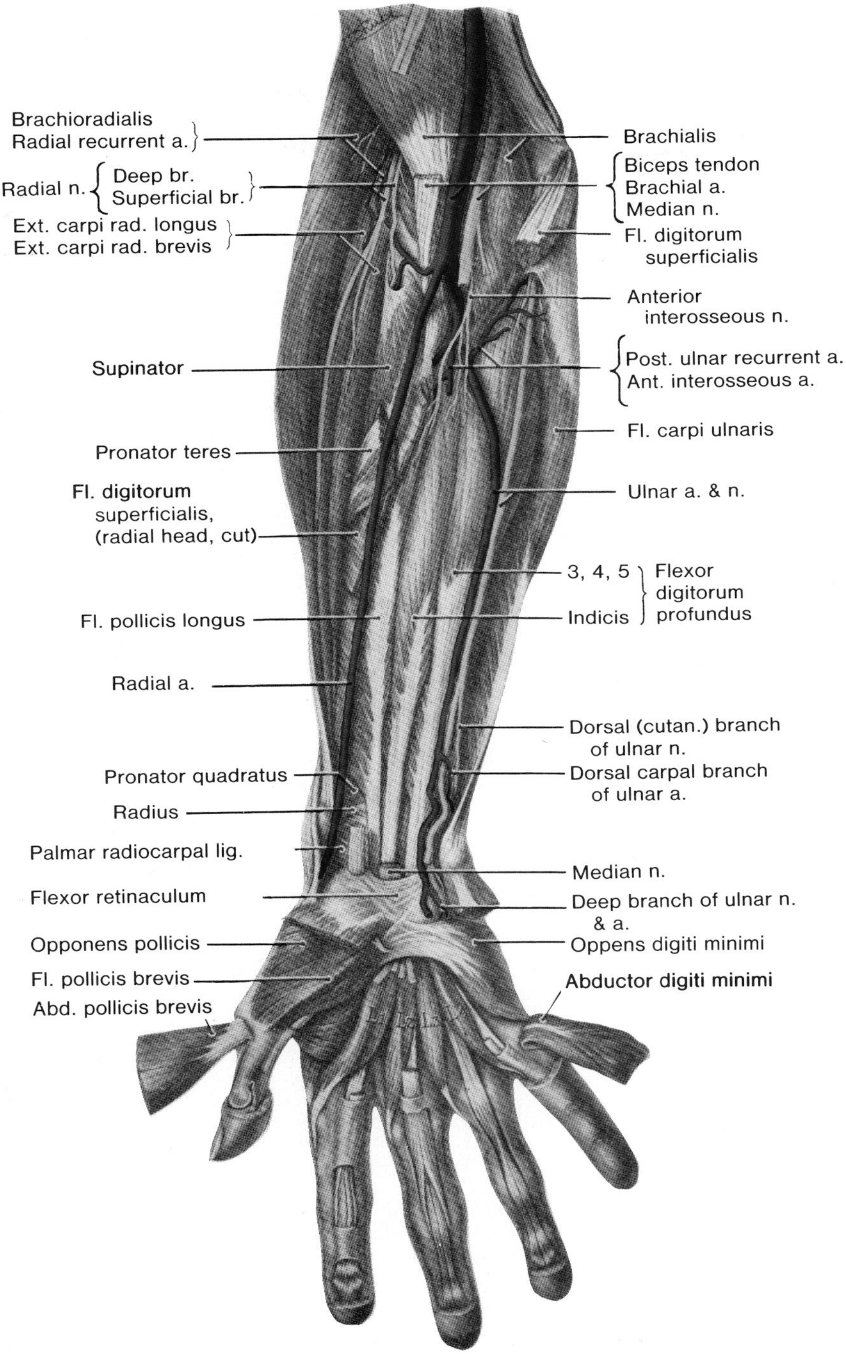

Figure 6-97. Drawing of a dissection of the deep flexors of the digits and related structures. Observe that the two deep digital flexor muscles, flexor pollicis longus and flexor digitorum profundus, form a sheet of muscle that arises from the flexor aspects of the radius, the interosseous membrane, and the ulna (see Figure 6-85). Note that the portion of the profundus for the index finger (*i.e.,* indicis) is free above the wrist and that the portions for digits 3, 4, and 5 are fused.

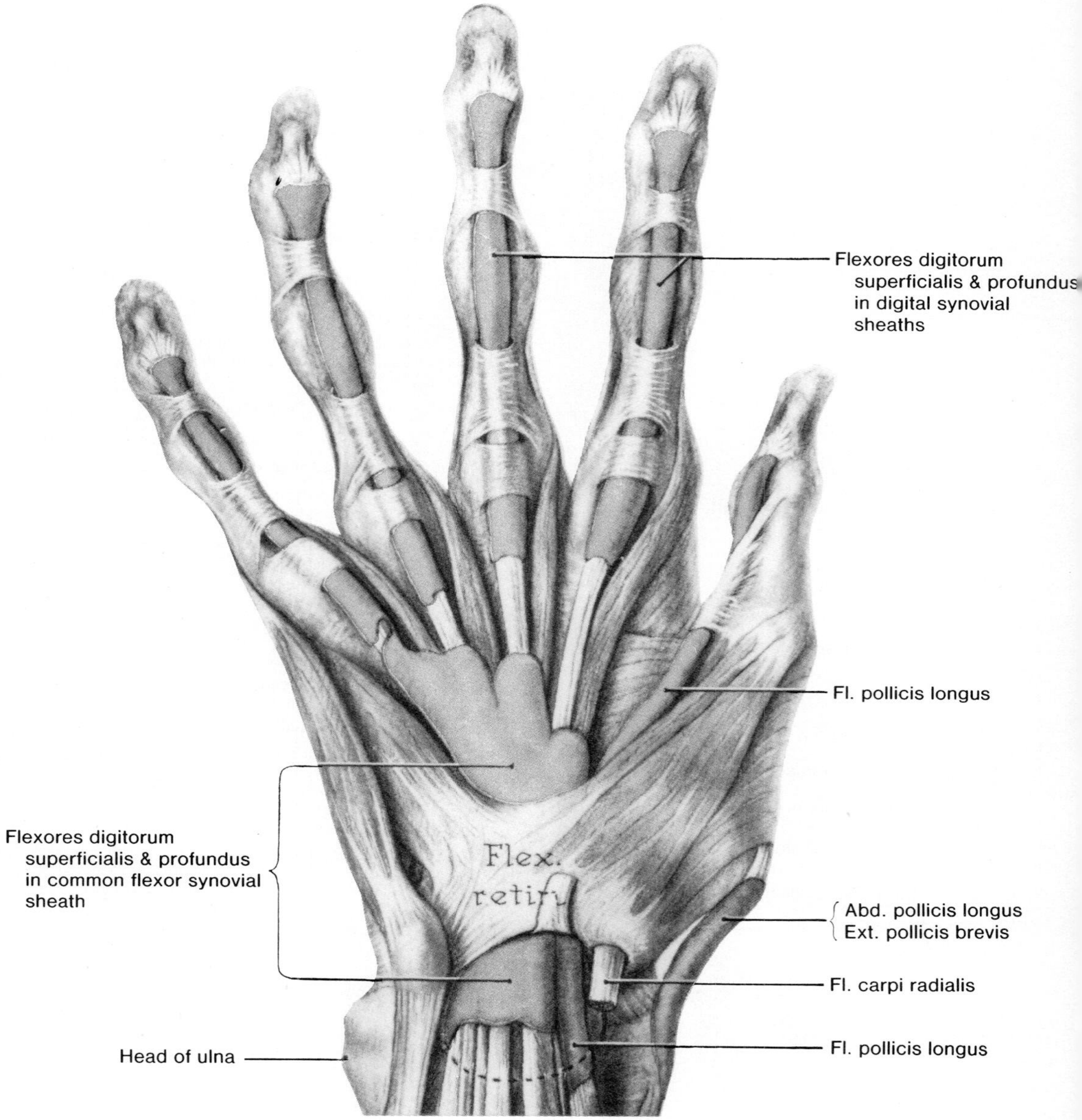

Figure 6-98. Drawing of a dissection of the synovial sheaths of the long flexor tendons of the digits. There are two sets: (1) proximal or carpal behind the flexor retinaculum, and (2) distal or digital behind the fibrous sheaths of the digital flexors. The carpal synovial sheaths of the flexors of the fingers, although developmentally separate, unite with one another to form a *common flexor synovial sheath*; the carpal sheath of the thumb tendon usually communicates with it. This common flexor sheath extends 1 to 2.5 cm proximal to and distal to the flexor retinaculum, varying distally with the extent of the site of friction and with the degree of mobility of the corresponding metacarpal bone. These are greatest in the marginal digits (thumb and little finger). Further, the marginal metacarpals being the shortest, the common flexor sheath extends to and is continuous with the digital sheaths of the thumb and little finger.

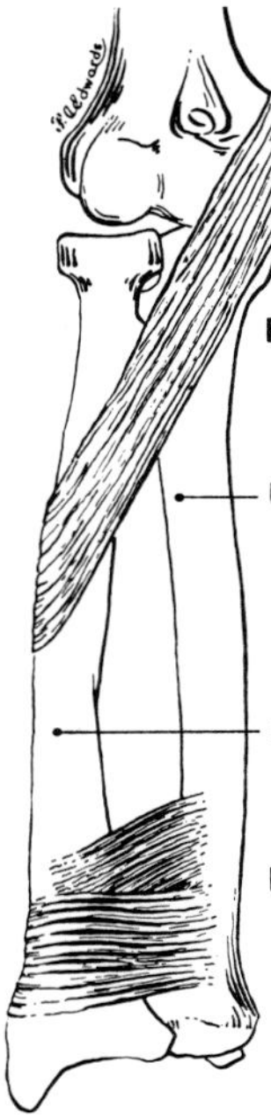

Figure 6-99. Drawing of the right pronator teres and pronator quadratus muscles. The pronator quadratus is the principal pronator of the forearm; it is reinforced by the pronator teres during rapid and/or forceful pronation. Observe that the pronator teres descends obliquely over the forearm bones and inserts into the summit of the main curve of the radius (for a better view of this, see Fig. 6-80). This arrangement enables the pronator teres to rotate the head of the radius in the anular ligament (Figs. 6-79*B* and 6-167).

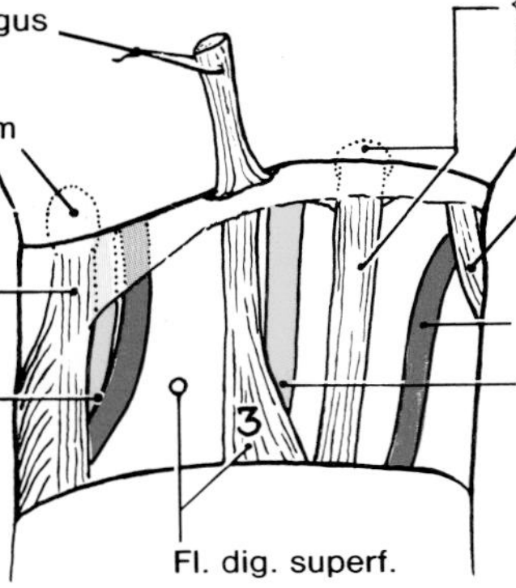

Figure 6-100. Drawing of the anterior surface of the wrist showing the structures present in this region. As the wrist is the favorite site for suicide attempts, these structures are commonly lacerated (Case 6-10).

by making the tendon of your palmaris longus stand out by flexing your wrist against resistance. Using your index finger, you should be able to palpate the stout median nerve, just lateral to the palmaris longus tendon (Figs. 6-93 and 6-94).

Branches of the Median Nerve. The median nerve has no branches in the arm. They arise in the forearm and hand as follows:

1. **Articular branches** pass to the elbow joint as the median nerve passes by it (Fig. 6-97).
2. **Muscular branches** supply the pronator teres, the pronator quadratus, and all the flexors *except* the flexor carpi ulnaris and the medial half of the flexor digitorum profundus; they are supplied by the ulnar nerve (Fig. 6-28).
3. **The anterior interosseous nerve** (Fig. 6-97) arises in the distal part of the cubital fossa and passes inferiorly on the interosseous membrane in company with the anterior interosseous branch of the ulnar artery (Fig. 6-101). It runs between the flexor digitorum profundus and the flexor pollicis longus to reach the pronator quadratus which it supplies. It passes deep to this muscle and ends by sending articular branches to the wrist joint.
4. **The palmar cutaneous branch** (Fig. 6-93) arises just above the flexor retinaculum and becomes cutaneous between the tendons of the palmaris longus and flexor carpi radialis muscles. It passes superficial to the flexor retinaculum to supply the skin of the lateral part of the palm (Figs. 6-29 and 6-102).

CLINICALLY ORIENTED COMMENTS

Median Nerve Injury. This nerve may be injured by wounds to the forearm. When it is severed in the elbow region, there is loss of flexion of the proximal interphalangeal joints of all the digits. There is also loss of flexion of the distal interphalangeal joints of the index and middle fingers. Flexion of the distal interphalangeal joints of

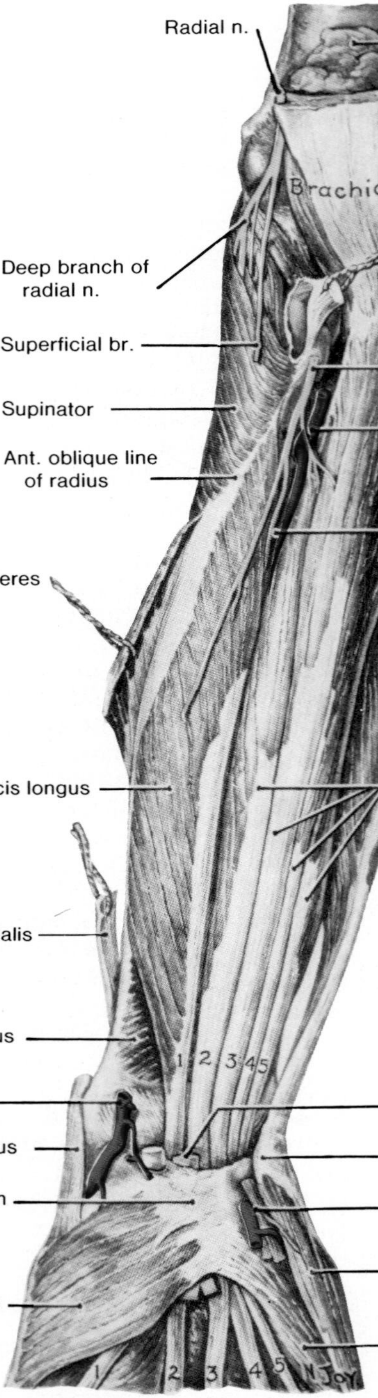

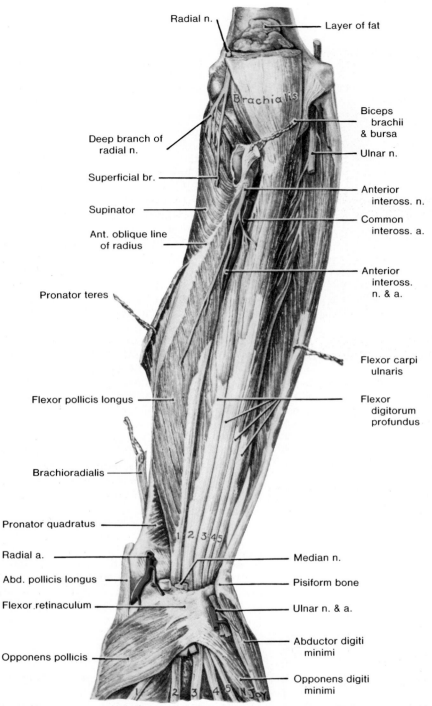

Figure 6-101. Drawing of a dissection of the muscles attached to the anterior aspect of the radius and ulna (Fig. 6-85). Observe that the anterior aspect of the ulna is covered by the brachialis (Fig. 6-90), which inserts into the coronoid process of the ulna (Fig. 6-80), and distal to this by the flexor digitorum profoundus. Note that the profundus also arises from the upper two-thirds of the medial aspect of the ulna. Observe that the anterior aspect of the radius is covered with the supinator above the anterior oblique line and distal to this with the flexor pollicis longus. Observe the five tendons of the deep digital flexors converging on the carpal tunnel and, after having traversed it, diverging to pass to the five terminal phalanges. Note that the biceps is inserted into the medial aspect of the radius, hence it can rotate it laterally (*i.e.*, supinate, Fig. 6-79*A*), whereas the pronator teres is attached to the lateral surface and can rotate it medially (*i.e.*, pronate, Fig. 6-79*B*).

the ring and little fingers is not affected because the part of the flexor digitorum profundus producing these movements is supplied by the ulnar nerve. The ability to flex the metacarpophalangeal joints of the index and middle fingers will be affected because the digital branches of the median nerve supply the first and second lumbrical muscles (Fig. 6-123).

Most commonly the median nerve is injured just proximal to the flexor retinaculum (Figs. 6-97 and 6-100) owing to the frequency of wrist slashing in suicide attempts (Case 6-10). Although severance of the palmaris longus tendon is common in these cases owing to its location superficial to the median nerve (Fig. 6-91), the loss of function of this muscle is not missed.

Carpal Tunnel Syndrome. The median nerve enters the palm through an osseofibrous carpal tunnel (Fig. 6-88), close to the deep surface of the flexor retinaculum (Fig. 6-97). The tendons of the long flexor muscles of the digits also pass through this rather restricted passage. Any lesion that significantly reduces the size of the carpal tunnel (*e.g.*, inflammation of the flexor retinaculum, anterior dislocation of the lunate bone, arthritic changes, or tenosynovitis of the tendons) may cause **compression of the median nerve**. As this nerve has two terminal branches (lateral and medial) that supply skin of the thumb, index, middle, and lateral half of the ring finger on their palmar surfaces and sides and on the dorsum of the terminal phalanges of the same digits (Fig. 6-29), there is often tingling (**paresthesia**), absence of tactile sensation (**anesthesia**), or diminished sensation (**hypoesthesia**) in these digits. Because the median nerve sends a palmar cutaneous branch superficial to the flexor retinaculum to supply most of the palm, there may be no sensory impairment of this area (Figs. 6-93 and 6-102).

Often a progressive loss of coordination and strength in the thumb occurs if the exciting cause is not alleviated, which results in difficulty in performing fine movements. As the thenar (G. palm of hand) muscles and the lateral two lumbrical muscles of the fingers are supplied by the median nerve, the usefulness of the thumb, index, and middle fingers may be diminished. In cases of severe compression, there may be wasting (atrophy) of the thenar muscles (Fig. 6-131). To relieve symptoms of the carpal tunnel syndrome, partial or complete division of the flexor retinaculum may be necessary.

The Ulnar Nerve (Figs. 6-73, 6-89 to 6-91, 6-93, 6-95, 6-97, and 6-100 to 6-103). After passing posterior to the medial epicondyle of the humerus, the ulnar nerve enters the forearm by passing between the heads of the flexor carpi ulnaris muscle (Fig. 6-101). It then descends deep to this muscle on the flexor digitorum profundus to accompany the ulnar artery near the middle of the forearm. It then passes on the medial side of this artery and the lateral side of the tendon of the flexor carpi ulnaris (Fig. 6-97). In the distal part of the forearm the ulnar nerve becomes relatively superficial, covered only by fascia and skin (Fig. 6-93). Near the pisiform bone it pierces the deep fascia and passes over the flexor retinaculum (Figs. 6-97 and 6-101), where it ends by dividing into superficial and deep branches (Fig. 6-102, 6-103, and 6-137).

Branches of the Ulnar Nerve. The ulnar nerve has no branches in the arm. They arise in the forearm and hand as follows:

1. **Articular branches** pass to the elbow joint while the nerve is in the groove between the olecranon and the medial epicondyle (Figs. 6-72 and 6-73).
2. **Muscular branches** supply the flexor carpi ulnaris and the medial half of the flexor digitorum profundus muscles (Figs. 6-95 and 6-97).
3. **The palmar cutaneous branch** arises from the ulnar nerve near the middle of the forearm and pierces the deep fascia in its distal third (Fig. 6-102) to supply skin on the medial part of the palm (Fig. 6-29).
4. **The dorsal cutaneous branch** (Fig. 6-97) arises in the distal half of the forearm and passes posteroinferiorly between the ulna and the flexor carpi ulnaris to become cutaneous and to supply the posterior surface of the medial part of the hand (Figs. 6-29, 6-103, and 6-137).

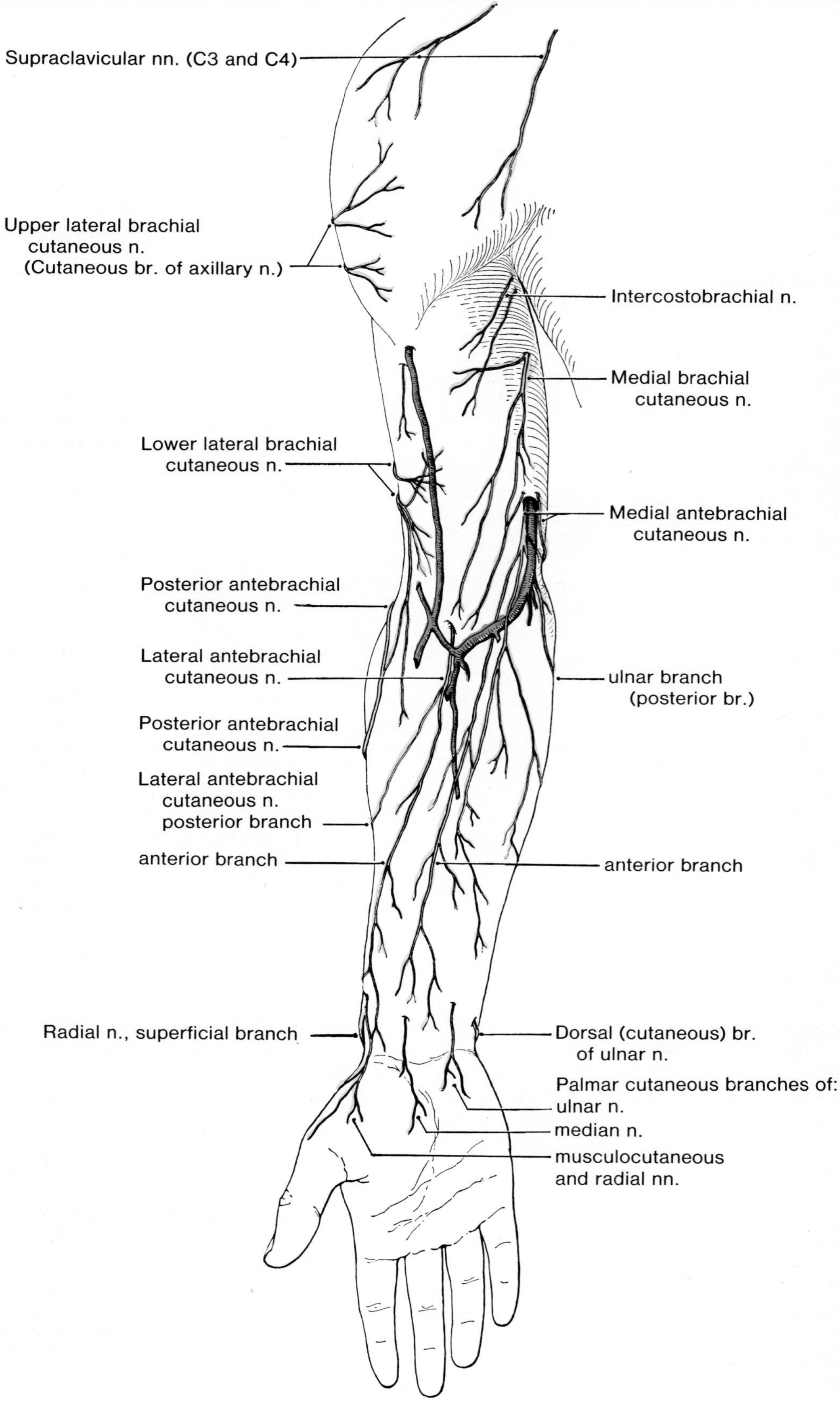

Supraclavicular nn. (C3 and C4)
Upper lateral brachial cutaneous n. (Cutaneous br. of axillary n.)
Intercostobrachial n.
Medial brachial cutaneous n.
Lower lateral brachial cutaneous n.
Medial antebrachial cutaneous n.
Posterior antebrachial cutaneous n.
Lateral antebrachial cutaneous n.
ulnar branch (posterior br.)
Posterior antebrachial cutaneous n.
Lateral antebrachial cutaneous n. posterior branch
anterior branch
anterior branch
Radial n., superficial branch
Dorsal (cutaneous) br. of ulnar n.
Palmar cutaneous branches of:
ulnar n.
median n.
musculocutaneous and radial nn.

CLINICALLY ORIENTED COMMENTS

Ulnar nerve injury may occur in wounds of the forearm, the most common site being where the nerve lies posterior to the medial epicondyle of the humerus (Figs. 6-72 and 6-101). Often this occurs when the elbow hits a hard surface (Case 6-5) and may result in extensive motor and sensory loss to the hand. There is impaired power of adduction and when an attempt is made to flex the wrist joint, the hand is drawn to the radial side by the flexor carpi radialis. Following ulnar nerve injury, patients are likely to have difficulty in making a fist because they cannot flex their fourth and fifth digits at the distal interphalangeal joints. This characteristic appearance of the hand is known as *main en griffe* or **clawhand** (Fig. 6-104).

The Radial Nerve (Figs. 6-84, 6-93, 6-95, 6-97, 6-102, 6-103, and 6-137). The radial nerve descends between the brachialis and brachioradialis muscles and crosses the front of the lateral epicondyle of the humerus. As it divides into its terminal branches, superficial and deep, it enters the cubital fossa deeply (Fig. 6-84).

The superficial radial nerve (Figs. 6-84, 6-95, and 6-97), the smaller of the two terminal branches, is the direct continuation of the radial nerve. It passes distally, anterior to the pronator teres muscle and under cover of the brachioradialis. In the lower one-third of the forearm, the superficial radial nerve passes posteriorly, deep to the tendon of the brachioradialis, and enters the posterior compartment of the forearm. It pierces the deep fascia 3 to 4 cm proximal to the wrist and supplies skin on the dorsum of the wrist, hand, thumb, and lateral one (or two) and one-half fingers (Figs. 6-29, 6-102, and 6-103).

In Figure 6-95, observe that the superficial branch of the radial nerve can be exposed from the elbow region to near the wrist without cutting a muscle or a tendon. It can also be exposed on the dorsal aspect of the hand by cutting only the tendon of the brachioradialis muscle.

The deep radial nerve (deep branch of radial), the larger of the two terminal branches, is entirely muscular and articular in its distribution. As it passes posteroinferiorly it gives branches to the extensor carpi radialis brevis and supinator muscles (Fig. 6-30). It then pierces the supinator, giving additional branches to it and curving around the lateral side of the radius to enter the posterior compartment of the forearm (Fig. 6-89).

On reaching the posterior aspect of the forearm, the deep radial nerve gives off many branches to the extensor muscles (Figs. 6-89 and 6-109). One of these branches, the **posterior interosseous nerve**, accompanies the posterior interosseous artery to supply the deep extensor muscles.

CLINICALLY ORIENTED COMMENTS

Radial nerve injury may occur in deep wounds of the forearm (Case 6-8). Severance of the deep radial nerve produces inability to extend the thumb and the metacarpophalangeal joints of the fingers. There is no loss of sensation because the deep radial is entirely muscular and articular in distribution. For details of the effects of this type of radial nerve injury, see the discussion of Case 6-8.

THE ANTERIOR ANTEBRACHIAL ARTERIES

The brachial artery ends opposite the neck of the radius in the lower part of the cubital fossa by dividing into its two terminal branches, the radial and ulnar arteries.

Figure 6-102. Drawing of the anterior aspect of the upper limb showing the cutaneous nerves of the five terminal branches of the brachial plexus (musculocutaneous, median, ulnar, radial, and axillary nerves). Note that the first four reach the hand. For an illustration of the distribution of the cutaneous nerves to the palm of the hand, see Figure 6-29.

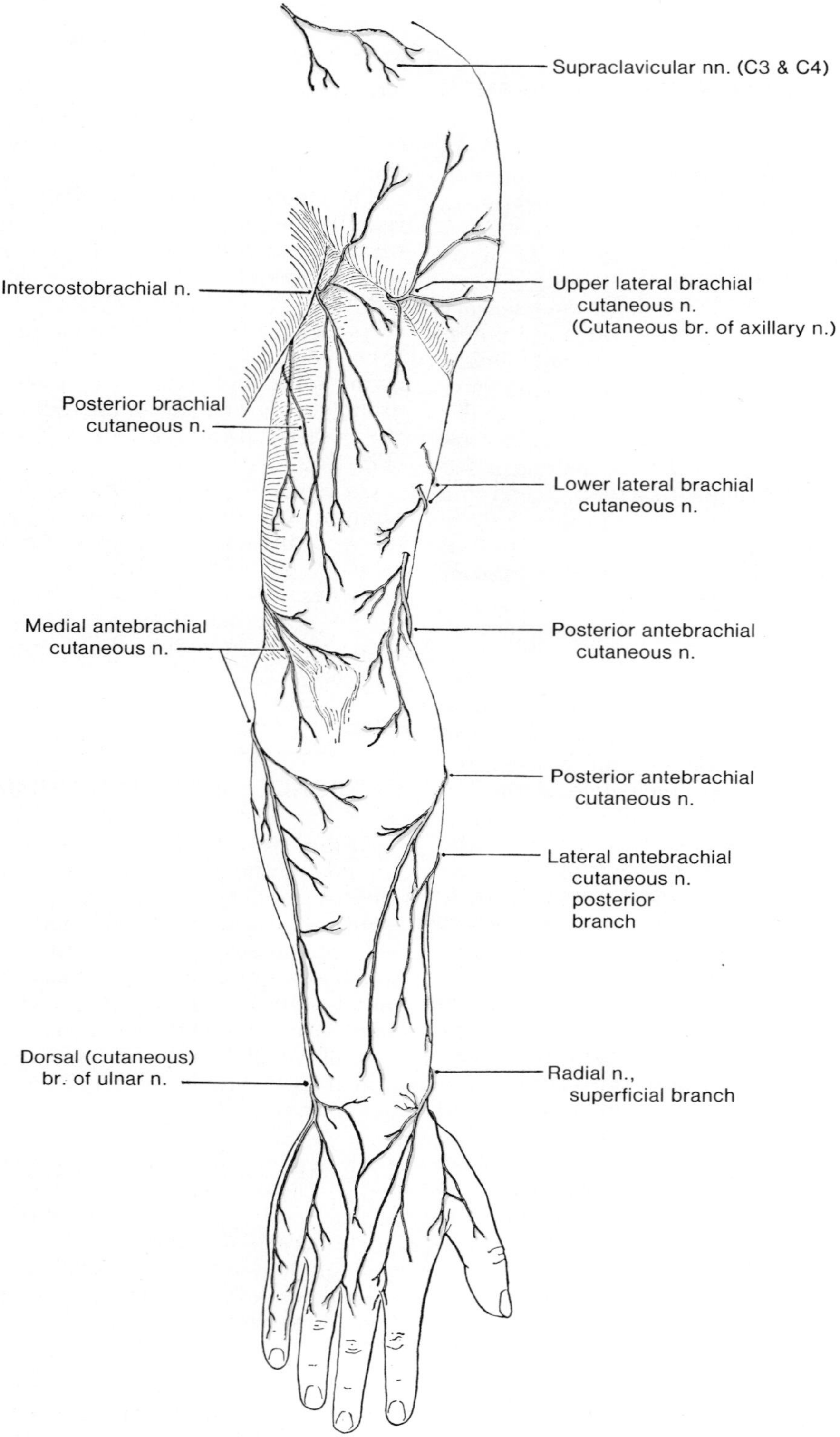

Figure 6-103. Drawing of the posterior aspect of the upper limb showing its cutaneous nerves. For an illustration of the distribution of the cutaneous nerves to the dorsum of the hand, see Figures 6-29 and 6-137.

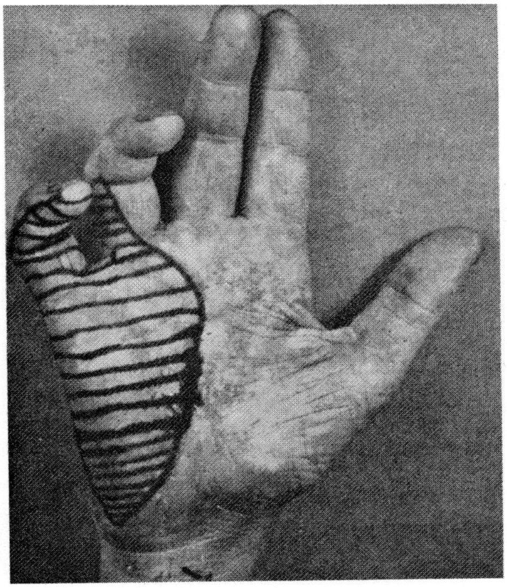

Figure 6-104. Photograph of a clawhand (main en griffe) resulting from severance of the ulnar nerve by a laceration at the wrist. Note that the ring and little fingers are hyperextended at the metacarpophalangeal joints because the medial two lumbrical muscles are paralyzed and the extensor digitorum is unopposed. This claw-like hand looks not unlike the hand in the act of playing the piano or scratching oneself.

The Radial Artery (Figs. 6-84, 6-95, and 6-97). The radial artery **begins in the cubital fossa,** just medial to the biceps brachii tendon *at the level of the neck of the radius* (*i.e.*, on the lateral side about 1 cm distal to the elbow crease). This artery is the smaller of the two terminal branches of the brachial and continues the direct line of this vessel (Fig. 6-97). Its course in the forearm is represented by a line connecting the mid-point of the cubital fossa to a point just medial to the tip of the styloid process of the radius (Fig. 6-97). Its proximal part is overlapped by the fleshy belly of the brachioradialis muscle which can be pulled laterally during dissection to reveal the entire length of the artery in the forearm (Fig. 6-95).

The radial artery lies on muscle until it comes into contact with the lower end of the radius, where it is covered only by superficial and deep fasciae and skin (Fig. 6-93). The radial artery leaves the forearm by winding around the lateral aspect of the radius and passing posteriorly between the lateral collateral ligament of the wrist joint and the tendons of the abductor pollicis longus and extensor pollicis brevis. As it **crosses the floor of the anatomical snuff box,** it lies on the scaphoid and the trapezium (Figs. 6-109 and 6-110). *The radial artery ends* by completing the **deep palmar arch** in conjunction with the ulnar artery (Fig. 6-138).

The branches of the radial artery in the forearm are as follows:

1. The **radial recurrent artery** (Fig. 6-95) arises from the lateral side of the radial, just distal to its origin, and ascends between the brachioradialis and brachialis muscles and on the supinator. It supplies these muscles and the elbow joint and anastomoses with the radial collateral artery, a branch of the profunda brachii, thereby participating in the *anastomoses of the elbow region* (Fig. 6-74).
2. The **muscular branches** supply muscles on the lateral side of the forearm.
3. The **palmar carpal branch**, a small artery, arises near the distal border of the pronator quadratus (Fig. 6-95) and runs across the wrist deep to the flexor tendons. Here it anastomoses with the carpal branch of the ulnar artery to form the **palmar carpal arch** (Fig. 6-105), which supplies the wrist region.
4. The **superficial palmar branch** (Figs. 6-95 and 6-105) arises just proximal to the wrist and passes through, sometimes over, the muscles of the thenar eminence (Fig. 6-127) which it supplies. It usually anastomoses with the terminal part of the ulnar artery to form a **superficial palmar arch** (Figs. 6-127 and 6-138).
5. The **dorsal carpal branch** (Fig. 6-108) runs medially across the dorsal surface of the wrist, deep to the extensor tendons, where it anastomoses with the dorsal carpal branch of the ulnar artery to form a **dorsal carpal arch** or rete.

CLINICALLY ORIENTED COMMENTS

The common place for taking the pulse is where the radial artery lies on the anterior surface of the distal end of the radius, lateral to the tendon of the flexor carpi radialis muscle (Figs. 6-92, 6-93, and 6-105). Here it is covered only by deep and superficial fasciae and skin. About two fingerbreadths of this artery can be compressed against the distal end of the radius. Because *this is traditionally where the pulse is taken,* you should practice taking your **radial pulse** and that of others. Do not use the pulp of your thumb when doing this because it has its own pulse which could be interpreted as the patient's pulse. If the pulse cannot be felt, try the other wrist because occasionally an aberrant radial artery (Fig. 6-91) makes the pulse difficult to palpate.

The Ulnar Artery (Figs. 6-84, 6-89 to 6-91, 6-93, 6-95, 6-97, and 6-100). The ulnar is the larger of the two terminal branches of the brachial artery. It describes a gentle curve as it passes from the **cubital fossa** to the ulnar side of the forearm (Fig. 6-97). Beginning at the level of the neck of the radius, just medial to the biceps tendon, it passes inferomedially deep to the pronator teres muscle (Fig. 6-90). In company with the median nerve, it passes between the ulnar and radial heads of the flexor digitorum superficialis (Figs. 6-89 and 6-95). About midway between the elbow and the wrist, it crosses posterior to the median nerve to reach the medial side of the forearm, where it lies on the flexor digitorum profundus (Figs. 6-91, 6-95, and 6-97).

In the distal two-thirds of the forearm the ulnar artery lies lateral to the ulnar nerve (Fig. 6-97). In the middle third, these structures are overlapped by the flexor carpi ulnaris muscle (Figs. 6-90 and 6-91).

At the wrist the ulnar artery and nerve lie lateral to the tendon of the flexor carpi ulnaris, where they are covered only by fascia and skin (Figs. 6-93 and 6-100). The **pulsations of the ulnar artery** can be felt where it passes anterior to the head of the ulna (Figs. 6-92 and 6-93). The ulnar artery leaves the forearm by passing superficial to the flexor retinaculum on the lateral side of the pisiform bone (Fig. 6-97). Like the radial, the ulnar artery is accompanied by venae comitantes.

The branches of the ulnar artery in the forearm are as follows:

1. The **anterior ulnar recurrent artery** (Fig. 6-74) arises from the ulnar just below the elbow joint and runs proximally between the brachialis and pronator teres muscles. It supplies these muscles and anastomoses with the inferior ulnar collateral artery, thereby participating in the **anastomoses of the elbow region** (Fig. 6-74).
2. The **posterior ulnar recurrent artery** (Figs. 6-74 and 6-97) arises distal to the anterior ulnar recurrent. It passes upward and runs posterior to the medial epicondyle, where it lies deep to the tendon of the flexor carpi ulnaris (Figs. 6-73 and 6-97). It supplies adjacent muscles and then takes part in the **anastomoses of the elbow region** (Fig. 6-74).
3. **The common interosseous artery** arises in the distal part of the cubital fossa (Figs. 6-97, 6-101, and 6-167) and divides into anterior and posterior interosseous arteries. The **anterior interosseous artery** passes distally on the interosseous membrane to the proximal border of the pronator quadratus (Figs. 6-101 and 6-167), where it pierces the membrane and continues distally to join the dorsal carpal arch (Fig. 6-108). The **posterior interosseous artery** passes backward between the bones of the forearm, just proximal to the interosseous membrane (Fig. 6-167). It supplies adjacent muscles and then gives off the **posterior interosseous recurrent artery** (Fig. 6-109) which passes upward, posterior to the lateral epicondyle, to participate in the **anastomoses of the elbow region** (Fig. 6-74).
4. The **muscular branches** supply muscles on the ulnar side of the forearm.
5. The **palmar carpal branch** is a small

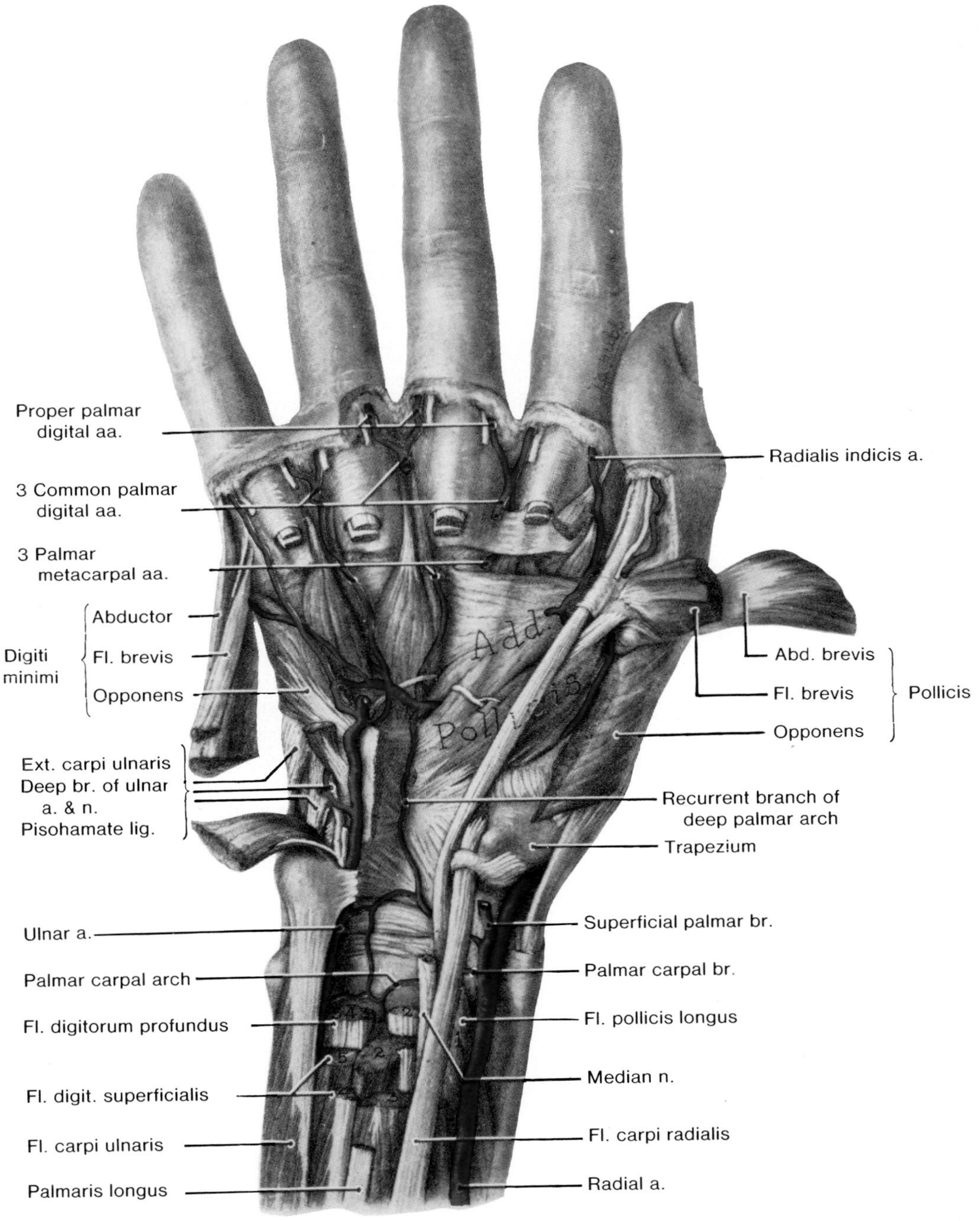

Figure 6-105. Drawing of a deep dissection of the palm of the hand showing its muscles and arteries. Observe the palmar carpal arch and its connections and the deep branch of the ulnar artery joining the radial artery to form the deep palmar arch.

branch that runs across the front of the wrist, deep to the tendons of the flexor digitorum profundus. It anastomoses with the palmar carpal branch of the radial artery to form the **palmar carpal arch** (Figs. 6-105, 6-138, and 6-139).

6. The **dorsal carpal arch** arises just proximal to the pisiform bone and passes across the dorsal surface of the wrist deep to the extensor tendons. It anastomoses with the deep carpal branch of the radial artery forming the **dorsal carpal arch** (Fig. 6-109).

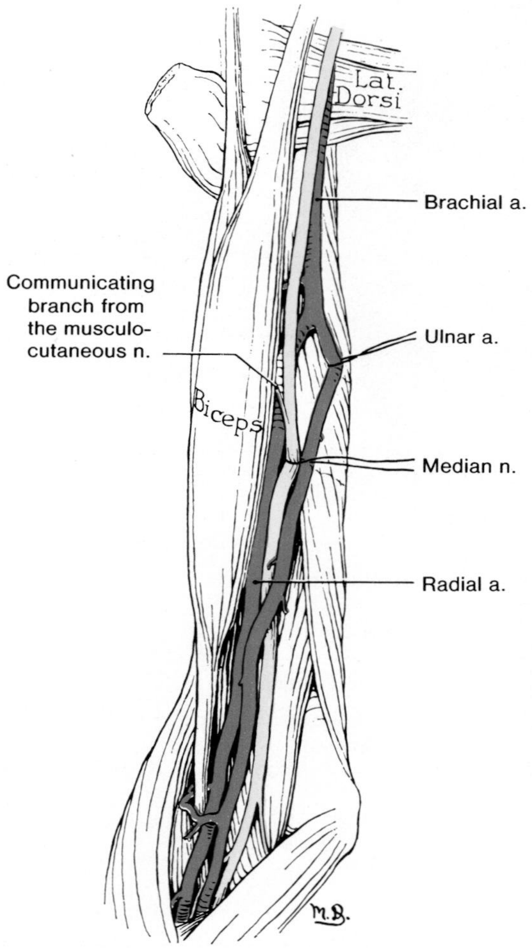

Figure 6-106. Drawing of a dissection of the arm and elbow regions showing a high division of the brachial artery into the radial and ulnar arteries. Note that the median nerve passes between these arteries.

CLINICALLY ORIENTED COMMENTS

Sometimes the brachial artery divides at a more proximal level than usual (Fig. 6-106). In other cases the ulnar artery passes superficial to the flexor muscles in the superficial fascia (Fig. 6-107). These variations must be kept in mind when performing **venesections** (incisions into a vein) at the elbow, *e.g.*, for inserting a metal cannula or polyethylene catheter into a vein for intravenous injection of fluids, blood, or medication. If an artery is mistaken for a vein and certain drugs are injected into it, the result may be disastrous, *e.g.*, gangrene (necrosis or death), resulting in partial or total loss of the hand.

THE POSTERIOR ANTEBRACHIAL MUSCLES

There are 11 muscles in the posterior part of the forearm and they are classified as **extensors**. They can be organized into functional groups as follows: (1) *muscles that extend the hand at the wrist* (extensor carpi radialis longus, extensor carpi radialis brevis, and extensor carpi ulnaris); (2) *muscles that extend the digits*, except the thumb (extensor digitorum, extensor indicis, and extensor digiti minimi); and (3) *muscles that are involved in extension of the thumb* (abductor pollicis longus, extensor pollicis brevis, and extensor pollicis longus). For purposes of description, these extensor muscles are usually divided into superficial and deep anatomical groups.

The Superficial Extensor Muscle Layer (Figs. 6-72, 6-84, 6-97, and 6-108). Four of the superficial extensors (extensor carpi radialis brevis, extensor digitorum, extensor digiti minimi, and extensor carpi ulnaris) arise from a flattened **common extensor tendon** (Figs. 6-72 and 6-85) which is attached to the front of the **lateral epicondyle**, the adjacent fascia, and the lateral supracondylar ridge of the humerus. This is known as **the common extensor origin**.

The brachioradialis and the extensor carpi radialis longus arise from the upper and lower parts of the supracondylar ridge, respectively. The brachioradialis, a flexor

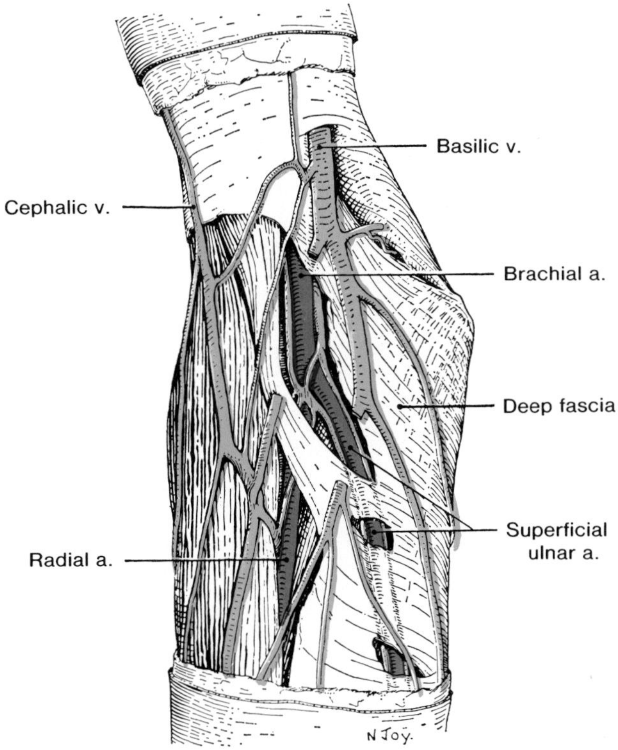

Figure 6-107. Drawing of a dissection of the elbow region showing a superficial ulnar artery descending superficial to the flexor muscles. This clinically important variation occurs in about 3% of people.

of the elbow joint, is included with the extensors because it is supplied by the radial nerve. It is described with the muscles of the **cubital region** (p. 747) because it forms the lateral boundary of this hollow in front of the elbow (Figs. 6-82 and 6-84).

The extensor tendons occupy the radial side as well as the dorsum of the wrist where they lie within synovial sheaths in bony grooves (Figs. 6-108 to 6-111). They are held in place by a strong fibrous band, called the **extensor retinaculum** (Fig. 6-108), which is attached laterally to the distal end of the radius and medially to the styloid process of the ulna and the triquetral and pisiform bones. *The extensor retinaculum prevents bowstringing of the long extensor tendons* when the wrist is hyperextended.

The Extensor Carpi Radialis Longus Muscle (Figs. 6-84, 6-89, 6-97, and 6-108 to 6-111). This muscle is partly overlapped by the brachioradialis with which it is often blended.

Origin (Fig. 6-85). Distal third of **lateral supracondylar ridge** of humerus and **lateral intermuscular septum.**

Insertion (Fig. 6-86). Dorsum of **base of second metacarpal** bone. Its flat tendon runs deep to the extensor retinaculum and passes through the anatomical snuff box (Figs. 6-108 to 6-111).

Nerve Supply (Fig. 6-30). **Radial** nerve (C6 and C7) *above the elbow.*

Actions. **Extends** and **abducts wrist.**

The Extensor Carpi Radialis Brevis Muscle (Figs. 6-84, 6-89, 6-97, and 6-108 to 6-111). As its name indicates, this muscle is shorter than the extensor carpi radialis longus which covers it.

Origin (Figs. 6-85, 6-86, 6-108, and 6-160). **Lateral epicondyle** of humerus by *common extensor tendon* and **radial collateral ligament** of elbow joint.

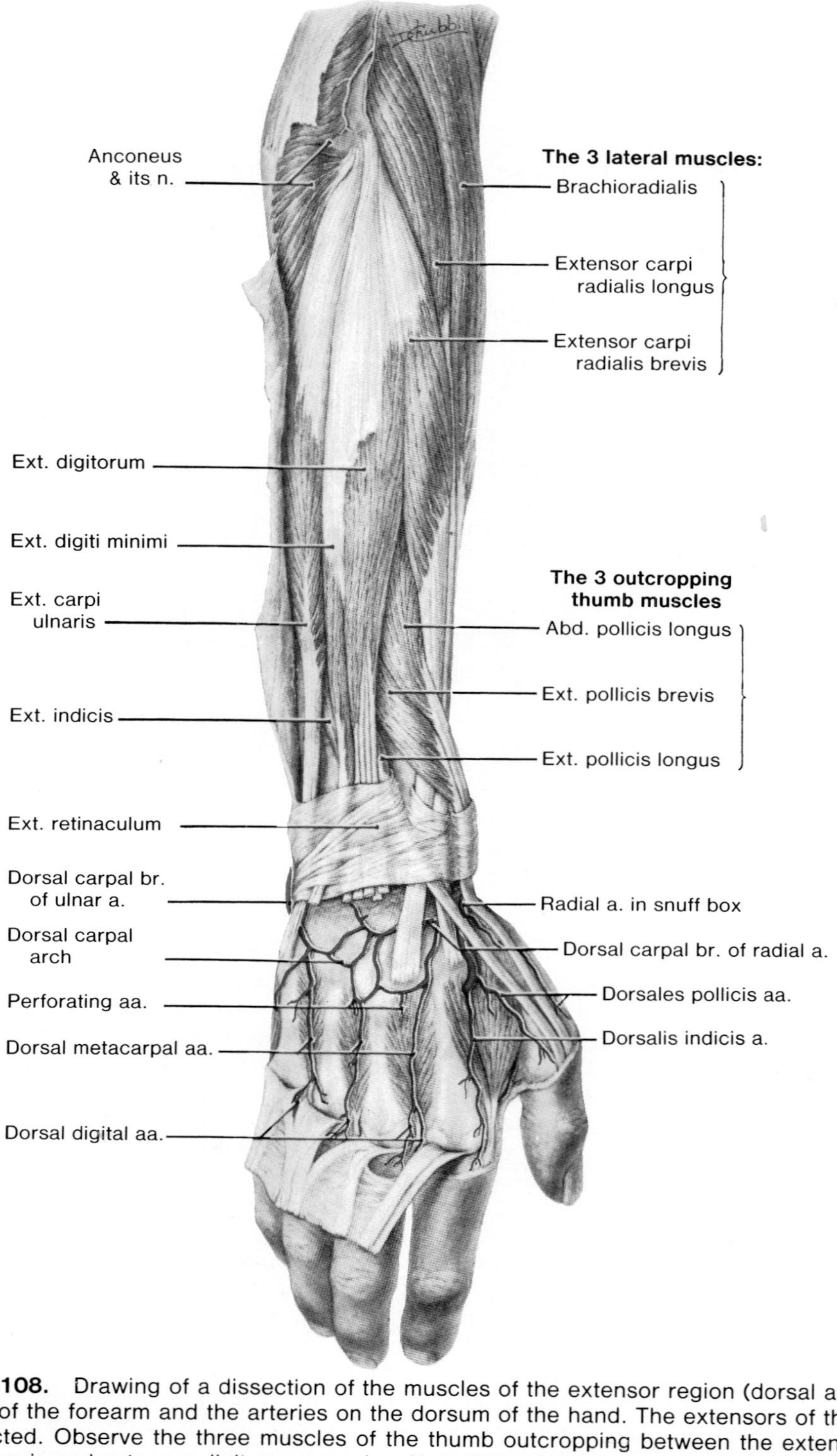

Figure 6-108. Drawing of a dissection of the muscles of the extensor region (dorsal and lateral aspects) of the forearm and the arteries on the dorsum of the hand. The extensors of the fingers are reflected. Observe the three muscles of the thumb outcropping between the extensor carpi radialis brevis and extensor digitorum muscles. Note the radial artery, the dorsal carpal branch of the ulnar, and their branches; all these are undisturbed by the removal of muscles because they lie on the skeletal plane (*i.e.*, on bone, ligament, or fascia). Observe the radial artery disappearing between the two heads of the first dorsal interosseous muscle, where it is in series with the perforating arteries. Note that no muscle is attached to the back of any carpal bones. The three extensors of the wrist span the carpal bones to reach the bases of metacarpals 2, 3, and 5.

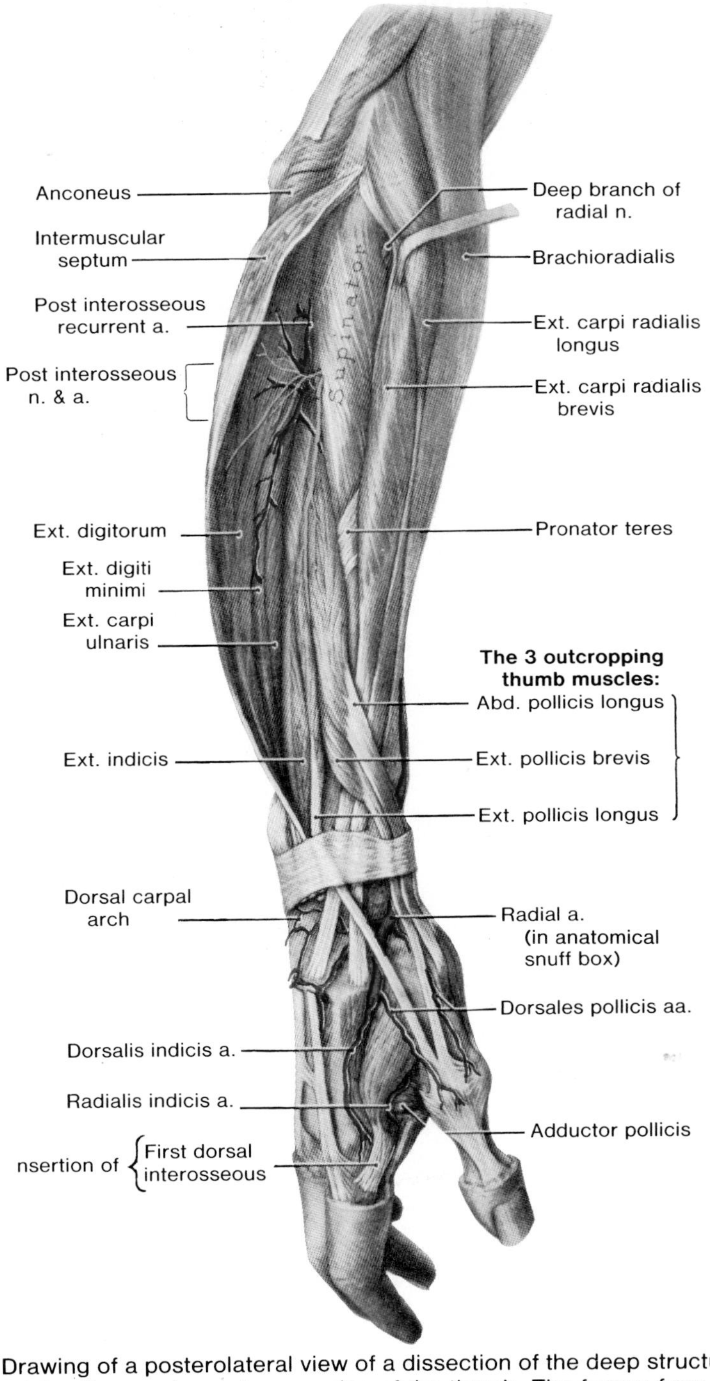

Figure 6-109. Drawing of a posterolateral view of a dissection of the deep structures at the back of the forearm and the three outcropping muscles of the thumb. The furrow from which the three muscles outcrop has been opened widely, up to the lateral epicondyle. It crosses the supinator and is a "*line of safety*" because the three laterally retracted muscles are supplied by the posterior interosseous nerve at its proximal end, whereas the others are supplied about 6 cm distal to the head of the radius. Observe that after the deep radial nerve emerges from the supinator, it is called the posterior interosseous nerve.

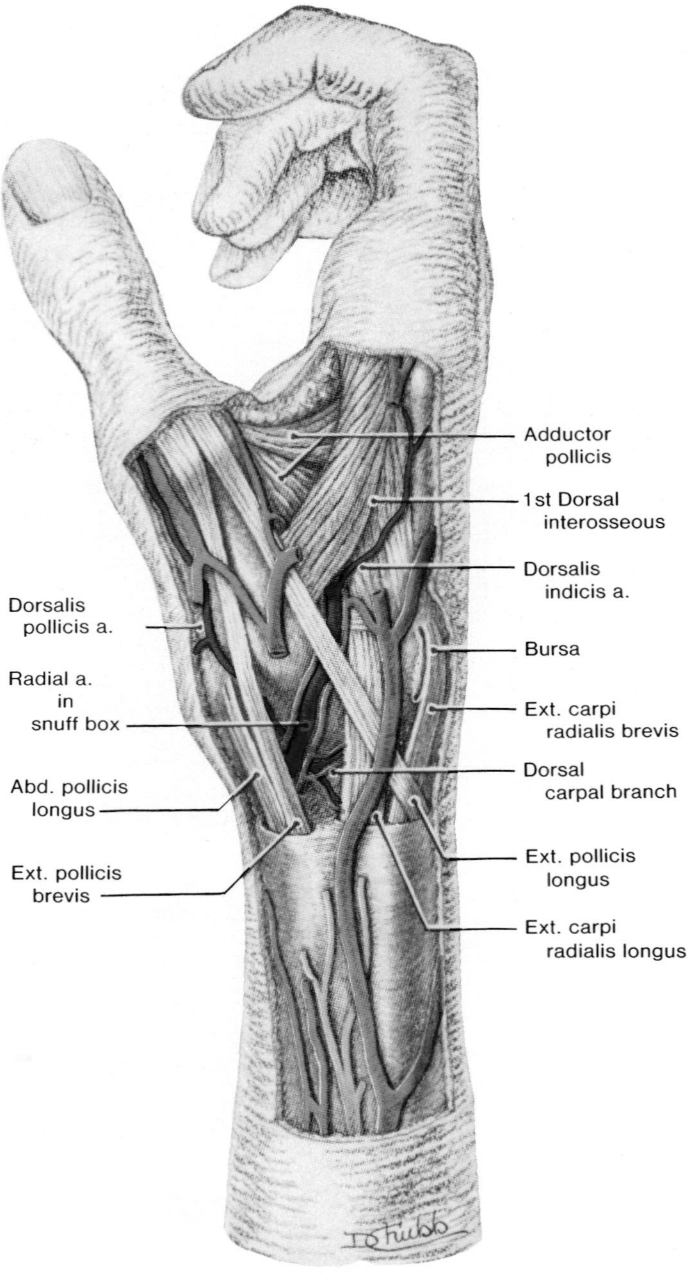

Figure 6-110. Drawing of a dissection of the radial aspect of the wrist. Observe the three long tendons of the thumb forming the sides of the triangular hollow known as the *anatomical snuff box*. The abductor pollicis longus and extensor pollicis brevis form the anterior boundary of the snuff box and the extensor pollicis longus forms its posterior boundary. Observe that the radial artery passes on the dorsal aspect of the carpus between the lateral collateral ligament (Fig. 6-172) and the tendons of the abductor pollicis longus and extensor pollicis brevis, and then crosses the scaphoid and trapezium in the floor of the snuff box. Compare this dissection with the photograph of this region (Fig. 6-113).

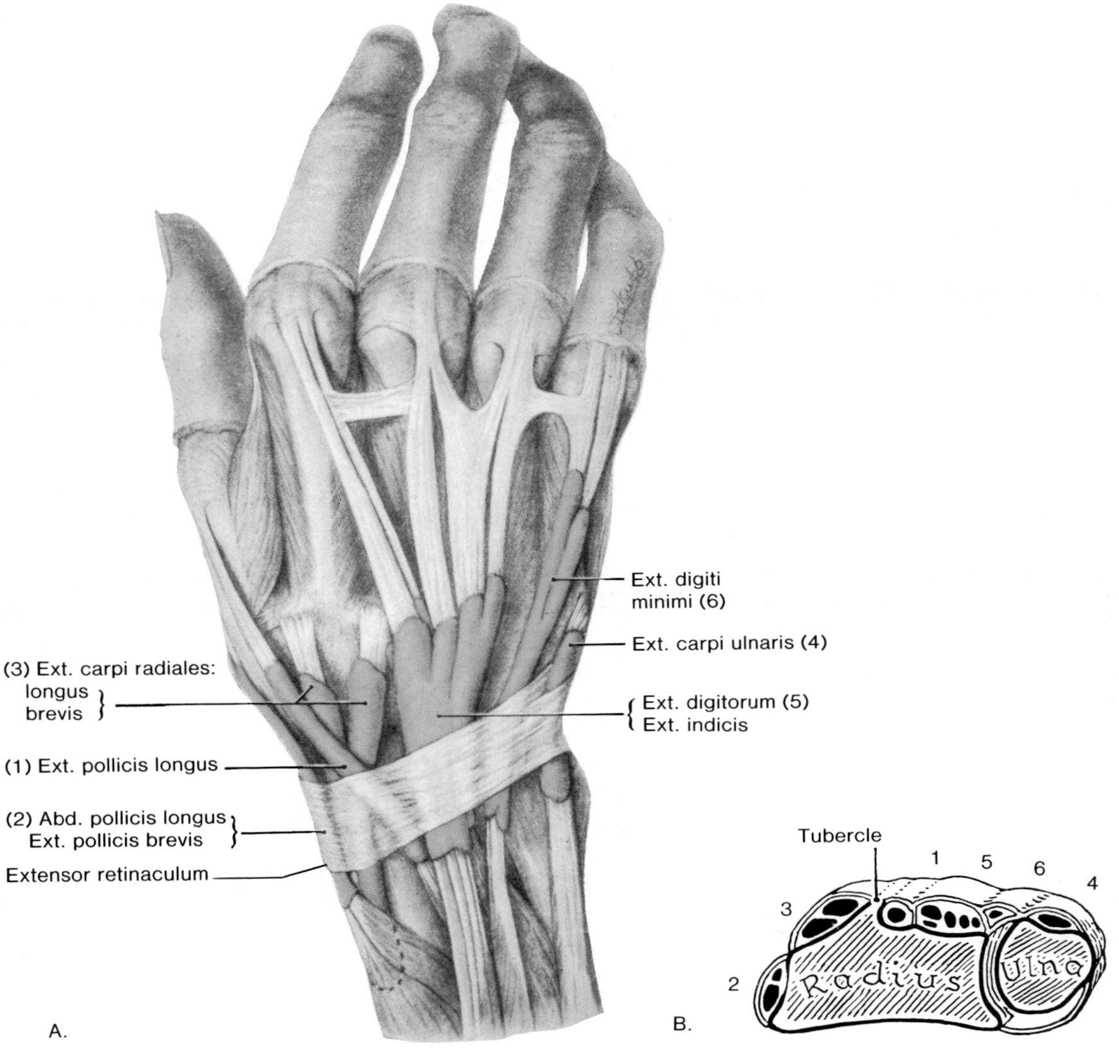

Figure 6-111. *A*, drawing of the synovial sheaths on the dorsum of the wrist. Observe that the six sheaths occupy six osseofibrous tunnels deep to the extensor retinaculum. They contain nine tendons: three for the thumb in sheaths (one and two); three for the extensors of the wrist in two sheaths (three and four); and three for the extensors of the fingers in two sheaths (five and six). The tendons of the extensors of the wrist are the strongest because they work synergically with the flexors of the digits. Note the bands proximal to the knuckles that connect the tendons of the digital extensors and thereby restrict independent action of the fingers. *B*, diagram of a cross-section of the tendons and their synovial sheaths on the dorsum of the distal ends of the radius and ulna.

Insertion (Fig. 6-86). Dorsal surface of **base of third metacarpal** bone. Its tendon passes deep to the extensor retinaculum and through the anatomical snuff box (Figs. 6-108 to 6-111).

Nerve Supply (Fig. 6-97). **Deep branch of radial** nerve (C7 and C8).

Actions. **Extends** and **abducts wrist.** This muscle and the extensor carpi radialis longus act synergistically (*i.e.*, together) to steady the wrist during flexion of the fingers.

The Extensor Digitorum Muscle (Figs. 6-89, 6-108, 6-109, and 6-111). This **principal extensor of the fingers** divides into four tendons proximal to the wrist which pass through a **common synovial sheath** deep to the extensor retinaculum (Figs. 6-111 and 6-114).

Origin (Fig. 6-86). **Lateral epicondyle** of humerus by *common extensor tendon* and **intermuscular septa.**

Insertion (Figs. 6-111, 6-112, and 6-114). **Extensor expansions of fingers.**

Nerve Supply (Fig. 6-109). **Posterior interosseous** nerve (C7 and C8), a branch of the radial.

Actions. **Extends fingers** at metacarpophalangeal and interphalangeal joints and **extends wrist** joint.

The Extensor Digiti Minimi Muscle (Figs. 6-108 and 6-109). This slender slip of muscle is a partially detached part of the extensor digitorum. Its tendon runs through a separate compartment in the extensor retinaculum (Fig. 6-111).

Origin (Figs. 6-85, 6-86, and 6-108). **Lateral epicondyle** of humerus by *common extensor tendon.*

Insertion (Figs. 6-111 and 6-114). **Extensor expansion of little finger.**

Nerve Supply (Fig. 6-109). **Posterior interosseous** nerve (C6 and C7), a branch of the radial.

Actions. **Extends little finger** at metacarpophalangeal and interphalangeal joints, allowing separate extension of little finger.

The Extensor Carpi Ulnaris Muscle (Figs. 6-89, 6-91, 6-108, 6-109, and 6-111). This long, thin muscle is located on the ulnar border of the forearm. Its tendon runs in a groove or pit between the head and the styloid process of the ulna (Fig. 6-80) within a special compartment of the extensor retinaculum.

Origin (Figs. 6-85, 6-86, and 6-108). **Lateral epicondyle** of humerus by *common*

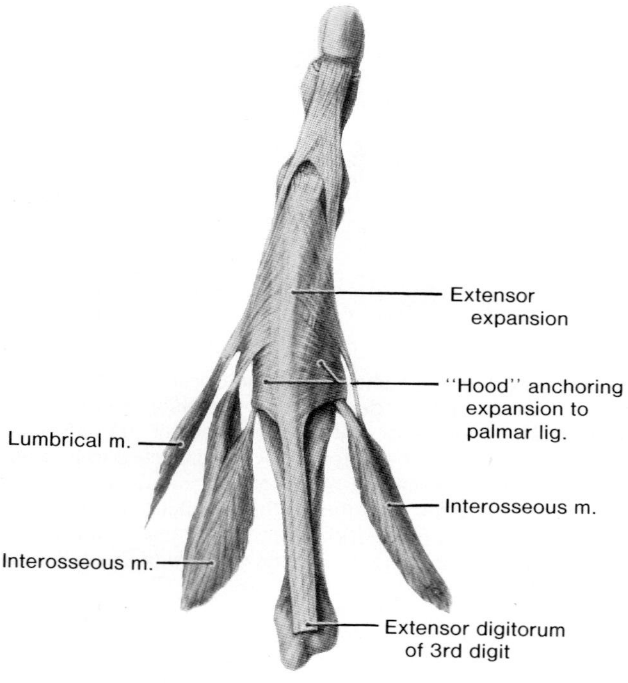

Figure 6-112. Drawing of a dorsal view of a dissection of the middle finger showing the dorsal extensor expansion (dorsal expansion). Observe that the expansion extends to the bases of the middle and distal phalanges and gives a strong areolar band to the base of the proximal phalanx (not in view here).

extensor tendon and **posterior border of ulna.**

Insertion (Figs. 6-86 and 6-111*A*). **Base of fifth metacarpal** bone.

Nerve Supply (Fig. 6-109). **Posterior interosseous** nerve (C7 and C8), a branch of the radial.

Actions. **Extends** and **adducts wrist.**

The Deep Extensor Muscle Layer (Figs. 6-108 to 6-111). The deep extensors of the forearm consist of three muscles acting on the thumb (abductor pollicis longus, extensor pollicis brevis, and extensor pollicis longus) and the extensor indicis. All these muscles originate from the radius, the ulna, and the interosseous membrane between them (Figs. 6-80, 6-86, and 6-167).

The abductor pollicis longus, extensor pollicis brevis, and extensor pollicis longus arise deep to the superficial extensors and appear from concealment (*i.e.*, crop out) along a furrow that divides the extensors into lateral and medial groups (Figs. 6-108 and 6-109); thus, they are referred to as the **three outcropping muscles**. The tendons of these muscles appear from under the lateral border of the extensor digitorum and pass superficial to the tendons of the extensor carpi radialis longus and brevis.

The abductor pollicis longus and the extensor pollicis brevis bound the anatomical snuff box anteriorly (Fig. 6-110), and the extensor pollicis longus bounds it posteriorly. Extend your thumb and examine your anatomical snuff box (Fig. 6-113). Put the tip of your finger into this depression and feel the pulsations of the radial artery as it crosses the floor of the snuff box (Fig. 6-110).

The Abductor Pollicis Longus Muscle (Figs. 6-108 to 6-111 and 6-114). This **long abductor of the thumb** (L. pollex) lies just distal to the supinator.

Origin (Fig. 6-86). **Posterior surfaces of ulna** and **radius**. Although deeply situated, it emerges at the wrist as one of the outcropping muscles (Fig. 6-108). Its tendon passes deep to the extensor retinaculum in a common synovial sheath with the tendon of the extensor pollicis brevis (Fig. 6-111). Distal to the retinaculum these tendons form the anterior boundary of the anatomical snuff box (Figs. 6-108, 6-110, and 6-113).

Insertion (Fig. 6-85). **Base of first metacarpal** bone.

Nerve Supply (Fig. 6-109). **Posterior interosseous** nerve (C7 and C8), a branch of the radial.

Actions (Figs. 6-129 and 6-134). **Abducts** and **extends thumb** at carpometacarpal joint.

The Extensor Pollicis Brevis Muscle (Figs. 6-108 to 6-111, 6-113, and 6-114). This **short extensor of the thumb** lies distal to the long abductor of the thumb (abductor pollicis longus).

Origin (Figs. 6-86 and 6-167). **Posterior surface of radius** and **interosseous membrane**. Its tendon lies in contact with the abductor pollicis longus tendon as they pass deep to the extensor retinaculum (Fig. 6-108). Deep to these tendons are **three important structures**: the *styloid process of the radius*; the *lateral collateral ligament* of the wrist joint (Fig. 6-172); and the *radial artery* crossing between the tendons and the ligament (Figs. 6-108 to 6-110).

Insertion (Fig. 6-86). **Base of proximal phalanx of thumb.**

Nerve Supply (Fig. 6-109). **Posterior interosseous** nerve (C7 and C8), a branch of the radial.

Action (Fig. 6-129). **Extends thumb** at carpometacarpal and metacarpophalangeal joints.

The Extensor Pollicis Longus Muscle (Figs. 6-108 to 6-111, 6-113 and 6-114). This **long extensor of the thumb** is larger and its tendon is longer than that of the extensor pollicis brevis.

Origin (Figs. 6-86 and 6-167). **Posterior surface of middle third of ulna** and **interosseous membrane.** Its tendon passes through a special compartment of the extensor retinaculum (Fig. 6-111), where it turns laterally around the **dorsal tubercle of the radius** (Fig. 6-81) to form the posterior boundary of the anatomical snuff box (Figs. 6-108 to 6-111, and 6-113).

Insertion (Fig. 6-85). **Base of distal phalanx of thumb.**

Nerve Supply (Fig. 6-109). **Posterior interosseous** nerve (C7 and C8), a branch of the radial.

Action (Fig. 6-129). **Extends metacarpophalangeal** and **interphalangeal joints of thumb.**

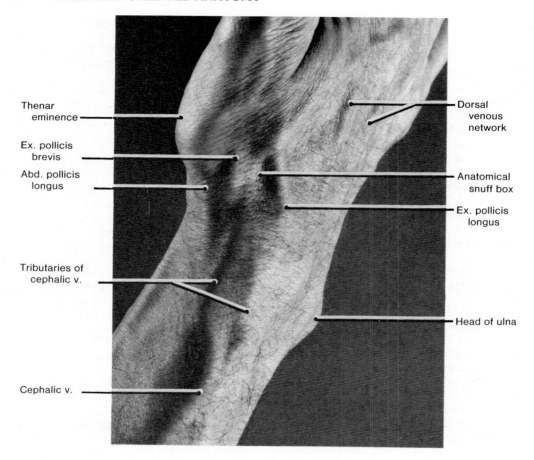

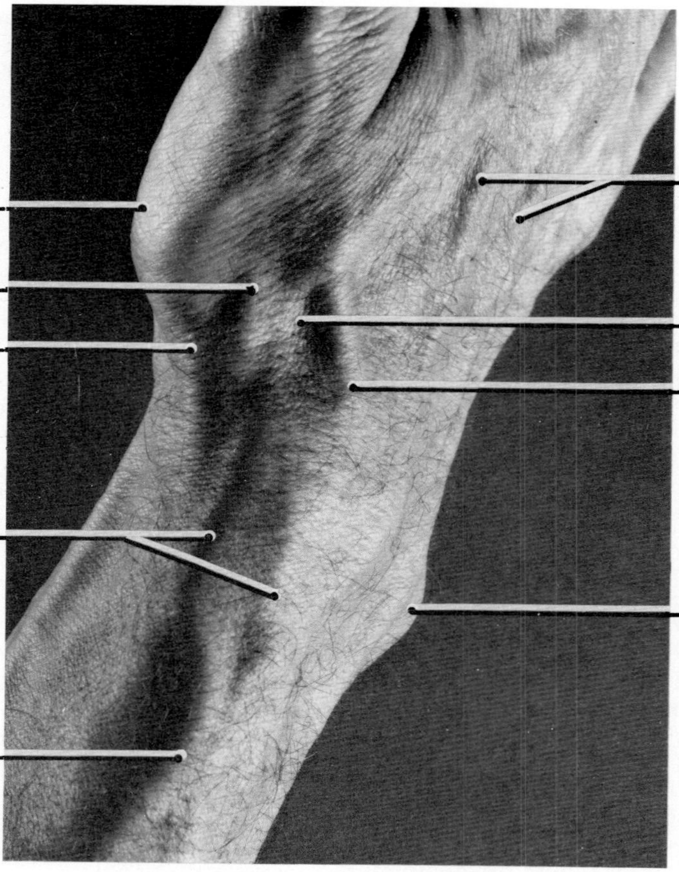

Figure 6-113. Photograph of a dorsolateral view of the forearm and hand of a 46-year-old man showing the principal surface landmarks. Observe the hollow called the *anatomical snuff box* because of the use to which it was once put. The abductor pollicis longus and extensor pollicis brevis bound the snuff box anteriorly and the extensor pollicis longus bounds it posteriorly. Compare this photograph with the dissections of the radial aspect of the wrist (Figs. 6-110 and 6-116). Note that the tendons of the abductor pollicis longus and extensor pollicis brevis diverge in this man as they proceed distally. If you have difficulty distinguishing the one from the other on your wrist, move your thumb anteriorly and posteriorly and insert your fingernail between them when you see them move. The cephalic vein usually lies in the superficial fascia just posterior to the styloid process of the radius. The cephalic vein and its tributaries are clinically important because they are used for venipuncture (*e.g.*, for obtaining blood or giving transfusions).

The Extensor Indicis Muscle (Figs. 6-108, 6-109, 6-111, 6-114, and 6-120). This narrow, elongated muscle lies medial to and alongside the extensor pollicis longus in the forearm.

Origin (Figs. 6-86 and 6-167). **Posterior surface of ulna** and **interosseous membrane.** Its tendon passes deep to the extensor retinaculum within the same synovial sheath as the tendons of the extensor digitorum (Fig. 6-111).

Insertion (Fig. 6-114). **Extensor expansion of index finger.** Opposite the second metacarpal bone, its tendon joins the tendon of the extensor digitorum to the fingers.

Nerve Supply (Fig. 6-109). **Posterior in-**

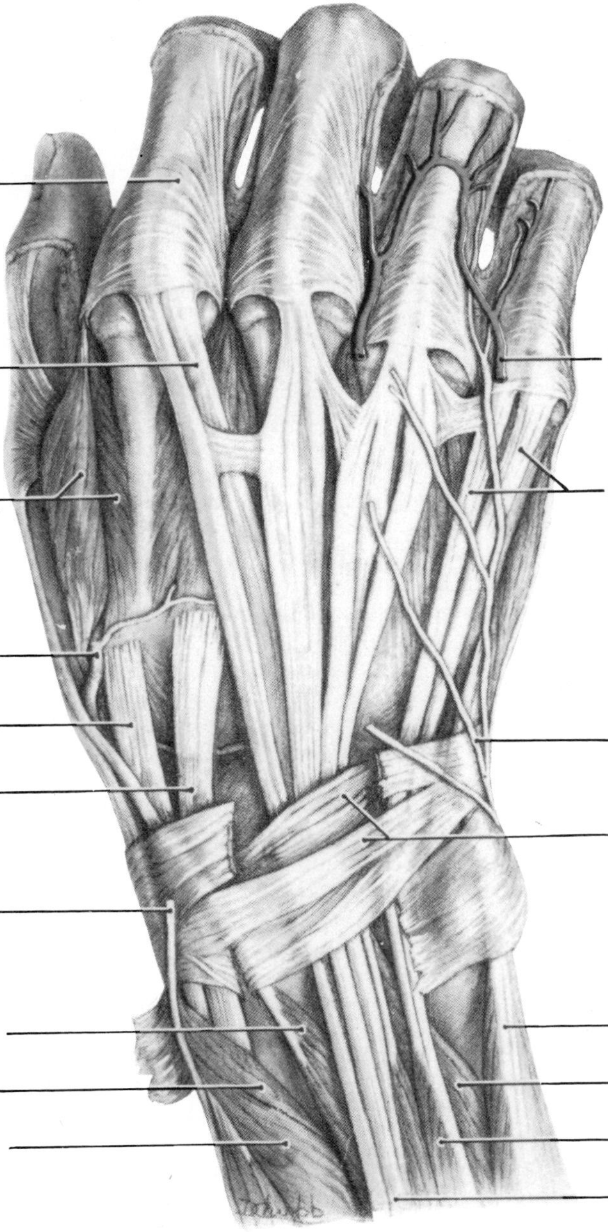

Figure 6-114. Drawing of a dissection of the extensor tendons passing deep to the extensor retinaculum on the dorsum of the hand. Observe that this strong band stretches obliquely from one ridge on the radius to another. Medially it passes distal to the ulna to be attached to the pisiform and triquetrum (Fig. 6-87*A*). Note the bands proximal to the knuckles that connect the tendons of the digital extensor and thereby restrict the independent action of the fingers.

terosseous nerve (C7 and C8), a branch of the radial.

Action. **Extends index finger**.

CLINICALLY ORIENTED COMMENTS

"**Tennis elbow**," or **lateral epicondylitis** (inflammation of the lateral epicondyle of the humerus and the tissues around it), results from premature *degeneration of the common extensor origin* of the superficial extensor muscles (*i.e.*, the origin of the common extensor tendon, Figs. 6-85 and 6-86). *Tennis elbow is characterized clinically by tenderness and pain around the lateral epicondyle* (Fig. 6-115) and by radiation of pain down the forearm. The pain is aggravated by activities that put tension on the common extensor tendon (*e.g.*, dorsiflexion of the hand).

This condition is common in persons who play tennis because of the repeated strenuous contraction of the extensor muscles, especially during the backhand stroke. This repeated movement *strains the common extensor tendon* of these muscles and produces inflammation of the lateral epicondyle. This condition is not confined to those who play tennis. It may develop following an injury to the elbow or any continuous activity that involves extensive use of the superficial extensor muscles of the forearm.

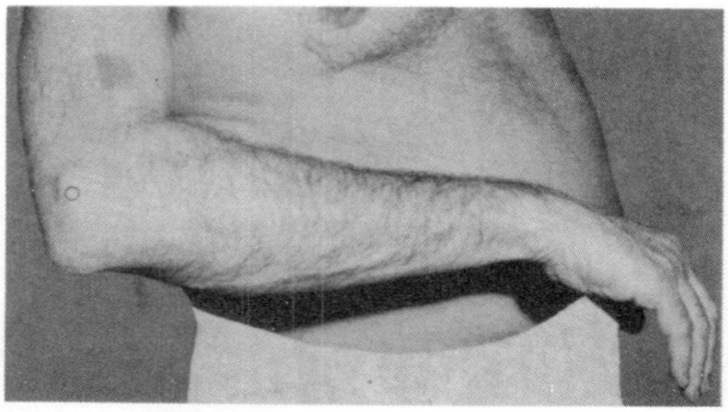

Figure 6-115. Photograph of the upper limb of a man with lateral epicondylitis ("tennis elbow"). The *circle* marks the point of local tenderness over the lateral epicondyle of his humerus.

THE POSTERIOR ANTEBRACHIAL NERVES

After entering the cubital fossa, the **radial nerve** divides into deep and superficial branches (Fig. 6-84). The **deep branch of the radial** supplies the extensor carpi radialis brevis muscle and the supinator muscle before entering the latter muscle. When it emerges from the supinator, the deep branch is referred to as the **posterior interosseous nerve** (Fig. 6-109). It passes deep to the extensor pollicis longus muscle and lies on the interosseous membrane (Fig. 6-167), where it is accompanied by the **posterior interosseous artery**. It terminates on the dorsum of the wrist. The posterior interosseous nerve supplies the extensor digitorum, the extensor digiti minimi, the extensor carpi ulnaris, the extensor indicis, and the three outcropping thumb muscles (Fig. 6-109).

The **superficial branch of the radial** nerve (Fig. 6-95) passes distally, deep to the brachioradialis. At the wrist it divides into four or five digital nerves (Figs. 6-103 and 6-137). The superficial radial nerve, **entirely cutaneous**, supplies the lateral two-thirds of the posterior surface of the hand and the posterior surface of the lateral two and one-half fingers over the proximal phalanx (Figs. 6-29, 6-102, and 6-103). The area of skin it supplies is subject to variation.

THE POSTERIOR ANTEBRACHIAL ARTERIES

The back of the forearm and the hand are supplied by the **posterior interosseous artery** (Fig. 6-109). It arises in the front of the forearm from the common interosseous branch of the ulnar artery (Fig. 6-167). It passes backward between the radius and ulna, just proximal to the interosseous membrane, and appears at the back of the forearm between the supinator and the abductor pollicis longus muscles (Fig. 6-109). It then descends between the superficial and deep muscles. As it reaches the back of the wrist, it becomes very small and ends by anastomosing with the termination of the anterior interosseous artery and with the **dorsal carpal arch** (Figs. 6-117 and 6-139).

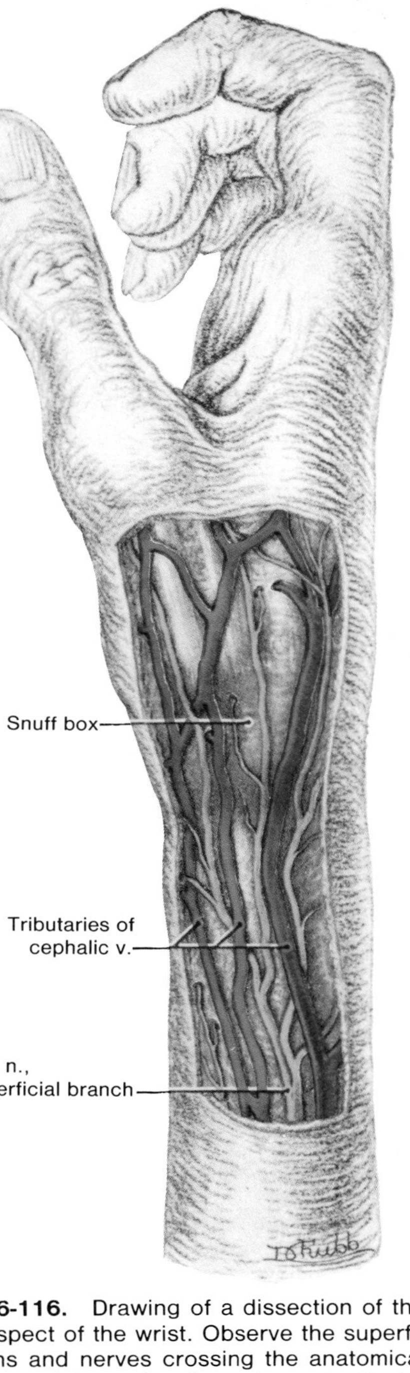

Figure 6-116. Drawing of a dissection of the radial aspect of the wrist. Observe the superficial veins and nerves crossing the anatomical snuff box and the perforating veins and articular nerves piercing the deep fascia. The branches of the superficial radial nerve are sometimes injured during puncture of the tributaries of the cephalic vein for intravenous transfusion. This may result in anesthesia of the skin between the dorsal surfaces of the thumb and index finger (Fig. 6-181*A*). See the cephalic vein and its tributaries in the photograph of this region (Fig. 6-113).

THE WRIST OR CARPUS

The wrist or carpus is the region between the forearm and the hand (*i.e.*, distal to the forearm). A "wrist" watch is usually not worn around the wrist; commonly the strap or band encircles the distal end of the forearm, just proximal to the head of the ulna (Figs. 6-83 and 6-92). Movements of the hand occur primarily at the wrist joint. The wrist or **carpal bones** are illustrated in Figures 6-1, 6-87, and 6-122, and the **wrist joint** is described subsequently.

The antebrachial fascia (deep fascia of the forearm) is thickened posteriorly at the wrist to form the transverse band known as the **extensor retinaculum** (Fig. 6-108). It retains the extensor tendons in position, thereby increasing their efficiency. The antebrachial fascia is also thickened anteriorly at the wrist to form the **flexor retinaculum** (Fig. 6-95), a fibrous band that converts the anterior concavity of the carpus into a carpal tunnel (Fig. 6-88) through which the flexor tendons pass.

Observe the transverse **wrist creases** (Figs. 6-93 and 6-121). The distal wrist crease indicates the proximal border of the flexor retinaculum (Fig. 6-101), and the proximal wrist crease roughly indicates the level of the wrist joint (Fig. 6-122).

CLINICALLY ORIENTED COMMENTS

When a person falls on the outstretched hand with the forearm pronated, the main force of the fall is transmitted via the carpus to the distal ends of the forearm bones, particularly the radius, and then proximally to the humerus, scapula, and clavicle. During such falls fractures may occur in the wrist, forearm, or clavicle.

In old people, particularly women, the radius tends to break about 2.5 cm proximal to the wrist joint (**Colles' fracture**). In this

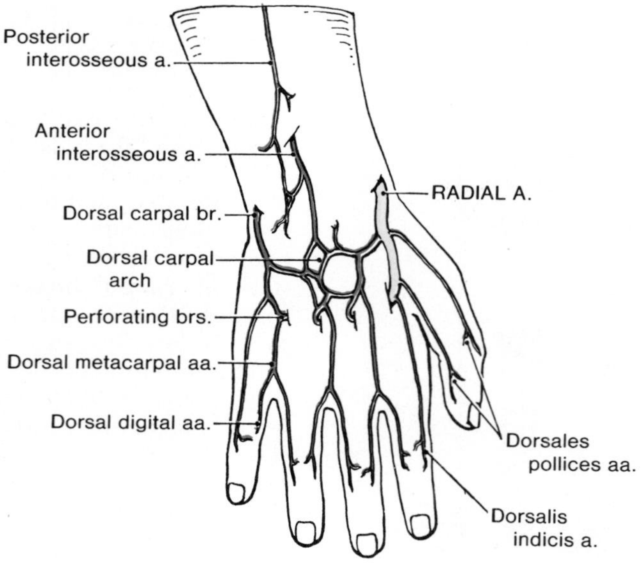

Figure 6-117. Diagram of the arteries of the dorsum of the forearm and hand. Note the radial artery emerging from the anatomical snuff box. Compare with the dissection of the radial aspect of the wrist (Fig. 6-110). Observe that the deep carpal branch of the radial anastomoses with the deep carpal branch of the ulnar to form the dorsal carpal arch (rete).

injury the distal fragment of the radius is often comminuted (broken into pieces) and the fragments are usually displaced backward and upward, producing shortening (Case 6-11). When there is a single fragment it may be impacted (*i.e.*, the jagged ends of the bone are driven into each other). Displacement of the distal part of the radius often breaks off the ulnar styloid process owing to the pull of the articular disc connecting the radius and the ulna (Figs. 6-170 and 6-172).

Fracture of the scaphoid bone is a common carpal injury, especially when the person falls on the palm of the hand with the wrist abducted. Commonly the bone fractures at its narrow "waist," producing two fragments (Fig. 6-118). As the scaphoid lies in the floor of the anatomical snuff box, suspicious clinical **signs of fracture of the scaphoid** (Figs. 6-118 and 6-190) are tenderness in the snuff box or tenderness on the anterior aspect of the wrist over the tubercle of the scaphoid (Fig. 6-87*A*).

Often an apparent "**sprained wrist**" is really a fractured scaphoid bone (Case 6-9). Of all upper limb fractures, a broken scaphoid is the easiest to overlook.

THE HAND

The hand or manus forms the distal part of the upper limb; it includes the wrist or carpus, the hand proper (metacarpus), and the digits (thumb and fingers). Because of the importance of manual dexterity in many occupational and recreational activities, a good understanding of the structure and function of the hand is essential for all who are involved in maintaining or restoring its various activities (free motion, power grip, precision handling, and pinching).

The skeleton of the hand has been described previously and is illustrated in Figures 6-1, 6-87, and 6-122.

CLINICALLY ORIENTED COMMENTS

Fractures and dislocations in the hand are common and, because hand function is so closely related to anatomical form, disability can result if normal relationships are not restored.

Street fighters commonly fracture the distal end of the shaft of their fifth meta-

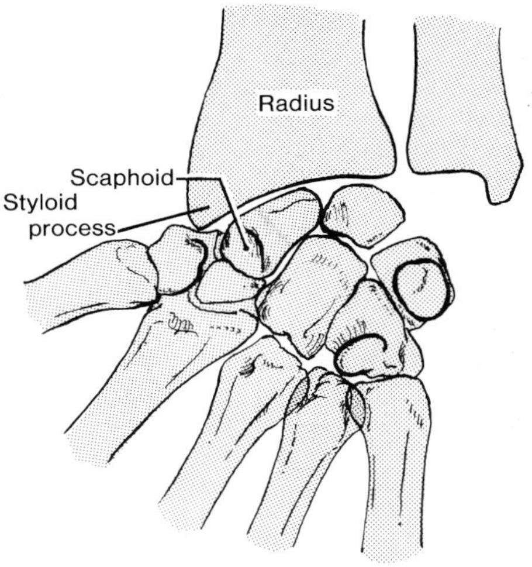

Figure 6-118. Drawing illustrating a fracture of the scaphoid bone; the *arrow* indicates the fracture line. When a person falls on the extended hand with the wrist abducted as shown, the scaphoid may be fractured by the impact of the capitate (*C*) driving it against the styloid process of the radius. Nonunion of the proximal fragment followed by aspectic necrosis is common. The anatomical basis of the death of this bone fragment is that the scaphoid is usually supplied by two nutrient arteries, one to the proximal and one to the distal half; however, occasionally both vessels supply the distal half. Fracture in these cases leaves the proximal half with no blood supply and necrosis follows.

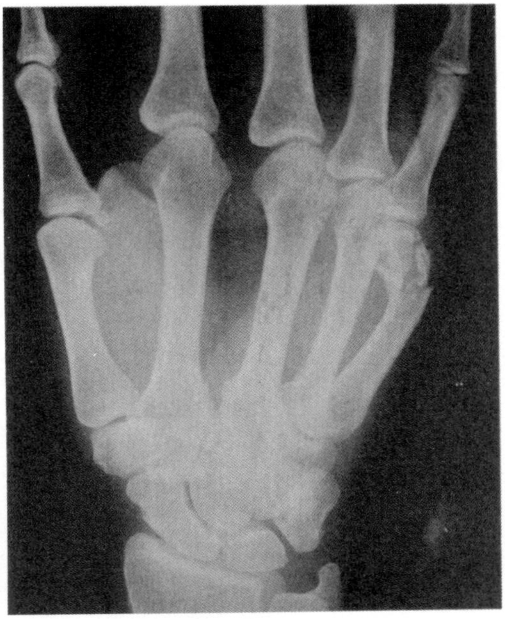

Figure 6-119. Radiograph of a slightly oblique view of the right hand showing an angulated fracture of the distal end of the body (''neck'') of the fifth metacarpal bone.

carpal bone; this region is referred to clinically as the neck of the bone (Fig. 6-119). In this type of fracture the head of the metacarpal is bent toward the palm, giving the appearance that the bone is shortened. Although commonly called a **boxer's fracture**, it is better referred to as street fighter's fracture because it results from an unskillful punch with the clenched fist. Because a trained boxer punches so that the second and third metacarpals take the strain, he rarely fractures the more mobile fifth metacarpal.

SURFACE ANATOMY OF THE HAND

The Dorsum of the Hand (Fig. 6-120). The skin on the back of the hand is thin and loose. If this aspect of the hand is examined with the wrist extended (dorsiflexed) and the fingers abducted, the extensor tendons often stand out clearly, particularly in thin persons. These tendons are not visible far beyond the knuckles (Fig. 6-120) because they flatten to form the extensor expansions (Fig. 6-114). The knuckles that become visible when a fist is made are produced by the heads of the metacarpal bones (Fig. 6-87*A*).

Under the loose subcutaneous tissue, you can easily palpate the metacarpal bones. Hair is present on the dorsum of the hand and the proximal parts of the digits. A prominent feature of the dorsum of the hand is the **dorsal venous network** (Figs. 6-82 and 6-141). To display it, compress the vessels at your wrist for a minute or so, as you open and close your hand.

The Palm of the Hand (Fig. 6-121). The skin on the palm is relatively thick and is richly supplied with **sweat glands**, but it contains no hairs or sebaceous glands. It presents several more or less constant curved **longitudinal** and **transverse flexion creases** or lines where skin is firmly bound down to the underlying deep fascia (Fig. 6-123). Usually four major palmar

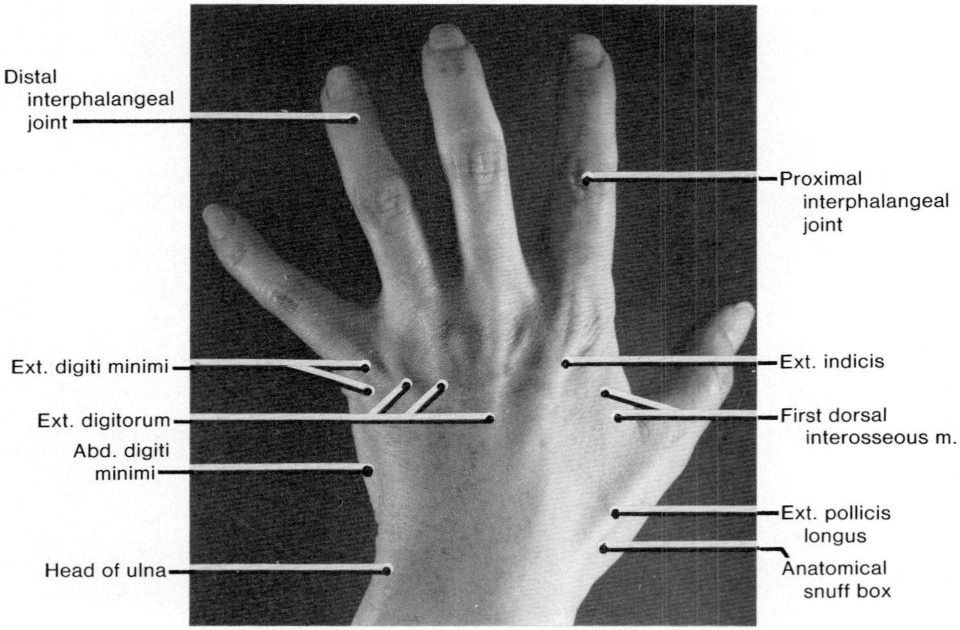

Figure 6-120. Photograph of the dorsum of the hand of a 36-year-old woman with her fingers abducted and her thumb extended. Observe the extensor tendons and the location of the anatomical snuff box. Compare with the dissection of the tendons on the dorsum of the hand shown in Figure 6-114.

creases form a variable M-shaped pattern (Fig. 6-121). These creases indicate where folding of the skin occurs during flexion of the hand. Observe that the longitudinal creases deepen when your thumb is opposed (Fig. 6-129) and that the transverse creases deepen when you flex your metacarpophalangeal joints.

The Palmar Flexion Creases (Fig. 6-121). Some creases are useful surface landmarks. The **radial longitudinal crease** partially encircles the *thenar eminence* (ball of thumb) formed by the short muscles of this digit. The **midpalmar crease** begins at the distal transverse crease and ends on the *hypothenar eminence* (ball of little finger), formed by the short muscles of the fifth digit.

The **proximal transverse crease** commences on the radial (lateral) border of the palm, in common with the radial longitudinal crease (Fig. 6-121) and superficial to the head of the second metacarpal bone (Fig. 6-122). It extends medially and slightly proximally across the palm, superficial to the shafts of the third, fourth, and fifth metacarpal bones.

The **distal transverse crease** begins at or near the cleft between the index and middle fingers (Fig. 6-121) and crosses the palm with a slight convexity, superficial to the heads of the second, third, and fourth metacarpal bones (Fig. 6-122).

The Digital Flexion Creases (Fig. 6-121). Each of the medial four digits usually has three transverse flexion creases. The **proximal flexion crease** is located at the root of the finger, about 2 cm distal to the metacarpophalangeal joint. There are two **middle flexion creases**, the proximal one lying over the proximal interphalangeal joint (Figs. 6-121 and 6-122). The **distal flexion crease** lies proximal to the distal interphalangeal joint.

The thumb, having but two phalanges, has only two flexion creases. Like the other digital creases, they deepen when the digits are flexed. The proximal flexion crease crosses the thumb obliquely, proximal to the first metacarpophalangeal joint (Fig. 6-

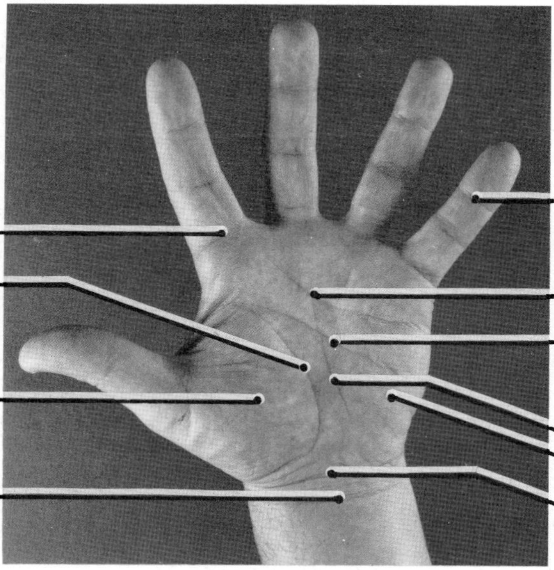

Figure 6-121. Photograph of the palmar surface of the hand of a 53-year-old man showing its surface landmarks. The distal skin crease on the wrist crosses (medial to lateral) the pisiform, the tubercle of the scaphoid (Fig. 6-87*A*), and the styloid process of the radius. Compare with the radiograph shown in Figure 6-122.

122). The distal flexion crease on the thumb, comparable in position to the middle digital creases on the fingers, lies proximal to the interphalangeal joint.

It is common knowledge that the ridges on the fingers are known as **fingerprints** and that they are used for identification because of their unique patterns. Their real function is to reduce slippage when grasping objects.

CLINICALLY ORIENTED COMMENTS

Because the skin is firmly bound to the underlying connective tissue and to the structures deep to it at the various skin creases (Fig. 6-123), these creases are avoided in planning surgical incisions. In addition, scar tissue may form where an incision crosses a crease and subsequently reduce the range of movement permitted at the nearby joint.

The science of studying deviations in dermal configurations and skin creases is known as **dermatoglyphics**. It can be a valuable extension of the conventional physical examination of patients with certain congenital malformations and genetic diseases. For example, persons with the **Down syndrome** often have only one transverse palmar crease, usually referred to as a **simian crease** (Fig. 6-124*B*). Less than 1% of the general population has this crease.

In patients with the **trisomy 18 syndrome**, the little finger frequently has only one interphalangeal digital crease. Examination of the palmar and digital creases in patients suspected of having chromosomal abnormalities is often helpful in deciding whether or not chromosomal investigations are indicated.

The Deep Fascia of the Palm (Fig. 6-123). The deep fascia of the palm is continuous proximally with the antebrachial fascia and at the borders of the palm with the fascia on the dorsum of the hand. It is thin over the thenar and hypothenar eminences (**thenar** and **hypothenar fasciae**) but is thick in the palm where it forms the **palmar aponeurosis** (Fig. 6-123) and in the

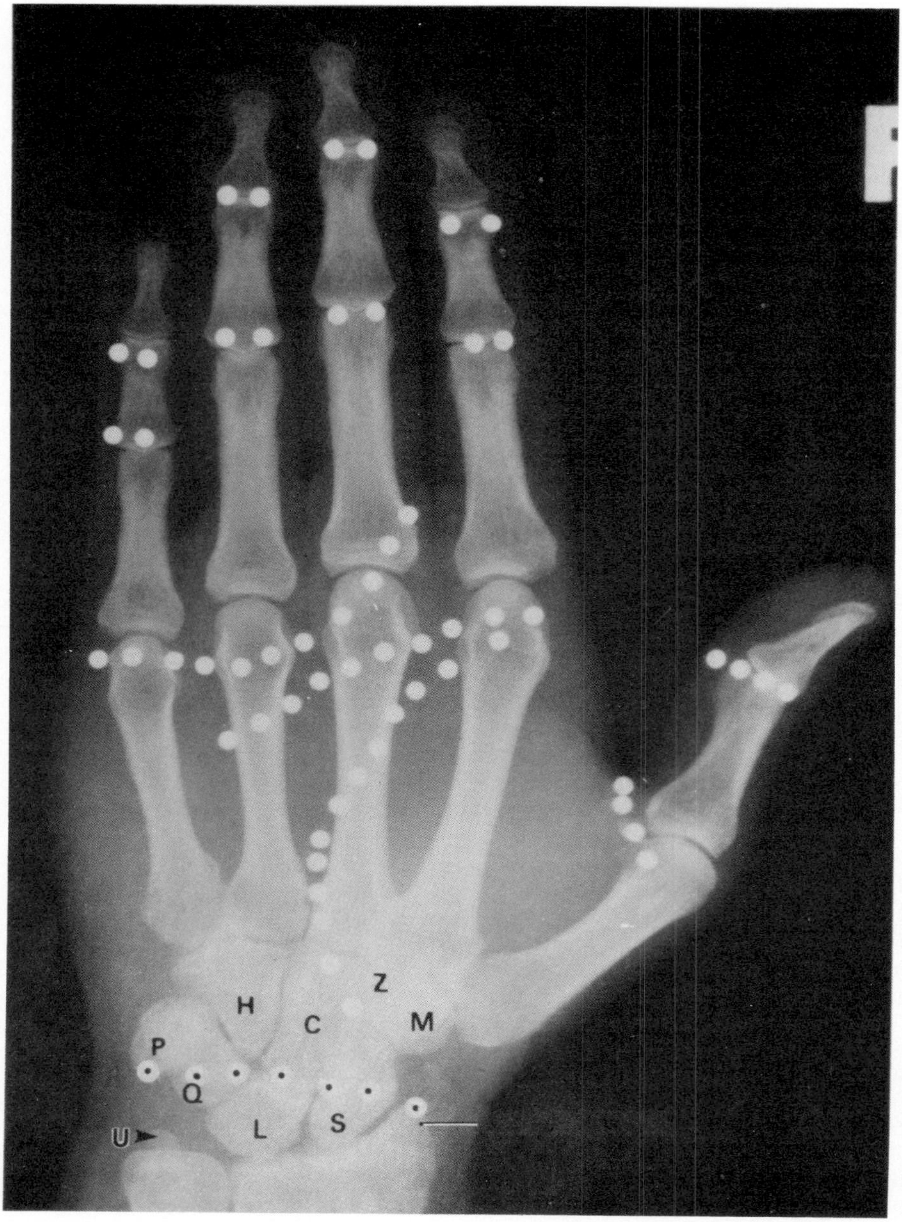

Figure 6-122. Radiograph of the left hand (posteroanterior projection) showing the posterior surfaces of the fingers and the *lateral surface of the thumb* (Fig. 6-120). Place your hand palm down on a table and you will see why this occurs. Observe the two rows of carpal bones. In the distal row note the hamate (*H*), the capitate (*C*), the trapezoid (*Z*), and the trapezium (*M*) which forms a saddle-shaped joint with the metacarpal (*I*). In the proximal row note the scaphoid (*S*), the lunate (*L*), and the pisiform (*P*) superimposed on the triquetrum (*Q*). Observe the ulnar styloid process (*U* with *arrow*). Lead shot has been placed along the palmar and digital flexion creases to show their relationship to the joints. Note that the distal wrist crease (*black dots* inside white circles) shown in Figures 6-93 and 6-121 crosses the pisiform, the joint between capitate and lunate, the tubercle of the scaphoid, and the radial styloid process.

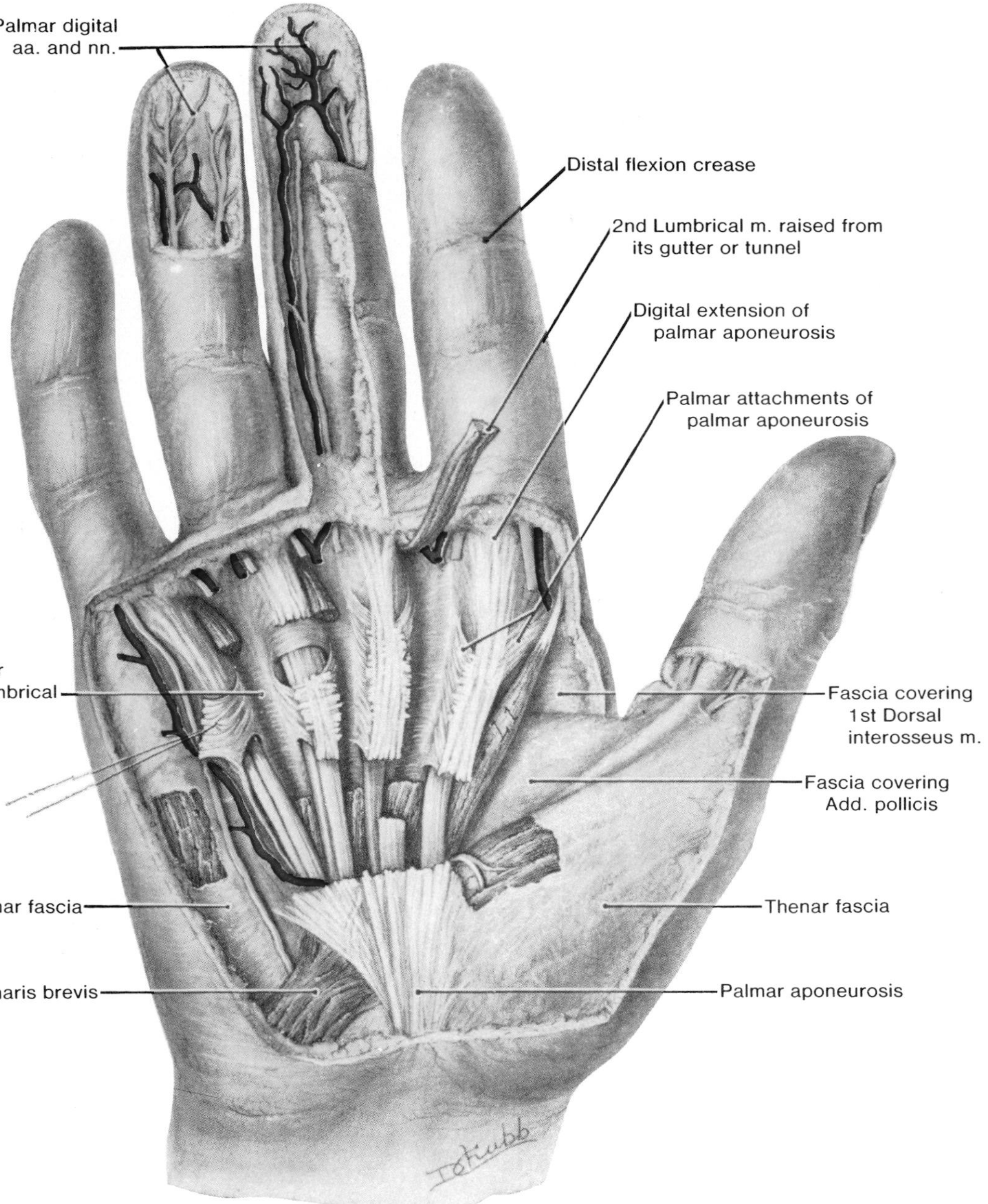

Figure 6-123. Drawing of a dissection of the palm showing the palmar digital vessels and nerves and the attachments of the palmar aponeurosis. Observe the two sets of tunnels in the distal half of the palm: (1) those for the long flexor tendons and (2) those for the lumbrical muscles and digital vessels and nerves. The former are continued into the fingers; the latter open on the dorsum of the hand behind the web. In a finger, note the digital artery and nerve lying on the side of the fibrous digital sheath and the absence of fat deep to the digital flexion creases. Observe the four palmar spaces: (1) a *thenar space* behind the thenar fascia; (2) a *hypothenar space* behind the hypothenar fascia; (3) a *middle space* behind the palmar aponeurosis; and (4) an *adductor space* between the adductor pollicis and the first dorsal interosseous muscles. The middle space contains the superficialis and profundus tendons, the lumbricals, and the digital vessels and nerves.

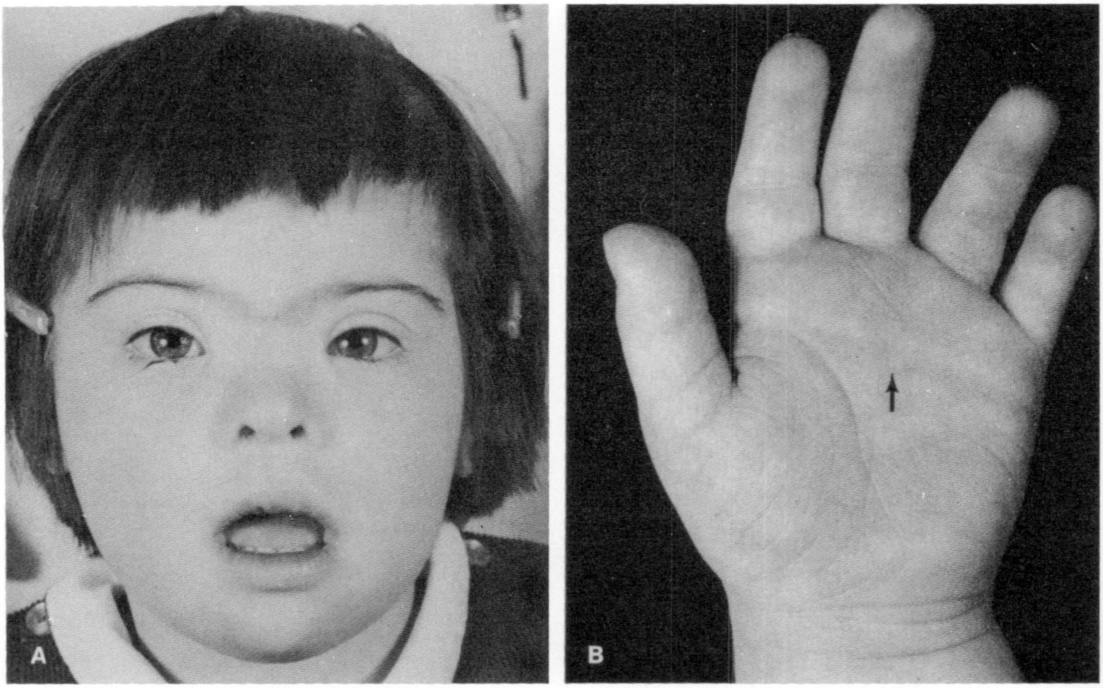

Figure 6-124. *A*, photograph of a 3-year-old girl showing the typical facial appearance associated with the Down syndrome. Note the flat broad face, oblique palpebral fissures, epicanthus, speckling of the iris, and the furrowed lower lip. *B*, the typical short broad hand of this child shows the characteristic single transverse palmar or simian crease (*arrow*).

fingers where it forms the **fibrous digital sheaths** (Fig. 6-125).

The Palmar Aponeurosis (Figs. 6-90, 6–123, and 6–126). This strong, well defined, triangular part of the deep fascia covers the soft tissues of the hand and overlies the long flexor tendons of the palm. Its apex is anchored to the **flexor retinaculum** (Fig. 6-97) and is where the palmaris longus muscle inserts (when present, Fig. 6-90). The base of the palmar aponeurosis divides at the roots of the fingers into four longitudinal bands or slips which fuse with the fibrous digital sheaths (Figs. 6-123 and 6-125).

Verify the resistance of the palmar aponeurosis by exerting pressure in the center of your palm. Compare this resistance to that over the thenar and hypothenar eminences. Owing to the thickness of the palmar aponeurosis, it is difficult to palpate the tendons in the palm (Fig. 6-126).

CLINICALLY ORIENTED COMMENTS

Dupuytren's contracture is a progressive fibrosis (increase of fibrous tissue) of the palmar aponeurosis resulting in the formation of abnormal bands of fibrous tissue that extend from the aponeurosis to the bases of the phalanges (Fig. 6-128). These bands may pull the fingers into such marked flexion at the metacarpophalangeal joints that they cannot be straightened. The condition is often familial (L. family).

Usually the ring and little fingers are affected initially. In more advanced cases the proximal interphalangeal joints of these fingers are also flexed so that the distal phalanges are pulled against the palm. The index finger is rarely involved. The etiology (cause) of this disease is unknown, but there appears to be a hereditary predisposition (*i.e.*, multiple genetic factors appear to be involved).

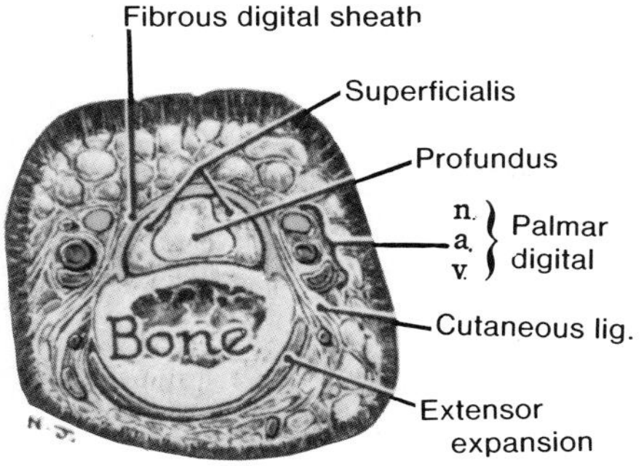

Figure 6-125. Drawing of a cross-section through the proximal phalanx of a finger. Note the osseofibrous tunnel containing the tendons of the flexors of the digit. Observe that the skin is thickest on the palmar surface and that the palmar digital nerves and vessels are applied to the fibrous sheath, not to the bone. Note the ligaments that attach the skin to the bone.

Fascial Compartments of the Palm (Fig. 6-126). A fibrous **medial septum** extends deeply from the medial border of the palmar aponeurosis to the fifth metacarpal bone. Medial to this septum is the **medial (hypothenar) compartment** containing the three hypothenar muscles (concerned with movements of the little finger), blood vessels, and nerves.

Similarly a fibrous **lateral septum** extends deeply from the lateral border of the palmar aponeurosis to the first metacarpal bone. Lateral to this septum is the **lateral (thenar) compartment** containing the thenar muscles (concerned with movements of the thumb), blood vessels, and nerves.

Between the thenar and hypothenar compartments is the **intermediate (central) compartment** containing the flexor

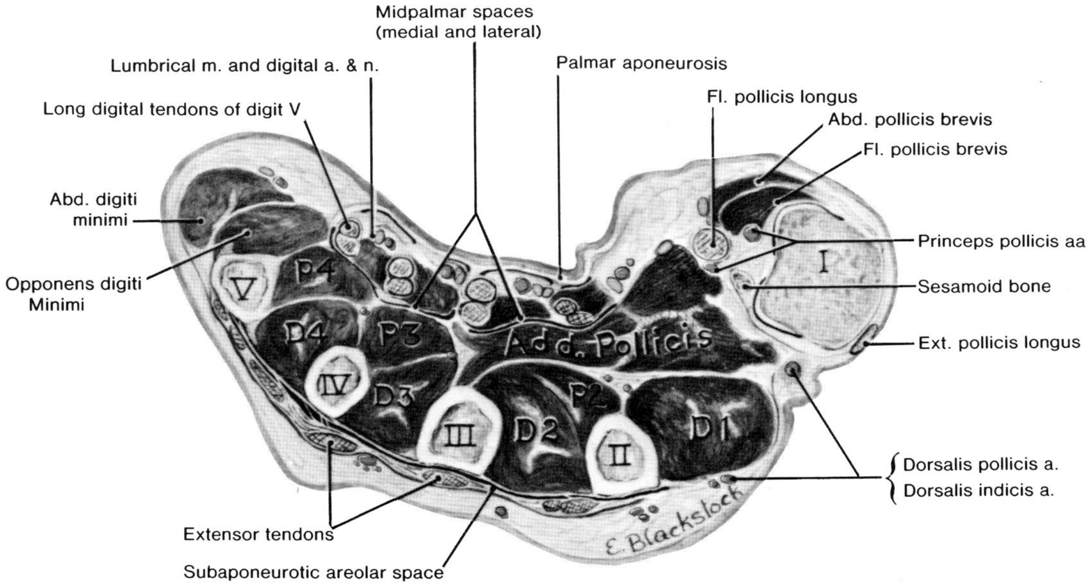

Figure 6-126. Drawing of a cross-section through the middle of the palm, passing through the head of the first metacarpal bone and therefore distal to the opponens pollicis muscle. Observe the fascial compartments of the palm: (1) a lateral *thenar compartment* containing vessels, nerves, and the thenar muscles; (2) an intermediate *central compartment* containing vessels, nerves, and the flexor tendons and their sheaths; (3) a medial *hypothenar compartment* containing vessels, nerves, and the hypothenar muscles; and (4) an *adductor compartment* containing the adductor pollicis muscle. Observe the dorsal interosseous muscles (D1 to D4) filling the spaces between the five metacarpal bones and the palmar interossei (P2 to P4). The first palmar interosseous muscle (formerly called the deep head of flexor pollicis brevis) is not visible here. Also observe the long flexor tendons (superficial and deep) of the four fingers, the four lumbricals, and the palmar digital nerves and arteries.

tendons and their sheaths, the superficial palmar arch, and branches of the median and ulnar nerves (Fig. 6-126).

From the lateral border of the palmar aponeurosis, another fibrous septum passes obliquely backward to the third metacarpal bone. This creates potential medial and lateral **midpalmar spaces**.

The **adductor compartment** (Fig. 6-126) is the deepest muscular plane of the palm of the hand. It contains the adductor pollicis muscle.

CLINICALLY ORIENTED COMMENTS

The potential fascial spaces of the palm are clinically important because they may become infected (*e.g.*, following a puncture wound of the hand). If the infection occurs between the interosseous muscles and the metacarpal bones, the spread of pus is restrained by the septum connected to the third metacarpal bone (Fig. 6-126). Thus, depending on the site of infection, pus will accumulate in the thenar, hypothenar, or adductor space. Owing to the widespread use of antibiotics, infection rarely spreads from one of these fascial spaces, but an untreated and uncontrolled infection can spread proximally from the fascial spaces into the forearm, anterior to the pronator quadratus and its fascia.

THE HAND MUSCLES

All the **intrinsic muscles** of the hand are on the palmar aspect and are innervated by branches from the ulnar or the median nerve (Figs. 6-126 and 6-127). They can be divided into three groups: (1) the thumb or **thenar muscles** in the thenar compartment; (2) the little finger or **hypothenar muscles** in the hypothenar compartment; and (3) the **lumbrical muscles** in the central compartment and the **interosseous muscles** in the intervals between the metacarpal bones (Figs. 6-131 and 6-133).

The long flexor tendons of the extrinsic muscles that arise in the forearm and pass to the digits are in the central compartment of the palm with the four lumbrical muscles. These slender muscles arise from the sides of the tendons of the flexor digitorum profundus as they traverse the palm (Fig. 6-131).

The Short Muscles of the Thumb (Figs. 6-127 and 6-130). The three thenar muscles (abductor pollicis longus, flexor pollicis brevis, and opponens pollicis), supplied by the recurrent branch of the median nerve, are chiefly responsible for the movement termed **opposition of the thumb** (Fig. 6-129). A fourth muscle (adductor pollicis), supplied by the deep branch of the ulnar nerve, adducts the thumb and is active during later stages of opposition.

The Thenar Muscles (Figs. 6-129 to 6-131, 6-134, and 6-135). These three short muscles of the thumb in the **thenar compartment** of the palm (Fig. 6-126) produce the **thenar eminence** (Fig. 6-121). They are all supplied by the recurrent branch of the median nerve (Figs. 6-93 and 6-127) and aid in performing opposition, the most important movement of the thumb (Fig. 6-129).

The Abductor Pollicis Brevis Muscle (Figs. 6-126, 6-127, and 6-131). The abductor pollicis brevis is a thin, relatively broad muscle that forms the anterolateral part of the thenar eminence.

Origin (Figs. 6-97 and 6-131). **Flexor retinaculum**, **scaphoid**, and **trapezium.**

Insertion (Figs. 6-85 and 6-131). Lateral side of **base of proximal phalanx of thumb.**

Nerve Supply (Fig. 6-127). Recurrent branch of **median** nerve (T1).

Actions (Fig. 6-129). **Abducts thumb** (*e.g.*, when depressing a key during piano playing) and assists the opponens pollicis muscle during the early stages of opposition of the thumb.

The Flexor Pollicis Brevis Muscle (Figs. 6-127, 6-130, and 6-131). The flexor pollicis brevis is located medial to the abductor pollicis brevis which partly overlaps it.

Origin (Figs. 6-97 and 6-131). **Flexor retinaculum** and **trapezium.**

Insertion (Figs. 6-85, 6-127, 6-130, and 6-131). Radial side of **base of proximal phalanx of thumb**, medial to abductor pollicis brevis.

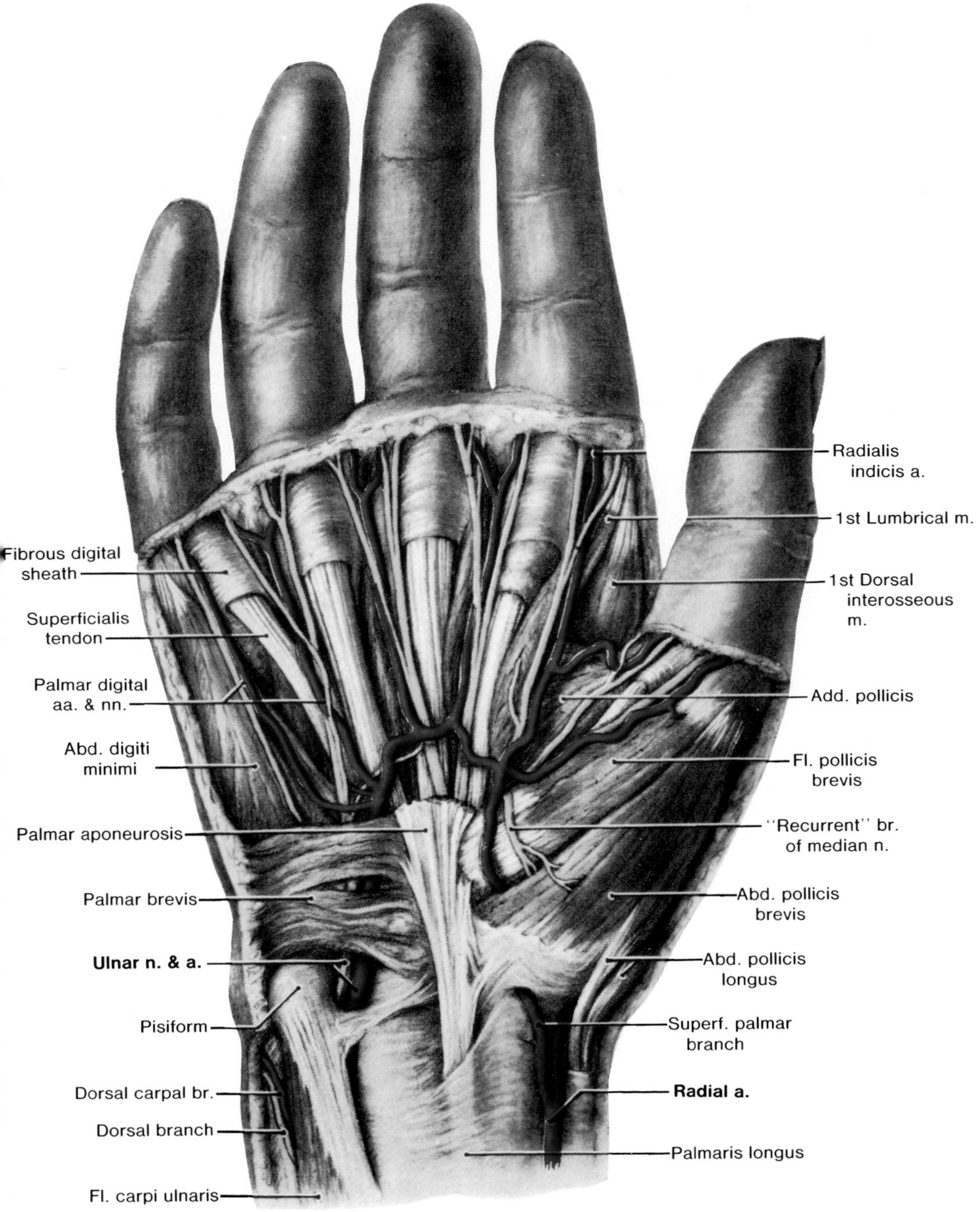

Figure 6-127. Drawing of a superficial dissection of the palm. The skin and superficial fascia are removed as are the palmar aponeurosis and the thenar and hypothenar fasciae (Fig. 6-123). Observe the superficial palmar arch formed by the ulnar artery. Note that the prominent *pisiform bone protects the ulnar nerve and artery* as they pass into the palm.

Nerve Supply (Fig. 6-127). Recurrent branch of **median** nerve (T1).

Actions (Fig. 6-129). **Flexes thumb** at carpometacarpal and metacarpophalangeal joints and **aids in opposition** of thumb.

The Opponens Pollicis Muscle (Figs. 6-97, 6-130, and 6-131). This muscle lies deep to the abductor pollicis brevis and lateral to the flexor pollicis brevis.

Origin (Figs. 6-97 and 6-131). **Flexor retinaculum** and **trapezium.**

Insertion (Figs. 6-85 and 6-97). Whole length of **lateral half of palmar surface of first metacarpal** bone.

Nerve Supply (Fig. 6-127). Recurrent branch of **median** nerve (T1).

Actions (Fig. 6-129). **Draws thumb toward center of palm** and **rotates it medially** at the carpometacarpal joint. This is called **opposition** and is the most important movement of the thumb. In Figure 6-129, note that the tip of the thumb is brought into contact with the palmar surface of the little finger. The thumb can also be opposed to the other fingers. Opposition involves extension initially, then abduction, flexion, and medial rotation, and usually adduction.

Eight muscles appear to be involved in opposing the thumb, but the five in bold type are primarily involved: extensor pollicis brevis, extensor pollicis longus, abductor pollicis longus, **flexor pollicis longus, adductor pollicis**, and the three thenar muscles (**abductor pollicis brevis, flexor pollicis brevis**, and **opponens pollicis**).

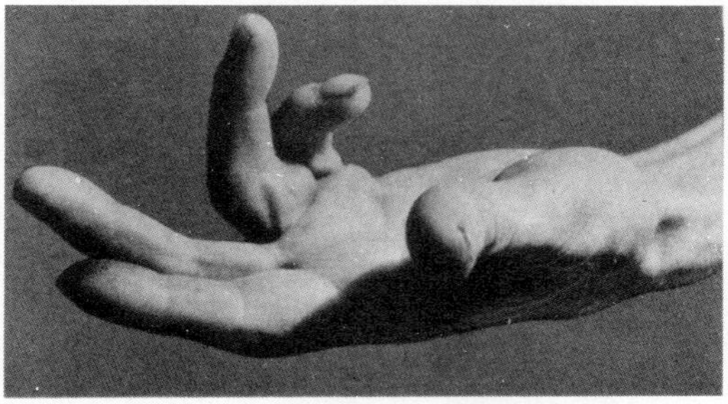

Figure 6-128. Photograph of the hand of a 56-year-old man with *Dupuytren's contracture.* Note the marked flexion of the ring and little fingers at the metacarpophalangeal and proximal interphalangeal joints.

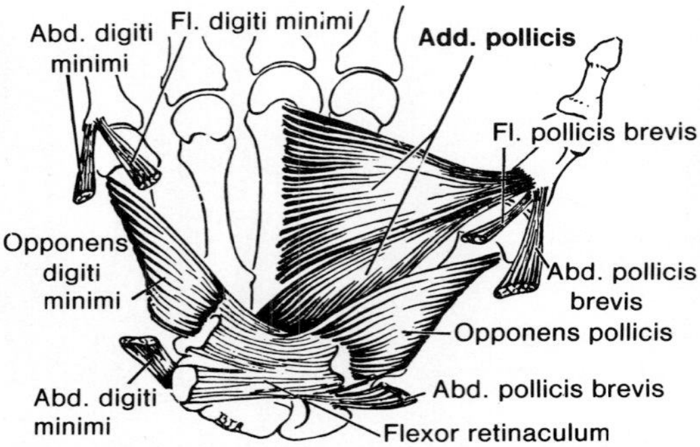

Figure 6-130. Drawing illustrating the three thenar muscles, the three hypothenar muscles, and the adductor pollicis muscle in the right hand.

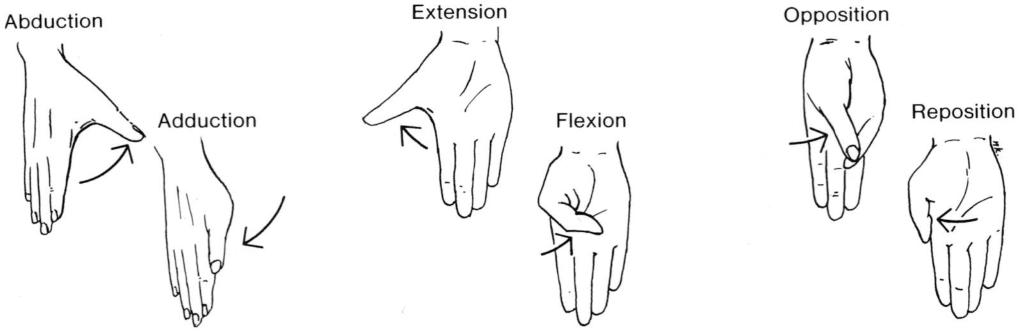

Figure 6-129. Drawings illustrating most movements of the thumb. Circumduction is also possible and medial rotation occurs during the complex movement termed opposition. Because the metacarpal of the thumb is set at a right angle to those of the other digits, all movements of the thumb take place at right angles to the corresponding movements of the fingers. Movements of the thumb are very important; you are unable to do much with your hand without them. Thumb movements account for about 50% of the hand's operations; imagine going a day without using your thumb!

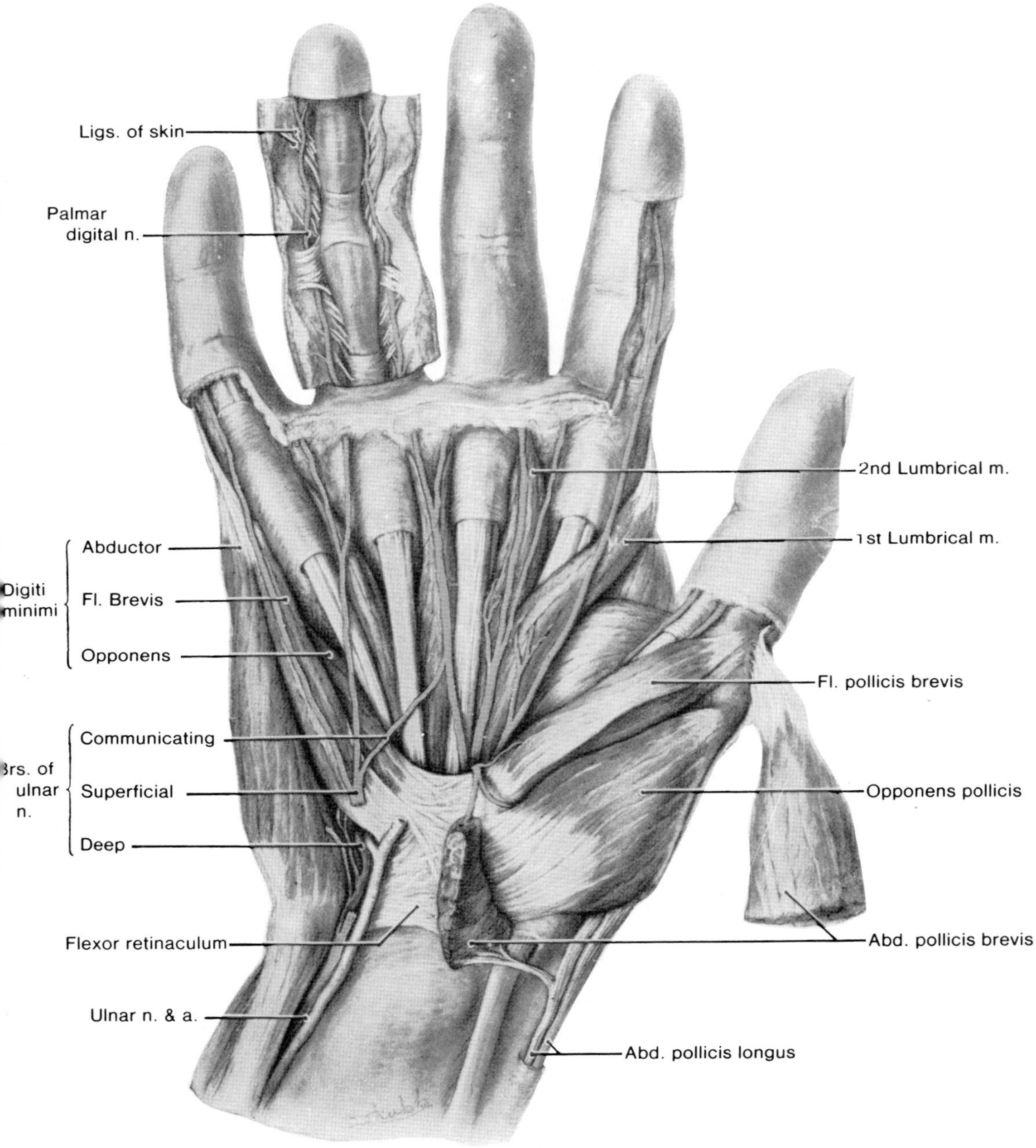

Figure 6-131. Drawing of a superficial dissection of the palm showing the three thenar and the three hypothenar muscles arising from the flexor retinaculum and from the four marginal carpal bones united by it. Note the four lumbrical muscles arising from the radial sides of the four profundus tendons and inserting into the radial sides of the extensor expansions of the corresponding digits (Fig. 6-132). Observe that the median nerve supplies five muscles (three thenar and two lumbrical) and provides cutaneous branches to three and one-half digits including parts of their dorsal aspects. Note that the ulnar nerve supplies all other short muscles in the hand and provides cutaneous branches to one and one-half digits. See Figure 6-29 for an illustration of the distribution of the cutaneous nerves to the palm of the hand.

CLINICALLY ORIENTED COMMENTS

Because of the complexity of the movement called opposition of the thumb, it may be affected by most nerve injuries in the upper limb. Obviously, injuries to the nerves supplying the intrinsic muscles of the hand, especially the median nerve, have the most severe effects on this movement.

If the median is severed in the forearm or at the wrist, the most common injury site, the thumb cannot be opposed; however, it is important to know that the intact abductor pollicis longus and adductor pollicis muscles, supplied by the posterior interosseous and ulnar nerves, respectively, may combine to imitate the action of opposition. For the other effects of median nerve injury, see Case 6–10.

The recurrent branch of the median nerve supplying the thenar muscles lies superficial (Figs. 6-93 and 6-127) and may be severed by relatively minor lacerations of the palm that involve the thenar eminence. If this nerve is severed, the thenar muscles are paralyzed and the thumb loses much of its usefulness; *i.e.*, the patient would be unable to oppose the thumb normally. Here again, the intact abductor pollicis longus and adductor pollicis may combine to imitate this action.

Injury to the median nerve at the wrist (*e.g.*, during wrist slashing) results in paralysis of the thenar muscles, the first two lumbrical muscles (Fig. 6-133), and probably sensory impairment in the digits supplied by this nerve (Fig. 6-29). As stated previously, the chief effect of lesions here is inability to oppose the thumb. In a few weeks wasting or **atrophy of the thenar muscles** may occur, producing a characteristic flattening of the thenar eminence, often referred to as "**ape hand**."

The Adductor Pollicis Muscle (Figs. 6-105, 6-109, 6-110, 6-126, 6-127, and 6-130). This fan-shaped muscle lies in the interosseous adductor compartment and has *two heads of origin* that are separated by a gap through which the radial artery passes.

Origin (Fig. 6-85). *Oblique head*, **bases of second** and **third metacarpal bones, capitate**, and **adjacent carpal bones.** *Transverse head*, anterior surface of **third metacarpal** bone.

Insertion (Fig. 6-85). Medial side of **base of proximal phalanx of thumb.** The two heads converge and insert by a tendon that contains a sesamoid bone.

Nerve Supply. Deep branch of **ulnar** nerve (T1).

Actions (Figs. 6-129 and 6-134). **Adducts thumb** and **assists in opposition** of thumb.

The Short Muscles of the Little Finger (Figs. 6-127, 6-130, and 6-131). The three **hypothenar muscles** are concerned with movements of the little finger. This digit is not nearly so mobile as the thumb.

The Hypothenar Muscles (Figs. 6-123, 6-126, 6-127, 6-130, and 6-131). These three short muscles of the little finger lie in the **hypothenar compartment** with the fifth metacarpal bone and produce the **hypothenar eminence** or ball of the little finger (Fig. 6-121). They are all supplied by the deep branch of the **ulnar nerve.**

The Abductor Digiti Minimi Muscle (Figs. 6-120 and 6-131). This is the most superficial of the three muscles forming the hypothenar eminence (Fig. 6-111).

Origin (Fig. 6-85). **Pisiform** bone, **tendon of flexor carpi ulnaris**, and pisohamate ligament.

Insertion (Figs. 6–85, 6–97, and 6–130). **Medial side of base of proximal phalanx of little finger** and extensor expansion.

Nerve Supply. Deep branch of **ulnar** nerve (T1).

Actions. **Abducts little finger** and helps to flex its metacarpophalangeal joint. To feel this muscle, lay your hand on the table and abduct your little finger against resistance as you palpate the medial border of your hand.

The Flexor Digiti Minimi Brevis Muscle (Fig. 6-131). This muscle is variable in size and lies lateral to the abductor digiti minimi.

Origin (Figs. 6-87*A* and 6-131). **Hook of hamate** and **flexor retinaculum.**

Insertion (Figs. 6-85 and 6-131). Medial side of **base of proximal phalanx of little finger**. Its tendon is fused with that of the abductor digiti minimi.

Nerve Supply. Deep branch of **ulnar** nerve (T1).

Action. **Flexes little finger** at metacarpophalangeal joint.

The Opponens Digiti Minimi Muscle (Figs. 6-97, 6-130, and 6-131). The opponens digiti minimi muscle lies deep to the abductor and flexor of the little finger.

Origin (Figs. 6-97 and 6-130). **Hook of hamate** and **flexor retinaculum.**

Insertion (Figs. 6-85 and 6-97). Whole length of **medial half of palmar surface of fifth metacarpal** bone.

Nerve Supply. Deep branch of **ulnar** nerve (T1).

Actions (Fig. 6-129). **Draws fifth metacarpal bone forward** and **rotates it laterally**, thereby deepening the hollow of the palm and bringing the little finger into opposition with the thumb.

The Palmaris Brevis Muscle (Figs. 6-90 and 6-127). This small, thin, quadrilateral muscle lies beneath the skin on the ulnar side of the palm. It overlies the three hypothenar muscles and is relatively unimportant, except that it covers and protects the ulnar nerve and artery.

Origin (Figs. 6-90 and 6-127). **Flexor retinaculum** and **palmar aponeurosis**.

Insertion (Figs. 6-123 and 6-127). **Skin on medial side of palm.**

Nerve Supply. Superficial branch of **ulnar** nerve (T1).

Actions. **Wrinkles skin on medial side of palm** and **deepens hollow of hand**, thereby aiding the palmar grip.

The Short Muscles of the Hand (Figs. 6-123, 6-126, 6-127, and 6-131 to 6-133). There are 12 muscles included in this group (four lumbrical and eight interosseous muscles). The lumbricals act only on the fingers, but the interossei act on all five digits (*i.e.*, the four fingers and the thumb).

The Lumbrical Muscles (Figs. 6-123, 6-127, 6-131, and 6-132). The four slender lumbricals (L. *lumbricus*, earthworm), one for each finger, were named because of their elongated, worm-like form.

Origin (Figs. 6-131 and 6-132). **Tendons of flexor digitorum profundus** as they traverse the palm. The lateral two lumbricals usually arise by one head and the medial two by two heads.

Insertion (Fig. 6-132). Radial side of **extensor expansions**, distal to metacarpophalangeal joints.

Nerve Supply. Lateral two by **median** nerve (T1) and *medial* two by deep branch of **ulnar** nerve (T1).

Actions. **Flex digits at metacarpophalangeal joints** because they pass anterior to their central axes and **extend interphalangeal joints**, because they pass posterior to their central axes.

The Interosseous Muscles (Figs. 6-123, 6-126, 6-127, 6-132, and 6-133). **Eight interossei muscles** occupy the spaces between the metacarpal bones. At one time the first palmar interosseous muscle was called the deep head of the flexor pollicis brevis and only seven interossei were described. The interossei are **arranged in two layers**, four palmar and four dorsal muscles. As their name indicates, they are located in the spaces *between bones* (*i.e.*, the metacarpals).

Origin (Fig. 6-133). *Dorsal interossei,* **adjacent sides of two metacarpal bones.** *Palmar interossei,* **palmar surfaces of first, second, fourth, and fifth metacarpal bones.**

Insertion (Figs. 6-85, 6-86, and 6-132). **Extensor expansions of digits** and **bases of proximal phalanges.**

Nerve Supply. Deep branch of the **ulnar** nerve (T1).

Actions (Fig. 6-134). **Dorsal interossei abduct fingers** (**DAB** is the key, *i.e.*, **D**orsal **AB**duct) and **palmar interossei adduct fingers** (**PAD** is the key, *i.e.*, **P**almar **AD**uct). They also act with the lumbrical muscles.

It is important to understand that the median plane or axial line of the hand passes through the third digit or "middle" finger (Fig. 6-134) and that adduction of the fingers is movement toward this imaginary line and that abduction is movement away from it. Therefore you can abduct your middle finger to either side of this imaginary line. Adduction restores it to the axial line.

The Long Flexor Tendons of the Extrinsic Muscles of the Hand (Figs. 6-98, 6-131, and 6-133). Some information about the course and insertion of the tendons is given with the description of the flexor muscles of the forearm (p. 754). Revise your

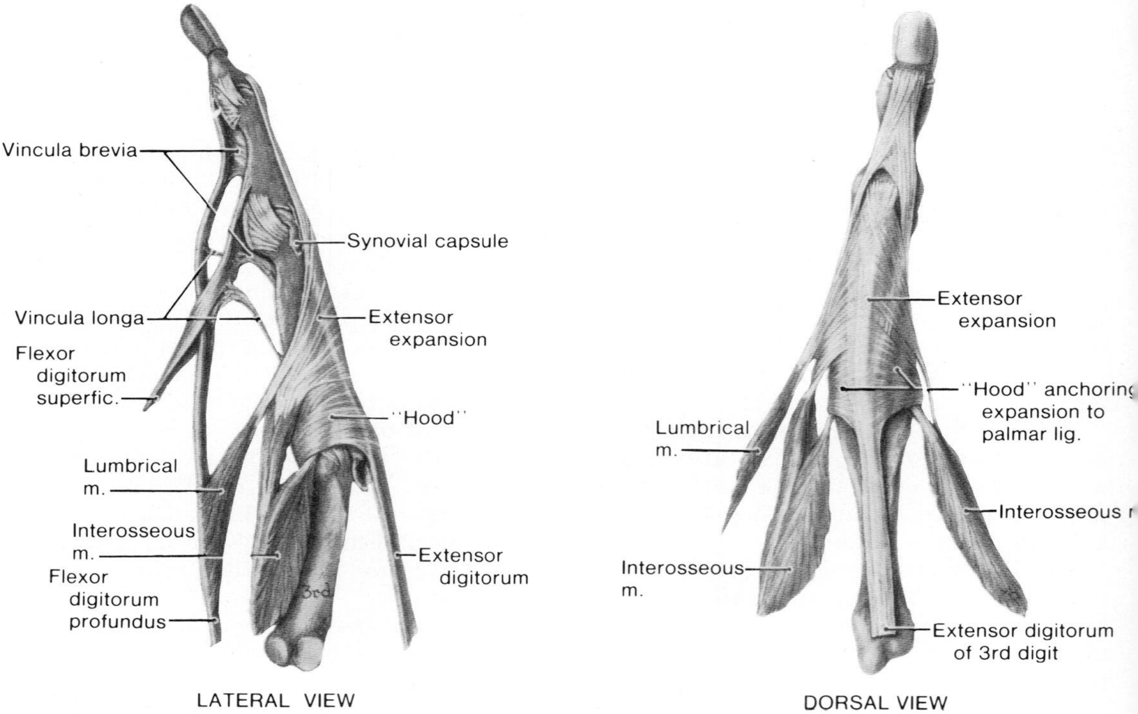

Figure 6-132. Drawings of dissections of the middle finger to show its dorsal extensor expansion. This fascial expansion is a unique structure on the dorsal aspect of each digit through which the extensor tendons, the interosseous muscles, and the lumbrical muscles gain insertion. Observe the interossei inserted in part into the bases of the proximal phalanx and in part into the extensor expansion. Note that the lumbrical muscle is inserted wholly into the radial side of the extensor expansion. Observe the "hood" covering the head of the metacarpal which is moored to the palmar ligament; thus, medial, lateral, and posterior bowstringing of the extensor tendon and extensor expansion is prevented. Note that the extensor expansion extends to the bases of the middle and distal phalanges.

knowledge of the flexor tendons of the fingers. Recall that the tendons of the flexor digitorum superficialis and flexor digitorum profundus pass in a common sheath deep to the flexor retinaculum (Figs. 6-98 and 6-101). They then pass deep to the palmar aponeurosis (Figs. 6-123 and 6-126) and enter the osseofibrous digital tunnels (Figs. 6-125 and 6-127). In Figure 6-133, observe that there are two tendons in each **osseofibrous tunnel**. In order that these tendons can slide freely over each other during movements of the fingers, each tendon is covered with synovial membrane and is contained in a **common synovial sheath** (Figs. 6-96 and 6-98).

Near the base of the proximal phalanx, the tendon of the flexor digitorum superficialis splits and surrounds the tendon of the flexor digitorum profundus (Figs. 6-132 and 6-133). The halves of the tendon of the flexor digitorum superficialis insert into the margins of the shaft of the middle phalanx. The tendon of the flexor digitorum profundus, after passing through the split in the tendon of the flexor digitorum superficialis, passes distally to insert into the base of the distal phalanx (Figs. 6-85, 6-132, and 6-133).

The long tendons are supplied with blood by small blood vessels that pass from the periosteum of the phalanges within special folds of connective tissue called **vincula tendinum** (Fig. 6-96). There are two kinds of vincula (L. fetter or chain): *vincula brevia* and *vincula longa* (Fig. 6-132). These bands connect the tendons of the

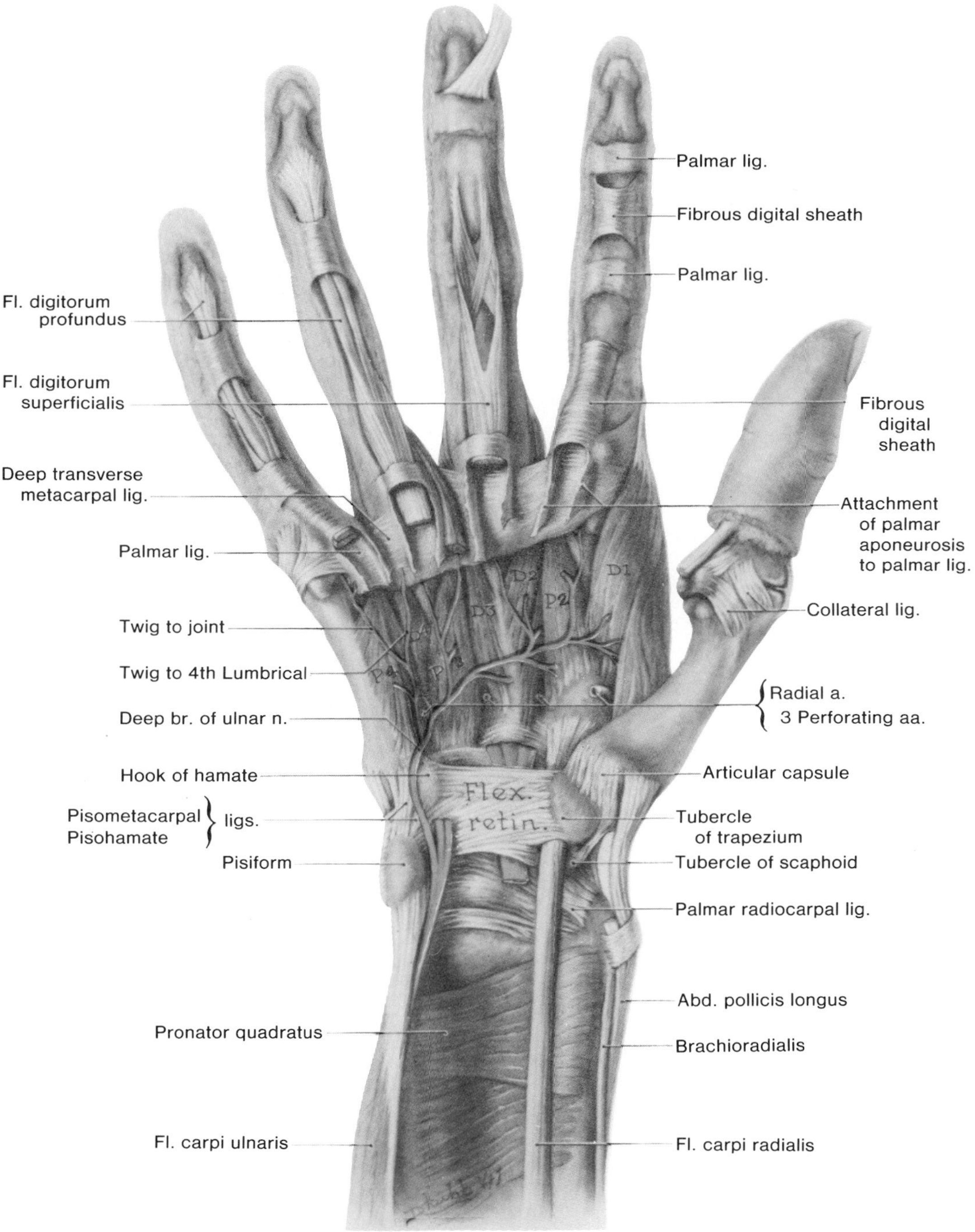

Figure 6-133. Drawing of a deep dissection of the palm, the digits, and the ulnar nerve. The first palmar interosseous muscle, together with the small muscles of the thumb, has been removed. Observe the interosseous muscles located in the spaces between the metacarpals and the deep branch of the ulnar nerve passing medial to the hook of the hamate to be distributed to the hypothenar muscles, all the interossei, two lumbricals, the adductor pollicis, and several joints.

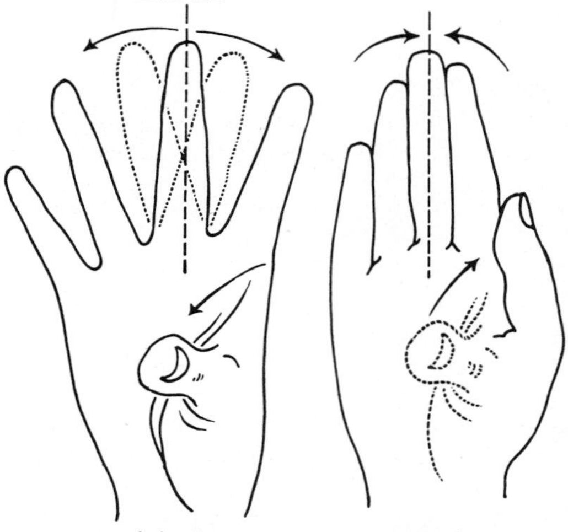

Figure 6-134. Drawings illustrating abduction and adduction of the digits (thumb and fingers). Note that abduction of the fingers is movement away from the axial line and adduction of them is movement toward it. Observe that in abduction of the thumb, it stands anteriorly away from the palm at a right angle and that adduction closes the thumb on the index finger. These and other movements of the thumb are also shown in Figure 6-129.

flexor digitorum superficialis and flexor digitorum profundus to the fibrous digital sheaths in the fingers (Figs. 6-125 and 6-132). The vincula are the remains of primitive mestotendons that connect the tendons to the fibrous digital sheath (Fig. 6-96).

The tendon of the flexor pollicis longus passes to the thumb, deep to the flexor retinaculum, within its own synovial sheath, and passes within the osseofibrous digital tunnel in the thumb. At the head of the metacarpal it runs between two sesamoid bones, one in the combined tendon of the flexor pollicis brevis and the abductor pollicis brevis, and the other in the tendon of the adductor pollicis (Fig. 6-127).

CLINICALLY ORIENTED COMMENTS

The synovial sheaths of the flexor tendons of the hand may become infected (*e.g.*, by entry of a foreign object into a finger). **Tenosynovitis** (inflammation of the tendon and its sheath) occurs, the finger swells, and movement of it is painful. As the tendons of the index, middle, and ring fingers nearly always have separate synovial sheaths (Fig. 6-98), the infection is usually confined to the finger concerned. In neglected infections, however, the proximal ends of these sheaths may rupture and infection may spread to the midpalmar fascial spaces (Fig. 6-126).

As the synovial sheaths of the thumb and little finger are often continuous with the **common flexor synovial sheath**, tenosynovitis in these digits may spread to this sheath (Fig. 6-98). Because there are variations in the connections between the common sheath and the digital sheaths, the degree of spreading of infections from the fingers depends upon whether or not there are connections between them.

In summary, an infection of the synovial sheath of the thumb or little finger may spread to the palm, wrist, and even into the forearm, whereas infections of the other digits are more likely to remain localized.

NERVES OF THE HAND

The median, ulnar, and radial nerves supply the hand. The territories that they supply vary, but in general the ulnar and median nerves supply the palmar surface and the sides of the hand and the digits, and the radial nerve supplies the lateral side of the dorsum of the hand and the digits.

The Median Nerve (Figs. 6-29, 6-93, 6-102, and 6-135 to 6-137). In the distal third of the forearm, the median nerve usually gives off a **palmar cutaneous branch** which pierces the deep fascia and enters the palm of the hand superficial to the flexor retinaculum (Figs. 6-93 and 6-102). It supplies a small area of skin on the palm and adjacent thenar eminence (Fig. 6-29).

The median nerve enters the hand by passing through the carpal tunnel deep to the flexor retinaculum and superficial to the flexor tendons to the index finger (Fig. 6-97). The site of the nerve can be located on the surface in the middle of the anterior aspect of the wrist in the interval between the tendons of the flexor carpi radialis and

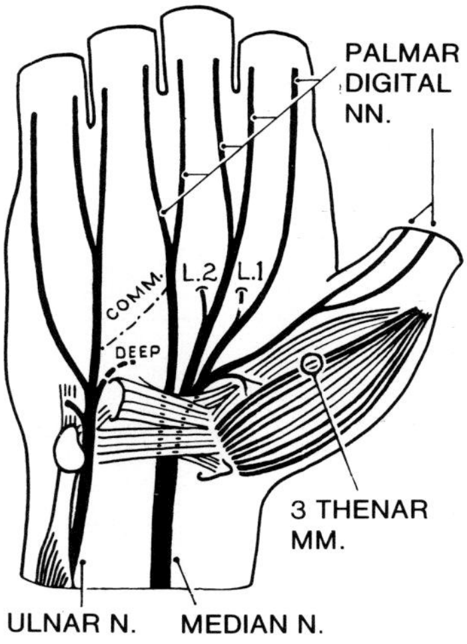

Figure 6-135. Diagram illustrating the nerves supplying the palm of the hand. Note that the median is distributed to five muscles (three thenar and two lumbricals) and provides cutaneous branches to three and one-half digits. The ulnar nerve supplies all other short muscles in the hand and provides cutaneous branches to one and one-half digits. The areas of skin on the palm of the hand supplied by these nerves are illustrated in Figures 6-29 and 6-136.

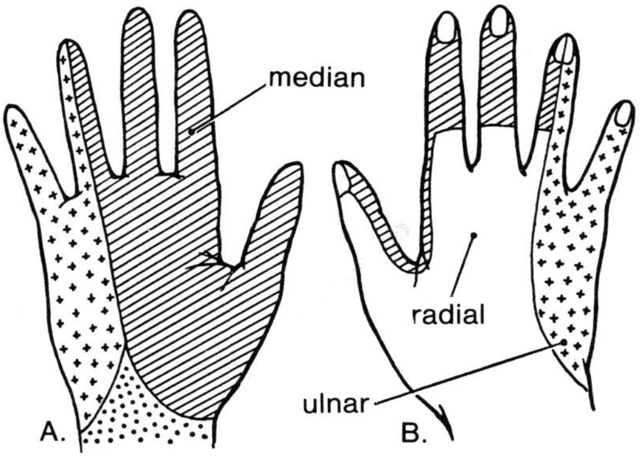

Figure 6-136. Drawings showing the usual distribution of cutaneous nerves to the palm (*A*) and the dorsum (*B*) of the hand. When the radial nerve is injured the sensory deficit is surprisingly small and may be absent. Usually there is a small area of anesthesia on the dorsal surface of the hand between the bases of the first and second metacarpals (Fig. 6-181*A*). The explanation for this is that the musculocutaneous nerve may supply the same area of skin as the radial or replace the branches of the radial to the dorsal surface of the thumb.

flexor digitorum superficialis, usually overlapped by the palmaris longus tendon (Figs. 6-90 to 6-93).

The median nerve supplies a **recurrent branch** to the three thenar muscles (Figs. 6-28, 6-93, and 6-127). This large nerve divides into two terminal branches, a lateral and a medial. The **palmar digital branches** of the median arise from these terminal divisions in the proximal part of the hollow of the hand (Figs. 6-131 and 6-135). They supply the skin of the thumb, index, middle, and lateral half of the ring finger on their palmar surfaces and sides and on the dorsum of the terminal phalanx of these digits (Figs. 6-136 and 6-137). Motor fibers of the digital branches of the median nerve supply the lateral two lumbrical muscles to the second and third digits (Fig. 6-131).

CLINICALLY ORIENTED COMMENTS

Median nerve injury frequently occurs just proximal to the flexor retinaculum, the common site for suicide attempts (Fig. 6-100). The chief effect of lesions here is usually **inability to oppose the thumb** because the median nerve supplies the three thenar muscles and the lateral two lumbricals (Case 6-10). To appreciate the seriousness of this injury, try using a pair of scissors without your thumb. Patients usually are able to initiate opposition of the thumb owing to the action of their intact abductor pollicis longus and adductor pollicis muscles.

As discussed previously, the median nerve may be compressed in the carpal tunnel by pathological conditions affecting the carpal bones or the long flexor tendons (see the **carpal tunnel syndrome**, p. 767).

The Ulnar Nerve (Figs. 6-93, 6-97, 6-127, 6-131, 6-133, and 6-135 to 6-137). The ulnar nerve enters the hand by passing anterior to the flexor retinaculum. As it does so, it divides into two terminal branches, superficial and deep, at the level of the pisiform bone (Fig. 6-133).

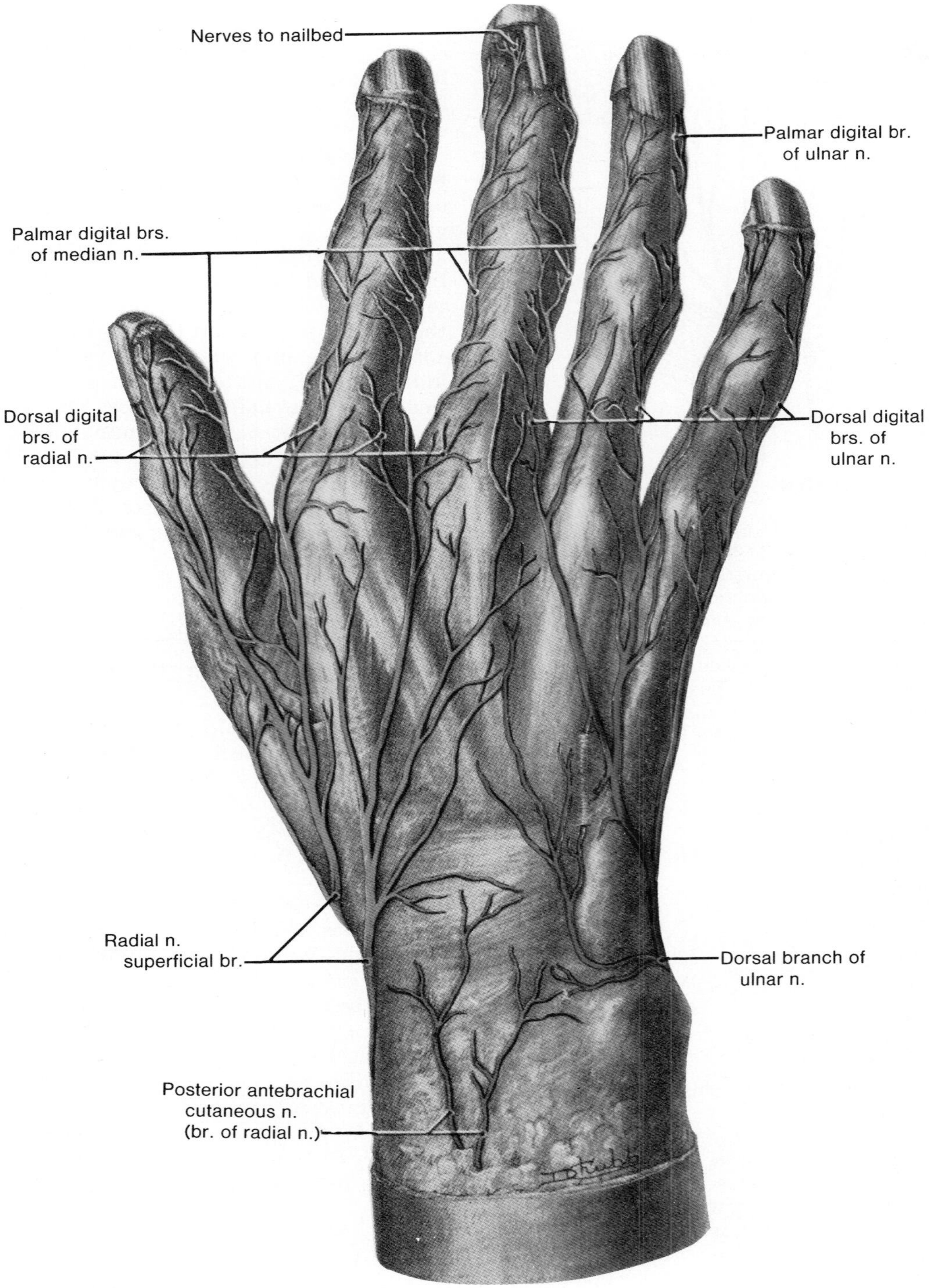

Figure 6-137. Drawing of a superficial dissection of the dorsum of the hand showing its cutaneous nerves. Observe that the radial nerve and the dorsal branch of the ulnar nerve are distributed nearly equally and symmetrically on the dorsum of the hand and digits. The radial nerve supplies the radial half of the dorsum and two and one-half digits; the dorsal branch of the ulnar nerve is distributed similarly on the ulnar half. Note that the palmar digital branches of the median and ulnar nerves alone supply the distal halves of the three middle digits, including the nailbeds. See Figures 6-29 and 6-136 also.

The superficial branch supplies the palmaris brevis muscle and skin on the ulnar side of the hand (Fig. 6-102). It divides into two **palmar digital nerves** which supply the palmar surface and the medial half of the ring finger and motor branches to the medial two lumbrical muscles (Figs. 6-135 to 6-137).

The deep branch passes through the hypothenar muscles (Figs. 6-105 and 6-135) medial to the hook of the hamate (Fig. 6-133) and is distributed to the three hypothenar muscles, all the interossei, the adductor pollicis, and several joints (wrist, intercarpal, carpometacarpal, and intermetacarpal).

CLINICALLY ORIENTED COMMENTS

Ulnar nerve injury is common because this nerve lies superficially in the distal part of the forearm and at the wrist (Fig. 6-97). It may be injured by lacerations at these sites, producing a sensory alteration in the medial part of the hand and in the little and part of the ring fingers (Figs. 6-136). There is also impaired power of adduction (Fig. 6-186) and abduction of the fingers owing to paralysis of the interossei (Fig. 6-133). Some adduction of the fingers may be possible on flexion of the fingers by the long flexor tendons. Adduction of the thumb is lost owing to paralysis of the adductor pollicis, but other movements of the thumb are normal.

The Radial Nerve (Figs. 6-102, 6-103, and 6-137). The terminal branches, superficial and deep, of the radial arise in the cubital fossa (Fig. 6-97). *They supply no muscles in the hand.* The **deep branch** is entirely muscular (supinator and extensor muscles in the forearm) and articular in its distribution. The **superficial branch** is the direct continuation of the radial nerve along the anterolateral side of the forearm and is entirely sensory. It pierces the deep fascia near the dorsum of the wrist to supply skin and fascia over the lateral side of the dorsum of the hand, the dorsum of the thumb, and proximal parts of the lateral two and one-half fingers (Figs. 6-136 and 6-137).

CLINICALLY ORIENTED COMMENTS

Although the radial nerve supplies no muscles in the hand, **radial nerve injury** in the arm and the forearm produces serious disability of the hand. The characteristic handicap in all injuries to this nerve is **inability to extend the wrist.** The hand is flexed at the wrist and lies flaccid, a condition known as **wrist-drop** (Case 6-6 and Fig. 6-181). The fingers are also flexed at the metacarpophalangeal joints. The interphalangeal joints can be extended weakly through the action of the intact lumbrical and interosseous muscles which are supplied by the median and ulnar nerves.

As the radial nerve has only a small area of exclusive cutaneous supply on the hand, the extent of anesthesia is minimal even in serious radial nerve injuries and is usually confined to a small area on the lateral part of the dorsum of the hand (Fig. 6-181*A*).

ARTERIES OF THE HAND

The radial and ulnar arteries provide a good supply of blood to the hand (Fig. 6-117). The **arterial arcades** (L. arcs) formed by anastomoses between them give off branches to the tendons, fascia, and soft tissues of the fingers.

The Radial Artery (Figs. 6-101, 6-108 to 6-110, 6-117, 6-127, and 6-138). The radial artery leaves the forearm by curving around the lateral aspect of the wrist to reach the dorsum of the hand. Just before passing from the anterior to the posterior surface of the wrist, the radial artery gives off a **superficial palmar branch** (Fig. 6-127). This vessel passes through the thenar muscles and runs superficial to the long flexor tendons, where it joins the **superficial palmar arch,** the continuation of the ulnar artery (Figs. 6-127 and 6-138).

As the radial artery curves dorsally over the wrist (Fig. 6-105), it passes deep to the tendons of the abductor pollicis longus and extensor pollicis brevis muscles (Figs. 6-109

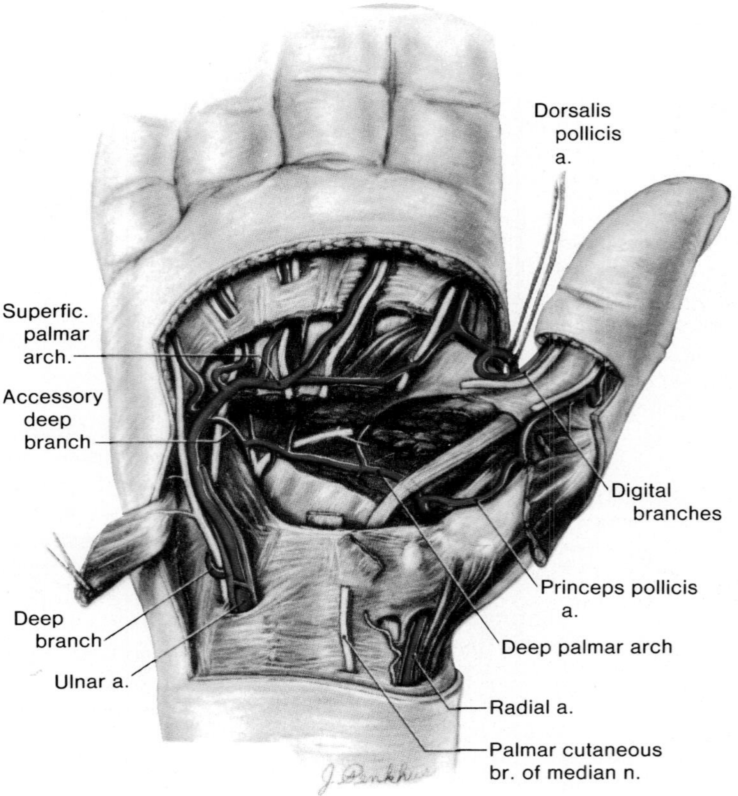

Figure 6-138. Drawing of a deep dissection of the palm of the hand showing the deep branch of the ulnar artery joining the radial artery to form the deep palmar arch.

and 6-110). It then crosses the floor of the anatomical snuff box and enters the palm by passing between the heads of the first dorsal interosseous muscle (Figs. 6-108 and 6-110). The radial artery then gives off the **princeps pollicis** and **radialis indicis arteries** (Figs. 6-105, 6-108 to 6-110, and 6-138), the digital arteries to the thumb and the lateral side of the index finger, respectively.

The radial artery then passes between the two heads of the adductor pollicis muscle and joins the deep branch of the ulnar artery to form the **deep palmar arch** (Figs. 6-105, 6-138, and 6-139). It is located between the long flexor tendons and the metacarpal bones.

The Ulnar Artery (Figs. 6-95, 6-97, 6-105, 6-127, and 6-138). The ulnar artery enters the palm on the radial side of the ulnar nerve, superficial to the flexor retinaculum of the wrist. In so doing, it passes lateral to the pisiform bone and then gives off a deep palmar branch before continuing across the palm as the superficial palmar arch (Figs. 6-97 and 6-138).

The deep palmar branch of the ulnar artery passes through the hypothenar muscles and anastomoses with the radial artery, thereby completing the **deep palmar arch** (Figs. 6-105 and 6-138). **The superficial branch** of the ulnar artery passes laterally across the palm between the long flexor tendons and the palmar aponeurosis to form the **superficial palmar arch** (Figs. 6-127 and 6-138). It anastomoses with the superficial palmar branch of the radial artery.

The Palmar Arterial Arches (Figs. 6-105, 6-127, and 6-138). A clear understand-

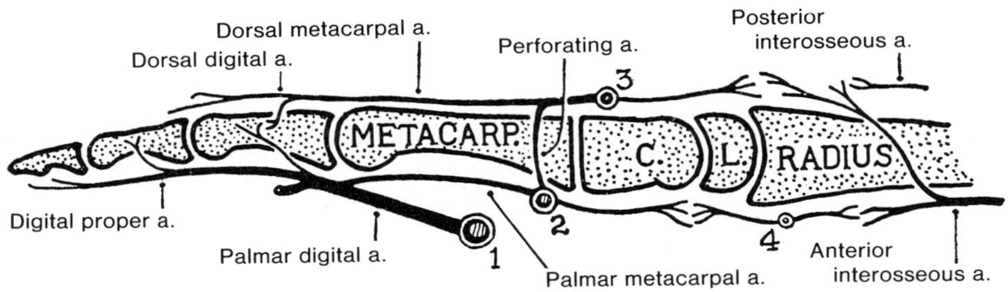

Figure 6-139. Drawing of the arteries of the hand showing the four transversely placed arterial arches numbered in order of size. *1*, the superficial palmar arch lying deep to the palmar aponeurosis (Fig. 6-138); *2*, the deep palmar arch (Fig. 6-105); *3*, the dorsal carpal arch (Fig. 6-117); *4*, the palmar carpal arch.

ing of these arches is important because of the frequency of lacerations of arteries in the hand.

The Superficial Palmar Arch (Figs. 6-127 and 6-138). This arterial arch is **formed mainly by the ulnar artery** and is located distal to the deep palmar arch. It is convex toward the fingers and the middle of its convexity lies deep to the center of the proximal transverse crease of the palm (Fig. 6-121). The superficial palmar arch gives rise to four **palmar digital arteries** which anastomose with the palmar metacarpal arteries and continue distally to supply the digits (Figs. 6-105, 6-123, 6-127, 6-138, and 6-139).

The Deep Palmar Arch (Figs. 6-138 and 6-139). This arterial arch is formed by the radial artery and the deep palmar branch of the ulnar artery, but the **radial artery forms the main part.** The deep arch lies across the metacarpal bones, just distal to their bases; thus, it is about a fingerbreadth closer to the wrist than the superficial palmar arch. The convexity of the deep arch is also directed toward the fingers.

The deep palmar arch gives rise to three **palmar metacarpal arteries,** three **perforating arteries,** and several **recurrent branches** (Figs. 6-105, 6-138, and 6-139).

Surface Anatomy of the Palmar Arches. As the names indicate, the **deep palmar arch** lies deeper in the palm than the superficial palmar arch. To visualize its location, make a cup in your palm. The summit of the deep arch lies deep to the proximal rim of the cup which is just distal to the bases of the metacarpals (Fig. 6-122).

The **superficial palmar arch,** the larger of the two, lies deep to the center of the cup in your palm, about a fingerbreadth distal to the convexity of the deep palmar arch (Fig. 6-138). It lies deep to the palmar aponeurosis (Fig. 6-127) at the level of the distal surface of the extended thumb.

CLINICALLY ORIENTED COMMENTS

Because of the number of arteries in the hand, bleeding is usually profuse when it is lacerated. Usually both ends of the bleeding artery must be tied in order to stop the hemorrhage because there are four transversely placed arterial arches that communicate with each other (Fig. 6-139).

In **lacerations of the arterial arches,** it is useless to ligate only one of the forearm arteries because of their numerous communications. Often simultaneous clamping of the ulnar and radial arteries proximal to the wrist fails to stop all bleeding. To obtain a **bloodless operating field** in the hand for treating complicated injuries, it is necessary to compress the brachial artery and its branches proximal to the elbow (*e.g.,* using a pneumatic tourniquet). This prevents blood from reaching the arteries of the forearm and hand through the anastomoses around the elbow (Fig. 6-74).

VEINS OF THE HAND

The superficial and deep palmar arterial arches are accompanied by **venae comi-**

tantes, known as the superficial and deep venous arches, respectively.

The **dorsal digital veins** drain into three **dorsal metacarpal veins** which unite to form a **dorsal venous network** located superficial to the metacarpus (Fig. 6-140). This network is prolonged proximally as the **cephalic vein,** which winds upward from this network around the radial border of the forearm to its anterior surface (Figs. 6-76 and 6-77).

JOINTS OF THE UPPER LIMB

As the **pectoral girdle** (clavicle and scapula) connects the upper limb to the trunk, its articulations are included with those of the upper limb.

THE STERNOCLAVICULAR JOINT

This articulation is a **saddle type of synovial joint.** It is the only bony articulation between the upper limb and the trunk (Fig. 6-142). The function of the clavicle is to hold the upper limb away from the trunk, *i.e.,* it acts as a strut for holding the shoulder out from the chest to give the arm maximum freedom of motion.

CLINICALLY ORIENTED COMMENTS

Uncommonly the clavicle is incomplete or absent in some people, a normal occurrence in many animals (*e.g.,* the dog). This human congenital abnormality is often associated with delayed ossification of the skull. The combined condition, known as **cleidocranial dysostosis,** is characterized by drooping and excessive mobility of the shoulders (Fig. 6-142). Sometimes only the middle of the clavicle is absent and the two ends are joined by fibrous bands. In some cases the muscles that attach to the clavicle are also defective.

The Articular Surfaces (Figs. 6-141 and 6-143). The enlarged medial end of the clavicle articulates in a shallow socket formed by the superolateral part of the manubrium sterni and the medial part of the first costal cartilage (cartilage of first rib). Both articular surfaces are covered with fibrocartilage, but the layer on the clavicle is thicker than that on the sternum.

The sternoclavicular joint can be readily palpated because the medial end of the clavicle lies above the manubrium sterni (Figs. 6-2, 6-25, and 6-141). Put your thumb in the **jugular notch** of the sternum and your index and middle fingers over the medial end of the clavicle. Determine its free movement by elevating and depressing your shoulder and then by protracting and retracting it.

Movements of the Joint. Despite the saddle-like form of its articular surfaces, the sternoclavicular joint moves in many directions like a ball and socket joint. Verify this by elevating and depressing your shoulder, moving it forward and backward, and by rotating your humerus. Elevate your arm as far as possible and verify by palpation that your clavicle is raised to about a 60° angle from its usual position (Fig. 6-143).

The Articular Disc (Fig. 6-144). This is a strong, thick, nearly circular, fibrocartilaginous disc inside the joint which divides it into two synovial cavities. It is attached superiorly to the medial end of the clavicle and inferiorly to the sternum and first costal cartilage at their junction. The articular disc is continuous with the anterior and posterior sternoclavicular ligaments and acts like a ligament in preventing medial displacement of the clavicle. It is also an important shock absorber of forces transmitted along the length of the clavicle.

The Articular Capsule (Fig. 6-144). *The fibrous capsule* surrounds the whole joint, including the epiphysis at the medial end of the clavicle. Although thin inferiorly, other parts of the capsule are strong because they are reinforced in front and behind by the **anterior** and **posterior sternoclavicular ligaments,** respectively, and superiorly by an **interclavicular ligament.** The interclavicular ligament, extending across the jugular notch of the sternum, may be homologous with the wishbone of chickens. The sternoclavicular and

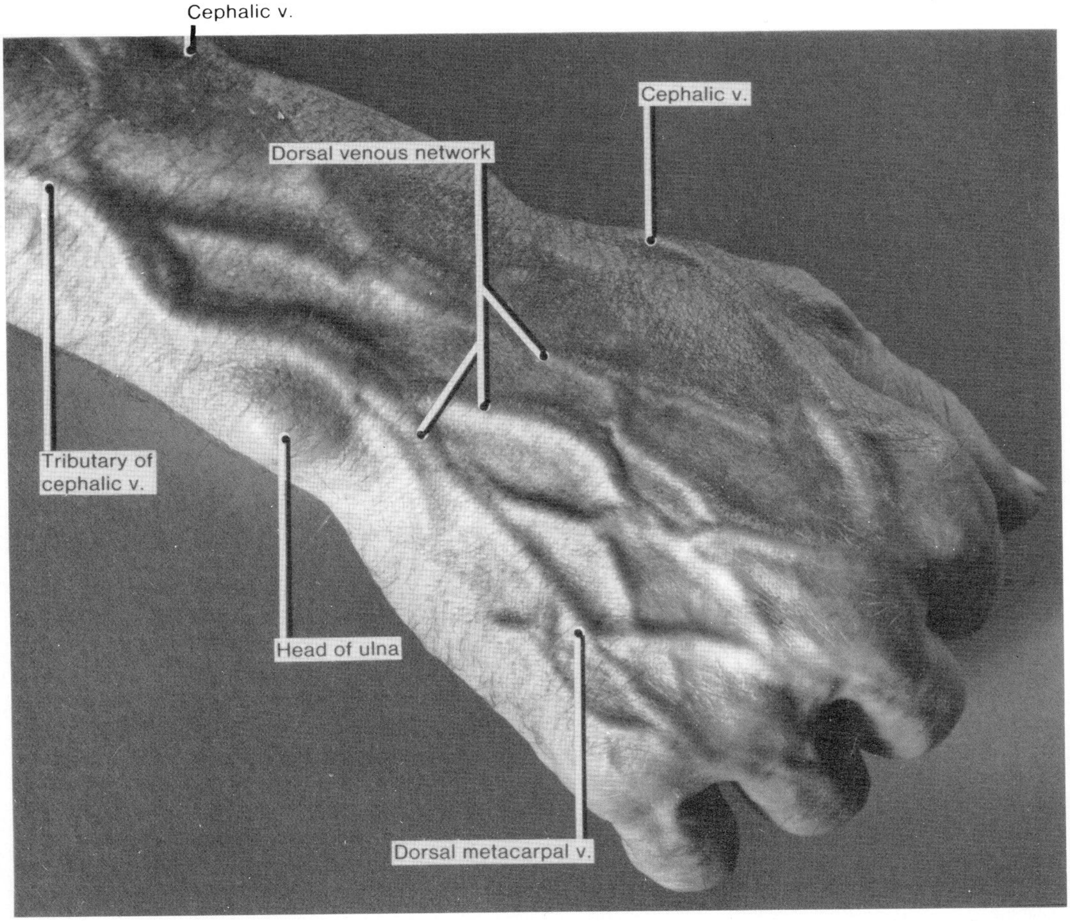

Figure 6-140. Photograph of the dorsum of the hand and distal end of the forearm of a 46-year-old man showing the superficial veins and the head of the ulna. Observe that the cephalic vein winds upward from the dorsal venous network around the radial border of the forearm (Fig. 6-116), receiving tributaries from both surfaces. *Understand that the superficial venous network and its drainage are variable.*

interclavicular ligaments are intrinsic ligaments (*i.e.,* they are thickenings of the fibrous capsule).

The synovial capsule lines the fibrous capsule. Because the articular disc divides the joint into two cavities (Fig. 6-143), there are two synovial membranes. The lateral one reflects from the articular margin of the medial end of the clavicle to the margins of the disc. The medial one lines the capsule between its sternal attachments and the disc.

The Costoclavicular Ligament (Figs. 6-25 and 6-144). This extrinsic ligament ascends from the first costal cartilage to the upper margin of the medial end of the clavicle. This strong ligament, reinforcing the joint laterally, limits elevation of the clavicle.

Stability of the Joint. Because the bony surfaces involved are rather incongruent and the surrounding muscles offer little support, the sternoclavicular joint depends on its ligaments and articular disc for stability. A blow on the side of the shoulder or a fall on the outstretched upper limb

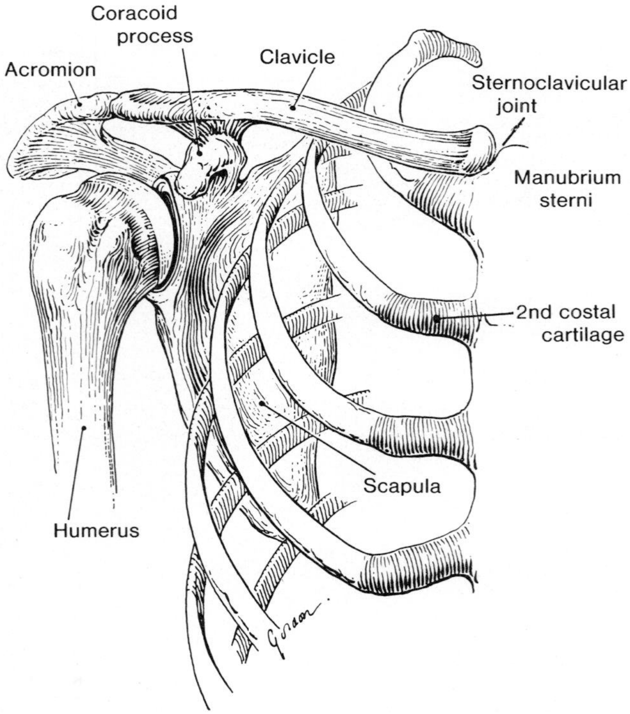

Figure 6-141. Drawing of the bones of the right shoulder region. Note that the clavicle is the only bone uniting the upper limb to the axial skeleton and that the superior part of the medial end of the clavical lies above the manubrium sterni. For the surface anatomy of this region, see Figure 6-2.

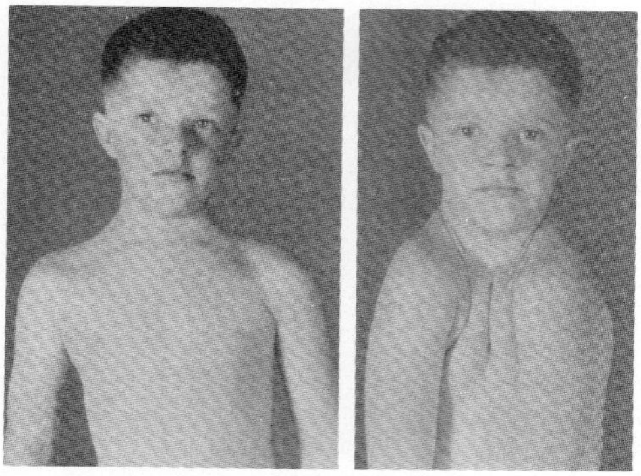

Figure 6-142. Photographs of an 8-year-old boy with a congenital abnormality known as *cleidocranial dysostosis.* It is characterized by absence or rudimentary development of the clavicles and an abnormal shape of the skull. Owing to the congenital absence of clavicles, this boy has excessive mobility of the shoulders and can almost bring them together; however, there is no significant disability and no treatment was necessary.

imparts its force to the clavicle, which transmits it to the sternum. It is the strong articular disc which is largely responsible for preventing medial displacement of the clavicle (*i.e.,* it prevents the medial end of the clavicle from being pushed out of its socket and superior to the manubrium).

When the clavicle is depressed (*e.g.,* when carrying a heavy object in the hand), there is a tendency for its medial end to be forced out of its socket. This is resisted by the strong sternoclavicular ligaments and the articular disc (Fig. 6-144).

Excessive protraction and elevation of the clavicle are also restrained by the sternoclavicular ligaments and probably by the subclavius muscle (Fig. 6-23).

Blood Supply (Fig. 6-46). The articular arteries are branches of the internal thoracic and suprascapular arteries.

Nerve Supply. The articular nerves are branches of the medial supraclavicular nerve and the nerve to the subclavius.

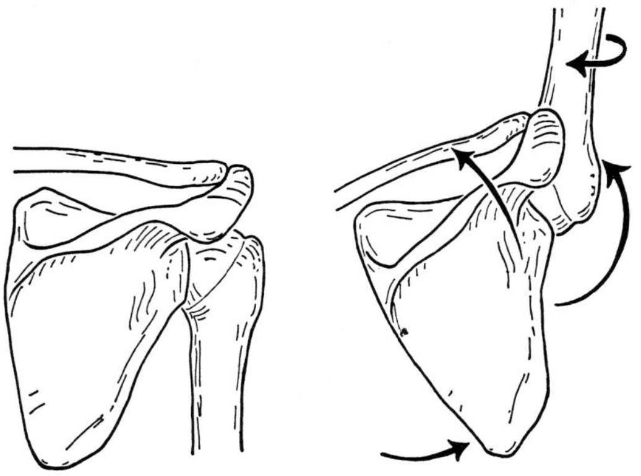

Figure 6-143. Drawing of the pectoral girdle and humerus showing that as the arm is elevated the clavicle rotates and is raised to about a 60° angle from its anatomical position. In this posterior view note that the bones of the pectoral girdle (clavicle and scapula) move with the arm and that the humerus rotates laterally as it is elevated.

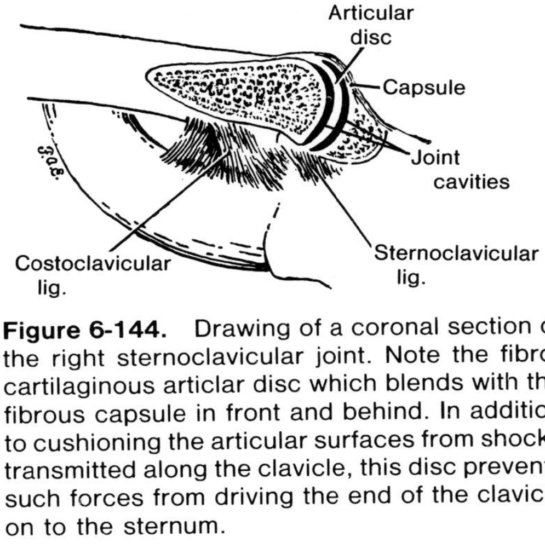

Figure 6-144. Drawing of a coronal section of the right sternoclavicular joint. Note the fibrocartilaginous articlar disc which blends with the fibrous capsule in front and behind. In addition to cushioning the articular surfaces from shocks transmitted along the clavicle, this disc prevents such forces from driving the end of the clavicle on to the sternum.

CLINICALLY ORIENTED COMMENTS

The rarity of dislocation of the sternoclavicular joint indicates its strength, which depends upon its ligaments and articular disc. Even when a hole is worn out of the central part of the disc with old age, the joint rarely dislocates.

When a blow is received to the acromion of the scapula or when a force is transmitted from the upper limb during a fall on the outstretched hand, the clavicle may break near the junction of its middle and lateral thirds (Fig. 6-65), but dislocation of the sternoclavicular joint rarely occurs.

THE ACROMIOCLAVICULAR JOINT

This articulation is a **plane type of synovial joint** between the lateral end of the clavicle and the medial border of the acromion of the scapula. It is located 2 to 3 cm medial to the acromion, which often forms a visible prominence known as the point of the shoulder (Fig. 6-2).

The Articular Surfaces (Figs. 6-145 to 6-147 and 6-153). The small oval articular facet on the lateral end of the clavicle, facing inferolaterally, articulates with a similar facet on the anterior part of the medial surface of the outer end of the acromion, facing superomedially. Both articular surfaces are covered with fibrocartilage; this is said to be an exception to the rule that the articulating surfaces of synovial joints are covered by hyaline cartilage.

Movements of the Joint (Fig. 6-143). The acromioclavicular joint allows the ac-

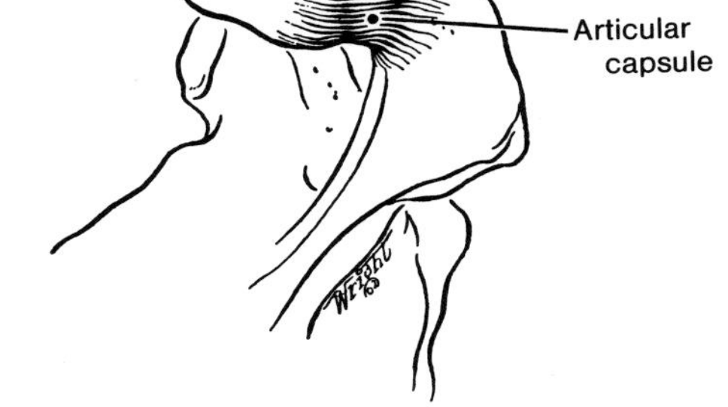

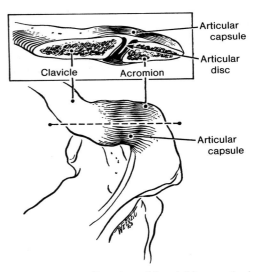

Figure 6-145. Drawing of the right acromioclavicular joint from above and unopened. *Inset above* is a coronal section of the joint showing its wedge-shaped articular disc.

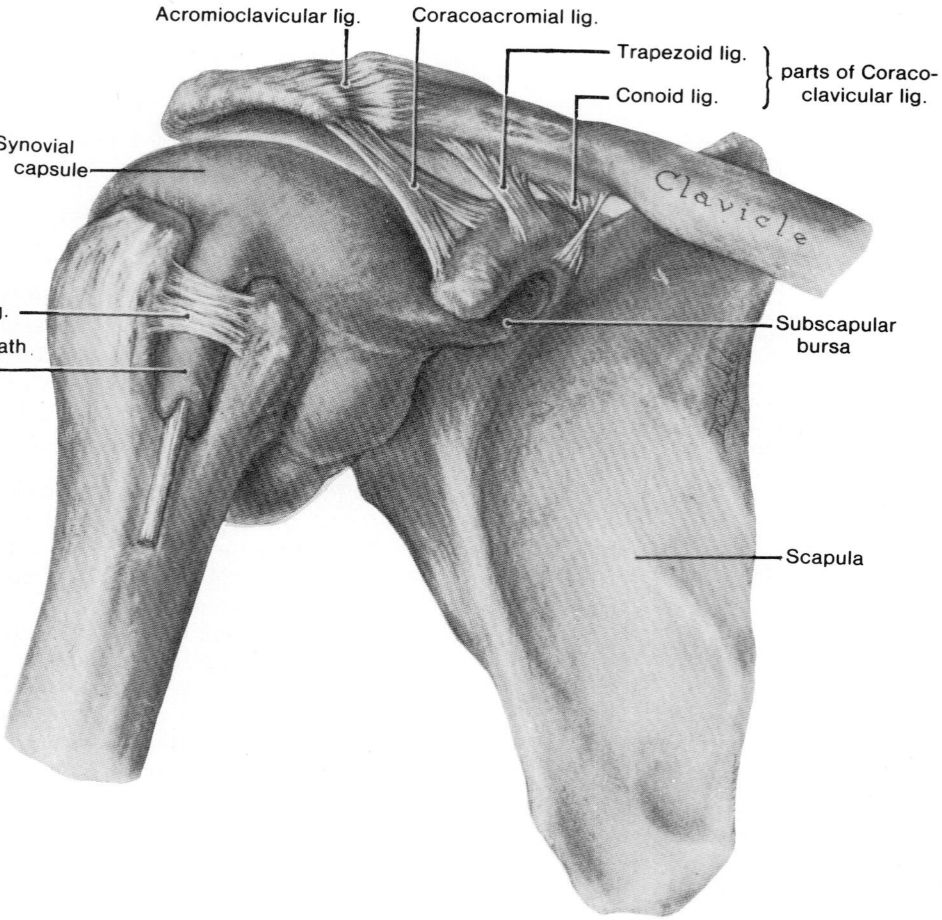

Figure 6-146. Drawing of the synovial capsule of the shoulder joint and of the ligaments at the lateral end of the clavicle. Observe that the capsule cannot extend on to the lesser and greater tubercles of the humerus because the four short muscles (subscapularis, supraspinatus, infraspinatus, and teres minor) are inserted there, but it can and does extend inferiorly on to the surgical neck of the humerus. Note that the synovial capsule has two prolongations: (1) where it forms a synovial sheath for the tendon of the long head of the biceps in its osseofibrous tunnel, and (2) below the coracoid process where it forms a bursa between the subscapularis tendon and the margin of the glenoid cavity. Observe that the conoid and trapezoid ligaments are directed so that the clavicle holds the scapula laterally.

romion, and thus the scapula, to rotate on the clavicle and to glide forward and backward. When the arm is elevated, the clavicle rotates on the acromion. These movements are associated with those at the sternoclavicular joint.

The Articular Disc (Fig. 6-145). A wedge-shaped, incomplete, fibrocartilaginous articular disc projects into the joint from the superior part of the capsule. This disc partially divides the joint cavity into two parts.

The Articular Capsule (Fig. 6-145). *The fibrous capsule* encloses the joint and is attached to the margins of its articular surfaces. The capsule is strengthened superiorly by the **acromioclavicular ligament** (Fig. 6-146). This quadrilateral intrinsic ligament extends from the superior part of the lateral end of the clavicle to the

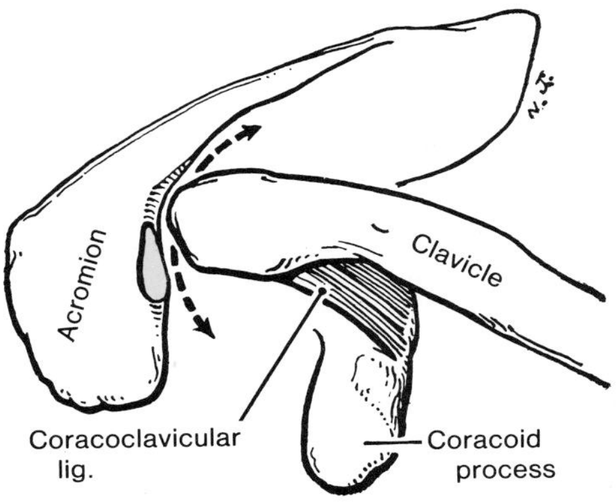

Fiugre 6-147. Drawing showing the relationship of the clavicle to the acromion and coracoid process of the scapula. Observe the powerful coracoclavicular ligament which binds the acromial end of the clavicle to the coracoid process. This ligament helps to prevent dislocation of the acromial end of the clavicle. So long as the coracoclavicular ligament is intact, the acromion cannot be driven under the clavicle. This ligament does not, however, prevent protraction and retraction of the acromion.

superior surface of the acromion. Its fibers interlace with the aponeuroses of the trapezius and deltoid muscles.

The synovial capsule lines the inner surface of the fibrous capsule.

The Coracoclavicular Ligament (Figs. 6-146 and 6-147). This powerful ligament anchors the lateral part of the clavicle to the coracoid process of the scapula. It is the strongest of the ligaments that hold the clavicle to the scapula. It consists of two parts, *conoid* and *trapezoid ligaments,* which are directed in such a way that they enable the clavicle to hold the scapula and the upper limb laterally.

Stability of the Joint (Figs. 6-145 and 6-146). The coracoclavicular ligament, an extrinsic ligament of the acromioclavicular joint, is principally responsible for providing stability to the articulation. Owing to the flatness and orientation of the articular surfaces, dislocation of the joint occurs when the coracoclavicular ligament ruptures.

Blood Supply (Figs. 6-41 and 6-46). The articular arteries are branches of the suprascapular and thoracoacromial arteries.

Nerve Supply. The articular nerves are branches of the lateral supraclavicular, pectoral, and axillary nerves.

CLINICALLY ORIENTED COMMENTS

In contact sports such as football and hockey, it is not uncommon for dislocation of the acromioclavicular joint to occur as the result of a fall on the shoulder or from being "driven into the boards" (Case 6-3). This injury, often inaccurately called a "**shoulder separation**," is serious when both the acromioclavicular and coracoclavicular ligaments are torn. When the coracoclavicular ligament ruptures, the shoulder falls away from the clavicle owing to the weight of the upper limb. The fibrous capsule of the acromioclavicular joint also ruptures and the acromion then passes inferior to the lateral end of the clavicle which produces an obvious subcutaneous prominence.

THE SHOULDER JOINT

The shoulder joint or glenohumeral (scapulohumeral) articulation is a **ball and socket type of synovial joint** which permits a wide range of movement.

The Articular Surfaces (Figs. 6-148 and 6-149). The roughly hemispherical **head of the humerus** (the ball) articulates with the shallow **glenoid cavity** (the socket) of the scapula. Both articular surfaces (glenoid cavity and head of humerus) are covered with a layer of hyaline cartilage.

The shallow glenoid cavity accepts little more than a third of the large humeral head (Fig. 6-153), but it is deepened slightly and enlarged by a fibrocartilaginous rim (Fig. 6-149), called the **glenoidal (glenoid) labrum** (L. lip). It is triangular in cross-section with a thin, sharp, free margin and a base that is attached to the glenoid cavity. The superior portion of the glenoidal labrum blends with the tendon of the long head of the biceps brachii muscle (Fig. 6-149).

Movements of the Joint. *The shoulder joint has more freedom of movement than*

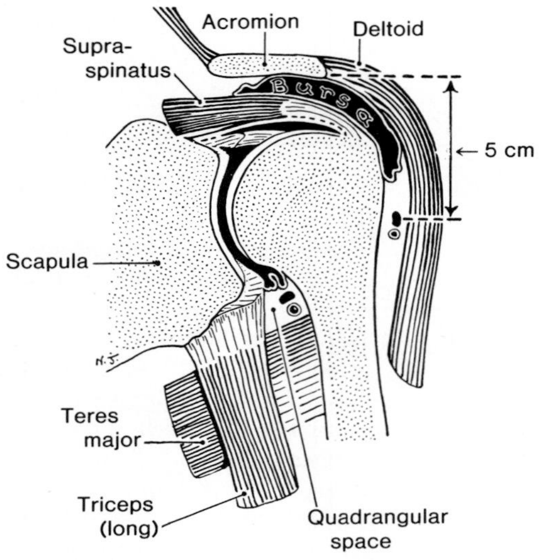

Figure 6-148. Drawing of a coronal section of the shoulder region. Observe that the shoulder joint is a ball-and-socket type of synovial joint. The ball is the head of the humerus and the socket is the glenoid cavity of the scapula.

any other joint in the body owing to the laxity of its articular capsule and the large size of the humeral head compared with the small size of the glenoid cavity. It is a **multiaxial joint** that allows movements around three axes, permitting flexion-extension, abduction-adduction, circumduction, and rotation (medial or lateral). In Figure 6-150, note that flexion and extension are parallel to the median plane of the body. Although not illustrated, understand that abduction and adduction are at right angles to the median plane.

When the upper limb is elevated 40 to 60°, the humerus rotates laterally, carrying its greater tuberosity posterior to the acromion. This prevents this bony prominence from striking the outer edge of the acromion; in addition, the scapula rotates so that the glenoid cavity faces superiorly (Fig. 6-143). As a result of these movements of the shoulder joint, involving the humerus and the scapula, the upper limb can be elevated to a fully vertical position (180°).

The Articular Capsule (Figs. 6-146, 6-148, 6-151, and 6-152). *The fibrous capsule* enclosing the shoulder joint is thin and loose; thus, it allows a wide range of movement. It is attached to the scapula just proximal to the margin of the glenoid cavity and to the anatomical neck of the humerus. Inferiorly its attachment passes along the surgical neck (Fig. 6-67*A*).

The inferior part of the capsule, its weakest area, is lax and lies in folds when the arm is adducted (Fig. 6-148), but it becomes taut when the arm is abducted. There are two apertures (openings) in the articular capsule of the shoulder joint. One opening between the tubercles of the humerus is for passage of the tendon of the long head of the biceps brachii muscle while it is in the intertubercular sulcus in the humerus (Fig. 6-151). The other opening in the articular capsule is situated anteriorly, below the coracoid process. It allows communication between the **subscapular bursa** and the synovial cavity of the joint (Figs. 6-45, 6-146, and 6-151).

The synovial capsule lines the fibrous capsule and is reflected from it on to the glenoidal labrum and the neck of the humerus as far as the articular margin of the head. The synovial capsule forms a tubular sheath for the tendon of the long head of the biceps brachii (Fig. 6-146), where it passes into the joint cavity and lies in the intertubercular sulcus, extending as far as the surgical neck of the humerus.

Intrinsic Ligaments of the Capsule (Figs. 6-146, 6-149, 6-151, and 6-152). These thickenings of the fibrous capsule strengthen the shoulder joint.

The glenohumeral ligaments (Fig. 6-152) are three thickenings (strengthening bands) of the anterior part of the fibrous capsule. The superior, middle, and inferior glenohumeral ligaments run from the supraglenoid tubercle of the scapula to the lesser tuberosity and the anatomical neck of the humerus. These ligaments are frequently indistinct or absent.

The transverse humeral ligament (Fig. 6-146) is a special band of transverse fibers of the fibrous capsule that is attached to the greater and lesser tubercles of the humerus and forms a bridge over the superior end of the intertubercular sulcus. It holds the tendon of the long head of the biceps in this groove as it emerges from the capsule of the shoulder joint.

The coracohumeral ligament (Fig. 6-149) is continuous posteriorly with the fibrous capsule and is partly separated from it. This sturdy ligament passes from the lateral side of the base of the coracoid process of the scapula to the anatomical neck of the humerus adjacent to the greater tubercle. It strengthens the fibrous capsule, particularly when the arm is adducted, at which time the capsule and this ligament are under tension.

Accessory Ligament of the Shoulder Joint and the Coracoacromial Arch. There is one scapular ligament, the **coracoacromial ligament,** that affords protection to the shoulder joint.

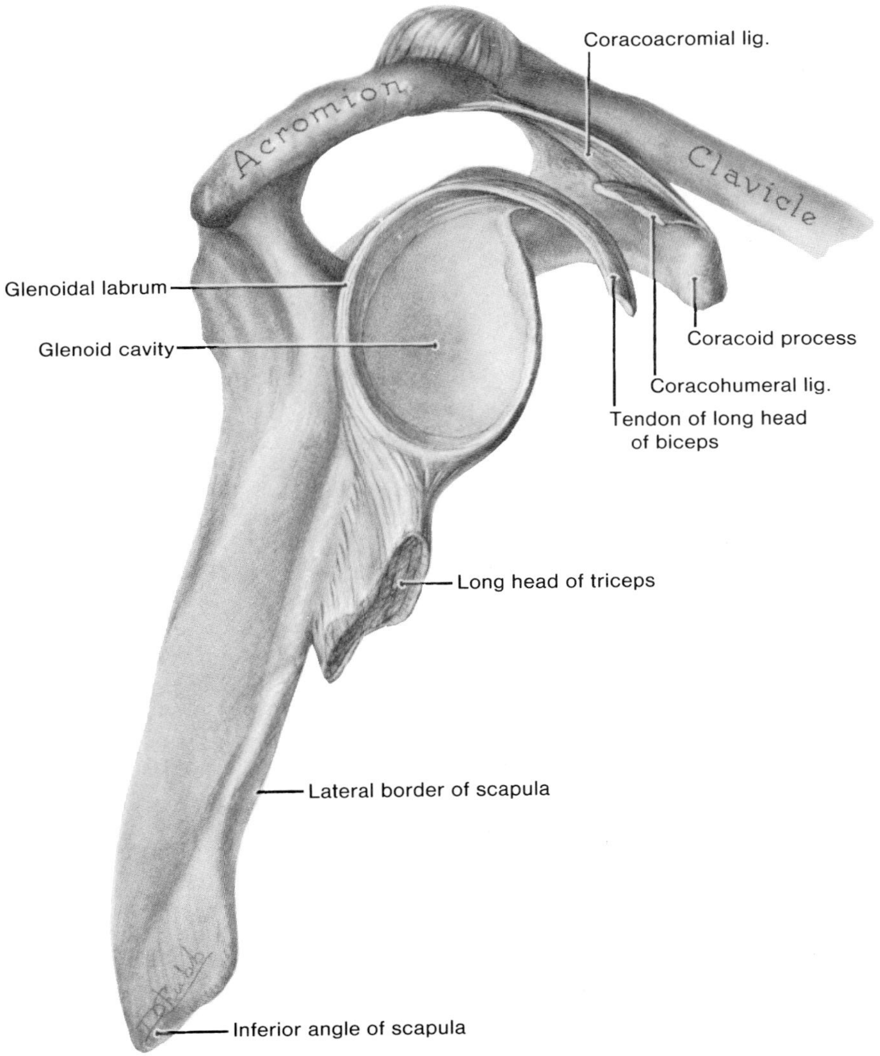

Figure 6-149. Drawing of the clavicle and scapula (pectoral girdle) showing a lateral view of the glenoid cavity. Observe that the glenoid cavity is deepened by the *glenoidal labrum*, a dense fibrocartilaginous lip (L. labrum) that is attached to the rim of the glenoid cavity. Note that the cavity is overhung by the resilient *coracoacromial arch* formed by the coracoid process, the coracoacromial ligament, and the acromion. This arch prevents upward displacement of the head of the humerus.

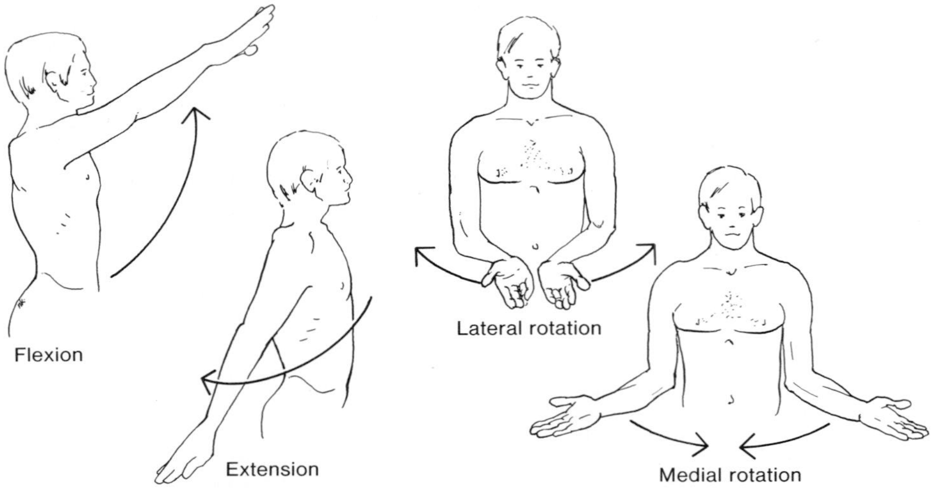

Figure 6-150. Drawings illustrating some movements at the shoulder joint. The joint also permits abduction-adduction and circumduction. As the shoulder joint is the ball-and-socket type of synovial joint, movement is permitted in every direction.

The Coracoacromial Arch (Figs. 6-61 and 6-149). The coracoid process, the coracoacromial ligament, and the acromion form a protective coracoacromial arch for the shoulder joint. When force is transmitted upward along the humerus (*e.g.,* when standing at a desk and partly supporting your body with your outstretched upper limbs), the head of the humerus is pressed against this arch, which prevents upward displacement of the head of the humerus from the glenoid cavity. The **supraspinatous muscle** passes under the coracoacromial arch and lies between the deltoid muscle and the articular capsule of the shoulder joint (Fig. 6-148). The supraspinatous tendon, passing between the arch and the humerus, is separated from the arch by the **subacromial bursa** (Figs. 6-61 and 6-148).

The Coracoacromial Ligament (Figs. 6-61, 6-146, and 6-149). This strong, triangular ligament, with the coracoid and the acromion of the scapula, forms a protective shelf over the shoulder joint. Its base is attached to the lateral border of the coracoid process and its apex is inserted into the tip of the acromion (Fig. 6-146). Superiorly the coracoacromial ligament is covered by the deltoid muscle (Fig. 6-60); inferiorly is the subacromial bursa (Fig. 6-61).

Stability of the Joint. The free movement of the shoulder joint is attained at the expense of stability. The shallowness of the glenoid cavity and the laxity of the fibrous capsule result in a considerable loss of stability. The strength of the joint results mainly from the muscles which surround it, particularly the **rotator cuff muscles** (supraspinatus, infraspinatus, teres minor, and subscapularis). They are attached near the articular areas and are closely related to the fibrous capsule of the joint (Fig. 6-58).

Although these muscles have separate functions, they work as a group in holding the head of the humerus in the glenoid cavity (Figs. 6-58 and 6-60). They give stability to the shoulder joint in several positions, especially when the arm is abducted. The supraspinatus muscle and the coracoacromial arch guard the shoulder joint above (Figs. 6-60, 6-149, and 6-151); the infraspinatus and teres minor muscles stabilize the shoulder joint below, and the subscapularis protects it in front (Figs. 6-32 and 6-63). In Figure 6-151, observe that no tendons support the joint inferiorly; consequently, this is where it is likely to dislocate (Fig. 6-155).

Bursae About the Shoulder Joint (Figs. 6-61, 6-148, and 6-151). There are several bursae (flattened connective tissue sacs containing capillary films of synovial fluid) in the vicinity of the shoulder joint where tendons rub against bone, ligaments, or other tendons, and where skin moves over a bony prominence.

The Subscapular Bursa (Figs. 6-45, 6-146, and 6-151). This large bursa is between the tendon of the subscapularis muscle and the neck of the scapula. It protects this tendon where it passes under the root of the coracoid process and over the neck of the scapula. It usually communicates with the cavity of the shoulder joint through an opening in its fibrous capsule; thus, it is really an extension of the joint cavity.

The Subacromial Bursa (Figs. 6-61, 6-148, and 6-151). This large bursa is described with the supraspinatus muscle (p. 723). It lies between the deltoid muscle and the supraspinatus tendon and the fibrous

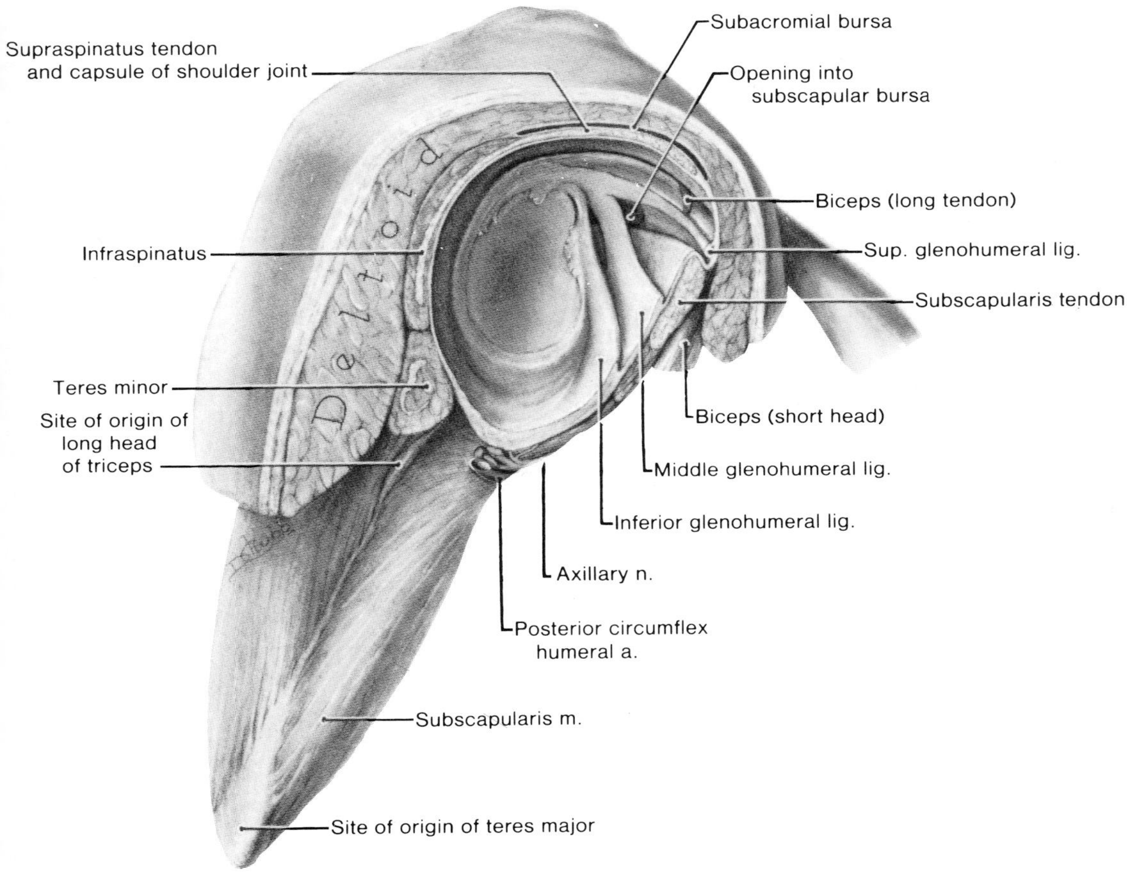

Figure 6-151. Drawing of a dissection of the right glenoid cavity as viewed from the anterolateral aspect. Observe the articular capsule of the joint, thickened in front by the three glenohumeral ligaments which converge from the humerus to be attached with the long tendon of the biceps brachii muscle to the supraglenoid tubercle of the scapula. Note the four short *rotator cuff muscles* (teres minor, infraspinatus, supraspinatus, and subscapularis) crossing the joint and blending with the capsule. Their prime function is to hold the head of the humerus in the glenoid cavity of the scapula. Observe the subacromial bursa between the acromion and the deltoid muscle above and the tendon of the supraspinatus muscle below. For a superolateral view of the large subacromial bursa, see Figure 6-61. Note the subscapularis bursa opening above and below the middle glenohumeral ligament.

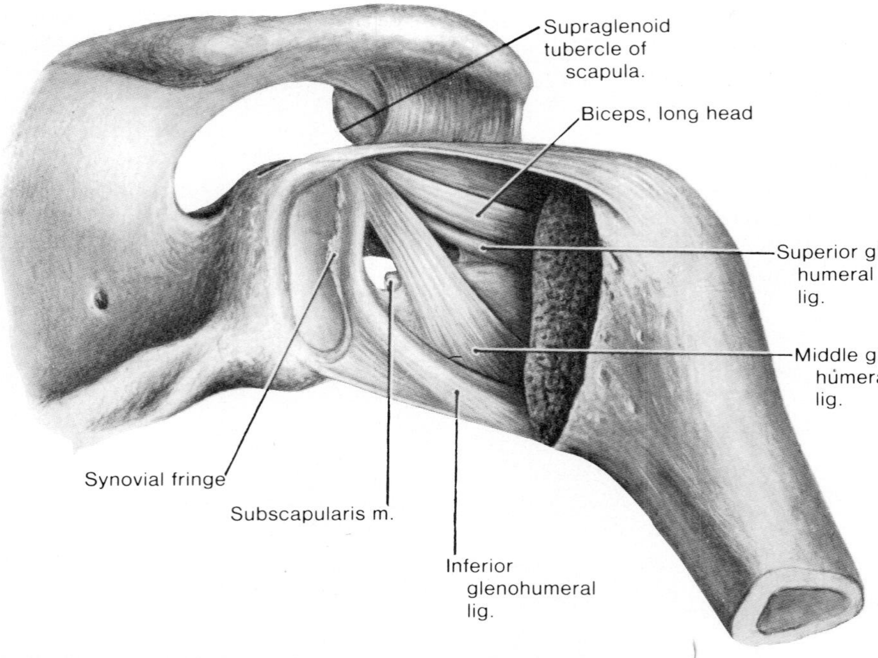

Figure 6-152. Drawing of a dissection of the interior of the left shoulder joint, exposed from behind by cutting away the posterior part of the articular capsule and sawing off the head of the humerus. Observe the three thickenings of the anterior part of the fibrous capsule, called the *glenohumeral ligaments*, which may be viewed from within the joint when the synovial capsule is removed. Note how these three ligaments and the long tendon of the biceps brachii muscle converge on the supraglenoid tubercle of the scapula. Observe the slender superior ligament parallel to the biceps tendon; the middle ligament free medially owing to the fact that the subscapularis bursa communicates with the joint cavity both above and below this ligament; and the inferior ligament contributing largely to the anterior lip of the glenoidal labrum, much as the biceps contributes to the posterior lip (Fig. 6-149). Note the synovial fringe that overlies the anterior part of the glenoidal cavity.

capsule of the shoulder joint. Its size varies in different people and it does not normally communicate with the joint cavity. It extends inferior to the acromion and the coracoacromial ligament (Fig. 6-61), between them and the supraspinatus, and facilitates movement of the deltoid muscle over the fibrous capsule of the shoulder joint and the supraspinatus tendon.

Blood Supply (Figs. 6-31 and 6-58). The articular arteries to the shoulder joint are branches of the anterior and posterior circumflex humeral arteries from the axillary and of the suprascapular artery from the subclavian.

Nerve Supply. The articular nerves are branches of the suprascapular, axillary, and lateral pectoral nerves.

CLINICALLY ORIENTED COMMENTS

Calcific Supraspinatus Tendinitis (Fig. 6-154). Deposition of calcium in the supraspinatus portion of the musculotendinous rotator cuff is common. This condition, known as **calcific supraspinatus tendonitis,** usually produces no symptoms. Deposition of calcium in the supraspinatous tendon (Fig. 6-154*B*) causes increased local pressure and may cause pain during abduction of the shoulder joint (Fig. 6-154*A*). The calcium deposit may irritate the underlying subacromial bursa producing an inflammatory reaction known as **subacromial bursitis** which causes increasing pain. So long as the shoulder joint is adducted, there is usually no pain, because in this position the painful lesion is away from the acromion. In most patients pain occurs during the 50 to 130° of abduction (Fig. 6-154*A*) because during this arc the supraspinatus tendon is in intimate contact with the inferior surface of the acromion.

Rupture of the Rotator Cuff (Fig. 6-64). When an older person strains to lift something (*e.g.*, a window that is stuck), a previously degenerated musculotendinous rotator cuff may rupture. Often this also tears the articular capsule of the shoulder joint; as a result, the joint cavity communicates with the subacromial bursa. In these cases the patient has reduced power of abduction of the shoulder joint (the action performed by the supraspinatous and deltoid) and when attempting to do so, shrugs the shoulder. If the arm is passively abducted to about 90°, however, the patient can maintain the arm in the abducted position owing to the action of the deltoid muscle.

Dislocation (Subluxation) of the Shoulder (Fig. 6-155). Because of the great freedom of movement and instability of the shoulder joint, it is more often dislocated than any other joint in adults. The dislocation may result from direct or indirect injury.

Anterior dislocation of the shoulder joint occurs most often in young adults, particularly athletes (Case 6-4). It is usually caused by forced extension and lateral rotation of the shoulder (*e.g.*, when a quarterback's arm is hit from behind just as he is ready to release the ball). The head of the humerus is driven anteriorly, and usually the fibrous capsule and glenoidal labrum are avulsed (stripped off) from the anterior aspect of the glenoid cavity. Unable to use

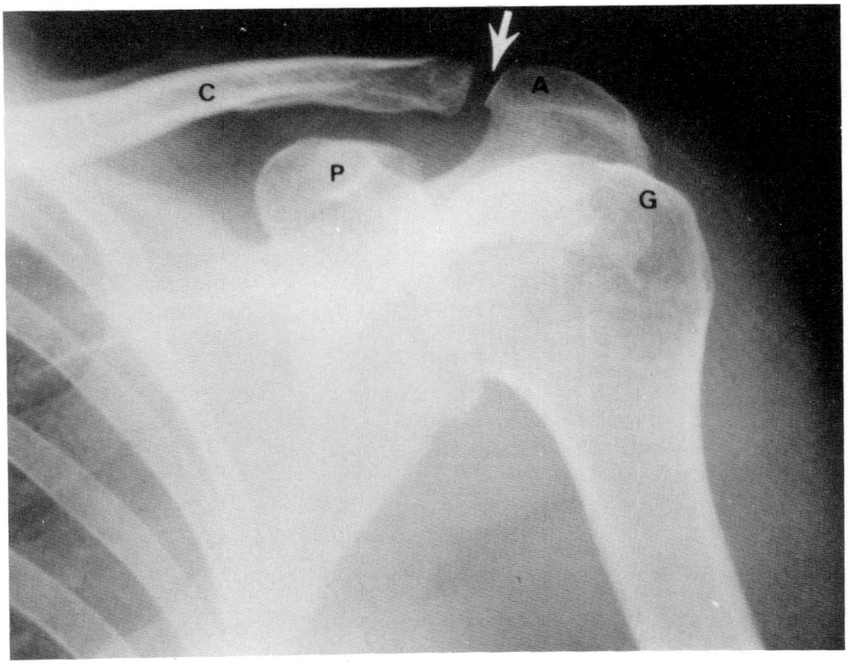

Figure 6-153. Radiograph of the left shoulder with the arm at the side and the humerus rotated (anteroposterior projection; *i.e.*, an AP). The *white arrow* indicates the acromioclavicular joint. The apparent space represents the cartilages on the ends of the clavicle and the acromion and the articular disc (Fig. 6-145). Examine the shoulder (glenohumeral) joint and observe the relatively small part of the head of the humerus that is within the glenoid cavity of the scapula. This partly accounts for the instability of the articulation. *C*, clavicle. *A*, acromion. *P*, coracoid process. *G*, greater tubercle of humerus.

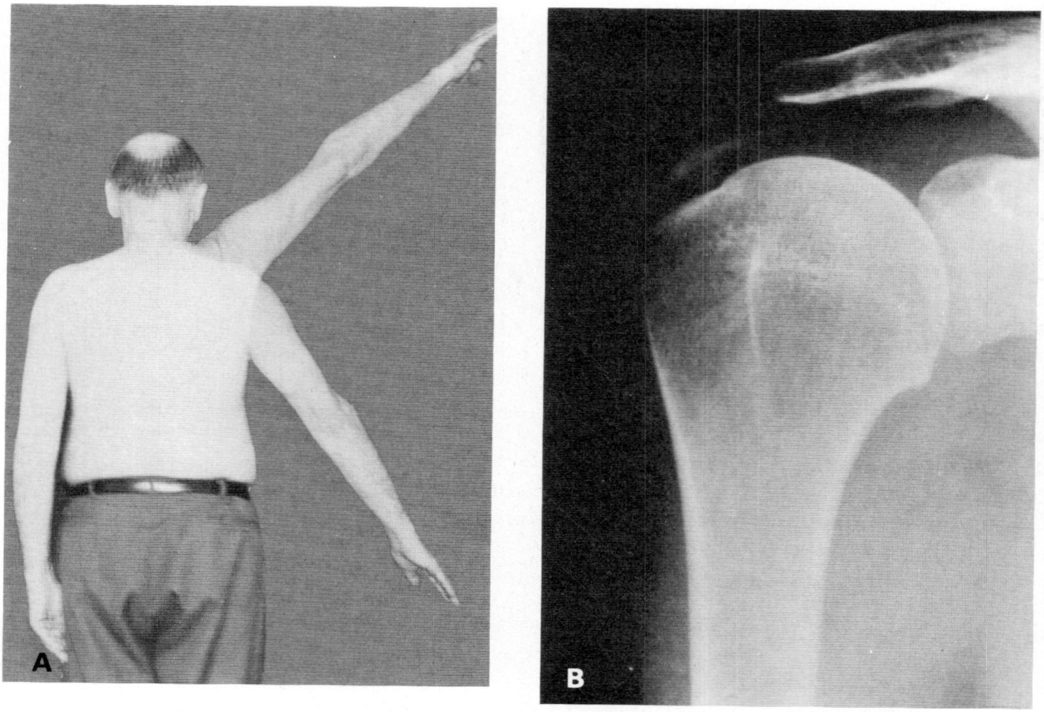

Figure 6-154. *A,* double exposure photograph of a middle-aged man demonstrating the painful arc syndrome associated with calcific supraspinatus tendinitis in the right shoulder. Abduction of the shoulder joint from about 50 to 130° causes severe pain owing to the tendinitis and associated subacromial bursitis. *B,* radiograph of the right shoulder joint (frontal projection). Note the calcium deposits in the region of the musculotendinous rotator cuff close to its insertion into the humerus.

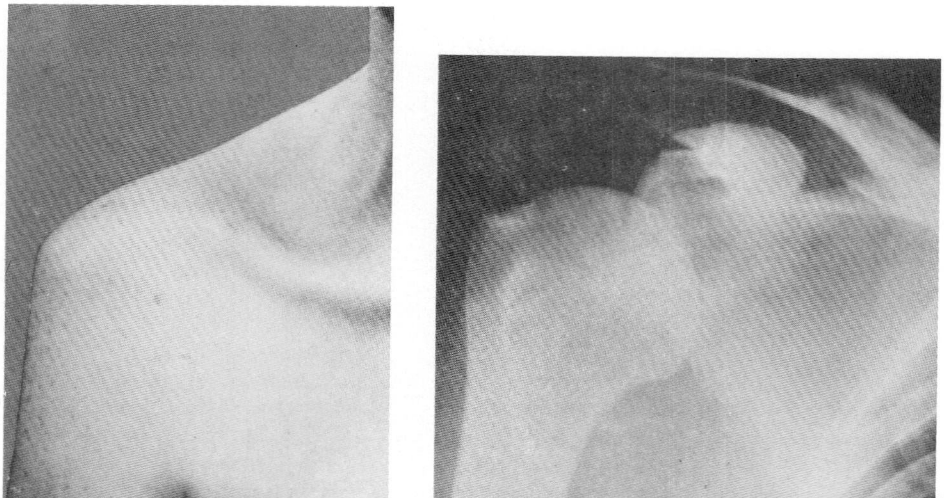

Figure 6-155. *A,* photograph of a young man with an anterior (inferomedial) dislocation of the right shoulder. Observe that the shoulder appears square and that its normal round contour is absent. *B,* radiograph of the shoulder anteroposterior (AP), projection, showing that the humeral head is not in articulation with the glenoid cavity, but is lying in a subcoracoid position.

the arm, the patient commonly supports it with the other hand. The diagnosis is confirmed by radiographic examination (Fig. 6-155). The axillary nerve is often injured when the shoulder is dislocated because it is in close relation to the lowest part of the articular capsule of this joint.

THE ELBOW JOINT

This articulation is essentially a **hinge type of synovial joint** formed by the distal end of the humerus with the radius and the ulna (Fig. 6-156). Although the joint cavity and the ligaments of the elbow joint are continuous with the cavity and the ligaments of the proximal radioulnar joint, the latter articulation is considered separately (p. 829).

The Articular Surfaces (Figs. 6-156 and 6-157). The spool-shaped **trochlea** and the spheroidal **capitulum** of the humerus articulate with the **trochlear notch of the ulna** and the proximal surface of the **head of the radius,** respectively. The articular surfaces, covered with hyaline cartilage, are most fully in contact when the forearm is in a position midway between pronation and supination and is flexed to a right angle.

Extend your elbow joint completely and palpate the medial and lateral epicondyles of the humerus and the olecranon of the ulna (Fig. 6-83). Recall that in this position these epicondyles and the tip of olecranon are in a straight line. Note that they form the points of an equilateral triangle during flexion. In partial flexion you can easily palpate part of the olecranon fossa of the humerus (Fig. 6-157*B*).

Using an articulated skeleton of the upper limb, verify that the elbow joint consists of three different articulations (Figs. 6-1 and 6-157):

1. **The humeroulnar articulation** is between the trochlea of the humerus

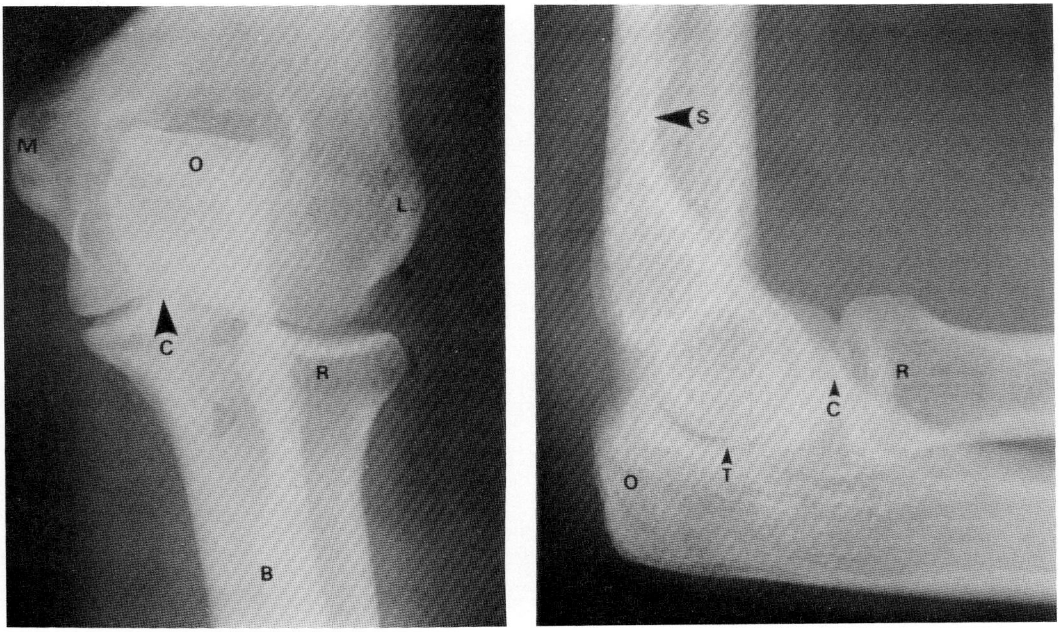

Figure 6-156. Radiographs of the elbow region (anteroposterior, *i.e.*, AP, projection on the *left* with the elbow extended and a lateral projection on the *right* with the elbow flexed). *On the humerus* observe the medial (*M*) and lateral (*L*) epicondyles and the supracondylar ridge (*S*). *On the ulna* observe the olecranon (*O*), the coronoid process (*C*), and the trochlear notch (*T*). Observe the head (*R*) and the radial tuberosity (*B*) of the radius. Compare the lateral view of the elbow with Figure 6-160.

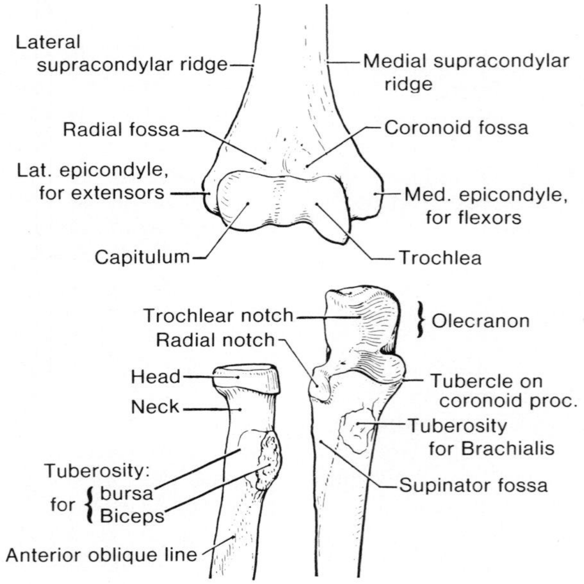

A. ANTERIOR VIEW

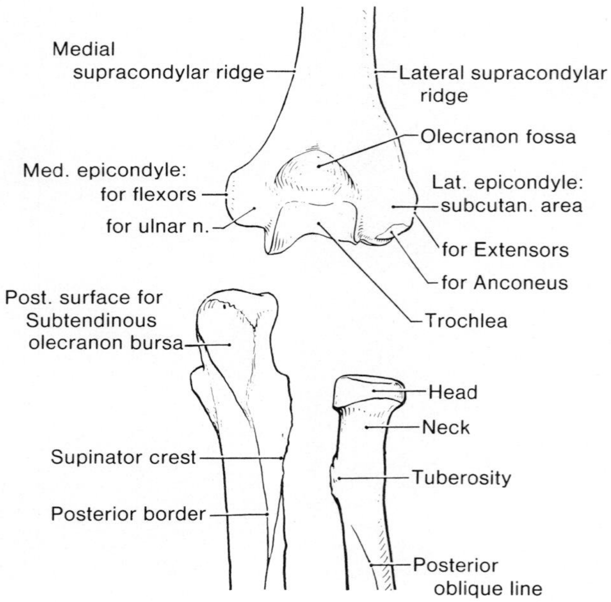

B. POSTERIOR VIEW

Figure 6-157. Drawings illustrating the bones of the elbow region. At the elbow joint the trochlea and capitulum of the distal end of the humerus articulate with the trochlear notch of the ulna and the head of the radius, respectively.

and the trochlear notch of the ulna; it is a simple **hinge joint** permitting flexion and extension. Observe that the trochlea does not fit closely into the trochlear notch in the proximal end of the ulna (Fig. 6-157*A*). Palpate the head or distal end (Fig. 6-140) of your right ulna with your left index finger and then feel the head of the ulna move as you pronate and supinate your forearm and hand (Fig. 6-173) by pretending you are driving a screw with a screwdriver.

2. **The humeroradial articulation** is between the capitulum of the humerus and the facet on the head of the radius. The capitulum fits into the slightly cupped surface of the head of the radius. In movements of the elbow joint the humeroradial articulation acts as a **hinge joint**, but in movements of the proximal radioulnar joint it acts as a pivot joint.
3. **The proximal radioulnar joint** is between the circumference of the head of the radius and the radial notch of the ulna; it is a **pivot joint** permitting rotation of the radius about the ulna.

The three articulations in the elbow region are sometimes referred to as the cubital articulation (joint).

Movements of the Joint. (Fig. I-10*B*). The elbow can be flexed or extended. **Flexion** is limited by apposition of the anterior surfaces of the forearm and arm and by tension of the posterior muscles and the collateral ligaments. When the supinated forearm is fully flexed, the fingers lie over the medial half of the clavicle and not over the acromion of the scapula. Several muscles may produce flexion of the elbow joint. In slow flexion of the elbow joint and in maintaining flexion against gravity, the **brachialis,** the **biceps brachii,** and the **pronator teres** muscles are primarily involved (Figs. 6-73 and 6-158). In fast flexion, the **brachioradialis** is also involved, and it is most effective when the forearm is in the midprone position.

Extension is limited by impingement of the olecranon process of the ulna on the olecranon fossa of the humerus (Figs. 6-156 and 6-157) and by tension of the anterior muscles and the collateral ligaments. The muscles producing extension of the elbow joint are the **triceps brachii** and the anconeus (Fig. 6-72).

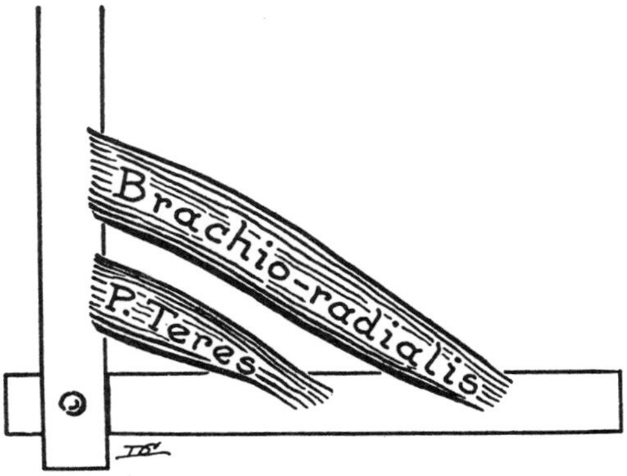

Figure 6-158. Schematic diagram of the elbow region showing that the brachioradialis is more advantageously situated than the pronator teres for producing flexion of the forearm. *H,* humerus. *R,* radius. In addition to flexing the forearm, the pronator teres pronates it (Fig. 6-173*B*).

When your forearm is fully extended and supinated, as in the anatomical position, verify that your arm and forearm are not in the same line. Normally the forearm is directed somewhat laterally, forming a "**carrying angle**" of about 163°. Because of this natural angle, one has difficulty touching the thighs with the hands when standing in the anatomical position (Figs. I-3*A* and 6-83).

The Articular Capsule. *The fibrous capsule* completely encloses the joint. Its anterior and posterior parts are thin and weak, but its sides are strengthened by the radial and ulnar collateral ligaments. The fibrous capsule is attached to the proximal margins of the **coronoid** and **radial fossae** anteriorly (Fig. 6-157*A*), but not quite to the upper limit of the **olecranon fossa** posteriorly (Fig. 6-157*B*). Distally the fibrous capsule is attached to the margins of the **trochlear notch,** the anterior border of the **coronoid process**, and the **anular ligament** (Figs. 6-157 and 6-159).

The Collateral Ligaments (Figs. 6-160 and 6-161). These strong, triangular bands are medial and lateral thickenings of the

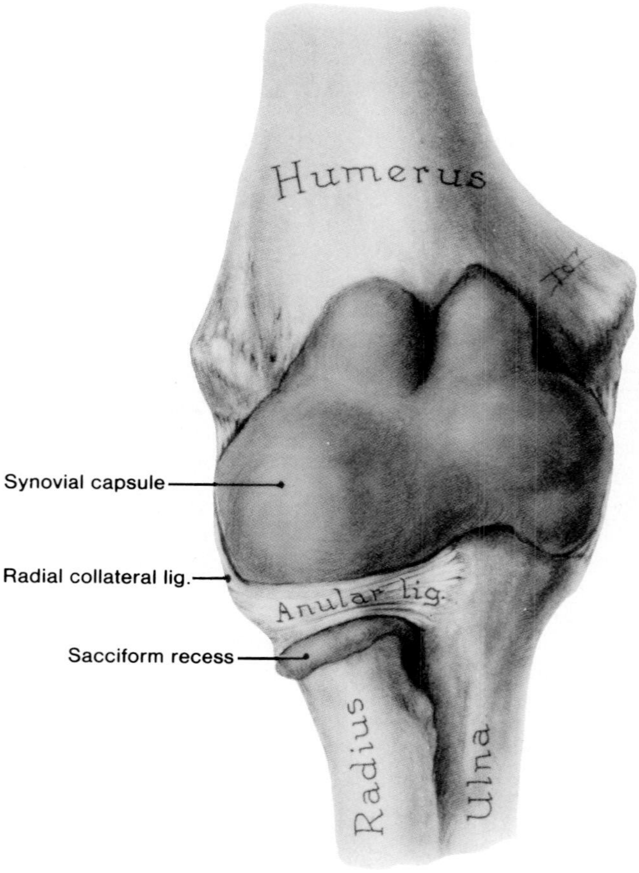

Figure 6-159. Drawing of the synovial capsule which lines the fibrous capsule of the elbow joint. The joint cavity was distended with wax and then the fibrous capsule was removed, leaving the synovial capsule. Note the saccular recess of the joint cavity between the head of the radius and the anular (annular) ligament; hence, the joint cavity of the elbow is continuous with the joint cavity of the proximal radioulnar joint.

fibrous capsule; hence, they are intrinsic ligaments.

The radial collateral ligament (lateral ligament) is a strong triangular or fan-shaped band (Fig. 6-160). Its **apex** is attached proximally to the **lateral epicondyle** of the humerus and its **base** blends with the **anular ligament** of the radius (Figs. 6-159 and 6-160), which is attached to the margins of the radial notch in the ulna (Figs. 6-157*A* and 6-160).

The ulnar collateral ligament (medial ligament) is also triangular in shape (Fig. 6-161). It is composed of anterior and posterior parts connected by a relatively weak oblique band (Fig. 6-161). Its **apex** is attached to the **medial epicondyle** of the humerus. The strong cord-like **anterior part** is attached to the medial edge of the **coronoid process** of the ulna and the weak fan-like **posterior part** is attached to the medial edge of the olecranon.

As the ulnar nerve passes posterior to the medial epicondyle it is closely applied to the ulnar collateral ligament (Fig. 6-162), as it enters the forearm between the heads of the flexor carpi ulnaris muscle.

The synovial capsule (Figs. 6-159 and 6-162) lines the fibrous capsule and is reflected on to the humerus, lining the coro-

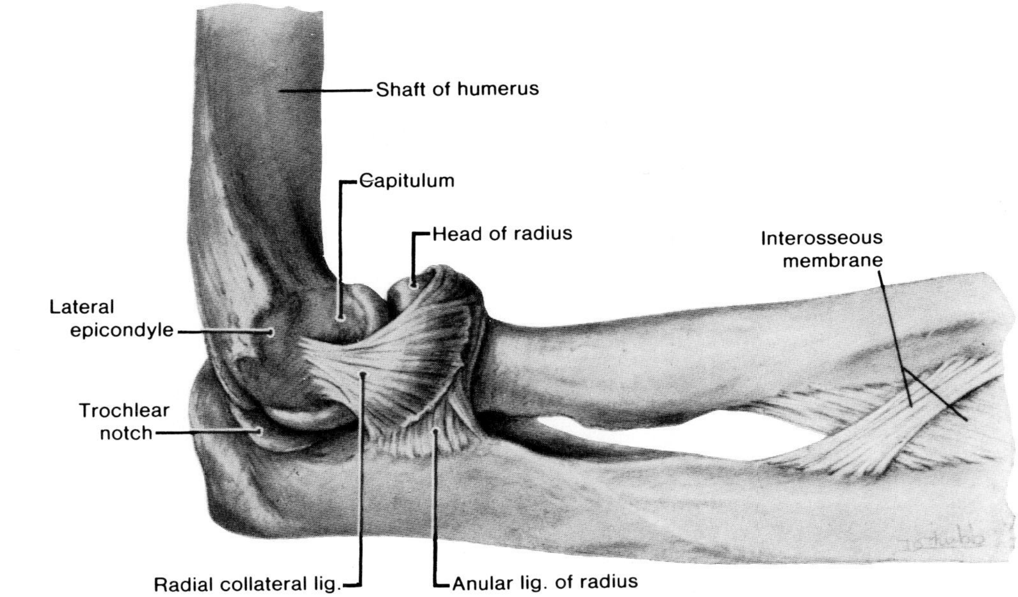

Figure 6-160. Drawing of the bones of the arm (humerus) and forearm (ulna and radius) in articulation at the elbow joint. Observe that the fan-shaped radial collateral ligament is attached to the anular liagment of the radius. Note the anular ligament encircling the head of the radius and attaching to the margins of the radial notch of the ulna.

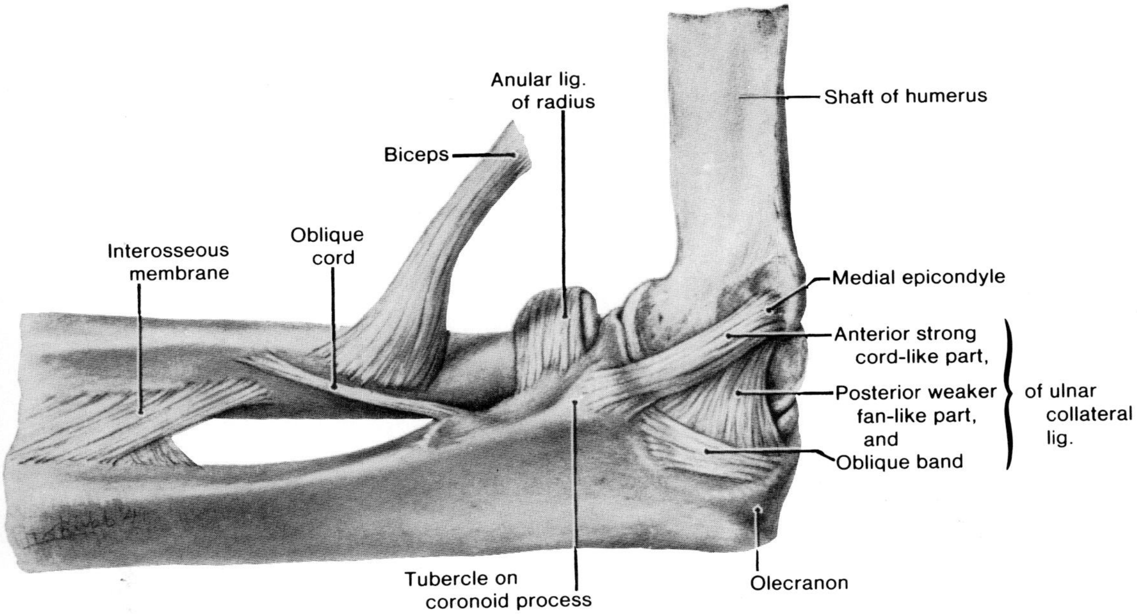

Figure 6-161. Drawing of the bones of the arm and forearm in articulation at the elbow jont. Observe the ulnar collateral ligament and verify that its strong anterior cord-like part becomes taut in extension, and that its posterior fan-like part is taut in flexion (as here). Understand that the oblique fibers merely deepen the socket for the trochlea of the humerus. Recall that the humeroulnar head of the flexor digitorum superficialis arises from the end of the anterior strong part of the ulnar collateral ligament (Fig. 6-95).

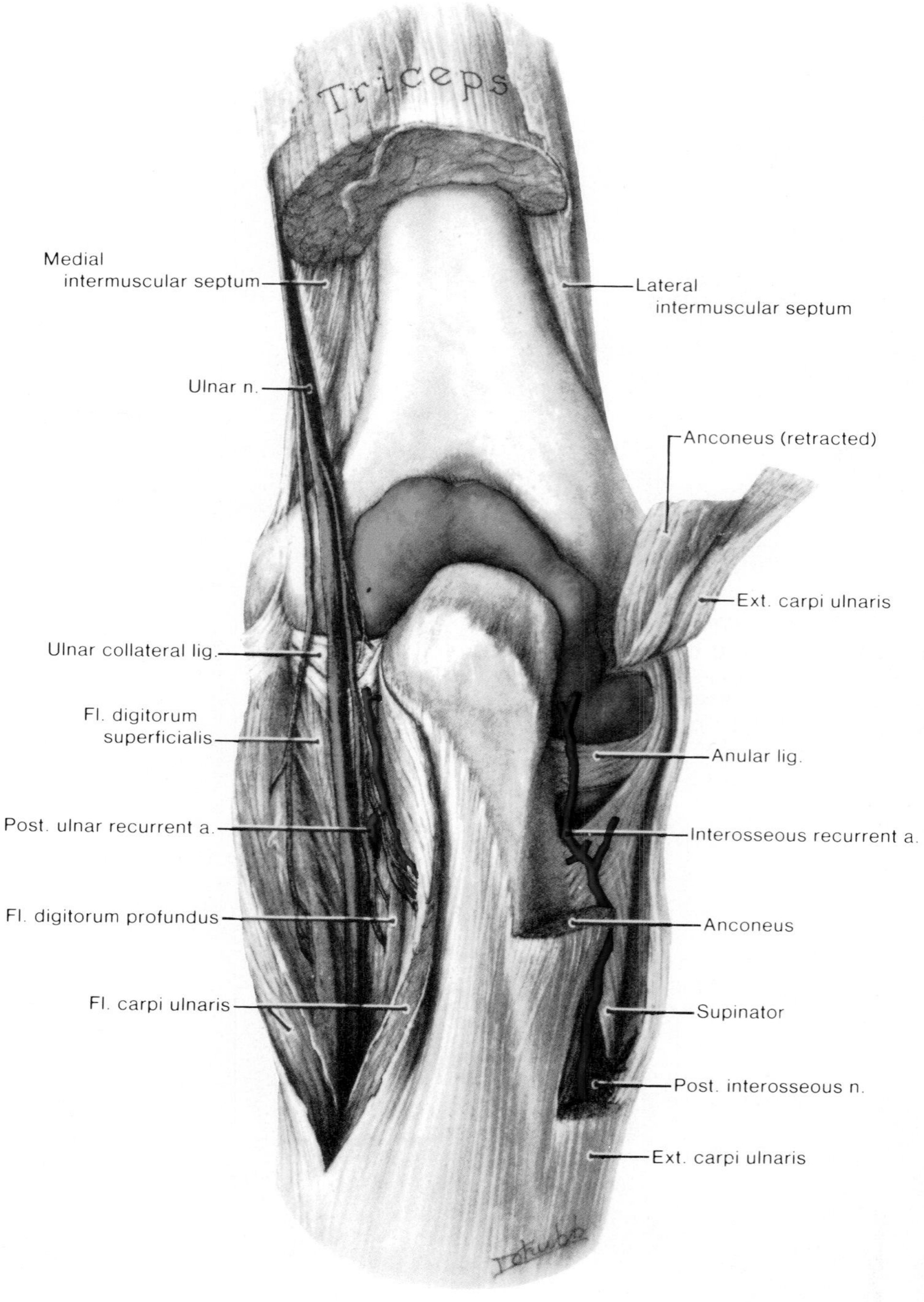

Figure 6-162. Drawing of a dissection of the elbow from behind with the distal portion of the triceps muscle removed. Observe the ulnar nerve descending (1) subfascially within the posterior compartment of the arm, applied to the medial head of the triceps, and behind the medial epicondyle; (2) applied to the ulnar collateral ligament of the joint; and (3) between the flexor carpi ulnaris and the flexor digitorum profundus muscles. Observe the synovial capsule (*blue*) protruding below the anular ligament.

noid and radial fossae anteriorly (Figs. 6-157*A* and 6-159) and the olecranon fossa posteriorly (Figs. 6-157*B* and 6-162). It is continuous below with the synovial membrane of the proximal radioulnar joint (Fig. 6-159).

Stability of the Joint. The elbow joint in adults is quite stable because of the hinge-like arrangement formed by the spanner-shaped (jaw-like) trochlear notch of the ulna into which the spool-shaped trochlea of the humerus fits. In addition, the joint is strengthened by very strong ulnar and radial collateral ligaments (Figs. 6-160 and 6-161). The elbow joint of children is not so stable owing to the late fusion of the epiphyses of the ends of the bones involved in the articulation.

Bursae About the Elbow Joint. Only a few of the many bursa around the elbow are clinically important. There are two olecranon bursae. The **subcutaneous olecranon bursa** (Fig. 6-163) is located in the subcutaneous connective tissue over the olecranon, whereas the *subtendinous olecranon bursa* is located between the tendon of the triceps brachii muscle and the olecranon, just proximal to its insertion into the olecranon (Figs. 6-86 and 6-157*B*).

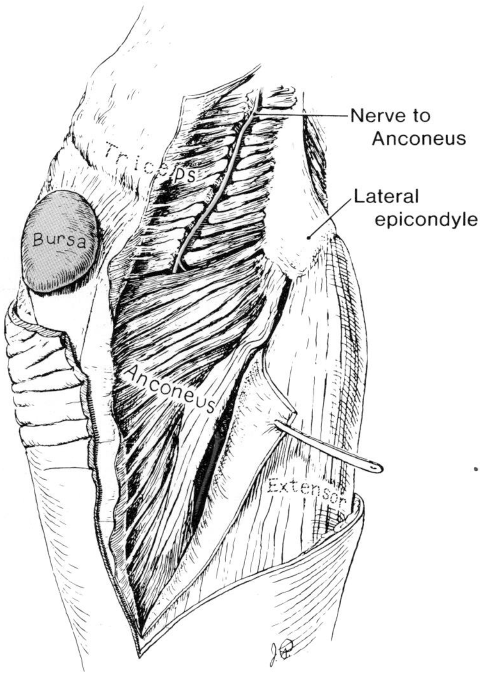

Figure 6-163. Drawing of a dissection of the posterolateral aspect of the elbow. Observe the subcutaneous olecranon bursa lying upon the tendinous expansion of the triceps muscle.

CLINICALLY ORIENTED COMMENTS

The subcutaneous olecranon bursa is exposed to injury from falls on the elbow and to infection from skin abrasions. As a result of repeated excessive friction, this bursa may become inflamed, producing a friction bursitis [*e.g.*, "student's elbow" (Fig. 6-164) or miner's elbow].

Inflammation of the subtendinous olecranon bursa, although much less common, may result from excessive friction between the triceps tendon and the olecranon, *e.g.*, resulting from repeated flexion-extension of the forearm as occurs during certain assembly line jobs. The pain would be most severe on flexion because of pressure on the inflamed bursa by the triceps tendon.

The **radioulnar bursa** lies between the extensor digitorum and the radiohumeral joint and the supinator muscle. The **interosseous bursa** lies posterior to the supinator muscle and is lateral to the tendon of the biceps brachii muscle and medial to the

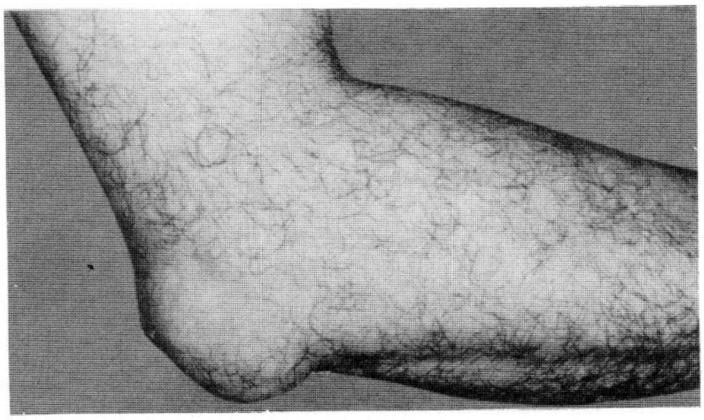

Figure 6-164. Photograph of a student's right elbow exhibiting enlargement of the superficial olecranon bursa. This condition, known as olecranon bursitis ("student's elbow") may result from the repeated microtrauma of friction (*e.g.*, against a desk top) or from a single direct trauma.

ulna. The **bicipitoradial bursa** lies between the biceps tendon and the anterior part of the tuberosity of the radius.

CLINICALLY ORIENTED COMMENTS

Radioulnar bursitis may result from the irritation of repeated or violent extension of the wrist with the forearm pronated (Fig. 6-173*B*), as occurs especially during the backhand stroke in tennis (see tennis elbow, p. 784). Pain occurs on elbow extension with the forearm pronated.

In **bicipitoradial bursitis** pain occurs when the elbow joint is flexed and the forearm is supinated (Fig. 6-173*A*). Recall that the biceps is a strong flexor-supinator of the forearm.

Blood Supply (Fig. 6-74). The articular arteries are derived from the **anastomoses of the elbow region** which are formed by collateral branches of the brachial and recurrent branches of the ulnar and radial arteries.

Nerve Supply. The articular nerves are derived mainly from the musculoculocutaneous and radial nerves, but the ulnar, median, and anterior interosseous nerves occasionally supply articular branches.

CLINICALLY ORIENTED COMMENTS

Knowledge of the normal carrying angle of the forearm is essential for aligning the arm and forearm after fracture of the elbow. In addition, an increase in the carrying angle of the upper limbs is one of the clinical characteristics of females with the **Turner syndrome** who have an XO sex chromosome complement. When standing in the anatomical position, their extended forearms deviate markedly to the radial side of the axis of the upper limb, a condition known as **cubitus valgus.** These females also exhibit short stature, a broad chest, webbing of the neck, and sexual immaturity.

Fracture-separation of the proximal radial epiphysis (Fig. 6-165) can result when a young person falls and exerts a compression and abduction force on the elbow joint. The anatomical basis for the injury is the late fusion (14 to 17 years) of the proximal epiphysis with the shaft of the radius.

Avulsion of the medial epicondyle of the humerus in children can result from a fall that causes severe abduction of the extended elbow joint. The resulting traction on the ulnar collateral ligament avulses the medial epicondyle and carries it distally. The anatomical basis of this avulsion is that the epiphysis for the medial epicondyle does not fuse with the distal end of the humerus until about the 20th year. A fallacious diagnosis of fracture of the medial epicondyle could be made by a person unaware of this late fusion.

A **traction injury of the ulnar nerve** is a frequent complication of the abduction type of avulsion of the medial epicondyle (Case 6-5).

Posterior dislocation of the elbow joint may occur in children when they fall on their hands with their elbows flexed.

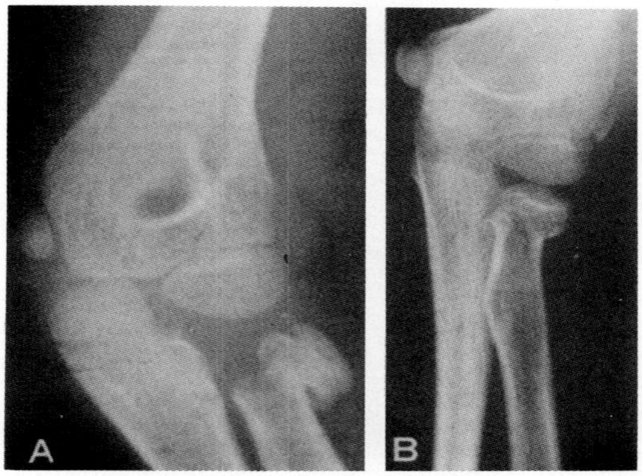

Figure 6-165. *A*, radiograph of the elbow region of a child showing a fracture-separation of the proximal radial epiphysis. Note that the head of the radius is displaced and is not in contact with the capitulum of the humerus. *B*, radiograph taken after reduction of the fracture-dislocation showing the radial head in its normal position.

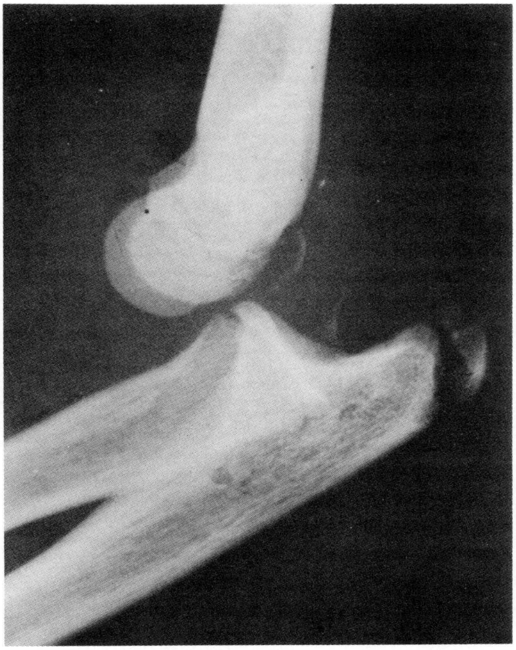

Figure 6-166. Radiograph of the elbow region of a child showing a posterior dislocation of the elbow joint. Note that the distal end of the humerus has been driven anteriorly and is not in articulation with the radius and ulna. Note the apparently separated fragment of bone at the proximal end of the olecranon. This is not a fracture but rather the epiphysis of the proximal end of the ulna which still has not fused with the olecranon. This occurs at 14 to 16 years.

The distal end of the humerus is driven through the weak posterior portion of the fibrous capsule as the radius and ulna dislocate posteriorly (Fig. 6-166).

THE RADIOULNAR JOINTS

The radius and ulna articulate at their proximal and distal ends at synovial joints, called the proximal and distal radioulnar joints. These articulations are the **pivot type of synovial joint** which produces the movements of pronation and supination (Figs. 6-79 and 6-173). In addition the shafts of the radius and ulna are connected by an interosseous membrane and an oblique cord (Figs. 6-161 and 6-167). The interosseous membrane and the oblique cord are sometimes regarded as a nonsynovial middle radioulnar joint.

The interosseous membrane is a strong, broad, thin, fibrous sheet which stretches between the interosseous borders of the radius and the ulna, commencing 2 to 3 cm distal to the tuberosity of the radius (Fig. 6-167). In addition to providing a flexible attachment between the forearm bones, it provides an origin for the deep muscles of the forearm. A thin fibrous layer, called the **quadrate ligament,** extends between the neck of the radius and the ulna, distal to the radial notch. It supports the synovial membrane at this site.

The *oblique cord* is an unimportant fibrous band that extends inferolaterally from the lateral border of the tuberosity of the ulna to the radius, just below its tuberosity and the insertion of the biceps brachii muscle (Fig. 6-161). The oblique cord is not always present and is not known to be of much functional significance.

The Proximal (Superior) Radioulnar Joint (Fig. 6-167). This articulation is the **pivot type of synovial joint** which allows movement of the radius on the ulna.

The Articular Surfaces (Figs. 6-157*A*, 6-159, 6-162, 6-167, and 6-168). The circumference of the **radial head** articulates with the **radial notch** of the ulna. The bony surfaces are covered with hyaline cartilage which allows free movement. The head of the radius is held in position by the strong **anular ligament**, a U-shaped fibrous collar which encircles it. It is attached to the anterior and posterior margins of the radial notch (Figs. 6-157*A*, 6-167, and 6-168) and forms about four-fifths of the osseofibrous ring that is completed by the radial notch. In Figure 6-168, observe that the anular ligament is cup-shaped (*i.e.,* wide above and narrow below).

The Articular Capsule. The **fibrous capsule** encloses the joint and is continuous with the capsule of the elbow joint. The proximal border of the anular ligament also blends with the fibrous capsule of the elbow joint.

The **synovial capsule** (Figs. 6-159, 6-162, and 6-168) lines the fibrous capsule. This synovial membrane is a downward prolongation of the synovial capsule of the

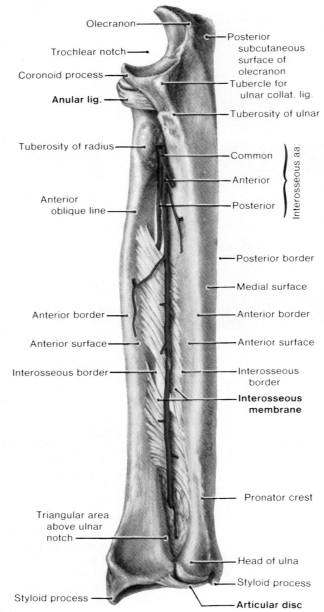

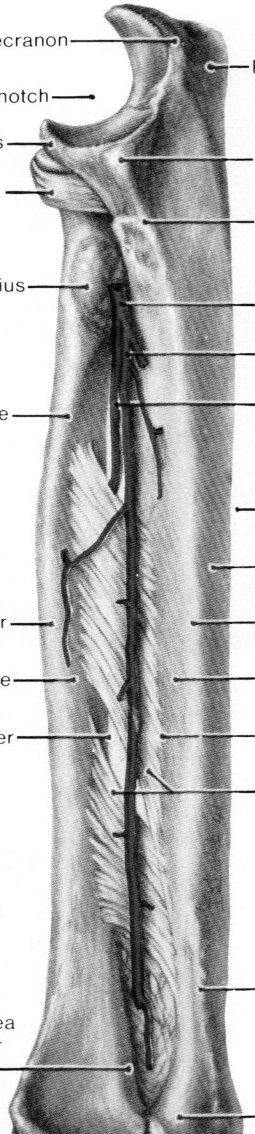

Figure 6-167. Drawing of a dissection of the radius and ulna showing the radioulnar articulations and the interosseous arteries. The ligament of the proximal radioulnar joint is the anular ligament; the bond of union at the distal joint is the articular disc. Observe the interosseous membrane and the general direction of its fibers which are attached to the interosseous borders of the radius and ulna. Note that the posterior interosseous artery passes backward above the superior border of the interosseous membrane and runs inferiorly to supply muscles on the posterior surface of the forearm and hand. Observe that the anterior interosseous artery descends on the anterior surface of the interosseous membrane to supply muscles on the anterior surface of the forearm. Note that it pierces the interosseous membrane about 5 cm above the distal end of the radius and descends to the dorsum of the carpus where it joins the posterior carpal arch (Fig. 6-117). Observe the *nutrient arteries* of the radius and ulna which are derived from the anterior interosseous artery.

elbow joint. In Figure 6-162, observe that the deep surface of the anular ligament is lined with synovial membrane which continues distally in a sac-like manner on the proximal part of the neck of the radius (Fig. 6-159). This arrangement allows the radius to rotate within the anular ligament without tearing the synovial capsule. *The synovial cavities of the elbow and proximal radioulnar joints are in free communication with each other.*

CLINICALLY ORIENTED COMMENTS

Preschool children, especially 1 to 3 year-olds, are particularly vulnerable to an injury usually known as "**pulled elbow**" (Fig. 6-169). Synonyms for this common condition are subluxation of the head of the radius, partial dislocation of the radial head, "slipped elbow," and "nursemaid's elbow." The last term is a poor one because it implies that it is the nursemaid that is injured when it is she or the mother who often injures the child's elbow.

The history of these cases is typical (Case 6-7). The child is suddenly lifted up by the extended arm with the forearm pronated (*e.g.,* when lifting children into a bus or pulling them away from danger). The child cries out and refuses to use the limb, which he/she protects by holding it with the elbow flexed and the forearm pronated.

Although it is commonly assumed that the sudden jerk pulls the head of the radius out of the cup-shaped anular ligament because it is no larger than the neck of the radius, this is incorrect. The child's radial head (although not so large as an adult's radial head) is still larger than the neck of the radius. The sudden pull while the forearm is pronated tears the distal attachment of the anular ligament, where it is only loosely attached to the neck of the radius by a thin layer of fibrous tissue. In children under 7 years, this attachment is especially weak; consequently, when a child's arm is jerked the radial head is pulled distally, partially out of the torn anular ligament. The proximal part of the ligament may become trapped between the head of the radius and the capitulum of the humerus.

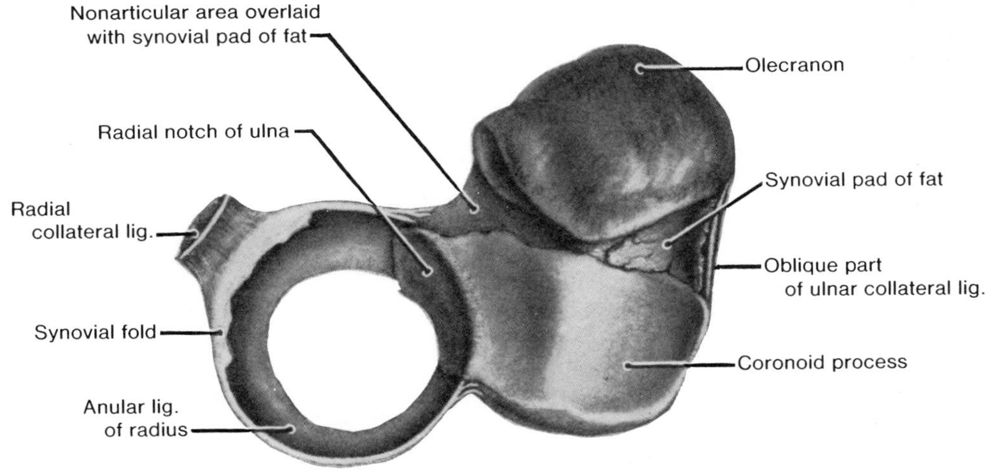

Figure 6-168. Drawing of a dissection of the socket for the head of the radius and the trochlea of the humerus, from above. Study this illustration and Figures 6-160 to 6-162, verifying that the anular ligament keeps the head of the radius applied to the radial notch of the ulna (Fig. 6-157*A*). The anular ligament and the radial notch of the ulna form a cup-shaped osseofibrous ring that prevents the radial head from being pulled distally through its socket. Note that the anular (L. ring) ligament is bound to the humerus by the radial collateral ligament of the elbow and that a crescentic synovial fold occupies the angular space between the head of the radius and the capitulum of the humerus (Fig. 6-162).

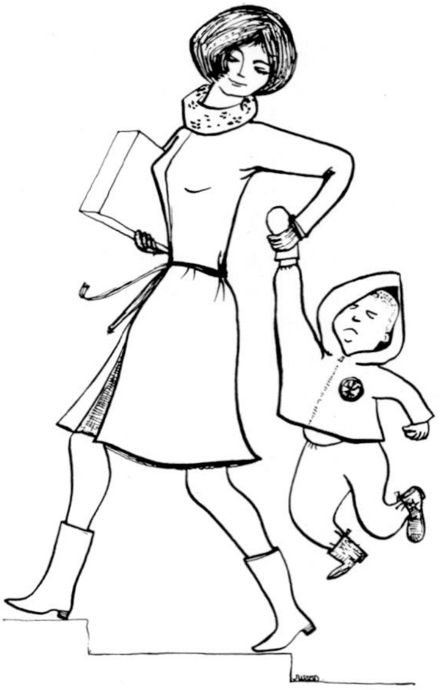

Figure 6-169. Illustration showing how a "pulled elbow" may occur in a child. This is a common injury in preschool children. The sudden pull or jerk results in transient subluxation (dislocation) of the head of the radius.

The Distal (Inferior) Radioulnar Joint (Figs. 6-167 and 6-170 to 6-172). This articulation is a **pivot type of synovial joint.**

The Articular Surfaces (Fig. 6-157). The rounded side of the **head of the ulna** articulates with the ulnar notch in the **distal end of the radius.** These surfaces are covered with hyaline cartilage.

The Articular Disc (Figs. 6-167, 6-170, and 6-171). This fibrocartilaginous disc binds the lower ends of the ulna and radius together and is the main uniting structure of the joint. Its **base** is attached to the medial edge of the ulnar notch of the radius and its **apex** is attached to the lateral side of the base of the styloid process of the ulna. The proximal surface of this triangular disc articulates with the distal aspect of the head of the ulna. Hence, the joint cavity is L-shaped in vertical section (Figs. 6-170 and 6-171). The disc separates the cavity of the distal radioulnar joint from the cavity of the wrist joint.

The Articular Capsule (Fig. 6-170). The **fibrous capsule** encloses the joint. Relatively weak transverse bands extend from the radius to the ulna across the anterior and posterior surfaces of the joint as intrinsic ligaments.

The **synovial capsule** (Figs. 6-170 to 6-172) lines the fibrous capsule and the proximal surface of the articular disc and extends proximally a short distance between the radius and ulna as the **sacciform recess.** This redundancy of the synovial capsule accommodates the twisting of the membrane that occurs as the distal end of the radius travels around the fixed lower end of the ulna during pronation of the forearm (Fig. 6-173*B*).

Movements of the Radioulnar Joints (Fig. 6-173). Movements at these joints contribute to pronation and supination of the forearm. The axis for these movements passes proximally through the center of the head of the radius and distally through the site of attachment of the apex of the articular disc to the head of the ulna. It is mainly the radius that rotates; its proximal end rotates within the osseofibrous ring formed by the anular ligament and the radial notch on the ulna (Figs. 6-167 and 6-168). Distally the end of the radius rotates around the fixed end of the ulna (Fig. 6-173) to which it is attached by the articular disc (Fig. 6-172).

When the forearm is fully supinated, the

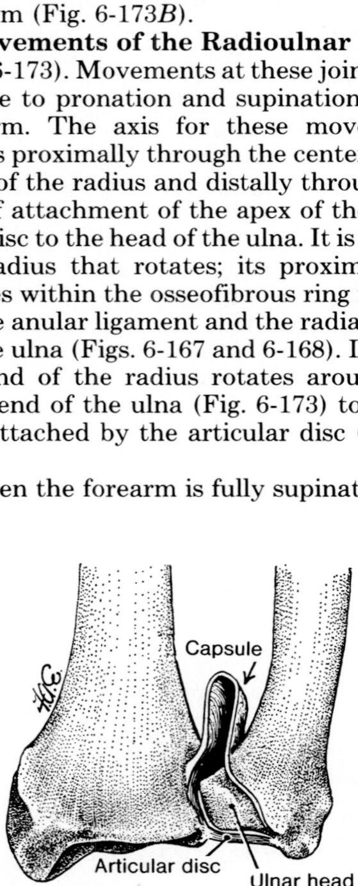

Figure 6-170. Drawing of the right distal radioulnar joint viewed from the front with the anterior part of the capsule removed to show its interior. Note that the joint cavity is L-shaped owing to the upward extension of the capsule (sacciform recess) between the radius and the ulna (see Fig. 6-171 also). Understand that the articular disc, not the capsule, is the chief uniting structure of the joint.

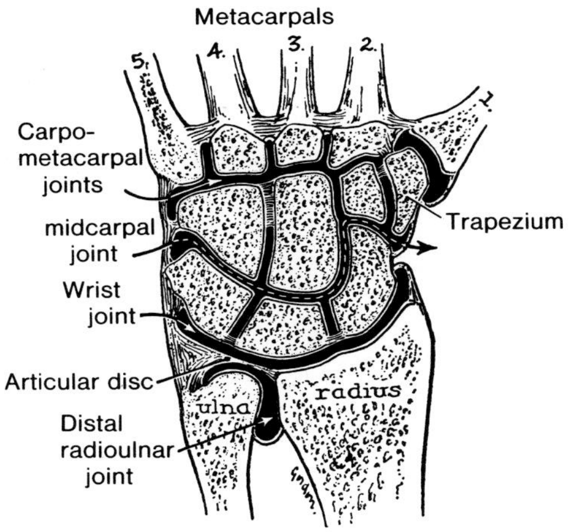

Figure 6-171. Drawing of a coronal section of the forearm and hand showing the distal radioulnar, wrist, intercarpal, carpometacarpal, and intermetacarpal joints. Note that the cavities of the distal radioulnar and wrist joints are separated by the articular disc of the distal radioulnar joint. Observe the important carpometacarpal joint of the thumb where the first metacarpal bone articulates with the trapezium by a saddle-shaped joint with a loose capsule. These features allow the thumb a considerable range of movement (Fig. 6-129).

radius and the ulna are parallel (Fig. 6-173*A*), and during full pronation these bones are crossed (Fig. 6-173*B*). **Supination,** the action used to drive a screw, is more powerful than **pronation,** the action used to extract a screw. Verify this by trying to drive a screw with your other hand.

Pronation and supination are special movements occurring at the radioulnar joints. Pronation is the movement of the forearm which results in the hand facing posteriorly, whereas supination is the movement which results in the palm facing anteriorly (in the anatomical position). These movements can occur in three different ways: (1) *the usual way* (Fig. 6-79) is by rotating the distal end of the radius over the distal end of the ulna while at the same time abducting the ulna with the anconeus so that the ulna takes the place of the distal end of the radius; (2) another way (Fig. 6-173) is by rotating the distal end of the radius over the stationary distal end of the ulna (*e.g.,* when doing the butterfly stroke in swimming); and (3) an unusual way is by rotating the ulna over the proximal end of the stationary radius by laterally rotating the humerus, as occurs in abducting the arm while keeping the hand facing forward (*e.g.,* when throwing a baseball or cricket ball overhand).

Several muscles are involved in supination, but the **principal supinators** of the forearm are the *biceps brachii* and the *supinator* muscles. The biceps is the most powerful supinator and is particularly important when force is required, especially when the forearm is flexed (*e.g.,* driving a large screw into hard wood). Verify that the biceps is a strong supinator by supinating your forearm against resistance with the elbow flexed to 90°. As you do this, palpate your biceps with your other hand.

The **principal pronators** of the forearm are the *pronator teres* and the *pronator quadratus* muscles. The activity of the pronator quadratus is reinforced by the pronator teres during rapid and forceful pronation.

Blood Supply (Figs. 6-74 and 6-167). The articular arteries supplying the **proximal radioulnar joint** are derived from the anastomoses in the elbow region. Those supplying the **distal radioulnar joint** are derived from the anterior and posterior interosseous arteries.

Nerve Supply. The articular nerves to the proximal radioulnar joint are derived mainly from the musculocutaneous, median, and radial nerves. The nerves to the distal radioulnar joint are derived from the anterior and posterior interosseous nerves.

THE WRIST JOINT

The wrist or radiocarpal joint is between the distal end of the radius and the carpus; it is an *ellipsoid type of synovial joint.*

The Articular Surfaces (Figs. 6-122, 6-171, and 6-174). The distal end of the radius and the articular disc of the distal radioulnar joint articulate with the proximal row of carpal bones (scaphoid, lunate, and triquetrum). In Figure 6-174, observe that the convex surfaces formed by the carpal bones fit into the concave surfaces of the distal end of the radius and the articular disc.

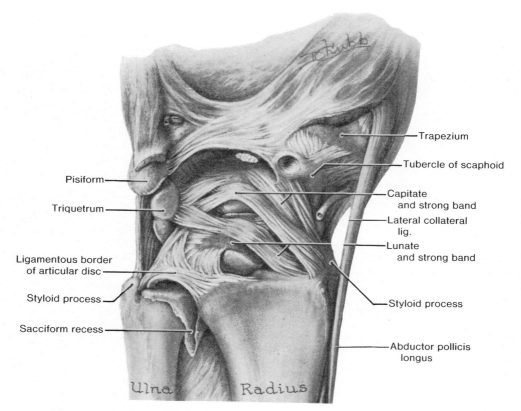

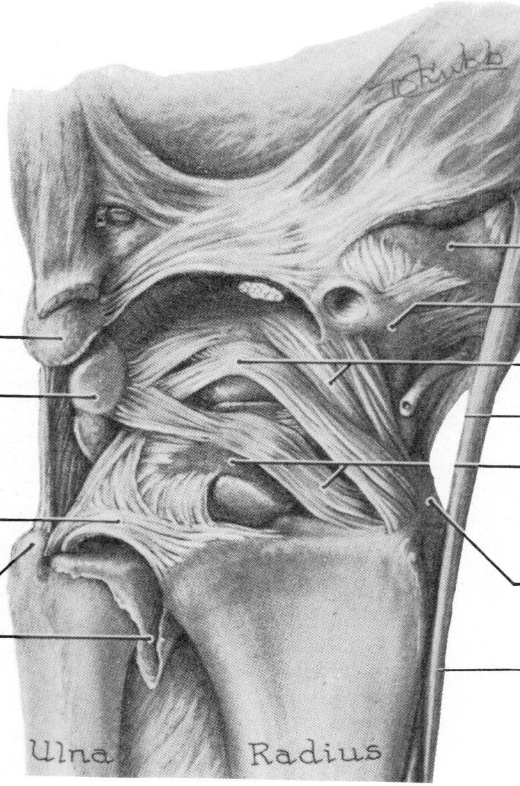

Figure 6-172. Drawing of a dissection of the forearm and wrist with the hand forcibly extended, showing an anterior view of the ligaments of the distal radioulnar, radiocarpal, and intercarpal joints. Observe the sacciform recess of the synovial capsule of the distal radioulnar joint and the ligamentous anterior border of the triangular articular disc. Note the anterior or palmar ligaments passing from the radius to the two rows of carpal bones; they are strong and so directed that the hand follows the radius during supination (Fig. 6-173*A*). The dorsal ligaments take the same direction; hence the hand follows during pronation also (Fig. 6-173*B*).

Movements of the Joint. In Figure 6-174, note that the carpal bones form a much larger surface than do the radius and the articular cartilage. This arrangement allows the movements of adduction, abduction, flexion, extension, and circumduction to occur (Fig. 6-175).

Rotation of the wrist joint proper is impossible because the articular surfaces are ellipsoid in shape; however, pronation and supination of the forearm and hand compensate for this lack of movement.

Much of the apparent movement at the radiocarpal joint occurs between the proximal and distal rows of carpal bones at the midcarpal joint (Fig. 6-171).

As no forearm muscles (except part of the flexor carpi ulnaris) insert into the carpus, its movements result from the action of muscles whose tendons pass over it.

The principal **flexor muscles of the wrist** are the flexor carpi radialis, the flexor carpi ulnaris, and the palmaris longus (Fig. 6-90). These muscles are aided by the flexor digitorum superficialis, the flexor digitorum profundus, and the flexor pollicis longus (Figs. 6-95 and 6-97).

The principal **extensor muscles of the wrist** are the extensor carpi radialis longus, the extensor carpi radialis brevis, and the extensor carpi ulnaris (Fig. 6-108). These muscles are aided by the extensor digitorum, the extensor indicis, the extensor digiti minimi, and the extensor pollicis longus.

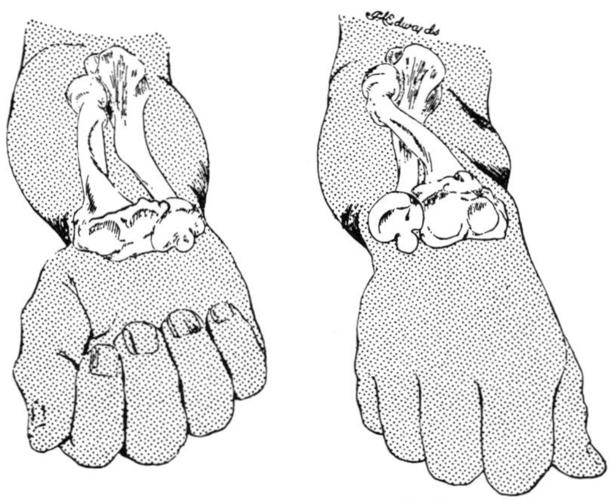

Figure 6-173. Drawings of the forearm and hand showing movements at the radioulnar joints. In pronation the distal end of the radius is carried anteriorly and medially around the distal end of the ulna until the palm faces dorsally and the shafts of the radius and ulna are crossed in the form of an X. Note that the crossing occurs in the proximal part of the forearm. When the forearm is fully supinated as in *A*, the thumb is directed laterally and the radius and ulna are parallel. Pronation and supination are also illustrated in Figure 6-79.

The principal **abductors of the wrist** are the flexor carpi radialis and the extensor carpi radialis longus and brevis. These muscles are aided by the abductor pollicis longus and the extensor pollicis longus and brevis (Fig. 6-109).

The principal **adductors of the wrist** are the flexor carpi ulnaris and the extensor carpi ulnaris (Figs. 6-90 and 6-108).

Adduct and abduct your wrist, noting that adduction is freer than abduction. This occurs because the ulnar styloid process does not extend as far distally as the radial styloid. Using your thumb and index finger, palpate the radial and ulnar styloid processes. Verify that the radial styloid is about 1 cm distal to the ulnar styloid. This normal relationship is essential knowledge for the orthopaedist reducing a **Colles' fracture** of the distal end of the radius (Case 6-11).

The Articular Capsule (Fig. 6-171). *The fibrous capsule* encloses the joint and is attached proximally to the distal ends of the radius and ulna and distally to the proximal row of carpal bones. It is strengthened by dorsal and palmar radiocarpal ligaments, which run obliquely downward and medially from the radius, and by radial and ulnar collateral ligaments (Fig. 6-172).

The synovial capsule (Figs. 6-171 and 6-174) lines the fibrous capsule and is attached to the margins of the articular surfaces. It presents numerous folds, especially dorsally. Normally the joint cavity of the radiocarpal joint does not communicate with either the distal radioulnar or the midcarpal joint (Fig. 6-171); however, perforation of the articular disc of the distal radioulnar joint, which may occur with age, results in communication between the two joints (Fig. 6-174).

Blood Supply (Figs. 6-138 and 6-139). The articular arteries are derived from the dorsal and palmar carpal arches.

Nerve Supply. The articular nerves are derived from the anterior interosseous branch of the **median** nerve, the posterior interosseous branch of the **radial** nerve, and the dorsal and deep branches of the **ulnar** nerve. This is a good illustration of **Hilton's law** (*i.e.,* nerves that supply muscles acting on a joint usually send sensory fibers to it).

CLINICALLY ORIENTED COMMENTS

Wrist fractures (Colles' fracture, Case 6-11), involving the distal end of the radius, are the most common type of fracture in persons over 50 years; they occur more frequently in women. This fracture commonly results when the person slips or trips and, in attempting to break a fall, lands on the open hand with the forearm pronated. The distal end of the radius fractures and the fragment or fragments are displaced upward (superiorly), causing shortening of the radius (Fig. 6-191*C*). The distal fragment is usually tilted backward and slightly to the lateral side. This dorsal displacement produces a characteristic hump described as the "**dinner fork**" **deformity** (Fig. 6-191*A*).

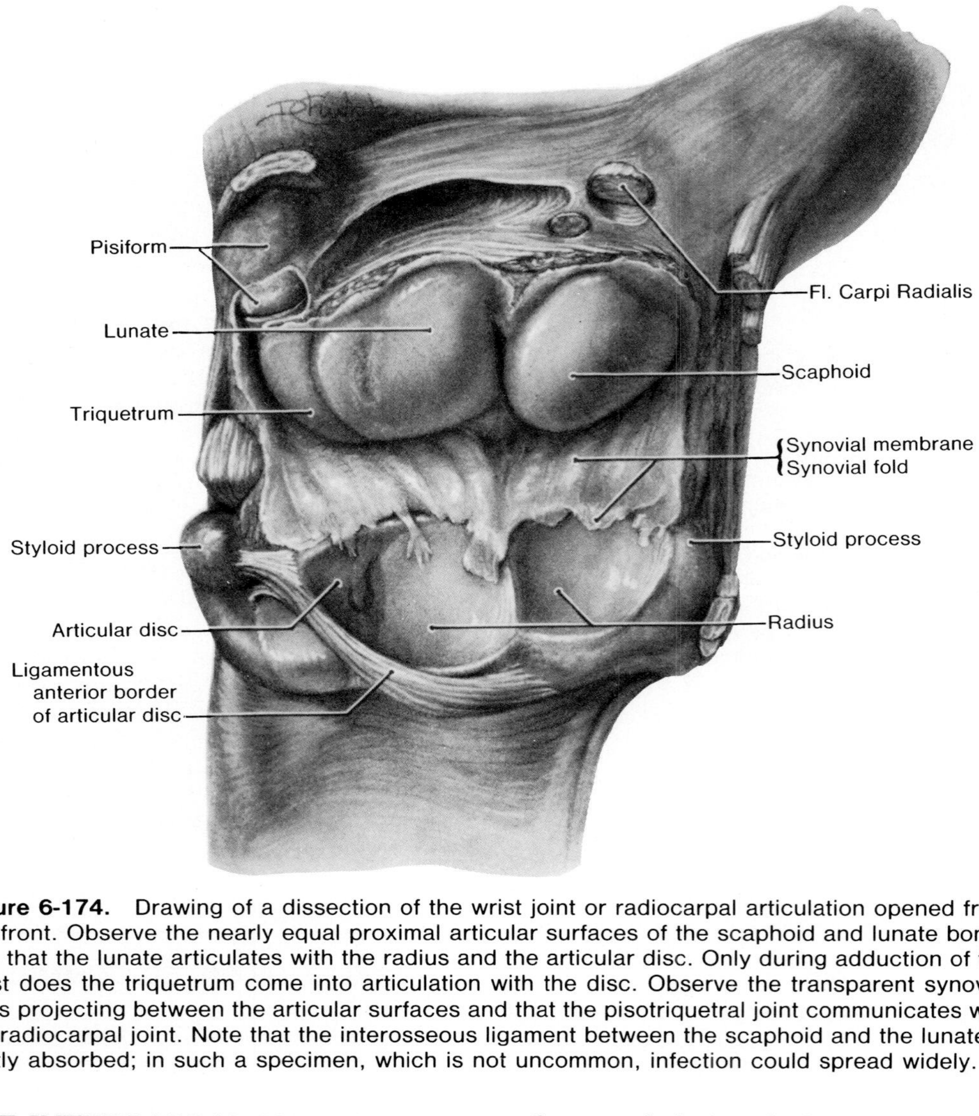

Figure 6-174. Drawing of a dissection of the wrist joint or radiocarpal articulation opened from the front. Observe the nearly equal proximal articular surfaces of the scaphoid and lunate bones and that the lunate articulates with the radius and the articular disc. Only during adduction of the wrist does the triquetrum come into articulation with the disc. Observe the transparent synovial folds projecting between the articular surfaces and that the pisotriquetral joint communicates with the radiocarpal joint. Note that the interosseous ligament between the scaphoid and the lunate is partly absorbed; in such a specimen, which is not uncommon, infection could spread widely.

THE INTERCARPAL JOINTS

These joints between the bones of the carpus are the *plane (gliding) type of synovial joint.*

The Articular Surfaces (Figs. 6-171, 6-176, and 6-177). These joints are between the bones of the proximal row, the bones of the distal row, and the bones of the two rows forming the transverse **midcarpal joint.** The pisiform bone rests on the palmar surface of the triquetrum forming a separate synovial joint with it, called the *pisotriquetral joint.*

Osteoarthristis of the pisotriquetral joint is particularly disabling to typists and pianists.

Movements of the Joints. Movements of the intercarpal joints occur with and increase the range of movements at the radiocarpal joint. Movement of the head of the capitate in its socket and the gliding movement of the bones on each side of it result in considerable flexion of the hand. The midcarpal joint also increases the range of abduction of the hand. Extension of the wrist joint and flexion of the intercarpal joints improve the grasp of the hand.

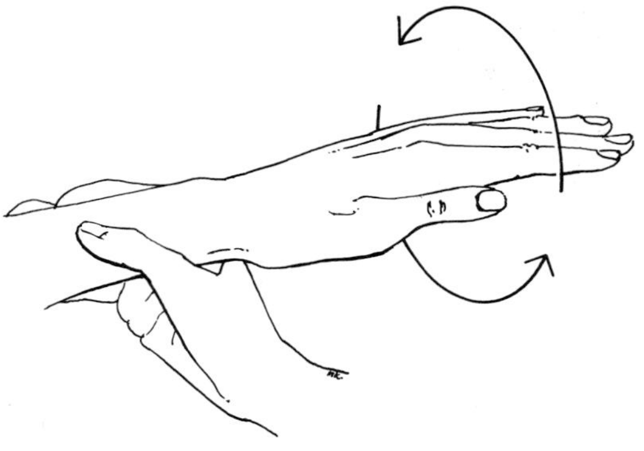

Figure 6-175. Drawing of the forearm and hand illustrating circumduction of the wrist joint. It is easier to circumduct the wrist when it is held because this prevents the movement of the forearm bones.

The Articular Capsule (Figs. 6-171, 6-172, and 6-177). *The fibrous capsule* encloses these joints and helps to unite the bones. The bones of each row are connected to each other by dorsal, palmar, and interosseous ligaments. The two rows are connected by dorsal, palmar, medial, and lateral ligaments.

The synovial capsule (Figs. 6-174 and 6-177) lines the fibrous capsule and is attached to the margins of the articular surfaces. In Figure 6-171 observe that the cavity of the midcarpal joint is part of the general joint cavity which extends between the bones of each row. The common joint space includes the bases of the metacarpal bones, where it is called the carpometacarpal and intermetacarpal joints (Fig. 6-171).

Blood Vessels (Figs. 6-108, 6-138, and 6-139). The articular arteries are derived from the palmar and dorsal carpal arches.

Nerve Supply. The articular nerves are derived from the anterior interosseous nerve of the **median**, the posterior interosseous of the **radial**, and the dorsal and deep branches of the **ulnar** nerve.

THE CARPOMETACARPAL AND INTERMETACARPAL JOINTS

These are *plane synovial joints* that permit a small amount of gliding movement. They share a common joint cavity with the intercarpal joints (Fig. 6-171). The bones are united by dorsal, palmar, and interosseous ligaments.

The Carpometacarpal Joint of the Thumb (Fig. 6-171). This is a separate *saddle type of synovial joint.*

The Articular Surfaces (Fig. 6-176). The trapezium articulates with the saddle-shaped base of the first metacarpal bone.

Movements of the Joint. This saddle joint permits angular movements in any plane and a restricted amount of axial rotation. Only ball and socket joints (*e.g.,* the shoulder articulation are more mobile. The following thumb movements are possible: **flexion** (flexor pollicis brevis and opponens pollicis), **extension** (extensor pollicis longus and brevis), **abduction** (abductor pollicis longus and brevis), **adduction** (adductor pollicis), and **opposition** (opponens pollicis). The functional importance of the thumb lies in its ability to be opposed to the fingers (Fig. 6-129).

The Articular Capsule. The **fibrous capsule** encloses the joint and is attached to the margins of the articular surfaces. The looseness of the capsule facilitates its important movement of opposition (Fig. 6-129).

The **synovial capsule** lines the fibrous capsule and forms a separate joint cavity from the rest of the carpus (Fig. 6-171).

Blood Supply (Figs. 6-108 and 6-138). The articular arteries are derived from the dorsal and palmar metacarpal arteries and from the dorsal and deep palmar arches.

Nerve Supply. The articular nerves are branches of those supplying the intercarpal joints which are derived from the anterior interosseous of the **median**, the posterior interosseous of the **radial**, and the dorsal and deep branches of the **ulnar** nerve.

THE METACARPOPHALANGEAL JOINTS

These articulations are the *condyloid (knuckle-like) type of synovial joint* that allows movement in two directions.

Articular Surfaces (Figs. 6-171 and 6-178). The heads of the metacarpal bones articulate with the bases of the proximal phalanges. The unique feature of their bony surfaces is that they both have oval articular surfaces.

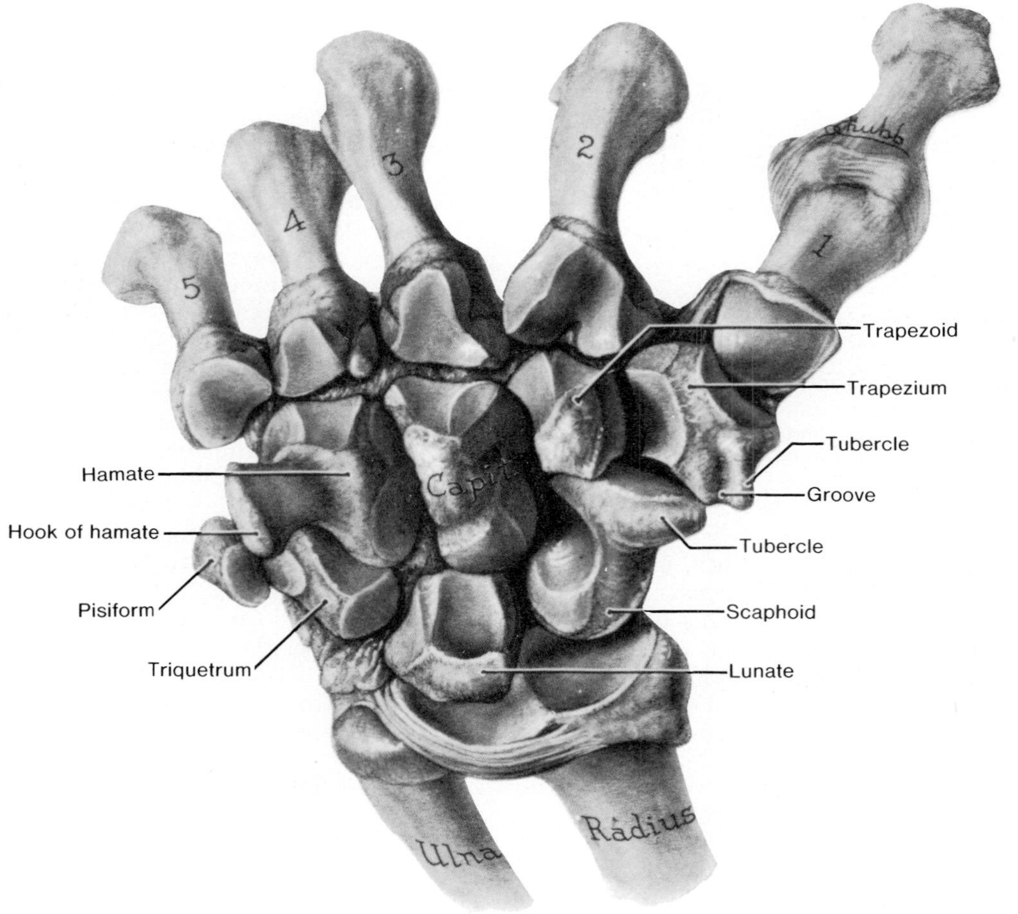

Figure 6-176. Drawing of an anterior view of the carpal bones and the bases of the metacarpal bones. Observe that the radius supports two proximal carpal bones (scaphoid and lunate) and that these in turn support three distal carpal bones (trapezium, trapezoid, and capitate) and articulate with the apex of the hamate. Note that the four distal carpals support the five metacarpals and that the capitate articulates with three metacarpals (second, third, and fourth). Observe that the second metacarpal articulates with three carpal bones (trapezium, trapezoid, and capitate).

Movements of the Joints (Fig. 6-179). The following movements occur at these articulations: flexion, extension, abduction, adduction, and circumduction. The metacarpophalangeal joint of the thumb does not allow a significant amount of abduction and adduction. These movements occur at its carpometacarpal joint.

The Articular Capsule (Fig. 6-178). The *fibrous capsule* encloses each joint and is strengthened on each side by a triangular **collateral ligament.** It extends downward and forward from the sides of the head of the proximal bone to the sides of the base of the distal bone.

The **palmar ligaments** are very strong, thick plates that are firmly attached to the phalanx and loosely to the metacarpal (Fig. 6-178). The palmar ligaments of the second to fifth joints are united by the **deep transverse metacarpal ligaments** which hold the heads of the metacarpals together (Fig. 6-133). The lumbrical muscles pass on the palmar surface of these deep transverse ligaments (Fig. 6-105) and the interossei pass posterior to them (Fig. 6-133).

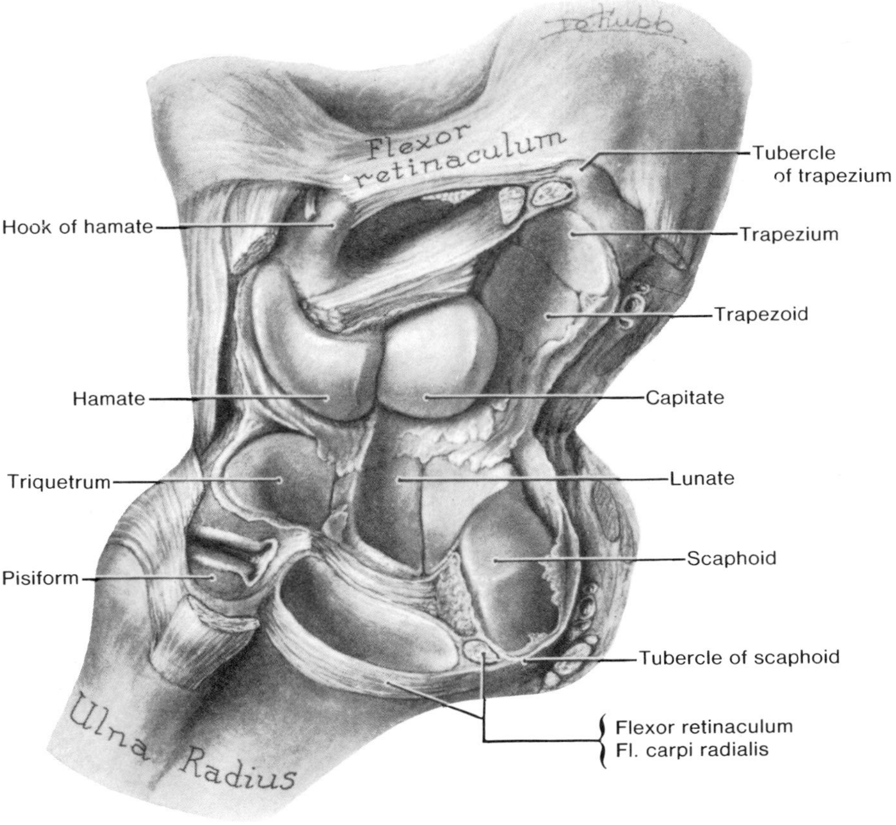

Figure 6-177. Drawing of a dissection showing the surfaces of the midcarpal joint. The flexor retinaculum has been divided and the midcarpal joint has been exposed by extending the wrist. Observe the surfaces of the opposed bones: the trapezium and trapezoid together presenting a concave, oval surface to the scaphoid; the capitate and hamate together presenting a convex surface to the scaphoid, lunate, and triquetrum which is slightly broken by the linear facet on the apex of the hamate for its counterpart on the lunate. Note the synovial folds projecting into the joint.

The *synovial capsule* lines the fibrous capsule and is attached to the margins of the articular surfaces.

Blood Supply (Figs. 6-123, 6-125, 6-138, and 6-139). The articular arteries are branches of the digital arteries arising from the superficial palmar arch.

Nerve Supply (Figs. 6-123 and 6-131). The articular nerves are derived from the digital nerves.

THE INTERPHALANGEAL JOINTS

These joints join the head of one phalanx and the base of the more distal one and are structurally similar to the metacarpophalangeal joints (Fig. 6-178). They are the **hinge type of synovial joint** which permits only flexion and extension owing to the pulley-like form of the articular surfaces. They are reinforced dorsally by the **extensor expansions** of the fingers (Fig. 6-132). The articular arteries and nerves are derived from the adjacent digital arteries and nerves (Figs. 6-123, 6-125, and 6-131).

CLINICALLY ORIENTED COMMENTS

Sudden tension on a long extensor tendon which inserts into a phalanx may

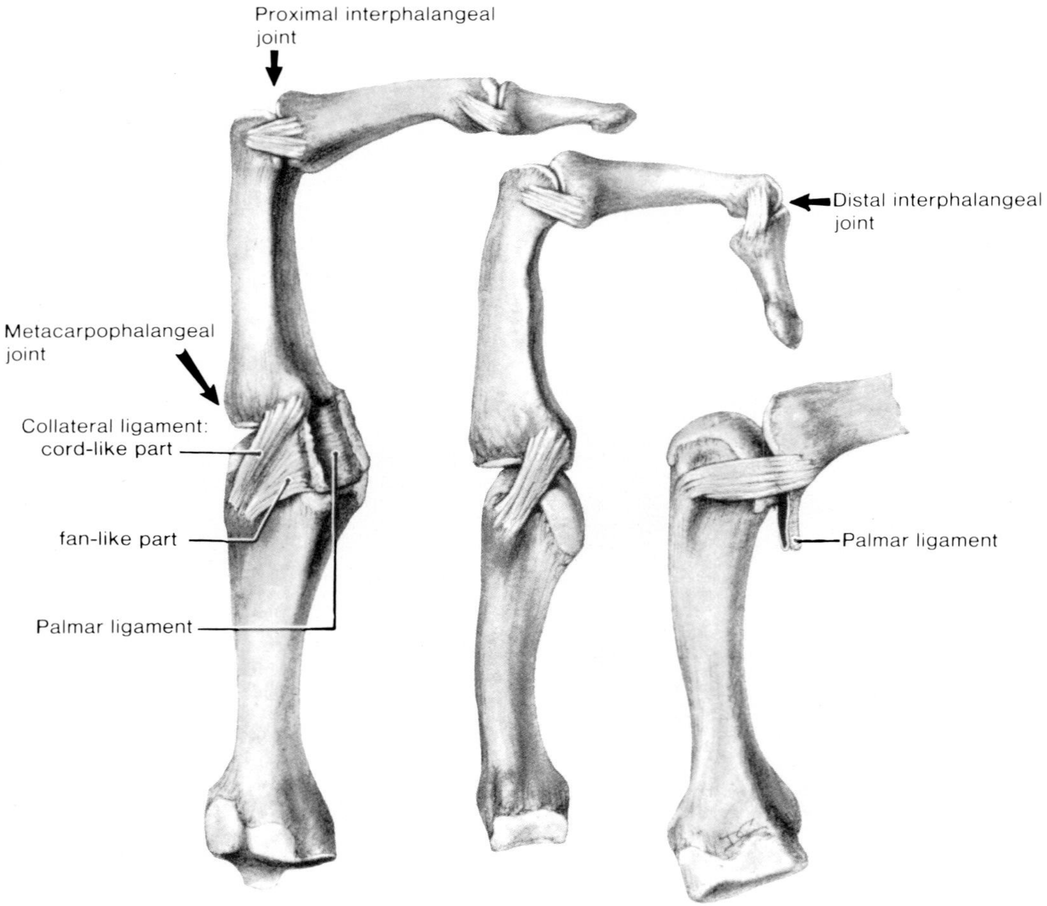

Figure 6-178. Drawings of dissections of the metacarpophalangeal and interphalangeal joints. Observe the palmar ligament, the fibrocartilaginous plate hanging from the base of the proximal phalanx. It is fixed to the head of the metacarpal by the weaker, fan-like part of the collateral ligament. The palmar ligament moves like a visor across the head of the metacarpal. The extremely strong, cord-like parts of the collateral ligaments of this joint are attached eccentrically to the metacarpal heads. These ligaments are slack during extension and taut during flexion; hence the fingers cannot be abducted unless the hand is open. Observe that the interphalangeal joints have corresponding ligaments and that the distal ends of the first and second phalanges are flattened anteroposteriorly.

avulse (strip off) part of its bony insertion. The most common type of this injury is called the **mallet finger** (baseball finger or cricket finger). The distal interphalangeal joint is suddenly forced into extreme flexion (*e.g.,* when a ball is caught improperly). This avulses part of the insertion of the long extensor tendon into the base of the distal phalanx. As a result the patient is unable to extend the distal interphalangeal joint (Fig. 6-180).

PATIENT ORIENTED PROBLEMS

Case 6-1. A 20-year-old man complained that he was unable to raise his right arm. He held it limp at his side with the palm facing backward like a waiter hinting for a tip (Fig. 6-35). During questioning he stated that he had been *thrown from his motorcycle* about 2 weeks previously and that he had hit his shoulder against a tree. He also

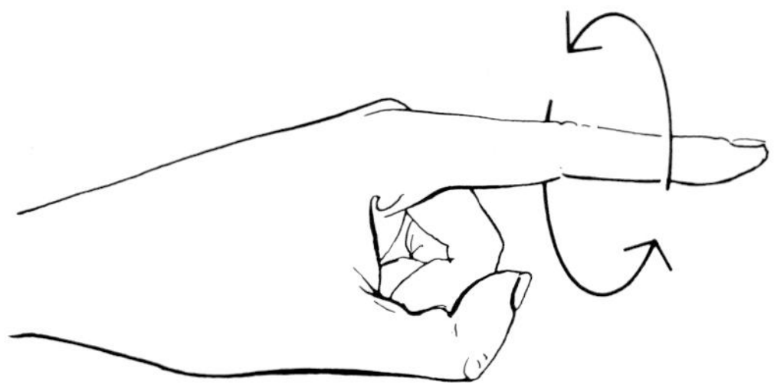

Figure 6-179. Drawing of the hand illustrating circumduction of the index finger occurring at the second metacarpophalangeal joint. Circumduction is a combination of flexion-extension and abduction-adduction. Note that a cone of movement occurs and that rotation is not a component of circumduction.

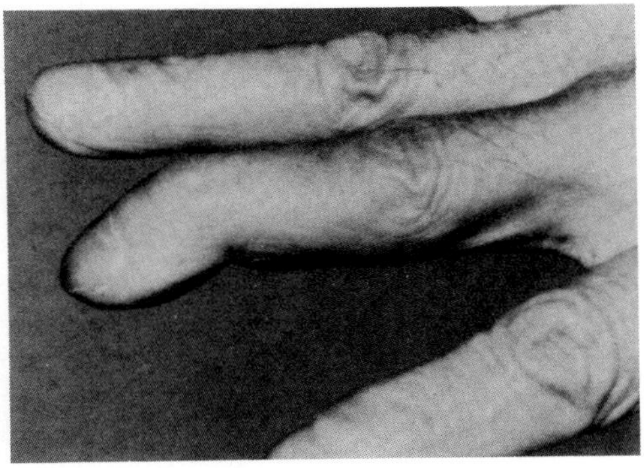

Figure 6-180. Photograph of a mallet (baseball, cricket) finger resulting from avulsion of the attachment of the long tendon of the extensor digitorum from the base of the distal phalanx of the middle finger (Fig. 6-112).

recalled that his neck felt sore shortly after the accident.

On examination it was found that he was unable to flex, abduct, or laterally rotate his arm. In addition there was *loss of flexion of the elbow* joint. A lack of sensation was detected on the lateral surface of his arm and forearm.

Problems. Using your anatomical knowledge of the nerve supply to the upper limb, discuss the probable cause of this patient's loss of motor and sensory function. What muscles are paralyzed? Is he likely to recover use of his paralyzed limb? *These problems are discussed on page 845.*

Case 6-2. A 22-year-old man sustained a *knife wound* that severely affected movements of his right upper limb. Following emergency procedures to stop the bleeding, he was given a neurological examination. Among the *principal findings* were absence of the triceps reflex, inability to extend the elbow joint, paralysis of all the extensor muscles of the forearm, **wrist-drop** (Fig. 6-181*A*), inability to extend the digits at the metacarpophalangeal joints, and weakness of extension of the interphalangeal joints. Obviously there was severe nerve damage.

Problems. What nerve has been severed? Where is the lesion located? What area of skin would you test for anesthesia? Would the presence of sensation in most of this area affect your diagnosis? *These problems are discussed on page 845.*

Case 6-3. One of your classmates injured his shoulder during an interfaculty hockey game when he was driven heavily into the boards, hitting the point of his shoulder. As you assisted him to the dressing room, you noted that his injury was very painful. When his sweater and shoulder pads were removed, you observed that the lateral end of his clavicle produced an abnormal prominence. At first you thought he may have what sports broadcasters call a "**shoulder pointer**." Later the team doctor informed you that your classmate had a dislocation of the acromioclavicular joint ("**shoulder**

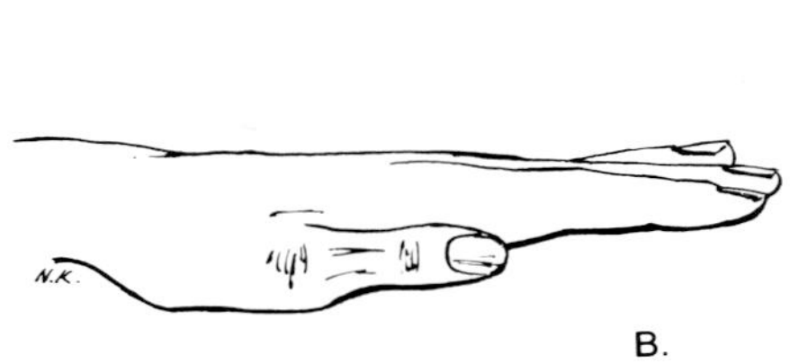

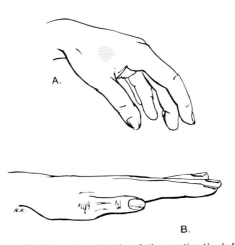

Figure 6-181. *A*, sketch of the patient's left hand showing the wrist drop and the area of sensory loss. *B*, the patient is unable to extend his wrist and fingers as shown here.

separation") and would be out of the lineup for several weeks. The engineering student who "boarded" him asked you to explain the injury.

Problems. Explain what sportswriters mean by the terms "*shoulder pointer*" and "*shoulder separation.*" How would you explain the structure of the shoulder joint to an engineering student? What ligaments would be torn? What makes the patient's shoulder fall? Why was the acromial extremity of his clavicle so prominent? *These problems are discussed on page 845.*

Case 6-4. The quarterback of your football team dropped back to pass but was "trapped" and tackled as he was attempting to throw the ball. He fell on his outstretched hand with his arm abducted. He was later helped to the sidelines holding his injured arm with his other hand. It was soon announced that he had a **dislocated shoulder.** Knowing that you are a medical student, your friends asked you to explain the quarterback's injury.

Problems. Discuss the injury in layman's terms. In your account, answer the following questions. What group of muscles is responsible for holding the head of the humerus in the glenoid cavity? Where is the weakest part of the fibrous capsule of the shoulder joint? What would be the appearance of the patient's shoulder if he had sustained an anterior dislocation? *These problems are discussed on page 846.*

Case 6-5. A 12-year-old boy fell off his skateboard, hitting his elbow on the sidewalk. Because the boy was suffering considerable elbow pain and some numbness in his hand, his mother took him to a doctor. The boy told the doctor, "I fell on my funny bone and right away my little finger began to tingle."

The doctor noted that the boy showed no response to pin-prick over the little finger and ulnar border of the palm and was unable to grip a piece of paper placed between his fingers. Suspecting a fracture of the elbow and peripheral nerve damage, the doctor arranged to have the boy's elbow radiographed. The radiographs showed a slight *separation of the epiphysis* of the medial epicondyle of the humerus.

Problems. Using your knowledge of peripheral nerves and the muscles supplied by them, explain the numbness of the boy's little finger and his inability to hold a piece of paper between his fingers. Discuss the probable injury in this case. Drawing on your knowledge of degeneration and regeneration of peripheral nerves, make an attempt to forecast the probable degree of recovery of the boy's motor and sensory functions that may occur. *These problems are discussed on page 847.*

Case 6-6. A young man who was kicked very hard in the posterior midhumeral region of his left arm presented with signs of tenderness, swelling, deformity, and abnormal movement of his left upper limb.

The physical examination revealed a **wrist-drop,** an *inability to extend the fingers* at the metacarpophalangeal joints, and loss of sensation on a small area of skin on the dorsum of the hand proximal to the thumb and index finger (Fig. 6-181*A*). There was also weakness of extension of the interphalangeal joints. Measurement of the limb indicated that there was some shortening.

Radiographs showed the presence of a **fracture of the humerus** in the midshaft, just distal to the attachment of the deltoid muscle, and that the proximal fragment of bone was abducted and the distal fragment displaced proximally (2 cm shortening).

Problems. Using your anatomical knowledge, determine what peripheral nerve has been severed and what artery may have been torn. Would elbow flexion be weakened? Explain the observed effects of this peripheral nerve injury. Why are the fragments of humerus displaced in the manner described? *These problems are discussed on page 848.*

Case 6-7. As a mother was entering a bus she lifted her 3-year-old boy up the steps by the hand (Fig. 6-169). The child immediately cried with pain and refused to use his right upper limb, which he protected by holding it with the elbow flexed and the forearm pronated.

Fearing that something must be broken, she took the child to the hospital. The intern's examination revealed a painful limitation of supination of the forearm. Radiographs of the elbow were difficult to obtain and were not helpful. On further questioning of the mother by the senior resident, she recalled jerking the child's arm as she entered the bus because he was "acting up." She thought she heard a "click" and said that it was this sound which made her think the elbow might be broken.

Recognizing the common clinical features, the resident made a diagnosis of dislocation (**subluxation**) **of the head of the radius** or, as he told the mother, *pulled elbow.* He effected an immediate cure by firm, passive supination of the forearm with the elbow flexed; no anesthesia was required. Within moments the child's pain was relieved and he soon began to use the limb again.

Problems. What is the anatomical basis of pulled elbow or transient subluxation of the radial head? Name the joint involved. What anatomical fact predisposes dislocation of the radial head in children under 7 years? *These problems are discussed on page 849.*

Case 6-8. A 14-year-old boy fell and cut his forearm on a large sliver of glass. He was rushed to the emergency department with a deep penetrating cut on the posterolateral aspect of his right forearm, just distal to the neck of the radius (Fig. 6-182).

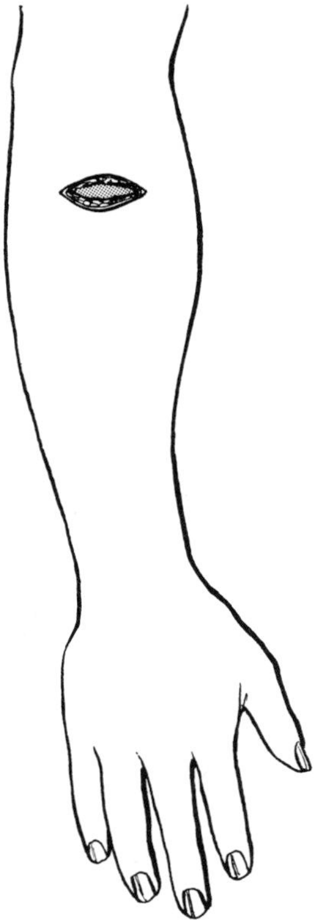

Figure 6-182. Sketch of the boy's right upper limb to show the site of the wound.

The significant *clinical findings* included inability to extend the thumb and the metacarpophalangeal joints of the fingers, impairment of abduction of the thumb, normal opposition of the thumb and supination of the forearm, and no loss of sensation.

Problems. What peripheral nerve was severed? Explain the anatomical basis of the boy's disabilities, mentioning the muscles affected. Would wrist extension and adduction be normal? *These problems are discussed on page 849.*

Case 6-9. While you were playing touch football, you fell on your open hand with the wrist dorsiflexed and radially deviated. You told your friends that you had just sprained your wrist and did not pay much attention to the injury for about 2 weeks. You sought medical advice then because the wrist pain was still present.

When the doctor deeply palpated your "snuff box," there was localized tenderness. You experienced most pain on the radial side of your wrist, particularly when he asked you to dorsiflex it. Suspecting a fracture, he took radiographs of your wrist which revealed a small **hairline fracture** of one of the carpal bones.

Problems. Which carpal bones lie in the floor of the anatomical snuff box? The distal end of which forearm bone is in the floor of this depression? Which of the carpal bones was most likely fractured? *These problems are discussed on page 850.*

Case 6-10. A 15-year-old girl was rushed to the emergency room of a hospital while you were visiting the chief resident. The girl had *slashed her wrists* with a razor blade, proximal to the flexor retinaculum. The moderate bleeding from the left wrist was soon stopped with slight pressure. The small spurts of blood coming from the radial side of the right wrist were more difficult to stop. Examination of her left hand and wrist revealed that her hand movements were normal and that there was no anesthesia (loss of sensation).

The following observations were made on her right wrist and hand: two superficial tendons and a large midline nerve were cut; she could adduct her thumb but was unable to oppose it; she had lost some fine control of the movements of her second and third digits; and there was anesthesia over the lateral half of her palm and digits.

Problems. Which tendon was almost certainly severed? What nerve was cut? Which tendon may have been severed? What superficial artery appears to have been lacerated? Would flexion of her wrist be affected? Discuss the anatomical basis of the clinical findings. *These problems are discussed on page 850.*

Case 6-11. An elderly lady who was walking in front of you slipped on a patch of ice and *fell on the palm of her outstretched hand.* She told you that she heard her wrist crack and that it was very sore. As you helped her to her feet, you noticed that the dorsal aspect of her wrist was unduly prominent and resembled a dinner fork.

In view of these signs and symptoms, you decided to take her to a nearby doctor. When you informed the doctor that you were a first year medical student, he explained that the appearance of her wrist was typical of this kind of fracture and described it as a **"dinner fork" deformity.** He presented you with the following questions.

Problems. What bone in the forearm or wrist is commonly fractured in persons over the age of 50, particularly women? What do you call this kind of fracture? Explain the cause of the dinner fork appearance of the patient's wrist. *These problems are discussed on page 852.*

Case 6-12. A patient reported to her doctor that she had detected a *lump in her breast* several months ago but fearing that it was cancer had delayed doing anything about it.

Inspection revealed localized retraction of skin in the superolateral quadrant of the left breast and the skin in this area was finely dimpled like an orange peel (referred to clinically as *peau d'orange*).

Palpation revealed a hard mass in the superolateral quadrant that was attached to the skin and to the tissues deep to it. The skin over the mass had a leathery feel and a group of enlarged lymph nodes was felt in the axilla.

Xeromammograms revealed a jagged, rounded density in the breast and that the skin overlying the mass was thickened (Fig. 6-183). A diagnosis of **breast cancer** (carcinoma of the breast) was made.

Problems. Name the deep structure to

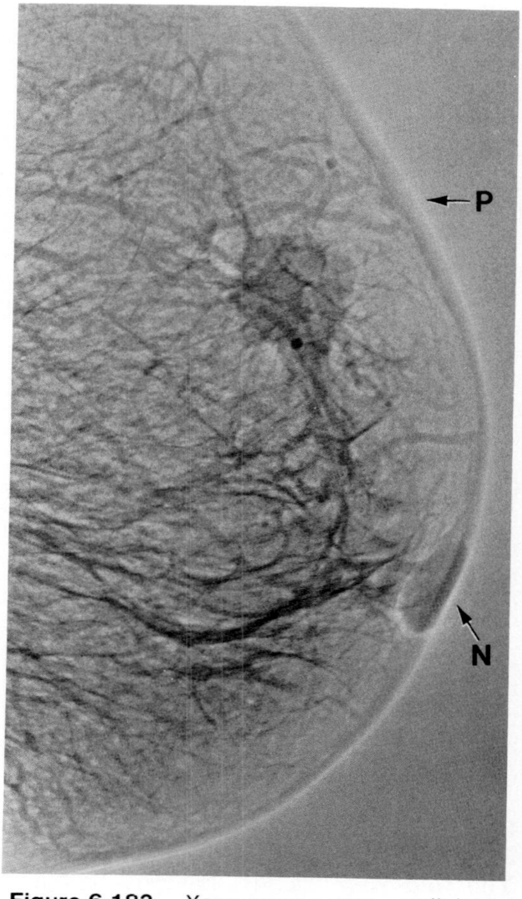

Figure 6-183. Xeromammogram, mediolateral projection. The carcinoma appears as a jagged, rounded density. Note the overlying skin thickening (*P*, peau d'orange) secondary to impaired lymph drainage. The jagged appearance of the cancer resulted from the infiltration of malignant cells along the suspensory ligaments and the lymphatics. *N* indicates the nipple.

which the tumor would be fixed. What probably caused the leathery thickening of the skin over the tumor? Explain the anatomical basis of the skin retraction. Based on your anatomical knowledge, where do you think the most common sites for metastases from a carcinoma of the breast would be? Which group of lymph nodes would be primarily involved in the present case? What other nodes might be involved? *These problems are discussed on page 852.*

DISCUSSION OF PATIENT ORIENTED PROBLEMS

Case 6-1. When the patient was thrown from his motorcycle and hit a tree, his right shoulder was pulled violently away from his head (Fig. 6-33). This pulled on the upper trunk of the brachial plexus (Fig. 6-26), stretching or tearing the ventral primary rami of cervical nerves 5 and 6 and may have pulled some rootlets out of the spinal cord (Fig. 5-57). As a result, the nerves arising from these rami and the upper trunk are affected and the muscles supplied by them are paralyzed. The muscles involved are the deltoid, biceps, brachialis, brachioradialis, supraspinatus, infraspinatus, teres minor, and supinator (Figs. 6-28 and 6-30).

The patient's arm was medially rotated because the infraspinatus and teres minor muscles (lateral rotators of the shoulder) were paralyzed. His forearm was pronated because the supinators were paralyzed, notably the biceps. Flexion of his elbow was weak because of paralysis of the brachialis and biceps muscles. The inability of the patient to flex his shoulder resulted from paralysis of the deltoid and coracobrachialis muscles and probably the clavicular head of the pectoralis major muscle. Loss of abduction of the shoulder resulted from paralysis of the supraspinatus and deltoid muscles.

The paralysis will be permanent if the rootlets making up the rami (C5 and C6) have undergone **avulsion** (*i.e.,* pulled out of the spinal cord). As these rootlets cannot presently be sutured back into the cord, the axons of the nerves will not regenerate and the muscles supplied by them will soon undergo **atrophy** (wasting). Movements of the shoulder and elbow will be greatly affected, *e.g.,* the patient will always have difficulty lifting a glass to his mouth with his right arm. The *loss of sensation in his arm* resulted from damage to sensory fibers of C5 and C6 that are conveyed in the upper lateral cutaneous nerve of the arm (from axillary), the lower lateral cutaneous nerve of the arm (from radial), and the lateral cutaneous nerve of the forearm (from musculocutaneous). (See Figs. 4-160, 6-102 and 6-104.)

Case 6-2. The radial nerve has been severed in the axilla close to its orgin from the brachial plexus because all heads of the triceps muscle are paralyzed, as indicated by absence of the **triceps reflex.** The radial nerve is seldom injured in the axilla; however, it is often damaged where it passes obliquely across the posterior aspect of the humerus in the **radial groove.**

Following injury to the radial nerve in the axilla, there should be loss of sensation on the posterior surface of the lower part of the arm, along a narrow strip on the back of the forearm, on the dorsum of the hand, and on the base of the thumb. However, because of the overlapping of the areas of distribution of the cutaneous nerves, the area of impaired sensation may be surprisingly small (Fig. 6-181*A*). Often the only area of total anesthesia is on the dorsal surface of the hand between the bases of the first and second metacarpals. Even the absence of anesthesia in this area is not necessarily indicative of an intact nerve because other nerves may be supplying the same area of skin.

Case 6-3. A "shoulder pointer" is a sportswriter's term for a contusion over the "point of the shoulder," *i.e.,* over the bony prominence of the acromion of the scapula.

To explain a "shoulder separation," first you should make a simple diagram of the scapula and the clavicle, showing the ligaments attaching these bones together (Fig. 6-145). Emphasize that it is the **coracoclavicular ligament** which provides most stability to the acromioclavicular joint. You should explain that the scapula and clavicle are parts of the upper limb and make up what is called the **pectoral girdle,** and that the clavicle articulates laterally with the acromion of the scapula to form the acromioclavicular joint. Emphasize that this joint is not the shoulder joint.

Explain that the scapula and clavicle are held together by the acromioclavicular and the coracoclavicular ligaments (Fig. 6-146). Point out that the coracoclavicular is the stronger of these ligaments.

In discussing your classmate's injury, you should explain that when he hit the boards with the "point of his shoulder" (acromion of the scapula), the acromioclavicular and coracoclavicular ligaments were torn (Fig. 6-184). As a result, the shoulder fell under the weight of the upper limb and the acromion was pulled inferiorly relative to the clavicle. Also the lateral end of the clavicle was displaced upward relative to the acromion and so produced an obvious prominence.

Make it clear that the expression "**separation of the shoulder**" is a misnomer by explaining that it is the acromioclavicular joint that is separated, not the shoulder joint. Rupture of the acromioclavicular ligament alone is not a serious injury, but when combined with rupture of the corcoclavicular ligament, the dislocation is complicated because the scapula and the clavicle are separated and the scapula and arm are displaced downward.

Case 6-4. First you should make a simple diagram of the shoulder joint (similar to Fig. 6-143), pointing out the relationship of the humerus and the scapula to each other. You should then explain that the shoulder (glenohumeral) joint is a very mobile ball and socket joint that permits a greater range of movement than any other joint in the body. In addition, the articular surface of the glenoid cavity of the scapula is smaller than the head of the humerus. Use your fist and cupped hand to illustrate this. Explain that to acquire this mobility, the fibrous capsule of the joint is relatively loose, particularly inferiorly. Point out that the capsule is reinforced by four **rotator cuff muscles** (supraspinatus, infraspinatus, teres minor, and subscapularis) and that it is weakest inferiorly where it is not supported by these muscles. Emphasize that the main stability of the shoulder joint and the normal relationship of the head of the humerus to the glenoid cavity is maintained by the rotator cuff muscle tendons which fuse with the fibrous capsule of the joint.

Using your fist and cupped hand, illustrate that when the quarterback fell on his outstretched hand with his arm abducted, the head of the humerus was driven infe-

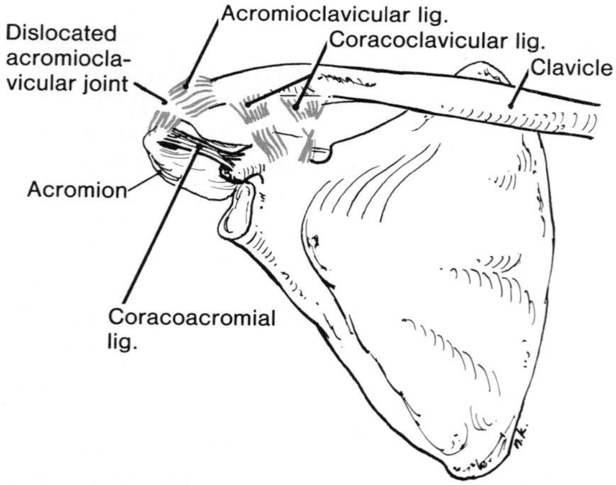

Figure 6-184. Diagram illustrating dislocation of the acromioclavicular joint ("separation of shoulder"), following tearing of the acromioclavicular and coracoclavicular ligaments. Obviously rupture of these ligaments will result in the clavicle slipping above the acromion. It will also be pulled posteriorly by the trapezius muscle.

riorly out of the glenoid cavity and came to lie below it. Describe why the patient's shoulder would appear square (*i.e.,* lose its normal round contour) when the head of the humerus was dislocated. Explain that during this process the inferior part of the capsule was torn and the associated muscles were stretched or torn. Mention that the inferior rim of the glenoidal labrum is often detached, which may lead to recurrent dislocation. You could also tell your friends that a shoulder dislocation may *stretch the axillary nerve*, resulting in partial or complete paralysis of the deltoid muscle, and that this would affect abduction of the arm. You should emphasize that dislocation of the shoulder is not what the sports writers call a "shoulder separation" (see Case 6-3).

Case 6-5. The ossifying medial epicondyle of the humerus is extracapsular and does not completely fuse with the side of the diaphysis until the 20th year (Fig. 6-185). Although an epiphyseal separation is sometimes called "an epiphyseal fracture" or a fracture-dislocation, it is best to refer to this injury as a **separation of the epiphysis** for the medial epicondyle (Fig. 6-185). Had this accident occurred in a person over 20, a fracture of the medial epicondyle might have occurred. Because the epiphyseal cartilage plate is weaker than the surrounding bone in children and adolescents, a direct blow that causes a fracture or a ligamentous tear in adults is likely to cause an **epiphyseal cartilage plate injury** in children.

As the ulnar nerve passes posterior to the medial epicondyle (Fig. 6-72), between it and the olecranon process of the ulna, it is particularly vulnerable to injuries at the elbow. In the present case it is likely that the ulnar nerve was crushed and that the axons were damaged at the site of the injury; however, the connective tissue sheaths (endoneurial tubes) and **neurolemmal sheaths** (of Schwann) probably remained intact. This kind of injury causes paralysis of muscles and some loss of sensation in the area of skin supplied by the ulnar nerve (Fig. 6-29).

Appreciation of light touch is usually lost over the medial one and one-half fingers in front and behind and response to pin-prick is lost over the little finger and ulnar border of the palm. Undoubtedly it was these sensory changes that first suggested ulnar nerve injury to the doctor. Knowing that the interosseus muscles are supplied by the ulnar nerve, he probably decided to test them for weakness by placing a piece of paper between the boy's fully extended fingers and asking him to grip it as tightly as possible while he pulled on it (Fig. 6-186). *Inability to adduct the medial four digits* is a classic sign of paralysis of the palmar interosseous muscles and of ulnar nerve damage.

Had the doctor tested other movements he would likely have detected inability to abduct the medial four digits (paralysis of

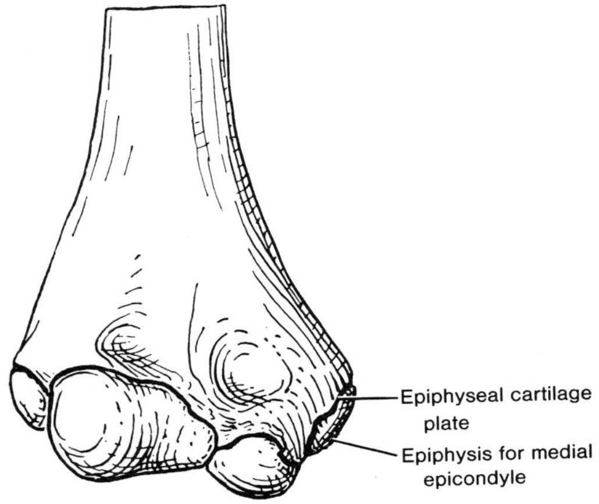

Figure 6-185. Anterior view of the distal end of the humerus of a child showing the epiphysis for the medial epicondyle. It appears about the 6th year and does not fuse with the diaphysis of the humerus until about the 20th year.

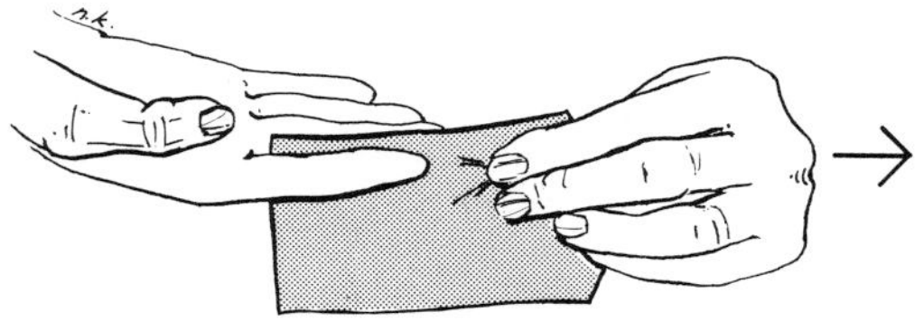

Figure 6-186. Demonstration of the test for determining weakness of the interosseous muscles. The examiner is attempting to pull the paper away from the patient in the direction of the *arrow.*

the dorsal interossei), loss of adduction of the thumb (paralysis of the adductor pollicis), weakness of flexion of the ring and little fingers at the metacarpophalangeal joints (paralysis of the medial two lumbricals), impaired flexion and adduction of the wrist (paralysis of the flexor carpi ulnaris), and a poor grasp in the ring and little fingers and inability to flex the distal interphalangeal joints of the fourth and fifth digits (paralysis of the lumbricals, the interossei, and the part of the flexor digitorum profundus supplying these fingers).

Because all but five of the intrinsic muscles of the hand are supplied by the ulnar nerve, lesions of it at the elbow or wrist have their primary effect in the hand. As the nerve was only crushed, the nerve does not require suturing since new axons can grow down into the part of the nerve distal to the injury within the original endoneurial tubes and neurolemmal sheaths and reinnervate the paralyzed muscles. Hence after a crush injury, as in this case, restoration of function should occur in a few months' time with proper physiotherapy.

Case 6-6. The inability of the patient to extend his hand at the wrist indicates **damage to the radial nerve** proximal to the elbow. As the fracture is in the midshaft of the humerus, it is likely the radial nerve was damaged where it passes diagonally across the back of the humerus in the radial groove (Fig. 6-187). The nerve is particularly susceptible to injury in this location because of its close relationship to the humeral shaft.

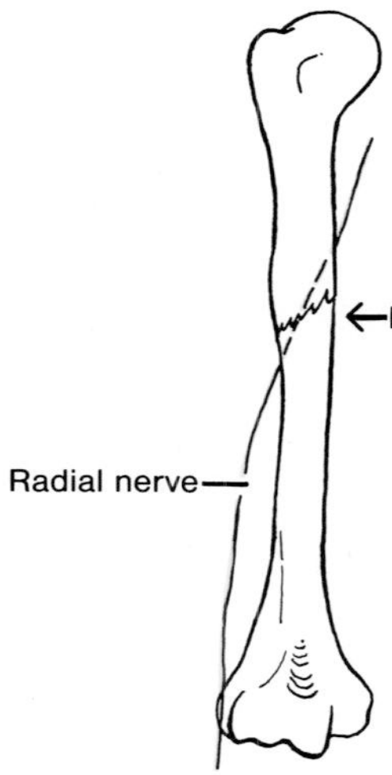

Figure 6-187. Drawing of the anterior aspect of the right humerus showing the radial nerve passing obliquely downward across the back of the humerus in the radial groove. Because of its close relationship to this bone (Fig. 6-74), it may be severed by the bone fragments. The profunda brachii artery, a branch of the brachial, which follows the radial nerve closely along the radial groove, may also be torn by the fragments of bone.

Severing the radial nerve totally paralyzes the extensor muscles of the forearm and hand. As a result, extension of the wrist is impossible and the hand assumes the flexed position referred to clinically as **wrist-drop** (Fig. 6-181*A*). The radial nerve supplies no muscles in the hand but it supplies muscles whose tendons pass into the hand; hence, he cannot extend his metacarpophalangeal joints.

Because the lumbricals (supplied by the median and ulnar nerves) and the interossei (supplied by the ulnar nerve) are intact, the patient is able to flex his metacarpophalangeal joints and extend his interphalangeal joints; however, he would not have normal power of extension of his fingers. Elbow flexion would be very painful and would be weakened when the forearm is in the position midway between pronation and supination. Recall that the radial nerve innervates the brachioradialis muscle, a strong flexor of the elbow in this position.

The area of sensory loss is often minimal following radial nerve injury (Fig. 6-181*A*) because its area of exclusive supply is very small. The degree of sensory loss varies from patient to patient, depending on the extent to which the territory is overlapped by adjacent nerves. Sometimes there may be no detectable loss of sensation. Recall that the radial nerve arises from the posterior cord of the **brachial plexus** (C5 to C8 and T1) and is the largest branch of this plexus (Figs. 4-160 and 6-30).

The shortening of the patient's arm occurs because the broken fragments of bone are pulled apart. Contraction of the deltoid muscle abducts the proximal part of the humerus and the upward pull of the triceps, biceps, and coracobrachialis muscles pulls the distal fragment superiorly.

Although the profunda brachii artery accompanies the radial nerve through the radial groove (Fig. 6-78) and may be severed by bone fragments, the muscles and structures supplied by this artery (*e.g.,* the humerus) are not likely to show **ischemia** (deficiency of blood) because the radial recurrent artery anastomoses with the profunda brachii artery (Fig. 6-74). This communication should provide sufficient blood for the structures supplied by the damaged artery. This is one reason why the **anastomoses around the elbow** joint are so important clinically.

Case 6-7. The head of the radius fits into the radial notch of the ulna, forming the proximal radioulnar joint (Fig. 6-188). A strong fibrous anular ligament almost completely encircles the head of the radius, forming a U-shaped collar that holds it in contact with the radial notch of the ulna. The **anular ligament** is funnel-shaped, particularly in adults, being of a smaller circumference below than above (Fig. 6-168).

In children under the age of 7, the head of the radius is relatively smaller than in the adult and so the grip of the anular ligament is not so firm as in later life. In addition the capsule is lax and its distal attachment to the radius is thin and weak.

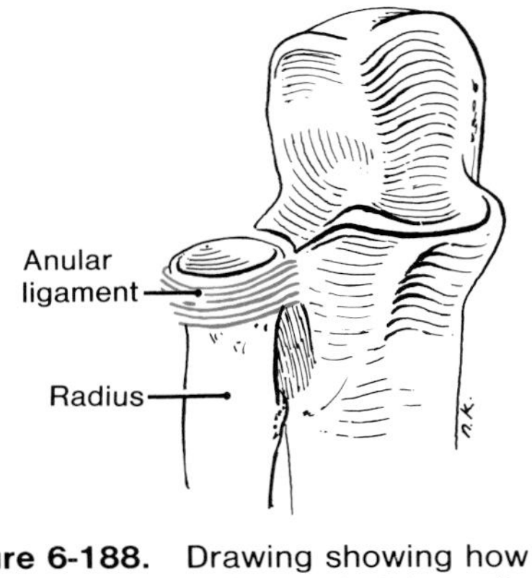

Figure 6-188. Drawing showing how the anular ligament holds the head of the radius against the radial notch of the ulna, thereby forming a pivot joint. Note that the head of the radius in children is only slightly larger than the neck of the radius.

The sudden pulling of the child's limb upward when the elbow joint was fully extended (Fig. 6-169) tore the anular ligament near its attachment to the radial neck. Then the small radial head pulled distally partially through this tear, out of the grasp of the ligament. This type of dislocation may also occur when a child is picked up by both hands and swung around in a circle or pulled by the legs when it is holding onto something (*e.g.,* the monkey bars).

Supination of the forearm with the elbow flexed reduces the dislocation and inserts the radial head into the collar-like anular ligament and in contact with the radial notch of the ulna (Fig. 6-80). This is achieved relatively easily in these cases because the head of the radius is not pulled completely out of the ligament. It is important to understand the *anatomical basis of subluxation of the radial head* and of its reduction, so you can explain the mechanism of its production to the parent in order to minimize the risk of recurrence of this injury.

Case 6-8. The site of the penetrating wound suggests that the **deep branch of the radial** nerve has been cut as it passes posteroinferiorly through the supinator muscle (Fig. 6-189). Having deduced this, you know that the nerve supply to the extensor carpi radialis longus is intact because its nerve arises from the radial before it divides into its two terminal branches (superficial and deep). In addition, because the nerves to the supinator and the extensor carpi radialis brevis usually arise from the deep branch before it enters the supinator, the nerve supply to these muscles has not been interrupted. Recall that when the deep branch emerges from the supinator muscle it is called the **posterior interosseous nerve.** Hence, all muscles supplied by it are paralyzed.

As this is a motor and articular nerve, there is no loss of sensation (**anesthesia**). However, the extensor digitorum, extensor digiti minimi, extensor carpi ulnaris, and all the outcropping muscles have been denervated. Abduction of the thumb is weakened but not lost because the abductor pollicis brevis is supplied by the recurrent branch of the median nerve. This muscle can ab-

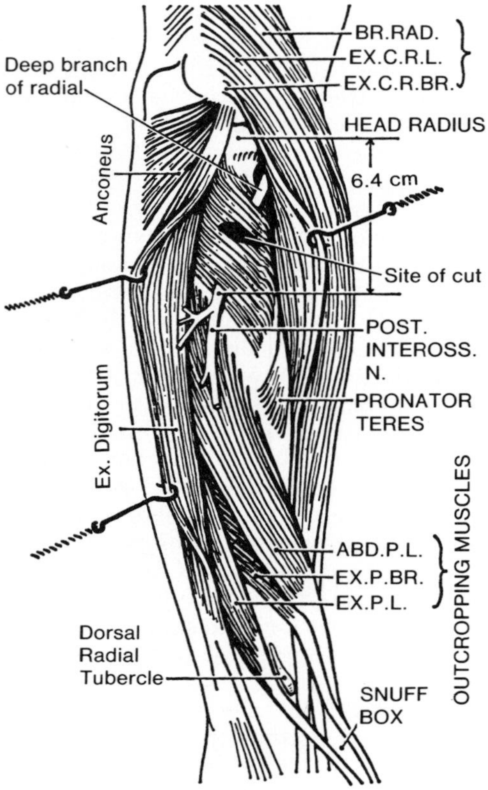

Figure 6-189. An exposure of the deep structures on the posterior aspect of the right forearm showing the site of the cut and where the deep branch of the radial nerve was cut. Refer to Figure 6-182 as you study this illustration and the site of the deep cut.

duct the thumb effectively, although weakness of this movement can be demonstrated with resisted or repeated abduction.

The patient can oppose his thumb because the thenar muscles (supplied by the median nerve) and adductor pollicis (supplied by the ulnar nerve) are functional. He cannot extend the metacarpophalangeal joints of his fingers, however, because his extensor digitorum and extensor indicis muscles are paralyzed. He would have some ability to extend the interphalangeal joints of his fingers because of his intact lumbrical muscles (supplied by the median and ulnar nerves). His wrist extension is weak because of paralysis of the superficial and deep extensors. Owing to paralysis of his extensor carpi ulnaris, adduction of his wrist would also be weakened. Although this movement can be produced by his intact flexor carpi ulnaris muscle (supplied by the ulnar nerve), adduction of the wrist is not normal.

Case 6-9. The two lateral marginal bones of the carpus (scaphoid and trapezium) lie in the floor of the anatomical snuff box (Fig. 6-110). This depression at the base of the thumb is limited proximally by the styloid process of the radius and distally by the base of the first metacarpal bone.

In Figure 6-190, observe the **fracture of the scaphoid** near the middle or "waist" of the bone, producing two fragments. This is the *most common type of carpal injury* and usually results from a fall on the hand, as in the present case. Because of the position of the scaphoid and its small size, it is a difficult bone to immobilize. Continued movement of the wrist often results in nonunion of the fragments. Often there is displacement and tearing of ligaments which may interfere with the blood supply to one of the fragments. **Ischemic necrosis** (death) of part of the bone may result. Usually the bone is supplied by two nutrient arteries, one to the proximal and one to the distal half. Occasionally both vessels supply the distal half so that the separated proximal half receives no blood. The resulting **ischemia** (poor blood supply) may result in delay or lack of union of the fragments.

The *characteristic clinical sign* of this fracture, as in this case, is acute tenderness in the anatomical snuff box, particularly when the wrist is dorsiflexed.

Case 6-10. Obviously the patient had not cut her wrist deeply on the left side; the slight bleeding was probably from severed superficial veins. On the right side, she would have certainly cut the tendon of the palmaris longus, if it was present (Fig. 6-93). She probably also cut the tendon of her flexor carpi radialis muscle.

In view of the clinical findings, it is obvious that her **median nerve** was also severed. At the wrist this nerve lies deep and lateral to the tendon of the palmaris longus muscle, just before it passes deep to the flexor retinaculum and enters the carpal tunnel (Figs. 6-90 to 6-93).

The slight spurting of blood in the right wrist suggests she probably cut the **superficial palmar branch** of her radial artery. This artery arises from the radial just proximal to the wrist. It passes through, occasionally over, the thenar muscles. Had she severed her radial artery, the bleeding would have been severe.

Cutting the median nerve at her wrist resulted in paralysis of the thenar muscles and the first two lumbricals. **Paralysis of the thenar muscles** explains the girl's inability to oppose her thumb. As the posterior interosseus nerve was not affected, she could abduct her thumb using her abductor pollicis longus, but there would be some impairment of this movement owing to paralysis of the abductor pollicis brevis. She could extend her thumb normally using her extensor pollicis longus and brevis muscles. As the nerve supply to her adductor pollicis muscle (deep branch of ulnar) is intact, she can also adduct her thumb. Because of the **paralysis of her first two lumbricals** and the loss of sensation over her thumb and adjacent two and one-half fingers and the radial two-thirds of her palm, fine control of movements of her second and third digits is lacking. Thus, by cutting her median nerve, this girl produced a serious disability of her right hand.

In a few weeks there will likely be atrophy (wasting) of the thenar region. Because of atrophy of these muscles and the action of her intact adductor pollicis muscle, her thumb will be held close to the base of the lateral surface of her index finger. Her index and middle fingers will probably be hyperextended at the metacarpophalangeal joints and slightly flexed at the interphalangeal joints owing to the paralysis of her first two lumbrical muscles.

Atrophy of the thenar muscles gives a characteristic flattening of the thenar region producing a deformity often referred to as "**ape hand.**"

The cutting of the tendons of the palmaris longus and flexor carpi radialis would also weaken flexion of her wrist. In addition, if she attempted to flex her wrist, her hand would be pulled to the ulnar side by the flexor carpi ulnaris (supplied by the ulnar nerve).

When the median nerve is severed at the

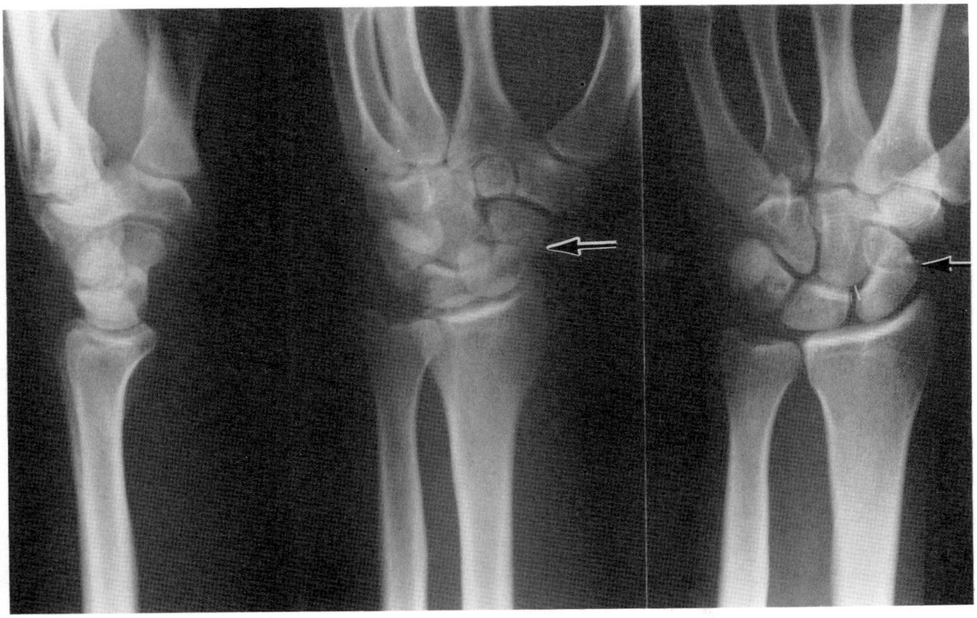

Figure 6-190. *Left to right,* lateral, oblique, and frontal radiographs of the left wrist showing a fracture of the scaphoid bone (*arrows*). In the frontal projection observe that there is some displacement of the distal fragment.

wrist, the anesthetic area covers the lateral portion of the palm, the palmar surface of the thumb, and the lateral two and one-half fingers, and extends onto the dorsal surface of these fingers (Fig. 6-29). Obviously the cut ends of the tendons and the median nerve would have to be brought together and fastened by sutures or held together by some other means. After a considerable time, function should be partially restored.

Case 6-11. The common injury of the forearm in elderly persons, particularly women, is fracture of the distal end of the radius, known as a **Colles' fracture** (Fig. 6-191). The doctor radiographed her wrist and showed you how the distal fragments of the radius had tilted posteriorly producing the "**dinner fork**" **deformity** of her wrist (Fig. 6-191*A*). The distal ends of the ulna and radius are at the same level (Fig. 6-191*C*), instead of the radial styloid being more distal than the ulnar styloid as is normal (Figs. 6-80 and 6-191*D*). There is also some degree of subluxation (dislocation) of the distal radioulnar joint.

The doctor asked you to stay while he reduced the fracture by manipulation and applied a plaster cast to hold the bone fragments in the correct position while the bone healed.

Case 6-12. Many carcinomas of the breast occur in the superolateral (upper and lateral) quadrant of the breast, which includes the axillary tail. In advanced cases the tumor is fixed to the **pectoralis fascia.** Interference with the lymphatic drainage of the breast very probably produced the leathery thickening and orange-peel appearance of the skin over the malignant tumor (**neoplasm**). The retraction of the skin is mainly caused by infiltration of cancer cells along the suspensory ligaments of the breast. This shortens the ligaments and causes them to invaginate or retract the skin.

The most common sites for metastases from a carcinoma of the breast are the axillary lymph nodes. Lymph vessels from the superolateral quadrant of the breast, the site of the tumor in the present case, mainly drain to the anterior or **pectoral group of axillary lymph nodes** (Fig. 6-47). It is very probable that the subscapular group of lymph nodes would also be in-

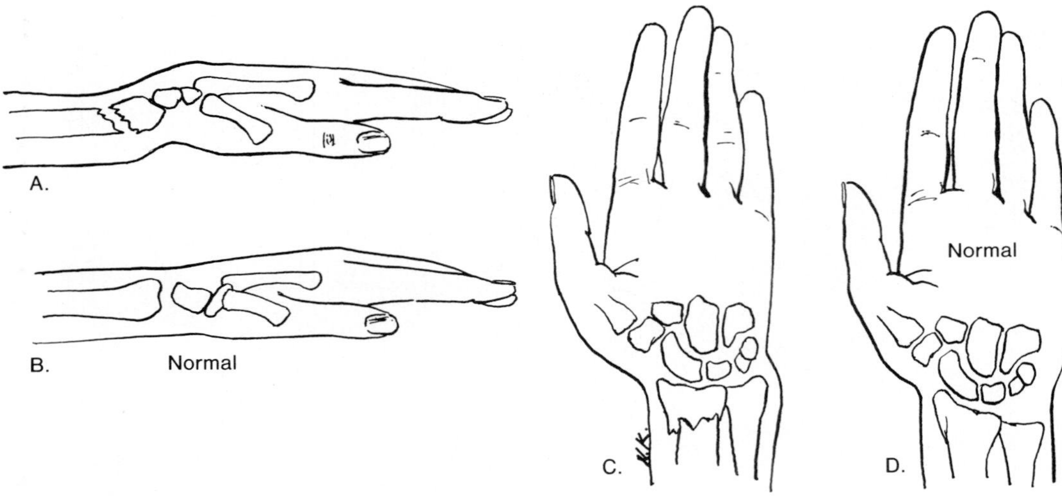

Figure 6-191. *A,* drawing of the patient's wrist showing an obvious jog just proximal to the wrist, producing the typical "dinner fork" deformity. This abnormality results from fracture of the distal end of the radius and posterior tilting of the distal fragment. Often the hand tends to be radially deviated owing to shortening of the radius. *B,* schematic drawing showing the normal position of the radius and carpal bones. *C,* anterior view of the wrist before reduction of the fracture. Note that the distal ends of the radius and ulna are at the same level. *D,* during reduction of the radial fracture, the shortening was corrected by placing the displaced fragment in its correct position. Observe that the radial styloid is now distal to the ulnar styloid.

volved. Although the metastatic spread of cancer cells would most likely be as described, it is possible for any group of axillary lymph nodes to be involved (Fig. 6-10). As lymph from the breast drains superiorly to the supraclavicular nodes, toward the other breast, to the parasternal lymph nodes, deep into the thorax, and inferiorly to the anterior abdominal wall, cancer cells may be carried to lymph nodes in any of these areas. *Cancer cells can also spread via the blood;* blood borne metastases may occur in the ovaries, the adrenal glands, the pituitary, the lungs, and the vertebral column.

SUGGESTIONS FOR ADDITIONAL READING

1. Anson, B. J., and McVay, C. B. *Surgical Anatomy,* Ed. 5, W. B. Saunders Co., Philadelphia, 1971.

   Anatomy is used in this book as the groundwork for surgical techniques. The rationale for operations, rather than the detailed steps of surgery, is stressed. Descriptions are given of common variations in the attachment of muscles, in the origin and branching of arteries, in the pattern of anastomosis and termination of veins, and in the course and relationship of nerves.

2. Ellis, H. *Clinical Anatomy. A Revision and Applied Anatomy for Clinical Students,* Blackwell Scientific Publications, Oxford, 1960.

   This classic book integrates the anatomy that is learned in the dissecting laboratory with that used on the wards and in the operating theaters. It highlights features of anatomy which are of clinical importance in medicine and surgery and gives practical applications to illustrate how clinical phenomena can be understood and remembered on simple anatomical grounds.

3. Haymaker, W., and Woodhall, B. *Peripheral Nerve Injuries. Principles and Diagnosis,* Ed. 2, W. B. Saunders Co., Philadelphia, 1953.

   This unique monograph deals in a terse manner with the fundamentals of diagnosis of peripheral nerve injuries. It contains good descriptions and excellent illustrations of the methods used in the assessment of muscle function in the upper limb and in other regions. It contains many photographs of patients who sustained nerve injuries during World War II and in the Korean conflict. Aids to the investigation of peripheral nerve injuries and characteristic clinical features of nerve injuries in the upper limb are clearly presented.

4. Healey, J. E. *A Synopsis of Clinical Anatomy,* W. B. Saunders Co., Philadelphia, 1969.

   This book presents many clinical applications of gross anatomy. The essential anatomy of each region is presented before clinical considerations are discussed, using very good illustrations. For example, the various surgical approaches for exposing the humeral head, neck, tubercles, and shaft for the open reduction of fractures are well described and illustrated, and the anatomical bases of the techniques are explained.

5. Salter, R. B. *Textbook of Disorders and Injuries of the Musculoskeletal System.* The Williams & Wilkins Company, Baltimore, 1970.

   This textbook was written especially for undergraduate medical students as an introduction to orthopaedics, rheumatology, metabolic bone disease, rehabilitation, and fractures. Many of the clinically oriented comments in the present chapter are based on clinical material in this book; hence, it should be consulted for additional information.

CHAPTER 7

The Head

Few complaints are more common than **headache** and **head pain**. The term headache is used to describe all painful sensations in the forehead, vertex, temples, and back of the head, whereas localized head pains are given specific names, *e.g.*, facial pain, **earache** (otolgia), sinus pain, and **toothache** (odontalgia). Headache often accompanies fever, tension, and/or fatigue, but sometimes it indicates a serious intracranial problem (*e.g.*, **brain tumor**, **subarachnoid hemorrhage**, or **meningitis**). For these reasons all medical and dental practitioners must have a sound knowledge of the anatomy of the head to understand the anatomical basis of certain types of headache and head pain.

THE SKULL

Intelligent study of any part of the head requires a good knowledge of the skeleton of the head and of the soft tissues associated with it. The skull is the most complex bony structure in the body because it (1) **encloses the brain** which is irregular in shape; (2) **houses the organs of special sense** for seeing, hearing, tasting, and smelling; and (3) **encloses the openings into the digestive and respiratory tracts**.

TERMINOLOGY

Five views or aspects of the exterior of the skull are used in anatomical descriptions; each is spoken of as a **norma**. In each case the description applies to the skull *in the anatomical position* and each view is from a position that is at right angles to one of the three planes of the body (frontal, median, and horizontal).

Norma Frontalis (Figs. 7-1 and 7-2). This view of the skull is from the front, or the anterior aspect, and is at right angles to the frontal plane. It features the anterior part of the calvaria (cranial vault) and the face.

Norma Occipitalis (Fig. 7-3). This view of the skull is from the back, or the posterior aspect, and is also at right angles to the frontal plane. Obvious features are the lambda, the external occipital protuberance, the posterior aspect of the mandible, and the mastoid processes.

Norma Verticalis (Figs. 7-4 and 7-5*B*). This view of the skull is from above, or the superior aspect, and is at right angles to the horizontal plane. Obvious features of this aspect are the cranial sutures, the bregma, and the lambda. In fetal and infant skulls, the sutures are formed by fibrous tissue, and the bregma and lambda are represented by the anterior and posterior fontanelles (fonticuli), respectively.

Norma Basalis (Fig. 7-6). This view of the cranium (*i.e.*, the skull with the mandible removed) is from below, or the inferior aspect, and is at right angles to the horizontal plane. Obvious features of this surface are the **foramen magnum**, the maxillary teeth, and the hard palate.

Norma Lateralis (Figs. 7-7 and 7-8). This view of the skull is from the side, or the lateral aspect, and is at right angles to the median plane. A very important feature of this aspect is the **pterion** in the area of the temporal fossa (temple), where four bones usually meet. Other features are the zygomatic arch, the external acoustic meatus, and the mandible.

Parts of the Skull. For purposes of description the skull is considered to be composed of *two parts*: the **calvaria** which

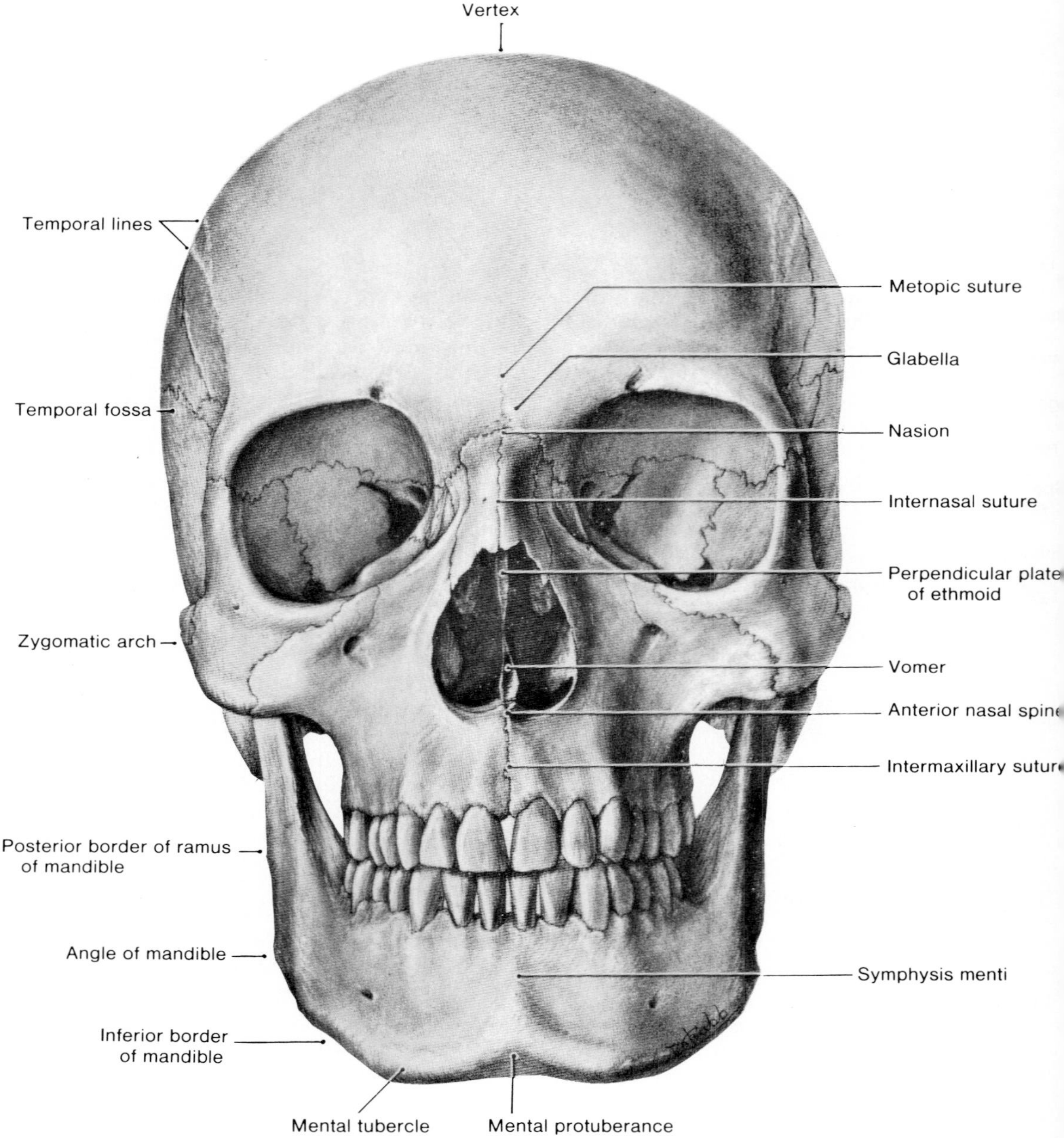

Figure 7-1. Drawing of an anterior view of an adult skull (*norma frontalis*) showing the marginal or outline features on the right side and midline features on the left side. The inferior part of the metopic suture persists (as here) in about 8% of people.

encloses the brain and the **face** which is attached to the anteroinferior part of the calvaria. Because the terms skull, cranium, and calvaria are used with different meanings by different people, their use in this book will be explained.

The term **skull** refers to the entire skeleton of the head (Figs. 7-1 to 7-3), and the

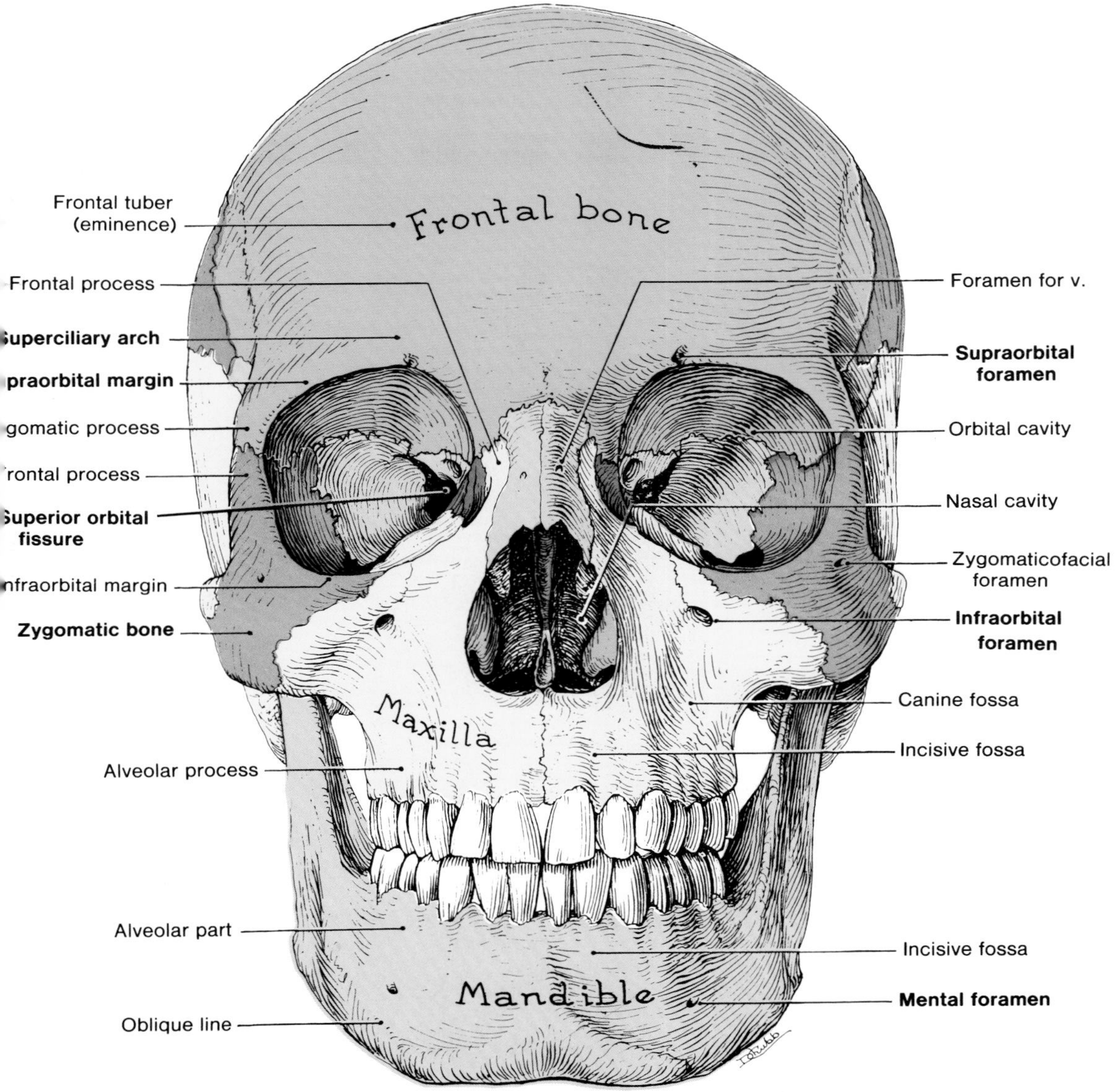

Figure 7-2. Drawing of the anterior aspect of an adult skull (*norma frontalis*) showing surface features on the right side and foramina, fossae, and cavities on the left side. Note that the skull exhibits a more or less oval outline, wider above than below. Verify that an imaginary vertical line passes through the supraorbital, infraorbital, and mental foramina. In a living person, this line also passes through the pupil of the eye when looking straight ahead.

cranium is the skeleton of the head excluding the lower jaw or mandible (Fig. 7-6). The calvaria is sometimes called the cranial vault or braincase. The term calvarium is often incorrectly used instead of calvaria. The roof of the calvaria, called the **skullcap**, is commonly removed during autopsies and anatomical studies so the contents and interior may be examined (Fig. 7-9). The floor of the calvaria (internal surface of base of skull) shows three regions: the anterior, middle, and posterior **cranial**

fossae (Fig. 7-9). *Fossa* is a Latin word meaning a ditch or trench. Examine the interior of the base of a dried skull, noting the many **foramina** (L. apertures). Hold the skull up to a light and observe the numerous thin areas of bone in its base. Because of these foramina and thin areas, *the base of the skull is fragile and fractures of it are common,* **but not so frequent as in the superior part of the calvaria.**

Study of the skull as a whole is more practical than study of its 22 bones (28 if

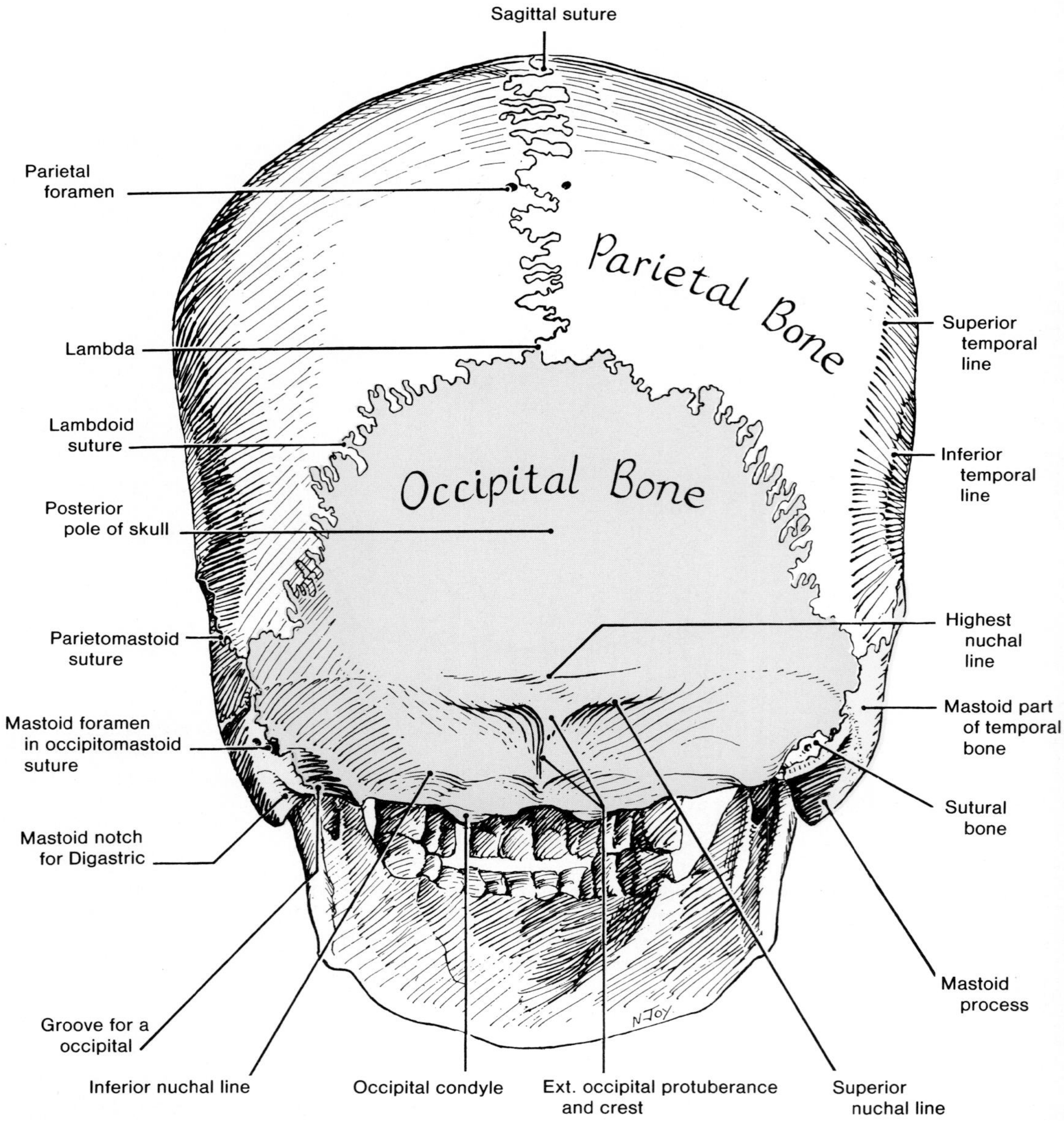

Figure 7-3. Drawing of a posterior view of an adult skull (*norma occipitalis*). Note that the outline of the skull is horseshoe-shaped from the tip of one mastoid process over the vertex (Fig. 7-1) to the other process. The occipital bone (*blue*) forms much of the back and base of the cranium. The external occipital protuberance is usually easy to palpate, particularly in males.

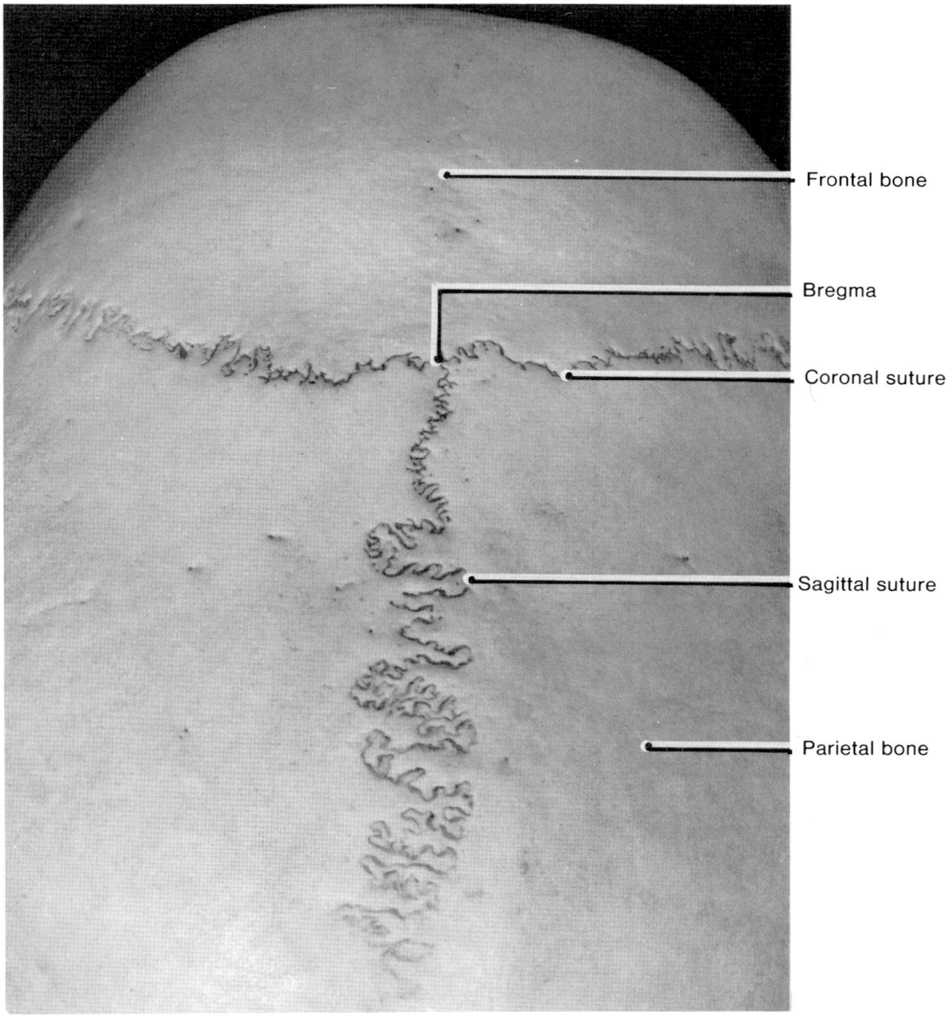

Figure 7-4. Photograph of the superior aspect of an adult skull (*norma verticalis*) showing a close-up view of the sagittal and coronal sutures of the calvaria (Figs. 7-3 and 7-8). The meeting place of the coronal and sagittal sutures is called the bregma (also see Fig. 7-7). In the fetal skull (Fig. 7-5) it is the site of the anterior fontanelle, a membrane-filled gap. Note the variation in the form and in the degree of interlocking of the cranial bones. Observe that the sutures are serrated like the teeth of a saw and that some projections from the edge of one bone are surrounded by bone from the edge of the opposing bone, not unlike the pieces of a jigsaw puzzle. Although there is no bony union, the bones are locked together in such a way that they cannot be spread apart.

the three pairs of small ear bones or auditory ossicles are included); 7 of the 22 are facial bones. These bones are firmly bound together, with the exception of the mandible and the ossicles, to form the skull. Some bones form part of the base, some part of the calvaria, and some part of the face.

Anatomical Position of the Skull. All anatomical descriptions of the skull refer to it with the head in the anatomical position with the eyes directed forward. To place a dried skull so that it approximates this position, it must be oriented so that the **infraorbital margin** (Fig. 7-2) and the su-

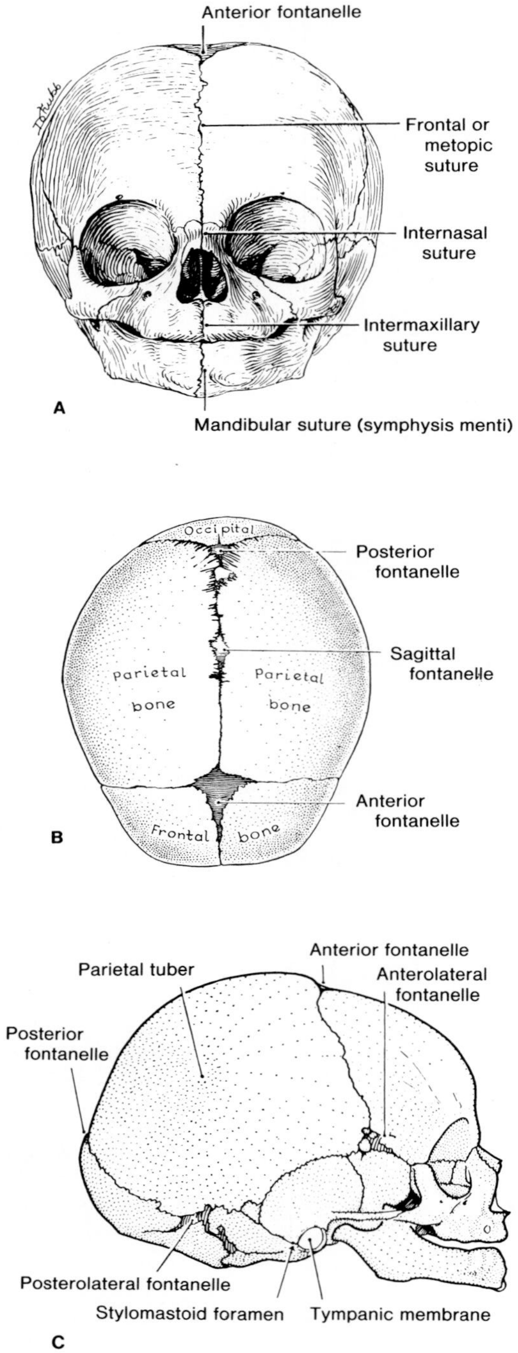

Figure 7-5. Drawings of the fetal skull showing its fontanelles, bones, and connecting sutures. *A*, anterior aspect (*norma frontalis*). Note that the face is very small because the teeth have not erupted and the paranasal air sinuses are rudimentary. The frontal or metopic suture between the right and left frontal bones is usually obliterated by the 6th year. If present after this, it is referred to as a persistent metopic suture (Fig. 7-1). *B*, superior aspect (*norma verticalis*) showing the anterior fontanelle (resembling an arrowhead) and other fontanelles. These fontanelles, particularly the anterior one, are clinically important. *C*, lateral view (*norma lateralis*). Note that the mastoid process (Fig. 7-7) has not developed at this stage. It develops during the 2nd year as the mastoid air cells form (Fig. 7-187). Observe that the angle of the mandible is obtuse at birth.

perior margin of the external acoustic meatus (Fig. 7-7) lie in the same horizontal plane. This orbitomeatal or **Frankfort plane** was universally accepted as the standard guide for examining skulls at a convention of anthropologists held in Frankfort in 1882. You can put a skull in this plane by placing a 5-cm block under the **foramen magnum** with the point of the chin (L. *mentum*) resting on the table. Observe that the **vertex** (Fig. 7-1) is the highest part of the skull when it is in the anatomical position.

Other common terms used to describe parts of the skull are the **forehead** (brow, frons) for the frontal region, the **occiput** (back of head) for the occipital region, and the **temple** (side of head) for the temporal region above the zygomatic arch.

The Calvaria (Figs. 7-1 to 7-5). The upper dome-like part of the cranium is formed anteriorly by the frontal bone and posteriorly by the parietal bones and the superior part of the occipital bone. These bones articulate with each other at **sutures** (L. seams), where they are held together by fibrous tissue. Sutures are confined to the skull and their names indicate the bones between which they lie or the plane of the body in which they run (*e.g.*, coronal suture runs in the coronal plane).

On a skullcap note that the sutures where the cranial bones join are serrated like the teeth of a saw (L. *serra*, saw). Observe also that these serrations are more pronounced on the external surface than on the internal surface of the calvaria.

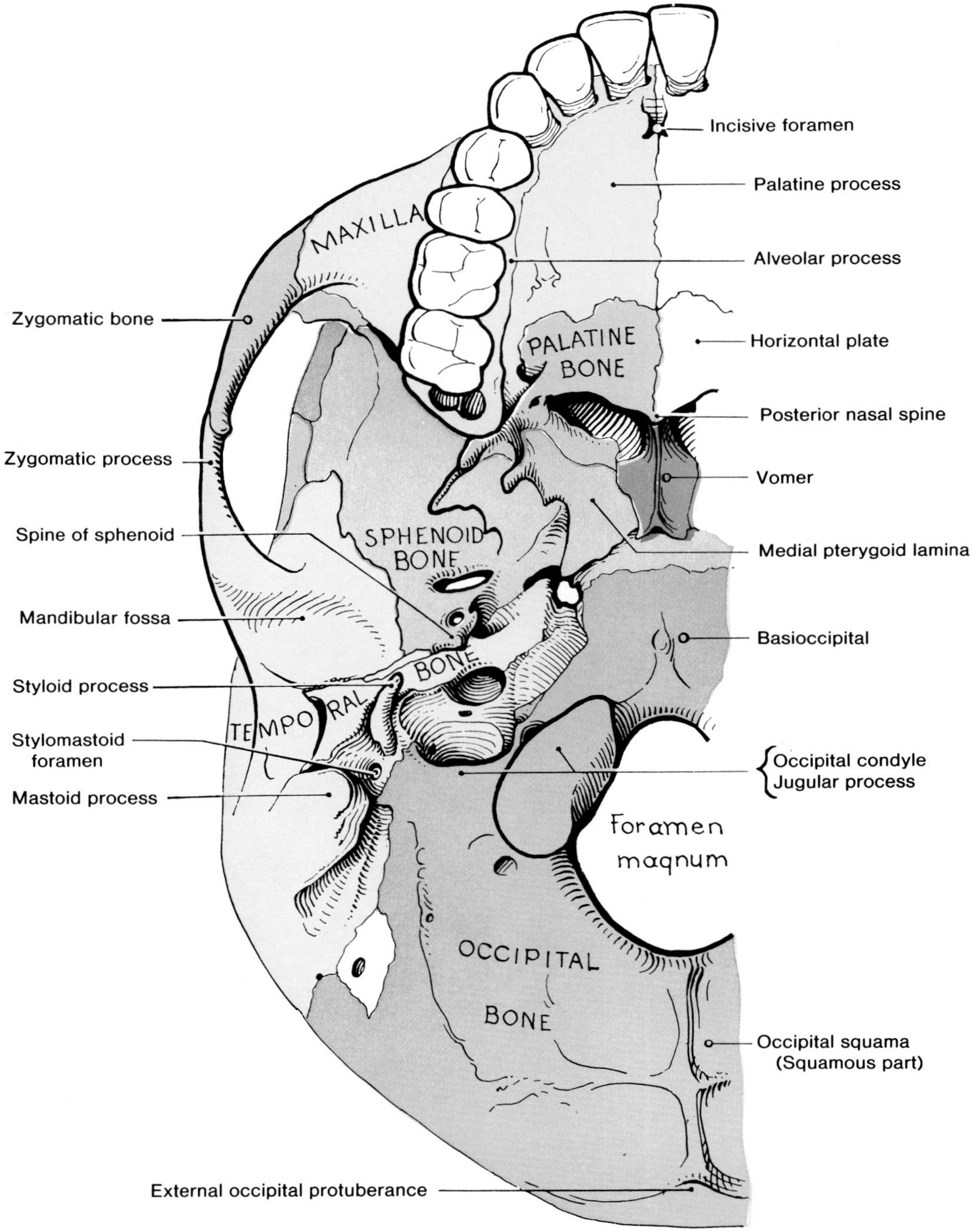

Figure 7-6. Drawing of slightly more than half of the external surface of the base of the skull (*norma basalis*). The various bones taking part in its formation are colored differently.

CLINICALLY ORIENTED COMMENTS

Synostosis, or obliteration of sutures by bone, does not usually begin until middle age, except for the frontal or **metopic suture** between the two parts of the developing frontal bone (Fig. 7-5*A*), which begins to fuse during infancy (up to 2 years). The obliteration of the other sutures commences during the 30s on the inner surface and during the 40s on the outer surface of the calvaria, but *the time of closure of sutures is subject to wide variations*. Premature closure of the cranial sutures results in skull deformities (Figs. 7-10 and 7-11).

The walls of the cranial cavity vary in thickness in different regions of the skull and in skulls of different persons. Check this statement by examining both sides of your dried specimen and those of your colleagues. The skull tends to be thinnest in areas that are well covered with muscles, *e.g.*, the squama (L. a scale) temporalis or squamous part of the temporal bone (Fig. 7-6) and the posteroinferior part of the skull behind the foramen magnum. You can observe these thin areas if you remove the skullcap and hold the remainder of the skull up to a light.

Most bones of the calvaria consist of inner and outer tables (cortices) of compact

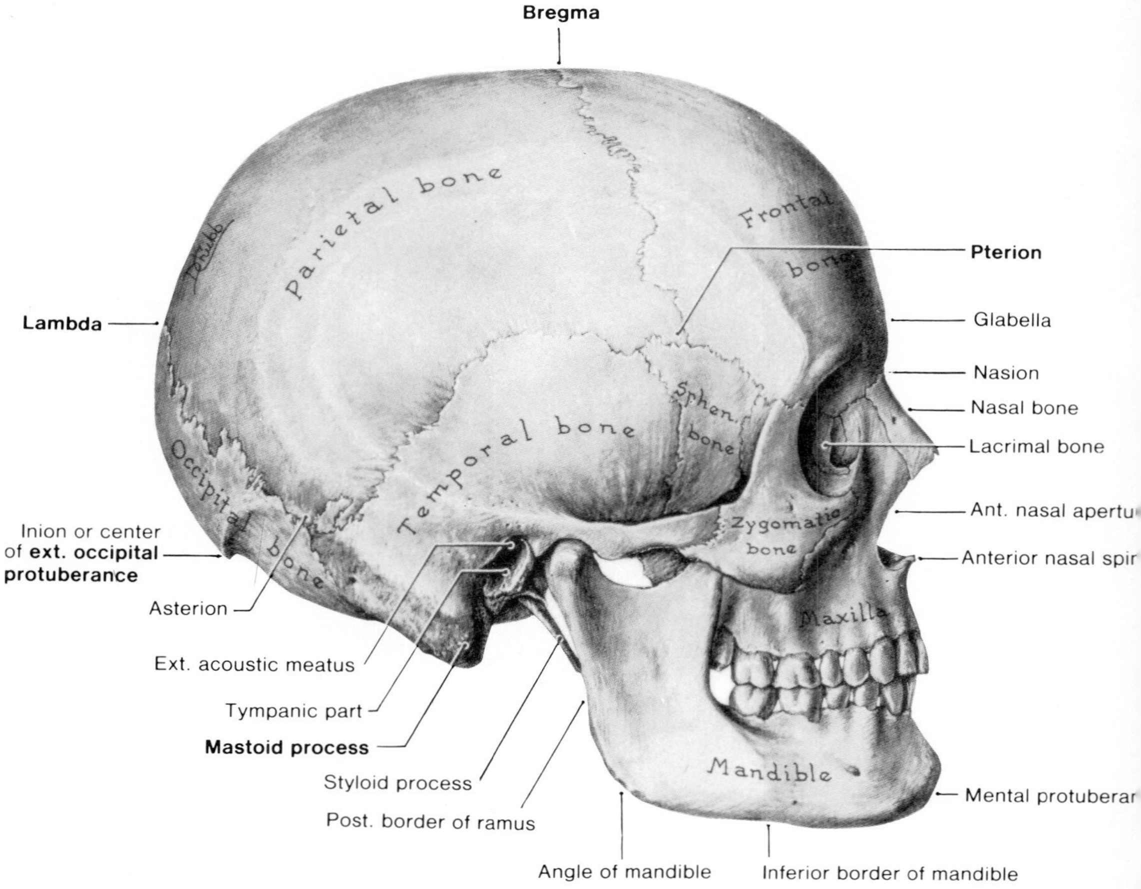

Figure 7-7. Drawing of a lateral view of an adult skull (*norma lateralis*) naming the bones and various outline features. Observe that the center of the pterion is about two fingerbreadths above the zygomatic arch.

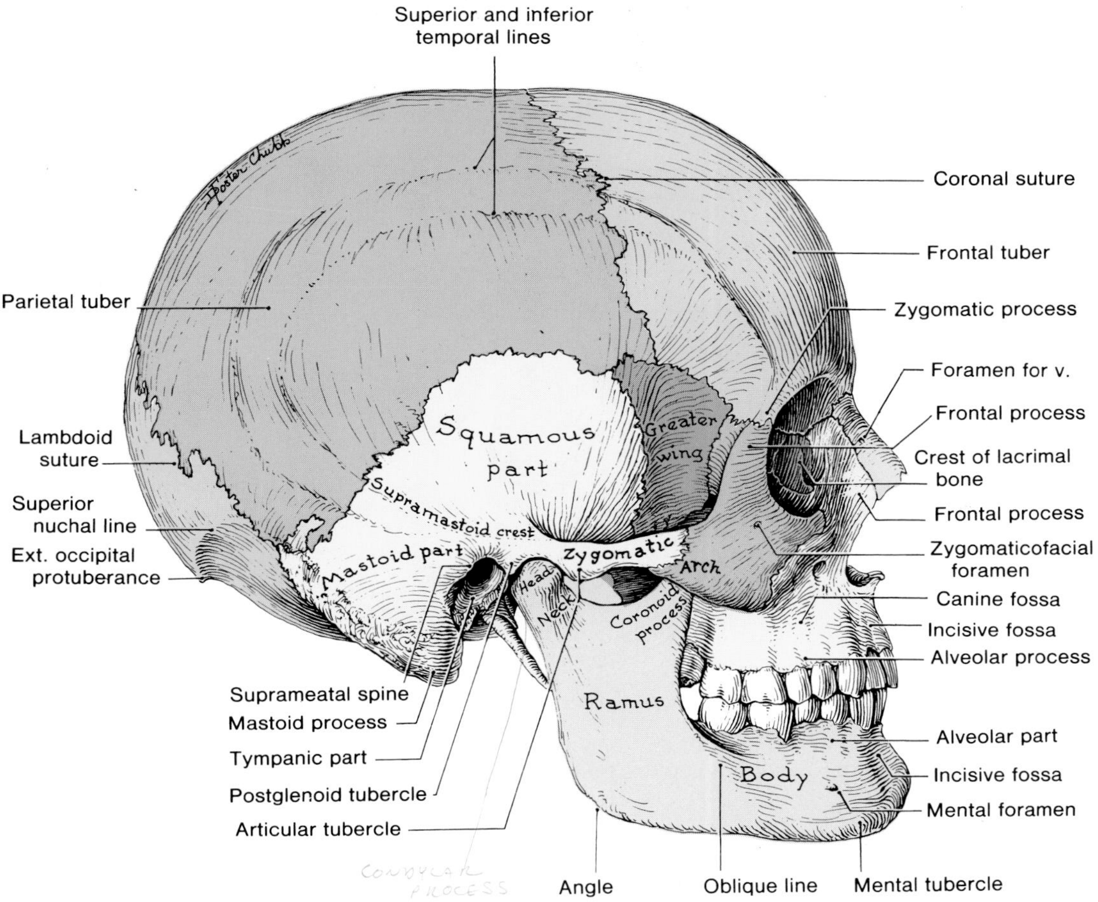

Figure 7-8. Drawing of an adult skull from the side (*norma lateralis*). Note that the temporal process of the zygomatic bone (*yellow*) and the zygomatic process of the temporal bone (*pink*) are united at an oblique suture to form the zygomatic arch. Zygomatic is an appropriate adjective because it is derived from the Greek word *zygotus*, meaning yoked. Observe that this arch forms a bridge that extends horizontally backward from the zygomatic (cheek) bone to the superior attachment of the auricle to the head. Verify that it is subcutaneous throughout; in emaciated persons this arch appears unusually prominent.

bone, separated by spongy **diploë** (Fig. 7-43*A*); it is cancellous bone containing **red bone marrow** during life, through which run the channels formed by the **diploic veins** (Fig. 7-46). Examine the diploë in the skullcap from your specimen. It is not red in the dried skull because the protein was removed during preparation of the specimen. Also observe that the inner table is thinner than the outer table and that in some areas of the skull there is a thin plate of compact bone with no diploë.

CLINICALLY ORIENTED COMMENTS

Hard blows to the head in areas where the calvaria is thin (*e.g.*, in the temporal fossa, particularly in the region of the **pterion**, Fig. 7-7) are likely to produce fractures. Fractures involving the bony grooves in the inner table formed by blood vessels (Fig. 7-15) are liable to tear the vessels, resulting in **intracranial bleeding**, a serious complication (Case 7-5). In depressed fractures

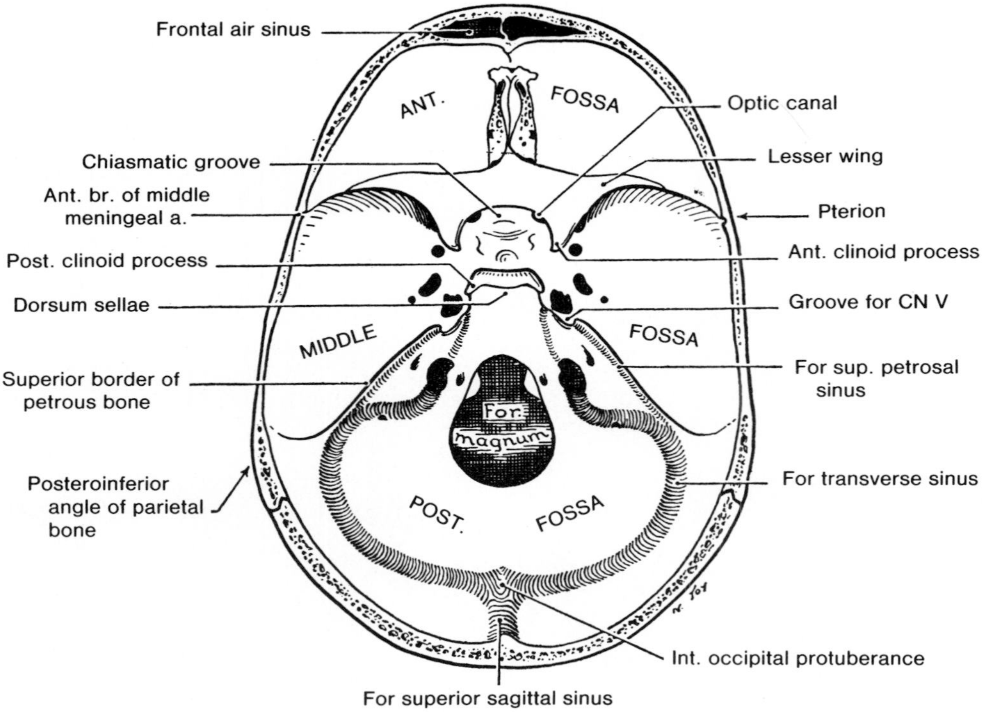

Figure 7-9. Drawing of the floor of the cranial cavity (interior of base of the skull) showing the anterior, middle, and posterior cranial fossae.

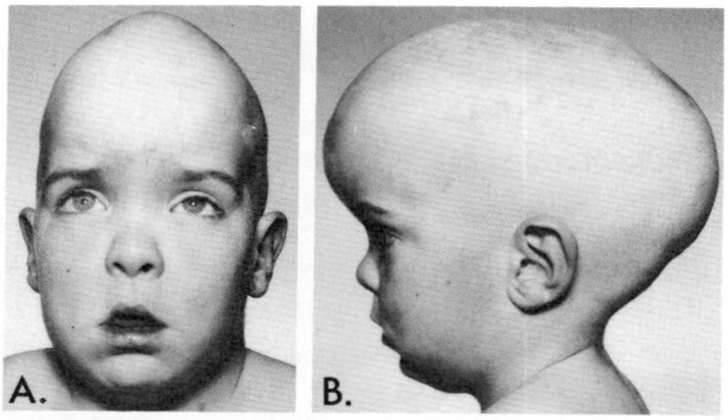

Figure 7-10. Photographs of a boy with scaphocephaly resulting from premature closure of the sagittal suture. *A*, anterior view. *B*, lateral view.

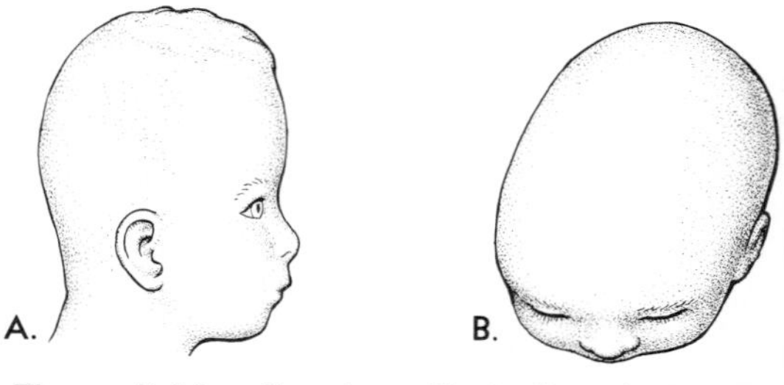

Figure 7-11. Drawings illustrating skull malformations. *A*, turricephaly (tower head) resulting from premature closure of the lambdoid and coronal sutures. *B*, plagiocephaly resulting from premature closure of the coronal or the lambdoid sutures on the right side.

of the skull, the inner table of the calvaria is often more extensively fractured than the outer table.

The Frontal Bone (Figs. 7-1, 7-2, 7-4, 7-5, and 7-7 to 7-9). The forehead (frons) is formed by the smooth, broad, convex plate of bone called the **frontal squama**. In fetal and newborn skulls the two halves of the frontal squama are divided by a **metopic** (G. forehead) or **frontal suture** (Fig. 7-5*A*). In most people the halves of the frontal bone begin to fuse during infancy and the suture between them is usually not visible after the 6th year.

CLINICALLY ORIENTED COMMENTS

In about 8% of adult skulls (Fig. 7-1), the remains of the frontal or metopic suture are visible and may be mistaken in radiographs for a fracture line by inexperienced observers (Fig. I-19). In addition, one could misdiagnose the age of a child's skull if this was the only criterion used.

The frontal bone forms the thin roof of the orbit (eye socket). Just superior to and parallel with each **supraorbital margin** (Fig. 7-2) is a ridge, the **superciliary arch**, which overlies the frontal air sinus (Figs. 7-16 and 7-18); it is more pronounced in males. Between these arches there is a slight, smooth midline protuberance called the **glabella** (Fig. 7-1); this term derives from the Latin word *glabellus* meaning smooth and hairless. The slight prominences of the forehead on each side, above the superciliary arches, are called the **frontal tubers** or **eminences** (Figs. 7-2 and 7-8).

The **supraorbital foramen** (occasionally a notch), which transmits the supraorbital vessels and nerve, is located in the medial part of the supraorbital margin (Fig. 7-2). You can easily determine the location of this foramen, about 2 cm from the midline, by exerting pressure in this area on yourself. Compression of the **supraorbital nerve** as it emerges from this foramen (Fig. 7-31) causes considerable pain, a fact that is used by anesthetists to determine the depth of anesthesia and by doctors attempting to arouse a moribund (L. dying) patient.

The frontal bone articulates with the two parietal bones at the **coronal suture** (Figs. 7-4 and 7-8). It may help you to remember the plane of this suture if you observe that the crown-like ornament, known as a tiara, fits over the coronal (L. crown) suture. As the coronal suture is in a frontal plane, the terms frontal plane and coronal plane are used interchangeably.

The frontal bone also articulates with the **nasal bones** at the **frontonasal suture** (Figs. 7-1, 7-2, and 7-7). At the point where this suture crosses the **internasal suture** in the median plane, there is a useful anatomical point of reference called the **nasion** (L. *nasus*, nose). This depression is at the root of the nose where it joins the calvaria. The frontal bone also articulates with the zygomatic (malar or cheek) bone, the lacrimal bones (Figs. 7-7 and 7-8), the ethmoid bone, the sphenoid bone, and often the temporal bones.

CLINICALLY ORIENTED COMMENTS

As the superciliary arches of the frontal bone are relatively sharp ridges of bone, a blow to them often lacerates the skin over them and causes bleeding. Bruising of the skin over an arch causes tissue fluid and blood to accumulate in the surrounding connective tissue which gravitate into the upper eyelid, resulting in swelling and a "**black eye.**"

The Parietal Bones (Figs. 7-3 to 7-5, 7-7, and 7-8). The two parietal (L. wall) bones form the superior part of the sides of the calvaria. On the outside of these smooth convex bones there is a slight elevation near the center called the **parietal tuber**, or **eminence**. The middle of the lateral surfaces of the parietal bones is crossed by two curved lines, the superior and inferior **temporal lines** (Figs. 7-1, 7-3, and 7-8). The superior one indicates the attachment of the **temporal fascia** (Fig. 7-35), whereas the inferior one marks the superior limit of the **temporalis muscle** (Fig. 7-114).

The parietal bones articulate with each other in the midline at the **sagittal suture**. The sagittal (L. *sagitta*, arrow) suture was probably given this name because of its resemblance to an arrow in the skull of a newborn (Fig. 7-5*B*). The diamond-shaped membranous interval at the junction of the coronal, sagittal, and frontal sutures known as the **anterior fontanelle** (F. fountain) resembles an arrowhead. The **median plane** (Fig. I-4) passes through the sagittal suture; hence, the terms midsagittal plane and median plane are interchangeable. The junction of the sagittal and coronal sutures is called the **bregma** (Figs. 7-4 and 7-7).

The inverted V-shaped suture between the parietal bones and the occipital bone is called the **lamboid suture** (Figs. 7-3 and 7-8) because of its resemblance to the 11th letter (lambda, λ) of the Greek alphabet. The joint where the two parietal bones and the occipital bone join is a useful reference point called the **lambda** (Fig. 7-3). It can be felt as a depression in some people.

CLINICALLY ORIENTED COMMENTS

In fetal and infant skulls, the bones of the calvaria are separated by dense connective tissue membranes at fibrous joints called **sutures** (Fig. 7-5). The large fibrous areas where several sutures meet are called **fontanelles** (fonticuli). The softness of the bones and the looseness of their connections at these sutures enable the calvaria to undergo changes of shape during birth called **molding**. The frontal bone becomes flat and the occipital bone becomes drawn out as one parietal bone slightly overrides or overlaps the other. The bony and cartilaginous base of the skull is deformed little, if any, during **parturition** (birth). Within a day or so after birth, the shape of the calvaria returns to normal.

The loose construction of fetal and newborn calvariae also allows the skull to enlarge during infancy and childhood. The increase in the size of the cranium is greatest during the first 2 years of life, the period of most rapid postnatal growth of the brain. A person's cranium normally increases in capacity until about the 15th or 16th year; after that, the cranium usually increases slightly in size because its bones thicken for 3 to 4 years.

The **anterior fontanelle** (Fig. 7-5*A*), called the "soft spot" by laymen, is usually obliterated by the end of the 2nd year and its former site is indicated in the adult skull by the **bregma** (Figs. 7-4 and 7-7). The site of closure of the **posterior fontanelle** is indicated by the **lambda** of the adult skull (Figs. 7-3 and 7-7).

The anterior fontanelle, the larger of the two main fontanelles, is frequently used clinically. During parturition it is palpated to determine the position of the fetal head in a vertex (head) presentation. During infancy it is used to estimate intracranial pressure (*e.g.*, tenseness suggests increased intracranial pressure, as occurs with **meningitis** (inflammation of the membranes covering the brain). The state of closure of the anterior fontanelle may also be used to estimate the degree of brain development. Blood may also be withdrawn from the underlying **superior sagittal sinus** (Figs. 7-42 and 7-59) by inserting a needle through the anterior fontanelle.

Several rare **skull deformities** may result from premature closure of the cranial sutures. The type of skull deformity formed depends upon which of the various sutures closes prematurely. If the sagittal suture closes early, the skull becomes long and narrow with a ridge along the closed sagittal suture, a condition called **scaphocephaly** (Fig. 7-10). Premature closure of the lambdoid and coronal sutures results in a tower-like skull, called **turricephaly**, or a sharp, pointed head, known as **acrocephaly** (Fig. 7-11*A*). If the lambdoid or coronal suture on one side closes prematurely, the skull is asymmetrical (Figs. 7-11*B*), a condition known as **plagiocephaly**.

The Temporal Bones (Figs. 7-1, 7-3, 7-5 to 7-8, and 7-15). The sides and the base of the skull are formed partly by the temporal bones. Each temporal bone consists of four morphologically distinct parts that fuse together during development (squamous, petromastoid, tympanic parts, and styloid process). The flat **squamous part** (squama temporalis) of the temporal bone lies beside the temporal lobe of the brain. The **petromastoid part** encloses the internal ear and the mastoid air cells and forms part of the base of the skull. The **tympanic part** forms the bony **external acoustic meatus** (auditory meatus) and part of the bony wall of the tympanic cavity, which are concerned with the transmission of sound waves. The slender, pointed **styloid process** (Figs. 7-6 and 7-7) gives attachment to certain ligaments and muscles (*e.g.*, the stylohyoid muscle which elevates the hyoid bone).

The temporal bones articulate at sutures with the parietal, the occipital, the sphenoid, and the zygomatic bones. The **zygomatic process** of the temporal bone unites with the **temporal process** of the zygomatic bone to form the **zygomatic arch** (Fig. 7-8). These arches lie at the widest parts of the face. The head of the mandible articulates with the **mandibular fossa** on the inferior surface of the squamous part of the temporal bone. Anterior to this fossa is the **articular tubercle** (Fig. 7-8).

Explanatory Note. There are different views about the meaning of the term **zygoma** (G. *zygotus*, yoked). In some books the term zygoma is an abbreviation for the zygomatic process of the temporal bone; however, most books use it

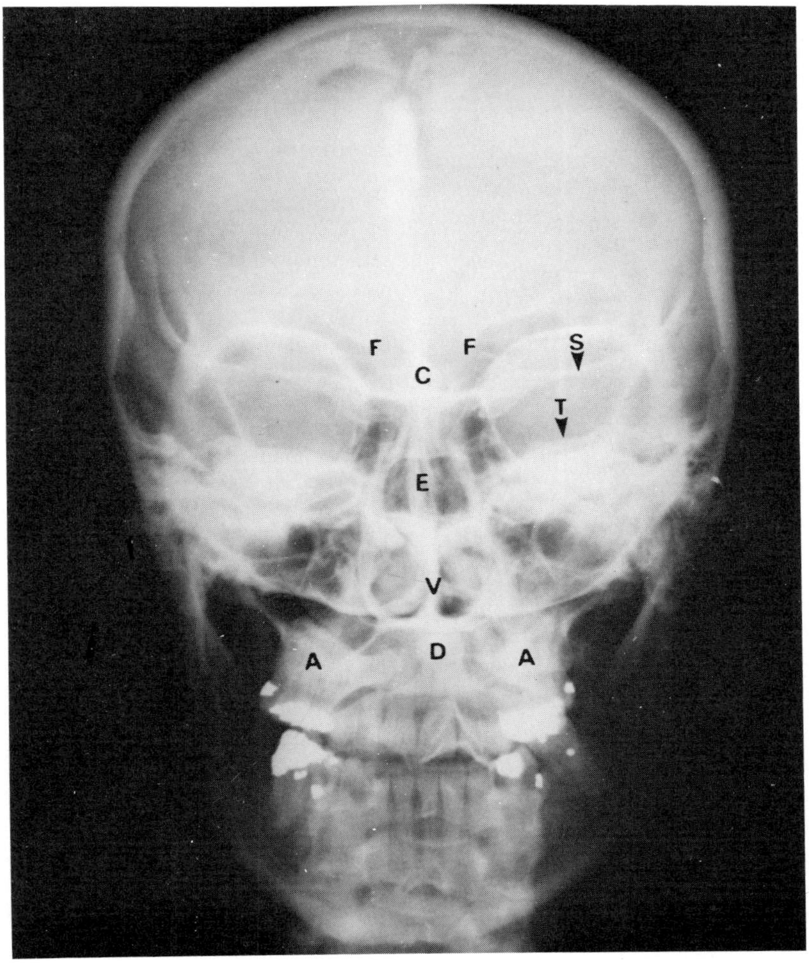

Figure 7-12. Posteroanterior (PA) radiograph of the skull. Observe that (1) the orbital outline is divided into three horizontal parts by the lesser wings of the sphenoid (*S*) and the upper surface of the petrous part of the temporal bone (*T*); (2) the bony nasal septum is formed by the perpendicular plate of the ethmoid (*E*) and the vomer (*V*); (3) the crista galli (*C*) and the frontal sinuses (*F*) are recognizable; and (4) the dens (*D*) is superimposed on the facial skeleton as are the lateral masses of the atlas (*A*).

correctly to indicate the **zygomatic arch**, made up of the zygomatic and temporal processes of the temporal and zygomatic bones that are yoked together. A few books consider the term zygoma to be synonymous with the zygomatic bone. Because of the many uses of the term zygoma, it is not used in this book or in the *Nomina Anatomica*, the international guide to nomenclature. If you see or hear this term, you can usually determine what part of the skull is meant by the context in which it is used.

The Sphenoid Bone (Figs. 7-6 to 7-8, 7-13, and 7-14). This wedge-shaped bone (G. *sphēn*, wedge) in the base of the skull anterior to the temporal bones resembles a bat with its wings outstretched. *The sphenoid bone is a key bone in the cranial skeleton because it articulates with eight bones* (frontal, parietal, temporal, occipital, vomer, zygomatic, palatine, and ethmoid). Its main parts are the central **body** and the **greater** and **lesser wings** which spread out from the body. The upper surface of the body of the sphenoid is shaped like a Turkish saddle (L. *sella*, a saddle); hence, its name **sella turcica** (Fig. 7-47*A*). In the sella turcica or **hypophysial fossa** lies the *hypophysis cerebri* or *pituitary gland* (Fig. 7-63). Inside the body of the sphenoid bone there are right and left sphenoidal air sinuses (Fig. 7-84). The floor of the sella turcica forms the roof of these sinuses when they are well developed.

CLINICALLY ORIENTED COMMENTS

Study of the sella turcica in radiographs is important because it may reflect local pathological changes such as a **pituitary tumor** or a localized dilation **(aneurysm) of the internal carotid artery**. Decalcification of the dorsum sellae is one of the signs of a generalized increase in intracranial pressure.

An irregularly H-shaped confluence of sutures in the anterior part of the external surface of the temporal fossa outlines a clinically important area known as the **pterion** (Figs. 7-1 and 7-7). Here four bones usually meet: the frontal, the sphenoid, the parietal, and the squamous part of the temporal bone. *The pterion is an important anatomical landmark for physicians and surgeons* because it indicates the location of the anterior branch of the **middle meningeal artery** or occasionally the middle meningeal artery itself. You can easily see the imprint of this artery on the inner surface of the calvaria crossing the pterion (Figs. 7-15 and 7-52).

To determine the site of the pterion on the skull of a living person, place your thumb behind the frontal process of the zygomatic bone (Fig. 7-14) and two fingers above the zygomatic arch. The angle formed by your fingers and thumb indicates the pterion and the location of the anterior branch of the middle meningeal artery. You should be aware that *there are numerous variations in the intracranial branching of the middle meningeal artery*. Compare the internal markings of this artery and its branches on the two sides of your dried calvaria with those of your colleagues.

When **skull fractures** occur in the region of the pterion, the anterior branch of the middle meningeal artery and/or its accompanying veins may be torn, resulting in intracranial (usually extradural) hemorrhage (Case 7-5).

The pterion is also a useful landmark for locating parts of the brain. An oblique line drawn from the frontozygomatic suture to the pterion (Fig. 7-7) is level with the inferior edge of the frontal lobe. The posterior end of this line is close to the anterior end of the lateral sulcus of the brain (Figs. 7-51*B* and 7-76); moreover, the **motor speech area** (Broca's area) of the brain lies about one fingerbreadth above this oblique line on the left side of the head in all or nearly all right-handed persons.

The Occipital Bone (Fig. 7-3). This bone forms much of the base and back of the skull. It has a large oval opening in it called the **foramen magnum** through which the cranial cavity communicates with the vertebral canal. It consists of a squamous part, a basilar part, and two lateral parts. On the inferior surfaces of the lateral parts are the **occipital condyles**, where the skull articulates with the *atlas*, the first cervical vertebra.

Other Bones of the Cranium (Figs. 7-1 to 7-3 and 7-5 to 7-8). The previously described cranial bones are the principal ones. Other bones in the *Nomina Anatomica* classified as part of the cranium are the unpaired **vomer** and **ethmoid** and the paired inferior **nasal conchae, lacrimals,** and **nasals**. These bones are often included

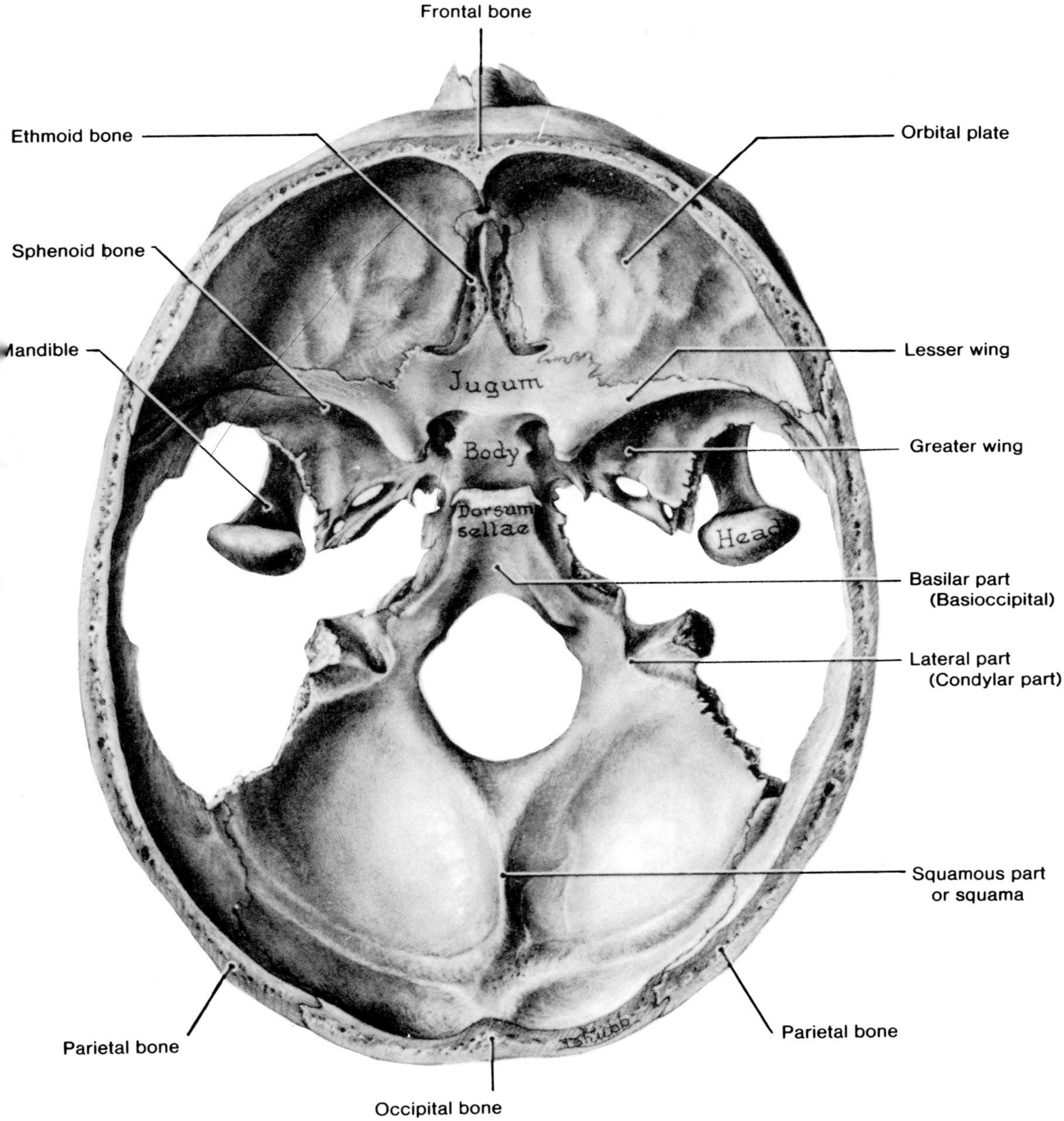

Figure 7-13. Drawing of the interior of the base of an adult skull from which the temporal bones have been removed. Observe that the splenoid bone resembles a bat or bird with its wings outstretched.

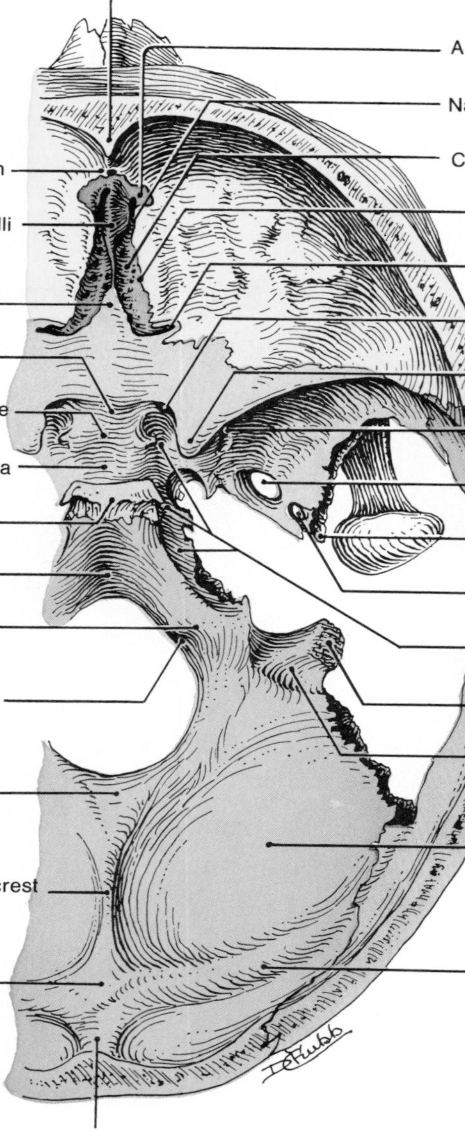

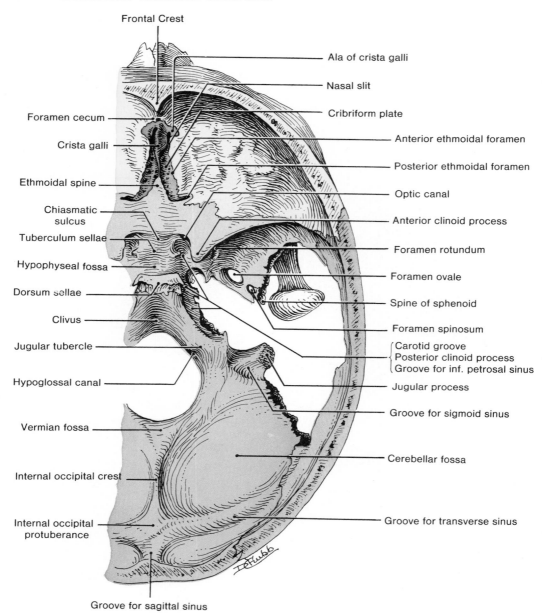

Figure 7-14. Drawing of slightly more than the right half of the interior of the base of the adult skull. Observe the many features in the median plane. Note particularly the crista galli and cribriform plate (*red*) in the anterior cranial fossa (*yellow*). Most of the middle cranial fossa (*blue*) is missing because the temporal bones have been removed. Note the large cerebellar fossa in the posterior cranial fossa (*green*) in which the cerebellar hemisphere lies (Fig. 7-76). Note the clivus (L. slope), a downward sloping surface from the dorsum sellae to the foramen magnum. Observe that it is composed of part of the body of the sphenoid bone and part of the basilar part of the occipital bone.

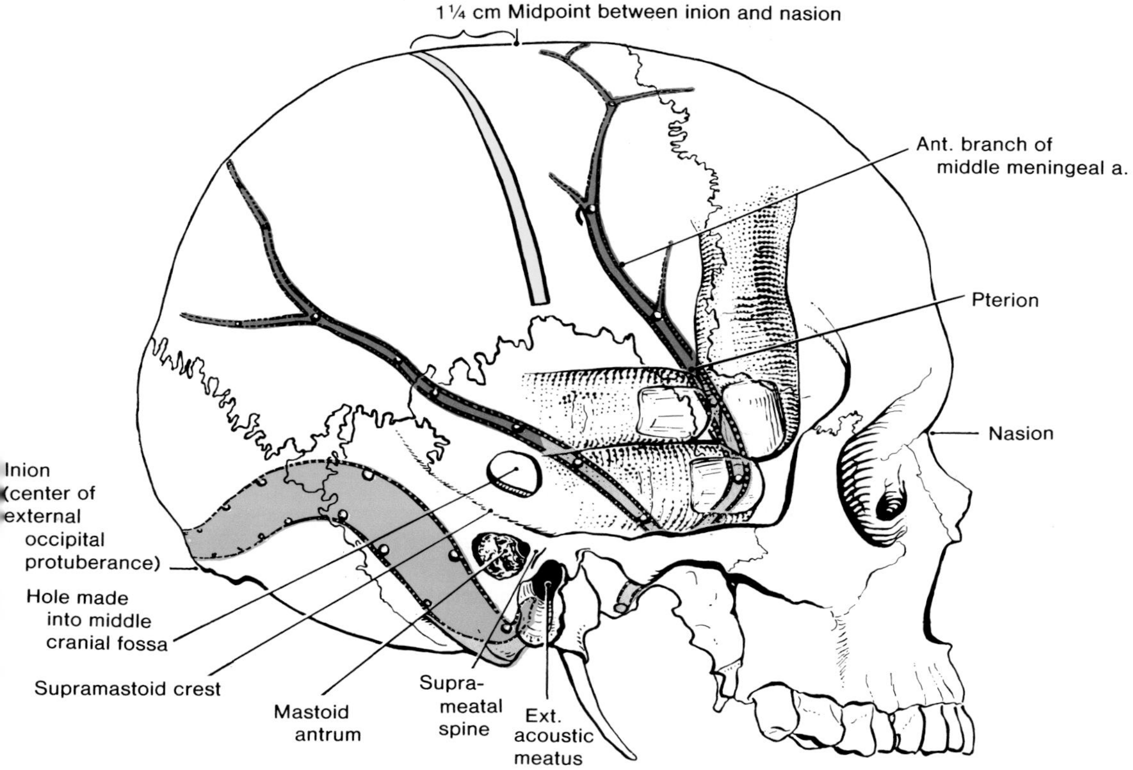

Figure 7-15. Drawing of an adult cranium showing its surface anatomy. The middle meningeal artery and the dural venous sinuses were related to the exterior of the cranium by drilling holes along the grooves produced by these structures on the inside of the cranium. The angle formed by the thumb and fingers indicates the site of the anterior branch of the middle meningeal artery (*red*). *Observe that it crosses the pterion.* The location of the central sulcus of the brain (Fig. 7-76) is shown in *yellow* and the transverse and sigmoid sinuses are shown in *blue*.

with the facial skeleton. The **nasal bones** may be easily felt because they form the bridge of the nose; its right and left halves are joined at the **internasal suture**. These and other bones forming parts of the skull are discussed subsequently with the orbit and the nasal cavities.

CLINICALLY ORIENTED COMMENTS

The mobility of the lower portion of the nose (supported only by cartilages) serves as a partial protection against injury (*e.g.*, a punch in the nose); however, a hard blow to the bony portion of the nose may fracture the nasal bones, producing a **broken nose**). Often the bones are displaced sideways and/or backward.

The outer table of bone forming the calvaria of a living person is somewhat resilient, unlike that in a dried skull from which the proteins have been removed. This elasticity, especially in infants and children, tends to prevent many blows to the head from producing **skull fractures**. Furthermore, in places where the bone is very thin (e.g., the temporal squama, Fig. 7-19), the overlying muscles afford some assistance in cushioning blows (Fig. 7-114).

Fractures of the skull are almost always caused by external violence. **Linear (fissured) fractures** are the most frequent type. The fracture usually occurs at the point of impact, but fracture lines may radiate away from it in two or more directions. The directions of the radiating fracture lines are determined by the thick and thin areas of the skull. Sometimes there is no fracture at the point of impact, but one occurs at the opposite side of the skull (a **contrecoup fracture**); this French word means counter-blow.

Depressed fractures of the calvaria are invariably caused by direct violence. Usually the inner table of the skull is more extensively fractured than the outer table. In infants and children, depressed fractures are similar to the indentation that occurs in a ping-pong ball when it is pressed with the thumb. Using appropriate techniques, the depressed fragments can be elevated, but in many cases one of the fragments has to be removed.

THE FACIAL SKELETON

Most of the facial skeleton is formed by the upper (paired **maxillae**) and lower (unpaired **mandible**) jaws (Figs. 7-2 and 7-16). The other facial bones are the paired **zygomatic**, **palatine**, inferior nasal conchae, and nasal bones.

The calvaria of the newborn infant is large compared with the face (Fig. 7-5). The relatively small facial skeleton results from the small size of the jaws and the almost complete absence of the maxillary and other **paranasal air sinuses** (Figs. 7-16 and 7-18). As the teeth erupt and these sinuses develop during infancy and childhood, the facial bones enlarge. The growth of the maxillae between the ages of 6 and 12 years accounts for the vertical elongation (increase in height) of the face.

The Maxillae (Figs. 7-1, 7-2, 7-5, and 7-6). The skeleton of the face between the mouth and the eyes is formed by the two maxillae which are united in the median plane at the **intermaxillary suture** to form the entire upper jaw. This suture is also visible in the hard palate (Fig. 7-17), where the palatine processes of the maxillae unite.

Each adult maxilla consists of a hollow **body** containing a large **maxillary sinus** (Figs. 7-16 and 7-18); a **zygomatic process** that articulates with the zygomatic bone; a **frontal process** that articulates with the frontal and nasal bones; a **palatine process** which articulates with its mate on the other side to form most of the hard palate (Fig. 7-17); and an **alveolar process** that bears the upper or maxillary teeth. The maxillae also articulate with the vomer, lacrimal, sphenoid, palatine bones, and the inferior nasal conchae.

The body of the maxilla presents a **nasal surface** that contributes to the lateral wall of the nasal cavity (Fig. 7-2); an **orbital surface** which forms most of the floor of the orbit; an **infratemporal surface** (Fig. 7-19) that forms the anterior wall of the infratemporal fossa; and an **anterior surface**, facing partly anteriorly and partly anterolaterally, which is covered with facial muscles (Fig. 7-31). The relatively large **infraorbital foramen**, which faces downward and medially, is located about 1 cm below the infraorbital margin (Fig. 7-2); it transmits the infraorbital vessels and nerve.

CLINICALLY ORIENTED COMMENTS

To anesthetize the infraorbital nerve (Fig. 7-20), a local anesthetic agent is injected around the mouth of the infraorbital foramen; sometimes it is also necessary to inject into the foramen. Examine this foramen on a dried skull, noting that the needle has to be inserted upward, backward, and laterally. When inserting a needle into a patient, care must be taken not to inject the anesthetic agent into the infraorbital vessels that also pass through this foramen.

In old age, or earlier if the teeth are lost, the bone of the alveolar processes of the maxillae is absorbed. As a result, the maxillae become smaller (*i.e.*, decreased in height) and the shape of the face changes. Owing to absorption of the alveolar processes of the jaws, there is a marked reduction in the height of the lower face which produces deep creases in the facial skin that pass backward from the corners of the mouth.

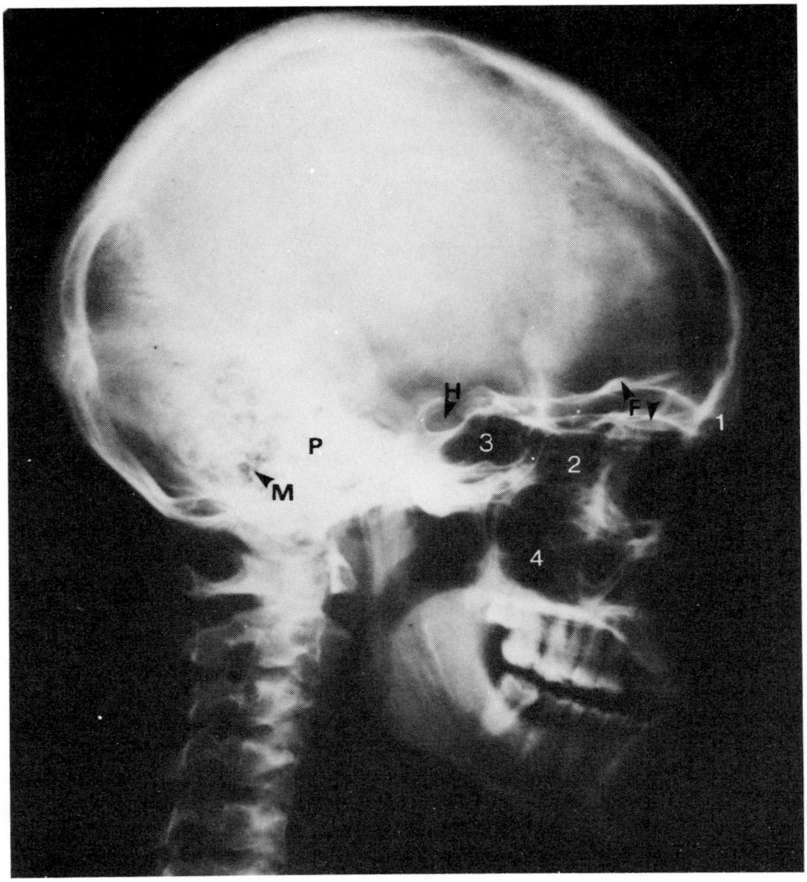

Figure 7-16. Lateral radiograph of the skull. Observe the paranasal air sinuses: (1) frontal, (2) ethmoidal, (3) sphenoidal, and (4) maxillary. Also note the hypophysial fossa (*H*), the great density of the petrous parts of the temporal bones (*P*), and the mastoid air cells (*M*). The right and left orbital plates of the frontal bone (*F*) are not superimposed, thus the floor of the anterior cranial fossa appears as two lines.

The Mandible (Figs. 7-1, 7-2, 7-5, 7-7, and 7-19 to 7-25). The mandible (lower jaw) is the *largest and strongest bone of the face*. The lower or mandibular teeth project upward from their alveoli (sockets) in the alveolar part of the mandible. The mandible (L. *mandere*, to masticate) consists of a horizontal part or **body** and two vertical oblong parts, the **rami**. Viewed from above, the mandible is horseshoe-shaped (Fig. 7-141), whereas each half is L-shaped when viewed from the side. The rami and the body meet posteriorly at the **angles** of the mandible. The bodies of the two sides are fused at the **symphsis menti**; this fusion occurs during the 2nd year of life. Inferior to the second premolar tooth on each side there is a **mental foramen** for transmission of the mental (L. chin) vessels and nerve.

In the anatomical position, the rami of the mandible are almost vertical, except during infancy (Fig. 7-5*C*) and in edentulous (toothless) persons (Fig. 7-24). Each ramus has two processes: an anterior, sharp **coronoid process** for attachment of the temporalis muscle, and a posterior **condylar process**, the head of which articulates with the **mandibular fossa** of the temporal bone as part of the temperomandib-

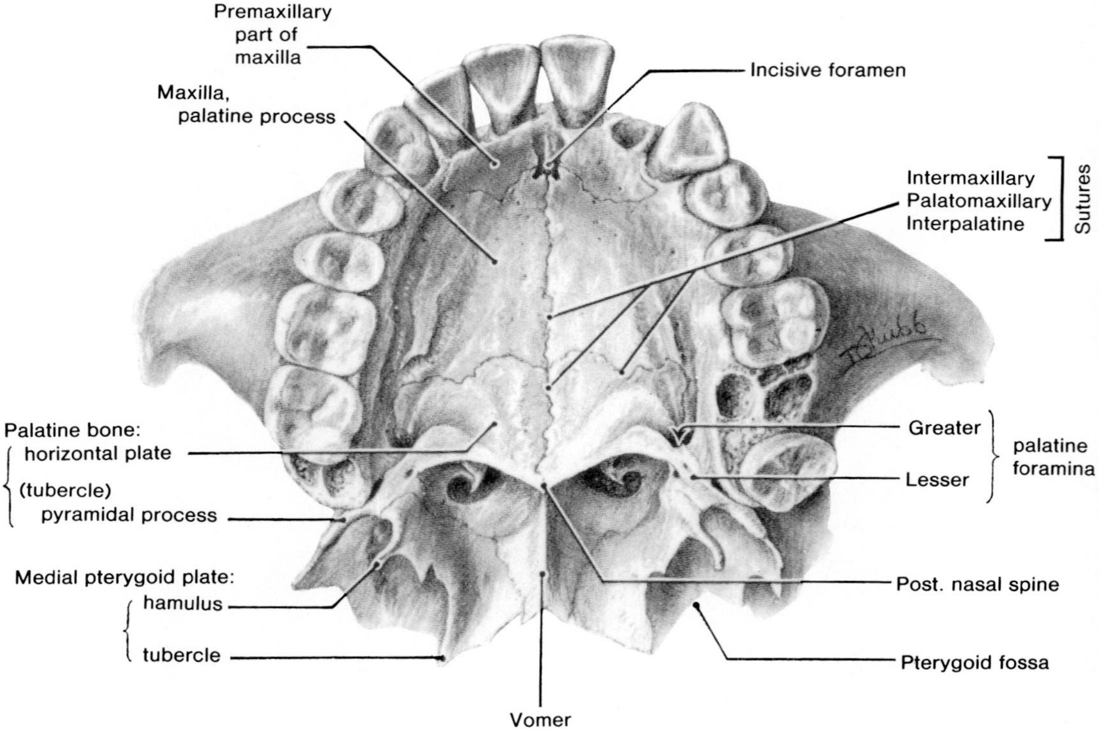

Figure 7-17. Drawing of an inferior view of the bony palate and the aveolar arch. The palate forms the arched roof of the mouth. It consists of a hard a and soft palate (Fig. 7-147). Note that the hard palate is composed of the palatine processes of the maxillae and, united to them posteriorly, the horizontal portions of the palatine bones.

ular joint (Fig. 7-19). Put the tip of your forefinger anterior to the **tragus** (Fig. 7-179) of your auricle (L. external ear) and open your mouth widely. Verify that the head of the mandible glides downward and forward. Insert your fingertip into the mandibular fossa into which the head fits. If you press firmly you will be unable to close your jaw because you prevent the head from sliding upward and backward in the fossa.

Below the head is the neck of the condylar process, which is separated from the coronoid process by the **mandibular notch** (Figs. 7-19 and 7-21). On the internal (medial) surface of the ramus of the mandible is the **mandibular foramen** (Fig. 7-22), the entrance to the **mandibular canal**. This canal transmits the inferior alveolar vessels and nerve to the roots of the teeth (Fig. 7-20). Branches of these vessels and the **mental nerve** emerge from the mandibular canal at the **mental foramen** (Fig. 7-31), which faces upward and backward. For this reason injections into this foramen have to be made from the posterosuperior aspect of it. *Verify this on a dried mandible.*

Anterior to the mandibular foramen there is a thin projection (spur) of bone, called the **lingula** of the mandible (L. *lingua*, tongue), that somewhat overlaps the foramen like a tongue or shield (Fig. 7-22). Running downward on the inner surface of the mandible from the mandibular foramen is a small **mylohyoid groove**, indicating the course taken by the mylohyoid nerve and vessels. These structures arise from the inferior alveolar nerve and vessels before they enter the mandibular foramen.

The internal surface of the mandible is divided into two areas by the **mylohyoid line** (Fig. 7-22), which commences behind the third molar tooth. Above the anterior

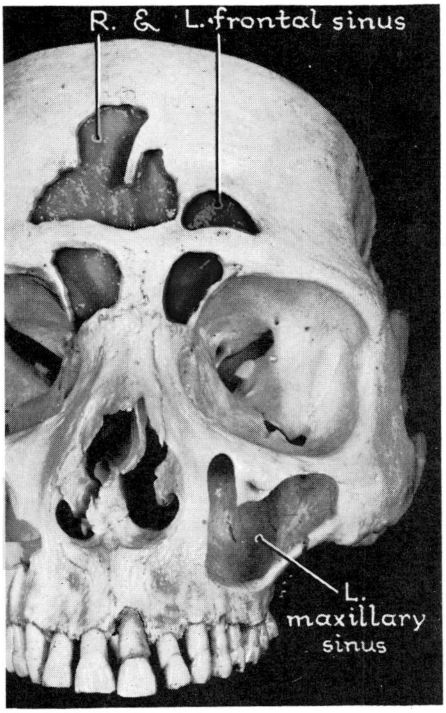

Figure 7-18. Photograph of an anterior view of an adult skull (*norma frontalis*) that has been specially prepared to demonstrate the paranasal air sinuses. Observe the crooked bony nasal septum in this specimen. This deformity may have resulted from an injury but more likely resulted from flattening of the nose during passage through the birth canal (lower end of the uterus and vagina (Fig. 3-106)).

ends of the mylohyoid lines on the internal surface in the small irregular elevation midline are called the **mental spines** (tubercle). Often there are upper and lower spines.

CLINICALLY ORIENTED COMMENTS

The size and shape of the mandible and the number of teeth it bears change with age. **In the newborn**, the mandible consists of two halves united in the median plane (**symphysis menti**) by fibrous tissue at the mandibular suture (Fig. 7-5*A*). The body of the newborn's mandible is a mere shell (Fig. 7-23), enclosing in each half five primary teeth in their sockets (alveoli) like peas in a pod. The teeth usually begin to erupt in infants of about 6 months (Table 7-4). The body of the mandible elongates, particularly posterior to the mental foramen, to accommodate the eight secondary teeth (Fig. 7-25), which begin to erupt during the 6th year. Eruption of the teeth is not complete until early adulthood, but the third molars ("wisdom teeth") may be malposed and impacted so they are unable to erupt properly (Case 7-8).

In old age or earlier, with loss of teeth, the bone of the alveolar part of the mandible becomes absorbed and the mental and mandibular foramina come to lie near the upper border of the body of the bone (Fig. 7-24). In some cases the mental foramen and part of the mandibular canal may disappear, exposing part of the **inferior alveolar nerve** to injury. Pressure of a **dental prosthesis** (G. addition, attachment), *e.g.*, a denture, on an exposed nerve in an edentulous jaw may produce pain during eating.

The bones of the face are often fractured by direct violence (*e.g.*, during fights or when the face crashes into a car's dashboard). The common sites of **fractures of the mandible** are illustrated in Figure 7-26. Usually there are two fractures and they are frequently on opposite sides; thus, if one fracture is observed, a search should be made for another. For example, a hard blow to the jaw often fractures the neck of the mandible and the body in the region of the opposite canine tooth. Displacement of bone fragments at the fracture lines results in **malocclusion** (deviation from the normal contact of the teeth).

The Zygomatic Bones (Figs. 7-2 and 7-7). The prominence of the cheek (L. *mala*), the anterolateral rim of the orbit and much of the infraorbital margins of the orbits, is formed by the zygomatic (malar) bone. These prominences (eminences) are what laymen call the *cheek bones.*

The zygomatic bone articulates with the frontal, maxilla, sphenoid, and temporal bones. The frontal process of the zygomatic

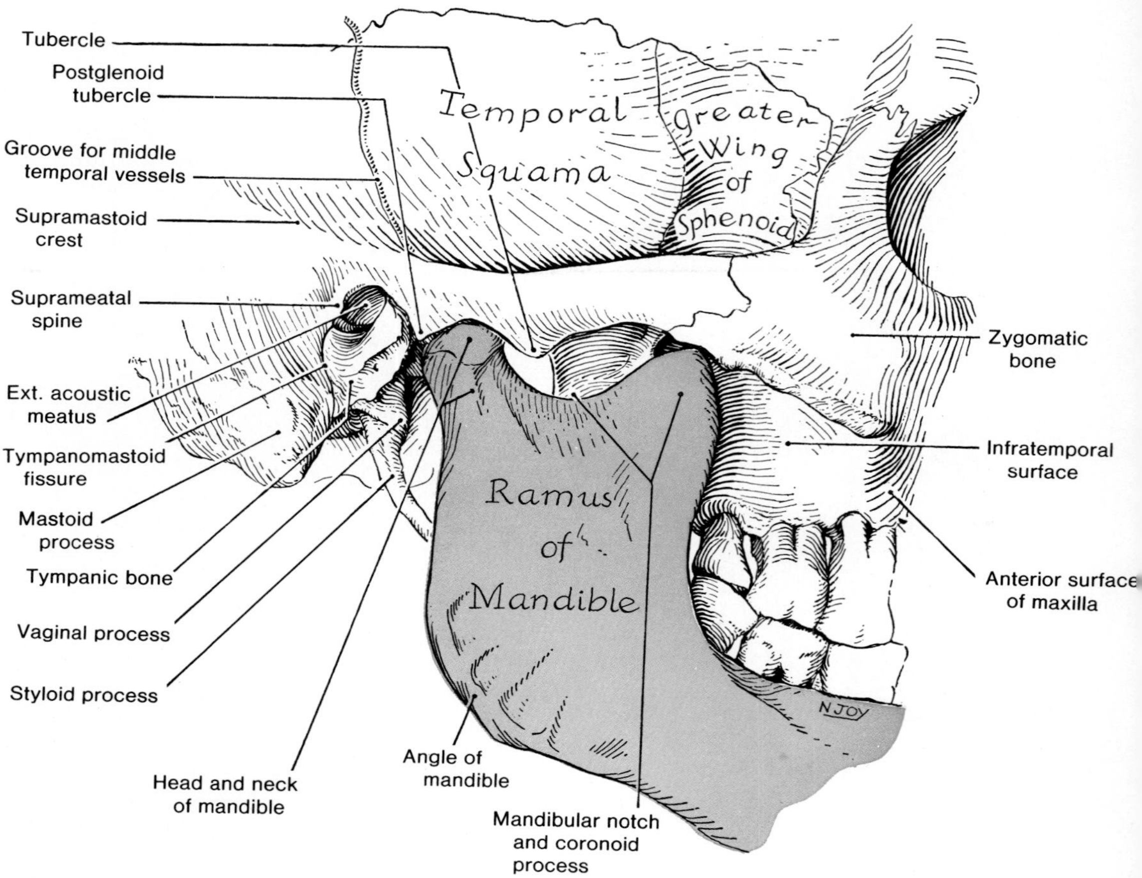

Figure 7-19. Drawing of a lateral view of part of the skull, primarily to show the infratemporal surface of the maxilla and its relationship to the infratemporal fossa. The inconsistent groove for the middle temporal vessels is sometimes mistaken for a fracture in radiographs.

bone passes upward, forming the lateral border of the orbit and articulating with the frontal bone at the outer edge of the supraorbital margin (Fig. 7-2). The **maxilla** lies mainly below and medial to the zygomatic bone. The zygomatic bone articulates medially with the greater wing of the **sphenoid bone**. The site of their articulation may be observed on the lateral wall of the orbit of a dried skull (Fig. 7-2). On the anterolateral aspect of the zygomatic bone, near the inferior orbital border, there is a small **zygomaticofacial foramen** (often double) for the nerve and vessels of the same name. The posterior (temporal) surface of the zygomatic bone, near the base of its frontal process, is pierced by a small **zygomaticotemporal foramen** for the nerve of the same name. The zygomaticofacial and zygomaticotemporal nerves, leaving the orbit through the previously mentioned foramina, enter the zygomatic bone through one (occasionally two) small **zygomaticoorbital foramina** that pierce its orbital surface.

The **temporal process** of the zygomatic bone unites with the **zygomatic process** of the temporal bone to form the **zygomatic arch** (Figs. 7-6 and 7-8). This arch can be easily palpated on the side of the head, posterior to the zygomatic (malar) eminence and inferior to the temporal region (temple). The zygomatic arches are prominent in emaciated (L. to make thin) persons. The zygomatic arch also forms one of the useful landmarks for determining the location of the pterion (Fig. 7-15). A horizontal plane passing inward from this arch separates the temporal fossa above from the infratemporal fossa below (Fig. 7-19).

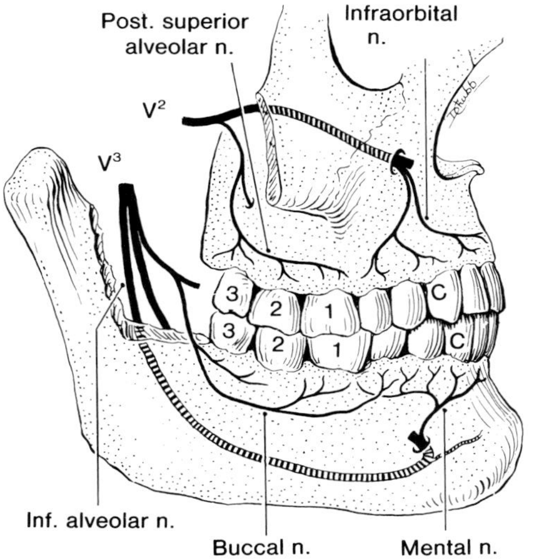

Figure 7-20. Drawing illustrating the distribution of the maxillary and mandibular divisions (CN V^2 and CN V^3) of the trigeminal nerve. The ophthalmic division of this fifth cranial nerve (CN V^1) is not shown; it is sensory to the eyeball and cornea.

CLINICALLY ORIENTED COMMENTS

You may hear the term **malar flush**; this is redness of the skin of the zygomatic (malar) eminences that often occurs in tuberculosis, mitral stenosis (narrowing of the left atrioventricular opening), and sometimes in rheumatic and other fevers.

The common variants of **fractures of the maxilla and zygomatic bones** were classified by Le Fort, a Paris surgeon. These fractures are remarkably constant and are classified into three types that are described and illustrated in Figure 7-27.

THE FACE

The term **facies** (L. face) refers to the appearance of the face. Some diseases produce a typical facies (*e.g.*, the mask-like, expressionless facies of patients with **Parkinson's disease** or Parkinson's syndrome, a disturbance of motor function) that is an objective and verifiable sign of

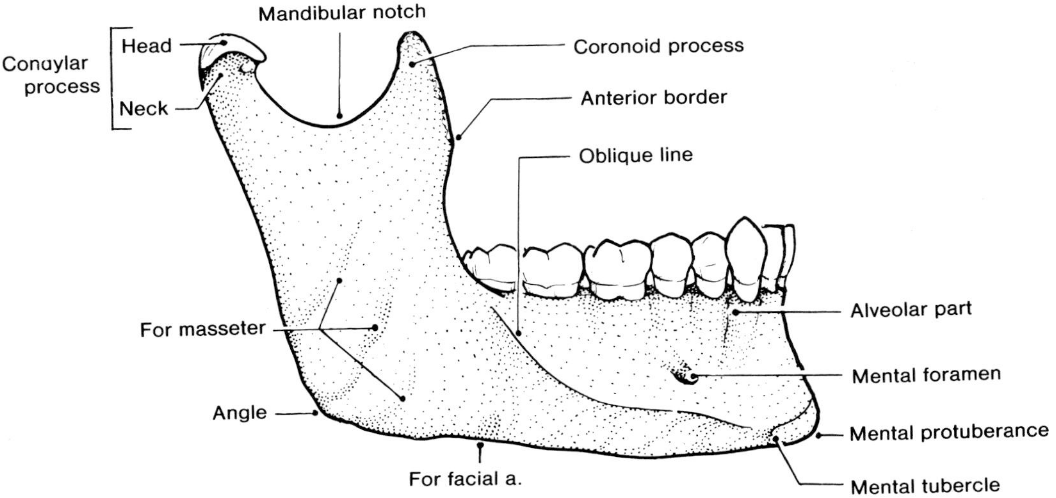

Figure 7-21. Drawing of the lateral (external) aspect of the right half of an adult mandible. Because the ramus of the mandible is covered by the masseter muscle (also see Fig. 7-134), only its posterior border can be easily palpated. The neck of the mandible lies just anterior to the lobule of the auricle.

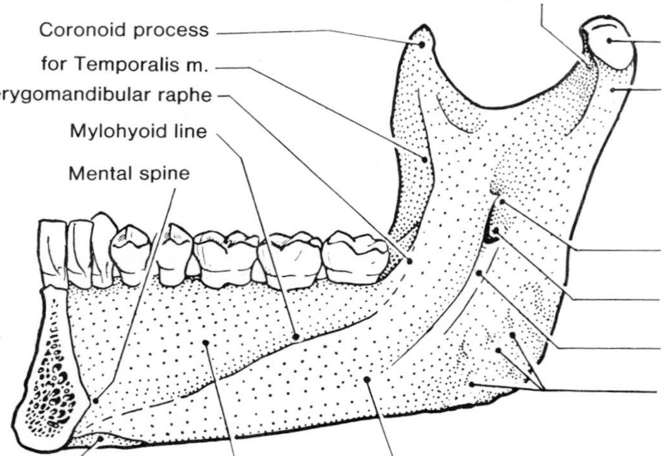

Figure 7-22. Drawing of the medial (internal) aspect of the right half of an adult mandible. The inferior alveolar nerve enters the mandibular canal via the mandibular foramen and runs close to the roots of the teeth (Fig. 7-20). The tongue-like lingula is a clinically important bony landmark that is used when injecting an anesthetic agent into the foramen for anesthesia of the nerve (*e.g.*, prior to dental procedures).

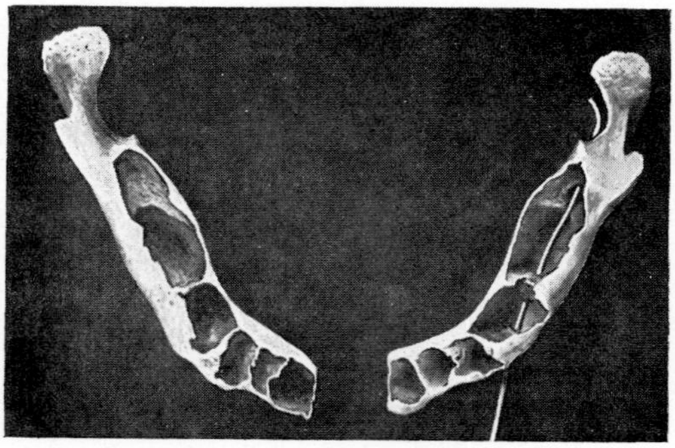

D MANDIBLE AT BIRTH FROM ABOVE

Figure 7-23. Photograph of a superior view of the mandible at birth. Understand that during life the halves of the mandible are united by fibrous tissue at the mandibular suture or symphysis menti (Fig. 7-5*A*). The two halves of the mandible fuse during the 2nd year. Note that each half of the mandible has sockets (alveoli) for five primary teeth. *On the left*, the course of the inferior alveolar nerve is indicated by a wire passing through the mandibular canal.

the disease. In general usage, the term face (facies) refers to the anterior and anterolateral aspects of the head which includes the eyes, nose, mouth, chin, cheeks, and jaws.

At birth the face is small compared with the rest of the head (Fig. 7-5*A* and *C*), as discussed previously, because the jaws have not developed fully and because of the almost complete absence of air sinuses in the facial bones. As these structures develop during infancy and childhood (Fig. 7-18), the face becomes longer, the zygomatic prominences (cheek bones) more prominent, and the cheeks less prominent.

Muscles of the Face (Figs. 7-28, 7-29, and 7-31). *The muscles of facial expression are attached to the skin of the face* and lie in the subcutaneous tissue; thus, they enable us to move our skin and change our **facial expression**. Clinically it is essential to know that *all muscles of facial expression are supplied by the facial nerve* (**CN VII**).

The facial muscles surround the facial orifices (openings) of the mouth, eyes, nose, and ears and act as **sphincters** (G. a band or lace) and **dilators**, *i.e.*, they close and open the orifices. Developmentally the facial muscles arise from the second branchial arch (hyoid arch) as part of a subcutaneous muscle sheet in the neck known as the **platysma** (Figs. 7-29, 9-8, and 9-9). It spreads out as a sheet over the face during

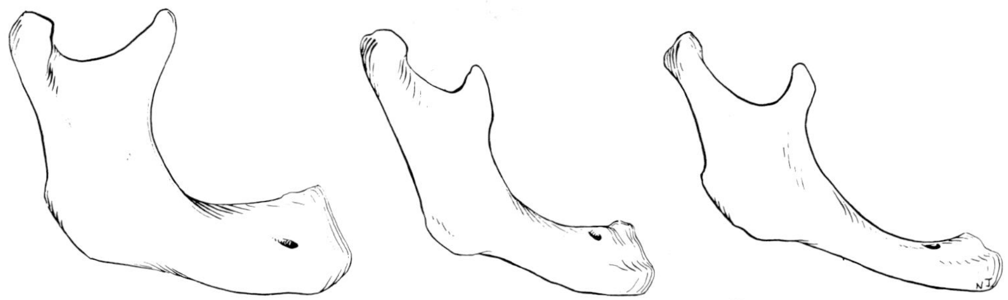

Figure 7-24. Drawings of lateral views of the right side of edentulous (toothless) mandibles showing how the position of the mental foramen varies with the extent of absorption of the alveolar process. *A*, several months after removal of all the permanent mandibular teeth. Observe that the angle between the body and the ramus is about normal, *i.e.*, approaches a right angle (also see Fig. 7-21). Note that the mental foramen is about midway between the upper and lower borders of the bone. *B*, several years after loss of the teeth. Observe that much of the alveolar bone has been absorbed and that the angle of the mandible has increased. Note that the mental foramen is now near the upper border of the mandible. *C*, many years after loss of the mandibular teeth showing that the alveolar part is entirely absorbed (an example of disuse atrophy) and that the body of the mandible consists entirely of the inferior part. The mental foramen now lies at the upper border of the mandible. Note that the angle between the body and the ramus has further increased and that the neck of the condyle is bent backward. Because of the exposed position of the mental nerve emerging from the mental foramen, probably a dental prosthesis (false teeth) would exert pressure on it producing pain in the skin of the chin and the lower lip, including the labial gingiva (gum) in this region.

development, bringing branches of the facial nerve (CN VII) with it. Because of their common origin, the facial muscles are often fused and their fibers of insertion into the skin are frequently intermingled. Although they are difficult to dissect, contractions of them are easily observed and they are used to express one's feelings. This is one reason why physicians observe their patient's facies carefully.

CLINICALLY ORIENTED COMMENTS

Because there is no definite deep fascia and the superficial fascia between the cutaneous attachments of facial muscles is loose, **facial lacerations** tend to gape (part widely); thus, the skin must be sutured (L. *sutura*, a sewing) with great care to prevent scarring. The looseness of the superficial fascia also enables much fluid and blood to accumulate in the loose connective tissue following contusion or bruising of the face. Similarly, facial inflammation causes considerable swelling (*e.g.*, the swelling resulting from a bee sting on the bridge of the nose can close both eyes).

Muscles of the Forehead (Figs. 7-28 and 7-35). The **frontalis** is part of a scalp muscle called the occipitofrontalis (Fig. 7-43*B*). The frontalis muscle elevates the eyebrows (*e.g.*, as occurs with a surprised look) and produces the tranverse wrinkles in the forehead when you frown.

Muscles of the Mouth (Figs. 7-28, 7-29, 7-31, 7-32, and 7-35). There are many muscles that alter the shape of the mouth and the lips (*e.g.*, as occurs during whistling, speaking, and mimicry). Some of them will be mentioned because they produce common oral movements which are affected when a lesion of the facial nerve is present (Case 7-1).

The **depressor anguli oris**, as its name indicates, depresses the corner of the mouth. Posterior fibers of the platysma assist with this movement. The **zygomaticus major**, extending from the zygomatic bone to the angle of the mouth, draws the angle of the mouth upward and laterally as in laughing.

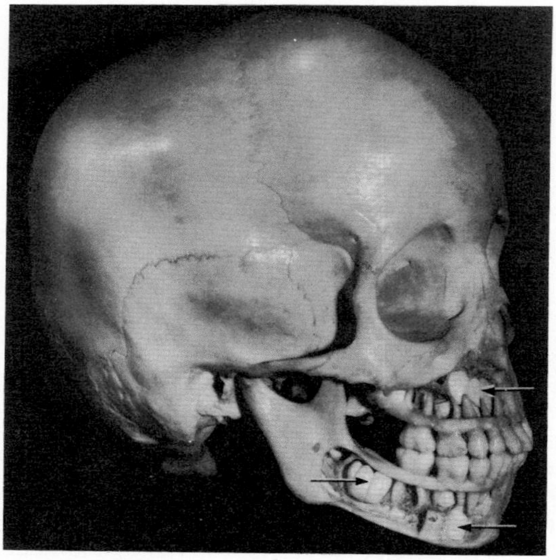

Figure 7-25. Photograph of the skull of a 4-year-old child. Alveolar bone has been ground away and the jaws have been dissected to show the relations of the developing permanent teeth (*arrows*) to the deciduous teeth. Between the 6th and 12th years, the 20 primary teeth are shed as the permanent teeth erupt. By the age of 12, 28 permanent teeth are present. The last four (the third molars or "wisdom teeth") erupt during adolescence, early adulthood, or never.

The **levator labii superioris**, descending from the lower margin of the orbital opening (infraorbital margin) to the upper lip (L. *labium*, lip), raises the upper lip. You may be able to use this muscle to evert (L. to turn out) your upper lip as chimpanzees often do.

The orbicularis oris is the important sphincter muscle of the mouth. Its fibers, lying within the lips, encircle the mouth and blend with other facial muscles, particularly the buccinator. The orbicularis oris **closes the mouth**, **purses the lips** as in whistling and sucking, and plays an important role in articulation and mastication (chewing). In association with the buccinator muscle, it helps to hold food between the teeth during chewing.

Muscles of the Cheek (Figs. 7-28, 7-31, and 7-32). The **buccinator** (L. trumpeter) is a thin, flat muscle that aids mastication by pressing the cheeks against the teeth during chewing. This muscle was given its unusual name because it also compresses the cheeks (L. *buccae*) during blowing, as occurs when a musician plays a wind instrument.

Muscles of the Eyelids (Figs. 7-28, 7-31, 7-32, and 7-35). The function of the eyelid is to protect the eye and to keep the cornea moist.

The orbicularis oculi is the important sphincter muscle of the eye. Its fibers sweep in concentric circles around the orbital margin and in the eyelids. Contraction of its fibers narrows the orbital opening and encurages the flow of tears by helping to empty the lacrimal (tear) sac. This sphincteric muscle **consists of three parts:** (1) a thick *orbital part* for closing the eyes to protect against the glare of light and dust in the air; (2) a thin *palpebral part* (L.

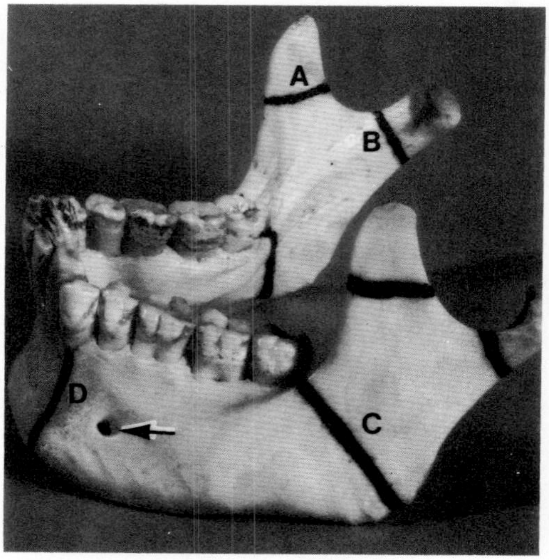

Figure 7-26. Photograph of a lateral view of an adult mandible from the left side, indicating the common sites of fracture. *Usually there are two fractures*, frequently on opposite sides. *A*, fractures of the coronoid process are usually single. *B*, fractures of the neck are often transverse and may be associated with dislocation of the temporomandibular joint on the same side (see Fig. 7-136*C*). *C*, fractures of the angle of the mandible are usually oblique and they may involve the alveolus (socket) of the third molar tooth. Fractures through the alveoli are (or potentially are) compound fractures. *D*, fractures of the body of the mandible frequently pass through the alveolus of the canine tooth. The *arrow* indicates the mental foramen.

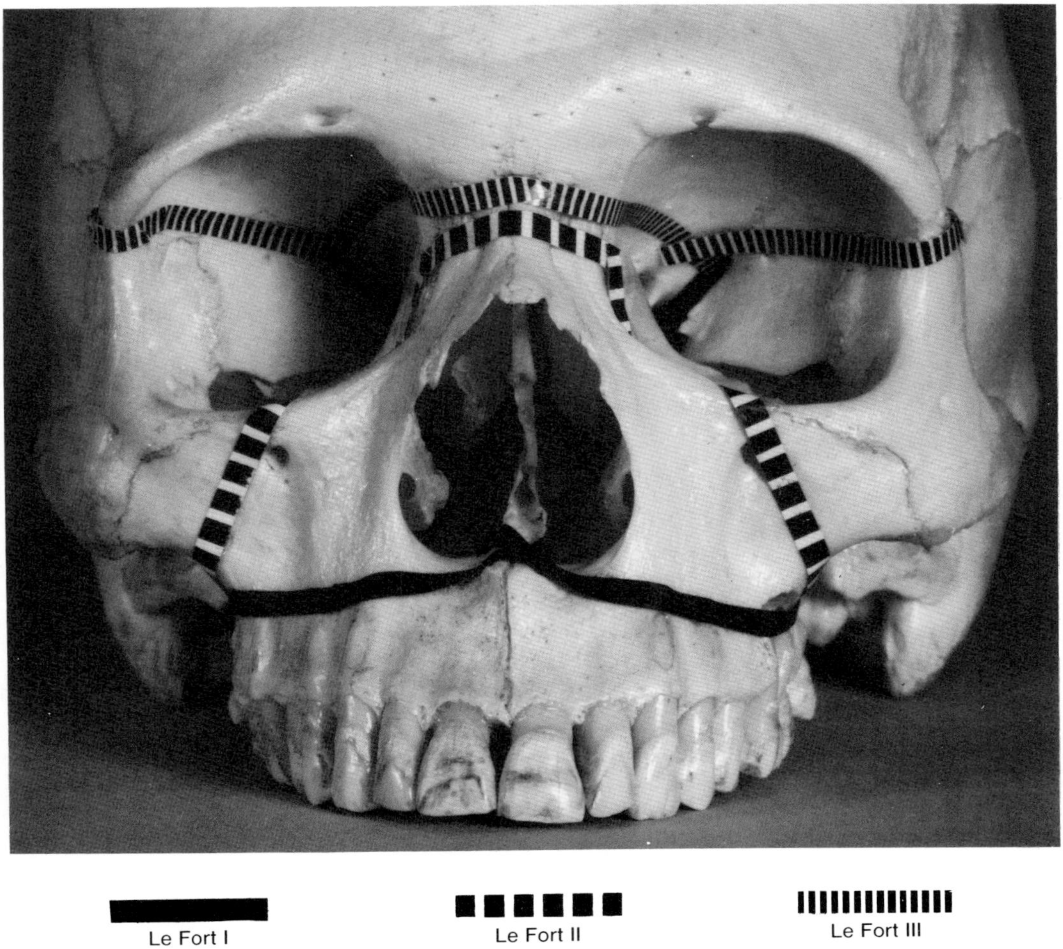

Figure 7-27. Photograph of a skull showing the common variants of fractures of the maxillae and concurrent fracturing of other bones. *A*, **Le Fort I.** A horizontal fracture of the maxillae, located just above the alveolar process, crossing the bony nasal septum and the pterygoid plates of the sphenoid bone (also see Fig. 7-123). The upper jaw (maxillae) becomes movable. *B*, **Le Fort II.** A fracture that passes from the posterolateral parts of the maxillary sinuses, upward and medially through the infraorbital notch, the lacrimals, or ethmoid to the bridge of the nose. As a result, the entire central pyramid of the face, including the hard palate and the alveolar processes, is separated from the rest of the skull. *CSF rhinorrhea* (leakage of cerebrospinal fluid from the nose) is common because of fracturing of the ethmoid bone and tearing of the meninges (membranes) covering the brain. *C*, **Le Fort III.** A horizontal fracture that passes through the superior orbital fissures, the ethmoid and nasal bones, and extends laterally through the greater wings of the sphenoid bone and the frontozygomatic sutures. As there is concurrent fracturing of the zygomatic arches, the maxillae and zygomatic bones are separated from the rest of the skull.

palpebra, eyelid) for closing the eyelids lightly to keep the cornea from drying; and (3) a *lacrimal part* for drawing the eyelids and the **lacrimal puncta** medially (Fig. 7-97). This third part lies deep to the palpebral part and is often considered to be part of it. It encloses the **lacrimal canaliculi** and passes posterior to the **lacrimal sac** (Fig. 7-100).

When all parts of the orbicularis oris contract, the eyes are firmly closed and the adjacent skin becomes wrinkled. Similar

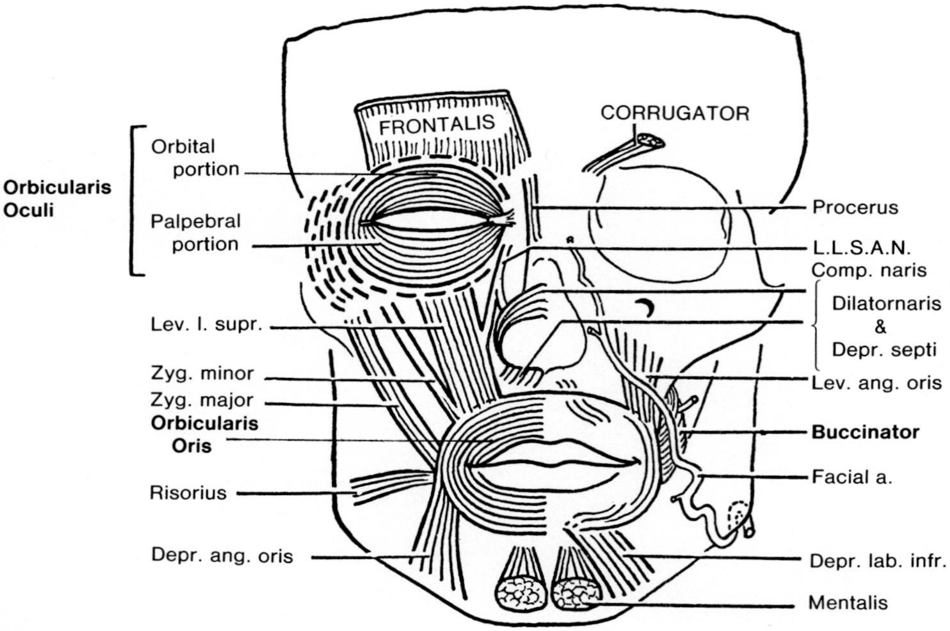

Figure 7-28. Diagram illustrating the facial muscles (muscles of facial expression), all of which are supplied by the facial nerve (CN VII). In general they arise from bones or fascia of the head and insert into the skin. The deeper muscles and the course of the facial artery are shown on the left. *The most important muscles are printed in bold type. L.L.S.A.N.,* levator labii superioris alaeque nasi. Plastic surgeons have a detailed knowledge of all the facial muscles and their variations. (For a drawing of a dissection of these muscles, see Fig. 7-31.)

wrinkling occurs when a person scrutinizes something. By 30 to 35 years these folds or creases around the eyes become permanent and are frequently called "crow's feet." Their presence in children and young adults may indicate a visual defect.

The **levator palpebrae superioris** muscle (Fig. 7-31), as its name indicates, **raises the upper eyelid**. It is supplied by the oculomotor nerve (CN III).

CLINICALLY ORIENTED COMMENTS

Injury to the facial nerve (CN VII) or to some of its branches produces paresis (weakness) or paralysis (loss of voluntary movement) in all or some of the facial muscles on the affected side. *The facial nerve is most often affected as it passes through the facial canal* in the petromastoid part of the temporal bone. In some cases the pressure on the nerve results from a viral infection that produces swelling (edema) of the nerve.

Paralysis of the facial nerve for no obvious reason, known as **Bell's palsy**, often occurs after exposure to a cold draft (Case 7-1). Patients with this condition are unable to close their lips and eye on the affected side; thus, they are unable to whistle, to blow a wind instrument, or to chew effectively. Because their buccinator muscle is also paralyzed, food dribbles out that side of the mouth or collects in the vestibule of the mouth.

Incomplete (paresis) or complete paralysis of the facial muscles is particularly noticeable around the mouth because the corner sags on the affected side. Complete paralysis of the entire side of the face indicates that the nerve has been injured between its origin in the brain stem and its point of branching in the parotid gland.

Paresis of some or all of the facial muscles suggests injury to one or more branches of the facial nerve within or beyond the parotid gland (Figs. 7-34 and 7-41), because there is some overlapping of the nerve supply to the muscles of the forehead.

In persons with **paralysis agitans (Parkinson's disease**, Parkinson's syndrome) resulting from neuronal degeneration in the **substantia nigra** (a large motor nucleus in the midbrain), emotional changes of facial expression are typically lost. This gives patients a mask-like, expressionless facies.

Muscles of the Nose (Figs. 7-28 and 7-31). All muscles around the nose are supplied by the facial nerve (CN VII). The **procerus** is a small slip of muscle that is continuous with the scalp muscle, occipitofrontalis (Fig. 7-43*B*). It passes from the forehead over the bridge of the nose where it is inserted into the skin. The procerus **draws the medial angle of the eyebrow down**, producing transverse wrinkles over the bridge of the nose. This probably reduces the glare of bright sunlight.

Figure 7-29. Drawing of a dissection of the platysma muscle. Observe that it is an extensive sheet of vertical muscle fibers that lies in the subcutaneous tissue of the neck and lower face. Note that it extends from in front of the upper two ribs obliquely upward in the neck and is inserted into the margin of the mandible. Observe that its fibers cross the mandible and blend with the other facial muscles (also see Fig. 7-31). This muscle is used chiefly to tense the skin of the neck. For more information on this muscle, see Chapter 9 and Figures 9-8 and 9-9.

The **nasalis** consists of transverse (compressor naris) and alar (dilator naris) parts. The *compressor naris* passes from the maxilla above the incisor teeth to the dorsum of the nose; it **compresses the anterior nasal aperture** (nostril). The dilator naris arises from the maxilla above the transverse part and inserts into the alar cartilages of the nose (Fig. 7-164). It **widens the anterior nasal aperture**. Observe the action of the nasalis in yourself in a mirror as you take a deep breath or in a person after a fast run. *Marked action of the dilator naris in sick infants strongly suggests respiratory distress, e.g.*, as occurs with pneumonia.

The **depressor septi**, often regarded as part of the dilator naris, arises from the maxilla above the central incisor tooth and inserts into the mobile part of the nasal septum. It assists the dilator naris in widening the nasal aperture during deep inspiration.

Sensory Nerves of the Face (Figs. 7-30 and 7-32). The innervation of the skin of the face is largely through the three branches of the **trigeminal nerve (CN V)**. Some skin over the angle of the mandible and anterior and posterior to the auricle is supplied by the **great auricular nerve** (from the cervical plexus). Although unimportant, some cutaneous fibers of the facial nerve probably also supply skin on both sides of the auricle.

The Trigeminal Nerve (Figs. 7-30 and 7-31). The trigeminal or **fifth cranial nerve** (CN V) is the largest of the 12 cranial nerves. It is *the principal general sensory nerve to the head*, particularly the face, and is the **motor nerve to the muscles of mastication** (masseter, temporalis, and the two pterygoids).

The cell bodies of most primary sensory neurons of the trigeminal nerve are located in the **trigeminal ganglion** (also called

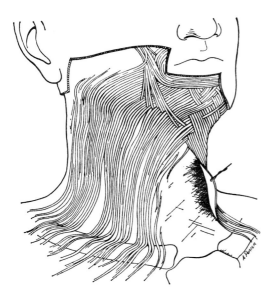

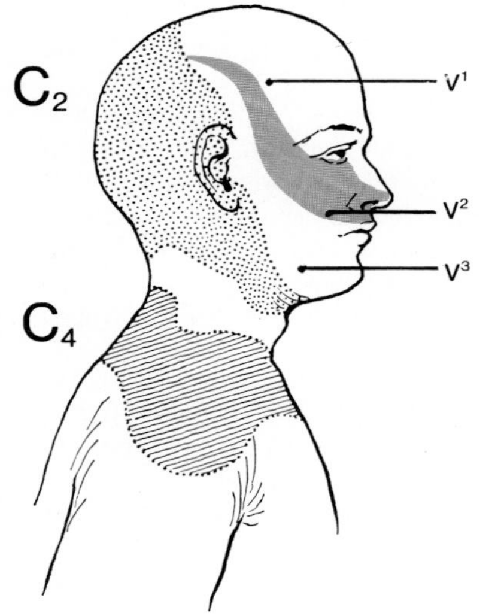
C2
C4
V1
V2
V3

A.

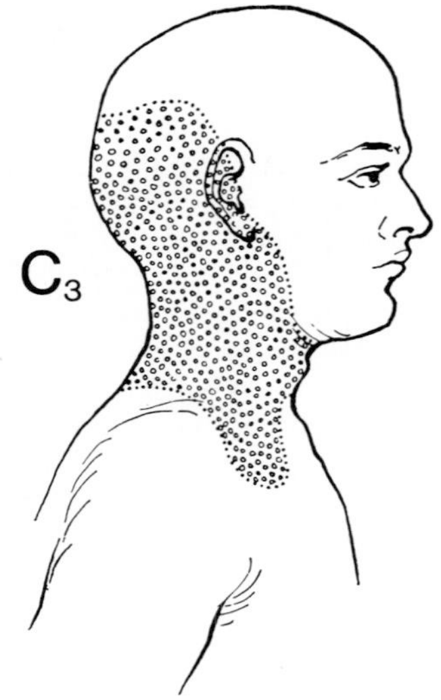
C3

B.

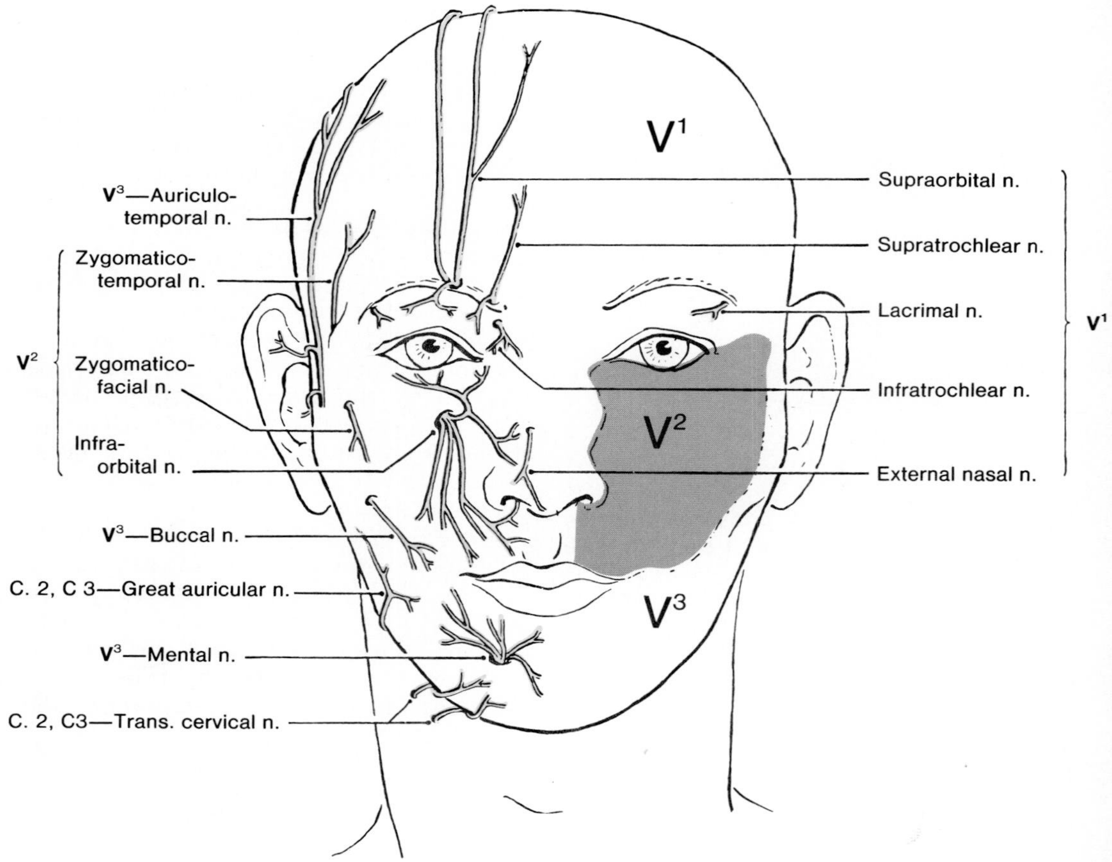
V1
V2
V3
V3—Auriculo-temporal n.
Zygomatico-temporal n.
V2
Zygomatico-facial n.
Infra-orbital n.
V3—Buccal n.
C. 2, C 3—Great auricular n.
V3—Mental n.
C. 2, C3—Trans. cervical n.
Supraorbital n.
Supratrochlear n.
Lacrimal n.
V1
Infratrochlear n.
External nasal n.

C.

semilunar or Gasserian ganglion); the other cell bodies are in the **mesencephalic nucleus** (the midbrain nucleus of this nerve). The peripheral processes of the unipolar cells in the trigeminal ganglion form the **ophthalmic** (CN V^1), the **maxillary** (CN V^2), and the sensory part of the **mandibular** nerve (CN V^3).

The Ophthalmic Nerve (Figs. 7-30 and 7-31). **CN V^1**, the **superior division of the trigeminal**, is the smallest of the three branches of this nerve and is **wholly sensory**. It supplies the area of skin derived from the embryonic frontonasal prominence (process). The ophthalmic nerve divides into **three branches**, the *nasociliary*, the *frontal*, and the *lacrimal*, just before entering the orbit through the superior orbital fissure. Five branches from these nerves take part in the sensory supply to the skin of the forehead, upper eyelid, and nose.

The nasociliary nerve supplies the tip of the nose via the external nasal branch of the anterior ethmoidal nerve, and the root of the nose via the infratrochlear nerve.

The frontal nerve, the direct continuation of the ophthalmic nerve *divides into two branches*. The **supratrochlear nerve** supplies the middle part of the forehead and the **supraorbital nerve** emerges through the supraorbital foramen (or notch) to supply the lateral part of the forehead and the front of the scalp.

The lacrimal nerve emerges over the upper lateral orbital margin to supply the lateral part of the upper eyelid.

The Maxillary Nerve (Figs. 7-30 and 7-31). **CN V^2**, the intermediate division of the trigeminal, has three cutaneous branches that supply the area of skin derived from the embryonic maxillary prominence (process).

The infraorbital nerve passes through the infraorbital foramen to supply skin of the **ala** (L. wing) **of the nose**, the **upper lip**, and the **lower eyelid**.

The zygomaticofacial nerve, a small branch of the maxillary, emerges from the zygomatic bone through a small foramen with the same name as the nerve. It supplies the skin of the face over the zygomatic bone (*i.e.*, zygomatic or malar prominence).

The zygomaticotemporal nerve emerges from the zygomatic bone through a foramen of the same name and supplies the skin over the temporal region.

CLINICALLY ORIENTED COMMENTS

For local anesthesia of the face, the infraorbital nerve is often infiltrated with an anesthetic agent at the **infraorbital foramen** (Fig. 7-31) or inside the canal (*e.g.*, for treatment of wounds of the upper lip or for repairing the upper incisor teeth). You can easily determine the site of emergence of this nerve by exerting pressure on your zygomatic bone in the region of the infraorbital foramen and nerve. Pressure on the nerve causes considerable pain.

The Mandibular Nerve (Figs. 7-30 and 7-31). **CN V^3**, the **inferior division of the trigeminal**, has three sensory branches that supply the area of skin derived from

Figure 7-30. Drawing of the sensory nerves of the head, neck, and face. *A* and *B* show the distribution of the cutaneous areas (dermatomes) supplied by spinal nerves. In *A* observe that the trigeminal nerve (CN V) is responsible for general sensation from the skin of the face, the forehead, and the scalp as far posterior as the vertex. In *C* the distribution of the three divisions of the trigeminal nerve (CN V) correspond *roughly* to the three embryological regions of the face. Thus the superior or first division, the ophthalmic nerve (V^1) supplies the skin and tissues derived from the frontonasal prominence (process); the intermediate or second division, the maxillary nerve (V^2), supplies the *pink colored area* of skin and other tissues derived from the maxillary prominence (process); and the inferior or third division, the mandibular nerve (V^3) supplies the skin and other tissues derived from the mandibular prominence (process). Note that some cutaneous branches [*e.g.*, auriculotemporal nerve (V^3)] have spread backward in the scalp as the head developed.

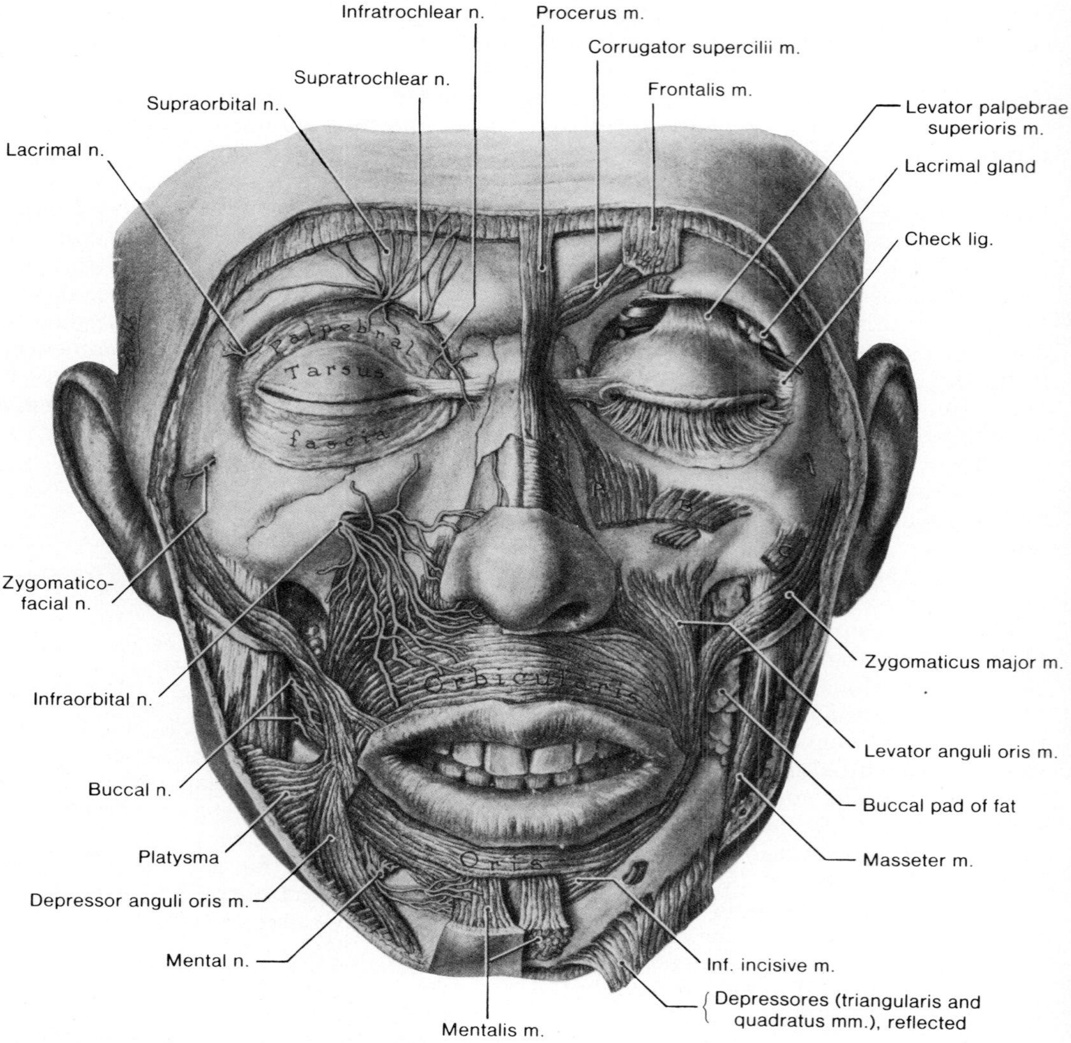

Figure 7-31. Drawing of a dissection of the face showing the cutaneous branches of the trigeminal nerve (*yellow*) and several facial muscles. A *greenish colored pin* has been inserted behind the aponeurosis of the levator palpebrae superioris muscle to demonstrate its fan-shaped attachment to the superior tarsus (thin plate of condensed fibrous tissue in the eyelid). Some fibers of this tendon insert into the skin of the upper eyelid. *A*, levator labii superioris alaeque nasi. *B*, levator labii superioris. *C*, zygomaticus major.

the embryonic mandibular prominence (process) of the first branchial arch. It also supplies motor fibers to the **muscles of mastication** (chewing). Of the three divisions of the trigeminal, *CN* V^3 *is the only division of the trigeminal nerve that carries motor fibers.*

The mental nerve, a branch of the *inferior alveolar nerve*, emerges through the mental foramen and divides into three branches that supply the skin of the chin and the skin and mucous membrane of the lower lip and gingiva (gum).

The buccal nerve (L. *bucca*, cheek) is a small branch of the mandibular that emerges from deep to the ramus of the mandible and supplies the skin of the cheek over the buccinator muscle. It also supplies the mucous membrane lining the cheek and the posterior part of the buccal surface of the gingiva.

The auriculotemporal nerve (Figs. 7-32, 7-116, and 7-118), the third sensory branch of the mandibular, passes medial to the neck of the mandible and then turns upward posterior to its head in front of the auricle. *It crosses over the root of the zygomatic process* of the temporal bone deep to the superficial temporal artery. As its name suggests, it supplies parts of the auricle, the external acoustic meatus, the tympanic membrane (eardrum) and skin in the temporal area.

CLINICALLY ORIENTED COMMENTS

Dentists frequently anesthetize the **inferior alveolar nerve** before repairing or removing the premolar or molar teeth of the mandible (Fig. 7-20). As the mental nerve is one of the two terminal branches of the inferior alveolar nerve, it is understandable why one's chin and lower lip on the affected side also lose sensation.

Trigeminal neuralgia (tic douloureaux) is a condition characterized by sudden attacks of excruciating pain in the distribution of one of the divisions of the tri-

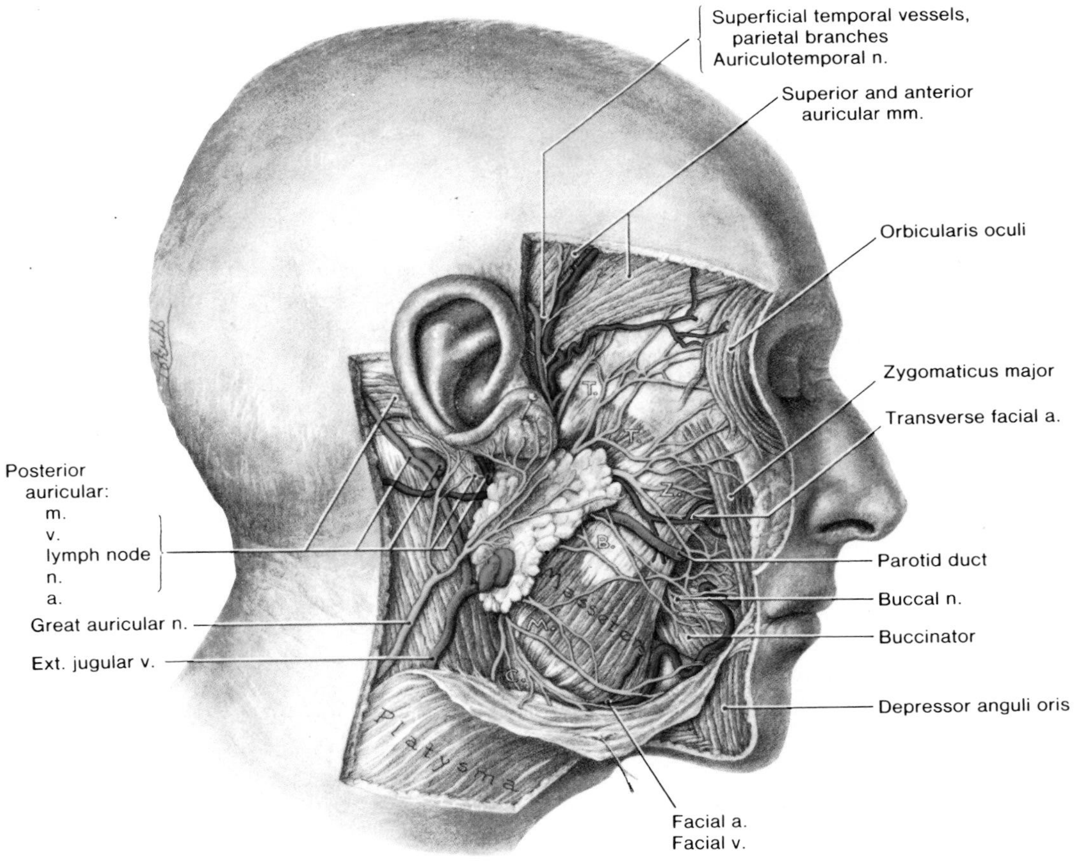

Figure 7-32. Drawing of a lateral view of a dissection of the right side of the head showing the great auricular nerve (C2 and C3) and the terminal branches of the facial nerve (CN VII): *T*, temporal, *Z*, zygomatic, *B*, buccal, *M*, mandibular and *C*, cervical. Obviously the facial nerve, motor to the muscles of facial expression, is in jeopardy during surgery of the parotid gland. The masseter is a muscle of mastication that is derived from mesenchyme of the second branchial arch and is supplied by the nerve of that arch (CN V^3).

geminal nerve, usually CN V^2. The cause of the condition is unknown, but current views are mentioned in the discussion of **Case 7-2**, as are present procedures for alleviating the pain.

The sensory and motor nuclei of the trigeminal nerve may be involved in degenerative or other lesions in the brain stem, or intracranial portions of the nerve may be affected by trauma or a tumor. If the motor fibers are affected, the muscles of mastication will be weakened or paralyzed, causing deviation of the mandible to the affected side on opening the mouth.

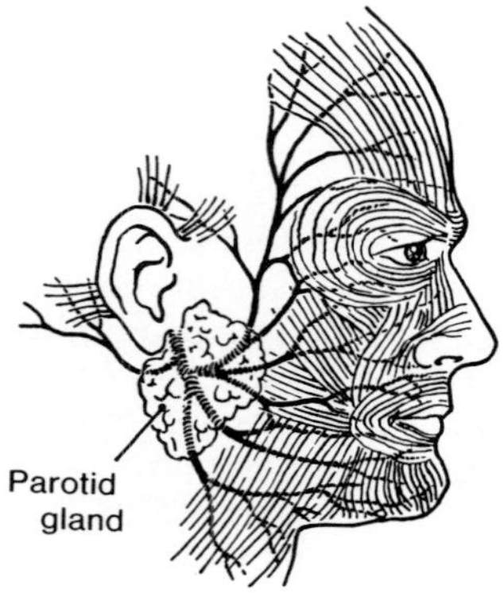

Figure 7-34. Drawing of a lateral view of a deep dissection of the right side of the face of an adult male exposing the stem of the facial nerve descending from the stylomastoid foramen and curving forward to penetrate the deep part of the parotid gland. Observe that within the parotid gland the facial nerve divides into numerous radiating branches which spread from the scalp to the neck. Note its distribution to the facial and scalp muscles.

Motor Nerves of the Face (Figs. 7-31 and 7-32). CN VII supplies the muscles of facial expression and CN V^3 supplies the muscles of mastication.

The Facial Nerve (Figs. 7-32 to 7-34 and 7-116 to 7-118). **CN VII** supplies the superficial muscles of the neck (*i.e.*, the platysma), the face, the auricle, the muscle of the scalp, and certain other muscles derived from mesoderm of the embryonic second branchial arch. It is the *sole motor supply to the muscles of facial expression* and is sensory to the taste buds in the anterior two-thirds of the tongue. It also conveys general sensation from a small area around the external acoustic meatus and is secretomotor to the submandibular, sublingual, and intralingual salivary glands.

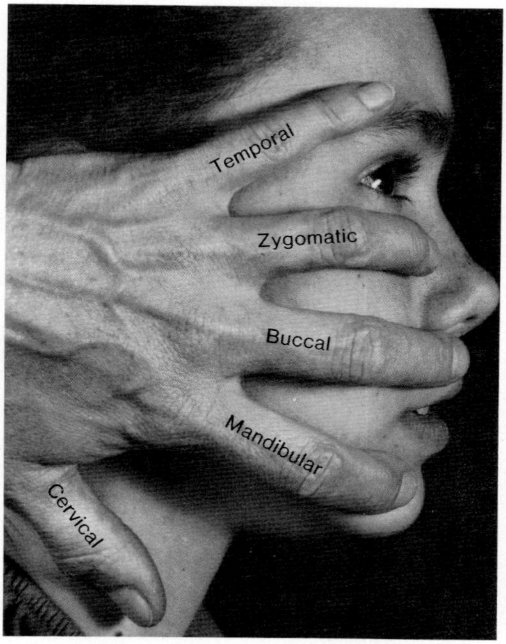

Figure 7-33. Photograph of a lateral view of the face of a 12-year-old girl illustrating a simple method for remembering the general course of the five main branches of the facial nerve (CN VII) that are motor to the muscles of facial expression. (For details, see Fig. 7-32).

The facial nerve emerges from the skull through the **stylomastoid foramen** (Fig. 7-6), between the mastoid and styloid processes of the temporal bone, and almost immediately enters the **parotid gland**. It runs superficially within this gland before giving rise to **five terminal branches** (*temporal, zygomatic, buccal, mandibular*, and *cervical*) which emerge from the superior, anterior, and inferior margins of the gland. These branches spread out like the abducted fingers of the hand (Figs. 7-32 to 7-34) to supply the **muscles of facial expression**, or mimetic (G. imitative) muscles.

The motor component of the facial nerve,

supplying muscles of facial expression and certain other muscles, is the most important part of the nerve clinically. The motor nucleus of the facial nerve is located in the pons.

The main clinical tests for the facial nerve concern the facial muscles; hence, you should have a general idea where the five major branches of the facial nerve go (Figs. 7-32 and 7-33). *The names of the nerves indicate the regions they supply.*

The **temporal branches** cross the zygomatic arch to supply all the superficial muscles above it. [The deeper temporalis muscle (Fig. 7-114), the major muscle of the temporal region that closes the jaw, is supplied by CN V^3, the mandibular division of the trigeminal nerve.]

The **zygomatic branches** pass over the zygomatic bone to supply muscles in the infraorbital region. The **buccal branches** pass horizontally external to the masseter to supply the buccinator and the muscles of the upper lip. The **mandibular branch** supplies the muscles of the lower lip and chin and the **cervical branch** supplies the platysma, the superficial muscle of the neck (Fig. 7-29).

CLINICALLY ORIENTED COMMENTS

If the **motor nucleus of the facial nerve** is involved in a disease process or a lesion in the brain stem, there will be paralysis of the ipsilateral (L. same side) muscles of facial expression. In time the facial muscles atrophy (waste away).

Peripheral facial paralysis may be caused by chilling of the face, middle ear infections, tumors, fractures, and other disorders. About 75% of all facial nerve lesions are of this type. The types of signs and symptoms depend upon the location of the lesion. For the clinical characteristics of a lesion outside the stylomastoid foramen, see Case 7-1.

As the facial nerve runs superficially within the parotid gland, it may be infiltrated by malignant cells (*e.g.*, from a **carcinoma of the parotid**). This commonly results in incomplete paralysis (**paresis**) of the facial muscles. Benign (nonmalignant) tumors usually do not infiltrate and cause facial nerve paralysis, but care must be taken to preserve the facial nerve and its branches (Fig. 7-34) during excision of a benign tumor. On rare occasions, parotid inflammation (*e.g.*, mumps) may temporarily affect the facial nerve.

As the **mastoid process** is not present at birth, the facial nerve may be easily injured by forceps during delivery of a baby. Similarly, as the mastoid process that usually protects the facial nerve is not well developed in children, the facial nerve may be more easily injured at its site of emergence from the skull than it is in adults.

In view of the fan-like distribution of the branches of the facial nerve (Fig. 7-32), it is unwise from an anatomical standpoint to make vertical incisions in the parotid gland (*e.g.*, for drainage of pus). Short incisions, parallel to the courses of the branches in the area concerned, are less likely to produce a noticeable effect on the functioning of the facial muscles. Weakness rather than complete paralysis of a muscle(s) usually results from injury to the branches of the facial nerve because of their overlapping distribution.

Following one common type of **stroke**, or cerebrovascular accident (**CVA**), one side of the body is paralyzed; however, there is usually some preservation of movement of muscles of the forehead on the paralyzed side. The explanation for this is that the upper part of the motor nucleus of the facial nerve is bilaterally controlled from the cerebral cortex; hence, forehead muscles are relatively spared in a unilateral brain lesion above the level of origin of the motor component of the nerve that supplies the muscles of facial expression.

Arteries of the Face (Figs. 7-32, 7-35, and 7-36). The face is richly supplied with arteries.

The Facial Artery. This vessel, the **chief artery of the face**, arises from the **external carotid** and appears at the inferior border of the mandible, just anterior to the

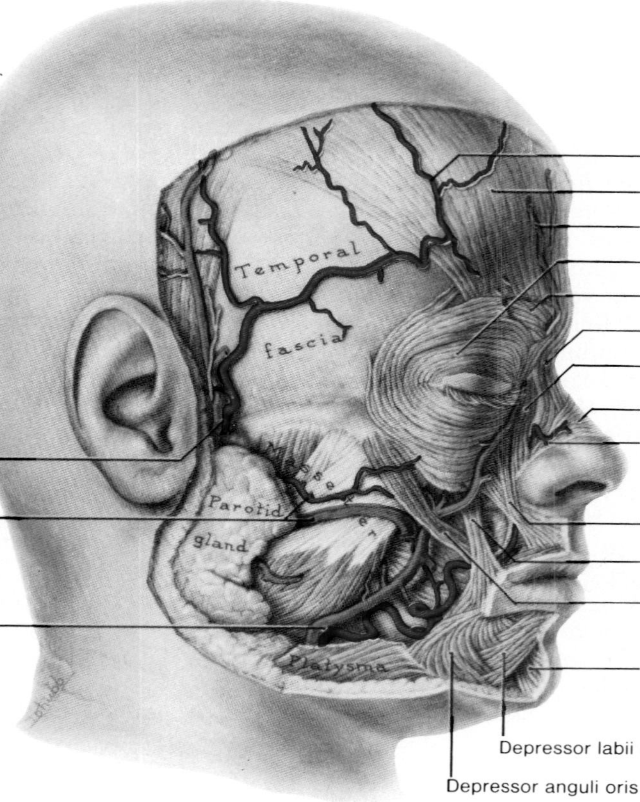

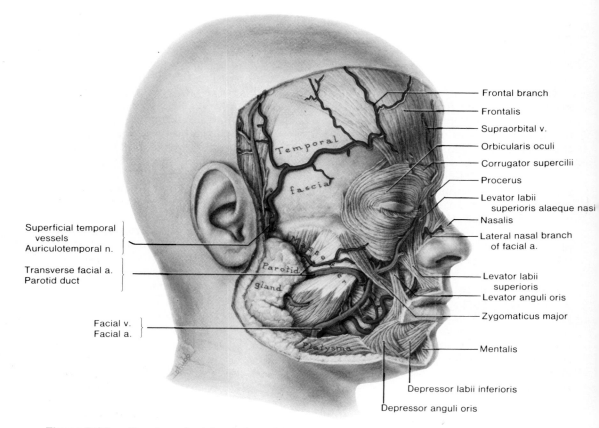

Figure 7-35. Drawing of a lateral view of a dissection of the face of a young man exposing the muscles of facial expression (all supplied by CN VII) and the arteries of the face. The masseter muscle, one of the muscles of mastication that is a powerful closer of the jaw, is also shown; it is supplied by CN V^3 (mandibular division of the trigeminal nerve).

masseter muscle. As it crosses the inferior border of the mandible, it usually grooves the bone (Fig. 7-21). Because the artery is superficial and lies immediately beneath the platysma, its pulsations can be easily felt here in most people.

In its course over the face to the **inner canthus** (medial angle) of the eye (Fig. 7-97), the facial artery crosses successively the mandible, the buccinator, the maxilla, and the levator anguli oris but lies deep to the zygomaticus major and levator labii superioris (Figs. 7-31 and 7-35). Near the termination of its sinuous course, it passes about a fingerbreadth lateral to the angle of the mouth and ends by sending branches to the lip and the side of the nose. The part of the facial artery that runs along the nose to the inner angle of the eye is often called the *angular artery*.

CLINICALLY ORIENTED COMMENTS

There are numerous communications (anastomoses) between the branches of the facial artery and other arteries of the face; hence, compressing the facial artery against the mandible on one side does not stop all bleeding from a lacerated facial artery or one of its branches. In **lacerations of the lip**, pressure must be applied on both sides of the cut to stop the bleeding (*e.g.*, by compressing both parts of the cut lip between the index finger and the thumb). In general, *facial wounds bleed freely and heal quickly*.

Because branches of the external carotid artery anastomose so freely with each other and with those of the external carotid artery on the other side, one external carotid can be clamped in order to minimize bleeding and thus facilitate extensive surgery on one side of the head. Owing to the numerous anastomoses, there would be little or no impairment of functional circulation or wound healing. Clamping an external carotid artery will sometimes (but not always) control intractable nasal hemorrhage.

The Superficial Temporary Artery (Figs. 7-32, 7-35, and 7-36). This large vessel is the *smaller of the two terminal branches of the external carotid* artery; the other terminal branch is the **maxillary artery**. The superficial temporal artery begins deep to the parotid gland, behind the neck of the mandible, and ascends superficial to the posterior part of the zygomatic process of the temporal bone to enter the **temporal fossa** (Figs. 7-1 and 7-7). It ends in the scalp by dividing into frontal and parietal branches. Pulsations of this artery can be felt when it is compressed against the zygomatic process anterior to the auricle and are often visible, particularly in thin elderly persons.

The Transverse Facial Artery (Figs. 7-32, 7-35, and 7-36). This small artery of the face *arises from the superficial temporal artery* before it emerges from the parotid gland. It crosses the face, superficial to the masseter muscle, about a fingerbreadth inferior to the zygomatic arch in company with one or two branches of the facial nerve. It divides into numerous branches which supply the parotid gland and its duct, the

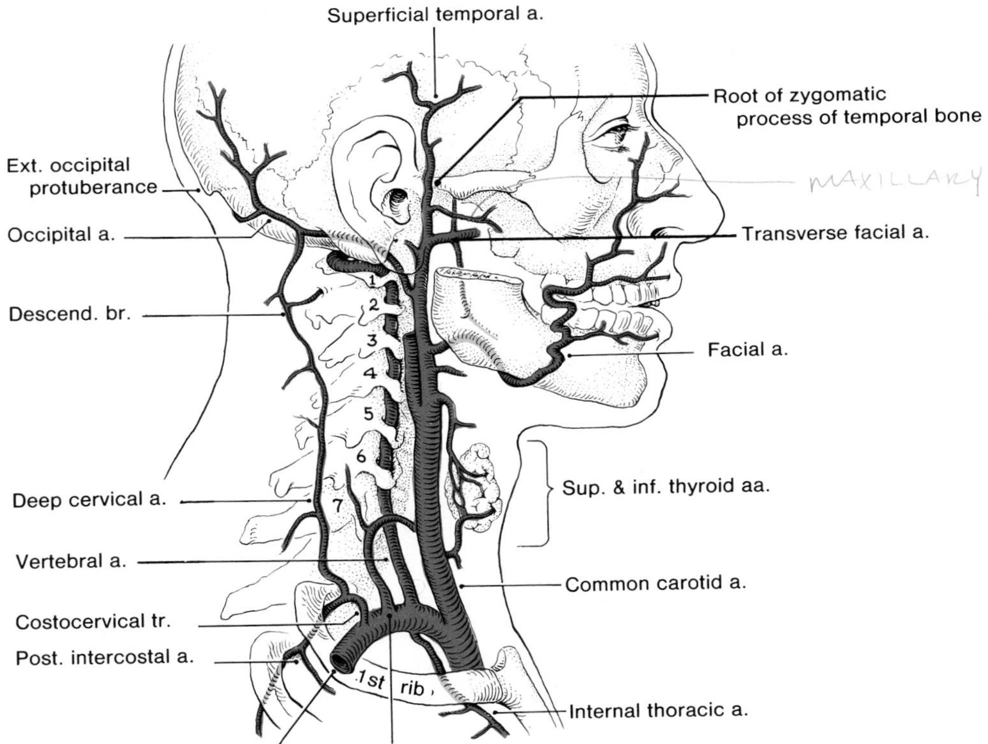

Figure 7-36. Diagram showing the arteries of the head. Note particularly the tortuous course of the facial artery. The temporal pulse can be taken anterior to the auricle where the superficial temporal artery crosses the root of the zygomatic process of the temporal bone. The facial pulse may be felt where the facial artery turns around the lower border of the mandible. Observe the important vertebral artery arising from the first part of the subclavian artery and ascending through the foramina transversaria of the upper six cervical vertebrae. Note that on reaching the base of the skull, it winds around the lateral mass of the atlas (C1).

masseter, and the skin of the face before anastomosing with branches of the facial artery.

CLINICALLY ORIENTED COMMENTS

The pulse of the superficial temporal and facial arteries are often taken by physicians when it is not convenient to take the pulse at the usual sites (*e.g.*, the lower end of the radius). Anesthetists, sitting at the head of the operating table, often take the **temporal pulse** just in front of the tragus of the ear where the superficial temporal artery crosses the root of the zygomatic process of the temporal bone (Fig. 7-35), but the **facial pulse** can also be palpated where the facial artery winds around the lower border of the mandible (Fig. 7-36). Because of the clinical importance of these pulses, be certain that you can detect them quickly on yourself and others.

Veins of the Face (Figs. 7-32, 7-35, 7-37, 7-38, and 7-41). These veins anastomose freely and are drained by veins accompanying the arteries of the face.

The Facial Vein. This vessel provides the **major venous drainage of the face**. It begins at the medial angle (inner canthus) of the eye (Fig. 7-97) by the union of the supraorbital and the supratrochlear veins. The superior part of the facial vein near the medial angle of the eye is often called the **angular vein**. The facial vein runs downward and backward through the face, posterior to the facial artery, but it takes a straighter and more superficial course than the artery. Inferior to the margin of the mandible, the facial vein is joined

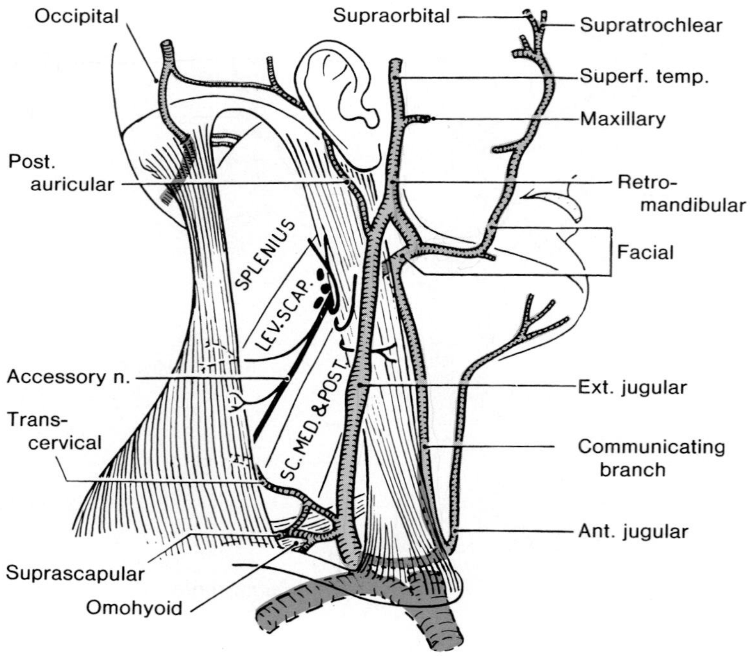

Figure 7-37. Diagram of the superficial veins of the right side of the head and neck. Observe that the facial vein passes deeply at the anterior margin of the sternocleidomastoid muscle and crosses the external carotid artery (not shown) to enter the internal jugular vein (Fig. 7-74). Observe that the facial vein is formed by the union of the supraorbital and supratrochlear veins at the medial angle of the eye. The first part of the facial vein near this angle is often referred to clinically as the angular vein.

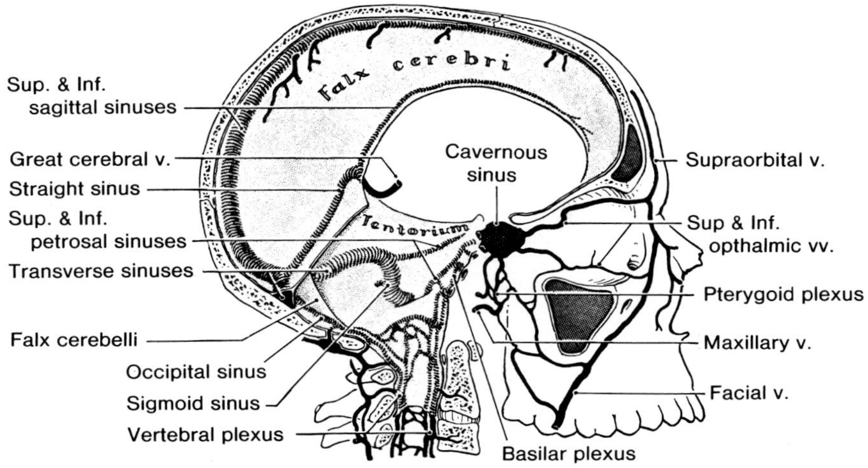

Figure 7-38. Diagram of the venous sinuses of the dura mater. The cavernous sinuses are situated one on each side of the sphenoid bone. The cavernous sinus drains into the transverse sinus through the superior petrosal sinus. Note particularly that the cavernous sinus communicates with the veins of the face via the ophthalmic veins and the pterygoid plexus.

by the anterior branch of the **retromandibular vein**, which is formed by the junction of the maxillary and superficial temporal veins. The facial vein ends by draining into the internal jugular vein deep to the sternocleidomastoid muscle (Fig. 7-37).

The facial vein makes clinically important connections with the cavernous sinus (Fig. 7-38) through the **superior ophthalmic vein** and also through the **pterygoid plexus** via the deep facial vein.

CLINICALLY ORIENTED COMMENTS

Blood from the inner canthus of the eye, the nose, and the lips usually drains downward through the facial vein, especially when the patient is erect. However, as *the facial vein has no valves*, blood may run through it in the opposite direction when pressure conditions are different and enter the cavernous sinus, one of the cranial venous sinuses (Fig. 7-38). In patients with **thrombophlebitis of the facial vein**, pieces of an infected clot (embolus) may extend or pass into the intracranial venous system. Here it may produce **thrombophlebitis of the cortical veins** or of the cavernous sinuses (Case 7-3). Infection of the facial veins spreading to the dural venous sinuses may be initiated by squeezing pustules on the side of the nose and upper lip. Consequently, this triangular area is often called **the danger triangle of the face** (Fig. 7-203).

The Superficial Temporal Vein (Figs. 7-32, 7-35, 7-37, and 7-38). This vein drains the forehead and scalp and receives tributaries from the veins of the temple and face. In the region of the temporomandibular joint, it enters the parotid gland and unites with the maxillary vein to form the retromandibular vein.

The Retromandibular Vein (Figs. 7-37, 7-41, and 9-21). This vein is *formed by the union of the superficial temporal and maxillary veins*, posterior to the neck of the mandible. It descends within the parotid gland, superficial to the external carotid artery, but deep to the facial nerve. It divides into an anterior branch that unites with the facial vein and a posterior branch that joins the posterior auricular vein to become the external jugular vein.

Lymphatic Drainage of the Face (Figs. 7-32, 7-39, 7-41, and 9-21). The lym-

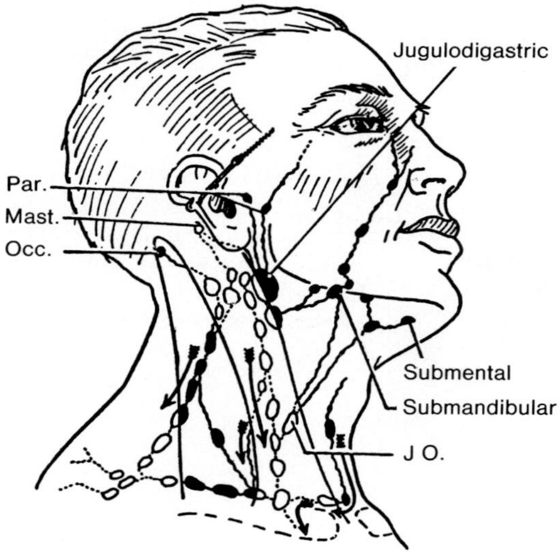

Figure 7-39. Diagram of the lymphatics of the head and neck illustrating the lymphatic drainage of the face. Note that there is a wide band or ring of superficial lymph nodes around the junction of the head and the neck composed as follows: occipital, retroauricular (mastoid), parotid, submandibular, and submental. Note that lymph from the anterior part of the face drains via the submandibular and submental lymph nodes into the jugulo-omhyoid (*JO*) node.

phatic vessels in the forehead and the anterior part of the face accompany the other facial vessels and drain into the three to six **submandibular lymph nodes** located along the submandibular gland and the inferior border of the mandible. A few buccal and mandibular nodes occur along the course of the lymph vessels. The vessels from the lateral part of the face, including the eyelids, drain downward toward the **parotid nodes**. The superficial parotid nodes drain into the deep parotid nodes which in turn drain into the **deep cervical lymph nodes**.

Lymphatics in the upper lip and in the lateral parts of the lower lip drain into the **submandibular lymph nodes**, whereas lymphatics in the central part of the lower lip and in the chin drain into the **submental lymph nodes**, from which lymph may drain directly into the **jugulo-omohyoid lymph nodes**.

CLINICALLY ORIENTED COMMENTS

The lymph vessels and nodes draining an infected area of the face may become inflamed, resulting in an acute or chronic **lymphangitis** (inflammation of lymph vessels) or **lymphadenitis** (inflammation of lymph nodes). Blockage of lymphatic channels may also occur as a result of the spread of malignant (cancer) cells, a process known as **lymphogenous metastasis**. Knowledge of the lymphatic drainage of the face enables one to predict where cancer cells may spread (*e.g.*, a squamous cell carcinoma of the lower lip as in Case 7-4).

The Parotid Gland (Figs. 7-32, 7-34, 7-35, 7-40, and 7-116). Although part of the digestive system, this gland is in the face and shall also be considered here. The parotid (G. *para*, near + *otis*, the ear) is wedged between the ramus of the mandible and the mastoid process. It occupies the side of the face anterior and inferior to the

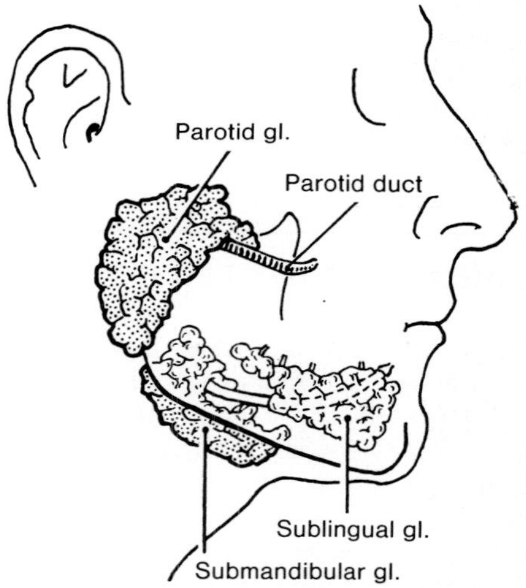

Figure 7-40. Diagram illustrating the location of the three salivary glands. Note that the parotid gland (the largest of them) is wrapped around the neck of the mandible. The parotid duct is a thick-walled tube that drains the saliva from the gland and carries it to the vestibule of the mouth.

auricle. You can determine its general location by making a triangle, the angles of which are at the mastoid process, the angle of the mandible, and the midpoint of the zygomatic arch.

In living persons the parotid is an irregular, lobulated, yellowish mass closely related to the ramus of the mandible. It has a very irregular shape because, during development, it grew into the cervical fascia and became moulded into a more or less triangular shape as it was wedged between the mandible and the mastoid process. It also encloses structures in the area it invaded (*e.g.*, the facial nerve).

The parotid gland is the largest of the paired salivary glands and, like the other two, develops as an outgrowth from the mouth (buccal cavity). As viewed superficially, the parotid gland is somewhat triangular with its apex posterior to the angle of the mandible and its base along the zygomatic arch, overlapping the posterior part of the masseter muscle.

The parotid duct (Fig. 7-32), about 5 cm long, passes horizontally forward from the anterior edge of that part of the gland lying lateral (external) to the masseter muscle. It passes anteriorly across this muscle and at its anterior border it turns medially and **pierces** the **buccinator** muscle. It opens into the mouth cavity on the inside of the cheek, usually at the level of the crown of the **upper second molar tooth**. To locate the approximate course of the parotid duct, place your index finger along the lower border of the **zygomatic arch** and then point it toward the upper lip (Fig. 7-42). The parotid duct courses along the lower border of your finger and ends approximately at your fingertip.

If you tense your **masseter muscle** by clenching your teeth, you may be able to palpate the thick-walled parotid duct in your cheek, about a fingerbreadth below the zygomatic arch, as you roll it with your finger over the anterior border of the masseter muscle. The gland itself is more difficult to palpate because it is covered by a dense layer of deep cervical fascia which is continuous with that over the adjacent muscles and the periosteum of the zygomatic arch.

Look into someone's mouth with a flashlight and observe the opening of the parotid duct opposite the second upper molar tooth. If the person is asked to suck a lemon slice, you may be able to see clear saliva flowing out of the duct. Where the duct opens into the mouth, note that there is a small papilla. You should be able to feel this papilla in your mouth with your finger and possibly with your tongue.

Structures in the Parotid Gland (Figs. 7-32, 7-34, 7-40, and 7-41). The vessels, nerves, and lymph nodes in and around the parotid have been described; thus, only summary notes on them are given here.

Parotid lymph nodes are located superficial and deep to the parotid fascia and within the gland. Consequently, to ensure removal of all cancerous nodes associated with a **malignant parotid tumor**, often the surgeon removes the entire gland.

Other structures in and around the parotid gland are the **facial nerve**, the **retromandibular vein**, the **external carotid artery**, and the **great auricular** and **au-**

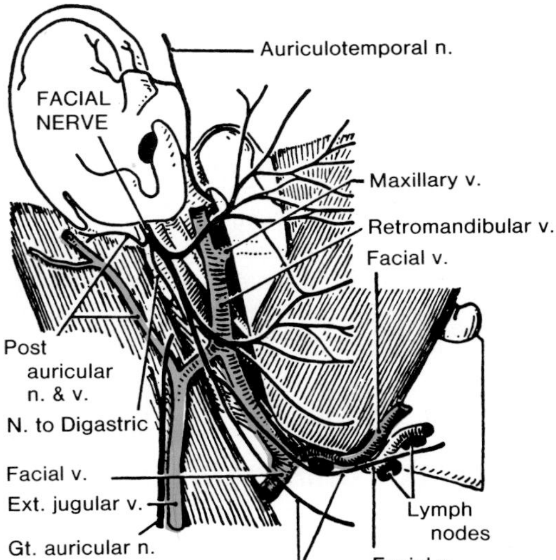

Figure 7-41. Drawing of a dissection of the parotid region showing the location of the facial nerve and veins. The facial nerve and its branches are foremost in importance and are in jeopardy during surgery of the parotid gland. Compare with the superficial dissections illustrated in Figures 7-32 and 7-34.

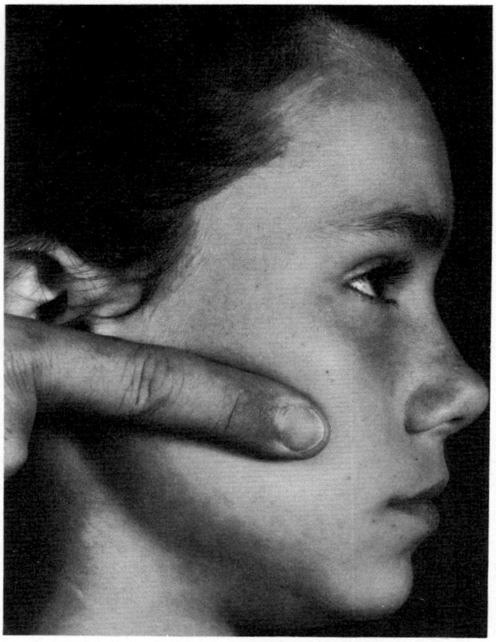

Figure 7-42. Photograph of a lateral view of the right side of the face of a 12-year-old girl illustrating how to determine the course of the parotid duct. The examiner's finger is placed along the inferior border of her zygomatic arch and parallel with it. The parotid duct runs along the inferior border of the finger and ends internally opposite the second upper molar tooth (indicated by the tip of the finger). With the jaws clenched you can palpate the duct by rolling it with the fingertip against the anterior border of the underlying masseter muscle.

riculotemporal nerves. These nerves supply sensory fibers to the parotid and to the skin overlying it.

CLINICALLY ORIENTED COMMENTS

As the facial nerve passes into the substance of the parotid gland and divides into numerous branches, it is in jeopardy during surgery in the parotid region (*e.g.*, for removal of a **carcinoma of the parotid**). Injury to this nerve results in partial or complete paralysis of the ipsilateral muscles of facial expression.

During illness, particularly debilitating ones, a bacterial infection may spread from the mouth along the parotid duct to the gland. The parotid may also become infected via the blood stream [*e.g.*, as occurs in **mumps** (*epidemic parotiditis* or *parotitis*), an acute communicable viral disease affecting the salivary glands, particularly the parotid].

Infection of the parotid gland causes inflammation (**parotiditis**). Severe pain soon occurs because the gland is invested with a capsule derived from a dense layer of **deep cervical fascia** which limits swelling. The pain results from stretching of the parotid capsule. Often the pain is worse during chewing because the gland is wrapped around the posterior border of the ramus of the mandible and is compressed against the mastoid process when the mouth is opened.

The mumps virus may also cause inflammation of the parotid duct, producing redness of its papilla. As mumps (an old English word meaning lumps) may be confused with a **toothache**, often redness of the papilla of the parotid duct is an early sign indicating disease involving the parotid gland and not the teeth. Sucking a lemon is also used as a **test for parotiditis** because lemon juice (being acid) stimulates the secretion of saliva (*i.e.*, it is a **salivant**). This increases the swelling of the gland and stimulates the sensory (pain) nerve fibers in its capsule.

Parotid gland disease often causes pain in the auricle, the external acoustic meatus, the temple, and the temporomandibular joint because the pain may be referred to these structures from the parotid gland by the **auriculotemporal nerve** (Fig. 7-32), a superficial branch of the mandibular division of the trigeminal nerve (CN V^3). It supplies sensory fibers to the skin of the temple and carries parasympathetic motor fibers to the gland to which they are **secretomotor.**

A **radiopaque material** (*e.g.*, Pantopaque) can be injected into the duct system of the parotid gland via a cannula inserted into the parotid duct. This technique, followed by radiography, is called **sialography**. By studying **parotid sialograms**, parts of the duct system displaced or dilated by disease can be detected. The parotid duct may become blocked by a **calculus** (L. a pebble), resulting in pain in the parotid gland which is made worse by eating. Again, sucking a lemon slice is painful because of the build-up of saliva in the proximal part of the duct.

THE SCALP

The scalp consists of five layers of soft tissue covering the calvaria (Fig. 7-43). It extends from the superior part of the neck at the back of the head to the forehead and eyebrows in front and to the level of the zygomatic arches laterally.

CLINICALLY ORIENTED COMMENTS

The scalp is of clinical importance mainly because it covers the calvaria which en-

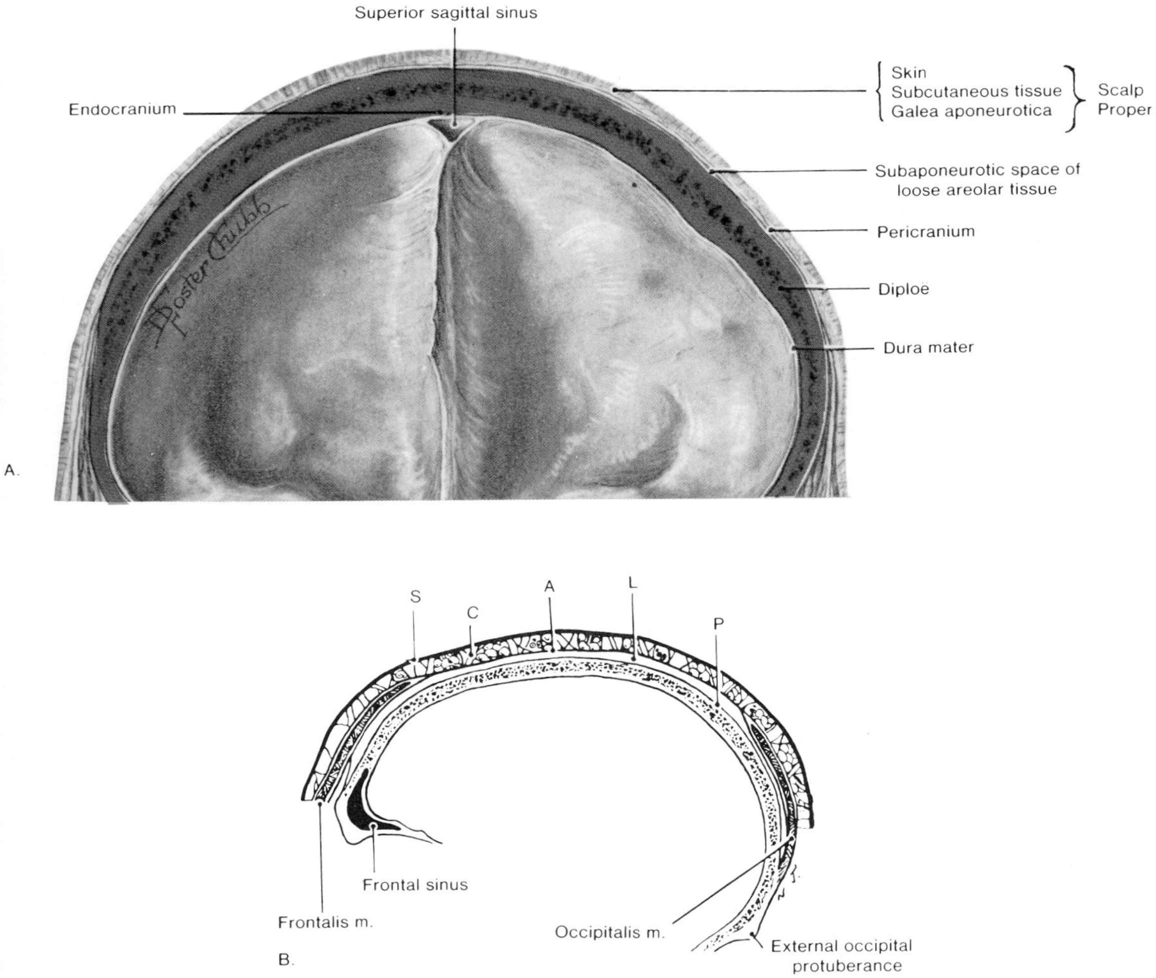

Figure 7-43. Sections through the scalp and the calvaria. *A*, a coronal section showing the layers of the scalp and the dura mater. *B*, a sagittal section showing the key to remembering the five layers of the scalp as demonstrated. *S*, skin; *C*, connective tissue (dense subcutaneous); *A*, aponeurosis epicranalis including frontalis and occipitalis muscles at its anterior and posterior ends, respectively; *L*, loose connective tissue; *P*, pericranium (periosteal layer).

closes the brain. *Scalp lacerations are the most common type of head injury requiring surgical care.* Scalp wounds bleed profusely because arteries enter all around the periphery of the scalp and they do not retract because the scalp is tough; hence, unconscious *patients may bleed to death from scalp lacerations* if the bleeding is not controlled. If scalp wounds are not treated appropriately, a scalp infection may develop and spread into the underlying cranial bones, causing **osteomyelitis**, and thence into the cranial cavity, producing an **extradural abscess** (collection of pus) or **meningitis** (inflammation of the membranes covering the brain).

LAYERS OF THE SCALP

The scalp consists of **five layers** (Fig. 7-43), but clinically the first three (the scalp proper) are usually regarded as a single layer because they remain firmly bound together when a scalp flap is turned down during a **craniotomy** (surgical opening of the cranium) or is torn off in accidents. It is difficult, if not impossible, to separate the skin and the subcutaneous tissues of the scalp from the dense connective tissue of the **epicranial aponeurosis** or galea aponeurotica (L. *galea*, helmet).

The scalp proper is composed of three fused layers (Fig. 7-43*A*). It is separated from the pericranium (periosteum of the cranium) by loose connective tissue (areolar tissue) that forms a cleavage plane. Because of this potential areolar space, the scalp is fairly mobile. Verify this by massaging your scalp or by moving your scalp on your skull by contracting your **epicranius muscle** (particularly the occipitofrontalis part of it). As your scalp moves, note in the mirror that your eyebrows and the skin over the root of your nose rise and your forehead wrinkles. As this scalp muscle (occipitofrontalis) is used to express surprise, it is included as a muscle of facial expression. Do not be upset if you are unable to move all of your scalp; few people can. The looseness of the scalp proper explains why a person can be scalped so easily (*e.g.*, during automobile or industrial accidents).

Each letter of the word **S C A L P** serves as a memory key for one of the **five layers of the scalp** (Fig. 7-43): (1) **S***kin*; (2) **C***onnective tissue*; (3) **A***poneurosis epicranalis*; (4) **L***oose connective* tissue; and (5) **P***ericranium* (periosteal layer).

1. Skin (Figs. 7-43 to 7-45). *The scalp skin is thick*, particularly in the occipital region, and contains many sweat and sebaceous glands. Hair covers the scalp in

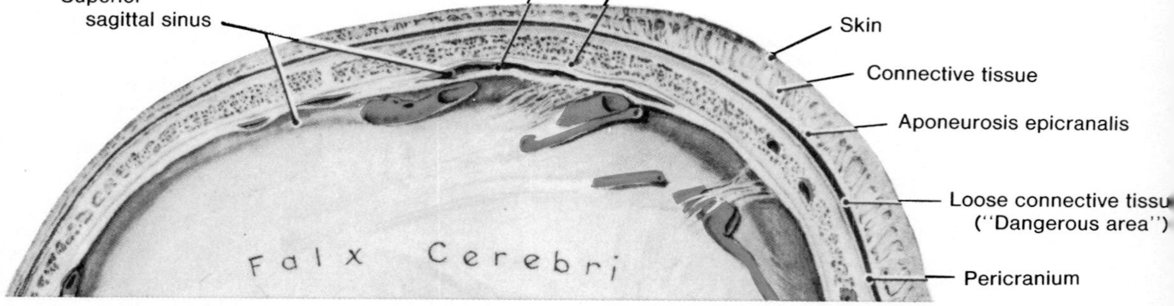

Figure 7-44. Median section of the upper part of the head showing the scalp proper (first three layers) separated from the pericranium by loose connective tissue (potential space). Emissary veins pass through apertures in the cranium (Fig. 7-71) and establish communication between the dural venous sinuses (*e.g.*, the superior sagittal sinus) inside the cranium and the veins external to it. If lacerated, blood from these veins travels freely within the loose connective tissue layer and is limited only by its attachments (highest nuchal line posteriorly and zygomatic arches laterally). Anteriorly this blood may enter the eyelids because the frontalis attaches to skin, not bone.

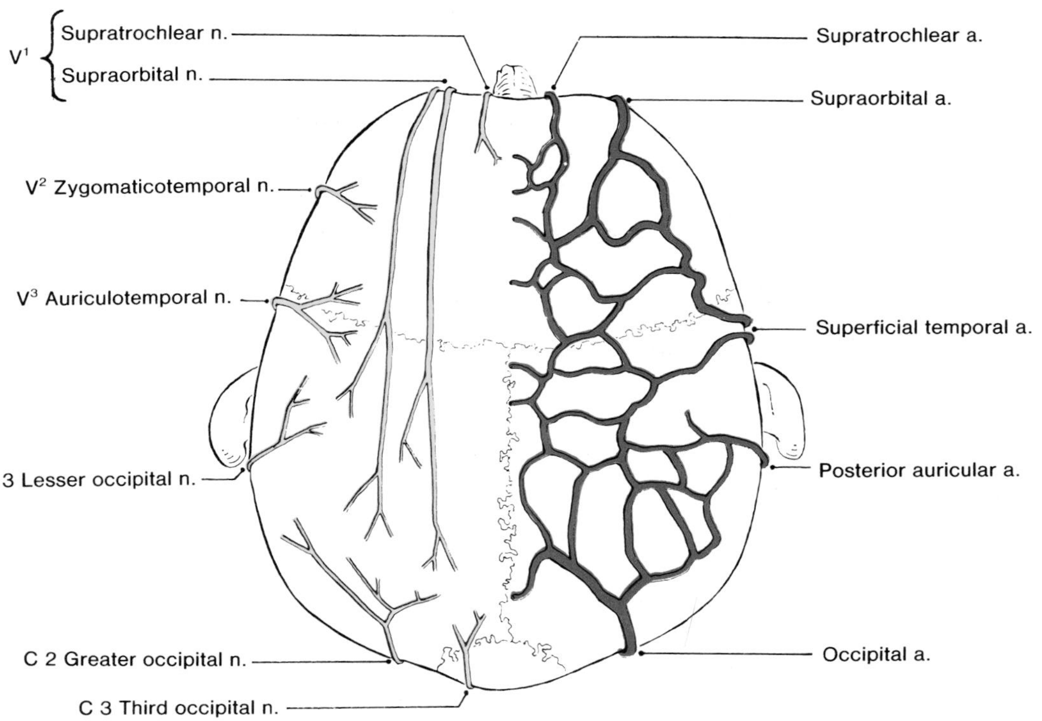

Figure 7-45. Diagram showing the arteries and nerves of the scalp. Note that the arteries anastomose freely. The supraorbital and supratrochlear arteries are derived from the internal carotid artery via the ophthalmic artery. The other three arteries are branches of the external carotid artery. Because of the rich anastomosis of arteries, bleeding from scalp wounds is usually profuse. The nerves appearing in sequence are: CN V^1, CN V^2, and CN V^3 (branches of the trigeminal nerve); ventral rami of C2 and C3; and dorsal rami of C2 and C3. (For anterior and lateral views of the sensory nerves of the face and scalp, see Fig. 7-30.)

most people. The skin has an abundant arterial supply and a good venous and lymphatic drainage.

CLINICALLY ORIENTED COMMENTS

The ducts of the **sebaceous glands** associated with hair follicles may become obstructed, resulting in the retention of secretions and the formation of **sebaceous cysts** (*wens*). These cysts may also be derived from the outer hair root sheath of the hair follicle. As these cysts are in the skin and do not invade the subcutaneous tissue, they *move freely with the scalp*. Sebaceous cysts are more common in the scalp than elsewhere.

Sometimes synthetic fiber hairs are sewn into the scalp or a hairpiece (toupee) is attached to it with sutures. Generally these procedures are unacceptable owing to the high incidence of scalp infection that follows. **Hair transplanting** done by **dermatologists** (physicians who specialize in the diagnosis and treatment of skin lesions) rarely become infected. A small punch is used to remove hair-bearing skin from the base of the hairline and these hair plugs are then implanted into the bald area, where they remain viable because they are self-produced, *i.e.*, **autogenous grafts**.

2. Connective Tissue (Figs. 7-43 to 7-45). This is a thick, subcutaneous layer of connective tissue which is **richly vascu-**

larized and well supplied with nerves. Its collagenous and elastic fibers crisscross in all directions, attaching the skin to the epicranial aponeurosis. **Fat** is enclosed in lobules between the fibers, much as it is in the palms of the hands and the soles of the feet. The amount of subcutaneous fat in the scalp is relatively constant, varying little in **emaciation** or **obesity**, but seems to decrease with advancing age.

CLINICALLY ORIENTED COMMENTS

Properly treated scalp lacerations normally heal quickly. Superficial infections of the scalp tend to remain superficial owing to the density of the fibrous tissue in the connective tissue layer.

3. Aponeurosis Epicranialis (Figs. 7-43 and 7-44). The epicranial aponeurosis (galea aponeurotica) is *a strong membranous sheet that covers the calvaria.* The term galea (L. helmet) was used to indicate the helmet-like nature of the epicranial aponeurosis. It contains the epicranius muscle, consisting of frontal and occipital bellies which are located in the forehead and occipital regions, respectively. During early development, the **epicranius** was part of a broad sheet of muscle that was continuous with the muscles of facial expression and the platysma. Hence, it is supplied by the **facial nerve** (CN VII), the nerve of the second branchial arch in the embryo.

The epicranius in man is aponeurotic except in front and behind. It consists of the **occipitofrontalis**, a broad musculoaponeurotic layer that covers the calvaria from the highest nuchal line posteriorly (Fig. 7-3) to the level of the eyebrows anteriorly. It consists of four parts: two occipital bellies (**occipitalis**) and two frontal bellies (**frontalis**) connected by the epicranial aponeurosis (**galea aponeurotica**).

Each **occipital belly** arises from the lateral two-thirds of the **highest nuchal line** of the occipital bone and the mastoid part of the temporal bone and ends in the galea (Fig. 7-43). Each **frontal belly** arises from the galea and inserts into the skin and dense subcutaneous connective tissue at about the level of the eyebrows. *The frontalis has no bony attachment.* All four parts of the occipitofrontalis are supplied by the facial nerve (CN VII), the occipitalis by posterior auricular branches, and the frontalis by temporal branches.

The galea is attached posteriorly to the external occipital protuberance (Figs. 7-3 and 7-43*B*) and to the **highest nuchal line**. It is continuous laterally with the fascia over the temporalis muscle (**temporal fascia**), which is attached to the zygomatic arch (Fig. 7-35).

CLINICALLY ORIENTED COMMENTS

The galea aponeurotica is a clinically important layer of the scalp. Owing to its strength, a superficial cut in the skin does not gape because its margins are held together by this aponeurosis. When suturing a superficial laceration, deep sutures are not necessary because the galea does not allow separation. Careful suturing of the galea following **craniotomy** (surgical opening of the cranium) or deep lacerations prevent disruption of the skin incision.

Scalp wounds gape widely when the galea is split or cut because of the pull of the frontal and occipital parts of the epicranius muscle in different directions (anteriorly and posteriorly, respectively); obviously transverse lacerations gape most widely. Bleeding from scalp wounds is severe because the arteries cannot retract in the dense connective tissue.

4. Loose Connective Tissue (Figs. 7-43 and 7-44). This subaponeurotic "space" or layer is somewhat like a collapsed sponge because it contains innumerable potential spaces that are capable of becoming distended with fluid. This loose areolar tissue allows free movement of the scalp proper (the first three layers) as one sheet; it is easily torn in deep scalp lacerations.

CLINICALLY ORIENTED COMMENTS

The loose connective tissue (subaponeurotic layer) is sometimes called the **dangerous area** or space because pus or blood in it can spread easily. Infection in it can also be transmitted to the cranial cavity via **emissary veins** that pass from this space through apertures in the cranial bones (*e.g.*, the **parietal foramina**, Fig. 7-71). Emissary veins connect with the intracranial venous sinuses (*e.g.*, the superior saggital sinus, Fig. 7-44). Infections in the loose connective tissue layer may produce inflammatory processes in the emissary veins, leading to **thrombophlebitis** of the intracranial venous sinuses and later of the cortical veins. **Cortical infarction** (production of an area of necrosis or death of cells in the cerebral cortex) could follow. Cortical infarcts may produce permanent neurological defects.

Awareness of the limits of the loose connective tissue (*subaponeurotic space*) *is important* so that the possible spread of an infection can be anticipated. **Posteriorly**, it is unable to spread into the neck because the occipitalis and the galea are attached to the highest nuchal line of the occipital bone (Fig. 7-3). **Laterally**, it is unable to spread beyond the zygomatic arches because the galea is continuous here with the temporal fascia, which is attached to the zygomatic arch. (Fig. 7-35). **Anteriorly**, fluid can enter the eyelids and the root of the nose because the frontalis is inserted into the skin and dense subcutaneous tissue, not into the frontal bone.

5. Pericranium (Figs. 7-43 and 7-44). This is the periosteum of the cranium and is attached to its outer surface by connective tissue fibers known as **Sharpey's fibers**. They penetrate the bones of the calvaria and *anchor the periosteum to the bones*. The pericranium can be stripped fairly easily from the cranial bones of living persons, except where it is continuous with the fibrous tissue of the sutures. Here the pericranium passes inward to be continuous with the endocranium on the inside of the calvaria. *The pericranium is a dense layer of specialized connective tissue* that has relatively poor osteogenic properties in adults.

CLINICALLY ORIENTED COMMENTS

During birth, bleeding sometimes occurs between the pericranium and the calvaria, usually over one parietal bone. The bleeding is from the rupture of multiple, minute periosteal arteries that enter and nourish the bone. The resulting swelling which develops several hours after birth is called a **cephalhematoma**. This *blood cyst of the scalp* in infants does not spread beyond the margins of the bone concerned because the pericranium is closely bound to the fibrous tissue connecting the edges of the bones at the cranial sutures.

Cephalhematoma should not be confused with **caput succedaneum**, which is an edematous swelling of the soft tissues of the scalp that may develop during birth. This condition occurs in the area that presents into the birth canal (usually the scalp in the region of the lambda), as this region is the only part of the infant that is not being compressed by the walls of the birth canal (cervix of uterus and vagina, Fig. 3-22). This swelling, being in the subcutaneous tissue, is not localized to any particular bone as occurs with a cephalhematoma.

Because *the adult pericranium has poor osteogenic properties*, there is very little regeneration if bone loss occurs. Surgically produced **bone flaps** are usually put back into place and wired to the calvaria. Traumatic defects in the adult skullcap usually do not fill in, necessitating the insertion of a metal or plastic plate to protect the brain.

NERVES AND VESSELS OF THE SCALP

Nerves of the Scalp (Figs. 7-30 and 7-45). The sensory innervation of the scalp, from in front backward, is via nerves that are branches of all three divisions of the

trigeminal nerve (CN V) and of the **cervical plexus** (C2 and C3). The area of distribution of the trigeminal and cervical nerves is usually about equal.

Arteries of the Scalp (Fig. 7-45). The vascular supply is from the **external carotid artery** via the occipital, posterior auricular, and superficial temporal arteries and from the **internal carotid artery** via the supratrochlear and the supraorbital arteries. *All these arteries anastomose freely with each other.*

The arteries are in the dense subcutaneous connective tissue layer (second layer) of the scalp. Very few branches of these arteries cross the subaponeurotic loose connective tissue layer (fourth layer) of the scalp to supply the calvaria. Its bones are supplied mainly by the middle meningeal arteries, but they receive some blood from pericranial vessels that enter the cranium through **Volkmann's canals** (vascular canals in bones).

Veins of the Scalp (Figs. 7-32, 7-35, 7-37, and 7-38). The **vena comitantes** accompany the arteries and have the same names. The **supraorbital** and **supratrochlear veins** (visible on the forehead of some people) unite at the medial angle of the eye to form the **facial vein**. At this point it communicates with the **superior ophthalmic vein**, thus making an important link which may allow facial infections to reach the **cavernous sinus** (Fig. 7-38). The **superficial temporal vein** joins the **maxillary vein** posterior to the neck of the mandible to form the **retromandibular vein**. The **posterior auricular vein** drains the scalp behind the ear and often receives a mastoid emissary vein from the **sigmoid sinus** (Fig. 7-38), an intracranial venous sinus.

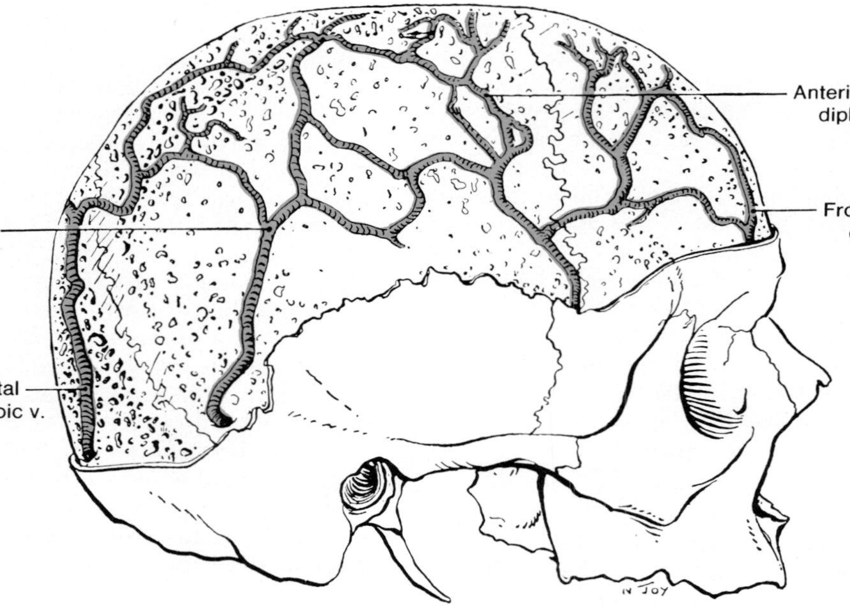

Figure 7-46. Drawing of the diploic veins which have been displayed by filing away the outer table of compact bone, thereby opening the channels that contained them. Of the four paired diploic veins, the frontal diploic vein opens into the supraorbital vein at the supraorbital notch; the anterior temporal diploic vein opens into the sphenoparietal sinus; the posterior temporal and the occipital diploic veins both open into the transverse sinus (Fig. 7-69), but they may open into veins of the scalp. The connections of the diploic veins with intracranial and extracranial venous channels allow an infection to spread from the scalp, through the skull to the meninges (Fig. 7-59) and the brain. There are no accompanying diploic arteries. The blood supply for the bones of the skull is derived from the meningeal and pericranial arteries.

Lymphatic Drainage of the Scalp (Figs. 7-39 and 9-66). Most lymph from the scalp and forehead drains to the **superficial collar** or **ring of lymph nodes**, located at the junction of the head and neck, but some vessels drain directly into the **deep cervical lymph nodes**. Lymph vessels from the frontal region just above the root of the nose drain into the **submandibular group**, one of the deep group of lymph nodes. The occipital region drains into the **occipital nodes**, the temporoparietal region into the **retroauricular nodes**, and the frontoparietal region into the superficial **parotid lymph nodes.** *Lymph from the entire scalp eventually drains into the deep cervical group of lymph nodes.*

CLINICALLY ORIENTED COMMENTS

As the nerves and vessels of the scalp enter from below (Fig. 7-45) and ascend through the connective tissue layer (second layer of the scalp) into the skin, surgical pedicle flaps of the scalp are made so that they remain attached inferiorly in order to preserve the nerves and vessels and promote good healing. The term **pedicle flap** is used to describe a detached mass of tissues cut away from underlying parts but attached at the edge containing its blood vessels and nerves.

The anastomoses of blood vessels are so numerous in the scalp that partially detached portions of the scalp can usually be replaced without necrosis (death of tissue) occurring. **Accidental scalping** can occur during automobile accidents (*e.g.*, when the head goes through a windshield), or during industrial accidents (*e.g.*, when a person's long hair becomes entangled in machinery). Scalping does not result in necrosis of the cranial bones because their blood is supplied by the pericranial and **middle meningeal arteries** (Fig. 7-59).

The abundant blood supply of the scalp often leads to **extensive hemorrhage** when it is lacerated because *the vessels are unable to retract* or contract owing to the denseness of the subcutaneous connective tissue surrounding them. However, if the skin adjacent to a scalp laceration is compressed between the fingers and the cranium, bleeding can usually be stopped. In **extensive scalp wounds**, hemorrhaging can be temporarily stopped by applying a *tourniquet around the base of the scalp.* This procedure applies the anatomical knowledge that the vessels enter the scalp from below (Fig. 7-45).

INTERIOR OF THE CRANIUM

Removal of the skullcap (top of calvaria) exposes the **meninges** (G. membranes) enveloping the brain (Figs. 7-59 and 7-61). This is done routinely in autopsies by pulling the anterior half of the scalp over the face and the posterior half over the nape or back of the neck and cutting the skullcap horizontally, about 5 cm above the **external acoustic meatus** (Fig. 7-7). Following section of the cranial nerves and all attachments of the meninges to the cranium, the brain can be removed intact by severing the spinal cord just below the foramen magnum.

THE CRANIAL FOSSAE

When the skullcap and then the brain are removed, the superior aspect of the base of the skull is exposed (Figs. 7-9 and 7-47). This bowl-shaped area that supports the brain has three levels or downward steps called the **anterior, middle, and posterior cranial fossae** (L. depressions). On a dried skull note that each fossa is at a slightly lower level than the one rostral (nearer the nose) to it. The posterior cranial fossa is the largest and the deepest of the three fossae. The floors of the fossae are irregular owing to upward projections of some bones in the base of the skull. These floors also reflect some features of parts of the brain that are related to it.

Anterior Cranial Fossa (Figs. 7-47 to 7-51). The anterior extremities of the frontal lobes of the cerebral hemispheres, known as the **frontal poles**, occupy the anterior cranial fossa, the shallowest of the three fossae. This fossa is largely formed by the **frontal bone**; most of its floor is composed of the convex **orbital parts** of this

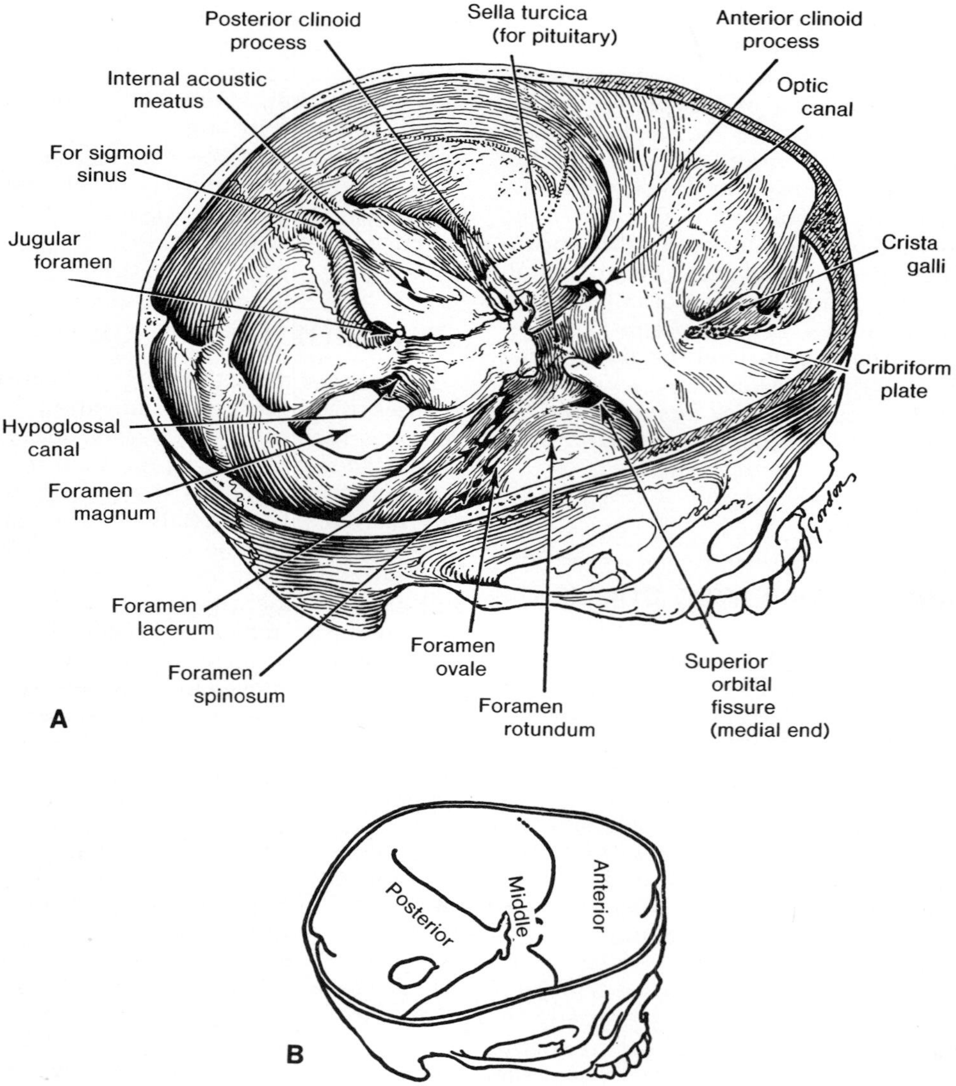

Figure 7-47. Drawing of the internal surface of the base of the skull showing the three cranial fossae indicated in sketch *B*. (For the relationship of the brain to these fossae, see Fig. 7-76.)

bone which constitute the bony roof of the **orbits** (F. circles) or eye sockets. The orbital plates show sinuous, shallow depressions called convolutional impressions or *brain markings*, which are formed by the **orbital gyri** (convolutions) of the frontal lobe of the brain. Between these convolutional impressions, low sinuous ridges are produced by the sulci (L. furrows) between the gyri on the inferior surface of the frontal lobe (Fig. 7-78).

The **crista galli** (L. *crista*, crest + *gallus*, a cock) is a median process or crest resembling a cock's comb that extends upward from the **ethmoid** bone (Fig. 7-50). On each side of the crista galli there is a perforated **cribriform plate** (L. *cribrum*, sieve) through the foramina of which the *olfactory nerves* pass to enter the **olfactory bulbs** (Fig. 7-48). The crista galli, together with the **frontal crest**, gives attachment to a midline septum (fold) of dura mater,

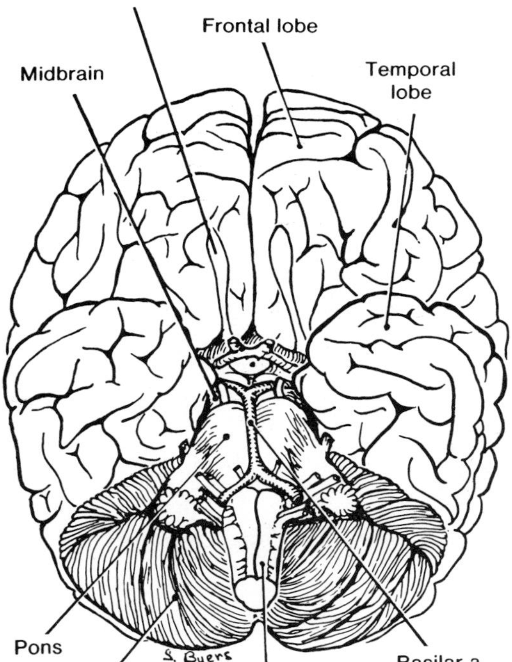

Figure 7-48. Drawing of the inferior surface of the brain that rests on the floors of the cranial fossae. Each fold or rounded elevation of the cerebral cortex (L. bark) is known as a gyrus and the intervening furrow is known as a sulcus.

called the **falx cerebri** (Figs. 7-44, 7-60, 7-61, and 7-62), which lies between the cerebral hemispheres of the brain.

The **lesser wings of the sphenoid** bone articulate with the orbital plates of the frontal bone and form the posterior part of the floor of the anterior cranial fossa. The lesser wings present sharp posterior margins, called **sphenoidal ridges**, which overhang the anterior part of the middle cranial fossa and project into the anterior part of the lateral sulci of the cerebral hemispheres (Fig. 7-51*B*). Each lesser wing ends medially in an **anterior clinoid process** (Fig. 7-50) which gives attachment to a dural septum called the **tentorium cerebelli** (Figs. 7-61 and 7-62). The anterior clinoid process (G. *klinē*, bed + *eidos*, resemblance) reminded Greek anatomists of bedposts for the bed (**hypophysial fossa**) in which the **pituitary gland** (*hypophysis cerebri*) rests (Fig. 7-63).

The central and lowest part of the floor of the anterior cranial fossa is formed by the **cribriform plates** (previously described) of the ethmoid bone.

Middle Cranial Fossa (Figs. 7-47, 7-50, and 7-52). The rounded anterior extremities of the temporal lobes of the cerebral hemispheres (Fig. 7-48), known as the **temporal poles** (Fig. 7-51*A*), fit into the middle cranial fossa, which is posterior to and deeper than the anterior cranial fossa.

The middle cranial fossa is marked off from the posterior cranial fossa by a median rectangular bony projection, the **dorsum sellae** (L. seat or saddle), at whose outer corners are knob-like projections called the **posterior clinoid processes**. The dorsum sellae is a square portion of bone on the body of the *sphenoid bone*, posterior to the *sella turcica* (described subsequently).

More laterally, the middle cranial fossa is also separated from the posterior cranial fossa by crests or prominences formed by the superior borders of the petrous parts of the **temporal bones**. Examine the floor of the middle cranial fossa and note that the part formed by the sphenoid (G. wedge) bone resembles a butterfly. The body of the "butterfly" is formed by the body of the sphenoid bone and its wings are formed by the greater wings of this bone. The remainder of the floor of the middle cranial fossa is formed by the **petrous** and **squamous parts of the temporal bone**.

The midline saddle-like prominence of the sphenoid bone, between the anterior and posterior clinoid processes, is known as the **sella turcica** (L. Turkish saddle). It is composed of three parts: (1) anteriorly an olive-shaped swelling, the **tuberculum sellae** (the pommel or knob-like protuberance at the front of a saddle); (2) a seat-like depression, called the **hypophysial fossa**, for the **hypophysis cerebri** (pituitary gland; and (3) the back of the "saddle" known as the **dorsum sellae**.

Posterior Cranial Fossa (Figs. 7-47, 7-52, and 7-53). This fossa lodging the cerebellum, pons, and medulla is formed largely by the inferior and anterior parts of the **occipital bone**, but the body of the sphenoid and the petrous and mastoid parts of

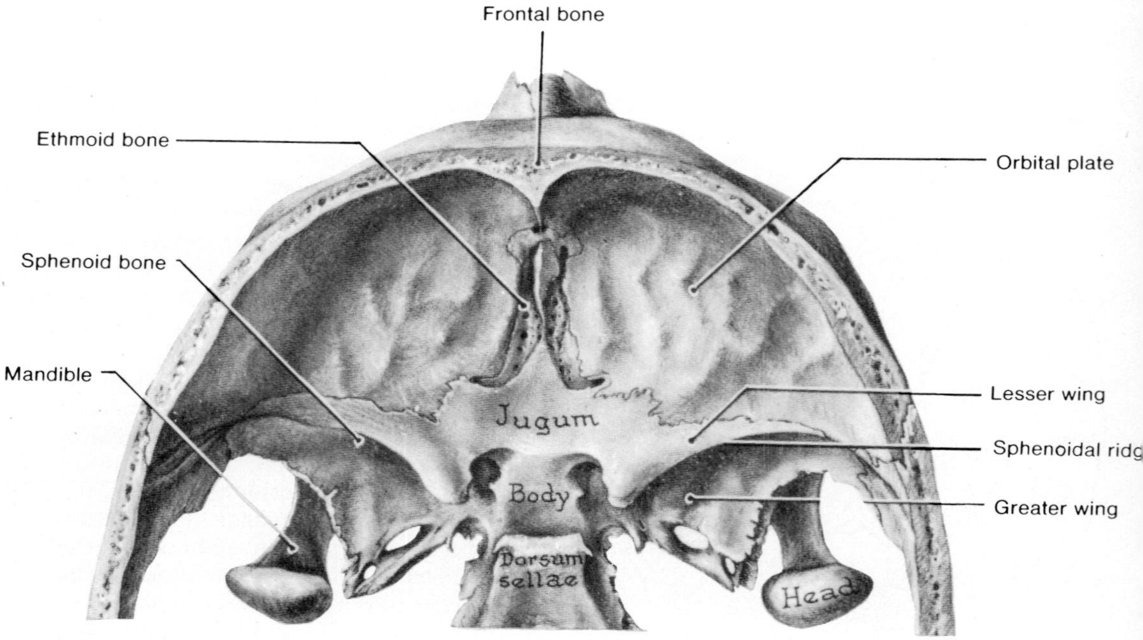

Figure 7-49. Drawing of the interior of the base of the anterior half of the cranium showing the anterior cranial fossa and the anterior part of the middle cranial fossa. The temporal bones have been removed so the heads of the mandible may be seen. Observe the sinuous shallow depressions in the orbital part of the frontal bone produced by the orbital gyri of the frontal lobes of the brain (Fig. 7-78).

the temporal bones also contribute to its formation.

The **occipital lobes** of the cerebral hemispheres (Fig. 7-51*B*) lie on the **tentorium cerebelli** (Fig. 7-62) above the posterior cranial fossa. In Figure 7-53 observe the broad grooves formed by the **transverse sinuses** which lie between diverging folds of the peripheral attachments of the tentorium (Figs. 7-38, 7-61, and 7-69). The groove for the right sinus is usually larger (Fig. 7-53) because the superior sagittal sinus commonly enters the sinus on that side. The **tentorium** (L. tent), a tent-shaped dural septum, roofs over most of the posterior cranial fossa, intervening between the occipital lobes of the cerebral hemispheres and the cerebellum (Figs. 7-61 and 7-63). Between the anteromedial parts of the right and left leaves of the tentorium is an oval opening, called the *tentorial incisure* (notch), for the brain stem as it passes from the middle to the posterior cranial fossa (Figs. 7-61 and 7-64).

In the midline below the grooves for the transverse sinus, there is often a prominent bony ridge, the *internal occipital crest* (Fig. 7-53), which partly divides the posterior cranial fossa into two **cerebellar fossae** for the cerebellar hemispheres. This crest ends above and behind in an irregular elevation called the **internal occipital protuberance**, which more or less matches the **external occipital protuberance** (Figs. 7-3 and 7-7). The site of these protuberances is a strong part of the skull.

The **vermis** (L. worm) or midline portion of the cerebellum (Fig. 7-65) lies in the **vermian fossa** (Fig. 7-53). Directly anterior to this fossa is the largest opening in the base of the skull, the **foramen magnum**, through which the spinal cord passes to join the medulla. Rostral to the foramen magnum, the basilar part of the occipital bone rises to meet the base or body of the sphenoid bone (**basisphenoid**). This inclined bony surface called the **clivus** (L. slope) is located anterior to the pons and medulla of the brain stem (Figs. 7-50 and 7-57).

CRANIAL FORAMINA

Many **foramina** or apertures (L. openings), perforate the cranial base. Most of them are for transmission of the 12 cranial nerves but some are for the passage of blood vessels. The presence of so many foramina and thin areas of bone in the floor of the cranium makes the base of the skull fragile and vulnerable to fracture. Hold the base of the skull up to a light and observe the foramina, the sutures (**synchondroses**), and the paper-thin areas of bone. You can easily see where fractures and widening (**diastases**) of sutures are most likely to occur.

Foramina in the Anterior Cranial Fossa (Figs. 7-47 and 7-50). The sieve-like appearance of the **cribriform plates** of the ethmoid on each side of the crista galli is caused by the numerous small foramina in them. Axons of **olfactory cells** in the olfactory epithelium in the roof of each nasal cavity converge to form about 20 small bundles, the **fila olfactoria** of the olfactory nerve (Fig. 7-167). These bundles of axons pass through the tiny foramina in the cribriform plates of the ethmoid to enter the olfactory bulbs of the brain.

The foramina which transmit the **anterior ethmoidal nerve** and artery to the nasal cavity are located lateral to the anterior end of a slit-like fissure in the anterior end of the cribriform plate on each side. Both these structures entered the cranial cavity after arising from the nasociliary nerve and ophthalmic artery in the orbit. There are other foramina for the posterior ethmoidal nerves and arteries which are small and relatively unimportant clinically.

Between the frontal crest and the crista

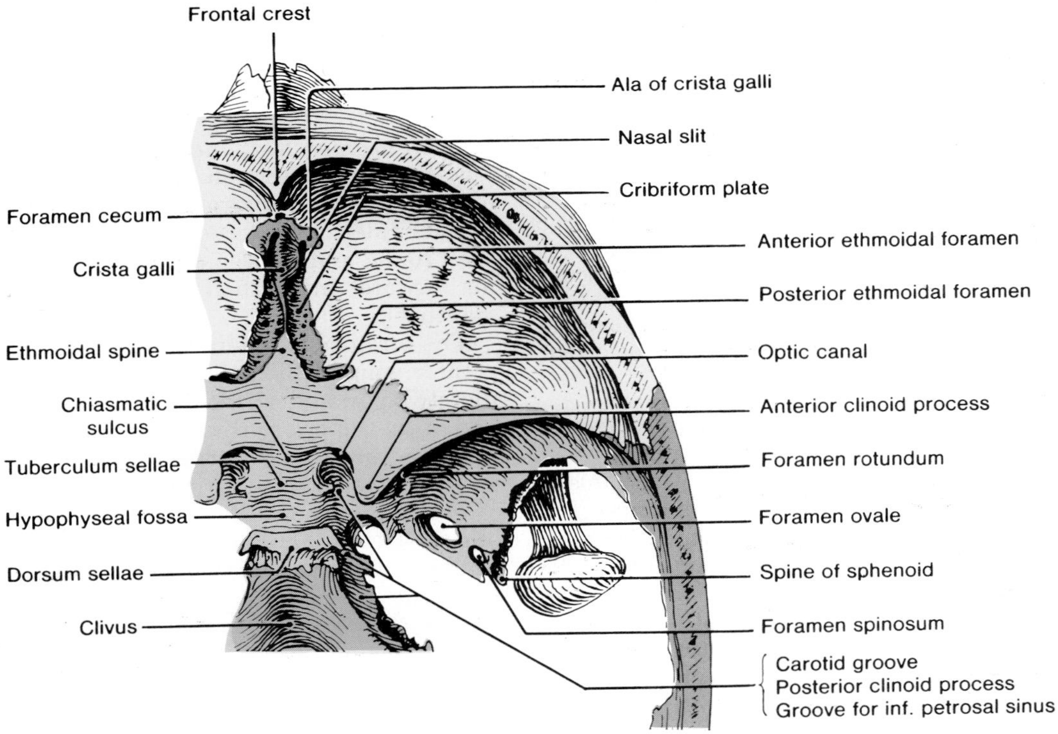

Figure 7-50. Drawing of the interior of the base of the skull showing the right anterior cranial fossa and the anterior part of the right middle cranial fossa. The temporal bone has been removed; thus, the head of the mandible is visible. Note the foramina in the cribriform plate through which the olfactory nerves pass to the olfactory bulbs (Fig. 7-48).

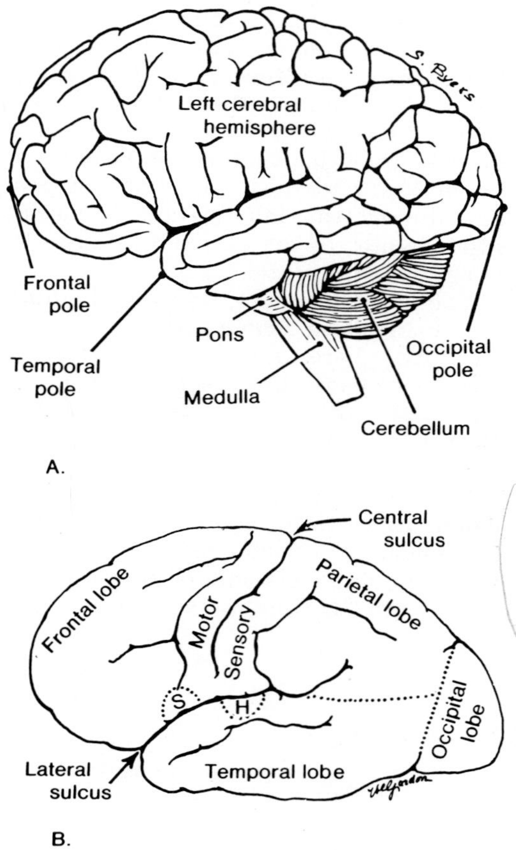

Figure 7-51. Drawings of the lateral aspect of the brain. *A* shows the cerebral hemisphere, its poles, and other parts of the brain. *B* indicates the lobes and the main sulci on the lateral aspect of the hemisphere. The location of centers for hearing (*H*) and speech (*S*) are also indicated.

galli there is often a small **foramen cecum** (Fig. 7-50), through which an emissary vein passes from the superior sagittal sinus to the veins of the frontal sinus and nose. It is present in children and in some adults but is relatively unimportant clinically.

Foramina in the Middle Cranial Fossa (Figs. 7-47, 7-50, 7-52, 7-54, and 7-55). In the anteromedial part of the middle cranial fossa, the **optic canals** (foramina) establish communication with the orbits. The optic canals are traversed by the **optic nerves** (CN II) and the **ophthalmic arteries.** Observe these canals from the orbital cavities. While doing this, place your finger in the middle cranial fossa and cover one of the optic canals. Sometimes these canals are so short they are best called foramina.

On each side of the base of the body of the sphenoid bone (**basisphenoid**) in the greater wing of the sphenoid bone there is an important **crescent of foramina.** Only the *four constant foramina* and the nerves and vessels traversing them warrant special note.

The Superior Orbital Fissure (Figs. 7-2, 7-54, and 7-55). This elongated slit between the greater and lesser wings of the sphenoid bone forms a *communication between the middle cranial fossa and the orbit.* This large fissure is usually not visible in photographs or drawings of the interior of the cranium (*e.g.*, Figs. 7-50, 7-52, and 7-56) when the skull is in the anatomical position, because the backwardly projecting lesser wing of the sphenoid forms a roof over it. To observe the fissure well, the skull must be tipped forward and sideways.

The superior orbital fissure is traversed by four cranial nerves (CN III, CN IV, nasociliary, frontal, and lacrimal branches of CN V, and CN VI) and the ophthalmic vein(s).

The Foramen Rotundum (Figs. 7-50 and 7-54 to 7-56). Although the name of this foramen (L. *rotundus*, round) indicates that it is circular, it is frequently oval rather than round and is often a short canal leading forward rather than a foramen (L. an aperture).

The foramen rotundum is located in the greater wing of the sphenoid bone, immediately below and a little behind the medial end of the superior orbital fissure. It transmits the **maxillary nerve** (Fig. 7-55), the second division of the trigeminal (CN V^2).

The Foramen Ovale (Figs. 7-47*A*, 7-50, and 7-54 to 7-56). This is the next largest aperture along the crescent of foramina. As its name indicates it is oval in form. It passes through the greater wing of the sphenoid bone, posterior and slightly lateral to the foramen rotundum, before opening into the **infratemporal fossa** (Figs. 7-123 to 7-125). It transmits the **mandibular nerve** (Fig. 7-55), the third division of the trigeminal (CN V^3).

The Foramen Spinosum (Figs. 7-47*A*, 7-50, 7-55, and 7-56). This is the smallest of

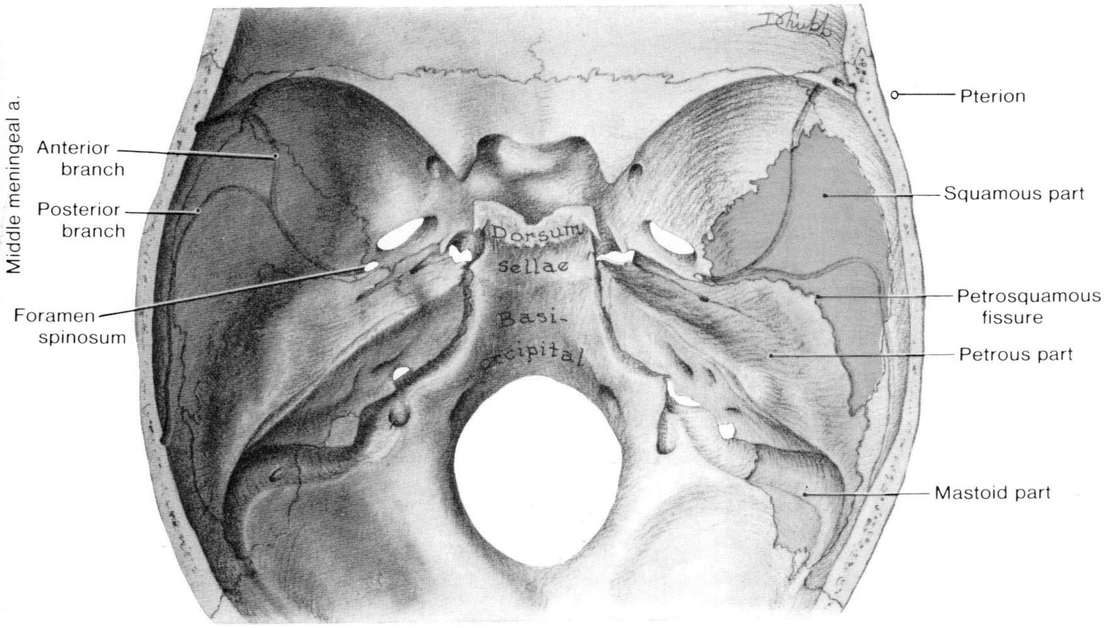

Figure 7-52. Drawing of the interior of the base of the skull showing the middle cranial fossa and most of the posterior cranial fossa. The parts of the temporal bone are colored. Observe the bone markings formed by the branches of the middle meningeal artery; usually a corresponding vein runs in the groove with the artery. These vessels run between the dura mater and the skull and may be torn when there is a blow to the temple in the region of the pterion, particularly if the bones are fractured (Case 7-5). This bleeding is known as an extradural hemorrhage.

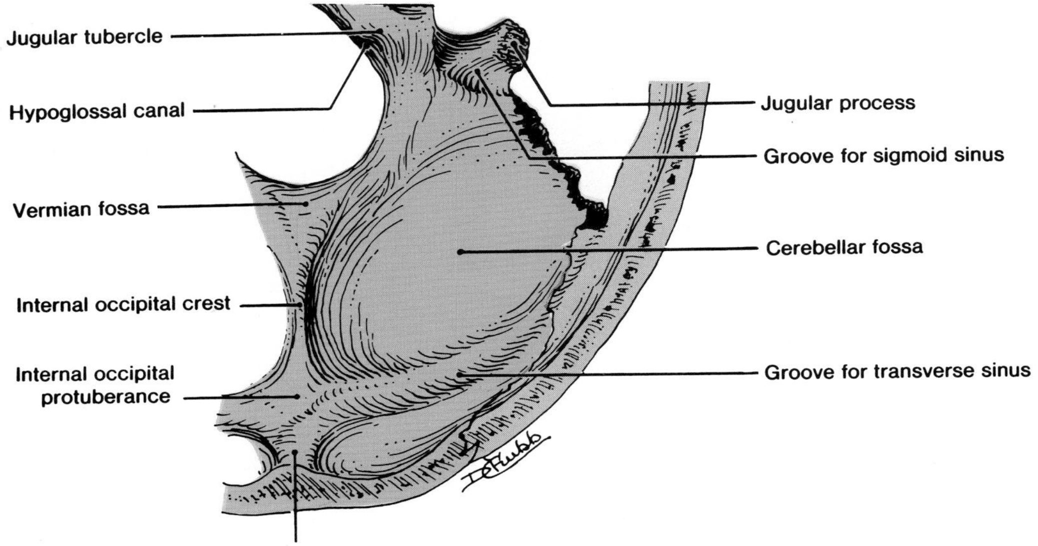

Figure 7-53. Drawing of the interior of the base of the skull showing most of the right posterior cranial fossa. The small part of the fossa formed by the temporal bone (Fig. 7-52) is not shown because the temporal bone has been removed from this specimen.

the important foramina in the crescent of foramina. It was named the foramen spinosum because it enters the skull close to the spine of the sphenoid. The foramen spinosum, located posterolateral to the foramen ovale, transmits the **middle meningeal artery**.

The Foramen Lacerum (Figs. 7-47*A* and 7-56). This ragged foramen (really a canal) is not part of the crescent of foramina. It is

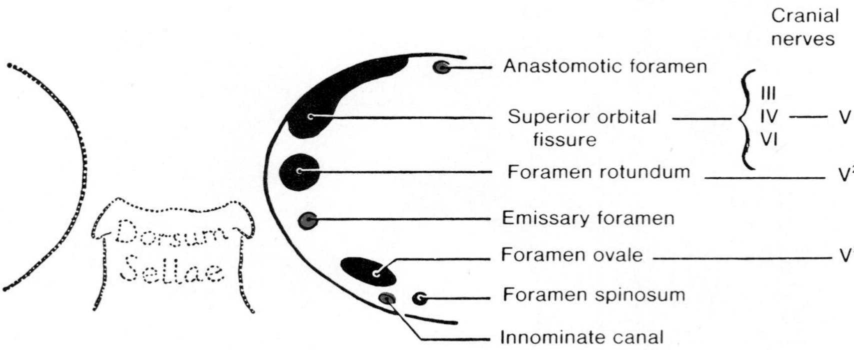

Figure 7-54. Diagram illustrating the crescent of foramina in the middle cranial fossa. The four foramina which are constant are shown in *black*, whereas those that are inconstant are *red*. These foramina all open from the sphenoid bone into the middle cranial fossa and are also shown in the drawing of this fossa (Fig. 7-56).

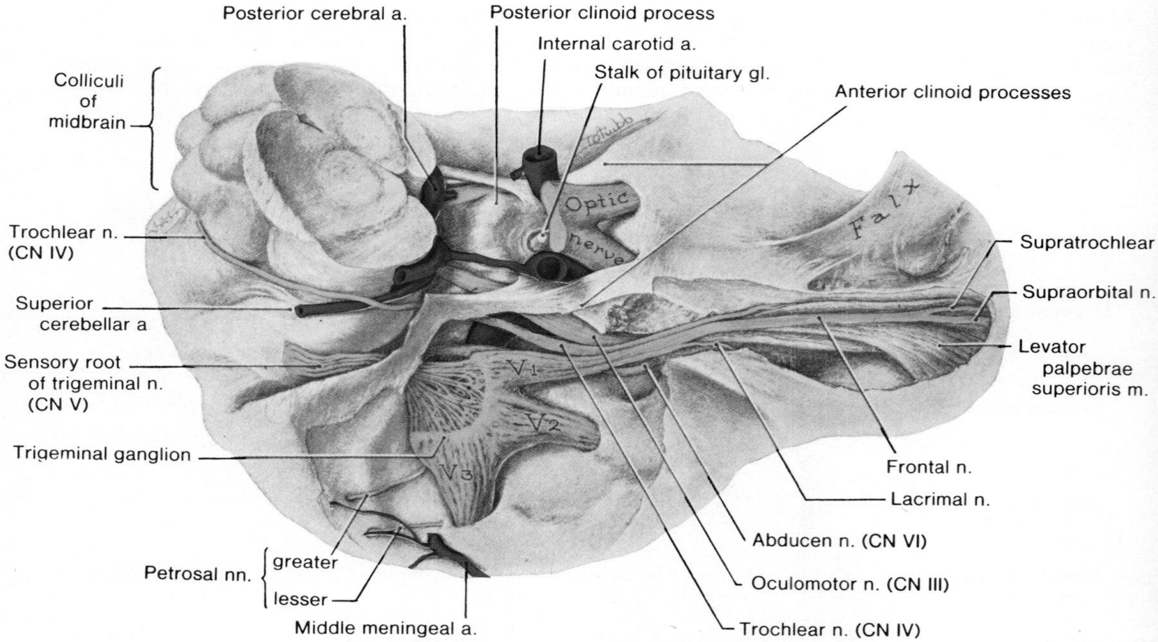

Figure 7-55. Drawing of a dissection of the nerves in the right middle cranial fossa. The roof of the orbit has been partly removed and the tentorium has been removed on the right side to show the trochlear nerve (CN IV) and the sensory root of the trigeminal (CN V). It may help you to orientate this drawing if you place the left hand side of the illustration toward you. The large trigeminal ganglion forms an impression on the anterior surface of the petrous part of the temporal bone (Fig. 7-56). This ganglion occupies a recess called the trigeminal cave (Fig. 7-88) in the dura mater covering the trigeminal impression. Observe the mandibular nerve CN V^3 passing through the foramen ovale to enter the infratemporal fossa (Fig. 7-125).

located between the basisphenoid and the apex of the petrous part of the temporal bone, posteromedial to the foramen ovale. The carotid and pterygoid canals open into the foramen lacerum, which is filled with cartilage, except in dried skulls. The superior end of the foramen lacerum contains the **internal carotid artery** and its accompanying sympathetic and venous plexuses as they enter the cavernous sinus (Fig. 7-38).

Hiatuses for the Petrosal Nerves (Fig. 7-56). Extending backward and laterally from the foramen lacerum there is a narrow groove (sulcus) for the **greater petrosal nerve** on the anterior surface on the petrous part of the temporal bone. At the lateral end of this sulcus there is a small hiatus (slit) or foramen, called the **greater petrosal hiatus** (foramen). It transmits the greater petrosal nerve as it leaves the **geniculate ganglion** of the facial nerve (CN VII).

Sometimes there is also a groove for the **lesser petrosal nerve**, but its hiatus (foramen) is usually so small that it cannot be identified with certainty.

Foramina in the Posterior Cranial Fossa (Figs. 7-56 to 7-58). There are four clinically important foramina and canals in the posterior cranial fossa.

The Foramen Magnum (Figs. 7-47, 7-52, and 7-57). This large foramen is *unique for at least three reasons*: (1) it is the largest foramen in the skull; (2) the junction of the medulla and the spinal cord occurs within it (Fig. 7-63); and (3) it is unpaired. This foramen, usually oval, lies at the lowest part of the posterior cranial fossa, midway between the mastoid processes which are at

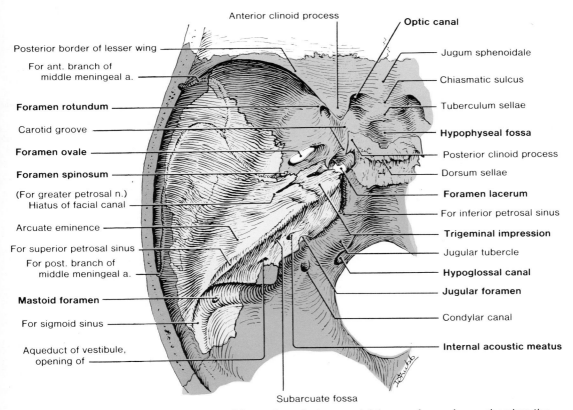

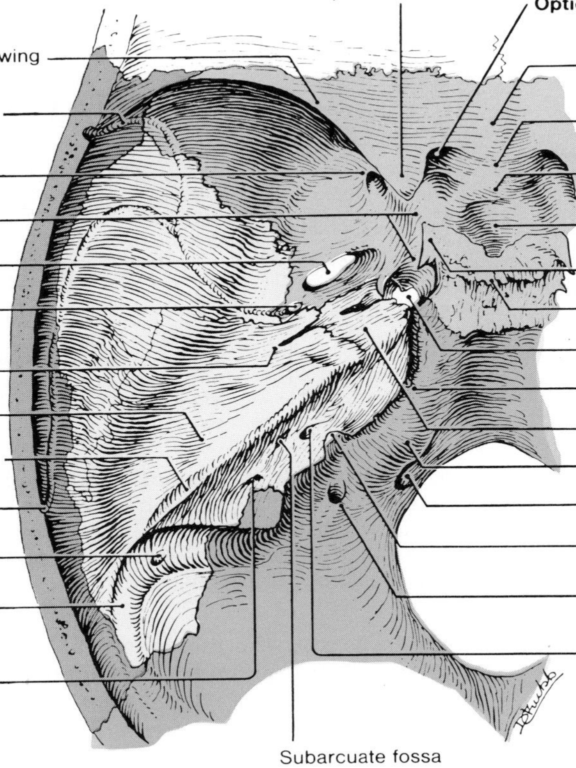

Figure 7-56. Drawing of the left middle and posterior cranial fossae from above showing the location of several foramina. Note the distinct impression posterolateral to the foramen lacerum formed by the trigeminal ganglion (the ganglion of CN V). This trigeminal impression is on the anterior surface of the petrous part of the temporal bone.

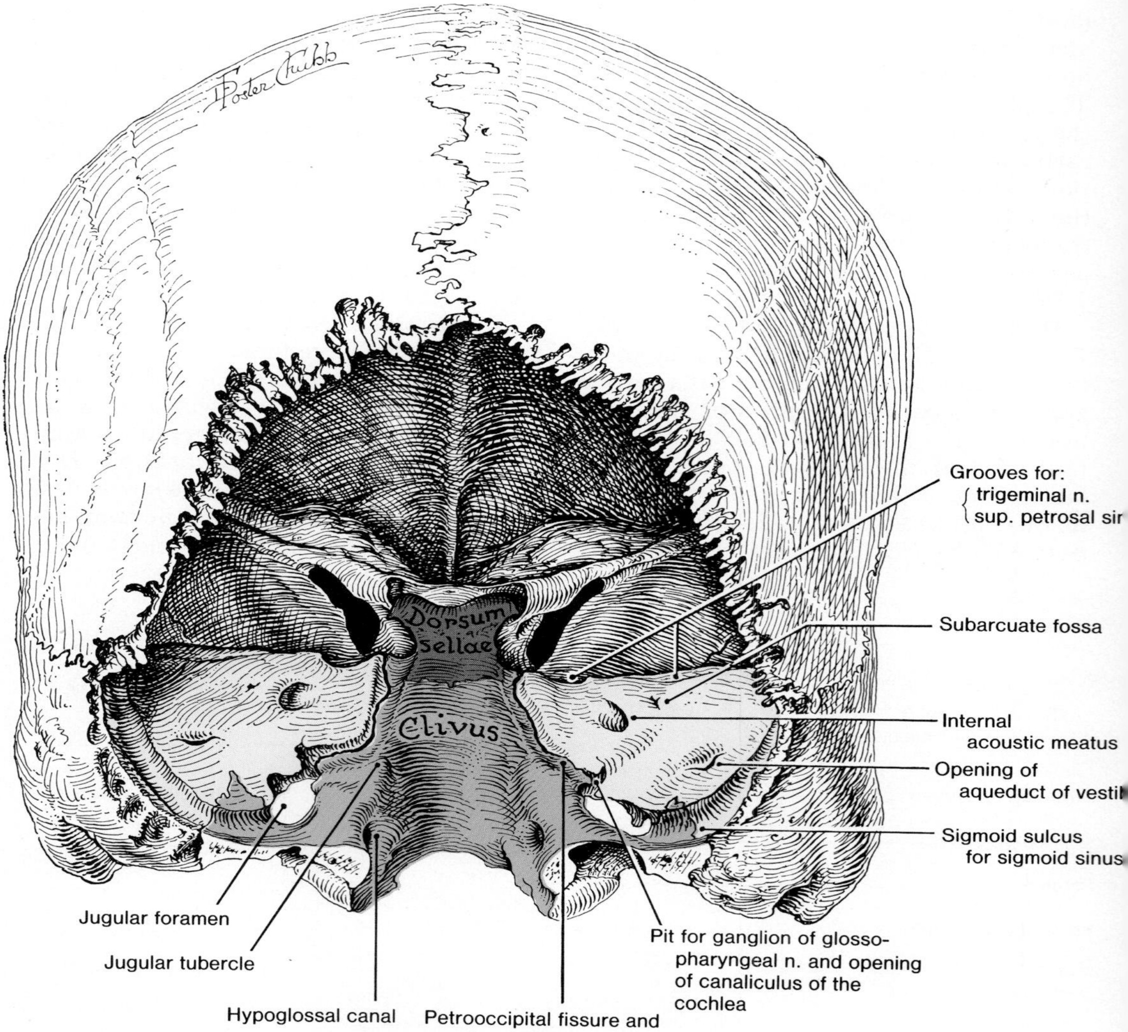

Figure 7-57. Drawing of the posterior aspect of the posterior cranial fossa after removal of the squamous part of the occipital bone. Observe the flat plate of bone known as the dorsum sellae on the body of the sphenoid bone. It forms the posterior wall of the sella turcica or hypophysial fossa. The clivus is a sloping piece of bone that is formed by the basilar part of the occipital bone (basiocciput) and the body of the sphenoid bone (basisphenoid).

the same level. The posterior cranial fossa communicates with the vertebral canal via the foramen magnum.

Structures passing through the foramen magnum are: (1) the junction of the medulla and spinal cord; (2) the spinal roots of the accessory nerves (CN XI) pass upward through it; (3) the meningeal branches of the upper cervical nerves (C1 to C3); (4) the meninges; (5) the **vertebral arteries** ascending to supply parts of the brain (Fig. 7-36); and (6) the anterior and posterior **spinal arteries** descending to supply the upper part of the spinal cord.

The Jugular Foramen (Figs. 7-57 and 7-58). This is an interosseous foramen located between the occipital bone and the petrous part of the temporal bone. It lies at the

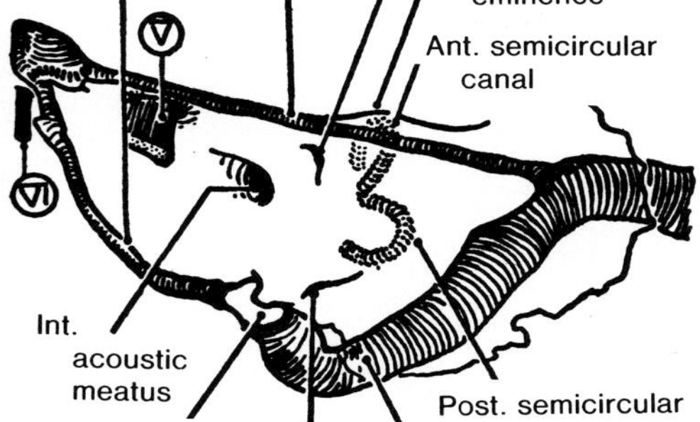

Figure 7-58. Diagram of the posterior surface of the petrous part of the right temporal bone showing the jugular foramen, the internal acoustic meatus, and some of the cranial venous sinuses.

posterior end of the **petrooccipital suture**. The posterior part of the jugular foramen contains the superior bulb of the internal jugular vein (Fig. 7-74) into which the **sigmoid sinus** enters (Figs. 7-38 and 7-58). The *jugular glomus* is a small ovoid body consisting of *chemoreceptor tissue* which is enclosed in the adventitia of the jugular bulb. Anteromedial to this vein, several structures descend through this foramen: (1) the glossopharyngeal (**CN IX**); (2) the vagus (**CN X**); (3) the accessory (**CN XI**); and (4) the inferior petrosal sinus on its way to the upper end of the internal jugular vein (Figs. 7-72 and 7-74).

The Hypoglossal Canal (Figs. 7-53, 7-56, and 7-57). This canal transmits the **hypoglossal nerve** (CN XII). Its internal opening lies between the jugular foramen and the occipital condyle. Look into the foramen magnum of a dried skull from below and note that the **hypoglossal canal** passes laterally and forward. The inner end of this canal is frequently divided into two canals by a bony septum which separates the two roots of the hypoglossal nerve. Pass a coarse thread through the canal and you will understand how CN XII reaches the tongue to supply its intrinsic muscles.

The Condylar Canal (Figs. 7-56 and 7-57). This canal at the lower end of the groove for the sigmoid sinus is inconstant. It transmits an emissary vein from the sigmoid sinus to the vertebral veins in the neck. The canal passes downward and backward to emerge just posterior to the occipital condyle.

The Internal Acoustic Meatus (Figs. 7-56 to 7-58). This opening lies above the anterior part of the **jugular foramen** in the petrous part of the temporal bone. Running to it in a transverse direction from the brain stem are the **facial** (CN VII) and **vestibulocochlear** (CN VIII) nerves, the **nervous intermedius**, and the labyrinthine vessels. The internal acoustic meatus is closed laterally by a perforated plate of bone which separates it from the internal ear. Observe this important meatus on a dried skull.

CLINICALLY ORIENTED COMMENTS

Fractures of the anterior part of the skull (*e.g.*, "**a facial smash** " sustained by the passenger beside the driver during a head-on collision) may involve the **cribriform plate** of the ethmoid bone and may tear the **meninges** (Figs. 7-59 and 7-61), allowing cerebrospinal fluid (CSF) to escape. The CSF drains from the nose or back into the pharynx depending on the patient's posture. A **CSF leak** indicates a compound fracture and that **meningitis** (inflammation of the membranes enclosing the brain) may develop.

Fractures of the middle part of the skull may extend downward into the floor of the middle cranial fossa and involve important structures; *e.g.*, fracture of the petrous part of the temporal bone with resultant **otorrhagia** (bleeding from the ear) and/or **CSF otorrhea** (discharge of CSF from the ear). These conditions could result in meningitis.

The most important intracranial structure to consider in skull fractures is the brain. The various types of skull fracture have been discussed previously (p. 871). Review Figure 7-27 and those comments and think about the damage that might result, keeping in mind the blood vessels

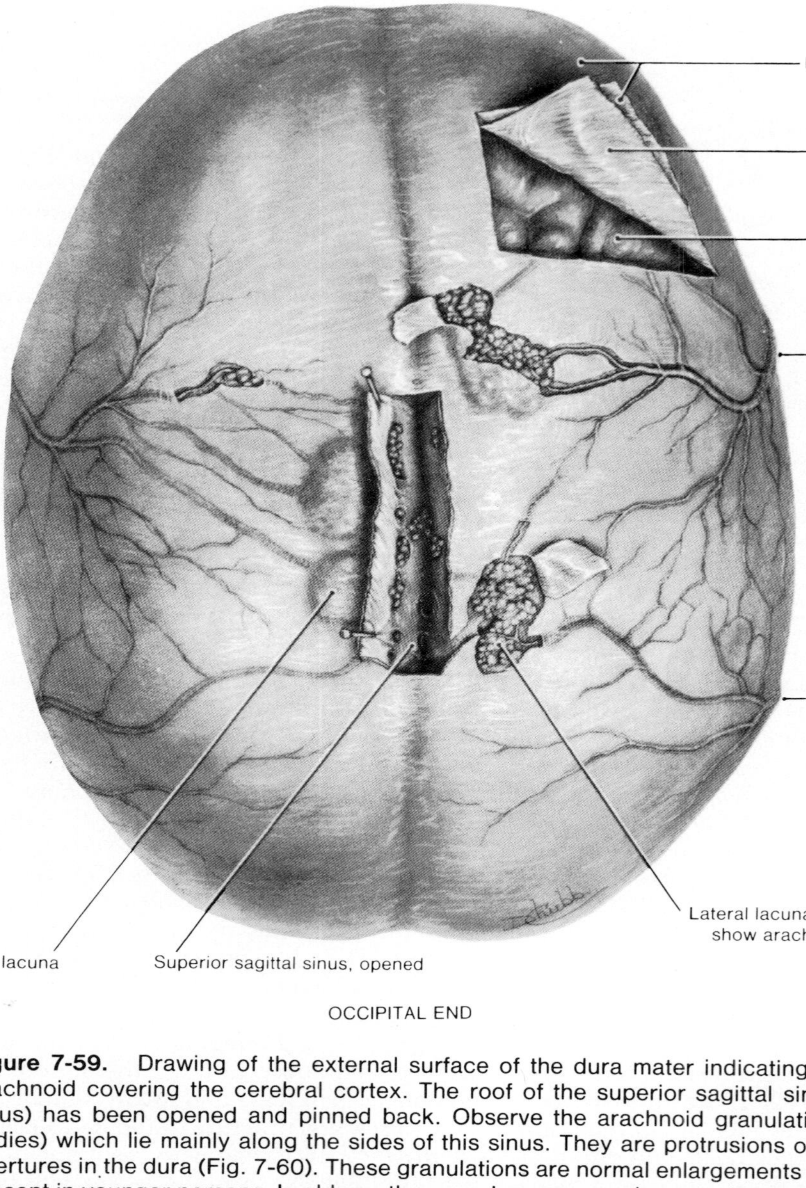

Figure 7-59. Drawing of the external surface of the dura mater indicating the location of the arachnoid covering the cerebral cortex. The roof of the superior sagittal sinus (a dural venous sinus) has been opened and pinned back. Observe the arachnoid granulations (small granular bodies) which lie mainly along the sides of this sinus. They are protrusions of arachnoid through apertures in the dura (Fig. 7-60). These granulations are normal enlargements of the arachnoid villi present in younger persons. In old age they may become very large and even erode the inner table of calvarial bone (Fig. 7-71). When the brain and its meninges were removed from the skull, the internal periosteum (endocranium) was also stripped from the calvaria. Near the frontal end of this specimen, an angular flap of the internal periosteum and the dura mater has been turned anterolaterally. Some authors consider the internal periosteum to be the outer layer of the dura.

and nerves traversing the many foramina in the cranial fossae. During your clinical studies you will learn the symptoms and signs resulting from fractures in each of the three cranial fossae. In view of the possible consequences, it is *no wonder safety rules for many workers require that hard hats be worn!*

CRANIAL MENINGES AND CSF

A clear understanding of the membranes (L. *meninges*) *and their relationship to CSF is an essential basis for the understanding of intracranial disease*, including head injuries.

The soft and jelly-like fresh brain tends to flatten when removed from the skull. In the living body, this vital organ is *enveloped by three membranes* (Fig. 7-59): (1) an outer thick, **tough dura mater** (L. *dura*, hard + *mater*, mother); (2) an exceedingly thin, intermediate, **cobweb-like arachnoid mater** (G. *arachne*, spider + *eidos*, resemblance); and (3) a delicate, adherent **vascular pia mater** (L. *pius*, tender). These three membranes covering the brain are known collectively as the **cranial meninges** (Fig. 7-59); they are continuous with the **spinal meninges** (covering the spinal cord) at the foramen magnum.

The main function of the cranial meninges and the CSF is to provide support and protection for the brain in addition to that afforded by the calvaria.

CLINICALLY ORIENTED COMMENTS

The tough, tenacious **dura mater** is occasionally called the pachymenix (G. *pachys*, thick + *menix*, membrane); hence, you may hear the term **pachymeningitis**, meaning inflammation of the dura mater. Since the advent of antibiotics, this condition is rare.

The pia mater and the arachnoid develop from a single layer of mesoderm that surrounds the embryonic brain. During development fluid-filled spaces develop within this layer which divide it into two layers. The spaces give rise to the subarachnoid space containing CSF. The embryonic origin of the pia mater and arachnoid mater from one layer is reflected by the numerous connective tissue fibers, called **trabeculae** (L. beams), passing between them (Fig. 7-60).

The pia and arachnoid together are referred to as the **leptomeninges** (G. *leptos*, slender + *meninges*, membranes). Later, when you hear of **leptomeningeal arteries**, you will realize that they supply the leptomeninges. Also, when your clinical instructors refer to pia-arachnitis, **leptomeningitis**, or simply meningitis, you should realize that all these terms mean the same thing (*i.e.*, inflammation of the pia-arachnoid or leptomeninges).

The Dura Mater (Figs. 7-59 to 7-63). This is a thick, tough membrane consisting

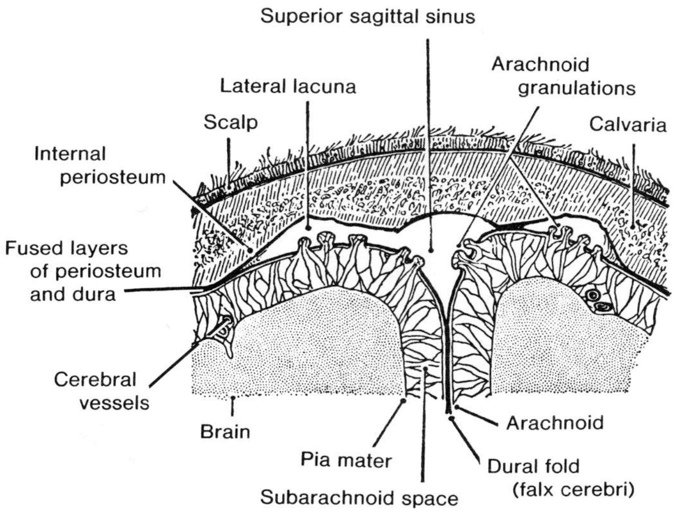

Figure 7-60. Diagram of a coronal section through the upper part of the head showing the relationship of the meninges to the calvaria and the brain. Note the midline groove in the calvaria for the superior sagittal sinus.

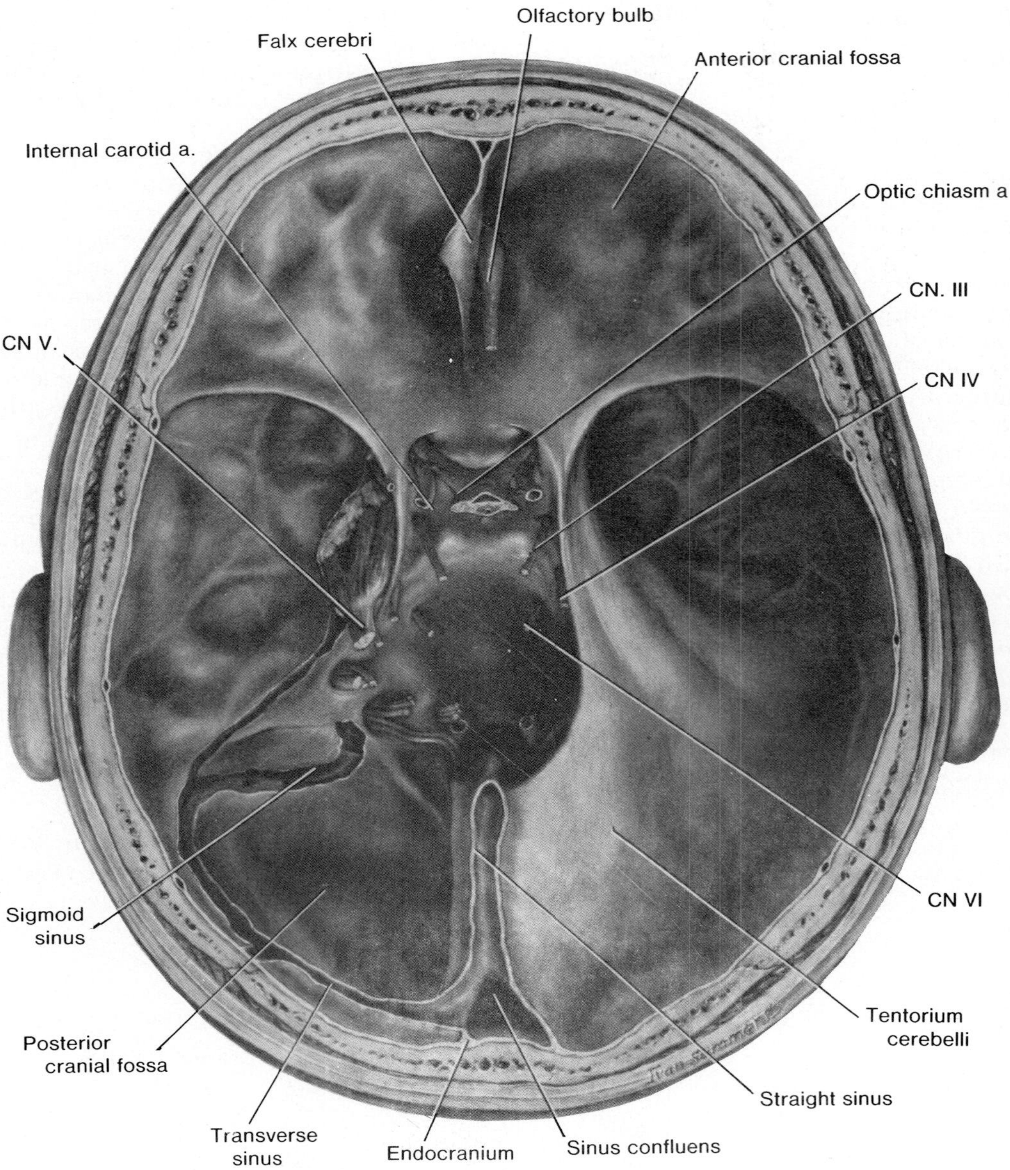

Figure 7-61. Drawing of the interior of the base of the skull showing the dura mater. Observe that the dura and the endocranium are separated by the venous sinuses (*e.g.*, at the sinus confluens or confluence of the sinuses). The falx cerebri has been cut close to its anterior attachment and most of it has been removed. The tentorium cerebelli has been cut away on the left to expose the posterior cranial fossa.

of collagenous connective tissue. Test its strength by trying to tear it! You will find when you remove the upper part of the **calvaria** during dissection to expose the brain that the skullcap can be pried loose from the membranes without difficulty. When you do this, you also strip the internal periosteum (endocranium) from the inner surface of the bones of the calvaria.

Although the cranial dura consists of only

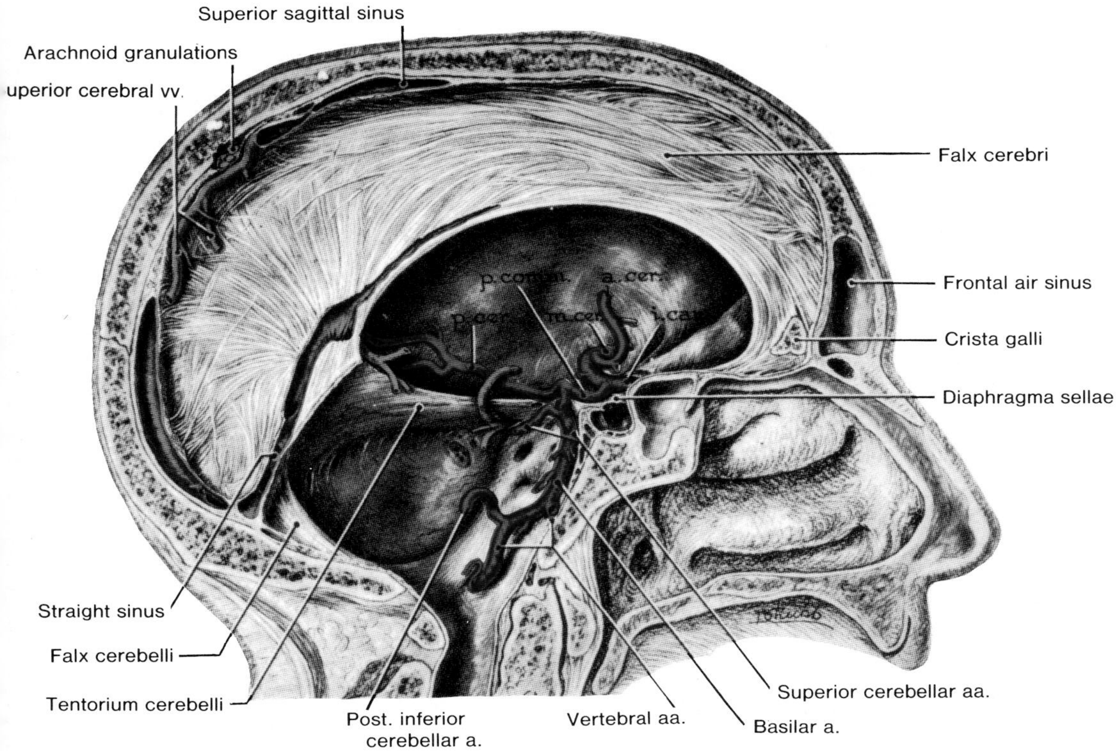

Figure 7-62. Drawing of a median section of the head showing the four folds (septa) of the dura mater: two sickle-shaped folds, the falx cerebri and the falx cerebelli, which lie vertically in the median plane; and two roof-like folds, the tentorium cerebelli and the diaphragma sellae. The tentorium is a wide, sloping tent-like fold of dura mater that covers the cerebellar hemispheres. The tentorium is traversed by the midbrain and the diaphragma sellae by the stalk of the hypophysis cerebri (Fig. 7-79). Note the two paired arteries that supply the brain, the internal carotid and the vertebral arteries.

one layer (like the spinal dura), it is sometimes described as consisting of two layers because the dura adheres so closely to the internal periosteum, except where there are dural venous sinuses and lateral venous lacunae. It also extends inwardly to form dural folds or septa, *e.g.*, the falx cerebri (Fig. 7-60). *It is important that you understand that the so-called "outer layer of dura"* is really the internal periosteum of the calvaria. It is attached to the bones of the calvaria by collagenic **Sharpey's fibers** that penetrate the cranial bones. It is also attached to the outer pericranium where these fibers traverse the cranial sutures (*e.g.*, the sagittal suture). This endosteal layer is continuous with the outer periosteum of the cranial bones at the margins of the foramen magnum and the smaller foramina for nerves and vessels.

The cranial dura, referred to as the meningeal layer of the dura by those who describe it as consisting of two layers, is continuous with the spinal dura at the foramen magnum. This true dura also provides **tubular sheaths** for the cranial nerves as they pass through the foramina in the floors of the **cranial fossae** (Fig. 7-61). Once outside the cranium, the dural sheaths fuse with the epineurium of the cranial nerves. The dural sheaths extend approximately to the ganglia; *e.g.*, the trigeminal (semilunar) ganglion of the fifth cranial nerve (CN V) is surrounded by an extension of the meninges. The dura-enclosed space at the **trigeminal impression** in the petrous part

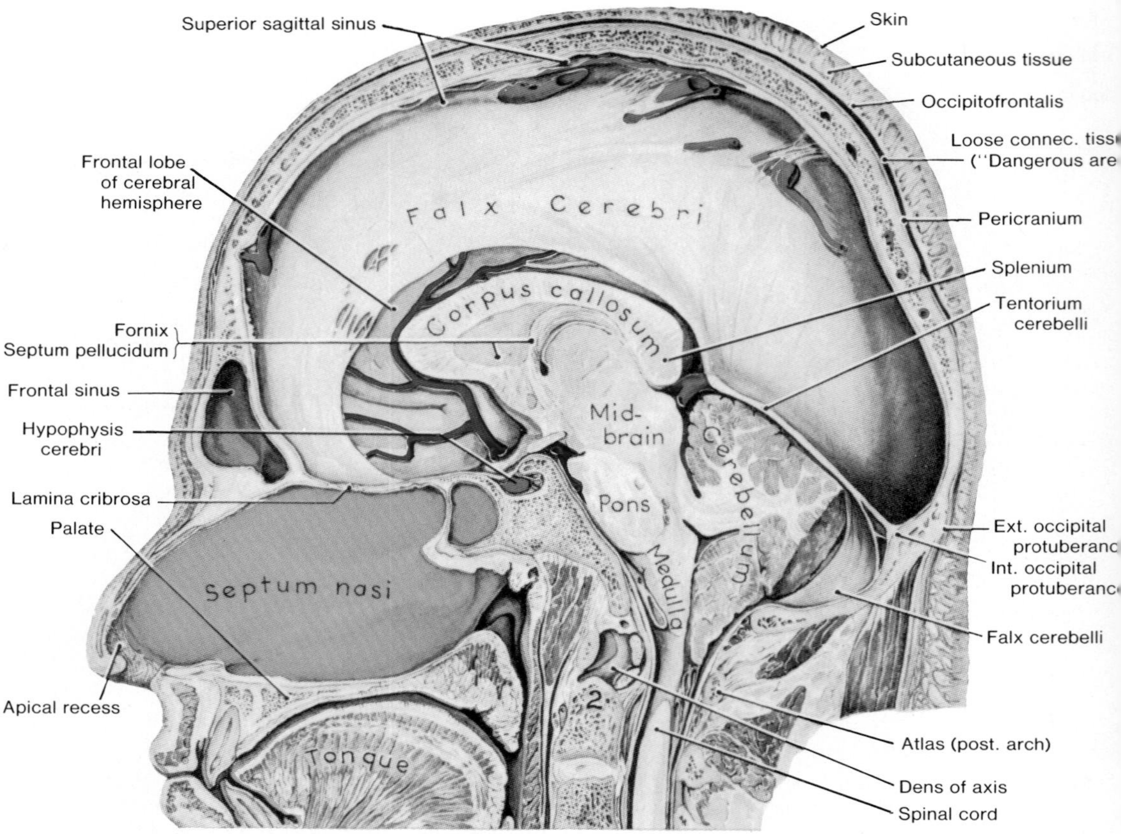

Figure 7-63. Drawing of a median section of the head. Note the attachments of the dural septa (reflections) and their relationship to the parts of the brain. There are two major septa, one vertical (falx cerebri) and one sloping like the roof of a tent (tentorium cerebelli). Note the superior sagittal sinus (a dural venous sinus) in the base of the falx cerebri. Observe that part of the cerebellum has herniated into the foramen magnum in this cadaveric specimen. Note that the sella turcica containing the hypophysis cerebri is roofed over by a fold of dura called the diaphragma sellae (not labeled, see Fig. 7-62).

of the temporal bone (Fig. 7-56), occupied by the trigeminal ganglion, is called the **trigeminal cave** (Figs. 7-88 and 7-133). The dural sheath of the optic nerve is continuous with the sclera of the eye; *this is clinically important*!

CLINICALLY ORIENTED COMMENTS

Part of the sensory root of the trigeminal nerve (CN V) is sometimes sectioned (**trigeminal rhizotomy**) to alleviate the pain of *trigeminal neuralgia* (tic douloureux). This syndrome is characterized by severe pains in the area of distribution of one or more branches of the trigeminal nerve. During trigeminal rhizotomy involving the mandibular nerve, the electrode passes through the cheek and the foramen ovale into the trigeminal cave occupied by the trigeminal ganglion (Fig. 7-133). Other methods of treating this condition are described in the discussion of Case 7-2.

The attachment of the dura mater to the bones in the floors of the cranial fossae (Fig. 7-61) is firmer than it is to the calvaria. Thus, a blow on the head can detach the dura from the calvaria without fracturing the bones, whereas a basal fracture usually tears the dura, resulting in leakage of CSF into the soft tissues of the neck, the nose, the ear, or the nasopharynx.

Dural Septa or Dural Reflections (Figs. 7-60, 7-62, and 7-63). During development of the brain, the dura is duplicated or reflected to form four inwardly projecting folds or septa. *The dural septa divide the cranial cavity into three intercommunicating compartments*, one subtentorial and two supratentorial, which provide support for parts of the brain, particularly the cerebral hemispheres.

The falx cerebri (L. *falx*, a sickle) is a large, sickle-shaped, vertical partition in the longitudinal fissure between the two cerebral hemispheres (Figs. 7-60 to 7-63). This large dural fold is attached in the median plane to the inner surface of the calvaria from the frontal crest of the frontal bone (Fig. 7-50) and the **crista galli** of the ethmoid bone anteriorly to the **internal occipital protuberance** posteriorly (Fig. 7-53). The falx cerebri is also attached to the midline of the **tentorium cerebelli**, another dural fold that lies between the occipital lobes of the cerebral hemispheres and the cerebellum (Figs. 7-61 to 7-63). At the superior convex border of the falx cerebri, its two layers separate to enclose the **superior sagittal sinus** (Figs. 7-43*A*, 7-59, and 7-60).

The falx cerebri increases in depth from the front to the back so that its free inferior edge comes close to the **splenium**, the thickened posterior end of the **corpus callosum** (Fig. 7-63). The **inferior sagittal sinus** (Fig. 7-69*A*) lies enclosed within the free inferior edge of the falx cerebri. Throughout life the falx cerebri forms a rigid partition between the cerebral hemispheres which reduces side-to-side movement of the brain.

The tentorium cerebelli (L. *tentorium*, tent) is a wide, crescentic, arched fold of dura mater that separates the occipital lobes of the cerebral hemispheres from the cerebellum (Figs. 7-61 to 7-63). The attachment of the falx cerebri to the midline portion of the tentorium holds the latter up like the ridge of a tent.

The tentorium is attached anterolaterally to the upper edges of the petromastoid parts of the temporal bones and to the **anterior** and **posterior clinoid processes** (Fig. 7-43*A*). Posteriorly, it is attached to the occipital bone along the grooves for the transverse sinuses which it encloses (Figs. 7-53 and 7-61). Its concave anteromedial border is free, and between it and the **dorsum sellae** of the sphenoid bone there is an opening ("door of the tent") called the **tentorial incisure** or notch (Figs. 7-64 and 9-53). This oval opening surrounds the midbrain as it passes from the middle to the posterior cranial fossa. It is also closely related to the anterior part of the superior surface of the **vermis** of the cerebellum (Fig. 7-65) and the *uncus* of each temporal lobe.

Fluid from the lateral ventricles of the brain passes *downward through the tentorial incisure* within the **cerebral aqueduct** (Fig. 7-80*A*) into the fourth ventricle. After leaving the ventricular system the CSF passes *upward through the tentorial incisure* in the subarachnoid space surrounding the midbrain. Hence, there are two chances of obstructing the flow of ventricular fluid and/or CSF at the tentorial incisure, and each produces a different type of **hydrocephalus** (excessive accumulation of ventricular fluid and/or CSF resulting in enlargement of the head).

The tentorium cerebelli prevents downward displacement of the occipital lobes when a person is erect.

CLINICALLY ORIENTED COMMENTS

The tentorial incisure, or tentorial notch, is slightly larger than is necessary to accommodate the midbrain; hence, when intracranial pressure above the tentorium is considerably higher than that below it (*e.g.*, when a tumor or an **intracranial hematoma** is present as in Case 7-6), part of the adjacent ipsilateral temporal lobe may herniate through the tentorial incisure. Often it is the **uncus** (L. a hook), the hooked extremity of the rostral end of the parahippocampal gyrus (Fig. 7-79), that herniates through the tentorial incisure. During **tentorial**

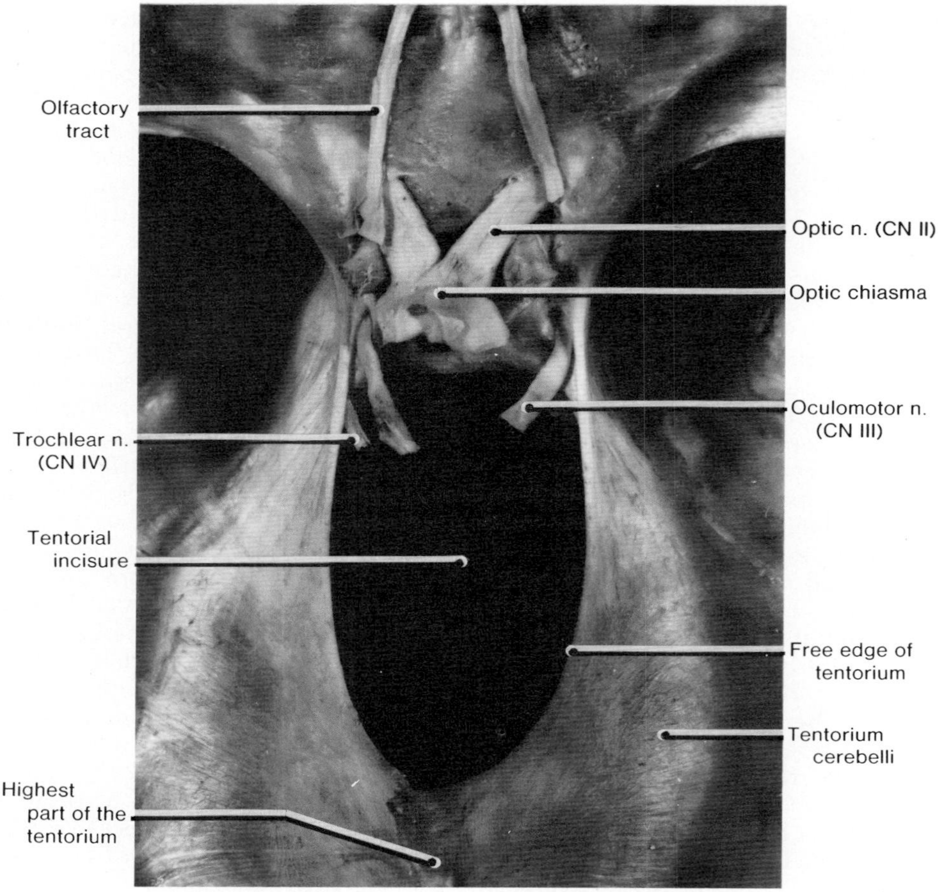

Figure 7-64. Photograph of a dissection of the tentorium cerebelli showing the typical shape of the tentorial incisure (notch), the opening in the tentorium cerebelli through which the brain stem extends from the middle to the posterior cranial fossa. (For orientation, see Figs. 7-61 and 7-88).

herniation the temporal lobe may be lacerated by the tough, taut tentorium, and the **oculomotor nerve** (CN III) may be stretched and/or compressed. Compression of CN III leads to **third nerve palsy** (*e.g.*, paralysis of pupillary constriction resulting in a fixed, dilated pupil; see Case 7-6).

Increased intracranial pressure may also force the cerebellar tonsils, the rounded lobules on the inferior surface of the cerebellar hemispheres (Fig. 7-65), downward and medially through the foramen magnum. **Herniation of the cerebellar tonsils** compresses the medulla containing the vital respiratory and cardiovascular centers, producing a lifethreatening situation.

The falx cerebelli (Figs. 7-62 and 7-63) is a small, sickle-shaped midline dural fold (septum) in the posterior part of the posterior cranial fossa, extending almost vertically upward to the inferior surface of the tentorium cerebelli. Its free edge projects slightly between the cerebellar hemispheres. The **occipital venous sinus** is located in its base (Fig. 7-38).

The diaphragma sellae is a small, circular, horizontal fold of dura that roofs over the **hypophysial fossa** in the sella turcica. The diaphragma is formed by the dura surrounding the hypophysis cerebri and encroaching around the stalk of this gland. It covers the **hypophysis cerebri** or pitui-

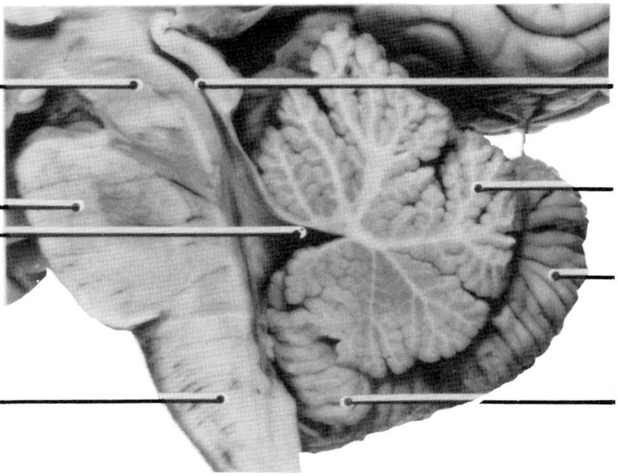

Figure 7-65. Photograph of a median section through the brain stem, fourth ventricle, and cerebellum. The cerebellar hemispheres, being lateral to the vermis that lies in the midline, are not cut in this median section.

tary gland (Fig. 7-63). The diaphragma has a central aperture for passage of the hypophysial veins and the hypophysial stalk or **infundibulum** (Fig. 7-79), connecting the hypothalamus and the hypophysis.

CLINICALLY ORIENTED COMMENTS

Tumors of the hypophysis cerebri (**pituitary tumors**) may extend upward through the opening in the **diaphragma sellae** and/or cause upward bulging of it. Pituitary tumors often expand the sellae and may produce endocrine symptoms early or late (*i.e.*, before or after enlargement of the sellae). Upward extension of the tumor causes visual symptoms owing to pressure on the **optic chiasma** (Fig. 7-79), the point of crossing of the optic nerve fibers.

The Arachnoid Mater (Figs. 7-59, 7-60, and 7-66). This is a delicate, transparent membrane composed of *cobweb-like tissue*. It forms the intermediate covering for the brain and is separated from the dura mater by a molecular film of fluid in the potential **subdural space**. The arachnoid does not form a close investment of the brain but passes over its small sulci (L. furrows or ditches) and the fissures without dipping into them. The term arachnoid is derived from Greek words meaning "resembling a spider's web."

The arachnoid is partly separated from the pia mater by the **subarachnoid space** containing CSF. Numerous trabeculae (delicate strands of connective tissue with mesenchymal epithelial cells on their surfaces) pass from the arachnoid to the pia (Fig. 7-66), giving it a cobweb-like structure.

The Pia Mater (Figs. 7-60, 7-64, and 7-66). Although this membrane (L. *pius*, tender) is very thin, it is thicker than the arachnoid. The pia, the innermost of the three layers of meninges, is a **highly vascularized connective tissue membrane** that adheres closely to the surface of the brain. It dips into all sulci and fissures, carrying blood vessels with it (Fig. 7-66). The cerebral veins run on the pia within the subarachnoid space. When branches of cerebral vessels penetrate the brain, the pia follows them for a short distance, forming a sleeve of pia mater. Hence, **perivascular spaces** (Virchow-Robin spaces) form which are continuous with the subarachnoid space. They extend in an increasingly attenuated form as far as the arterioles and venules in the brain.

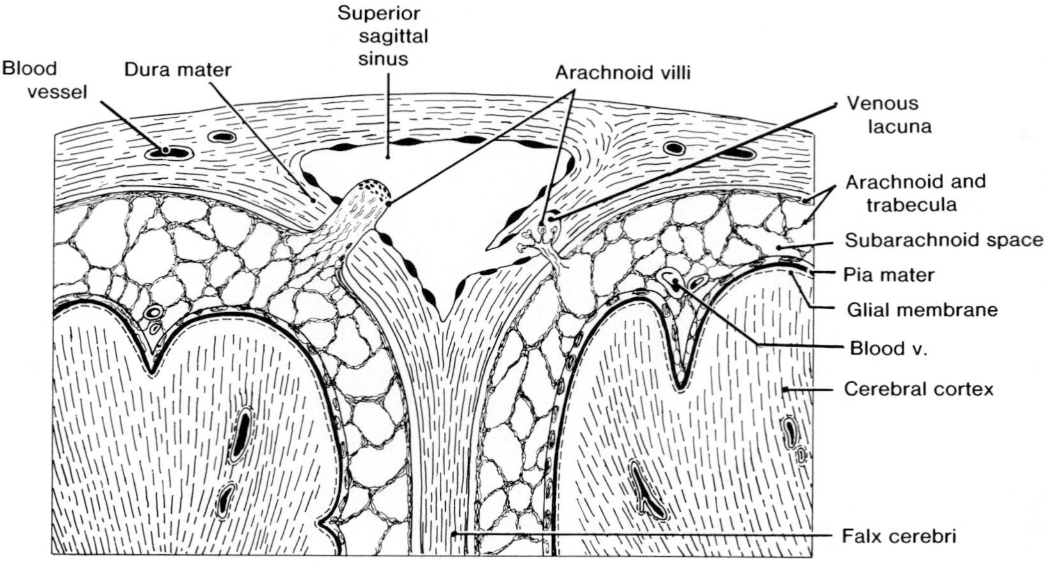

Figure 7-66. Diagram of the meningeal-cortical relationships. Note that the arachnoid does not form a close investment of the cerebral cortex and that it is attached to the pia by delicate strands (trabeculae). The subarachnoid space (containing CSF) is shown of greater width than is normal to illustrate the trabeculae crossing it and connecting the pia mater and arachnoid. Note that the pia is firmly anchored to the cerebral cortex. The main site of passage of CSF into venous blood is through the arachnoid villi projecting into the dural venous sinuses, especially the superior sagittal sinus and adjacent venous lacunae. Arachnoid villi that have become hypertropied with age (*e.g.*, the one on the left) are called arachnoid granulations.

CLINICALLY ORIENTED COMMENTS

Meningiomas (neoplastic growths of meningeal tissues) make up about 25% of primary intracranial tumors. As they enlarge they compress adjacent neural tissues. One common site for meningiomas is along the **sphenoidal ridge**, formed by the sharp posterior margin of the lesser wing of the sphenoid bone and the orbital plate of the frontal bone (Fig. 7-49).

Because the *central artery and vein of the retina cross the subarachnoid space* to become enclosed in the space around the posterior part of the optic nerve (Figs. 7-67 and 7-101), an increase in CSF pressure around the nerve slows the return of venous blood, resulting in **edema of the retina.** This is most apparent as a swelling of the optic papilla (**papilledema**). Thus, inspection of the **ocular fundi** (Fig. 7-102) is an important part of a neurological examination (Case 7-6).

In cases of **ruptured aneurysm** of the circulus arteriosus cerebri (Fig. 7-90), there is usually hemorrhage into the subarachnoid space. Blood in the CSF results in an increase in intracranial pressure. The increased pressure is transmitted to the *subarachnoid spaces around the optic nerves*, compressing the retinal vein where it runs in the subarachnoid space around the optic nerve (Figs. 7-67 and 7-101). This results in increased pressure in the retinal capillaries and **subhyaloid hemorrhages** between the retina and the vitreous body (Case 7-6).

Arteries and Veins of the Cranial Dura Mater (Figs. 7-59, 7-63, and 7-66). There are many **meningeal arteries** in the periosteum. *These arteries are inappropriately named* because they supply more blood to the bones of the calvaria than to the dura of the meninges. Only very fine branches are distributed to the dura.

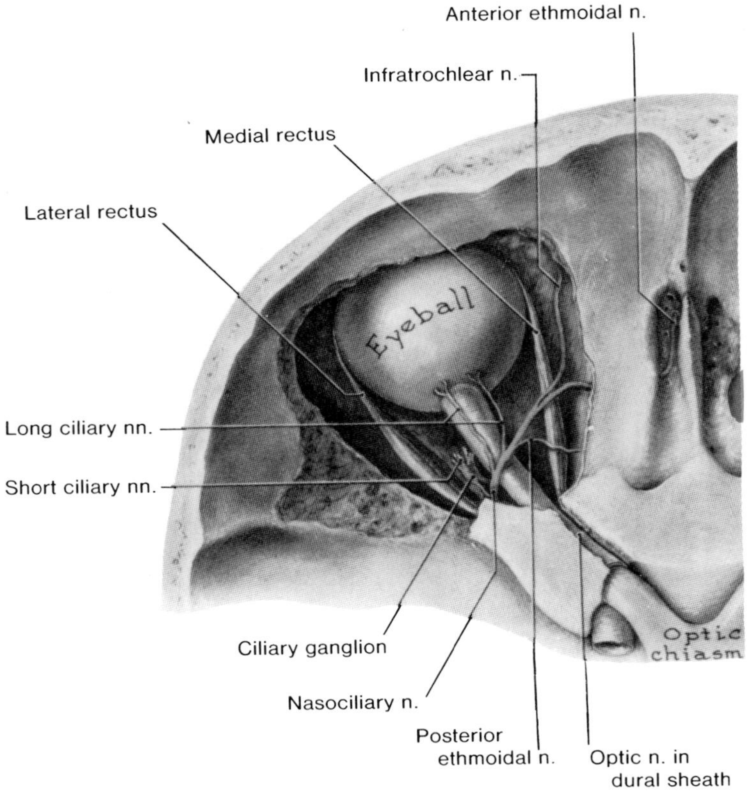

Figure 7-67. Drawing of a dissection of the left orbital cavity from above showing the nasociliary nerve and its branches to the ocular muscles. Observe the optic nerve in its dural sheath, which is continuous with the dura mater covering the brain.

As stated in the previous section, the arteries to the brain, branches of the paired internal carotid and vertebral arteries, lie in the pia mater within the subarachnoid space (Fig. 7-66).

The middle meningeal artery (Figs. 7-15, 7-55, and 7-59), a branch of the **maxillary**, is clinically important largely because it is often torn when the overlying skull is fractured. These vessels within the periosteum often *form distinct grooves on the inner surface of the calvaria* (Fig. 7-71). Examine the floor of the middle cranial fossa and the skullcap of a dried skull. Note the deep markings formed by the middle meningeal artery and its branches (Figs. 7-52, 7-56, and 7-71). By observing these grooves in the calvaria, you can see that this artery enters the cranial cavity through the **foramen spinosum** in the floor of the middle cranial fossa (Fig. 7-56) and soon divides into anterior and posterior branches. These branches ramify on the internal surface of the calvaria. It is obvious that a fracture in the temporal region of the skull (*e.g.*, the pterion) may tear one or more branches of this artery, producing an **extradural (epidural) hematoma** (Case 7-5). The meningeal arteries are accompanied by meningeal veins (Fig. 7-59), which may also be torn in fractures of the calvaria.

Sensory Nerve Supply to the Cranial Dura Mater (Fig. 7-68). *The rich sensory supply to the dura is largely through the three divisions of the trigeminal* (**CN V**), but sensory branches are also received from the vagus (**CN X**) and the upper three **cervical nerves** via the hypoglossal nerve. The sensory endings are more numerous in the dura mater along each side of the su-

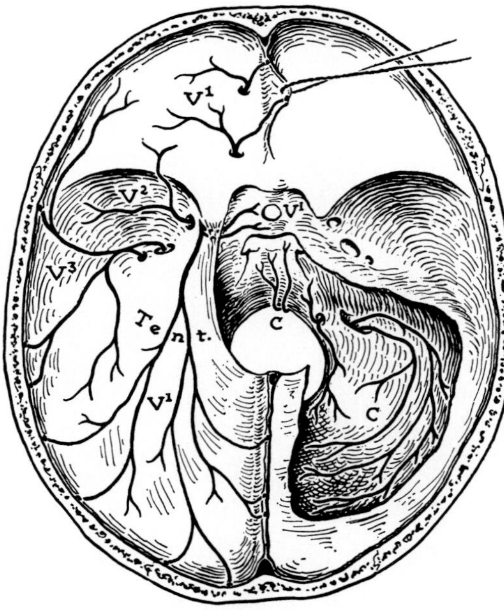

Figure 7-68. Drawing illustrating the nerves of the cranial dura mater. The nerves to the dura, the dural vessels, and the dural sinuses are derived mainly from the three divisions of the trigeminal nerve (CN V^1, CN V^2, and CN V^3), but branches are also received from the vagus (CN X) and the upper cervical nerves (*C*).

perior sagittal sinus and in the tentorium cerebelli than they are in the floor of the cranium.

CLINICALLY ORIENTED COMMENTS

The brain is insensitive to pain, but some of the large cerebral vessels have a sensory supply. Pulling on the arteries at the base of the skull or the veins in the vertex or at the base where they pierce the dura mater causes pain.

Although there are many causes of headache, distention of the scalp and/or meningeal arteries is believed to be one cause. *Many headaches appear to be dural in origin*; for example, the headache that occurs during and after a **lumbar puncture** (Fig. 5-69) for the removal of CSF is thought to result from stimulation of sensory endings in superior parts of the dura. When CSF is removed, the brain sags slightly, pulling on the dura mater, which is thought to cause pain. It is for this reason that, following lumbar punctures for removal of CSF, patients are asked to keep their heads down to minimize or prevent headaches.

The Meningeal Spaces. The extradural (epidural) space is outside the dura and is between the bone and the periosteum. Because the dura is attached initimately to the periosteum of the cranium (Fig. 7-59), the **extradural space** is only a potential one which becomes real when blood accumulates in it from torn meningeal vessels (**extradural hemorrhage**) resulting from a fractured skull.

The subdural space is deep to the dura mater, *i.e.*, between the dura and the arachnoid. It is also a potential space with only a thin film of subdural fluid in it. It is not obliterated except at places where it is pierced by arteries, veins, and nerves.

CLINICALLY ORIENTED COMMENTS

Air or oil injected into the **spinal subdural space** in the lumbar region (Fig. 5-69) may enter the **cranial subdural space**, but this is inadvertent, not intentional.

Head injuries may be associated with various types of **intracranial bleeding** (hemorrhage).

Extradural (Epidural) Hemorrhage. Bleeding between the dura and the periosteum of the calvaria (*i.e.*, outside the dura) may follow a blow to the head. Typically there is a **brief concussion** (loss of consciousness) followed by a **lucid interval** of some hours (Case 7-5). This is followed by drowsiness and **coma** (profound unconsciousness). Usually there is a tearing of meningeal vessels, (*e.g.*, the middle meningeal artery is often torn in fractures of the squama of the temporal bone). *The artery most commonly injured is the middle meningeal artery* or one of its branches, often the anterior one (Fig. 7-59). Similarly, the superior sagittal sinus (Fig. 7-63) may be torn in fractures of the upper part of the calvaria.

Although veins and venous sinuses may be torn, the bleeding is usually arterial. Because the periosteum is firmly attached to bone, there is a slow, gradual, localized accumulation of blood (**hematoma**). As the fluid mass increases in size, compression of the brain occurs necessitating evacuation of the fluid and occlusion of the bleeding vessel(s).

The formation of an extradural hematoma above the **tentorium cerebelli** causes a rise in supratentorial pressure which, if high enough, produces herniation of the temporal lobe (usually the uncus) through the tentorial incisure adjacent to CN III. This causes **third nerve palsy** and dilation of the pupil on the affected side. If the pressure rises very high, the cerebellar tonsils may be forced through the foramen magnum, compressing the medulla with possible fatal effects owing to interference with its respiratory and cardiovascular centers.

Subdural Hemorrhage. Bleeding between the dura and the arachnoid often follows a blow which jerks the brain inside the skull. Such a displacement of the brain is greatest in elderly people in whom some shrinkage of the brain has occurred. The hemorrhage commonly results from tearing of **cerebral veins** where they enter the superior sagittal sinus (Fig. 7-62). Subdural hemorrhage is usually classified as acute or chronic. At first the subdural blood is spread over the cerebral hemispheres, but after a few days or weeks it localizes, most often under the **parietal tuber** (Fig. 7-8). Being hypertonic, the collection of blood slowly expands; this explains why symptoms may not occur for weeks after a trivial injury.

Subarachnoid Hemorrhage. Bleeding into the subarachnoid space usually occurs following rupture of a saccular or **berry aneurysm** on an intracranial artery (Case 7-7 and Fig. 7-91). These thin-walled outpouchings occur chiefly at bifurcations of the arteries at the base of the brain (Fig. 7-90), at areas where two pulse waves meet (*e.g.*, where the wave from the internal carotid artery meets the wave from the posterior cerebral artery). Subarachnoid hemorrhages are also associated with skull fractures and cerebral lacerations. *Subarachnoid hemorrhage results in meningeal irritation*, which is indicated by severe headache, stiff neck, and often loss of consciousness.

Intracerebral Hemorrhage. Bleeding into the brain from an artery, often one of the **striate branches of the middle cerebral artery** (Fig. 7-89) going to the corpus striatum (basal ganglia), is frequent in hypertension. One of these arteries was named the **artery of cerebral hemorrhage** by Charcot because he observed that it hemorrhages into the region of the internal capsule, producing a **paralytic stroke**. The paralysis occurs because of interruption of motor pathways from the motor cortex to the brain stem and the spinal cord.

The Venous Sinuses and Venous Lacunae of the Dura Mater (Figs. 7-38, 7-63, and 7-69). These sinuses and lacunae are **venous channels** (spaces) located *between the dura and the internal periosteum* lining the cranium, usually along the lines of attachment of the dural septa. They are lined with endothelium that is continuous with that of the cerebral veins entering them (Fig. 7-62). These venous sinuses have no valves and no muscular tissue in their walls; *they drain all the blood from the brain*. Several of the sinuses are triangular in cross-section (Fig. 7-66) because their bases are on bone and their side walls are formed by the origins of the dural folds.

The Superior Sagittal Sinus (Figs. 7-38, 7-43*A*, 7-59, 7-60, 7-62, 7-63, 7-69*A* and 7-70) lies in the midline along the attached border of the falx cerebri. It begins at the **crista galli** and runs the entire length of the superior attached portion of the falx cerebri, before ending at the **internal occipital protuberance** (Fig. 7-63). Examine the inner surface of a dried skullcap and observe the prominent longitudinal groove formed by the posterior two-thirds of the superior sagittal sinus, particularly at the posterior end where it is usually about 1 cm wide (Fig. 7-62).

In about 60% of cases the *superior sagittal sinus ends by becoming the right*

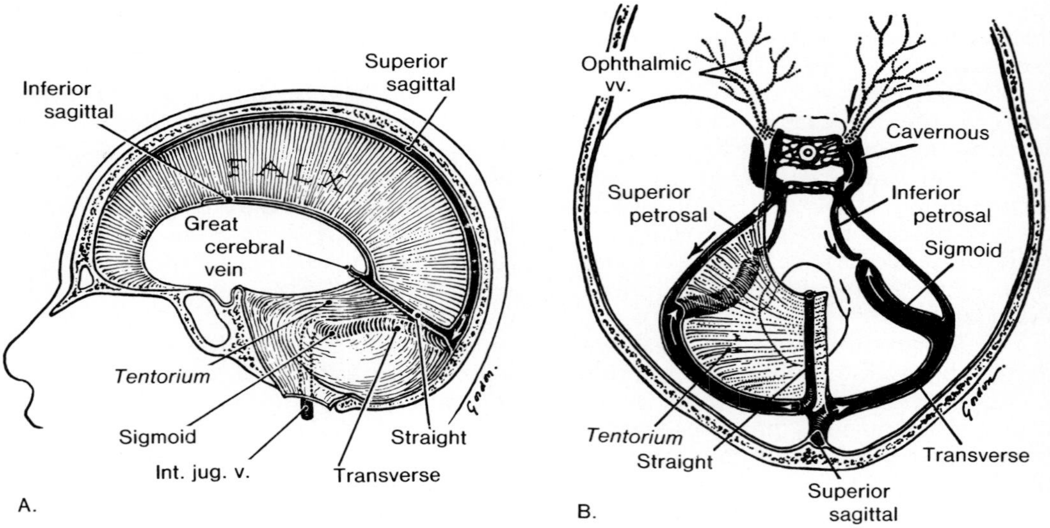

Figure 7-69. Semischematic diagrams of the venous sinuses of the dura mater. *A*, in falx cerebri and tentorium cerebelli. *B*, opened from above. *Arrows* show the direction of the blood flow. See Figures 7-38 and 7-70 for other views of these sinuses.

transverse sinus (Figs. 7-69 and 7-70). In other cases, it turns to the left and ends in the left transverse sinus or bifurcates and ends in both. Examine the posterior cranial fossa of several dried skulls and determine by examining the groove in each made by the transverse sinus (Figs 7-9 and 7-13) how the superior sagittal sinus ended in the person from whom the skull was obtained. *Note that the jugular foramen is larger on the side with the deeper groove for the transverse sinus.*

The termination of the superior sagittal sinus shows a dilation, known as the **confluence of the sinuses** or **confluens sinuum** (Fig. 7-70). Occasionally you will hear this dilation referred to as the *torcular Herophili* (L. winepress of Herophilus, an early anatomist and surgeon). Five sinuses often communicate at the confluence; however, considerable variation in venous pathways occurs in the vicinity of the confluens sinuum.

The superior sagittal sinus is triangular in cross-section (Figs. 7-43*A* and 7-60), the superior wall being formed by the internal periosteum lining the calvaria and the lateral walls by the dura. It becomes larger as it passes posteriorly and receives more and more **superior cerebral veins** (Fig. 7-62). They enter the sinus in a forward direction. This results from their fixation to the superior sagittal sinus in early fetal life, but their more distal parts were carried posteriorly by subsequent growth of the brain. The superior sagittal sinus communicates on each side via slit-like openings with several venous lacunae, called **lateral lacunae**, into which some of the **arachnoid villi** project (Figs. 7-59, 7-60, and 7-66).

The main site of passage of CSF into venous blood is through the **arachnoid villi**, especially those projecting into the superior sagittal sinus and the adjacent venous lacunae. *Hypertrophied aggregations of arachnoid villi,* associated with advancing age, are called **arachnoid granulations** (Pacchionian bodies). These granulations often produce erosion or pitting of the inner surface of the upper portions of the frontal and parietal bones as they invade them (Fig. 7-71).

The superior sagittal sinus also communicates with veins in the scalp via **emissary veins** which pass through the *parietal foramina* (Fig. 7-71).

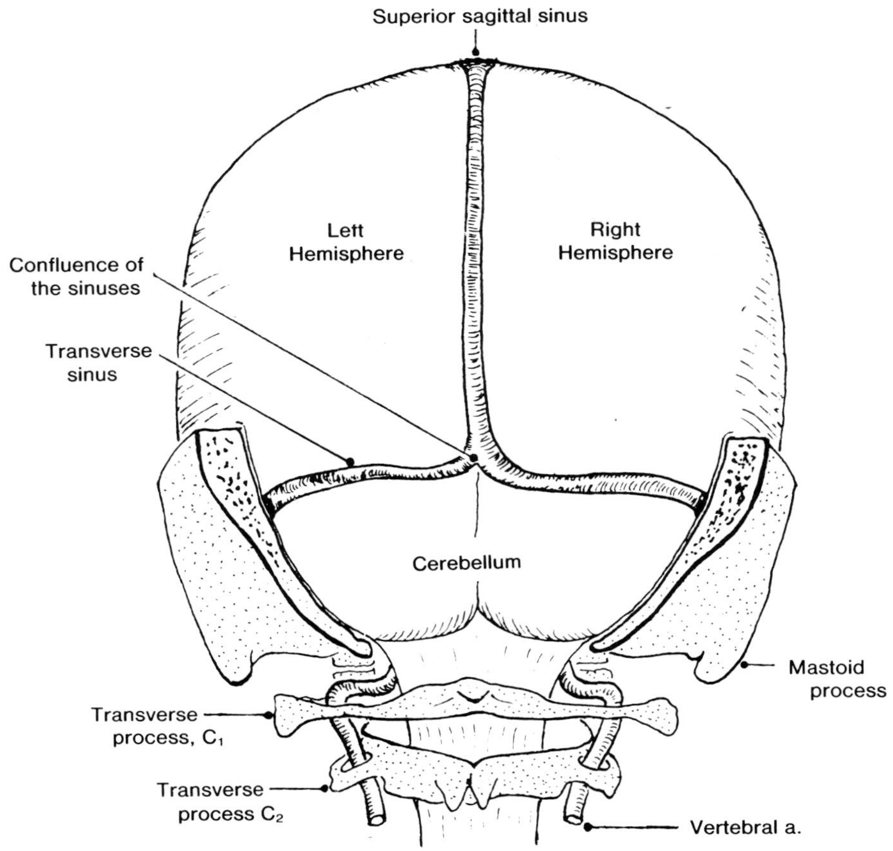

Figure 7-70. Schematic drawing of a posterior view of some of the venous sinuses of the dura mater. The calvaria and a large wedge of the occipital bone have been removed. The straight and occipital sinuses (not shown) also enter the confluence of sinuses (confluens sinuum). Observe the vertebral arteries passing through the foramen transversaria in the transverse processes of the axis (C2) and the atlas (C1). Note that once they pass through these foramina they turn posteriorly and then medially. They enter the skull through the foramen magnum and join to form the basilar artery (Fig. 7-90).

The Inferior Sagittal Sinus (Figs. 7-38 and 7-69), much smaller than the superior one, occupies the posterior two-thirds of the free inferior edge of the **falx cerebri**. It ends by joining with the **great cerebral vein** (of Galen) to form the straight sinus (Fig. 7-62). It receives cortical veins from the medial aspects of the cerebral hemispheres.

The Straight Sinus (Figs. 7-61, 7-62, 7-69, and 7-70) is formed by the union of the inferior sagittal sinus with the great cerebral vein. It runs downward and backward along the line of attachment of the **falx cerebri** to the tentorium cerebelli and becomes continuous with one of the transverse sinuses, usually the left.

The Transverse Sinuses (Figs. 7-9, 7-38, 7-69*B*, and 7-70) pass laterally from the confluence of the sinuses in the attached border of the tentorium, grooving the occipital bones and the posteroinferior angles of the parietal bones (Fig. 7-53). They then leave the tentorium and change their name to the sigmoid sinus because they curve downward and then medially in an S-shaped curve (Fig. 7-56).

The Sigmoid Sinuses (G. *sigma*, the

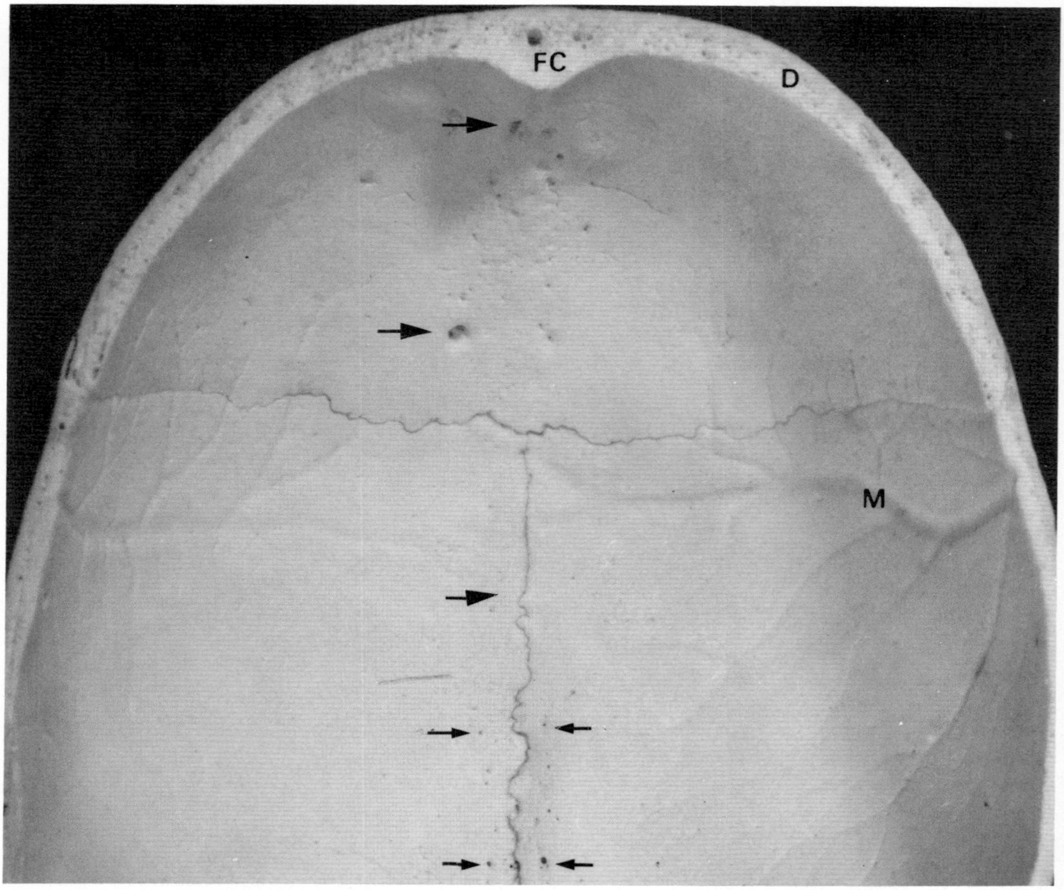

Figure 7-71. Photograph of the internal surface of an adult skullcap showing parts of the frontal and parietal bones. Note the coronal suture between the frontal and the parietal bones and the sagittal suture between the parietal bones. Observe the pits in the frontal bone (*large arrows*) produced by arachnoid granulations (hypertrophied aggregations of arachnoid villi). On each side of the sagittal suture, note the parietal foramina (*small arrows*), through which emissary veins passed to connect the superior sagittal sinus with veins in the diploë and the scalp (Fig. 7-46). The spongy diploë (*D*), or cancellous bone, that contained red marrow in life is visible in the frontal region of the sectioned calvaria. Note also the sinuous groove (*M*) formed by the anterior branch of the middle meningeal artery (also see Figs. 7-14, 7-52, and 7-59). Note the frontal crest (*FC*) to which the falx cerebri is attached (also see Fig. 7-50).

letter S) follow S-shaped courses in the posterior cranial fossa (Figs. 7-61, 7-69, and 7-72), forming deep grooves in the inner surface of the posterior part of the mastoid parts of the temporal bones and the superior surfaces of the jugular tubercles of the occipital bone (Fig. 7-57). The sigmoid sinuses then turn anteriorly and enter venous enlargements called **superior bulbs** of the jugular veins, which occupy the **jugular foramina**. These large bulbs or the jugular veins just below (Fig. 7-74) receive the inferior petrosal sinuses and continue downward as the **internal jugular veins.** *All the venous sinuses of the dura mater eventually deliver most of their blood to the sigmoid sinuses and thence to the internal jugular veins,* except for the inferior petrosal sinuses which enter these veins directly (Fig. 7-74). It is worth noting here

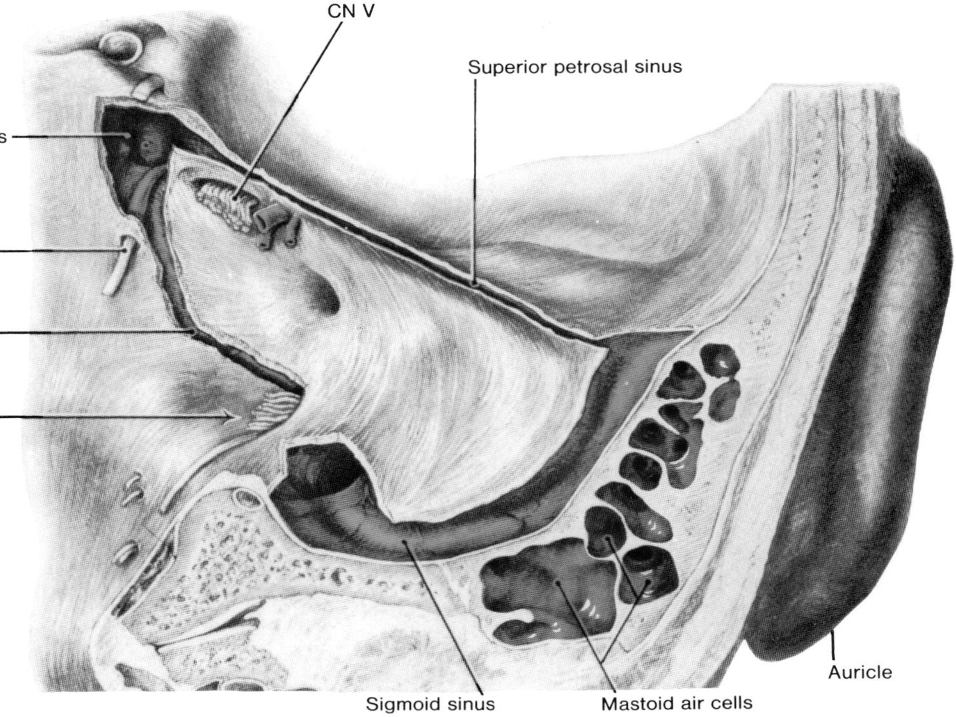

Figure 7-72. Drawing of a dissection of the anterior wall of the right posterior cranial fossa, as seen from behind. Some of the venous sinuses of the dura mater are illustrated. Note that the posterior surface of the petrous part of the temporal bone is encircled by three sinuses, sigmoid, superior petrosal, and inferior petrosal, and that these sinuses have no valves. The two petrosal sinuses drain the cavernous sinus. Observe the mastoid air cells (air-filled spaces) lined with mucus membrane (*pink*) in the diploë of the mastoid process of the temporal bone. Observe the sigmoid sinus, cranial nerves IX, X, and XI, and the inferior petrosal sinus entering the jugular foramen.

that in the erect position, pressure in the veins of the head is negative.

The Occipital Sinus (Fig. 7-38), the smallest of the dural venous sinuses, begins near the posterior margin of the foramen magnum as two or more venous channels around the edges of this large aperture. These usually join to form an unpaired sinus that lies in the attached border of the **falx cerebelli.** The occipital sinus communicates below with the **internal vertebral plexus** and ends above in the confluence of the sinuses.

The Cavernous Sinuses (L. *caverna*, cave or grotto) are about 2 cm long and 1 cm wide (Figs. 7-38, 7-69*B*, 7-72, and 7-73). They are located on each side of the sella turcica and the body of the **sphenoid** bone. They were named cavernous sinuses because of their cave-like appearance resulting from the many blood channels formed by numerous trabeculae. Each sinus extends from the superior orbital fissure in front to the apex of the petrous part of the temporal bone behind, where it is joined to the posterior **intercavernous sinus** and the **superior** and **inferior petrosal sinuses** (Fig. 7-69*B*). Each cavernous sinus receives blood from the superior and inferior **ophthalmic veins,** the superficial **middle cerebral vein** running along the lateral fissure of the cerebral hemisphere, and the **sphenoparietal sinus.** The latter sinus lies beneath the edge of the lesser wing of the sphenoid bone. The cavernous sinuses communicate with each other through **intercavernous sinuses** that pass anterior and posterior to the hypo-

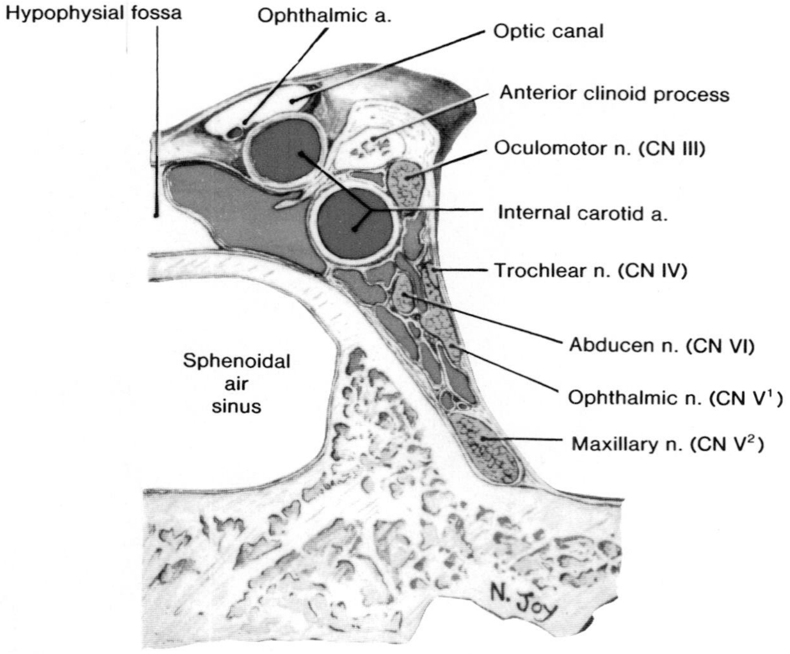

Figure 7-73. Drawing of a coronal section of the cavernous sinus. Observe that this dural venous sinus is situated at the side of the sphenoidal air sinus and of the hypophysial fossa. Note that the cranial nerves III, IV, V^1, and V^2 are in a sheath in the lateral wall of the cavernous sinus. Observe that the internal carotid artery and the abducent nerve pass through the sinus and so are vulnerable in thrombosis of the cavernous sinus. Note that the internal carotid artery, having made a hairpin bend, is cut twice, once in the cavernous sinus and again above the cavernous sinus in the subarachnoid space. Refer to Figure 7-38 for help in interpreting this drawing.

physial stalk or **infundibulum**. They drain posteriorly and inferiorly via the superior and inferior petrosal sinuses and the pterygoid plexuses.

Located in the lateral wall of each cavernous sinus, from superior to inferior, are the following structures (Fig. 7-73): (1) the oculomotor nerve (**CN III**); the trochlear nerve (**CN IV**); the ophthalmic and maxillary divisions of the trigeminal nerve (**CN V^1** and **CN V^2**). *Inside each cavernous sinus* are the **internal carotid artery,** with its sympathetic plexus, and the abducent nerve (**CN VI**).

The Superior Petrosal Sinuses (Figs. 7-38, 7-69, and 7-72) are *small channels draining the cavernous sinuses.* They run from the posterior ends of the cavernous sinuses to the **transverse sinuses,** at the points where they curve downward to form the **sigmoid sinuses** (Fig. 7-70). Each superior petrosal sinus lies in the attached margin of the **tentorium cerebelli**, running in a small groove on the superior margin of the petrous part of the temporal bone (Fig. 7-56).

The Inferior Petrosal Sinuses (Figs. 7-38, 7-69*B*, and 7-74), also small, *drain the cavernous sinuses directly into the internal jugular veins,* just below the skull. Commencing at the posterior end of the cavernous sinus, each inferior petrosal sinus runs backward, laterally, and downward in a groove between the petrous part of the temporal bone and the basilar part of the occipital bone. It passes into the jugular foramen and may enter the **superior bulb** of the internal jugular vein, but it usually traverses the foramen and enters the vein below the skull. It receives cerebellar and labyrinthine (internal auditory) veins.

The Basilar Plexus (sinus) consists of

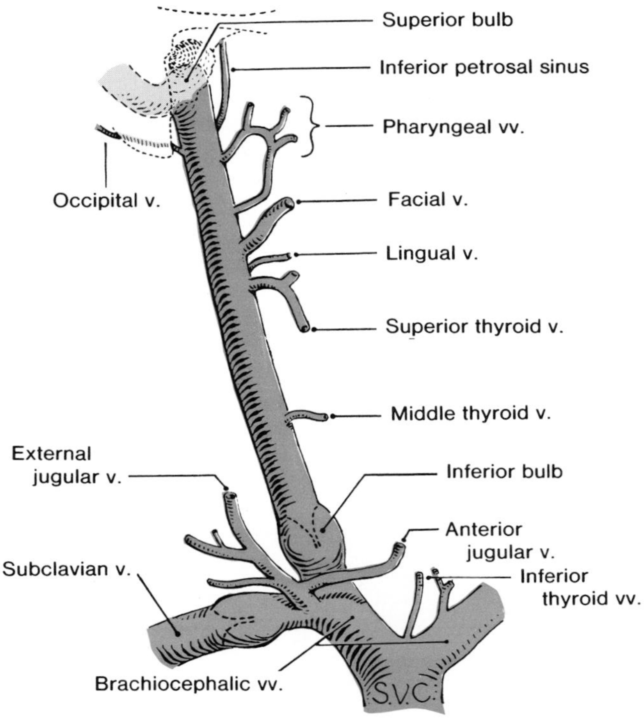

Figure 7-74. Drawing of an anterior view of the right internal jugular and its tributaries. It begins at the superior margin of the jugular foramen and dilates within it to form the superior bulb (jugular bulb). Note that the inferior petrosal sinus joins the internal jugular vein just below the skull. Recall that it drains the posterior end of the cavernous sinus and passes through the jugular foramen to reach the internal jugular vein (Figs. 7-69 and 7-73).

several interconnecting venous channels on the **clivus** (Figs. 7-57 and 7-69), the posterior surfaces of the basiocciput, and the basisphenoid. It connects the two inferior petrosal sinuses and communicates below with the **internal vertebral venous plexus** (Fig. 5-64).

Emissary Veins. These connect the intracranial venous sinuses with veins outside the cranium. Although they are valveless and blood may flow in both directions, the flow is usually away from the brain. The size and number of emissary veins vary. Only those which are clinically important are mentioned. In children (and some adults) a *frontal emissary vein* passes through the foramen cecum (Fig. 7-50), connecting the superior sagittal sinus with the veins of the frontal sinus and/or with those of the nasal cavities.

The parietal emissary veins, one on each side, pass through parietal foramina in the calvaria (Fig. 7-71) and connect the **superior sagittal sinus** with the veins external to it, particularly those in the scalp. They may also communicate with the diploic veins (Fig. 7-46).

A **mastoid emissary vein** connects each sigmoid sinus through the mastoid foramen with the occipital or the posterior auricular vein. A *posterior condylar emissary vein* may be present and pass through the condylar canal (Figs. 7-56 and 7-57), connecting the sigmoid sinus with the suboccipital plexus of veins.

CLINICALLY ORIENTED COMMENTS

Although most blood leaves the skull and the brain via the internal jugular veins, there are several other routes (*e.g.*, the emissary veins) that are important clinically.

The **basilar plexus** and the **occipital sinus**, via the foramen magnum, communicate with the **internal vertebral plexuses** (Fig. 7-38); consequently, blood may pass to or from the **vertebral venous system** (Fig. 5-64). As these venous channels are valveless, compression of the thorax, abdomen, or pelvis, as occurs during heavy coughing and straining, may force venous blood from these regions into the dural venous sinuses and into the vertebral system. As a result, tumors and abscesses of the head or inside the thorax, abdomen, or pelvis may spread to the vertebrae and the brain (Case 1-2, a patient with **bronchogenic carcinoma,** and Case 3-5, a patient with **prostatic cancer**).

These connections of the vertebral plexuses with the dural venous sinuses also explain how a blood clot (*e.g.*, from the pelvic veins after childbirth) can reach the dural venous sinuses without passing through the heart and lungs. Within a sinus, the thrombus (clot) may block it, possibly leading to venous infarction of the cerebral cortex.

Infections outside the skull may pass via **emissary veins** or their walls into the venous sinuses of the dura mater. An infection in the scalp can be transmitted to the superior sagittal sinus via the **parietal emissary veins.** The bacteria may produce inflammatory processes in the walls of the emissary veins that could cause **thrombophlebitis of the dural venous sinuses** and later of the cortical veins. **Cortical infarction** (death of nervous tissue) could follow.

The facial vein connects with the cavernous sinus through communications with the ophthalmic veins or with its tributary, the supraorbital. Thus, **thrombophlebitis of the facial vein** may extend into the dural sinuses (Case 7-3). Thrombophlebitis in one cavernous sinus commonly spreads to the other because they are connected by **intercavernous sinuses.** Furthermore, thrombosis could spread from the cavernous sinus into the superior petrosal sinus, the transverse sinus, the sigmoid sinus, and the jugular vein(s). In cases of **mastoiditis** (uncommon since the advent of antibiotics), thrombosis of the sigmoid sinus is common owing to its proximity to the mastoid air cells (Fig. 7-72).

Excision of an internal jugular vein is sometimes necessary (*e.g.*, in radical neck dissection to remove the **deep cervical lymph nodes** draining certain malignant tumors of the head and neck). In most cases the circulatory complications are minimal because the connections between the dural venous sinuses and veins outside the skull (*e.g.*, the vertebral venous plexus and the facial veins) enlarge enough to carry the blood from intracranial structures.

Although emissary veins cannot enlarge quickly because their size is limited by the foramina in the bones, they can enlarge and carry considerable blood in certain conditions (*e.g.*, *chronic increase in intracranial pressure*).

When a dural venous sinus is torn in association with a skull fracture, bleeding may persist instead of diminishing as in most other vessels. The reason for this is that the patient is usually lying down, which increases the pressure in the venous sinuses. In addition the dural venous sinuses (being only endothelial-lined spaces between the dura and the internal periosteum) are noncontractile. If there is bleeding into the subdural or extradural spaces it will continue. If it is an open fracture (*i.e.*, compound), blood may drain through the wound.

The fact that the **cavernous sinus envelops the internal carotid artery** and several cranial nerves is of clinical significance. In fractures of the base of the skull, the internal carotid artery may tear within this sinus, producing an **arteriovenous fistula.** In such cases arterial blood rushes into the cavernous sinus, enlarging it and forcing blood out of all the connecting veins (Fig. 7-38), especially the ophthalmic veins, which normally drain the orbital cavity. As a result the eye protrudes (**exophthalmos**) and the conjunctiva is engorged (**chemosis**) on the side of the torn artery. In these circumstances, the bulging eye pulsates in synchrony with the radial pulse (Fig. 6-92); because of this, the condition is often called **pulsating exophthalmos**.

Because cranial nerves III, IV, V^1, V^2, and VI lie in the lateral wall of the cavern-

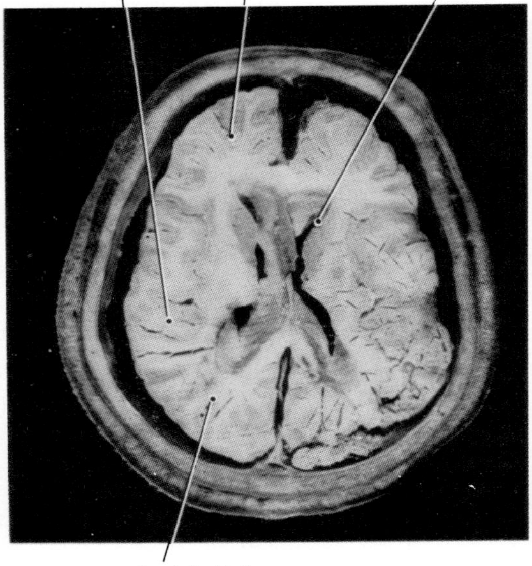

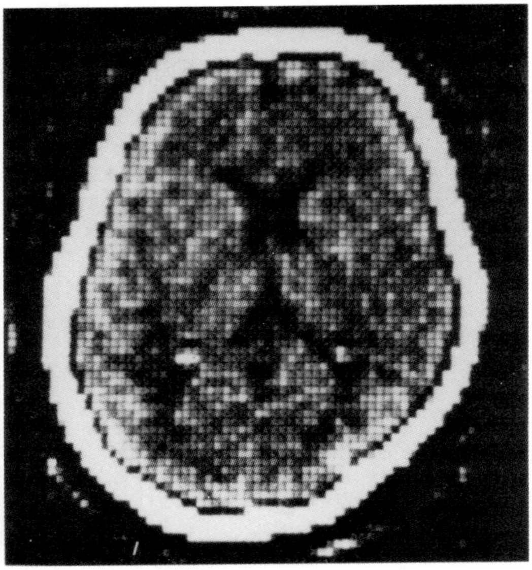

Figure 7-75. *A*, horizontal section through the head of a cadaver. *B*, computerized tomograph (CT scan) of a living person's head scanned in a horizontal plane at the same level. Note (1) the reduced density (*dark*) in the area of the cerebral ventricles; (2) the reduced density in the subarachnoid spaces outside the brain; (3) the dense (*white*) skull outline; and (4) the intermediate density of the brain.

ous sinus, they may also be affected when injuries or infections of this sinus occur.

THE BRAIN

GROSS FEATURES

The gross features of the brain are described in this anatomy book to help you *understand the relationship of the brain to the meninges and to the calvaria.* A clear understanding of these relationships is needed so that you will know when an intracranial lesion has altered the appearance of structures within the head (*e.g.,* **displacement of the pineal** gland or distortion of the cerebral arteries or ventricles in radiographs). In addition, the analysis of computerized tomograms (**CT scans**) of the head depends mainly on a knowledge of transverse sections of this region (Fig. 7-75).

Normally the brain is wholly within the cranial cavity, but space-occupying lesions may result in displacement of parts of it through the foramen magnum (Case 7-6). When the skullcap is removed and the dura mater reflected (Fig. 7-76), you can observe the convolutions (**gyri**) and grooves (**sulci**) of the **cerebral cortex** through the delicate pia-arachnoid (Fig. 7-59). *The complicated folding of the surface of the cerebral hemispheres greatly increases the surface area of the brain.* The cortex of the cerebral hemispheres consists of gray matter composed of nerve cells and fibers. The folds are known as convolutions or **gyri** (L. *gyros,* circle), and the intervening grooves are called **fissures** or **sulci** (L. a furrow).

Major Fissures and Sulci (Figs. 7-76 and 7-77). There are *six main fissures and sulci*: (1) the **longitudinal cerebral fissure**; (2) the **transverse cerebral fissure**; (3) the **lateral sulcus** (fissure); (4) the **central sulcus**; (5) the **parietooccipital** sulcus; and (6) the **calcarine sulcus.**

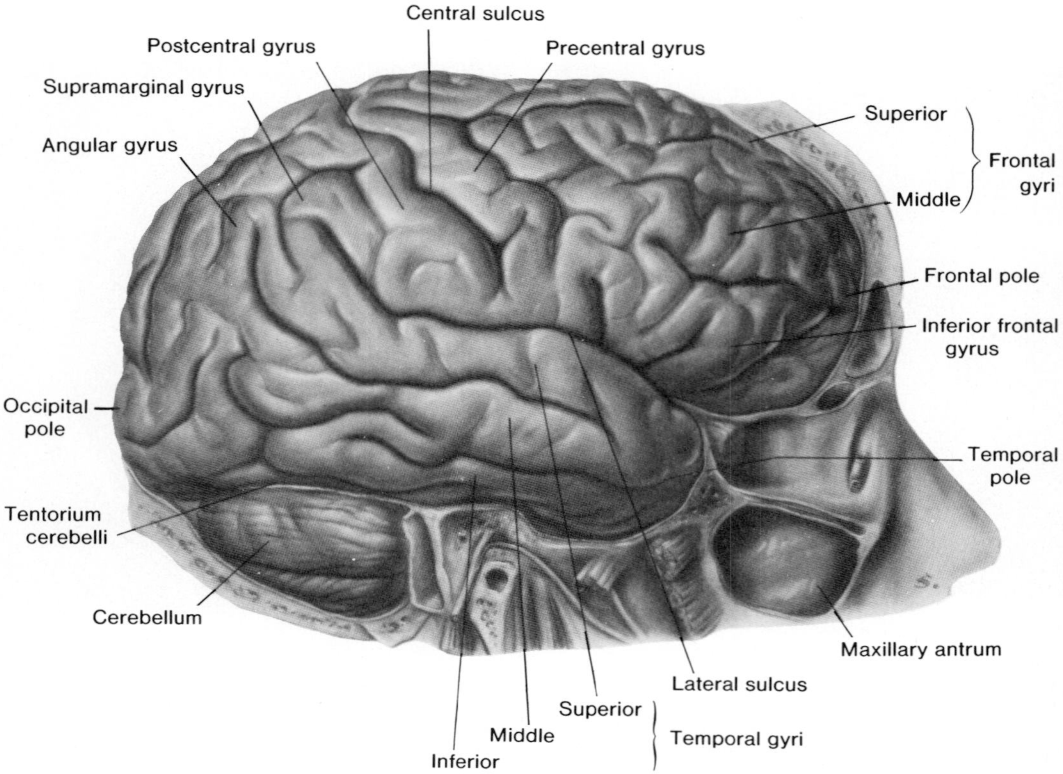

Figure 7-76. Lateral view of the brain exposed in the skull to show its relationship to the cranial cavity. Observe that (1) the frontal poles occupy the anterior cranial fossa; (2) the temporal poles are lodged in the middle cranial fossa; and (3) the cerebellum, pons, and medulla are located in the posterior cranial fossa. Consequently, in frontal impacts the frontal and temporal poles of the hemispheres may be bruised, whereas in occipital impacts the occipital poles and cerebellum may be damaged.

The longitudinal cerebral fissure (sagittal fissure) partially separates the cerebral hemispheres (Figs. 7-78 and 7-79) and *in situ* contains the **falx cerebri** (Fig. 7-62). This dural septum separates the occipital and parietal lobes but only the periphery of the frontal lobes. The longitudinal fissure separates the cerebral hemispheres in the frontal and occipital regions, but between these parts the fissure extends only as low as the **corpus callosum** (Figs. 7-63 and 7-77).

The transverse cerebral fissure separates the cerebral hemispheres above from the cerebellum, midbrain, and diencephalon below. The **tentorium cerebelli** lies in the posterior part of this fissure (Fig. 7-76).

The lateral sulcus (fissure) begins inferiorly on the inferior surface of the cerebral hemisphere as a deep furrow (Fig. 7-51*B*) and extends posteriorly, separating the frontal and temporal lobes (Figs. 7-76 and 7-78). Posteriorly, the lateral sulcus separates parts of the parietal and temporal lobes.

The central sulcus (Fig. 7-51*B*) is a prominent groove running from about the middle of the superior margin of the cerebral hemisphere downward and forward, stopping just short of the lateral sulcus (Fig. 7-76). *The central sulcus is an important landmark for the cerebral cortex* because the **motor cortex** (precentral gyrus) lies anterior to it and the **general sensory cortex** (postcentral gyrus) lies posterior to it. The superior end of the central sulcus is

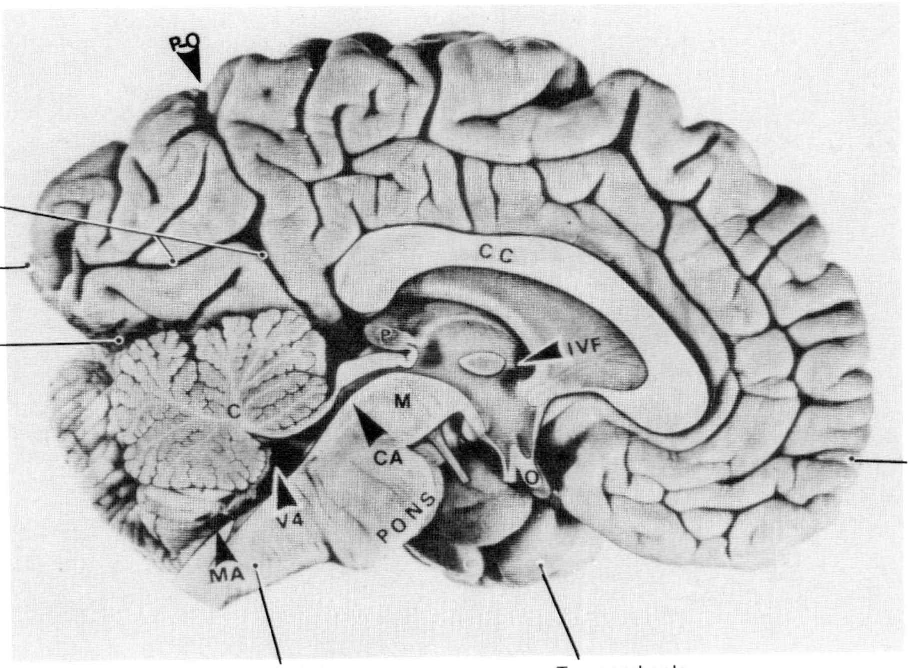

Figure 7-77. Photograph of a median section of a brain. Note (1) the parietooccipital sulcus (*P-O*) separating the parietal and occipital lobes; (2) the cerebellum (*C*) below the occipital lobe; (3) the corpus callosum (*CC*), a broad curved band of fibers, connecting the two cerebral hemispheres; (4) the optic chiasma (*O*); (5) the brain stem; (6) the interventricular foramen (*IVF*) connecting the lateral and third ventricles; (7) the median aperture (*MA*) of the fourth ventricle (*V4*), which connects the ventricular system with the subarachnoid space; and (8) the cerebral aqueduct (*CA*) which runs through the midbrain (*M*) connecting the third and fourth ventricles. The poles of the cerebral hemispheres are also illustrated in Figure 7-51*A*.

located 1 cm behind the midpoint of a line joining the **inion** (center of external occipital protuberance) and the **nasion** (Fig. 7-15), and its inferior end is about 5 cm above the external acoustic meatus.

The parietooccipital sulcus (fissure), as its name indicates, separates the parietal and occipital lobes on the medial aspect of the brain (Fig. 7-77). It extends from the calcarine sulcus to the superior border and continues for a short distance on the superolateral surface.

The calcarine sulcus on the medial surface (Fig. 7-77) commences near the occipital pole and runs anteriorly, taking a curved course and joining the parietooccipital sulcus at an acute angle.

Main Lobes of the Cerebral Hemispheres. There are *four main lobes* of the cerebral hemispheres; sometimes the insula (Fig. 7-80*B*) is described separately as a fifth lobe.

The frontal lobes (Figs. 7-48, 7-51, and 7-75 to 7-77), the largest of all the lobes, form the anterior parts of the cerebral hemispheres. They lie in front of the central sulci and above the lateral sulci. Their lateral and superior surfaces extend posterior to the coronal suture. The basal surfaces of the frontal lobes rest on the **orbital part** of the frontal bone in the **anterior cranial fossa** (Figs. 7-49 and 7-76). The **olfactory bulbs** rest on the **cribriform plates** (Fig. 7-53). The **orbital gyri** (Fig. 7-78) form impressions in the orbital plates of the frontal bone.

The parietal lobes (Fig. 7-51*B*) are related to the internal aspects of the posterior

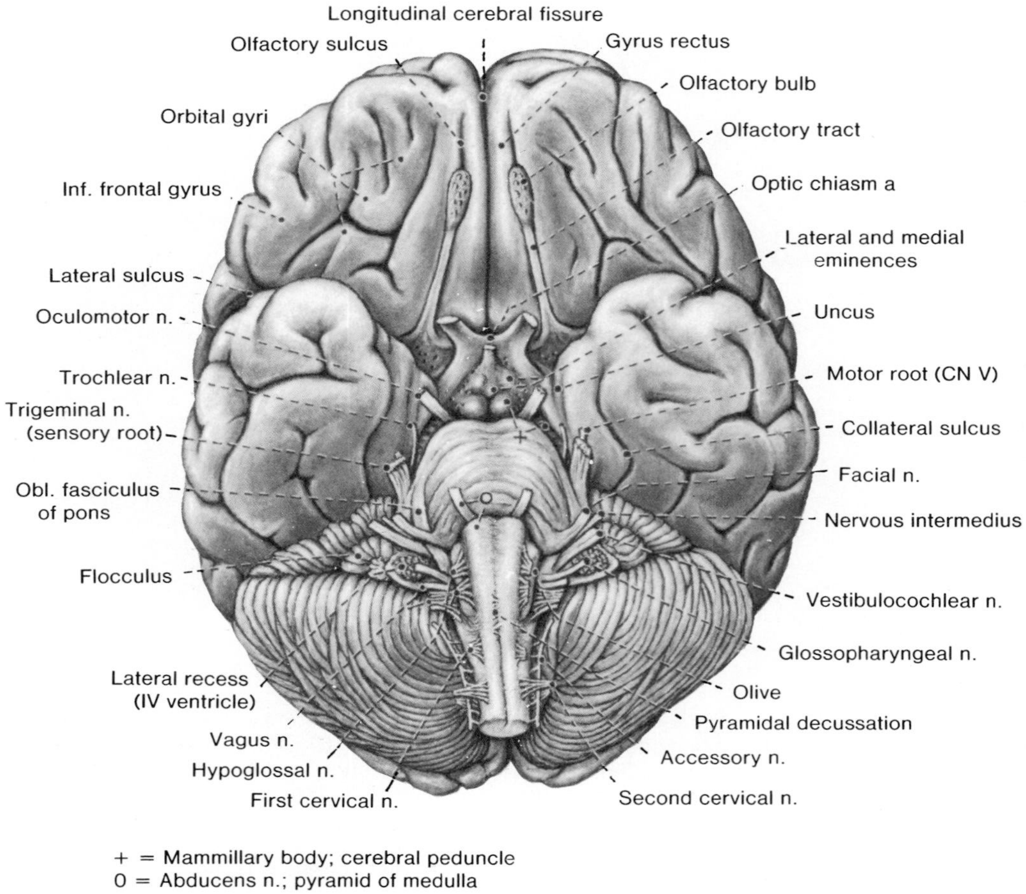

Figure 7-78. Drawing of the inferior surface of the brain.

and superior parts of the parietal bones. Each parietal lobe is bounded anteriorly by the central sulcus and posteriorly by the upper part of the line joining the parietooccipital fissure and the **preoccipital notch.** The inferior boundary of each lobe is indicated by an imaginary line extending from the posterior ramus of the lateral sulcus to the inferior end of the posterior boundary.

The temporal lobes (Figs. 7-48, 7-51*B*, and 7-76) lie inferior to the lateral sulci. Their convex anterior ends, called the **temporal poles,** fit into the anterior and lateral parts of the middle cranial fossa. Their posterior parts lie against the middle one-third of the lower part of the parietal bone.

The occipital lobes (Fig. 7-51*B*) are relatively small and are located posterior to the parietooccipital sulci (Fig. 7-77). They rest on the **tentorium cerebelli,** above the posterior cranial fossa (Figs. 7-62 and 7-76). Although small, *the occipital lobes are important because they contain the visual cortex.*

Major Parts of the Brain. To understand the origin of cranial nerves and the structure of the ventricular system (a series of spaces within the brain), the major divisions of the brain must be understood. As the names of some structures are derived from embryonic terms, a basic knowledge of brain development is also required.

The brain develops from the walls of vesicles that develop from the cranial end of the **neural tube.** The names of some walls of the secondary brain vesicles are

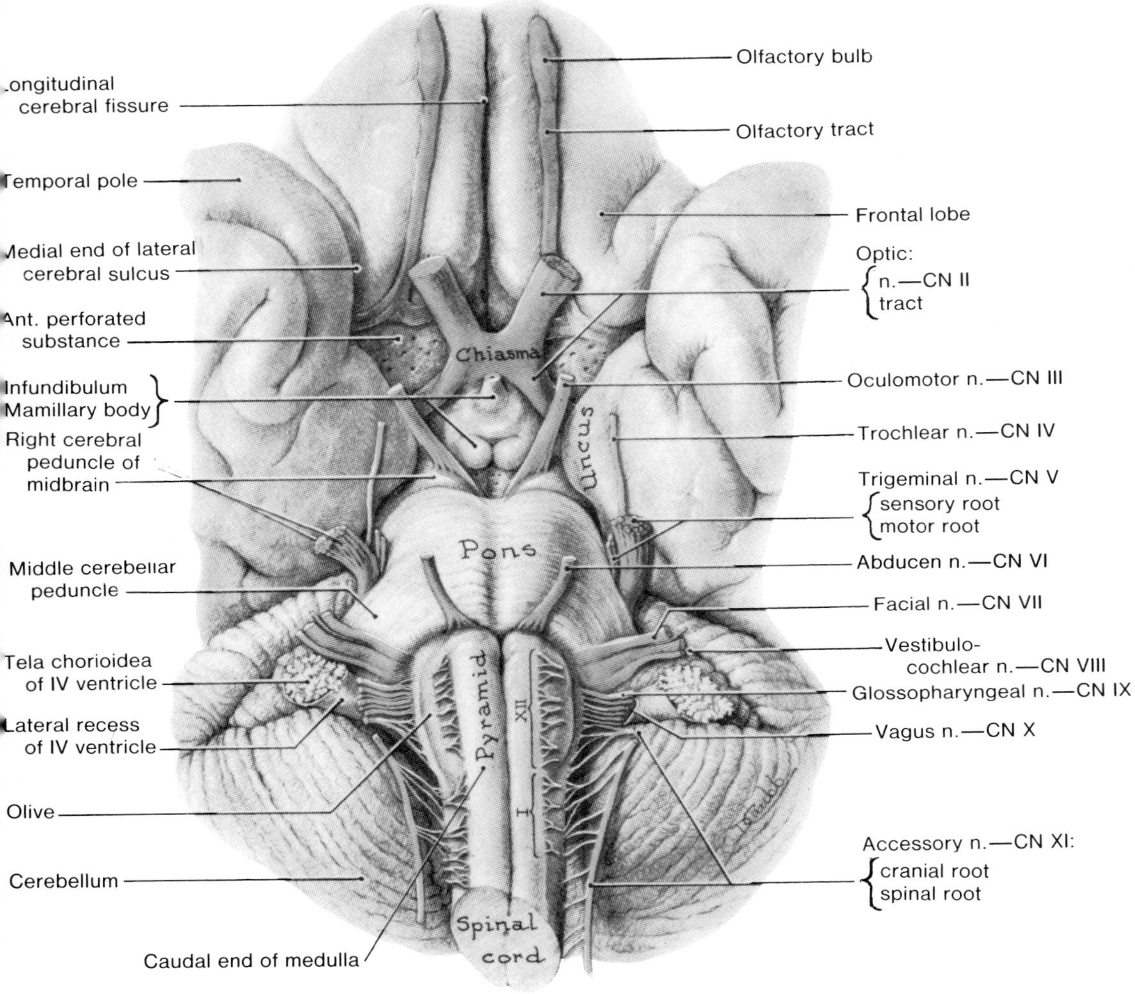

Figure 7-79. Drawing of the inferior surface of the brain showing the superficial origin of the 12 cranial nerves. The olfactory bulbs, into which the olfactory nerves (CN I) end, are related to the cribriform plates (Fig. 7-50). The infundibulum and mammillary bodies are in the middle cranial fossa, as are the temporal lobes lateral to them. The pons, medulla, and cerebellum are in the posterior cranial fossa (Fig. 7-76). *I*, indicates rootlets of the first cervical segment of the spinal cord

used to describe parts of the mature brain (*e.g.*, **telencephalon** and **diencephalon**, derivatives of the embryonic forebrain, and **mesencephalon,** the name of the midbrain). Encephalon is derived from the Greek word *enkephalos*, meaning brain. It forms the basis of many medical terms (*e.g.*, **encephalitis,** inflammation of the brain and **encephalocele,** herniation of the brain). The Latin word for the brain is **cerebrum** and it is used to refer to derivatives of the **telencephalon** (*e.g.*, the cerebral hemispheres). The term does not include the diencephalon, the brain stem (midbrain, pons, and medulla), or the cerebellum.

At one time the term cerebrum was considered to consist of all parts of the brain derived from the forebrain (*i.e.*, telencephalon and diencephalon). The *Nomina Anatomica* now rec-

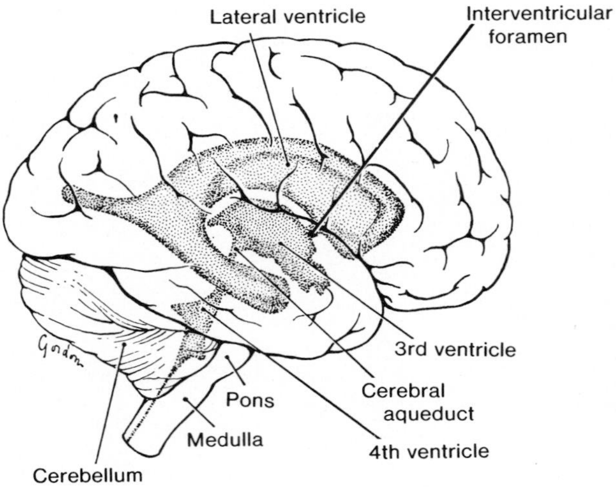

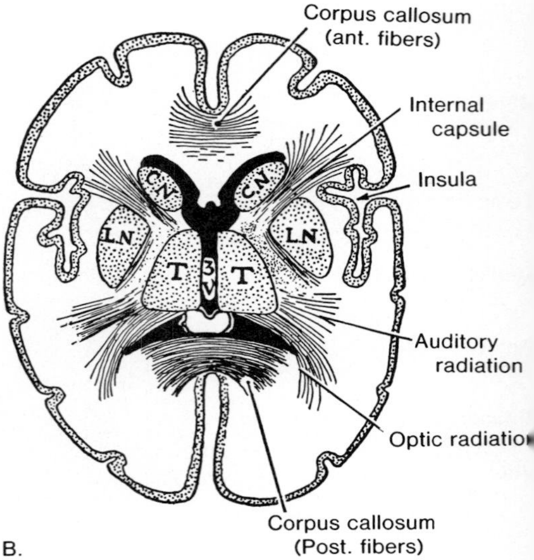

Figure 7-80. *A*, drawing of a schematic lateral view of the right side of the brain illustrating the ventricular system. *B*, diagramatic horizontal section of the brain. Between the right and left thalami (*T*) is the third ventricle (*3V*). The internal capsule separates the thalamus (*T*) and the caudate nucleus (*CN*) from the lentiform nucleus (*LN*) which lies deep to the insula in the depth of the lateral sulcus (Fig. 7-76). The corpus callosum consists of nerve fibers interconnecting the cerebral hemispheres. The body of the corpus callosum (Figs. 7-82 and 7-84), its largest part, would be visible in horizontal sections superior to this one.

ommends that it refer only to derivatives of the telencephalon (*i.e.*, mainly the cerebral hemispheres and basal ganglia).

The cerebrum occupies the anterior and middle cranial fossae and extends posteriorly over the tentorium cerebelli to the internal occipital protuberance (Figs. 7-53 and 7-76). The **cerebral hemispheres** form the largest part of the cerebrum and of the entire brain. A cerebral hemisphere consists mainly of an outer layer of gray matter (the **cerebral cortex**) and an inner mass of white matter (the **medullary center**). A cavity in each cerebral hemisphere, known as the **lateral ventricle** (Figs. 7-75 and 7-80*A*), is part of the ventricular system of the brain. Within the cerebral hemisphere, there are several masses of gray matter known collectively as the **basal ganglia.** The largest of these is the **corpus striatum**, consisting of the **caudate** and **lentiform nuclei** (Fig. 7-80*B*). The corpus striatum is a major center in the **extrapyramidal motor system,** as opposed to the **pyramidal motor system** (the motor cortex and the corticobulbar and corticospinal tracts).

The diencephalon forms the central core of the brain and is surrounded by the cerebrum (cerebral hemispheres and basal ganglia). Only the basal or inferior surface of the diencephalon is exposed to view in the diamond-shaped area containing the **infundibulum** and the **mammillary bodies** (Fig. 7-79). The two **thalami** (Fig. 7-80*B*) make up four-fifths of the diencephalon. Although the **hypothalamus** forms only a small part of the diencephalon, it is very important to life.

The cavity of the diencephalon is the narrow **third ventricle** lying between the right and left thalami (Fig. 7-80*B*). CSF enters the third ventricle from each lateral ventricle through the **interventricular foramina** (Figs. 7-77 and 7-80*A*).

The Midbrain (Figs. 7-79, 7-80, and 7-84). This is the smallest part of the brain. Very little of it is visible in an unsectioned brain. The midbrain is at the junction of the middle and posterior cranial fossae, lying partly in each and in the opening of the tentorium (tentorial incisure, Fig. 7-64). The cavity of the midbrain is reduced to a narrow canal, termed the **cerebral aqueduct**. It contains no choroid plexus (Fig. 7-82) but conducts CSF from the lateral and third ventricles to the fourth ventricle. The posterior brain mass or cerebellum is attached to the midbrain by *superior cerebellar peduncles* (L. little feet).

The Pons (Figs. 7-51*A* and 7-79). This Latin word meaning **bridge** is appropriate for this part of the brain because all of it that is visible from the inferior and lateral surfaces is a wide, transverse band of nerve fibers. Although it looks somewhat like a bridge between the cerebellar hemispheres, it is not. *These fibers connect one cerebral hemisphere with the opposite cerebellar hemisphere.* The cavity in the pons forms the superior (upper) part of the **fourth ventricle.** The inferior part of this ventricle is formed by the cavity of the medulla. *The fourth ventricle is largely roofed by the cerebellum* (Figs. 7-77 and 7-80*A*) and it receives **CSF** from the lateral and third ventricles via the cerebral aqueduct. The pons lies in the most anterior part of the posterior cranial fossa, posterior to the upper part of the **clivus** and the posterior surface of the **dorsum sellae** (Figs. 7-47 and 7-57).

The Medulla (Figs. 7-79, 7-80*A*, and 7-84). *This is the most caudal part of the brain stem* (midbrain, pons, and medulla). It is located in the posterior cranial fossa with its ventral aspect facing the clivus (Fig. 7-57). *The medulla is continuous with the spinal cord at the foramen magnum,* but the transition is gradual. The distinctive characteristics of its ventral surface are the elongated **pyramids,** containing the corticospinal tracts from the cerebral cortex. Often the **decussation of the pyramids** is recognizable in the anterior median fissure. The medulla contains the **cardiovascular** and **respiratory centers** for automatic control of heart beat and respiration, respectively.

The cavity of the medulla forms the inferior (lower) part of the **fourth ventricle** (Figs. 7-77 and 7-80*A*). This rhomboid-shaped cavity, posterior to the pons and the medulla, extends from the **cerebral aqueduct** to the **obex** (L. barrier), a dimple indicating where the fourth ventricle may be continuous with the central canal of the spinal cord. *CSF enters the fourth ventricle via the cerebral aqueduct* and leaves it through three openings in its roof, one median and two lateral (Figs. 7-77 and 7-80*A*). The **median aperture** (foramen of Magendie) is just dorsal to the inferior part of the medulla and the **lateral apertures** (foramina of Luschka) are located at the ends of the lateral recesses of the fourth ventricle. *All three apertures open into the subarachnoid space and are the only communications between the ventricular system and the subarachnoid space.* If these foramina are occluded, all the ventricles become enlarged (**internal hydrocephalus**, Fig. 7-86) because of continued production of CSF in them.

The Cerebellum (Figs. 7-65 and 7-76 to 7-80*A*). This part of the brain overlies the posterior aspect of the pons and medulla and extends laterally beneath the tentorium cerebelli, occupying most of the **posterior cranial fossa.** The cerebellum (L. little brain) consists of a midline portion, the **vermis** (L. worm), and two lateral lobes, or **cerebellar hemispheres.** These hemispheres lie behind the petrous parts of the temporal bones and rest on the concavities of the lower parts of the occipital bones (Fig. 7-53).

CLINICALLY ORIENTED COMMENTS

Brain injuries are commonly associated with head injuries. The main purpose of the calvaria and the CSF is to protect the brain. Helmets are used by motorcycle riders, construction workers, soldiers, some athletes, and others for additional protection. *Various terms are used to describe injuries to the brain resulting from trauma.*

Cerebral Concussion. A concussion is an abrupt but **transient loss of consciousness** immediately following a blow to the head or a sudden stopping of the moving head resulting in the brain hitting the stationary skull (Fig. 7-81). When a person is hit (*e.g.*, by a club or baseball), they may be stunned and fall to the ground for a few seconds. The concussion appears to result from a mechanical disturbance of cerebral cells because there is no **visible bruising of the brain** on gross or microscopic examination. However, repeated cerebral concussions, as may occur in alcoholics and professional fighters, lead to **cerebral atrophy**; thus, some submicroscopic damage appears to occur with each concussion. The **punchdrunk syndrome,** caused by repeated cerebral concussion, is characterized by weakness in the lower limbs, unsteadiness of gait, slowness of muscular movements, tremors of the hands, hesitancy of speech, and slow cerebration.

Cerebral Contusion (L. *contusio,* a bruising). In this injury there is **visible bruising of the brain** owing to trauma and blood leaking from microscopic vessels. The pia mater is stripped from the brain in the injured area and may be torn, allowing blood to enter the subarachnoid space. Contusions are frequently found at the frontal, temporal, and occipital poles (Figs. 7-51 and 7-77). The bruising results either from the sudden impact of the moving brain against the stationary skull (Fig. 7-81) or the skull against the brain when there is a blow to it. The living calvaria is somewhat flexible and may sometimes bend without breaking. **A contusion usually results in an extended loss of consciousness** (several minutes to many hours).

Blows to the forehead tend to produce contusions of the frontal and perhaps the temporal poles, whereas *blows to the back of the head* generally produce contusions of the occipital poles. When the moving head strikes a stationary object (*e.g.,* when a hockey player falls backward striking his **occiput,** *i.e.*, the back of his head), there is a tendency for localization of contusions to that part of the brain underlying the part of the skull that received the impact. Contusion is soon followed by **edema** (swelling) of the brain, which contributes to a rise in intracranial pressure, a serious complication that may result in death.

Cerebral Laceration (L. *lacero,* to tear). *Tearing of the brain* is often associated with a depressed skull fracture or a gunshot wound and results in rupture of large blood vessels with bleeding into the brain and the subarachnoid space. This leads to **cerebral hematoma,** edema, and an increase in local and general intracranial pressure.

Cerebral Compression. Pressure on the brain may be produced by: (1) intracranial collections of blood or other fluid; (2) obstruction to the circulation or absorption of CSF; (3) intracranial tumors or abscesses; and (4) edema of the brain. *Cerebral compression is associated with increased intracranial pressure.* A marked increase in intracranial pressure results in herniation of parts of the brain. Often the **uncus** of the temporal lobe (Figs. 7-78 and 7-79) herniates through the **tentorial incisure,** causing pressure on the midbrain and kinking of the oculomotor nerve (CN III) on the edge of the tentorium. This results in **third nerve palsy,** usually commencing with progressive enlargement of the pupil and fixation of it to light. In some cases the **cerebellar tonsils** herniate through the foramen magnum (Fig. 7-63), compressing the medulla and disturbing the

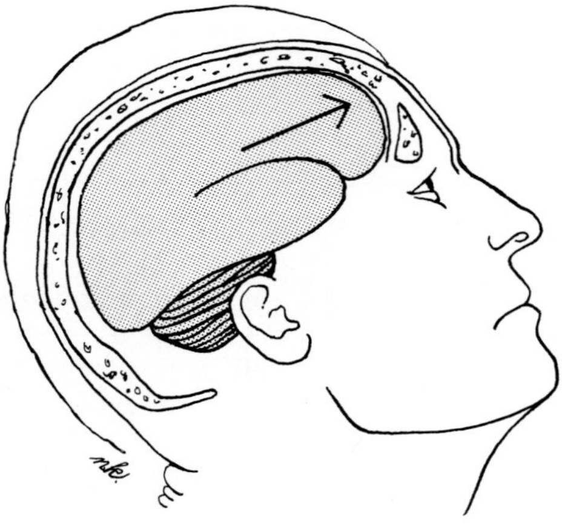

Figure 7-81. Schematic drawing of the head illustrating one way a cerebral concussion may occur. A sudden stopping of the moving head results in the brain hitting the inside of the stationary skull. This produces an abrupt but transient loss of consciousness, called a cerebral concussion.

vital cardiovascular and respiratory centers. *Tonsillar herniation* carries the tonsils and the median aperture of the fourth ventricle into the superior part of the vertebral canal. This compromises the flow of fluid out of the fourth ventricle or upward in the subarachnoid space or both. **Internal hydrocephalus** results. Immediate surgical intervention is usually necessary to relieve the high intracranial pressure.

THE VENTRICULAR SYSTEM AND CSF

Formation of CSF (Figs. 7-82 and 7-83). *The main source of CSF is the choroid plexuses of the lateral, third, and fourth ventricles.* The **choroid plexus** is located in the roofs of the third and fourth ventricles and on the floors of the bodies and inferior horns of the lateral ventricles. *The choroid plexus in the lateral ventricles is the largest and most important.* It is continuous with the choroid plexus in the roof of the third ventricle via the interventricular foramina. The **lateral apertures** of the fourth ventricle are also partially occupied by parts of the choroid plexuses which protrude through them and secrete CSF into the **subarachnoid space.**

Each choroid plexus (G. *choroid,* delicate membrane + *eidos,* resemblance) is composed of highly vascular pia mater, called **tela choridea** (L. *a web* + G. *chorioeidēs,* like a membrane), covered by a simple cu-

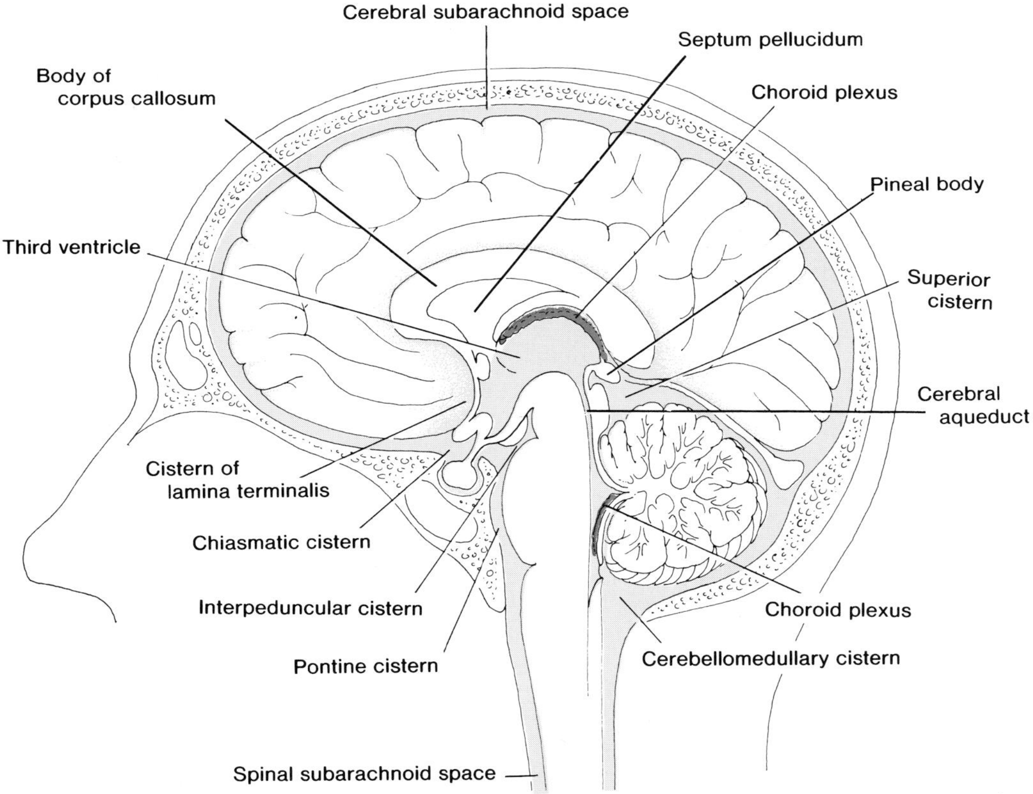

Figure 7-82. Diagram of the subarachnoid spaces and cisterns (*blue*) as seen in a median section of the brain. The superior cistern (located dorsal to the midbrain) together with the subarachnoid space at the sides of the midbrain are referred to clinically as the cisterna ambiens. The superior cistern is important because it contains internal cerebral veins which join caudally to form the great cerebral vein (of Galen). It also contains the posterior cerebral and superior cerebellar arteries. The choroid plexuses in the roof of the third and fourth ventricles are shown in *red.*

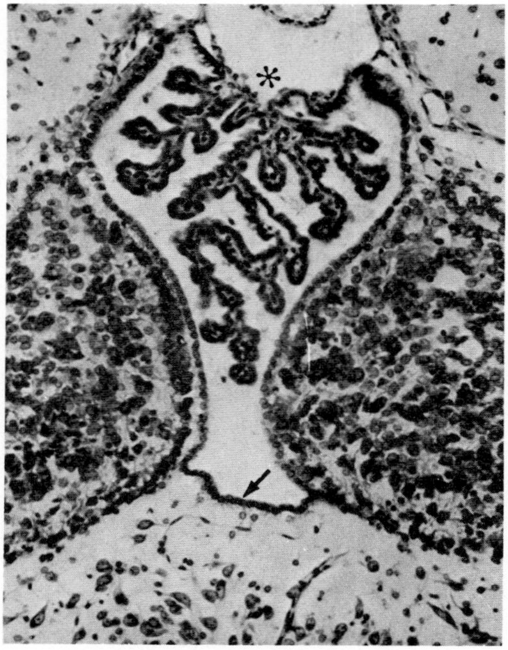

Figure 7-83. Photomicrograph showing tufts of choroid plexus hanging from the roof (*asterisk*) of the third verticle. The *arrow* points to the ependymal cells lining this ventricle. Modified ependymal cells cover the tela choroidea (vascular pia) of the choroid plexus. Rat brain ×130.

boid or low columnar epithelium (Fig. 7-83). Its epithelial cells have numerous long **microvilli.**

The flow of CSF is from the lateral ventricles into the third ventricle via the **interventricular foramina** and then into the fourth ventricle via the **cerebral aqueduct** of the midbrain. CSF passes from the ventricular system through the **median** and **lateral apertures** of the fourth ventricle into the subarachnoid space around the brain, spinal cord, and cauda equina (Fig. 5-65).

Ventricular fluid and CSF are not the same. The fluid in the ventricles is more dilute and has a different protein content than the CSF in the subarachnoid space.

The Subarachnoid Cisterns (Figs. 7-82 and 7-84). At certain places, mainly at the base of the brain, the arachnoid is widely separated from the pia mater forming large spaces or **pools of CSF**, called **subarachnoid cisterns** (L. underground cisterns or reservoirs for water). These cisterns communicate freely with each other, with the subarachnoid space of the spinal cord, and over all surfaces of the cerebral hemispheres.

The cerebellomedullary cistern (cisterna magna) is located in the space between the cerebellum and the lower part of the medulla. It receives CSF from the **median aperture** of the fourth ventricle and is continuous with the **subarachnoid space** of the spinal cord.

The pontine cistern is the extensive space along the ventral and lateral surfaces of the pons containing the basilar artery and some of the cranial nerves (Figs. 7-84 and 7-90). It is continuous inferiorly with the cerebellomedullary cistern and superiorly with the interpeduncular cistern.

The interpeduncular cistern, between the cerebral peduncles (Figs. 7-78 and 7-79), contains the posterior part of the **arterial circle** (circle of Willis) where the major arteries supplying the cerebrum are joined to one another at the base of the brain (Fig. 7-90). The interpeduncular cistern is continuous anteriorly with the **cistern of optic chiasma** which continues forward and upward as the **cistern of the lamina terminalis.** This cistern continues into the shallow **cistern of the corpus callosum** which is located above this large commissure.

The cistern of the lateral sulcus (lateral fissure), containing the **middle cerebral artery** (Fig. 7-90), is located in front of each temporal lobe where the arachnoid covers the **lateral sulcus** (Fig. 7-76).

The superior cistern, or cistern of the great cerebral vein (Fig. 7-82), lies between the splenium of the corpus callosum and the superior surface of the cerebellum. It contains the great cerebral vein (of Galen) and the **pineal gland.** Because this cistern lies dorsal to the **inferior** and **superior colliculi** (corpora quadrigemina), it is often referred to clinically as the *quadrigeminal cistern.*

CLINICALLY ORIENTED COMMENTS

The pineal gland (about 5 × 7 mm in size) is an endocrine gland that has the

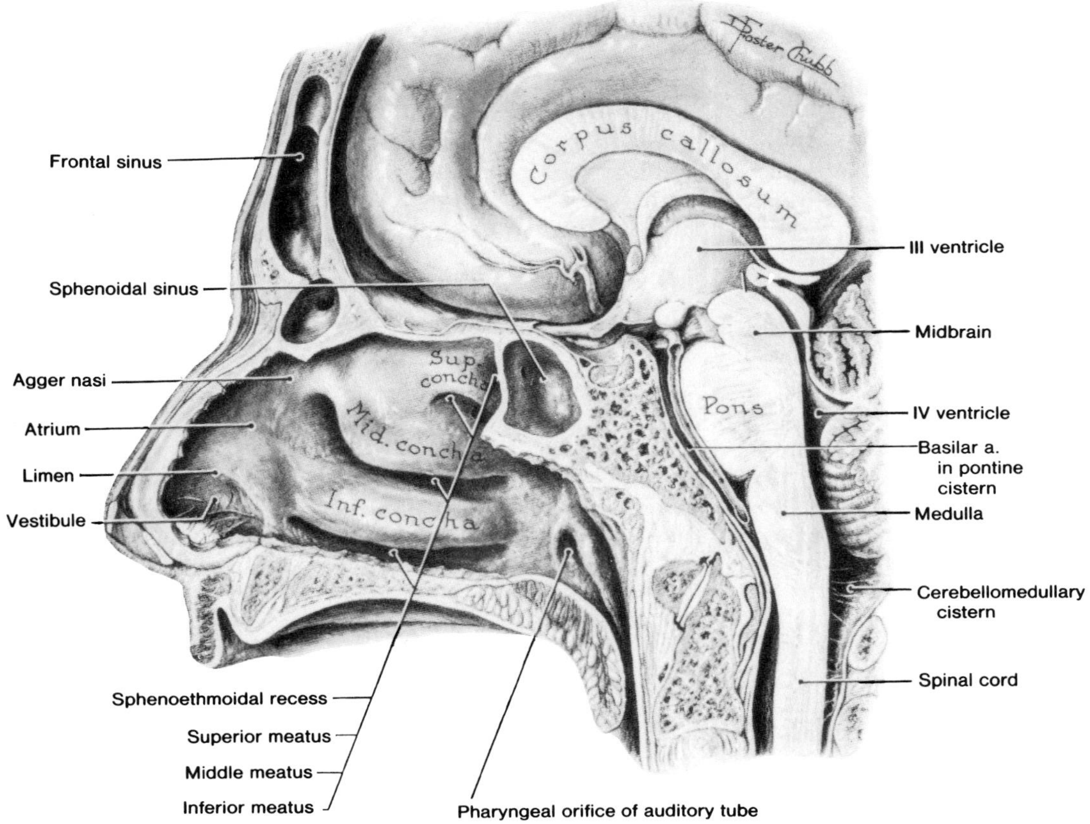

Figure 7-84. Drawing of median section of the head showing the lateral wall of the nasal cavity, the brain, and the spinal cord. The midbrain, pons, and medulla collectively are referred to as the brain stem. Note that the basilar artery in the pontine cistern has been sectioned longitudinally.

shape of a pine cone. It serves as a *useful neuroradiological and neurosurgical landmark.* It becomes calcified in adolescence and is visible on ordinary skull radiographs of approximately 75% of North American adults. Charts showing its usual position on lateral skull radiographs are used to diagnose upward, downward, forward, or backward displacement of the pineal gland in patients with suspected expanding intracranial lesions. Side to side displacement of the pineal gland is measured with a ruler.

Although samples of CSF for laboratory studies are usually obtained by **lumbar puncture** (Fig. 5-69), CSF may be obtained from the cerebellomedullary cistern [*e.g.*, in a person with a spina bifida cystica in the lumbar region (Fig. 5-71) in whom a lumbar puncture is not practical]. For a discussion of **cisternal puncture,** see page 647. Samples of ventricular fluid are obtained via anterior **fontanelle puncture** in infants (Fig. 7-5*B*) or through burr holes drilled in the calvaria of adults. The subarachnoid space or the ventricular system are also entered for measuring or monitoring CSF pressure, injecting antibiotics, or administering contrast media for radiography (**ventriculography**).

Circulation of CSF (Figs. 7-80*A* to 7-82). CSF produced in the lateral and third ventricles passes via the cerebral aqueduct into the fourth ventricle, where more CSF is produced by the choroid plexuses in its roof. CSF escapes from the fourth ventricle through its median and possibly its lateral apertures into the subarachnoid space and enters the cerebellomedullary and pontine cisterns. From these cisterns some CSF passes inferiorly around the spinal cord and posterosuperiorly over the cerebellum, but most of it flows upward through the tentorial incisure in the subarachnoid space around the midbrain (**cisterna interpeduncularis,** right and left **cisterna ambiens,** and the **superior cistern**). The cisterna ambiens is located on the dorsal surface of the midbrain.

From these cisterns, the CSF spreads upward through the sulci and fissures on the medial and superolateral surfaces of the cerebral hemispheres. This flow of CSF over the cerebrum is probably aided by pulsations of the cerebral arteries and of the cerebral hemispheres.

CSF also passes into the extensions of the subarachnoid space around the cranial nerves, the most important of which is that surrounding the optic nerves (Figs. 7-67 and 7-101).

Absorption of CSF (Figs. 7-59, 7-62, and 7-66). *The main site of absorption or passage of CSF into venous blood is through the arachnoid villi,* which are protrusions of the arachnoid into the dural venous sinuses, especially the **superior sagittal sinus** and its adjacent **lateral lacunae.**

The rate of CSF absorption is pressure dependent and the arachnoid villi appear to act as one-way "valves." When CSF pressure is greater than venous pressure, the valves open and CSF passes into the blood in the venous sinuses; however, when venous pressure is higher than CSF pressure, the valves close, preventing blood from entering the CSF.

Some CSF appears to be absorbed by the ependymal lining of the ventricles (**ependyma**), in the spinal subarachnoid space, and through the walls of capillaries in the pia mater. In addition, some CSF is probably absorbed into the lymphatics adjacent to the subarachnoid space around cerebrospinal nerves, (*e.g.*, the optic nerves, Fig. 7-101).

CLINICALLY ORIENTED COMMENTS

By replacing some CSF by contrast media of various types, certain *parts of the brain can be outlined by radiography.* Air may be used to replace CSF, to demonstrate the ventricular system and the subarachnoid spaces, and to detect or exclude any displacement or deformities of their walls.

Ventriculography (Fig. 7-85). Before taking radiographs, a hole is made in the posterior part of the frontal or one of the parietal bones with a **trephine** (a cylindrical or crown saw) or a burr. Then a special **ventricular needle** or **cannula** is passed through the hole and a relatively safe part of the cerebrum into one lateral ventricle. *Air is then exchanged for ventricular fluid,* the needle or cannula removed or replaced by a fine caliber soft catheter, the head bandaged, and a series of radiographs made. By suitably positioning the patient's head, air can be moved into various parts of the ventricular system if there is no obstruction. Sometimes **radiopaque oil** is injected and, with or without fluoroscopic control, the oil is maneuvered into the third ventricle, the cerebral aqueduct, or the fourth ventricle, depending on the site of the lesion under investigation.

Encephalography (*Pneumoencephalography or Radiography of the Brain Outlined by Air*). Lumbar puncture is performed with the patient sitting up (Fig. 5-69), the CSF pressure is measured, and (if it is not abnormally high) air is injected and CSF removed alternately in small amounts. *The air bubbles pass rapidly upward in the spinal subarachnoid space and enter the cerebellomedullary cistern and the fourth ventricle* because the patient's head is strongly flexed. Frontal and lateral films are usually made at this time to show structures in the posterior cranial fossa. Later more air is injected with the head less flexed. The air passes upward in the ventricular system, partly draining it, and also upward around the brain stem through the tentorial incisure and finally onto the medial and dorsolateral surfaces of the cerebr ʾ hemispheres. The lumbar needle is re-

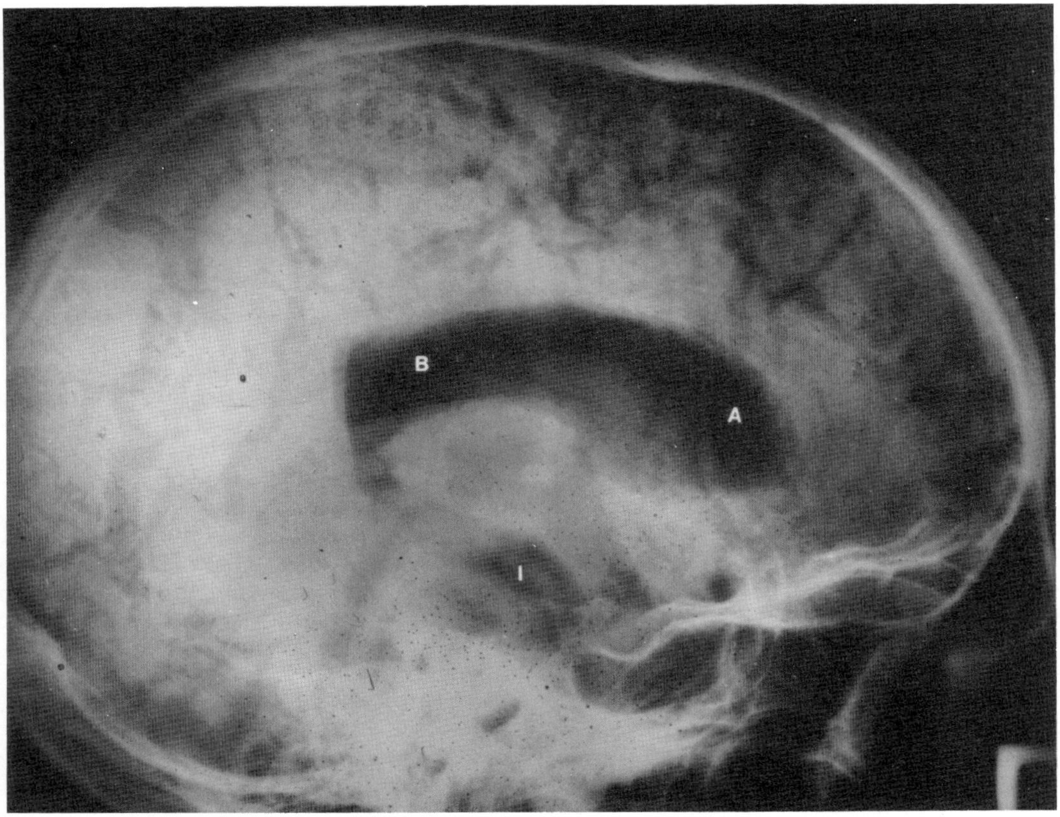

Figure 7-85. Brow-up lateral radiograph of the head after lumbar injection of air (*pneumoencephalogram*). Compare with Figure 7-80*A*. Note that the anterior horns (*A*) and bodies (*B*) of both lateral ventricles are filled with air and the right and left images overlap. One inferior horn (*I*) is also filled with air. The posterior horns are filled with fluid because the patient is in the *supine position* (lying on the back); if the patient is put in the *prone position* (lying face down), air will fill these horns. Air is also present in the third ventricle, the cerebral aqueduct, and the fourth ventricle but is difficult to see because these parts of the ventricular system are narrow. Note that some air is visible in the basal cisterns and in some frontal sulci.

moved and the patient lies down on the x-ray table while a series of radiographs are taken. By suitably positioning the patient's head, air can be made to outline the ventricular system of the brain [*e.g.*, in **brow-up films** (Fig. 7-85), air outlines anterior parts of the ventricular system and subarachnoid spaces, whereas in **brow-down films,** air outlines the posterior parts of the ventricular system].

Radiographic study of the brain by ventriculography or encephalography enables radiologists to locate atrophic or space-occupying lesions (*e.g.*, a brain tumor). These methods may also be used to determine the site of an obstruction in the circulation of CSF.

Hydrocephalus (Fig. 7-86). Overproduction of CSF, obstruction of its flow, or interference with its absorption results in an excess of CSF, a condition known as **hydrocephalus** (G. *hydór*, water + *kephalē*, head).

Meningitis (inflammation of the meninges) produces pus in the subarachnoid spaces over the brain and in the cisterns

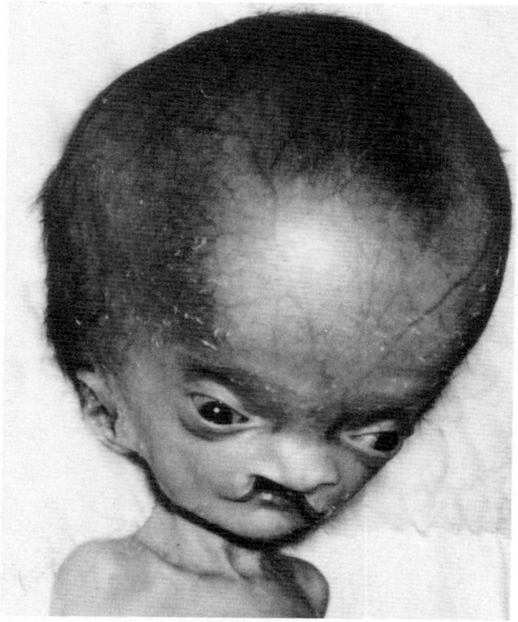

Figure 7-86. Photograph of an infant with hydrocephalus (excess of CSF) and bilateral cleft lip.

that results in obstruction of CSF circulation.

A tumor may block the cerebral aqueduct, stopping the flow of CSF to the fourth ventricle. Hydrocephalus often results from **congenital aqueductal stenosis** in which the cerebral aqueduct is narrow or consists of several minute channels.

Blockage of CSF circulation results in dilation of the ventricles above the point of obstruction and in pressure on the cerebral hemispheres (Fig. 7-86). This squeezes the brain between the ventricular fluid and the bones of the calvaria. In infants the internal pressure results in expansion of the brain and the calvaria because the sutures and fontanelles are still open. It is possible to form an artificial drainage system (**ventriculoatrial shunt**) to allow the CSF to escape, thereby lessening damage to the brain.

Hydrocephalus usually refers to internal hydrocephalus in which all or part of the ventricular system is enlarged. All ventricles are enlarged if the apertures of the fourth ventricle or the subarachnoid spaces are blocked, whereas the lateral and third ventricles are dilated when the cerebral aqueduct is obstructed. Although rare, obstruction of one interventricular foramen can produce dilation of one lateral ventricle.

Functions of CSF. The CSF, along with the meninges and the calvaria, *protects the brain by providing a cushion against blows to the head.* As the brain is slightly heavier than CSF, the gyri on the basal surface of the brain are in contact with the cranial fossae in the floor of the cranial cavity (Fig. 7-47) when a person is erect. Recall that the orbital gyri of the frontal lobes produce sinuous depressions in the orbital part of the frontal bone (Fig. 7-49). In many places at the base of the brain only the cranial meninges intervene between the brain and the cranial bones. In this position the CSF is in the subarachnoid cisterns and in the sulci on the superior and lateral parts of the brain; hence, *CSF separates the upper part of the brain from the calvaria.* The brain is kept from sagging by the cerebral veins as they enter the dural venous sinuses (Fig. 7-69). Of course the relations of CSF to the calvaria and to the brain are reversed when a person stoops or does a headstand.

There are small rapidly recurring changes in intracranial pressure owing to the heartbeat as well as slow recurring changes resulting from unknown causes. In addition, *there are momentarily large changes in intracranial pressure during coughing and straining.* Any change in the volume of the intracranial contents (brain, ventricular fluid, and blood) will be reflected by a change in intracranial pressure. This is called the **Monro-Keller doctrine.**

CLINICALLY ORIENTED COMMENTS

Subarachnoid hemorrhage (bleeding into the subarachnoid space) often impedes CSF circulation by partly obstructing the cisterns, the sulci, and the arachnoid villi. This results in an increase in intracranial pressure (Case 7-6).

Contusions of the brain resulting from acceleration or deceleration are frequent at the base of the brain and at the frontal, temporal, and occipital poles, partly because of the paucity of CSF at these areas when a person is in the erect position. This allows the brain to strike the cranial bones with only the meninges intervening (Fig. 7-81).

Fractures of the floor of the middle cranial fossa may result in *leakage of CSF* from the ear (**CSF otorrhea**) if the meninges above the middle ear and mastoid antrum (Fig. 7-188) are torn and the tympanic membrane (eardrum) is also ruptured. **Fractures of the anterior cranial fossa** may involve the cribriform plate (Fig. 7-50), resulting in leakage of CSF through the nose (**CSF rhinorrhea**). This indicates that the subarachnoid space is in communication with the outside via the nose as the result of a tear in the meninges. These conditions present a risk of **meningitis** from infection spreading from the ear or the nose, especially if the nose is blown.

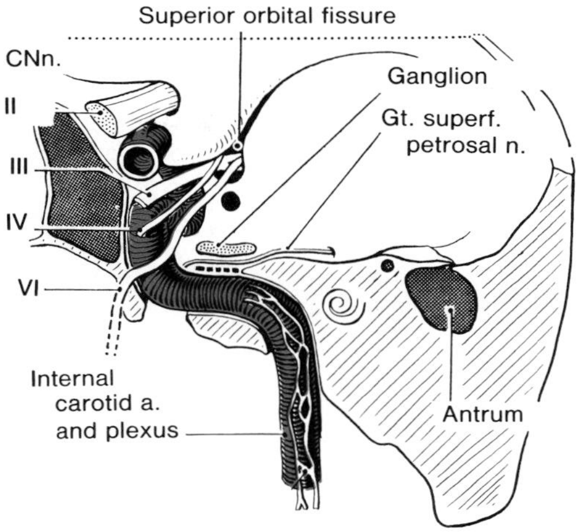

Figure 7-87. Drawing showing the course of the internal carotid artery in the temporal bone. Note that it takes an inverted L-shaped course from the undersurface of the petrous part of the temporal bone to its apex. At the upper end of the foramen lacerum, it enters the cavernous sinus, turns anteriorly, makes a hairpin turn, and enters the subarachnoid space.

ARTERIAL SUPPLY OF THE BRAIN

The brain is supplied through an extensive system of branches from two pairs of vessels, the internal carotid and the vertebral arteries (Figs. 7-62 and 7-90).

The Internal Carotid Artery (Figs. 7-87 to 7-90). The internal carotid *arises in the neck from the common carotid* opposite the upper border of the thyroid cartilage. This **cervical part** ascends almost vertically to the base of the skull where it turns into *the carotid canal* in the petrous part of the temporal bone. This **petrous part** enters the middle cranial fossa through the superior portion of the **foramen lacerum** and then runs forward *in the cavernous sinus.* This **cavernous part** is covered by the endothelium of this sinus. At the anterior end of the sinus, the internal carotid *makes a hairpin turn* and leaves the sinus to enter the subarachnoid space (Fig. 7-73). This **cerebral part** (supracavernous or supraclinoid part) of the artery immediately gives off the important **ophthalmic artery** and then passes below the optic nerve. Finally it turns obliquely upward, lateral to the **optic chiasma** (Fig. 7-88), for a variable distance before branching into the **anterior** and **middle cerebral arteries** at the medial end of the lateral sulcus (Figs. 7-89 and 7-90). The sinuous course taken by the cavernous and cerebral parts of the internal carotid artery forms a U-shaped bend often called the "**carotid siphon**" (G. a bent tube). Within the cranial cavity, the internal carotid artery and its branches supply the **hypophysis cerebri** (pituitary), the **orbit,** and much of the supratentorial part of the brain.

The Vertebral Artery (Figs. 5-38, 7-36, 7-90*A*, 9-24, and 9-34). The vertebral artery begins in the root of the neck as a **branch of the first part of the subclavian artery.** It ascends vertically through the foramina transversaria of C6 to C3 vertebrae and then *inclines laterally in the foramen transversarium of C2* (axis). Above this foramen it ascends vertically into the foramen transversarium of C1 (atlas). It then bends backward at right angles and *winds around the upper part of the lateral mass*

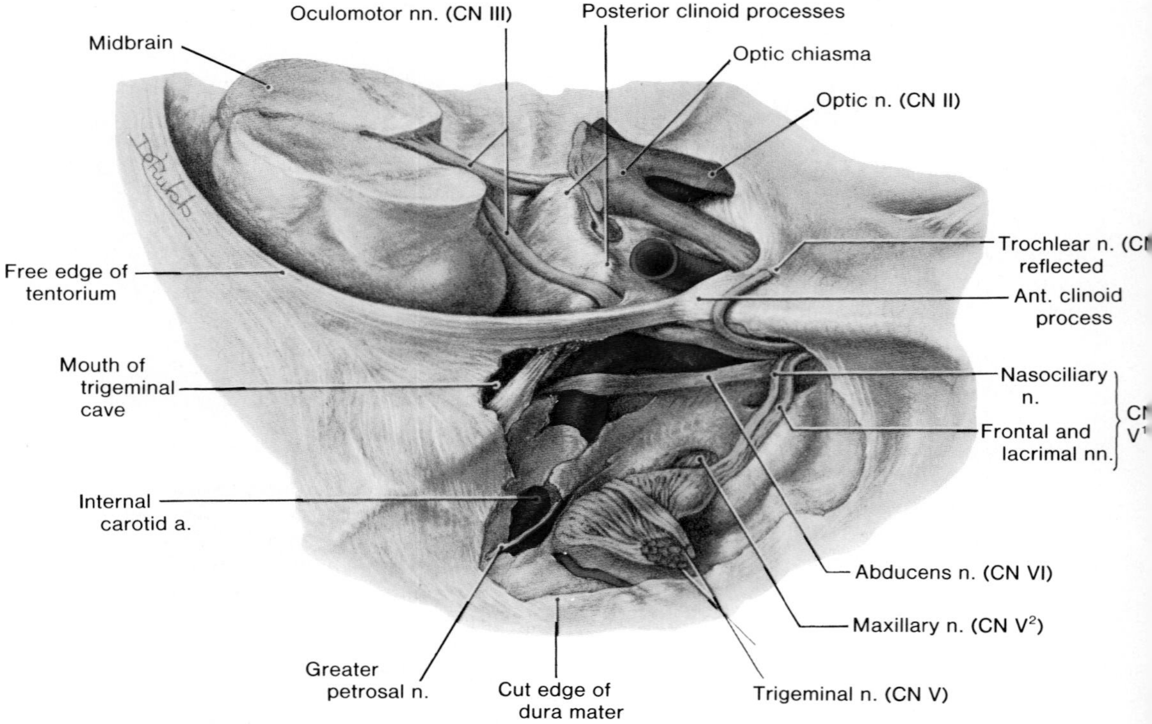

Figure 7-88. Drawing showing the nerves in the middle cranial fossa and the sinuous course of the internal carotid artery. The trigeminal nerve is divided and turned forward and laterally from the mouth of the trigeminal cave. Observe the midbrain and the oculomotor nerves in the tentorial notch.

of the atlas. It pierces the posterior atlantooccipital membrane, the dura mater, and the arachnoid to enter the **subarachnoid space** of the cerebellomedullary cistern at the level of the **foramen magnum** (Figs. 7-82 and 7-84). The vertebral artery runs forward on the anterolateral surface of the medulla and unites with its fellow of the opposite side at the caudal border of the pons to form the basilar artery. For Clinically Oriented Comments on the unique course of these arteries, see Chapter 5 (p. 646).

The Basilar Artery (Figs. 7-84 and 7-90). As just stated, this artery is formed by the union of the two vertebral arteries. It runs within the **pontine cistern** to the upper border of the pons, where it ends by dividing into the two **posterior cerebral arteries.**

CLINICALLY ORIENTED COMMENTS

To investigate the vertebral and basilar arteries using **angiography** (Fig. 9-24), injections of contrast material are made into them by various routes [*e.g.*, via a femoral catheter advanced into the lower part of the vertebral artery or by retrograde injections into the brachial artery in the cubital fossa (Fig. 6-75)].

Occlusion (blockage) **or stenosis** (narrowing) **of one vertebral artery** results in the brain stem being dependent mainly on the other vertebral artery for blood. If that supply is reduced by injury or occasionally by prolonged turning of the head as occurs during backing up a car, brain stem symptoms may occur such as dizziness, fainting, spots before the eyes, and transient **diplopia** (double vision).

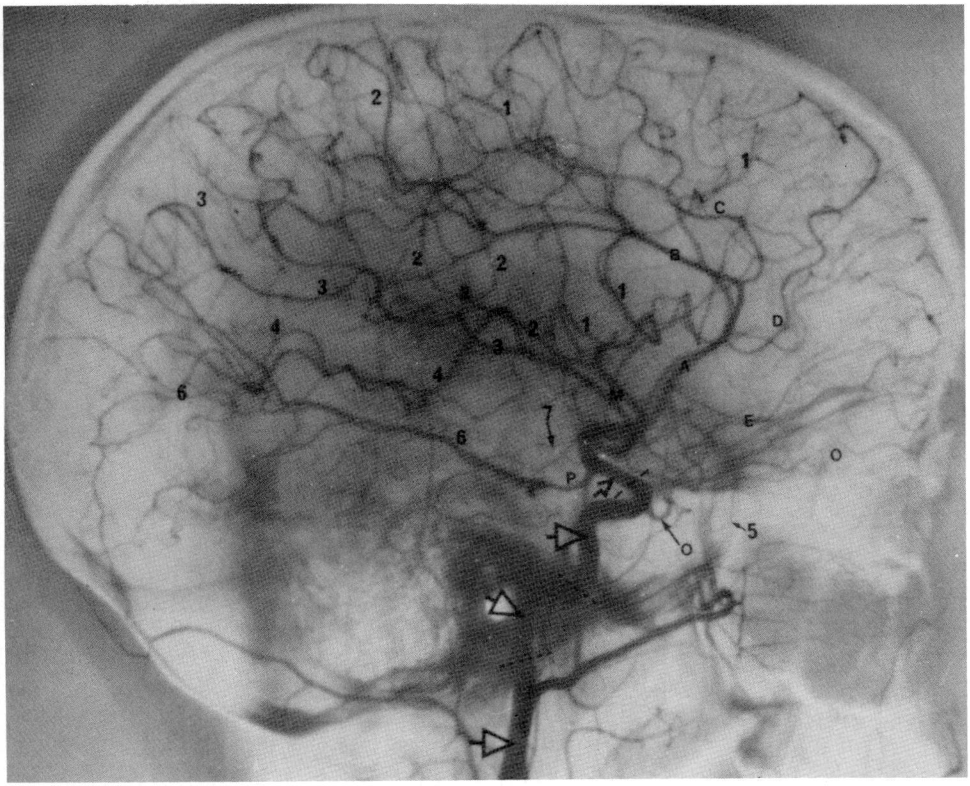

Figure 7-89. A common carotid arteriogram. This is a positive print of a radiograph with radiopaque material in the internal carotid artery. (Some external carotid branches are also seen.) *Four arrows* indicate parts of the internal carotid: *cervical*, before entering the skull; *petrous*, within the petrous part of the temporal bone; *cavernous*, within that venous sinus (note the hairpin turn below the broken line); and *supracavernous* or cerebral, within the cranial subarachnoid space. *A*, anterior cerebral artery; *B*, middle cerebral artery; *P*, posterior communicating artery connecting the internal carotid to the posterior cerebral artery. The letters and numbers of the smaller branches should be ignored at this time.

The Cerebral Arterial Circle (Figs. 7.55 and 7-90). The two **internal carotid arteries** and the two **vertebral arteries** are the four major arteries supplying blood to the brain. The cerebral arterial circle is *located at the base of the brain*, **principally in the interpeduncular fossa,** and extends from the superior border of the pons to the longitudinal fissure between the cerebral hemispheres. In Figure 7-90*B* observe that it encircles the **optic chiasma,** the **infundibulum,** and the **mammillary bodies** (Fig. 7-79).

The cerebral arterial circle forms a route through which blood may be distributed to any part of the cerebral hemispheres from either the internal carotid or the basilar arteries. It was described by Thomas Willis in 1664 and for many years was called the "circle of Willis."

The cerebral arterial circle is formed by the **anterior communicating,** the **anterior cerebral,** the **internal carotid** (short segment), the **posterior communicating,** the **posterior cerebral,** and the **basilar arteries** (Fig. 7-90*A*). Note that *the middle*

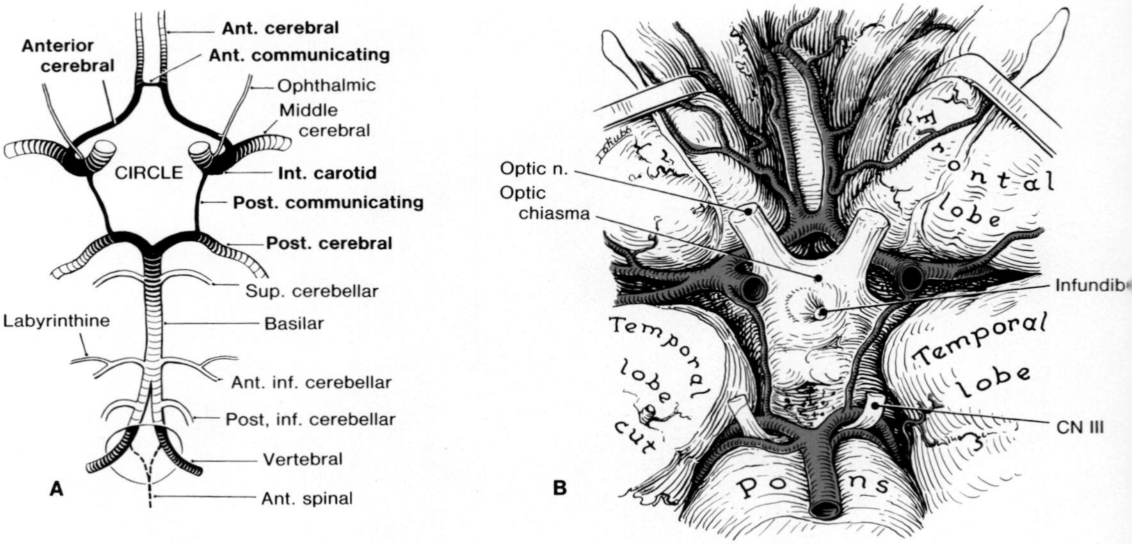

Figure 7-90. *A*, diagram showing the two internal carotid arteries and the two vertebral arteries that supply the brain. The internal carotids enter the cranium through the carotid canals of the temporal bones and the vertebrals through the foramen magnum. The names of *the arteries contributing to the circulus arteriosus cerebri appear in bold type. B*, drawing of the anastomosis of major arteries supplying the brain. They join together at the base of the brain to form the cerebral arterial circle. This diagram shows the classical arterial circle, similar to that drawn by Sir Christopher Wren in 1664, but there are many variations of this typical configuration.

cerebral artery is not part of the cerebral arterial circle; it is the continuation of the internal carotid artery.

Two types of branches, central and cortical, arise from the arterial circle and the main cerebral arteries. **Central arteries** penetrate the substance of the brain and supply deep structures (*e.g.*, the **basal ganglia** and the **internal capsule**, Fig. 7-80*B*), whereas **cortical branches** pass in the pia mater and supply the more superficial parts of the brain.

In general, each of the cerebral arteries, (anterior, middle, and posterior) supplies a surface and a pole as follows: (1) the **anterior cerebral** supplies most of the medial and superior surface and the frontal pole; (2) the **middle cerebral** supplies the lateral surface and the temporal pole; and (3) the **posterior cerebral** supplies the inferior surface and the occipital pole.

CLINICALLY ORIENTED COMMENTS

The anterior, middle, and posterior cerebral arteries communicate with each other via small terminal branches (anastomoses); thus, in case of occlusion of one of the three major cerebral arteries, the remaining two patent ones carry some blood to the area that would otherwise be bloodless. Unfortunately, not enough blood is supplied by these collateral routes in most cases to prevent **infarction** (microscopic area of necrosis) of at least part of the area supplied by the occluded artery.

In the typical arterial circle (Fig. 7-90*B*), there is little exchange of blood between the cerebral arteries via the anterior and posterior communicating arteries. However, *the arterial circle forms an important means of collateral circulation* in the event of obstruction of one of the major arteries entering the circle. In elderly persons, these anastomoses forming the circle are often inadequate when there is a **sudden arterial occlusion** in a large artery, such as one internal carotid. *Vascular insufficiency of the brain usually results in irreversible neurological damage in 5 minutes.* Vascular insufficiency to the whole brain (*e.g.*, resulting from cardiac arrest) results in unconsciousness in about 10 seconds.

For radiographic diagnostic purposes, radiopaque material is injected into any of the carotid or vertebral arteries in the neck by direct **arterial puncture** or by catheterization of them from a distant site such as the femoral artery. Thus, the condition of the extracranial and intracranial carotid and/or vertebral artery systems can be studied (Fig.7-89).

Variations in the size of the vessels forming the arterial circle and in the configuration of the circle are common, *e.g.*, the **posterior cerebral artery** is a branch of the internal carotid in about 20% of persons. Sometimes one anterior cerebral artery is very small and the anterior communicating artery is larger than usual to compensate for this.

Stroke or cerebrovascular accident (**CVA**) results from either *sudden hemorrhage into the brain* or *sudden stoppage of the blood supply to a part of the brain.* The latter occurrence leads to **infarction** (death of tissue) in the area of brain supplied by the blocked artery.

Hemorrhagic stroke follows from rupture of an arteriosclerotic artery or an **aneurysm** (localized dilation of an artery), resulting in bleeding into the brain substance (Figs. 7-91 and 7-92).

Thrombotic stroke may result from (1) **thrombosis** (G. a clotting), which is the formation of a **thrombus** or clot in an artery supplying part of the brain, or (2) from an **embolus** (G. a plug, wedge, or stopper), which is a mass of material that is carried from a distant site by the blood stream into a small artery. Emboli may be (1) **blood clots** (usually from the heart), (2) **masses of atheromatous material** (from ulcerated atheromata in large or medium sized arteries), (3) **aggregations of platelets** (swept off the walls of medium sized arteries), or (4) **gas bubbles**, either nitrogen (in divers or tunnel workers) or air (when large veins of the head and neck are opened at operation or during trauma).

Temporary strokes, called transient ischemic attacks (**TIAs**), often result from soft emboli which break up and/or slowly pass through small arteries producing **temporary neurological deficits**. Such attacks warrant immediate investigation to determine if a remedial cause is present that may be removed before a second possibly permanent episode occurs.

Abnormal dilation of arteries supplying the brain are the most commonly encountered aneurysms in the body. Usually the lesions are located where division points occur in the arteries at the base of the brain (Figs. 7-90 and 7-91). Pathologists classify aneurysms according to their form as saccular, fusiform, or tubular. Most aneurysms

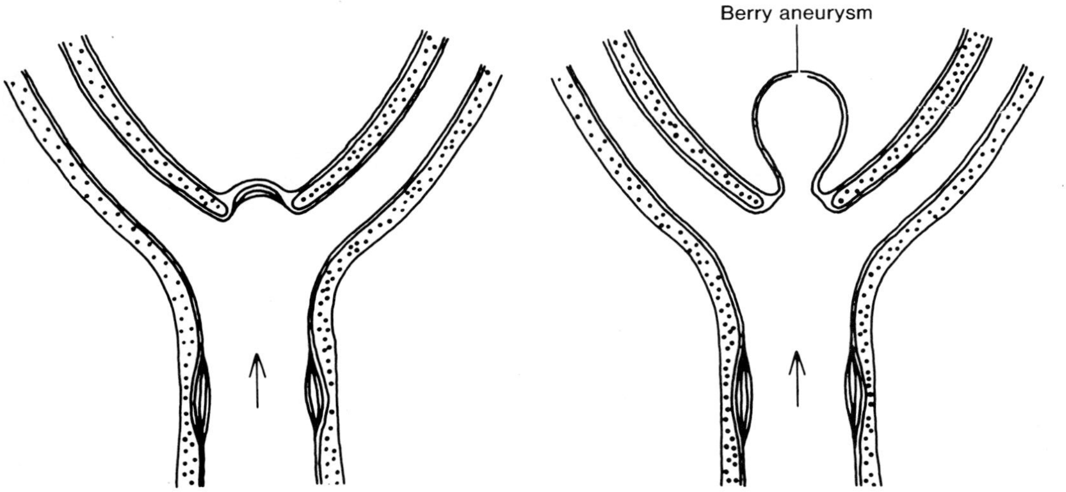

Figure 7-91. Diagrams illustrating the mechanism of development of a *berry aneurysm* at the site of a weakness in an arterial wall, usually at the bifurcation of an artery. Evagination of the wall occurs producing a saccular aneurysm or localized dilation.

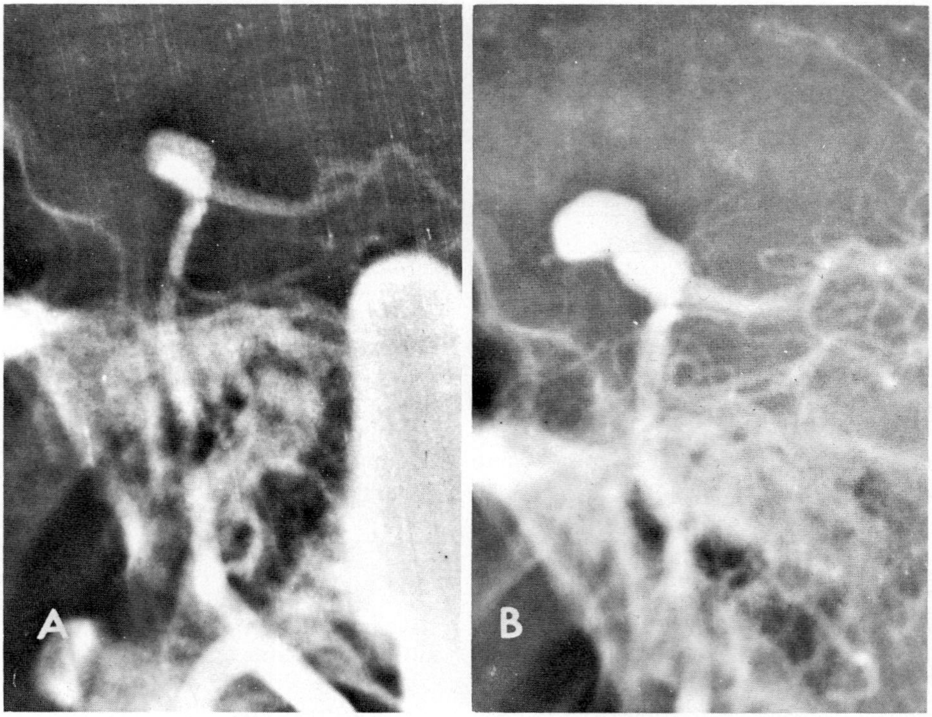

Figure 7-92. A cerebral angiogram demonstrating a berry aneurysm at the bifurcation of the basilar artery into the two posterior cerebrals. *A*, initial examination. *B*, 3 months later. Note its enlargement which probably indicates deterioration of the wall of the aneurysm and a danger of its rupture.

probably develop as the result of congenital weakness of the arterial wall, permitting a localized berry-like evagination to occur. The most common type of aneurysm is the saccular **berry aneurysm**, arising from the cerebral arterial circle and the medium-sized arteries at the base of the brain (Fig.7-92). In time, especially in persons with high blood presure (**hypertension**), the weak part of the wall of the artery may expand and rupture. If rupture occurs, blood escapes into the subarachnoid space (**spontaneous subarachnoid hemorrhage**), and/or into the brain substance (**intracerebral hemorrhage**), and/or into the subdural space (**subdural hemorrhage**). The sites where the blood collects and forms a **hematoma** depend on the relationship of the aneurysm to the cranial meninges.

An **unruptured cerebral aneurysm** is usually asymptomatic, but intermittent enlargements of it may cause symptoms (*e.g.*, throbbing headaches as in Case 7-6) and sometimes neurological signs (*e.g.*, **third nerve palsy** associated with an aneurysm of the posterior communicating artery). These headaches probably result from stretching of the meninges in most cases, but in others they may result from slight bleeding of the aneurysm into the subarachnoid space.

Sudden rupture of a cerebral aneurysm usually produces a very sudden severe, almost unbearable headache owing to gross bleeding into the subarachnoid space that produces a sudden increase in intracranial pressure and **meningeal irritation**. The pain may be so severe the patient is maniacle (wild, furious).

For other complications of a berry aneurysm (*e.g.*, third nerve palsy), see the discussion of Case 7-6. Rupture of a berry aneurysm is one of the causes of a "**stroke**," a term that connotes the abruptness with which the symptoms appear and with which the patient is struck down.

THE ORBIT AND THE EYE

The orbits of a skull appear as two recesses or **bony sockets** when viewed from the front (Fig. 7-1 and 7-93). The orbits almost surround the eyes (eyeballs, globes), protecting them and their associated muscles, nerves, and vessels, together with most of the lacrimal (tear) apparatus (Fig. 7-96).

THE BONY ORBIT

The orbit is shaped somewhat like a four-sided pyramid lying on its side, with its apex pointing posteriorly and its base anteriorly. It has a roof, a floor, a medial wall, and a lateral wall. Each of these is roughly triangular.

The bones forming the orbit are lined with periosteum, called the orbital periosteum or **periorbita**. At the optic canal and the superior orbital fissure, the periorbita is continuous with the periosteum lining the interior of the skull (**endocranium**). It is continuous over the orbital margins and through the inferior orbital fissure with the periosteum covering the external surface of the skull (**pericranium**). The periorbita forms a funnel-shaped sheath which encloses the orbital contents. The periorbita is tough and may be easily detached, especially from the roof and the medial wall of the orbit. This is important from a surgical viewpoint.

The Orbital Margin (Fig. 7-93). Three bones, the **frontal**, the **maxilla**, and the **zygomatic**, contribute about equally to the formation of the orbital margin. Study its make-up using a dried skull. By palpating the margins of your orbits, determine that the entire orbital margin may be felt and that all its margins are sharp and clear-cut,

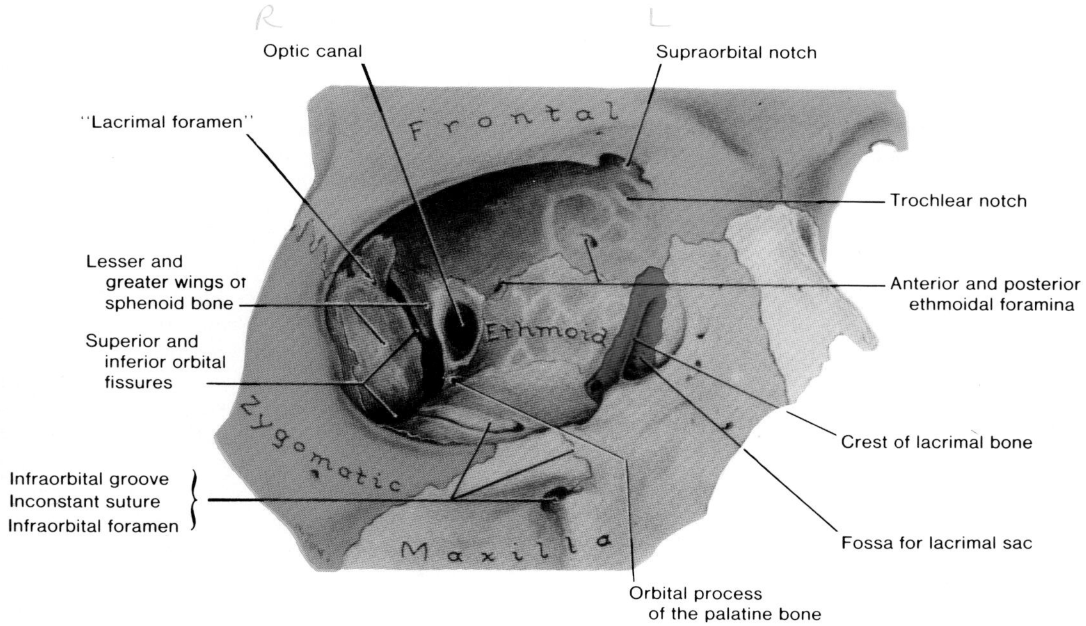

Figure 7-93. Drawing of the bony walls of the orbit (orbital cavity). The orbital margin (brim) surrounds its entrance. Note that the supraorbital margin is formed entirely by the frontal bone and that the lateral margin is formed almost entirely by the frontal process of the zygomatic bone but is completed above by the zygomatic process of the frontal bone. The zygomatic bone and the maxilla share in the formation of the infraorbital margin, whereas the medial margin is formed by the frontal bone above and the lacrimal crest of the frontal process of the maxilla below. The word ethmoid covers the thin orbital lamina (plate) that separates the orbit from the ethmoidal air sinuses (visible through it).

except the medial one. Note that only the medial part of the supraorbital margin is covered by a thick eyebrow in most people.

Observe on a dried skull, and palpate on yourself, the tubercle formed where the zygomatic and maxillary bones meet above the **infraorbital foramen**. This foramen transmits the nerve and vessels of the same name to the face. Familiarize yourself again with the **supraorbital notch** (or foramen, as the case may be). If a notch is present (Fig. 7-93), it can be felt by running your finger along the supraorbital margin. Recall that this notch (or foramen) transmits the **supraorbital nerve** and vessels (Fig. 7-31).

Walls of the Orbit (Figs. 7-93 and 7-94). Each orbit has four walls: superior (roof), medial, inferior (floor), and lateral. The medial walls are almost parallel to each other, with the upper parts of the nasal cavities separating them, whereas the lateral walls are at approximately right angles to each other.

The Superior Wall or Roof of the Orbit (Figs. 7-2, 7-49, 7-93, and 7-94). The roof is formed almost completely by the orbital part of the frontal bone. Posteriorly it is formed by the lesser wing of the **sphenoid bone**. The roof is a thin, translucent, gently arched plate of bone which intervenes between the orbit and the **anterior cranial fossa** when there is not an extension of the frontal sinus into the orbital part of the frontal bone (Fig. 7-94). Anteromedially, the roof separates the orbit from the **frontal sinus** (Figs.7-18 and 7-95), an air space in the vertical part of the frontal bone which extends into the orbital part of the frontal bone in some people (Figs.7-94 and 7-173).

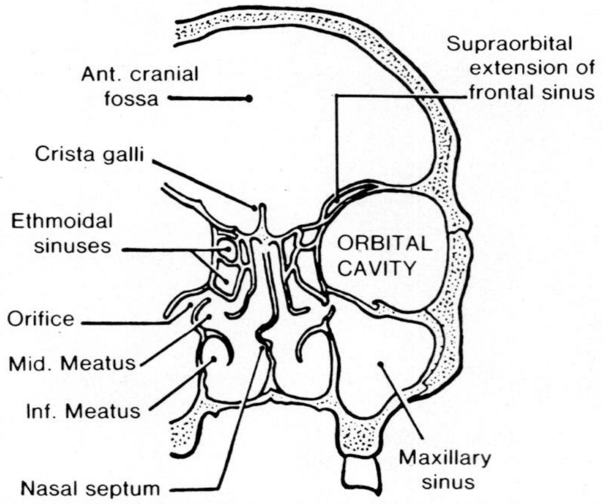

Figure 7-94. Drawing of part of a coronal section of the cranium showing the relations of the orbital cavity. Note that there is a supraorbital extension of the frontal sinus in this specimen. Note also that the orifice of the maxillary sinus is high on its medial wall.

The optic canal (Fig.7-93), located in the posterior part of the roof, transmits the **optic nerve** and its meninges, along with the **ophthalmic artery**. Note that the sphenoidal air sinuses lie medial to the optic canals (Fig.7-95).

The Medial Wall of the Orbit (Figs. 7-93 and 7-94). This paper-thin wall is formed by the **orbital lamina** or plate (lamina papyracea) of the ethmoid bone, along with contributions from the frontal, lacrimal, and sphenoid bones. There is a vertical **lacrimal groove** formed anteriorly by the maxilla and posteriorly by the lacrimal bone for the **lacrimal sac** and the adjacent part of the **nasolacrimal duct** (Fig. 7-100). The posterior edge of this groove is the **posterior lacrimal crest**, a vertical ridge on the lacrimal bone. The orbital lamina is a thin plate of bone that separates the orbits from the nasal cavity and the **ethmoidal sinuses** (ethmoidal air cells). Hold a dried skull up to a light and observe the complex honey-comb appearance of these cells through the paper-thin medial wall of the orbit (Fig. 7-93). Along the suture between the ethmoid and frontal bones, locate two small foramina, the anterior and posterior **ethmoidal foramina** which transmit vessels and nerves of the same name.

The Inferior Wall (Figs. 7-93 and 7-94). The thin inferior wall or floor of the orbit is formed mainly by the orbital surface of the maxilla and partly by the zygomatic bone and the orbital process of the palatine bone. The floor is partly separated from the lateral wall of the orbit by the **inferior orbital fissure** which transmits various structures, the most important being the **maxillary nerve** (CN V^2). The thin floor of the orbit forms the roof of the **maxillary sinus**.

The Lateral Wall of the Orbit (Figs. 7-

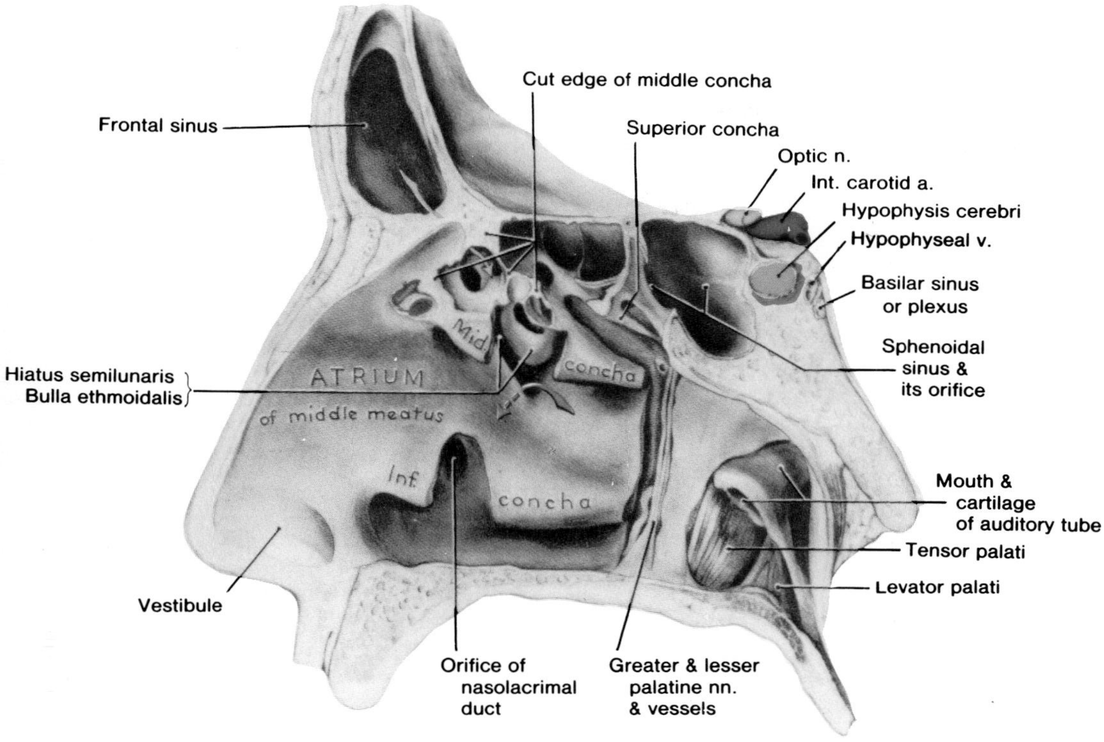

Figure 7-95. Drawing of the paranasal air sinuses. Note that the frontal sinus drains via its infundibulum (L. a funnel) into the upper part of the hiatus semilunaris (*yellow arrow*). Observe the opening in the maxillary sinus (*blue arrow*).

93 and 7-94). This wall is thick, especially the posterior part separating the orbit from the **middle cranial fossa**. The lateral wall is formed by the frontal process of the **zygomatic bone** and by the greater wing of the **sphenoid bone**. Anteriorly, the lateral wall lies between the orbit and the temporal fossa (Fig. 7-1). The lateral wall and the roof of the orbit are partially separated posteriorly by the **superior orbital fissure** which communicates with the middle cranial fossa and transmits the **oculomotor** (CN III), **trochlear** (CN IV), and **abducens** (CN VI) nerves and the terminal branches of the **ophthalmic nerve** (CN V^1), as well as the superior ophthalmic vein.

The apex of the orbit is at the medial ends of the superior and inferior orbital fissures. These fissures form a V-shaped area which encloses the orbital part of the greater wing of the sphenoid bone.

CLINICALLY ORIENTED COMMENTS

Because of the thinness of the medial and inferior walls of the orbital cavity, blows to the eye may produce **blow-out fractures** of these walls as the result of the sudden increase in intraorbital pressure. Because the medial wall of the orbit is so delicate, surgery of the ethmoidal sinuses (Fig. 7-94) must be performed with extreme care.

Although the superior wall (roof) of the orbit is stronger than the medial and inferior walls, it is thin enough to be translucent and may be readily penetrated. Thus, a sharp object, even a pencil, may pass through it into the frontal lobe of the brain.

One type of prefrontal **lobotomy** or **leukotomy** (G. *leukos*, white + *tomē*, a cutting) used in the past in attempting to modify the behavior of severely psychotic patients involved driving a sterile instrument (**leukotome**) through the roof of the orbit and sectioning fiber connections forming the white matter in the anterior part of the frontal lobe.

An object accidentally pushed through the anteromedial part of the roof of the orbit is likely to penetrate the **frontal sinus** (Fig. 7-95), whereas an object pushed through its floor will probably enter the **maxillary sinus** (Fig.7-94). Similarly, a foreign object (*e.g.*, a piece of wire or a bullet) penetrating the eye in an anteroposterior direction could traverse the superior orbital fissure and enter the middle cranial fossa. Because the petrous part of the temporal bone is so hard, it might stop the bullet which would remain in the middle cranial fossa.

Owing to the closeness of the optic nerve to the sphenoidal and posterior ethmoidal sinuses (Fig. 7-95), **malignant tumors** in these sinuses may erode the thin bony walls and compress the optic nerve and the orbital contents. The easiest entrance to the orbit for a tumor in the middle cranial fossa is through the **superior orbital fissure**, whereas tumors in the temporal or infratemporal fossa gain access through the **inferior orbital fissure**. Tumors in the orbit produce bulging of the eyeball (**proptosis** or **exophthalmos**).

Although the lateral wall of the orbit is nearly as long as the medial wall, it does not reach so far forward; thus, nearly 2.5 cm of the eyeball is exposed when the pupil is turned medially as far as possible. Check this by putting your finger on the bridge of someone's nose and asking the person to look at your finger. You now know why the lateral side affords the best approach for operations on the eyeball.

A person attempting suicide by shooting through the temple could destroy the optic nerve and/or the eyeball, but miss the brain. Verify on a dried skull that the brain would be about 2 cm posterior to the frontozygomatic suture, which is marked by a notch on its posterior surface.

THE ORBITAL CONTENTS

The most important contents of the orbit are the eyeball and the optic nerve, CN II (Fig. 7-96). The orbit also contains the muscles of the eyeball, their nerves and vessels, the lacrimal gland, and other nerves.

Terminology. The terms eye, eyeball, oculus, bulbus oculi, bulb, and globe all refer to the same structure, *i.e.*, the **visual organ**. The eye is called an **oculus** in Latin and **ophthalmos** in Greek; hence, the terms **oculist** and **ophthalmologist** are interchangeable and indicate physicians who specialize in **ophthalmology**, the branch of medical science that deals with the eye. You will see many other terms derived from these Latin and Greek words, *e.g.*, **oculomotor** (related to or causing movements of the eye) and **ophthalmoscope** (an instrument for examining the interior of the eye).

The Living Eye and Associated Structures (Figs. 7-96 and 7-97). The "white of the eye" or front of the **sclera** (G. hard) is continuous with the **dura mater** covering the optic nerve and the brain (Fig. 7-101). This tough opaque part of the external tunic of the eye appears slightly blue in infants and children and has a yellow hue in many older people.

The anterior transparent part of the eye is the **cornea** (L. horny, *i.e.*, horn-like structure); it is continuous at its margins with the sclera (Figs. 7-97 and 7-101). The dark circular aperture that you see through the cornea is the **pupil**. This opening is surrounded by a circular, pigmented diaphragm known as the **iris**. The white sclera that you see in a mirror, or when looking at someone else's eye, is covered by a thin, moist, mucous membrane called the **bulbar (ocular) conjunctiva**. As it is transparent, you can see the white sclera beneath it. The conjunctiva is reflected off the sclera on to the deep surface of the eyelids (**palpebrae**), lining them to their margins where it becomes continuous with the skin.

Turn someone's lower eyelid downward and examine the **palpebral conjunctiva**. It is normally red and very vascular; thus, it is commonly examined in cases of suspected **anemia**, a blood condition that is commonly manifested by pallor of the mucous membranes. As the bulbar conjunctiva is continuous with the anterior epithelium of the cornea and with the palpebral con-

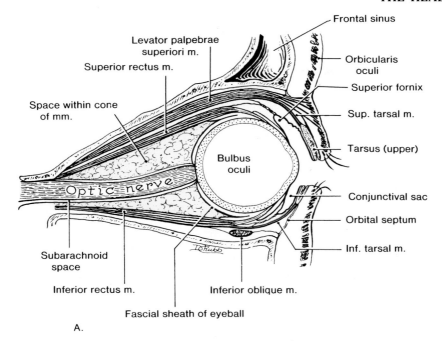

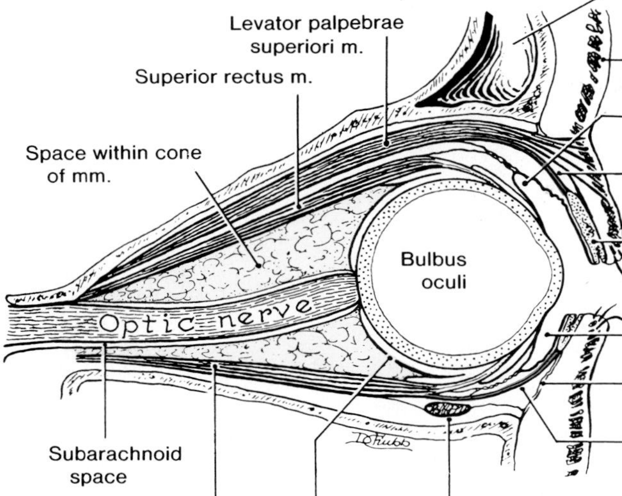

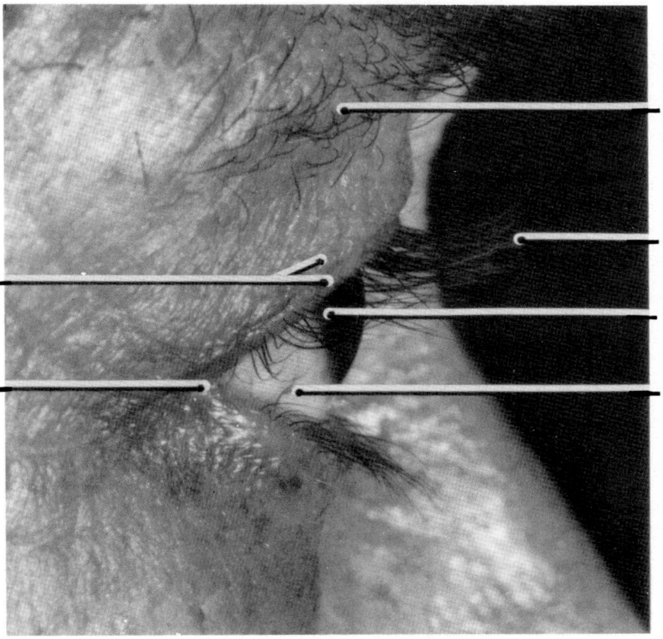

Figure 7-96. *A*, drawing of a sagittal section of the orbit and its contents. Note that the eyeball is sunken or retracted in this cadaveric specimen owing to embalming and loss of fluid. *B*, photograph of a lateral view of the eye of a 46-year-old man. The most prominent anterior bulge is produced by the transparent cornea, which becomes continuous at its margins with the white sclera.

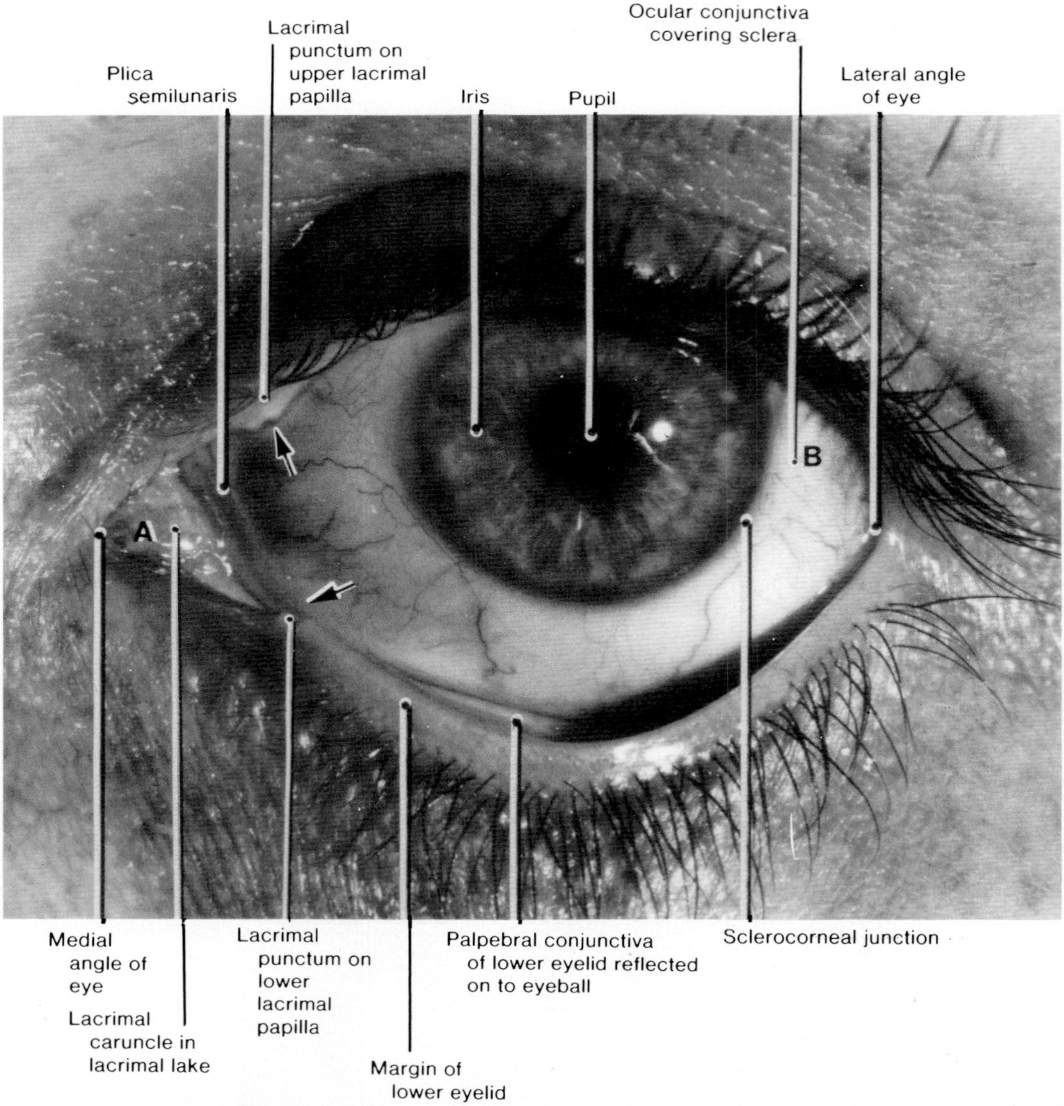

Figure 7-97. Photograph of the left eye of a 36-year-old woman with her eyelids slightly everted to show the structures at the medial angle (canthus). Note the pupil, which is an aperture in the surrounding iris. The pupil appears black because you are looking through the pupil toward the pigmented back of the eye. Understand that you are looking through the transparent cornea to see the iris and pupil. Observe the fine vascular network of the ocular conjunctiva covering the sclera. The line of reflection of the conjunctiva from the eyelids on to the eyeball is called the conjunctival fornix; hence, there are superior and inferior fornices (Fig. 7-96*A*). The white spot on the iris is a highlight from the photographer's lamps. Note that her upper eyelid partly covers her iris; this is normal. The *arrows* indicate the lacrimal puncta on the upper and lower lacrimal papillae. *A*, lacrimal caruncle in lacrimal lake. *B*, ocular conjunctiva covering the sclera.

junctiva, it forms a **conjunctival sac** (Fig. 7-96). The opening between the eyelids, called the palpebral fissure, is the mouth of the conjunctival sac; hence, when it is closed, the conjunctivae form a closed sac. Sensory innervation of the conjunctiva is from the trigeminal nerve (CN V) through the infratrochlear, maxillary, and lacrimal nerves.

CLINICALLY ORIENTED COMMENTS

The bulbar conjunctiva is colorless, except when its vessels are dilated and congested (*e.g.*, **bloodshot eyes**). This **hyperemia of the conjunctiva** is caused by local irritations (*e.g.*, dust, chlorine, and smoke) and infections (*e.g.*, pinkeye).

Subconjunctival hemorrhage is common and is manifested by bright or dark red patches under and in the bulbar conjunctiva. It may result from injury or inflammation. The conjunctiva is frequently inflamed owing to infection, a condition called conjunctivitis. **Acute conjunctivitis** is common in children, especially in newborn infants who have prophylactic silver nitrate instilled into their eyes in case they were exposed to venereal disease during birth.

Examine your eyes in a mirror and then those of a colleague. Note that from the front (Fig. 7-97) most of the eyeball appears to be in the orbit, but from the side much of it protrudes between the eyelids, *i.e.*, through the **palpebral fissure** (Fig. 7-96*B*).

The eyelids *protect the eyes* from injury and excessive light and they *keep the cornea moist.* Look into a mirror and slowly move your finger toward your eye. Note that your eyelids close. Verify that the upper eyelid is larger and more movable than the lower one and that *the upper eyelid partly covers the iris* (Fig. 7-97), whereas the entire lower half of the eye is normally uncovered. The eyelids are essentially movable folds of skin, covered externally by thin skin and internally by the *highly vascular palpebral conjunctiva* (Figs. 7-97 and 7-98). This is reflected on the eyeball up to the cornea, forming deep recesses known as the superior and inferior *fornices* (Fig. 7-96*A*).

Each eyelid is strengthened by a dense connective tissue band, about 2.5 cm wide, called the **tarsal plate** (Fig. 7-98). In the connective tissue between this plate and the anterior surface are palpebral fibers of the **orbicularis oculi muscle** (Figs. 7-96*A* and 7-98). Embedded in the tarsal plate are a number of **tarsal glands** (meibomian glands), the fatty secretion of which lubricates the edges of the eyelids, preventing them from sticking together and sealing them when the eyelids are closed.

The eyelashes (cilia) are in the margins of the eyelids (Figs. 7-96 to 7-98) and are arranged in two or three irregular rows. The large sebaceous glands associated with these hairs are known as **ciliary glands** (of Zeiss). Between the hair follicles are large apocrine type sweat glands called **glands of Moll**.

The place where the two eyelids meet is

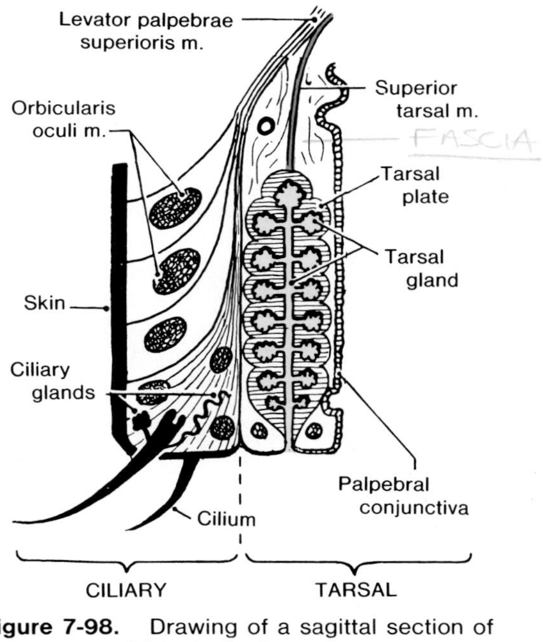

Figure 7-98. Drawing of a sagittal section of an upper eyelid (palpebra).

called the **angle**, or **canthus** (G. corner of eye); thus, each eye has a medial and a lateral angle or canthus (Figs. 7-96 and 7-97). When the eyelids are closed the **palpebral fissure** is nearly in the horizontal plane, except in certain races (*e.g.*, Mongolian) where there is a slight upward slant of the palpebral fissure toward the nose because the medial ends of the upper eyelids project upward and medially. Furthermore, the medial canthi of their eyes are covered by an extra skin fold called the **epicanthal fold** (Fig. 7-99). Slanted palpebral fissures and inner epicanthal folds are also present in persons with the **Down syndrome** or the trisomy 21 chromosomal abnormality (Fig. 6-124*A*) and with several other syndromes (*e.g.*, the **cri du chat syndrome**), resulting from a terminal deletion of chromosome number 5.

In your medial angle observe the reddish area known as the **lacrimal lake**, or lacus lacrimalis (Fig. 7-97), within which there is a small hillock, the **lacrimal caruncle** (L. a small fleshy mass). Lateral to the caruncle is a vertical curved fold of conjunctiva called the **semilunar fold**, or plica semilunaris. This fold slightly overlaps the eyeball and is a *remnant of the nictitating membrane present in some animals* (*e.g.*, amphibians).

Evert the edge of your lower eyelid and locate at its medial end a small black dot or pit, the **lacrimal punctum** (L. a point), on the summit of a small elevation called the **lacrimal papilla** (Figs. 7-97 and 7-100). There is a similar punctum and papilla on the upper eyelid. The punctum is the opening of a slender canal called the **lacrimal canaliculus** (little canal), which carries the tears to the **lacrimal sac**. From here, they are conducted to the nose via the **nasolacrimal duct**. The lacrimal sac has some fibers of the orbicularis oris muscle posterior to it which insert into the posterior **lacrimal crest** (Fig. 7-93). When they contract the lacrimal sac is squeezed, forcing the tears into the nasolacrimal duct, which opens into the nasal cavity (Fig. 7-95). Observe that the puncta face posteriorly and so are able to suck up the tears (Fig. 7-100). Press your fingertip between your nose and the medial canthus of your eye. You should feel a horizontal cord, the **medial palpebral ligament** (Fig. 7-100). It connects the eyelids, including their muscle, to the medial margin of the orbit. If you pull your eyelid laterally, this ligament may raise a small skin fold. A similar **lateral palpebral ligament**, although lighter, attaches the eyelids to the lateral margin of the orbit. The two palpebral ligaments are connected by **tarsal plates**, or tarsi (Figs. 7-98 and 7-100). Because of these plates, the eyelids can be everted. Verify that it is easy to evert the lower eyelid but difficult to evert the upper eyelid because its tarsal plate is rigid. Hence, when it is everted (*e.g.*, over a match stick), it tends to stay that way until it is turned downward.

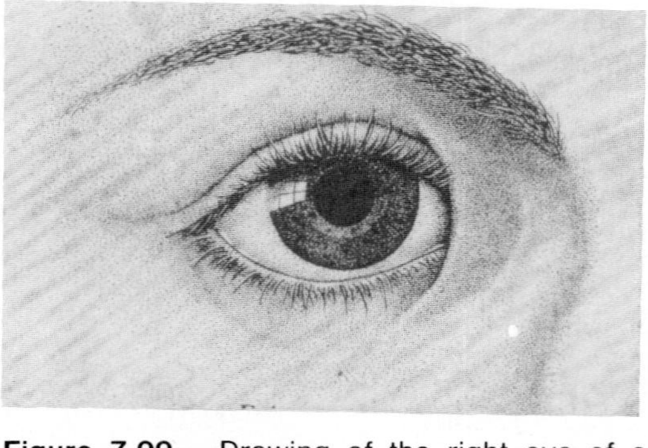

Figure 7-99. Drawing of the right eye of a Mongoloid person with a large inner epicanthal fold. Note that it obscures the medial canthus or angle of the eye. Some people have this fold removed by a plastic surgeon.

The **palpebral fascia** is a thin fibrous membrane which connects the tarsal plates to the margins of the orbit and with them forms an orbital septum. This septum passes posterior to the lacrimal sac and is pierced by the levator palpebrae superioris muscle.

On the deep surface of your eyelids you may be able to see the **tarsal glands** (Fig. 7-98) because they appear as yellowish streaks through the conjunctiva lining the eyelids. The ducts of these glands open on the flat free margin of the eyelid near the posterior edge (Fig. 7-98). Note that the **eyelashes (cilia)** project from the anterior edge of the eyelid.

Lacrimal fluid (tears) is produced by a small, almond-shaped **lacrimal gland**, located in the upper and lateral part of the orbit (Figs. 7-100 and 7-104). Its three to nine excretory ducts open into the **superior fornix of the conjunctival sac** (Fig.

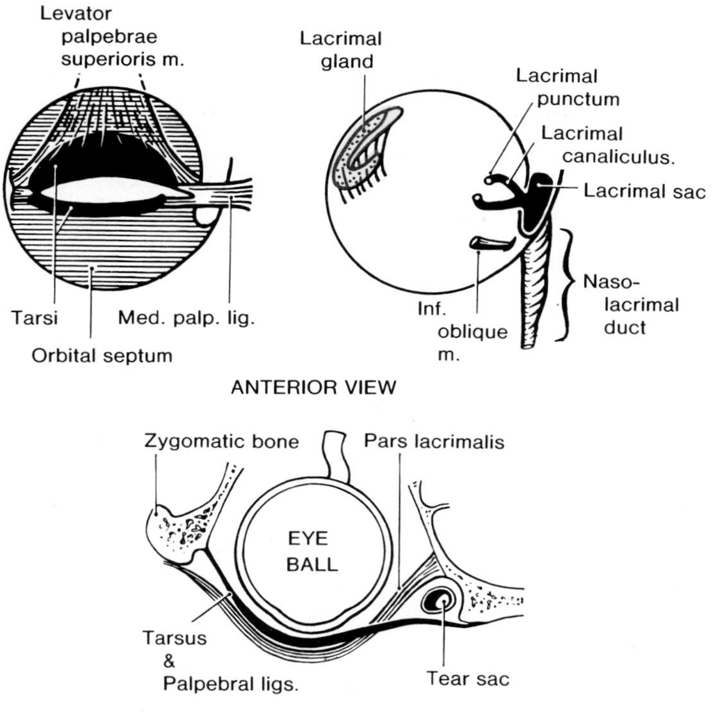

Figure 7-100. Drawings illustrating the parts of the lacrimal apparatus. Tears are secreted from the lacrimal gland into the superolateral angle of the conjunctival sac and, after passing over the cornea, they drain into the lacrimal puncta in the upper and lower eyelids (see Fig. 7-97). The puncta open into the lacrimal canaliculi (little canals) through which the lacrimal fluid is transported to the lacrimal sac. Medially the superior and inferior canaliculi usually meet to form a common canaliculus (1 to 3 mm long) which carries the tears to the lacrimal sac (*upper right*). This sac drains into the nasolacrimal duct, which empties into the inferior meatus of the nose (Fig. 7-84).

7-96*A*). In addition to the main gland, there are numerous accessory glands. As the lacrimal fluid drains into the lacrimal sac, it moistens the corneal surface. When the cornea becomes dry, the eye blinks and the eyelids carry a film of lacrimal fluid over the cornea, somewhat like the windshield wipers on a car. In this way, foreign material (*e.g.*, dust particles) is also carried to the medial canthus of the eye. When you cry, the excess tears cause overflowing of the lacrimal lakes and tears to roll down your cheek.

CLINICALLY ORIENTED COMMENTS

Awareness of the normal position of the eyelids is clinically important because their pattern changes when the nerves that control their movement or tone are compressed or injured.

In **third nerve palsy** (Cases 7-5 and 7-6), the upper eyelid droops (**ptosis**) and cannot be voluntarily raised. This results from damage to the superior division of the **oculomotor nerve** (CN III), which supplies the **levator palpebrae superioris** muscle (Figs. 7-31 and 7-98). You can tell by its name that this muscle normally elevates the upper lid.

When the facial nerve (CN VII) is damaged, the eyelids cannot be closed owing to paralysis of the **orbicularis oculi muscle**, which closes the eyelids. In this case the levator palpebrae superioris (acting alone) keeps the upper eyelid elevated, even during sleep (Case 7-1).

When the facial nerve is paralyzed the

eyelids cannot be closed and protective blinking of the eye is lost. As a result, tears cannot be washed across the cornea. Irritation of the unprotected eyeball results in excessive lacrimation. Excessive tearing also occurs when the lacrimal drainage apparatus is obstructed or when the lower eyelid is lax and everted, thereby preventing the tears from reaching the inferior lacrimal punctum (Fig. 7-100).

Any of the glands in the eyelid may become inflamed and swollen owing to infection or obstruction of their ducts. If the ducts of the sebaceous glands become obstructed or inflamed, a painful swelling known as a **sty** protrudes from the eyelid. They are common in children and nearly always are caused by staphylococcal infection.

Cysts of these glands, called **chalazia**, may also form. An obstruction of a tarsal gland produces a **tarsal chalazion** that protrudes toward the eyeball and rubs against it as the eyelids blink. Such an inflammation can be more painful than a sty.

The Eyeball (Bulbus Oculi). The main features of the externally visible parts of the living eye have been discussed.

The eyeball is like a miniature camera 2.5 cm long suspended in the anterior half of the orbital cavity in such a way that the six ocular muscles in the orbit can move the eye in all directions (Fig 7-109). In Figure 7-96*A* observe that the eyeball projects more than a centimeter beyond the base of the orbit; thus, there is about 4 cm behind the eyeball that are occupied by muscles, nerves, and fat. *Do not be misled by the position of the eyeballs in cadavers*; they are sunken owing to dehydration and atrophy of the fat and muscles in the orbit. Sunken eyes are also characteristic of emaciated and/or dehydrated people owing to the scantiness of fat in their orbital cavities. The eyeball has three concentric coats:

1. External or Fibrous Coat (Fig. 7-101). This supporting coat of the eye consists of a white opaque posterior five-sixths, the **sclera**, and a transparent anterior one-sixth, the **cornea**.

2. Middle or Vascular Coat (Fig. 7-101). This vascular and heavily pigmented layer consists, from posterior to anterior, of the **choroid**, the **ciliary body**, and the **iris**.

The choroid is a dark brown membrane located between the sclera and the retina. It forms the largest part of the middle coat and lines most of the sclera. It terminates anteriorly in the ciliary body. The choroid is firmly attached to the retina, but it can be easily stripped from the sclera. It contains many venous plexuses and layers of capillaries that are responsible for nutrition of the adjacent layers of the retina.

The ciliary body connects the choroid with the circumference of the iris and is continuous posteriorly with the choroid. The ciliary body has protrusions or folds on its internal surface called **ciliary processes**. These secrete **aqueous humor**, a watery fluid that fills the **anterior** and **posterior chambers** of the eye, which are the spaces in front of and behind the iris. The direction of flow of the aqueous humor is shown by the arrow in Figure 7-101. Externally the ciliary body contains **ciliary muscle**, which on contraction permits the **lens** to bulge by relaxing its **suspensory ligament**.

The iris is a contractile diaphragm situated in front of the lens which has a central, circular aperture termed the **pupil**. During waking hours, the size of the pupil is continually varying in order to regulate the amount of light entering the eye through the lens. The iris is between the cornea and the lens.

Eye color depends on the amount and the distribution of pigment in the iris. The pupil appears black because one looks through the pupil toward the back of the eye (**optic fundus**, Fig. 7-102) which is heavily pigmented. In persons with blue eyes, the pigment is limited to the posterior surface of the iris, whereas in persons with dark brown eyes the pigment is scattered throughout the connective tissue of the iris.

3. Internal or Retinal Coat (Fig. 7-101). The **retina** or nervous layer of the eyeball is a very thin, delicate membrane in which the fibers of the optic nerve are spread out. It is covered externally by the choroid and internally by the **vitreous body**.

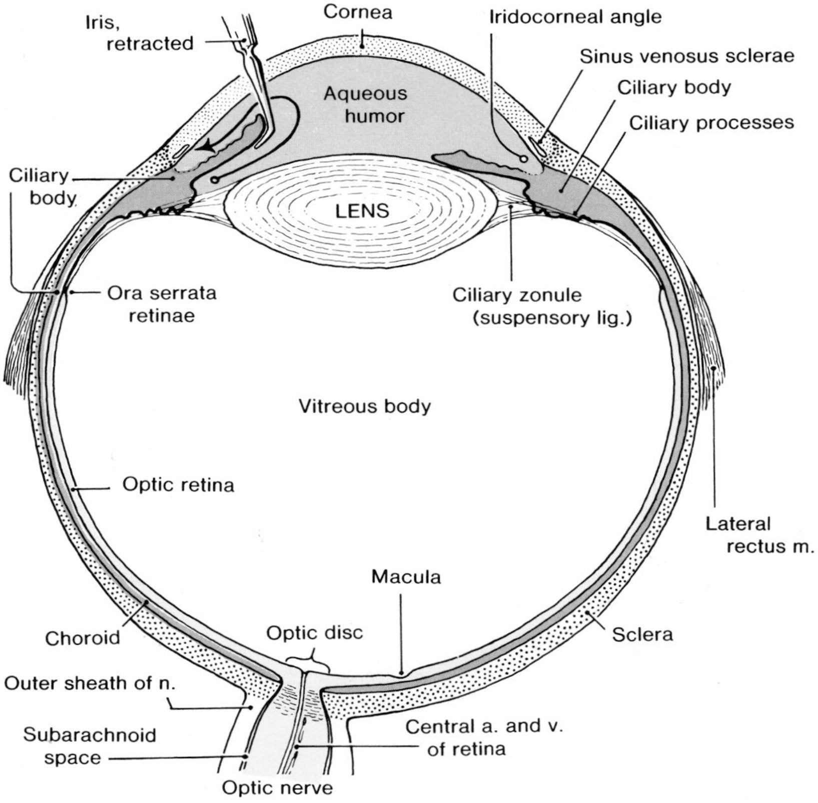

Figure 7-101. Drawing of a horizontal section of the eyeball. Observe its *three coats*: (1) external or fibrous coat (sclera and cornea); (2) middle or vascular coat (choroid, ciliary body, and iris); and (3) internal or retinal layer. The *four refractive media* are: (1) the cornea; (2) the aqueous humor; (3) the lens; and (4) the vitreous body.

The retina is composed of two layers: an outer **pigment cell layer** and an inner **neural layer**, the light-sensitive retina. The neural layer of the retina ends at the posterior edge of the ciliary body in a wavy border called the **ora serrata**. A thin, insensitive layer continues anteriorly onto the ciliary body and the iris.

In the posterior portion of the interior of the eye, called the **optic fundus**, there is a circular, depressed, white to pink area in the retina known as the **optic papilla** or **optic disc** (Figs. 7-101 and 7-102). This is where the optic nerve enters the eyeball. Because the papilla contains only nerve fibers and no photoreceptor cells, it is insensitive to light; thus, it is sometimes referred to as the **blind spot**. Just lateral to the optic disc is a small, oval, yellowish area called the **macula lutea** (L. yellow spot). The central depressed part of the macula, known as the **fovea centralis**, is the area of most acute vision. The retina is more adherent to the choroid at the optic disc and the ora serrata than elsewhere.

The retina is supplied by the **central artery of the retina**, a branch of the **ophthalmic artery**, which enters the eyeball with the optic nerve (Fig. 7-101). Pulsation is usually visible in the retinal arteries through an **ophthalmoscope** (Fig. 7-102). A corresponding system of retinal veins unites to form the **central vein of the retina**. The retinal arteries and veins usu-

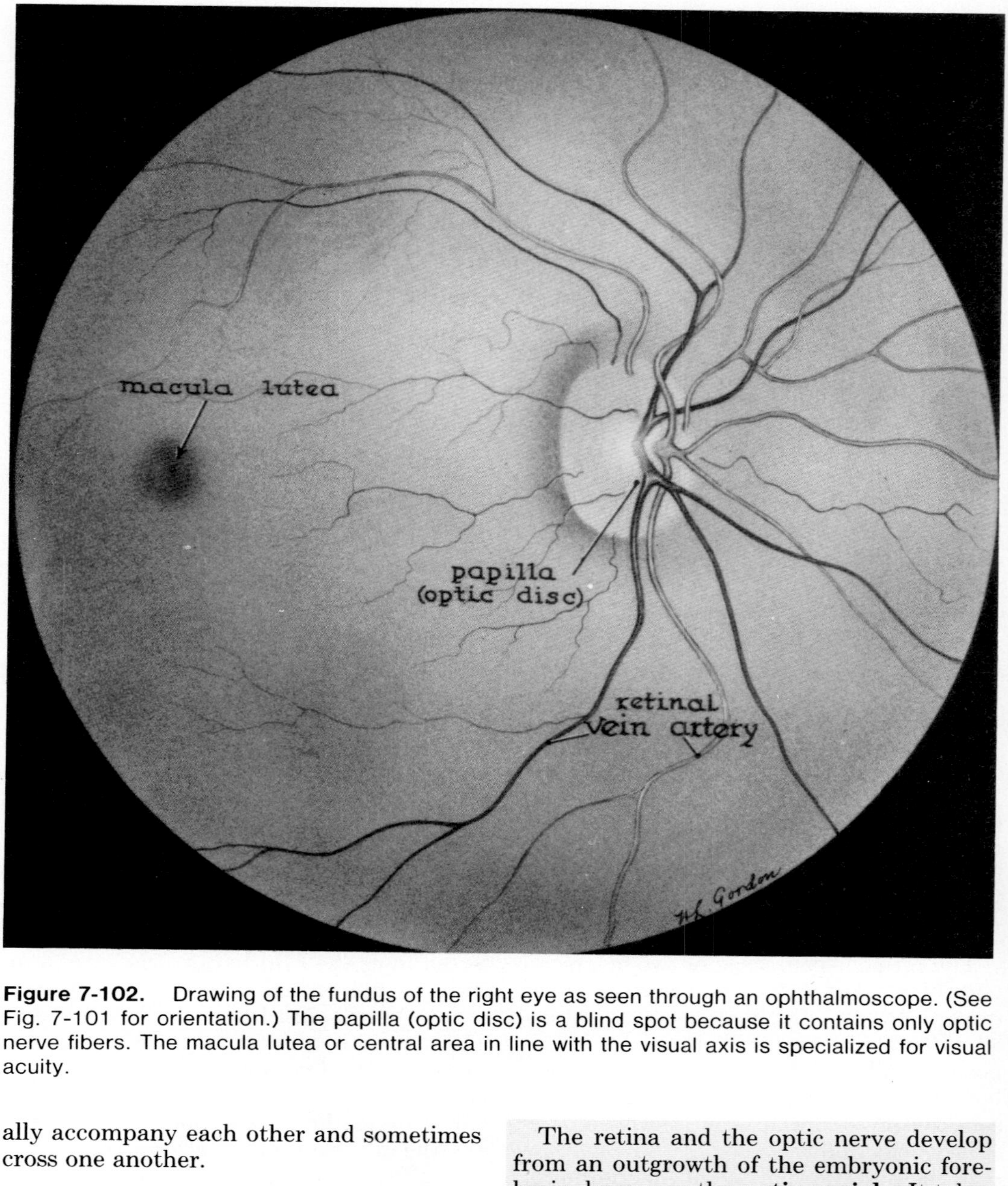

Figure 7-102. Drawing of the fundus of the right eye as seen through an ophthalmoscope. (See Fig. 7-101 for orientation.) The papilla (optic disc) is a blind spot because it contains only optic nerve fibers. The macula lutea or central area in line with the visual axis is specialized for visual acuity.

ally accompany each other and sometimes cross one another.

CLINICALLY ORIENTED COMMENTS

One **sign of hypertension** (high blood pressure) is nicking of the retinal veins where the retinal arteries cross them; this is visible through an **ophthalmoscope**.

The retina and the optic nerve develop from an outgrowth of the embryonic forebrain, known as the **optic vesicle**. It takes its covering of meninges with it; hence, the meningeal layers and the subarachnoid space extend around the optic nerve to its attachment to the eyeball (Fig. 7-101). The central artery and vein of the retina, branches of the ophthalmic artery and vein, run within the anterior part of the optic nerve and cross the extension of subarachnoid space around it. Consequently, an increase in CSF pressure slows venous return from the retina, causing **edema** (G. a swelling) as the result of fluid accumulation. This is obvious on **ophthalmoscopy** as a swelling of the optic papilla (*i.e.*, **papilledema**). Inspection of the ocular fundus or optic fundus (**funduscopy**) is an essential part of a neurological examination.

As the **pigment epithelium** of the retina develops from the outer layer of the **optic cup,** a derivative of the optic vesicle, and the **neural layer** develops from the inner layer, they may separate. During the early fetal period (up to 20 weeks), these layers of the retina are separated by an **intraretinal space.** Although the pigment layer becomes firmly fixed to the choroid, its attachment to the neural layer is not so firm. Thus, **detachment of the retina** which may follow a blow to the eye is actually separation of the pigment layer from the neural layer.

Refractive Media. On their way to the retina, light waves pass through a number of structures with different densities: the cornea, the aqueous humor, the lens, and the vitreous body (Fig. 7-101). These structures constitute the refracting media of the eye.

The cornea, consisting chiefly of a special kind of dense connective tissue, is transparent and forms the anterior part of the outer coat of the eye. The degree of curvature of the cornea varies in different people and is greater in young than in old persons.

CLINICALLY ORIENTED COMMENTS

Because the cornea is exposed to the exterior, it is subject to cuts, abrasions, and other kinds of trauma. For example, a stick poked into the eye may tear the cornea or produce a **corneal abrasion.** These are painful and may take several months to heal.

In **facial nerve paralysis** (Case 7-1), the orbicularis oculi muscle is paralyzed and the eyelids remain open. As a result, there is no blinking to keep the cornea moist and the tears run uselessly out of the eye. *A dry cornea becomes ulcerated* and if not treated the eyesight may be lost. Ointment applied to the eye will slow the drying process, but sometimes the eyelids have to be sutured together to keep the cornea moist until the facial nerve regenerates.

Homologous corneal transplants can be done for patients with scarred or opaque corneas with considerable success. The surface epithelium is regenerated by the host and covers the transplant in a few days. Some persons who donate their bodies for anatomical studies also arrange to have their eyes removed shortly after death so that their corneas may be transplanted to persons who need them. In such persons the donated stromal cells live for at least a year after the donor's death.

The aqueous humor is a clear watery fluid in the anterior and posterior chambers of the eye. After passing through the pupil from the posterior chamber into the anterior chamber, the aqueous humor, which is continuously produced by the **ciliary processes,** is drained off through spaces at the **iridocorneal angle** (filtration angle) in the **pectinate ligament** of the iris (Fig. 7-101). These spaces, visible through an instrument known as a **slitlamp,** open into a circular venous canal, called the **sinus venosus sclerae** (canal of Schlemm, Figs. 7-101 and 7-103). This sinus drains via aqueous veins into the scleral plexuses.

CLINICALLY ORIENTED COMMENTS

If the rates of production and absorption become unequal or there is **blockage of the sinus venosus sclerae,** the pressure of the aqueous humor rises, producing a condition known as **glaucoma.** The presence of the **rubella virus** in the embryo during the critical stages of eye development can result in abnormal formation of the sinus venous sclerae and **congenital glaucoma** (Fig. 7-104*A*).

The biconvex lens lies behind the iris and in front of the vitreous body. It is normally transparent. The curvatures of the surfaces of the lens, particularly the anterior surface, are constantly varying in order to focus near or distant objects on the retina.

As one gets older, the lens becomes harder and more flattened. In old age, the lens gradually acquires a yellow tint. These changes gradually reduce the person's focussing power, a condition known as **presbyopia.** In some old people there is also a loss of transparency of the lens; this opaqueness of the lens is known as a **senile cataract.**

Many lens opacities are inherited, but some are caused by noxious agents affecting early development of the lens. **Congenital cataract** (Fig. 7-104*B*) may develop in an embryo when the mother contracts **German measles** (rubella) during early pregnancy when the lens is developing.

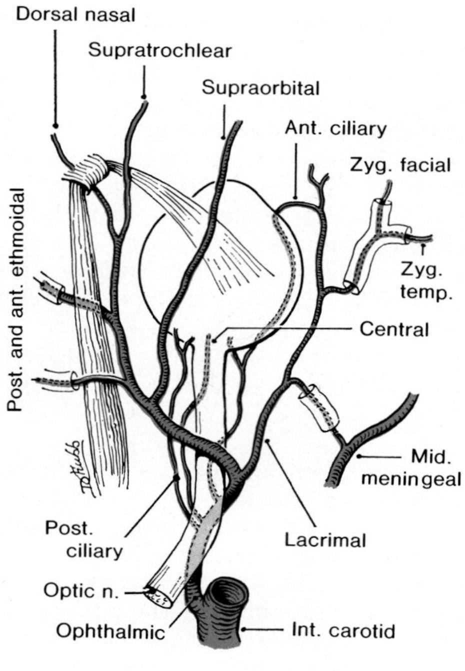

Figure 7-103. Diagram of the ophthalmic artery and its numerous branches supplying the orbital contents. Note its relationship to the optic nerve with which it enters the orbit via the optic canal.

The vitreous body consists of a transparent, jelly-like substance in which there is a meshwork of fine fibrils. This colorless, transparent gel occupies the **vitreous chamber,** the space between the lens and the retina (Fig. 7-101). It consists of about 99% water and constitutes about four-fifths of the eyeball. In contrast to the aqueous humor, *the vitreous body is not continuously replaced.* It forms during the embryonic period and is not exchanged.

At the periphery of the vitreous body there is a **vitreous (hyaloid) membrane** which is formed by a condensation of fibrils. A narrow passage, called the **hyaloid canal** (Cloquet's canal), runs from the optic disc to the lens. In the fetus this canal was

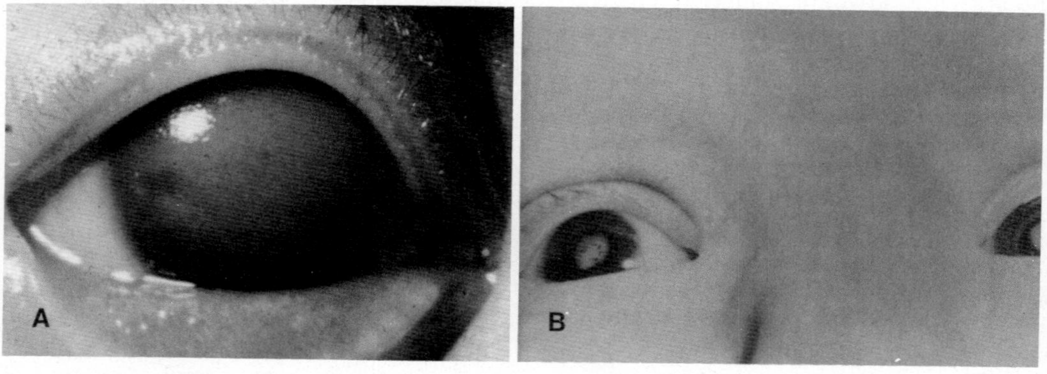

Figure 7-104. Photographs of the eyes of infants whose mothers contracted German measles during early pregnancy. *A*, congenital glaucoma. *B*, congenital cataracts.

traversed by the hyaloid artery. A remnant of this vessel may be visible during ophthalmoscopic examinations as a very small corkscrew-like structure hanging from the posterior aspect of the lens.

The Fascial Sheath of the Eyeball (Bulbar Fascia, Vagina Bulbi, Tenon's Capsule). This cup-like fascia forms a thin sheath around the eyeball, except for its corneal part, and separates it from the fat and other contents in the orbit (Fig. 7-96*A*). The fascial sheath is attached to the sclera posteriorly, close to the optic nerve, and anteriorly, just behind the cornea (**corneoscleral junction**). The tendons of the muscles that rotate the eyeball within the fascial sheath pierce it on their way to their places of insertion. The fascial sheath also blends with the fascial sheaths of the ocular muscles. There is a potential space between the eyeball and the fascial sheath which allows the eyeball to move inside this cup-shaped fascia.

There are triangular expansions from the sheaths of the medial and lateral rectus muscles (to be described later) which are attached to the lacrimal and zygomatic bones, respectively. As they check (prevent excessive movement) the actions of these muscles, they are called the medial and lateral **check ligaments.** There is also a check ligament associated with the levator palpebrae superioris muscle (Figs. 7-105 and 7-108).

The fascial sheath is perforated behind by the ciliary nerves (Fig. 7-105) and vessels and fuses with the sheath of the optic nerve. A thickening of the lower part of the fascial sheath of the eyeball, called the **suspensory ligament of the eye**, is attached to anterior parts of the medial and lateral walls of the orbit. As it is a sling-like ham-

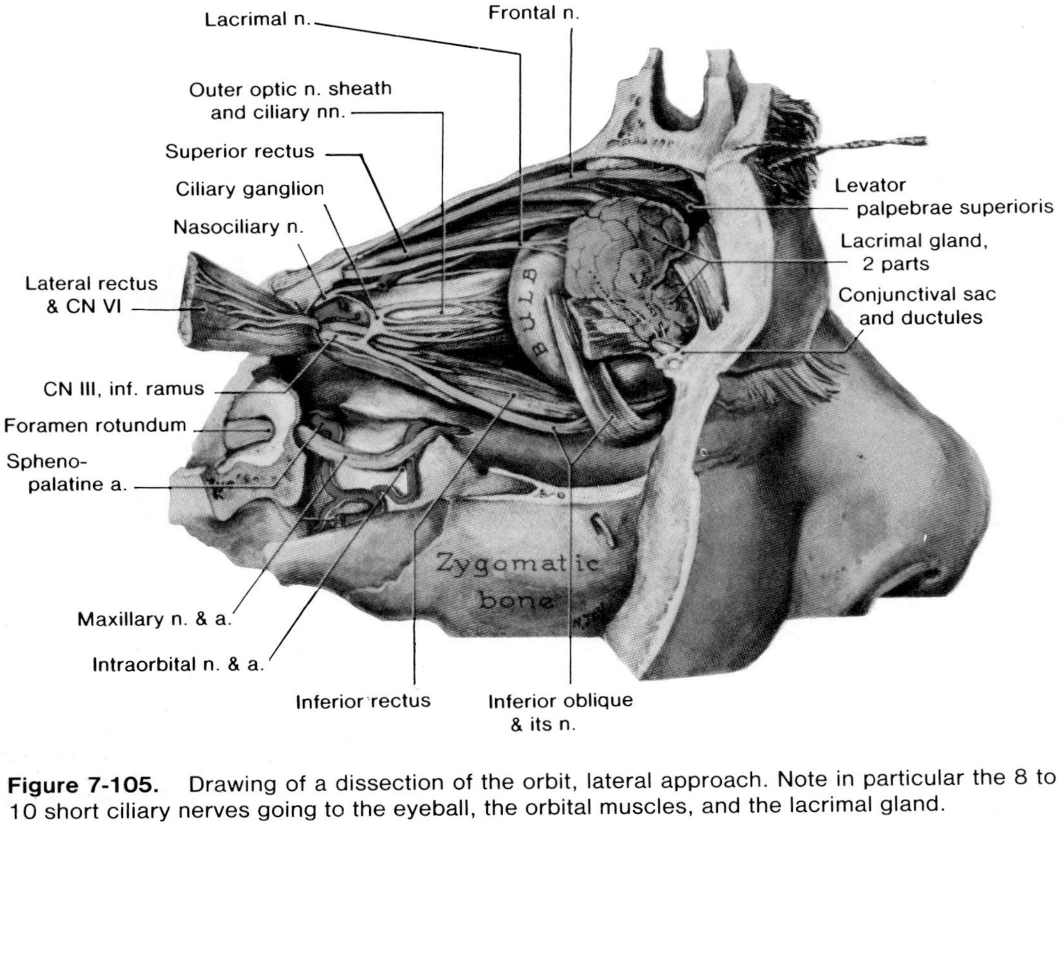

Figure 7-105. Drawing of a dissection of the orbit, lateral approach. Note in particular the 8 to 10 short ciliary nerves going to the eyeball, the orbital muscles, and the lacrimal gland.

mock below the eyeball, it supports this organ.

CLINICALLY ORIENTED COMMENTS

The cup-like fascial sheath of the eyeball helps to form a socket for an artificial eye when the eyeball is removed (**enuclation**). After this operation, the eye muscles cannot retract far because their fascial sheaths are attached to the fascial sheath of the eyeball. Because the suspensory ligament of the eye supports the eyeball, it is preserved when surgical removal of the floor of the orbit is carried out.

The Muscles of the Orbit (Extraocular or Extrinsic Ocular Muscles). There are seven voluntary muscles of the orbit, all of which move the eyeball except the levator palpebrae superioris, which elevates the upper eyelid (Fig. 7-31). The **six ocular muscles** are capable of rotating the eyeball in any direction. There are four straight (L. *rectus*) and two oblique muscles.

Levator Palpebrae Superioris Muscle (Figs. 7-31, 7-96, 7-98, 7-99, 7-106, and 7-109). This thin, triangular-shaped muscle elevates the upper eyelid. *The levator palpebrae superioris muscle does not insert into the eyeball and so cannot move it.* It arises from the inferior surface of the **lesser wing of the sphenoid** bone, above and anterior to the optic canal. This thick muscle *fans out into a wide aponeurosis* that inserts into the **skin of the upper eyelid.** The inferior part of this aponeurosis contains some smooth muscle fibers that are called the **superior tarsal muscle** (Figs 7-96*A* and 7-98). These involuntary muscle fibers insert into the tarsal plate.

The levator palpebrae superioris is innervated by the superior branch of the oculomotor nerve (CN III), whereas the superior tarsal muscle is innervated by sympathetic fibers from the **superior cervical ganglion**. The superior tarsal muscle presumably assists the levator palpebrae superioris muscle in elevating the eyelid and is responsible for the wide-eyed stare of a frightened person.

CLINICALLY ORIENTED PROBLEMS

Injury to sympathetic fibers from the superior cervical ganglion to the superior tarsal muscle (*e.g.*, inadvertently during thyroidectomy) and/or excision of this ganglion during surgery (*e.g.*, during removal of a malignant tumor in the neck) results in a slight lowering (**ptosis**) of the upper eyelid owing to loss of tone and/or paralysis of the **superior tarsal muscle**. In these cases, more of the iris is covered by the upper eyelid than is usual (Fig. 7-97). This type of ptosis (G. a falling) of the eyelid is a characteristic of the **Horner syndrome**, which also includes pupillary constriction. Patients with **hemisection of the cervical region of the spinal cord** also have Horner syndrome on the side of the lesion owing to interruption of descending **autonomic fibers** in the lateral white column of the spinal cord.

In **third nerve palsy** (Cases 7-5 and 7-6), the levator palpebrae superioris is involved and the upper eyelid is in complete ptosis, *i.e.*, the eye is completely closed and the upper lid cannot be raised voluntarily.

In **seventh nerve paralysis**, the levator palpebrae superioris muscle, acting unopposed because the **orbicularis oculi** muscle, used for gentle closing of the eye is paralyzed, elevates the upper eyelid, keeping the eye open (even during sleeping). Protective blinking is lost and irritation of the unprotected and dry cornea results, which could lead to ulceration of the cornea. (See discussion of Case 7-1.)

The Rectus Muscles (Superior, Inferior, Medial, and Lateral). The **four** rectus (L. straight) muscles arise by a tough tendinous cuff, called the **common tendinous ring** (common ring tendon), which surrounds the optic canal and the junction of the superior and inferior orbital fissures (Figs. 7-106 and 7-107). *From their common origin,* the four recti run forward close to the walls of the orbit and *insert into the eyeball,* just behind the **sclerocorneal junction**. Each muscle passes forward in the position implied by its name. All the recti are supplied by the **oculomotor nerve** (CN III), except the lateral rectus, which is supplied

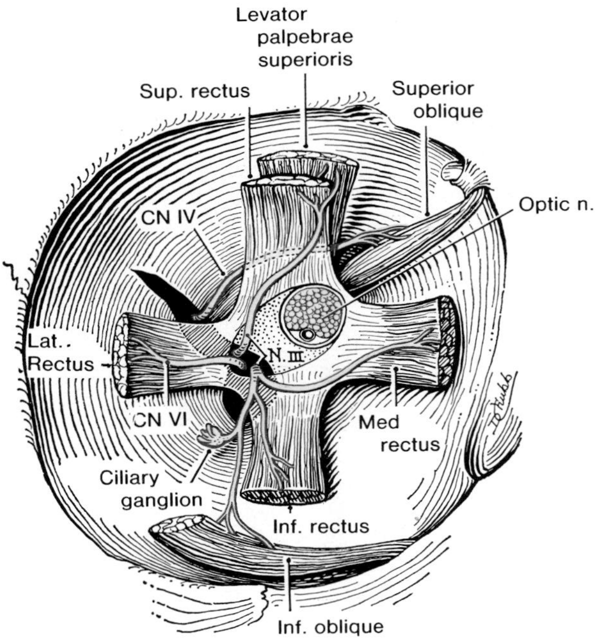

Figure 7-106. Dissection of the orbit showing the common tendinous ring and the motor nerves of the orbit. Observe the large optic nerve surrounded by its meningeal layers. Note the four rectus muscles arising from the fibrous cuff known as the common tendinous ring that encircles the dural sheath of the optic nerve (CN II), the abducent nerve (CN VI), and the upper and lower divisions of the oculomotor nerve (CN III). The nasociliary nerve (not shown) also passes through this cuff, but the trochlear nerve (CN IV) clings to the bony roof of the cavity and is outside the common tendinous ring. CN IV and CN VI supply one muscle each and CN III supplies the remaining five orbital muscles: two via its upper division and three via its lower division. The oculomotor nerve (CN III) via the ciliary ganglion supplies parasympathetic fibers to the ciliary muscle and the sphincter pupillae muscle.

by the **abducens nerve** (CN VI). Note that the lateral and medial recti lie in the same horizontal plane, whereas the superior and inferior recti lie in the same vertical plane.

The Oblique Muscles, Superior and Inferior (Figs. 7-105 to 7-110). **The superior oblique muscle** is fusiform and *arises from the body of the sphenoid* superomedial to the common tendinous ring and passes forward above and medial to the superior and medial recti. It ends in a round tendon which runs through a fibrocartilaginous loop called the **trochlea** (Fig. 7-108), which is attached to the superomedial angle of the orbital wall. After passing through the trochlea, the tendon of the superior oblique turns posterolaterally and *inserts into the sclera* at the posterosuperior aspect of the lateral side of the orbit.

The inferior oblique muscle is a thin, narrow muscle that *arises from the floor of the orbit* (orbital surface of the maxilla) lateral to the nasolacrimal canal (Fig. 7-106). It passes laterally and posteriorly, inferior to the inferior rectus muscle, and inserts into the sclera at the posteroinferior aspect of the lateral side of the orbit (Fig. 7-109).

Summary of the Nerve Supply of the Muscles of the Orbit (Fig. 7-109). All three cranial nerves supplying the muscles of the eyeball (the oculomotor, **CN III**; the trochlear, **CN IV**; and the abducens, **CN VI**) enter the orbit through the **superior orbital fissure**. Cranial nerves IV and VI each supply one muscle, whereas CN III supplies the remaining five muscles. **CN IV** supplies the superior oblique (SO); **CN VI** supplies the lateral rectus (LR); and **CN III**

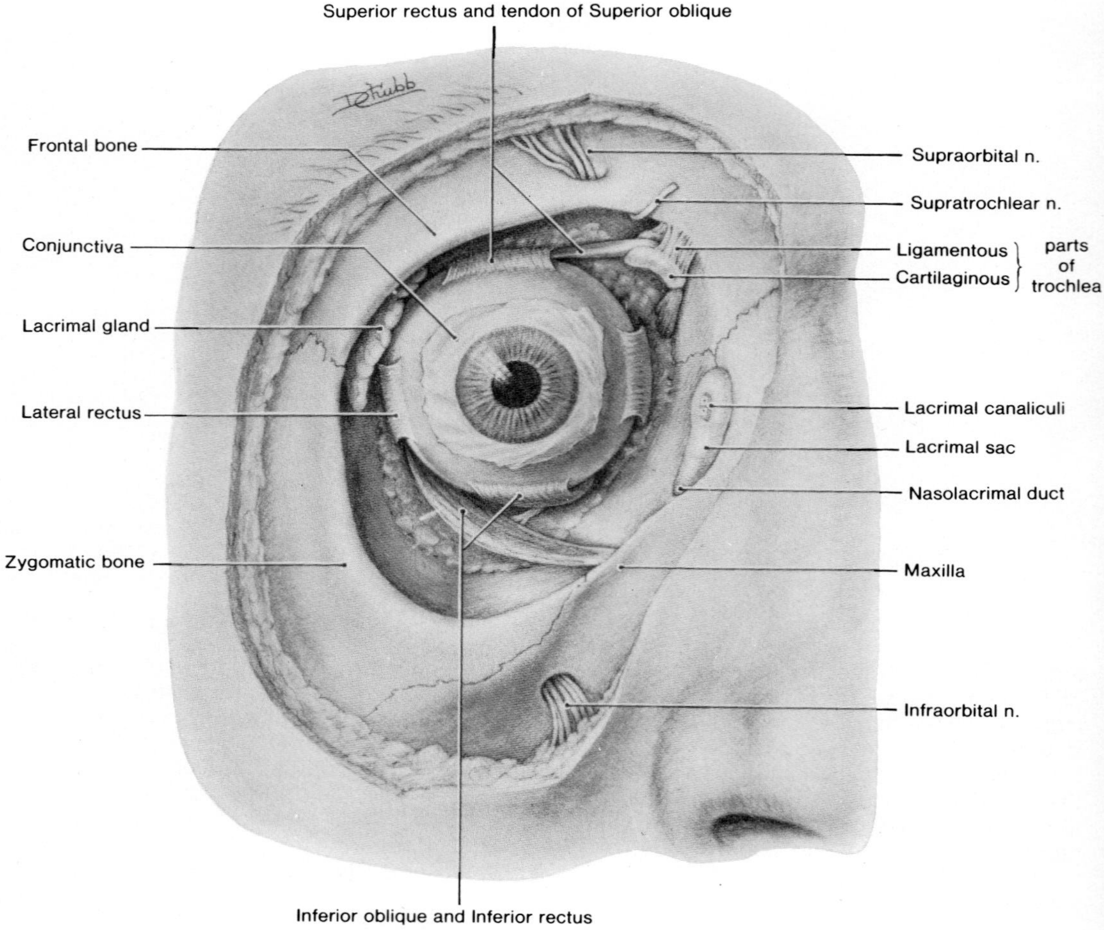

Figure 7-107. Drawing of a dissection of the orbital cavity from the front. The eyelids, orbital septum, levator palpebrae superioris, and some fat have been removed. Observe the aponeurotic insertion of the four rectus muscles, inserted 6 to 8 mm behind the sclerocorneal junction. Note the superior and inferior oblique muscles crossing inferior to the corresponding superior and inferior rectus muscles and the tendon of the superior oblique running through a cartilaginous pulley or trochlea, which is fixed by ligamentous fibers just behind the superomedial angle of the orbital margin.

supplies the levator palpebrae superioris (muscle of eyelid, not of eyeball), superior rectus (SR), medial rectus (MR), inferior rectus (IR), and inferior oblique (IO). Hence, all three nerves carry fibers which are motor to extraocular muscles (muscles of the eyeball). *In summary*, all orbital muscles are supplied by CN III except the superior oblique and the lateral rectus, which are supplied by CN IV and VI, respectively (*i.e.*, SO IV, LR VI, all others III). The following "formula" is worth committing to memory: $SO_4(LR_6)_3$.

Actions of the Six Ocular Muscles (Fig. 7-110). The six extraocular muscles rotate the eyeball in the orbit about three axes (sagittal, horizontal, and vertical). Verify that the four rectus muscles are arranged around the orbital axis, not around the anteroposterior, sagittal, or optic axis; thus, medial, superior, and inferior recti, respectively, are adductors.

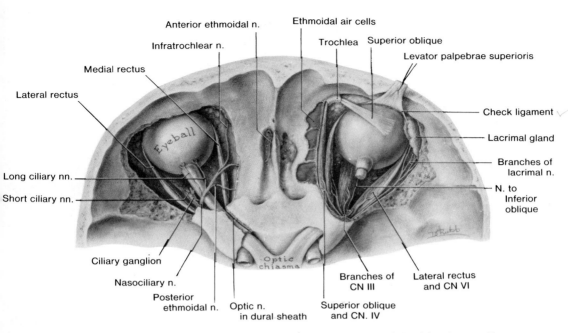

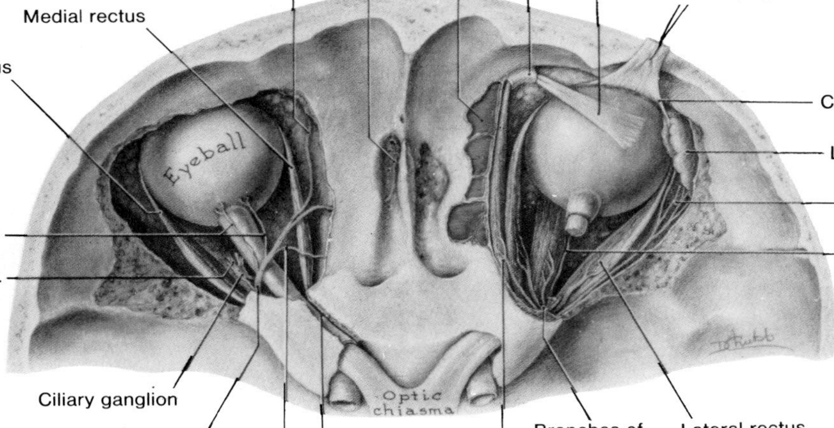

Figure 7-108. Dissection of the orbital cavities from above. On the *right side*, observe the nerves to the six ocular muscles (the four recti and the two obliqui), the trochlear to obliquus superior, the abducent to rectus lateralis, and the oculomotor to the remaining four eye muscles and also to the levator palpebrae superioris muscle.

Do not try to memorize the actions of the ocular muscles. Be able to make simple sketches like those in Figure 7-110 and you can easily work them out. *Study Table 7-1.*

CLINICALLY ORIENTED COMMENTS

Knowing the actions of the ocular muscles is important not only for understanding their effect on the field of vision but also for clinical testing of the cranial nerves supplying them.

The paralysis of one or more muscles owing to injury of the nerves supplying them results in **diplopia** (double vision). Paralysis of a muscle of the eyeball is noted by the limitation of movement of the eye in the field of action of the paralyzed muscle and by the production of two images when an attempt is made to use the paralyzed muscle.

When the abducens nerve is paralyzed, the patient is unable to abduct the eye on the affected side (see Case 8-3 and Fig. 8-25). Usually there is also double vision. You can produce this by preventing abduction of your eye with your finger. Two images are then seen; this is called **diplopia** .

For **clinical testing**, each muscle is examined in its position of greatest efficiency, *i.e.*, when its action is at a right angle to the axis around which it is moving the eyeball. The patient is asked to look: upward and outward to test the superior rectus; downward and outward to test the inferior rectus; upward and inward to test the inferior oblique; downward and inward to test the superior oblique; inward to test the medial rectus; and outward to test the lateral rectus.

The eyes of patients with **Graves' disease** (a form of hyperthyroidism) commonly protrude, a condition known as **exophthalmos** or **proptosis** (G. a falling forward), as exhibited in Case 9-5. The association of hyperthyroidism and exophthalmos was first described by Dr. Graves, but the cause of this protrusion is not precisely

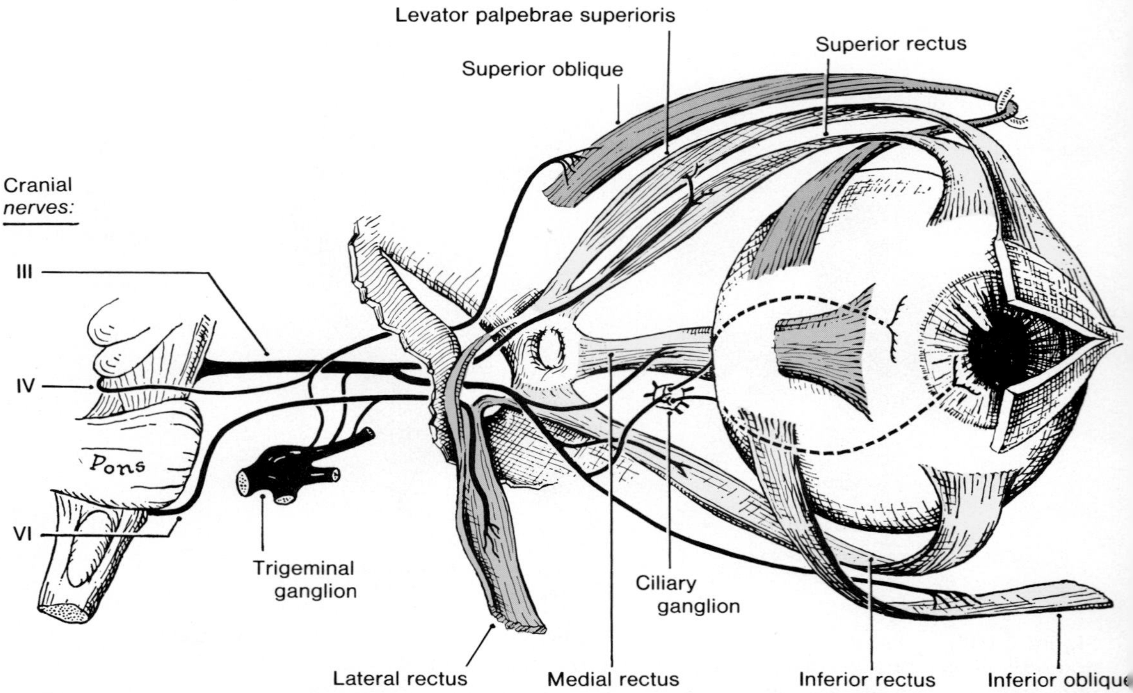

Figure 7-109. Diagram illustrating the distribution of the oculomotor (CN III), trochlear (CN IV), and abducent (CN VI) nerves to the muscles of the eyeball, which enter the orbit through the superior orbital fissure. Note that CN IV supplies the superior oblique, CN VI supplies the lateral rectus, and CN III supplies the remaining five muscles. The ciliary ganglion is a parasympathetic ganglion. Its postsynaptic fibers pass in the short ciliary nerves (– – – –) to the eyeball.

known. A considerable increase in the size of the orbital muscles can be observed in CT scans, but no increase in orbital fat is obvious.

Orbital Vessels. The orbital contents are supplied chiefly by the **ophthalmic artery**. The infraorbital artery, the continuation of the maxillary, also contributes to the supply of this region. Venous drainage is through the two **ophthalmic veins**, superior and inferior, which pass through the superior orbital fissure to enter the **cavernous sinus** (Figs. 7-38 and 7-111).

The Ophthalmic Artery (Fig. 7-112). The ophthalmic artery, a branch of the internal carotid as it emerges from the **cavernous sinus**, passes through the optic foramen within the dural sheath of the **optic nerve** (Figs. 7-111 and 7-113). It runs forward close to the superomedial wall of the orbit, giving off branches to structures in the orbit and to the ethmoid bone.

The central artery of the retina (Fig. 7-101), one of the smallest but most important branches of the ophthalmic, arises below the optic nerve (Fig. 7-112). It runs within the dural sheath of the optic nerve until it approaches the eyeball and then it pierces the optic nerve; it runs within it to emerge through the optic disc (Fig. 7-101). It spreads over the internal surface of the retina and supplies it. Twigs of this artery anastomose with the ciliary arteries, but *its terminal branches are essentially end arteries.*

CLINICALLY ORIENTED COMMENTS

Because the retinal artery is essentially an end artery, obstruction of it by an **em-**

bolus or by **thrombosis** leads to instant and **total blindness** in the eye concerned.

The ciliary arteries, branches of the ophthalmic (Figs. 7-111 and 7-112), supply the sclera, choroid, ciliary body, and iris. Two long posterior ciliary arteries pierce the sclera and supply the ciliary body and the iris. Several short posterior ciliary ar-

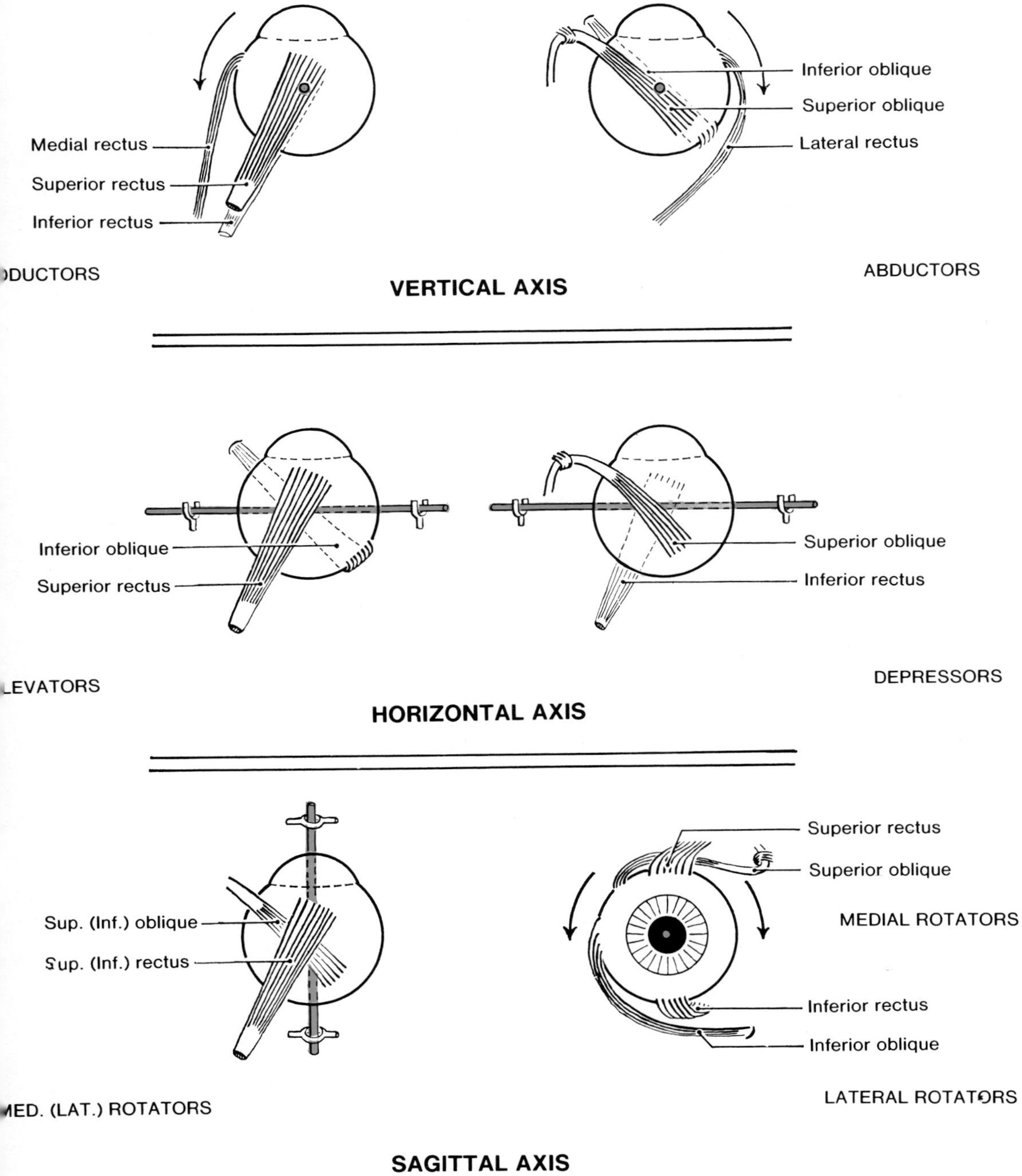

Figure 7-110. Diagrams illustrating the actions of the six ocular muscles. The right eyeball is represented in each instance.

Table 7-1
Actions and Nerve Supply of the Ocular Muscles

Muscle	Action(s) on Eyeball	Nerve Supply
Medial rectus	**adducts**	CN III
Lateral rectus	**abducts**	CN VI
Superior rectus	**elevates, adducts,** and rotates medially	CN III
Inferior rectus	**depresses, adducts,** and rotates laterally	CN III
Superior oblique	**depresses medially rotated eye,** abducts, and rotates medially	CN IV
Inferior oblique	**elevates medially rotated eye,** abducts, and rotates laterally	CN III

Notes:

1. The medial rectus and the lateral rectus move the eyeball in one axis only, whereas each of the other four muscles moves it in all three axes (see Fig. 7-109).
2. Cranial nerves IV and VI each supply one muscle, whereas CN III supplies the other four muscles.
3. The two oblique muscles protrude the eyeball, whereas the four rectus muscles retract it.
4. The superior and inferior oblique muscles are used with the medial rectus muscle in turning both eyes inward for near vision. This movement, accompanied by pupillary constriction, is known as **accommodation** and is used when examining a near object or when reading.

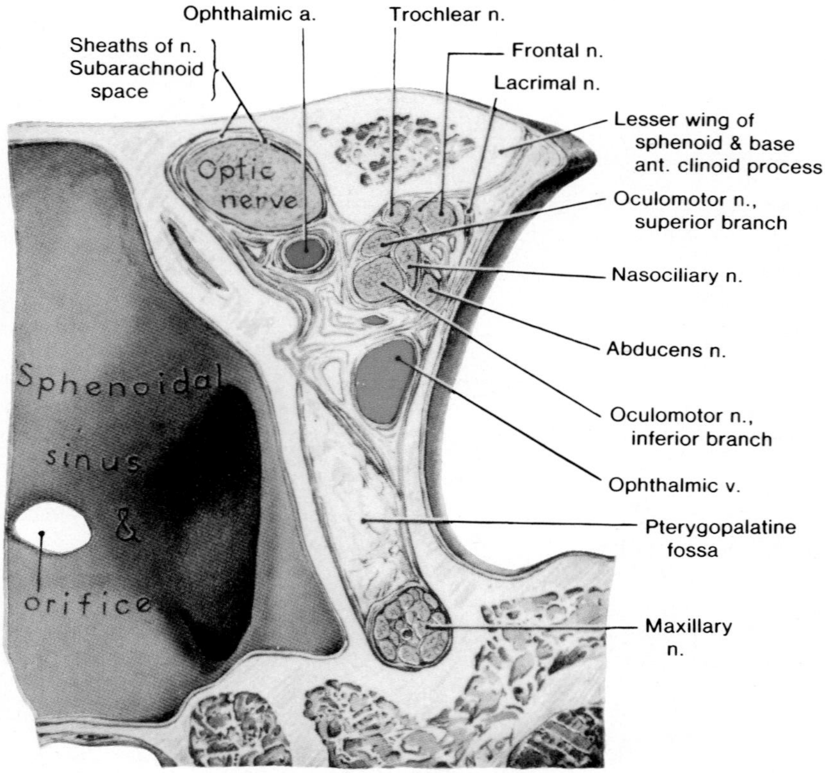

Figure 7-111. Drawing of a coronal section of the apex of the orbital cavity. Observe the optic nerve surrounded by its sheaths (extensions of the cranial meninges), the subarachnoid space, and the ophthalmic artery, a branch of the internal carotid artery, as they enter the optic canal. Note that the nerves to the orbit are crowded together as they pass through the medial end of the superior orbital fissure. Note also the ophthalmic vein, about to open into the cavernous sinus. (See Fig. 7-38 for orientation.)

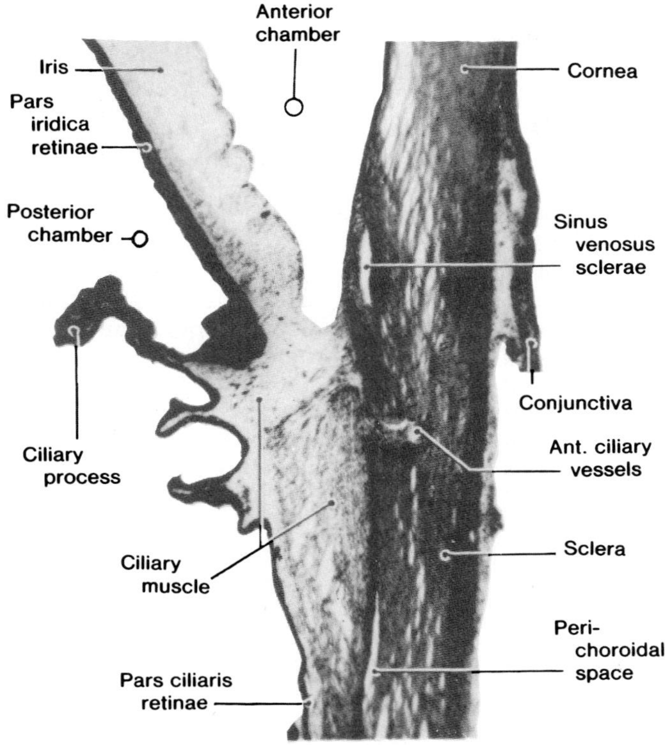

Figure 7-112. Photomicrograph of a section of the iridocorneal region. The aqueous humor in the anterior chamber escapes into anterior ciliary veins through the sinus venous sclerae, a ring-like venous sinus or canal near the anterior edge of the sclera.

teries pierce the sclera and supply the choroid.

The lacrimal artery (Fig. 7-112) supplies the lacrimal gland, the conjunctiva, and the eyelids. A **recurrent meningeal branch** anastomoses with the middle meningeal artery, hence, an anastomosis between branches of the internal and external carotid arteries.

The muscular branches to the eye muscles frequently arise from a common trunk and accompany the branches of the oculomotor nerve. Muscular branches also give rise to **anterior ciliary arteries**, which give branches to the conjunctiva and then pierce the sclera to supply the iris.

Five other branches of the ophthalmic artery leave the orbit with correspondingly named nerves and anastomose with branches of the external carotid artery. They are the *supraorbital, supratrochlear*, and *dorsal nasal arteries* which end on the forehead or face and the anterior and posterior *ethmoidal arteries* (Fig. 7-112) which enter the skull but end in the nasal mucosa.

The Ophthalmic Veins (Fig. 7-38). There are two ophthalmic veins, superior and inferior. The **superior ophthalmic vein** anastomoses with the facial vein; *as it has no valves, blood can flow in either direction*. It crosses above the optic nerve, passes through the superior orbital fissure, and ends in the cavernous sinus.

The **inferior ophthalmic vein** begins as a plexus on the floor of the orbit, communicates through the inferior orbital fissure with the **pterygoid plexus** (Fig. 7-38), crosses below the optic nerve, and ends either in the superior ophthalmic vein or in the cavernous sinus.

The **central vein of the retina** (Fig. 7-

101) usually enters the cavernous sinus directly, but it may join one of the ophthalmic veins, usually the superior ophthalmic.

CLINICALLY ORIENTED COMMENTS

Because the cavernous sinuses of the dura mater communicate with the veins of the face via the valveless superior and inferior ophthalmic veins, **thrombophlebitis** of the facial veins, resulting from infections of the face in the area drained by these veins, may spread to the cavernous sinus (Case 7-3). As the central vein of the retina enters either the cavernous sinus or the superior ophthalmic vein, thrombosis may sometimes extend along the central vein of the retina and produce thromboses in the small retinal veins. For this reason pustules or furuncles (boils) *on the face* should never be squeezed.

The Optic Nerve (Figs. 7-79, 7-87, 7-88, 7-96*A*, 7-101, 7-108, 7-111, and 7-113). This is the second cranial nerve and the nerve of sight. CN II is considered in detail in Chapter 8. It is about 5 cm in length and extends between the **optic chiasma** (G. a crossing) and the eyeball. The optic nerve is slightly longer than the distance it travels; thus, it permits free movement of the eyeball. *Most of the fibers of the optic nerve are afferent and arise from ganglion cells in the retina* (Fig. 8-6). The fibers lie internal or deep to the ganglion cells in the retina and converge on the optic disc (Fig. 7-101). The optic nerve passes backward and medially within a cone formed by the extraocular muscles and leaves the orbit through the optic canal to enter the optic chiasma slightly above and anterior to the tuberculum sellae.

During eye development the optic nerve carried forward sheaths of dura mater, arachnoid, and pia mater. These meninges enclose extensions of the subdural and sub-

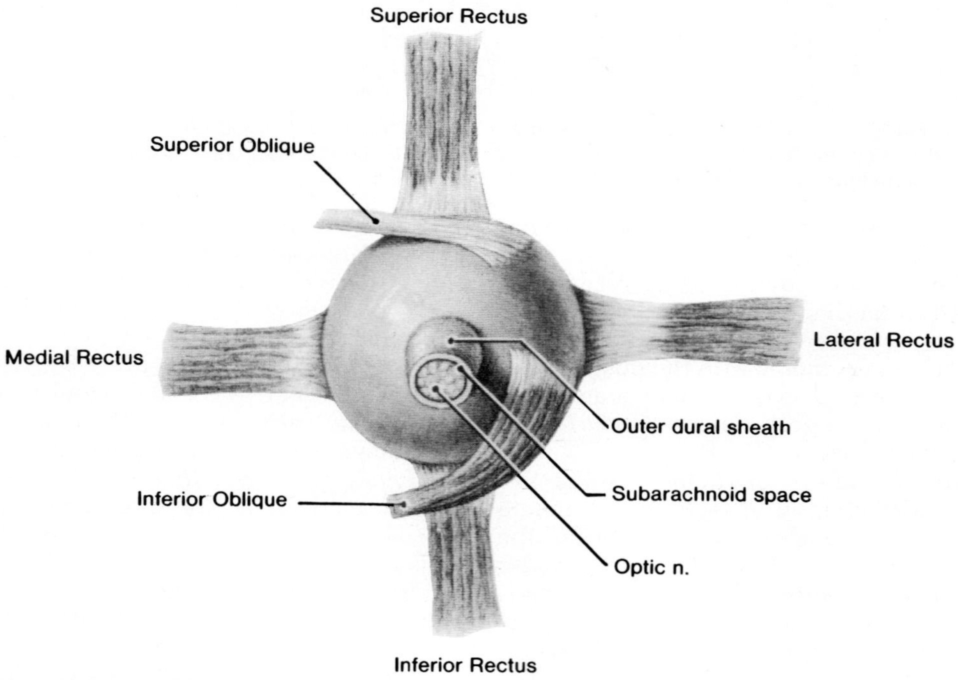

Figure 7-113. Drawing of a posterior view of the eyeball showing the insertions of the superior and inferior oblique muscles. Observe that the optic nerve is surrounded by a dural sheath and a subarachnoid space that are extensions from the meninges and subarachnoid space covering the brain.

arachnoid spaces (Figs. 7-96*A*, 7-101, and 7-113) as far as the eyeball.

PAROTID, TEMPORAL, AND INFRATEMPORAL REGIONS

THE PAROTID REGION

This region is mainly the space between the mastoid process of the temporal bone and the neck and ramus of the mandible. It contains the **parotid gland** (which surrounds part of the posterior edge of the ramus) as well as the structures related to this gland.

The Parotid Gland and the Parotid Bed (Figs. 7-114 to 7-119). The parotid gland and the parotid duct were described previously with the face (p. 894). The **parotid bed** occupied by the parotid gland is a small space between the mastoid process posteriorly and the ramus of the mandible anteriorly. **Superiorly**, it is bounded by the floor of the *external acoustic meatus* and the *zygomatic process* of the temporal bone. **Medially** (deeply), there is the *styloid process* and its associated muscles. **Laterally** (superficially), the space is bounded by the superficial layer of the parotid fascia and skin.

The posterior wall of the parotid bed extends between the mastoid and styloid processes; thus, the muscles attached to them (sternocleidomastoid, posterior belly of the digastric, and the stylohyoid) are

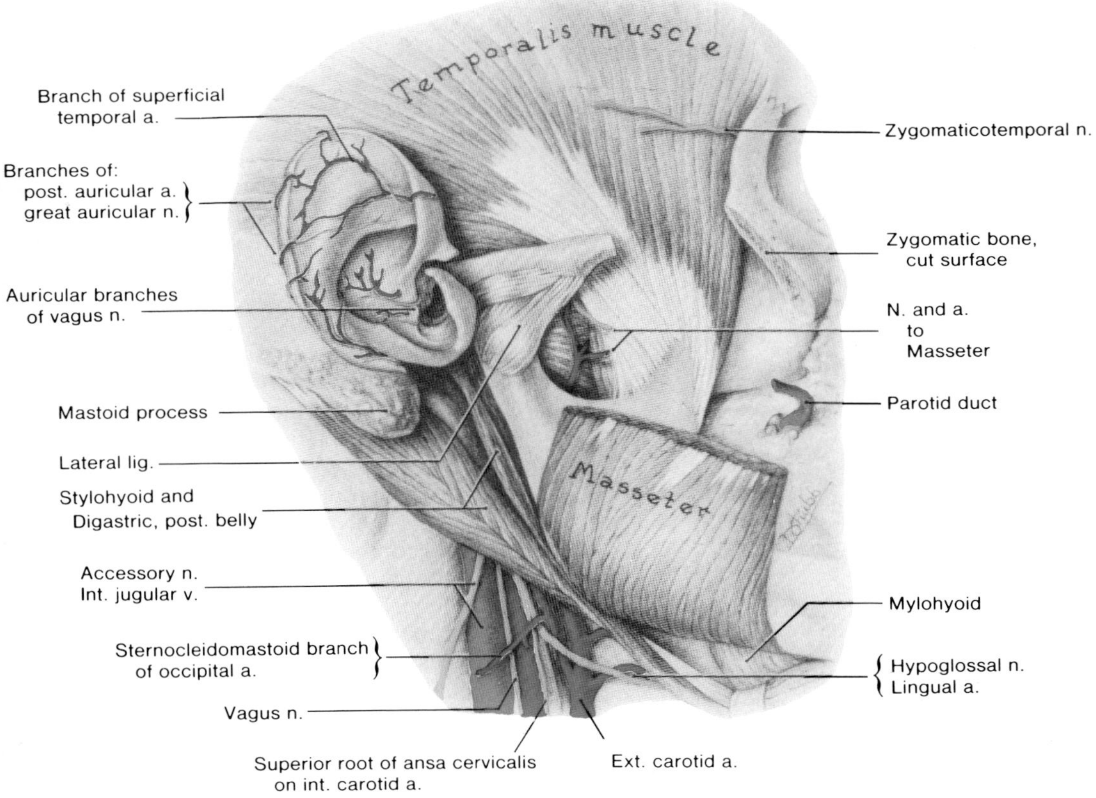

Figure 7-114. Drawing of a dissection of the parotid bed, the temporalis muscle, and the auricular vessels and nerves. The sternocleidomastoid, splenius capitus, and longissimus capitus muscles have been removed from the mastoid process. Note the posterior belly of the digastric muscle arising deep to the mastoid process and passing deep to the angle of the mandible. This muscle is closely related to the parotid gland as shown in Figure 7-115.

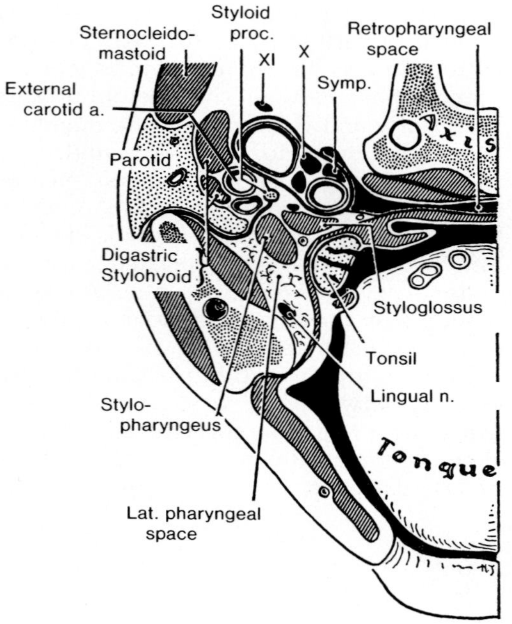

Figure 7-115. Drawing of a cross-section at the level of the parotid gland. Observe that this gland fills its wedge-shaped bed and that the digastric and stylohyoid muscles intervene between it and the great vessels and nerves of the neck. Note also the masseter muscle inserted into the outer surface of the ramus of the mandible and the medial pterygoid muscle inserted into its inner surface. (The other structures shown in this drawing are described in Chap. 9 and illustrated in Fig. 9-62.)

closely related to the parotid gland (Figs. 7-114 and 7-115).

The anterior wall of the parotid bed is formed by the ramus of the mandible and the two muscles (masseter and medial pterygoid) attached to it (Fig. 7-115). The **parotid gland**, enclosed within fascia called the **parotid sheath**, occupies all the space available to it in the area around the posterior margin of the mandible.

Structures Within the Parotid Gland (Figs. 7-32, 7-41, and 7-115 to 7-117). From superficial to deep, structures traversing the parotid gland are the **facial nerve**, the **retromandibular vein**, and the **external carotid artery**. There are also parotid lymph nodes on or deep to the parotid fascia and within the gland.

The facial nerve (CN VII) is unique in traversing the parotid gland, an event of considerable clinical significance. During its early development, the gland lies between the two major branches of the facial nerve. As the gland enlarges, it overlaps these branches and superficial and deep parts of the gland fuse intimately with each other between and around the branches of the facial nerve (Fig. 7-117).

The facial nerve emerges from the stylomastoid foramen and can be exposed in the notch between the mastoid process and the external acoustic meatus (Fig. 7-118). Beyond this, the nerve enters the posterior part of the parotid gland and divides almost at once into upper and lower divisions, which give rise to temporal, zygomatic, and buccal branches and to mandibular and cervical branches, respectively (Fig. 7-32). The branches of the facial nerve emerge on the anterior aspect of the periphery of the parotid gland (Fig. 7-117) and lie on the lateral surface of the **masseter muscle** (Fig. 7-116). From here, they pass to the muscles of facial expression which they supply.

The retromandibular vein (Figs. 7-37 and 7-41), formed by the union of the temporal and maxillary veins, descends in the parotid gland, superficial to the external carotid artery but deep to the facial nerve (Fig. 7-116). Blood drains from the parotid gland into the retromandibular vein, which joins the posterior auricular to form the external jugular vein via its posterior branch and the facial vein via its anterior branch.

The external carotid artery (Figs. 7-115 and 7-118) enters the deep surface of the parotid gland, where it lies deep to the facial nerve and the retromandibular vein. At the neck of the mandible, the external carotid artery divides into the **superficial temporal** and **maxillary arteries**. The external carotid and its branches supply blood to the parotid gland.

Nerves Near the Parotid Gland (Figs. 7-32, 7-41, 7-116, and 7-117). The **auriculotemporal nerve**, a branch of the mandibular division of the trigeminal nerve (CN V^3), is in the parotid space but passes superior to the upper part of the parotid gland. It communicates with the facial nerve, usually via two branches.

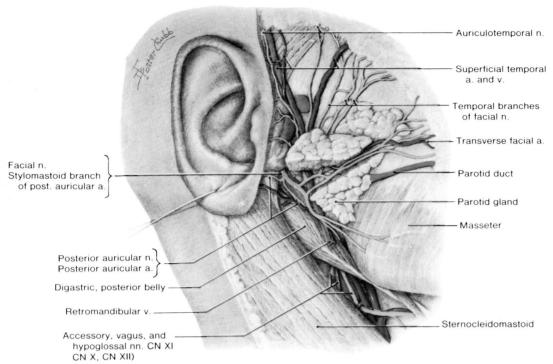

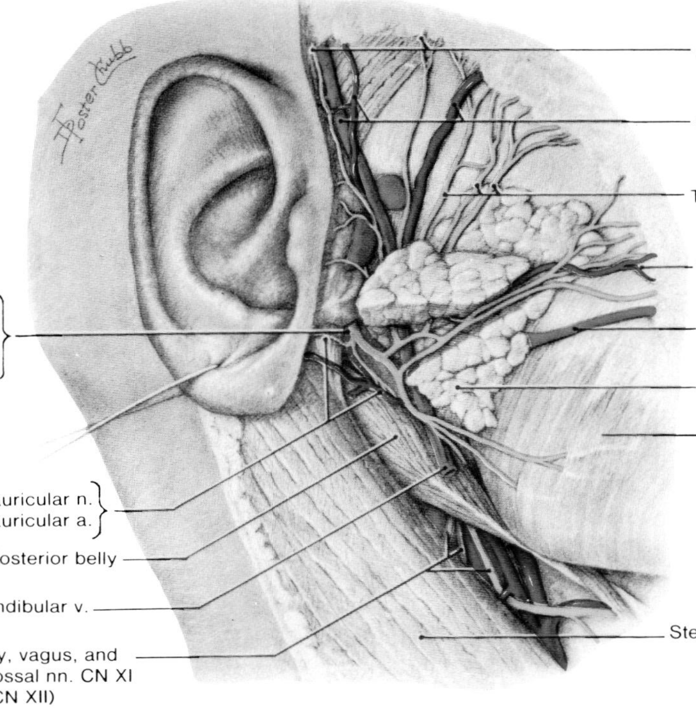

Figure 7-116. Drawing of a dissection of the parotid region. Part of the parotid gland has been removed to expose the facial nerve (CN VII). (For a more superficial dissection, see Fig. 7-41.) Observe the stem of the facial nerve descending from the stylomastoid foramen and then curving forward to penetrate the deep part of the parotid gland.

The great auricular nerve (C2, C3), a superficial ascending branch of the **cervical plexus** (Fig. 9-33), passes external to the parotid gland where it divides into an anterior and a posterior branch, but it usually does not enter the parotid gland.

Vessels of the Parotid Gland (Figs. 7-37, 7-116, 7-118, and 7-133). The parotid gland is supplied by the **external carotid artery** and its terminal branches (superficial temporal and maxillary arteries) that arise within the gland.

The veins drain into the *retromandibular vein* and then into the **external jugular vein** (Fig. 7-37).

Nerve Supply to the Parotid Gland (Fig. 7-119). The **parasympathetic** component of the glossopharyngeal nerve (**CN IX**) supplies secretory fibers to the parotid gland via the **otic ganglion.** Stimulation of these fibers produces a thin, watery saliva. Sensory nerve fibers pass to the gland via the great auricular and the auriculotemporal nerves. Sympathetic fibers also pass to the gland via a nerve plexus associated with the external carotid artery.

Lymph Drainage of the Parotid Gland (Figs. 7-39, 7-116, and 7-133). The parotid lymph nodes are located on or deep to the parotid fascia and within the gland. They receive lymph from the forehead, the lateral parts of the eyelids, the temporal region, the lateral surface of the auricle, and the anterior wall of the external acoustic meatus. The nodes within the gland also receive lymph from the middle ear. Lymph from the parotid nodes drains into the superficial and deep **cervical lymph nodes.**

THE TEMPORAL REGION

The Temporal Fossa (Figs. 7-1, 7-8, and 7-120 to 7-122). The temporal lines curve backward from the frontal process of the zygomatic bone and then curve forward to the posterior end of the zygomatic arch.

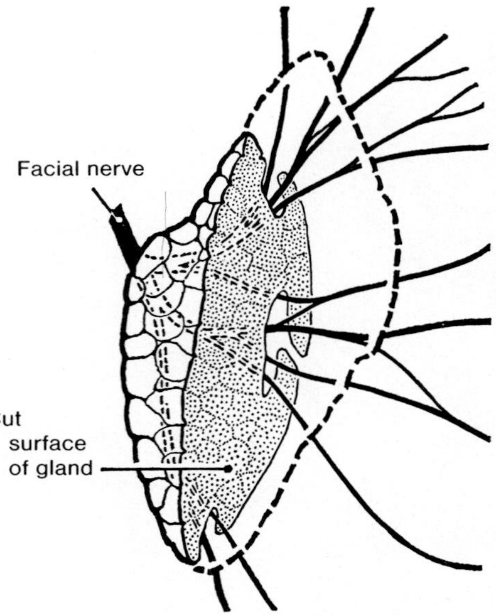

Figure 7-117. Diagram of the facial nerve showing its close relationship to the parotid gland. Observe that it enters the deep surface of the gland and divides into five terminal branches within it, which radiate forward and appear at the border of the gland as numerous smaller branches (also see Fig. 7-116).

The superior temporal line surrounds the **temporal fossa** and gives attachment to the **temporal fascia**. This strong membrane stretches over the temporal fossa and the **temporalis muscle**. Inferiorly it splits into two layers, superficial and deep. The superficial layer is attached to the upper margin of the zygomatic arch and the deep layer passes medial to the arch to become continuous with the fascia deep to the masseter muscle.

The floor of the temporal fossa, which gives origin to the temporalis muscle, is usually formed by portions of four bones: parietal, frontal, greater wing of the sphenoid, and squamous part of the temporal bone. The area where these bones meet is called the **pterion** (Figs. 7-7 and 7-15); see page 868 for a discussion of this clinically important area and Case 7-5.

The temporal fossa contains the fan-shaped **temporalis muscle**, the "handle" of which passes deep to the zygomatic arch. Note that the temporal fossa is deepest where the **temporalis** is thickest (*i.e.*, anteroinferiorly, Fig. 7-114), where it inserts into the coronoid process of the mandible and the anterior surface of the ramus (Fig. 7-22).

The masseter muscle is quadrilateral and consists of three superimposed layers that blend anteriorly. It covers the lateral surface of the ramus of the mandible but not the neck region (Fig. 7-21).

THE INFRATEMPORAL REGION

The infratemporal fossa is an irregularly shaped space behind the maxilla (Figs. 7-114, 7-123, and 7-124). This fossa communicates with the temporal fossa via the interval between the zygomatic arch and the skull, which is traversed by the temporalis (temporal) muscle and by the deep temporal nerves and vessels.

Bony Boundaries of the Infratemporal Fossa (Figs. 7-120 to 7-126). The **lateral wall** of this fossa is the *ramus of the mandible.* Its **medial wall** is formed by the *lateral pterygoid plate.* Follow the posterior free border of this plate upward to the foramen ovale in the roof of the infratemporal fossa. The rounded **anterior wall** of the infratemporal fossa, formed by the *infratemporal surface of the maxilla,* is limited superiorly by the inferior orbital fissure and medially by the pterygomaxillary fissure. Hold a dried skull up to a light and observe the eggshell thickness of this wall formed by the posterior wall of the maxillary sinus. The **posterior wall** of the infratemporal fossa is formed by the *anterior surface of the condylar process* (head and neck) of the mandible and the styloid process of the temporal bone.

The flat roof of the infratemporal fossa is formed mainly by the inferior surface of the *greater wing of the sphenoid bone.* The roof is separated from the temporal fossa by a ragged edge called the *infratemporal crest* (Fig. 7-123). Observe the **foramen ovale** in the roof of the fossa (Fig. 7-47*A*) and that the lateral pterygoid plate is the bony guide to this foramen (Fig. 7-123) which transmits the mandibular division of the trigeminal nerve (CN V^3). The **inferior boundary of** the infratemporal fossa is the point where the medial ptery-

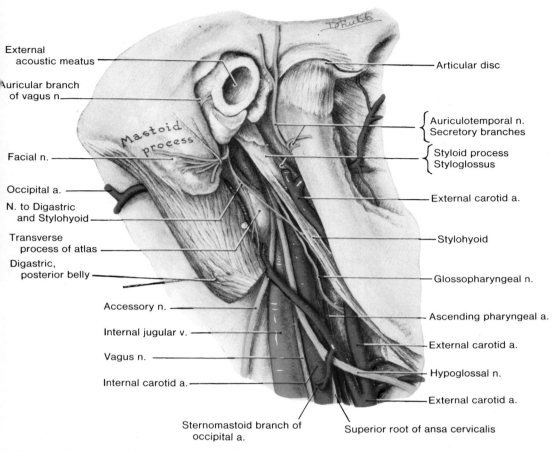

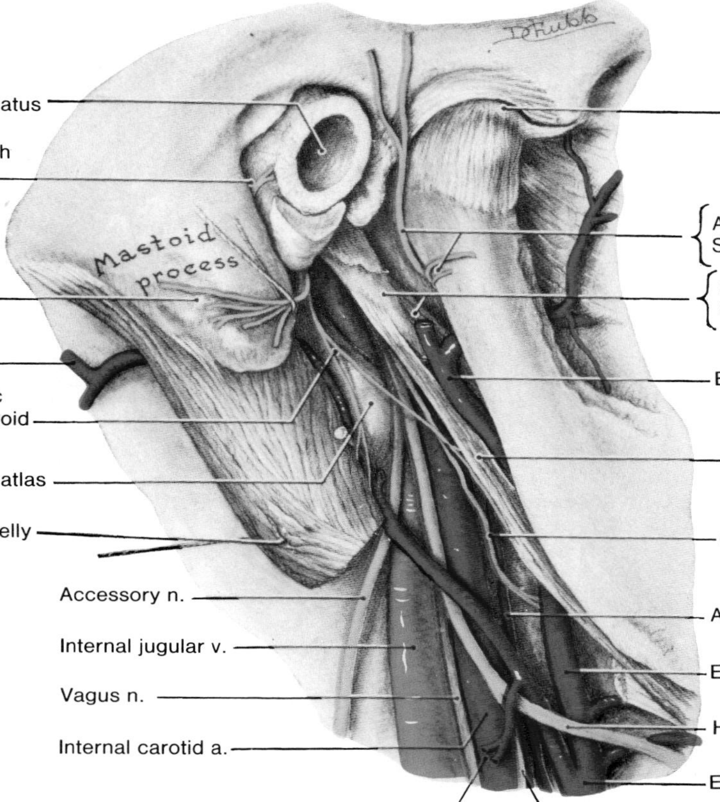

Figure 7-118. Drawing of a dissection of the structures deep to the parotid bed. The facial nerve, the posterior belly of the digastric, and the nerve to it are retracted. Observe the internal jugular vein, the internal carotid artery, and the last four cranial nerves crossing in front of the transverse process of the atlas and deep to the styloid process.

goid muscle inserts into the medial aspect of the mandible near the angle (Fig. 7-124).

Contents of the Infratemporal Fossa (Figs. 7-124 to 7-127). This fossa contains the lower part of the **temporalis muscle**, the medial and lateral **pterygoid muscles**, the **maxillary artery**, the **pterygoid venous plexus**, the **mandibular** and **chorda tympani nerves**, the **otic ganglion,** the **inferior alveolar**, **lingual**, and **buccal nerves**.

The temporalis muscle, which moves the mandible and acts on the temporomandibular joint, is discussed subsequently.

The Maxillary Artery (Figs. 7-124 to 7-127). This vessel, the larger of the two terminal branches of the **external carotid**, arises posterior to the neck of the mandible. Usually it passes through the infratemporal region, superficial or deep to the **lateral pterygoid muscle** (or even to the mandibular nerve). The maxillary artery is divided into three parts by the lateral pterygoid muscle.

The branches of the first part of the maxillary artery which pass through foramina or canals are: (1) the **deep auricular artery** to the external acoustic meatus; (2) the **anterior tympanic artery** to the tympanic membrane (eardrum); (3) the middle and (4) accessory **meningeal arteries** to the cranial cavity via the foramen

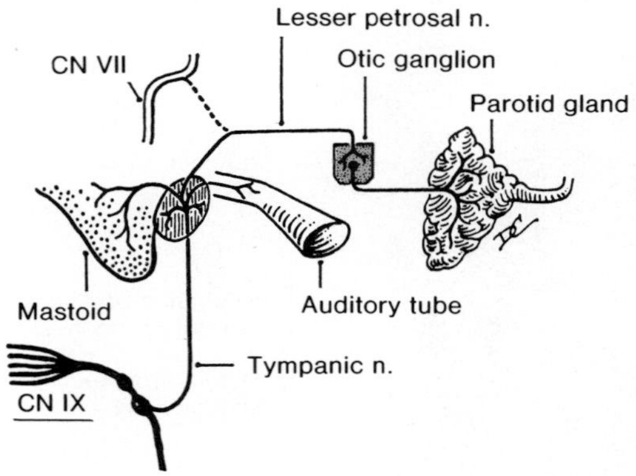

Figure 7-119. Diagram showing the glossopharyngeal nerve (CN IX) sending secretomotor fibers to the parotid gland via its tympanic branch, the lesser petrosal nerve, the otic ganglion, and the auriculotemporal nerve.

spinosum and the foramen ovale, respectively; and (5) the **inferior alveolar artery** to the mandible, gingivae (gums), and the teeth. The middle meningeal artery is of considerable surgical importance (Fig. 7-59).

The branches of the second part of the maxillary artery supply muscles by masseteric, deep temporal, pterygoid, and buccal branches (Fig. 7-126). The artery then passes through the pterygomaxillary fissure and enters the **pterygopalatine fossa**.

The branches of the third or pterygopalatine part of the maxillary artery arise just before and after it enters the pterygopalatine fossa: (1) posterior superior alveolar, (2) middle superior alveolar, (3) infraorbital, (4) descending palatine, (5) artery of the pterygoid canal, (6) pharyngeal, and (7)

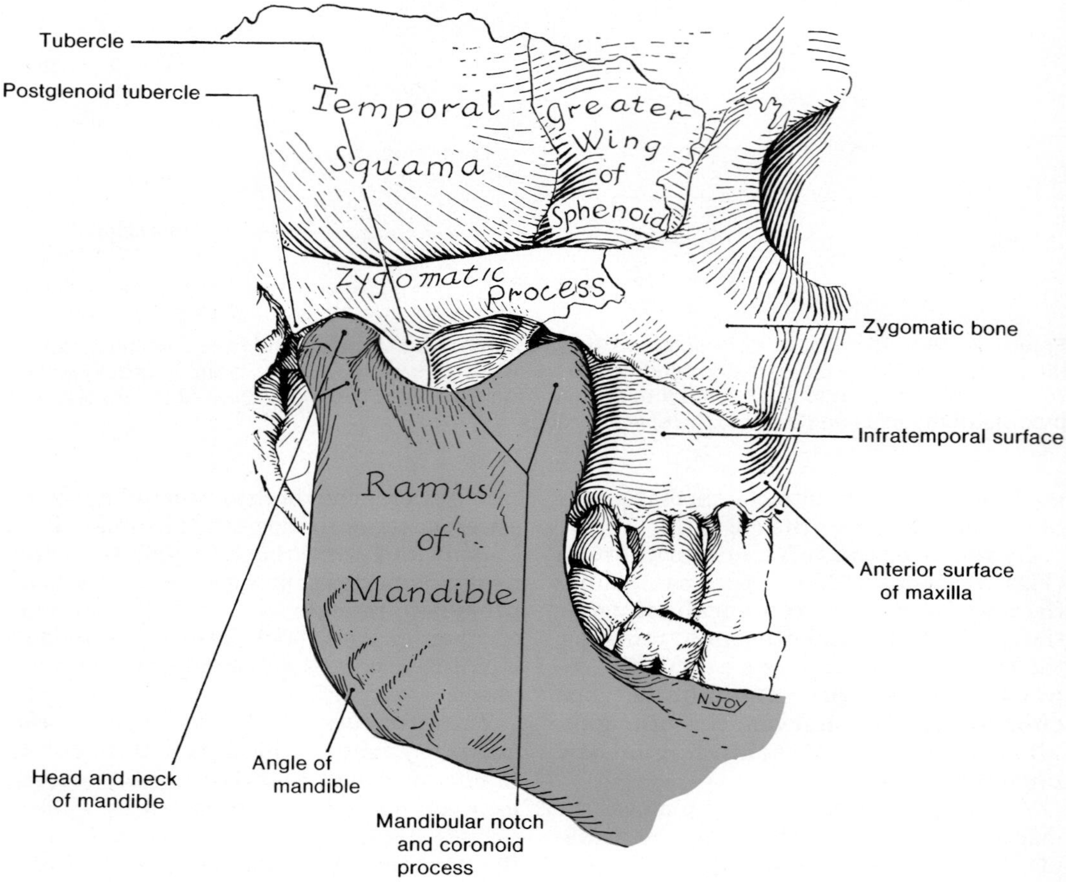

Figure 7-120. Drawing of part of the skull to show the lateral wall of the infratemporal fossa formed by the ramus of the mandible.

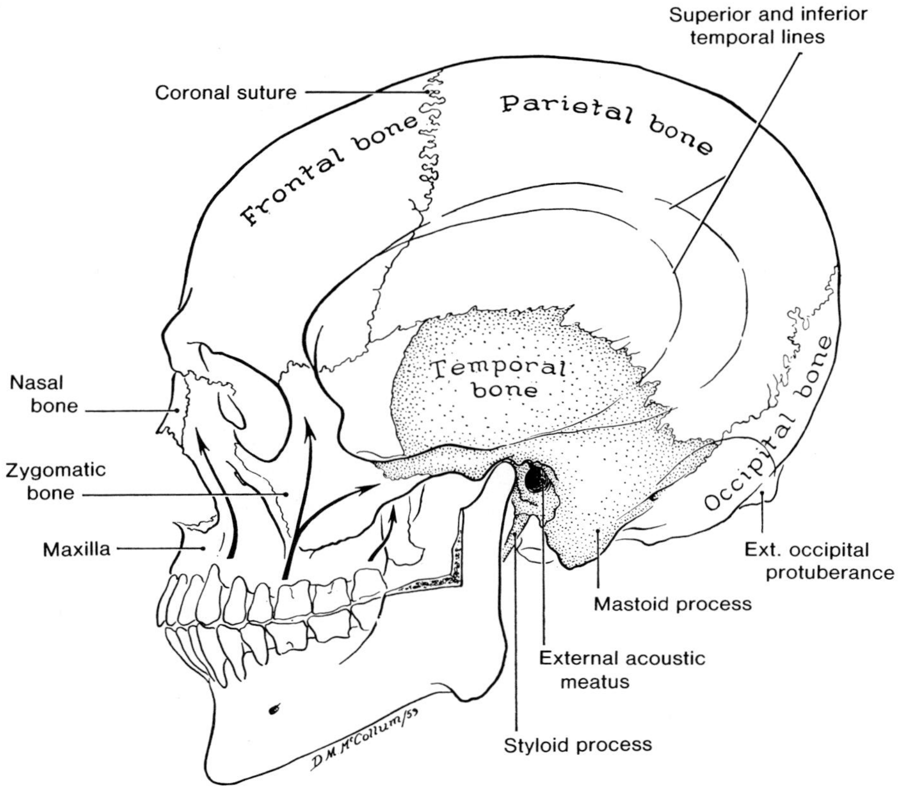

Figure 7-121. Drawing of the skull from the side (norma lateralis) showing the bony landmarks of the temporal and masseteric regions. The coronoid process of the mandible has been removed to show the pterygoid process of the sphenoid bone. The superior temporal line surrounds the temporal fossa and gives attachment to the temporal fascia. The *short arrow* indicates the anteroinferior and deepest part of the infratemporal fossa.

sphenopalatine. These arteries, accompanied by branches of the maxillary nerve, pass through bony canals or foramina.

The Pterygoid Plexus. This important venous plexus is located partly between the temporalis and the lateral pterygoid muscles and partly between the two pterygoid muscles. It has connections with the facial vein via the cavernous sinus (Fig. 7-38).

The Mandibular Nerve (CN V^3) (Table 7-2). All nerves of the infratemporal region except the **chorda tympani**, a branch of the facial (CN VII), are derived from this lowest division of the trigeminal nerve. Descending through the foramen ovale into the infratemporal fossa from the medial part of the middle cranial fossa (Figs. 7-47*A* and 7-55), the mandibular nerve divides at once into sensory and motor fibers (Fig. 7-128). Branches supply the four **muscles of mastication** (temporalis, masseter, and medial and lateral pterygoids) but not the buccinator, which is supplied by CN VII. The area of facial skin derived from the mandibular prominence (process) of the embryonic first branchial arch which CN V^3 supplies is illustrated in Figure 7-30. The three sensory branches of the mandibular nerve to the face are the **auriculotemporal**, **inferior alveolar**, and **buccal nerves** (Fig. 7-128). The mandibular nerve also supplies sensory fibers to the gingiva of the mandible via the lingual (medial side) and buccal (lateral side) nerves. The mandibular teeth are supplied by the inferior alveolar nerve.

The Auriculotemporal Nerve (Figs. 7-32, 7-116, 7-118, 7-124, 7-127, and 7-128). This nerve encircles the middle meningeal artery and breaks up into numerous branches, the

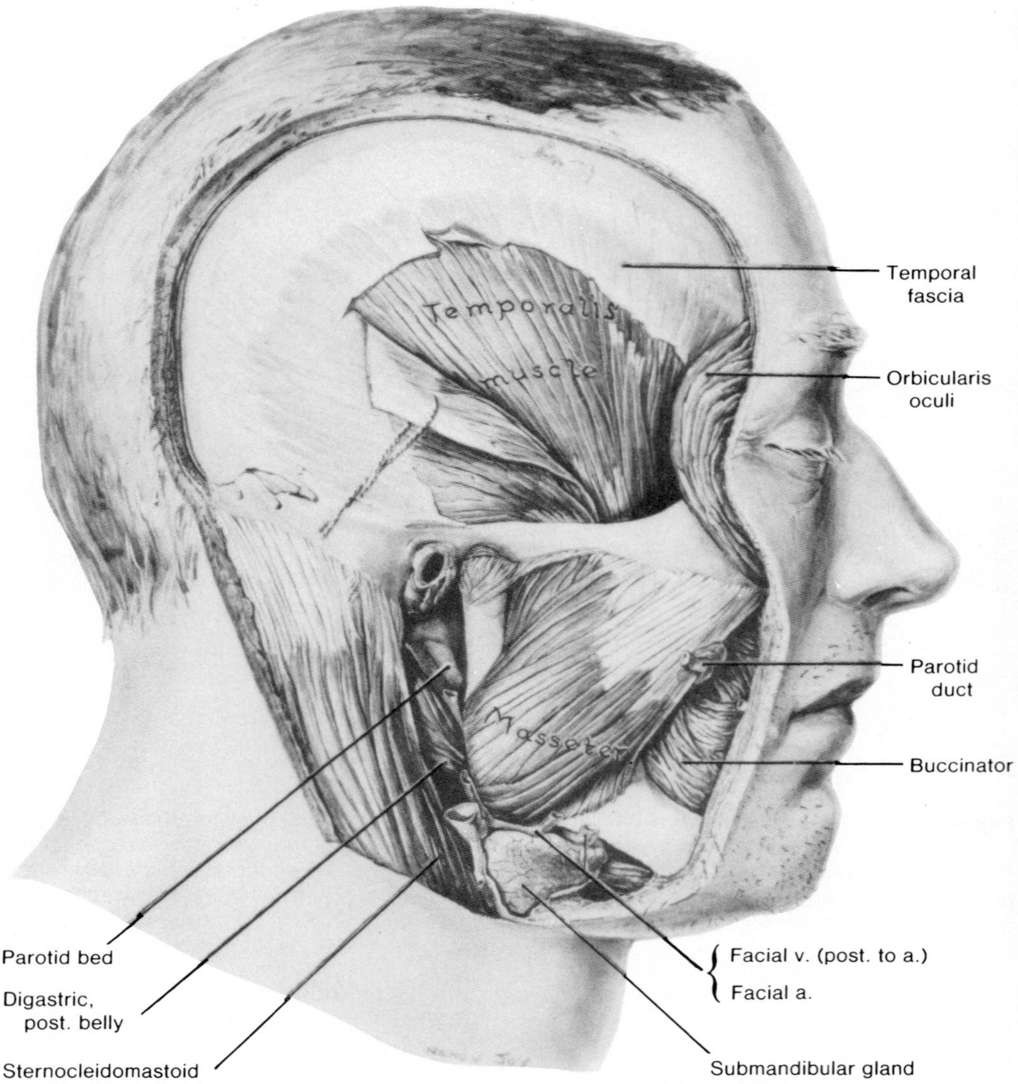

Figure 7-122. Drawing of the large muscles on the side of the head. Observe the temporalis and masseter muscles. Both are supplied by the trigeminal nerve and both close the jaw. The temporalis arises in part from the overlying temporal fascia.

largest of which passes backward medial to the neck of the mandible to supply sensory fibers to the **auricle** and the **temporal region**. It sends articular fibers to the **temporomandibular joint** and secretomotor fibers (parasympathetic) to the **parotid gland**.

The Buccal Nerve (Figs. 7-124, 7-125, 7-127, and 7-128). This long sensory nerve usually runs between the two heads of the lateral pterygoid muscle and descends through the deep fibers of the temporalis muscle, where its branches spread out over the lateral surface of the buccinator muscle. It supplies sensory fibers to the skin and the mucous membrane of the cheek, as well as to the lateral surface of the gingiva.

The Inferior Alveolar Nerve (Figs. 7-124, 7-125, and 7-127 to 7-129). This nerve, *commonly anesthetized in dental practice*, enters the mandibular foramen, passes through the mandibular canal, and appears on the face as the **mental nerve**. While in the canal, it sends nerves to all teeth in the mandible on its side.

The **mental nerve**, a branch of the inferior alveolar nerve, innervates the skin of the chin and the lower lip.

The **incisive nerve**, the terminal part of the inferior part of the alveolar nerve, after it has given off the mental nerve, continues within the mandible and supplies the canine and incisor teeth.

The Lingual Nerve (Figs. 7-124 and 7-127 to 7-129). This long nerve, lying anterior to the inferior alveolar nerve, is sensory to the tongue, the floor of the mouth, and the gingivae. It enters the mouth between the medial pterygoid muscle and the ramus of the mandible, passing anteriorly under the mucosa just below the third molar tooth.

CLINICALLY ORIENTED COMMENTS

Because the **lingual nerve** passes forward submucously just below the third molar tooth (Fig. 7-129), care must be taken not to damage it during operative procedures in the mouth (*e.g.*, removal of the third molar or "wisdom" tooth).

The **inferior alveolar nerve**, as it runs through the mandibular canal, passes close to the roots of the teeth (Fig. 7-130). Hence, it may be injured during removal of a malposed and impacted third molar tooth, as in Case 7-8).

Local anesthesia may be applied to the mandibular nerve, a procedure called a **mandibular nerve block**, as it emerges from the foramen ovale and enters the infratemporal fossa. The injection needle is passed about 5 cm through the mandibular

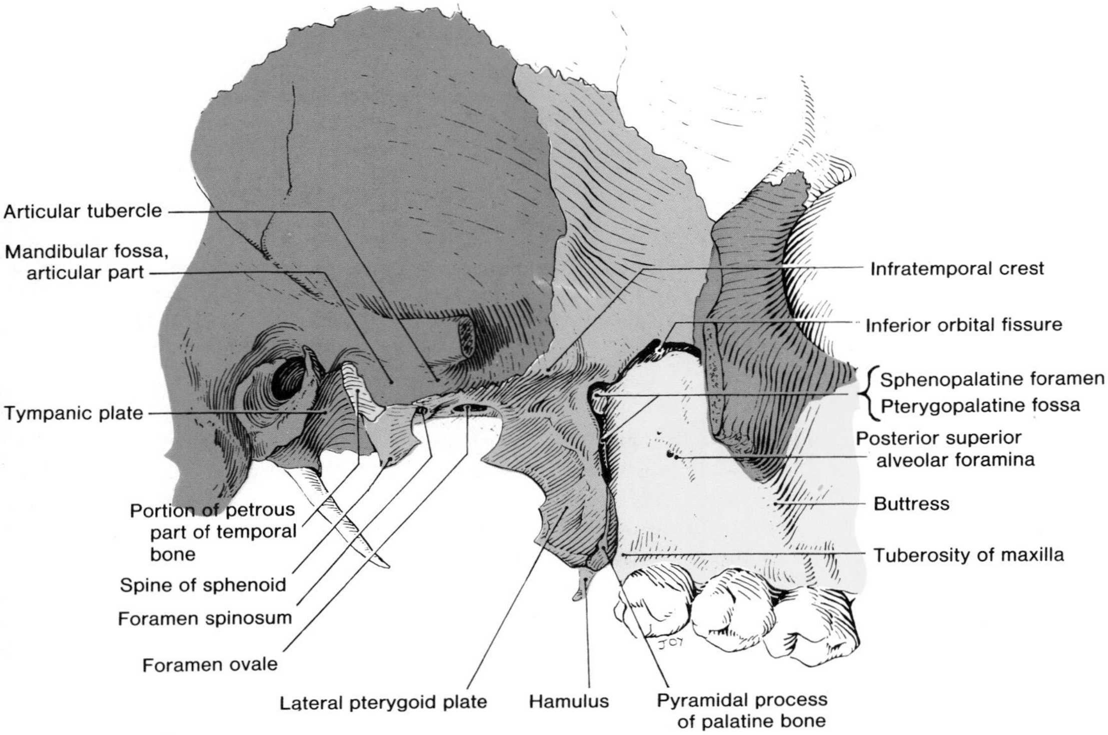

Figure 7-123. Drawing of part of the lateral side of the skull showing the roof and the medial and lateral walls of the infratemporal fossa. The ramus of the mandible which forms the lateral wall of the fossa is not illustrated. Note that the posterior free border of the lateral pterygoid plate, when followed superiorly, leads to the foramen ovale in the roof of the fossa.

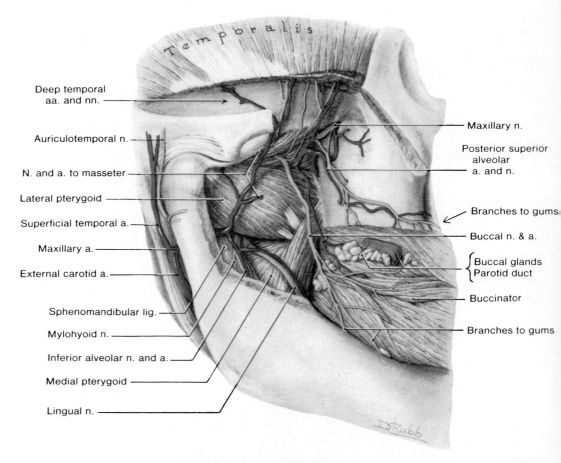

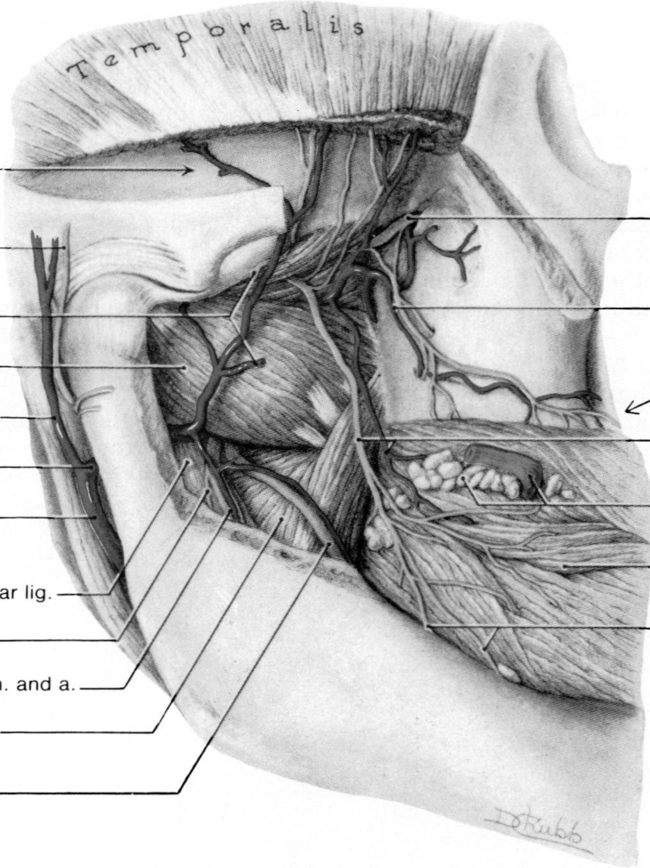

Figure 7-124. Drawing of a superficial dissection of the infratemporal region. Observe the maxillary artery (also see Fig. 7-125), the larger of the two end branches of the external carotid, running forward deep to the neck of the mandible. Note that it disappears deep to the lateral pterygoid muscle and reappears between its two heads before plunging into the pterygopalatine fossa.

notch (Fig. 7-120) into the fossa (**extraoral approach**), where the local anesthetic agent is injected. The following nerves are usually anesthetized: the auriculotemporal, the inferior alveolar, the lingual, and the buccal. Thus, all areas of skin innervated by the mandibular nerve and its branches are anesthetized.

Commonly dentists and oral surgeons plan only to block some branches of the mandibular nerve to the mandible (*e.g.*, only the **inferior alveolar** and **lingual nerves**). This nerve block anesthetizes these nerves and their subdivisions. The areas anesthetized are the body and inferior portion of the ramus of the mandible, the mandibular teeth and gingivae, and the mucous membrane of the anterior two-thirds of the tongue. The needle is inserted intraorally through the buccal mucosa and the buccinator muscle. The anesthetic solution is injected into the loose connective tissue and fat, immediately medial to the ramus of the mandible near the mandibular foramen.

The chorda tympani nerve (Figs. 7-125, 7-127, and 7-128) is a branch of the facial (CN VII). It leaves this nerve in the facial canal and crosses the medial aspect of the tympanic membrane to join the lingual nerve from behind, near the inferior border of the lateral pterygoid muscle.

The Otic Ganglion (Fig. 7-119). This parasympathetic ganglion is located in the infratemporal fossa, just below the foramen ovale, medial to the mandibular nerve and posterior to the medial pterygoid muscle. **Preganglionic parasympathetic fibers,** derived mainly from the **glossopharyngeal nerve** (CN IX), synapse in the otic ganglion. Postganglionic parasympathetic fibers, which are secretory to the parotid gland, pass from this ganglion to the auriculotemporal nerve.

THE TEMPOROMANDIBULAR JOINT

The temporomandibular joint (TM joint) is a **synovial joint** formed by the articu-

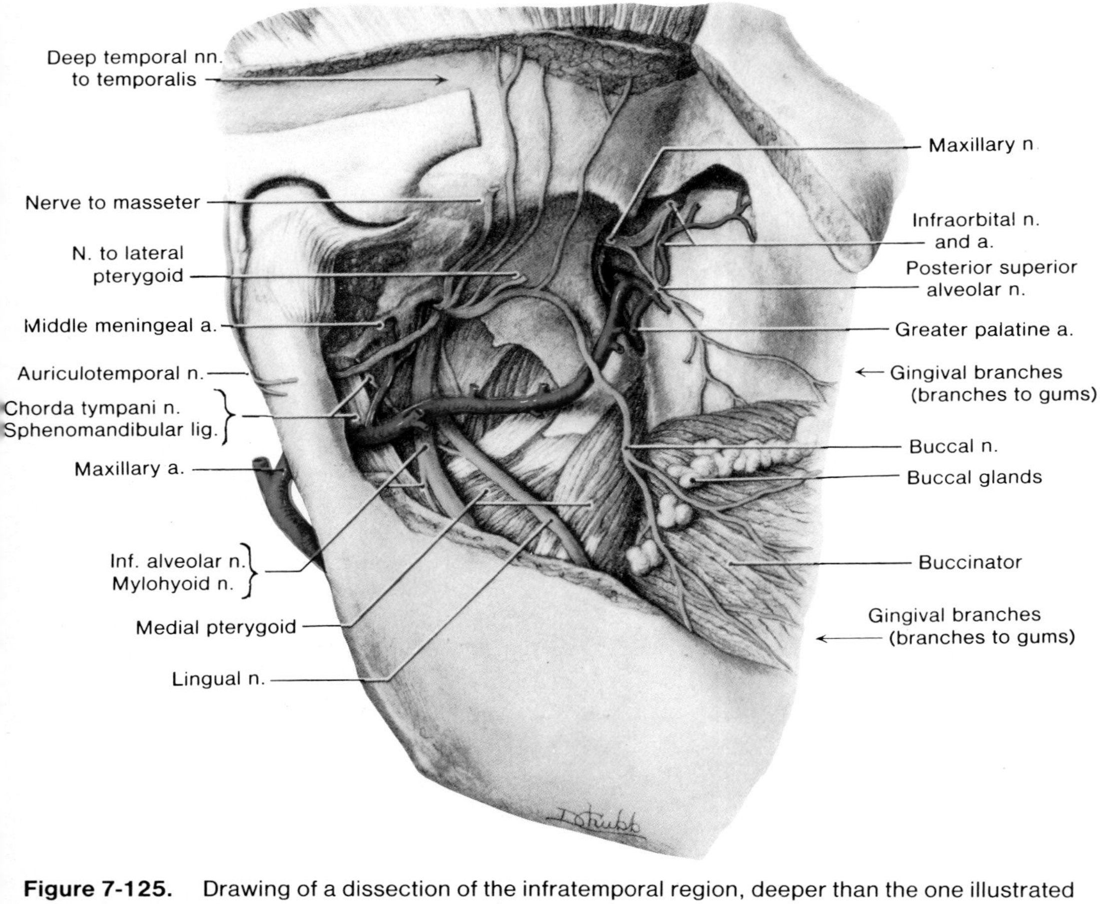

Figure 7-125. Drawing of a dissection of the infratemporal region, deeper than the one illustrated in Figure 7-124. The lateral pterygoid muscle and most branches of the maxillary artery have been removed. Observe the maxillary artery and the auriculotemporal nerve passing between the ligament and the neck of the mandible. Note that the mandibular nerve (CN V^3) enters the infratemporal fossa through the roof via the foramen ovale. Observe the inferior alveolar and lingual nerves descending on the medial pterygoid muscle, the former giving off the mylohyoid nerve (to the mylohyoid and anterior belly of digastric), the latter receiving the chorda tympani which carries secretory fibers and fibers of taste. Note the nerves to the muscles of mastication: masseter, temporalis, and lateral pterygoid (labeled) and the nerve to the medial pterygoid (not labeled). Note that the buccal branch of the mandibular nerve (CN V^3) is sensory. The buccal branch of the facial nerve (CN VII) is the motor supply to the buccinator.

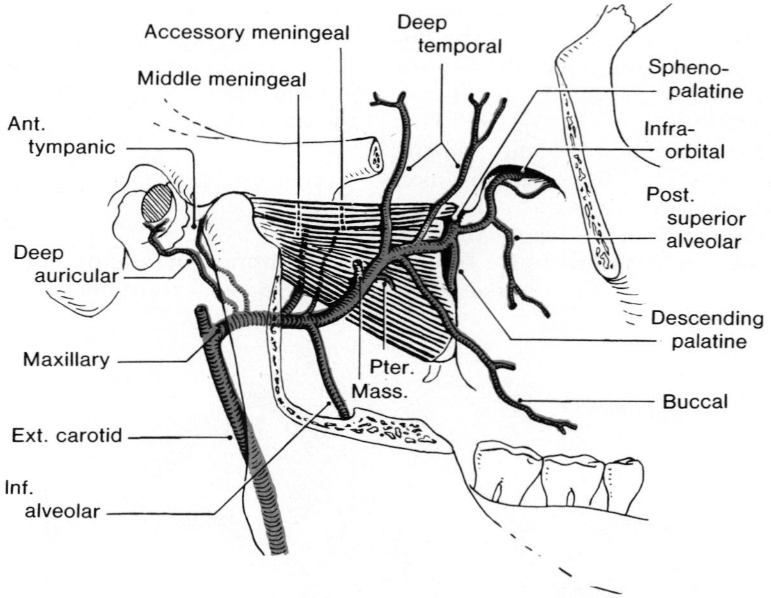

Figure 7-126. Diagram of the maxillary artery, the larger of the two terminal branches of the external carotid artery, that arises at the neck of the mandible and is divided into three parts by the lateral pterygoid muscle.

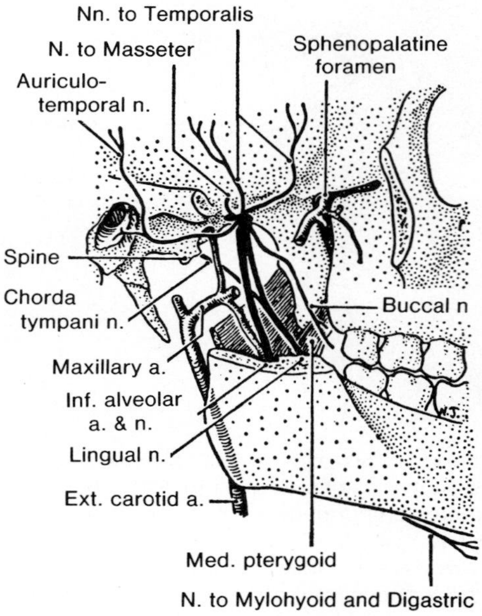

Figure 7-127. Diagram showing the distribution of the mandibular nerve (CN V^3). The maxillary artery is also shown.

lation of the **head of the mandible** with the **mandibular fossa** and the **articular tubercle** of the temporal bone (Figs. 7-131 to 7-133).

The two bones involved (mandible and temporal) are separated by an oval, fibrocartilaginous **articular disc** which completely divides the joint cavity into upper and lower compartments. The articular disc of the TM joint is fused with the articular capsule surrounding the joint, and through this attachment it is bound above to the limits of the temporal articular surface and below to the neck of the mandible. It is more firmly attached to the mandible than to the temporal bone. Thus, when the head of the mandible slides forward on the articular tubercle as the mouth is opened, the articular disc slides forward against the posterior surface of the articular tubercle.

The fibrous capsule of the TM joint is attached to the margins of the articular area on the temporal bone and around the neck of the mandible. This fibrous capsule is thickened laterally to form the **lateral**

Table 7-2
Branches of the Mandibular Nerve (CN V^3)

Muscular Branches	Sensory Branches	Other Branches
Temporalis and Masseter	Auriculotemporal	Taste
Medial and Lateral pterygoids	Inferior alveolar	Secretory
Tensor veli palantini and Tensor tympani	Lingual	Articular
Mylohyoid and Digastric (anterior belly)	Buccal	

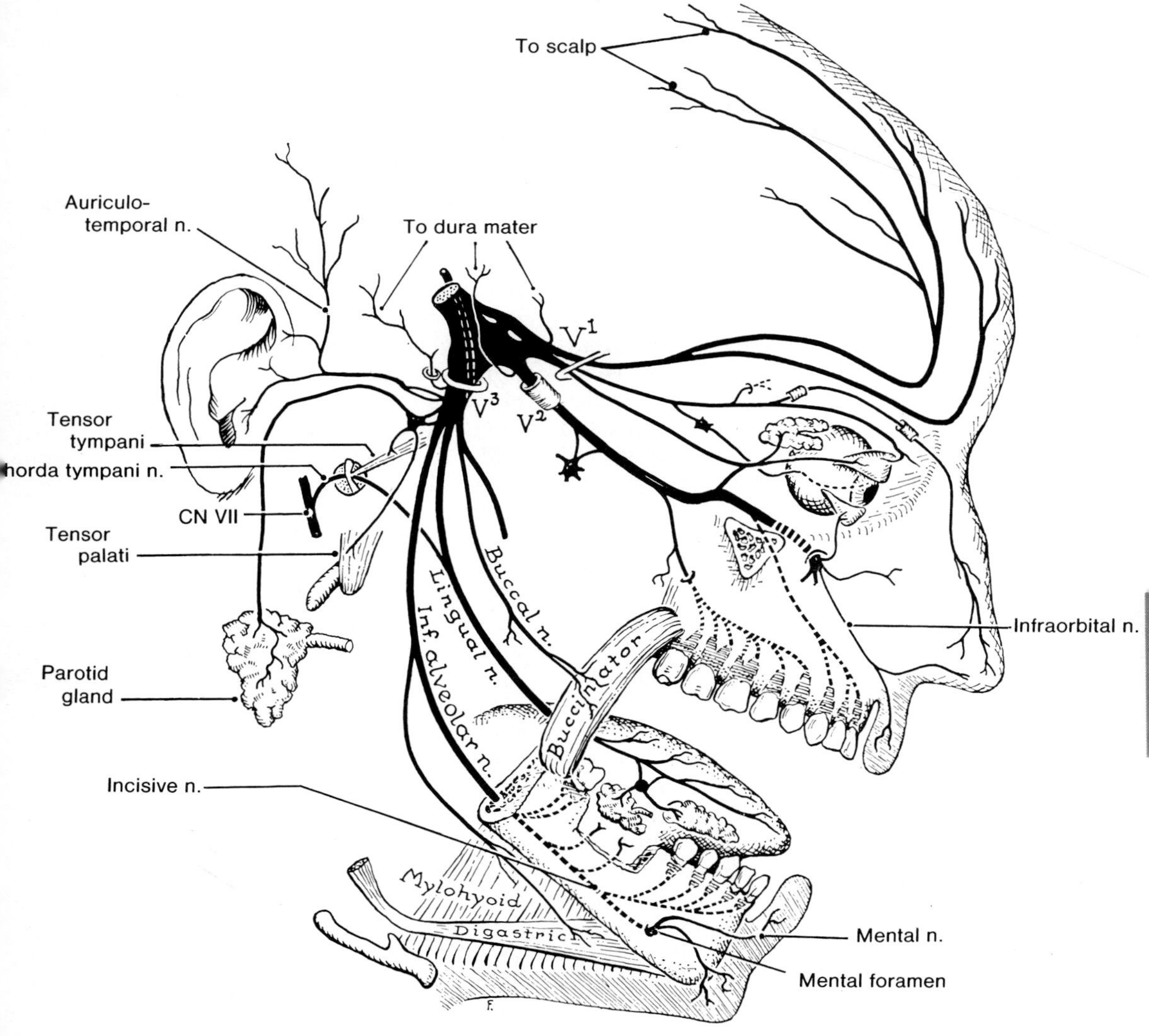

Figure 7-128. Diagram showing the distribution of the trigeminal nerve (CN V). The inferior alveolar nerve, a branch of the mandibular nerve (CN V^3), enters the mandible via the mandibular foramen and runs in the mandibular canal below the teeth, as far as the mental foramen.

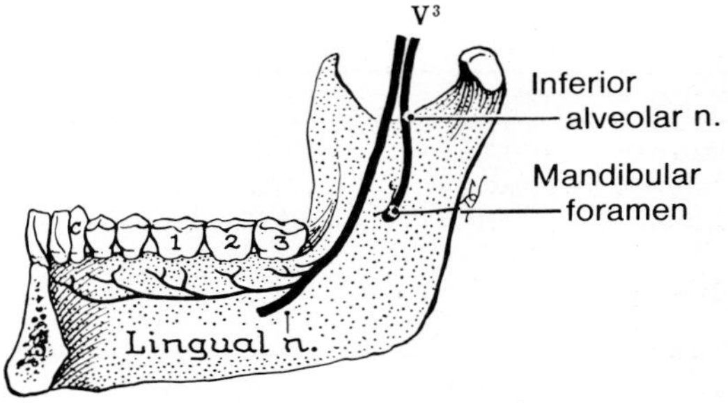

Figure 7-129. Drawing of the medial aspect of the mandible to show the inferior alveolar and lingual nerves, branches of the mandibular division of the trigeminal nerve (CN V^3). The inferior alveolar nerve passes through the mandibular canal in the mandible, whereas the lingual nerve passes under the mucosa.

ligament (Fig. 7-114). The base of this triangular ligament is attached to the zygomatic process of the temporal bone and the articular tubercle. Its apex is fixed to the lateral side of the neck of the mandible.

Two other ligaments connect the mandible to the skull, but they provide little if any strength to the TM joint. The **stylomandibular ligament**, a thickened band of deep cervical fascia, runs from the styloid process to the angle of the mandible and separates the parotid and submandibular salivary glands. The **sphenomandibular ligament** (Figs. 7-125 and 7-133), a remnant of the first branchial arch cartilage (**Meckel's cartilage**), is a long membranous band that lies medial to the TM joint and runs from the spine of the sphenoid bone to the **lingula** on the medial aspect of the mandible (Fig. 7-22).

Although the **fibrous capsule** and the **lateral ligament** are the only *true ligaments of the TM joint* (*i.e.*, the ones supporting it), the muscles acting on the TM joint are largely responsible for maintaining the joint. As with any joint maintained mainly by muscles, the TM joint is relatively easily dislocated (Fig. 7-136).

The synovial membrane lines the fibrous capsule and is reflected upward on to the neck of the mandible to the margin of the articular cartilage.

Movements of the Temporomandibular Joint. Two movements occur at the TM joint, a forward gliding and a hinge-like rotation. When the mandible is depressed during opening of the mouth, the head and articular disc move forward on the articular surface until the head lies inferior to the **articular tubercle** (Fig. 7-132).

You can appreciate this gliding movement by placing your index finger in front of the tragus of your ear (Fig. 7-179), just below the posterior end of the zygomatic process of the temporal bone. Note that when the mouth is opened widely, the head of the mandible moves downward and forward with the articular disc. Now, with your index finger on the joint, place your thumb on the angle of your mandible. Verify that as the condyle moves forward, the angle moves backward.

As this forward gliding occurs, the head of the mandible rotates on the lower surface of the articular disc in the inferior compartment of the joint (Fig. 7-132*B*). This permits simple chewing or grinding movements over a small range. Verify this by placing your index fingers over your TM joint on each side and then pretend you are chewing a piece of steak. During this kind of chewing, both types of movement of the TM joint occur, *i.e.*, forward gliding and hinge-like rotation of the head of the mandible.

The axes of these two movements are different. In simple opening of the mouth, the axis of the forward gliding movement passes approximately through the mandibular foramen, whereas in hinge-like rotation the axis is through the head of the mandible. Because of these axes of movement, the vessels and nerves entering the mandible are not excessively stretched when the mouth is wide open.

In **protraction** (protrusion) and **retraction** of the mandible, the head and the articular disc slide forward and backward on the articular surface of the temporal bone, both sides moving together. The **grinding movement** occurs when protraction and retraction of the mandible alternate on the two sides. Palpate the head of your mandible by placing your little finger into the cartilaginous portion of your **external acoustic meatus** (L. a passage). *First*, open and close your mouth; *second*, protract and retract your mandible; and finally, alternate protraction and retraction on the two sides. As you palpate, try to detect the considerable amount of movement and rotation of the head of the mandible that occurs during chewing.

Muscles Acting on the Temporomandibular Joint (Table 7-3). The mandible

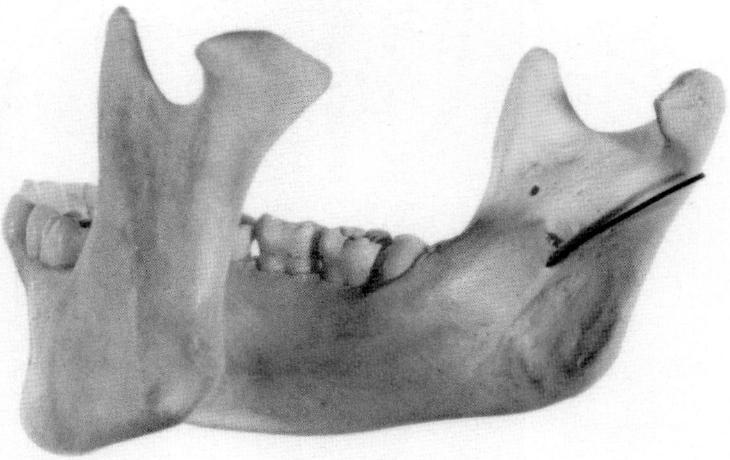

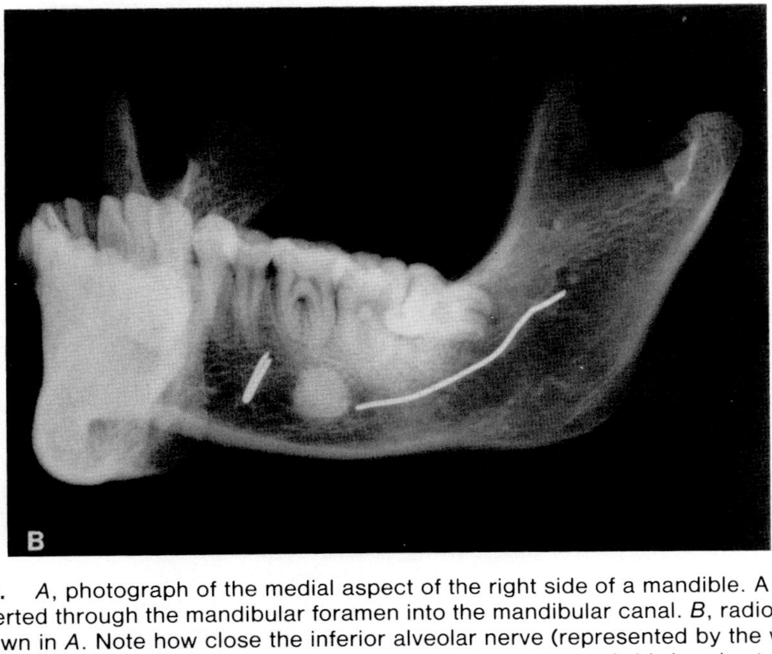

Figure 7-130. *A*, photograph of the medial aspect of the right side of a mandible. A copper wire has been inserted through the mandibular foramen into the mandibular canal. *B*, radiograph of the mandible shown in *A*. Note how close the inferior alveolar nerve (represented by the wire) passes to the roots of the molar teeth. Observe the malposed and impacted third molar tooth and the direction of the emerging wire from the mental foramen (upward and backward). For another view of this impacted tooth, see Figure 7-141.

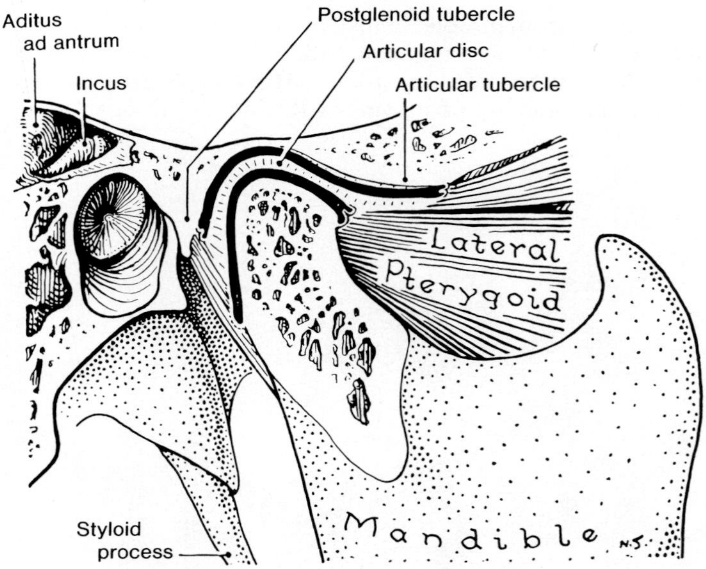

Figure 7-131. Drawing of a sagittal section of the temporomandibular joint. Note the mandibular fossa and the condyle on the head of the mandible. When the mouth opens, the head passes forward to a point directly below the articular tubercle in normal persons (Fig. 7-132).

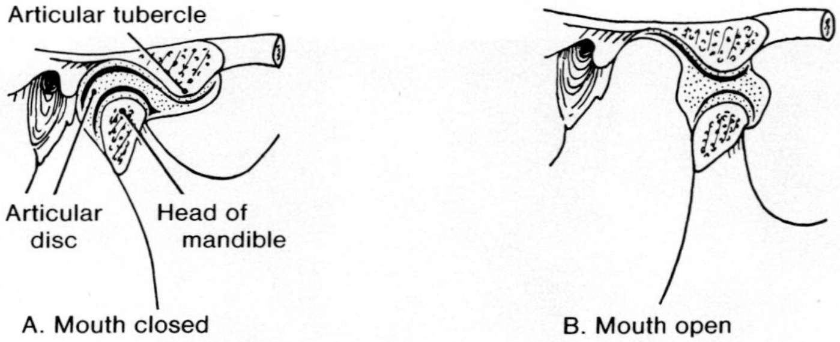

Fig 7-132. Drawings of sagittal sections of the temporomandibular joint to show the changing relationship between the head of the mandible and the temporal bone when the mouth is opened (*B*). Observe that the head of the mandible, together with the articular disc, slides forward to the articular tubercle while the head of the mandible rotates on the disc.

may be depressed or elevated, protracted or retracted; considerable rotation also occurs. These movements are controlled mainly by the muscles acting on the TM joint. The various movements result from cooperative activity of several muscles bilaterally or unilaterally. These movements, summarized in Table 7-3, result chiefly from the action of the **muscles of mastication** (temporalis, masseter, and medial and lateral pterygoids). Note that the temporalis, masseter, and medial pterygoid produce the biting movement (*i.e.*, elevate the mandible and close the mouth). The mandible is protracted by the lateral pterygoids with help from the medial pterygoids and retracted largely by the posterior fibers of the temporalis. Gravity is sufficient to depress the mandible, but if there is resistance (*e.g.*, a person wearing a chin strap), the mylohoid and anterior digastric muscles (Fig. 7-128) are activated.

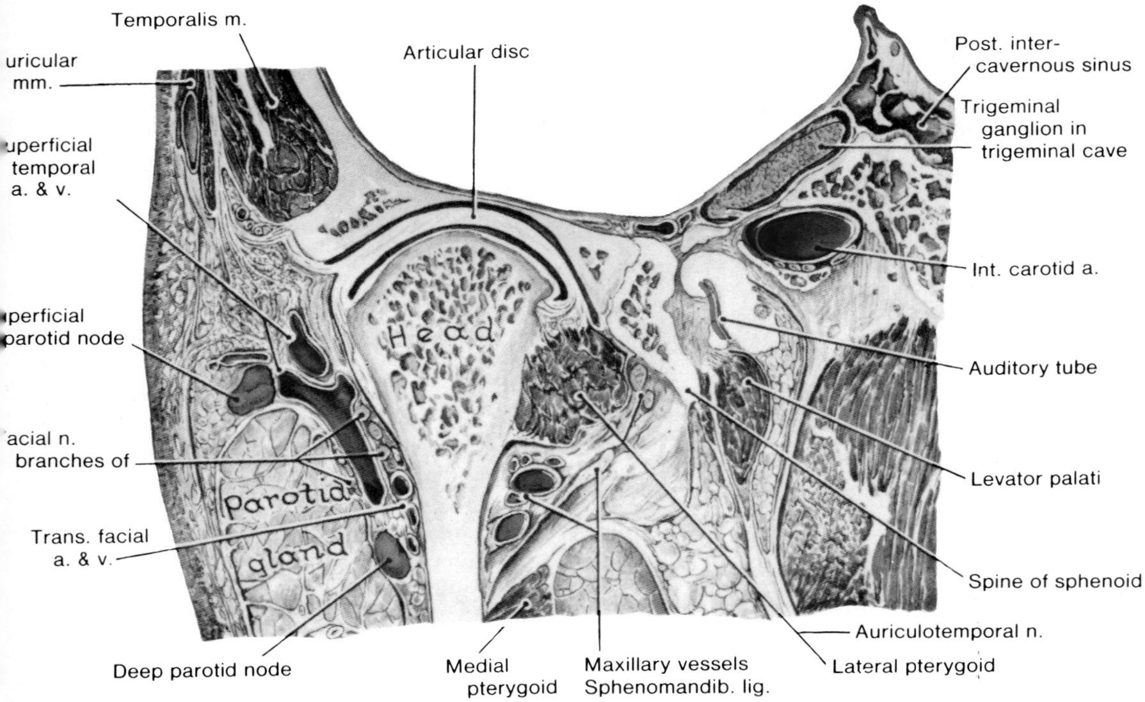

Figure 7-133. Drawing of a coronal section of the temporomandibular joint. Observe the articular disc attached to the neck of the mandible medially and laterally, partly in conjunction with the lateral pterygoid muscle. Note the articular disc dividing the articular cavity into upper and lower compartments and the lateral pterygoid muscle inserted in part into the front of the disc. Note also that the roof of the mandibular fossa, separating the head and the disc from the middle cranial fossa, is thin centrally but thick elsewhere. Also observe the maxillary vessels crossing the neck of the mandible on its medial side and the superficial and deep parotid lymph nodes.

Table 7-3
Movements of the Mandible and Chief Muscles Involved

Depress (Open Mouth)	Elevate (Close Mouth)	Protract (Protrude Chin)	Side-to-Side (Grinding, Chewing)
Digastric Mylohyoid Geniohyoid Infrahyoid Gravity	Temporalis Masseter Medial pterygoid	Masseter (deep part) Lateral pterygoid	Temporalis of same side Pterygoids of oppposite side Masseter

The Temporalis Muscle (Figs. 7-114, 7-122, 7-133, and 7-134). This extensive fan-shaped muscle, covering the temporal region, is a powerful masticatory (biting) muscle that can easily be seen and felt during closure of the mandible.

Origin. Floor of **temporal fossa** and **temporal fascia.**

Insertion. **Coronoid process** and anterior border of **ramus of mandible.**

Actions. **Elevates mandible** (closes mouth) and **retracts mandible** (posterior fibers) after protraction.

Nerve Supply. Deep temporal branches of the **mandibular** nerve (CN V^3).

The Masseter Muscle (Figs. 7-114, 7-116,

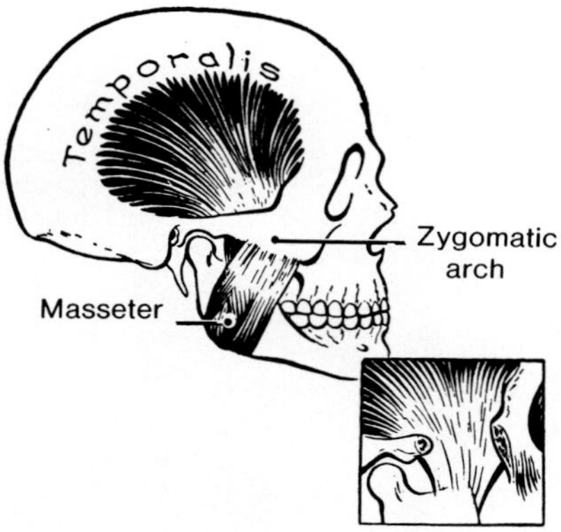

Figure 7-134. Sketch of the right temporalis and masseter muscles. A smaller sketch (lower right) shows the insertion of the temporalis into the coronoid process of the mandible.

7-122, and 7-134). This quadrangular muscle covers the lateral aspect of the ramus and coronoid process of the mandible. The Greek word *masētēr* means masticator or chewer. Place your fingers on your cheek and tense your masseter by clenching your teeth. You should have no difficulty feeling this muscle because of its proximity to the skin.

Origin (Fig. 7-122). Inferior margin and deep surface of **zygomatic arch**.

Insertion (Figs. 7-21 and 7-134). Lateral surface of **ramus** and **coronoid process** of mandible.

Actions. **Elevates mandible, clenches teeth,** and **helps to protract mandible**.

Nerve Supply (Figs. 7-114 and 7-124). **Mandibular** (CN V^3) via a branch that enters its deep surface.

The Lateral Pterygoid Muscle (Figs. 7-124, 7-126, 7-131, 7-133, and 7-135). This short, thick muscle has *two heads of origin.*

Origin (Figs. 7-123 and 7-135). *Upper head,* **infratemporal ridge** and infratemporal surface of **greater wing of sphenoid** bone; *lower head,* lateral surface of **lateral pterygoid plate**.

Insertion (Figs. 7-22 and 7-135). Front of **neck of mandible** and articular disc and capsule of TM joint.

Actions. Acting together the lateral pterygoids **protrude mandible** and **depress chin**. Acting alone and alternately, they produce **side-to-side movement** of mandible.

Nerve Supply. **Mandibular** (CN V^3) via a branch from anterior trunk that enters its deep surface.

The Medial Pterygoid Muscle (Figs. 7-124, 7-125, 7-133, and 7-135). This thick, quadrilateral muscle also has *two heads of origin* which embrace the lower head of the lateral pterygoid. Note that the medial pterygoid is located deep to the ramus of the mandible.

Origin (Figs. 7-123 and 7-135). *Deep head* (most of the muscle), medial surface of **lateral pterygoid plate**. *Superficial head,* **tuberosity of maxilla**.

Insertion (Figs. 7-22 and 7-135). Medial surface of mandible, near angle.

Actions. **Assists in elevating** and **protruding mandible**. Acting alone, it pulls the chin to opposite side; when muscles act alternately, they produce a grinding motion.

Nerve Supply. Branch from **mandibular** nerve (CN V^3).

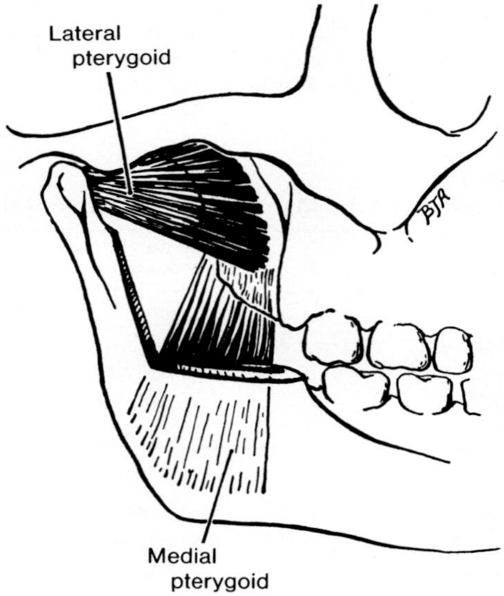

Figure 7-135. Sketch showing the origin and insertion of the medial and lateral pterygoid muscles. Note that each arises from the lateral pterygoid plate (Fig. 7-123).

CLINICALLY ORIENTED COMMENTS

The **temporomandibular joint** usually dislocates anteriorly (Fig. 7-136*C*). During normal opening of the mouth, the head of the mandible and the articular disc move forward to the **articular tubercle** of the zygomatic process of the temporal bone (Fig. 7-136*B*). During yawning or taking a large bite, contraction of the lateral **pterygoid muscles** may cause the heads of the mandible to dislocate, *i.e.*, pass anterior to the articular tubercle beneath the zygomatic arch (Fig. 7-136*C*). In this position, the mandible remains wide open and the person is unable to close it.

Dislocation of the TM joint could also occur during extraction of teeth if the mandible were depressed excessively. Most commonly, the TM joint is dislocated by a blow to the chin when the mouth is wide open (*e.g.*, when a person is laughing, gaping, or yawning). The displacement is usually bilateral and the mandible projects with the mouth fixed in an open position.

Fractures of the mandible (Fig. 7-26) may be accompanied by dislocation of the TM joint(s), a possibility that is not to be overlooked in treating these fractures.

Because of the close relationship of the facial (CN VII) and the auriculotemporal (branch of CN V^3) nerves to the TM joint (Figs. 7-116, 7-128, and 7-133), care must be taken during operations on the joint to preserve branches of the facial nerve overlying it and articular branches of the auriculotemporal nerve that enter the posterior part of the joint. Injury to the trunk of the facial nerve causes **facial paralysis** similar to that which occurs in Bell's palsy (Case 7-1), resulting from inflammation of the nerve. Injury to branches of the facial nerve causes paralysis of the muscles of facial expression innervated by them.

Injury to the articular branches of the auriculotemporal nerve supplying the TM joint, associated with traumatic dislocation and rupture of the articular capsule and/or the lateral ligament, leads to **joint laxity** and instability of the joint.

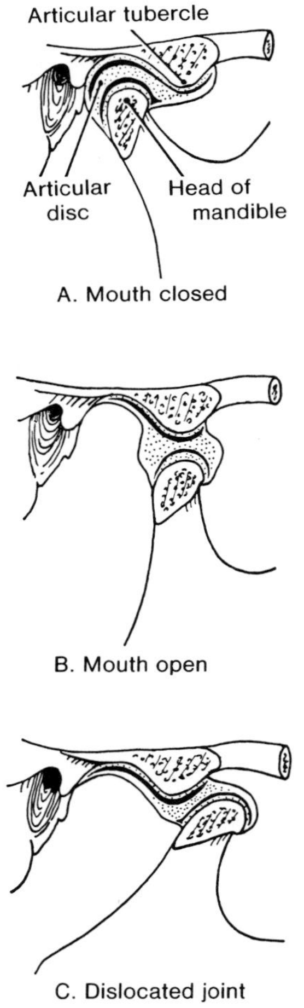

Figure 7-136. Diagrams illustrating the changing position of the head of the mandible and the temporal bone when *A*, the mouth is closed, *B*, the mouth is open, and *C*, the temporomandibular joint is dislocated. Note that the head of the mandible and the articular disc slide forward over the articular tubercle as the head rotates on the disc.

THE MOUTH, TEETH, PALATE, AND TONGUE

THE MOUTH

The mouth is the *first part of the digestive tube* and it is also used in breathing. The **oral cavity** (mouth cavity) consists of a smaller outer part, the **vestibule**, and a larger inner part, the **oral cavity proper**.

The oral cavity is bounded externally by the cheeks and the lips. The aperture between the lips is called the **oral orifice** or opening of the mouth. The horseshoe-shaped space external to the teeth is called the **vestibule** (buccal cavity) of the mouth. The space bounded externally by the teeth and the **gingivae** (gums) is referred to as the **oral cavity proper**. The roof of the oral cavity is formed by the **hard** and **soft palates** and the median, conical process, the **uvula** (L. a grape), in which the soft palate ends (Figs. 7-137, 7-147, and 7-151).

Posteriorly, the oral cavity communicates with the oral part of the pharynx (**oropharynx**), bounded by the soft palate above, the **epiglottis** below, and the palatoglossal folds laterally (Fig. 7-147).

Put your index finger in the vestibule of your mouth and palpate the anterior (facial) and infratemporal surfaces of the **maxilla**, the inferior margin of the zygomatic arch, and the anterior border of the **ramus** of the mandible up to the **coronoid** process (Fig. 7-120). Alternately clench and relax your teeth while your finger is in your vestibule and feel the anterior margin of the **masseter muscle** and the tendon of the temporalis muscle (Figs. 7-114 and 7-134).

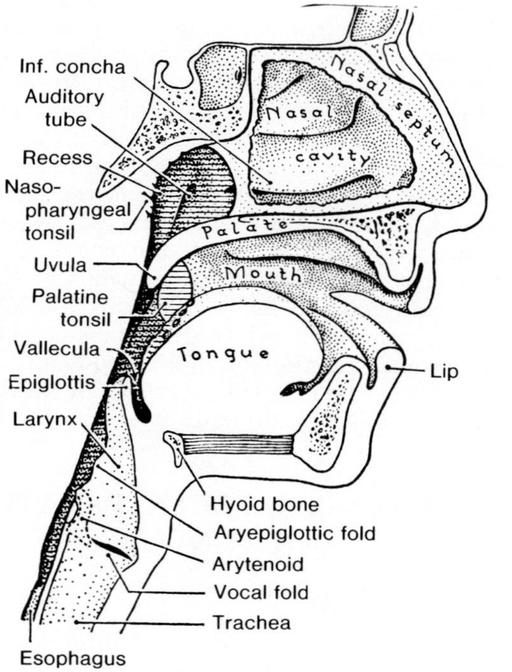

Figure 7-137. Drawing of a sagittal section of the anterior part of the head and neck showing the nose, mouth, pharynx, and larynx.

The Lips (Figs. 7-31, 7-137, 7-138, and 7-145). These muscular folds surrounding the oral orifice are covered externally by skin and internally by mucous membrane. In between these layers are the muscles of the mouth (*e.g.*, **orbicularis oris muscle**) and the upper and lower labial branches of the facial arteries. Recall that the labial arteries anastomose with each other to form an arterial ring. The pulsations of these arteries (Fig. 7-36) can be palpated by grasping the lip lightly between the index finger and the thumb. **Labial salivary glands** are located around the orifice of the mouth between the mucous membrane and the orbicularis oris muscle. These small glands resemble mucous salivary glands in structure. Their ducts open into the vestibule.

The upper and lower lips are attached to the gingivae in the median plane by raised folds of mucous membrane, called the **frenula** (L. *frenum*, a bridle) of the lips. You can see these when you draw your lower lip downward and pull your upper lip upward. They can be easily felt with your finger or by putting the tip of your tongue into the vestibule at the front of your mouth.

The junction of the upper lip and the cheek is clearly demarcated by the **nasolabial sulcus**, running laterally from the margin of the nose to the angle of the mouth. This sulcus is particularly obvious during smiling (Fig. 7-138*B*) and in old persons. A similar groove, the **mentolabial sulcus** indicates the junction of the lower lip and the chin. The upper lip has a median shallow vertical groove called the **philtrum** (G. *philtron*, a love-charm). Examine your lip, identifying the following: the cutaneous zone, the vermilion border (red zone), and the mucosal zone. The **vermilion border** (to which lipstick is sometimes applied) between the outer skin and inner mucosa is a *distinctive characteristic of humans*. It appears red because of the presence of capillary loops close to the surface composed of thin skin.

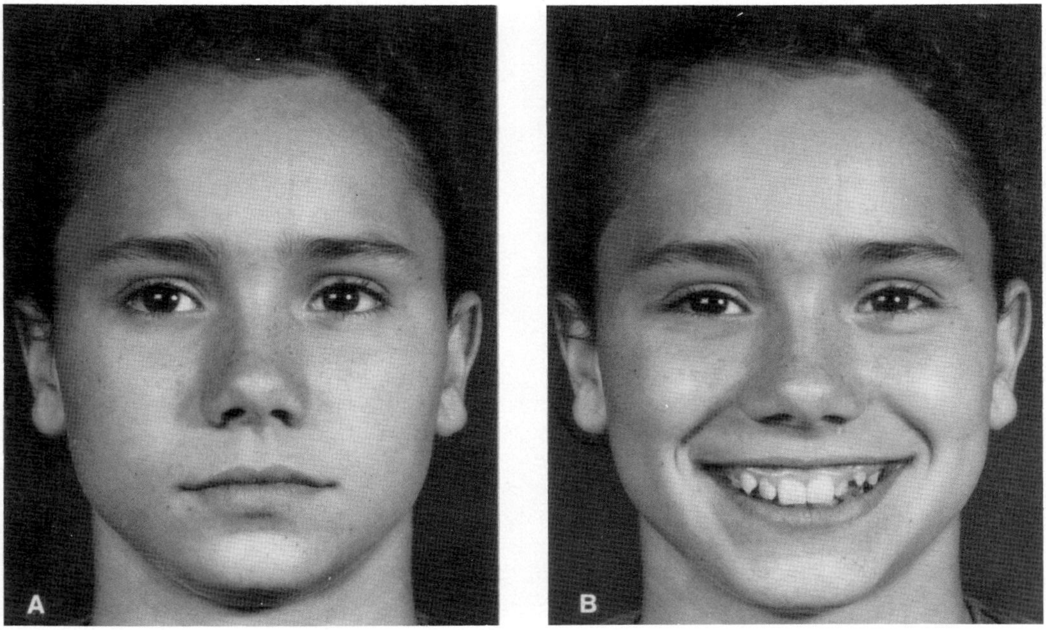

Figure 7-138. Photographs of the face of a 12-year-old girl primarily to show the mouth, teeth, chin, lips, and nose. In *A*, note the philtrum (median vertical groove) and in *B*, note the nasolabial sulcus dividing the upper lip and the cheek and the mentolabial groove dividing the lower lip and the chin. Observe that the philtrum is not so obvious during smiling because of relaxation of the orbicularis oris muscle (Fig. 7-31). Note that her permanent central incisor teeth, which erupted when she was 7-years-old, are large relative to her face, which is still growing.

The sensory nerves of the upper and lower lips are the **infraorbital** and **mental nerves**, branches of the maxillary (CN V^2) and mandibular (CN V^3) nerves, respectively (Fig. 7-128). **Lymph vessels** from both lips drain into the **submandibular lymph nodes** (Figs. 7-39 and 7-41). In addition, lymph from the central part of the lip drains into the **submental lymph nodes**.

CLINICALLY ORIENTED COMMENTS

Pustules of the upper lip are potentially dangerous because the infection may extend intracranially via the superior labial vein, the angular vein, and the superior orbital vein (Fig. 7-35) and enter the **cavernous sinus** (Fig. 7-38). See Case 7-3 for discussion of the *danger triangle of the face* (Fig. 7-203) and the condition known as **thrombophlebitis of the cavernous sinus** (*i.e.*, infection of the walls of this dural venous sinus accompanied by thrombus formation in it). Structures lying in and around it may be involved (Figs. 7-72 and 7-73).

Persons with facial palsy (paralysis of facial nerve) are unable to whistle because the air blows out through the paralyzed lips on that side. When persons with unilateral facial paralysis are asked to show their teeth, the nasolabial fold does not form on the injured side and the angle of the mouth on that side does not rise (Fig. 7-199). This results from paralysis of the facial muscles, including the oribicularis oris supplied by the facial nerve (Case 7-1).

Cleft lip ("Hare Lip") is a congenital malformation of the upper lip that occurs once in 800 to 900 births (Fig. 7-139). The clefts vary from a small notch in the vermilion border to ones that extend through the lip into the nose. In severe cases the cleft extends deeper and is continuous with a cleft in the palate. Cleft lip may be unilateral or bilateral. Unilateral cleft lip is the more common deformity and results from failure of the maxillary prominence (process) on the affected side to merge with the medial nasal prominence during the embryonic period of facial development.

Many **oral cancers** (usually squamous cell carcinomas) occur on the lips, primarily the lower one (Fig. 7-200). A major etiologic (causative) factor appears to be extensive exposure to intense sunlight. Using your knowledge of the lymphatic drainage of the lips, you can predict that these tumors will metastasize to the submandibular and/or submental lymph nodes depending on the site of the lesion (Case 7-4).

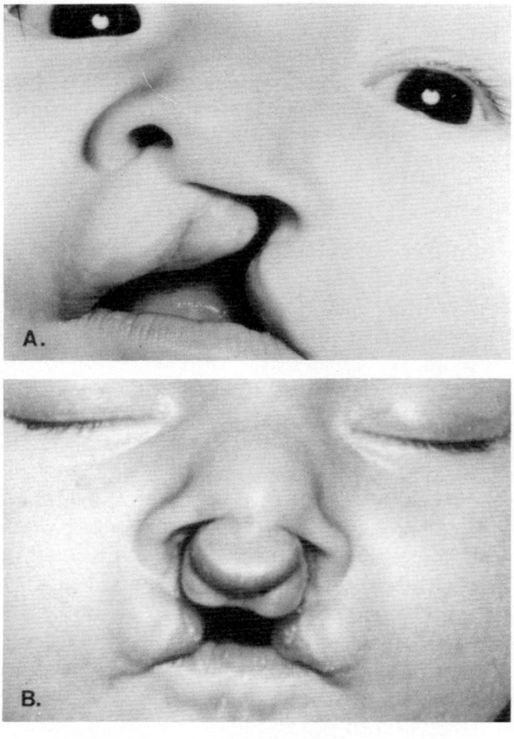

Figure 7-139. Photographs of infants with clefts of the upper lip. *A*, unilateral. *B*, bilateral. In both cases there is loss of continuity of the orbicularis oris muscle (Fig. 7-31).

The Cheeks (L. buccae). The lateral walls of the mouth, formed by the cheeks, have essentially the same structure as the lips, with which they are continuous. The muscle of the cheek is the **buccinator** (Figs. 7-32, 7-122, and 7-125), which is covered by fascia. Superficial to this fascia is the **buccal fat pad** that gives the cheeks a rounded contour, particularly in infants.

The **buccal glands** (Figs. 7-124 and 7-125) are small mucous glands that are situated between the mucous membrane and the buccinator muscle. There are groups of these glands around the terminal part of the parotid duct which runs forward from the gland, *external to the masseter muscle* (Fig. 7-122), and opens on a small papilla on the oral surface of the cheek *opposite the crown of the second upper molar tooth* (Figs. 7-32, 7-35, 7-40, and 7-42).

The sensory nerves of the cheeks are branches of the maxillary and mandibular nerves (CN V^2 and CN V^3). They supply the skin of the cheek and the mucous membrane lining the cheek (Fig. 7-30).

CLINICALLY ORIENTED COMMENTS

In paralysis of the facial nerve, which supplies the muscles of the cheeks and the lips, food tends to accumulate in the vestibule of the mouth on the affected side. In addition, these patients are unable to puff out the cheek on the paralyzed side and saliva and food dribble out of the corner of the mouth (Case 7-1).

The Gingivae (Gums). The gingivae are composed of fibrous tissue which is covered with a mucous membrane. They are attached to the margins of the alveolar processes of the jaws and to the necks of the teeth (Fig. 7-142). In addition to their nerve supply from the nerves supplying the teeth, the gingivae receive nerve fibers from adjacent sensory nerves (buccal, infraorbital, greater palatine, and mental; Fig. 7-128).

THE TEETH

Ten deciduous teeth (primary or "milk" teeth) usually develop in each jaw of children (Fig. 7-140 and Table 7-4). The first tooth usually erupts at 6 to 8 months and the last by 20 to 24 months. As everyone knows, this process is called "teething or cutting of the teeth." The deciduous teeth are usually shed (lost) from the 6th to the 12th year, as they are replaced by the permanent teeth (Figs. 7-24 and 7-140).

Eruption of the permanent teeth (commonly 16 in each jaw) is usually complete by the 18th year, except for the third molars ("wisdom" teeth). If they are malposed and/or impacted (Fig. 7-141), they may not erupt. Table 7-4 (*for reference only*) gives the average times for the eruption and shedding of deciduous teeth and the eruption of permanent teeth.

The 16 teeth in each adult jaw (Fig. 7-141) consist of two **incisors** (cutters), one **canine** (piercer), two **premolars**, and three **molars** (grinders). Each tooth has a **crown** above the gingiva, a **neck** embedded in the gingiva, and a **root** fixed in an alveolus (socket) in the alveolar process of the jaw by a fibrous, **periodontal membrane** (Fig. 7-144). Most of the tooth is composed of **dentine** which is covered by

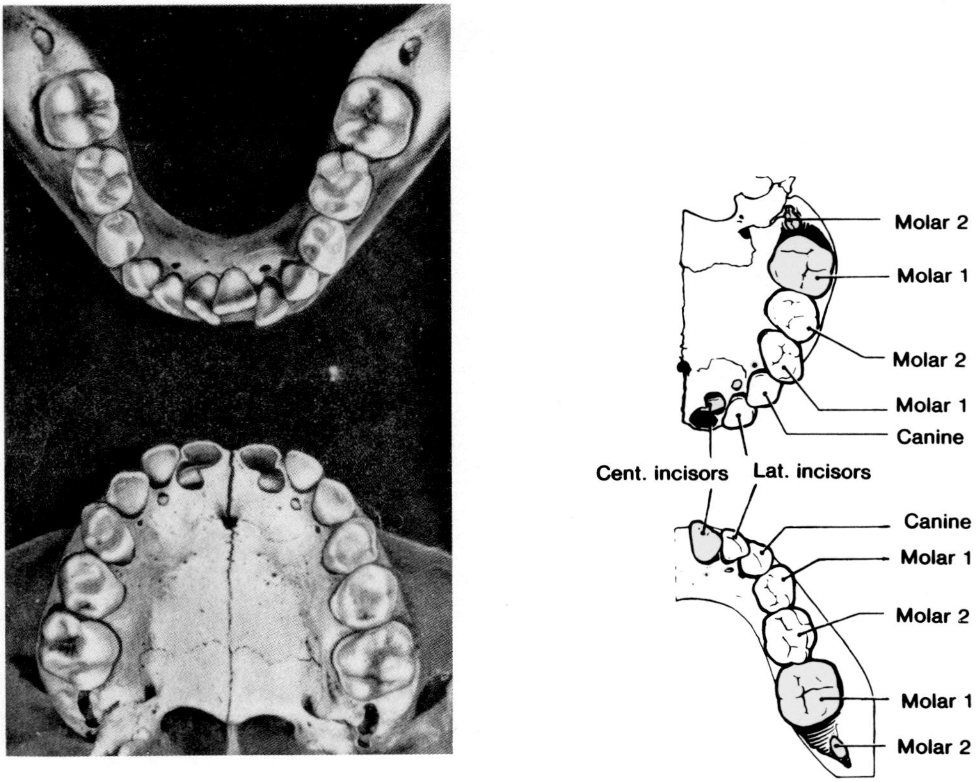

Figure 7-140. *Left*, photographs of the jaws of a child 6 to 7 years old. Note that the upper deciduous central incisors are absent (*i.e.*, they have been shed). *Right*, drawings of halves of these jaws giving the names of the teeth. Permanent teeth are colored *yellow*. The permanent first molars (6-year molars) are fully erupted and that the deciduous central incisors have been shed. Note that the lower central incisors have nearly fully erupted, whereas the upper central incisors have not erupted, but the buds of the permanent incisors are beginning to move downward into the empty sockets.

Table 7-4
Order and Time of Eruption of Teeth and Time of Shedding of Deciduous Teeth

	Deciduous Teeth				
	Medial Incisor	Lateral Incisor	Canine	First Molar	Second Molar
Eruption (months)	6 to 8	8 to 10	16 to 20	12 to 16	20 to 24
Shedding (years)	6 to 7	7 to 8	10 to 12	9 to 11	10 to 12

	Permanent Teeth							
	Medial Incisor	Lateral Incisor	Canine	First Premolar	Second Premolar	First Molar	Second Molar	Third Molar
Eruption (years)	7 to 8	8 to 9	10 to 12	10 to 11	11 to 12	6 to 7	12	13 to 25

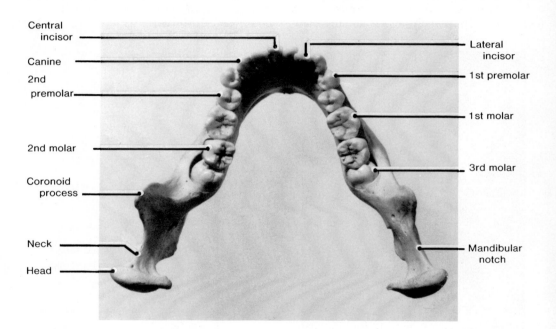

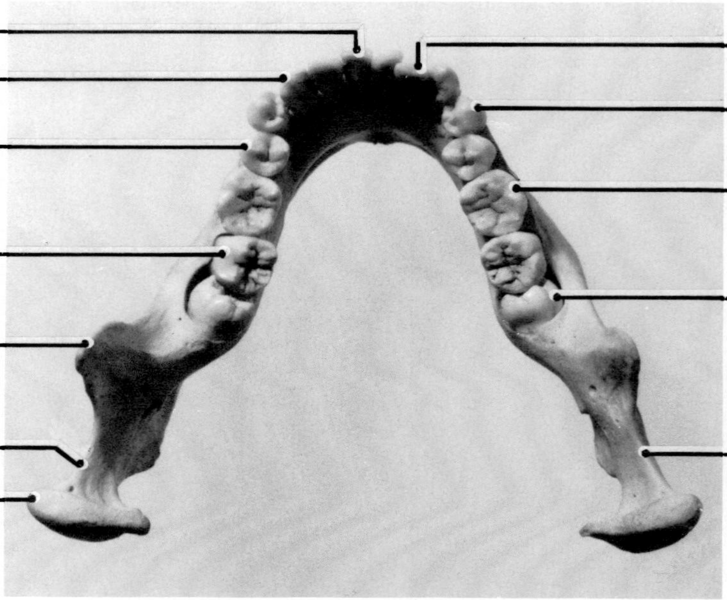

Figure 7-141. Photograph of a superior (occlusal) view of a mandible showing the permanent teeth of an adult male. Note that the third molar is malposed (*i.e.*, pointing anteriorly) and probably would not have erupted because it is also impacted.

enamel over the crown and **cementum** over the root (Fig. 7-142). The **pulp cavity** contains connective tissue, blood vessels, and nerves and is continuous with the periodontal tissue through the **root canal** and the apical foramen.

For purposes of description, incisor and canine teeth have lingual (tongue side) and labial (lip side) surfaces and incisal (cutting) edges. The premolar and molar teeth have buccal (cheek side), lingual, and occlusal (chewing) surfaces. *Teeth vary considerably in shape* (Fig.7-143). The **incisors** (cutters) have chisel-like edges (Fig. 7-141) and usually the upper ones overlap the lower ones. The **canines** (L. *canis*, a dog) are conical but poorly developed in man compared to carnivorous (flesh-eating) an-

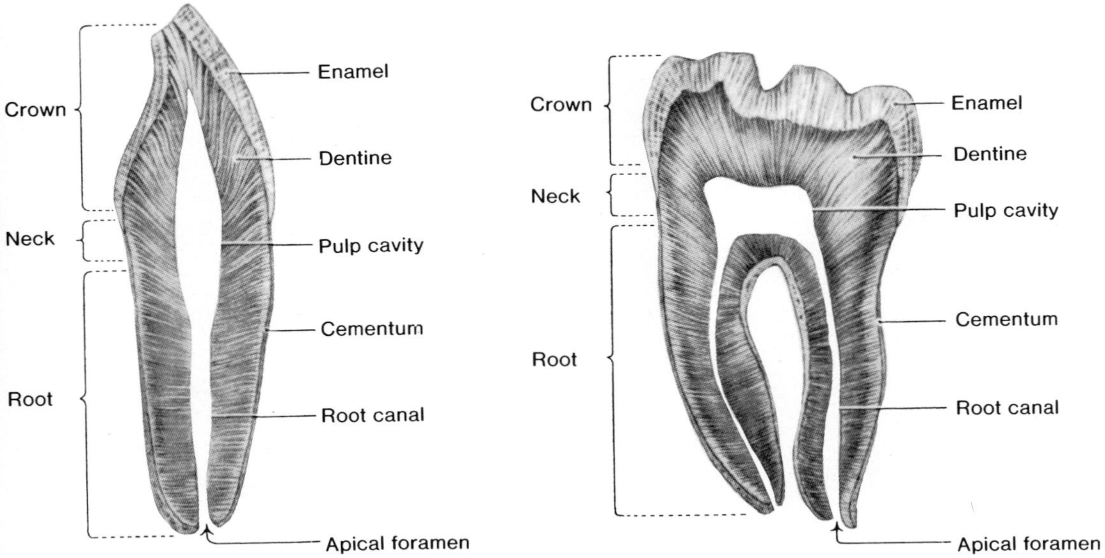

Figure 7-142. Drawings of longitudinal sections of *A*, an incisor tooth, and *B*, a molar tooth illustrating their parts.

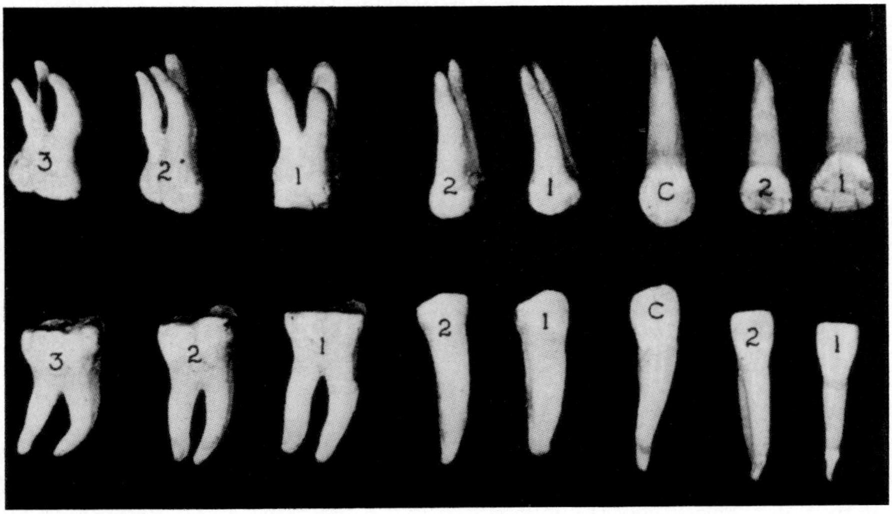

Figure 7-143. Photograph of a buccal view of adult maxillary (upper) and mandibular (lower) teeth. Note that the shapes of teeth vary and that their roots differ. The names of the teeth are given in Figure 7-141.

imals. As premolars have two cusps (L. points) on the crown, they are often referred to as **bicuspids**, whereas upper molars have four cusps and the lower ones five.

The roots of the teeth vary, as is shown in Figure 7-143. The root of a tooth is separated from the cortical plate of its socket, composed of compact bone, by the

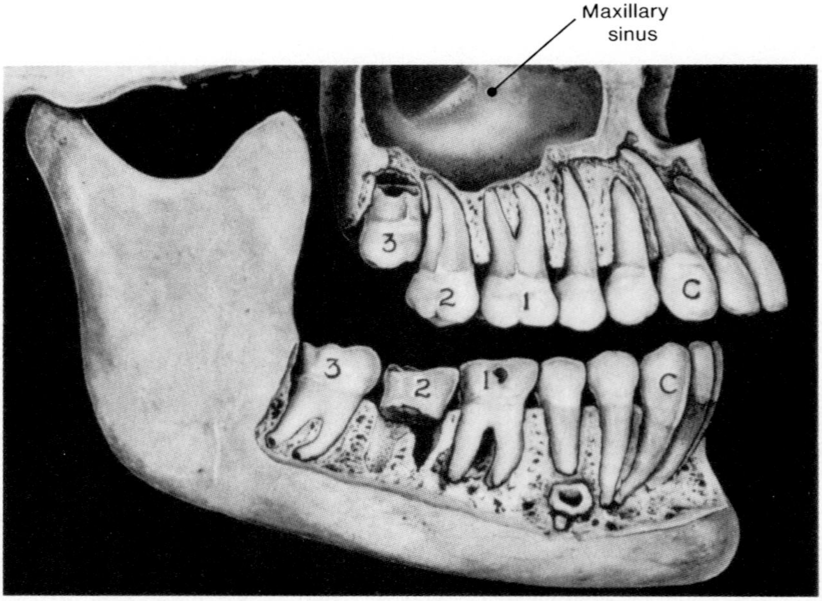

Figure 7-144. Photograph of the permanent teeth on the right side of an adult. The alveolar bone has been ground away to expose the roots of the teeth. Note that the upper canine tooth has the longest root and that the roots of the upper three molars almost penetrate into the maxillary sinus (antrum). The roots of the second lower molar have been removed to show the cribriform (sieve-like) nature of the wall of the socket owing to collagen fibers (Sharpey's fibers) of the periodontal membrane entering the bone.

periodontal membrane of densely packed collagen fibers which attaches the tooth to the bony alveolus. The cortical plate can be seen as a radiopaque line, the **lamina dura**, in radiographs (Fig. 7-130*B*).

CLINICALLY ORIENTED COMMENTS

As doctors have numerous opportunities to detect dental problems (and may have to deal with them), a basic knowledge of the teeth and how diseases affect them is required. Disease that occurs while the teeth are developing can produce distinctive abnormalities that may be useful diagnostic signs. **Congenital syphilis** affects differentiation of the permanent teeth, resulting in **barrel-shaped incisor teeth** which often have central notches in their incisal edges (Hutchinson's incisors). A *marked delay in the eruption of teeth* commonly indicates some nutritional disturbance or general disease. **Transverse ridges on the teeth** indicate temporary arrests of tooth development. These localized disturbances of calcification can often be correlated with periods of illness, malnutrition, or trauma (*e.g.*, **neonatal lines** on the teeth resulting from a traumatic birth).

Discoloration of the teeth has been observed following administration of all the **tetracycline antibiotics** before and after birth. Tetracyclines become incorporated into the teeth and may produce brownish-yellow discoloration. As enamel is not completely formed on the first and second molar teeth until the 8th year, tetracycline therapy can affect the teeth of unborn infants and of children up to 8 years of age.

Chronic infections of the pulp cavity of a tooth lead to infection in the periodontal ligament, destroying it and the lamina dura (the compact layer of bone lining the alveolus). The abscess (circumscribed pus cavity) that forms causes swelling of the adjacent soft tissues ("**gum boil**"). Pus may escape from the abscess and pass between the periosteum and the soft tissues or between the periosteum and the jaw. For example, an abscess associated with a third lower molar tooth may penetrate the tissues at the angle of the mandible, where it may form a large abscess in the submandibular region. Pus from abscesses of the upper molar teeth may extend into the nasal cavity or perforate the maxillary sinus (Fig. 7-144). Note that the roots of the upper molar teeth are closely related to the floor of this sinus. As a consequence, pulpal infection may cause **sinusitis** or sinusitis may stimulate nerves entering the teeth and simulate toothache.

Pus from abscesses of the upper canine teeth often open into the facial region, just below the medial canthus of the eye. Such swelling may obstruct drainage from the **angular vein** and allow infected material to pass via the superior ophthalmic vein to the cavernous sinus (Fig. 7-38).

Trigeminal neuralgia (tic douloureaux) is a syndrome of the trigeminal nerve (CN V) characterized by extremely severe, unilateral, stabbing pain of the face (Case 7-2), usually in the lips, gums, cheek, or chin. It may be confused with diseases of the jaws, teeth, or sinuses.

Receding Gingivae. As people get older their teeth *appear* to get longer owing to the recession of their gums, hence the expression "*long in the tooth.*" Gingival recession exposes the sensitive cementum of the teeth (Fig. 7-142). This process occurs faster in persons who do not have the **tartar** (white, brown, or yellowish-brown deposit), which forms at or below the gingival margin of the teeth, removed by the procedure called **scaling**.

Periodontitis or inflammation of the periodontium (connective tissue attaching the tooth to the alveolar bone) results in inflammation of the gingivae and may result in absorption of alveolar bone and recession of the gingivae. As a consequence of gingival recession, exposure of the periodontal membrane occurs allowing microorganisms to invade and destroy it. **Granulation tissue** (vascular connective tissue forming projections on the gingival surface) and foreign matter collect in the space formerly occupied by the periodontal membrane. The gingivae become inflamed and may bleed readily if pressed; sometimes pus exudes, a condition often called **pyorrhea alveolaris** (G. *pyon*, pus + *rhoia*, a flow). Periodontitis and pyorrhea are a common cause of **halitosis**.

Toothache or pain in a tooth results from involvement of the pulp cavity or periodontal membrane as a result of caries (cavities), infection, or trauma.

THE PALATE

The palate forms the roof of the mouth and the floor of the nasal cavities (Fig. 7-137). Hence, it separates the oral cavity from the nasal cavities and the nasal part of the pharynx or nasopharynx (Fig. 7-145). It consists of two regions, the anterior two-thirds or bony part, called the **hard palate**, and the mobile posterior one-third or fibromuscular part, known as the **soft palate**.

Examine someone's mouth (Fig. 9-61) and the hard palate on a skull (Fig. 7-146). Note that it is arched anteroposteriorly and transversely and verify that the arch of the palate is more pronounced anteriorly in the hard palate region. The depth and breadth of the palatine vault is subject to considerable variation. Verify this by examining several dried skulls.

The Hard Palate (Figs. 7-145 to 7-148). The hard palate is formed by the palatine processes of the maxillae and the horizontal plates of the palatine bones. Anteriorly and laterally, the hard palate is bounded by the alveolar processes (Fig. 7-2) and the gingivae. Posteriorly it is continuous with the soft palate. On the bony palate of a dried skull, observe the pit called the **incisive foramen** lying posterior to the upper central incisor teeth. Within this foramen you may observe two to four foramina. The two constant ones are the orifices of the incisive canals which transmit the **nasopalatine nerves** (Fig. 7-167) and the terminal

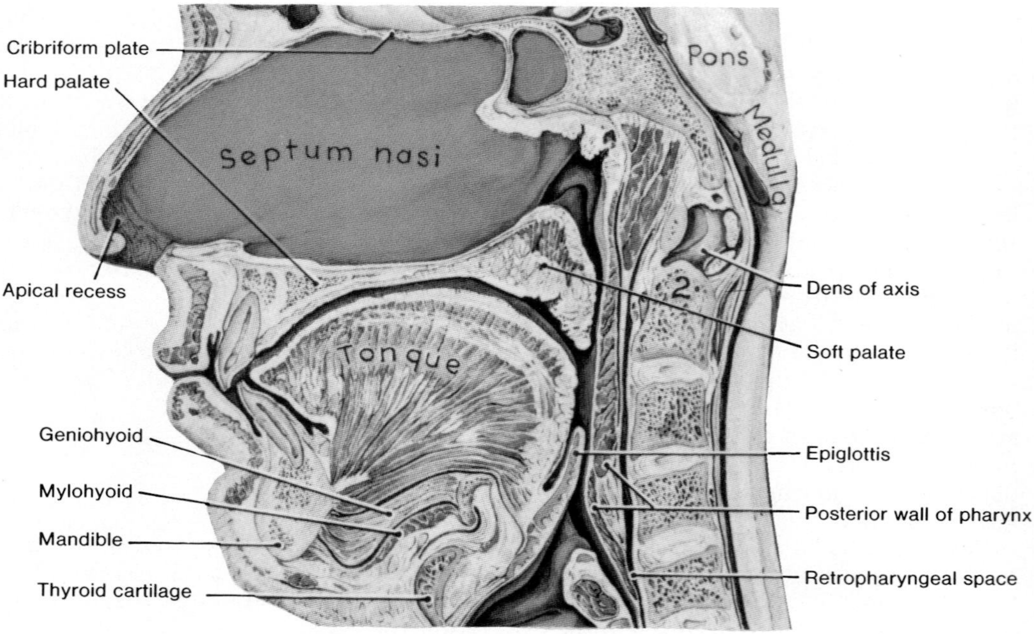

Figure 7-145. Drawing of a median section of part of the head showing the nasal septum, palate, tongue, pharynx, jaws, lips, and various other structures.

branches of the **nasopalatine arteries**. These vessels anastomose with the **sphenopalatine arteries** in the nose (Fig. 7-148).

In hard palates from young people (Figs. 7-140 and 7-146*A*), a suture line is usually visible between the premaxillary part of the maxilla (sometimes called the incisive bone) and the palatine processes of the maxillae. This suture represents the site of fusion of the median and lateral palatine processes during the 12th week of prenatal development. In clefts of the anterior palate, the defect passes along the site of this suture line (Fig. 7-152*B*).

Medial to the third molar tooth, observe the **greater palatine foramen** piercing the lateral border of the bony palate (Fig. 7-146). It is the lower orifice of the **greater palatine canal**. The greater palatine vessels and nerve emerge from this foramen and run anteriorly in two grooves on the palate. The **lesser palatine foramina** transmit the lesser palatine nerves and vessels to the soft palate and adjacent structures.

The hard palate is covered by mucous membrane which is intimately connected to the periosteum (Fig. 7-147). Deep to the mucosa are mucus secreting **palatine glands**. The orifices of the ducts of these glands give the mucous membrane of the palate an orange-peel appearance. Verify that there is no muscle under the hard palate (Fig. 7-145). What might appear to be muscles are the brownish palatine mucous glands.

In the mucous membrane of the anterior part of someone's hard palate, observe three or four **transverse palatine folds (rugae)** of mucous membrane and the **palatine raphe** (Fig. 7-147). Feel these structures in your mouth with the tip of your tongue and finger.

CLINICALLY ORIENTED COMMENTS

Dentists anesthetize the **nasopalatine nerve** by injecting an anesthetic agent into the **incisive foramen** (Figs.7-147 and 7-148). The needle is inserted posterior to the

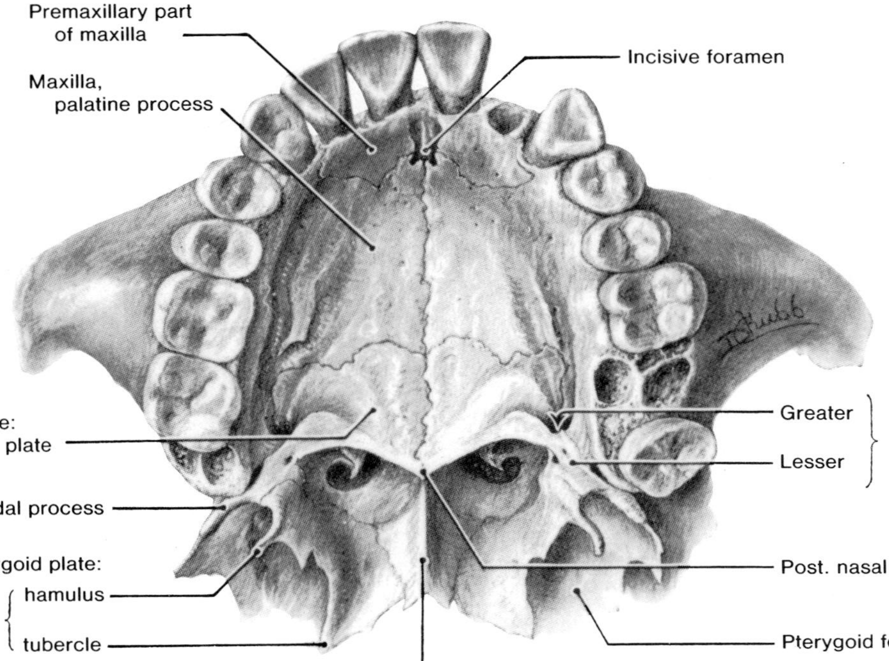

A.

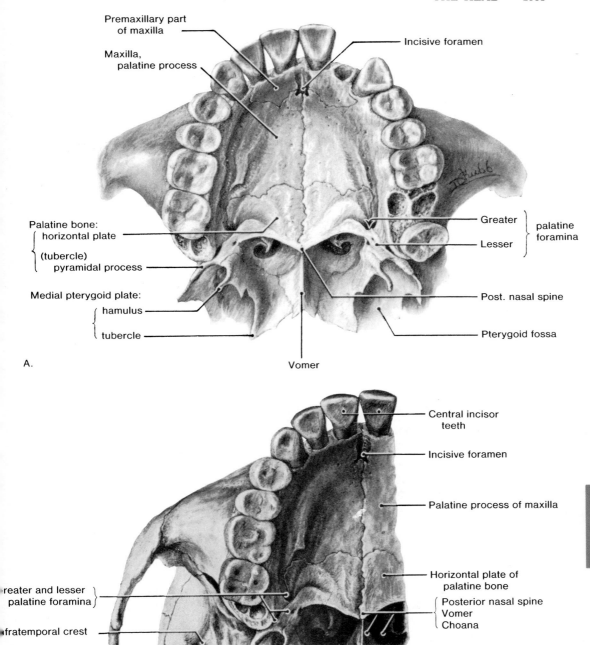

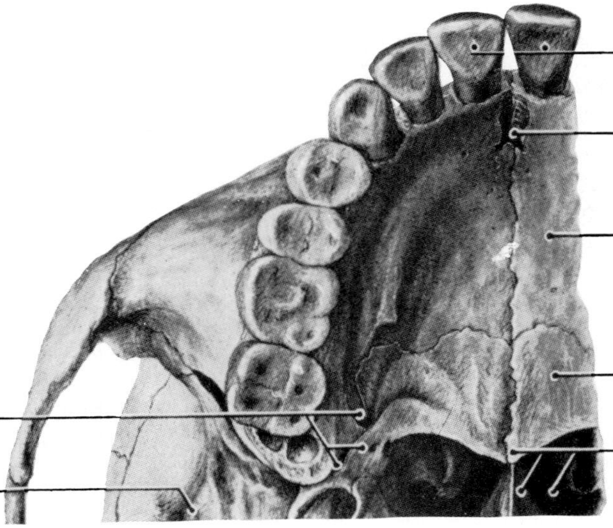

B.

Figure 7-146. Drawings of the hard palate and maxillary teeth. Observe that the hard palate is formed by the palatine processes of the maxillae and the horizontal plates of the palatine bones. Note the sutures between these processes and plates and between the maxillae and the palatine bones. The suture between the premaxillary part of the maxilla (sometimes called the incisive bone) and the fused palatine processes of the maxillae is usually visible only in skulls from young persons (*A*); hence, it is not visible in the hard palates of most dried skulls which are taken from older adults (*B*).

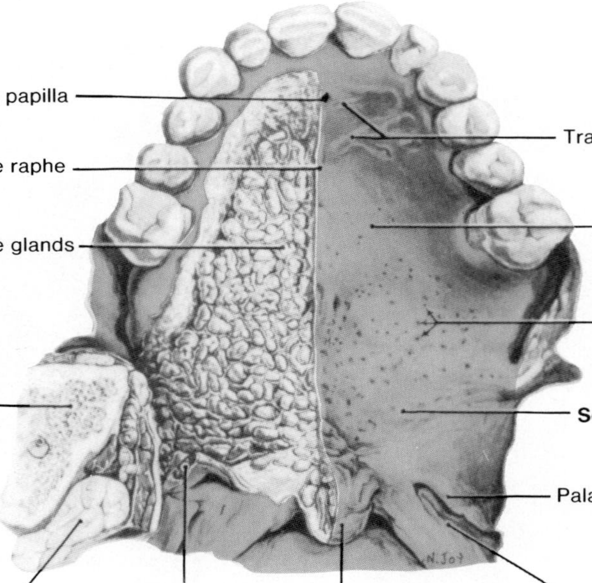

Figure 7-147. Drawing of the palate of an adult. Note that the second and third molars are missing and that the epithelium has been removed on the right side of the palate. Observe the transverse palatine folds (rugae) and the orifices of the ducts of the palatine glands, which give the mucous membrane an orange-peel appearance. Note that the palatine glands form a very thick layer in the soft palate (Fig. 7-145) but not in the hard palate. Observe that the palate ends posteriorly in the uvula and on each side in the palatopharyngeal arch. Observe the palatoglossus muscle and the palatoglossal arch extending from the under surface of the soft palate to the pharynx. (For a color view of the soft palate, see Fig. 9-61.)

incisive papilla, a slight elevation of the mucosa that covers the foramen at the anterior end of the palatine raphe (Fig. 7-147). This injection is given before performing certain operative procedures (*e.g.*, preparing an incisor tooth for capping or extracting an incisor tooth).

The Soft Palate (Figs. 7-145, 7-147, and 9-61). The soft palate, or velum palatinum (L. *velum*, sail or veil), is the curtain-like posterior part of the palate, a movable muscular fold that is attached to the posterior edge of the hard palate. It extends posteroinferiorly to a curved free margin from which a conical process, the **uvula**, hangs (Fig. 9-61). During swallowing the soft palate moves posteriorly against the wall of the pharynx, thereby preventing regurgitation of food into the nasal cavities.

Laterally the soft palate is continuous with the wall of the pharynx and is joined to the tongue and the pharynx by folds, called the **palatoglossal** and **palatopharyngeal arches**, respectively. The **palatine tonsil** is located in the triangular interval between these arches. The palatopharyngeal arch and the palatine tonsils (Figs. 7-147, 9-31, and 9-61) are described in Chapter 9 with the oropharynx to which they belong.

The soft palate is strengthened by the **palatine aponeurosis**, formed by the *expanded tendon of the tensor veli palatini muscle* (Figs. 7-148 to 7-150). This aponeurosis, attached to the posterior margin of the hard palate, is thick anteriorly and very thin posteriorly. *All other muscles of the soft palate are attached to the palatine aponeurosis.* The anterior part of the soft palate contains little muscle and consists

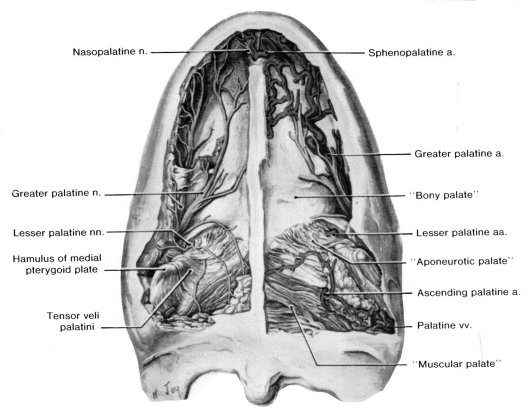

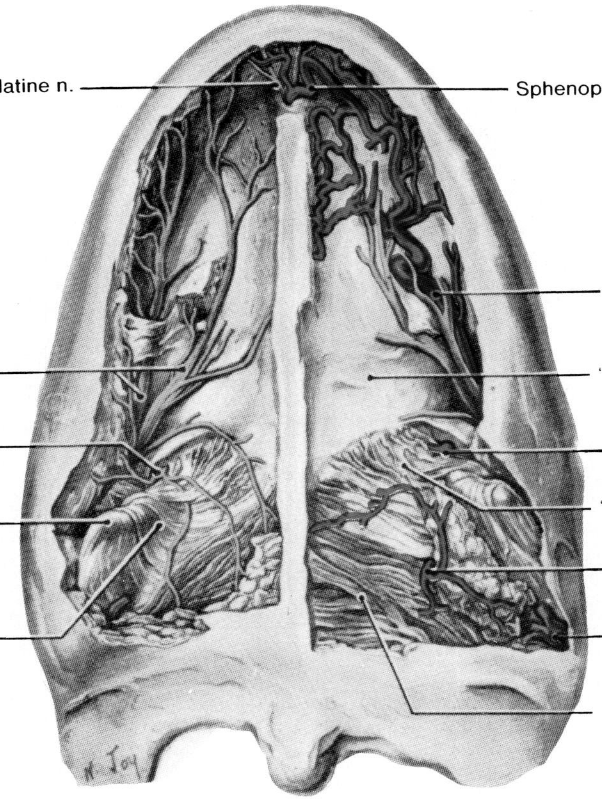

Figure 7-148. Drawing of a dissection of the inferior surface of the palate. Observe that the palate has bony, aponeurotic, and muscular parts. Note the tensor veli palatini muscle hooking around the hamulus of the medial pterygoid plate of the sphenoid bone to join the palatine aponeurosis. Also observe the the palatine vessels and nerves.

mainly of the aponeurosis, whereas the posterior part is muscular.

The Palatal Muscles (Figs. 7-148 to 7-150). The **five muscles of the palate**, arising from the base of the skull and descending to the palate, produce various movements of the soft palate. The posterior part may be raised so that it becomes a horizontal continuation of the plane of the hard palate and is in contact with the posterior wall of the pharynx. The soft palate can also be drawn down so that its undersurface is in contact with the posterior part of the upper surface of the tongue. During quiet breathing the soft palate is curved backward and downward. Movements of the palate during speech and swallowing are discussed in Chapter 9.

The Levator Veli Palatini (levator palati), a cylindrical muscle (Figs. 7-148 to 7-150), arises from the undersurface of the **petrous part of the temporal bone** and the medial side of the **auditory tube.** It runs inferiorly, spreading out in the soft palate where it inserts into the **palatine aponeurosis**. As its name indicates, it *elevates the soft palate*.

The Tensor Veli Palatini (tensor palati), a thin triangular muscle (Figs. 7-146, 7-148, and 7-151), arises from the **scaphoid fossa** at the base of the medial pterygoid process, the **spine of the sphenoid bone**, and the lateral side of the **auditory tube**. As it passes inferiorly, the tendon of this muscle hooks around the **hamulus** of the medial pterygoid plate before inserting into the **palatine aponeurosis**. The hamulus, or hook-like lower end of the medial pterygoid plate, can be palpated in the mouth by pressing upward a little anterior to the

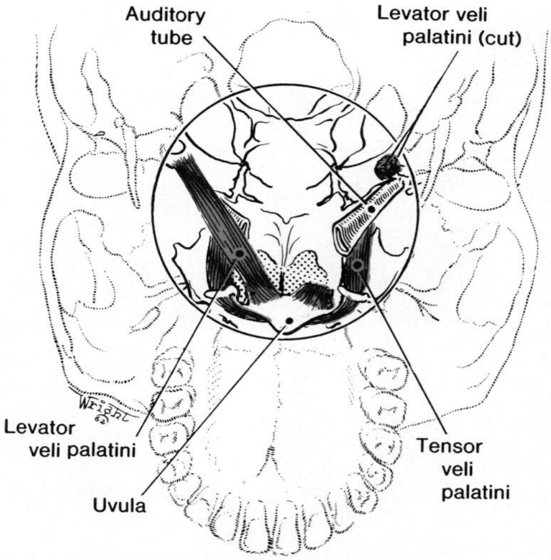

Figure 7-149. Diagram of the base of the skull showing the relationship of two of the palatal muscles (levator veli palatini and tensor veli palatini) to the auditory tube. This tube passes between these two muscles.

palatoglossal arch, *i.e.*, immediately posterior to the lingual surface of the third upper molar tooth (Fig. 7-146*A*).

The tensor veli palatini, as its name indicates, **tenses the soft palate**. Acting together, the two levator veli palatini muscles raise the soft palate as the two tensor veli palatini muscles tense it. This forces the soft palate against the posterior wall of the pharynx, a movement which occurs during swallowing.

The Palatoglossus Muscle arises from the palatine aponeurosis, passes inferiorly in the palatoglossal arch and inserts into the side of the tongue (Fig. 7-147). The palatoglossus elevates the posterior part of the tongue and draws the soft palate down on to the tongue. These movements tend to close off the oral cavity from the oral part of the pharynx (*i.e.*, close the oropharyngeal isthmus).

The Palatopharyngeus Muscle arises from the posterior border of the hard palate and from the palatine aponeurosis and passes in the **palatopharyngeal arch** (Fig. 7-147). It inserts into the posterior border of the thyroid cartilage and the side of the pharynx and esophagus. The palatopharyngeus tenses the soft palate and pulls the walls of the pharynx upward, forward, and **medially** during swallowing.

The Musculus Uvulae (Figs. 7-146 and 7-147), consisting of two small slips of mus-

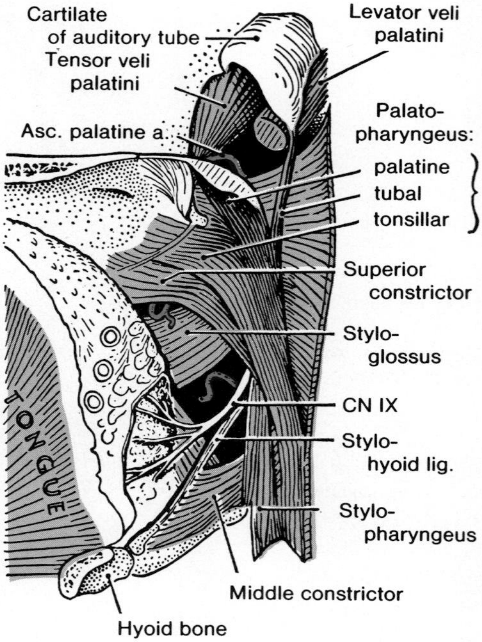

Figure 7-150. Drawing of a dissection of the side wall of the pharynx from within.

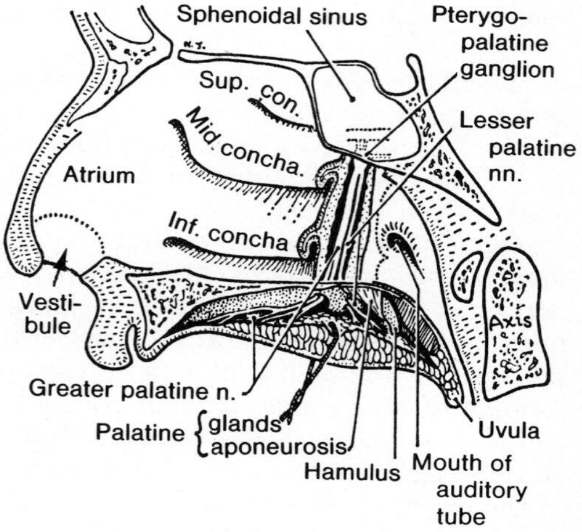

Figure 7-151. Drawing of a dissection of a sagittal section of part of the head showing particularly the sensory nerves of the palate, which are branches of the pterygopalatine ganglion.

cle, arises from the posterior nasal spine and the palatine aponeurosis and inserts into the **uvula**. *It assists in closing the nasopharynx during swallowing.*

Innervation of the palatal muscles is through the **pharyngeal plexus** by fibers derived from the cranial part of the accessory nerve (**CN XI**), except for the tensor veli palatini, which is supplied by the mandibular nerve (**CN V**^{3}).

Vessels and Nerves of the Palate (Figs. 7-148, 7-150, and 7-151). The palate has a rich blood supply from branches of the maxillary artery, chiefly the **greater palatine artery**, a branch of the descending palatine artery. This artery passes through the **greater palatine foramen** and runs anteriorly and medially. Try to palpate the greater palatine artery, medial to the third upper molar tooth, as it emerges from the foramen and runs anteriorly in a groove in the palate. The **lesser palatine artery** enters via the lesser palatine foramen and anastomoses with the **ascending palatine artery**, a branch of the facial. The two palatine arteries supply the soft palate.

The sensory nerves, branches of the pterygopalatine ganglion (Figs. 7-151 and 7-167), are the greater and lesser palatine nerves which accompany the arteries through the greater and lesser palatine foramina, respectively. The **greater palatine nerve** supplies the gingivae, the mucous membrane, and the glands of the hard palate. The **lesser palatine nerve** supplies the soft palate. The **nasopalatine nerve**, another branch of the pterygopalatine ganglion, emerges from the incisive foramen (Figs. 7-146 and 7-167) and supplies the mucous membrane of the anterior part of the hard palate (Fig. 7-148).

CLINICALLY ORIENTED COMMENTS

About once in 2500 births, infants are born with a **cleft palate** (Fig. 7-152) that may or may not be associated with a **cleft lip.** The cleft may involve only the uvula or it may extend through the entire palate. In severe cases associated with cleft lip, the cleft extends through the alveolar process and the whole palate (Fig 7-152*B*). In these infants the nasal and mouth cavities communicate; thus, they lack the power to suck. An **artificial palate** (prosthesis) is used until the palate can be repaired surgically.

The embryological basis of cleft palate is failure of the mesenchymal masses of the lateral palatine processes to fuse with each other, with the nasal septum, and/or with the posterior margin of the primary palate (primordium of the anterior part of the palate bearing the incisor teeth).

Paralysis of the soft palate sometimes results from *diphtheria*, a rare but prevent-

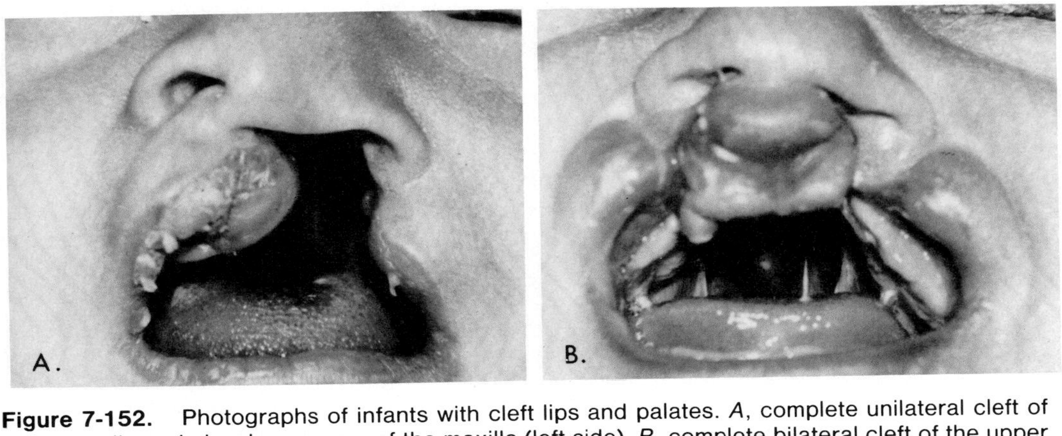

Figure 7-152. Photographs of infants with cleft lips and palates. *A*, complete unilateral cleft of the upper lip and alveolar process of the maxilla (left side). *B*, complete bilateral cleft of the upper lip and alveolar process of the maxilla, associated with a bilateral cleft of the anterior palate.

able disease. A **neurotoxin** is produced that destroys nerve cells and can lead to temporary or permanent paralysis of muscles. When the palatal muscles are affected the soft palate will not rise during swallowing. As a result, food and fluids may be forced into the nasopharynx and run out of the nose.

THE TONGUE

The tongue is a highly mobile muscular organ concerned with mastication (chewing), taste, deglutition (swallowing), articulation (speech), and oral cleansing. It is situated partly in the mouth and partly in the oropharynx (Figs. 7-137 and 7-145). It is mainly composed of muscle (Fig. 7-154) and is covered by a mucous membrane on its dorsum, tip (apex), and sides.

Gross Features of the Tongue (Fig. 7-153). The dorsum of the oral (anterior two-thirds) and pharyngeal (posterior one-third) parts of the tongue are separated by a V-shaped furrow called the **sulcus terminalis.** At the apex of this sulcus is a small median pit, the **foramen cecum,** which is the remnant of the opening of the embryonic *thyroglossal duct.* The thyroid gland in the embryo was attached to the tongue by this duct which normally disappears leaving only this small median pit. Only rarely does this duct persist and open at this foramen.

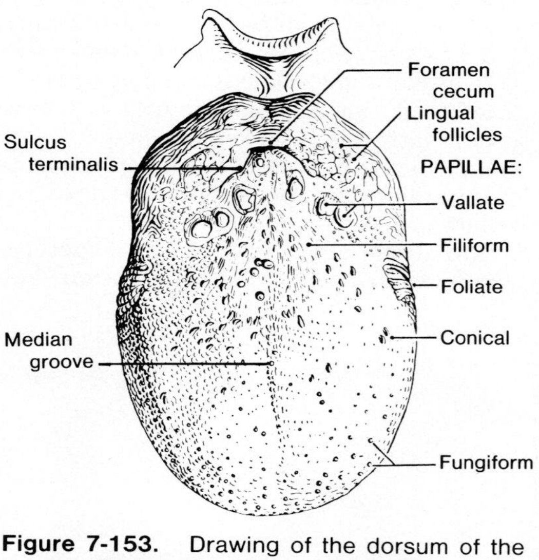

Figure 7-153. Drawing of the dorsum of the tongue. Observe the foramen cecum, the patent upper end of the embryonic thyroglossal duct, and the V-shaped sulcus terminalis, the limbs of which diverge from the foramen slightly behind the vallate papillae. This sulcus demarcates the developmentally different pharyngeal or posterior one-third of the tongue from the oral or anterior two-thirds. These parts differ in the structure of their mucous membrane and in their nerve supply (related to their different developmental origin).

The oral part (anterior two-thirds) of the tongue is freely movable but is loosely attached to the floor of the mouth by the **frenulum.** On each side of the frenulum observe the **deep lingual vein** under the mucous membrane. It begins at the tip and runs posteriorly near the median plane. It lies immediately deep to the mucous membrane on the inferior surface. All the veins of one side of the tongue unite at the posterior border of the hyoglossus muscle to form the lingual vein, which joins either the facial vein or the internal jugular vein. Note that the inferior surface and the sides of the tongue are covered with smooth, thin mucous membrane.

On the dorsum of the oral part of your tongue, observe the **median groove** (sulcus); it is inconspicuous in some people. The **dorsal lingual veins** drain the dorsum and sides of the tongue and join the **lingual veins,** which accompany the lingual artery.

Lingual Papillae and Taste Buds (Fig. 7-153). The mucous membrane on the oral or anterior two-thirds of the tongue is rough owing to the presence of numerous papillae which contain **taste buds.** The following are the main types.

The filiform papillae are numerous and thread-like and are arranged in rows parallel to the sulcus terminalis. Feel these papillae on your tongue, verifying that they are rough or scaly.

The fungiform papillae are small and mushroom-shaped. Examine your tongue in a mirror and observe these on the tip and margins of your tongue. They usually appear as bright pink or red spots.

The vallate papillae (7 to 12) are relatively large (1 to 2 mm in diameter) and are

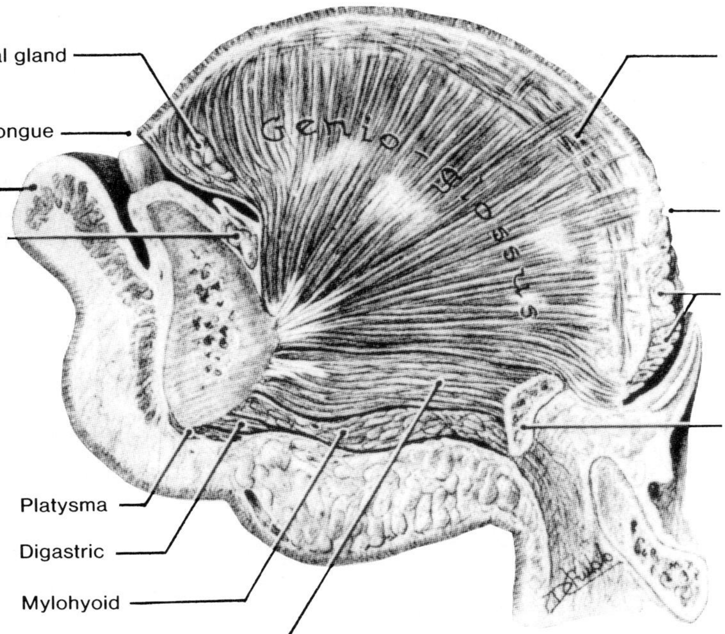

Figure 7-154. Drawing of a median section of the tongue and the floor of the mouth. Observe that the tongue is composed mainly of muscles, extrinsic that alter the position of the tongue and intrinsic that alter its shape. In this illustration, extrinsic muscles are represented by the genioglossus and intrinsic ones by the superior longitudinal muscle.

the largest ones, lying just anterior to the sulcus terminalis. They appear like flat-topped, short cylinders sunken into the mucosa and surrounded by a deep trench. The walls of this trench are studded with taste buds. You can see the vallate papillae on your tongue, but they are easier to observe on someone else's.

The pharyngeal part (posterior one-third) of the tongue lies behind the palatoglossal arches (Fig. 7-147). Its mucous membrane has no papillae; however, the underlying nodules of **lymphoid tissue** give the pharyngeal surface of the tongue a *cobblestone appearance.* These lymphoid masses or lingual follicles are collectively known as the **lingual tonsil** (Fig. 7-153).

CLINICALLY ORIENTED COMMENTS

When quick absorption of a drug is desired (*e.g.*, nitroglycerine that is used as a vasodilator in angina pectoris), it is placed under the tip of the tongue where it dissolves and enters the lingual veins in less than 1 minute.

Occasionally the lingual frenulum extends almost to the tip of the tongue and interferes with its protrusion. This **"tongue-tie"** condition is known as **ankyloglossia.** Usually the frenulum grows sufficiently during the 1st year of life so that surgical correction is unnecessary. **Fissured (scrotal) tongue** is present in some people, particularly those with the **Down syndrome** (Fig. 6-124).

Thyroglossal duct cysts may form anywhere along the course followed by the thyroglossal duct through the substance of the tongue during descent of the thyroid gland (Fig. 9-47). Usually the thyroglossal duct atrophies and disappears, but remnants of it may persist and give rise to cysts within the tongue. In very rare instances, the developing thyroid gland fails to descend, resulting in a **lingual thyroid.**

Muscles of the Tongue (Figs. 7-145 and 7-154 to 7-157). The tongue is divided into halves by a fibrous **lingual septum** that lies deep in the median groove (Fig. 7-153). In each half of the tongue, there are four extrinsic and four intrinsic muscles.

The Extrinsic Muscles (Figs. 7-154 to 7-157). This group of four muscles (genioglossus, hyoglossus, styloglossus, and palatoglossus) originate outside the tongue and insert into it. These muscles mainly move the tongue but they can alter its shape as well. The **hyoid bone** (Fig. 7-155) is attached to the posterior part of the tongue and moves with it.

The genioglossus muscle is a bulky, fan-shaped muscle that **arises** by a short tendon ("the handle") from the **superior mental spine** (Figs. 7-22 and 7-154) and fans out as it enters the tongue from below. Its fibers are inserted into the entire dorsum of the tongue. The genioglossus muscle **protrudes the tongue.**

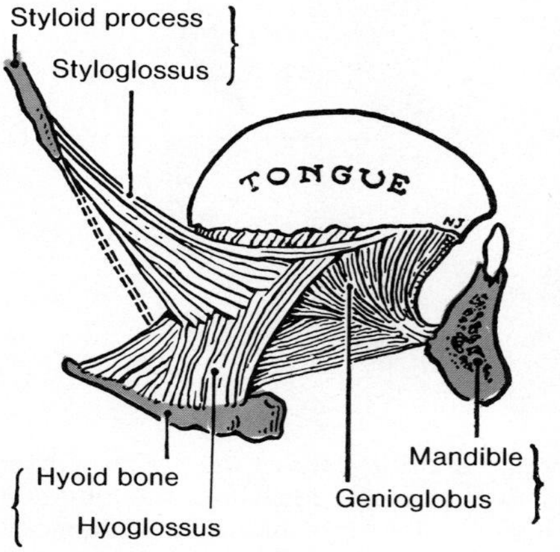

Figure 7-155. Drawing of the three extrinsic muscles of the tongue showing their bony origins, shapes, and directions.

CLINICALLY ORIENTED COMMENTS

If the genioglossus muscle is paralyzed, the tongue has a tendency to fall back and to obstruct the vital airway of the oropharynx, presenting the risk of suffocation. Total relaxation of the genioglossus muscles occurs during general anesthesia; therefore, the tongue of the anesthetized patient must be prevented from relapsing by exerting forward pressure on the mandible and inserting a curved airway which extends from the lips to the laryngopharynx. It does not enter the larynx or trachea.

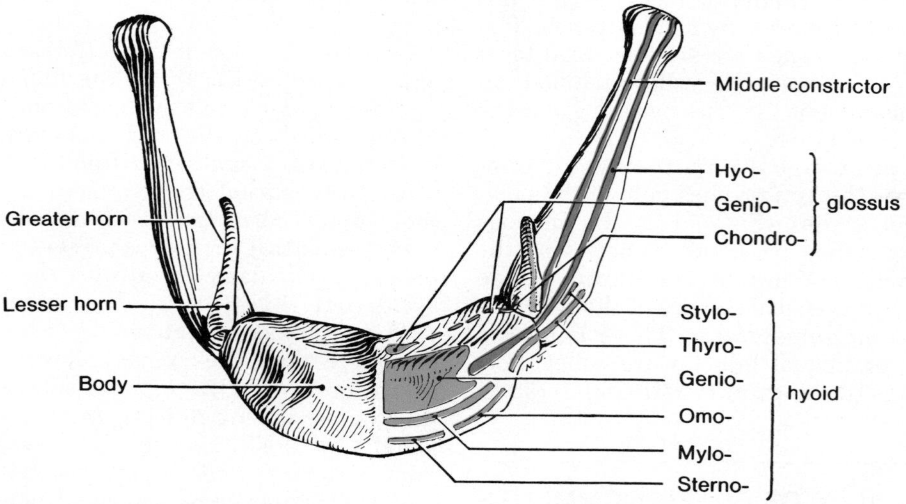

Figure 7-156. Drawing of the hyoid bone showing its parts and the sites of attachments of muscles. Observe that the hyoid is a horseshoe-shaped bone with a central body and greater and lesser horns. The origin of muscles is shown in *red* and the insertion of muscles is indicated in *blue*.

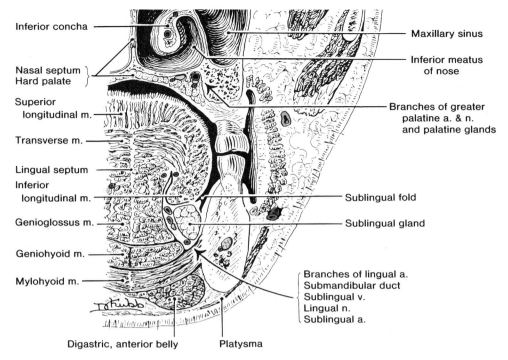

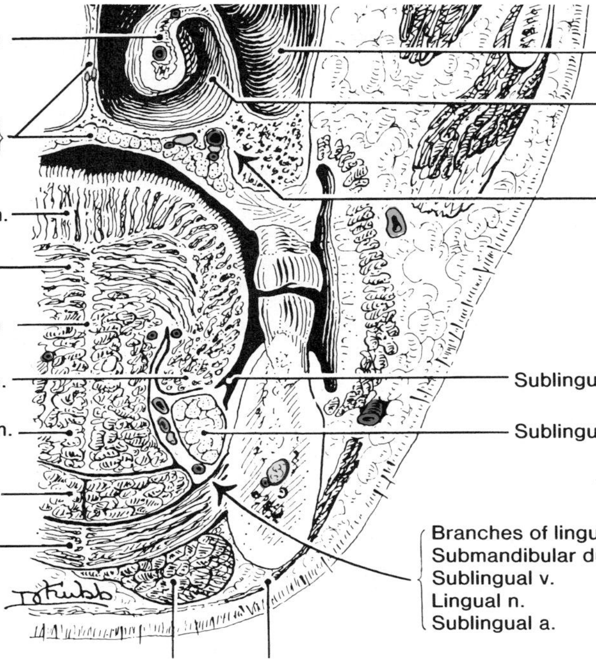

Figure 7-157. Drawing of a coronal section through the lower nose and mouth region, particularly to show the intrinsic muscles of the tongue and the muscles in the floor of the mouth.

The hyoglossus muscle is thin and quadrilateral in shape (Fig. 7-155). It arises from the body and greater horn of the **hyoid bone** and passes upward and forward to be inserted into the side of the tongue. The hyoglossus **depresses the tongue.**

The styloglossus muscle (Fig. 7-155) is a small, short muscle that arises from the anterior border of the **styloid process** near its tip and from the **stylohyoid ligament** and inserts into the side of the tongue. Note that its fibers interdigitate with those of the hyoglossus. The styloglossus **retracts the tongue.**

The palatoglossus muscle (Fig. 7-147) originates in the soft palate and enters the lateral part of the tongue with the styloglossus. It passes almost transversely through the tongue with the transverse intrinsic muscle fibers. Acting with the styloglossus, the palatoglossus **elevates the posterior part of the tongue.**

The Intrinsic Muscles (Figs. 7-154 and 7-157). There are four pairs of intrinsic muscles: superior and inferior longitudinal, transverse, and vertical. The intrinsic muscles are *mainly concerned with altering the shape of the tongue.*

The superior longitudinal muscle (Fig. 7-157) forms a thin layer deep to the mucous membrane on the dorsum of the tongue, running from the tip to the root. It arises from the submucous fibrous layer and the fibrous **lingual septum** and inserts mainly into the mucous membrane. This muscle **curls the tip** and **sides of the tongue superiorly,** making the dorsum of the tongue concave.

The inferior longitudinal muscle (Fig. 7-157) consists of a narrow band close to the inferior surface of the tongue. It extends from the tip to the root of the tongue and some of its fibers attach to the hyoid bone. This muscle **curls the tip of the tongue inferiorly,** making the dorsum of the tongue convex.

The transverse muscle (Fig. 7-157), lying inferior to the superior longitudinal muscle, arises from the fibrous **lingual**

septum of the tongue and runs laterally to its right and left margins. Its fibers are inserted into the submucous fibrous tissue. This muscle **narrows** and **increases the height of the tongue.**

The vertical muscle runs inferolaterally from the dorsum of the tongue. It **flattens and broadens the tongue.** Acting with the transverse muscles, the vertical muscles **increase the length of the tongue.**

Nerves of the Tongue. The muscles and the mucous membrane of the tongue have separate nerve supplies. The reason for this difference is embryological; the mucous membrane is derived from the floor of the primitive pharynx, whereas most of its muscles originate from the **occipital myotomes.** Myoblasts (primitive muscle cells) from these myotomes migrate into the tongue and give rise to its muscles. The hypoglossal nerve (CN XII) accompanies these myoblasts during their migration.

Innervation of the Muscles of the Tongue (Figs. 7-158 and 7-159). All the muscles of the tongue except the palatoglossus are supplied by CN XII, the **hypoglossal** nerve. The **palatoglossus,** although an extrinsic muscle of the tongue, is more closely associated with the soft palate. Like most muscles of the soft palate, it is supplied by nerve fibers from the **pharyngeal plexus** via the **vagus nerve** (CN X).

The hypoglossal nerve (CN XII) is the *motor nerve of the tongue* (Figs. 7-158, 7-161, and 9-22). It descends from the medulla through the hypoglossal canal (Fig. 7-47*A*) and passes laterally between the internal jugular vein and internal and external carotid arteries. It then curves anteriorly to enter the tongue, runs forward on the lower part of the hyoglossus muscle, and passes on to the lateral aspect of the genioglossus muscle. It continues forward in the substance of the tongue as far as the tip, distributing branches to the tongue muscles.

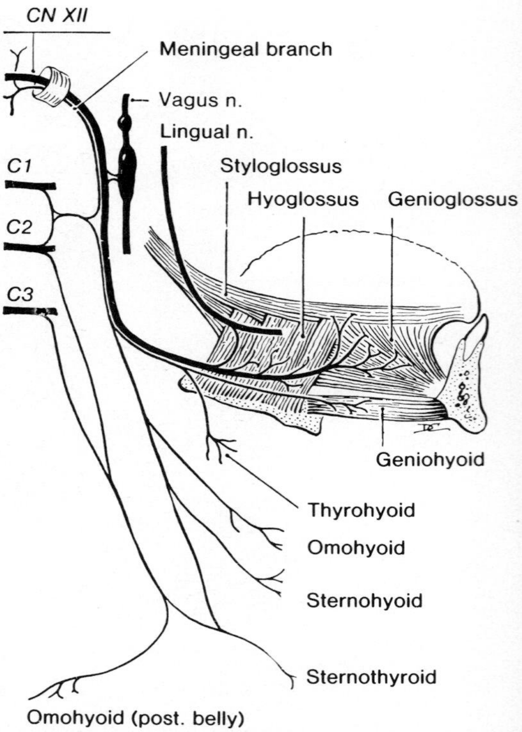

Figure 7-158. Diagram showing the distribution of the hypoglossal nerve (CN XII). This efferent nerve supplies all the intrinsic and extrinsic muscles of the tongue except the palatoglossus, which is supplied by the pharyngeal plexus via CN X. Note the connection between the hypoglossal and lingual nerves.

CLINICALLY ORIENTED COMMENTS

Section or injury of the hypoglossal nerve results in paralysis and eventual atrophy of one side of the tongue. The tongue deviates to the paralyzed side during protrusion because of the action of the unaffected genioglossus muscle on the other side. Hence, asking a person to stick out the tongue is *a good test of the function of the hypoglossal nerve (Fig. 8-24).*

Sensory Nerves of the Tongue (Fig. 7-159). The nerve supply to the mucous membrane of the tongue is complex because of its origin from the floor of the embryonic pharynx, which is *associated with the embryonic branchial apparatus.*

For general sensation, the mucosa of the *anterior two-thirds* of the tongue is

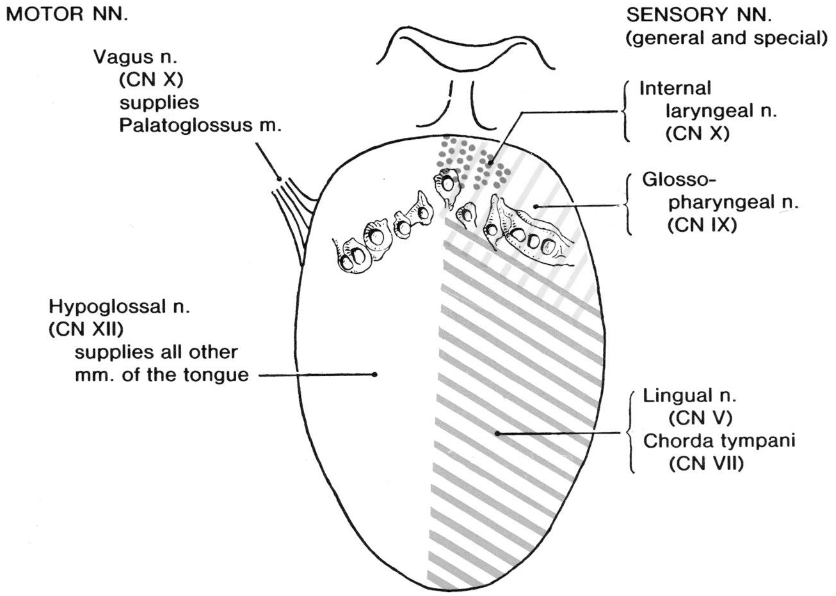

Figure 7-159. Diagram illustrating the nerve supply to the tongue.

supplied by the lingual branch of the **mandibular division of the trigeminal** (CN V^3), the nerve of the first branchial arch. **For special sensation** (taste), the anterior two-thirds of the tongue, except for the vallate papillae, is supplied by the **chorda tympani** from the facial (CN VII), the nerve of the second branchial arch. The chorda tympani joins the lingual branch of the mandibular nerve (CN V^3) and runs forward in its sheath (Fig. 7-128).

The mucosa of the **posterior one-third** of the tongue is supplied by the lingual branch of the **glossopharyngeal** (CN IX), the nerve of the third branchial arch, for general and special (taste) sensation, including the vallate papillae. Twigs of the internal branch of the superior laryngeal nerve of the **vagus** (CN X), the nerve of the posterior branchial arches, supplies a small area of the mucosa of the tongue just anterior to the epiglottis.

The sensory nerves to the tongue also carry **parasympathetic secretomotor fibers** to the glands buried in the substance of the tongue. Parasympathetic fibers from the chorda tympani travel with the lingual nerve to the **submandibular** and **sublingual salivary glands** (Fig. 7-157). These fibers synapse in the **submandibular ganglion** that hangs from the lingual nerve and rests on the hyoglossus muscle.

Arteries to the Tongue (Figs. 7-160, 9-27, and 9-29). The arterial supply to the tongue is chiefly through the **lingual artery,** which arises from the external carotid opposite the tip of the greater horn of the hyoid bone. On entering the tongue, the lingual artery passes deep to the hyoglossus muscle on each side, sending **dorsal lingual branches** to the tongue muscles and to the mucosa of the posterior one-third of the tongue. At the tip of the tongue, the terminal part of the lingual artery, called the **deep lingual artery** (profunda linguae artery) forms an anastomotic loop by joining the artery on the other side. The **sublingual artery** arises from the lingual artery at the anterior border of the hyoglossus muscle. It runs anterosuperiorly to supply the sublingual gland and adjacent muscles.

Veins of the Tongue. Two veins accompany the lingual artery (venae comitantes). The **deep vein,** the principle one of the tongue, begins at the tip and runs posteriorly in the median plane. *All veins of one*

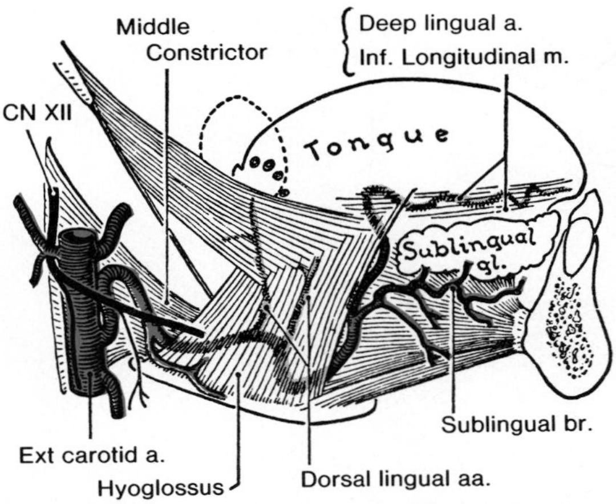

Figure 7-160. Drawing of the lingual artery and its branches. Note the dorsal lingual branches to the posterior part and the deep lingual artery to the anterior part of the tongue.

side of the tongue unite to form the **lingual vein,** which joins either the facial vein or the internal jugular vein.

The Submandibular and Sublingual Glands (Figs. 7-157 and 7-161). These are two of the three large paired salivary glands; the other is the parotid gland (Fig. 7-116), which is the largest one.

The submandibular gland (Fig. 7-161) lies partly above and partly below the posterior half of the base of the mandible and partly superficial and partly deep to the mylohyoid muscle. The **submandibular duct** arises from the portion of the gland that lies between the mylohyoid and hyoglossus muscles. This duct passes deep and then superficial to the lingual nerve to open by one to three orifices on a small, sublingual papilla beside the frenulum of the tongue.

The arterial supply of the submandibular gland is from the submental branch of the facial artery. The veins accompany the arteries. The submandibular gland is supplied by parasympathetic, secretomotor fibers from the *submandibular ganglion.*

The sublingual gland (Figs. 7-157, 7-160, and 7-161) is the smallest of the three paired salivary glands and is the most deeply situated. It lies in the floor of the mouth between the mandible and the genioglossus muscle. The glands on each side unite to form a horseshoe-shaped glandular mass around the frenulum. Numerous small ducts (10 to 12) open into the floor of the mouth, forming a linear series along the summit of the sublingual fold. Sometimes one of the ducts opens into the submandibular duct.

The arteries supplying the sublingual glands are branches of the sublingual and submental arteries (Fig. 7-160). The secretory nerves accompany those of the submandibular gland.

CLINICALLY ORIENTED COMMENTS

Calculi (L. pebbles) may form in the ducts of the salivary glands and produce pain, particularly during eating, because the saliva cannot escape from the gland. Calculi, usually *composed of calcium salts of inorganic or organic acids or other material,* can be detected on plain radiographs.

The parotid and submandibular salivary glands may be examined radiographically following the injection of contrast media into their ducts. This type of radiograph, called a **sialogram,** demonstrates the salivary ducts and some of the alveoli. Because of the small size of the ducts of the sublingual glands, injections of contrast medium cannot be made into them.

THE PTERYGOPALATINE FOSSA, NOSE, AND PARANASAL SINUSES

THE PTERYGOPALATINE FOSSA

The pterygopalatine fossa is a small, elongated, **pyramidal space** below the apex of the orbit (Figs. 7-123 and 7-162). The upper larger end is continuous with the **superior orbital fissure** and its lower end is closed except for the palatine foramina. Laterally it opens into the infratemporal fossa and thus can be partly inspected without separating the bones.

The pterygopalatine fossa was given its name because it is located between the

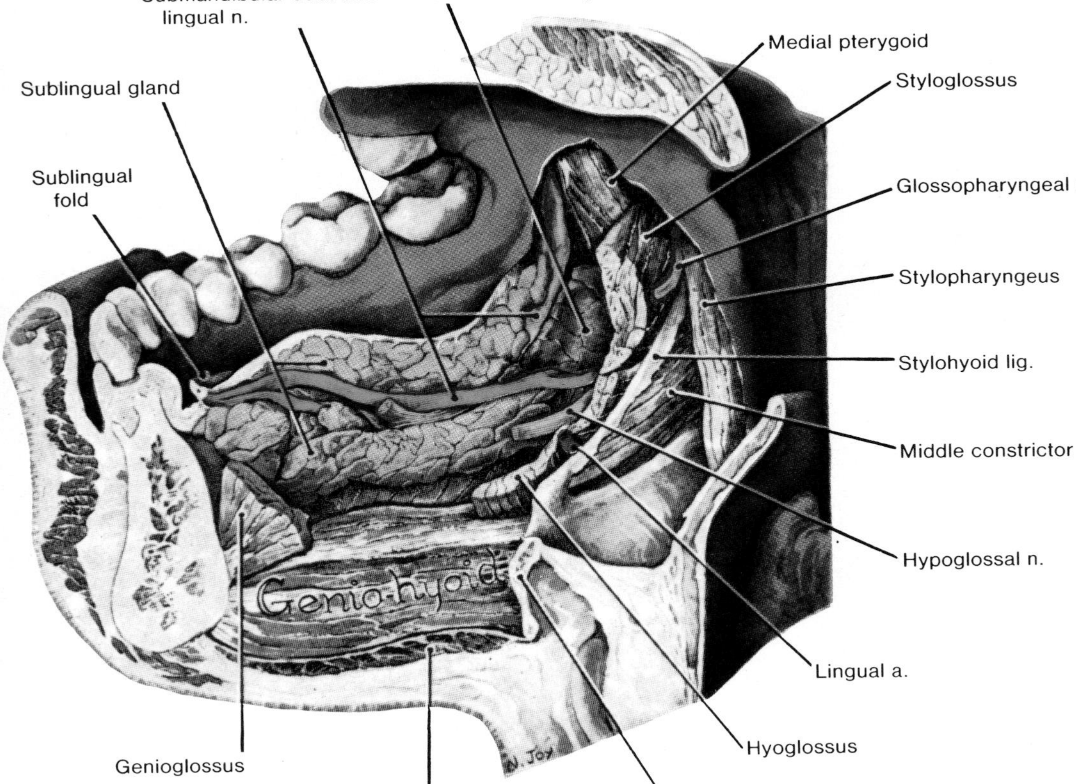

Figure 7-161. Drawing of a dissection of the floor of the mouth from which the tongue has been excised. Note the deep or oral part of the submandibular gland in the angle between the lingual nerve and the submandibular duct, which separates it from the sublingual gland. The orifice of the duct is at the anterior end of the plica sublingualis (sublingual fold). Also observe that the submandibular duct adheres to the medial side of the sublingual gland and here receives (as it sometimes does) a large accessory duct from the lower part of the sublingual gland. This communication is of importance in sialography (radiographic demonstration of the salivary ducts) because the sublingual duct that sometimes opens into the submandibular duct may be injected, resulting in visualization of some of the sublingual ducts as well as the submandibular duct.

pterygoid process of the sphenoid bone posteriorly and the **palatine** bone medially. The maxilla lies in front and the fragile vertical plate of the palatine bone forms its medial wall. Its **roof,** which is incomplete, is formed by the greater wing of the sphenoid bone.

The pterygopalatine fossa has several communications (Fig. 7-162): (1) **laterally** with the infratemporal fossa through the **pterygomaxillary fissure;** (2) **medially** with the nasal cavity through the **sphenopalatine foramen;** (3) **anteriorly** with the orbit through the **inferior orbital fissure;** and (4) **posterosuperiorly** with the middle cranial fossa through the foramen rotundum.

Contents of the Pterygopalatine Fossa (Figs. 7-125 and 7-163). This fossa contains the terminal branches of the **maxillary artery,** the **maxillary nerve,** and the **pterygopalatine ganglion.** The most important of these is the maxillary nerve. The maxillary nerve (CN V^2) *enters the*

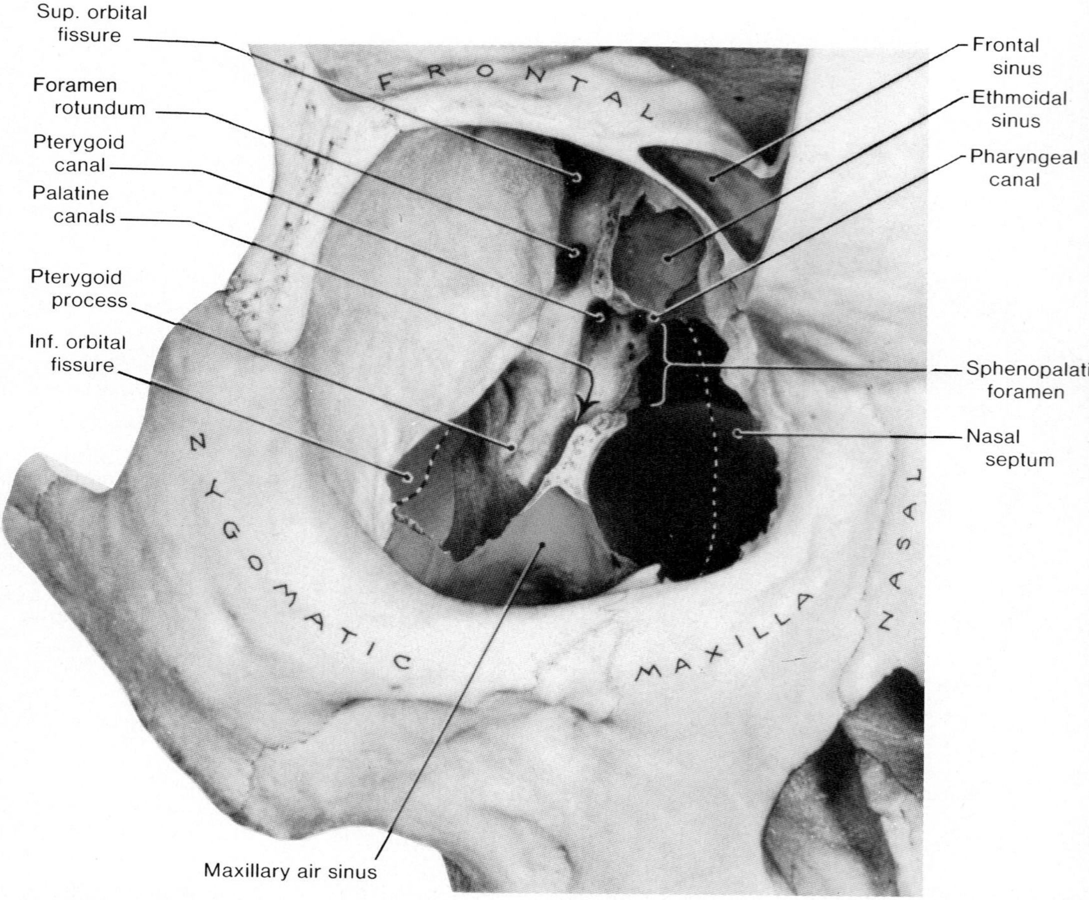

Figure 7-162. Photograph of an anterior view of the pterygopalatine fossa which has been exposed through the floor of the orbit and the maxillary sinus. For a lateral view (from the infratemporal fossa), see Figure 7-123.

pterygopalatine fossa through the foramen rotundum (Figs. 7-47 and 7-55) and runs forward and laterally in the posterior wall of the fossa (Fig. 7-163). Verify this course of the maxillary nerve by passing a bristle or hair through the foramen rotundum of a dried skull. Note that this **purely sensory nerve** runs forward across the upper part of the fossa. Within the fossa, the maxillary nerve gives off the **zygomatic nerve,** which divides into zygomaticofacial and zygomaticotemporal branches (Fig. 8-12). The nerves emerge from the zygomatic bone through foramina of the same name and supply the lateral region of the cheek and the temple (Fig. 7-30).

While in the fossa, the maxillary nerve also gives off two pterygopalatine nerves which suspend the **pterygopalatine ganglion** (Figs. 7-163 and 7-167); this *parasympathetic ganglion* is situated in the upper part of the fossa. Fibers of the maxillary nerve pass through this ganglion without synapsing. The parasympathetic fibers to the ganglion come from the facial nerve (CN VII) via the greater petrosal nerve. The sensory fibers that pass through the pterygopalatine ganglion without synapsing supply the nose, the palate, the tonsil, and the gingivae.

The maxillary nerve leaves the pterygopalatine fossa through the inferior orbital fissure as the **inferior orbital nerve.** In the orbit it passes through the infraorbital groove and canal in the floor of the orbit. The infraorbital nerve appears on the face through the **infraorbital foramen** (Figs. 7-30, 7-31, and 7-128) and supplies the skin of the lower eyelid, the side of the nose, and the anterior portion of the cheek. Just before it enters the orbit and during its passage through it, the maxillary nerve gives off the **superior alveolar nerves** which supply the upper (Fig. 7-124) or maxillary teeth.

The third or pterygopalatine part of the **maxillary artery** passes through the *pterygomaxillary fissure* into the pterygopalatine fossa (Fig. 7-125), where it lies in front of the pterygopalatine ganglion. It breaks up into branches which accompany all the nerves in the fossa and receive the same names. The **posterior superior alveolar artery** is given off from the maxillary artery as it enters the pterygopalatine fossa (Fig. 7-125). It descends on the infratemporal surface of the maxilla and supplies the molar and premolar teeth and the lining of the maxillary sinus. The **infraorbital artery,** often arising in conjunction with the posterior superior alveolar artery, enters the orbital cavity.

THE NOSE

The nose is the superior part of the respiratory tract and contains the peripheral organ of smell (Figs. 7-168, 8-2, and 8-3).

The External Nose. Noses vary considerably in size and shape mainly as a result of differences in the nasal cartilages and the depth of the glabella (Fig. 7-1). The nose projects forward from the face to which its root is joined just below the forehead. The **dorsum of the nose** extends from the root to the **apex** (tip). The inferior surface of the nose is pierced by two apertures, called **anterior nares** (nostrils), which are separated from each other by the **nasal septum** (Fig. 7-165). Each naris is bounded laterally by the **ala** (L. wing) or side of the nose. The posterior apertures or **choanae** open into the nasopharynx (Fig. 9-58).

The Skeleton of the Nose (Figs. 7-164 to 7-166). The immovable **bridge** or upper bony part of the nose consists of **nasal bones,** the frontal processes of the **maxillae,** and the nasal part of the **frontal bone.** The movable lower cartilaginous part of the nose consists of five main cartilages and a few smaller ones. *The nasal cartilages are composed of hyaline cartilage* and are connected with one another and with the nasal bones by the continuity of the perichon-

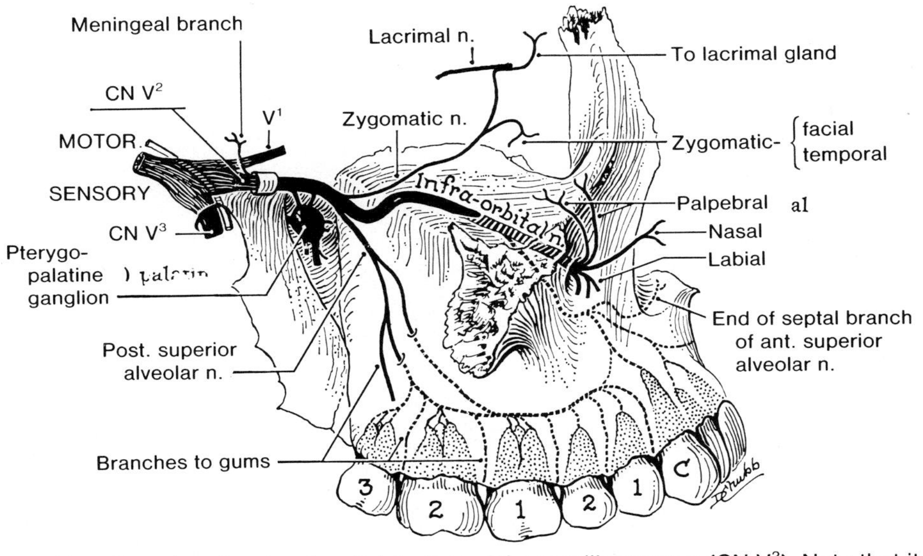

Figure 7-163. Drawing showing the distribution of the maxillary nerve (CN V^2). Note that it gives off two pterygopalatine nerves which suspend the pterygopalatine ganglion in the pterygopalatine fossa.

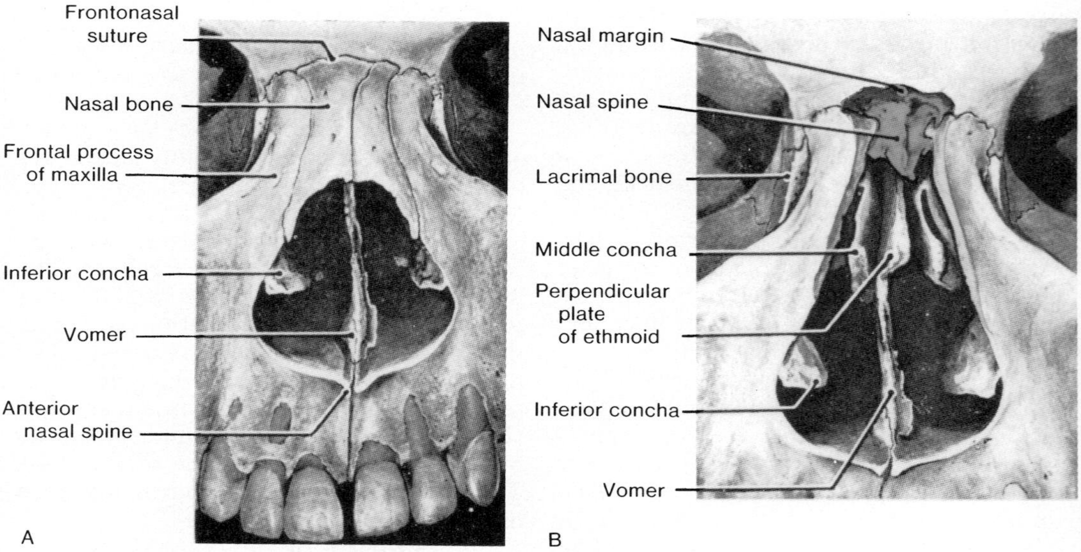

Figure 7-164. Drawings of the bones of the nose. In *A*, observe that the bony anterior nasal aperture formed by the maxillae and the nasal bones is sharp. In *B*, the nasal bones have been removed to show the areas on the frontal processes of the maxillae (*yellow*) and on the frontal bone (*blue*) that articulate with and buttress the nasal bones.

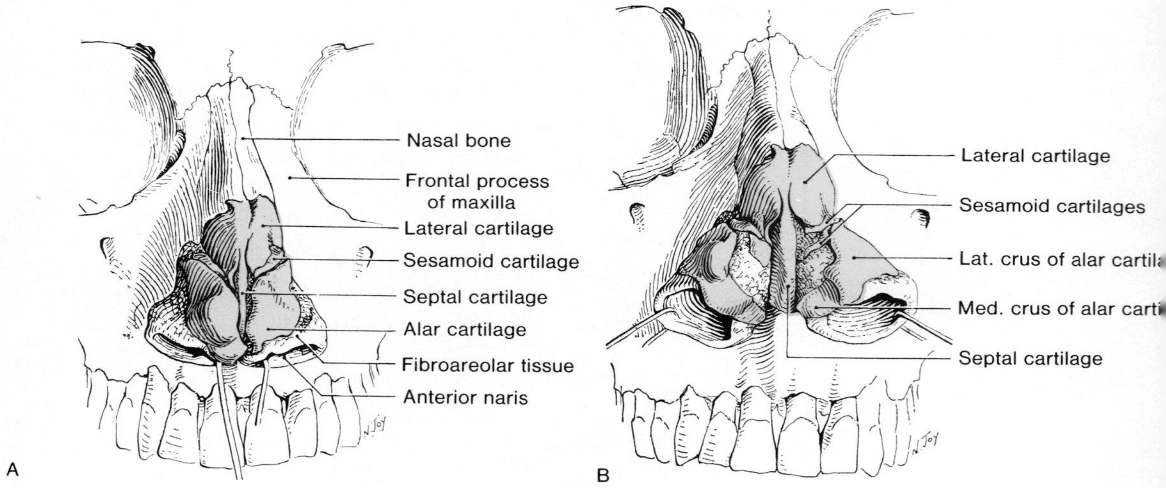

Figure 7-165. Drawings of the cartilages of the nose (*yellow*). In *A*, the alar cartilages have been pulled down to expose the sesamoid cartilages. In *B*, the alar cartilages are separated by dissection and retracted laterally.

drium and the periosteum, respectively. The U-shaped alar nasal cartilages are free and movable. The alar cartilages can dilate or constrict the external nares by muscular contraction. The muscles acting on the external nose have been described and illustrated (Fig. 7-28).

Structure of the Nasal Septum (Figs. 7-145 and 7-166). This **partly bony** and **partly cartilaginous** septum divides the cavity of the nose into two narrow **nasal cavities.** The bony part is usually located in the median plane until the 7th year; thereafter it often bulges to one or other side, more frequently to the right. *The nasal septum has three main components: (1) the* **perpendicular plate** of the ethmoid; (2) the **vomer;** and (3) the **septal cartilage.** Observe the bony parts on a dried skull, particularly a bisected one. Note that the perpendicular plate forming the upper part of the septum is very thin and descends from the **cribriform plate** of the ethmoid bone. The **vomer,** a thin flat bone, forms the posteroinferior part of the septum of the nose. It articulates with the perpendicular plate of the ethmoid and the septal cartilage (Fig. 7-166).

Immediately above the anterior naris, the nasal septum is covered with skin which contains a number of stiff hairs (Fig. 7-172) called **vibrissae** (F. *vibro*, to quiver). The rest of the nasal septum is covered with mucous membrane. The lower two-thirds of this mucosa is called the **respiratory area** and the upper one-third is the **olfactory area** (Fig. 7-168). Air passing over the respiratory area is warmed and moistened as it passes to the lungs. The olfactory area, yellowish in living persons, contains the *peripheral organ of smell.* Sniffing draws air to the olfactory area.

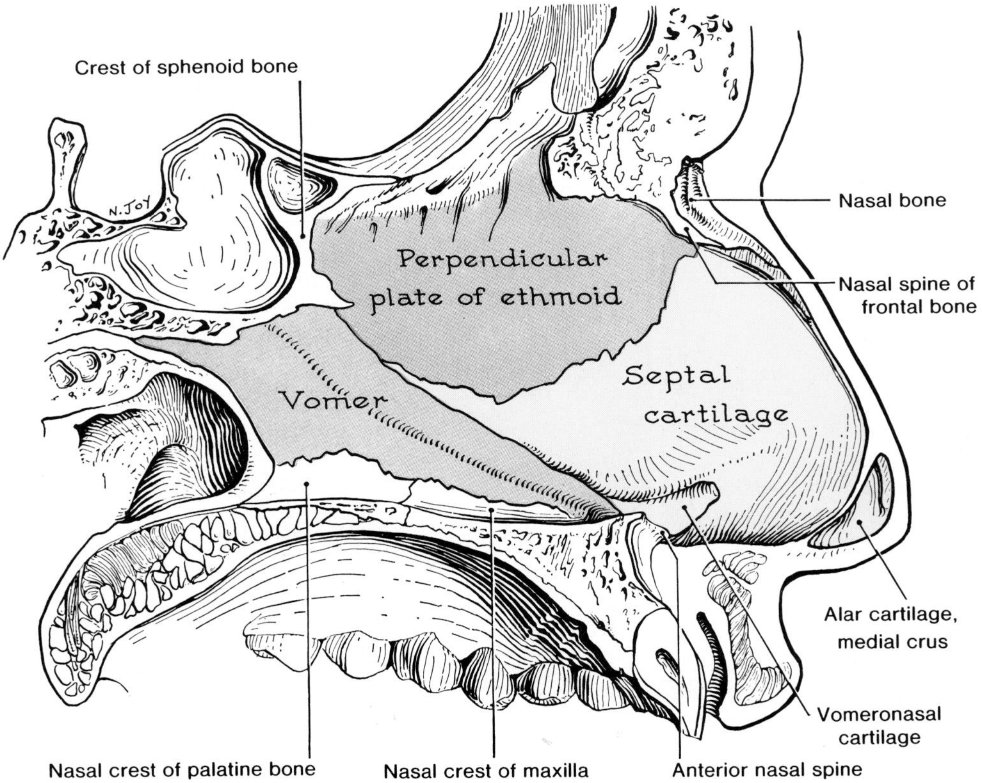

Figure 7-166. Drawing of the anterior part of a bisected skull showing the septum of the nose. Note that, like the palate, the nasal septum has a hard part (here partly bony and partly cartilaginous) and a soft or mobile part. The skeleton or basis of the hard septum consists of three parts: perpendicular plate of ethmoid, septal cartilage, and vomer. Around the circumference of these, the adjacent bones (frontal, nasal, maxillary, palatine, and sphenoid) make minor contributions. The soft or mobile part of the septum is composed of the alar cartilages, covered by skin and soft tissues between the tip of the nose and the anterior nasal spine.

Nerves of the Nasal Mucosa (Figs. 7-167 and 7-168). The **olfactory mucosa,** covering an area of about 2.5 cm^2 in the roof and lateral wall of each nasal cavity, contains many sensory **olfactory cells.** Axons from these cells converge to form the **olfactory nerves** (CN I), which pass from the nasal cavity via foramina in the **cribriform plate** of the ethmoid bone (Fig. 7-50). The olfactory nerve bundles, about 20 on each side, enter the ventral surface of the **olfactory bulbs** (Figs. 7-79, 7-167 and 8-3).

The **respiratory area,** the lower two-thirds of the nasal mucosa, is supplied chiefly by the trigeminal nerve (Figs. 7-167 and 7-168). The mucous membrane of the **nasal septum** is supplied chiefly by the **nasopalatine nerve** (from CN V^2); its anterior portion is supplied by the **anterior ethmoidal nerve** (from CN V^1). The lateral wall of the nasal cavity is supplied by nasal branches from the maxillary nerve (CN V^2), by branches of the greater palatine nerve, and by the anterior ethmoidal nerve.

Arteries of the Nasal Mucosa (Fig. 7-172). There is a rich blood supply to the mucosa of the nasal cavity. The **sphenopalatine,** a branch of the *maxillary artery,* supplies most of the blood to the mucosa, the lateral wall, and the septum of the nasal cavity. It enters via the sphenopalatine foramen and sends branches to posterior re-

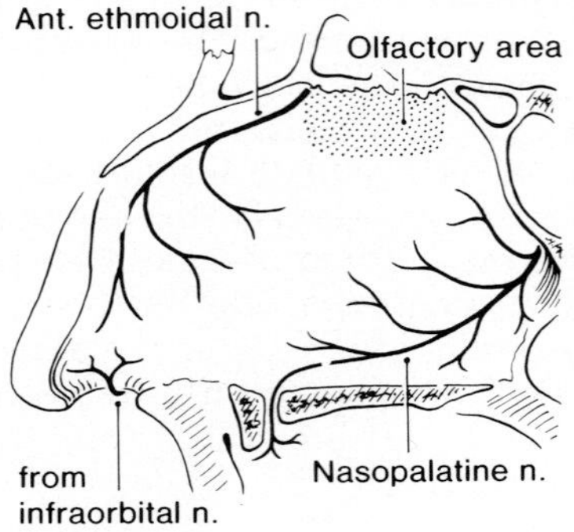

Figure 7-168. Diagram showing the nerves of the nasal septum. The nasopalatine nerve emerges from the pterygopalatine ganglion (Fig. 7-167) and enters the nasal cavity through the sphenopalatine foramen. Note that the nasopalatine nerve ends by passing through the incisive foramen (Figs. 7-146 and 7-148) to supply the anterior part of the hard palate.

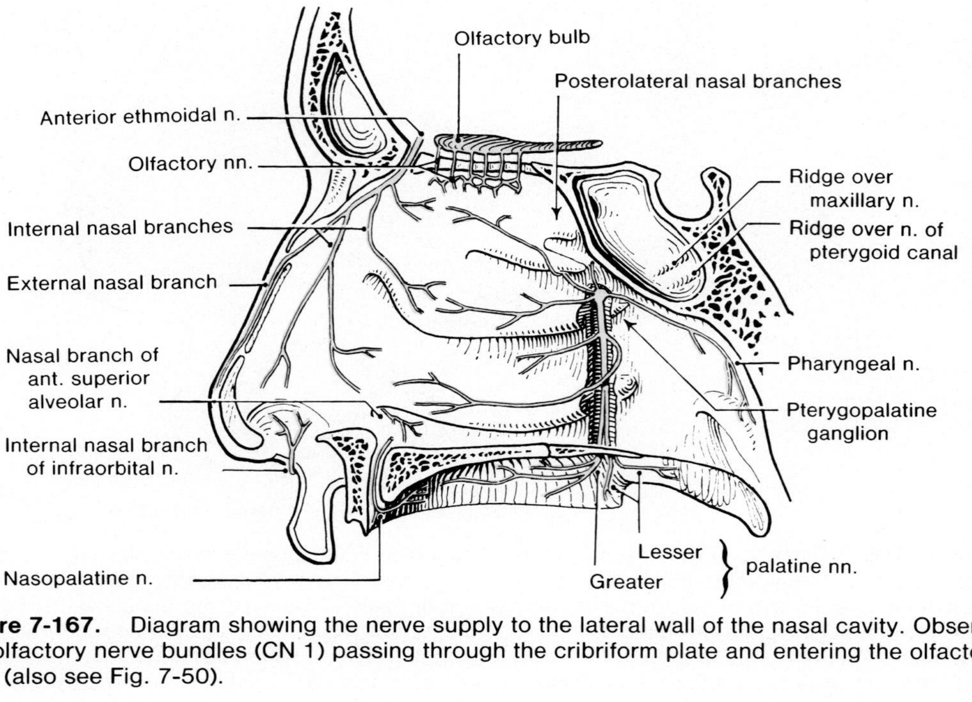

Figure 7-167. Diagram showing the nerve supply to the lateral wall of the nasal cavity. Observe the olfactory nerve bundles (CN 1) passing through the cribriform plate and entering the olfactory bulb (also see Fig. 7-50).

gions of the lateral wall and the septum. The **greater palatine,** another branch of the maxillary artery, passes through the incisive foramen to supply the nasal septum. The sphenopalatine and greater palatine arteries anastomose on the nasal septum.

The anterior and posterior **ethmoidal arteries,** branches of the **ophthalmic artery,** supply the anterosuperior part of the mucosa of the lateral wall and the septum of the nasal cavity. Three branches of the **facial artery** also supply anterior parts of the nasal mucosa.

Veins of the Nasal Mucosa. The veins of the nasal cavity form a rich venous network or plexus beneath the nasal mucosa, especially over the lower part of the septum. Some of the veins open into the sphenopalatine vein, others join the facial vein, and some empty into the ophthalmic veins and drain into the cavernous sinus (Fig. 7-38).

The Nasal Cavities (Figs. 7-137, 7-164, 7-169 to 7-171, and 7-177). The right and left cavities of the nose are situated above the hard palate and are separated from each other by the nasal septum. They extend from the **anterior nares** to the **posterior nares (choanae)** that open posteroinferiorly into the **nasopharynx.** The first part of the nasal cavity is called the **vestibule** (Fig. 7-170).

Each choana, bounded by bone, is about 2.5 cm high and the floor is about 1.3 cm wide. Each cavity is about 5 cm in height and 5 to 7 cm in length and has a roof, a floor, and medial and lateral walls.

The roof of each nasal cavity is curved and narrow except at the posterior end. It is divided into three parts, frontonasal, ethmoidal, and sphenoidal, which indicate the bones forming them, The **olfactory nerves (CN I)** pass through the foramina in the cribriform plate of the ethmoidal part (Fig. 7-167). **The floor** is wide in comparison with the roof and is formed by the palatine process of the **maxilla** and the horizontal process of the *palatine bone.*

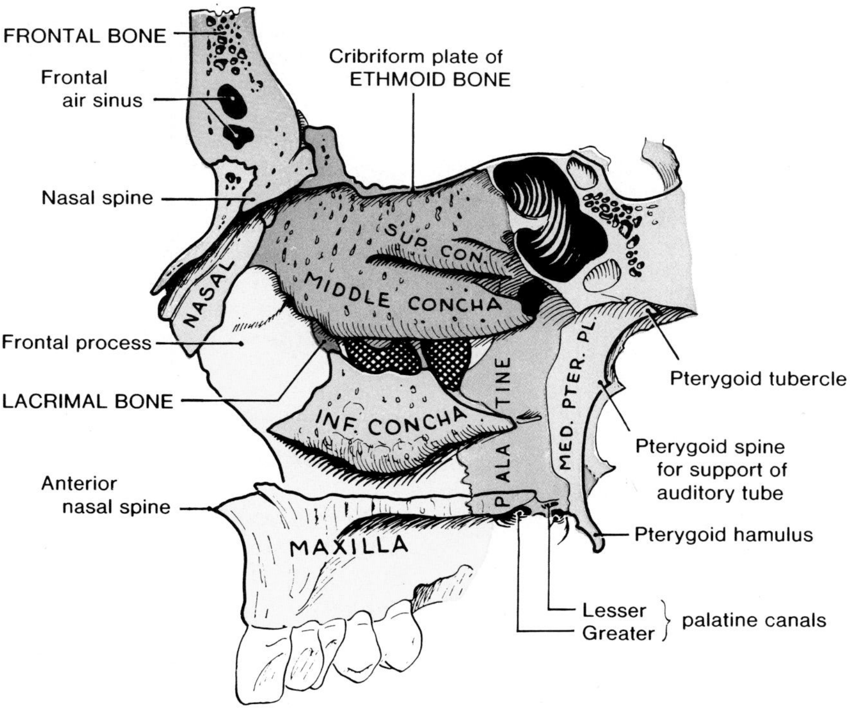

Figure 7-169. Drawing of a sagittal section of part of a skull to show the bones in the lateral wall of the nasal cavity.

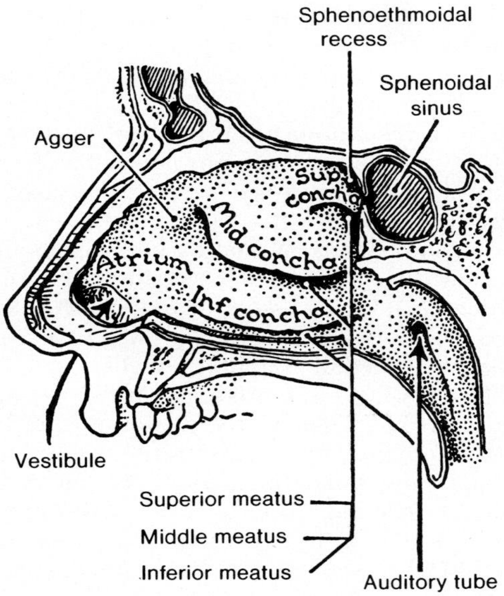

Figure 7-170. Drawing of a sagittal section of the nose and palate to show the lateral wall of the nasal cavity. Observe the entrance to the nose, called the vestibule, which is located above the nostril (naris) and in front of the inferior meatus. The atrium, above the vestibule and in front of the middle meatus, is lined with mucous membrane. Note the inferior and middle conchae, extending downward and medially from the lateral wall and dividing it into three nearly equal parts. They cover the inferior and middle meatuses, respectively. About 1.5 cm posterior to the inferior concha, note the pharyngeal orifice of the auditory tube.

The medial wall of the nasal cavity, formed by the bony nasal septum, is usually smooth. **The lateral wall** is uneven owing to three longitudinal, scroll-shaped elevations or *turbinates* (L. shaped like a top), which are called superior, middle, and inferior **nasal conchae** (L. shells). They are named according to their position on the wall. The superior and middle conchae are parts of the ethmoid bone, whereas the inferior concha is separate, *i.e.*, the **turbinate bone.** The inferior and middle conchae project medially and inferiorly, producing air passageways called the inferior and middle **meatuses** (L. passages). The short superior concha conceals the superior meatus. The space posterosuperior to the superior concha into which the *sphenoidal sinus* opens is called the **sphenoethmoidal recess.**

The superior meatus is a narrow passageway between the superior and middle nasal conchae into which the **posterior ethmoidal sinuses** open by one or more orifices.

The middle meatus is longer and wider than the superior meatus. The anterosuperior part of this meatus leads into a funnel-shaped opening, called the **infundibulum,** through which it communicates with the frontal sinus. The passage that leads downward from the frontal sinus to open into the infundibulum of the middle meatus is called the **frontonasal duct** (Fig. 7-171). There is one for each frontal sinus and, as there may be several frontal sinuses on each side, there may be several frontonasal ducts.

When the middle concha is raised or removed, a rounded elevation, called the **ethmoidal bulla** (L. a bubble), is visible (Fig. 7-171). This bulge is formed by the **middle ethmoidal sinuses** (Fig. 7-175) which open on the surface of this bulla. Below the bulla is a semicircular groove called the **hiatus semilunaris.** Anteriorly and above, the frontal sinus opens into the hiatus and near to this are the openings of the anterior ethmoidal sinuses (Fig. 7-174). The maxillary sinus opens into the middle meatus.

The inferior meatus (Fig. 7-170) is a horizontal passage, below and lateral to the inferior nasal concha. The *nasolacrimal duct* (Fig. 7-100) opens into the anterior part of this meatus. Usually the orifice of this duct is wide and circular.

CLINICALLY ORIENTED COMMENTS

Fractures of the nose are common; usually the fractures are transverse. If the injury results from a direct blow, the horizontal plate of the ethmoid bone is often fractured.

The nasal mucosa becomes swollen **(rhinitis)** during upper respiratory infections and with some allergies (*e.g.*, hayfever). Swelling of this membrane occurs readily because of its vascularity. When

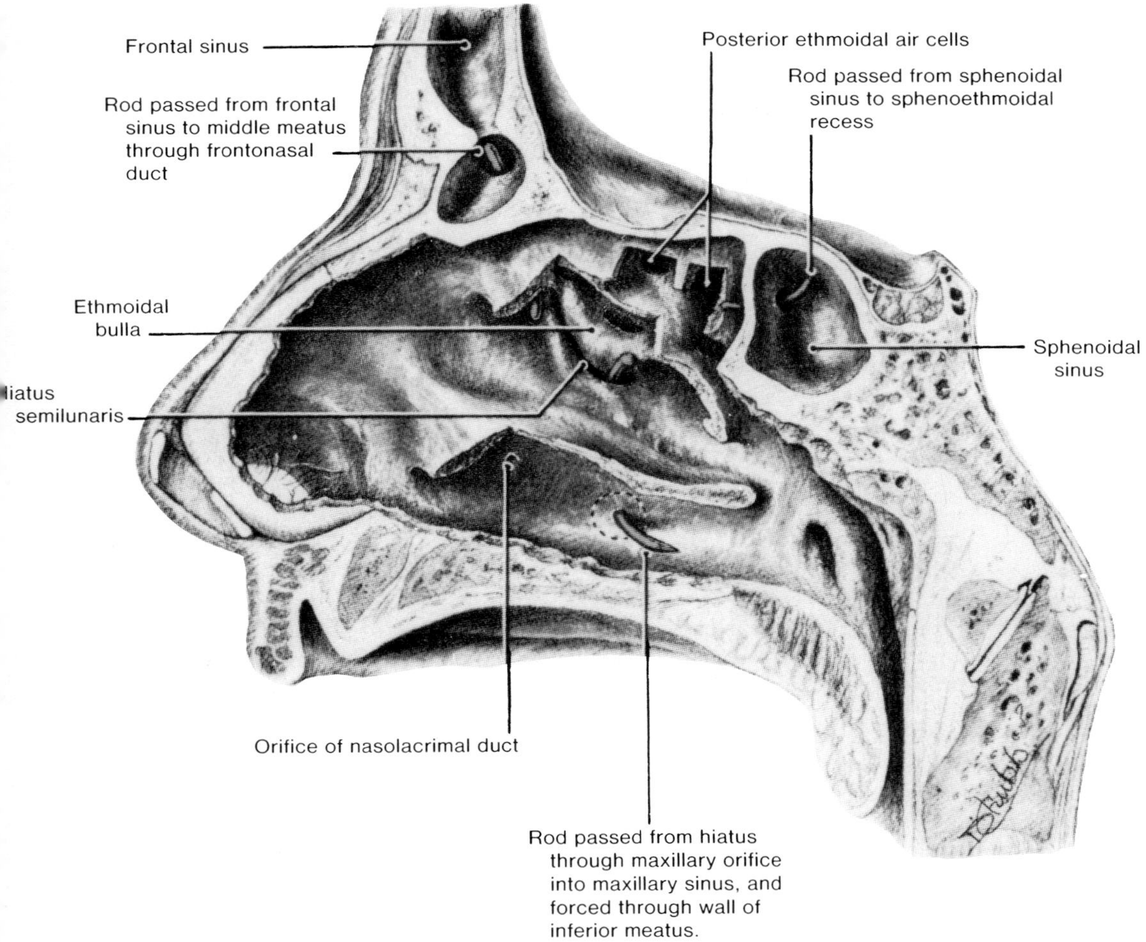

Figure 7-171. Drawing of a dissection of the lateral wall of the nasal cavity. Parts of the superior, middle, and inferior conchae are cut away. Observe the sphenoidal sinus in the body of the sphenoid bone and its orifice above the middle of its anterior wall that opens into the sphenoethmoidal recess. Note the orifices of the posterior ethmoidal cells opening into the superior meatus. Also observe the orifice of the nasolacrimal duct, a short distance below and lateral to the inferior concha.

swelling is associated with increased mucus secretion, the common "stopped-up nose" or "runny nose" occurs. Spread of infection from the nose and paranasal sinuses to the meninges, although rare, is dangerous.

The skin of the nose contains many sebaceous glands which may become infected and blocked. As discussed previously, *infections about the nose* may spread to the cavernous sinus via connections between the facial and ophthalmic veins (Fig. 7-38); hence, the nose is part of the danger triangle of the face (Fig. 7-203 and Case 7-3).

Because of its other relations, infections of the nasal cavities may spread into: (1) the anterior cranial fossa via the **cribriform plate** of the ethmoid bone; (2) the nasopharynx and retropharyngeal soft tissues; (3) the middle ear via the **auditory tube** (Fig. 7-170); (4) the paranasal air sinuses (see subsequent section); and (5) the lacrimal apparatus and conjunctiva.

Although nasal discharge is commonly associated with acute upper respiratory tract infections, *nasal discharge associated with a head injury* may actually be

CSF **(CSF rhinorrhea)** *owing to fracture of the cribriform plate and tearing of the meninges.* This condition may be diagnosed by injecting a radioactive tracer into the CSF and later detecting it in pledgets of cotton in each nostril. **CSF leakage** may also result from a fracture of the sphenoid sinus or of the petromastoid part of the temporal bone. In this case, the CSF leaks via the middle ear through the auditory tube.

Epistaxis (nosebleed) is relatively common owing to the richness of the blood supply to the nasal mucosa (Fig. 7-172). In most cases the cause of the bleeding is trauma and the bleeding is located in the anterior third of the nose. Mild epistaxis often results from **nose picking,** which tears the rich network of veins around the anterior nares. However, epistaxis is also associated with infections (*e.g.*, typhoid fever) and hypertension. **Spurting of blood** results from rupture of arteries, particularly at the site of anastomosis of the sphenopalatine and greater palatine arteries. If nasal bleeding is so abundant that it cannot be stopped by usual treatments, the external carotid artery is sometimes clamped and/or ligated in the neck, as it is the source of blood passing to the nose via the maxillary and sphenopalatine arteries (Fig. 7-114).

The cartilaginous nasal septum may be displaced at birth or it may deviate from the median plane as a result of injury (Fig. 7-18). In some cases the deviation is so great that the septum may produce unilateral obstruction of the nasal passage.

PARANASAL SINUSES

The paranasal sinuses are air-filled extensions of the nasal cavities **(pneumatic areas)** in the following cranial bones: frontal, ethmoid, sphenoid, and maxilla (Fig. 7-173). The sinuses are named according to the bones in which they are located. They vary considerably in size and form in different people and in different races (*e.g.*, the frontal sinuses are generally small in oriental people).

Most of the sinuses are rudimentary or absent in newborn infants. There are no frontal or sphenoidal sinuses present at birth, but there are usually a few ethmoidal air cells and tiny maxillary sinuses. They enlarge and invade adjacent bones (frontal and sphenoid) during childhood and adolescence. Growth of the sinuses is important in altering the size and shape of the face and in adding resonance to the voice.

The paranasal sinuses are lined with mucous membrane which is continuous with that of the nasal cavities. The mucosa of the sinuses is, however, thinner, less vascular, and not so adherent to the bony walls of the sinuses. Mucus secreted by the glands in the mucous membrane passes into the nasal cavities through the meatuses (Fig. 7-170).

The Frontal Sinuses (Figs. 7-16, 7-18, and 7-170 to 7-176). These air chambers are located between the outer and inner tables of the **frontal bone,** posterior to the **superciliary arches** (on which the eyebrows are set) and the root of the nose. The size of the superciliary arches varies in degree of development; however, *the prominence of the superciliary arches is no indication of the size of the subjacent frontal sinuses.* Only a radiographic examination or **transillumination** (discussed subsequently) can reveal their actual size in any given person. Usually the frontal sinuses are detectable in radiographs of children by the 7th year.

Understand also that (1) *the right and left frontal sinuses are rarely of equal size* in the same person; (2) the *septum between the right and left sinuses is rarely situated entirely in the median plane.* Often a frontal sinus has two parts: (1) a **vertical part** *in the squamous part* of the frontal bone, and (2) a **horizontal part** *in the orbital part* of the frontal bone. One or both parts may be large or small. When the supraorbital part is large, its roof forms the floor of the anterior cranial fossa and its floor forms the roof of the orbit.

Examine the frontal sinuses in a bisected skull and explore the cavities with a bristle. Attempt to find their openings into the nose. *The frontal sinuses vary in size* from about 5 mm (pea size) to large spaces extending laterally into the greater wing of the sphenoid bone. The frontal sinuses may be multiple on each side and each of these

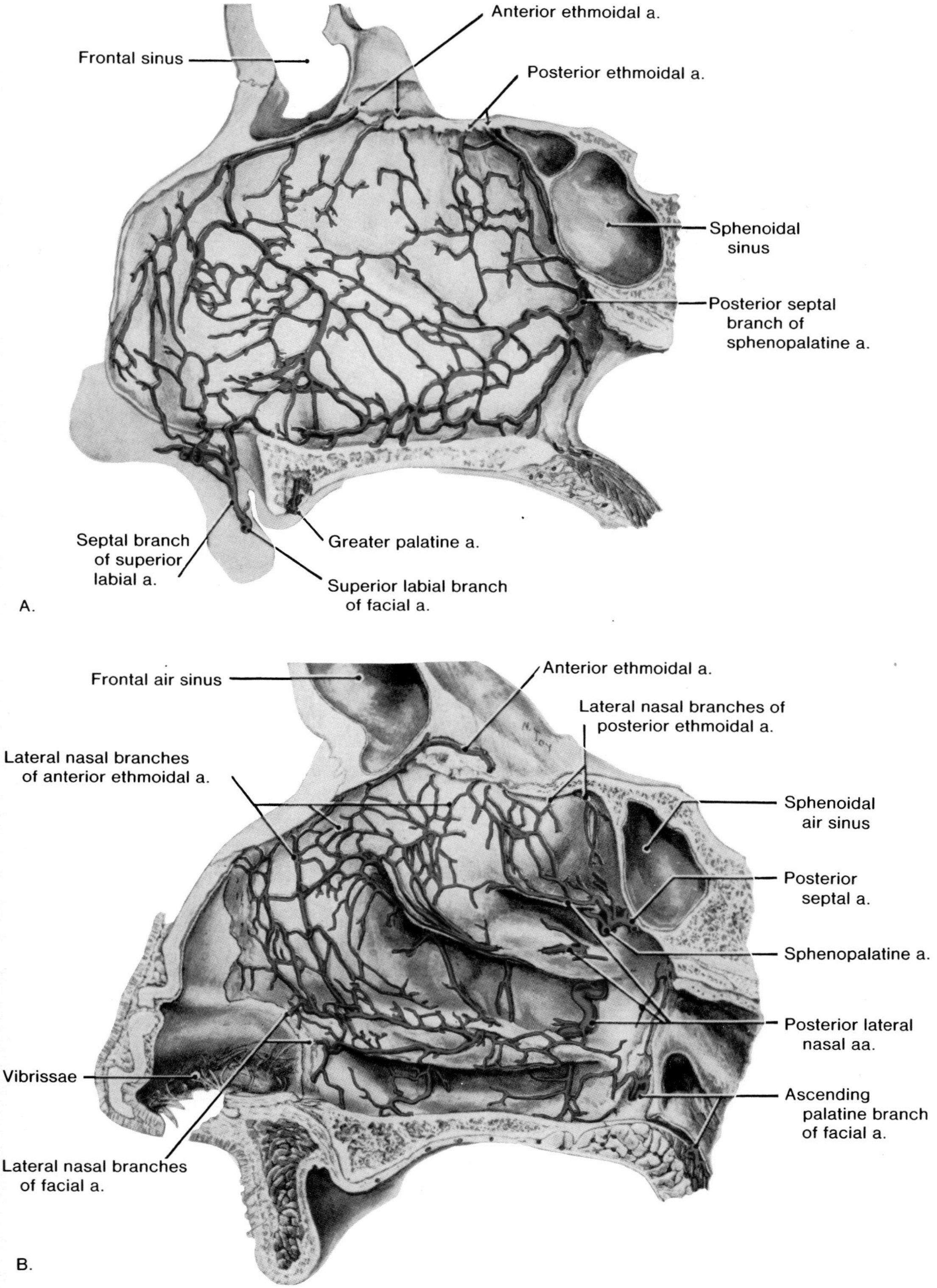

Figure 7-172. Drawings of the medial wall of the nasal septum (*A*) and of the lateral wall of the nasal cavity (*B*) to show the arterial supply to the mucosa. The sphenopalatine artery is the main supply. Entering through the sphenopalatine foramen (Fig. 7-148), it sends lateral nasal branches forward on both surfaces of the conchae, partly in bony canals. Note the posterior septal artery which crosses the roof of the nose below the anterior part of the floor of the sphenoidal sinus and anastomoses through the incisive foramen.

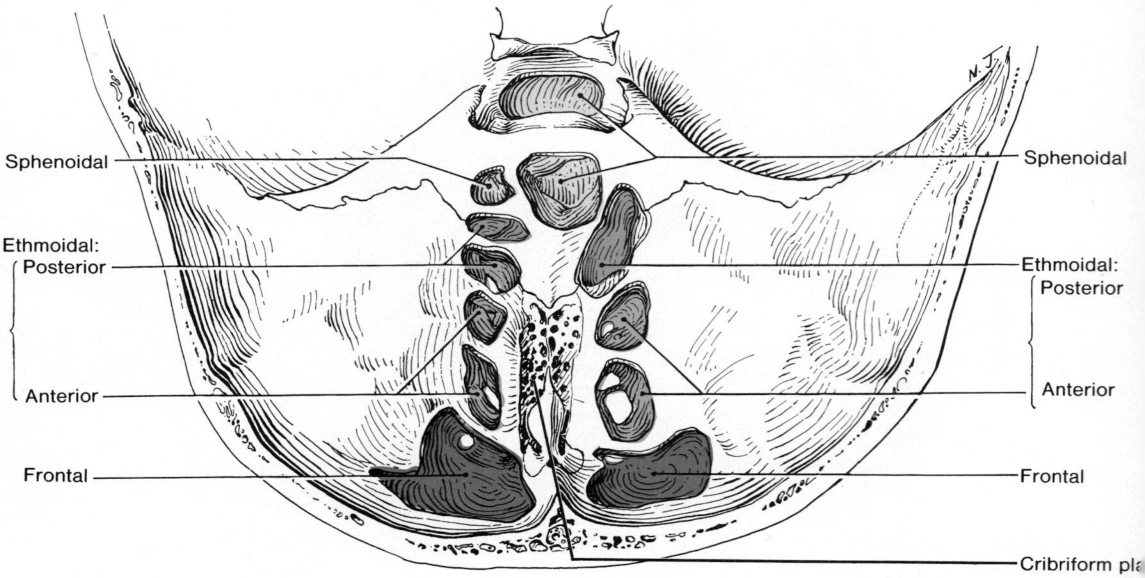

Figure 7-173. Drawing of the floor of the anterior cranial fossa showing the paranasal air sinuses surrounding the cribriform plates (also see Fig. 7-50). The exposed parts of the frontal sinuses are the supraorbital portions.

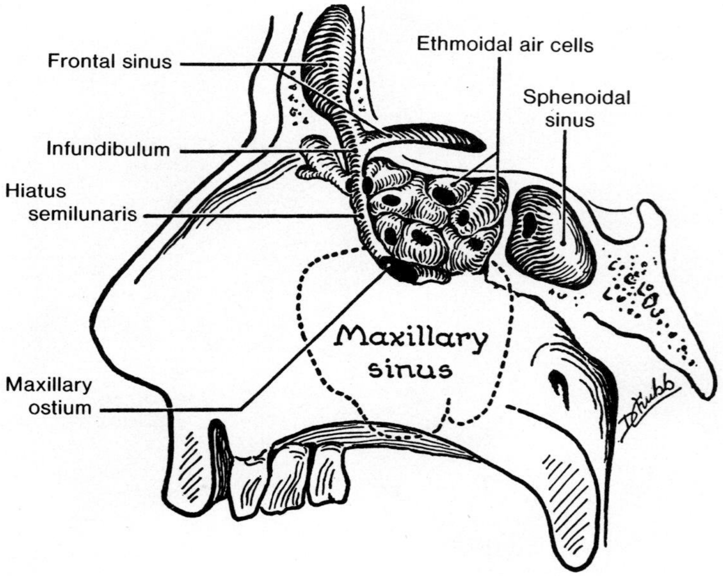

Figure 7-174. Schematic drawing of the paranasal air sinuses. Understand that fluid in the frontal sinus would tend to flow through the infundibulum, along the hiatus, and into the maxillary sinus because the orifice of the former sinus is at its floor and of the latter sinus at its roof. The sphenoidal ostium is in the upper half of its anterior wall. The ethmoidal ostia are variable.

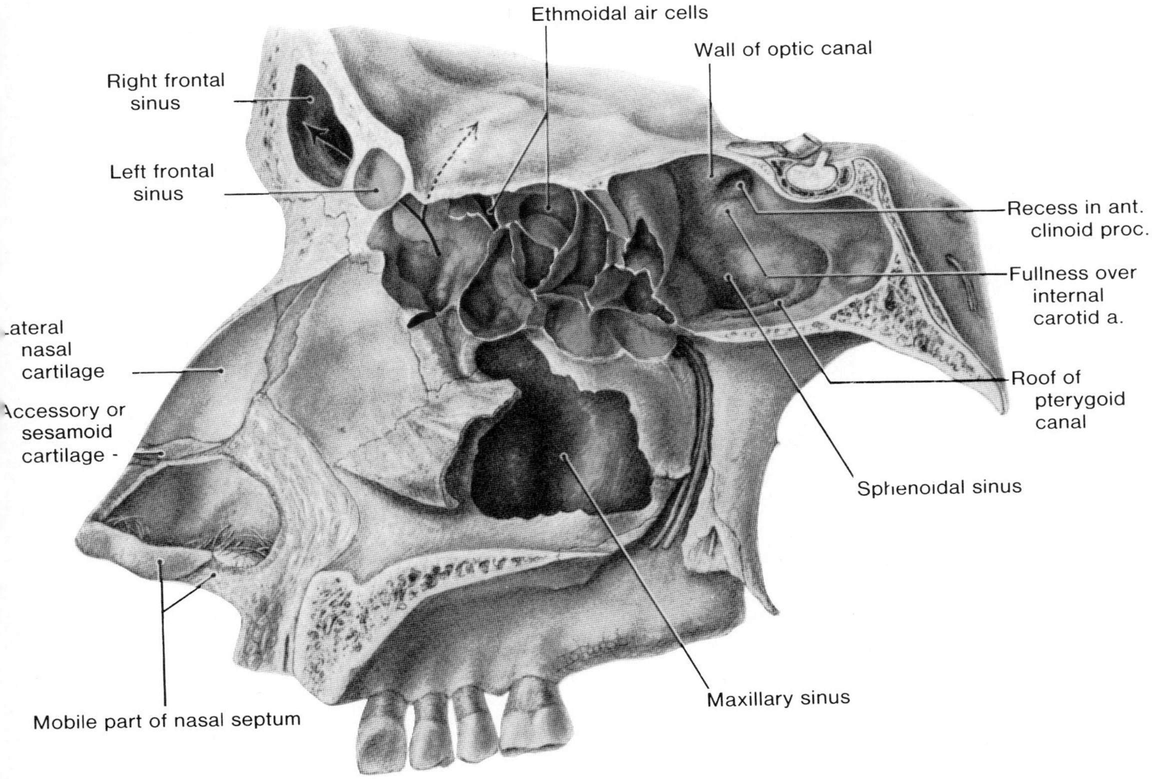

Figure 7-175. Drawing of a sagittal section of the nasal cavity and palate. Bone has been removed to show the paranasal sinuses (opened). The ethmoidal cells (*pink*), collectively called a sinus, appear like a honeycomb. An anterior ethmoidal cell (*blue*) is invading the diploë of the frontal bone to become a frontal sinus. It is ethmoidal in origin but frontal in location. An offshoot (*broken arrow*) invades the orbital plate of the frontal bone. The sphenoidal sinus (*blue*) in this specimen is very extensive, extending (1) backward below the hypophysis cerebri to the clivus, (2) laterally below the optic nerve into the anterior clinoid process, and (3) downward to the pterygoid process but leaving the pterygoid canal rising as a ridge on the floor of the sinus. The maxillary sinus (*yellow*) is pyramidal in shape. Its base contributes to the lateral wall of the nasal cavity, its apex is in the zygomatic process, and its orifice is at its highest point. In "blow-out fractures" of the orbit resulting from a blow to the eyeball, the thin medial or ethmoidal wall (Fig. 7-93) and the floor (maxillary sinus) of the orbit are the walls that most often fracture. As a consequence, orbital tissues may enter the ethmoid and maxillary sinuses.

may have a separate **frontonasal duct** (Fig. 7-171) that drains via the infundibulum into the middle meatus. Usually the frontal sinus drains via one duct on each side into the middle meatus.

The Ethmoidal Sinuses (Figs. 7-16, 7-171, 7-173, and 7-174 to 7-177). The **ethmoidal air cells** form the labyrinth of the **ethmoid bone,** located between the nasal cavity and the orbit. The number varies from 3 to 18. The cells are larger when the number is small. Hold a skull up to a light and observe these thin-walled air cells through the delicate orbital lamina of the ethmoid bone (Fig. 7-93), which forms the medial wall of the orbit.

Usually the ethmoidal air sinuses are not visible in radiographs before the age of 2 years and they do not grow rapidly until 6 to 8 years after puberty. For purposes of description, the ethmoidal air sinuses are divided into **anterior, middle,** and **pos-**

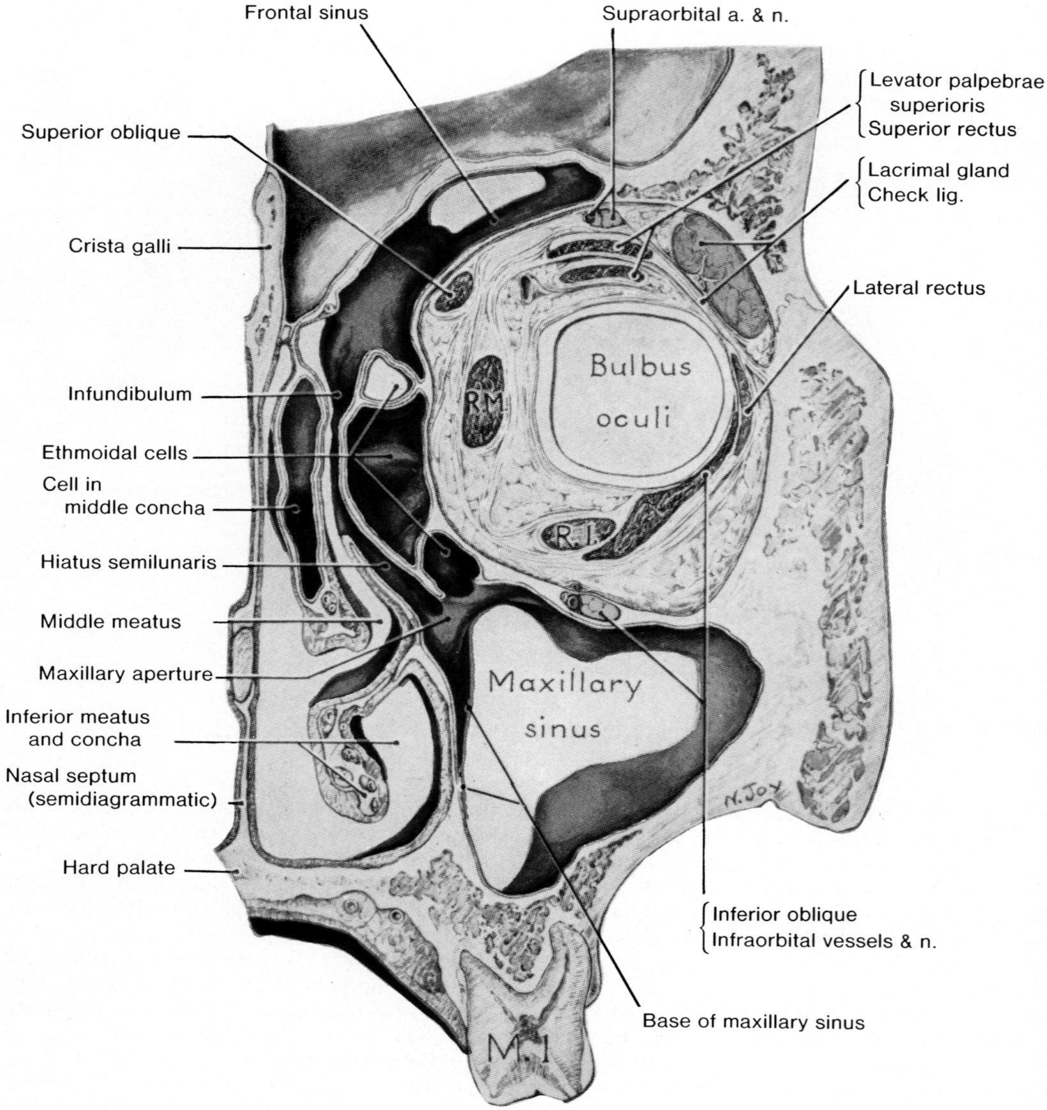

Figure 7-176. Drawing of a coronal section of the right side of the head from behind, showing the orbital contents, the nasal cavities, and the paranasal sinuses. Observe the eyeball within the somewhat circular orbital cavity that has a stout, thick, lateral bony wall and a roof, medial wall, and floor that are surrounded with paranasal air sinuses (frontal, ethmoidal, and maxillary). See the note about "blow-out fractures" of the orbit given in the legend of Figure 7-175. The middle concha in this specimen contains an air cell. This specimen also shows the horizontal part of the frontal sinus producing two plates of bone between the frontal lobe of the brain and the orbit. Note the entrance to the frontal sinus through the infundibulum, which is at the lowest point of the sinus. Observe the entrance to the maxillary sinus through the hiatus semilunaris, which is at the level of the roof of the sinus. The lowest point of the sinus is below the level of the floor of the nasal cavity. Note that the nasal wall of the sinus is very thin in the inferior meatus, well above the floor of the nose. Also note the relationship of the sinus to the first molar tooth (*M.1*).

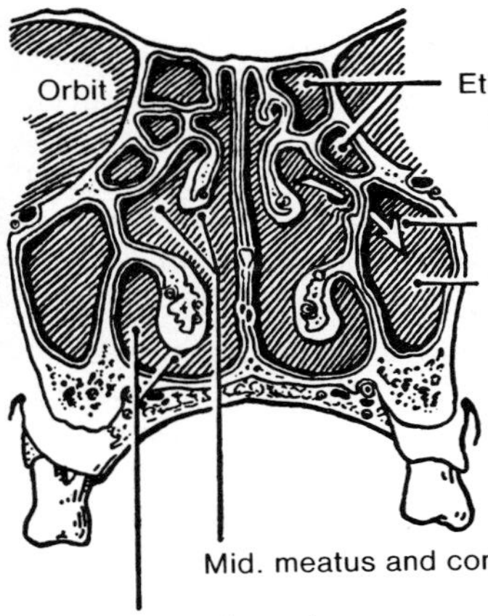

Figure 7-177. Drawing of a coronal section of the nasal cavities showing their relationship to the paranasal air sinuses. Note the high position of the aperture of the maxillary sinus.

terior groups which drain onto the surface of the superior meatus, the **ethmoidal bulla,** the **hiatus semilunaris,** and the **infundibulum** (Fig. 7-171). The middle ethmoidal cells are sometimes called "bullar cells" because they form the ethmoidal bulla.

The Sphenoidal Sinuses (Figs. 7-15, 7-170, 7-174, and 7-175). These often unequal air cavities in the **sphenoid bone** are located posterior to the upper part of the nasal cavity. The two sphenoidal sinuses are *separated by a bony septum* which is usually not in the median plane; hence, when you bisect a skull you may have to break down the septum to expose the sinus on one side. The sphenoidal sinuses are related to the optic nerves and optic chiasma, the hypophysis cerebri, the internal carotid artery, the cavernous sinuses (Fig. 7-73), and the intercavernous sinuses.

Although it is sometimes stated that the sphenoidal sinuses are present at birth (although minute), this is not generally accepted because *they are not observable in skull films of newborn infants.* The current view is that sphenoidal sinuses are derived from a posterior ethmoidal cell which begins to invade the sphenoid bone at about 2 years of age. In some people more than one posterior ethmoidal cell invades the sphenoid bone, giving rise to multiple sphenoidal sinuses that open separately into the **sphenoethmoidal recess.** Hence, the sphenoidal sinuses occupy a variable amount of the sphenoid bone; they are very large in the specimen shown in Figure 7-175. They may extend into the wings of the sphenoid and the pterygoid processes and even into the basiocciput (Fig. 7-57).

The Maxillary Sinuses (Figs. 7-16 and 7-174 to 7-177). This pair of sinuses in the maxillae is *the largest of the paranasal air sinuses.* They are pyramidal-shaped cavities occupying the entire bodies of these large bones. The apex of each cavity extends toward and often into the zygomatic bone (Figs. 7-7 and 7-175). The base of the maxillary sinus forms the lower part of the lateral wall of the nasal cavity. The roof of the maxillary sinus is formed by the floor of the orbit and its narrow floor is formed by the alveolar process of the maxilla. The roots of the maxillary teeth, particularly the first two molars, often produce conical elevations in the floor of the maxillary sinus (Fig. 7-144).

The maxillary sinuses are very small at birth and grow slowly until puberty. They are not fully developed until all the permanent teeth have erupted (up to 25th year). The maxillary sinus drains into the middle meatus of the nasal cavity through an aperture in the upper part of its base (Figs. 7-176 and 7-177). Because of the location of this opening, it is impossible for fluid in the sinus to drain when the head is erect, until the sinus is nearly full.

Blood and Nerve Supply of the Paranasal Sinuses (Figs. 7-30, 7-31, 7-45, and 7-168). The **supraorbital artery** and **nerve** are the main supply to the *frontal sinus.* The *ethmoidal sinuses* are supplied by the **anterior** and **posterior ethmoidal vessels** and **nerves** and the orbital branches of the pterygopalatine ganglion. The *sphenoidal sinuses* are supplied by the **posterior ethmoidal vessels** and **nerves** and the orbital branches of the pterygopalatine ganglion. The innervation to the *maxillary sinus* is from twigs that leave the anterior, middle, and posterior superior **alveolar** and **infraorbital nerves.** The blood supply is via the **facial, infraorbital,** and **greater palatine vessels.**

CLINICALLY ORIENTED COMMENTS

As each paranasal sinus is continuous with the nasal cavity through an aperture that opens into a meatus of the nasal cavity, infection may spread from the nose, producing *inflammation and swelling of the mucosa* **(sinusitis)** and local pain. Often these changes in the mucosa result in blockage of the opening of the sinus into the nasal cavity. Acute infections of the frontal or maxillary sinuses often result in localized tenderness to pressure over the infected sinus. The frontal sinus may be palpated by pressing the finger upward at the medial end of the superior orbital margin. If you put your finger in your orbit you are unable to put it much behind the lacrimal bone. The ethmoidal sinuses may be palpated with the thumb in one inner canthus and the index finger in the other and pushing backward, posterior to the lacrimal bone, and squeezing. If you try this on a colleague, do so carefully, keeping in mind the fragile medial wall of the orbit overlying these cells. Because of the proximity of the sinuses to the nose, there is a tendency after a cold for multiple sinuses to become inflamed **(pansinusitis).**

As the ethmoidal air cells are separated from the orbital cavity by only the thin orbital plate of the ethmoid bone (Fig. 7-176), infection may spread from these sinuses into the orbit, producing **orbital cellulitis.** Although rare, this condition is apt to be dangerous.

Usually the paranasal sinuses are radiolucent, but diseased sinuses show varying degrees of opacity. Radiographs may also reveal thickening of the mucous membranes and fluid in the sinuses.

The maxillary and frontal sinuses can also be examined by **transillumination** in a dark room. To examine the maxillary sinuses, a very bright light is placed in the patient's mouth. A normal sinus is revealed as a red glow on the cheek. A diseased sinus does not transilluminate. To examine the frontal sinus, the light is placed against the superomedial angle of the orbit and, if a normal frontal sinus is present, a red glow appears on the forehead over the vertical part of the sinus.

Pus formation (suppuration) in the paranasal sinuses is not uncommon. Pus running down from the frontal or anterior ethmoidal sinuses may be directed into the opening of the maxillary sinus by the hiatus semilunaris. Verify that this could occur by examining Figures 7-171 and 7-177. One can often determine whether pus is coming from the frontal or the maxillary sinus by placing the patient's head down. Pus from the maxillary sinus, but not the frontal sinus, will usually drain in this position.

Infection can spread into the maxillary sinus from an abscessed molar tooth (Fig. 7-176). During extraction of a molar tooth, the mucous membrane of the maxillary sinus covering its projecting root may be torn, with the result that the empty alveolus (tooth socket) connects the maxillary sinus to the mouth. This communication is referred to as an **oroantral fistula** and usually remains open until closed surgically.

Because the superior alveolar nerves, branches of the maxillary nerve (CN V^2), supply both the teeth and the mucous membrane of the maxillary sinus, inflammation in the sinus is frequently accompanied by the sensation of toothache, especially when bone is absent in the lower part of the wall of this sinus.

The maxillary sinus is the one most commonly involved in infection, probably because its aperture is located high above the floor of the sinus (Figs. 7-176 and 7-177) and is **poorly located for natural drainage** of the sinus. In addition, when the mucous membrane of the sinus is congested, the opening may be obstructed. Gravity drainage from the maxillary sinus is best when one is lying on the side opposite the affected sinus. Surgical drainage may occasionally be necessary and is done by opening the lateral wall of the inferior meatus of the nasal cavity.

Infants and children commonly put peanuts, candies, and small toys into their noses. Because of the shelf-like conchae and the deep meatus (Fig. 7-177) it is easy for these foreign bodies to become impacted. To locate such objects, the nasal cavities are examined with a **speculum** inserted through the external nares **(anterior rhinoscopy).** The posterior nasal apertures **(choanae)** may also be examined by a special mirror placed in the nasopharynx **(posterior rhinoscopy).** *Patients with fractures of the frontal and/or nasal bones,* are usually warned against blowing their noses because of the possibility of expelling air from the frontal sinuses and/or nasal cavities into the subcutaneous tissues or into the cranium or orbit.

THE EAR

The ear consists of three anatomical parts: external, middle, and internal. The external and middle parts are concerned mainly with the transference of sound waves from the exterior to the internal ear, which contains the **vestibulocochlear organ** concerned with equilibration and hearing.

THE EXTERNAL EAR

The external ear is composed of the **auricle** (pinna) and the **external acoustic meatus** (auditory meatus, ear canal), the medial end of which is closed by the **tympanic membrane** (eardrum).

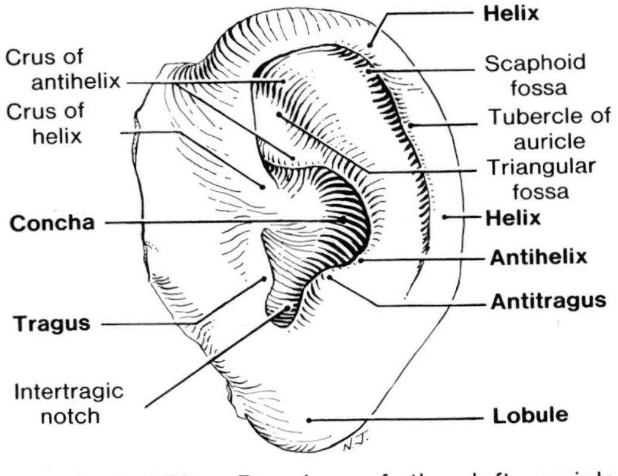

Figure 7-178. Drawing of the left auricle showing its many parts. The *terms in common clinical use are in bold type.*

The Auricle (Figs. 7-178 to 7-180). Many names are used to describe the depressions and elevations of the auricle, but only a few of them are commonly used by most clinicians. The curved outer *rim of the auricle* is called the **helix** and inside it a less complete curved elevation, the **antihelix.** The two are separated by a curved depression, the **scaphoid fossa.** The central depression leading to the **external acoustic meatus** is called the **concha** (L. a shell) because of its shell-like appearance. The **tragus** (G. a goat), so-named because hairs project from it which thicken in older men (like a goatee), is a tongue-like projection of cartilage of the auricle that overlaps the opening of the external acoustic meatus. The lobule (ear lobe) is familiar to everyone; it may hang free or be attached to the skin of the neck.

The auricle acts as a collecting trumpet for sound waves (although not so effectively as in most animals), directing them into the relatively narrow external acoustic meatus. The shape of the auricle varies considerably in different people and in some they are low set and/or slanted. Normally the auricle is at the level of the eye and nose.

The framework of the auricle consists of a single piece of yellow elastic cartilage, except the lobule which consists of fibrofatty tissue. Auricular muscles are unimportant in man and the ability to move them is inconsequential, but amusing. Both surfaces of the auricle are covered with thin skin containing hairs, sweat glands, and sebaceous glands.

CLINICALLY ORIENTED COMMENTS

A small, pinhead-sized, blind depression, called a **preauricular pit,** is sometimes found in a triangular area anterior to the tragus (Fig. 7-179). A deep pit is referred to as a **preauricular sinus;** usually they have pinpoint openings. An obstructed sinus may give rise to a **preauricular cyst.**

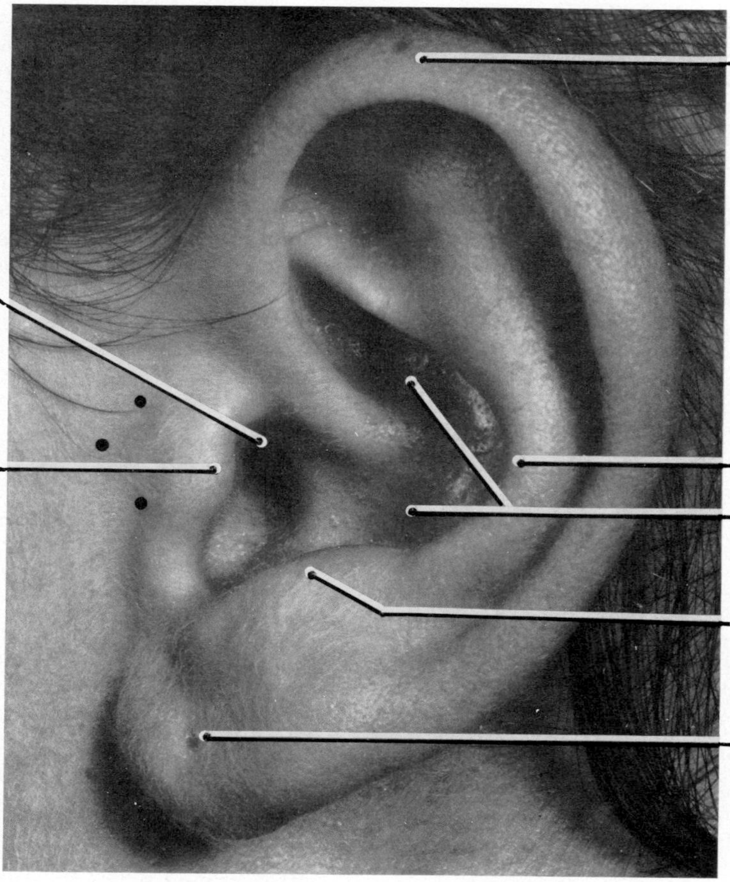

Figure 7-179. Photograph of the left auricle of a 12-year-old girl. Note that her lobule has been pierced (indicated by end of pointer) for an earring. The names given here are commonly used in clinical descriptions of the external ear (other terms are given in Fig. 7-178). The black dots anterior to her tragus indicate the common sites for preauricular pits and appendages (tags).

Most pits and sinuses probably result from imperfect fusion of the separate swellings (**auricular hillocks**) that develop around the margins of the **first branchial groove** and fuse to form the auricle. The groove becomes the **external acoustic meatus.**

Auricular appendages or tags are most often observed anterior to the tragus. They result from the development of more than the usual six auricular hillocks. Minor malformations of the auricle are common, but serious ones are rare. *There is considerable normal variation in the appearance and position of the auricle*; anything esthetically acceptable is in the normal range. Some variations give diagnostic signs of the existence of congenital abnormalities (*e.g.*, low set, malformed ears are characteristic of infants with trisomy 18, a numerical chromosomal abnormality that is accompanied by mental retardation and often by congenital malformations of the heart and kidneys).

The External Acoustic Meatus (Figs. 7-179 and 7-180). The external acoustic meatus is a slender canal that extends from

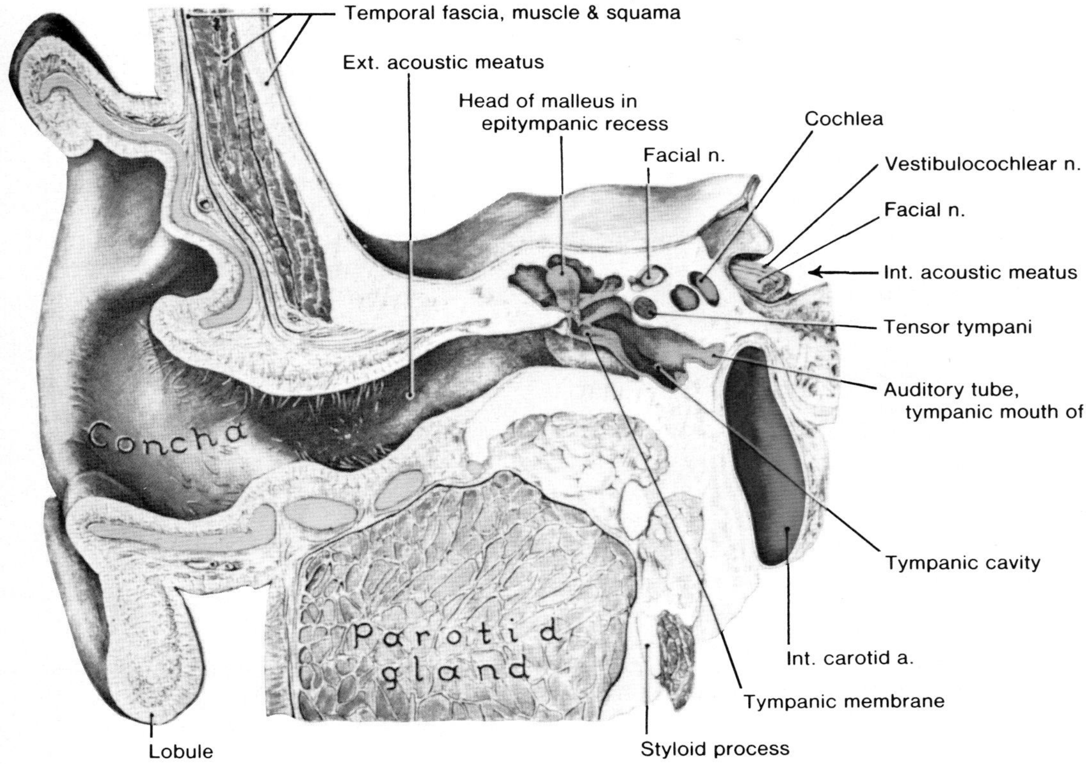

Figure 7-180. Drawing of an anterior view of a coronal section of the right ear. The inner ear is tinted *blue*; the mucous membrane of the middle ear is *pink*. The external acoustic meatus is one-third cartilaginous (*yellow*) and two-thirds bony. It is narrowest near the tympanic membrane owing to the rise on the floor, hence the "well" where fluid can collect at the medial end of the meatus during swimming. The cartilaginous or mobile part of the external acoustic meatus is lined with thick skin and has hairs and many ceruminous glands that secrete wax (cerumen). The bony part of the external acoustic meatus is lined with a thin epithelium that also forms the outermost layer of the tympanic membrane. Note the obliquity of the tympanic membrane which meets the roof of the meatus at an obtuse angle and the floor at an acute one. The handle of the malleus (an ear bone or ossicle) is attached to the innermost layer of the tympanic membrane (Figs. 7-181 and 7-182).

the concha to the tympanic membrane (about 2.5 cm in an adult). The lateral third of this S-shaped passage is cartilaginous, whereas the medial two-thirds is bony. *In infants, the external acoustic meatus is almost entirely cartilaginous.*

The skin of the auricle, containing hairs and glands, is continued into the external acoustic meatus and covers the external surface of the tympanic membrane, but it is very thin and hairless here. In the outer cartilaginous part of the meatus in particular, there are numerous modified sweat glands, called **ceruminous glands,** that secrete **cerumen** (ear wax).

The lateral end of the external acoustic meatus is its widest part. It is about the width of the little finger, explaining the French name *l'auriculaire* (little finger), which some people use to clean the meatus. The external meatus becomes narrow at the medial end of the cartilaginous portion, particularly at the **isthmus,** which is about 4 mm from the tympanic membrane.

CLINICALLY ORIENTED COMMENTS

The external acoustic meatus is directed somewhat anteriorly as well as medially. As the stethoscope tips are angulated to conform to this shape, you should put the **stethoscope** to your auricles with the tips pointing forward. The anatomy of the external acoustic meatus also has to be considered when using an **auriscope** to examine the meatus and the tympanic membrane.

The Tympanic Membrane (Fig. 7-181). This thin, semitransparent, oval membrane (about 1 cm across) is at the medial end of the external acoustic meatus, separating it from the middle ear. It is a thin, fibrous membrane covered with very thin skin externally and mucous membrane internally. In the adult it is oblique, sloping medially from top to bottom. In a living person, the *tympanic membrane normally appears pearly gray and shiny.* Its parts and their relationship to the auditory ossicles of the middle ear are illustrated in Figures 7-180 to 7-182. It shows a concavity towards the meatus with a central depression, the **umbo,** formed by the handle of the malleus, one of three middle ear bones, called **auditory ossicles** (Fig. 7-181). From the umbo a bright area, the cone of light, radiates anteroinferiorly. *The tympanic membrane moves in response to air vibrations that pass to it via the external acoustic meatus.*

Blood Supply of the External Ear and Tympanic Membrane (Figs. 7-34 and 7-36). The lateral surface of the auricle is supplied by the **superficial temporal artery.** Branches of this artery also supply the external acoustic meatus which is supplied by the **deep auricular artery,** a branch of the maxillary. The deep auricular also supplies the external surface of the tympanic membrane. The medial side of the auricle is supplied by the **posterior auricular artery,** a branch of the external carotid.

Nerve Supply of the External Ear and Tympanic Membrane (Fig. 7-32). The nerve supply to most of the auricle is through the **great auricular nerve.** The auriculotemporal branch of the mandibular (CN V^3) supplies part of the lateral surface of the auricle and the **lesser occipital nerve** supplies part of its medial surface. Most of the external acoustic meatus and the external surface of the tympanic membrane are supplied by the auriculotemporal nerve, but some innervation is supplied by a small auricular branch of the **vagus** (CN X). This nerve may also contain some glossopharyngeal and facial nerve fibers.

CLINICALLY ORIENTED COMMENTS

To visualize the external acoustic meatus and the tympanic membrane, an **otoscope** or **auriscope** (L. *auris,* ear + *skopeō,* to view) is usually used, but sometimes a reflecting mirror and **speculum** are preferred. Because the external acoustic meatus curves downward and anteriorly, the auricle has to be pulled upward, backward, and a little laterally in order to straighten the meatus as much as possible. In children the meatus is shorter and not so curved; thus, one usually needs to pull backward and slightly downward on the auricle to straighten the meatus.

Foreign objects (*e.g.,* peanuts, insects) may have to be removed from the meatuses of infants and children. Paper and organic objects like beans, peas, and peanuts may absorb moisture, swell, and become impacted. Although cerumen is a normal content of the external acoustic meatus, it may have to be removed by syringing in order to visualize the tympanic membrane. In some cases the meatus may become blocked with cerumen, resulting in symptoms of impaired hearing, noises in the ear, and pain.

The vagal connections of the external acoustic meatus explain the occurrence of reflex coughing, sneezing, and occasionally nausea that occur when the meatus is syringed or a foreign body is being removed from it. For the same reason (although unlikely), a foreign object such as a dog hair in the meatus could cause a persistent cough in a patient whose throat appears normal.

Rupture of the eardrum (tympanic membrane) is one of several causes of **middle ear deafness.** Perforation of the tympanic membrane may result from foreign bodies, pressure (*e.g.*, during scuba diving), or infection. Severe bleeding and/or escape of CSF through a ruptured tympanic membrane and the external acoustic meatus **(CSF otorrhea)** may occur following a severe blow on the head. Either of these conditions is indicative of a skull fracture and results from the close relation of the tympanic cavity, mastoid antrum, mastoid air cells, and the bony external acoustic meatus to the meninges of the brain (Fig. 7-183). Understand that a skull fracture may pass through the external acoustic meatus and cause bleeding and/or loss of CSF via the ear with an intact eardrum.

On rare occasions it is necessary to incise the tympanic membrane to allow pus to escape from the middle ear. Because the upper half of the tympanic membrane is much more vascular than the lower half, incisions are made posteroinferiorly through the membrane. This site also avoids the **chorda tympani nerve** and the auditory ossicles.

THE MIDDLE EAR

The middle ear or **tympanic cavity** is an air-containing space within the junction of the petrous and mastoid parts of the temporal bone. It is separated from the external acoustic meatus by the tympanic membrane (Fig. 7-182). The vibrations of this membrane are transmitted through the tympanic cavity by the chain of three auditory ossicles.

The tympanic cavity is lined with a mucous membrane which is continuous with that lining the auditory tube (pharyngotympanic or Eustachian tube), the mastoid air cells, and the mastoid antrum. *The tympanic cavity consists of two parts* (Figs. 7-180, 7-182, and 7-183*B*): the **tympanic cavity proper** opposite the tympanic membrane and the **epitympanic recess** above the level of the membrane.

Contents of the Middle Ear (Figs. 7-180, 7-182, and 7-183). The middle ear contains the **auditory ossicles** (malleus, incus, and stapes); the **stapedius** and **tensor tympani** muscles; the **chorda tympani** nerve (a branch of the facial, CN VII), and the **tympanic plexus** of nerves.

Walls of the Tympanic Cavity (Fig. 7-183). The tympanic cavity is shaped like a narrow, six-sided box which has convex medial and lateral walls. It has the *shape of a biconcave lens or red blood cell in cross-section.* It is 15 mm in vertical diameter, 2 mm across at the center, 4 mm at the floor, and 6 mm at the roof. The general shape of the tympanic cavity is shown diagrammatically in Figure 7-183*B*.

The Roof or Tegmental Wall (Fig. 7-183). The roof of the tympanic cavity is formed by a thin plate of bone, the **tegmen tympani** (L. *tegmen*, a cover or roof). It separates the tympanic cavity from the dura mater on the floor of the middle cranial fossa. The tegmen tympani also roofs the mastoid antrum.

The Floor or Jugular Wall (Fig. 7-183). The floor of the tympanic cavity is thicker than the roof, but it is formed by a layer of bone which may be thick or thin. It separates the cavity from the superior bulb of the internal jugular vein **(superior jugular bulb).** In Figure 7-183*B* note that as the internal jugular vein and the internal carotid artery pass upward within the carotid sheath, they diverge at the floor of the tympanic cavity. The **tympanic nerve,** a branch of the glossopharyngeal (CN IX), passes through an aperture in the floor of the tympanic cavity and branches to form the tympanic plexus (Fig. 7-187).

The Lateral Wall or Membranous Wall (Figs. 7-183 and 7-184). The lateral wall of the tympanic cavity is formed almost entirely by the tympanic membrane. Superiorly it is formed by the lateral bony wall of the **epitympanic recess.** The handle of

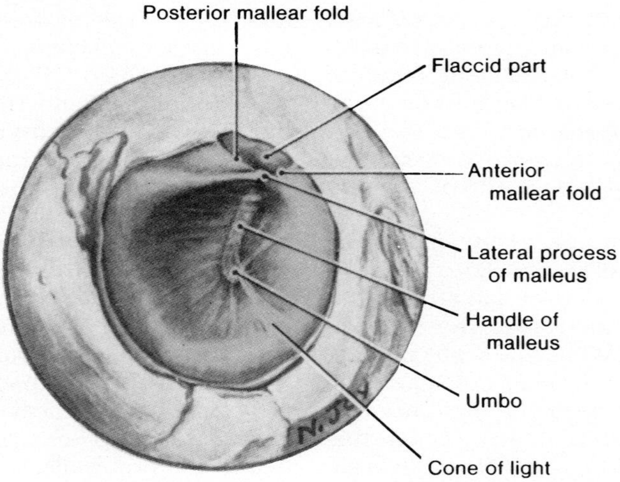

A.

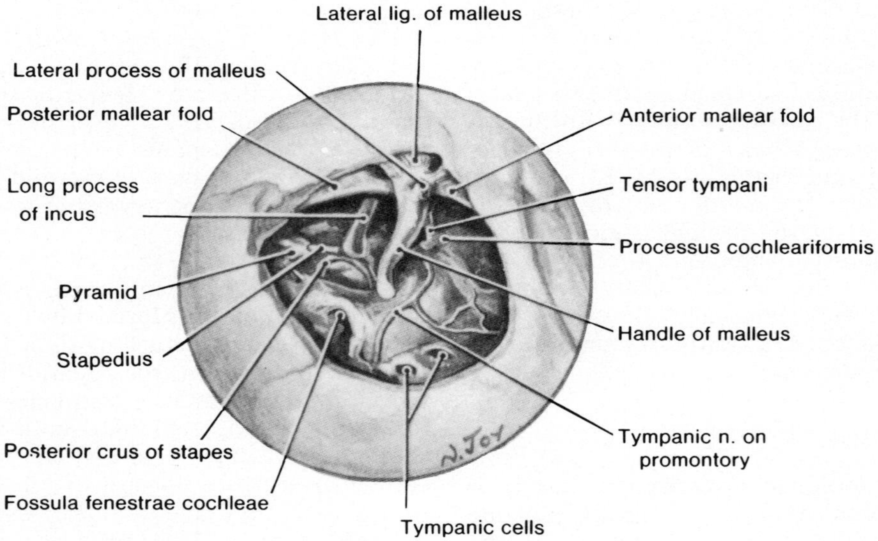

B.

Figure 7-181. *A*, drawing of a lateral view of the right tympanic membrane. *B*, drawing of inferolateral view of the tympanic cavity after removal of the tympanic membrane. Observe that the tympanic membrane is oval rather than round and is shaped like a funnel with a rolled rim and a depressed part, called the umbo, at the tip of the handle of the malleus which is situated anteroinferior to the center of the membrane (Fig. 7-182). Above the lateral process of the malleus (prominentia) the membrane is thin and is called the flaccid part (pars flaccida). The flaccid part lacks the radial and circular fibers present in the remainder of the membrane (tense part). The junction between the two parts, flaccid and tense, is marked by an anterior and a posterior line which run from the prominentia to the free ends of the horseshoe-shaped tympanic ring. The cone of light is a reflection of light from the membrane. Observe the tendon of the stapedius in *B* passing the neck of the stapes on which it pulls.

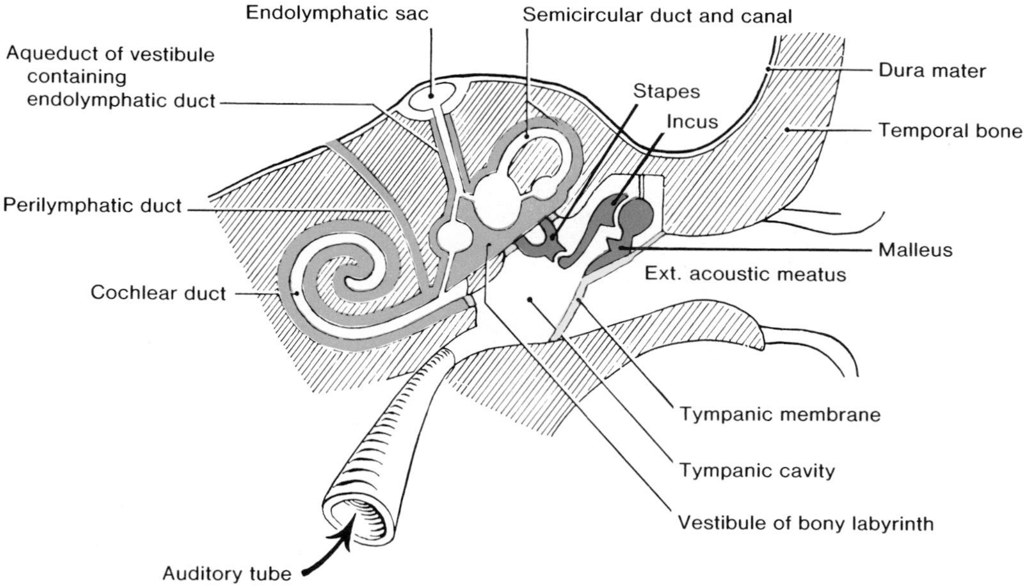

Figure 7-182. Diagram showing the three parts of the ear. The middle ear or tympanic cavity lies between the tympanic membrane and the internal ear. Three ossicles (*red*), malleus, incus, and stapes, stretch from the lateral to the medial wall of the tympanic cavity. Of these,the malleus is attached to the tympanic membrane; the stapes is attached by an anular ligament to an oval opening in the wall of the bony vestibule of the inner ear, called the fenestra vestibuli; and the incus connects these two ossicles. The auditory tube opens into the anterior wall of the tympanic cavity; the aditus ad antrum opens from the epitympanic recess backward to the mastoid antrum. The internal ear is contained in the petrous part of the temporal bone. It is usually described in two parts, a bony labyrinth and a membranous labyrinth. The bony labyrinth is a series of interconnected spaces and canals containing the organs for hearing and balancing. The organ of hearing is housed in a spiral tube, the cochlea, the base of which connects with the vestibule, the globular middle part of the bony labyrinth. The organ of equilibrium or balance is in three semicircular canals and structures in the vestibule. The bony labyrinth is filled with a fluid called perilymph which is continuous with the CSF through a small duct. Inside the bony labyrinth and largely surrounded by perilymph is a complicated system of tubes and spaces containing endolymph which bathes the special end organs for hearing and balancing.

the malleus, an auditory ossicle, is incorporated in the tympanic membrane and its head extends into the epitympanic recess.

The Medial Wall or Labyrinthine Wall (Figs. 7-182, 7-183, and 7-185). This bony wall separates the middle ear (tympanic cavity) from the inner ear, consisting of a membranous labyrinth (semicircular ducts and cochlear duct) encased in a bony labyrinth. *The medial wall exhibits several important features.* Centrally, opposite the tympanic membrane, there is a rounded **promontory** (L. an eminence) formed by the large first turn of the **cochlea** (Fig. 7-185). The **tympanic plexus** of nerves, lying on the promontory, is formed by fibers of the facial and glossopharyngeal nerves (CN VII and CN IX, respectively) that pass through an aperture in the floor of the tympanic cavity within the tympanic nerve (Fig. 7-187).

The medial wall has two small apertures or windows (Fig. 7-186). The **fenestra vestibuli** is closed by the **base** (footplate) of the stapes, which is bound to its margins by an **anular ligament.** Through this window, vibrations of the stapes are transmitted to the perilymph within the bony labyrinth of the inner ear (Fig. 7-182). The **fenestra cochleae,** below the fenestra ves-

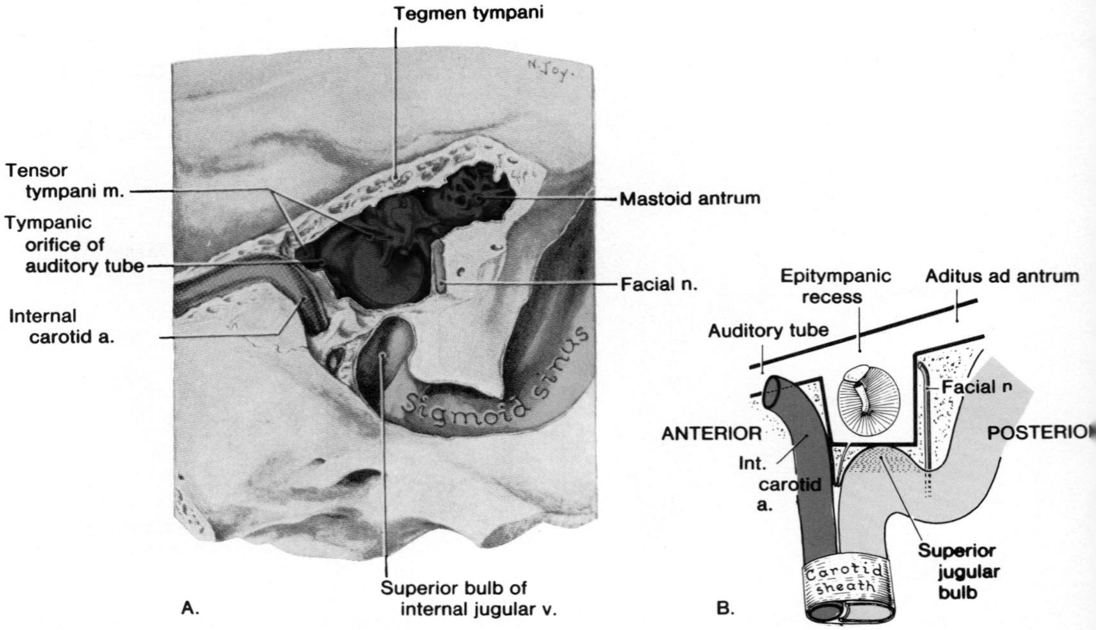

Figure 7-183. *A*, drawing of a dissection of the middle ear (done with a drill) to show the walls of the tympanic cavity. Note that the tegmen tympani forms the roof of the mastoid antrum and part of the middle ear. Also observe the internal carotid artery (the main feature of the anterior wall), the internal jugular vein (the main feature of the floor), and the facial nerve (the main feature of the posterior wall). *B*, inset drawing that simplifies the dissection shown in *A* and emphasizes the relations of the tympanic cavity. These figures show an unusually high position of the jugular bulb near (or in relation to) to the floor of the middle ear.

tibuli, is closed by a **secondary tympanic membrane.** This membrane allows the perilymph to move slightly in response to impulses from the base of the stapes. Thus, both apertures are related to the cavity of the inner ear; see the legend of Figure 7-182 for a general description of their roles in the over-all scheme of the ear.

CLINICALLY ORIENTED COMMENTS

In **otosclerosis** (G. *ous* (*ōt*), ear + *sklērosis*, hardening), there is a new formation of spongy bone around the stapes and fenestra vestibuli, resulting in progressively increasing deafness. This bony overgrowth may stop movement of the base of the stapes and/or the membrane of the fenestra cochleae. If either or both of these are immobilized, they must be freed to restore the hearing.

The Posterior Wall or Mastoid Wall (Fig. 7-183). This wall of the tympanic cavity has several openings in it. In its upper part, there is the **aditus to the mastoid antrum** (aditus ad antrum), which leads posteriorly from the **epitympanic recess** into the mastoid antrum and beyond into the **mastoid air cells.** Inferiorly there is a pinpoint aperture on the apex of a tiny, hollow projection of bone called the **pyramidal eminence** or pyramid (Fig. 7-187). The pyramid contains the stapedius muscle and the aperture transmits its tendon, which enters the tympanic cavity and inserts into the stapes. Lateral to the pyramid, there is an aperture (Fig. 7-184) through which the **chorda tympani nerve,** a branch of the facial (CN VII), enters the tympanic cavity.

The Anterior Wall or Carotid Wall (Figs. 7-183, 7-184, and 7-188). The anterior wall of the tympanic cavity is narrow because the medial and lateral walls converge anteriorly. There are two openings in the

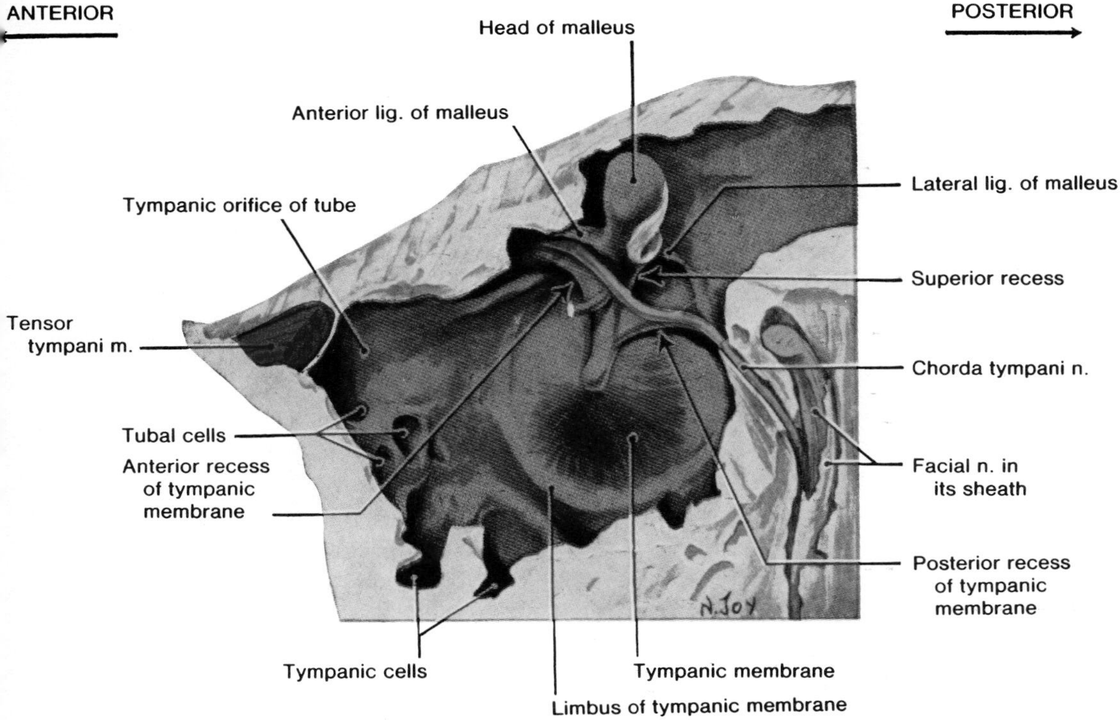

Figure 7-184. Medial view of a dissection of the right middle ear to show the lateral wall of the tympanic cavity. Observe that the lateral wall is formed almost entirely by the tympanic membrane. Note that this membrane has a greater vertical than horizontal diameter and that the handle of the malleus is incorporated in the membrane, its end being at the umbo (Fig. 7-181). Note the facial nerve within its tough periosteal tube and the chorda tympani leaving the facial nerve. Note the head of the malleus in the epitympanic recess. Here its posterior surface articulates within the body of the incus. Also note the chorda tympani nerve passing forward across the medial aspect of the upper part of the tympanic membrane. *It is incorporated in the tympanic membrane.*

anterior wall. The upper opening communicates with a canal occupied by the **tensor tympani** muscle (Fig. 7-191), the tendon of which inserts into the handle of the malleus and keeps the tympanic membrane tense. Below, the tympanic cavity communicates with the nasopharynx via the **auditory tube.** It runs downward, medially, and forward to open into the nasopharynx posterior to the inferior meatus of the nasal cavity (Fig. 7-170).

CLINICALLY ORIENTED COMMENTS

Inflammatory conditions in the tympanic cavity (*i.e.*, **otitis media**) sometimes spread through the thin tegmen tympani, causing inflammation of the meninges **(meningitis)** and brain **(cerebritis** and **brain abscess).** In infants and children the unossified *petrosquamous fissure* (Fig. 7-52) may allow direct spread of infection from the tympanic cavity to the cranial meninges. In the adult, veins pass through the *petrosquamous suture* to the **superior petrosal sinus** (Fig. 7-69 *B*); thus, infection can spread via them to the dural venous sinuses.

Earache is a common symptom which has multiple causes, some in the ear and others at a distance. **Otitis externa** (inflammation of the external acoustic meatus) is one cause. In adults with this condition, movement of the tragus results in increased pain because the cartilage in it is continuous with that in the external acoustic meatus (Fig. 7-180). In **otitis media** (middle ear infection), movement of the

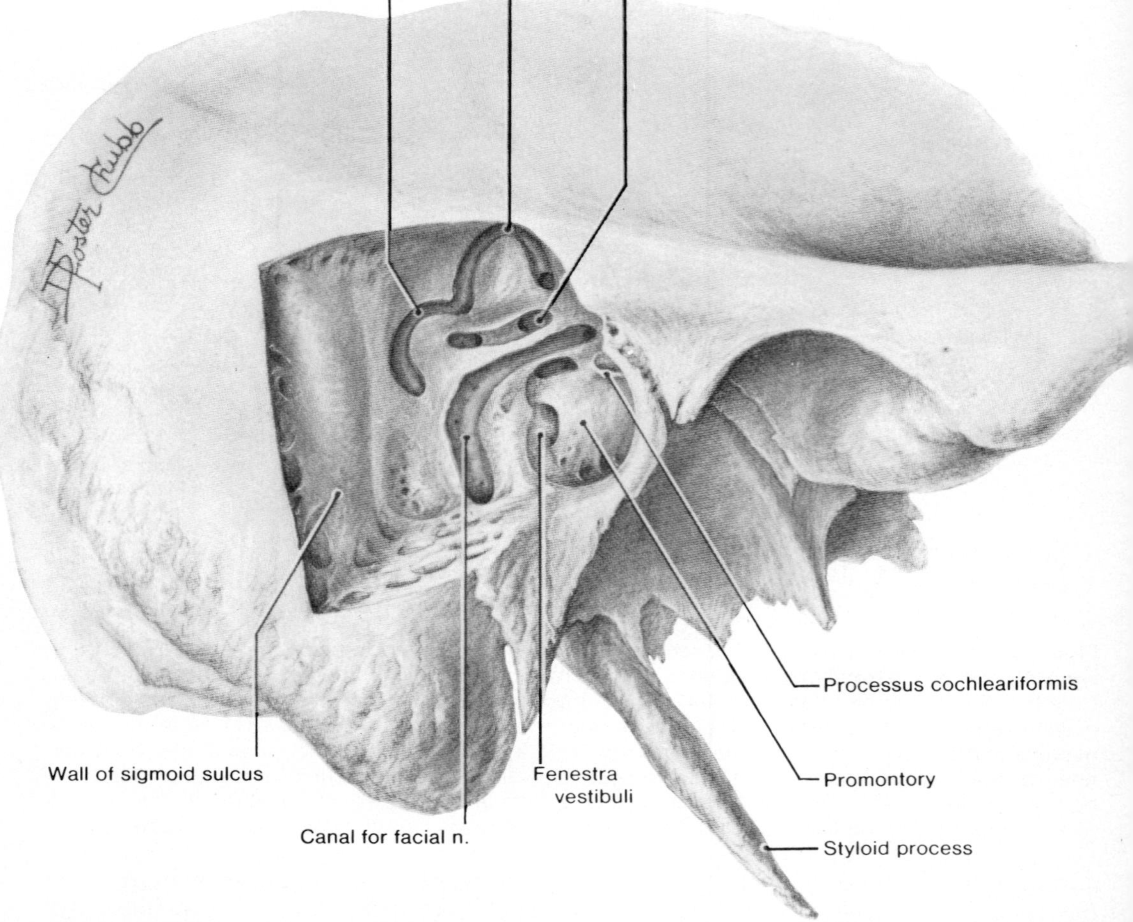

Figure 7-185. Drawing of a dissection showing a lateral view of the medial wall of the tympanic cavity and the semicircular canals. The posterior wall of the external acoustic meatus and the mastoid antrum have been removed between the fenestra vestibuli (oval window) and the lateral semicircular canal. Note the following features of the medial or labyrinthine wall of the tympanic cavity: (1) the promontory lying 2 mm deep to the umbo (Fig. 7-181) and overlying the basal turn of the cochlea; (2) the processus cochleariformis at the end of the canal for the tensor tympani that acts as a pulley for the tensor; (3) the fenestra vestibuli close behind the pulley and medial to it; and (4) the facial canal (opened) running horizontally backward between the vestibular window and the lateral semicircular canal to the junction of the medial and posterior walls, then descending in the posterior wall to its orifice, the stylomastoid foramen.

tragus does not increase the pain in adults but may do so in infants and children. In these young patients, the external acoustic meatus is almost entirely cartilaginous so that movement of the tragus is transmitted to the tympanic membrane.

Earache may be referred pain from distant lesions, e.g., the mouth **(dental abscess** or **cancer of tongue)** via the mandibular nerve (CN V^3) or the pharynx or larynx via the vagus nerve (CN X). Some patients will refer to **temporomandibular**

joint disease as ear pain because of the proximity of this articulation to the tragus of the ear.

The Auditory Tube (Figs. 7-180, 7-182 to 7-184, 7-186, and 7-188). This *funnel-shaped tube connects the nasopharynx to the tympanic cavity* and beyond that to the mastoid air cells through the mastoid antrum. Its wide end is toward the nasopharynx where it opens posterior to the inferior meatus of the nasal cavity (Fig. 7-84). It is 3.5 to 4 cm long; its posterior one-third is bony and the other two-thirds are cartilaginous. The bony part lies in a groove on the inferior aspect of the base of the skull, between the petrous part of the temporal bone and the greater wing of the **sphenoid** bone. Locate this groove on a dried skull (Fig. 7-189).

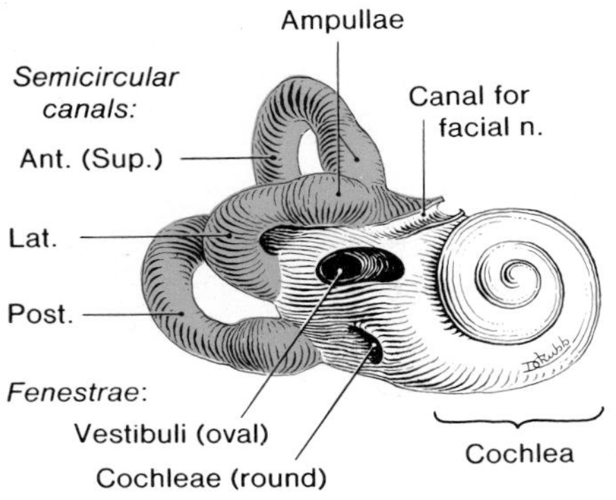

Figure 7-186. Drawing of a lateral view of the right bony labyrinth.

The auditory tube is lined by mucous membrane that is continuous posteriorly with that of the tympanic cavity and anteriorly with that of the nasopharynx. **The function of the auditory tube** is to *equalize pressure in the middle ear with the atmospheric pressure*, thereby allowing free movement of the tympanic membrane. By allowing air to enter or leave the cavity, it balances the pressure on both sides of the membrane.

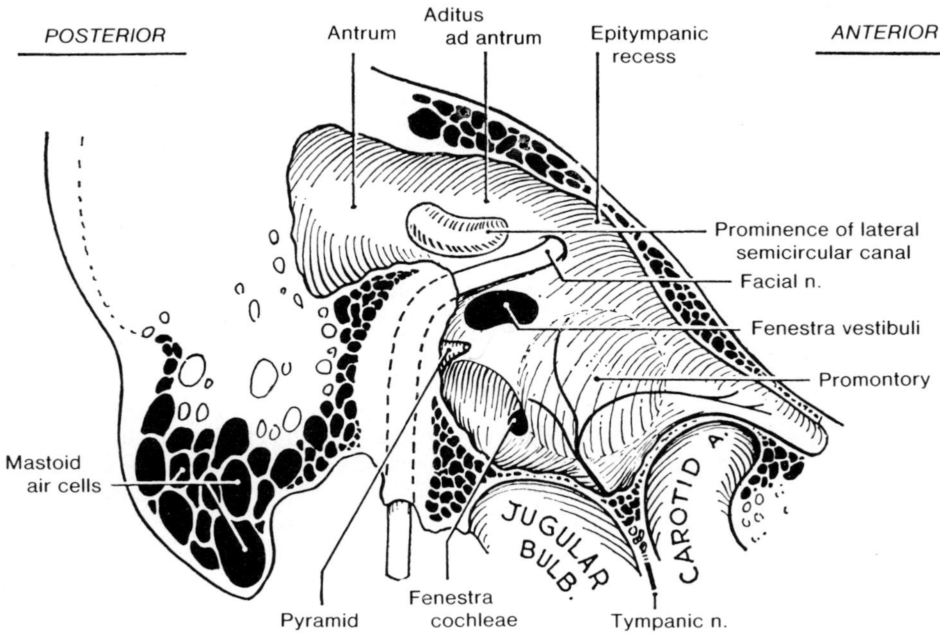

Figure 7-187. Drawing of the medial wall of the tympanic cavity. Note the tiny elevation on the posterior wall, called the pyramid (pyramidal eminence), which contains the small stapedius muscle. The jugular bulb is unusually close to the floor of the middle ear in this specimen.

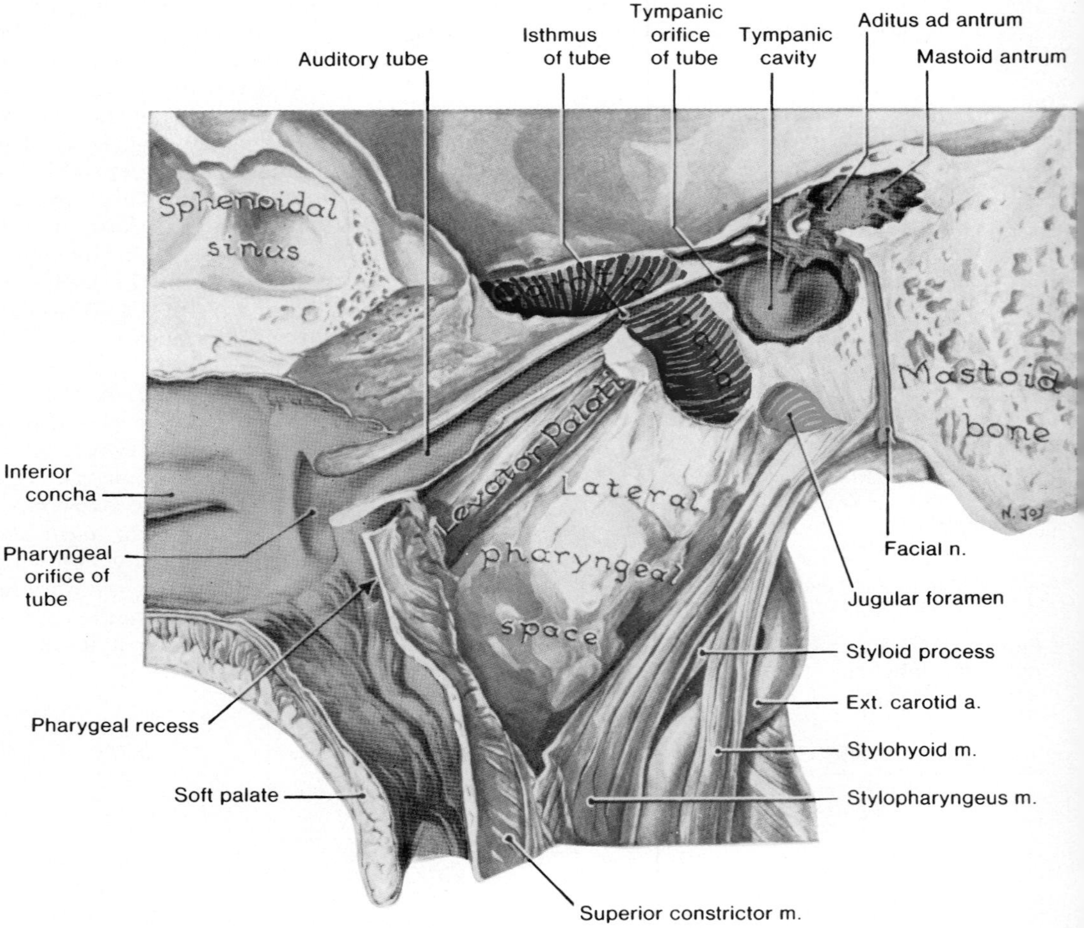

Figure 7-188. Drawing of a dissection that exposes the auditory tube from the medial or pharyngeal aspect. Observe that this tube passes upward, backward, and laterally from the nasopharynx to the tympanic cavity. Note the funnel-shaped pharyngeal orifice of the tube, situated posterior to the inferior concha of the nose. Observe the bony part of the tube (passing lateral to the carotid canal) narrows at the isthmus where it joins the cartilaginous part. Note the course of the facial nerve and its relationship to the mastoid antrum and the mastoid air cells.

The cartilaginous part of the auditory tube remains closed except during swallowing or yawning. The tube is opened by the simultaneous contraction of the tensor veli palatini (Fig. 7-149) and salpingopharyngeus muscles which are attached to opposite sides of the tube.

CLINICALLY ORIENTED COMMENTS

The auditory tube forms a route through which infections may pass from the nasopharynx to the tympanic cavity. It is easily blocked by swelling of its mucous membrane, even by mild infections, because the walls of its cartilaginous part are normally in apposition. When the auditory tube is blocked, the residual air in the tympanic cavity is usually absorbed into the mucosal blood vessels. This results in the lowering of pressure in the tympanic cavity, retraction of the tympanic membrane, and interference with its free movement. As a result hearing is affected. Under these circumstances fluid may exude into the tympanic cavity (a condition erroneously called **ser-**

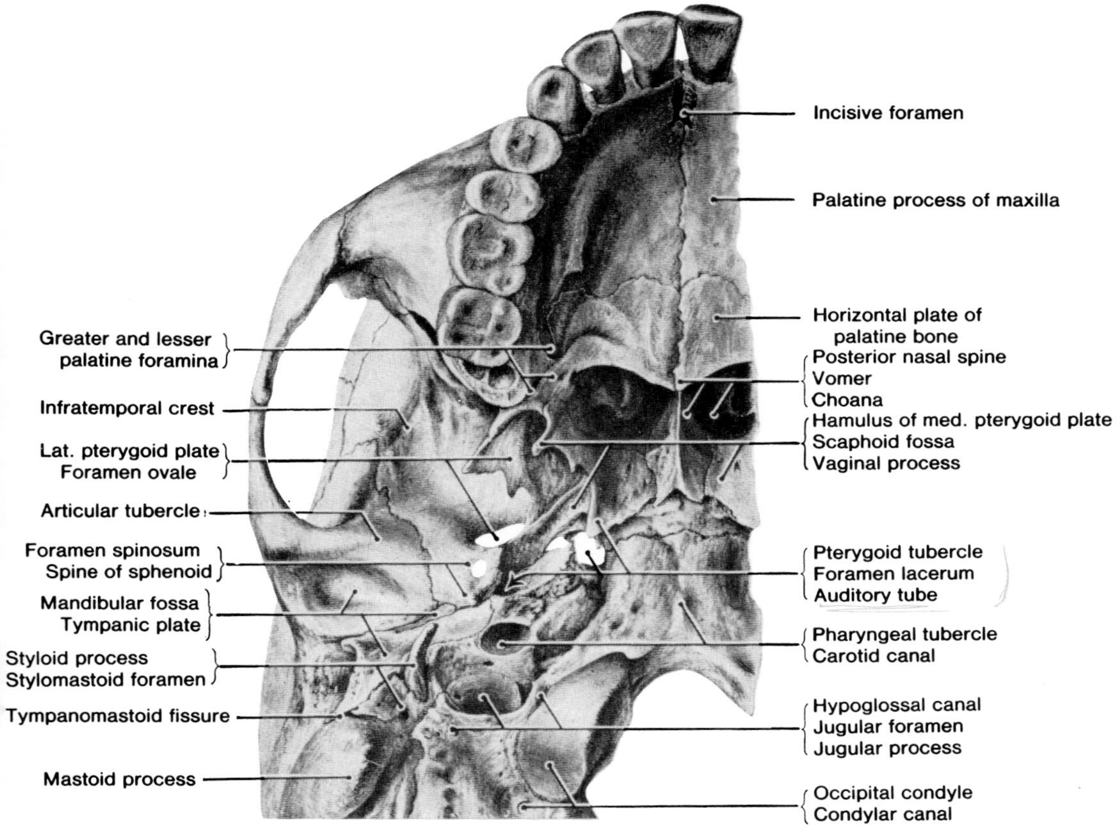

Figure 7-189. Drawing of the exterior of the base of the skull. Observe the groove for the auditory tube between the petrous part of the temporal bone and the greater wing of the sphenoid bone. Note the mastoid process.

ous otitis). Impaired hearing may result from inhibited movement of the tympanic membrane.

Auditory Ossicles (Figs. 7-180 to 7-184 and 7-190). These little movable ear bones **(malleus, incus,** and **stapes)** *form a chain across the tympanic cavity from the tympanic membrane to the fenestra vestibuli* (oval window). The malleus is attached to the tympanic membrane and the stapes occupies the fenestra vestibuli. The incus is located between these two bones and articulates with them. The ossicles are covered with the mucous membrane lining the tympanic cavity.

The Malleus (L. a hammer). Its rounded superior part, the **head,** lies in the epitympanic recess and its **neck** lies against the flaccid part of the tympanic membrane (Fig. 7-181). The **handle** of the malleus (Figs. 7-181*B* and 7-190) is embedded in the tympanic membrane and so moves with it. Its head **articulates with the incus** and the tendon of the tensor tympani muscle inserts into its handle. *The chorda tympani nerve crosses the medial surface of the neck of the malleus.*

The Incus (L. an anvil). Although named because of its resemblance to a blacksmith's anvil, it also resembles a premolar tooth (Fig. 7-143). Its **large body** lies in the epitympanic recess where it articulates with the head of the malleus (Figs. 7-182 and 7-183). Its **long process** articulates with the stapes and its short one is connected by a ligament to the posterior wall of the tympanic cavity.

The Stapes (L. a stirrup). The **base**

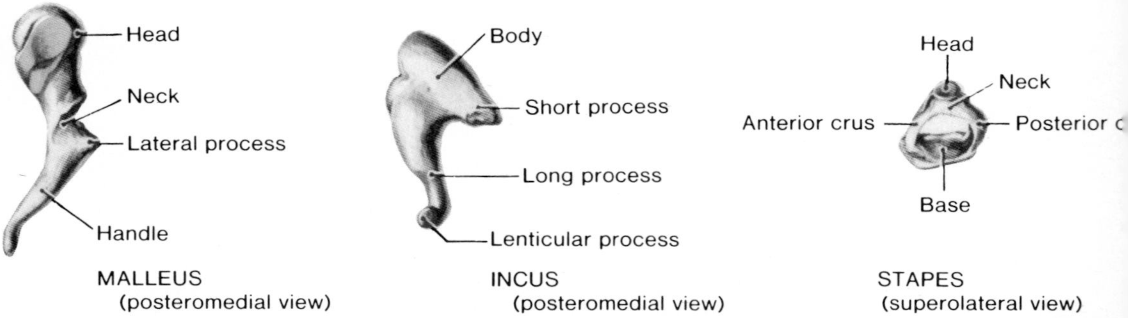

Figure 7-190. Drawings of the auditory ossicles (enlarged about five times). The three ossicles form a chain or jointed arch between the tympanic membrane and the fenestra vestibuli, as shown in Figure 7-182.

(footplate) of this little bone, the smallest ossicle, **fits into the fenestra vestibuli** on the medial wall of the tympanic cavity (Figs. 7-182 and 7-186). Its **head,** directed laterally, articulates with the lenticular process of the incus. In the living state, the opening between the **crura** (Fig. 7-190) is closed by a membrane (Fig. 7-181*B*).

The malleus functions as a lever with the longer of its two arms attached to the tympanic membrane. The base of the stapes is considerably smaller than the tympanic membrane (Fig. 7-194). As a result of these factors, *the vibratory force of the stapes is about 10 times that of the tympanic membrane.* Thus, **the ossicles increase the force but decrease the amplitude of the vibrations transmitted from the tympanic membrane.**

CLINICALLY ORIENTED COMMENTS

Abnormal development of the malleus and incus is often associated with abnormal transformation of the first branchial arch into adult structures. This is understandable when one recalls that these two auditory ossicles develop from the dorsal ends of the first branchial arch cartilage. Understandably, infants with the **first arch syndrome** have multiple malformations (deformed auricle, abnormal development of the cheek and mandible, and hearing defects).

Muscles Moving the Auditory Ossicles and the Tympanic Membrane. Two muscles are associated with movements of the auditory ossicles and the tympanic membrane.

The tensor tympani muscle (Figs. 7-183, 7-184, and 7-191) is only about 2 cm long.

Origin (Fig. 7-191). Superior surface of cartilaginous part of **auditory tube**, adjacent greater wing of **sphenoid bone**, and petrous part of **temporal bone**.

Insertion (Figs. 7-185 and 7-191). Its tendon turns around the processus cochleariformis before inserting into the **handle of malleus**.

Nerve Supply. **Mandibular** nerve (CN V^3) via fibers that pass through otic ganglion.

Action. Pulls handle of malleus medially; thus it **tenses tympanic membrane** and reduces the amplitude of oscillations. This tends to prevent damage to the inner ear when exposed to loud sounds.

The stapedius is a tiny muscle in the pyramidal eminence (pyramid).

Origin (Fig. 7-187). **Pyramidal eminence** on posterior wall of tympanic cavity. Its tendon enters the tympanic cavity by traversing a pinpoint foramen in the apex of the pyramid.

Insertion (Fig. 7-181*B*). **Neck of stapes.**

Nerve Supply. **Facial** nerve (CN VII).

Actions. **Pulls stapes posteriorly** and **tilts its base in fenestra vestibuli**, thereby tightening the anular ligament and reducing the oscillatory range. The stape-

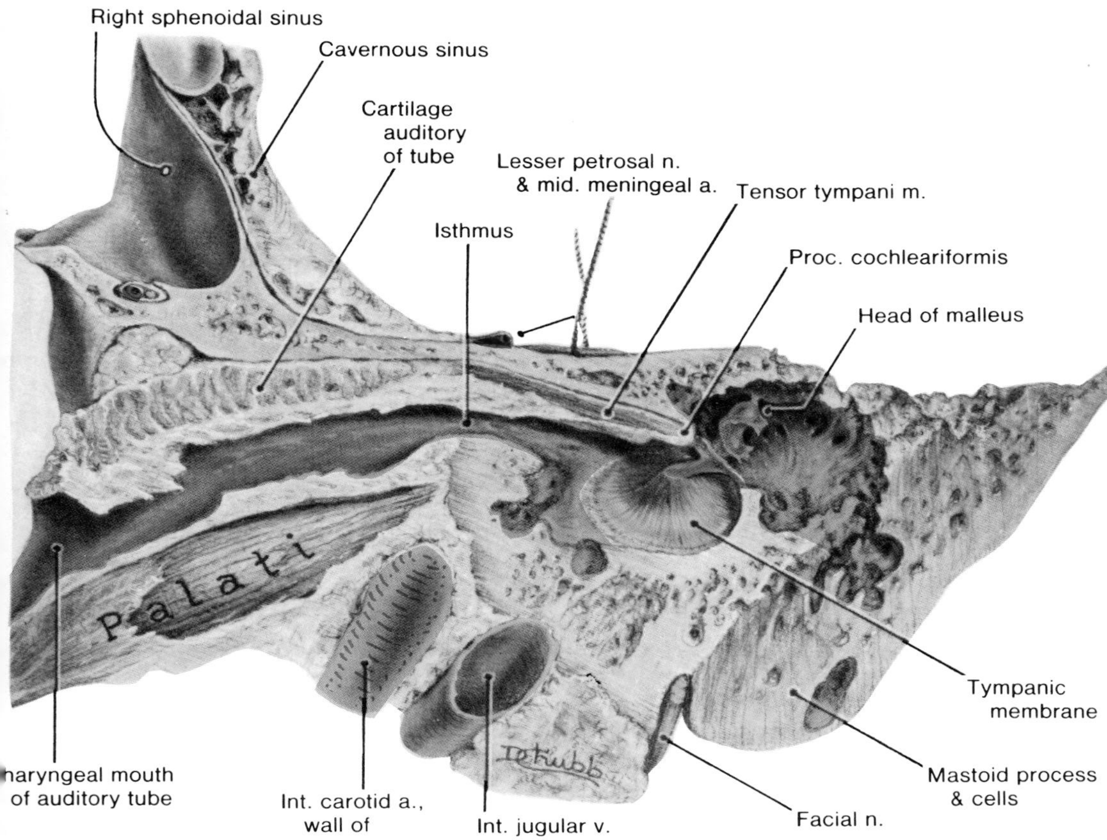

Figure 7-191. Drawing of a dissection of the auditory tube and the tympanic cavity. The medial part of a longitudinally split specimen is shown. Note the tensor tympani muscle arising from the auditory tube and adjacent bones. Its tendon is shown turning around the processus cochleariformis before inserting into the handle of the malleus.

dius **prevents excessive movement of stapes.**

CLINICALLY ORIENTED COMMENTS

The tympanic muscles or muscles of the auditory ossicles have a protective action in that they dampen (check) large vibrations resulting from loud noises. Thus, paralysis of the stapedius muscle resulting from a lesion of the facial nerve or other injury is associated with excessive acuteness of hearing **(hyperacusia)**. This condition results from the uninhibited movement of the stapes.

Congenital fixation of the stapes results in severe conduction deafness at birth. This deformity appears to result from failure of normal differentiation of the anular ligament which attaches the base of the stapes to the fenestra vestibuli (Fig. 7-194). As a result, the stapes becomes fixed to the bony labyrinth and is immovable.

Otosclerosis, a common type of progressive **conduction deafness** in adults, results from the formation of bone around the stapes and the fenestra vestibuli (Fig. 7-192*A*). To restore hearing, a **stapedectomy** (removal of stapes) and insertion of

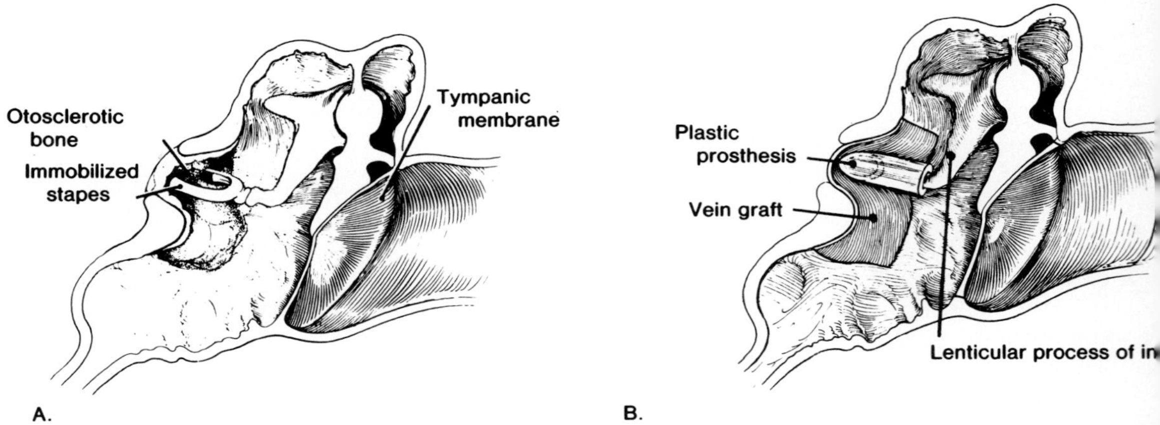

Figure 7-192. *A*, diagram illustrating immobilization of the stapes owing to otosclerosis. *B*, illustration showing a stapedectomy, one of many techniques for correction of a lesion produced by otosclerosis. The stapes and fenestra vestibuli have been replaced with a vein graft and a plastic prosthesis connects the graft to the incus. The vein graft usually covers the fenestra cochlea (round window) also because it is often closed by the same bony overgrowth. Hence, it must be opened (*i.e.*, cleared of bone) to permit perilymph to move back and forth, moving the hairs in the organ of Corti and the basilar membrane (Fig. 7-195).

a prosthesis may be performed (Fig. 7-192*B*).

The Mastoid Antrum and Air Cells (Figs. 7-183, 7-187, 7-188, and 7-191). The mastoid antrum is a spherical air sinus (cavity), slightly smaller than the tympanic cavity. It is located in the petromastoid part of the temporal bone posterior to the **epitympanic recess**. It is connected to the tympanic cavity by the **aditus to the mastoid antrum** and is separated from the middle cranial fossa by a thin roof, the **tegmen tympani**. In some people the **sigmoid sinus** is very close behind it. Its floor has a number of apertures through which the mastoid antrum communicates with the **mastoid air cells**. Anteroinferiorly the mastoid antrum is related to the canal for the facial nerve. The lateral wall of the antrum is only 1 mm thick at birth but increases about 1 mm a year until it is about 15 mm thick. At birth, unlike the paranasal air sinuses, the mastoid antrum is well developed and is almost adult size. *No mastoid air cells or mastoid processes are present at birth.* (Compare Figs. 7-5*C* and 7-7.) As the mastoid process forms, mastoid air cells invade it from the mastoid antrum. By 2 years of age these cells have bulged the bone outward and downward, forming a small mastoid process, the internal structure of which resembles a honeycomb (Fig. 7-72).

CLINICALLY ORIENTED COMMENTS

Infections of the mastoid antrum and the mastoid air cells always begin in the middle ear (*otitis media*). Infections may spread upward toward the middle cranial fossa via the petrosquamous suture in young children or because of **osteomyelitis** (bone infection with necrosis) of the tegmen tympani. Extradural pus is produced and occasionally a **temporal lobe abscess** forms. In other patients the infection may spread posteriorly into the posterior cranial fossa, producing osteomyelitis of the bone forming the sigmoid sinus groove, thrombophlebitis of the sigmoid sinus, and occasionally a **cerebellar abscess**.

Since the advent of antibiotics, mastoiditis as a complication of middle ear infection is rare. In **operations for mastoiditis**, surgeons have to be fully aware of the course of the facial nerve (Figs. 7-183, 7-184, and 7-188) so that it will not be injured.

One access to the tympanic cavity is through the mastoid antrum. In a child, only a thin plate of bone needs to be removed from the lateral wall of the antrum in the suprameatal region to expose the tympanic cavity. In adults, however, bone must be penetrated for 15 mm or more to reach the mastoid antrum. At present most mastoidectomies are **endaural** (within the ear), *i.e.,* via the posterior wall of the external acoustic meatus.

Pneumatization (formation of mastoid air cells) may be arrested during childhood; thus, in about 20% of persons very few mastoid air cells are visible in radiographs. In rare cases no mastoid air cells are visible; when these kinds of mastoid processes have been sectioned, they have been found to contain diploë (Fig. 7).

THE INTERNAL EAR

The internal ear (**vestibulocochlear organ**) is concerned with the reception of sound and the maintenance of balance. It is buried in the petrous part of the temporal bone (Figs. 7-182 and 7-185) and consists of sacs and ducts, the **membranous labyrinth**, containing endolymph, and the end organs for hearing and balancing. The latter are in a series of channels and spaces in the temporal bone. The membranous labyrinth is surrounded by *perilymph* and both are enclosed in a **bony labyrinth** that is visible on radiographs.

The Bony Labyrinth (Figs. 7-186 and 7-193). The bony (osseous) labyrinth has three parts: the **cochlea**, the **vestibule**, and the **semicircular canals**. It occupies much of the lateral portion of the petrous part of the temporal bone.

The Cochlea (Figs. 7-193 to 7-195). The bony cochlea (L. a snail shell) contains the *part of the internal ear that is concerned with hearing* (*i.e.,* membranous cochlea or cochlear duct). It somewhat **resembles a snail's shell** that makes two-and-one-half turns around a bony pillar or core, called the **modiolus**, (L. the nave of a wheel), in

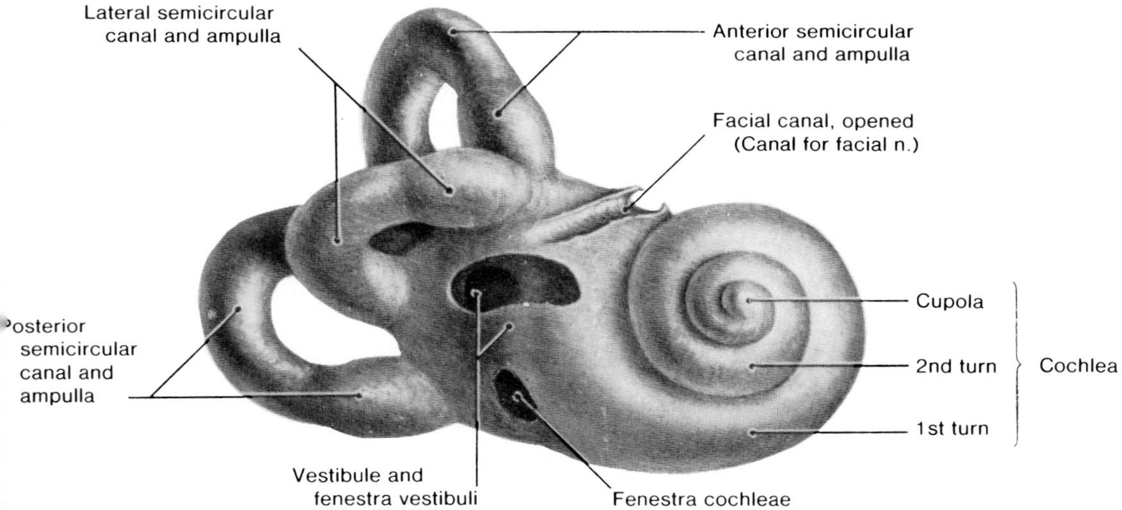

Figure 7-193. Drawing of a lateral view of the right side of the bony labyrinth, as it would appear if it was possible to dissect it from the petrous part of the temporal bone. Observe the three parts of the bony labyrinth: cochlea in front, vestibule in the middle, and the semicircular canals behind. Note that the cochlea makes 2½ coils. In life the fenestra vestibuli (oval window) and fenestra cochlea (round window) are closed by the foot piece of the stapes and the secondary tympanic membrane, respectively. Observe also the three semicircular canals: anterior, posterior, and lateral. Note that the anterior and posterior canals are set at a right angle to each other and that the lateral canal is set horizontally and at a right angle to the other two. Each canal forms about two-thirds of a circle and has an ampulla at one end. The lateral canal is shortest and the posterior canal is the longest.

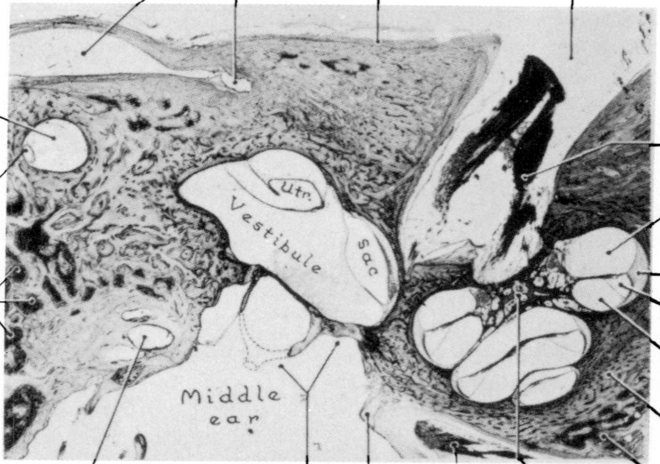

Figure 7-194. Drawing of a cross-section of the bony and membranous labyrinths. Note that the stapes was broken during preparation and that its foot piece is held in the fenestra vestibuli by the anular ligament. Observe the structures in the cochlear canal.

which there are canals for blood vessels and nerves (Figs. 7-194 and 7-195). It is the large first or basal turn of the cochlea that produces the **promontory** on the medial wall of the tympanic cavity (Fig. 7-185).

The axis of the modiolus is across the long axis of the petrous part of the temporal bone; thus, the apex of the cochlea, called the **cupola**, points anterolaterally (Fig. 7-193). A small shelf of bone, the **osseous spiral lamina**, protrudes from the central core of the cochlea, called the **modiolus**, like the thread on a screw. This starts at the vestibule (Fig. 7-195) and continues to the apex. The **basilar membrane** is attached to the osseous spiral lamina.

The modiolus is pierced by several longitudinal channels which turn outward toward the spiral lamina and enter the **spiral canal** of the modiolus. This canal runs in the base of the spiral lamina and contains the sensory **cochlear (spiral) ganglion** (Fig. 7-195). Cells in this ganglion send their peripheral processes to the **spiral organ** (of Corti), concerned with hearing.

The cochlear canal (canal in bony cochlea) *is divided by two membranous partitions into three spiral scala* (L. a stairway) or spaces: the **scala vestibuli** above; the **scala media** or **cochlear duct** in the middle; and the **scala tympani** below (Figs. 7-194 and 7-195).

The scala vestibuli is so-named because it opens into the vestibule of the bony labyrinth (Fig. 7-182). Through its opening, perilymph can be exchanged freely between the vestibule and the scala vestibuli (Fig. 7-194). The scala tympani, which also contains perilymph, is related to the tympanic cavity at the fenestra cochleae (round window), which is closed by the **secondary tympanic membrane**. The scala vestibuli communicates with the scala tympani through a small aperture, the **helicotrema**, at the apex of the cochlea.

The perilymph in the scalae of the bony labyrinth is similar in composition to CSF. This similarity is understandable because there is a narrow connection between the perilymphatic spaces of the bony labyrinth

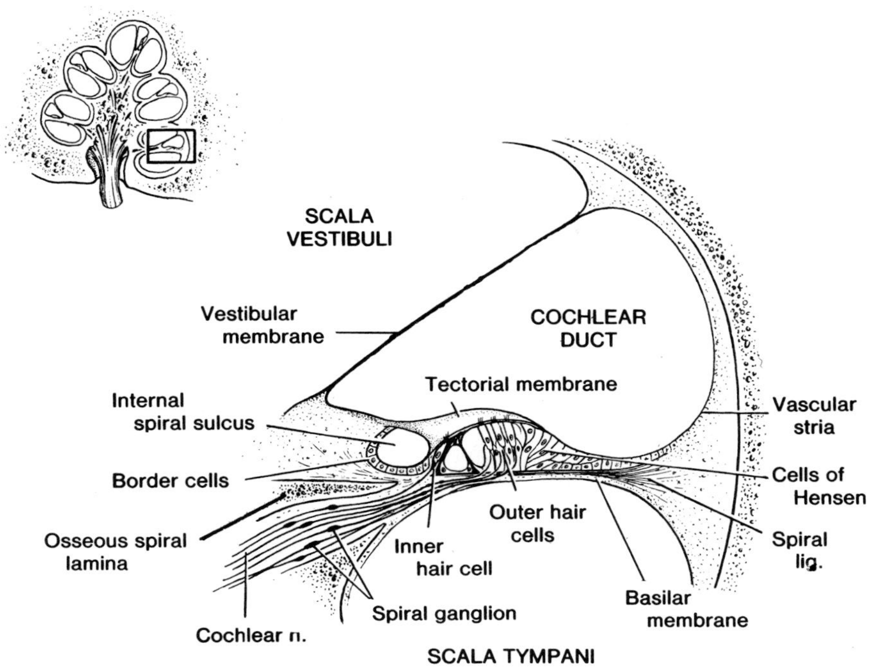

Figure 7-195. Drawing of a radial section through the cochlea showing the cochlear duct, the basilar membrane, the spiral organ (of Corti), and the tectorial membrane. In the *upper left* is a small drawing of an axial section of the cochlea. The large drawing shows details of the area enclosed in the rectangle.

and the subarachnoid space called the **perilymphatic duct** (Fig. 7-182). This connection consists of a canal in the petrous part of the temporal bone, running from the scala tympani in the basal turn of the cochlea to an extension of the subarachnoid space around the glossopharyngeal, vagus, and accessory nerves (CN IX, CN X, and CN XI, respectively, Fig. 7-182).

The Vestibule (Figs. 7-182 and 7-193). The vestibule is the small, oval, bony chamber (about 5 mm in length), containing the **utricle** and **saccule**, parts of the balancing apparatus (Fig. 7-197). The utricle and saccule are endolymph-containing dilations of the membranous labyrinth which are enclosed by the vestibule of the bony labyrinth. The vestibule is continuous anteriorly with the bony cochlea, posteriorly with the bony semicircular canals, and with the posterior cranial fossa by the **aqueduct of the vestibule** (Fig. 7-182). This aqueduct extends to the posterior surface of the petrous part of the temporal bone, where it opens posterolateral to the internal acoustic meatus (Figs. 7-56 and 7-57). It contains the **endolymphatic duct** and two small blood vessels. This duct emerges through the bone of the posterior cranial fossa and expands into a blind pouch, the **endolymphatic sac** (Figs. 7-182 and 7-197). It is located under cover of the dura mater on the posterior surface of the petrous part of the temporal bone. *The endolymphatic sac is a storage reservoir for excess endolymph* formed by the blood capillaries within the membranous labyrinth.

To visualize the relationship of the vestibule to the **tympanic cavity**, examine Figures 7-182 and 7-193. When the stapes is removed, the vestibule communicates with the tympanic cavity through the **fenestra vestibuli**. The five orifices of the semicircular canals are in the posterior part of the vestibule.

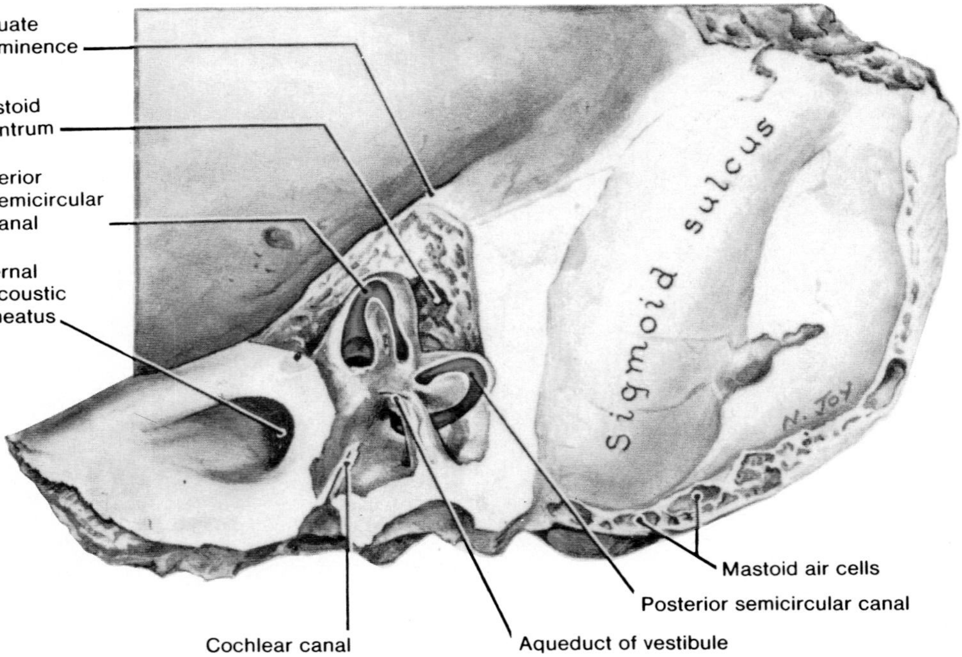

Figure 7-196. Drawing of a dissection of the semicircular canals, posterosuperior view. Observe the anterior semicircular canal, set vertically below the arcuate eminence and making a right angle with the posterior surface of the petrous bone. Note that the posterior semicircular canal is nearly parallel to the posterior surface of the bone, only 5 mm from the sigmoid sulcus, the groove containing the sigmoid sinus. Observe the aqueduct of the vestibule containing the endolymphatic duct. Note the canaliculus of the cochlea containing the perilymphatic duct (aqueduct of the cochlea) which opens into the subarachnoid space at the apex of the depression for the ganglion of CN IX.

The Semicircular Canals (Figs. 7-182, 7-185, 7-186, 7-193, and 7-196). The three semicircular canals (anterior, posterior, and lateral) lie posterosuperior to the vestibule into which they open. The canals are set at right angles to each other and occupy three planes in space. Each canal forms about two-thirds of a circle and is about 1.5 mm in diameter, except at one end where there is a swelling called the **ampulla**. The three semicircular canals have only five openings into the vestibule because the anterior and posterior canals have one stem common to both.

The anterior (superior) canal lies at a right angle to the posterior surface of the petrous part of the temporal bone and is closely related to the floor of the middle cranial fossa. It forms a transversely rounded elevation, called the **arcuate eminence** (Figs. 7-56 and 7-196), on the superior surface of the petrous process, just medial to the tegmen tympani.

The posterior canal lies in the long axis of the petrous part of the temporal bone, immediately deep to the posterior (cerebellar) surface. Note its location in Figure 7-185 and its proximity to the sigmoid sinus (Fig. 7-196).

The lateral canal is horizontal and its arch is directed horizontally backward and laterally (Fig. 7-185). It lies deep to the medial wall of the **aditus to the mastoid antrum** and runs above the *canal for the*

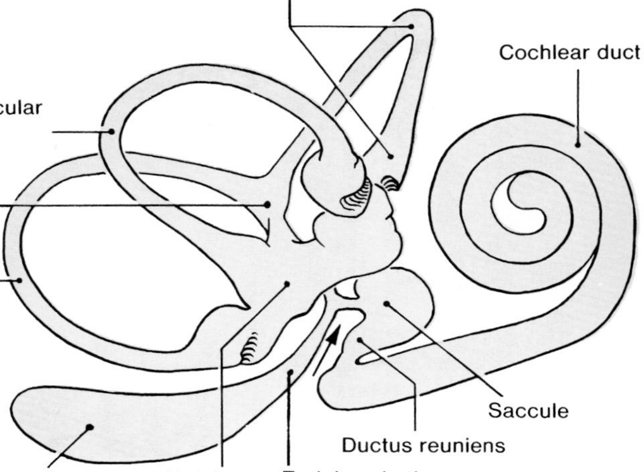

Figured 7-197. Drawing of a lateral view of the membranous labyrinth, right side. The membranous labyrinth is contained within the bony labyrinth (Fig. 7-193). It is a closed system of ducts and chambers filled with endolymph and bathed in perilymph. Observe its three parts—the duct of the cochlea, within the cochlea; the saccule and the utricle, within the vestibule; and the three semicircular ducts, within the three semicircular canals. One end of the duct of the cochlea is closed; the other end communicates with the saccule through the ductus reuniens. Note that the utricle communicates with the saccule via the utriculosaccular duct (*arrow*).

facial nerve (CN VII). The lateral semicircular canal of one ear is in the same plane as that in the other.

CLINICALLY ORIENTED COMMENTS

In one type of operation performed to restore hearing, an additional opening is made into the internal ear (**fenestration**). The opening is made into the lateral semicircular canal at its ampullary end. This operation produces another fenestra (window) between the tympanic cavity and the internal ear and is performed when the stapes in the fenestra vestibuli has become immovable owing to **otosclerosis** (Fig. 7-192*A*).

Examine Figure 7-185, noting the following important bony landmarks. The lateral canal produces a prominent bulge, the **prominence of the lateral semicircular canal**. Obviously it has to be differentiated from the **prominence of the facial canal** that lies below it. The facial nerve produces this bulge after it leaves the geniculate ganglion.

The Membranous Labyrinth (Fig. 7-197). Although some of the following material has been mentioned in the description of the bony labyrinth, the membranous labyrinth will be described separately because of its importance.

The membranous labyrinth is a series of communicating membranous sacs and ducts (Fig. 7-197) that are contained in the cavities of the bony labyrinth (Figs. 7-182 and 7-193). The membranous labyrinth generally follows the form of the bony labyrinth but is much smaller. The membranous labyrinth contains a watery fluid called **endolymph**, which differs in composition from the **perilymph** around it in the bony labyrinth. In these terms "lymph" does not indicate a relationship to the usual fluid called lymph. The term derives from the Latin word meaning clear spring water and is used in this sense here (*e.g.*, perilymph).

The membranous labyrinth consists of: (1) two small communicating sacs, the **utricle** and the **saccule**, in the vestibule; (2) **three semicircular ducts** in the semicircular canals; and (3) the **cochlear duct** in the cochlea. The vestibular parts of the membranous labyrinth are *suspended in the bony vestibule by trabeculae of connective tissue*; however, the cochlear duct is firmly attached along two sides of the wall of the cochlear canal. Except at the ampullae, *the semicircular ducts are much smaller than the semicircular canals,* but the convexity of each duct is adherent to the bony canal in which it is located.

Examine Figures 7-182 and 7-197, verifying that the various parts of the membranous labyrinth form a closed system of sacs and ducts which communicate with one another. Note that the semicircular ducts open into the utricle through five openings and that the utricle communicates with the saccule through the **utriculosaccular duct**, which also joins the *endolymphatic duct.* The saccule is continuous with the cochlear duct through a narrow communication known as the **ductus reuniens**.

The Utricle and the Saccule (Fig. 7-197). Each of these dilations has a specialized area of sensory epithelium called a macula. The **macula utriculi** is in the floor of the utricle, parallel with the base of the skull, whereas the **macula sacculi** is vertically placed on the medial wall of the saccule. The **hair cells** in the maculae are innervated by fibers of the vestibular division of the **vestibulocochlear nerve** (CN VIII). The primary sensory neurons are in the **vestibular ganglion** (Scarpa's ganglion), located at the bottom of the **internal acoustic meatus** (Fig. 7-196). The maculae are *primarily static organs for signaling the position of the head in space,* but they also respond to quick tilting movements and to linear acceleration and deceleration. **Motion sickness** results mainly from prolonged, fluctuating stimulation of the maculae.

The Semicircular Ducts (Fig. 7-197). Each duct has an expansion or **ampulla** at one end containing a sensory area called a **crista ampullaris**. *The cristae are sensors of movement,* recording movements of the endolymph in the ampulla that result from rotation of the head in the plane of the duct. The **hair cells** of the cristae, like those of the maculae, are supplied by primary sensory neurons whose cell bodies are in the **vestibular ganglion**.

The Cochlear Duct (Figs. 7-194 and 7-195). The duct of the cochlea is a spiral, blind tube which is firmly fixed to the inner and outer walls of the cochlear canal. It is triangular in transverse section and lies between the **osseus spiral lamina** and the outer wall of the cochlear canal. Its roof is formed by the **vestibular membrane** and its floor by the **basilar membrane** and the outer part of the osseus spiral lamina.

The receptor of auditory stimuli is the **spiral organ** (of Corti), situated on the basilar membrane. This complex sensory organ developed from the epithelium of the cochlear duct. Sound waves in the air pass into the external acoustic meatus, causing movements of the tympanic membrane and auditory ossicles. Stronger waves are transmitted to the perilymph at the fenestra vestibuli by the base of the stapes. Vibrations of the perilymph are transmitted to the **basilar membrane**, displacement of which, in response to acoustic stimuli, causes bending of the hair-like projections of the sensory hair cells of the spiral organ. These cells are in contact with the **tectorial membrane** and are innervated by peripheral fibers of bipolar primary sensory neurons in the **spiral ganglion**, situated about the modiolus of the cochlea. The central processes of these cells form the **cochlear nerve**, part of the vestibulocochlear nerve (**CN VIII**).

CLINICALLY ORIENTED COMMENTS

Persistent exposure to excessively loud sounds is known to cause degenerative changes in the spiral organ at the base of the cochlea, resulting in **high tone deafness**. This type of hearing loss commonly occurs in workers who are exposed to loud noises and do not wear protective ear muffs (*e.g.,* persons working for long periods around jet engines or farm tractors). **Acoustic trauma disease** is sometimes called "boiler-maker's disease" because it used to be detected in workers in boiler factories owing to injury to the cochlear nerve incident to riveting the inside of a boiler. Injury to ear by imbalance in pressure between ambient (surrounding) air and the air in the middle ear is called **otic barotrauma** (*baro* is a combining form relating to pressure). This type of injury occurs in flyers, divers, caisson workers, and battered infants. Some parents who beat their children "box their ears," thereby injuring them.

The Internal Acoustic Meatus (Figs. 7-194, 7-196, and 7-198). The internal acoustic meatus is a *narrow canal that runs directly laterally for about 1 cm within the petrous part of the temporal bone.* The opening of the meatus is in the posteromedial part of this bone (Fig. 7-57), opposite the **external acoustic meatus**, at a depth of about 5 cm. It is closed laterally by a thin, perforated plate of bone which separates it from the internal ear. Through this plate pass the facial nerve (CN VII), branches of the vestibulocochlear nerve (CN VIII), and small blood vessels. The **vestibulocochlear nerve** divides near the lateral end of the internal acoustic meatus into an anterior or **cochlear portion** and a posterior or **vestibular portion**. As has been described, *the cochlear nerve is the nerve of hearing* and *the vestibular nerve is the nerve of balance.*

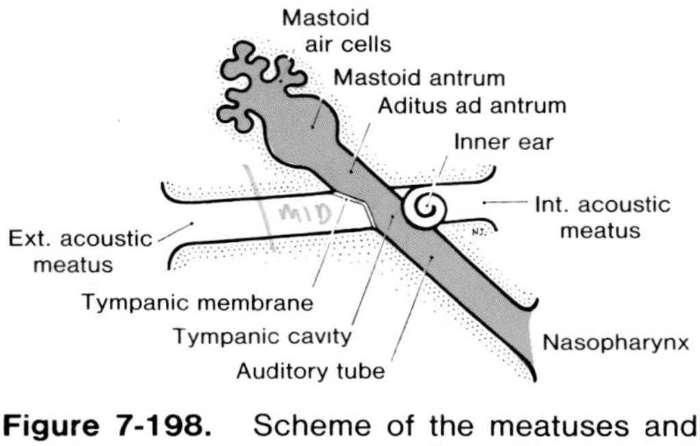

Figure 7-198. Scheme of the meatuses and the airway. Observe that the line of the external and internal meatuses intersect at the tympanic cavity with the line of the airway from the mastoid cells to the nasopharynx.

CLINICALLY ORIENTED COMMENTS

An abnormal increase in the amount of endolymph, called hydrops of the internal ear or Ménière's disease (syndrome), produces **recurrent vertigo** (dizziness) accompanied in later stages by **tinnitus** (L. a jingling) or noises in the ear and deafness. The pathological changes resulting from dilation of the endolymphatic system are **degeneration of the hair cells** in the maculae of the vestibule and in the spiral organ. The relation of these changes to paroxysms (sudden onsets) of vertigo (dizziness) is unknown. There are **other causes of vertigo**, e.g., **labyrinthitis** (inflammation of the membranous labyrinth), trauma (causing hemorrhage into the inner ear), certain **brain stem infarcts** (areas of necrotic nerve tissue), and **tumors** of the vestibulocochlear nerve.

PATIENT ORIENTED PROBLEMS

Case 7-1. The wife of a 45-year-old commercial traveler was awakened by the unusual nature of his snoring and was puzzled when she noticed that he was sleeping with his left eye open. In the morning she observed that the left side of his face was drooping. Whe he tried to look at his teeth, he found that his lips were also paralyzed on that side (Fig. 7-199). He was also unable to whistle or to puff out his cheek because the air blew out through his paralyzed lips on the left side. He also found that he was unable to raise his eyebrow or to frown on that side.

During breakfast he had trouble chewing his food, as it dribbled out of the left side of his mouth. Fearing that he may have poliomyelitis or have had a mild stroke during

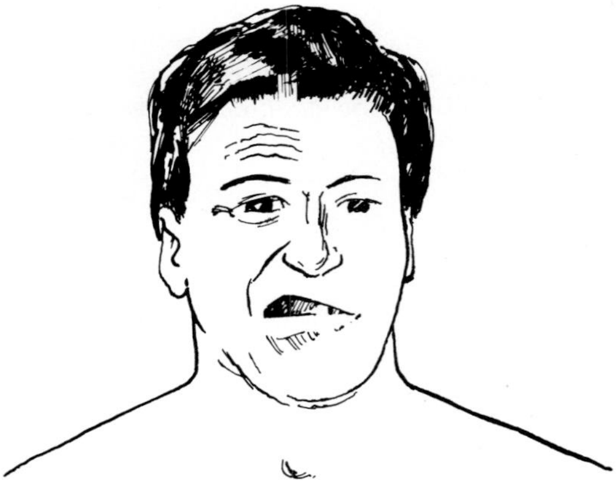

Figure 7-199. The appearance of the patient's face when he tried to examine his teeth is shown. Paralysis of the left side of his face is obvious as shown by the lack of wrinkling on that side, and the failure to expose the left teeth. Note that the skin of his forehead does not wrinkle either.

the night, he made an appointment to see his doctor.

During his examination the doctor made the following observations: at rest the left side of his face appeared flattened and expressionless; there were no lines on the left side of his forehead; there was sagging in the left lower half of his face, and saliva drooled from the left corner of his mouth. In addition there was a loss of taste sensation on the anterior two-thirds of the left side of his tongue and an absence of voluntary control of left facial and left platysma muscles. When the patient smiled, the lower portion of his face was pulled to the normal side and the right corner of his mouth was raised, but the left corner was not.

During questioning the patient related how he had driven home late the night before and, because of drowsiness, had rolled the window down part way. He also recalled that he had had a head cold and an ear infection a few days previously and that the doctor who treated him had described his illness as a viral infection.

Problems. Paralysis of what nerve would produce the signs exhibited by this patient? Why did his left eye remain open, even when he was sleeping? Why was there loss of taste sensation on the anterior two-thirds of the left side of his tongue? Where is the lesion of the nerve probably located? *These problems are discussed on page 1059.*

Case 7-2. A 62-year-old man complained to his dentist about sudden short bouts of excruciating pain on the left side of his face. They were of about 2 months' duration and had been increasing in severity. Following examination, the dentist informed him that there was no dental cause for the pain. He stated that it was probably a neurological disorder and that he should see a physician.

The man explained to the doctor that the **stabbing pains**, lasting 15 to 20 seconds, occurred several times during the day and were so severe that he had once contemplated suicide. He said the onset of pain seemed to be **triggered by chewing** or by a draft (of wind) affecting his upper lip. When the doctor asked him to point out the area where the pains occurred, he carefully pointed to his left upper lip, left cheek, and under his left eye. He said the pain also radiated to his lower eyelid, the lateral side of his nose, and the inside of his mouth. The doctor applied firm steady pressure over the patient's left cheek and over his infraorbital area but detected no tenderness indicative of inflammation of the maxillary sinus or defects in the orbital rim caused by a lesion of the maxilla. *Radiographs of the skull showed nothing abnormal.*

On evaluation, the doctor detected an acuteness of sensitivity to touch (**hyperesthesia**) on the left upper lip and to pin prick over the entire left maxillary region, but he found no abnormality of sensation in the forehead or mandibular regions.

Problems. What branch of what nerve supplies the area of skin and mucous membrane where the **paroxysms** (sudden recurring attacks) of stabbing pain were felt? Where does this nerve leave the skull? What are its branches and how are they distributed? *These problems are discussed on page 1060.*

Case 7-3. The mother of a 12-year-old girl explained to her family physician that her daughter had had **severe fever**, chills, and a headache for the last 2 days, with some **blurring of vision** in her left eye.

On examination the doctor noted redness and swelling (edema) of the girl's left eyelids and conjunctiva and slight protrusion of the left eye (**exophthalmos**). He also detected impairment of movement of her left eye and, during opthalmoscopy, he observed **thrombosis** (clotting of blood) in the retinal veins. He also noted that she had **acne vulgaris** (inflammatory disease of the sebaceous glands) and that one **nodulocystic lesion** between her nose and left eye was badly inflammed.

Following consultation with an ophthalmologist, a diagnosis of **thrombophlebitis** (septic thrombosis) of the cavernous sinus and ophthalmic veins secondary to infection of the pustule on her face was made.

Problems. How did the infection of the face spread to the **cavernous sinus**? Is there an anatomical basis for the spread of infection to the cavernous sinus on the other side? Why is there **thrombosis of the retinal veins**? Why was movement of her left eye impaired? What is the basis of the exophthalmos and the edema of the eyelids and conjunctiva? *These problems are discussed on page 1061.*

Case 7-4. A 55-year-old farmer complained to his doctor about a sore that had been on his lower lip for 6 months. He stated that he first thought it was a cold sore and then he became worried because this one looked different and did not respond to his usual treatment with salve.

On examination an ulcerated, indurated (hardened) lesion was present on the central portion of his lower lip (Fig. 7-200). His face was darkly tanned. Systematic palpation of the lymph nodes of his neck revealed enlarged, **hard submental lymph nodes**. None of the submandibular or deep cervical lymph nodes was enlarged. Examination of a small biopsy from the edge of the lesion revealed a **squamous cell carcinoma** (malignant tumor of epithelial origin).

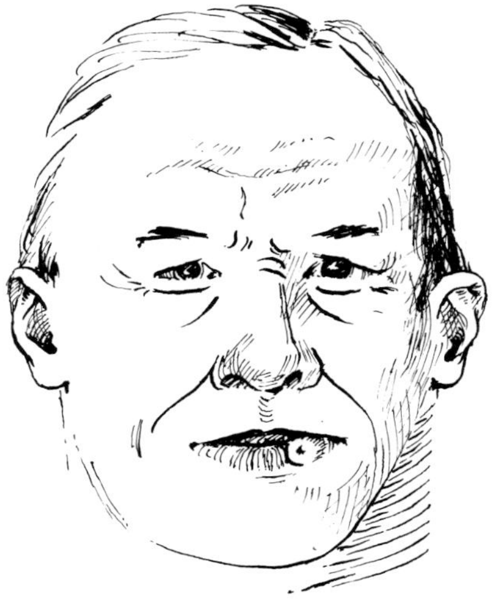

Figure 7-200. Drawing of the patient showing the lesion on his lower lip.

Problems. Where are the **submental lymph nodes** located? Between the bellies of which muscle do they lie? What structures, in addition to the central portion of the lip, do afferent lymph vessels of these nodes drain? To which lymph nodes do lymph vessels from lateral portions of the lip pass? If the cancer had spread from the submental lymph nodes, where would you expect to find **metastases** (new tumors). *These problems are discussed on page 1062.*

Case 7-5. A 22-year-old medical student was struck by a puck on the left "temple" (temporal fossa) during an interfaculty hockey game. He fell to the ice unconscious but *regained consciousness in about 1 minute.* There was some bleeding from a laceration located two fingerbreadths above his left zygomatic arch that extended from the top of his ear almost to his eyebrow.

As you helped him to the bench, he said that he felt rather weak and unsteady. Realizing that he may have sustained a skull fracture, you asked a classmate to call a doctor while you took him to the dressing room. The deep tendon reflexes in his arms and legs were equal. His pupils were equal in size and both contracted to light. As you waited, you observed that the injury site started to swell, but your friend otherwise seemed well.

In about half an hour he said that he was sleepy and wanted to lie down. His *left pupil was moderately dilated* and reacted sluggishly to light. By the time the doctor arrived he was unconscious. The pupil on the left was widely dilated and did not respond to light, whereas the pupil on the right was slightly dilated but showed a normal reaction to light. The doctor said, "We must get him to the hospital right away!"

In hospital, skull radiographs were made and a **CT scan** (computerized tomographic scan) was done. As the doctor was almost certain that there was intracranial hemorrhage, he called a neurosurgeon.

When the neurosurgeon arrived, the radiologist reported that there was a **fracture of the temporal squama** posterior to the pterion and that the CT scan showed an extradural (epidural) hematoma (Fig. 7-201).

Problems. Where is the **temple**? Define the area known as the **pterion**. In what part of the **temporal fossa** is it located? Why is it clinically important? What artery was most likely torn? What other vessel may have been torn? Where would the blood collect? *These problems are discussed on page 1062.*

Case 7-6. While cleaning the bathtub, a 49-year-old woman developed a **throbbing headache** which lasted for about 30 minutes and then slowly faded away. Similar headaches occurred occasionally for the next week. Then one day as she was lifting a heavy chair, she experienced a **sudden, severe headache** which was accompanied by nausea, vomiting, and a general feeling of weakness. It was decided that she should see her doctor immediately.

Examination revealed **nuchal rigidity** (stiff neck) and an elevation in blood pressure. Visualization of the optic fundus through the ophthalmoscope showed **subhyaloid hemorrhages** (bleeding between the retina and the vitreous body). Her deep tendon reflexes were symmetrical and all modalities (forms) of sensation were normal.

On the basis of these clear signs and symptoms, the doctor made a diagnosis of **subarachnoid hemorrhage**. He suggested that it was probably caused by rupture of an **aneurysm** (circumscribed dilation) of the arterial circle (Fig. 7-202).

Arteriograms showed a saccular aneurysm of the anterior communicating artery. A **lumbar puncture** (Fig. 5-69) demonstrated bloody CSF. After centrifugation, the supernatant fluid was **xanthochromatic** (yellow-colored).

Problems. Where would blood from the **ruptured aneurysm** most likely go? How do you explain anatomically the formation of **subhyaloid hemorrhages**? Why was the supernatant part of the CSF xanthochromatic? *These problems are discussed on page 1063.*

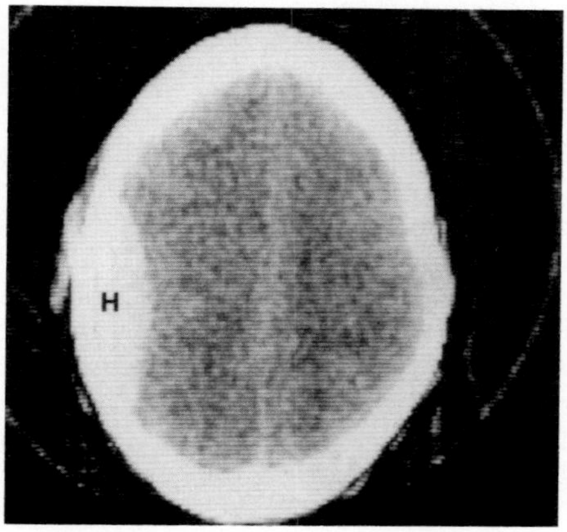

Figure 7-201. Computerized tomographic (CT) scan showing an extradural (epidural) hematoma (*H*) in the left middle cranial fossa.

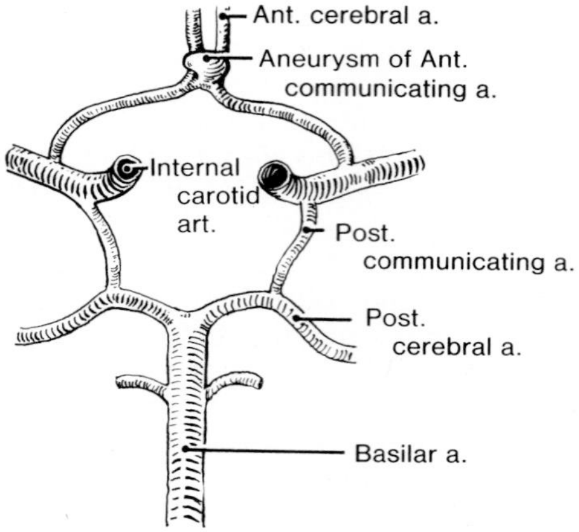

Figure 7-202. Drawing of the arterial circle (circle of Willis) showing a saccular (berry) aneurysm of the anterior communicating artery.

Case 7-7. A 23-year-old man went to a dentist to have a badly **decayed inferior third molar** ("wisdom") tooth extracted. The dentist explained that there was likely to be considerable pain associated with removal of the tooth and informed the patient that he was going to inject a "local" (anesthetic agent) to desensitize the tooth and associated soft tissues. When agreeing to the extraction, the patient requested that plenty of anesthetic be used because he was extremely sensitive to pain.

The dentist inserted the needle through the mucous membrane on the inside of the patient's mouth where the needle came to rest near the **lingula**, a bony projection on the medial surface of the ramus of the mandible. In a few minutes the patient stated that his gum (gingiva), lip, chin, and tongue on the affected side were numb (anesthetized). During the extraction procedure the patient said he felt pain; hence, the dentist injected more anesthetic. The tooth was removed without further incident.

As the patient was preparing to leave, he happened to look in the mirror. He found that he was **unable to close his eye and lips** on the affected side and that his mouth sagged on this side, particularly when he attempted to expose his teeth. He also found that his ear lobule was numb. When he reported these unusual symptoms, the dentist drew a sketch of the nerves of the face and explained that because of the large amount of anesthetic injected, other nerves in addition to those supplying the teeth had been anesthetized. He assured the patient that all these effects would disappear in 3 to 4 hours.

Problems. Name the nerve supplying the lower molar and premolar teeth. Why was the patient's chin, lower lip, and tongue on the injected side also anesthetized? When anesthetizing this nerve, what others might be affected? What probably caused the patient's **facial paralysis** and loss of sensation in part of his ear? *These problems are discussed on page 1064.*

Case 7-8. A 38-year-old female went to her dentist for a routine 6-month check-up. Her only complaint was some tenderness of the gums around the back teeth in her right mandible.

On examination the dentist observed redness of the **gingivae** (gums) around her right lower molar teeth and that her third molar ("wisdom") tooth had not erupted fully. He radiographed this region and observed on the radiograph that her **third molar tooth was malposed and impacted**, similar to that shown in Figure 7-130. He strongly advised that the tooth be extracted and explained that during this procedure there was a chance that the nerve supplying the tooth might be damaged.

The extraction was performed under local anesthesia. During the operation the tooth had to be broken into several pieces. In order to remove all the fragments, parts of the bone had to be chipped away.

The patient returned the next day, complaining that her right **lower lip was still numb**. The dentist explained that, although the nerve supplying her lower lip must have been damaged during removal of her tooth, sensation should return to her lip in a few months.

After 6 months, the patient still complained of abnormal sensation (**paresthesia**) in her right lower lip and that this interfered with her enjoyment of kissing. She planned to consult her lawyer about the possibility of a malpractice suit.

Problems. **What nerve was injured** during extraction of the patient's third molar tooth? What is its origin and course through the mandible? **Why is this nerve vulnerable** during oral surgery? What is the name of the branch of this nerve that supplies the side of the lower lip and the chin? Where does this nerve emerge from the mandible? Will complete sensation ever return to the patient's lower lip? *These problems are discussed on page 1064.*

DISCUSSION OF PATIENT ORIENTED PROBLEMS

Case 7-1. Sudden facial paralysis often follows exposure to the cold; thus, **Bell's palsy** is the most probable diagnosis in this case. The characteristic facial appearance results from a lesion of the facial nerve (CN

VII). In the present patient, the motor supply to the muscles of the left face, forehead, and eyelids were most severely affected (Fig. 7-199). **Paralysis of the muscles of facial expression** on the left side explains the expressionless look on that side of his face and his inability to whistle, puff his cheek, or close his left eye.

When the facial nerve is paralyzed, the levator palpebrae superioris (acting unopposed) causes the eye to remain open, even during sleep. The drooling and difficulty in chewing result from paralysis of the orbicularis oris and buccinator muscles. Loss of taste sensation on the anterior two-thirds of the left side of his tongue is understandable anatomically because this region of the tongue receives taste fibers via the **chorda tympani** branch of CN VII. This symptom also indicates that the nerve lesion is proximal to the origin of this nerve in the facial canal (Figs. 7-185 and 7-188).

Because of **paralysis of the orbicularis oculi muscle**, the lacrimal puncta are no longer in contact with the cornea, and as a result, tears tend to flow over the left lower lid onto the cheek. In addition, the cornea may dry out during sleep (if an ointment is not used) because the eyelids on the affected side remain open. **Drying of the cornea** can also occur during the day owing to the inability to blink; this dryness could result in **corneal ulceration**.

The site of the lesion is most likely in the facial canal in the petrous part of the temporal bone. The **paresis** (muscle weakness) or paralysis of the facial muscles are thought to be caused by inflammation of the nerve above the stylomastoid foramen. The etiology (causation) is generally thought to be a **viral infection** which causes edema (swelling) of the nerve and compression of its fibers in the **facial canal** or at the stylomastoid foramen. If the lesion is complete, all the facial muscles on that side are affected equally; voluntary, emotional, and associated movements are all affected.

In most cases the nerve fibers are not permanently damaged and nerve degeneration is incomplete. As a result, recovery is slow but generally good (see CN VII in Chap. 8). Some **facial asymmetry** may persist (*e.g.*, sagging of the left corner of his mouth).

Case 7-2. The area of skin and mucosa in which the stabbing pain was felt is supplied by the **maxillary nerve** (Fig. 7-30), the second division of the trigeminal nerve (CN V^2). This wholly sensory nerve leaves the skull through the **foramen rotundum** and, at its termination as the infraorbital nerve, gives rise to branches that supply the ala or side of the nose (nasal branches), the lower eyelid (palpebral branches), and the skin and mucous membrane of the cheek and upper lip (superior labial branches). Branches of the maxillary nerve also innervate the teeth in the maxilla and the mucous membranes of the nasal cavities, palate, mouth, and tongue.

The symptoms described by this patient are characteristic of the clinical condition known as **trigeminal neuralgia** (tic douloureaux). It occurs most often in middle-aged and elderly persons. The pain may be so intense that the patient winces, hence the term "tic" (twitch). In some cases *the pain may be so severe that mental changes occur; there may be depression and even suicide.* The maxillary nerve distribution (Fig. 7-42), as in the present case, is most frequently involved, then the mandibular, and least frequently the ophthalmic. The **paroxysm**, as in the present case, is of sudden onset and is often set off by touching the face, brushing the teeth, drinking, or chewing. Often there is an especially sensitive "*trigger zone,*" *e.g.,* the left upper lip in the present case.

At present, *the cause of trigeminal neuralgia is unknown.* Some persons believe the condition is caused by a pathological process affecting neurons in the trigeminal (semilunar) ganglion, whereas others believe neurons in the nucleus of the spinal tract may be involved. Medical and/or surgical treatment is used to alleviate the pain. Only the anatomical aspects of these treatments will be discussed here.

Attempts were made to *block the nerve at the infraorbital foramen* by using alcohol; this usually gives temporary relief of pain. The simplest surgical procedure is **avulsion** (pulling out) or *cutting of the branches of the nerve at the infraorbital* *foramen* (Fig. 7-31). **Radiofrequency selective coagulation of the trigeminal ganglion** via a needle electrode passing through the cheek and the foramen ovale is also used. To prevent regeneration of nerve fibers, the sensory root of the **trigeminal nerve** may be partially cut between the ganglion and the brain stem (**rhizotomy**). Although the axons may regenerate, they do not do so within the brain stem. Attempts are made to differentiate and cut only the sensory fibers to the division of the trigeminal nerve involved (Fig. 8–20).

The same result may be achieved by *sectioning the spinal tract of CN V* (**tractotomy**). After this operation the sensation of pain, temperature, and simple (light) touch are lost over the area of skin and mucous membrane supplied by the maxillary nerve (Fig. 7-30). This may be annoying to the patient who does not recognize the presence of food on the lip and cheek or feel it within the mouth on the side of the nerve section, but these disabilities are preferable to the excruciating pain. If sensation is lost in the eye, traumatic lesions (*e.g.,* scarring) of the cornea, followed by inflammation (**keratitis**), may occur which sometimes result in loss of vision in that eye.

In younger patients, "decompression" of the trigeminal ganglion may be done by removing the dura mater over it in the **trigeminal cave** (Figs. 7-88 and 7-133), and then massaging it. This often relieves the pain for several years without affecting other sensations.

Case 7-3. The **cavernous sinuses of the dura mater**, located one on each side of the body of the sphenoid bone, *communicate with tributaries of the facial vein* via the superior and inferior ophthalmic veins and via the pterygoid plexus (Fig. 7-38). The central vein of the retina usually opens into the cavenous sinus directly, but it may enter the superior ophthalmic vein. In the present case, the infection near the nose between the eye and the upper lip, the so-called **danger triangle of the face** (Fig. 7-203), probably reached the cavernous sinus via thrombosed left facial and superior ophthalmic veins.

Thrombophlebitis of the facial veins (sometimes called infective thrombosis) is propogated along veins via the lymphatics in their walls or by bits of infected clot (embolus) passing further along the veins. When a vein is occluded at some point, blood flow along it stops or is reversed.

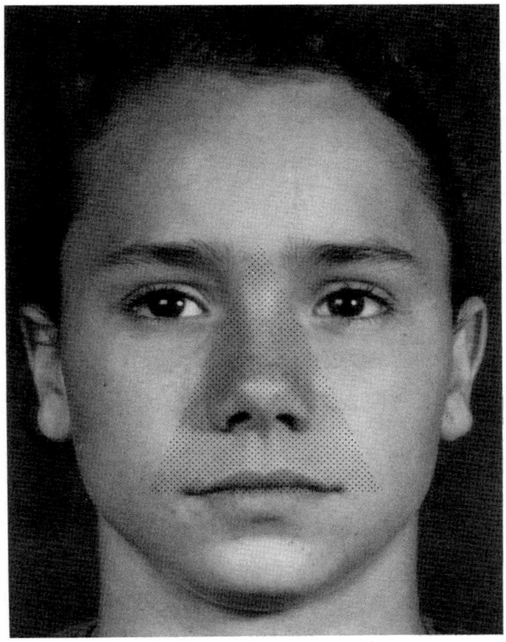

Figure 7-203. Photograph of a 12-year-old girl illustrating the danger triangle of the face. Veins in this area communicate with the superior ophthalmic veins which drain into the cavernous sinus posterior to the orbit.

Infection can spread from one cavernous sinus to the one on the other side because these sinuses are connected by intercavernous sinuses (Fig. 7-69*B*). As the **central vein of the retina** opens into the cavernous sinus or the superior ophthalmic vein, thrombosis can extend along the central vein of the retina and produce thromboses in the small retinal veins. As the facial vein has no valves and communicates with the cavernous sinus by two routes (Fig. 7-38), **thrombophlebitis of the facial vein** can spread to the intracranial venous system, including the cortical veins of the brain. This could result in **cortical infarcts** (areas of necrosis) and **meningitis**. Squeezing pustules may force bacteria into lymphatics or veins with serious consequences.

Suppuration (formation of pus) in the upper nasal cavities and the paranasal sinuses, especially the ethmoid and sphenoidal sinuses, may also lead to thrombophlebitis of the cavernous sinus, with risk of subsequent meningitis.

Thrombophlebitis of the cavernous sinus results in poor drainage of blood from it into the superior and inferior petrosal sinuses (Fig. 7-69). The **ocular signs** and symptoms in the present case were caused by *enlargement of the cavernous sinus and inflammatory edema of its walls.* Within the lateral wall of the sinus are the nerves supplying the extraocular muscles (CN III, CN IV, and CN VI) concerned with eye movements. As the ophthalmic and maxillary divisions of CN V pass forward in the cavernous sinus close to its lateral wall (Fig. 7-73), these fibers may also be involved. The **exophthalmos** and edema of the eyelids and conjunctiva result from the poor return of blood from the orbit owing to the closure of the ophthalmic veins and **stagnation of blood in the cavernous sinus**. The edema of the eyelids and conjunctiva result from inflammatory exudate and fluid escaping from the vessels associated with these structures.

Case 7-4. Carcinomas of the lip most commonly involve the lower lip. *Overexposure to sunshine over many years,* as occurs in outdoor workers such as farmers, is a common feature of the history in these cases. Chronic irritation from pipe smoking appears to be a factor also and may be related to long-term contact with tobacco tar.

The **submental lymph nodes** lie on the fascia covering the mylohyoid muscle between the anterior bellies of the right and left digastric muscles. The central part of the lip, the floor of the mouth, and the tip of the tongue drain to the submental lymph nodes, whereas lateral parts of the lip drain to the **submandibular lymph nodes** (Fig. 7-39).

If cancer cells had spread further, metastases would have developed in the submandibular lymph nodes because efferents from the submental lymph nodes pass to them. In addition, lymph vessels from the submental lymph nodes pass directly to the **jugulo-omohyoid node**. As the submandibular nodes are situated beneath the deep cervical fascia in the submandibular triangle, the patient's chin may have to be lowered to slacken this fascia before these enlarged nodes can be palpated.

Because all parts of the head and neck drain into a main chain of lymph nodes called the **deep cervical nodes** (Fig. 7-39), they might also be sites of metastases. As the jugulo-omohyoid node drains the submental and submandibular lymph nodes, it could be involved in the spread of tumor cells from a carcinoma of the lip. It is located where the omohyoid muscle crosses the internal jugular vein.

Case 7-5. The **temple** is the area between the temporal line (Fig. 7-8) and the zygomatic arch, where the skull is thin and is covered by the temporalis muscle and the temporal fascia. The blood vessels of the temple are very numerous. The **pterion** is a somewhat variable H-shaped area (Fig. 7-7) that lies deep to the temporalis muscle where four bones approach each other or meet (frontal, parietal, temporal, and sphenoid). It is an important bony landmark because it indicates the location of the **anterior branch of the middle meningeal artery** (Fig. 7-15). The center of the pterion is 4.0 cm superior to the zygomatic arch and 3.5 cm posterior to the frontozygomatic suture. It lies in the anterior part of the temporal fossa.

The thin squamous part of the temporal bone is grooved by the **middle meningeal artery** and its branches (Fig. 7-71). The temporal squama is easy to fracture and the broken pieces may tear the artery and its branches as they pass upward on the outer surface of the dura mater. This results in a slow accumulation of blood in the extradural space (Fig. 7-201), forming an **extradural hematoma** (epidural hematoma). The hematoma forms relatively slowly because the dura is firmly attached to the bone by **Sharpey fibers** which resist stripping of the dura from the bone to a certain extent.

The **middle meningeal artery**, a branch of the first part of the maxillary artery enters the skull through the **foramen spinosum**. It divides within the first

4 or 5 cm of its intracranial course into an anterior branch passing upward from the **pterion**, more or less parallel to the coronal suture of the skull (Fig. 7-15). The posterior branch passes backward and upward, its exact site depending on its point of origin. In the present case, the anterior branch of the middle meningeal artery was almost certainly torn. This artery is usually accompanied by a **meningeal vein** which may have also been torn.

The lucid interval which followed the patient's recovery from the brief loss of consciousness resulting from cerebral concussion occurs because of the slow formation (up to 12 hours) of the extradural hematoma. In addition, this kind of a space-occupying intracranial lesion can be tolerated for a short time because some blood and CSF are squeezed out of the cranium through the veins and the subarachnoid space. However, as the cranium is nonexpansile, the intracranial pressure soon rises, producing drowsiness and then **coma** (G. *koma,* deep sleep).

The increased intracranial pressure forces the supratentorial part of the brain, usually the uncus, through the **tentorial incisure** (Fig. 7-64), squeezing the oculomotor nerve (CN III) between the brain and the sharp, free edge of the tentorium. Compression of this nerve causes **third nerve palsy**, which results in a dilated, nonreacting pupil on the side of the lesion. An extradural hemorrhage in the characteristic position, illustrated by the present case, primarily causes **compression of the temporal lobe** underlying the pterion. Immediate surgical intervention is necessary to relieve the intracranial pressure so that further compression of the brain will not occur, which could cause death by interfering with the **cardiac and respiratory centers** in the medulla.

Case 7-6. Unruptured **saccular aneurysms** are usually asymptomatic. In the present case the initial headaches were probably caused by **intermittent enlargement of the aneurysm** or by slight bleeding from it (the so-called "**warning leak**"). Her subsequent severe, almost unbearable headache, was the result of gross bleeding from the aneurysm into the subarachnoid space. **Blood in the CSF** causes meningeal irritation which produces a headache. As the anterior communicating artery is in the longitudinal fissure, rostral to the optic chiasma (Fig. 7-90), blood escaping from the ruptured aneurysm would enter the **chiasmatic cistern** and other subarachnoid spaces around the brain and the spinal cord. This explains why there was blood in the CSF obtained by lumbar puncture.

Some authorities would recommend against a **lumbar puncture** in a case of subarachnoid hemorrhage that is so obvious as the present case because of the possibility of causing herniation of the brain. The lowering of CSF pressure in the spinal subarachnoid space by removing CSF might cause downward movement of the brain resulting in herniation (*e.g.,* of part of the *cerebellar tonsils* (Fig. 7-65).

Rupture of an aneurysm of the anterior communicating artery into the adjacent part of one frontal lobe may cause symptoms of a mass lesion in one hemisphere. In some cases, the **intracranial hematoma** may break into the ventricular system, causing an acute expansion of the ventricle and probably death.

Blockage of subarachnoid spaces by large amounts of blood in the CSF could impair circulation of this fluid, resulting in a further increase in intracranial pressure. This could force the medial part of the temporal lobe, usually the uncus, through the **tentorial notch** and the cerebellar tonsils through the foramen magnum. Herniation of the uncus leads to **third nerve palsy**, which is indicated by drooping of the upper eyelid (**ptosis**) and paralysis of pupillary constriction, resulting in a fixed dilated pupil. (*Fixed* means not reacting to light or accomodation). Herniation of the cerebellar tonsils compresses the medulla containing the vital respiratory and cardiovascular centers and produces a life-threatening situation. Surgical intervention would be required to lower this pressure (*e.g.,* ventricular drainage via a burr hole in the skull will sometimes reduce the intracranial pressure).

The **subhyaloid hemorrhages** observed during *funduscopy* resulted from the abrupt rise in intracranial pressure transmitted to the subarachnoid space around the optic nerve. This compressed and obstructed the central retinal vein where it crosses this space, resulting in increased pressure in the retinal capillaries and **hemorrhages between the retina and the vitreous body**. After centrifugation of the CSF, the supernatant fluid was yellow because it contained serum bilirubin and products of hemolized red blood cells.

Case 7-7. The **inferior alveolar nerve** supplies the lower molar and premolar teeth (Fig. 7-128) and then branches to form (1) an **incisive nerve** that supplies the canine and incisor teeth, and (2) a **mental nerve** that supplies the skin of the chin and the lower lip on that side. Hence, the **inferior alveolar nerve** supplies all teeth in one half of the mandible. Anesthetization of this nerve also anesthetizes the chin and lower lip because the mental nerve supplying these structures, as just stated, is a terminal branch of the inferior alveolar nerve.

As the **lingual nerve** descends just anterior to the inferior alveolar nerve near the mandibular foramen (Fig. 7-129), it was also anesthetized. This is advantageous because in addition to supplying the tongue, the lingual nerve also supplies sensory fibers to the mandibular gingiva.

Because of the relatively large amount of anesthetic solution that was injected, it must have spread into the parotid gland. Paralysis of the muscles of facial expression resulted from anesthetization of branches of the **facial nerve** (CN VII). As the parotid gland and these nerves occupy the space around the posterior margin of the ramus of the mandible, they could easily be affected as the anesthetic agent infiltrated the area. Probably the injection was made posteriorly so that the anesthetic solution passed through the **stylomandibular ligament**, a sheet of fascia condensed between the parotid and the submandibular glands which is continuous with the fascia covering the parotid gland. Like the anesthesia of the teeth and gums, these effects on the muscles of facial expression and of mastication would disappear in a few hours.

His ear lobule was numb because the intermediate branches of the **great auricular nerve** were also anesthetized. The anterior branches of this nerve supply skin on the posteroinferior part of the face and its intermediate branches supply the inferior part of the auricle on both surfaces.

Case 7-8. The **inferior alveolar nerve** appears to have been injured during extraction of the patient's tooth. It is a large trunk traversing the mandibular canal, close to the roots of the lower teeth. While in this canal it gives branches to the teeth (Fig. 7-129). In the region between the premolar teeth, the inferior alveolar nerve divides into a mental and an incisive branch. The **mental nerve** emerges at the mental foramen to supply the skin of one side of the chin and the mucous membrane on one side of the lower lip (Fig. 7-31).

The inferior alveolar nerve is a branch of the **mandibular nerve**, the lowest division of the trigeminal nerve (CN V). This division of the nerve (V^3) supplies all structures derived from the mandibular prominence of the embryonic first branchial arch.

As the inferior alveolar nerve passes close to the molar teeth (Figs. 7-129 and 7-130), and in some cases the anterior and posterior roots of the third molar develop around the inferior alveolar nerve, this nerve was probably injured during chipping away of the bone and/or by compression as fragments of the tooth were levered from the bone.

The woman's lawyer advised her not to sue the dentist for two reasons. First, the dentist had warned her before the operation that the nerve might be injured and second, this complication of this operation is well known and unavoidable; thus, there was no malpractice.

In most cases *regeneration of the inferior alveolar nerve occurs within 6 months*; hence, sensation should return to the lip if the nerve was merely crushed. If the nerve was severed and the cut ends were separated, restoration of sensory function is unlikely. Although peripheral nerve fibers regenerate, their chances of reinnervating the original structures are poor when the severed ends are separated or if scar tissue or bone intervenes. In the present case, the woman has altered sensation (**paresthesia**) in her right lower lip, 14 years after the operation. She takes special care to wipe her mouth during eating because she cannot be certain that particles of food are not left on that side of her lower lip.

SUGGESTIONS FOR ADDITIONAL READING

1. Barr, M. L. *The Human Nervous System: Anatomic Viewpoint,* Ed. 3, Harper & Row Publishers, Inc., Hagerstown, Maryland, 1979.

This textbook is recommended for obtaining the sound basis of neurological anatomy necessary for the interpretation of signs and symptoms of lesions in the head, particularly in the brain.

2. Carpenter, M. B. *Core Text of Neuroanatomy,* Ed. 2, The Williams & Wilkins Company, Baltimore, 1978

Another highly recommended textbook for 1st year students that presents a synthesis of basic concepts of neuroanatomy. Good attempts are made to correlate the structure and function of the nervous system and to demonstrate clinical applications of the structures concerned.

3. Hanaway, J. L., Scott, W. R., and Strother, C. M. *Atlas of the Human Brain and the Orbit for Computed Tomography,* Warren H. Green, Inc., St. Louis, 1977.

CT scans are commonly used for visualizing cross-sectional anatomy of the brain, the ventricular system, and the subarachnoid cisterns. This atlas shows cross-sections of the head with CT scans. It is recommended for persons learning computed tomography of the head for the first time. The quality of the illustrations is very good.

4. Lemire, R. R., Loeser, J. D., Leech, R. W., and Alvord, E. C. Jr., *Normal and Abnormal Development of the Human Nervous System,* Harper & Row, Inc., Hagerstown, Maryland 1975.

A comprehensive reference book on normal and abnormal development of the central nervous system, with particular emphasis on the brain. Most chapters begin with an analysis of normal development and end with a detailed consideration of abnormal development. The discussions will be of special interest to students aspiring to become pediatricians, neuroscientists, geneticists, and embryologists.

5. Moore, K. L. *The Developing Human. Clinically Oriented Embryology,* Ed. 2, W. B. Saunders Co., Philadelphia, 1977.

This text has a style similar to that used in the present book. Students wishing details of normal and abnormal development of the head briefly referred to in the present text should consult this book.

6. Norman, D., Korobkin, M., and Newton, T. D. (Eds.) *Computed Tomography,* The C. V. Mosby Company, St. Louis, 1977.

This compilation of current knowledge on CT scanning includes considerable practical information that will enable beginners to understand the physical foundations of this relatively new diagnostic technique. It illustrates clearly that CT scanning is an extremely useful diagnostic tool for the initial evaluation of patients with acute head trauma. Numerous demonstrations of the use of this technique in determining the presence or absence of neurological lesions are given.

7. Tavares, J. M., and Wood, E. H. *Diagnostic Neuroradiology.* Ed. 2, vols. 1 and 2, The Williams & Wilkins Company, Baltimore, 1976.

Skull films are routinely used for study of the skull and the brain. Various other techniques used in the radiological study of patients with neurological disorders and for systematically seeking an intracranial cause for a disturbance are described and fully discussed. Although written by and for neuroradiologists, it will give others an insight into this complex specialty.

8. Thorn, G. W., Adams, R. D., Braunwald, E., Isselbacher, K. J., and Petersdorf, R. G. In *Harrison's Principles of Internal Medicine,* Ed. 8, McGraw-Hill Company, New York, 1977.

This comprehensive book gives detailed accounts of most clinically oriented material mentioned in the present anatomy book. As medicine is an ever-changing science and actual clinical problems are usually more complex than those presented herein as examples of clinically oriented anatomy, you are urged to expand your knowledge about these problems by reading this and other clinical texts.

CHAPTER 8

The Cranial Nerves

The 12 pairs of cranial nerves are attached to the brain (Figs. 7-79, 8-1, and 8-7) and traverse openings in the skull (L. *cranium*) to enter the face and neck (Figs. 7-50, 7-52, and 7-54). The 12 pairs of cranial nerves, along with the 31 pairs of spinal nerves, comprise most of the **peripheral nervous system** (*PNS*); hence, *clinical examination of these nerves is essential for a complete study of the nervous system.*

The cranial nerves serve a variety of functions (Tables 8-1 and 8-2) concerned with the *specialized sense organs* of (1) **olfaction** (smell), (2) **vision,** (3) **gustation** (taste), (4) **audition** (hearing), and (5) **equilibrium** (balance), and the *specialized motor activities* of (1) **oculomotion** (eye movement), (2) **mastication** (chewing), (3) **deglutition** (swallowing), (4) **respiration,** (5) **vocalization** (speaking), and (6) **facial expression.**

The cranial nerves are named and numbered in a craniocaudal sequence as follows (Fig. 8-1 and Tables 8-1 and 8-2): *The Olfactory Nerve* (**CN I**), *The Optic Nerve* (**CN II**), *The Oculomotor Nerve* (**CN III**), *The Trochlear Nerve* (**CN IV**), *The Trigeminal Nerve* (**CN V**), *The Abducens Nerve* (**CN VI**), The *Facial Nerve* (**CN VII**), *The Vestibulocochlear Nerve* (**CN VIII**), *The Glossopharyngeal Nerve* (**CN IX**), *The Vagus Nerve* (**CN X**), *The Accessory Nerve* (**CN XI**), and *The Hypoglossal Nerve* (**CN XII**). The name and/or the number may be used. The cranial nerves have also been described in other parts of this book (Chaps. 1 to 3, 7, and 9). The purpose of the present chapter is to consider them as a group.

The cranial nerves provide input to the brain from (1) the **special sense organs** of *smell* (CN I), *sight* (CN II), *hearing and balance* (CN VIII), and *taste* (CN VII, CN IX, and CN X); and (2) the **general sensory receptors** for *pain and temperature, simple* and *fine touch, pressure, position sense,* and *vibration* (CN V, CN VII, CN IX, and CN X).

The cranial nerves convey the output of the brain to the voluntary muscles concerned with movements of the head, eyes, mouth, face, tongue, pharynx, and larynx. *The cranial nerves are also the major outlet for the parasympathetic nervous system,* which is concerned with conservation and restoration of the body's energy resources (*e.g.*, it decreases the rate and force of the heart beat).

The motor or efferent fibers of the cranial nerves *arise within the brain* from aggregations of neurons (nerve cells) called **motor nuclei.** *The motor nuclei of cranial nerves lie in the brain stem* (midbrain, pons, and medulla, Fig. 8-20) and are acted upon by nerve impulses from many sources (*e.g.*, the **cerebral cortex** and the **sense organs**). The nerve fibers **(axons)** of motor neurons in the cranial nerve nuclei leave the brain in the cranial nerves and pass to (1) **striated muscles** (*e.g.*, via CN XII to the muscles of the tongue, Fig. 8-23) and (2) **autonomic ganglia** where they synapse with cells that relay impulses to smooth muscle, the heart, and glands (Fig. I-63).

The sensory or afferent fibers of cranial nerves *arise from neurons outside the brain.* These nerve cells may be aggregated into groups called **cranial sensory ganglia** on the trunks of the cranial nerves (*e.g.*, the *trigeminal ganglion*, Fig. 7-55), or they may be located in **peripheral sense organs** (*e.g.*, the nose, eye, and internal ear). *The central processes of the sensory cells enter the brain* and terminate by synapsing with groups of neurons called **sen-**

Table 8-1
Summary of the Cranial Nerves

No.	Name	Special Sense	Sensory	Motor	Parasympathetic
CN I	Olfactory	*			
CN II	Optic	*			
CN III	Oculomotor			*	*
CN IV	Trochlear			*	
CN V	Trigeminal		*	*	
CN VI	Abducent			*	
CN VII	Facial	*	*	*	*
CN VIII	Vestibulocochlear	*			
CN IX	Glossopharyngeal	*	*	*	*
CN X	Vagus	*	*	*	*
CN XI	Accessory			*	
CN XII	Hypoglossal			*	

Note that four sensory modalities may be carried by the cranial nerves and that three nerves carry special sense only (CN I, CN II, CN VIII) and have no motor component. Note also that four nerves (CN III, CN VII, CN IX, and CN X) carry parasympathetic fibers to smooth muscles and glands.

sory nuclei (*e.g.*, the *spinal nucleus of CN V*, Fig. 8-20).

Myelination of Cranial Nerve Fibers. All the nerve fibers of the cranial nerves, except CN I, and most of the fibers in the **central nervous system (CNS)** acquire specialized sheaths. The primary sheaths of the peripheral fibers are formed by **Schwann cells** which extend along the fibers and wrap themselves around the axons as they grow peripherally during development. This forms the **neurolemma** (neurilemma), a delicate sheath of **neurolemma cells** (Schwann cells). For details of this process, see an embryology, neuroanatomy, or histology text.

The myelin sheaths surrounding the nerve fibers of cranial nerves within the brain have a different origin. They are formed by *neuroglial cells* called **oligodendrocytes** in the same manner as the Schwann cells in the peripheral parts of the nerves.

The development of the myelin sheath of cranial nerve fibers, a process called **myelination**, begins in some cases about 14 weeks after fertilization; however, myelination does not begin in the sensory part of CN V or in the cochlear division of CN VIII until about 22 weeks. *Myelination of the optic nerves (CN II) does not begin until just before birth* and is not completed until about 2 weeks thereafter. *In general, myelination begins first in those fibers that function earliest* and there is evidence that fibers become completely myelinated at about the time they begin to function fully.

CLINICALLY ORIENTED COMMENTS

Accurate localization of lesions affecting the various cranial nerves requires a combination of skill in neurological examination and a sound knowledge of the anatomy of the brain stem and the cranial nerves that emerge from it. To localize lesions within the brain stem, neurologists and neurosurgeons must know precisely where the cranial nerve nuclei are located and must be familiar with the course of the intramedullary portions of the cranial nerves. Knowledge of the peripheral distribution of the cranial nerves discussed in this chapter is also essential for diagnosing certain neurological conditions.

THE OLFACTORY NERVE (CN I)

The olfactory nerve is a special sensory nerve which is *attached to the telencephalon* (G. end brain), the anterior part of the brain from which the **cerebral hemispheres** develop (Figs. 7-79 and 8-1 to 8-

Table 8-2
An Overview of the 12 Cranial Nerves

Nerve	Efferent		Afferent		Special Senses
	Striated muscles	Smooth and cardiac muscles and glands	Skin	Mucous membranes and organs	
CN I					Smell (Fig. 8-3)
CN II					Sight (Fig. 8-8)
CN III	Supplies all muscles of eyeball except sup. oblique and lat. rectus (Fig. 8-10)	Muscles of lens and iris of eye		Proprioceptive fibers from eye muscles	
CN IV	Sup. oblique muscle of eyeball (Fig. 8-10)			Proprioceptive fibers from eye muscles	
CN V	Muscles of mastication and tensors of tympanum and palate (Fig. 8-11)	Carries parasympathetic ganglia for preganglionic nerve fibers of CN III, CN VII, and CN IX	Face and front of scalp	Teeth and mucous membranes of tongue, mouth, nose, and eye	Taste (fibers from chorda tympani) to ant. two-thirds of tongue
CN VI	Lat. rectus muscle of eyeball (Fig. 8-10)			Proprioceptive fibers from lat. rectus muscle	
CN VII	Muscles of facial expression (Fig. 8-15)	Nervus intermedius, glands of mouth, nose, and palate; lacrimal gland; submandibular and sublingual glands (see CN V)	External ear		Nervus intermedius, taste, ant. two-thirds of tongue
CN VIII					Hearing and equilibrium (Fig. 8-17)
CN IX	Stylopharyngeus muscle (Fig. 8-18)	Parotid gland (see CN V)		Eardrum, middle ear, pharynx, and tongue (post. one-third)	Taste, post. one-third of tongue
CN X	Muscles of pharynx (Fig. 8-19)	Organs in neck, thorax, and abdomen	Ext. acoustic meatus and eardrum	Organs in neck, thorax, and abdomen	Taste, epiglottis
CN XI	Soft palate, pharynx, and larynx; sternocleidomastoid and trapezius muscles (Fig. 8-22)				
CN XII	Extrinsic and intrinsic muscles of tongue (Fig. 8-23)				

4). Strictly speaking, the olfactory nerve, **serving the sense of smell**, does not arise from the brain; it arises from an appendage of the brain called the **olfactory bulb** (Figs. 8-1 to 8-4). The functional cells concerned with olfaction (L. *olfacere*, to smell) are called **olfactory cells** and are located in the *olfactory mucosa of the nose* (Figs.

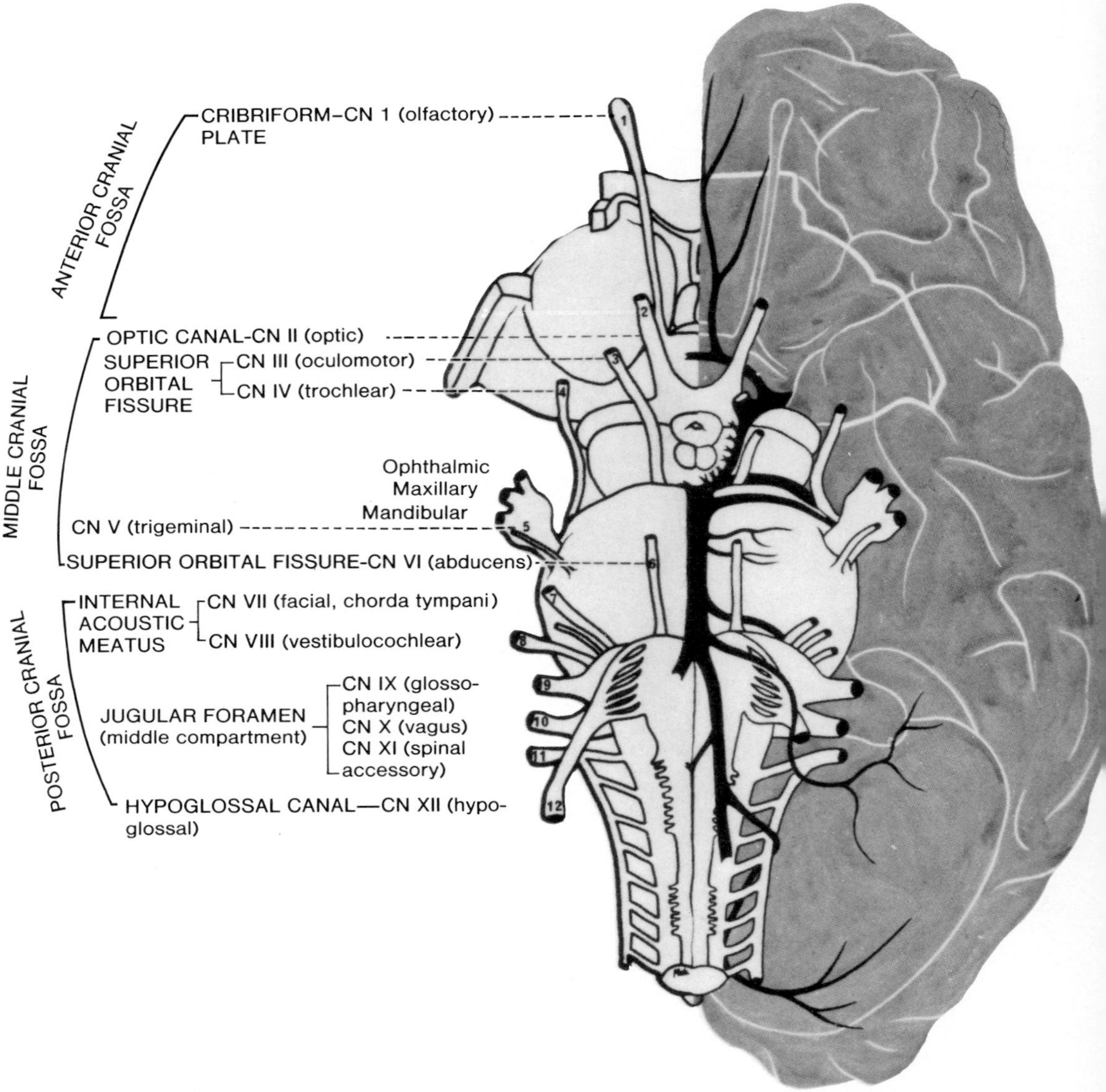

Figure 8-1. Diagram showing the cranial nerves leaving the base of the brain. CN I and CN II are not true cranial nerves but fiber tracts of the brain. Except for the spinal part of CN XI, which is derived from the upper cervical segments of the spinal cord, the caudal 10 cranial nerves emerge from the brain stem (midbrain, pons, and medulla) in which lie their nuclei of origin (see Fig. 8-20).

8-2 and 8-3). This region comprises the superior nasal concha and the opposed portion of the nasal septum (Figs. 7-167 and 7-168). *The olfactory cell is a primitive type of sensory receptor.* Its dendrite extends to the surface of the olfactory epithelium and ends as an exposed bulbous enlargement which has cilia up to 100 μ in length. Hence, the **odoriferous substance** has direct access to the neuron without the intervention of nonnervous tissue. It has been estimated that there are about 25 million olfactory cells in each half of the olfactory mucosa of young adults.

The olfactory cells are bipolar neurons which are modified to serve as sensory

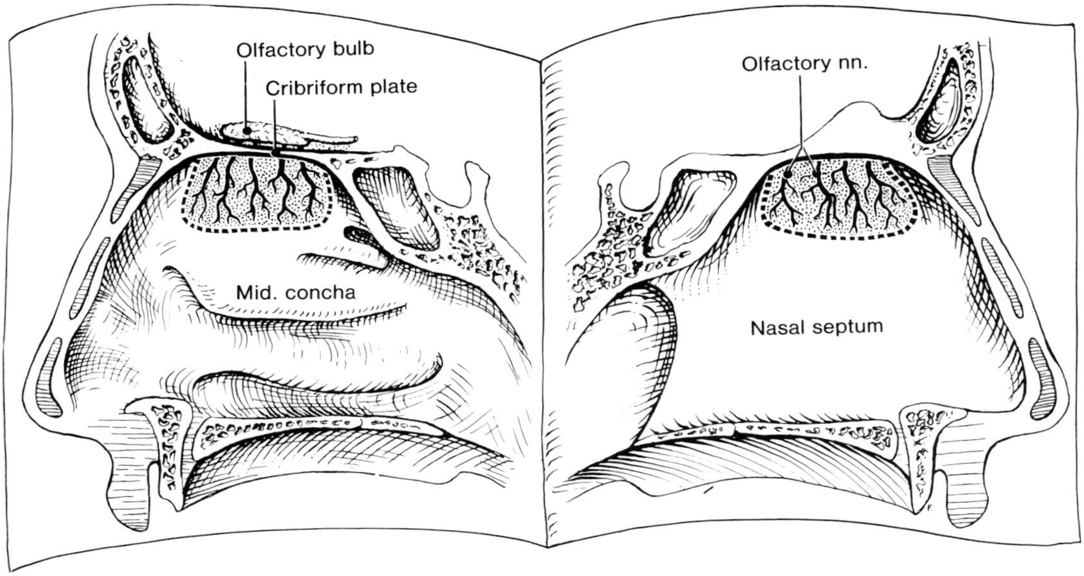

Figure 8-2. Drawings illustrating the scheme of distribution of the *olfactory nerve* (CN I). The olfactory area is usually much smaller than that shown here (see Fig. 1-15) and it is irregular in outline owing to the streamer-like invasion by nonolfactory, ciliated, columnar epithelium. The decrease in size is believed to result mainly from the destruction of the sensory olfactory neurons in the course of recurring infections of the nasal mucosa. A study of the olfactory nerves in 143 adults revealed that: (1) only 12% had a full complement of olfactory nerve fibers, (2) 8% had lost all fibers on one side, and (3) 5% had lost all fibers on both sides. There is considerable variation in the number of olfactory nerve fibers in individuals of a given age, but on the average there is a loss of about 1% of fibers per year during postnatal life, *i.e.*, at the age of 50 years the average person has lost 50% of fibers and at the age of 75 years, 75% of fibers.

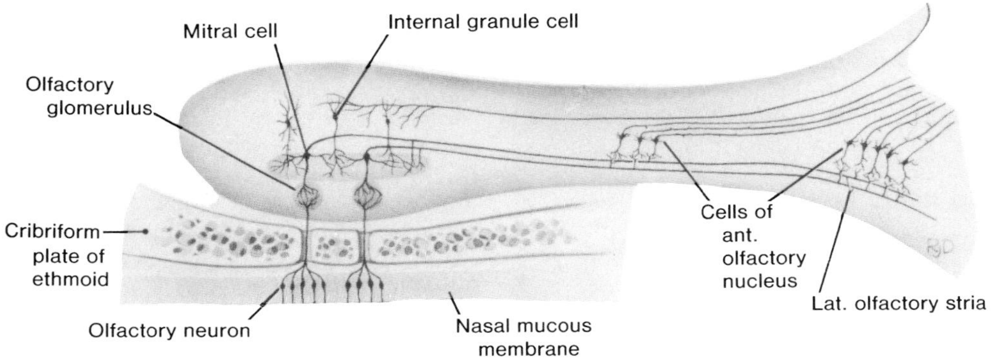

Figure 8-3. Diagram of the olfactory bulb and tract showing the relationship of the olfactory receptors and neurons in the nasal mucosa with cells in the olfactory bulb. The processes of olfactory neurons are located in the nasal mucous membrane and are in contact with the odor-producing chemicals in the inhaled air.

receptors and as conducting neurons. The axons of the olfactory cells constituting the olfactory nerves are collected into 18 to 20 bundles which pass through the foramina in the **cribriform plates** of the ethmoid bone in the anterior cranial fossa (Figs. 7-50 and 8-1, to 8-3). *The olfactory nerves are unmyelinated* and, after traversing the cribriform plates, they **pierce the dura mater and arachnoid** lining the inside of the

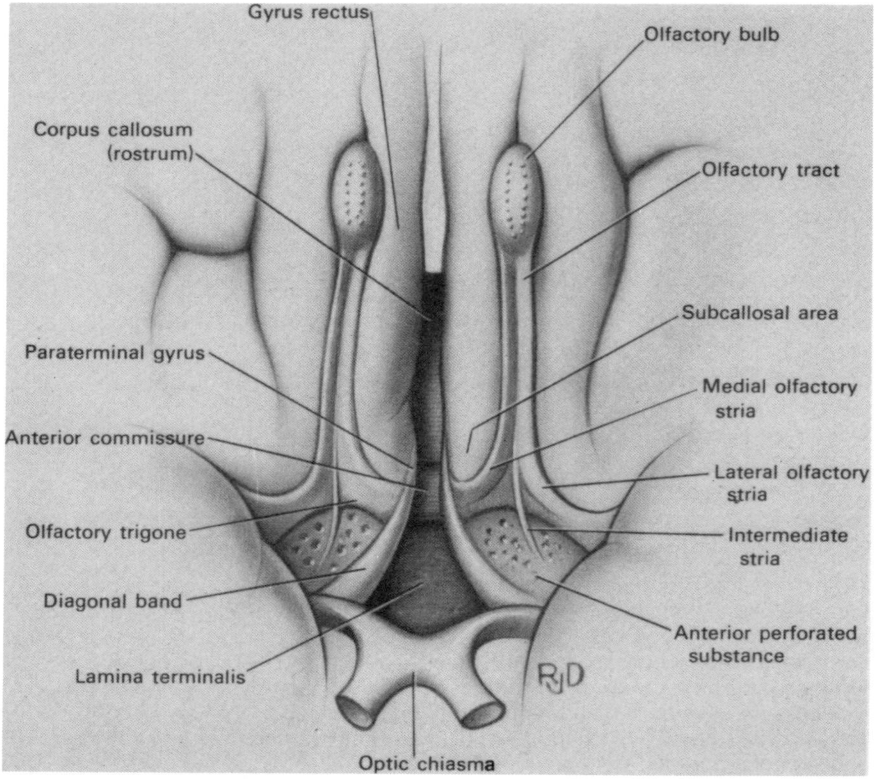

Figure 8-4. Diagram of the olfactory structures on the inferior surface of the brain (also see Fig. 7-79). The optic nerves and the optic chiasma have been retracted caudally to expose the olfactory area.

skull. Surrounded by a thin tube of pia mater, they cross the **subarachnoid space** containing cerebrospinal fluid (**CSF**) and enter the inferior aspects of the olfactory bulbs (Fig. 8-3).

In the *anterior cranial fossa*, the axons of the olfactory cells enter the olfactory bulb (Figs. 8-1 to 8-4), which lies above the cribriform plate. From the olfactory bulb the slender **olfactory tract** runs posteriorly to attach to the brain in front of the *anterior perforated substance* (Figs. 7-79 and 8-4). For details of the architecture and the central connections of the olfactory bulb, see a neuroanatomy text.

CLINICALLY ORIENTED COMMENTS

Unlike many mammals, we do not rely heavily on the *primitive sense of smell* for information about our environment. However, we are able to detect certain noxious substances and our sense of smell adds much to our enjoyment of food, wine, and each other (thanks to lotions and perfumes). *Even the newborn infant reacts to certain obnoxious smells by grimacing.* **Anosmia** (loss of sense of smell) is not, however, a serious handicap and occurs gradually with age at the rate of about 1% per year in most people (Fig. 8-2).

Disorders of olfaction (sense of smell) may result from conditions affecting (1) the *primary olfactory neurons* in the nasal mucous membrane, (2) the *secondary olfactory neurons* in the olfactory bulb and tract, or (3) their intracranial connections (Figs. 8-2 to 8-4). **Olfactory disorders may be caused by**: (1) *lesions of the nasal cavity*, *e.g.*, owing to inflammation; (2) *fractures of the anterior cranial fossa* (Fig. 7-50); (3) *tumors of adjacent parts of the brain*; (4)

meningitis (see Chap. 7); (5) *arteriosclerosis*; (6) certain *drug intoxications*; and (7) *cerebrovascular accidents* (*e.g.*, an effusion of blood into the base of the frontal lobe).

Unilateral anosmia may be of diagnostic significance in localizing brain lesions (*e.g., a tumor at the base of the frontal lobe*). Before **testing the olfactory nerves**, it must be determined that there is no obstruction of the nasal passages. With the eyes closed, the patient is asked to identify familiar odors (*e.g.*, coffee, wintergreen, and camphor). *Comparisons between the two sides are important*; thus, each nostril is tested separately by occluding the other one. **Unilateral brain lesions** do not usually result in a loss of the sense of smell unless both olfactory tracts are injured. Lesions of one olfactory tract produce **unilateral anosmia.** *Tumors of the inferior surface of the frontal lobe and trauma to the forehead are the common causes of neurogenic anosmia.*

Fractures of the cribriform plate of the ethmoid bone may tear olfactory nerve fibers and the meninges, resulting in the *discharge of CSF from the nose* (**CSF rhinorrhea**). For discussion of this condition, see the Clinically Oriented Comments on the nose (p. 1026).

THE OPTIC NERVE (CN II)

The optic nerve is a special sensory nerve but it is not a true nerve. *It is a fiber tract of the brain because developmentally the retina is a part of the brain.* The **optic nerve** extends from the retina of the eye (Figs. 7-96*A*, 7-101, and 8-5) and enters the cranial cavity through the *optic canal* (optic foramen) (Fig. 7-53), where it unites with its partner to form the **optic chiasma** (chiasm) (Figs. 7-79 and 8-4). Each nerve is composed of about one million axons of ganglion cells lying near the surface of the retina (Fig. 8-6).

The intraorbital part of the optic nerve is about 25 mm long and its intracranial part is about 10 mm long. *The optic nerve is enclosed by three sheaths which are continuous with the meninges* of the brain (Fig. 8-7). These sheaths extend as far as the back of the eyeball (Fig. 7-96*A*).

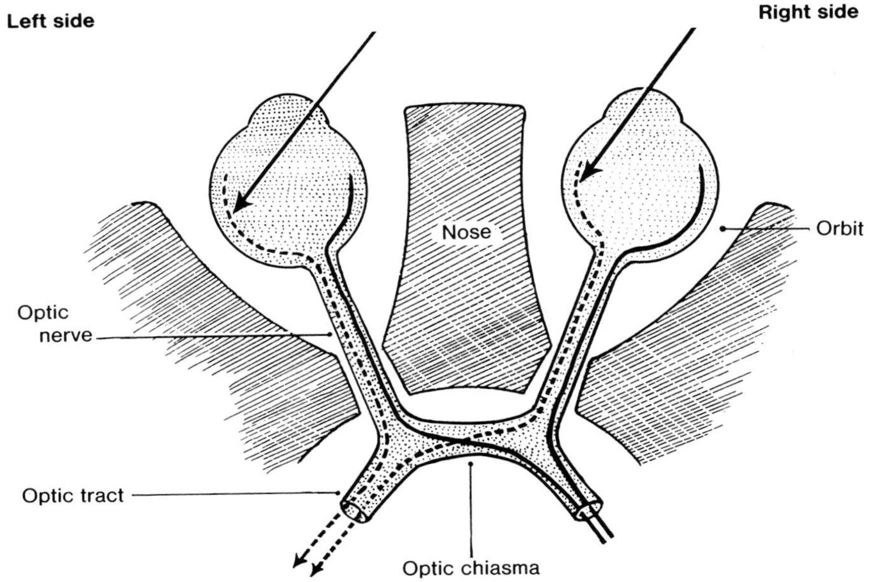

Figure 8-5. Scheme of distribution of the *optic nerves* (CN II). Rays of light from the right half of the visual field impinge on the left half of each retina and impulses set up there travel along nerve fibers that pass to the left optic tract. Similarly, rays of light from the left half of the visual field set up impulses that reach the right optic tract. Thus, the nerve fibers from the nasal half of each retina are the ones that cross in the optic chiasma; those from the temporal half of each retina remain uncrossed.

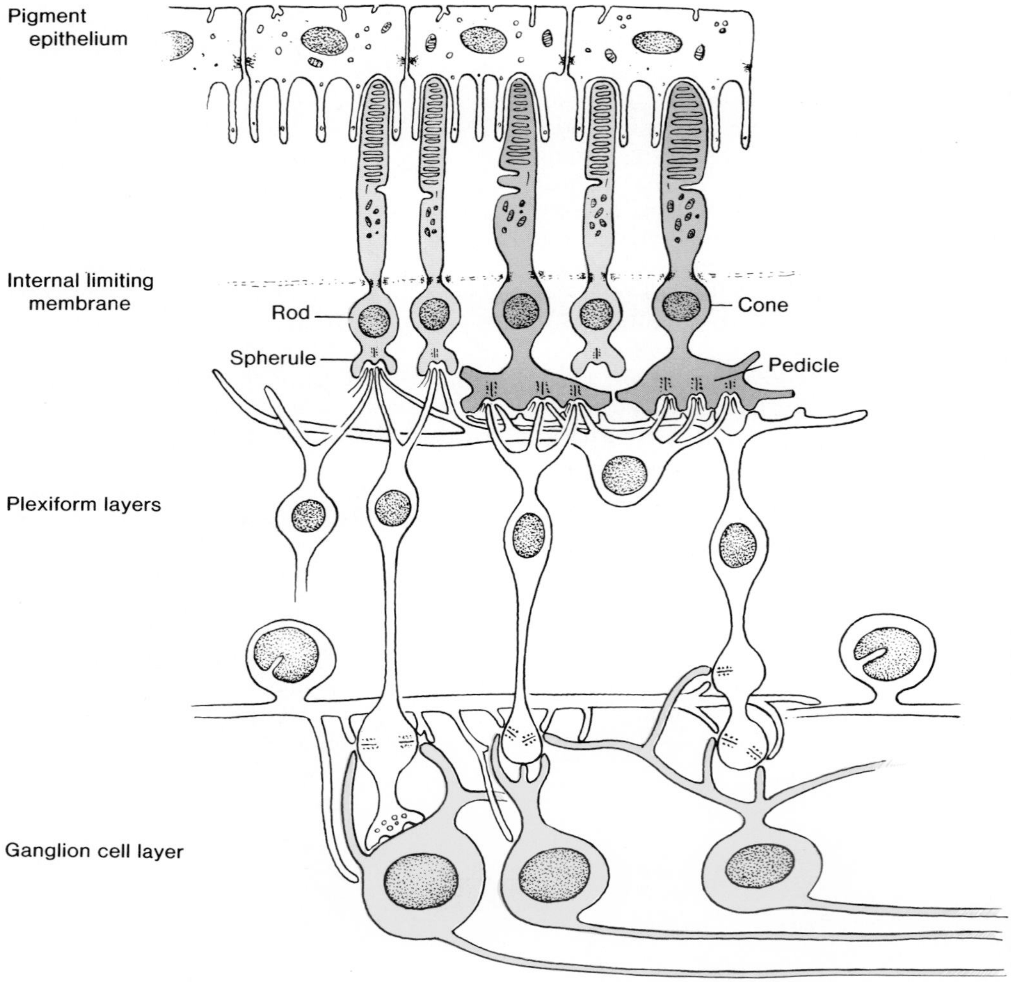

Figure 8-6. Schematic diagram of the ultrastructural organization of the retina. The rods are *blue* and the cones are *red.* The rods and cones of the retina react specifically to physical light. The cones are stimulated by relatively high intensity light and are responsible for sharp vision and color discrimination, whereas the more numerous rods react to low intensity light and function during twilight and in night vision.

The *thick outer sheath* is continuous with the **dura mater** of the brain and with the *sclera* of the eye (Figs. 7-101 and 7-113). The *thin intermediate sheath* is continuous with the **arachnoid** of the brain and is separated from the outer sheath by the **subdural space** and from the inner sheath by the **subarachnoid space** (Fig. 7-96*A*). The *vascular inner sheath* is continuous with the **pia mater** of the brain and closely invests the optic nerve. *The inner sheath (pial layer) sends connective tissue partitions and blood vessels into the nerve.*

The *central artery and vein of the retina pierce the dural and arachnoid coverings of the optic nerve about 1 cm behind the eyeball and, after a short course in the* **subarachnoid space**, *penetrate the optic nerve* and run within it to the inner aspect of the retina (Fig. 7-101). The investment

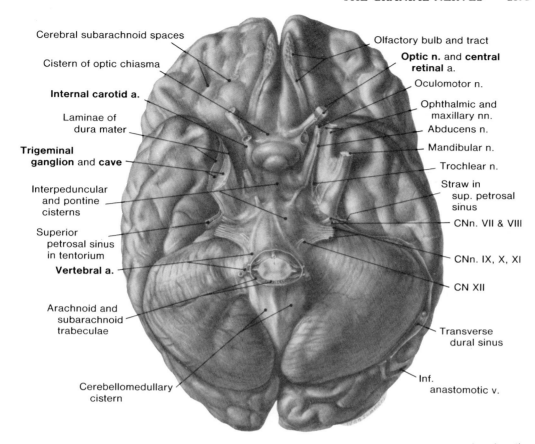

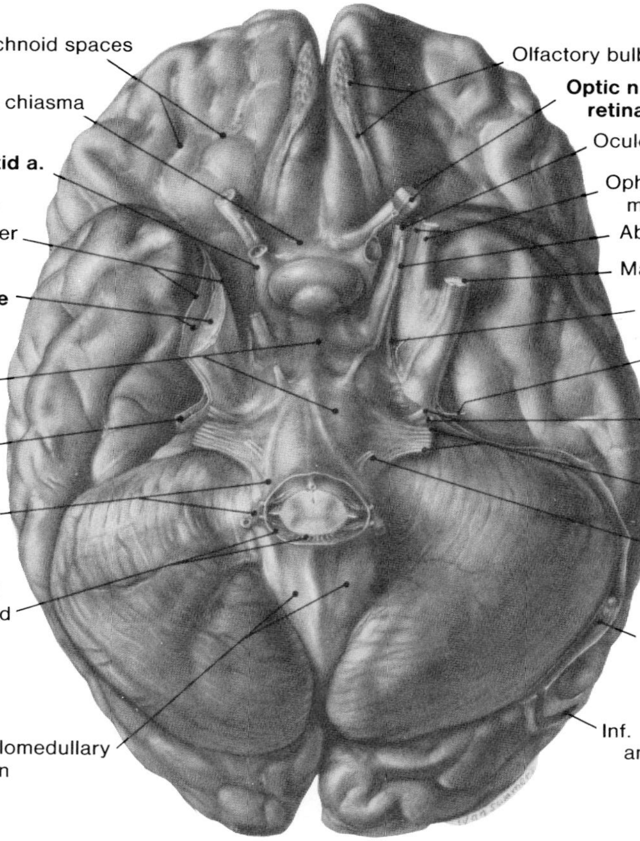

Figure 8-7. Drawing of an inferior view of the brain, cranial nerves, and meninges showing the location of the subarachnoid cisterns containing cerebrospinal fluid (CSF). For another view of these cisterns and a full discussion of CSF, see Figure 7-82 and Chapter 7.

from the pial or inner sheath of the optic nerve is carried on the central vessels of the retina as far as the **optic disc**.

Posterior to the optic chiasma, the optic nerves are continued as the **optic tracts** (Figs. 8-5 and 8-8) which pass to the *lateral geniculate bodies* and the *superior colliculi* (Fig. 7-55). Within the **optic chiasma** there is a *partial decussation of the optic nerve fibers.* Fibers from the nasal half of each retina cross to the opposite side (Fig. 8-8), whereas those from the temporal half of each retina are uncrossed. Thus, *fibers from the right half of the retina of both eyes form the right optic tract and those from the left halves form the left tract.* This crossing of nerve fibers results in the right optic tract conveying impulses from the left visual field and vice versa. The central connections of the optic nerve are indicated in Figure 8-8; for details consult a neuroanatomy text.

CLINICALLY ORIENTED COMMENTS

Because the retinal vessels are included in the anterior part of the optic nerve, an *increase in the pressure of CSF* around the nerve interferes with the return of venous blood. As a result, swelling or *edema of the optic disc* (**papilledema**) occurs (see Chap. 7). This is an important clinical sign of

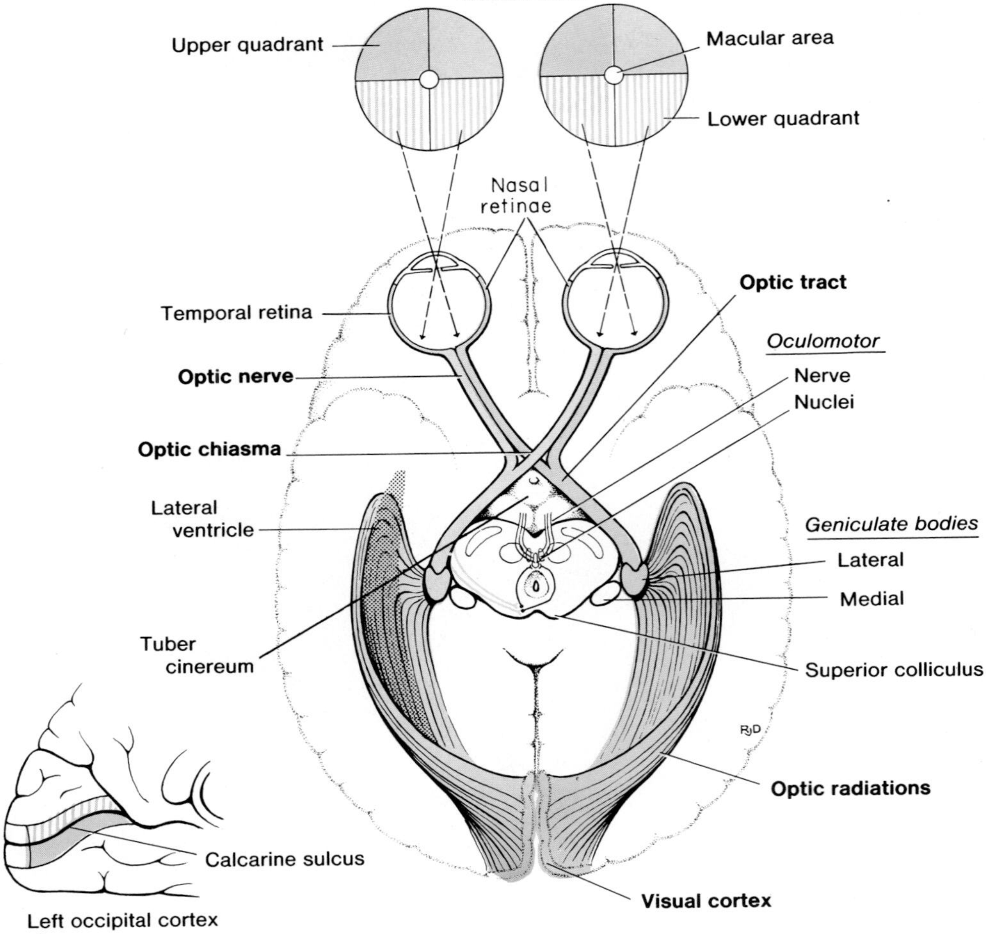

Figure 8-8. Diagram of the visual pathways viewed from the ventral surface of the brain. Understand that: (1) light from the superior half of the visual field falls on the inferior half of the retina; (2) light from the temporal half of the visual field falls on the nasal half of the retina; and (3) light from the nasal half of the visual field falls on the temporal half of the retina. The visual pathways from the retina to the visual cortex are shown; the plane of the visual fields has been rotated 90° toward you. The inset (*lower left*) shows the projection of the quadrants of the visual field upon the left calcarine or visual cortex. The macular area of the retina (Fig. 7-101) is represented nearest the occipital pole. Fibers mediating the light reflex leave the optic tract and project to the pretectal region; other fibers relay impulses indirectly to the visceral nuclei of the oculomotor complex (Fig. 8-20).

increase in intracranial pressure (*e.g.*, owing to a brain tumor, abscess, hemorrhage, hypertension, etc).

Inflammation of the meninges (**meningitis**) may involve the eyes because the sheaths of the optic nerves are continuous with those of the brain and the spaces between these sheaths communicate with the **subdural** and **subarachnoid spaces** (Figs. 7-96*A* and 7-101).

Injury to any part of the optic pathway results in visual defects, the nature of which depends on the location and extent of the injury (Fig. 8-9). **Severe degenerative disease** or a complete lesion of the optic nerve (*e.g.*, sectioning) causes **total**

blindness in the corresponding eye (Fig. 8-9*A*). *A lesion at the lateral border of the optic chiasma* results in nasal hemianopia or **nasal hemianopsia** (G. *hemi*, half + *an*, no + *opsis*, vision), *i.e.*, *loss of the nasal half of the visual field* of the eye on the same side as the lesion. A localized dilation or **aneurysm of the internal carotid artery** above the cavernous sinus could exert this kind of *pressure on the lateral border of the optic chiasma* and cause nasal hemianopsia (Fig. 7-55 and Case 8-4).

Interruption of an optic tract results in **homonymous hemianopsia** (Fig. 8-9*C*). Visual defects are described as *homonymous* when they are restricted to the same part of the visual field of each eye. *Complete interruption of decussating fibers in the optic chiasma* (*e.g.*, **chiasmal lesions** such as pituitary tumors) causes *bitemporal hemianopsia* or loss of the temporal half of the visual field of each eye (Fig. 8-9*D* and Case 8-5).

The optic nerve is peculiarly liable to neuritis (inflammation of a nerve). **Optic neuritis** results in **atrophy** (wasting of a nerve). *Retrobulbar neuritis* involving the optic nerve or tract is commonly caused by multiple sclerosis (*MS*). **Optic atrophy** results in *diminished visual acuity or blindness.* Primary (simple) optic atrophy is caused by processes that involve the optic nerve such as adjacent tumors.

THE OCULOMOTOR NERVE (CN III)

The oculomotor nerve is the somatic motor nerve *to four of the six muscles that move the eye* (Fig. 8-10) and to the muscle that raises the eyelid (*levator palpebrae superioris*, Figs. 7-31, 7-98, and 8-10). The oculomotor nerve was named because it *supplies most of the muscles that move the eye* (L. *oculus*, eye + *motor*, mover). It also contains parasympathetic fibers to the involuntary muscles that con-

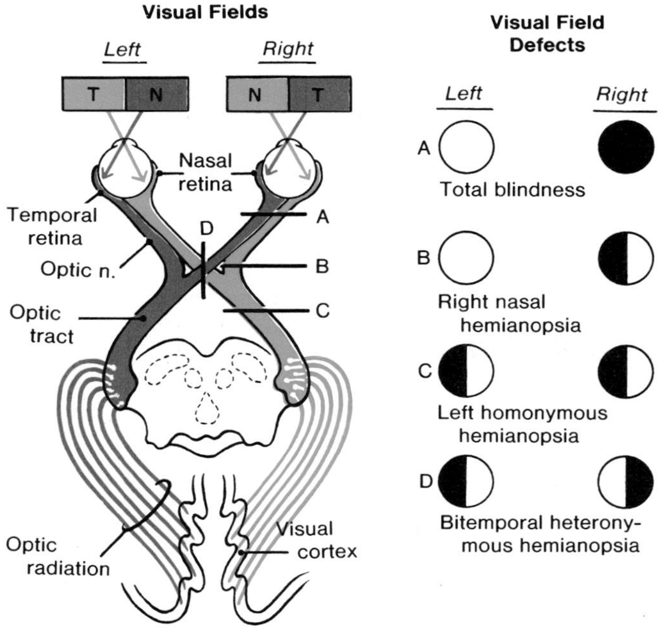

Figure 8-9. Diagrams showing the visual field defects caused by lesions affecting different parts of the visual pathway. *A* to *D* indicate lesions at various sites. The resulting visual field defects are shown on the right (*circles*). Loss of vision in half of the visual field of one eye is called hemianopsia (*B*). Loss of vision in the corresponding halves of both visual fields is called *homonymous hemianopsia* (*C*) and is further designated whether it is right or left. Loss of vision in the opposite halves of the opposite visual fields is called heteronymous hemianopsia (*D*).

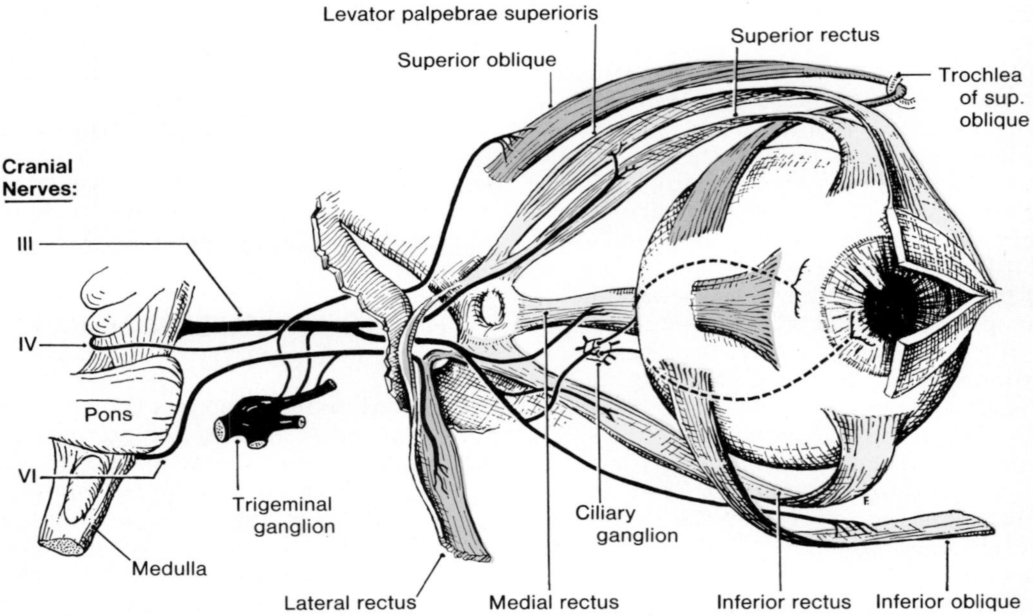

Figure 8-10. Scheme of distribution of the *oculomotor* (CN III), *trochlear* (CN IV), and *abducens* (CN VI) nerves. These three motor nerves, after receiving proprioceptive fibers from the trigeminal nerve (CN V), supply the orbital muscles. CN IV and CN VI each supply one muscle and CN III supplies the remaining five muscles. The trochlear nerve supplies the superior oblique, the muscle that passes through a trochlea or pulley (hence, its name); the abducens nerve supplies the lateral rectus, the muscle that abducts; and the oculomotor nerve supplies the levator palpebrae superioris, superior rectus, medial rectus, inferior rectus, and inferior oblique muscles. Via the ciliary ganglion, CN III supplies the ciliary muscle and the sphincter pupillae. Sympathetic fibers (not shown) from segments T1 and T2 pass via the superior cervical sympathetic ganglion on the walls of the carotid and ophthalmic arteries to supply the dilator pupillae and also involuntary muscle fibers in the upper and the lower eyelids.

strict the pupil of the eye and change the curvature of the lens (**accommodation**) for near vision.

The nucleus of the oculomotor nerve is a cylindrical cluster of cells that *lies in the midbrain* close to midline (Figs. 8-8 and 8-20). Its cells form five groups, one for each muscle it supplies. The oculomotor nucleus includes a *parasympathetic component*, the **Edinger-Westphal nucleus** (Fig. 8-20) for the *sphincter pupillae* and the *ciliary muscles* of the eye (see Chap. 7).

The oculomotor nerves emerge from the midbrain between the cerebral peduncles (Figs. 7-78, 7-79, 7-88, 8-1, 8-7, and 8-8) as a series of roots at the lateral borders of the **interpeduncular fossa.** These roots converge to form the nerves which pass *between the posterior cerebral and the superior cerebellar arteries* (Fig. 7-90*B*). They run forward in the **interpeduncular cistern** (Fig. 8-7) of the subarachnoid space on the *lateral sides of the posterior communicating arteries* (Fig. 7-90*B*). CN III pierces the dura mater lateral to the *posterior clinoid process* (Fig. 7-88) and comes to lie in the lateral wall of the **cavernous sinus** (Figs. 7-73 and 7-87). It then divides into a small superior and a large inferior division which traverse the superior orbital fissure (Fig. 7-87). The **superior division** of CN III supplies the *superior rectus* muscle and the *levator palpebrae superioris*; the **inferior division** supplies the *medial rectus*, *inferior rectus*, and *inferior oblique* muscles (Fig. 8-10).

CLINICALLY ORIENTED COMMENTS

CN III is tested with the other nerves (CN IV and CN VI) supplying the muscles for eye movement. **With involvement of CN III, the patient is unable to look up, down, or medially with the affected eye.** As CN III also supplies the muscles which constrict the pupil and the one that elevates the eyelid, *complete paralysis of CN III also results in dilation of the pupil* (owing to paralysis of the sphincter pupillae) and **ptosis** (drooping of the eyelid owing to paralysis of the levator palpebrae superioris, Figs. 7-98 and 8-26 and Case 8-6).

When all branches of the nerve are involved, it is probable that the lesion affects the peripheral course of the nerve. When only one ocular muscle is paralyzed, the lesion is probably in one of the several nuclei of the nerve (Figs. 8-8 and 8-20). *The most common causes of third nerve palsy are*: (1) **aneurysms** of the posterior communicating artery and/or the junction of the internal carotid and the posterior communicating artery (Fig. 7-90*A*); (2) **tumors** and *inflammatory lesions* in the region of the sella turcica (Fig. 7-50); and (3) pressure from **herniation of the uncus** (Fig. 7-79). See discussion of Case 7-6.

THE TROCHLEAR NERVE (CN IV)

The trochlear nerve is a motor nerve which supplies the *superior oblique muscle* of the eye (Fig. 8-10). It was named because of the **trochlea** (L. pulley) or *cartilaginous sling* through which its tendon passes on its way to its insertion into the posterolateral aspect of the sclera of the eyeball (Fig. 7-108).

The nucleus of the trochlear nerve is a small cluster of neurons (Fig. 8-20) near the floor of the **cerebral aqueduct** *at the level of the inferior colliculus* (Fig. 7-55). The nerve fibers of this nucleus have a very unusual course. They curve dorsally and caudally to cross the midline; hence, *each trochlear nerve has its nucleus on the opposite side of the brain.* After decussating, the fibers emerge as the trochlear nerves just inferior to the **inferior colliculi** (Fig. 7-55). *The trochlear nerves are the only motor nerves that arise from the dorsal aspect of the brain.* Because of its peculiar course, CN IV is very long and slender. It passes laterally and forward around the **cerebral peduncle** (Fig. 7-79), *between the posterior cerebral and the superior cerebellar arteries* (Fig. 7-90*B*). CN IV then runs in the subarachnoid space below the free edge of the **tentorium cerebelli** (Fig. 7-61) where it pierces the dura mater, just posterolateral to CN III (Figs. 7-64, 7-78, and 8-7). *Each trochlear nerve passes forward in the lateral wall of the cavernous sinus* (Figs. 7-73 and 7-87). Near the front of this sinus, CN IV crosses the oculomotor nerve (Fig. 7-55) and enters the orbit through the **superior orbital fissure** (Figs. 7-87 and 8-10). It then lies superior to the levator palpebrae superioris muscle and here enters the superior aspect of the superior oblique muscle (Fig. 8-10).

CLINICALLY ORIENTED COMMENTS

When the trochlear nerve is injured, the superior oblique muscle of the eye is paralyzed. The patient is *unable to look downward and inward* and when he/she attempts to do this, there is **diplopia** (double vision). Visual defects resulting from trochlear nerve injury may be difficult to detect, but patients frequently complain of *difficulty walking downstairs.*

THE TRIGEMINAL NERVE (CN V)

CN V is the principal sensory nerve for the head and is the motor nerve for the muscles of mastication. *The trigeminal nerve is the largest of the cranial nerves* and is the **sensory nerve** from the *face, teeth, mouth, nasal cavity,* and *paranasal sinuses* and from a large part of the *scalp* (Figs. 7-30 and 8-11). It also contributes sensory fibers to most of the *dura*

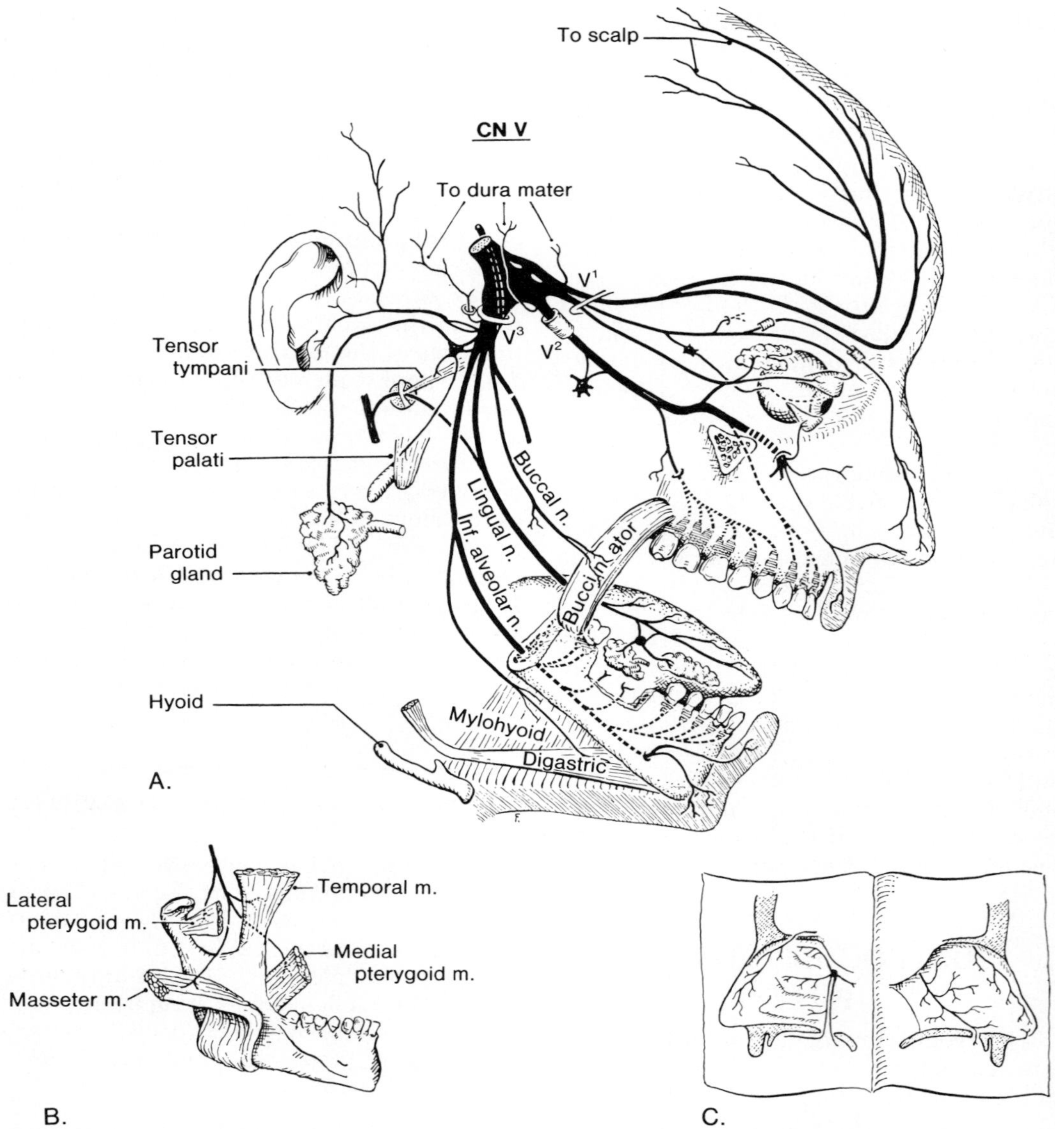

Figure 8-11. Drawings illustrating the scheme of distribution of the *trigeminal nerve* (CN V). In *A* observe its three divisions (V^1, V^2, and V^3). See Figure 7-30 for the cutaneous distribution of these nerves. Each division supplies not only the skin surface but the whole thickness of tissue from the skin surface to the mucous surface. Each of the divisions also sends a twig to the dura mater—V^1 to the tentorium cerebelli; V^2 and V^3 to the floor and side wall of the middle cranial fossa (see Fig. 7-68). Each of the three divisions is connected with a parasympathetic ganglion: V^1 with the ciliary, V^2 with the pterygopalatine, and V^3 with the submandibular and otic. These ganglia are excitor cell stations whose preganglionic fibers travel with nerves CN III, CN VII, and CN IX. The postganglionic fibers are distributed with the branches of CN V to smooth muscles of the eyeball and to glands. Note that the ophthalmic nerve (CN V^1) is sensory to: (1) the eyeball and the cornea via the ciliary nerves; hence, if paralyzed, the ocular conjunctiva is insensitive to touch; (2) the frontal, ethmoidal, and sphenoidal air sinuses via the supraorbital and ethmoidal nerves; and (3) the skin and conjunctival surfaces of the upper eyelid and to the skin and mucous surfaces of the external part of the nose. *B* illustrates the motor fibers passing to the muscles of mastication. *C* shows the sensory and secretory fibers to the nasal mucosa and the palate.

mater (Fig. 7-68). As mentioned, CN V is also the **motor nerve** to the *muscles of mastication* and to some other muscles (Figs. 7-114 and 8-11). The trigeminal was named (L. *trigeminus*, triplet) because it has *three large branches* (Figs. 7-30, 7-55, and 8-11), one to the area above and medial to the eye (sensory), one to the maxillary region (sensory), and one to the mandibular region (sensory and motor).

Most of the cell bodies of the sensory parts of CN V are located in the **trigeminal ganglion** (semilunar ganglion, Gasserian ganglion, Figs. 7-55, 8-10, and 8-11), but a few cell bodies are located in the **mesencephalic nucleus** in the midbrain (Fig. 8-20). Trigeminal ganglion cells are unipolar; *the peripheral processes of neurons in the trigeminal ganglion enter the three divisions of the nerve* and constitute the sensory components of the ophthalmic, maxillary, and mandibular divisions of the trigeminal nerve (Fig. 8-11). The **mandibular nerve** in particular also contains sensory fibers from the *mesencephalic nucleus,* which is *the only collection of primary sensory neurons within the CNS* (Fig. 8-20).

The central processes of neurons in the trigeminal ganglion *make up the large sensory root of the trigeminal nerve.* These fibers enter the lateral portion of the pons (Figs. 7-79 and 8-7) where they divide into ascending and descending fibers. The ascending fibers pass to the **chief sensory nucleus** (main or principal sensory nucleus, superior nucleus, Fig. 8-20). The descending fibers pass to the **spinal nucleus of the trigeminal nerve** (nucleus of the spinal tract) and contain the **pain and sensory components** of CN V. *The chief sensory nucleus of CN V receives position sense and tactile discrimination components.* Most of these sensory fibers enter the brain in CN V, but some enter via CN VII, CN IX, and CN X.

The motor nucleus of CN V lies at the midlevel of the pons, medial and ventral to the chief sensory nucleus. The efferent fibers from this nucleus leave the pons at the site of the entering sensory fibers (Fig. 8-18) and pass inferior to the trigeminal ganglion to become incorporated in CN V^3, the **mandibular nerve** (Fig. 8-11).

The three divisions of CN V are the **ophthalmic** (CN V^1), the **maxillary** (CN V^2), and the **mandibular** (CN V^3).

CN V^1, the ophthalmic nerve, passes to the superior part of the orbit through the *superior orbital fissure* (Figs. 7-55 and 8-11) and is distributed to the **conjunctiva,** the **cornea,** the upper **eyelid,** the **forehead,** the **nose,** and the **scalp** as far posteriorly as the vertex of the skull (Fig. 7-30).

CN V^2, the maxillary nerve, leaves the middle cranial fossa through the **foramen rotundum** (Figs. 7-54 and 7-55), crosses the *pterygopalatine fossa* (Fig. 8-12), passes through the **inferior orbital fissure**, crosses the floor of the orbit, and emerges through the *infraorbital foramen.* The **maxillary nerve** conveys tactile, pain, and temperature sensation from the *skin of the cheek* and the lateral aspect of the nose, the upper lip, teeth, and jaw (Fig. 8-13), and the mucosal surfaces of the uvula, hard palate, nasopharynx, and the inferior part of the nasal cavity.

CN V^3, the mandibular nerve, leaves the skull via the **foramen ovale** (Figs. 7-54, 7-55, and 8-11). This nerve *carries both sensory and motor impulses.* The sensory input is from the skin over the **mandible** (Fig. 7-30*C*), the **auricle,** the anterior part of the **external acoustic meatus** (Fig. 8-11), the homolateral side of the **tongue,** the **lower teeth** (Fig. 8-13), the **gingivae** (gums), the floor of the **mouth,** the *lower lip,* and the buccal surface of the **cheek.** *The motor supply of CN V^3 is to the muscles of mastication* (temporal, pterygoid, and masseter, Fig. 8-11).

CLINICALLY ORIENTED COMMENTS

A patient with his/her eyes closed who is unable to feel wisps of cotton touching the forehead, the cheeks, and the jaw has **anesthesia to light touch.** Other modalities of sensitivity may be tested using pinpricks and warm and cold objects (Fig. 8-14).

Lesions of the peripheral branches of the trigeminal nerve are not common, but may result from (1) **traumatic injury** to the face, (2) **tumors,** or (3) **fractures** of the

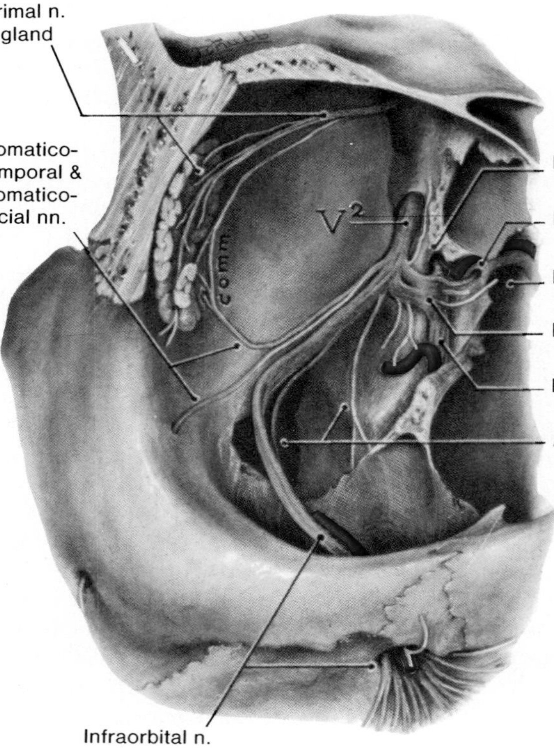

Figure 8-12. Drawing of a dissection of the maxillary nerve (CN V^2). Also see Figure 7-30*A* and *C*. This afferent nerve supplies the territory extending from the skin laterally (*pink area*) to the nasal septum medially, the lateral and medial branches of the nerve being separated by the maxillary sinus. The greater petrosal nerve, via the nerve of the pterygoid canal, brings parasympathetic fibers to the pterygopalatine ganglion in the pterygopalatine fossa which are relayed and distributed with branches of CN V^2 as secretomotor fibers (see Fig. 8-11).

bones of the skull or face. The **infraorbital nerve** (Fig. 7-30*C*) is commonly injured in fractures of the maxilla (Fig. 7-27) and the **mandibular nerve** may be damaged by a fracture of the ramus of the mandible (Fig. 7-26).

A lesion of the entire trigeminal nerve causes **anesthesia** of (1) the corresponding anterior half of the scalp (Fig. 7-30); (2) the face except for the area around the angle of the mandible; (3) the cornea and conjunctiva; and (4) the mucous membranes of the nose, mouth, and anterior two-thirds of the tongue (Fig. 7-159). *Paralysis and atrophy of the muscles of mastication* also occur so that when the mouth is opened the mandible moves to the paralyzed side.

Trigeminal neuralgia (tic douloureaux, facial neuralgia) manifests itself in a *characteristic clinical syndrome* (Case 7-2), **paroxysms of pain** localized to the peripheral area supplied by one or more divisions of CN V. The *sudden sharp attack of pain* lasts for a few seconds only and recurs with varying frequency. **The pain is usually severe** and is commonly described as stabbing or tearing. Usually there are *trigger zones* that set off the pain (*e.g.*, near the eye or nose). Between the **paroxysms of pain**, the patient is usually comfortable. Often a cold wind is sufficient to bring on a paroxysm of pain. In typical cases occurring after middle age, there are no neurological disturbances apart from the pain (*e.g.*, there are usually no areas of altered sensibility). *The etiology of trigeminal neu-*

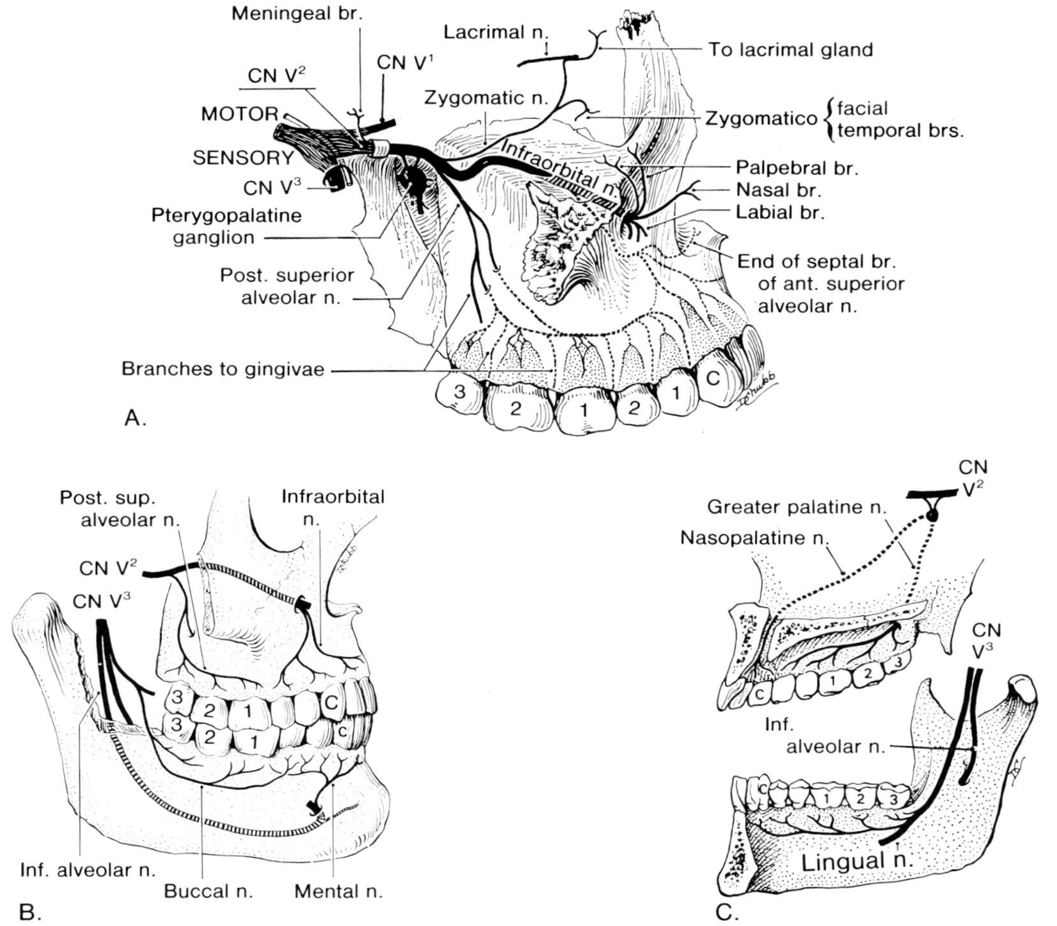

Figure 8-13. Drawings illustrating the distribution of CN V^2 and CN V^3. *A*, note that the maxillary nerve (CN V^2) is sensory (1) to the upper teeth and gingivae (gums); (2) to the face, both surfaces of the lower eyelid, the skin of the side and vestibule of the nose, and both surfaces of the upper lip; (3) via the pterygopalatine ganglion to the nasal cavity, palate, and roof of the pharynx; and (4) to the maxillary, ethmoidal, and sphenoidal air sinuses. Note also that secretory fibers from this ganglion pass with the zygomatic and then with the lacrimal nerve to the lacrimal gland. *B*, observe that the mandibular nerve (CN V^3) is motor (1) to the four muscles of mastication—but not to buccinator; (2) to the two tensores (tympani and palati) via the otic ganglion; and (3) to the mylohyoid and anterior belly of the digastric muscle. CN V^3 is sensory to: (1) the lower teeth and gums; (2) both surfaces of the lower lip by the mental nerve; (3) the auricle and temporal region by the auriculotemporal nerve, which also sends twigs to the external acoustic meatus and to the outer surface of the eardrum, and conveys secretory fibers from the otic ganglion to the parotid gland; (4) the mucous membrane of the cheek by the buccal nerve; and (5) the anterior two-thirds of the tongue, the floor of the mouth, and the gingivae by the lingual nerve which also distributes the chorda tympani. *C*, note that the mandibular nerve (CN V^3) supplies the lower gingivae by three branches and the lower teeth by one branch (inferior alveolar). The gingivae are also supplied by twigs that perforate the alveoli. The territory of any of these gingival and dental nerves may either be extended or contracted; *e.g.*, twigs of the mental and lingual nerves may cross the median plane to supply the gingivae of the opposite side, and the inferior alveolar nerves may decussate in the mandibular canal to supply the incisors of the opposite side.

ralgia is not clear. (For a discussion of possible causes and some current methods of treatment, see Chap. 7 and the discussion of Case 7-2.)

Herpes zoster, a virus infection, also affects the trigeminal ganglion (Figs. 7-55 and 8-7). Inflammation of the ganglion may result in necrosis of some ganglion cells and it usually produces typical *herpetic eruptions* in one or more of the three divisions of the nerve. **Herpes zoster of the face** usually involves the region supplied by the ophthalmic nerve (*herpes zoster ophthalmicus*); hence, the cornea is often involved (Case 8-8). No doubt it is the inflammatory changes affecting the ganglion cells and their fibers that cause the skin lesions. *In some cases* there is partial paralysis or **paresis of the ocular muscles** indicating that the infection has involved CN III, CN IV, or CN VI, the nerves supplying the muscles that move the eye (Fig. 8-10 and Tables 8-2 and 8-3).

Aneurysm of the internal carotid artery may involve CN V, particularly lesions below the *anterior clinoid process* (Fig. 7-55). When the aneurysm is located near the foramen lacerum (Fig. 7-47), it often affects all three divisions of the trigeminal nerve.

THE ABDUCENS NERVE (CN VI)

The abducens (L. abducting) **nerve is the motor nerve to the lateral rectus** muscle of the eye (Fig. 8-10), which turns the eye outward (*i.e.*, abducts it).

The nucleus of the abducens (abducent) nerve is a small cluster of neurons in the **caudal part of the pons** *in the floor of the fourth ventricle* near the midline (Fig. 8-20). Fibers from the **abducens nucleus** pass through the pons in a ventrocaudal direction and emerge from the brain stem at the *junction of the pons and the pyramid* of the medulla (Figs. 7-55, 7-79, and 8-7). The nerve leaves the pons just cranial to the **anterior inferior cerebellar artery** (Fig. 7-90) and then passes through the subarachnoid space (**pontine cistern**, Figs. 7-82 and 8-7) before piercing the dura mater. It *traverses the cavernous sinus* (Figs. 7-72 and 7-73) and *enters the orbit* through the **superior orbital fissure** (Fig. 7-55), where it supplies the lateral rectus muscle (Fig. 8-10).

CLINICALLY ORIENTED COMMENTS

Abducens paralysis is one of the most common eye palsies which probably results from its long intracranial course. When the abducens nerve is injured the patient has a **medial strabismus** or squint and he/she is unable to abduct the eye on the affected side (Fig. 8-25). As with involvement of CN III and CN IV, the patient will usually also complain of diplopia. With sixth nerve involvement, this visual defect occurs when the patient attempts to look laterally (Case 8-3).

The abducens nerve is sometimes injured in **fractures of the base of the skull** (*e.g.*, ones involving the cavernous sinus or the orbit).

THE FACIAL NERVE (CN VII)

The facial nerve is a mixed nerve, but it is *mainly motor.* It was given its name because its large motor branches spread over the face (Figs. 7-32 to 7-34).

The motor nucleus of the facial nerve is a fusiform cluster of cells in the **caudal part of the pons**, just dorsal to the *superior olive* (Figs. 7-79 and 8-20). The axons of cells in this **facial nucleus** have an unusual course in that they loop around the abducens nucleus (Fig. 8-20) before emerging at the **caudal border of the pons** (Fig. 8-7), between the rootlets of CN VI and CN VIII (Fig. 7-79). The nerve then enters the **lateral pontine cistern** and passes into the *internal acoustic meatus* along with CN VIII (Figs. 8-15 and 9-34). In the meatus, the motor and sensory roots of the nerve combine and then enter the **facial canal** in the temporal bone (Fig. 7-185). *The facial nerve leaves the skull through the stylomastoid foramen* and passes into the substance of the **parotid gland** (Fig. 7-34), where it divides into five branches

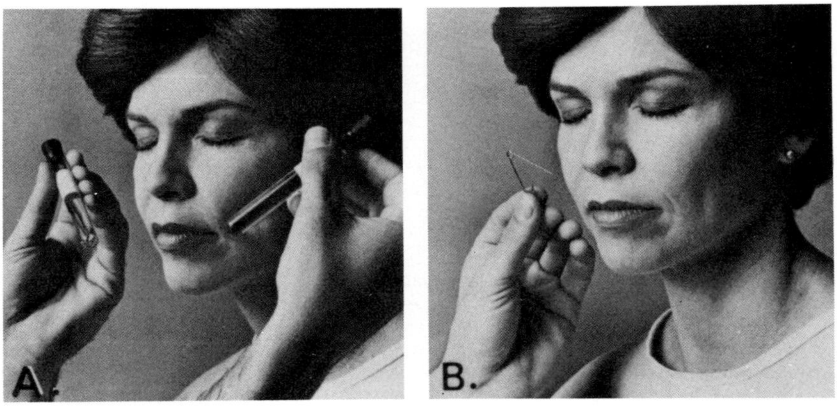

Figure 8-14. Photographs of a 33-year-old woman on whom the examiner is illustrating two of the ways the trigeminal nerve is tested during a neurological examination. Note that CN V tests are conducted with the patient's eyes closed. *A*, test tubes filled with warm and cold fluid are pressed alternately against her cheeks. Differences in response on opposite sides of the face indicate increased or decreased sensitivity to temperature. *B*, differences in response to pinpricks on opposite sides of the face indicate increased or decreased sensitivity to pain.

(Figs. 7-32 to 7-34) which *supply the muscles of facial expression.*

A secretomotor or **parasympathetic component** supplies the submandibular and sublingual salivary glands and the lacrimal gland (Fig. 8-15).

The facial nerve has two sensory components: (1) a **special sensory component** that supplies the taste buds on the anterior two-thirds of the tongue (Figs. 7-159 and 8-15), and (2) a **general sensory component** that supplies fibers to the external ear, tongue, and palate. *The sensory root, called the nervus intermedius, consists of the central processes of unipolar cells in the geniculate ganglion* (Fig. 8-15), which is located at the bend or genu of the facial canal. The peripheral processes of the cells for taste enter the **chorda tympani** branch of CN VII (Fig. 8-15), which joins the lingual branch of the mandibular nerve (Fig. 8-11). These fibers pass to the *taste buds in the anterior two-thirds of the tongue* (Fig. 7-159).

CLINICALLY ORIENTED COMMENTS

A *common lesion of the facial nerve is a type of facial paralysis called Bell's palsy* (Fig. 7-199). Usually there is sudden weakness (**paresis**) or *paralysis of the muscles of facial expression* on the affected side. (Refer to Case 7-1 for a typical history.) **The term Bell's palsy is usually reserved for a peripheral seventh nerve palsy of sudden onset,** often caused by exposure to cold or possibly from swelling of the geniculate ganglion. Bell's palsy is most common in the 20 to 50 age group and the symptoms and signs depend upon the location of the lesion. *The nerve is commonly affected as it traverses the facial canal in the petrous part of the temporal bone.* Most persons with Bell's palsy recover completely within 2 to 8 weeks; it may take 1 to 2 years in older patients. **Other types of CN VII paralysis** (palsy) may be caused by tumors, fractures, and meningitis.

All functions of the facial nerve are lost if the nerve is damaged proximal to the geniculate ganglion (Fig. 8-15). Hence, in addition to **facial paralysis**, there is *loss of sensation in the anterior two-thirds of the tongue* (Fig. 7-159) and in the palate on the affected side. There is also loss of secretion of the submandibular, sublingual, and lacrimal glands, including the mucous membrane on the side of the lesion.

When **testing the facial nerve**, the pa-

Table 8-3
Summary of Lesions Involving Cranial Nerves or Their Central Connections

Nerve	Frequency	Type and/or Site of Lesion	Abnormal Findings
CN I	Uncommon	Fracture of cribriform plate or in ethmoid area	Anosmia; CNS rhinorrhea
CN II	Common	Direct trauma to orbit or eyeball or fracture involving optic foramen	Loss of pupillary constriction
	Common	Pressure on optic pathway; laceration or intracerebral clot in temporal, parietal, or occipital lobes	Absence of blink reflex indicating visual field defect (Fig. 8-9; see Cases 8-4 and 8-5).
CN III	Common	Pressure of herniating uncus on nerve just before it enters cavernous sinus or fracture involving cavernous sinus; aneurysms	Dilated pupil, ptosis, eye turns down and out; direct pupil reflex absent (see Case 8-6)
CN IV	Uncommon	Course of nerve around brain stem or fracture of orbit	Inability to look down and in during convergence
CN V	Uncommon	Injury to terminal branches, particularly CN V^2 in roof of maxillary sinus (e.g., fracture of bones of face, Figs. 7-26 and 7-27); pathological processes affecting trigeminal ganglion (see Case 8-8)	Loss of pain and touch sensation; paresthesias; masseter and temporalis muscles do not contract; deviation of mandible to side of lesion when mouth is opened.
CN VI	Common	Base of brain or fracture involving cavernous sinus or orbit	Eye fails to move laterally; diplopia on lateral gaze (see Case 8-3)
CN VII	Common	Laceration or contusion of parotid region	Paralysis of facial muscles; eye remains open; angle of mouth droops; forehead does not wrinkle
	Common	Fracture of temporal bone	As above, plus associated involvement of cochlear n. and chorda tympani; dry cornea and loss of taste on ant. two-thirds of tongue
	Common	Intracranial hematoma ("stroke")	Forehead wrinkles because of bilateral innervation of frontalis muscle; otherwise paralysis of contralateral facial muscles
CN VIII	Common	Eighth nerve tumor (acoustic neuroma)	Progressive unilateral hearing loss; tinnitus (noises in ear; see Case 8-2)
CN IX	Rare	Brain stem or deep laceration of neck	Loss of taste on post. one-third of tongue; loss of sensation on affected side of soft palate
CN X	Rare	Brain stem or deep laceration of neck	Sagging of soft palate; deviation of uvula to normal side; hoarseness owing to paralysis of vocal fold (see Case 8-1)
CN XI	Rare	Laceration of neck	Sternocleidomastoid and upper fibers of trapezius muscles fail to contract; drooping of shoulder (see Case 8-7)
CN XII	Rare	Neck laceration often with major vessel damage; basal skull fractures	Protruded tongue deviates toward affected side (see Case 8-7); moderate dysarthria

tient is asked to look at the ceiling, wrinkle the forehead, frown, smile, and raise the eyebrows. To test the strength of the **orbicularis oculi muscles** (Figs. 7-28 and 7-32), the sphincter muscles of the eyelids, the patient is asked to try to keep his/her eyes closed while the examiner attempts to open them (Fig. 8-16). *When CN VII is damaged, the patient cannot close the eyelid* tightly on the affected side. In addition, when CN VII is injured, sounds are very loud in the affected ear owing to **paralysis of the stapedius** muscle supplied by CN VII (Fig. 7-181*B*).

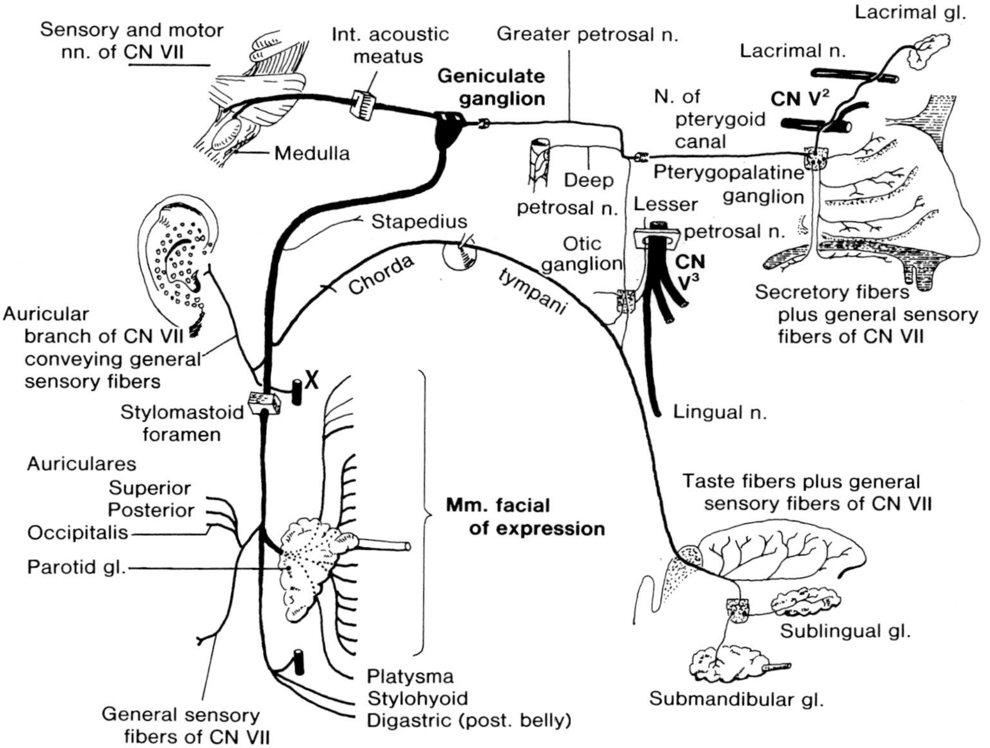

Figure 8-15. Diagram illustrating the distribution of the *facial nerve* (CN VII). Note that four modalities are carried by the facial nerve: (1) *motor* to the muscles of facial expression (the superficial muscles around the eye, nose, mouth, and ear; the scalp above; and the platysma, Fig. 7-35); it also supplies the stylohyoid muscle and the posterior belly of the digastric, as well as the stapedius; and (2) *special sense* (taste) fibers with cell stations in the geniculate ganglion pass from the palate through the pterygopalatine ganglion, the nerve of the pterygoid canal, and the greater petrosal nerve to the geniculate ganglion. Fibers from the anterior two-thirds of the tongue pass via two routes: (1) the chorda tympani to the facial nerve and then to the geniculate ganglion, and (2) by a branch of the chorda tympani that traverses the otic ganglion to join the greater petrosal nerve and then to the geniculate ganglion. Evidence of this double route is the fact that the chorda tympani may be cut without loss of taste, whereas cutting the greater petrosal nerve may result in loss of taste.

THE VESTIBULOCOCHLEAR NERVE (CN VIII)

The vestibulocochlear (acoustic) nerve is a special sensory nerve (Figs. 7-79, 8-7, and 8-17) consisting of *two kinds of sensory fiber in two bundles known as the vestibular and cochlear nerves.* The vestibular nerve comes from the **semicircular ducts** which detect movement of the head and record its position relative to the pull of gravity. The **cochlear nerve** is associated with hearing (Fig. 7-195).

The vestibulocochlear nerve is located posteroinferior to the facial nerve in the internal acoustic meatus (Figs. 8-1 and 9-34). It splits into its two divisions at the lateral end of this canal. The cochlear and vestibular nerves run together from the internal acoustic meatus through the lateral pontine cistern (Fig. 7-82) and enter the medulla (Figs. 7-79, 8-7, and 8-17).

The bipolar neurons of the **cochlear nerve** have their cell bodies in the **spiral ganglion**, which is situated about the *modiolus* of the cochlea in the petrous part of the temporal bone (Fig. 7-195). The peripheral processes of these cells end in relation to the *hair cells* of the spiral **organ of Corti** in the cochlear duct (Figs. 7-195 and 8-17). The central processes of these cells form the cochlear nerve, which enters the cranial cavity through the *internal acoustic meatus* (Fig. 7-196), where they end in the ventral and dorsal **cochlear nuclei** in the medulla (Figs. 8-17 and 8-20).

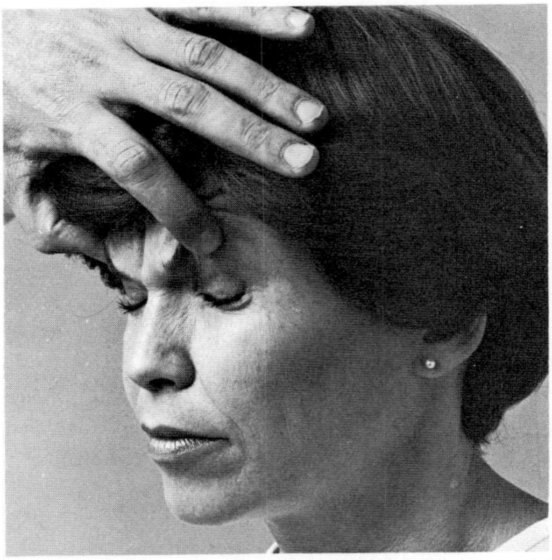

Figure 8-16. Photograph of a 33-year-old woman attempting to keep her eyes closed while the examiner attempts to open them. The neurologist is testing for paresis (weakness) of the orbicularis oculi muscles supplied by CN VII. When a facial nerve is paralyzed the patient is unable to close the eyelid on the affected side owing to paralysis of the orbicularis oculi, the sphincter muscle of the eyelid.

The peripheral processes of bipolar cells in the **vestibular ganglion**, located within the internal acoustic meatus, pass to the *cristae ampullares* of the semicircular ducts and the *maculae* of the utricle and the saccule (Figs. 7-197 and 8-17). The central processes of these vestibular ganglion cells form the **vestibular nerve**, which enters the medulla beside the fibers of the cochlear nerve (Figs. 7-79, 8-7, and 8-17). They terminate in **vestibular nuclei** which lie in the floor of the fourth ventricle.

CLINICALLY ORIENTED COMMENTS

Peripheral lesions usually involve both the cochlear and vestibular nerves. CN VIII is commonly injured in *fractures of the middle cranial fossa* which involve the **internal acoustic meatus** (Fig. 7-196). If the cochlear nerve is severed, *permanent deafness* results in the ear concerned. When the nerve is bruised or pressed upon by a **he-**

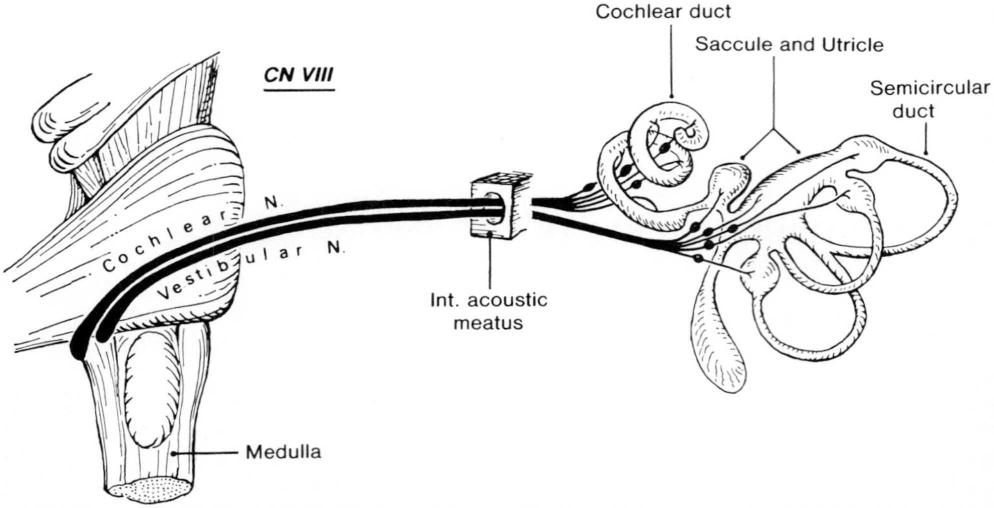

Figure 8-17. Scheme of the distribution of the *vestibulocochlear nerve* (CN VIII). This nerve has two parts: (1) the *choclear nerve* or nerve of hearing whose fibers transmit impulses from the spiral organ of Corti in the cochlear duct, and (2) the *vestibular nerve* or nerve of balance whose fibers transmit impulses from the maculae of the saccule and utricle and the ampullae of the three semicircular ducts (also see Figs. 7-194 and 7-195).

matoma, the deafness is usually temporary. *Other diseases and lesions that may involve CN VIII* are: meningitis, **tumors**, and certain virus diseases. Certain **antibiotics** may also affect CN VIII.

Central lesions also affect either the cochlear or vestibular nerves (*e.g.*, syphilis, **brain tumors**, and multiple sclerosis). *Symptoms of cochlear nerve involvement* are **tinnitus** (ringing, buzzing, and other noises in the ear) and **deafness** owing to interruption of the cochlear nerve pathway. *Symptoms of vestibular nerve involvement* are **vertigo** (dizziness) and **nystagmus** (rhythmic to and fro ocular movement with a slow movement away and a rapid return).

THE GLOSSOPHARYNGEAL NERVE (CN IX)

The glossopharyngeal nerve is a mixed nerve having sensory and motor components (Figs. 7-79 and 8-7). It was named according to its chief areas of distribution (Fig. 8-18), the **tongue** (G. *glossā*, tongue) and the **pharynx** (G. throat). Its sensory fibers convey (1) *special sensations* (taste) from the posterior one-third of the tongue; (2) *general sensations* (pain, temperature, and touch) from the back of the tongue (Fig. 7-159), the wall of the pharynx, and the middle ear (Fig. 8-18*A*); and (3) *chemoreceptors* and *pressure receptors* in the **carotid sinus** concerned with the regulation of respiration and blood pressure (Fig. 8-18*B*). *The glossopharyngeal nerve also carries motor fibers to the stylopharyngeus muscle* of the pharynx (Figs. 7-188 and 8-18*A*).

The glossopharyngeal nerve has two peripheral ganglia, a small *superior ganglion* in the **jugular foramen** (Fig. 7-57) and a larger *inferior ganglion* (petrosal ganglion) located in a notch in the lower border of the petrous part of the temporal bone.

CN IX is predominately a sensory nerve, but it also conveys preganglionic **parasympathetic fibers** to the **otic ganglion** (Fig. 8-18*A*). The postganglionic fibers accompany the *auricotemporal nerve* (Fig. 7-32) to the **parotid gland**.

The glossopharyngeal nerve is formed by several rootlets that leave the medulla posterior to the olive (Figs. 7-79, 8-1, 8-7, 8-18, and 8-20). It passes across the **posterior cranial fossa** and pierces the dura mater, leaving the skull through the **jugular foramen** (Figs. 7-56 and 7-72). After leaving the skull, CN IX passes forward between the internal jugular vein and the internal carotid artery (Fig. 9-22) to supply the **stylophagneus muscle** (Fig. 8-18*A*).

CLINICALLY ORIENTED COMMENTS

Isolated lesions of CN IX are rare. *Loss of the pharyngeal (gag) reflex and the carotid sinus reflex result from disturbances of this nerve.* The nerve is tested by touching the posterior wall of the pharynx with a wooden tongue depressor. As you can easily determine, the normal response is prompt contraction of the **pharyngeal muscles**, with or without gagging. *Stroking the affected side with the tongue depressor does not produce gagging if CN IX is injured* owing to loss of sensation in the trigger zone for eliciting this reflex.

Glossopharyngeal neuralgia, an uncommon syndrome, results in *paroxysmal attacks of severe pain* which usually start in the throat in the area of the **palatine tonsils** (Fig. 9-61). The onset of pain may be triggered by coughing and/or swallowing and frequently radiates to the area of the **auditory tube** (Fig. 8-18) and behind the auricle.

Because CN IX is closely related to CN VII, CN VIII, CN X, and CN XI (Fig. 9-34), they are commonly involved with lesions resulting from compression, inflammation, or trauma. **Jugular vein thrombophlebitis** (clotting) may also involve CN IX because of its proximity to the **jugular bulb** in the jugular foramen as it leaves the skull (Fig. 7-118).

THE VAGUS NERVE (CN X)

The vagus nerve, a mixed nerve, has the *most extensive distribution of any cranial nerve* (Fig. 8-19). It was named *vagus* (L. wandering) because of this extensive distribution and its *long meandering course.*

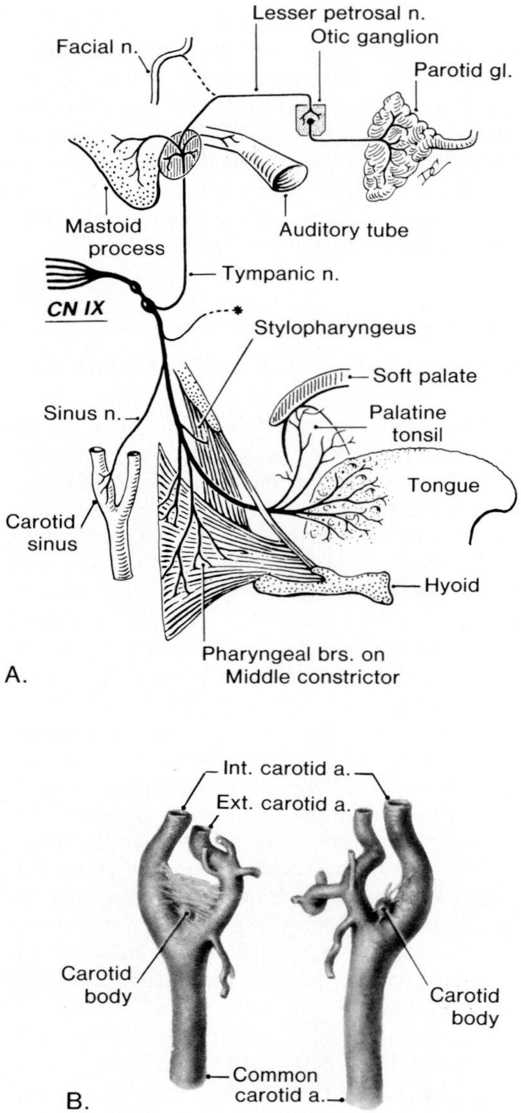

Figure 8-18. Scheme of distribution of the *glossopharyngeal nerve* (CN IX). In *A* note: (1) its *motor fibers* supply the stylopharyngeus muscle; (2) its *secretory fibers* travel via the tympanic and lesser petrosal nerves to the otic ganglion, from which they are relayed via the auriculotemporal nerve to the parotid gland; (3) its *general sensory fibers* supply almost the entire one-half of the pharyngeal wall, including the oropharyngeal isthmus (*i.e.*, the inferior surface of the soft palate, tonsil, pharyngeal arches, and posterior third of the tongue). They also supply the dorsum of the soft palate, the auditory tube, the tympanum, the medial surface of the eardrum, the mastoid antrum, and the mastoid air cells; (4) its *taste fibers* supply the posterior third of the tongue including the vallate papillae; and (5) the sinus nerve is afferent from the carotid sinus and carotid body. The *carotid sinus* responds to pressure changes within the artery; the *carotid body* (*B*) is believed to respond to chemical changes (concentration of CO_2) in the blood.

CN X has **one sensory** and **two motor nuclei** in the medulla (Fig. 8-20). *It is attached to the medulla by 8 to 10 rootlets* (Figs. 8-1 and 8-7) below the glossopharyngeal nerve in the groove between the **olive** and the *inferior cerebellar peduncle* (Figs. 7-79 and 8-20). The vagus exits from the cranial cavity via the **jugular foramen** (Fig. 7-72). *CN X is accompanied by and contained within the same sheath of dura mater and arachnoid as CN XI.* Within the jugular foramen, the vagus presents an enlargement known as the **superior ganglion.** After it leaves the jugular foramen, it exhibits another swelling called the **inferior ganglion.** The cells of both ganglia are *unipolar sensory neurons.* The superior ganglion contains the cell bodies of neurons concerned with *general somatic sensation,* whereas the cell bodies in the inferior ganglion are partly concerned with *special visceral sensations* (**taste from the epiglottis**) and partly with *general visceral afferent sensations* from the viscera (Fig. 8-20).

The vagus nerve passes vertically down the neck (Fig. 9-52) enclosed within the **carotid sheath** (Fig. 9-46), close to the *common carotid artery* and the *internal jugular vein.* For details of the course of the vagus in the neck, thorax, and abdomen, see Chapters 9, 1, and 2, respectively.

The vagus nerve has four kinds of fiber (Fig. 8-20): (1) **motor fibers to the striated muscles** of the larynx and pharynx; (2) **visceral motor (preganglionic) fibers** that carry impulses to the thoracic and abdominal viscera as far as the left colic flexure; (3) **sensory fibers from sense organs of pain** and possibly temperature and touch in the skin of the external acoustic meatus; (4) **visceral sensory fibers** that carry impulses from (a) *taste buds* in the epiglottis; (b) *stretch receptors* in the wall of the heart, aorta, and superior

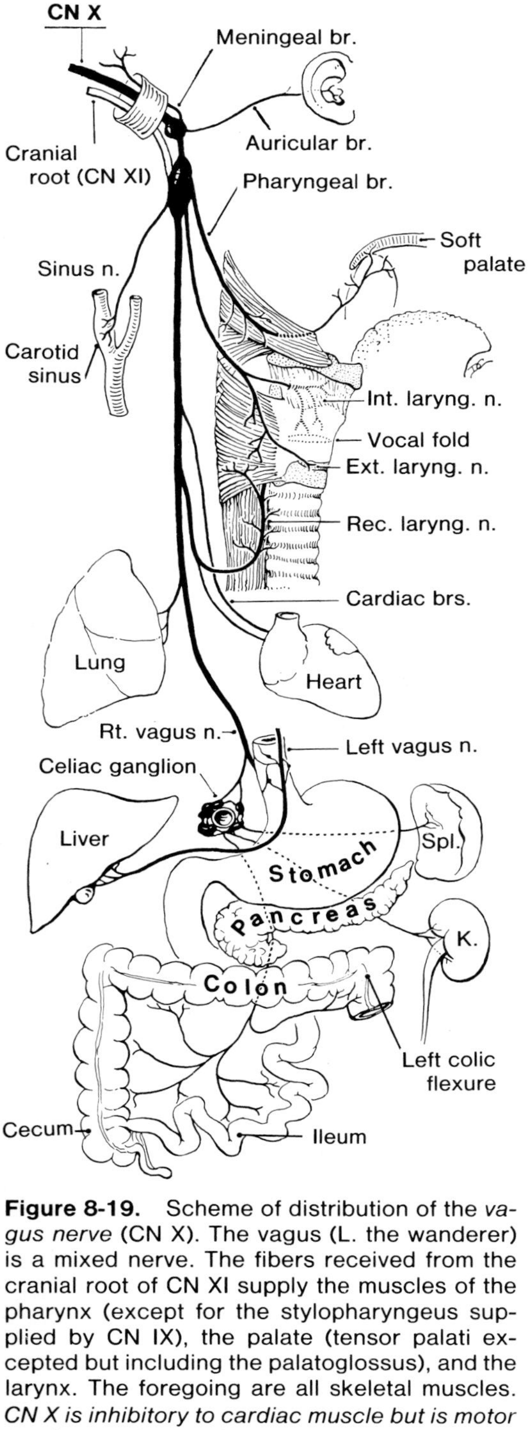

Figure 8-19. Scheme of distribution of the *vagus nerve* (CN X). The vagus (L. the wanderer) is a mixed nerve. The fibers received from the cranial root of CN XI supply the muscles of the pharynx (except for the stylopharyngeus supplied by CN IX), the palate (tensor palati excepted but including the palatoglossus), and the larynx. The foregoing are all skeletal muscles. *CN X is inhibitory to cardiac muscle but is motor to all smooth muscle, secretory to all glands, and afferent from all mucous surfaces in the following parts*—pharynx (inferior part), larynx, trachea, bronchi, lungs, esophagus, stomach, and intestines down to the left colic flexure; liver, gallbladder and bile passages, pancreas and pancreatic ducts, and perhaps spleen and kidney. It is also concerned with *taste* from the few taste buds in the epiglottis.

vena cava, and the bifurcation of the common carotid artery (these **stretch receptors** *regulate blood pressure and heart rate*); and (c) stretch receptors in the lung, *regulating the rate and depth of respiration*, and in the upper G.I. tract.

CLINICALLY ORIENTED COMMENTS

It is not easy to test the function of the vagus nerve despite its great size and many functions. Generally CN IX and CN X are tested together. *Normal function of the vagus nerve alone is indicated by the patient's ability to swallow and to speak clearly without hoarseness.* Symmetrical movement of the **vocal folds** (Fig. 9-76) and of the soft palate (Fig. 9-61) when the patient says "ah" also indicates intact vagus nerves.

Unilateral paralysis of the motor part of CN X produces paralysis of the palatal, pharyngeal, and laryngeal muscles on the same side as the lesion (Fig. 8-19). The voice is hoarse or brassy owing to *paresis (weakness) of the vocal fold.* The speech usually has a nasal twang when there is **paresis of the soft palate**, particularly when there are bilateral lesions. In unilateral involvement of CN X, swallowing is ordinarily not impaired, but *in bilateral lesions* there is (1) **dysphagia** (G. *dys*, difficult + *phagein*, to eat) or difficulty in swallowing and (2) **regurgitation** of fluids through the nose.

Unilateral lesions of the recurrent laryngeal nerve (Fig. 8-21) produce paresis or **paralysis of the vocal fold** on the same side, resulting in a *weak hoarse voice.* Injuries to these nerves may occur during surgical operations in the neck (*e.g.*, **carotid endarterectomy**; see Case 8-1 for details). Bilateral involvement of the recur-

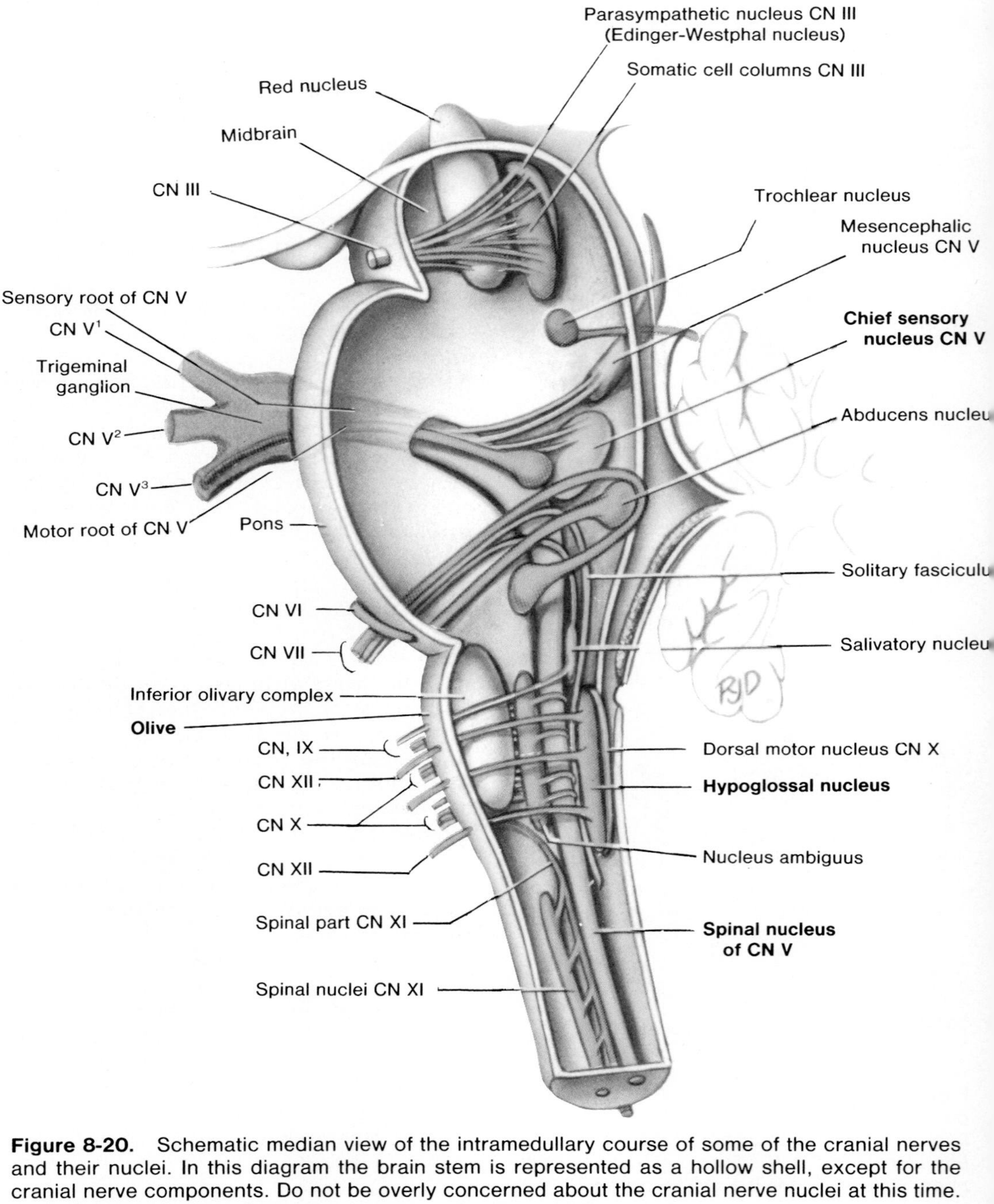

Figure 8-20. Schematic median view of the intramedullary course of some of the cranial nerves and their nuclei. In this diagram the brain stem is represented as a hollow shell, except for the cranial nerve components. Do not be overly concerned about the cranial nerve nuclei at this time. You will learn all about them in your neuroanatomy course.

rent laryngeal nerves produces variable signs and symptoms. **Hoarseness** is present and there may be **aphonia** (G. *a*, no + *phonē*, voice). If the nerves have been crushed or stretched, the paralysis is usually temporary.

Intramedullary lesions (Fig. 8-20), *e.g.*, hemorrhage, thrombosis, and tumors, can

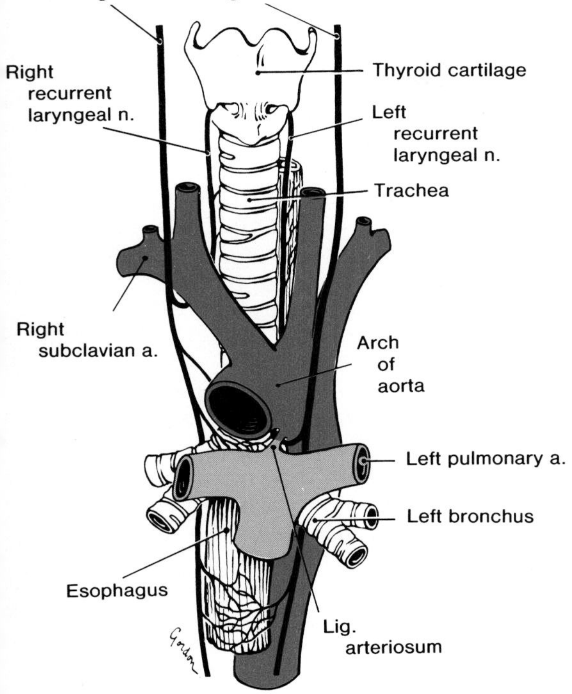

Figure 8-21. Drawing illustrating the course and relationship of the *vagus nerves* and their recurrent laryngeal branches. Observe that (1) *on the left side* the recurrent laryngeal *arises in the thorax* and recurs by hooking around the ligamentum arteriosum and the aortic arch, and (2) *on the right side* the recurrent laryngeal *arises in the root of the neck* and recurs by hooking around the right subclavian artery. The disappearance of the embryonic sixth aortic arch on the right side and its retention as the ligamentum arteriosum on the left side explains why the course of the recurrent laryngeal nerves differs on the two sides.

also affect vagal functions. In general, *lesions in the upper medulla* produce **dysphagia**, whereas *lesions in the lower medulla* cause **dysarthria** (G. *dys*, difficult + *arthroō*, to articulate) or disturbance of articulation owing to **paresis** or paralysis of the muscles concerned with speech. For the many other effects of lesions of the vagus nerves, consult a neurology text. [For notes on division of the vagus (**vagotomy**), see Chap. 2].

THE ACCESSORY NERVE (CN XI)

The accessory nerve is a motor nerve that *supplies muscles in the wall of the pharynx and larynx* and two superficial muscles of the neck (**sternocleidomastoid** and **trapezius**). *CN XI is a peculiar nerve made up of two parts* (Fig. 8-22); **its cranial root is accessory to the vagus** which it quickly joins. It is obvious how it received its name. *The accessory nerve is formed by the union of cranial and spinal roots*, but they are associated for only a very short part of their course.

The cranial root (part) of CN XI arises from cells in the most caudal part of the *nucleus ambiguus* (Fig. 8-20). The axons of these neurons emerge from the lateral surface of the medulla, *caudal to the rootlets*

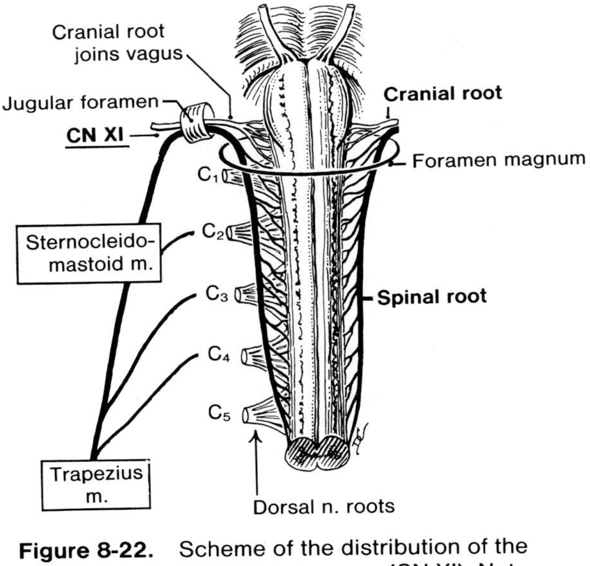

Figure 8-22. Scheme of the distribution of the spinal root of the *accessory nerve* (CN XI). Note that this root is joined by fibers from the ventral ramus of C2 and supplies the sternocleidomastoid muscle and is joined by fibers from the ventral rami of C3 and C4 and supplies the trapezius muscle. There is clinical evidence (both surgical and medical) that these contributions from C2 to C4 convey motor as well as sensory fibers. The spinal root of the accessory nerve usually passes through the spinal ganglion of C1 and may receive sensory fibers from it.

of the vagus nerve (Figs. 7-79, 8-7, and 8-20). The cranial root enters the **jugular foramen** (Fig. 7-72) where it combines temporarily with the spinal root. *Fibers of the cranial root join the vagus nerve* and supply the muscles of the **soft palate** and the intrinsic muscles of the **larynx.**

Explanatory Note. The cranial root of CN XI really should be considered as part of CN X because it is more closely associated with this nerve. *Fibers of the cranial root of CN XI join the vagus and are distributed through its branches.* Hence, it would be simpler, but contrary to convention, to consider the cranial root as part of the vagus and to leave the spinal root as CN XI. *Some neurologists do not consider the cranial root to be part of CN XI.* They assume it to be the inferior part of CN X because they believe it is confusing to consider it as part of CN XI just because it passes intracranially with the spinal root for a very short distance.

The spinal root (part) of CN XI arises from an elongated column of motor neurons in the anterior horn of the upper five or six segments of the **cervical region of the spinal cord** (Fig. 8-20). *The fibers of the spinal root emerge from the lateral aspect of the spinal cord* between the dorsal and ventral roots of upper cervical nerves (Figs. 7-79 and 8-7). The rootlets of the spinal root unite to form a common trunk which ascends in the **subarachnoid space** and enters the skull through the **foramen magnum**, behind the vertebral artery. It then passes upward and laterally to leave the posterior cranial fossa through the **jugular foramen** with the cranial root (Figs. 8-20, 8-22, and 9-34). The spinal fibers of CN XI form an external branch that supplies the **sternocleidomastoid** and **trapezius muscles** (Figs. 9-11 and 9-12).

CLINICALLY ORIENTED COMMENTS

Lesions of the accessory nerve are rare. The nerve may be damaged by traumatic injury, by tumors at the base of the skull, by *fractures running across the jugular foramen*, and by neck lacerations (Case 8-7).

Although contraction of one sternocleidomastoid muscle turns the head to one side, a unilateral lesion of CN XI usually does not produce an abnormality in the position of the head. However, **weakness in turning the head** to the opposite side against resistance can be detected. *Unilateral paralysis of the trapezius is evidenced by inability to elevate and retract the shoulder and by difficulty in elevating the arm above the horizontal.* The normal ridge formed by the trapezius is depressed and the scapula appears rotated (superior end laterally and downward; inferior end upward and inward). **Drooping of the shoulder** is an obvious sign (Case 8-7).

The functions of CN XI may be interfered with by *inflamed lymph nodes* in the neck (Fig. 9-21), resulting in **acute torticollis** (wryneck) or drawing of the head to one side. During extensive dissections in the **posterior triangle of the neck** (Figs. 9-12 and 9-16), *e.g.*, for the removal of diseased lymph nodes, *the accessory nerve is isolated in order to preserve it.*

THE HYPOGLOSSAL NERVE (CN XII)

The hypoglossal nerve is the motor nerve of the tongue, *supplying all its intrinsic and extrinsic muscles* (Figs. 7-159 and 8-23), except the palatoglossus (supplied by the pharyngeal branch of CN X). The hypoglossal nerve arises from the **hypoglossal nucleus** located in the posterior part of the floor of the fourth ventricle in the medulla (Fig. 8-20). Its 10 to 15 rootlets arise from the medulla *between the olive and the pyramid* (Figs. 7-79, 8-1, 8-7, and 8-20). The fibers pass anterolaterally and exit from the posterior cranial fossa of the skull via the **hypoglossal canal** (anterior condylar canal) in the *occipital bone* (Fig. 7-57). The rootlets unite to form CN XII after traversing this canal, which then passes posterior to the vagus, *picking up branches from C1 and C2 nerves* (Fig. 8-23) before coursing downward between the internal jugular vein and the internal carotid artery (Fig. 9-22). The hypoglossal nerve communicates with the sympathetic trunk, the vagus, and the lingual nerves (Fig. 8-23).

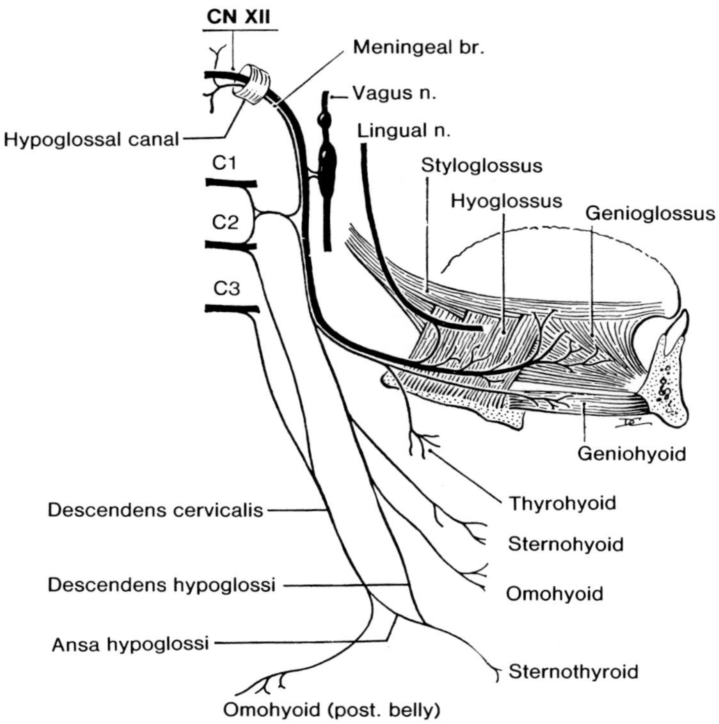

Figure 8-23. Scheme of the distribution of the *hypoglossal nerve* (CN XII). Note that this efferent nerve supplies all the intrinsic (longitudinal, transverse, and vertical) and extrinsic (styloglossus, hyoglossus, and genioglossus) muscles of the tongue, except the palatoglossus. Observe that it receives a mixed (motor and sensory) branch from the loop between the ventral rami of C1 and C2. The sensory or afferent fibers in part take a recurrent course and end in the dura mater of the posterior cranial fossa. Note that the motor or efferent branch supplies the geniohyoid and thyrohyoid muscles and (via the descendens hypoglossi nerve which unites with the descendens cervicalis nerve to form the ansa cervicalis) the remaining depressor muscles of the larynx.

CLINICALLY ORIENTED COMMENTS

Unilateral injury to the hypoglossal nerve or its nucleus results in unilateral **lingual paralysis** and *hemiatrophy of the tongue.* The surface of the paralyzed half of the tongue becomes **wrinkled** and it feels **flaccid.** When the patient protrudes ("sticks out") his/her tongue, it deviates toward the side of the lesion. **Dysarthria** (difficult speech) may also exist. The trunk of the nerve may be damaged where it passes through the hypoglossal canal or distal to this. The cause may be a tumor, fracture of the occipital bone, or traumatic wounds (*e.g.*, **neck laceration** usually associated with major vessel damage, Case 8-7).

Hypoglossal nuclear lesions are often bilateral owing to the close proximity of the right and left nuclei. In these cases the tongue lies motionless in the mouth and swallowing is very difficult.

To test CN XII the patient is asked to protrude the tongue (Fig. 8-24). Note is made of any lateral deviation, atrophy, or tremor of the tongue. The strength of the tongue is tested by asking the patient to move the protruded tongue from side to side against a tongue depressor.

PATIENT ORIENTED PROBLEMS

Case 8-1. A 67-year-old man suddenly noted *weakness and numbness of his left upper limb* without other symptoms. His

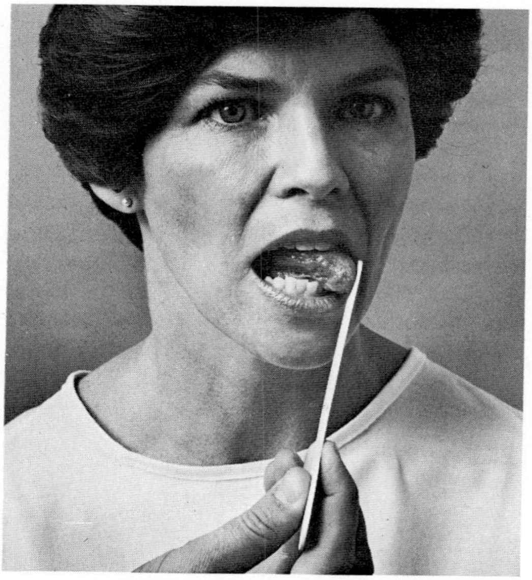

Figure 8-24. Photograph of a 33-year-old woman whose hypoglossal nerve is being tested. The strength of her tongue was determined by asking her to protrude her tongue and move it from side to side against the tongue depressor. If her left hypoglossal nerve was paralyzed it would deviate to the left as shown here and she would be unable to move her tongue to the right.

wife drove him to a hospital where the emergency physician examined him, making a provisional diagnosis of an **embolic stroke** involving the posterior part of the *frontal lobe* and the anterior part of the *parietal lobe* of his **right cerebral hemisphere.** He was admitted to hospital for further investigation.

After 2 days of *cardiovascular monitoring*, **cerebral angiograms** were performed by injecting radiopaque contrast material via a catheter inserted into his femoral artery. The **cerebral angiograms** revealed an *ulcerated atheroma at the origin of the right internal carotid* artery (see Fig. 9-24 for the site) and a moderately large **atheroma** at the origin of the left internal carotid artery.

Right carotid endarterectomy was performed under general anesthesia. After the operation the patient had a weak hoarse voice and **indirect laryngoscopy** (*i.e.*, using a mirror) revealed *paralysis of the right vocal fold* (cord). This paralysis was still present when the patient returned home a week after the operation to convalesce prior to returning for left carotid endarterectomy.

Problems. Define the terms **embolus** and **atheroma.** Using your gross and neuroanatomical knowledge, state on which side of the patient's brain the **embolus** became lodged in a small blood vessel? Which area of the brain was partially deprived of blood? *Explain what is meant by carotid endarterectomy* (discussed in Chap. 7). What nerve was injured during this operation? Describe the origin and course of this nerve. Is the paralysis of the patient's right vocal fold likely to be permanent? *These problems are discussed on page 1098.*

Case 8-2. A 58-year-old physician noticed that he was gradually becoming **hard of hearing** in his right ear. As it seemed to be getting worse, he consulted a neurologist.

Cochlear nerve tests showed that *hearing was greatly reduced* in the right ear. *Tests of vestibular function* performed by irrigating the external acoustic meatus of each ear with cold water showed **reduced vestibular function** on the right side. In addition, it was noted that the *right corneal reflex was diminished.* A computerized tomographic or **CT scan** revealed a mass projecting from the medial end of the **internal acoustic meatus.**

Problems. Which cranial nerve was *obviously* involved? What other cranial nerve was involved? Using your anatomical knowledge, determine which other cranial nerve could be involved in some cases? What would be the result of injury to this nerve? Which type of **skull fracture** could injure these nerves? *These problems are discussed on page 1099.*

Case 8-3. A 33-year-old woman was involved in an automobile accident during which she suffered **head injuries.** She was rushed to a hospital where the emergency physician performed a *neurological examination* which revealed that she had a medial or **convergent strabismus** and *diplopia* (double vision). When asked to follow the examiner's finger, the patient's *right* *eye failed to abduct* on right lateral gaze. Lateral and AP (anteroposterior) *radiographs of the skull* were then taken which showed a **linear fracture** *of the squamous part of the temporal bone* anteriorly, passing downward into the base of the middle cranial fossa. The **sphenoidal sinus** (Fig. 7-95) was airless, suggesting that the fracture passed across the base of the skull. Further radiographs of the base of the skull showed that the fracture line crossed the right *greater wing of the sphenoid bone* (Fig. 7-49) and ended in the lateral wall of the right sphenoidal sinus.

Problems. **Which orbital muscle is paralyzed**? What is its action? Which cranial nerve has been injured? Where is this nerve attached to the brain stem? Briefly describe its course. What anatomical feature makes this nerve so vulnerable to injury? *These problems are discussed on page 1099.*

Case 8-4. A 68-year-old man with a history of *arteriosclerosis* complained that he recently developed a **partial loss of sight** in his right eye. The family physician examined the patient's eyes during a physical examination, including *visual field tests.* He detected **right nasal hemianopsia** (Fig. 8-9*B*).

The patient was admitted to the hospital for **cardiovascular monitoring** and further ophthalmoscopic tests. *Cerebral angiograms* revealed a **berry aneurysm** (Fig. 7-91) of the right internal carotid artery, just above the right *anterior clinoid process* (Fig. 7-55). The **neuroradiologist** suggested that this vascular lesion was the probable cause for the patient's visual field defect.

Problems. Define right **nasal hemianopsia.** Which cranial nerve is involved? A lesion at what site of this nerve would produce the patient's symptoms? Briefly describe the cerebral part of the **internal carotid artery.** *These problems are discussed on page 1100.*

Case 8-5. A 38-year-old man complained of *failing eyesight.* An **ophthalmologist** found that he had a loss of the lateral halves of the fields of vision of both eyes and made a diagnosis of **bitemporal hemianopsia** (Fig. 8-9*D*). *Skull radiographs* demonstrated an **expanded sella turcica** (Fig. 7-56) and a *CT scan* showed a mass about 1.5 cm in diameter in the **suprasellar region.** A tentative diagnosis of a *neoplasm of the hypophysis cerebri* (pituitary gland) was made.

Problems. A lesion at which site of the visual pathway produces **bitemporal hemianopsia**? What is the relationship of the pituitary gland to this region of the **optic pathway**? Explain how a tumor of the hypophysis cerebri produces the visual defect observed? *These problems are discussed on page 1100.*

Case 8-6. The *chief complaint* of a 62-year-old woman was **severe headache** associated with **vomiting.** She said that her headache had been *constantly present for 3 days* and that it became worse when she coughed. She also mentioned an *alteration of vision in her right eye* and pointed out the **drooping of her right eyelid.**

The patient was admitted to the hospital where *stiffness of the neck* was noted. The **ophthalmoscopic examination** revealed: (1) *blurred optic discs* on both sides, but greater on the right; (2) *no pulsations of the retinal veins* (Fig. 7-102) of the right eye; (3) **dilation of the right pupil** which was not reactive to light on direct or consensual stimulation; (4) *ptosis of the right eyelid*; and (5) **inability to adduct the right eye** on left lateral gaze and to move this eye on upward or downward gaze.

Cerebral angiograms revealed an *aneurysm of the right posterior communicating artery* close to its junction with the internal carotid artery (see Fig. 7-90 for site).

Problems. The patient's husband asked the doctor to explain his wife's **headaches** and her **alteration of vision.** What do you think he would have said? *Which cranial nerve is involved*? Why do lesions of this nerve produce so many ocular symptoms? Name the muscles it supplies. *These problems are discussed on page 1100.*

Case 8-7. The neck of a 16-year-old hockey player was *deeply lacerated by a skate blade.* The 10-cm gash passed inferomedially across the *right anterior triangle of the neck* (Fig. 9-7), beginning about 6 cm below the **mastoid process** and extending through the *suprahyoid region.* The trainer was able to control the bleeding from the **lacerated superficial vessels** as he rushed the patient to a hospital. Under general anesthesia the wound was explored, the lacerated vessels were ligated, the nerves were sutured together, and then the wound was closed.

During a subsequent *neurological examination,* the following observations were made. The patient was *unable to rotate his head to the left side* or *shrug his right shoulder,* which was drooping slightly. *When he protruded his tongue, it deviated to the right side.*

Problems. What cranial nerves were injured? What muscles do they supply? What are the actions of these muscles? Where are the cell bodies of the motor neurons supplying these muscles located? *These problems are discussed on page 1101.*

Case 8-8. A 71-year-old woman experienced **tingling** and discomfort in her left frontonasal and maxillary regions. Soon afterwards she noted **redness** and slight **fever** on this side of her face. About 5 days after her initial symptoms, **skin eruptions** occurred in the same localized areas, including her *scalp.* Later **papules** (L. *papulae,* pimples) appeared which became vesicular, then pustular, and finally crusted. During the **eruptive period** she suffered *severe pain* in the left frontonasal and maxillary areas, *nausea,* and headaches. The **eruptive lesions** also appeared in the left side of her mouth and on her left cornea. There was marked **edema** beneath her eyes.

The condition was diagnosed as **herpes zoster**, *a disease of the nerves of the skin* and other tissues which they supply. Healing of the skin eruptions occurred after several weeks but the pain, **pruritus** (L. an itching) of her scalp, and *sensitivity of her left eye to light* persisted for several months. Anesthesia of the skin was present in the scarred areas of skin where the **herpetic eruptions** had occurred.

Problems. Which cranial nerve was involved? Which division(s) of this nerve was (were) affected? *List the areas to which these fibers supply branches.* Where are the cell bodies of these nerve fibers located? Describe the location of this aggregation or collection of neurons. Speculate on the cause of the anesthesia of the scarred areas of her face. *These problems are discussed on page 1101.*

DISCUSSION OF PATIENT ORIENTED PROBLEMS

Case 8-1. *Embolus* is a Greek term meaning a plug, wedge, or stopper. In the present case the *mass of atheromatous material* which formed the embolus resulting in the **embolic stroke** broke away from the *ulcerated atheroma* located at the origin of the right internal carotid artery. An **atheroma** (G. *athērē,* gruel + *oma,* tumor) is composed of *lipid deposits in the intima* of the artery and forms a yellow swelling on its endothelial surface. In the present case, **atheromatous material** broke free from the vascular lesion and was carried by the right internal carotid artery to the **right middle cerebral artery**, its larger terminal branch. This vessel ramifies over the lateral surface of the cerebral hemisphere (Fig. 7-89), including the **sensorimotor strip** surrounding the **central sulcus** of the brain (Figs. 7-51*B* and 7-76). *Occlusion of the cortical branches* of this artery therefore results in **contralateral paralysis** of muscles and *general sensory deficits.* The paralysis was in his left upper limb because the **right cerebral cortex controls movements on the left side** of the body. Because the anterior part of the parietal lobe of the cerebral cortex receives sensory input for cutaneous sensibility, the patient experienced *numbness in his left upper limb* on the extensor or posterior surface from the knuckles to the shoulder.

Carotid endarterectomy is a surgical operation which is performed for *removal of an atheroma from a carotid artery,* the right internal carotid in the present case. The artery is opened (**arteriotomy**) and its intima is stripped off along with the *atheromatous plaque* (F. *plaque,* plate). After the operation drugs are given to inhibit clot formation until the endothelium regrows on the artery.

Fibers of the patient's *right recurrent*

laryngeal nerve were injured during the operation, probably as the result of stretching during retraction of the **vagus nerve** (Fig. 9-84) from the operation site. *The recurrent laryngeal nerve arises from the vagus (CN X)* in front of the first part of the **subclavian artery** (Fig. 8-21). It then *hooks below the subclavian artery* before ascending obliquely to the side of the trachea behind the common carotid artery (Fig. 9-35). Hence, carotid endarterectomy may result in **trauma to the vagus nerve**, including fibers of the recurrent laryngeal nerve.

The recurrent laryngeal nerve supplies all the intrinsic muscles of the larynx (Figs. 9-49 and 9-84), except the cricothyroid, and distributes sensory branches to the mucous membrane below the level of the **vocal folds.** When fibers of the right recurrent laryngeal nerve were damaged in the present patient, *the right vocal fold became paralyzed*, producing a weak **hoarse voice.** Undoubtedly some fibers in his right recurrent nerve degenerated, but they underwent *slow regeneration* because the patient's voice returned almost to normal within 6 months.

Case 8-2. *CN VIII on the right side* was obviously involved in this case, producing a definite **loss of hearing** and some *disturbance of vestibular function.* The tumor on the vestibulocochlear nerve, called an **eighth nerve tumor** (often an *acoustic neuroma*), mainly affected the cochlear fibers of CN VIII which are concerned with hearing and take origin from the cells of the *spiral ganglion of the cochlea* (Fig. 7-195). Some of its vestibular fibers were also involved, as indicated by the abnormal vestibular function tests.

Because the *posterior root of CN V* is just a few millimeters above CN VIII (Fig. 9-34), an eighth nerve tumor may impinge on it, as in the present case, producing a **reduced corneal reflex**, without noticeable loss of sensation on the right side of the face supplied by the trigeminal nerve (Fig. 7-30*C*).

After leaving the medulla, CN VIII passes forward across the inferior border of the **cerebellar peduncle** in company with CN VII (Figs. 7-79 and 8-20). These nerves then enter the **internal acoustic meatus** (Fig. 9-34); hence, a lesion at the **medial orifice** of the internal acoustic meatus or within this canal in the **petrous part of the temporal bone** results in *varying degrees of hearing loss*, but CN VII involvement is not a common occurrence. **Injury to the facial nerve** results in *paresis or paralysis* of the *musculature* on the side of the lesion (**facial palsy**). CN VII is vulnerable to injury during removal of an eighth nerve tumor.

CN VII and CN VIII are closely related as they emerge from the medulla in the region of the internal acoustic meatus (Figs. 7-69, 8-7, and 9-34). After leaving the medulla they pass into the **internal acoustic meatus**; hence, the vestibulocochlear and facial nerves are frequently injured in *fractures of the middle cranial fossa* involving the mastoid or petrous parts of the temporal bone.

Case 8-3. The patient's **lateral rectus muscle** which abducts the eye is paralyzed (Fig. 8-25), indicating that the **abducens nerve** (CN VI) has been injured. *This is the only muscle supplied by this nerve.* The fibers of CN VI emerge from the inferior border of the pons in the sulcus between the caudal border of the pons and the cranial end of the medulla (Figs. 7-79, 7-55, and 8-7).

CN VI runs upward, forward, and laterally through the pontine cistern before piercing the *dura mater* about 1 cm below the root of the **dorsum sellae** of the sphenoid bone (Figs. 7-61 and 7-88). Once outside the dura, it runs superolaterally to the apex of the petrous part of the temporal

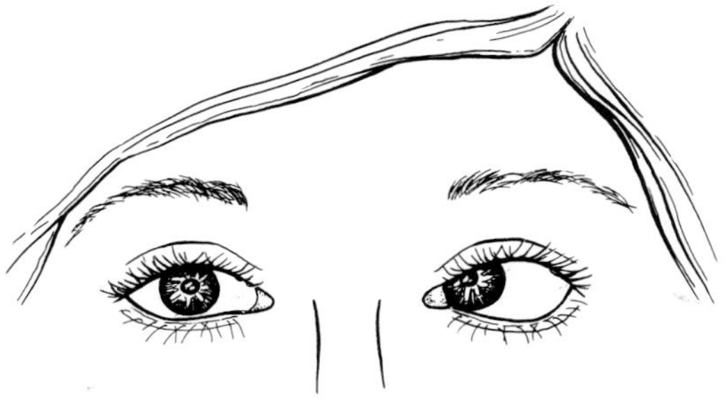

Figure 8-25. Drawing illustrating *paralysis of the right lateral rectus* muscle owing to injury to the abducens nerve. Observe that her right eye does not move laterally when she looks to her right.

bone and **enters the cavernous sinus** (Figs. 7-73 and 7-110). It leaves this sinus to enter the orbit through the **superior orbital fissure** (Figs. 7-55 and 7-88) with cranial nerves III, IV, and V^1.

CN VI has the longest intracranial course of all the cranial nerves which makes it vulnerable to **intracranial disease.** It is also vulnerable to injury in *fractures involving the base of the skull.* Its long course through the pontine cistern and its **sharp bend over the superior border of the petrous part of the temporal bone** also make it vulnerable to lesions that produce *downward displacement of the brain stem and stretching of CN VI.*

Case 8-4. *Right nasal hemianopsia* indicates that the patient has **no vision in the nasal half of the visual field** of the right eye (Fig. 8-9*B*) and that the lesion of the optic nerve is on the same side. A *localized dilation* or **aneurysm of the internal carotid artery** could exert pressure on the lateral border of the optic chiasma and cause nasal hemianopsia.

Fibers of the **right optic nerve** are involved in this case. This thick cylindrical nerve is *composed of myelinated nerve fibers which arise in the retina* (Figs. 7-101 and 8-6). It joins the anterolateral angle of the **optic chiasma** (Figs. 7-79 and 8-7), where the optic nerves meet anterior to the **infundibulum** (stalk of the hypophysis or pituitary, Figs. 7-90*B* and 8-8).

The internal carotid artery passes superiorly from its origin in the neck at the *bifurcation of the common carotid artery* (Figs. 9-22 and 9-24). It enters the **carotid canal** in the petrous part of the temporal bone (Fig. 7-73), passes through the **cavernous sinus** (Fig. 7-110), and perforates the dura mater medial to the *anterior clinoid process* (Figs. 7-55 and 7-88). It then **turns backward below the optic nerve.** The course of the internal carotid artery shows how an aneurysm of this vessel just above the anterior clinoid process could impinge on the lateral border of the optic chiasma.

Case 8-5. *Complete destruction* and/or failure of function of the optic chiasma results in **bilateral blindness. Tumors** (*e.g., meningiomas, pituitary tumors*) in the region of the optic chiasma *produce different visual field defects.* This variability results from variation in the **relation of the tumor to the chiasma** and of the chiasma to the anterior part of the arterial circle (Fig. 7-90).

A mass (**pituitary tumor** in this case) impinging on the *posterior edge of the optic chiasma* presses on the crossing fibers from the nasal halves of both retinae (Figs. 8-5 and 8-8) and produces *bitemporal hemianopsia.*

The optic chiasma (Figs. 7-79, 8-4, 8-5, and 8-8) is a *flattened bundle of optic nerve fibers* located at the junction of the anterior wall of the **third ventricle** with its floor (Fig. 7-82). Its anterolateral angles are continuous with the **optic nerves** and its posterolateral angles are continuous with the **optic tracts** (Figs. 7-79, 8-5, and 8-8). The *infundibulum,* passing from the pituitary gland to the floor of the third ventricle (**tuber cinereum**), touches or comes very close to the posterior edge of the optic chiasma (Fig. 7-79). *Neoplasms of the pituitary gland* result in an increase in the size of the **sella turcica**, the deep concavity which encloses the pituitary gland (Figs. 7-56 and 7-63). *The enlarging hypophysis exerts pressure on the inferior and/or posterior surface of the optic chiasma,* which causes **atrophy of the optic nerve fibers** coming from the lower nasal quadrants of the retinae (Fig. 8-5). As a result *the patient loses the upper temporal quadrants of his visual fields* (Fig. 8-9) *but retains his nasal fields.* In more advanced cases the entire temporal field on each side is lost.

Case 8-6. The doctor explained to the man that his wife has an **aneurysm** or circumscribed dilation of one of the major arteries supplying her brain. He drew a sketch of the **arterial circle** (of Willis), similar to that shown in Figure 7-90, explaining that this *arterial circle provides alternative routes of blood supply* when one of the major arteries leading to it is blocked. He further explained that *aneurysms usually develop where division points occur in the arteries* and drew a sketch similar to the one in Figure 7-91. He said that most aneurysms probably develop as the result of *congenital weakness of the arterial wall.*

The doctor explained to the husband that

in his wife's case, the aneurysm ruptured, allowing some blood to escape into the **subarachnoid space** around the brain and spinal cord that contains **CSF.** This produced the patient's severe headache by stretching and irritating the **meninges** or membranes covering the brain (Figs. 7-59 and 7-60). The meningeal irritation also produced some *spasm of the spinal muscles* resulting in her **stiff neck.**

The doctor also explained the patient's eye abnormalities to the husband (Fig. 8-26). He said that when the aneurysm enlarged, it impinged on the **oculomotor nerve**, which supplies all the muscles of the eye (*extraocular muscles*) except two (Fig. 8-10). As a result, the patient was *unable to look up, down, or medially with her right eye.* The **third nerve** also supplies the *sphincter of the iris* and the *ciliary muscle.* The doctor explained that the pupil of her right eye was larger than that on the normal side owing to the *absence of innervation of her sphincter pupillae*, the muscle that narrows the pupil (Fig. 7-97) when it contracts. When asked why her eyelid drooped, the doctor explained that the third nerve also innervates the muscle (**levator palpebrae superioris**, Fig. 7-96*A*) which elevates the upper eyelid. Thus, when it is paralyzed, the eyelid droops, a condition called ptosis.

Case 8-7. Fibers of the *accessory nerve* (**CN XI**) and of the *hypoglossal nerve* (**CN XII**) were severed by the neck laceration (Figs. 9-16, 9-21, and 9-22). The fibers of CN XI are motor to the **sternocleidomastoid** and **trapezius** muscles (Fig. 8-22), whereas the fibers of CN XII are motor to the intrinsic and extrinsic **muscles of the tongue** (Fig. 8-23).

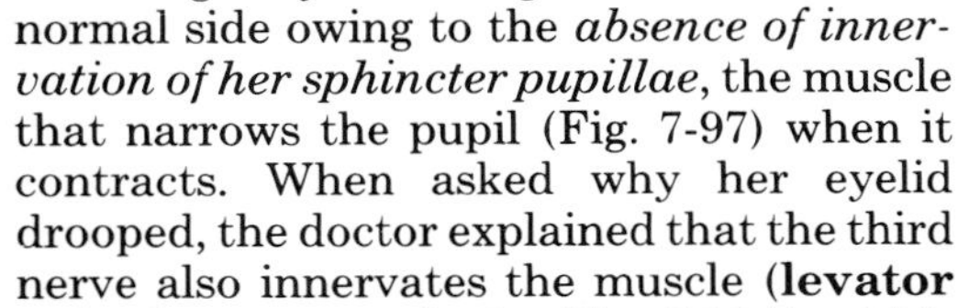

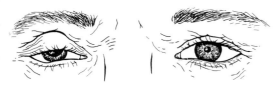

Figure 8-26. Drawing showing *right third nerve palsy.* Observe that her right upper eyelid droops (**ptosis**) owing to paralysis of the levator palpebrae superioris. Also observe that her *right pupil is dilated* owing to paralysis of the pupilloconstrictor fibers of CN III.

Acting individually, each *sternocleidomastoid muscle turns the head to the opposite side*; together they thrust the head forward to raise it from a pillow (see Chaps. 6 and 9). The *trapezius steadies, raises, and retracts the scapula*; it also rotates the scapula (see Chap. 6).

The motor neurons for the sternocleidomastoid and trapezius muscles are located in the ventral horns of the *spinal cord.* This elongated column of nerve cells, called the **spinal nucleus** of CN XI (Fig. 8-20), extends caudally as far as the *fifth cervical segment.* Arising as a series of rootlets from the side of the spinal cord, the **spinal root of CN XI** ascends in the *subarachnoid space* alongside the spinal cord and passes through the *foramen magnum,* where it joins the **cranial root** for a short distance (Figs. 8-20 and 8-22). Inside the skull it picks up a few rootlets from the caudal part of the **nucleus ambiguus** (Fig. 8-20). Having obtained all its fibers, it leaves the skull again through the **jugular foramen** (Fig. 7-72). Within this foramen its cranial and spinal fibers separate. The spinal fibers form an external branch which supplies the *sternocleidomastoid* and *trapezius* muscles (Figs. 8-22 and 9-11).

The **tongue muscles**, which move the tongue, are all supplied by CN XII except for the palatoglossus, which is supplied by the *vagus nerve* (Figs. 7-159 and 9-52). *The motor neurons for the tongue* muscles are located in the **hypoglossal nuclei** (Fig. 8-20) in the *floor of the fourth ventricle.* They are almost as long as the medulla. The nerve fibers from these nuclei course ventrally and *emerge as a series of rootlets between the pyramid and the olive* (Figs. 7-79 and 8-20).

This case illustrates why **surgical dissections of the neck** are conducted with great care and why the nerves are located and isolated before excision or incision of tissues is done (*e.g.*, removal of *cancerous lymph nodes*).

Case 8-8. *Herpes zoster is a sensory neuritis of viral cause, characterized by acute inflammation of sensory ganglia and fibers of craniospinal nerves.* It most commonly affects the thoracic (55%), cervical (20%), lumbar and sacral nerves (15%). Occasionally it affects the **trigeminal nerve.**

Based on the areas of the face affected, the fibers of CN V^1 and CN V^2 were involved in the present case (Fig. 7-30).

The trigeminal is the principal sensory nerve for the head and is the motor nerve for the muscles of mastication. Only the sensory fibers of the nerve were involved in this patient. Fibers of the **ophthalmic division (CN V^1)** were most severely affected, but those of **CN V^2** were also involved because the maxillary region of her face showed typical **herpetic eruptions.** The *inflammatory changes* causing irritation of the trigeminal ganglion cells and the fibers from it must have caused the **facial pain** which occurred before and after eruption of the vesicles. Destruction of the sensory twigs of CN V to the areas of erupted skin explains the loss of sensation (**anesthesia**) of the skin supplied by the ophthalmic and maxillary divisions of CN V.

The ophthalmic nerve, the superior division of CN V, is wholly sensory. *Herpes zoster* of the cranial nerves usually affects the **trigeminal ganglion.** Inflammation of the neurons in it may result in the death of some of them. The ensuing *scar formation in the ganglion* represents an abnormal irritant to the remaining neurons and probably explains the patient's facial pain (**postherpetic neuralgia**) many months after the eruptive stage. When **herpes** involves the region supplied by the ophthalmic nerve, the condition is referred to as *herpes zoster ophthalmicus* to indicate involvement of CN V^1.

CN V^1, the *ophthalmic nerve* (Fig. 8-11), supplies branches to (1) the *eyeball*, (2) the *conjunctiva*, (3) the *nasal mucosa* (superior part), and (4) the skin of the *nose, eyelids, forehead,* and *scalp* (Fig. 7-30*A* and *C*). **CN V^2**, *the maxillary nerve* (Fig. 8-11), supplies three cutaneous branches to a zone of skin, inferior and lateral to the eye (Fig. 7-30*A* and *C*).

The fibers of CN V^1 and CN V^2 and the sensory fibers of the other division of the trigeminal nerve (CN V^3) arise from neurons in the **trigeminal ganglion.** This large aggregation of neurons occupies a recess called the **trigeminal cave** (Figs. 5-38, 7-88, 7-133, and 8-7) in the dura mater covering the **trigeminal impression** (Fig. 7-56). This impression is on the anterosuperior surface of the apex of the petrous part of the temporal bone. On entering the pons the central processes of some cells in the trigeminal ganglion enter the *chief sensory nucleus of CN V* (Fig. 8-20); other processes descend to the *spinal nucleus of CN V.*

SUGGESTIONS FOR ADDITIONAL READING

1. Barr, M.L. *The Human Nervous System, An Anatomic Viewpoint*, Ed. 3, Harper & Row Publishers, Hagerstown, Maryland, 1979.

   A concise account of the cranial nerves with good illustrations of the cranial nerve nuclei and their connections. This widely accepted textbook of neuroanatomy has numerous clinical examples of lesions involving the cranial nerves.

2. Brodal, A. *Neurological Anatomy In Relation to Clinical Medicine*, Ed. 2, Oxford University Press, New York, 1969.

   This book gives a more detailed account of the cranial nerves than is required for most neuroanatomy courses. There is a thorough account of anatomical data which is of interest from a clinical point of view.

3. Carpenter, M. B. *Core Text of Neuroanatomy*, Ed. 2, The Williams & Wilkins Co., Baltimore, 1978.

   This widely used core text is beautifully illustrated. Several of these illustrations are included in the present book with the kind permission of the author and the publisher. Numerous clinical examples of cranial nerve lesions are included.

4. Chusid, J. G. *Correlative Neuroanatomy & Functional Neurology*, Ed. 17, Lange Medical Publications, Los Altos, California, 1979.

   This book is intended for the beginner in clinical neurology. It uses a concise format, charts, diagrams, and illustrations to present the material. Routine tests for the cranial nerves used in neurological examinations are described.

5. Mayo Clinic. *Clinical Examinations in Neurology*, Ed. 3, W. B. Saunders Co., Philadelphia, 1971.

   This book was written by 22 members of the Department of Neurology and the Department of Physiology and Biophysics in the Mayo Clinic at the University of Minnesota, Rochester, Minnesota. They present a factual outline of the practical components of the neurological examination.

6. Smith, C. G. *Basic Neuroanatomy*, Ed. 2, University of Toronto, Toronto, Ontario, 1971.

   This book presents a well organized concise account of the cranial nerves, their functional components, the course of their constituent fibers within the brain, and the location of their nuclei. The many three-dimensional drawings make it easy to understand the origin, course, and distribution of the cranial nerves.

CHAPTER 9

The Neck

The neck contains vessels, nerves, and other *structures connecting the head and the trunk* (*e.g.*, the carotid arteries, the jugular veins, the vagus nerves, the esophagus, and the trachea). It also contains very *important endocrine glands* (*e.g.*, the thyroid and parathyroids).

The common word collar is derived from the Latin word *collum*, meaning the neck. Many medical words are also derived from it; *e.g.*, **torticollis** (L. *tortus*, twisted + *collum*, neck) is the medical term for wryneck (Fig. 9-10). *Cervix* is another Latin word for the neck; hence the **cervical plexus** is a network of nerves in the neck and the cervical triangles are triangular areas of the neck.

As most lymphatic vessels in the head drain into deep **cervical lymph nodes**, their enlargement may indicate a tumor in the head, but it may be in the thorax or the abdomen because the neck connects the trunk and the head. There are several causes of **pain in the neck** (*e.g.*, inflamed lymph nodes, muscle strain, and protrusion of a cervical intervertebral disc).

This brief introduction indicates the clinical importance of the neck and the need for acquiring a clear understanding of its structure and functions. Many vital structures are crowded together in the neck, but there are good landmarks for helping you to locate them. Learn them well because missing one could result in a **misdiagnosis** or make a surgical procedure difficult and/or dangerous.

REGIONS OF THE NECK

SURFACE ANATOMY

The Posterior Aspect of the Neck. The surface anatomy of the back of the neck is described with the back (Chap. 5). Recall that the spinous process of the **axis** (C2) is the first bony point that can be felt in the midline below the external occipital protuberance and that the spinous process of the **vertebra prominens** (C7) is easily palpable and is usually clearly visible when the neck is flexed (Fig. 5-10). Recall that it is the bony landmark used when counting the vertebrae (see Chap. 5).

The Anterior and Lateral Aspects of the Neck (Figs. 9-1, 9-4, and 9-7). The **laryngeal prominence** ("Adam's apple")[1] is an important surface feature in the anterior midline of the neck. It is formed by the **thyroid cartilage** (Fig. 9-28), the largest one in the laryngeal skeleton (Fig. 9-73). The superior part of the thyroid cartilage is the most prominent and is more noticeable in men than in women and children and in some people more than in others. The sex difference in the angle formed by the **laminae** (plates) of the thyroid cartilage explains why the thyroid cartilage is indistinct in females. In Figure 9-2 note that the angle formed by the convergence of the laminae in the median plane is greater in females than in males. Also observe that each lamina in the male has a greater anteroposterior breadth than that in the female. Because of these anatomical differences, the superior border of the thyroid cartilage in most males projects anteriorly producing a distinct **laryngeal prominence** (Fig. 9-1). These sexual differences in the thyroid cartilages develop during puberty (13 to 16 years).

The thyroid cartilage (Fig. 9-72) lies at

[1] Supposedly this is where the forbidden fruit stuck in Adam's throat and is a fanciful way of accounting for the prominence of the male thyroid cartilage of the larynx. The anatomical basis for this sex difference is illustrated in Figure 9-2.

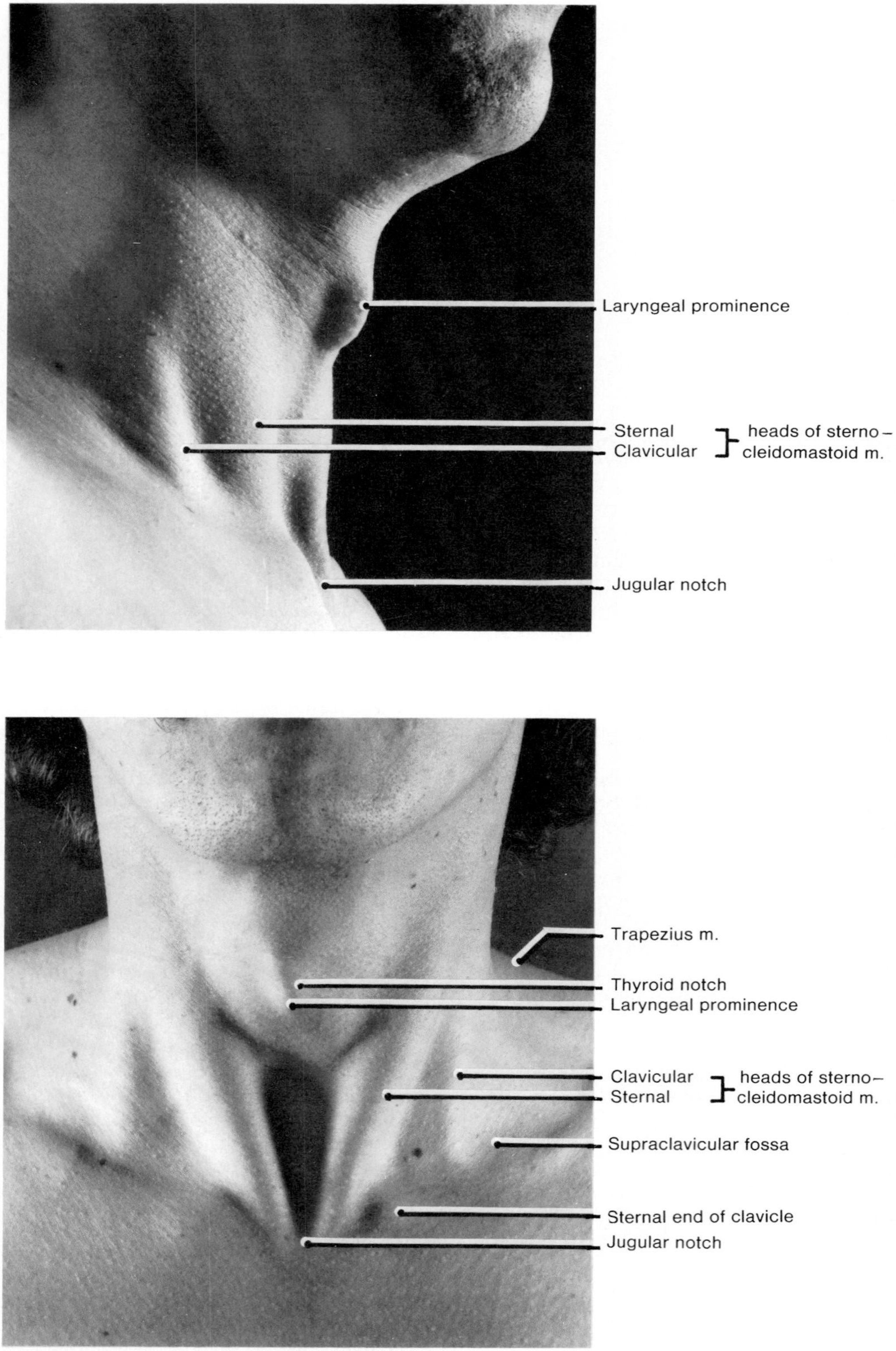

Figure 9-1. Surface features of the neck of a 28-year-old man. *A*, lateral view. *B*, anterior view. The laryngeal prominence is clearly visible in this person. The thyroid cartilage of the larynx is not prominent in most females (Fig. 9-38*B*). The anatomical basis of the laryngeal prominence in males is illustrated in Figure 9-28.

the level of the fourth and fifth cervical vertebrae and consists of two quadrilateral plates called laminae (Figs. 9-2 and 9-3), which can easily be felt. Grasp the laminae between your forefinger and thumb and move your thyroid cartilage from side to side. Also note that it rises when you swallow. Palpate the V-shaped **thyroid notch** on the superior border of your thyroid cartilage (Figs. 9-1*B* and 9-3*B*). The **vocal folds** (true vocal cords) lie about level with the midpoint of the anterior border of the thyroid cartilage (Figs. 9-76 to 9-79).

The hyoid bone (Figs. 9-4 and 9-5) lies just above the thyroid cartilage. This U-shaped bone is located at the level of the body of the third cervical vertebra. You can feel the body of the hyoid bone in the angle between the floor of the mouth and the front of the neck. It is *the first resistant structure felt in the midline below the chin* (Fig. 9-4). You can feel it more during swallowing. Grasp it between your forefinger and thumb and move it from side to side.

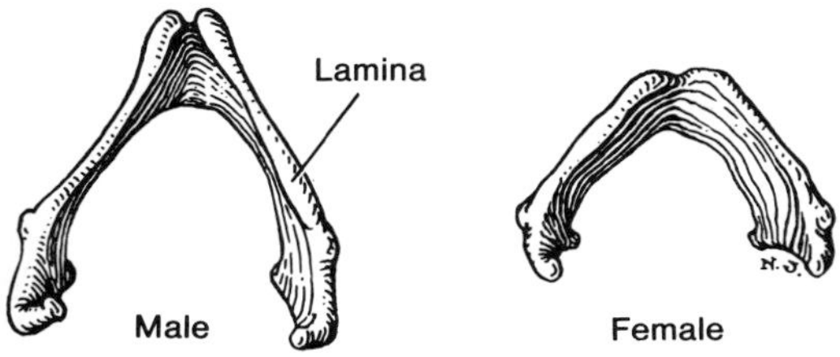

Figure 9-2. Drawings of male and female cartilages from above illustrating the sex difference in the angle at which the laminae meet. Note that the laminae in the male have greater anteroposterior breadths than those in the female. The above sex differences make the thyroid cartilage of the larynx more prominent in males than in females. Note the thyroid notch between the right and left laminae of the thyroid cartilage.

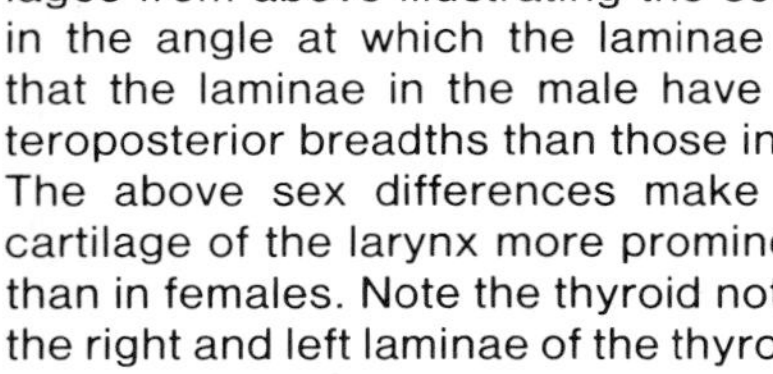

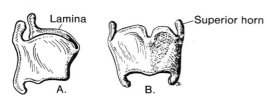

Figure 9-3. Drawings of the thyroid cartilage. *A*, from the right side. *B*, from the front. Observe the paired laminae, the thyroid notch (*arrow*), and the superior and inferiors horns.

You can palpate the tip of the **greater horn** (L. *cornu*) of one side of the hyoid if you steady the opposite side, as illustrated in Figure 9-5. Verify by palpation that the tips of the greater horns are fairly close to the anterior borders of the sternocleidomastoid muscles (Fig. 9-15).

CLINICALLY ORIENTED COMMENTS

The tip of the greater horn of the hyoid bone lies midway between the laryngeal prominence and the mastoid process (Fig. 9-4); thus, it is an important **surgical landmark for locating the lingual artery**, which arises from the external carotid posteroinferior to the tip of the greater horn of the hyoid (Figs. 9-6 and 9-31). Ligation of this artery is sometimes necessary, *e.g.*, during radical resection (L. cutting off) of the tongue because of the presence of a carcinoma (cancer) in it.

The tips of the transverse processes of the **atlas** (C1) can also be felt by deep palpation. Press upward with your forefinger between the angle of your mandible and a point 1 cm inferior and anterior to the tip of the mastoid process. As you do this, rotate your head slowly from side to side.

The cricoid cartilage is also part of the laryngeal skeleton; it lies inferior to the laminae of the thyroid cartilage (Figs. 9-4 and 9-73). It can easily be felt below the laryngeal prominence (Figs. 9-1 and 9-4). Extend your neck and run your fingertip down from your chin over your thyroid and cricoid cartilages. Note that after you pass the cricoid, your fingertip sinks in because the arch of the cricoid projects beyond the rings of the trachea (Fig. 9-4). In Figure 9-78 observe that the cricoid cartilage is *shaped like a signet ring* with its wide part (lamina) posterior and its narrow part (arch) anterior. Ensure that you can palpate the cricoid cartilage because it is a clinically important landmark, *e.g.*, in **tracheotomy** (Fig. 9-42). It lies at the level of the **sixth cervical vertebra** (Fig. 9-36), where the pharynx joins the esophagus and the larynx and the trachea join each other.

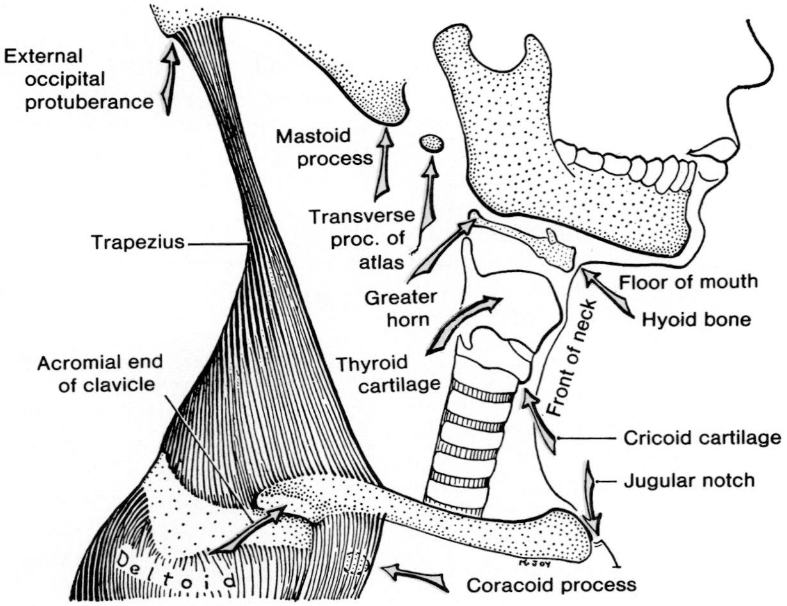

Figure 9-4. Drawing illustrating the bony landmarks of the neck. For a better view of the jugular notch, see Figure 9-1.

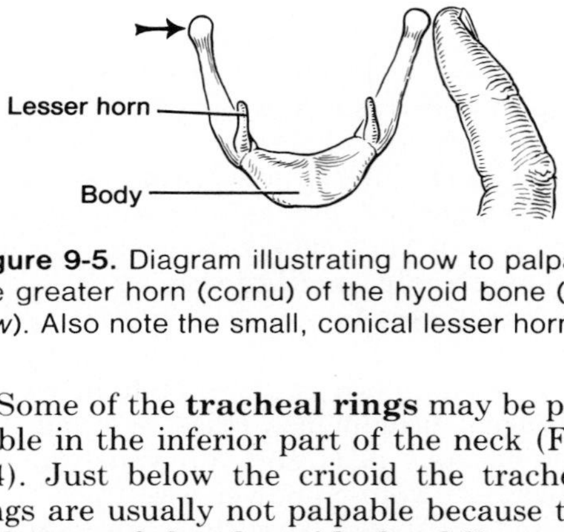

Figure 9-5. Diagram illustrating how to palpate the greater horn (cornu) of the hyoid bone (*arrow*). Also note the small, conical lesser horns.

Some of the **tracheal rings** may be palpable in the inferior part of the neck (Fig. 9-4). Just below the cricoid the tracheal rings are usually not palpable because the **isthmus of the thyroid gland** lies anterior to them (Fig. 9-43). Grasp the trachea between your forefinger and thumb, verifying that it is mobile and moves upward during swallowing.

The **lobes** of the **thyroid gland** are usually palpable, particularly in females in whom it enlarges during menstruation and pregnancy. Its isthmus, where the lobes are connected across the midline (Fig. 9-43), may be felt as a soft cushion-like mass about a fingerbreadth below the cricoid cartilage. The **isthmus of the thyroid** usually lies over the second and third tracheal rings. Feel it slip upward as you swallow and oscillate as you speak.

The **jugular notch** (suprasternal notch) is easily palpable between the medial ends of the clavicle and is clearly visible (Fig. 9-1*A*). It is a rounded depression in the superior border of the **manubrium sterni** (Fig. 9-30). Put your finger in the jugular notch and press posteriorly until you feel your **trachea**. If you let your finger slide laterally, it will encounter the narrow tendinous sternal head of the **sternocleidomastoid** (sternomastoid) muscle (Fig. 9-1). Let your finger pass over this tendon into a slight depression between the two heads of origin of the sternocleidomastoid. Run your finger over the clavicular head of this muscle and you will feel a large depression called the **supraclavicular fossa** (Fig. 9-1*B*); this fossa is clinically important [*e.g.*, it contains the **pressure point** for the subclavian artery (Fig. 9-13), which lies deep to it in the omoclavicular (subclavian) triangle (Fig. 9-15)].

The medial (sternal) ends of the **clavicle**

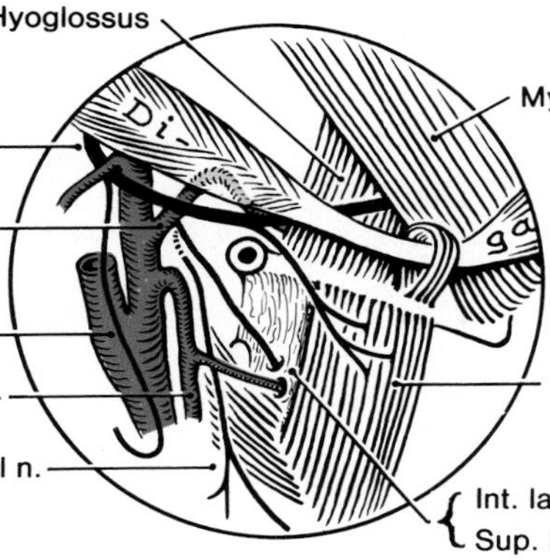

Figure 9-6. Drawing of the hyoid region of the anterior triangle of the neck (see Fig. 9-22 for a more extensive view of the area). The tip of the greater horn of the hyoid bone (*black dot*) is an important reference point for many muscles, nerves, and arteries in the neck (*e.g.*, note that the lingual artery arises from the external carotid just posterior to the tip of the greater horn).

are clearly visible at the root of the neck (Fig. 9-1*B*), particularly in thin persons. Palpate your clavicle, verifying that it is practically subcutaneous throughout its length. Observe its curves and general form on a skeleton as you palpate yours.

For purposes of description, the lateral aspect of the neck is divided into anterior and posterior triangles (Figs. 9-4 and 9-7). *Note the bony landmarks* forming the upper limit of the neck: the inferior margin of the **mandible**, the **mastoid process** of the temporal bone, and the **external occipital protuberance**.

Put your hand on your shoulder and then raise or shrug it as you feel the rounded edge of the large **trapezius muscle** (Figs. 9-1 and 9-7). Verify by palpation that it extends from the back of the head to the bones of the shoulder (*i.e.*, the **pectoral girdle** composed of the clavicle and the scapula).

The **trapezius** is a muscle of the upper limb that extends over the back of the neck in attaching the pectoral girdle to the skull and the vertebral column. The anterior border of the trapezius (Fig. 9-7) marks the posterior limit of the side of the neck and the midline of the neck demarcates its anterior limit.

The **sternocleidomastoid** muscle divides the lateral side of the neck into anterior and posterior triangles. Although you can define the boundaries of these triangles by palpation, they are also seen during dissection after the skin and the platysma muscle have been reflected (Fig. 9-15). *The sternocleidomastoid forms an important landmark in the neck* which stands out when contracted, forming a prominent ridge.

SUPERFICIAL AND LATERAL CERVICAL MUSCLES

The Platysma Muscle (Figs. 9-8 and 9-9). This wide, thin, subcutaneous sheet of muscle *lies in the superficial fascia.* The platysma (G. a flat plate) covers the superior part of the anterior triangle and the anteroinferior part of the posterior triangle. Its fibers blend superiorly with the facial muscles.

Origin (Fig. 9-8). **Fascia** and **skin** over pectoralis major and deltoid muscles.

Insertion (Fig. 9-8). **Inferior border of mandible** and **skin of lower face**.

Nerve Supply. **Cervical branch of facial** nerve (CN VII).

Actions (Fig. 9-9). **Tenses skin of neck** (*e.g.*, during shaving), **draws corners of mouth down**, and **assists in depressing mandible**. When the entire muscle contracts, it wrinkles the cervical skin in an oblique direction and widens the aperture of the mouth. It is *one of the muscles of facial expression* that we use to express

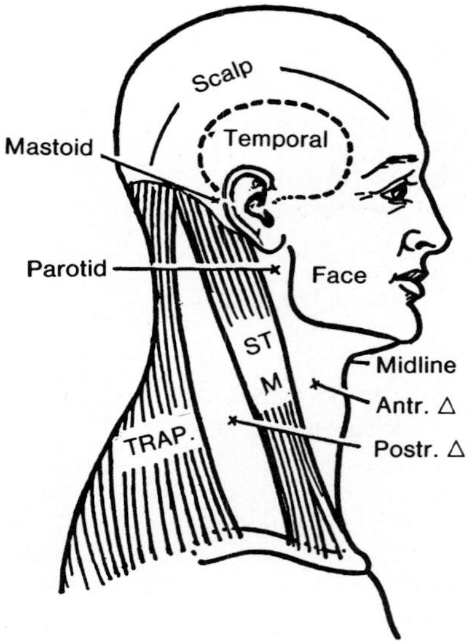

Figure 9-7. Drawing illustrating the superficial regions of the head and neck, particularly the anterior and posterior triangles. *ST M*, sternocleidomastoid muscle; *TRAP*, trapezius muscle.

sadness, horror, or fright. Men use this muscle to ease the pressure of a tight collar. It also acts during violent deep inspiration (*e.g.*, as occurs after a 200 m run).

CLINICALLY ORIENTED COMMENTS

Although the platysma is thin or absent in some people, it tenses the skin of the neck in most people. The platysma is well developed in animals (*e.g.*, horses) which use it to shake off flies. When very thin in man, the external jugular veins lie subcutaneously and are clearly visible, particularly when the intrathoracic pressure is raised (Fig. 9-38*B*).

If a well developed platysma is paralyzed owing to injury of the cervical branch of the facial nerve (*e.g.*, invasion by a malignant lesion in the parotid or submandibular area or by a laceration of the neck below the angle of the mandible), the skin tends to fall away from the neck in slack folds. Hence during surgical procedures performed in this region, *e.g.*, removal of a branchial cyst (Case 9-3), care is taken to preserve the mandibular and cervical branches of the facial nerve (Fig. 9-11). Injury to the mandibular branch produces a noticeable facial deformity, whereas damage to the cervical branch produces *unsightly postoperative defects* (*e.g.*, the skin of the neck droops in wrinkles). Similarly, surgeons carefully suture the edges of this muscle after neck surgery, *e.g.*, a thyroidectomy as in Case 9-5, to prevent gaping of the skin incision.

The Sternocleidomastoid Muscle (Figs. 9-1, 9-7, 9-11 to 9-15, and 9-28). The long name of this muscle indicates its origin and insertion. The "*cleido*" part of its name is derived from the Greek word *kleis* meaning clavicle. A long robust muscle, **the sternocleidomastoid is the key muscular landmark in the neck**. Running obliquely upward from the sternum and the clavicle to the lateral surface of the mastoid process, *it divides the side of the neck into anterior and posterior triangles* for purposes of description (Fig. 9-7); hence, swellings and other lesions in the neck can be described with reference to these **cervical triangles**. When it contracts, it stands out as a well defined prominence between the anterior and posterior triangles (Fig. 9-7).

To make your sternocleidomastoid stand out, put your chin upward and to one side. Palpate the anterior border of the rounded band of muscle on the other side. Begin at your **mastoid process** posterior to your **auricle** (external ear) and run your finger diagonally across your neck down to the sternoclavicular region. Verify that it has *two heads of origin*.

Origin (Figs. 9-1, 9-7, and 9-28). *Sternal head:* anterior surface of **manubrium sterni**. *Clavicular head:* upper surface of **medial third of clavicle**.

Insertion (Figs. 7-3, 9-4, 9-7, and 9-12). **Mastoid process** of temporal bone and **lateral half of superior nuchal line** of occipital bone.

Nerve Supply (Fig. 9-11). **Accessory (CN XI)** and ventral rumus of **second cervical nerve** directly.

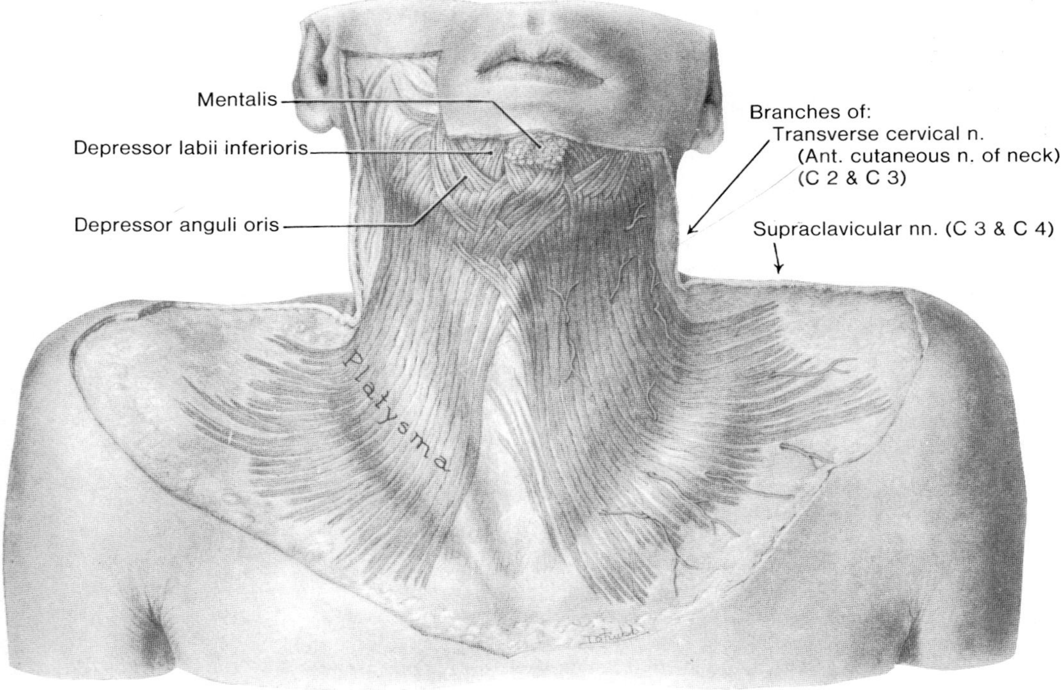

Figure 9-8. Drawing of a dissection of the platysma muscle. Observe that it spreads subcutaneously like a sheet and is pierced by cutaneous nerves. Note that it crosses the whole length of the inferior border of the mandible above and the entire length of the clavical below, extending downward to the level of the first or second rib. Observe that the platysma does not cover the median part of the neck, but overlies the superior part of the anterior triangle (Fig. 9-7) and most of the posterior triangle.

Actions. Acting alone, **tilts head to its own side** (laterally bends) and **rotates it** so the face is turned upward toward the opposite side. *Acting together,* they **flex the neck** (*e.g.*, when raising the head from a pillow against gravity).

CLINICALLY ORIENTED COMMENTS

Occasionally the sternocleidomastoid muscle is injured at birth, resulting in a condition known as **congenital torticollis** or wryneck (Fig. 9-10). There is fixed rotation and tilting of the head owing to *fibrosis and shortening of the sternocleidomastoid on one side.* Because torticollis or twisting of the neck is a correctable condition, it is rarely seen in an advanced form.

Most cases of torticollis result from tearing of fibers of the sternocleidomastoid when pulling the head during a difficult birth, particularly in a breech presentation (Case 9-1). Bleeding into the muscle may occur diffusely and/or in localized areas, the latter forming a small swelling (**hematoma**). Later a mass develops owing to **necrosis** (death) of muscle fibers and the formation of fibrous tissue (**fibrosis**) as part of the reparative or reactive process. Although this mass may disappear, it usually results in shortening of the muscle and torticollis by 3 to 4 years of age as the neck elongates. The shortening causes the typical lateral bending of the head to the affected side and the slight turning away of

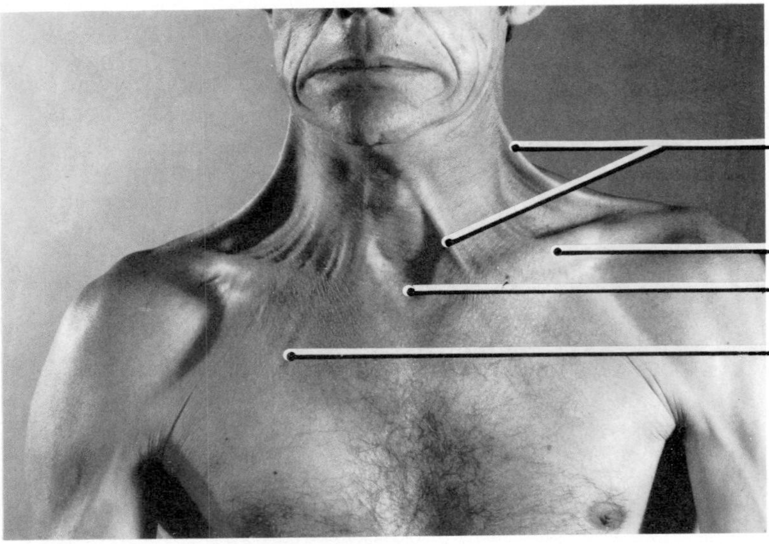

Figure 9-9. Photograph showing wrinkling of the skin in an oblique direction when the entire platysma is in action, as occurs during violent clenching of the jaws and drawing down of the corners of the mouth. Observe the fibers arising from the fascia and skin over the upper pectoral and anterior deltoid regions, particularly on the right. Note that the sheet of muscle passes over the clavicle and the front of the neck and that the clavicle stands out during contraction of the platysma. This muscle of facial expression may be used to indicate sadness and fright and to tense the skin of the neck (*e.g.*, during shaving).

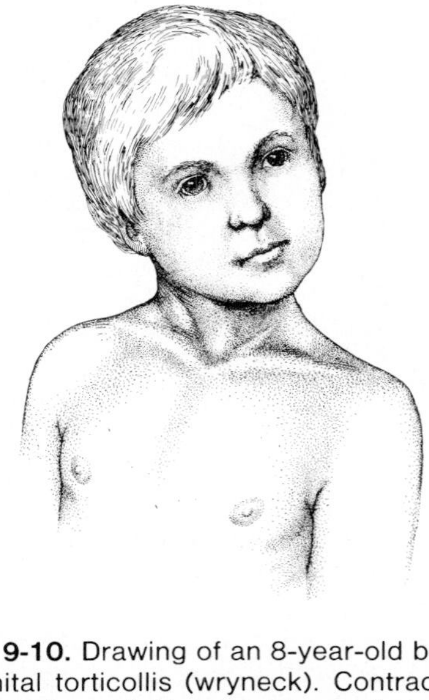

Figure 9-10. Drawing of an 8-year-old boy with congenital torticollis (wryneck). Contraction of the right sternocleidomastoid muscle resulting from fibrosis has drawn the head to the right and rotated it so that the chin points to the left.

the chin from the side of the short muscle (Fig. 9-10).

Usually daily turning and tilting of the head for several months (**physiotherapy**) stretches the affected muscle and corrects the condition, but in severe cases surgery and physiotherapy may be required to reduce the pull on the head. Failure to correct this abnormal condition will result in asymmetry of the skull, distortion of the face on the affected side, and an inability to turn the head normally.

POSTERIOR TRIANGLE OF NECK

Boundaries of Posterior Triangle (Figs. 9-7, 9-11, 9-12, and 9-15). The posterior cervical triangle is bounded *anteriorly* by the posterior border of the **sternocleidomastoid**, *posteriorly* by the anterior border of the **trapezius**, and *inferiorly* by the middle third of the **clavicle**. Thus, the clavicle forms the **base of the posterior**

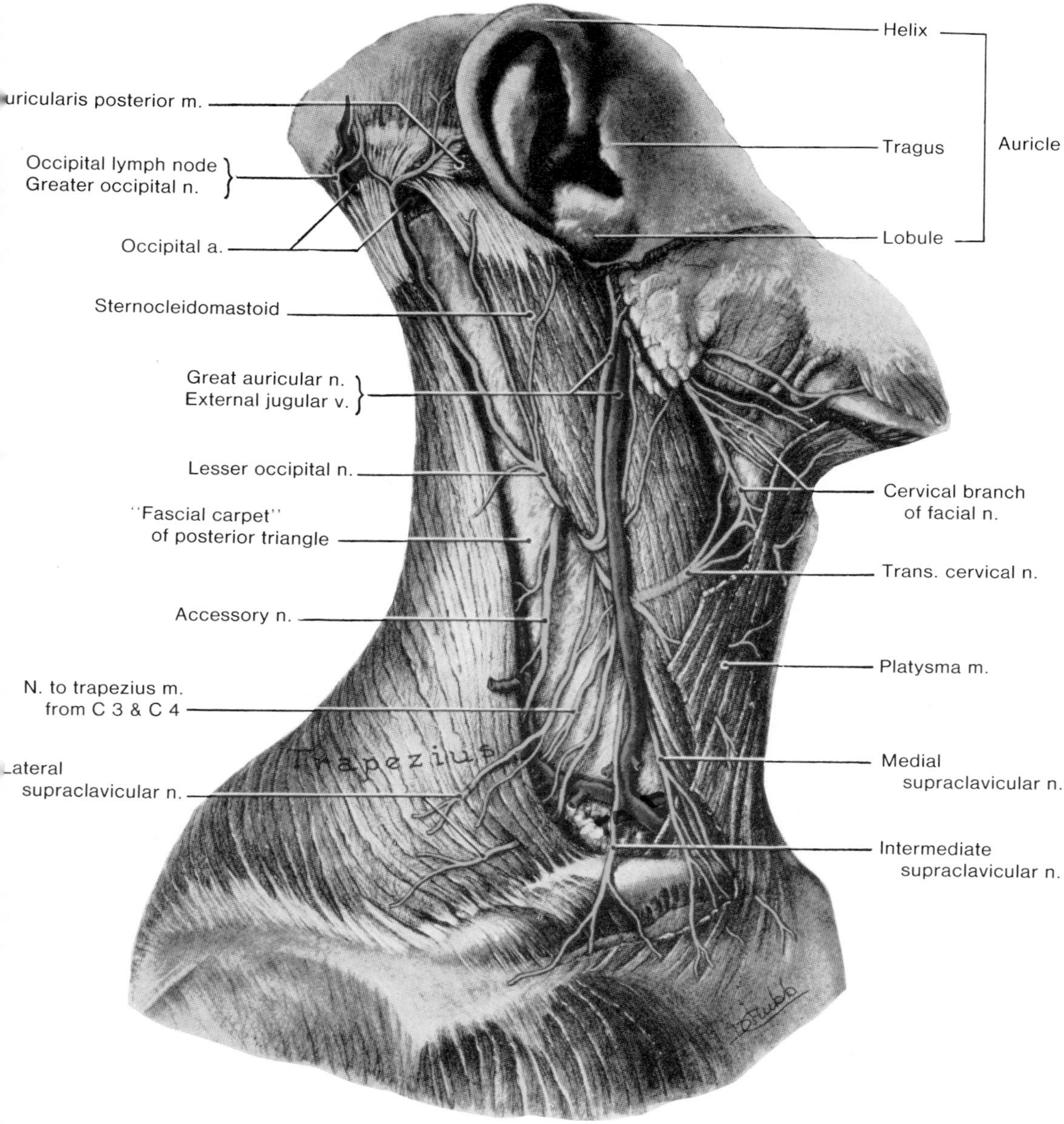

Figure 9-11. Drawing of a superficial dissection of the right side of the neck illustrating the posterior triangle. Observe its boundaries: anterior border of trapezius, posterior border of sternocleidomastoid, and middle third of clavicle (its base). The apex is where the aponeuroses of the two muscles blend a little below the superior nuchal line. The superficial fascia and the superficial layer of deep fascia have been removed. The deep cervical fascia is usually described as having two layers in some places, *e.g.*, where it splits to enclose the trapezius and sternocleidomastoid muscles and to form the roof and the floor of the posterior triangle. The fascial roof has been removed here, but the fascial floor of the posterior triangle is visible. This deep "fascial carpet" covers the muscular floor of the posterior triangle. Note the accessory nerve, the only motor nerve superficial to the "fascial carpet," descending within the deep fascia and disappearing two fingerbreadths or more superior to the clavicle.

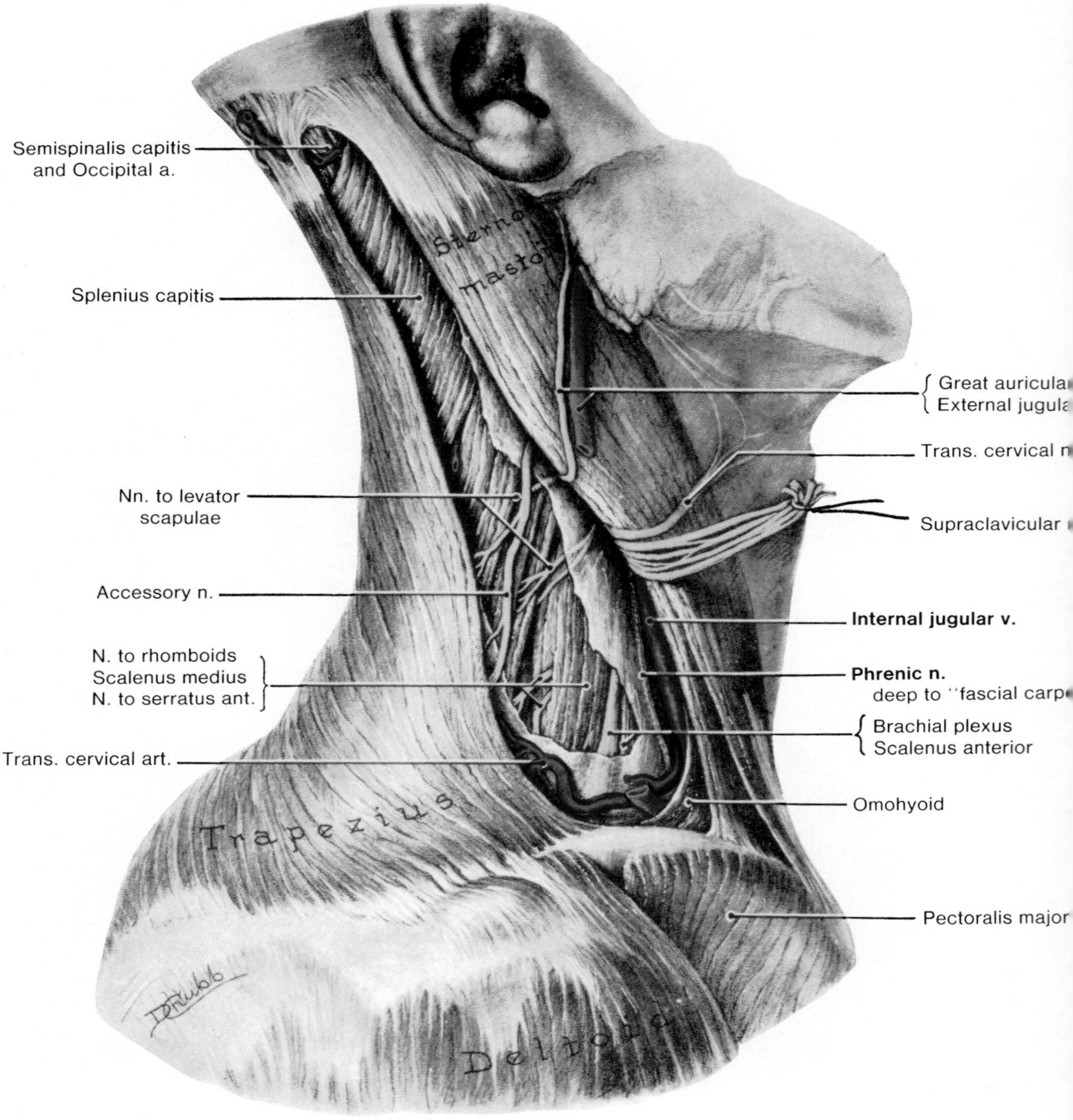

Figure 9-12. Drawing of a dissection of the right side of the neck showing the nerves deep to the deep "fascial carpet" on the floor of the posterior triangle. Observe the muscles forming the floor of the triangle (splenius capitis, levator scapulae, and scalenes). Note the accessory nerve to the sternocleidomastoid and the trapezius lying along the levator scapulae but separated from it by the "fascial carpet." Note the three motor nerves to upper limb muscles: to the levator scapulae (C3 and C4), to the rhomboids (C5), and to the serratus anterior (C5 and C6). Observe the two structures of surgical importance situated just beyond the geometrical confines of the triangle: (1) the phrenic nerve to the diaphragm (C3, **C4**, and C5); and (2) the internal jugular vein.

triangle, and the point where the borders of the sternocleidomastoid and trapezius muscles meet on the superior nuchal line forms the **apex of the posterior triangle**.

Roof of Posterior Triangle (Figs. 9-9 and 9-22). The posterior triangle is covered by deep fascia which covers the space between the trapezius and sternocleidomastoid muscles and splits to enclose these muscles and the posterior belly of the omohyoid muscle. Superficial to the **deep fascial roof** are the superficial fascia, the platysma, the superficial veins, the cutaneous nerves, and the skin.

Floor of Posterior Triangle (Figs. 9-11 to 9-13 and 9-38). From above downward, the floor of the posterior cervical triangle is formed by the **splenius capitis**, the **levator scapulae**, the three **scalene muscles** (scalenus posterior, scalenus medius, and scalenus anterior), and the first digitation of the **serratus anterior** muscle. This

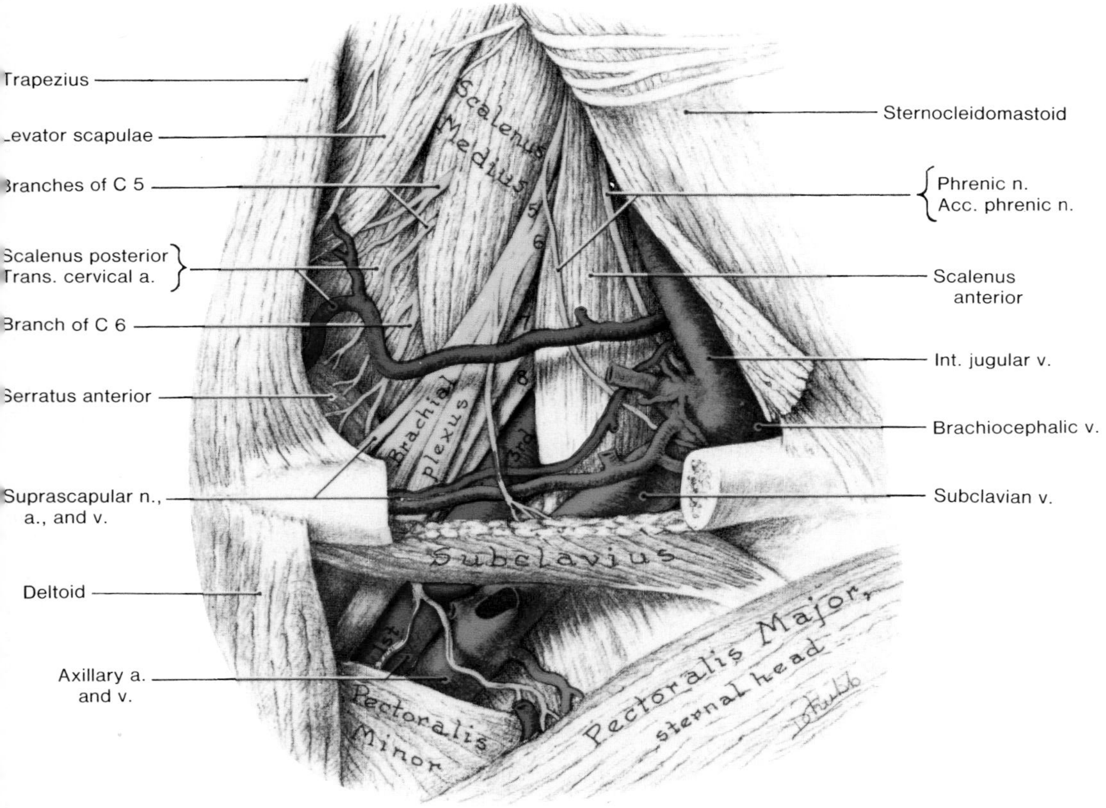

Figure 9-13. Drawing of a dissection of the right side of the neck and upper chest showing the brachial plexus and parts of the subclavian vessels in the posterior triangle of the neck. Observe the third part of the subclavian artery, the first part of the axillary artery, and the muscles forming the floor of the lower part of the triangle (scalene muscles and the first digitation of the serratus anterior). Note the brachial plexus and the subclavian artery appearing between the scalenus medius and scalenus anterior muscles and that the lowest root of the plexus (T1) is concealed by the third part of the artery. Observe that the subclavian vein hardly rises above the level of the clavicle and is separated from the second part of the subclavian artery by the scalenus anterior. Note that the internal jugular vein (usually the largest in the neck) is not in the posterior triangle but is very close to it.

muscular floor is covered by **cervical fascia**, which is a lateral prolongation of the prevertebral fascia (Figs. 9-40 and 9-50).

The **splenius capitus muscle**, the larger upper part of the splenius muscle (Fig. 5-46), arises from the **ligamentum nuchae** and the spinous processes of the **upper thoracic vertebrae** and runs superolaterally to insert into the **mastoid process** of the temporal bone and the lateral third of the **superior nuchal line** of the occipital bone, deep to the semispinalis muscle (Figs. 5-44 and 7-3). Acting together, they *extend the neck and the head on it.* They also slightly rotate the head.

The **levator scapulae muscle** arises from the transverse processes of the first four **cervical vertebrae**, passes deep to the trapezius, and inserts into the **medial border of the scapula** from the superior angle to the root of its spine (Fig. 6-49). As its name indicates, this muscle *elevates the scapula.*

The **scalenus posterior muscle** (often blended with scalenus medius) arises from the posterior tubercles of the transverse processes of the fourth, fifth, and sixth **cervical vertebrae** and inserts into the outer border of the **second rib**. It *elevates the second rib* and (acting from below) flexes the cervical region of the vertebral column.

The **scalenus medius muscle** arises from the posterior tubercles of the transverse processes of **all cervical vertebrae** and inserts into the upper surface of the posterior part of the **first rib**. It *helps to elevate the first rib* and (acting from below) flexes and *rotates the cervical region* of the vertebral column to the opposite side. In Figure 9-13 note that the *scalenus medius lies posterior to the roots of the brachial plexus* and the third part of the subclavian artery.

The **scalenus anterior** muscle *occupies a key position* in the inferior part of the neck. It arises from the anterior tubercles of the transverse processes of the **cervical vertebrae** (C3 to C6) and inserts into the **scalene tubercle** of the first rib (Fig. 9-33). It *assists in elevating the first rib* and (acting from below) flexes and rotates the cervical region of the vertebral column to the opposite side. *The scalenus anterior lies anterior to the roots of the brachial plexus* and the second part of the subclavian artery but posterior to the subclavian vein (Figs. 9-13, 9-14, and 9-33).

CLINICALLY ORIENTED COMMENTS

The scalenus anterior is a clinically important muscle because of its relationship to structures such as the subclavian artery, the brachial plexus, and the phrenic nerve (Figs. 9-13 and 9-14). Spasm or **hypertrophy of the scalenus anterior** muscle may lead to circulatory and neurological symptoms in the upper limb (**scalenus anticus syndrome** or scalenus neurocirculatory compression syndrome), similar to those produced by a **cervical rib** (Fig. 6-38). Transection of the scalenus anterior at its insertion is sometimes performed to alleviate the neurocirculatory compression.

There is a groove between the scalenus anterior and scalenus medius muscles which can be palpated just below the midpoint of the posterior border of the sternocleidomastoid muscle when the patient is in the supine position (*i.e.*, on the back) with the head turned away from the side to be examined. This groove is important because it indicates where the roots of the brachial plexus emerge from between these muscles to pass through the posterior triangle (Fig. 9-13) and where they are vulnerable to injury (*e.g.*, a stab wound).

Contents of the Posterior Triangle (Figs. 9-11 to 9-14). The posterior cervical triangle contains mostly vessels and nerves connecting the neck and the upper limb.

Veins in the Posterior Triangle (Figs. 9-11, 9-12, and 9-38). The **external jugular vein** begins near the angle of the mandible, just below the lobule of the auricle (ear lobe), by the union of the posterior division of the **retromandibular vein** with the **posterior auricular vein**. It crosses the sternocleidomastoid in the superficial fascia and then pierces the roof of the posterior triangle at the posterior border of this mus-

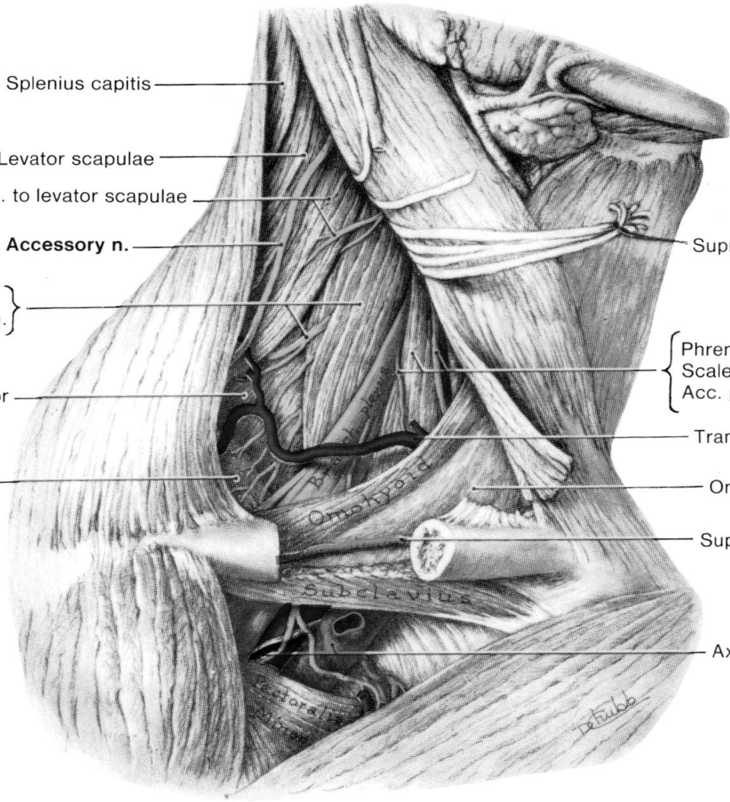

Figure 9-14. Drawing of a dissection of the right side of the neck and upper chest showing the muscles forming the floor of the posterior triangle. The deep fascia covering the floor (Fig. 9-11) and part of the clavicle have been removed. Note that the phrenic nerve that supplies the diaphragm is closely related to the anterior surface of the scalenus anterior muscle.

cle about 5 cm above the clavicle. The external jugular vein passes obliquely through the triangle and usually ends by emptying into the subclavian vein about 2 cm above the clavicle (Fig. 9-11). The external jugular vein drains most of the scalp and face on the same side.

CLINICALLY ORIENTED COMMENTS

When **venous pressure** is within the normal range, the external jugular vein is either invisible or observable for only a short distance above the clavicle when a person is lying in the supine position. However, when venous pressure is raised (*e.g.*, owing to **heart failure**), the external jugular vein becomes prominent throughout its course along the side of the neck. Consequently, routine observation of this vessel during physical examinations may give diagnostic signs of heart failure, obstruction of the superior vena cava (*e.g.*, by a tumor), enlarged supraclavicular lymph nodes, or increased intrathoracic pressure. Opera singers commonly exhibit bilateral enlargement of their external jugulars owing to the prolonged periods of high intrathoracic pressure required in their strenuous type of singing. Although uncommon, one or both external jugular veins may be absent. If present, they will become obvious when you compress their inferior ends just above the midpoints of the clavicles (Fig. 9-11) and when the person takes a deep breath and holds it (Fig. 9-38*B*).

Increased blood volume resulting from the administration of too much intravenous fluid will cause engorgement of the external and anterior jugular veins. For this reason, the neck of a patient receiving intravenous therapy is left uncovered so these signs of increased blood volume will be readily visible to all who care for the patient.

Should an external jugular vein be lacerated where it pierces the roof of the posterior triangle along the posterior border of the sternocleidomastoid about 5 cm above the clavicle (Fig. 9-11), air may be sucked into the vein during inspiration. This may occur because the vein does not retract (collapse) at this site owing to the attachment of its walls to the deep fascia. Consequently a **venous air embolism** fills the right heart with froth and practically stops blood flow through it. This results in **dyspnea** (difficult breathing), **cyanosis** (G. dark blue color), and sometimes death.

Arteries in the Posterior Triangle (Figs. 9-12 to 9-14). The third part of the **subclavian**, the large artery to the upper limb, begins about a fingerbreadth above the clavicle opposite the posterior border of the sternocleidomastoid. It lies hidden in the anteroinferior part of the posterior triangle, barely qualifying as one of its contents.

The **transverse cervical artery** (transverse colli) arises from the thyrocervical trunk (Figs. 9-29 to 9-33), a branch of the subclavian artery. It runs superficially lateralward across the posterior triangle, 2 to 3 cm above the clavicle (Fig. 9-40) deep to the omohyoid muscle, to supply muscles in the scapular region.

The **suprascapular artery** (Figs. 9-13 and 9-40), another branch of the thyrocervical trunk, passes inferolaterally across the lower part of the posterior triangle just superior to the clavicle. It then runs posterior to the clavicle to supply muscles around the scapula. Not infrequently this artery arises from the third part of the subclavian artery, lateral to the scalenus anterior, and passes anterior to the lower and middle trunks of the brachial plexus and posterior to the upper trunk.

The **occipital artery** (Figs. 9-11, 9-12, and 9-29), a branch of the external carotid, enters the apex of the posterior triangle before ascending over the posterior aspect of the head to supply the posterior half of the scalp.

Nerves in the Posterior Triangle (Figs. 9-11 to 9-15). The accessory nerve **(CN XI)** divides the posterior triangle into nearly equal upper and lower parts. The upper part contains only the lesser occipital nerve, which supplies the scalp, whereas the lower part contains numerous important nerves, *e.g.*, the ventral primary rami of the brachial plexus.

The accessory nerve enters the posterior triangle at or inferior to the junction of the superior and middle thirds of the posterior border of the sternocleidomastoid muscle (Figs. 9-11 and 9-12). It *passes posteroinferiorly* in the fascial roof of the posterior triangle and then disappears deep to the anterior border of the trapezius muscle at the junction of its upper two-thirds with its lower one-third.

The accessory nerve has spinal and cranial roots (*parts*). The **spinal root** is composed of fibers which arise from the cervical segments of the spinal cord (C1 to C5) and pass superiorly in the subarachnoid space to enter the posterior cranial fossa (Fig. 8-22) through the **foramen magnum**. Here it joins the **cranial root**, the fibers of which originate in the medulla and both leave the skull through the jugular foramen (Fig. 9-34). The spinal root of the accessory nerve then separates immediately from the cranial root and passes posteroinferiorly to supply the **sternocleidomastoid** (Fig. 8-22). It then crosses the posterior triangle superficial to the deep fascia covering its floor (Fig. 9-11) to supply the **trapezius** muscle. It passes deep to this muscle about 5 cm superior to the clavicle.

The **cervical plexus** (Figs. 9-11, 9-12, and 9-33) is a network of nerves formed by the communications between the ventral rami of the upper four cervical nerves. It lies deep to the internal jugular vein and the sternocleidomastoid muscle, immedi-

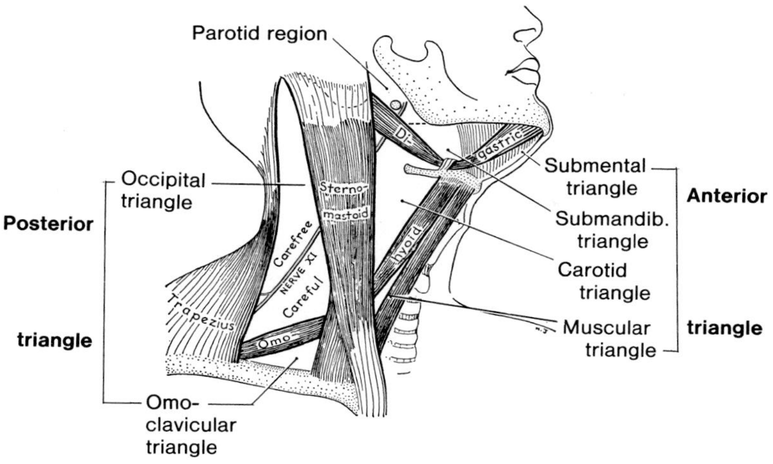

Figure 9-15. Drawing of the lateral aspect of the neck [right side] showing the triangles used for purposes of description. Note the important accessory nerve (CN XI) dividing the posterior triangle into nearly equal superior and inferior parts. The inferior part contains many important structures (Fig. 9-14); thus, careful surgical dissection is required so that these structures will be preserved. Note that the course of the accessory nerve is marked by two points: one slightly above the middle of the sternocleidomastoid muscle, and one about 5 cm above the clavicle at the anterior border of the trapezius. Observe that the inferior belly of the omohyoid muscle divides the posterior triangle into a large occipital triangle (superiorly) and a smaller supraclavicular triangle (inferiorly). The subclavian artery may be compressed against the first rib by deep pressure in the omoclavicular triangle (Fig. 9-15), which lies deep to the supraclavicular fossa (Fig. 9-1*B*).

ately *deep to the accessory nerve, CN XI.* Cutaneous branches from the cervical plexus emerge around the middle of the posterior border of the sternocleidomastoid to supply the skin of the neck and the scalp between the auricle and the external occipital protuberance (Fig. 7-30, *A* and *B*).

Nerves derived from the ventral rami of C2 to C4 via the cervical plexus:

The **lesser occipital nerve** (C2) ascends a short distance along the posterior border of the sternocleidomastoid (Fig. 9-11) before dividing into several branches that supply the skin of the neck and the scalp posterior to the auricle (Fig. 9-11). *The greater occipital nerve* is not in the posterior cervical triangle (Fig. 9-11). It is from the dorsal ramus of C2 and supplies the skin on the back of the scalp (Fig. 7-45).

The **great auricular nerve** (C2 and C3) curves over the posterior border of the sternocleidomastoid and ascends vertically toward the **parotid gland** (Figs. 9-11 and 9-12). It supplies branches to the skin of the neck and then divides into anterior and posterior branches that supply skin on the posterior aspect of the auricle and on an area extending from the mandible to the mastoid process.

The **transverse cervical nerve** (transverse colli, transverse nerve of the neck), from C2 and C3, passes transversely across the middle of the sternocleidomastoid to supply the skin over the anterior triangle of the neck (Fig. 9-11).

The **supraclavicular nerves** (C3 and C4) arise as a single trunk (Fig. 9-12) which divides into medial, intermediate, and lateral branches. They send small branches to the skin of the neck and then pierce the deep fascia just above the clavicle to supply skin over the front of the chest and the shoulder (Fig. 9-11). The medial and lateral supraclavicular nerves also supply the sternoclavicular and acromioclavicular joints, respectively.

The phrenic nerve, *the sole motor*

nerve supply to the diaphragm, arises from the ventral primary rami of the third, fourth, and fifth cervical nerves, but **mainly from C4**. It curves around the lateral border of the scalenus anterior muscle (Figs. 9-12 and 9-13) and descends obliquely across its anterior surface deep to the transverse cervical and suprascapular arteries (Fig. 9-40). It enters the thorax by crossing the origin of the internal thoracic artery between the subclavian artery and vein.

CLINICALLY ORIENTED COMMENTS

Severance of the phrenic nerve in the neck results in complete paralysis and atrophy of all the muscle of the corresponding half of the diaphragm. Injury to both nerves causes **dyspnea** (difficulty in breathing). Other lesions in the neck irritate the phrenic nerves causing **hiccups** (singultus).

The **supraclavicular part of the brachial plexus** is located in the posterior triangle, lying immediately anterior to the scalenus medius muscle and the first digitation of the serratus anterior muscle (Fig. 9-13). The infraclavicular part of this important plexus of nerves to the upper limb is located in the **axilla** (Fig. 6-25). The whole plexus is about 15 cm in length. The brachial plexus is formed by the ventral primary rami of the lower four cervical and the first thoracic nerves. There is often a small contribution from the fourth cervical and the second thoracic nerves. The plan of the brachial plexus and the nerves derived from it are discussed in Chapter 6 and illustrated in Figures 6-25 and 6-27.

Branches of the ventral primary rami of cervical nerves supply the rhomboid, the serratus anterior, and the nearby prevertebral muscles. Along the lateral border of the brachial plexus, the **suprascapular nerve** (Fig. 9-13) runs across the posterior triangle to supply the supraspinatus and infraspinatus muscles, which join the scapula to the humerus.

CLINICALLY ORIENTED COMMENTS

The region around the midpoint of the posterior border of the sternocleidomastoid muscle is often called the **nerve point of the neck** because several nerves lie superficially here, deep to the platysma (Fig. 9-11). **Slash wounds of the neck** may sever these relatively superficial nerves, resulting in loss of cutaneous sensation in the neck and posterior part of the scalp (Figs. 7-30, *A* and *B*). When extensive surgical dissections are done in the posterior cervical triangle, the accessory nerve is located and isolated in order to preserve it.

Cervical Nerve Blocks. For regional anesthesia prior to surgery, nerve blocks (temporary arrest of nervous impulses) are performed by injecting anesthetic solutions around the nerves from the cervical and brachial plexuses.

Cervical Plexus Block (Figs. 9-11 to 9-14). The anesthetic solution is injected at several points along the posterior border of the sternocleidomastoid muscle. The main point of injection is at the junction of the superior and middle thirds of this muscle, *i.e.*, around the accessory nerve. Because the phrenic nerve (supplying half of the diaphragm) is usually paralyzed by these blocks, they are not performed on patients with pulmonary and/or cardiac disease.

Brachial Plexus Block (Figs. 9-11 to 9-14). For anesthesia of the upper limb, the anesthetic solution is injected around the brachial plexus of nerves. The main point of injection is above the midpoint of the clavicle; the needle is directed medially and downward toward the first rib to infiltrate the brachial plexus. The subclavian artery is located by palpation prior to making the injections in order to avoid entering it.

Muscles in the Posterior Triangle (Figs.

9-12 to 9-14). The muscles in the floor of the posterior triangle have been discussed. The slender inferior belly of the strap-like **omohyoid muscle** (G. *omos*, shoulder), described with the infrahyoid muscles (Fig. 9-20), passes within the fascia of the roof from the anterior to the posterior triangle on its way to the scapula (Figs. 9-15 and 9-40). It runs one to two fingerbreadths above the clavicle to which it is attached by a fascial sling. This muscle, important as a landmark in the neck, can often be seen contracting when thin people speak.

Subdivisions of Posterior Triangle (Fig. 9-15). The inferior belly of the omohyoid muscle divides the posterior triangle into a large **occipital triangle** superior to it and a small **omoclavicular (subclavian) triangle** inferior to it. The occipital triangle was given this name because its superior part contains a portion of the occipital bone. The most important nerve crossing the occipital triangle is the **accessory nerve** (CN XI). The smaller omoclavicular triangle is indicated on the surface of the neck by the supraclavicular fossa (Fig. 9-1). The **external jugular vein** crosses the omoclavicular triangle superficially (Fig. 9-13) and the subclavian artery lies deep in it. These vessels are covered by the omohyoid fascia (Fig. 9-40*A*).

CLINICALLY ORIENTED COMMENTS

Pressure in the supraclavicular fossa will occlude blood flow in the subclavian artery where it passes over the superior surface of the first rib (Fig. 9-40*B*). In the event of **hemorrhage in the upper limb**, pressure in this fossa will control the bleeding because the subclavian artery supplies the upper limb.

The accessory nerve may also be used to divide the posterior triangle into a carefree area superiorly and a careful or dangerous area *inferiorly* (Fig. 9-15), indicating that care is essential during surgical dissection inferior to the nerve because of the presence of many vessels and nerves.

ANTERIOR TRIANGLE OF NECK

Boundaries of Anterior Triangle (Figs. 9-7 and 9-15). The anterior cervical triangle is bounded by the **anteromedian line** of the neck, the inferior border of the **mandible**, and the anterior border of the **sternocleidomastoid** muscle. The **apex** of the triangle is at the **jugular notch** and its **base** is formed by the **inferior border of the mandible** and a line drawn from the angle of the mandible to the mastoid process (Figs. 9-1 and 9-4). Practice outlining this important triangle with your forefinger.

The Hyoid Muscles (Figs. 9-15 to 9-18). The hyoid bone is held in place by several muscles that are attached to the mandible, the skull, the thyroid cartilage, and the scapula. *These muscles are primarily concerned with steadying or moving the hyoid bone and the larynx.* For purposes of description, they are divided into suprahyoid and infrahyoid muscles.

The Suprahyoid Muscles (Figs. 9-16 to 9-19). These muscles, as their group name indicates, lie superior to the hyoid bone. They include the mylohyoid, the geniohyoid, the stylohyoid, and the digastric muscles.

The Mylohyoid Muscles (Figs. 9-16 to 9-18). The two thin, flat mylohyoids form a supporting sling under the tongue that supports the floor of the mouth. The Greek word *mylē* means a mill and denotes the relationship of this muscle to the mouth where the food is ground.

Origin (Figs. 7-21 and 9-20). Entire length of **mylohyoid line of mandible**.

Insertion (Figs. 7-21 and 9-19). **Body of hyoid** bone and **median fibrous raphe**, extending from symphysis menti of mandible to body of hyoid.

Nerve Supply. **Mylohyoid** nerve, a branch of the inferior alveolar.

Actions. **Elevates hyoid** and **tongue** in swallowing and speaking and raises floor of mouth. Palpate it as you press the tip of your tongue against your upper incisor teeth.

The Geniohyoid Muscle (Figs. 9-16 and 9-18). This short narrow muscle is in con-

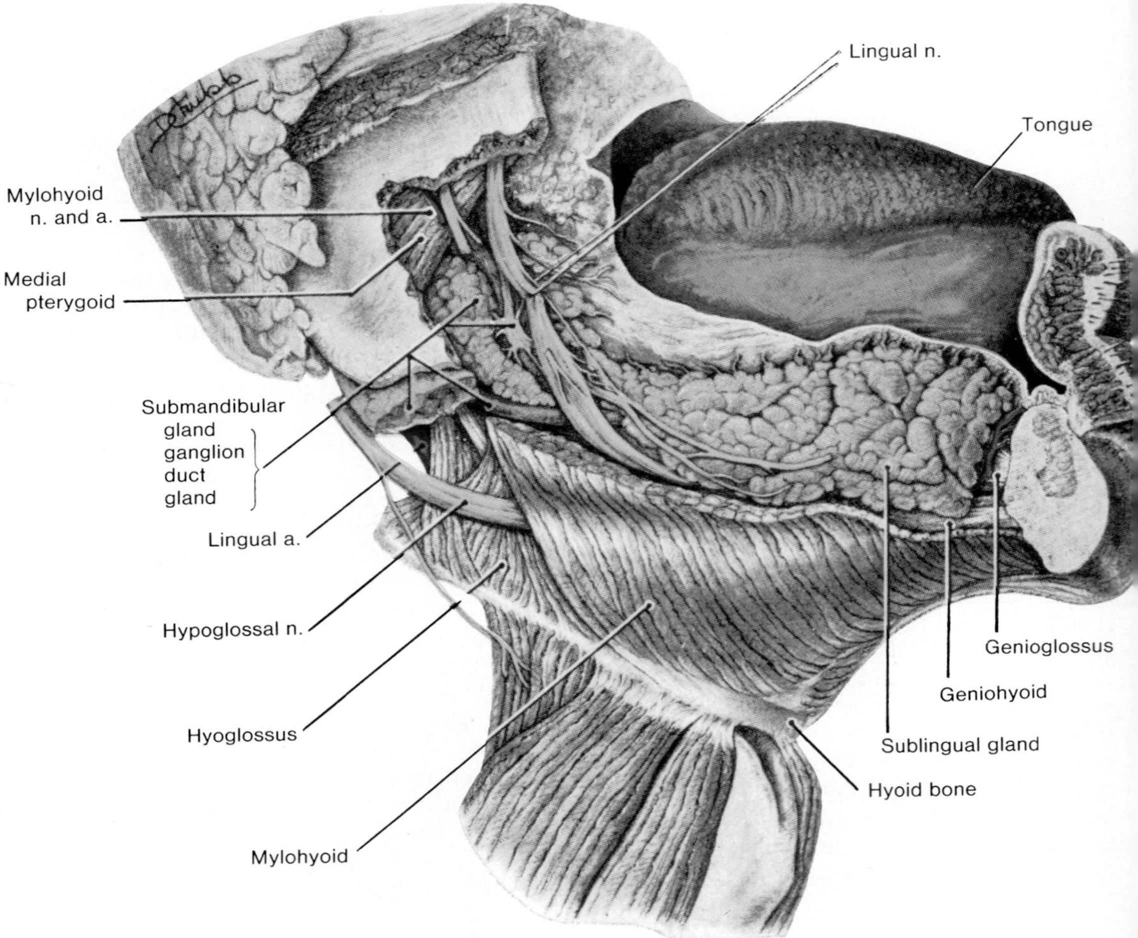

Figure 9-16. Drawing of a dissection of the suprahyoid region. The right half of the mandible and the superior part of the mylohyoid muscle are removed. Observe that the cut surface of the mylohyoid muscle becomes progressively thinner as it is traced forward. Note the mylohyoid nerve and artery (cut short) and the lingual nerve (clamped) between the medial pterygoid and the ramus of the mandible.

tact with its partner in the midline. The pair of muscles lies superior to the mylohyoids and reinforces the floor of the mouth.

Origin (Fig. 7-22). **Inferior mental spine of mandible**.

Insertion (Fig. 9-19). **Body of hyoid** bone.

Nerve Supply. Ventral ramus of first cervical nerve, *i.e.*, **C1 via hypoglossal** (CN XII).

Actions. **Pulls hyoid anterosuperiorly,** thereby shortening the floor of the mouth and widening the pharynx for receiving food during swallowing.

The Stylohyoid Muscle (Figs. 9-17 and 9-18). This small slip of muscle is nearly parallel to the posterior belly of the digastric muscle.

Origin (Figs. 7-7 and 9-17). **Styloid process** of temporal bone.

Insertion (Fig. 9-19). **Hyoid bone** at junction of body and greater horn.

Nerve Supply. **Facial** nerve (CN VII).

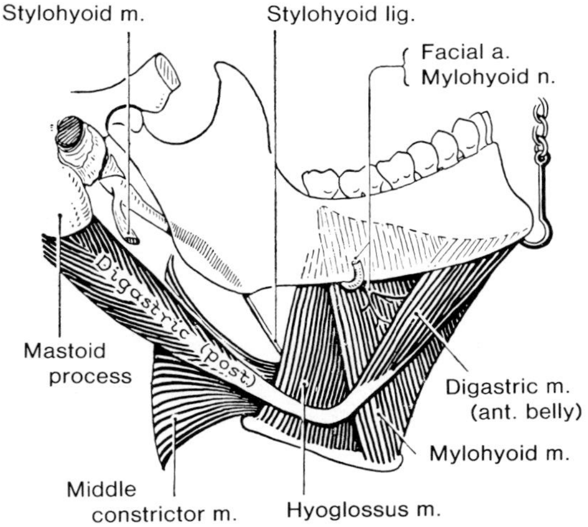

Figure 9-17. Drawing of the suprahyoid muscles showing that they are arranged in layers.

Actions. **Elevates** and **retracts hyoid** bone (*i.e.*, upward and backward), thereby elongating the floor of the mouth in swallowing.

The Digastric Muscle (Figs. 9-15 to 9-18 and 9-20). The name of this muscle indicates that it has **two bellies** (G. *gastēr*, belly or stomach). The bellies are joined by an intermediate tendon.

Origin and Insertion (Figs. 7-22, 9-17, and 9-22). *The anterior belly* arises from the **digastric fossa** on the inner surface of the lower border of the mandible, close to the symphysis. *The posterior belly* arises from the **mastoid notch** on the medial side of the mastoid process of the temporal bone. The two bellies descend toward the hyoid bone and are joined by an **intermediate tendon** which is connected to the hyoid bone by a strong loop of fibrous con-

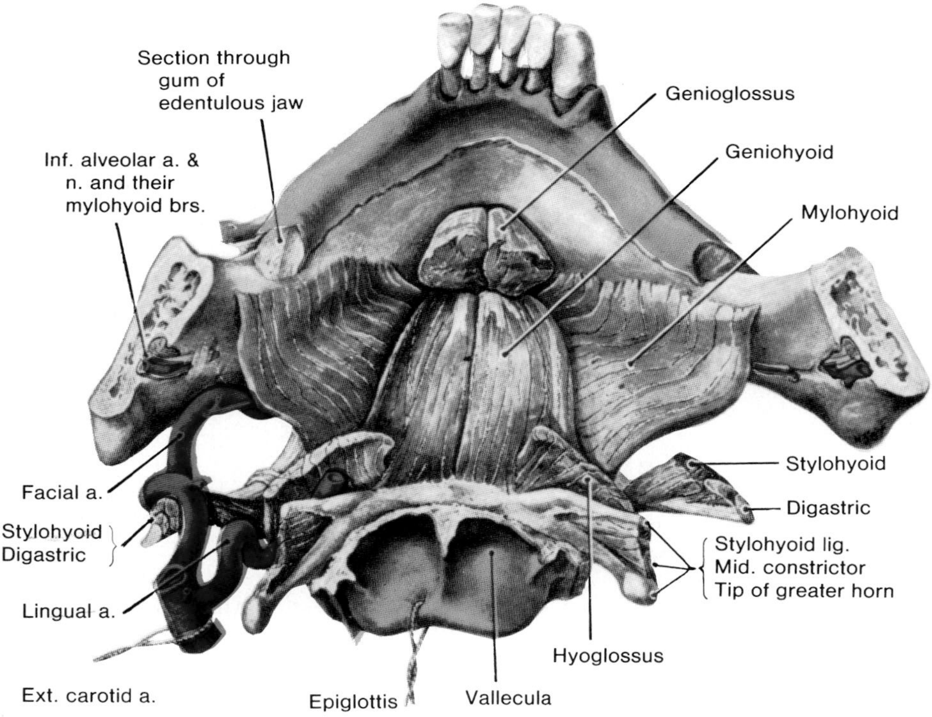

Figure 9-18. Drawing of a dissection showing the muscles of the floor of the mouth. Observe the paired, triangular geniohyoids occupying a horizontal plane, with their apex at the mental spine and their base at the body of the hyoid bone. The two mylohyoids form a muscular floor for the oral cavity which supports the tongue, the sublingual glands, and other structures shown in Figure 9-16. Note the mylohyoid arising from the whole length of the mylohyoid line of the mandible.

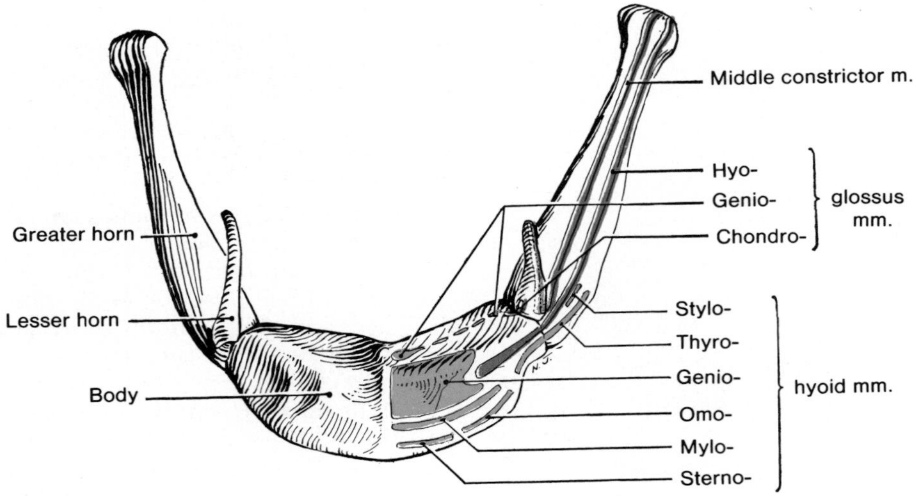

Figure 9-19. Drawing of the hyoid bone showing the sites of attachment of the hyoid muscles. *Red*, origins; *blue*, insertions. The term hyoid is derived from the Greek work *hyoeidēs*, which means shaped like the letter upsilon (*i.e.*, U-shaped). Note its greater and lesser horns (cornua).

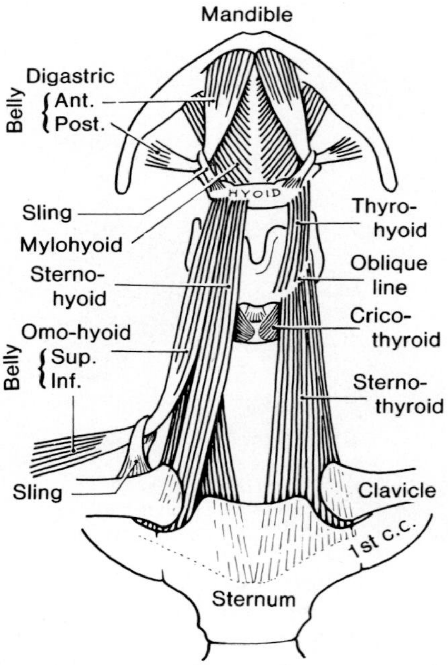

Figure 9-20. Drawing of the infrahyoid muscles (often called the strap muscles). Note that there are three flattened strap muscles in the anterior triangle.

nective tissue (Figs. 9-15 and 9-20). This fibrous pulley allows the tendon to slide backward and forward.

Nerve Supply. The two **bellies are supplied by different nerves**: the *anterior* by the **mylohyoid** nerve, a branch of the inferior alveolar nerve, and the *posterior* by the **facial** nerve (CN VII). This difference in nerve supply results from the derivation of the anterior and posterior bellies from the first and second branchial arches, respectively. CN V is the nerve to the first arch and CN VII supplies the second arch.

Actions. Acting together both bellies **raise the hyoid bone** and **steady it** during swallowing and speaking. *Acting from behind,* they **open the mouth and depress the mandible**. To feel the hyoid being elevated by the digastrics, grasp your hyoid between your thumb and forefinger as you swallow.

The Infrahyoid Muscles (Figs. 9-20 to 9-23 and 9-28). Because of their ribbon-like appearance, these muscles are often called the **strap muscles**. *All four of them act to depress the hyoid bone and the larynx* during swallowing and speaking.

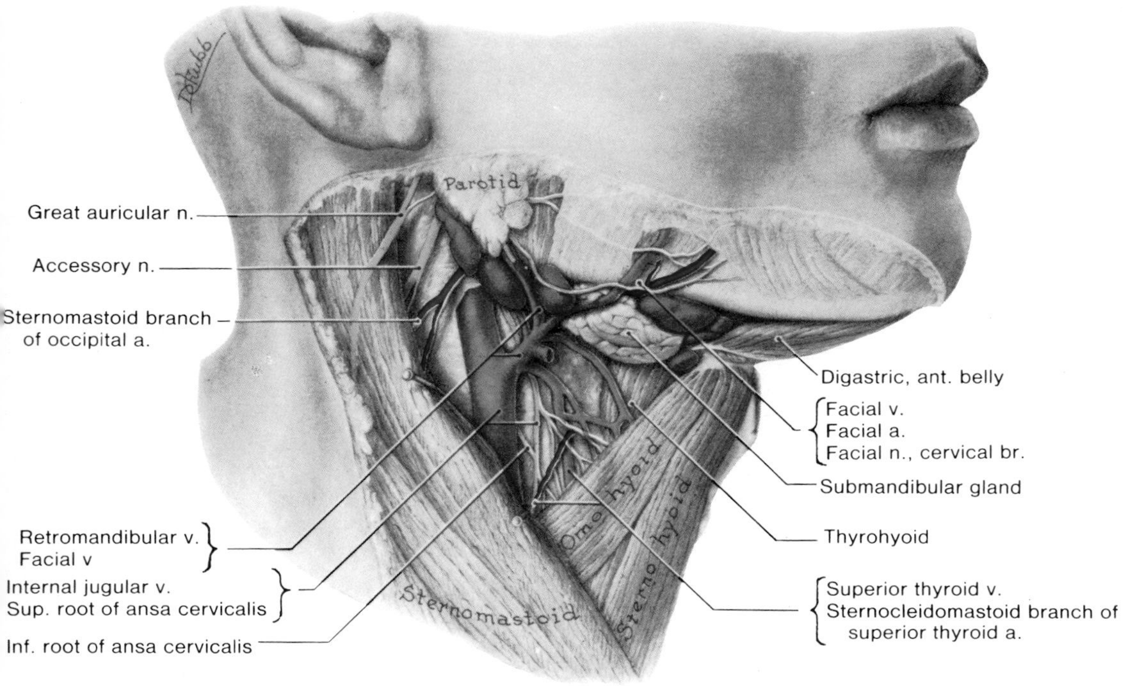

Figure 9-21. Drawing of a superficial dissection of the anterior triangle of the neck. Observe the submandibular gland, lymph nodes (*green*), and the cervical branch of the facial nerve in the submandibular (digastric) triangle. Note the retromandibular and facial veins running superficial to the submandibular gland.

The Sternohyoid Muscle (Figs. 9-20, 9-21, and 9-28). This thin narrow strap muscle is superficial, except inferiorly where it is covered by the sternocleidomastoid muscle.

Origin (Fig. 9-20). **Posterior surface of manubrium** sterni and **medial end of clavicle**.

Insertion (Fig. 9-19). Lower border of **body of hyoid bone**.

Nerve Supply (Fig. 9-22). Ventral rami of first three cervical nerves, *i.e.*, **C1 to C3 via ansa cervicalis** (L. *ansa*, a loop), a slender nerve root in the cervical plexus.

Action. **Depresses hyoid** bone after it has been elevated during swallowing.

The Sternothyroid Muscle (Figs. 9-20 and 9-22). This thin muscle is located deep to the sternohyoid and is shorter and wider than the sternohyoid muscle.

Origin (Fig. 9-20). **Posterior surface of manubrium** sterni and **first costal cartilage**.

Insertion (Fig. 9-20). **Oblique line of thyroid cartilage**.

Nerve Supply (Fig. 9-22). Branches from **ansa cervicalis**.

Action. **Depresses thyroid cartilage** after it has been elevated during swallowing and vocal movements.

The Thyrohyoid Muscle (Figs. 9-20 and 9-22). This muscle appears as the superior continuation of the sternothyroid muscle.

Origin (Fig. 9-20). **Oblique line of thyroid cartilage**.

Insertion (Fig. 9-19). **Lower border of body** and **greater horn of hyoid** bone.

Nerve Supply. Ventral ramus of **first cervical nerve** via the **hypoglossal** nerve (CN XII).

Actions. **Depresses hyoid** bone and **elevates thyroid cartilage**.

The Omohyoid Muscle (Figs. 9-14, 9-15, 9-20 to 9-23, and 9-40). Like the digastric

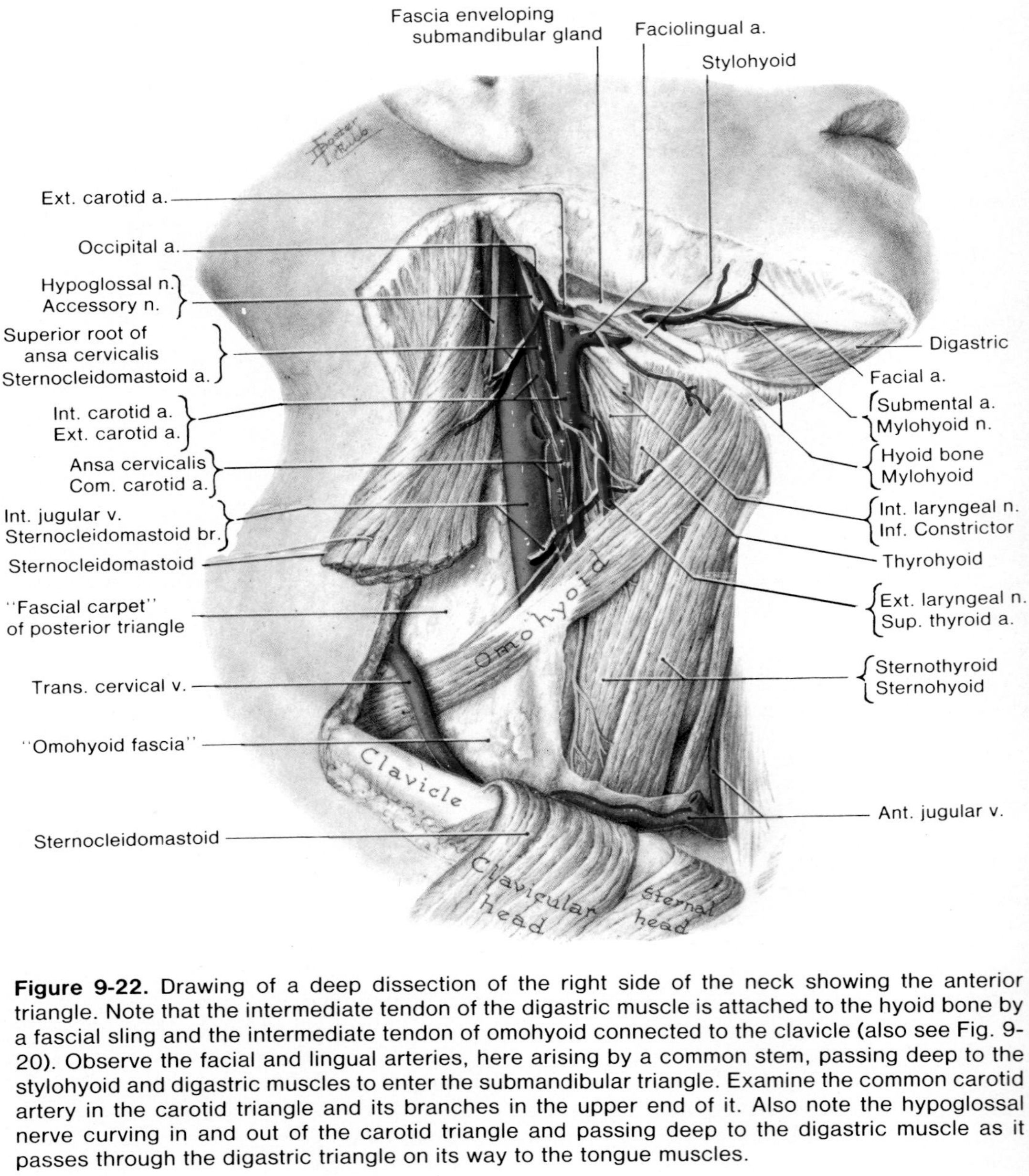

Figure 9-22. Drawing of a deep dissection of the right side of the neck showing the anterior triangle. Note that the intermediate tendon of the digastric muscle is attached to the hyoid bone by a fascial sling and the intermediate tendon of omohyoid connected to the clavicle (also see Fig. 9-20). Observe the facial and lingual arteries, here arising by a common stem, passing deep to the stylohyoid and digastric muscles to enter the submandibular triangle. Examine the common carotid artery in the carotid triangle and its branches in the upper end of it. Also note the hypoglossal nerve curving in and out of the carotid triangle and passing deep to the digastric muscle as it passes through the digastric triangle on its way to the tongue muscles.

this muscle has **two bellies** united by an intermediate tendon. It is connected to the clavicle by a **fascial sling**. The prefix *omo* in this muscle's name is derived from the Greek word meaning shoulder. *This muscle is an important landmark in the neck* and divides the posterior triangle into occipital and omoclavicular triangles.

Origin and Insertion (Figs. 9-15, 9-19, 9-21, and 9-22). *Inferior belly* arises from **upper border of scapula** and ends in **intermediate tendon**, from which the *su-*

perior belly arises and inserts into **lower border of hyoid** bone.

Nerve Supply (Figs. 9-21 and 9-22). Both bellies are supplied by the **ansa cervicalis.**

Actions. **Depresses, retracts,** and **steadies hyoid** bone in swallowing and speaking. In thin persons, the inferior belly can often be seen contracting during speech.

Subdivisions of Anterior Triangle (Fig. 9-15). In addition to the unpaired **submental triangle**, each anterior triangle is divisible into three smaller triangles: **submandibular, carotid**, and **muscular.**

The Submandibular Triangle (Figs. 9-15, 9-21, and 9-22). This **glandular area** on each side lies between the inferior border of the mandible and the anterior and posterior bellies of the digastric muscle; thus it is also called the digastric triangle.

The submandibular gland (Figs. 9-16 and 9-20) nearly fills the submandibular triangle. It wraps itself around the free posterior border of the mylohyoid muscle, not unlike a letter U on its side (⊂). This thin sheet of muscle separates the superficial and deep parts of the gland. The submandibular gland is about *half the size of the parotid gland* and is usually palpable as a soft mass between the body of the mandible and the mylohyoid muscle (Fig. 9-21). It is easily felt when you tense your mylohyoid by forcing the tip of your tongue against your upper incisor teeth. If it becomes inflamed (*e.g.*, owing to mumps), you can see the swelling formed by the enlarged gland.

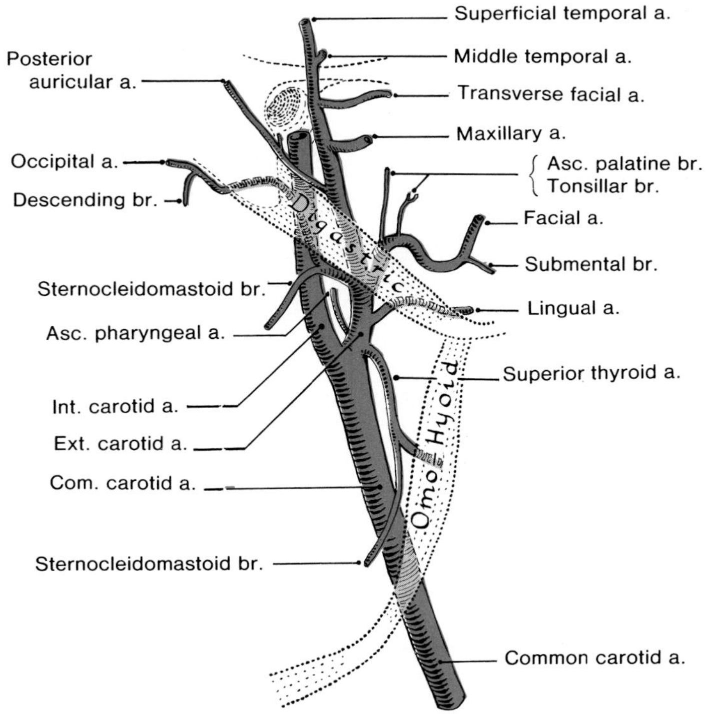

Figure 9-23. Diagram of the carotid arteries and their branches in the right side of the neck (for better orientation, see Fig. 9-22). Note that the common carotid divides into two terminal branches, the internal and the external, and that neither the common carotid nor the internal carotid gives off branches in the neck. The carotid triangle is of considerable surgical significance because it contains these parts of the carotid system of arteries (Fig. 9-15).

In Figure 9-21 note the position of the **submandibular lymph nodes**. They lie on the submandibular gland and along the lower border of the mandible (Fig. 9-66). Be certain you know what the normal submandibular gland feels like so you will later be able to differentiate it from enlarged lymph nodes, *e.g.*, owing to **metastases from a lip cancer** (Case 7-4). Tense your platysma as in Figure 9-9 and verify that the submandibular gland is deep to this superficial muscle. The **submandibular duct**, about 5 cm in length, passes from the deep process of the gland parallel to the tongue to open by one to three orifices into the oral cavity on the **sublingual papilla** at the side of the frenulum of the tongue (Figs. 7-161 and 9-16).

The **hypoglossal (CN XII) nerve** to the tongue muscles passes into the submandibular triangle (Figs. 9-16 and 9-22), as do the **mylohyoid nerve** and parts of the facial artery and vein.

The Carotid Triangle (Figs. 9-15 and 9-21 to 9-23). This **vascular area** is bounded by the superior belly of the **omohyoid**, the posterior belly of the **digastric**, and the anterior border of the **sternocleidomastoid**. It is an important area because the **common carotid artery** ascends into it, where its pulse can be auscultated (L. to listen to) with a stethoscope or palpated by placing the forefinger in the triangle and compressing the artery lightly against the transverse processes of the cervical vertebrae. At the level of the upper border of the thyroid cartilage, the common *carotid artery divides within the carotid triangle* into internal and external branches; thus, the triangle is important surgically.

The carotid sinus (Figs. 9-24, 9-29, and 9-36) is a slight dilation of the proximal part of the internal carotid artery which may involve the common carotid. This *blood pressure regulating area* is innervated principally by the glossopharyngeal nerve (CN IX) through a branch, the **carotid sinus nerve** (Fig. 8-18); however, it is also supplied by the vagus (CN X) and the sympathetic division of the autonomic nervous system. It *reacts to changes in arterial blood pressure* and effects appropriate modifications reflexly.

CLINICALLY ORIENTED COMMENTS

Although the common carotid artery can be occluded by compressing it against the carotid tubercle of the sixth cervical vertebra (Fig. 9-36) for control of hemorrhage in the neck, it is recommended that you not practice this on your colleagues because **syncope** may result (*i.e.*, the person may faint owing to deficiency of blood to the brain, **cerebral anemia**). *The carotid sinus responds to an increase in arterial pressure*, slowing the heart owing to parasympathetic outflow from the brain via the vagus nerve. Pressure on the sinus may also cause syncope, and if the person happens to have a **supersensitive carotid sinus**, it may cause cessation of the heart beat (temporary or permanent).

In elderly people with asymptomatic occlusion of one internal carotid artery owing to **atherosclerosis** (a type of arteriosclerosis or hardening of the arteries), occlusion of the common carotid on the other side will deprive the brain of a major source of blood and result in unconsciousness in 10 to 12 sec. As soon as the pressure is released, the patient should regain consciousness, but a permanent neurological deficit is likely to be produced if the artery is occluded for several minutes.

Carotid Endarterectomy. Atherosclerotic thickening of the intima of arteries supplying the brain will cause partial or complete obstruction of the blood flow. The resulting symptoms depend on the vessel obstructed, the degree of obstruction, and the collateral blood flow from other vessels, *e.g.*, the *cerebral arterial circle* (Fig. 7-90). The obstruction can be relieved partly or completely by opening the artery (**arteriotomy**) and stripping off the offending plaque with the adjacent intima. A common site for this operation, called a carotid endarterectomy, is the **internal carotid artery** just distal to its origin. After the operation drugs are used to inhibit clot formation at the operated area until the endothelium has regrown at the site. During this operation, several nerves in the carotid triangle, *e.g.*, the vagus and the **recurrent laryngeal nerves** (Figs. 9-22, 9-27, 9-30, 9-

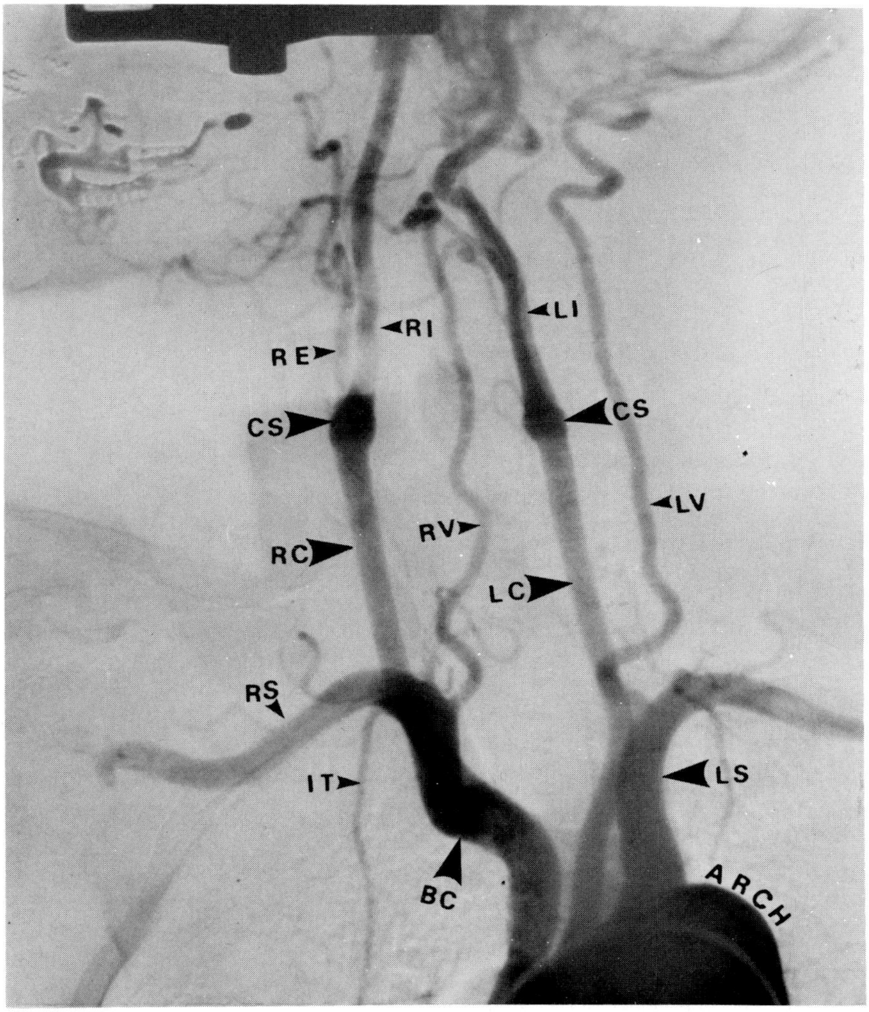

Figure 9-24. Arteriogram of the neck. The arteries were injected with a radiopaque material before the film was taken. Note that the brachiocephalic artery (*BC*) divides into right subclavian (*RS*) and right common carotid (*RC*) arteries, and that the common carotid divides into right external (*RE*) and right internal (*RI*) carotids. Observe the internal thoracic arising from the subclavian as is the right vertebral artery (*RV*). *On the left* observe the common carotid (*LC*), internal carotid (*LI*), and the tortuous course of the left vertebral artery (*LV*). On both sides observe the carotid sinus (*CS*). Distention of the wall of this pressure receptor stimulates nerve endings in it which results in a reflex showing of the heart and a fall in blood pressure. When this radiograph was taken the patient was lying supine in a right posterior oblique position (*i.e.*, right scapula on table and left shoulder elevated) with the face to the right.

46, and 9-84), may be injured and may produce an alteration in the voice (Case 8-1). Temporary paralysis of nerves may occur as the result of postoperative edema affecting them.

The carotid body (Fig. 9-25) is a small, flattened, ovoid mass of tissue located at the bifurcation of the common carotid artery. The carotid body is a *chemoreceptor that responds to changes in the chemical*

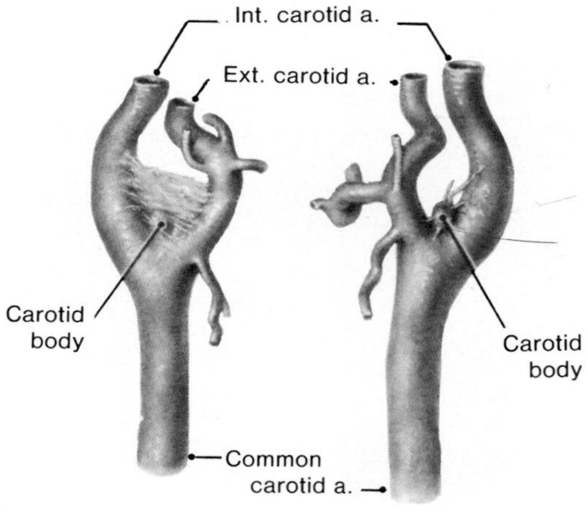

Figure 9-25. Drawing of two stages of a posterior view of a dissection of the carotid body. This particular body, black from engorged superficial veins, was easily recognized.

composition of the blood. It is supplied mainly by the carotid sinus nerve, a branch of CN IX, but is also supplied by CN X and sympathetic fibers. The carotid body responds to either increased carbon dioxide tension or to decreased oxygen tension in the blood.

The carotid sheath (Figs. 9-26, 9-41, 9-46 and 9-50) is a tubular, fascial condensation that extends from the base of the skull to the root of the neck. It is formed by fascial extensions of the cervical fascia, and its fibers fuse with the prevertebral fascia.

The carotid sheath encloses several clinically important structures: (1) the **common** and **internal carotid arteries** medially; (2) the **internal jugular vein** laterally; and (3) the **vagus nerve** (CN X) posteriorly. The superior root of the **ansa cervicalis** descends between the common carotid artery and the internal jugular vein and is sometimes embedded in the carotid sheath (Fig. 9-22).

Many **deep cervical lymph nodes** (Fig. 9-40*A*) lie along the carotid sheath and the internal jugular vein and between this vein and the common carotid artery. The cervical part of the ganglionated **sympathetic trunk** (Figs. 9-27 and 9-35) runs posterior to the carotid sheath.

The Muscular Triangle (Figs. 9-15, 9-20, 9-22, and 9-26). This **muscular area** is

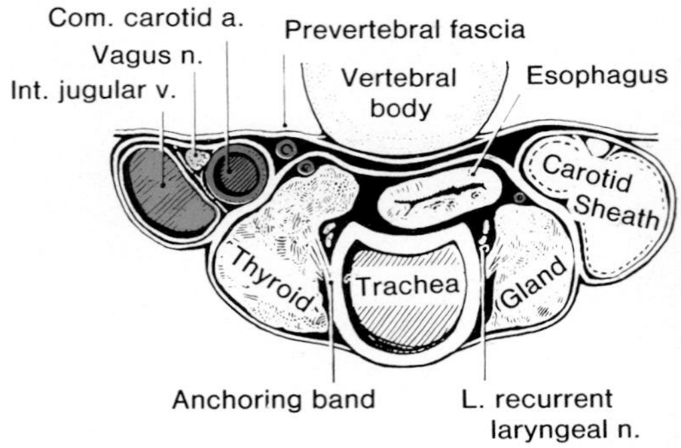

Figure 9-26. Drawing of a cross-section of the neck showing structures in its anterior part. Observe in particular the carotid sheath and its contents. This tubular condensation of cervical fascia is thicker around the artery than the vein. Observe that it both separates and encloses the common carotid artery, the internal jugular vein, and the vagus nerve.

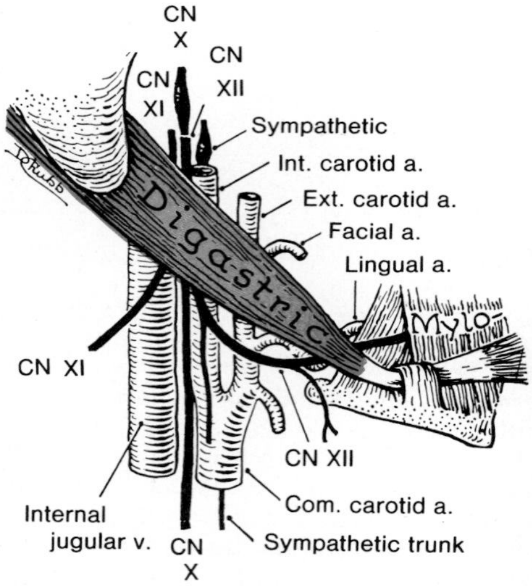

Figure 9-27. Drawing of structures in the carotid triangle (Fig. 9-15) related to the posterior belly of the digastric muscle. The carotid sheath has been removed. Note the key position of this muscle running from the mastoid process to the hyoid bone deep to the angle of the mandible. Observe that all the vessels and nerves cross deep to the posterior belly of this muscle. (Also see Fig. 9-22.)

bounded by the superior belly of the omohyoid (separating it from the carotid triangle), the anterior border of the sternocleidomastoid, and the midline of the neck. The muscular triangle contains the *four infrahyoid muscles and the neck viscera.*

The Submental Triangle (Figs. 9-15, 9-20 to 9-22, and 9-28). This **unpaired area** is bounded inferiorly by the body of the hyoid bone and laterally by the right and left anterior bellies of the digastric muscles. The **floor** of the triangle is formed by the two **mylohyoid muscles** which meet in a median fibrous raphe. The **apex** of the submental triangle is at the inferior end of the symphysis menti and its base is formed by the hyoid bone.

The submental triangle contains the submental lymph nodes (Figs. 9-15, 9-21, and 9-28). They receive lymph from the tip of the tongue, the floor of the mouth, the incisor teeth and associated gingivae, the central part of the lower lip, and the skin of the chin. Lymph from these nodes drains into the **submandibular** and **deep cervical lymph nodes** (Figs. 9-21, 9-40, and 9-66). It also contains small veins that unite to form the anterior jugular vein (Fig. 9-38).

CLINICALLY ORIENTED COMMENTS

Most **carcinomas (cancers) of the lip** occur on the lower lip and tend to spread via the lymphatics (Case 7-4). Depending on the site of the lesion, metastases spread to the submental nodes from the central part of the lower lip and to the submandibular nodes from other parts of the lip. In advanced cancers of the central part of the lip, the submandibular and deep cervical lymph nodes would also be involved because they receive lymph from the submental nodes (Figs. 9-21, 9-28, and 9-66).

A discharging **sinus** on the point of the chin often results from an *abscess of an incisor tooth.* The pus from the infected tooth passes to the apex of the **submental triangle** (inferior end of the symphysis menti), where it forms a sinus from which pus escapes.

Arteries of the Anterior Triangle (Figs. 9-24 and 9-29). Most arteries in the anterior triangle arise from the common carotid artery or one of its branches.

The Common Carotid Artery (Figs. 9-22, 9-24, 9-26, 9-27, 9-29, 9-30, and 9-35 to 9-37). The right common carotid begins at the bifurcation of the brachiocephalic trunk posterior to the right sternoclavicular joint. The left common carotid arises from the aortic arch and ascends into the neck posterior to the left sternoclavicular joint. Each common carotid artery ascends within the **carotid sheath** (Fig. 9-26) to the level of the superior border of the thyroid cartilage, where it terminates by dividing into internal and external carotid arteries.

The Internal Carotid Artery (Figs. 9-24, 9-27, and 9-47). This vessel is the direct continuation of the common carotid artery and *has no branches in the neck.* Its name indicates that it *supplies structures within the skull.* It arises from the common carotid artery at the level of the superior border of the thyroid cartilage and passes superiorly, almost in the vertical plane, to enter the **carotid canal** in the petrous part of the temporal bone (Fig. 7-189). A plexus of sympathetic fibers accompanies it (Fig. 7-87). During its course through the neck, the internal carotid lies on the longus capitis muscle and the sympathetic trunk (Figs. 9-27 and 9-33). The vagus nerve (CN X) lies posterolateral to it (Fig. 9-52).

The internal carotid artery enters the middle cranial fossa beside the dorsum sellae of the sphenoid bone (Fig. 7-13). Within the cranial cavity, the internal carotid and its branches supply the hyophysis cerebri, the orbit, and most of the supratentorial part of the brain (Figs. 7-89 and 7-90).

The External Carotid Artery (Figs. 9-24, 9-27, and 9-29). This vessel begins at the bifurcation of the common carotid at the level of the superior border of the thyroid cartilage. Its name indicates that it *supplies structures external to the skull.* It runs posterosuperiorly to the region between the

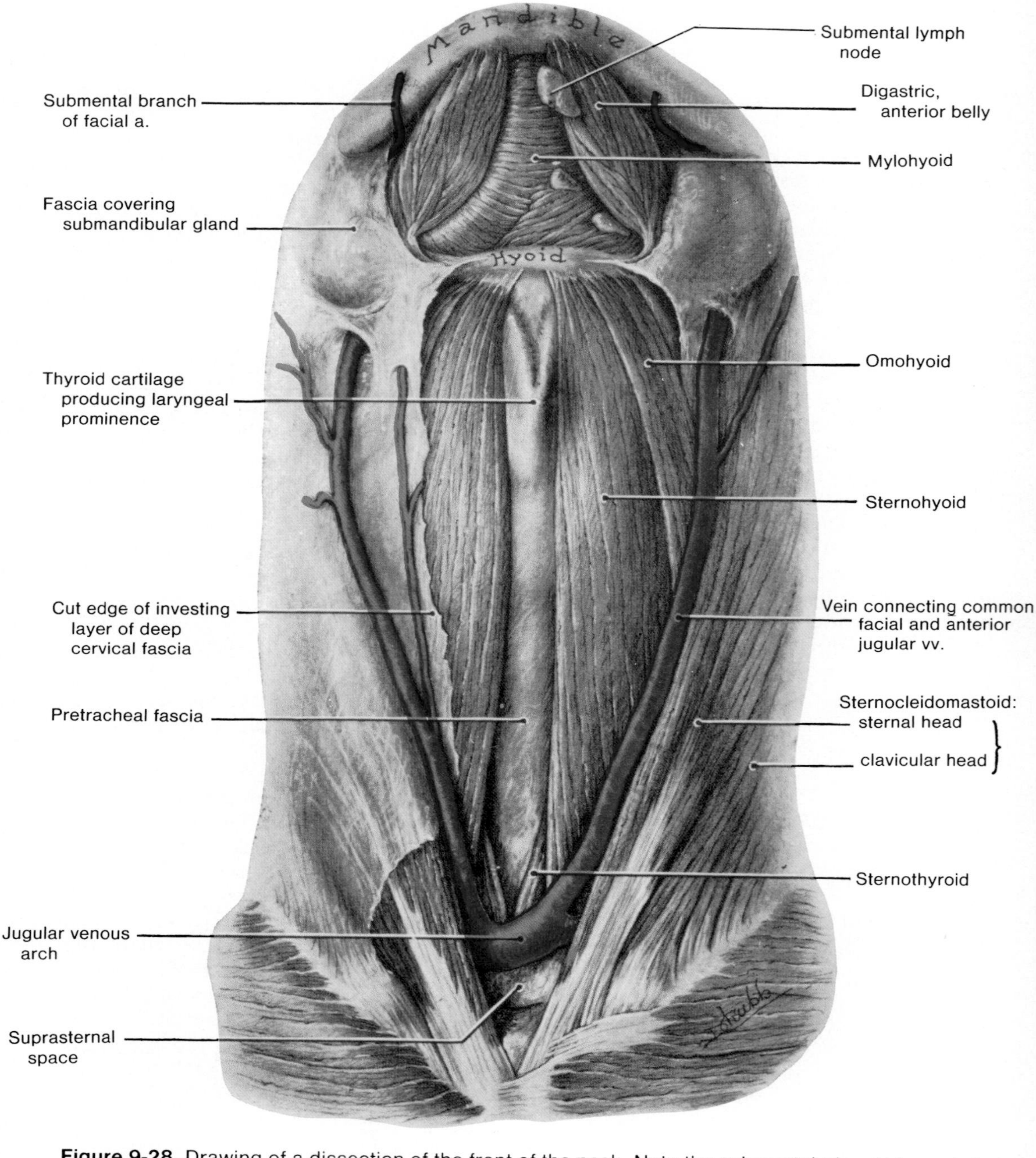

Figure 9-28. Drawing of a dissection of the front of the neck. Note the submental triangle bounded inferiorly by the body of the hyoid bone and laterally by the right and left anterior bellies of the digastric muscles. Observe that its floor is formed by the two mylohyoid muscles. Note that it contains some submental lymph nodes (actually the submental triangle is part of the floor of the mouth). Note the pronounced laryngeal prominence in this male specimen.

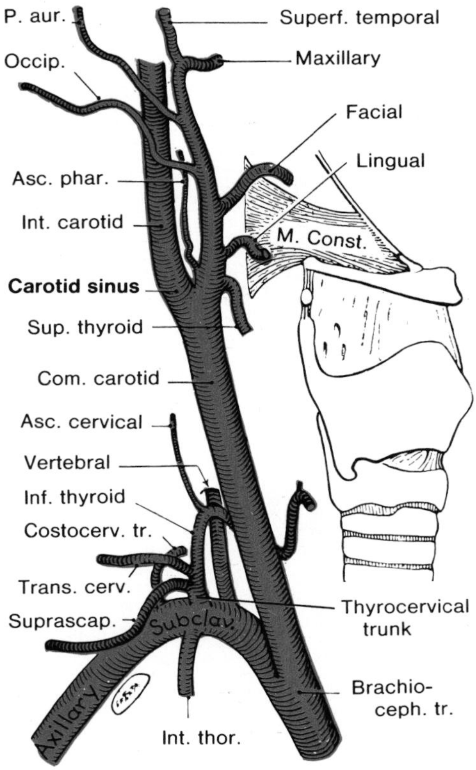

Figure 9-29. Drawing of the subclavian and carotid arteries and their branches. Note that the terminal part of the common carotid and the proximal part of the internal carotid artery are dilated for about 1 cm to form the carotid sinus. The walls of this region, which are important in blood pressure regulation, are especially elastic and contain many sensory nerve endings that respond to changes in blood pressure and bring about appropriate modifications reflexly.

neck of the mandible and the lobule of the auricle, where it terminates by dividing into two branches, the **maxillary** and **superficial temporal** arteries. The external carotid has several branches, some within the carotid triangle (Fig. 9-27), some outside it.

The stems of most of the **six branches of the external carotid** artery are in the *carotid triangle* (Fig. 9-23). The three important branches of this artery are described first and are set in **bold face** type.

The superior thyroid artery (Figs. 9-6 and 9-29), the most inferior of the three anterior branches of the external carotid, arises close to the origin of this vessel, just inferior to the greater horn of the hyoid. It runs anteroinferiorly deep to the infrahyoid muscles to reach the superior pole of the **thyroid gland** (Figs. 9-30 and 9-41). In addition to supplying the thyroid, it gives muscular branches to the sternocleidomastoid and the infrahyoid muscles. It also gives off the **superior laryngeal artery**, which pierces the thyrohyoid membrane in company with the internal laryngeal nerve and supplies the larynx (Fig. 9-30). Owing to its importance during **thyroidectomy** (p. 1152), note that the **external laryngeal nerve** (a branch of the superior laryngeal nerve) accompanies the superior thyroid artery during the early part of its course to the superior pole of the thyroid (Fig. 9-41). Observe that the artery loses this close relationship to the nerve as it approaches the thyroid gland. *This relationship is clinically important* (Case 9-5).

The lingual artery (Figs. 9-27 and 9-31) arises from the external carotid as it lies on the middle constrictor muscle of the pharynx. It arches upward and forward about 5 mm superior to the tip of the greater horn of the hyoid bone and then passes deep to the hypoglossal nerve (CN XII), the stylohyoid muscle, and the posterior belly of the digastric muscle and disappears deep to the hyoglossus muscle. At the anterior border of the hyoglossus, it turns superiorly and ends by becoming the **deep artery of the tongue** (profunda linguae artery).

The facial artery (Figs. 9-22, 9-23, 9-27, and 9-29) arises from the external carotid, either in common with the lingual artery or immediately superior to it. It passes vertically upward under cover of the digastric and stylohyoid muscles and the angle of the mandible. Looping anteriorly, it enters a deep groove in the submandibular gland and then hooks around the inferior border of the mandible to enter the face; here pulsations of the facial artery can easily be felt. In the neck the facial artery gives off its important **tonsillar branch** and branches to the palate and the submandibular gland.

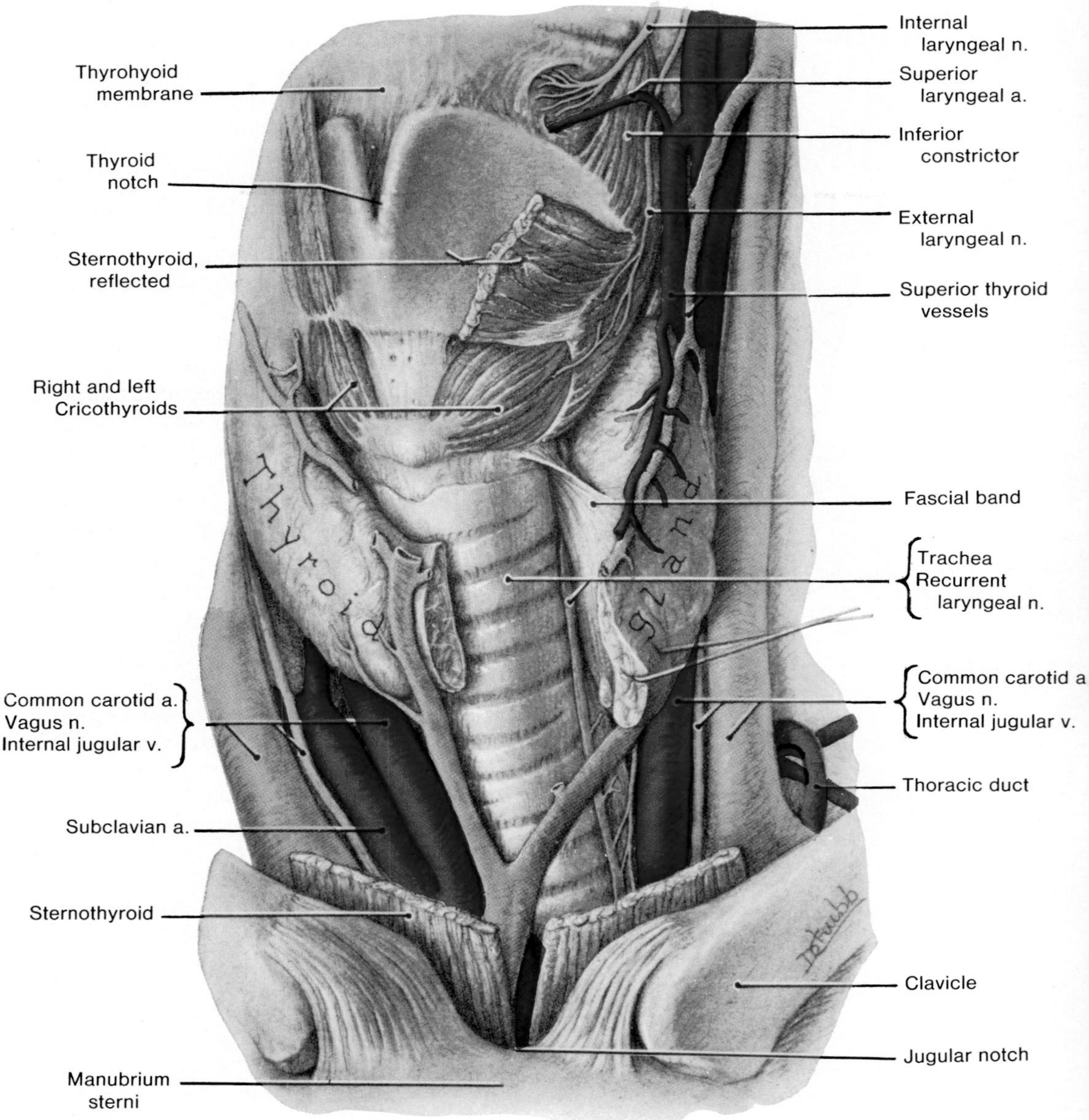

Figure 9-30. Drawing of a dissection of the front of the neck. The isthmus of the thyroid gland is divided and its left lobe is retracted. Observe the left recurrent laryngeal nerve on the side of the trachea, just in front of the angle between the trachea and esophagus and behind the retaining band. Note also the internal laryngeal nerve running along the upper border of the inferior constrictor muscle, piercing the thyrohyoid membrane, and dividing into several branches. Observe the external laryngeal nerve applied to the inferior constrictor, running along the anterior border of the superior thyroid artery, passing deep to the insertion of the sternothyroid, giving twigs to the inferior constrictor, and piercing it before ending in the cricothyroid muscle.

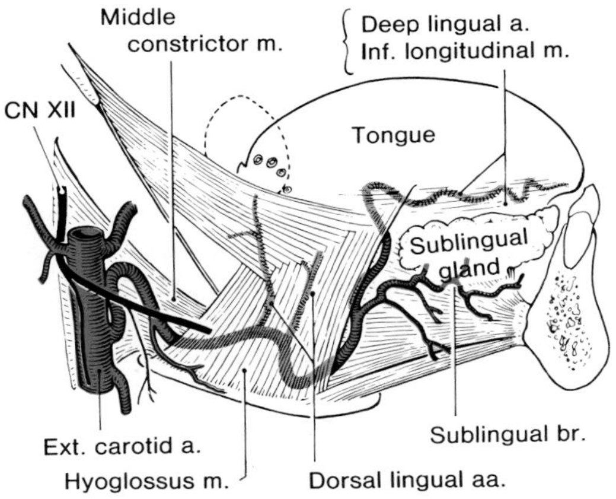

Figure 9-31. Drawing of the lingual artery. Note that it enters the submandibular triangle where it at once passes deep to the hyoglossus muscle. The terminal (third) deep part of the lingual artery that turns into the tongue is called the deep lingual (profunda linguae) artery.

The ascending pharyngeal artery (Fig. 9-29) is the first or second branch of the external carotid. This small artery ascends on the pharynx deep to the internal carotid and gives branches to the pharynx, prevertebral muscles, middle ear, and meninges.

The occipital artery (Figs. 9-22, 9-23, and 9-29) arises from the posterior surface of the external carotid, opposite the origin of the facial artery. It passes posteriorly along the lower border of the posterior belly of the digastric to end in the posterior part of the scalp. It is often palpable as it crosses the superior nuchal line between the trapezius and sternocleidomastoid muscles. During this course it passes superficial to the internal carotid artery and three cranial nerves (CN IX, CN X, and CN XI).

The posterior auricular artery (Figs. 9-23 and 9-29), a small posterior branch, arises from the external carotid at the su-

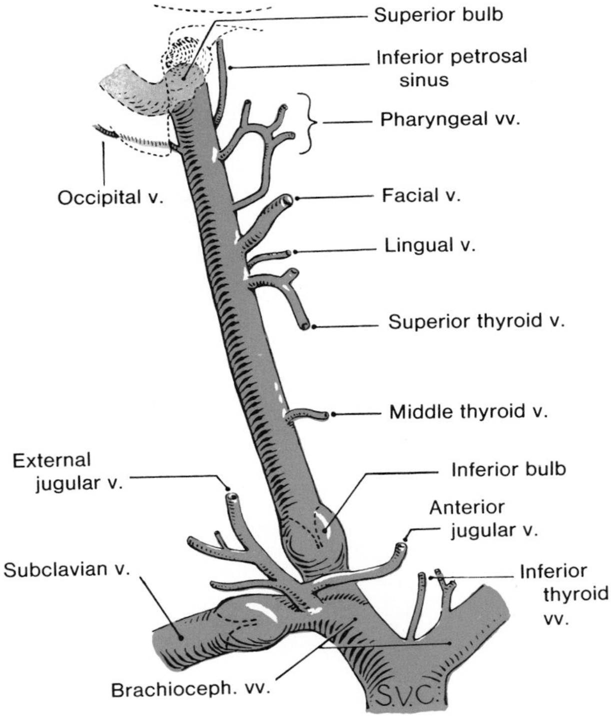

Figure 9-32. Diagram of the internal jugular vein and its tributaries. Note the dilation or bulb at each end of this large vein. The superior jugular bulb is separated from the floor of the middle ear by a bony plate. The inferior jugular bulb, like the corresponding bulb at the end of the subclavian vein, contains a biscuspid valve which prevents the retrograde flow of blood from the right atrium of heart. *S.V.C.*, superior vena cava.

perior border of the posterior belly of the digastric muscle. It ascends posterior to the external acoustic meatus and supplies the adjacent muscles, the parotid gland, the facial nerve, structures in the temporal bone, the auricle, and the scalp.

The Internal Jugular Vein (Figs. 9-12, 9-13, 9-21, 9-22, 9-26, 9-27, and 9-32). Usually the *largest vein in the neck*, the internal jugular drains blood from the brain, superficial parts of the face, and the neck. Its course corresponds to a line drawn from a point immediately below the external acoustic meatus to the medial end of the clavicle. It commences at the jugular foramen in the posterior cranial fossa (Fig. 7-57) as *the direct continuation of the sigmoid sinus*. From the dilation at its origin, called the **superior bulb**, the internal jugular runs inferiorly through the neck in the **carotid sheath** (Fig. 9-26). It shares this tubular condensation of fascia with the internal carotid artery (later with the common carotid) and the vagus nerve (CN X). The artery is medial, the vein lateral, and the nerve posterior in the angle between these vessels (Fig. 9-46). The internal jugular vein leaves the anterior cervical triangle by passing deep to the **sternocleidomastoid** (Fig. 9-21). Behind the sternal end of the clavicle, the internal jugular unites with the subclavian to form the **brachiocephalic vein** (Fig. 9-32). Near the termination of the internal jugular is the **inferior bulb**, which contains a bicuspid valve like that in the subclavian vein. The internal jugular vein is usually larger on the right side than on the left side because of the greater volume of blood entering it from the superior sagittal sinus via the sigmoid sinus (Fig. 7-38).

Deep cervical lymph nodes (Figs. 9-40, 9-46, and 9-66) lie along the course of the internal jugular vein, many on its superficial surface. These nodes may be small and scattered; thus they are often difficult to identify in dissections.

Tributaries of the Internal Jugular Vein (Fig. 9-32). This large vein is joined at its origin by the **inferior petrosal sinus** (Fig. 7-38), the facial, lingual, pharyngeal, superior and middle thyroid veins, and often by the occipital vein.

CLINICALLY ORIENTED COMMENTS

Superiorly the internal jugular vein lies posterolateral to the internal carotid artery, with cranial nerves CN IX to CN XII between them (Figs. 9-22, 9-30, and 9-33). When **thrombophlebitis** occurs in the superior bulb of the internal jugular vein (*e.g.*, associated with middle ear infection or **otis media**), these cranial nerves may cease to conduct impulses owing to pressure from the congested vein.

Pulsations of the internal jugular vein resulting from contraction of the right ventricle of the heart may be palpable and visible at the root of the neck (Fig. 9-40). Because there are no valves in the brachiocephalic vein or the superior vena cava, a wave of contraction passes up these vessels to the internal jugular vein. This **systolic venous pulse** is considerably increased in certain conditions (*e.g.*, disease of the mitral valve leading to increased pressure in the pulmonary circulation, right side of heart, and great veins).

All lymphatic vessels from the head and neck drain into the deep cervical lymph nodes (Fig. 9-66), many of which lie in the carotid sheath (Figs. 9-40 and 9-46), along the internal jugular vein, and between it and the common carotid artery. These nodes are very important when there are metastases from malignant tumors (*e.g.*, carcinoma of the mouth, larynx, or other structures in the head and neck). Removal of the **cancerous lymph nodes** is more difficult when they adhere closely to the internal jugular vein.

DEEP STRUCTURES OF THE NECK

Skeleton of the Neck. The cervical vertebrae and joints of the neck are described in Chapter 5 with the back (Fig. 5-18). Revise your knowledge of these bones, particularly the atlas and the axis, and review the joints associated with them. Recall that the joints between the atlas and the axis permit rotation, whereas those between the

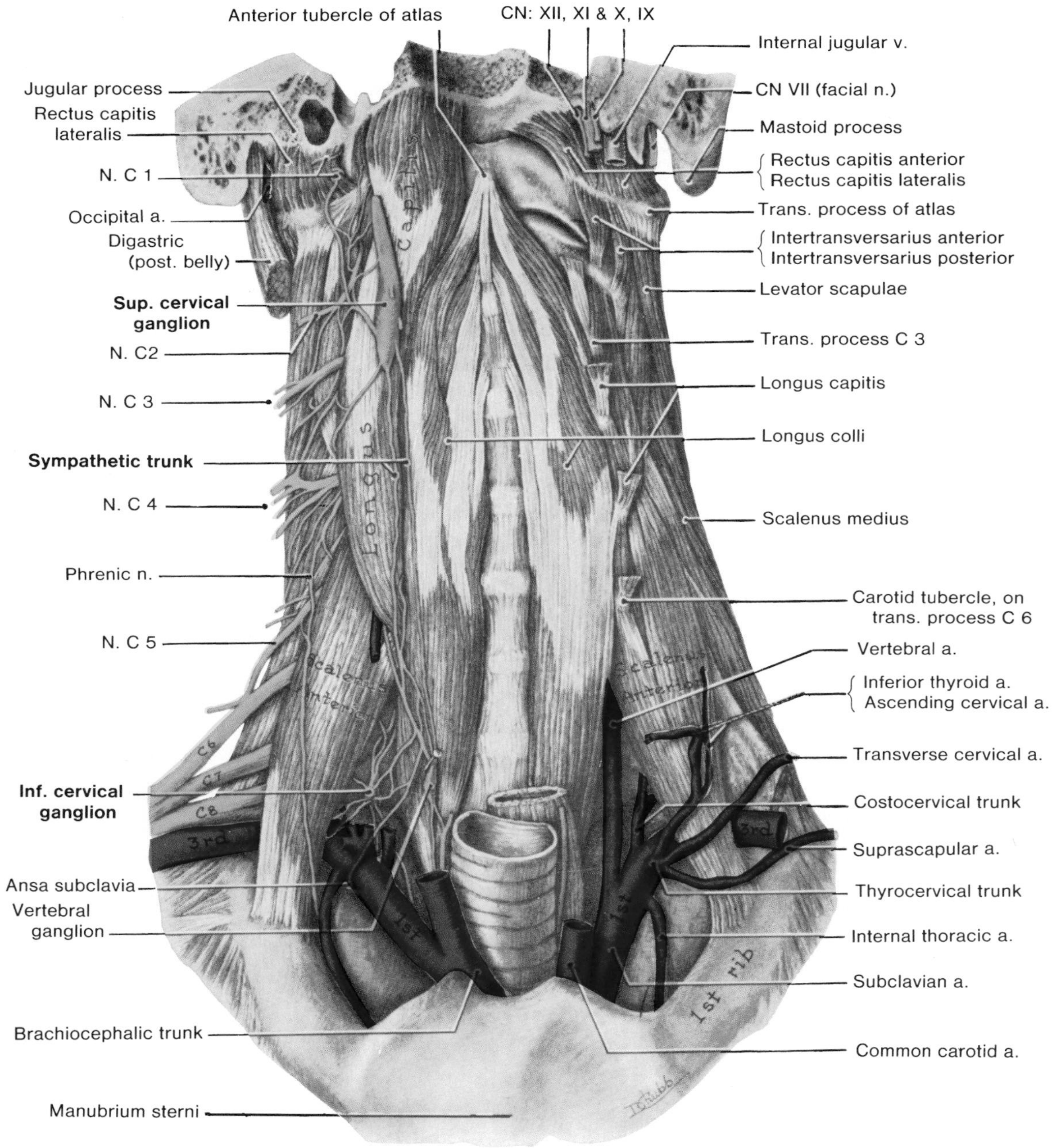

Figure 9-33. Drawing of a dissection of the prevertebral region and the root of the neck. The prevertebral fascia (Fig. 9-50) has been removed and the longus capitis muscle has been excised on the left side. Observe that three muscles, scalenus anterior, longus capitis, and longus colli, are attached to the anterior tubercles of the transverse processes of cervical vertebrae (C3 to C6). Note that the transverse process of the atlas is joined to the transverse process of the axis by the intertransverse muscles and is joined similarly to the occipital bone (*i.e.*, jugular process) by the rectus capitis lateralis, which morphologically is an intertransverse muscle. Note that the internal jugular vein crosses these structures. Observe the cervical plexus arising from ventral rami C1, C2, C3, and C4, and the brachial plexus from C5, C6, C7, C8, and T1. Note the sympathetic trunk, ganglia, and the gray rami communicantes. Examine the subclavian artery and its branches.

skull and the atlas are structured to allow nodding movements of the head on the cervical region of the vertebral column.

Muscles of the Neck. The superficial and lateral cervical muscles (**platysma, trapezius,** and **sternocleidomastoid**) were described previously (Figs. 9-8, 9-9, and 9-11 to 9-15), as were the hyoid muscles (Fig. 9-20) and the scalene muscles (Fig. 9-14), which form part of the floor of the posterior triangle.

The Anterior Vertebral Muscles (Figs. 9-33, 9-34, and 9-50). These deep prevertebral muscles are covered anteriorly by prevertebral fascia. They all **flex the neck** and **the head on it** and they are all supplied by the ventral primary rami of the cervical nerves.

The longus colli muscle (longus cervicis), the longest and most medial of the prevertebral muscles, extends from the anterior tubercle of the *atlas* to the body of the **third thoracic vertebra** (Fig. 9-33). It is also attached to the bodies of the vertebrae between these and to the transverse processes of the third to sixth cervical vertebrae.

The longus capitus muscle (Fig. 9-33), broad and thick above, arises from the anterior tubercles of the third to sixth **cervical transverse processes** and is inserted into the base of the **skull**.

The rectus capitus anterior (Fig. 9-33), a short wide muscle, arises from the anterior surface of the lateral mass of the **atlas** and inserts into the **base of the skull** just anterior to the occipital condyle.

The rectus capitis lateralis (Figs. 9-33 and 9-34), a short flat muscle, arises from the transverse process of the **atlas** and runs vertically to the **jugular process of the occipital bone**. This muscle and the rectus capitus anterior, in addition to flexing the head on the neck, help to stabilize the skull on the cervical region of the vertebral column.

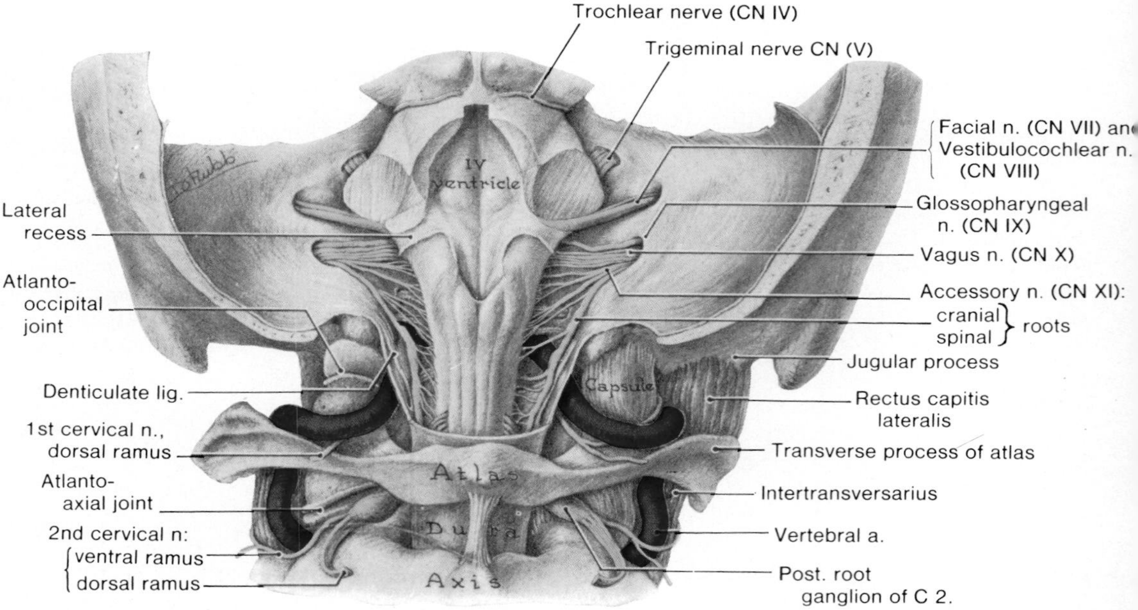

Figure 9-34. Dissection showing a posterior view of the cranial nerves. Observe that the transverse process of the atlas is joined to the jugular process of the occipital bone by the rectus capitis lateralis muscle, which morphologically is an intertransverse muscle. Note that the vertebral arteries are raised from their "beds" on the posterior arch of the atlas. The vertebral arteries join to form the basilar artery (also see Fig. 7-90).

THE ROOT OF THE NECK

The **thoracocervical region** (root of the neck) is the junctional area between the neck and the thorax. It includes **the thoracic inlet**, through which pass all structures going from the head to the thorax.

Boundaries of the Root of the Neck (Figs. 9-30, 9-33, and 9-37). The thoracocervical region is bounded *laterally* by the **first pair of ribs** and their costal cartilages, *anteriorly* by the **manubrium** sterni, and *posteriorly* by the body of the **first thoracic vertebra**.

Arteries at the Root of the Neck (Figs. 9-30, 9-33, and 9-37). The arteries in this junctional area originating from the arch of the aorta are the brachiocephalic (innominate) trunk on the right side and the common carotid and the subclavian arteries on the left.

The Brachiocephalic Trunk (Figs. 9-29, 9-33, 9-35, and 9-47). This great artery is *the largest branch of the arch of the aorta* and is 4 to 5 cm in length. It arises posterior to the center of the manubrium sterni and passes superiorly and to the right behind the right **sternoclavicular joint**, where it divides into the right common carotid and the right subclavian arteries. The brachiocephalic artery is covered anteriorly by the sternohyoid and sternothyroid muscles.

At first it lies on the trachea and then to its right side. *Usually the brachiocephalic artery has no branches* other than its terminal ones, but sometimes a small artery, the **thyroid ima** (L. lowest), arises from it and ascends anterior to the trachea to the isthmus of the thyroid gland (Fig. 9-43).

The Subclavian Artery (Figs. 9-33 and 9-35 to 9-37). This is the artery of the upper limb, but it also supplies branches to the neck and the brain.

The **right subclavian** is one of the terminal branches of the brachiocephalic trunk and arises behind the right sternoclavicular joint. The **left subclavian** arises from the arch of the aorta and enters the root of the neck by passing superiorly, posterior to the left sternoclavicular joint (Fig. 9-33).

Each subclavian artery arches superiorly, posteriorly, and laterally, grooving the pleura and the lung and then passes inferiorly behind the midpoint of the clavicle. As these arteries rise 2 to 4 cm into the root of the neck, they are crossed anteriorly by the scalenus anterior muscles (Figs. 9-33, 9-35, and 9-36).

Visualize the subclavian arteries in yourself by using your forefinger to make a curved line that starts at the sternoclavicular joint, rises above the clavicle, and then passes downward behind this bone.

For purposes of description, *the scalenus anterior muscle divides the subclavian artery into three parts*: the first part medial to the muscle, the second part posterior to it, and the third part lateral to it (Figs. 9-33 and 9-35).

Branches of the subclavian artery (Figs. 9-29, 9-36, and 9-37) are the vertebral, the thyrocervical trunk, and the internal thoracic *from the first part*; the costocervical trunk *from the second part*; and, occasionally the suprascapular and/or the dorsal scapular artery *from the third part*.

The Vertebral Artery (Figs. 9-33, 9-34, 9-36, 9-37, 9-39, and 9-40*B*). The **vertebral artery** arises from the first part of the subclavian and ascends through the foramina transversaria of the cervical vertebrae, except for the seventh. After winding around the lateral mass of the atlas, *the vertebral artery enters the skull through the foramen magnum* (Fig. 9-34). At the inferior border of the pons, the vertebral artery joins its fellow of the opposite side to form the **basilar artery** (Fig. 7-90), a very important artery supplying the brain.

The Thyrocervical Trunk (Figs. 9-29 and 9-35 to 9-37). The **thyrocervical trunk** arises from the first part of the subclavian artery, just medial to the scalenus anterior muscle. It gives rise to several branches, the largest and most important of which is the **inferior thyroid artery**, passing to the inferior pole of the thyroid gland. Other branches of the thyrocervical trunk are the *suprascapular artery* (except when it arises from the third part of the subclavian artery) supplying muscles around the scapula, and the *transverse cervical artery*, sending branches to the muscles in the posterior triangle of the neck.

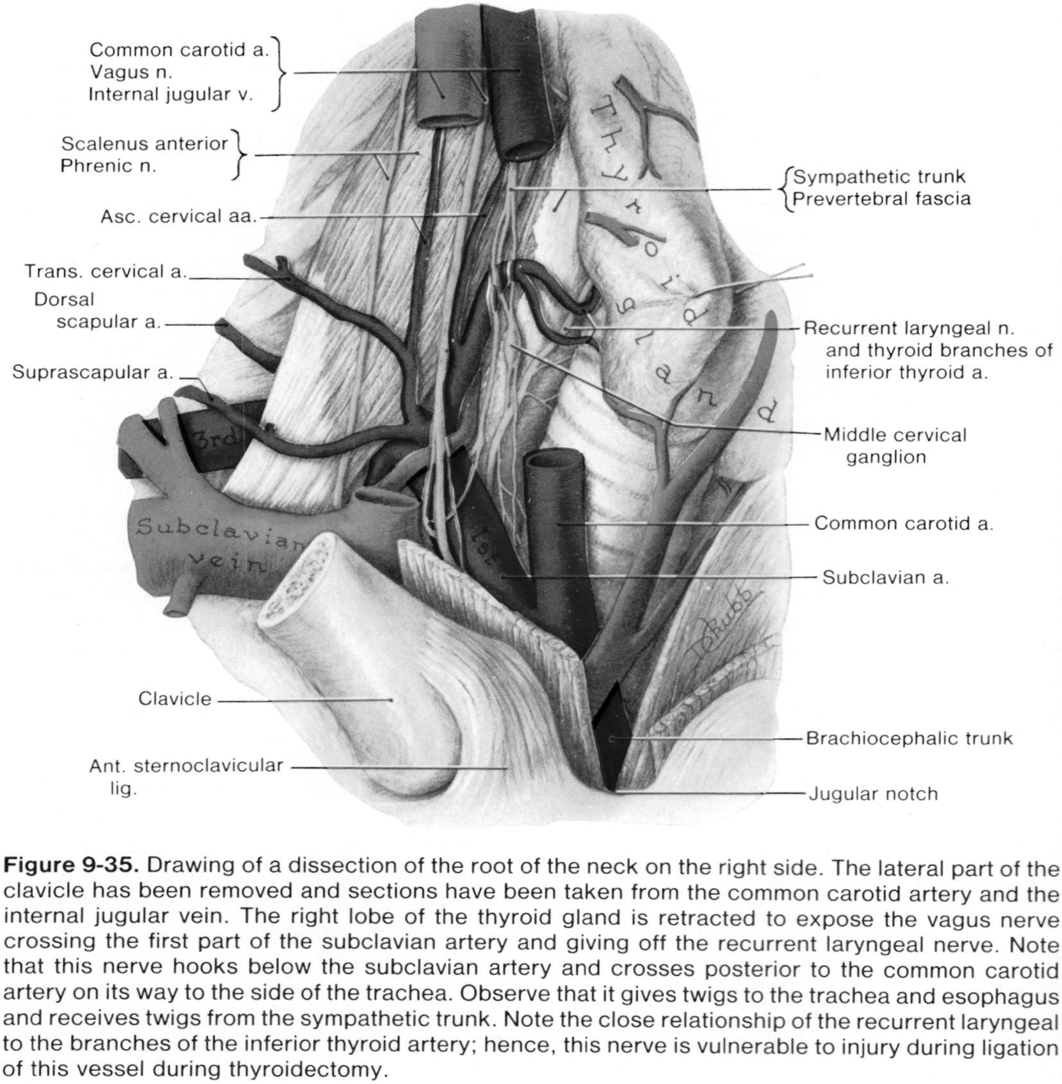

Figure 9-35. Drawing of a dissection of the root of the neck on the right side. The lateral part of the clavicle has been removed and sections have been taken from the common carotid artery and the internal jugular vein. The right lobe of the thyroid gland is retracted to expose the vagus nerve crossing the first part of the subclavian artery and giving off the recurrent laryngeal nerve. Note that this nerve hooks below the subclavian artery and crosses posterior to the common carotid artery on its way to the side of the trachea. Observe that it gives twigs to the trachea and esophagus and receives twigs from the sympathetic trunk. Note the close relationship of the recurrent laryngeal to the branches of the inferior thyroid artery; hence, this nerve is vulnerable to injury during ligation of this vessel during thyroidectomy.

The Internal Thoracic Artery (Fig. 9-33). The **internal thoracic artery** arises from the inferior aspect of the subclavian and passes inferomedially into the thorax. It runs parallel to the sternum (about 2.5 cm lateral to it) and gives off anterior intercostal branches to the first six intercostal spaces.

The Costocervical Trunk (Figs. 9-29 and 9-33). The **costocervical trunk** arises from the posterior aspect of the subclavian and passes superoposteriorly over the **cervical pleura**. It divides into the superior intercostal and deep cervical arteries, which supply the first two intercostal spaces and muscles in the neck.

Veins at the Root of the Neck (Fig. 9-37). The **external jugular** vein, receiving blood mostly from the scalp and the face, is described on page 1115 and is illustrated in Figures 9-11 and 9-38.

The Anterior Jugular Vein (Figs. 9-22,

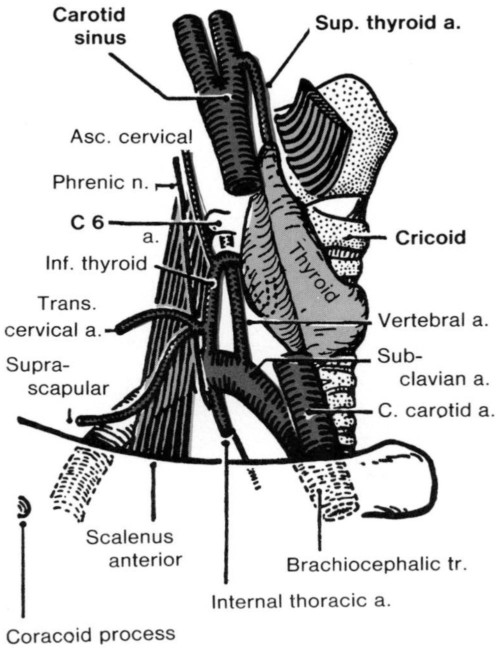

Figure 9-36. Drawing of the arteries in the root of the neck. Note that the course of the subclavian artery forms a curved line, extending from the sternoclavicular joint 2 to 4 cm above the clavicle and then crossing behind this bone near its middle. Also observe the scalenus anterior muscle which is used to divide the subclavian artery into three parts for descriptive purposes (Fig. 9-33).

9-28, and 9-38*A*). This vein is usually the smallest of the jugular veins and *is very variable.* The anterior jugular arises from the **submental venous plexus** and descends in the superficial fascia between the anteromedian line and the anterior border of the sternocleidomastoid muscle. At the root of the neck it turns laterally, posterior to this muscle, and opens into the termination of the external jugular or directly into the subclavian vein. Just above the sternum the right and left anterior jugular veins are united by the **jugular venous arch** (Fig. 9-28). The anterior jugular veins have no valves and may be represented by a single trunk descending in the midline of the neck. The anterior jugular vein, like the external jugular vein, can often be made visible by "blowing" with the mouth closed.

The Subclavian Vein (Figs. 9-13, 9-32, 9-35, and 9-38*A*). This large vein is *the continuation of the axillary vein.* It begins at the lateral border of the first rib and ends at the medial border of the scalenus anterior muscle, where it unites with the **internal jugular,** posterior to the medial end of the clavicle to form the **brachiocephalic vein**. The subclavian vein, lying in the concavity of the subclavian artery superior to the clavicle, has a bicuspid valve near its termination (Fig. 9-32). It usually has only one named tributary, the **external jugular vein**, which is often visible in the neck (Fig. 9-38*B*). Observe that the subclavian vein passes over the first rib parallel to the subclavian artery but is separated from it by the scalenus anterior muscle (Fig. 9-35).

The Internal Jugular Vein (Figs. 9-32, 9-35, 9-37, 9-40*A*, and 9-46). This vein, described previously, ends posterior to the medial end of the clavicle by uniting with the subclavian to form the **brachiocephalic vein**. Recall that throughout its course it is enclosed within the **carotid sheath**.

Nerves at the Root of the Neck (Figs. 9-30, 9-35, 9-37, and 9-39). Several important nerves are located at the root of the neck.

The Vagus Nerve (CN X). The vagus (L. wandering), so-named because of its wide distribution, leaves the skull through the **jugular foramen** and passes inferiorly in the posterior part of the **carotid sheath** (Figs. 9-26, 9-27, and 9-46) in the angle between and behind the internal jugular vein and the carotid artery (first internal and then common). On the right side it crosses the origin of the subclavian artery posterior to the brachiocephalic vein and the sternoclavicular joint to enter the thorax (Figs. 9-30 and 9-35).

The **recurrent laryngeal nerve** (Figs. 9-35, 9-39, 9-40*B*, 9-41, and 9-84), a branch of the vagus, hooks *around the subclavian artery on the right* side and *around the arch of the aorta on the left* side. Review the embryological basis for this difference. Both nerves then pass upward to reach the posteromedial aspect of the lower pole of the thyroid gland, where they ascend in the *tracheoesophageal groove* to supply all the

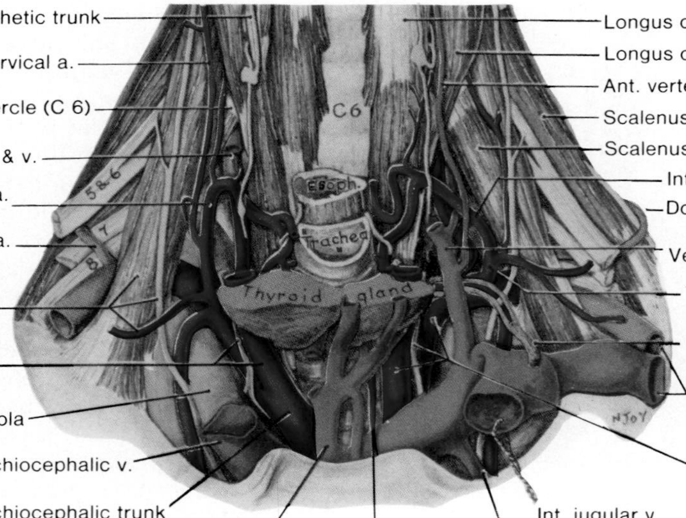

Figure 9-37. Drawing of a dissection of the root of the neck, viewed obliquely from above. Observe the "triangle of the vertebral artery," bounded laterally by the scalenus anterior and medially by the longus colli muscles. Note that the apex of the triangle is where these two muscles meet at the carotid tubercle (anterior tubercle of transverse process of C6), and the base of the triangle is formed by the first part of the subclavian artery. Observe the vertebral artery ascending from the base to the apex and dividing the triangle into two nearly equal parts.

intrinsic muscles of the larynx except the cricothyroid (Fig. 9-81).

The **cardiac nerves** (branches of the vagus, CN X) originate in the neck and thorax and run along the arteries to the aortic arch and the **cardiac plexuses**. When stimulated they slow the heartbeat, reducing its force, and in unusual cases may produce cardiac arrest. Cardiac branches also arise from the vagus where it lies on the subclavian artery and descend beside the trachea to the deep **cardiac plexus**.

The Phrenic Nerve (Figs. 9-33, 9-35, 9-40, and 9-46). This nerve, usually about 30 cm long, is the *sole motor nerve to the diaphragm*. It arises from the **fourth cervical nerve** (with contributions from the third and fifth cervical nerves). It is formed at the upper part of the lateral border of the scalenus anterior muscle, at the level of the superior border of the thyroid cartilage and superolateral to the internal jugular vein. It descends with this vein obliquely across the scalenus anterior, deep to prevertebral fascia and the transverse cervical and suprascapular arteries (Fig. 9-40*A*). *On the left* it crosses the first part of the subclavian artery, but *on the right* it lies on the scalenus anterior over the second part of this artery (Fig. 9-35). It crosses posterior to the subclavian vein on both sides and anterior to the internal thoracic artery to enter the thorax.

The unexpected innervation of the diaphragm by *cervical nerve roots* has an embryological explanation. During the 5th week of development, ventral rami from C3, C4, and C5 grow into the **septum transversum**, the primordium of the central tendon of the diaphragm, when it is in the cervical region. As the developing diaphragm migrates caudally, it carries the phrenic nerves with it.

CLINICALLY ORIENTED COMMENTS

Severance of the phrenic nerve in the root of the neck (or elsewhere) results in

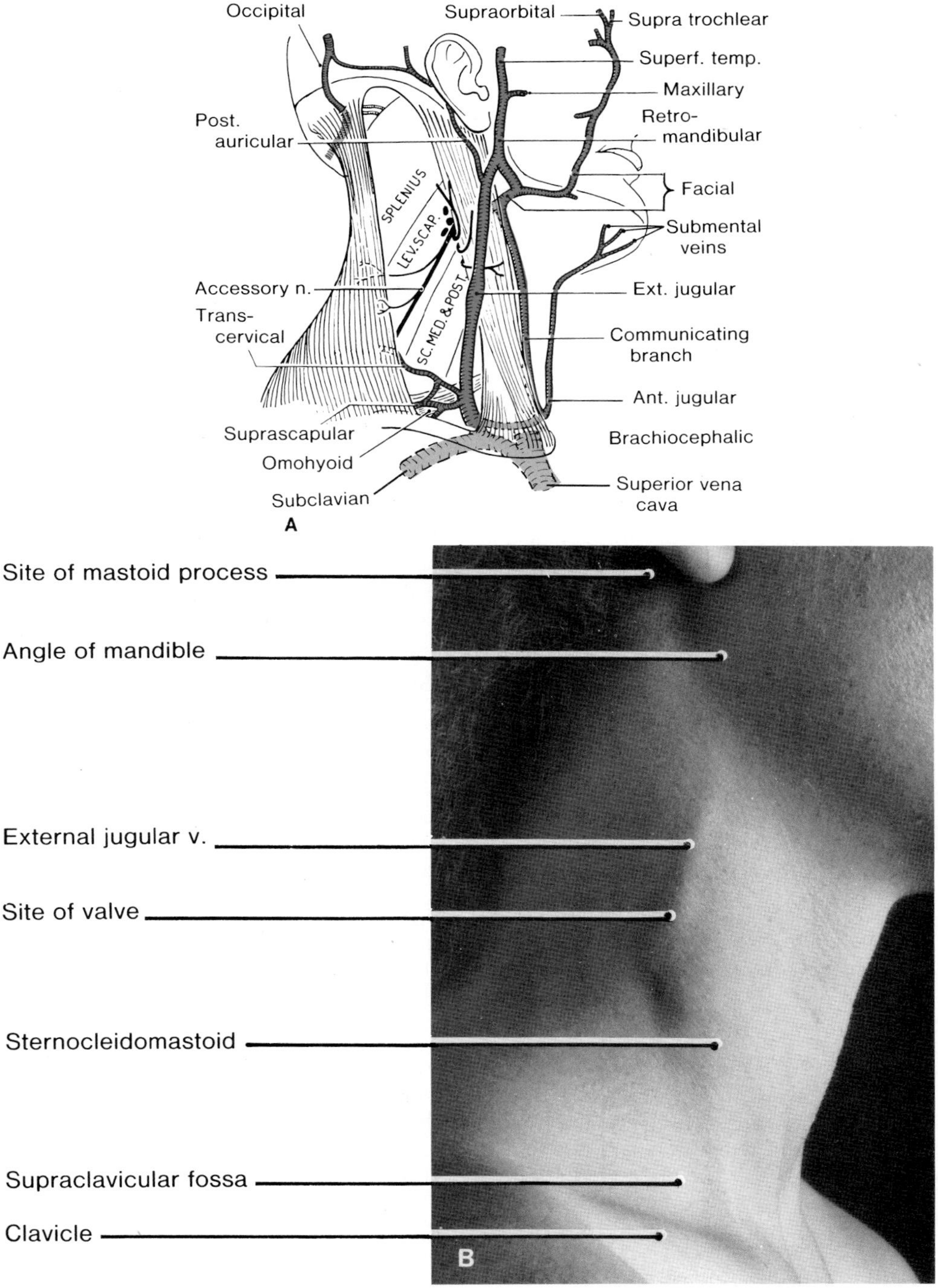

Figure 9-38. *A*, diagram illustrating the superficial veins of the right side of the neck. The size of the anterior jugular (usually the smallest of the jugulars) varies inversely with the external jugular. Note the accessory nerve (CN XI) descending through the posterior triangle of the neck (Fig. 9-11) and dividing it into nearly equal upper and lower parts. Note the muscles forming the floor of the posterior triangle. *B*, photograph of the right side of the neck of a 27-year-old woman. To make her external jugular vein stand out, she was asked to take a deep breath and to hold it. The slight swelling in her vein about 4 cm above the clavicle (also see *A*) indicates the site of one of the pairs of valves in this vein. You are unable to see the inferior part of her vein because it pierces the roof of the posterior triangle and passes through it.

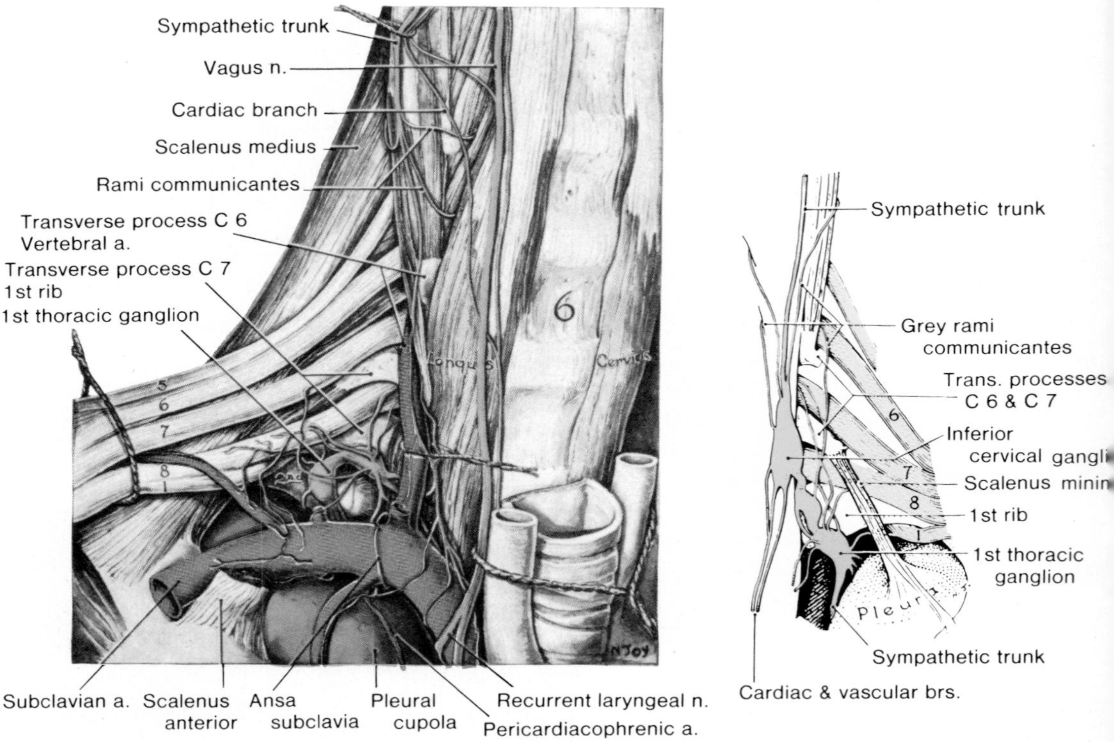

Figure 9-39. Drawing of a dissection of the neck on the right side. Observe that the lowest trunk of the brachial plexus (C8 and T1) has been raised from the groove it occupies on the first rib behind the subclavian artery. Note that the sympathetic trunk (retracted laterally) is sending a communicating branch to the vagus and that the gray rami communicantes (postganglionic fibers) pass to the roots of the cervical nerves. The cardiac branches are also shown. The vertebral artery has been retracted medially to uncover the stellate ganglion which rests behind it on the first and second ribs. The illustration on the right, a tracing of a photograph of the left side of the same specimen, reveals a very different pattern. Thus, the inferior cervical ganglion occupies its more usual position between the transverse process of C7 and the first rib. The ganglion (T1) lies on and below the first rib.

paralysis of the corresponding half of the diaphragm. Injuries to the lower cervical region of the spinal cord (*e.g.*, C7), severe enough to cause paraplegia or paralysis of the upper limbs (Case 5-9), do not affect breathing much because the phrenic nerves arise from more cranial segments of the spinal cord (C3, **C4**, and C5). Breathing would not be normal because the intercostal muscles would be paralyzed.

To produce temporary therapeutic **paralysis of one half the diaphragm** (*e.g.*, to interrupt a severe case of hiccoughs, *i.e.*, spasmodic, sharp contractions of the diaphragm), a phrenic nerve injection is sometimes done. The anesthetic solution is injected around the phrenic nerve where it lies on the anterior surface of the middle third of the scalenus anterior muscle, about one and one-half fingerbreadths above the clavicle (Fig. 9-40).

To produce a longer period of paralysis of half of the diaphragm or the hemidiaphragm, *e.g.*, for several months after the surgical repair of a diaphragmatic hernia, a **phrenic crush** is performed, where the phrenic nerve is crushed with a hemostat for up to 1 cm of its length. In some cases a **phrenicotomy** is performed, during which the phrenic nerve is sectioned. The phrenic nerve is exposed by making a 2 to 3 cm incision in a skin crease above the

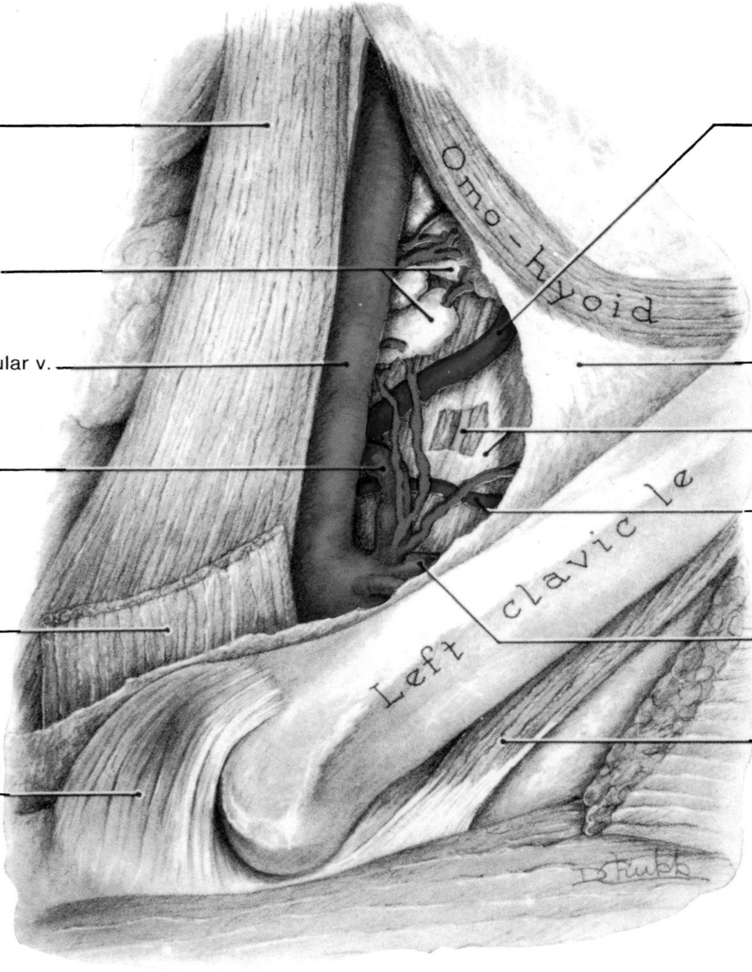

A.

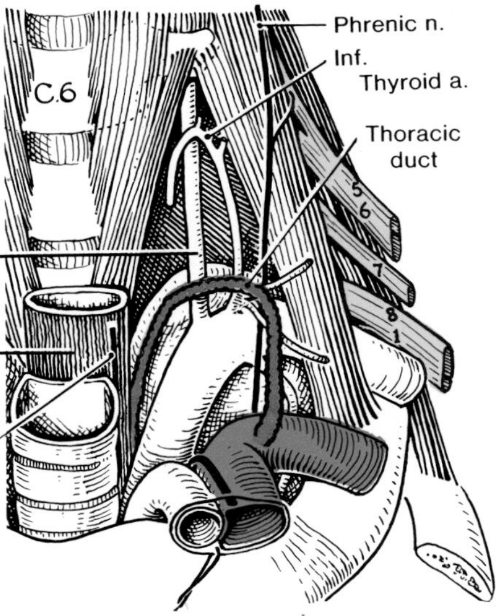

B.

Figure 9-40. *A*, drawing of a dissection of the root of the neck on the left side showing the deep cervical lymph nodes and the termination of the thoracic duct. Note the thoracic duct receiving a tributary from the nodes of the neck (jugular trunk) and ending in the angle between the internal jugular and subclavian veins. Observe that the deep nodes are arranged along the blood vessels, for the most part lateral and posterior to the internal jugular vein (Fig. 9-46). The inferior deep cervical nodes (*i.e.*, inferior to the omohyoid) shown here are often referred to as the supraclavicular or scalene nodes because they lie above the clavicle and on the scalenus anterior muscle. To produce temporary paralysis of the diaphragm, the phrenic nerve is crushed where it passes downward across the scalenus anterior muscle. *B*, deeper dissection showing the course of the thoracic duct in the neck. Observe the vertebral artery arising from the first part of the subclavian artery.

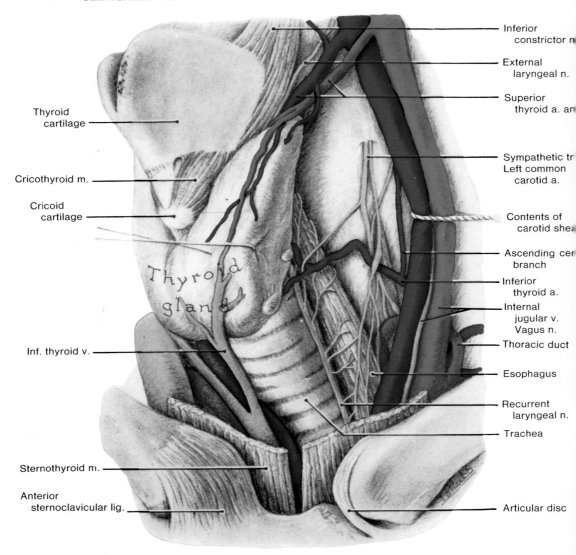

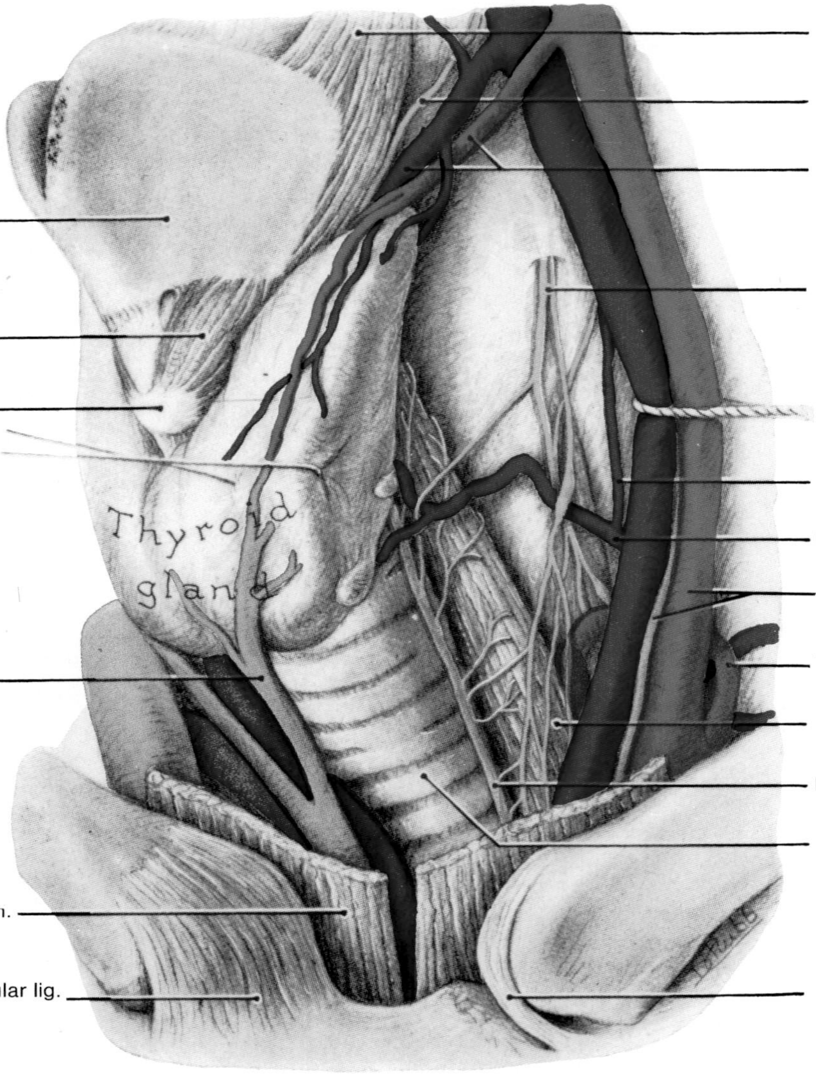

Figure 9-41. Drawing of a dissection of the root of the left side of the neck. Observe the esophagus, a thick muscular tube, which begins at the inferior border of the cricoid cartilage and passes to the left of the trachea. Note the recurrent laryngeal nerve ascending on the side of the trachea just in front of the angle between the trachea and esophagus giving twigs to the esophagus and trachea (not in view) and receiving twigs from the sympathetic trunk (also see Fig. 9-40*B*). Observe the thoracic duct passing from the side of the esophagus to its termination and arching immediately behind the three structures contained in the carotid sheath (internal jugular vein, common carotid artery, and vagus nerve), which are retracted.

clavicle posterior to the sternocleidomastoid muscle. The phrenic nerve is isolated, grasped, and cut where it passes across the scalenus anterior muscle posterior to the prevertebral fascia and between the transverse cervical and suprascapular arteries (Fig. 9-40*A*).

To produce permanent paralysis of the hemidiaphragm [*e.g.*, after **pneumonectomy** (removal of a lung) to allow the abdominal viscera to push the hemidiaphragm upward and to help obliterate the pleural space], a **phrenicectomy** is done by excising a portion of the phrenic nerve. Usually the nerve is avulsed, *i.e.*, the distal stump is pulled until it tears, but it may be pulled up for 3 to 4 cm and cut across.

An **accessory phrenic nerve** (Fig. 9-13) occurs in 20 to 30% of persons and is frequently derived from the fifth cervical nerve as a *branch of the nerve to the subclavius* muscle. It lies lateral to the main phrenic nerve and usually joins it in the root of the neck or in the superior part of the thorax; therefore, should an accessory phrenic nerve be present, sectioning or crushing of the phrenic nerve alone in the neck will not produce complete paralysis of the corresponding half of the diaphragm. However, **avulsion of the phrenic nerve** ruptures the accessory phrenic also and results in complete paralysis of the hemidiaphragm.

The Sympathetic Trunks (Figs. 9-27, 9-33, 9-35, and 9-39). These longitudinal strands of nerve fibers and **sympathetic ganglia** lie *anterolateral to the vertebral column* from the level of the first cervical vertebra to the front of the coccyx.

The sympathetic trunk in the neck receives no white rami communicantes (Fig. 9-33), but it contains three **cervical sympathetic ganglia** (superior, middle, and inferior) which receive their preganglionic fibers from the upper thoracic spinal nerves via white rami communicantes whose fibers leave the spinal cord in the ventral roots of thoracic spinal nerves.

From the sympathetic trunk in the neck, fibers pass to the structures as postganglionic fibers in cervical spinal nerves or leave as direct visceral branches (*e.g.*, to the thyroid gland). Branches to the head run with the arteries, especially the internal and external carotid arteries.

The **inferior cervical ganglion** (Figs. 9-33 and 9-39) lies at the level of the upper border of the neck of the first rib, where it is wrapped around the posterior aspect of the vertebral artery. It is usually fused with the first thoracic ganglion (and sometimes the second) to form a large ganglion known as the **cervicothoracic ganglion** (often called the **stellate ganglion** even though it is not star-shaped in humans). It lies anterior to the transverse process of the vertebra prominens (C7), just above the neck of the first rib on each side, posterior to the origin of the vertebral artery. Some postganglionic fibers from this ganglion pass into the seventh and eighth cervical nerves and to the heart and the **vertebral plexus** around the vertebral artery.

The **middle cervical ganglion** (Fig. 9-35) is small and lies on the anterior aspect of the inferior thyroid artery at about the level of the cricoid cartilage and the transverse process of C6, just anterior to the vertebral artery. Postganglionic branches pass from it to the fifth and sixth cervical nerves and to the heart and the thyroid gland.

The **superior cervical ganglion** (Fig. 9-33) is large and *2 to 3 cm long*. It is located at the level of the atlas and the axis, and because of its size it forms a good *landmark for locating the sympathetic trunk in the neck*. Postganglionic branches from it pass along the internal carotid artery and enter the cranial cavity. It also sends branches to the external carotid artery and into the upper four cervical nerves. Other postganglionic fibers pass to the **cardiac plexus** (Fig. 1-78).

CLINICALLY ORIENTED COMMENTS

If the sympathetic trunk is severed in the neck on one side, interruption of the sympathetic supply to the head on that side occurs. Patients have a sympathetic disturbance known as **Horner's syndrome** on the side of the interruption. It consists of (1) **pupillary constriction** owing to paralysis of the dilator pupillae muscle; (2) **ptosis** (slight lowering of the upper eyelid) owing to paralysis of the smooth muscle in the levator palpebrae superioris; (3) slight **endophthalmos** (sinking in of the eye), possibly resulting from paralysis of the orbitalis muscle, a scanty sheet of smooth muscle in the orbit; and (4) **vasodilation** and **absence of sweating** on the face and neck owing to lack of a sympathetic supply to the blood vessels and sweat glands. Patients with **hemisection of the spinal cord** in the cervical region also exhibit Horner's syndrome. In these cases, the disturbance results from interruption of descending autonomic fibers in the spinal cord.

Lymphatics at the Root of the Neck (Figs. 9-40*A* and 9-46). Several large lymph nodes are arranged within the carotid sheath along the blood vessels of the neck; particularly the internal jugular vein. Another group is found along the transverse cervical artery. All these are **deep cervical lymph nodes** because they are deep to the deep fascia. For descriptive purposes, they are often divided into superior and inferior groups according to their relationship to the point of crossing of the omohyoid over the internal jugular vein (Fig. 9-66).

The deep cervical lymph nodes receive lymph from the **superficial cervical lymph nodes** and from the entire head and neck. From the inferior end of the deep group of lymph nodes, a **jugular lymph trunk** emerges and joins the venous system near the junction of the internal jugular and the subclavian veins (Fig. 9-40). On the left side the jugular lymph trunk may empty into the **thoracic duct**(Figs. 1-48 and 9-30).

CLINICALLY ORIENTED COMMENTS

The deep cervical lymph nodes, particularly those located along the **transverse cervical artery** (Fig. 9-40), may become involved in the spread of cancer from the abdomen or thorax. As their enlargement may give the first clue to cancer in these regions, they are often referred to as the **cervical sentinel nodes**.

The Thoracic Duct (Figs. 9-30, 9-37, 9-40, and 9-41). This large lymphatic channel which drains lymph into the venous system passes upward from the thorax through the thoracic inlet at the left border of the esophagus. It then arches laterally in the root of the neck, posterior to the **carotid sheath** and anterior to the sympathetic trunk and the vertebral and subclavian arteries. It enters the left brachiocephalic vein at the junction of the subclavian and internal jugular veins (Figs. 1-48, 9-30, and 9-40).

The thoracic duct drains lymph from the entire body, except the right side of the head and neck, the right upper limb, and the right side of the thorax. These areas drain via the **right lymphatic duct**, a 1 to 2 cm long vessel which empties into the venous system at or near the junction of the right internal jugular and the right subclavian veins (Fig. 1-48).

CLINICALLY ORIENTED COMMENTS

Blockage of the thoracic duct owing to the permeation of tumor cells (*e.g.*, from an abdominal carcinoma) usually produces no symptoms. The lymph apparently enters the venous system via other lymphatic channels.

The malignant cells pass from an abdominal cancer via the thoracic duct into the root of the neck. Some tumor cells enter the venous system and others extend by retrograde permeation into the inferior deep cervical lymph (supraclavicular) nodes. The cancer cells proliferate here, forming **metastases** (new tumors). The **supraclavicular nodes**, particularly on the left side, may be enlarged with carcinoma of the bronchus, stomach, or any other abdominal organ.

THE CERVICAL VISCERA

The Esophagus (Figs. 9-26, 9-33, 9-40*B*, 9-41, 9-43, and 9-46). This thick, distensible, *muscular tube* (gullet) extends from the pharynx to the stomach (about 25 cm). It begins in the midline at the inferior border of the cricoid cartilage and ends anterior to the 11th thoracic vertebra, at which point it has deviated slightly to the left.

In the neck the esophagus lies between the trachea and the anterior longitudinal ligament on the anterior surfaces of the vertebral bodies (Fig. 9-40*B*). On the right it is in contact with the **cervical pleura** at the root of the neck, whereas on the left side, posterior to the subclavian artery, the thoracic duct lies between the pleura and the esophagus.

The Trachea (Figs. 9-26, 9-29, 9-30, 9-33, 9-36, 9-37, 9-41, 9-43, 9-46, and 9-51). The walls of this wide tube (windpipe) are supported by incomplete cartilaginous **tracheal rings** which are deficient posteriorly where the trachea is related to the esophagus. Here the wall of the trachea is flat. The cartilaginous rings keep the trachea patent (L. open). The trachea extends from the larynx to the roots of the lungs (about 12 cm). The isthmus of the **thyroid gland** usually lies over the second and third tracheal rings. Below the isthmus the jugular venous arch (Fig. 9-28), the inferior thyroid veins, and occasionally a **thyroid ima artery** lie anterior to the trachea.

The brachiocephalic trunk is related to the right side of the trachea at the root of the neck (Figs. 9-29 and 9-47). Occasionally the left brachiocephalic vein and the brachiocephalic trunk are located high enough to cover the trachea at the root of the neck. Lateral to the trachea are the common carotid arteries and the lobes of the thyroid gland (Fig. 9-26).

CLINICALLY ORIENTED COMMENTS

A surgical incision through the midline of the neck and the anterior wall of the

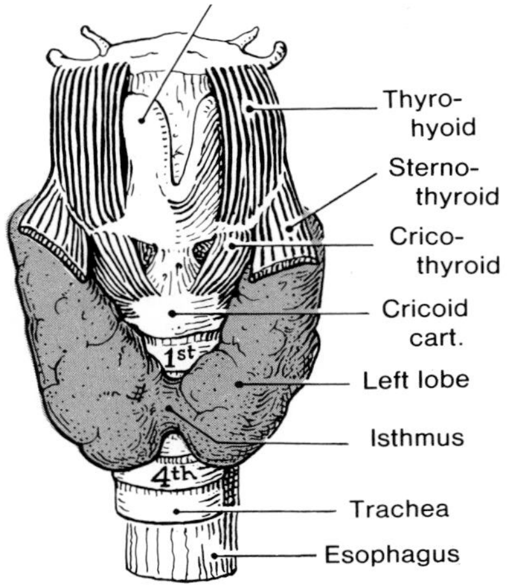

Figure 9-43. Drawing of a normal thyroid gland showing its relationship to the trachea, the esophagus, and the cricoid cartilage. The sternothyroid muscle has been cut to expose the thyroid gland. Note that the isthmus of the thyroid lies anterior to the second and third tracheal rings. In other persons it may extend lower and/or higher.

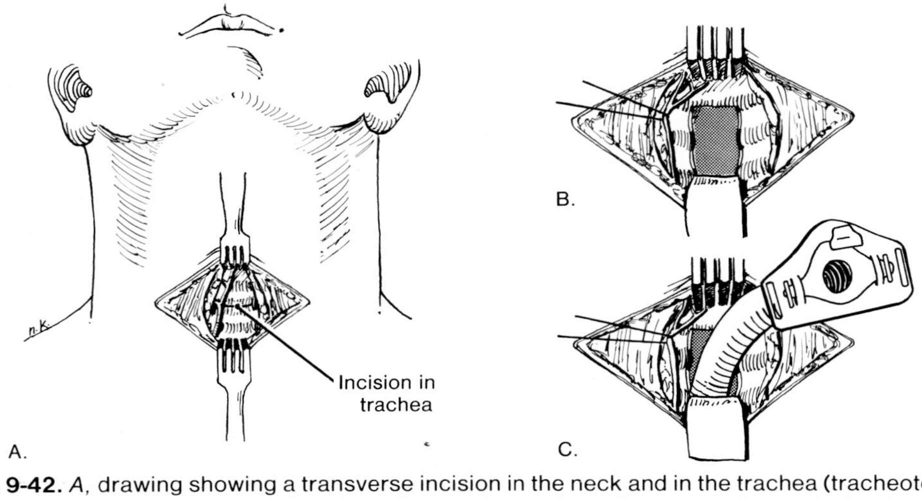

Figure 9-42. *A*, drawing showing a transverse incision in the neck and in the trachea (tracheotomy). *B*, the second and third tracheal rings have been cut, creating a larger opening and a tracheal flap that will be sewn to the skin. This facilitates removal and re-insertion of the tracheotomy tube. *C*, a tracheotomy tube has been inserted into the trachea.

trachea (**tracheotomy**, Fig. 9-42*A*), is often performed in patients with laryngeal obstruction in order to establish an adequate airway, either as an emergency lifesaving measure or as an elective procedure. A **tracheotomy tube** is inserted into the trachea to keep it patent.

Sometimes a round or square opening (Fig. 9-42*B*) rather than a slit is made and the tracheal mucosa is brought into continuity with the skin; this operation is referred to as a **tracheostomy** (L. *ostium*, mouth). If the anticipated duration of endotracheal intubation is short, a tracheotomy is usually performed, but when the supportive measures to maintain respiratory function are expected to be longer than 72 hr (*e.g.*, a patient in a **coma**), a tracheostomy is usually done (Fig. 9-42*C*). When a permanent opening in the trachea is necessary [*e.g.*, after removal of the larynx (laryngectomy) owing to cancer], the tracheotomy tube is removed when the skin and the epithelium of the trachea have united (*i.e.*, when an established tracheostomy has formed). The opening is covered with a gauze square for cosmetic purposes and to keep foreign bodies from entering the trachea.

Obstruction of the larynx can result from inhaled foreign bodies (*e.g.*, a piece of steak, Case 9-4), **laryngotracheobronchitis** (inflammation of the larynx, trachea, and bronchi), allergic reactions, tumors of the larynx, neurological disorders, **epiglotitis**, and the now rare (but serious) laryngeal diptheria.

Tracheotomy is also performed for the evacuation of excessive secretions (*e.g.*, resulting from a postoperative chest infection in a patient who is too weak to cough adequately) and for prolonged artificial ventilation (respiration) in patients with respiratory problems (*e.g.*, related to neurological disorders or drug overdosage).

Although one hears about **emergency tracheotomies** being performed without anesthesia and surgical instruments, *a tracheotomy is not a simple operation.* The common approach to the trachea through the skin, subcutaneous tissue, and deep cervical fascia is made by a transverse incision in the neck, usually midway between the laryngeal prominence and the jugular notch (Fig. 9-1). Surgical opinions vary concerning the best site for making the tracheal incision, but it is commonly made through the second and third tracheal rings. The first ring is not cut because of the danger of narrowing of the trachea during healing of this ring. As the isthmus of the thyroid gland covers the second and third tracheal rings (Fig. 9-43), it is retracted inferiorly or superiorly or divided between clamps.

Because of the shortness of the neck in infants, the incision may be made through the **cricothyroid ligament** (Fig. 9-70) in an emergency and the wound repaired after the immediate danger is over and a formal tracheotomy has been done.

During a tracheotomy inferior to the thyroid gland, *the following anatomical facts must be kept in mind* in order to avoid possible damage to important structures: (1) the **inferior thyroid veins** form a plexus in front of the trachea; (2) a small **thyroid ima** (lowest thyroid) artery may ascend to the lower border of the isthmus; (3) the **left brachiocephalic vein**, the jugular venous arch, and the pleurae (pleural sacs) may be encountered, particularly in infants and children; (4) the **thymus gland** covers the lower part of the cervical trachea in infants: and (5) the *trachea is small, mobile, and soft in infants* and children, making it easy to cut through its posterior wall and damage the esophagus.

The Thyroid Gland (Figs. 9-35 to 9-37, 9-41, 9-43, 9-44, 9-46, 9-47, 9-50, and 9-51). This **highly vascular endocrine gland,** brownish-red during life, consists of right and left lobes united by a narrow **isthmus** that extends across the trachea. The size of the thyroid gland varies greatly, but it usually weighs about 25 g. It is relatively larger and heavier in women in whom it becomes slightly larger during menstruation and pregnancy.

In about 50% of people, a **pyramidal lobe** is also present that ascends from the isthmus (Fig. 9-44). This lobe may be attached to the hyoid bone by fibrous or muscular tissue (levator glandulae thyroideae). In some cases it contains thyroid tissue (Fig. 9-44). The pyramidal lobe represents a persistent portion of the inferior

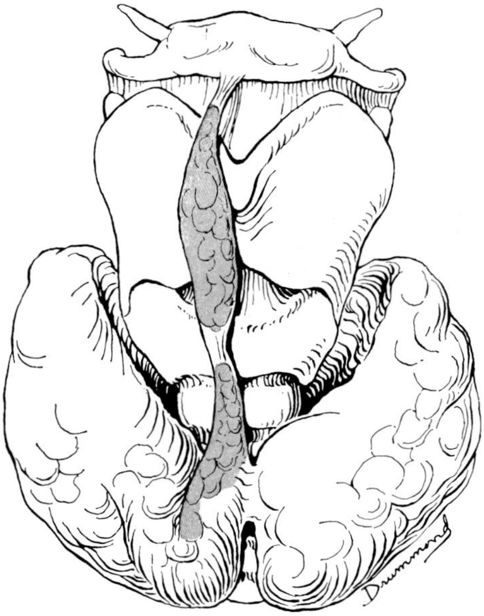

Figure 9-44. Drawing of a thyroid gland with a slender elongated process known as the pyramidal lobe, extending from the isthmus of the thyroid to the hyoid bone. In this case it contains accessory thyroid tissue (*blue*).

end of the **thyroglossal duct** (Fig. 9-45). In the embryo this duct opened into the foramen cecum of the tongue.

The thyroid gland lies deep to the sternothyroid and sternohyoid muscles. Its isthmus usually covers the second and third tracheal rings, but its size varies. Each lobe extends downward on each side of the trachea, often to the level of the sixth ring, and extends backward to the sides of the esophagus (Fig. 9-46).

The thyroid is surrounded by a **fibrous capsule**; external to this is a sheath of **pretracheal fascia** (Fig. 9-50) which is attached to the arch of the cricoid cartilage and to the thyroid cartilage. Hence, the thyroid gland moves with the larynx during swallowing and oscillates during speaking. Between the capsule and the pretracheal fascia (Fig. 9-46) lie the vessels supplying the gland.

Arterial Supply of the Thyroid Gland (Figs. 9-30, 9-35, 9-36, 9-41, 9-46, and 9-47). This **highly vascular organ** usually receives its blood from two rather large arteries.

The **superior thyroid artery**, the first branch of the **external carotid**, descends to the superior pole of the gland, pierces the pretracheal fascia, and then divides into two or three branches.

The **inferior thyroid artery**, a branch of the **thyrocervical trunk** (Fig. 9-29), runs superomedially posterior to the carotid sheath to reach the posterior aspect of the gland. It divides into several branches which pierce the pretracheal fascia to supply the lower pole of the thyroid gland.

Occasionally a third vessel, the small unpaired **thyroid ima artery** (L. lowest), supplies the thyroid gland. This small thyroid artery may arise from the aortic arch, the brachiocephalic artery, or the left common carotid artery. It ascends anterior to the trachea and *supplies the isthmus*.

CLINICALLY ORIENTED COMMENTS

The possible occurrence of a thyroid ima artery must be remembered by persons

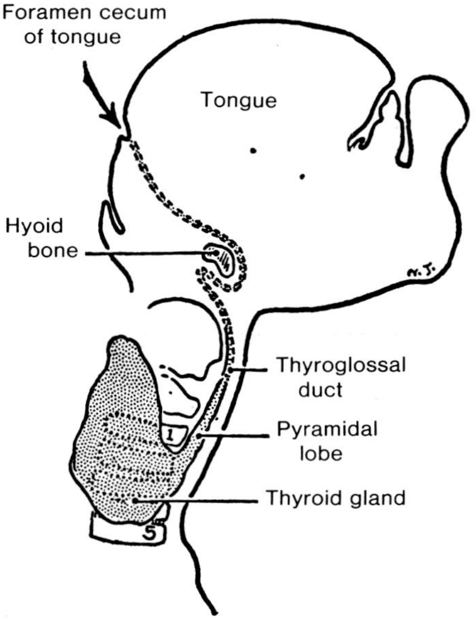

Figure 9-45. Drawing showing the course of the thyroid as it develops and descends through the neck. The thyroglossal duct usually degenerates, but sometimes it may persist and form a pyramidal lobe. Remnants of it may also persist and give rise to cysts or to a fistula.

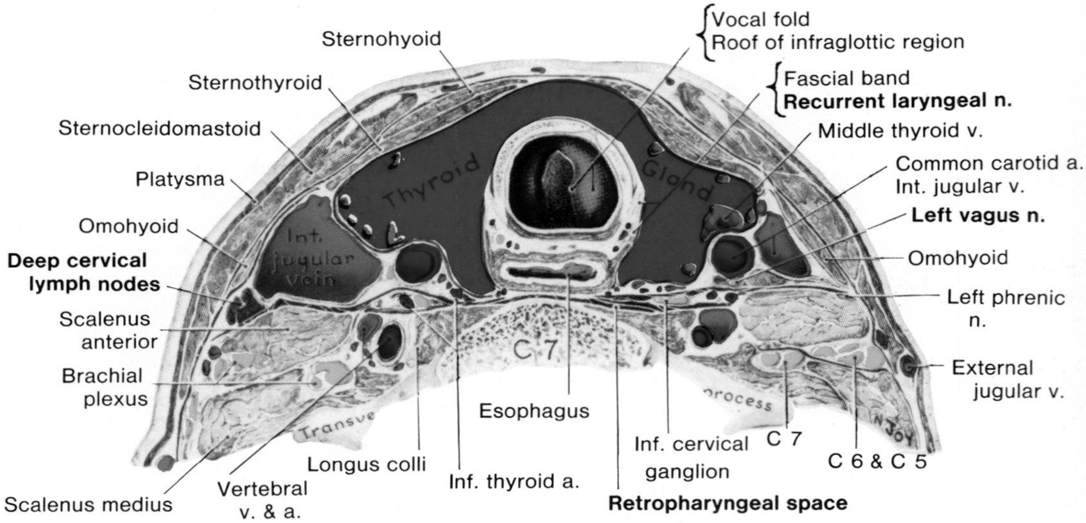

Figure 9-46. Drawing of a cross-section of the neck through the thyroid gland, viewed from below, showing the clinically important visceral compartment. Note that fascia surrounding the esophagus is separated from the prevertebral fascia by a retropharyngeal space. Observe the thyroid gland within its sheath, asymmetrically enlarged and covering the carotid sheath and its contents (common carotid artery, internal jugular vein, and vagus nerve) on the *right side.* Note the fascial band (sheath) that attaches the thyroid gland to the cricoid and thyroid cartilages. Observe the recurrent laryngeal nerve which is at risk during a thyroidectomy.

opening the trachea below the isthmus. As it runs anterior to the trachea, it is a potential source of serious bleeding.

As well as the named thyroid arteries, numerous small vessels pass to the thyroid from the pharynx and the trachea. Hence, the thyroid gland still oozes blood during a subtotal thyroidectomy even when the main arteries supplying it are ligated.

All the thyroid arteries anastomose freely on and in the substance of the thyroid gland (Fig. 9-47), but there is little anastomosis across the median plane except for branches of the superior thyroid artery.

Venous Drainage of the Thyroid Gland (Figs. 9-30, 9-35, 9-46, 9-47, and 9-59). Usually three pairs of veins drain the venous plexus on the surface of the gland. The **superior thyroid veins** drain the upper poles and the **middle thyroid veins** drain the lateral sides. The superior and middle thyroid veins empty into the internal jugular veins. The **inferior thyroid veins** (often several) drain the lower poles and empty into the *brachiocephalic veins.* Often they unite to form a single vein (Fig. 9-47) that opens into one of the brachiocephalic veins. As they *cover the anterior surface of the trachea* inferior to the isthmus of the thyroid gland, they are potential sources of bleeding during a tracheotomy.

Lymph Drainage of the Thyroid Gland (Figs. 9-37, 9-40, 9-46, and 9-49). The lymph vessels accompany the arteries and pass to the lower **deep cervical lymph nodes** and the paratracheal lymph nodes. Some lymph vessels may enter directly into the thoracic duct.

Nerve Supply to the Thyroid Gland (Figs. 9-33, 9-35, 9-39, and 9-41). The nerves are derived from the superior, middle, and inferior **cervical sympathetic ganglia.** They reach the gland via the cardiac and laryngeal branches of the vagus which run along the arteries supplying the gland. These postganglionic fibers are vasomotor and affect the gland indirectly through their action on the blood vessels.

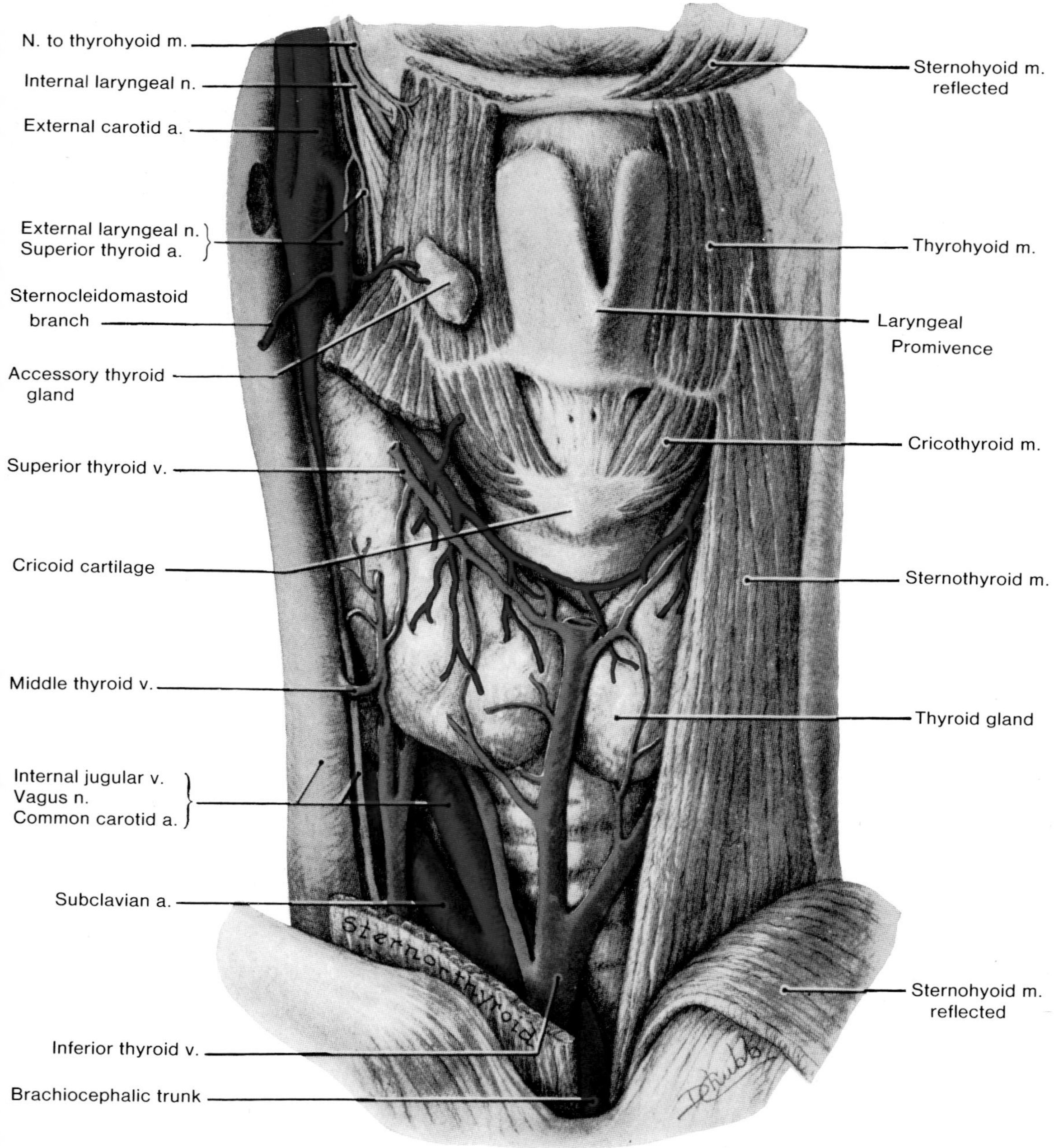

Figure 9-47. Drawing of a dissection of the front of the neck. Observe the two lobes of the thyroid gland which are united across the median plane by an isthmus (not visible here, see Fig. 9-43). Note the surface network of veins on the gland which is drained by the superior, middle, and inferior thyroid veins. Observe that the right lobe of the gland overlies the common carotid artery. In this specimen there is an accessory thyroid gland on the right, lying on the thyrohyoid muscle lateral to thyroid cartilage. The inferior thyroid veins have united to form a single vessel that ends in the right brachiocephalic vein (not shown).

CLINICALLY ORIENTED COMMENTS

Thyroglossal duct cysts may develop from remnants of the thyroglossal duct, anywhere along the course taken by the duct during descent of the thyroid gland during development (Figs. 9-45 and 9-48). The cysts may be in the tongue or in the midline of the neck, usually just below the hyoid bone (Case 9-2). In some cases an opening to the skin develops as a result of perforation following infection of a cyst. These **thyroglossal duct sinuses** usually open in the *midline of the neck* anterior to the thyroid cartilage (Fig. 9-48*A*).

Rarely the thyroid gland fails to descend during development resulting in a **lingual thyroid** gland or a high cervical thyroid gland (*e.g.*, in the region of the hyoid bone). **Accessory thyroid gland** tissue may also develop from remnants of the thyroglossal duct (Fig. 9-47).

Abnormal enlargement of the thyroid gland is called a **goiter** (Case 9-5). The enlarged gland may exert pressure on the trachea or the recurrent laryngeal nerves. In some cases of **hyperthyroidism** the enlarged thyroid gland may cause **stridor** (a harsh, high-pitched respiratory sound), **dyspnea** (difficult breathing), and **dysphagia** (difficulty in swallowing) as the result of compression of the trachea and esophagus. However, narrowing of the trachea is found more commonly with **carcinoma** of the thyroid gland and enlargement of a **retrosternal goiter** (extension of an enlarged thyroid gland behind the sternum).

It is sometimes necessary to remove the entire thyroid gland (*total thyroidectomy*), *e.g.*, during excision of a carcinoma of the thyroid gland. In the surgical treatment of **hyperthyroidism**, usually the posterior portion of each lobe of the enlarged thyroid is left (**subtotal thyroidectomy**). A sound knowledge of the anatomy of the thyroid gland and its relations is essential, otherwise serious complications may arise during and/or after thyroidectomy.

An enlarged thyroid gland may stretch the strap muscles (sternohyoid and sternothyroid) making them very thin. To obtain good exposure of the thyroid gland, it may be necessary to divide these muscles. To prevent injury to their nerves, the muscles are divided superiorly because the nerves enter inferior parts of the muscles (Fig. 9-22).

Injury to the recurrent laryngeal

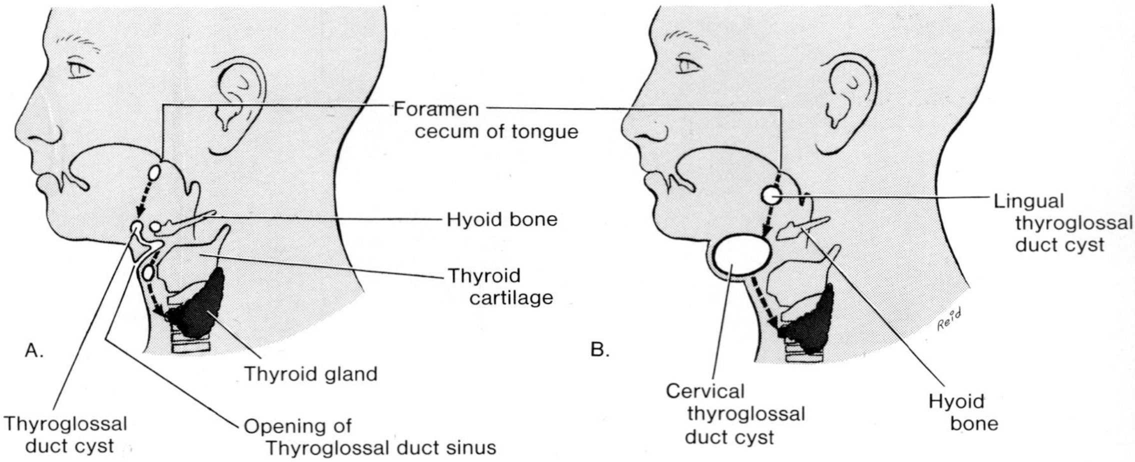

Figure 9-48. *A*, diagrammatic sketch of the head showing the possible locations of thyroglossal duct cysts. A thyroglossal duct sinus is also illustrated. --- indicates the course taken by the thyroglossal duct during descent of the thyroid gland from the foramen cecum to its final position in front of the trachea. *B*, similar sketch illustrating lingual and cervical thyroglossal duct cysts. Most cysts develop near the hyoid bone.

nerves is not common; however, as the risk of injuring them during surgery is ever present, a good knowledge of their relationship to the trachea, the carotid arteries, the thyroid gland, and the inferior thyroid arteries is essential (Figs. 9-30, 9-35, and 9-41). Near the lower pole of the thyroid gland, the **right recurrent laryngeal nerve** is intimately related to the **inferior thyroid artery**; it may cross anterior or posterior to the artery or it may pass between its branches. Because of this close relationship, *the inferior thyroid artery is ligated some distance lateral to the thyroid gland*, where it is not so close to the nerve. Although the danger of injuring the left recurrent laryngeal nerve is not so great, it must be remembered that the artery and the nerve are also closely associated near the lower pole of the thyroid gland (Fig. 9-41).

Damage to a recurrent laryngeal nerve may be partial or complete. *Temporary disturbance of phonation* (voice production) and laryngeal spasm not uncommonly follow partial thyroidectomy as the result of handling the nerves during the operation or from the pressure of accumulated blood and/or serous exudate after the operation.

Injury to the external laryngeal nerve is uncommon during thyroidectomy; however, as it is closely related to the **superior thyroid artery** during part of its course to the superior pole of the thyroid gland (Figs. 9-41 and 9-49), care must be taken not to damage it when the superior thyroid artery is ligated and sectioned. *Injury to this nerve results in the voice becoming monotonous* in character because the paralyzed cricothyroid muscle is unable to vary the length and tension of the **vocal fold** (Fig. 9-79). To avoid injuring this nerve, *the superior thyroid artery is ligated and sectioned near the superior pole of the thyroid gland* where it is not so closely related to the nerve as it is at its origin (Fig. 9-41).

Because an enlarged thyroid gland may itself be the cause of impaired innervation of the larynx as the result of compression, it is common practice to examine the vocal folds prior to an operation. In this way, damage to the larynx or its nerves resulting from a surgical mishap may be distinguished from a pre-existing injury.

The Parathyroid Glands (Figs. 9-49 and 9-52). There are *usually four* small (about 6 × 3 × 2 mm), but, vital, parathyroid glands. Yellowish-brown during life, these ovoid or lentiform (L. lens shaped) **endocrine glands** lie along the posterior border of the thyroid gland between its capsule and sheath of pretracheal fascia. Usually there are two glands associated with each lobe, but the total number usually varies between two and six. They are *named according to their positions* as the **superior** and **inferior parathyroid glands**. The superior ones are more constant in position than the inferior ones and they are usually located near the middle of the posterior surface of the lobes of the thyroid gland. *The inferior parathyroid glands are variable in position;* they are usually located near the inferior surface of the thyroid gland but may lie some distance below it. The best guide to them is their small arteries.

Blood Supply of the Parathyroid Glands (Fig. 9-49). These glands are usually supplied by the **inferior thyroid arteries**, but they may be supplied by the superior thyroid arteries or from the longitudinal anastomosis between the superior and inferior thyroid arteries.

Venous Drainage of the Parathyroid Glands (Fig. 9-47). The veins drain into the **thyroid plexus of veins** on the anterior surface of the thyroid gland and the trachea.

Lymph Drainage of the Parathyroid Glands (Figs. 9-40, 9-49, and 9-66). The lymph vessels drain with those of the thyroid gland into the inferior **deep cervical lymph nodes** and into the **paratracheal lymph nodes**. These lymph vessels end in the thoracic duct and the right lymphatic duct.

Nerve Supply of the Parathyroid Glands (Fig. 9-41). The nerves are derived from the **sympathetic trunk**, either directly from the superior or middle cervical sympathetic ganglia or from the plexus surrounding the superior and inferior thyroid arteries.

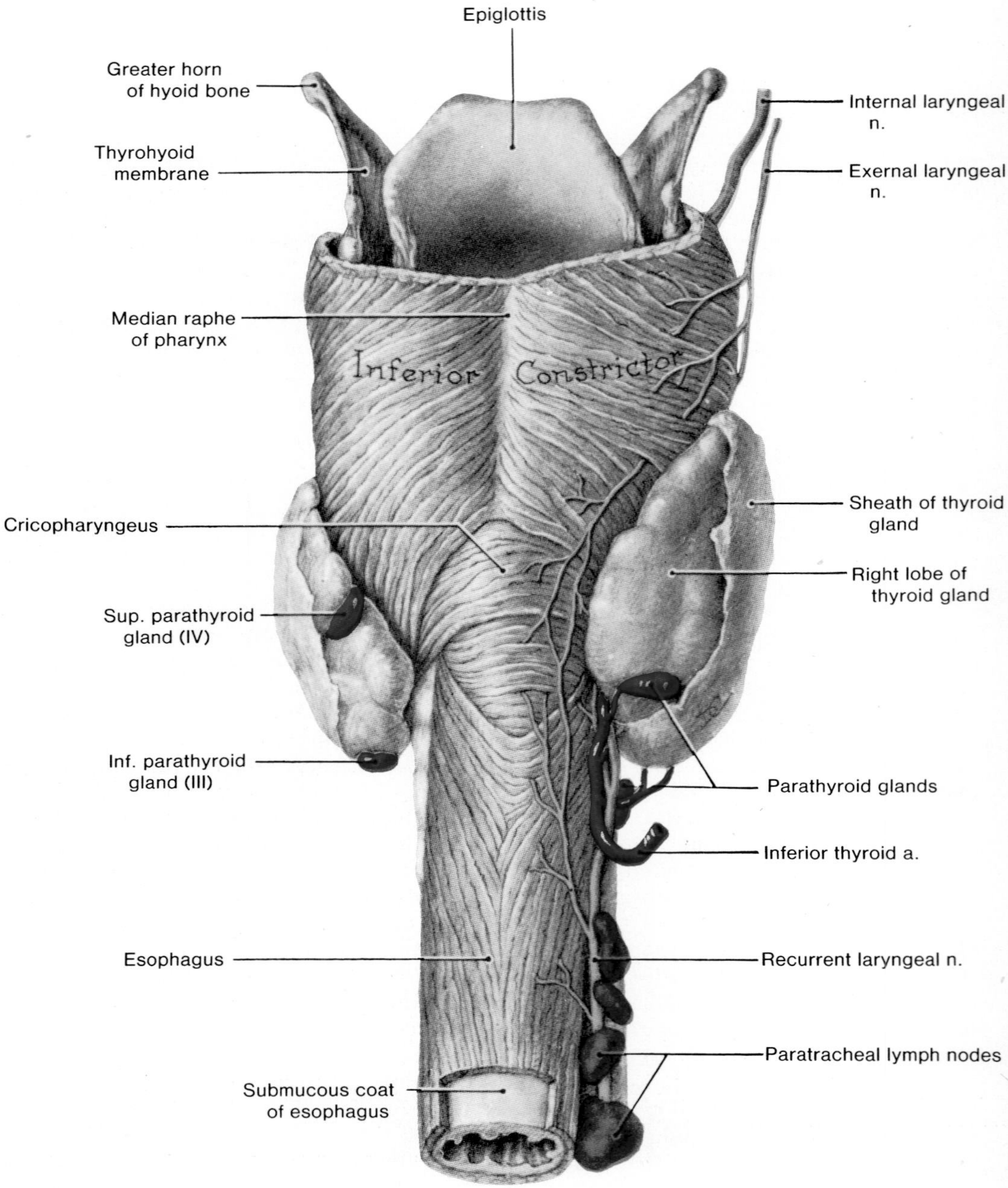

Figure 9-49. Drawing of a dissection of the posterior surface of the thyroid and parathyroid glands. Observe that the right and left lobes of the thyroid gland are unequal in size in this specimen. Note that these lobes are applied to the inferior constrictor muscle of the pharynx, the trachea, and the esophagus. Examine the parathyroid glands, noting that on the right side both parathyroids are rather low, the inferior gland being inferior to the thyroid gland. The Roman numerals after the superior and inferior parathyroid glands indicate that they developed from the IVth and IIIrd pharyngeal pouches, respectively. The inferior parathyroid glands (III) were pulled caudal to the superior parathyroid glands (IV) by the descending thymus gland, another derivative of the third pair of pharyngeal pouches. The continuation of the recurrent laryngeal nerve is known as the inferior laryngeal nerve. Note that it accompanies the inferior thyroid artery into the larynx.

CLINICALLY ORIENTED COMMENTS

An awareness of the close relationship between the parathyroid glands, the thyroid gland, and the recurrent laryngeal nerves is essential knowledge. The possibility of injuring the recurrent laryngeal nerves during thyroidectomy has been discussed previously. The small parathyroid glands are also in danger of being damaged or removed during this operation, but they are usually safe during subtotal thyroidectomy because the posterior rim of the thyroid is preserved. The variability in the position of these glands, particularly the inferior ones, creates a basic problem in thyroid and parathyroid surgery. The parathyroids may be as high as the thyroid cartilage and the inferior ones may be as low as the **superior mediastinum** (Fig. 1-49). An inferior parathyoid gland may even be within the substance of the inferior end of a lobe of the thyroid gland. These possible aberrant sites are of concern when searching for a tumorous parathyroid (*e.g.*, parathyroid adenoma) in hyperparathyroidism.

The variability in position of the inferior parathyroid glands has an embryological basis. They develop in association with the thymus gland and are carried caudally with it during its descent through the neck from the third pair of **pharyngeal pouches**. If the thymus fails to descend to its usual position, the inferior parathyroids usually lie at the level of the thyroid cartilage. If the inferior parathyroids do not disassociate from the thymus, they may be carried with it inferior to the thyroid and even into the thorax (*i.e.*, into the superior mediastinum, Figs. 1-49 and 9-51). Consequently it may be very difficult to distinguish between superior and inferior parathyroid glands or to find four of them; *rarely are there more than four.*

If the parathyroid glands atrophy or are inadvertently removed, the patient suffers from a severe *convulsive disorder* known as **tetany**.[2] The generalized convulsive spasms result from a lowered serum calcium level. There is nervousness, twitching, and spasms in the facial and limb musculature. If the respiratory and laryngeal muscles are also affected, death may occur if medical treatment is not given (*e.g.*, by injecting a calcium and/or a parathyroid extract). *To safeguard the parathyroid glands during thyroidectomy, the posterior portion of each lobe is usually not removed.* In rare instances when it is necessary to do a **total thyroidectomy** (*e.g.*, in malignant disease), the parathyroid glands are isolated with their blood vessels left intact.

[2] Note that *tetany* and *tetanus* are not the same conditions. Tetanus is an infectious disease in which tonic muscle spasm results in "lockjaw" and similar spasm of other muscle groups.

FASCIAL PLANES OF THE NECK

Although the layers of **cervical fascia** have been mentioned several times, their surgical importance warrants that they be discussed in more detail. For descriptive purposes the deep fascia of the neck is described in **three layers**: investing, pretracheal, and prevertebral.

The Investing Fascia (Figs. 9-28, 9-46, and 9-50). This superficial layer encircles the neck and *surrounds the structures in the neck.* It is attached superiorly to the **superior nuchal line** (Fig. 7-3), the mastoid process, the zygomatic arch, the inferior border of the **mandible**, the **hyoid**

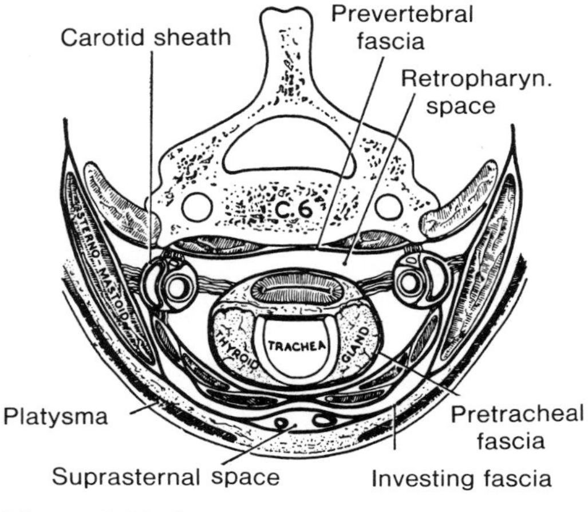

Figure 9-50. Drawing of a cross-section of the neck at the level of the sixth cervical vertebra illustrating the fascial layers. The retropharyngeal space between the prevertebral fascia and the digestive tract is a potential space (also see Figs. 9-46 and 9-51).

bone, and the spinous processes of the cervical vertebrae. Inferiorly it is attached to the **manubrium** sterni (Fig. 9-28), the **clavicle**, and the acromion and spine of the **scapula**. Immediately above the sternum the investing fascia divides into two layers which are attached to the anterior and posterior surfaces of the manubrium sterni, respectively. The interval between these two layers is called the **suprasternal space** (Figs. 9-28, 9-50, and 9-51). It encloses the sternocleidomastoid and trapezius muscles, the jugular venous arch (Fig. 9-28), and an occasional lymph node. *Together with the skin, the investing fascia also forms the roof of the anterior and posterior triangles of the neck* (Figs. 9-15 and 9-21).

CLINICALLY ORIENTED COMMENTS

The superficial investing layer of cervical fascia tends to prevent extension of **ab-**

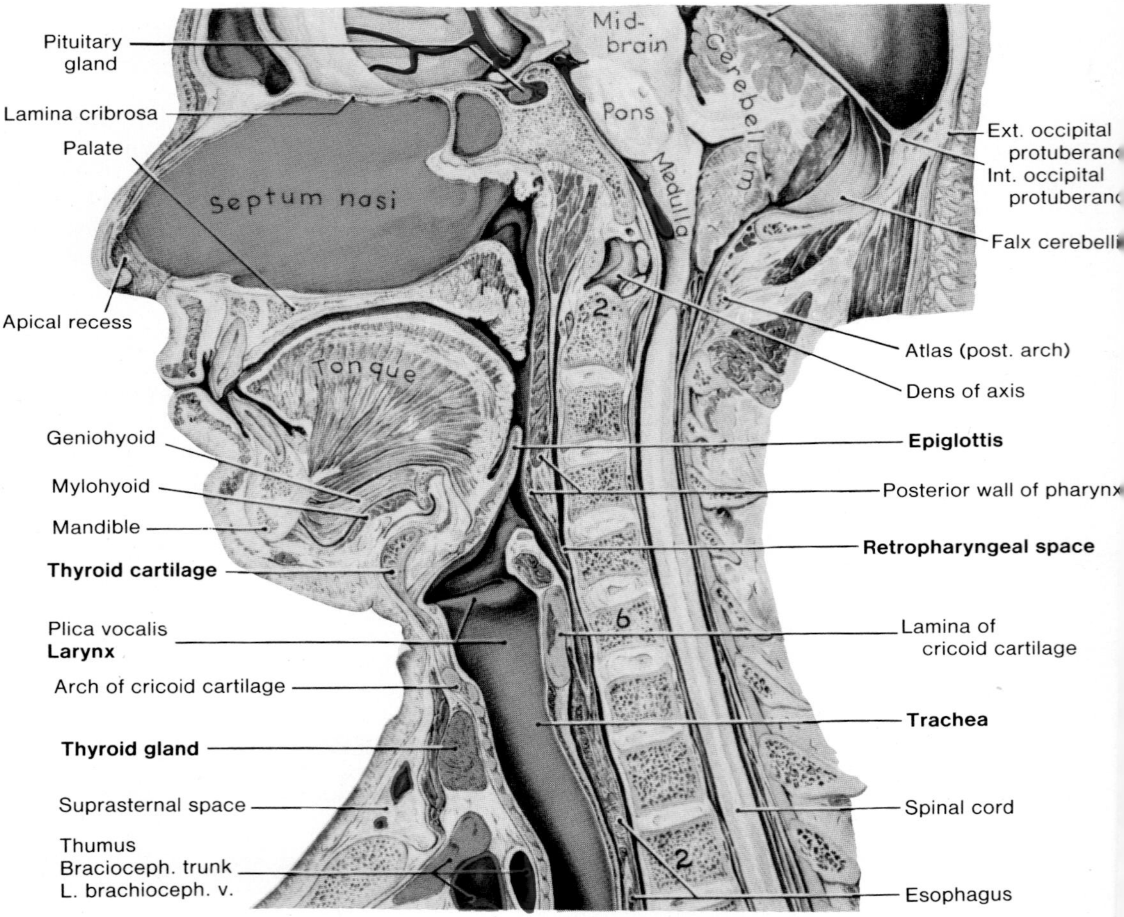

Figure 9-51. Drawing of a median section of the head and neck. Observe the pharynx extending from the base of the skull to the level of the body of the sixth cervical vertebra, where it is continuous with the esophagus. Note the lamina of the cricoid cartilage at the level of the body of the sixth cervical vertebra and that at its inferior border the larynx becomes the trachea and the pharynx becomes the esophagus. Observe the *retropharyngeal space* extending from the level of the atlas downward into the superior mediastinum. Observe the laryngopharynx (laryngeal portion of pharynx) lying behind the aperture and posterior wall of the larynx.

scesses (collections of pus) toward the surface. Pus beneath it usually extends laterally in the neck, but if the abscess is in the anterior triangle, the pus may pass inferiorly, producing a swelling in the suprasternal region. It could also pass into the mediastinum (Fig. 1-49).

The Pretracheal Fascia (Figs. 9-26, 9-28, 9-46, and 9-50). This thin layer of fascia, *limited to the front of the neck*, extends from the thyroid cartilage and the arch of the cricoid cartilage downward into the thorax. Note that it is more extensive than its name implies. It splits to enclose the thyroid gland, the trachea, and the esophagus and *blends laterally with the carotid sheath*.

CLINICALLY ORIENTED COMMENTS

Infections in the head or cervical region of the vertebral column can spread downward posterior to the esophagus into the mediastinum. They can also spread downward anterior to the trachea, entering the anterior part of the mediastinum (Fig. 1-49).

Air from a **ruptured trachea**, bronchus, esophagus, or so-called "spontaneous" **mediastinal emphysema** can pass upward into the neck. An unusual source of air in the face and neck is from a dentist's drill via a tooth socket. Similarly a small slit in the buccal mucosa, followed by hard blowing with the mouth closed, may result in subcutaneous **cervicofacial emphysema**. This unusual kind of swollen neck has been reported in glass blowers, players of wind instruments, and malingerers.

The Prevertebral Fascia (Figs. 9-26, 9-40, 9-46, and 9-50). This layer of fascia covers the **prevertebral muscles** and is continuous with the deep fascia (fascial carpet) covering the muscular floor of the posterior triangle of the neck. It is part of the strong "fascial sleeve" that envelops the deep muscles of the neck. It *extends from the base of the skull to the third thoracic vertebra* where it fuses with the anterior longitudinal ligament. It extends downward and laterally as the **axillary sheath** (Fig. 6-46) which surrounds the axillary vessels and the brachial plexus. The adjective "prevertebral" can be misleading; thus, you should observe that the prevertebral fascia *surrounds the vertebral column and the muscles related to it*.

CLINICALLY ORIENTED COMMENTS

Pus located posterior to the prevertebral fascia may perforate anteriorly in the **retropharyngeal space** (Figs. 9-46 and 9-51) but is more likely to extend into the lateral part of the neck beneath the deep fascia on the floor of the posterior triangle and form a swelling that points (L. *punctus*, to pierce) posterior to the sternocleidomastoid muscle (*i.e.*, perforates the deep fascia and enters the subcutaneous tissues).

The fascial planes are important to the surgeon because they form **lines of cleavage** through which the tissues may be separated and because they limit the spread of pus in infections of the neck.

The Retropharyngeal Space (Figs. 7-145, 9-46, 9-50, and 9-51). This consists of *loose connective tissue between the prevertebral fascia and the buccopharyngeal fascia* (fascia surrounding the larynx). It is a **potential space**, permitting movement of the pharynx, larynx, trachea, and esophagus in swallowing. This space is closed above by the base of the skull and on each side by the carotid sheath. It opens inferiorly into the superior mediastinum (Figs. 1-49 and 9-51).

CLINICALLY ORIENTED COMMENTS

The retropharyngeal space is of considerable surgical interest because of the structures related to it. Pus located posterior to the prevertebral fascia may perforate this layer and enter the retropharyngeal space, producing a bulge in the pharynx (**retropharyngeal abscess**). This causes difficulty in swallowing and speaking (Case 9-6). In addition, infections in this space may extend inferiorly into the mediastinum, producing **mediastinitis** (inflammation of the cellular tissue of the mediastinum).

THE PHARYNX

The pharynx is the *continuation of the digestive cavity from the mouth*. In its superior part it also receives the posterior openings of the nasal cavities, called **choanae**. The pharynx is a wide, **median fibromuscular tube** located posterior to the nasal and oral cavities and the larynx (Figs. 9-51 and 9-52). *It is the upper end of the respiratory and digestive tubes* and is continuous inferiorly with the esophagus. The pharynx conducts food to the esophagus and air to the larynx and lungs. For convenience of description, it is divided into **three parts**: (1) **the nasopharynx**, posterior to the nose and above the soft palate; (2) **the oropharynx**, posterior to the mouth; and (3) **the laryngopharynx**, posterior to the larynx.

The pharynx, about 15 cm long, *extends from* the **base of the skull** to the lower border of the **cricoid cartilage** anteriorly and to the lower border of the **sixth cervical vertebra** posteriorly. It is widest (about 5 cm) opposite the hyoid bone and narrowest (about 1.5 cm) at its inferior end, where it is continuous with the esophagus. The posterior wall of the pharynx lies against the **prevertebral fascia** (Fig. 9-50), with the potential **retropharyngeal space** between them (Fig. 9-51).

In Figure 9-51 observe that the pathways for food and air cross each other in the pharynx; hence, food sometimes enters the respiratory tract and causes choking (Case 9-4), and air may enter the digestive tract causing gas in the stomach that may result in **eructation** (belching).

Structure of the Pharynx. The pharyngeal wall is composed of five layers (coats). From within outward, they are (1) a **mucous membrane** that lines the pharynx and is continuous with all chambers with which it communicates; (2) a **submucosa**; (3) a **fibrous layer** forming the **pharyngobasilar fascia** (Figs. 9-52 and 9-53) which attaches to the skull; (4) a **muscular layer** composed of *inner longitudinal* and *outer circular parts*; and (5) a thin **areolar layer** forming the **buccopharyngeal fascia**. This fascia is continuous with the epimysial covering of the buccinator and pharyngeal muscles. This areolar layer permits movements of the pharynx and contains the pharyngeal plexus of nerves and veins.

The External Muscles of the Pharynx (Figs. 9-52 to 9-55). The outer circular part of the muscular layer in the wall of the pharynx is *formed by the paired superior, middle, and inferior constrictors* which overlap one another somewhat like roof tiles. The constrictor muscles are arranged so that the superior one is innermost and the inferior one is outermost. As their names indicate, they all *constrict the pharynx in swallowing*. They contract involuntarily in a way that results in contraction taking place sequentially from above downward. This action propels the food onward into the esophagus. *All three constrictors are supplied by the* **pharyngeal plexus of nerves** (Figs. 9-52 and 9-55) which lies on the lateral wall of the pharynx, mainly on the middle constrictor muscle. This plexus is formed by the pharyngeal branches of the vagus (*CN X*) and glossopharyngeal (*CN IX*) nerves.

The superior constrictor muscle (Figs. 9-52 to 9-55 and 9-57) is broad and arises from the posterior margin of the **medial pterygoid lamina** (plate), the **pterygomandibular raphe**, and the **mandible** posterior to the third molar tooth. The pterygomandibular raphe is a fibrous line of junction between the buccinator and the superior constrictor muscles (Fig. 9-54). Fibers of the superior constrictor curve backward around the pharynx to insert into the **median raphe of the pharynx** in the posterior wall.

The middle constrictor muscle (Figs. 9-52 to 9-56) arises from the inferior end of

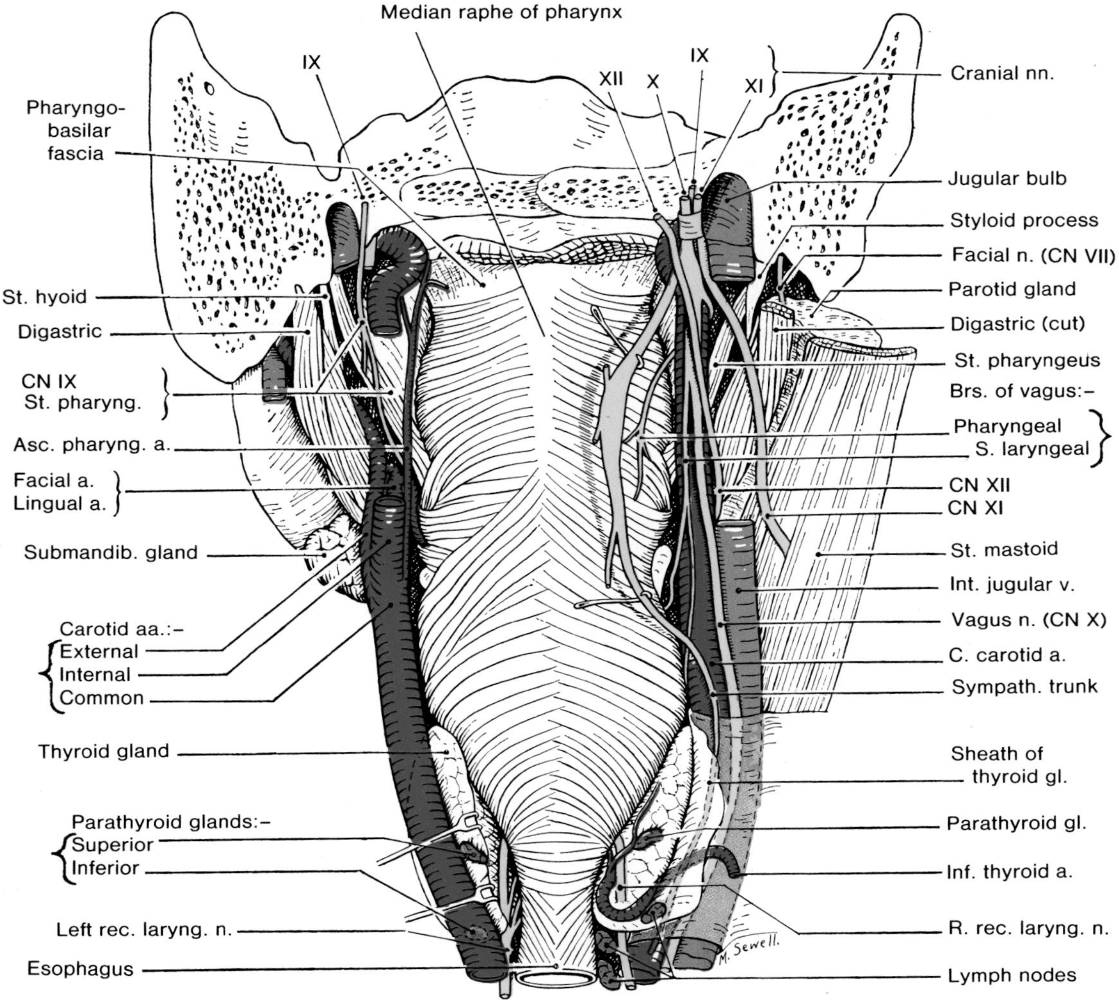

Figure 9-52. Drawing of a dissection of the posterior surface of the pharynx. Note that the pharynx begins at the skull and ends inferiorly in the esophagus. Observe the thyroid and parathyroid glands and that the parathyroids are closely applied to the posterior aspect of the thyroid. Although not visible, they are embedded in the posterior surface of the fibrous capsule of this gland. The parathyroids, particularly the inferior ones, may be located on the lateral or the anterior surface of the thyroid or be imbedded in it. Note that the left inferior parathyroid in this specimen is located posterior to the common carotid artery. *The inferior parathyroids are in an abnormal position in about 10% of persons.* Obviously a thorough knowledge of the parathyroids is necessary for their preservation during operations on the thyroid and in searching for a tumorous parathyroid.

the **stylohyoid ligament** and from the greater and lesser horns of the **hyoid** bone. Its fibers curve backward around the pharynx to insert into its **median raphe**.

The inferior constrictor muscle (Figs. 9-52 to 9-55 and 9-57) has a continuous origin from the oblique line of the **thyroid cartilage** and **fascia** over the cricothyroid muscle and the side of the **cricoid cartilage**. Its fibers pass upward, horizontally, and downward, overlapping those of the middle constrictor, to insert into the **me-**

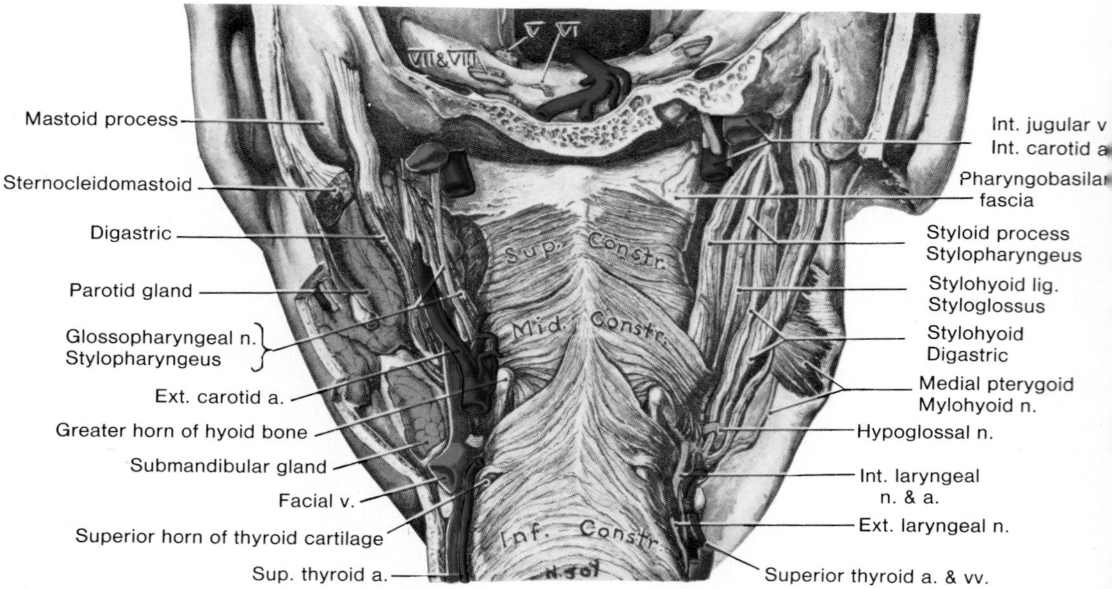

Figure 9-53. Drawing of a dissection of the posterior aspect of the pharynx and parotid gland. Observe the pharynogobasilar fascia which suspends the pharynx from the basioccipital bone. Note the three constrictor muscles nestled within each other like stacked roof tiles and that the posterior aspect of the pharynx is flat or slightly concave from side to side where it is applied to the prevertebral region. Note the stylopharyngeus muscle and the glossopharyngeal nerve (CN IX) passing from the medial side of the styloid process forward and medially through the gap between the superior and middle constrictor muscles.

dian raphe of the pharynx. The fibers arising from the cricoid cartilage (cricopharyngeus fibers) are believed to act as a sphincter, preventing air from entering the esophagus; they relax during swallowing.

The arrangement of the constrictor muscles leaves *four deficiencies or gaps in the pharyngeal musculature for structures to enter the pharynx* (Fig. 9-55).

1. **Above the superior constrictor** muscle, the levator palati, the auditory tube, and the ascending palatine artery pass through the gap between the superior constrictor and the skull (Fig. 9-54). Above the superior border of the superior constrictor, the pharyngobasilar fascia blends with the buccopharyngeal fascia to form, with the mucous membrane, the thin wall of the **pharyngeal recess** (Figs. 9-58 and 9-60).

2. **Between the superior and middle constrictors** (Fig. 9-53) lies the *gateway to the mouth*, through which pass the stylopharyngeus, the glossopharyngeal nerve (CN IX), the styloglossus muscle, the lingual nerve, the lingual artery, and the hypoglossal nerve (CN XII).

3. **Between the middle and inferior constrictors** (Fig. 9-55), the internal laryngeal nerve and the superior laryngeal artery and vein pass to the larynx.

4. **Below the inferior constrictor**, the recurrent laryngeal nerve and the inferior laryngeal artery pass upward into the larynx.

The Internal Muscles of the Pharynx (Figs. 9-53, 9-55, and 9-57). The internal, chiefly longitudinal layer consists of three muscles: the stylopharyngeus, the palatopharyngeus, and the salpingopharyngeus. They all elevate the larynx and pharynx in swallowing and speaking.

The Stylopharyngeus Muscle (Figs. 9-52, 9-53, and 9-55). This long thin, conical muscle arises from the medial aspect of the **styloid process** and descends downward between the external and internal carotid

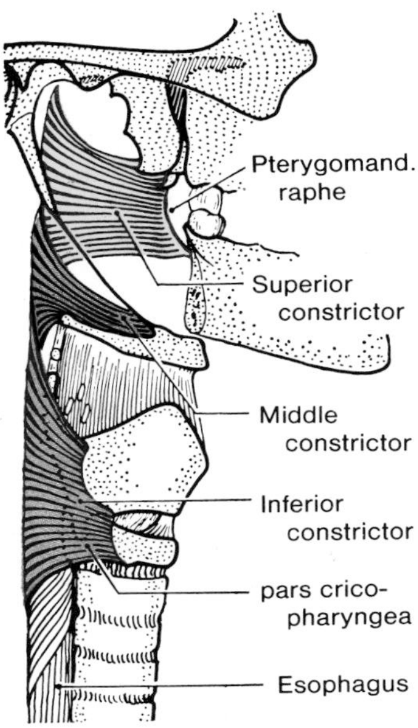

Figure 9-54. Drawing of a lateral view of the constrictor muscles of the pharynx showing their attachments and borders. Note that each constrictor is fan-shaped and the narrow ends of the fans are fixed anteriorly. Posteriorly they meet in the median raphe of the pharynx (Figs. 9-45 and 9-52). Observe the continuous origin of the inferior constrictor from the thyroid and cricoid cartilages.

arteries to enter the wall of the pharynx between the superior and middle constrictors.

Origin. Medial surface of the **styloid process**.

Insertion. Posterior and superior borders of **thyroid cartilage** and **palatopharyngeus** muscle with which it is continuous.

Nerve Supply. **Glossopharyngeal** nerve (CN IX). *The stylopharyngeus is the only muscle of the pharynx that is not supplied by the pharyngeal plexus* of nerves.

Actions. **Elevates larynx, raises pharynx**, and **expands sides of pharynx**, thereby aiding in pulling the pharyngeal wall over a bolus of food in swallowing.

The Palatopharyngeus Muscle (Figs. 9-57, 9-61, 9-62, and 9-65). This muscle and the overlying mucosa form the **palatopharyngeal arch**.

Origin (Fig. 7-148). Posterior border of **hard palate** and **palatine aponeurosis**.

Insertion. **Posterior border of thyroid cartilage** and sides of the pharynx and esophagus.

Actions. **Elevates larynx** and **wall of pharynx**, thereby shortening the pharynx in swallowing. It also produces a constriction of the palatopharyngeal arch.

The Salpingopharyngeus Muscle (Figs. 9-57 and 9-62). This slender muscle descends into the lateral wall of the pharynx and is covered by the **salpingopharyngeal fold** of mucous membrane.

Origin. **Cartilage of auditory tube** at its pharyngeal end.

Insertion. Descends vertically downward to join **palatopharyngeus** muscle.

Actions. **Elevates larynx** and **pharynx** and **opens auditory tube** (cartilaginous part) in swallowing.

Interior of the Pharynx (Figs. 9-57 to 9-62). The interior of the pharynx communicates with three cavities: the nose, the mouth, and the larynx; hence, it consists of three parts: the **nasopharynx**, the **oropharynx**, and the **laryngopharynx**. The soft palate, including the uvula, separates the nasopharynx above from the oropharynx below.

The Nasopharynx (Nasal Part of Pharynx). This part of the pharynx has a respiratory function. It lies above the soft palate and is a backward extension of the nasal cavities. The nose opens into the nasopharynx via two large posterior apertures called the internal nares or **choanae**; they are separated by the bony nasal septum (Fig. 9-58).

The **roof** and posterior wall of the nasopharynx form a continuous surface that lies below the body of the sphenoid bone and the basilar part of the occipital bone. In the mucous membrane of the roof and posterior wall of the nasopharynx, there is a *collection of lymphoid tissue* known as the **pharyngeal tonsil** (more precisely, the nasopharyngeal tonsil). When enlarged the pharyngeal tonsil is commonly called the "**adenoids**."

The pharyngeal orifice of the auditory tube (pharyngotympanic tube) is on the

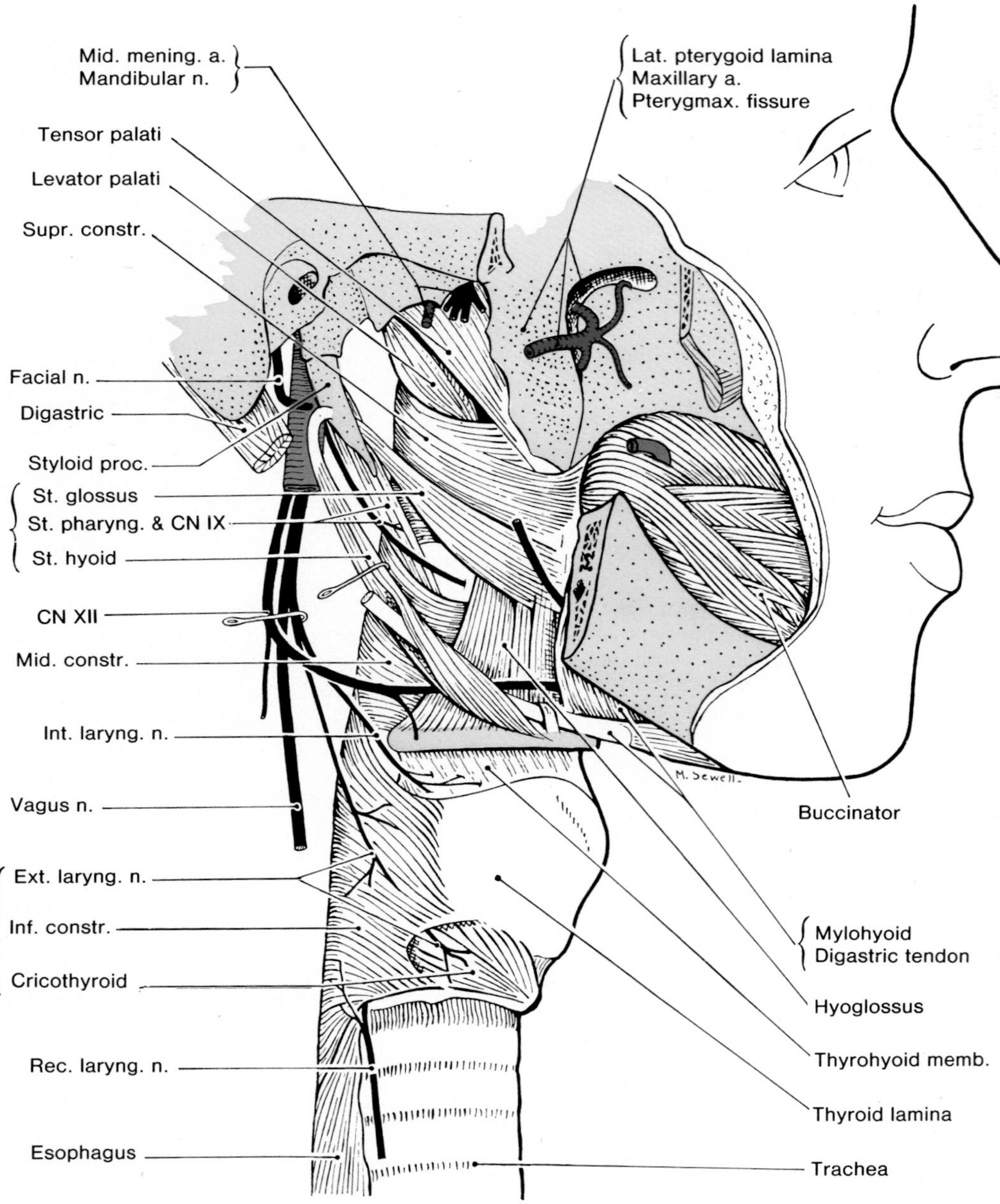

Figure 9-55. Drawing of a dissection of the right side of the head and neck showing the pharyngeal muscles and the buccinator. Observe that the superior constrictor and the buccinator arise from opposite sides of the pterygomandibular raphe, and that the middle constrictor is overlapped by the hypoglossus, which is in turn overlapped by the myohyoid. Observe the gaps between the constrictor muscles through which vessels and nerves pass. Note that the recurrent laryngeal nerve enters the pharyngeal wall below the free inferior border of inferior constrictor muscle.

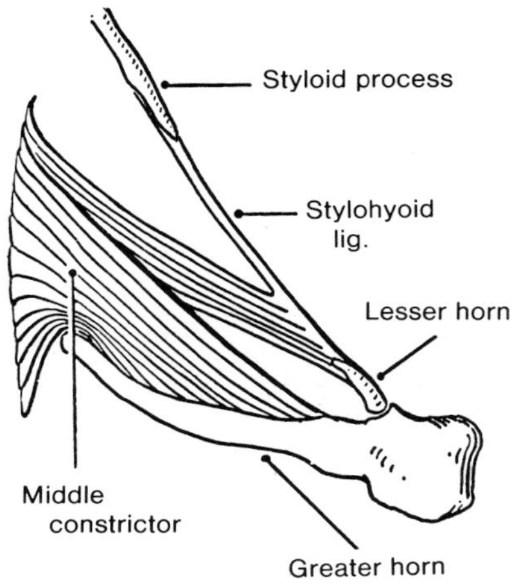

Figure 9-56. Drawing illustrating the angular origin of the middle constrictor muscle of the pharynx from the stylohyoid ligament and the horns of the hyoid bone.

lateral wall of the nasopharynx 1 to 1.5 cm posterior to the inferior concha (Fig. 9-59) at the level of the upper border of the palate. The tube is about 3.5 cm long (one-third osseous, two-thirds cartilaginous). Its orifice is directed downward and posterior to it, there is a hood-like *tubal elevation* called the **torus tubarius** (L. *torus*, swelling). It is produced by the projection of the cartilaginous part of the auditory tube. Extending downward from the torus of the tube is a vertical fold of mucous membrane known as the **salpingopharyngeal fold**. It covers the salpingopharyngeus muscle, which opens the auditory tube during swallowing (Figs. 9-57 to 9-59). The collection of lymphoid tissue in the submucosa behind the orifice of the auditory tube is known as the **tubal tonsil**.

Posterior to the torus tubarius and the salpingopharyngeal fold, there is a slit-like lateral projection of the pharynx called the **pharyngeal recess** (Fig. 9-59), which extends laterally and posteriorly.

CLINICALLY ORIENTED COMMENTS

Because of the close relationship of the pharyngeal tonsil to the choanae and the orifices of the auditory tubes, inflammation of it (**adenoiditis**) may lead to obstruction of these tubes and infection in the middle ear (Case 9-8). An enlarged pharyngeal tonsil (**adenoids**) can obstruct the passage of air from the nasal cavities through the choanae to the nasopharynx, making mouth breathing necessary. In chronic cases the patient develops a characteristic facial expression called **adenoid facies**. The open mouth and protruding tongue give the person a dull expression.

The auditory tube, connecting the nasopharynx with the tympanic (middle ear) cavity, *equalizes the pressure of the external air and that contained in the tympanic cavity*. It also provides a pathway for nasal and oral infections to spread to the middle ear and, in untreated cases, to the mastoid antrum and mastoid air cells (Fig. 7-191). Widespread use of antibiotics has made **mastoid infections** rare.

Infection from the adenoids may spread to the tubal tonsil (**tubal tonsillitis**) causing swelling and closure of the auditory tube. Infection spreading to the tympanic cavity causes **otitis media** (middle ear infection) which may result in a temporary or permanent hearing loss.

The Oropharynx (Oral Part of Pharynx). This part of the pharynx has a digestive function and is continuous with the mouth via the **oropharyngeal isthmus**. The oropharynx is bounded by the **soft palate** superiorly, the **base of the tongue** inferiorly, and laterally by the **pillars of the fauces** (L. throat). It extends from the soft palate to the superior border of the epiglottis (Figs. 9-51, 9-58, 9-59, and 9-61).

Examine someone's oropharynx using a flashlight and a tongue depressor. Have him/her open the mouth wide, stick out the tongue, and say "ah." Examine the pillars of the fauces and the palatine tonsils (Fig. 9-61). These pillars consist of two **palatine arches**. The anterior fold of mucous membrane, or **palatoglossal arch**, joining the palate to the side of the tongue, is formed by the palatoglossus muscle (Figs. 9-59 and 9-62). This arch forms a dividing line between the oral cavity and the oropharynx.

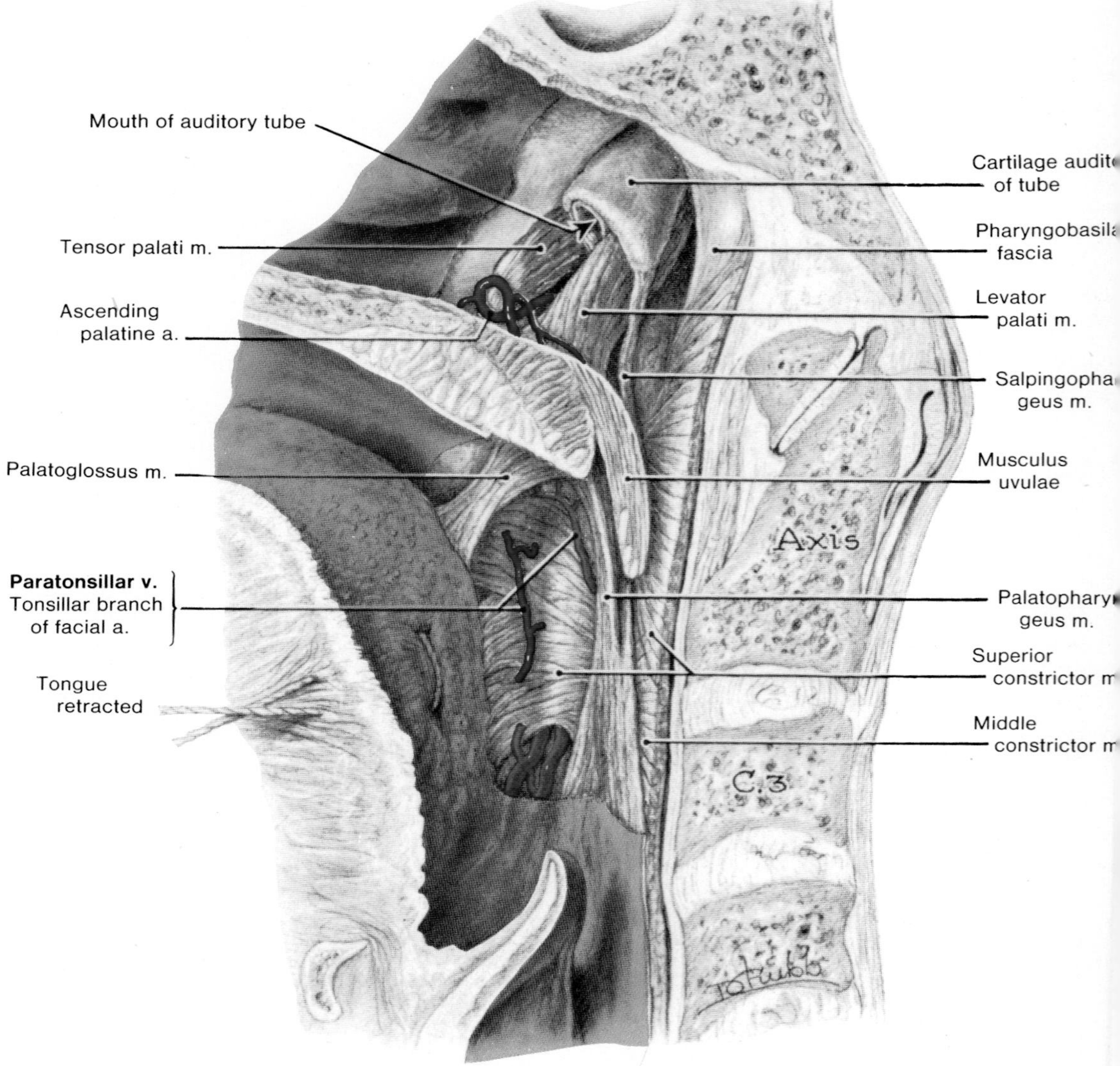

Figure 9-57. Drawing of a lateral view of a dissection of the interior of the pharynx. The palatine and pharyngeal tonsils and the mucous membrane are removed. Observe the remaining part of the submucous pharyngobasilar fascia which attaches the pharynx to the basilar part of the occipital bone. Examine the curved cartilage of the auditory tube, its free upper and posterior lips, and its pharyngeal orifice. Note the salpingopharyngeus muscle descending from the posterior lip to join the palatopharyngeus muscle. Observe the tonsillar bed from which a thin sheet of pharyngobasilar fascia has been removed to expose the palatopharyngeus and the superior constrictor. Note that the bed of the palatine tonsil extends far into the soft palate. The tonsillar branch of the facial artery is long and large here. The *paratonsillar vein*, descending from the soft palate to join the pharyngeal plexus of veins, is a close lateral relation of the tonsil and is the chief source of hemorrhage in tonsil operations (*e.g.*, tonsillectomies).

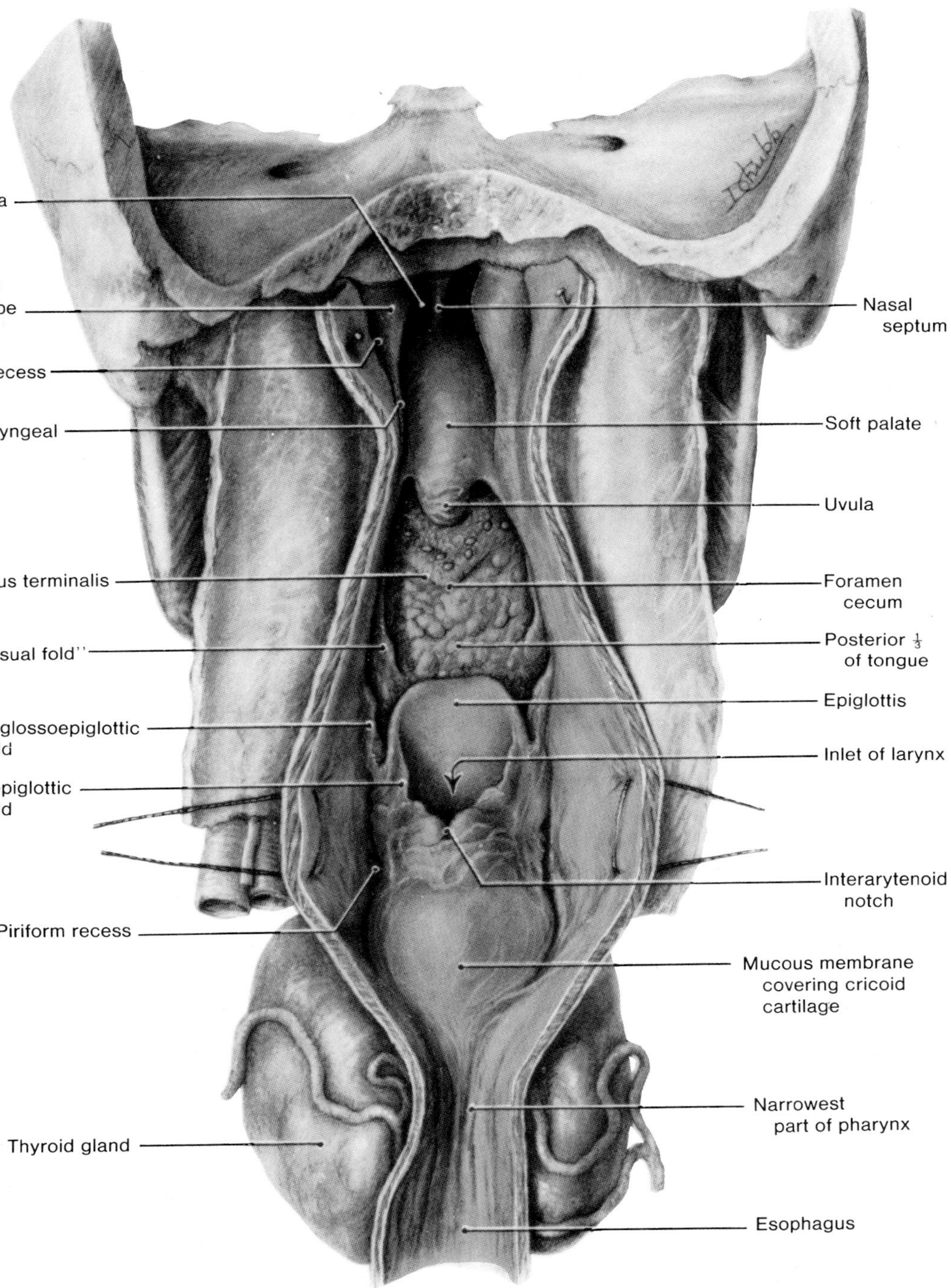

ure 9-58. Drawing of a posterior view of a dissection of the interior of the pharynx. Observe the rynx extending from the base of the skull to the inferior border of the cricoid cartilage, where it rows to become the esophagus. Note the three parts of the pharynx; nasal, oral, and laryngeal. The al part or *nasopharynx* lies above the level of the soft palate and is continuous in front through the anae with the nasal cavities. The oral part or *oropharynx* lies between the levels of the soft palate and larynx and communicates in front with the oral cavity. It has the posterior one-third of the tongue as anterior wall. Note that this part of the tongue is studded with lymph follicles, collectively called the ual tonsil and is demarcated from the anterior two-thirds by the foramen cecum and the V-shaped cus terminalis. The laryngeal part or *laryngopharynx* lies behind the larynx and communicates with cavity of the larynx through the inlet of the larynx. On each side of the inlet, and separated from it by aryepiglottic fold, observe a piriform recess.

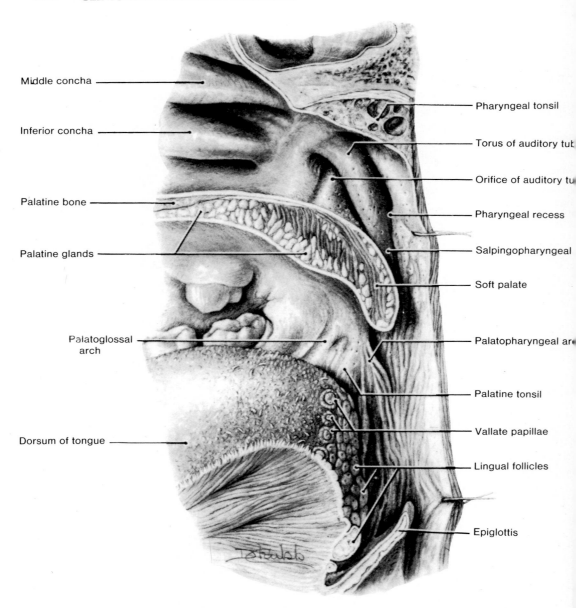

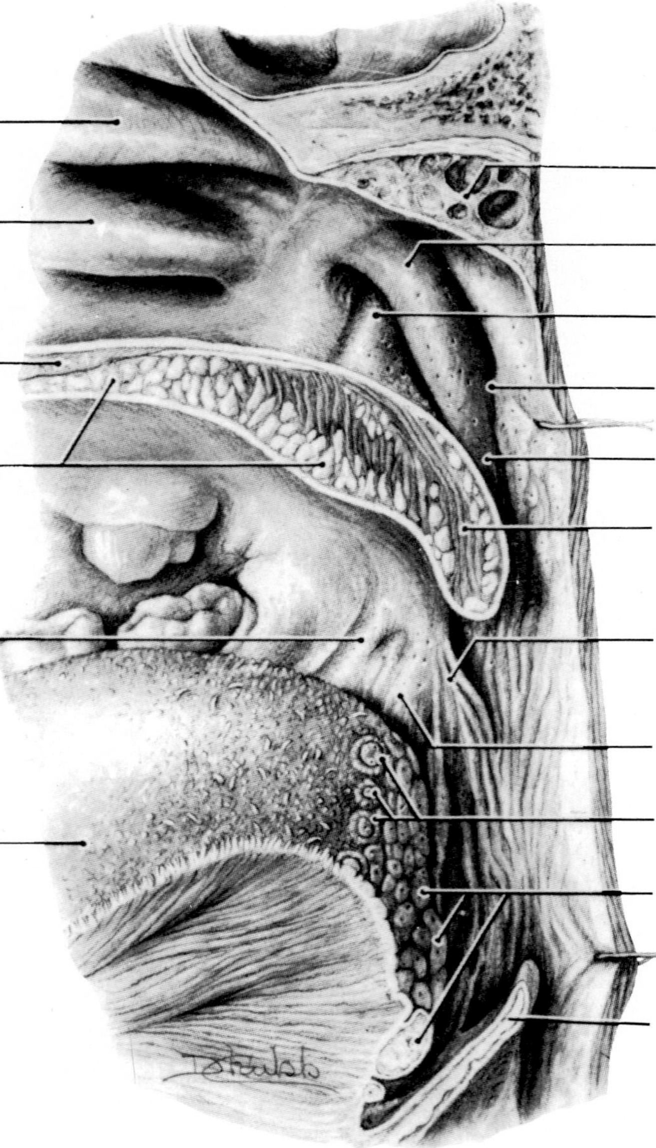

Figure 9-59. Drawing of a lateral view of a dissection of the pharynx. Observe the prominent torus (superior and posterior lips) of the auditory tube and the salpingopharyngeal fold which descends from the torus. Note the location of the orifice of the auditory tube (about 1.5 cm behind the inferior concha) and the deep pharyngeal recess behind the torus of the tube. Note the palatine tonsils which consist of masses of lymphoid tissue in the lateral walls of the oral part of the pharynx (also see Fig. 9-61). The tonsils reach their maximum size during early childhood and usually begin to diminish in size after puberty. Observe the lingual follicles which are known collectively as the lingual tonsil.

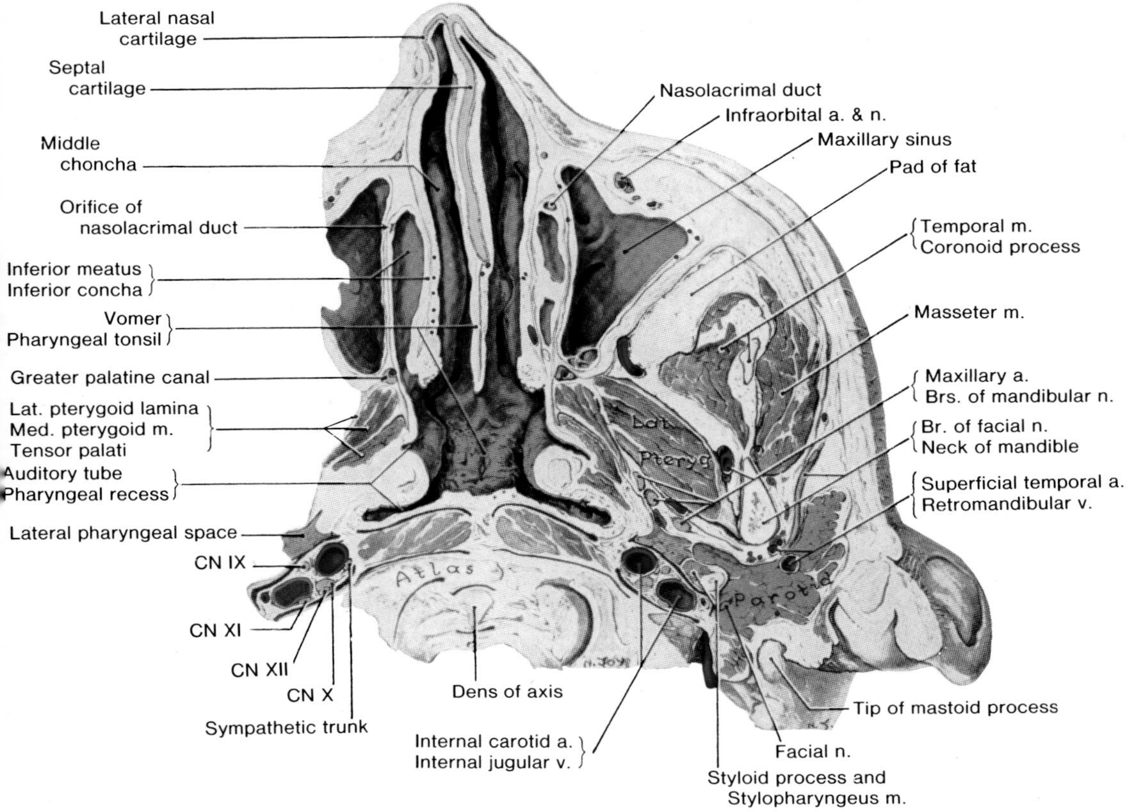

Figure 9-60. Drawing of a cross-section (from below) that passes through the nasal cavities and the nasopharynx. Observe the slightly enlarged pharyngeal tonsil ("adenoids") in the roof and posterior wall of the nasopharynx. Note the close relationship of the pharyngeal tonsil to the choanae and the orifices of the auditory tubes. Consequently, hypertrophy of the pharyngeal tonsils often interferes with the passage of air through the nose and obstructs the auditory tubes. This commonly results in mouth breathing and rhinitis (inflammation of the nasal mucous membrane). When these symptoms persist, the adenoids are sometimes removed (adenoidectomy).

The posterior fold of mucous membrane or **palatopharyngeal arch** (Fig. 9-61), passing downward from the soft palate into the lateral wall of the pharynx, is formed by the **palatopharyngeus** muscle (Fig. 9-57).

The palatine tonsils (Figs. 9-59 and 9-61 to 9-66), usually referred to as "*the tonsils*," lie on each side of the oropharynx in the triangular interval between the palatine arches or pillars of the fauces. Each palatine tonsil is a collection of lymphoid tissue under the mucous membrane of the oropharynx. The tonsil is called *palatine* because its upper one-third extends into the soft palate and owing to its relationship to the palatine arches.

Examine the tonsils in several persons of different ages, noting that they vary in size from person to person. In children the palatine tonsils tend to be large, whereas in older persons they are usually small and often inconspicuous. However, *the visible part of the tonsil is no guide to its actual size* because much of it may be hidden by the tongue and buried in the soft palate. Commonly the oval tonsil is about 2 cm in its greatest dimension and usually it does not completely fill the space between the

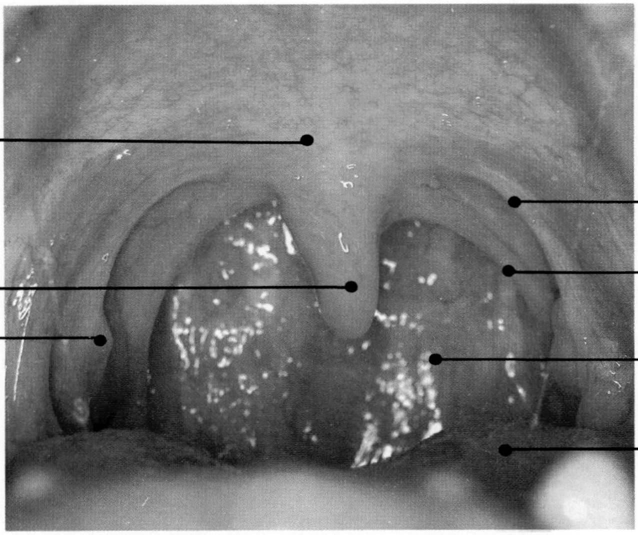

Figure 9-61. Photograph of the oral cavity of a young adult woman, taken with the mouth wide open and the tongue protruding. The oral cavity (L. *oris*, mouth) is lined by mucous membrane. Its roof is formed by the palate and its floor is largely occupied by the tongue. The fauces (L. throat) is the opening of the mouth into the pharynx. Note that its lateral walls are formed by two arches (often called the "pillars of the fauces") between which the palatine tonsils lie in the intratonsillar clefts.

palatine arches. Part of the remaining space, called the **intratonsillar cleft**, penetrates the tonsil and may pass into the soft palate (Fig. 9-63). This cleft is the remains of the second pharyngeal pouch in the embryo. The exposed free surface of the tonsil is characterized by the slit-like orifices of the mouths of the **tonsillar crypts**.

The tonsillar bed, in which the palatine tonsil lies, is between the palatoglossal and palatopharyngeal arches (Figs. 9-57, 9-59, and 9-61). The thin, fibrous sheet covering the tonsillar bed is part of the **pharyngobasilar fascia** (Fig. 9-52). The tonsillar bed is composed of two muscles, the palatopharyngeus and the superior constrictor (Figs. 9-57 and 9-62), which are part of the muscular coat of the pharynx.

The tonsillar artery, a branch of the facial, passes through the superior constrictor muscle and enters the lower pole of the tonsil (Figs. 9-63 to 9-65). The tonsillar bed also receives small arterial twigs from the ascending palatine, lingual, descending palatine, and ascending pharyngeal arteries (Fig. 9-29).

A large **external palatine vein** descends from the soft palate and passes close to the lateral surface of the tonsil before entering the **pharyngeal plexus of veins** (Fig. 9-65). One or more veins leave the lower part of the deep aspect of the tonsil. They open into the pharyngeal plexus and the facial vein.

The nerves of the tonsil are derived from a tonsillar plexus formed by a branch of the glossopharyngeal and vagus (CN IX and CN X) nerves. Other branches are from the **pharyngeal plexus**, a network of fine nerve fibers in the fascia covering the middle constrictor muscle (Figs. 9-52 and 9-55).

The **lymph vessels of the tonsil** pass laterally and downward to the lymph nodes near the angle of the mandible and the **jugolodigastric node** (Figs. 9-21 and 9-66). Because of the *frequent enlargement of this node in tonsillitis*, it is often referred to as the **tonsillar node**.

The palatine, lingual, and pharyngeal tonsils form a *circular band of lymphoid tissue* at the orophyngeal isthmus called the **tonsillar ring**. The anterior and lower part of the ring is formed by the **lingual tonsil**, a collection of lymphoid tissue in the posterior part of the tongue (Fig. 9-59). The lateral parts of the ring are formed by the palatine and tubal tonsils and the posterior and upper parts are formed by the pharyngeal tonsil. The tonsillar ring does not form a strong defense system against the spread of infection from the oral and nasal cavities to the lower respiratory organs.

CLINICALLY ORIENTED COMMENTS

Infection of the tonsils (**tonsillitis**) is often associated with a sore throat and **pyrexia** (G. feverishness). Usually the jugulodigastric lymph node (Fig. 9-66) in the deep cervical chain is enlarged and tender.

A **peritonsillar abscess** (collection of pus) or **quinsy** may develop in the loose connective tissue outside the capsule of the tonsil owing to proliferation of pyogenic organisms within the **intratonsillar cleft**. Airway obstruction may occur (Case 9-8).

Following frequent attacks of inflammation, the tonsils may be removed. **Tonsillectomy** is carried out by dissection (Fig. 9-64) or by a **guillotine operation**. In each case the tonsil and the fascial sheet covering the tonsillar bed are removed. Although some people consider tonsillectomy to be a simple operation, considerable bleeding and other complications can follow removal of the tonsils. Owing to its *abundant blood*

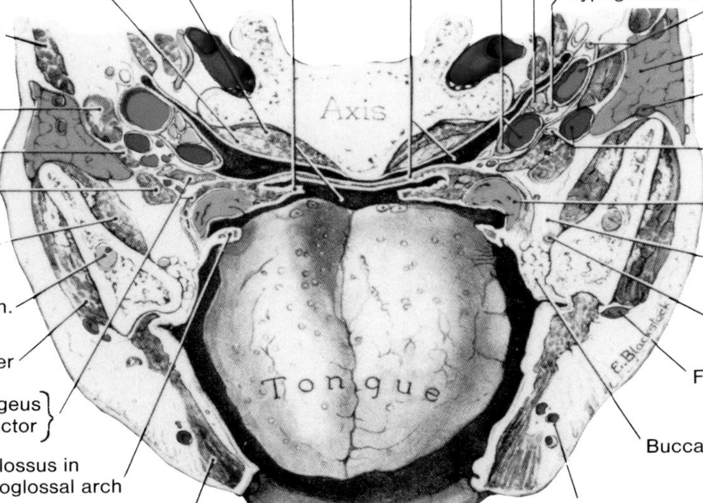

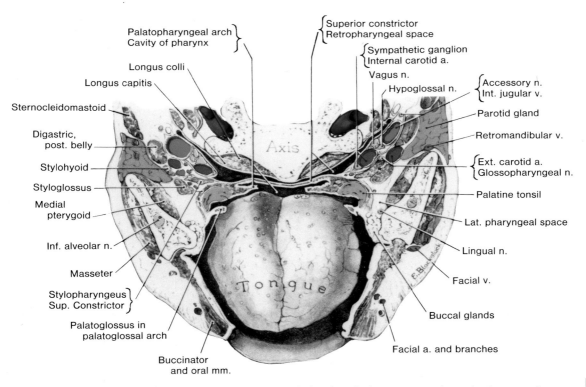

Figure 9-62. Drawing of a transverse section of the head that passes through the mouth. Understand that anterior to the ribbon-like palatoglossus muscle and its arch is the mouth and posterior to it is the pharynx. Observe the pharynx flattened anteroposteriorly and the tonsil in its wall. Note that the tonsillar bed is formed by the superior constrictor and palatopharyngeus muscles with an areolar space intervening and is limited in front and behind by the palatine arches. Observe the carotid arteries well behind the tonsillar bed. Examine the retropharyngeal space, here opened up, which allows the pharynx to contract and relax during swallowing. It is closed laterally at the carotid sheath and is limited posteriorly by the prevertebral fascia (also see Figs. 9-51 and 9-57).

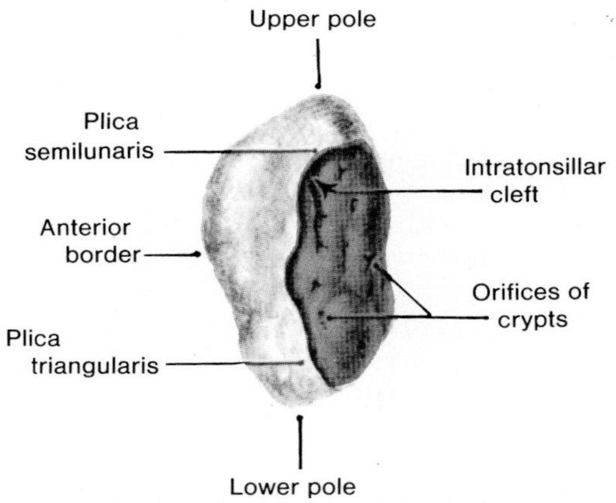

Figure 9-63. Drawing of a medial view of the palatine tonsil removed from its bed. Observe that its thin fibrous capsule extends around the anterior border and slightly over the medial surface as a thin, free fold which was covered with mucous membrane on both surfaces. The upper part of this fold is called the plica triangularis. On the medial or free surface, note the stellate orifices of the crypts that extend right through the organ to the capsule. Observe the intratonsillar cleft that extends toward the upper pole.

supply, bleeding may arise from the tonsillar artery or other arterial twigs, but more commonly bleeding comes from the paratonsillar **external palatine vein** (Fig. 9-65). This vein, which descends from the soft palate and passes into the areolar tissue, is *immediately related to the lateral surface of the tonsil.* Bleeding from this vessel is often the **chief source of hemorrhage** during operations on the tonsils.

The **glossopharyngeal** nerve to the tongue accompanies the tonsillar artery on the lateral wall of the pharynx (Fig. 9-65). As the wall is thin, this cranial nerve is vulnerable to injury. Also, edema about this nerve following tonsillectomy may result in temporary loss of taste. Careless removal of the tonsil could injure the **lingual nerve**. It does not supply the tonsil, but it passes lateral to the pharyngeal wall near the anterior part of the tonsil (Fig. 9-16).

Although the **internal carotid artery** (Fig. 9-62) should be safe during tonsillectomy, it could be injured if adjacent tissues are damaged in attempting to ensure that

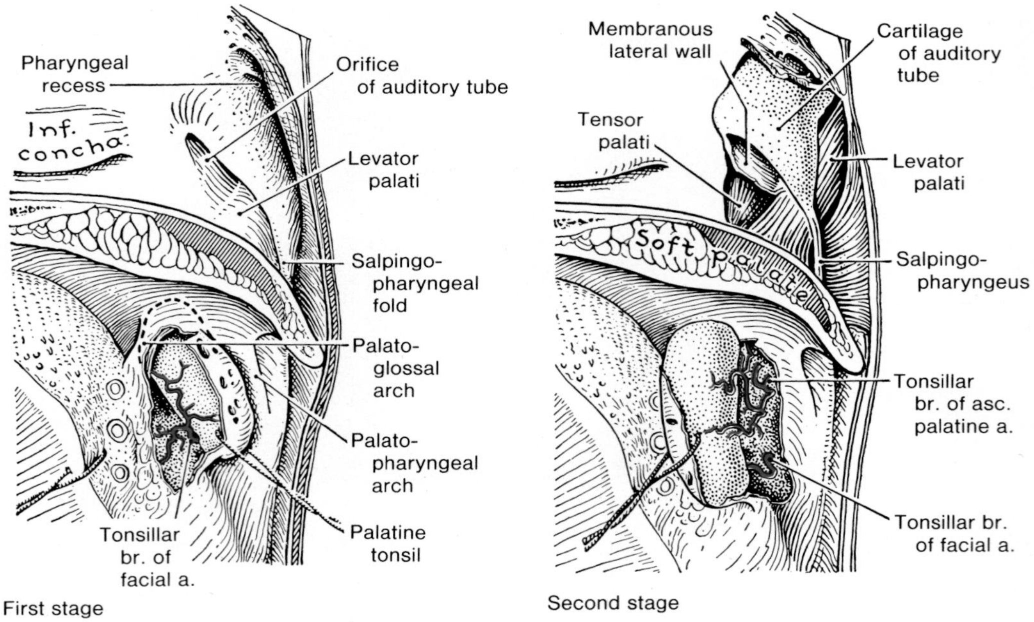

Figure 9-64. Drawings illustrating *one way* of removing the palatine tonsils (*i.e.*, a tonsillectomy). First the mucous membrane is incised along the palatoglossal arch and then the capsule of the tonsil is entered. With the point and the rounded handle of the knife, the anterior border of the tonsil is freed and the upper part, which extends far into the palate, is shelled out. The mucous membrane along the palatopharyngeal arch is then cut through. Bleeding from the tonsillar vessels, particularly the veins (Figs. 9-57 and 9-65) may occur at tonsillectomy.

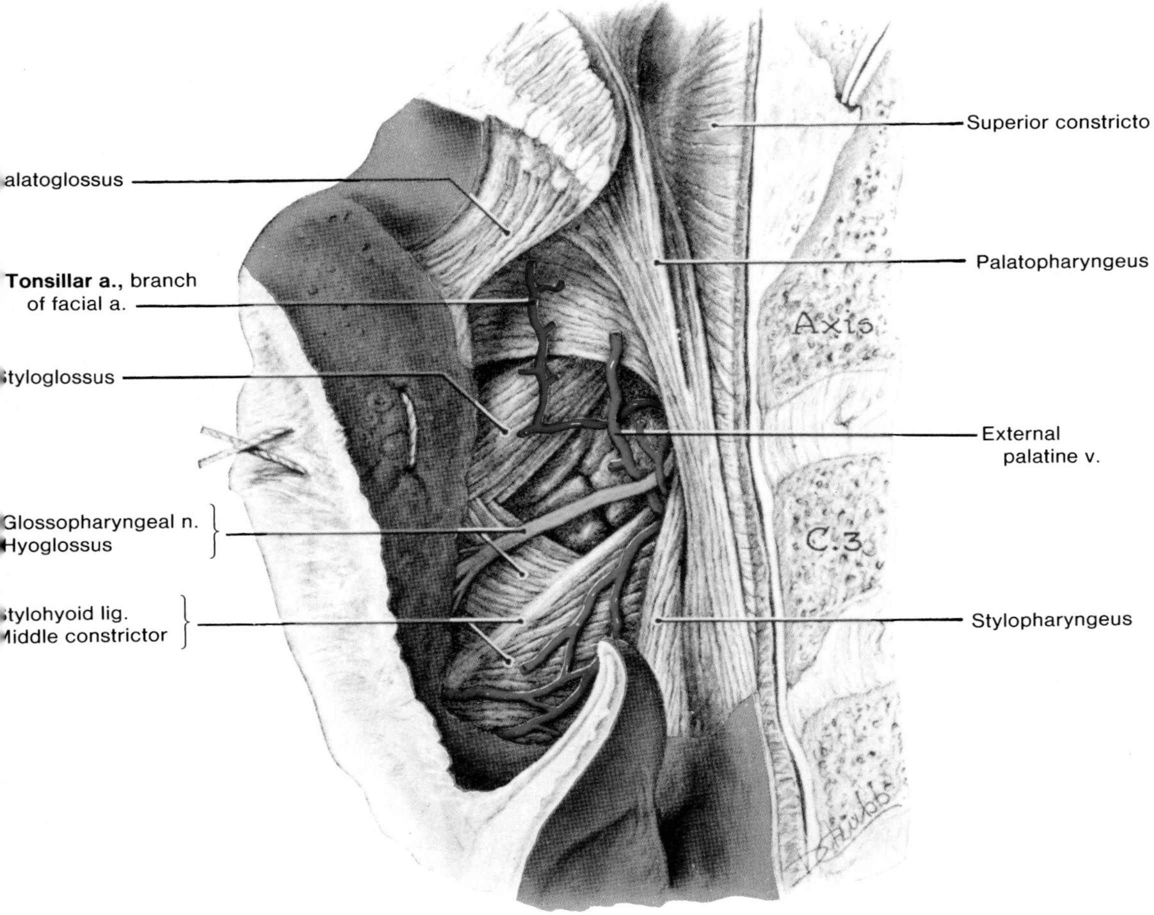

Figure 9-65. Drawing of a deep dissection of the tonsillar bed. The tongue is pulled forward and the inferior or lingual origin of the superior constrictor muscle is cut away. Observe the tonsillar branch of the facial artery, here sending a large branch (cut short) to accompany the glossopharyngeal nerve to the tongue. Lateral to this artery and the external palatine (paratonsillar) vein is the submandibular (salivary) gland. These veins may be a source of bleeding during tonsillectomy, particularly when they unite to form a large vein.

all tonsillar tissue is removed, especially when the internal carotid is tortuous and lies directly lateral to the tonsil. *Bleeding from the internal carotid artery results in severe hemorrhage* which can be controlled by compressing the common carotid artery against the anterior tubercle and the anterior surface of the sixth cervical transverse process.

Congenital sinuses and fistulae (Fig. 9-67) of the oropharynx generally result from failure of the second pharyngeal pouch and/or branchial groove to obliterate. **External branchial sinuses** frequently open externally along the anterior border of the sternocleidomastoid muscle, usually in the lower third of the neck. **Internal branchial sinuses** opening into the oropharynx are very rare, but usually they represent failure of the second pharyngeal pouch to obliterate normally. They open in the **intratonsillar cleft** (Figs. 9-63 and 9-67) and pass inferiorly through the neck for a variable distance between the external and internal carotid arteries.

A **branchial fistula**, opening into the intratonsillar cleft and on the side of the neck, usually results from persistence of

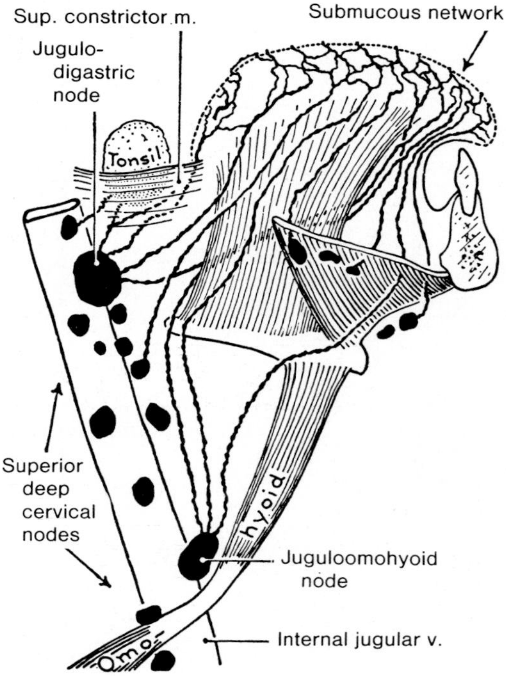

Figure 9-66. Diagram showing the lymphatics of the tongue and the tonsil. Note the jugulodigastric node, one of the highest nodes of the deep cervical chain. It is located at about the level of the hyoid bone and the posterior belly of the digastric muscle. It mainly drains the palatine tonsil and is often enlarged in cases of tonsillitis.

remnants of the second pharyngeal pouch and second branchial groove (Fig. 9-67). The fistula ascends from its cervical opening through the subcutaneous tissue, the platysma, and the deep fascia to enter the **carotid sheath**. It then passes between the internal and external carotid arteries on its way to its opening in the intratonsillar cleft.

The Laryngopharynx (Laryngeal Part of Pharynx). This part of the pharynx lies posterior to the larynx (Fig. 9-68) and extends from the upper border of the **epiglottis** to the lower border of the cricoid cartilage, where it narrows to become continuous with the esophagus. You may hear some clinicians refer to the laryngopharynx as the hypopharynx.

Posteriorly the laryngopharynx is related to the bodies of the fourth to sixth cervical vertebrae. Its posterior and lateral walls are formed by the middle and inferior constrictor muscles, with the palatopharyngeus and stylopharyngeus internally (Fig. 9-53). The laryngopharynx communicates with the cavity of the larynx through the **inlet of the larynx** (laryngeal aditus).

The piriform recess (Fig. 9-68) is a deep depression of the laryngopharyngeal cavity on each side of the inlet of the larynx. This rather deep, mucosa-lined fossa (L. a trench or ditch) is separated from the inlet of the larynx by the **aryepiglottic fold**. Laterally the recess is bounded by the medial surfaces of the thyroid cartilage and the thyrohyoid membrane (Fig. 9-70). In Figure 9-69 observe that branches of *the internal laryngeal and the recurrent laryngeal nerves lie deep to the mucous membrane of the piriform recess.*

Innervation of the Pharynx (Figs. 9-33, 9-49, 9-52, and 9-69). The motor and most of the sensory supply to the pharynx is derived from the **pharyngeal plexus of nerves** on the surface of the pharynx. This plexus is formed by pharyngeal branches of the vagus nerves (**CN X**), the glossopharyngeal nerves (**CN IX**), and sympathetic branches from the **superior cervical ganglion** (Figs. 9-33 and 9-52).

The motor fibers in the pharyngeal plexus are from the cranial root of the accessory nerve (CN XI) and are carried by the vagus to all muscles of the pharynx and soft palate, except the stylopharyngeus (CN IX) and the tensor veli palatini (CN V).

The sensory fibers in the pharyngeal plexus, derived from the glossopharyngeal nerve (CN IX), supply most of the mucosa of all three parts of the pharynx. The sensory nerve supply of the mucous membrane of the nasopharynx is mainly from the maxillary nerve (CNV^2), a purely sensory nerve.

CLINICALLY ORIENTED COMMENTS

Foreign bodies (*e.g.*, chicken bones and "safety pins") entering the pharynx may

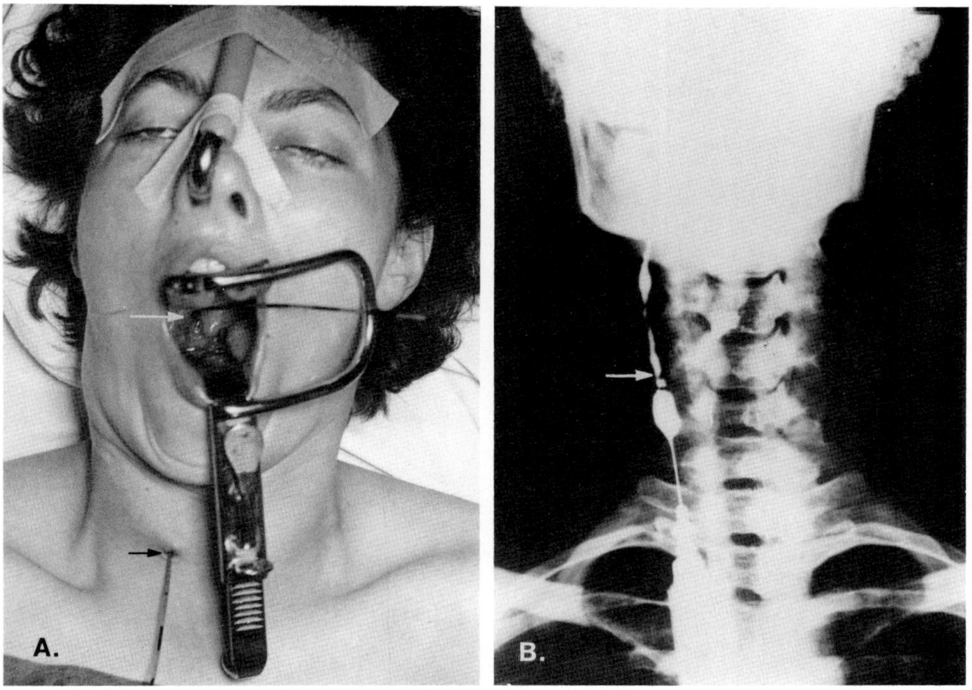

Figure 9-67. *A*, photograph of a woman with a branchial fistula. The catheter enters the fistula in the intratonsillar cleft (*white arrow*) and leaves via an opening in the neck (*black arrow*). *B*, radiograph taken following injection of radiopaque material into the inferior end of the fistula. Note the course of the fistula through the neck.

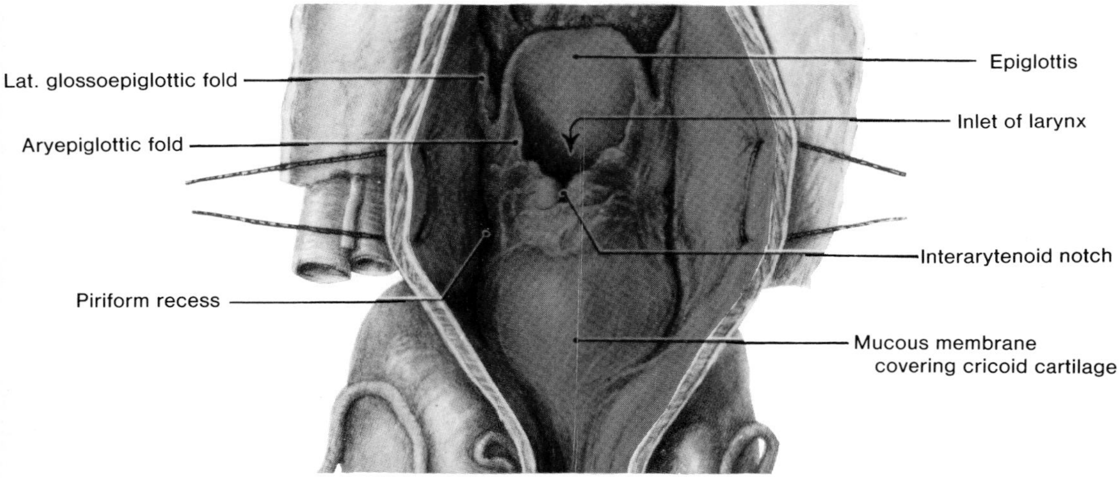

Figure 9-68. Drawing of a dissection of the posterior aspect of the laryngeal part of the pharynx (laryngopharynx). Note that it extends from the upper border of the epiglottis to the lower border of the cricoid cartilage and that it decreases rapidly in width from above downward. Observe that the laryngopharynx communicates with the cavity of the larynx via the laryngeal inlet.

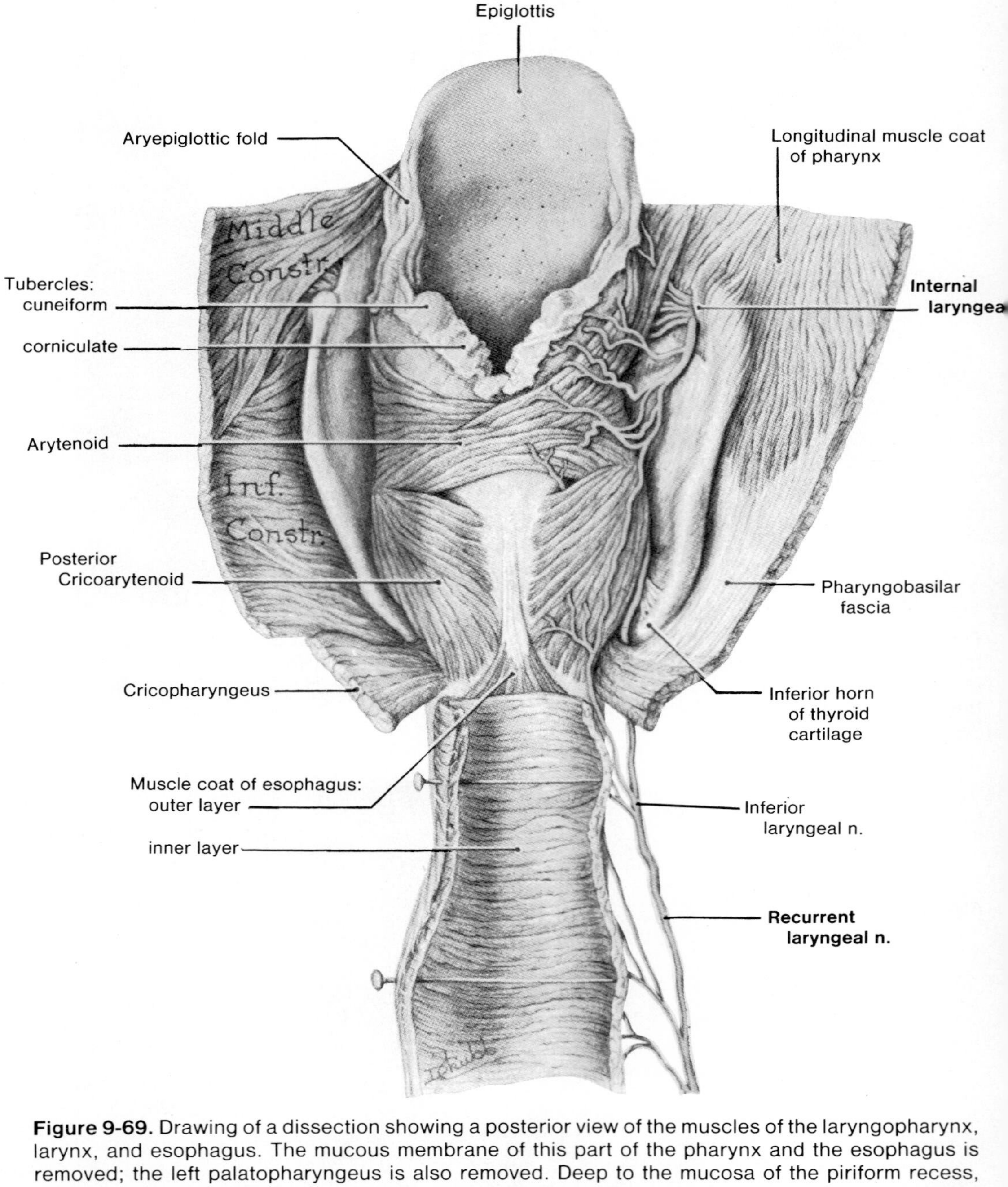

Figure 9-69. Drawing of a dissection showing a posterior view of the muscles of the laryngopharynx, larynx, and esophagus. The mucous membrane of this part of the pharynx and the esophagus is removed; the left palatopharyngeus is also removed. Deep to the mucosa of the piriform recess, observe the continuation of the recurrent laryngeal nerve, called the inferior laryngeal nerve. Note that is ascends under the inferior border of the inferior constrictor muscle of the pharynx and divides into anterior and posterior branches. Within the larynx it communicates with the internal laryngeal branch of the superior laryngeal nerve and supplies all the intrinsic muscles of the larynx except the cricothyroid. It also supplies the mucous membrane of the larynx below the vocal folds.

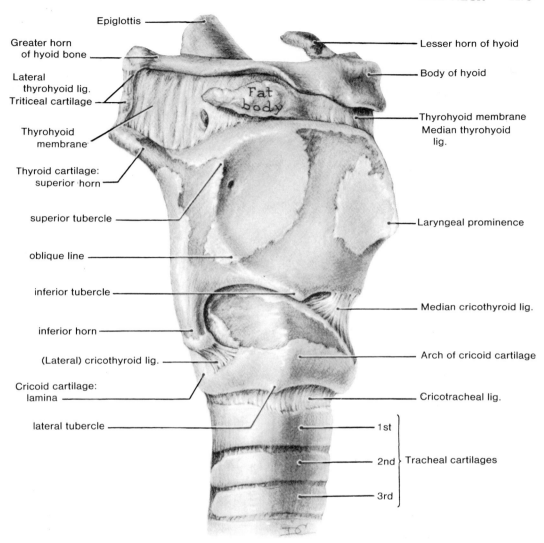

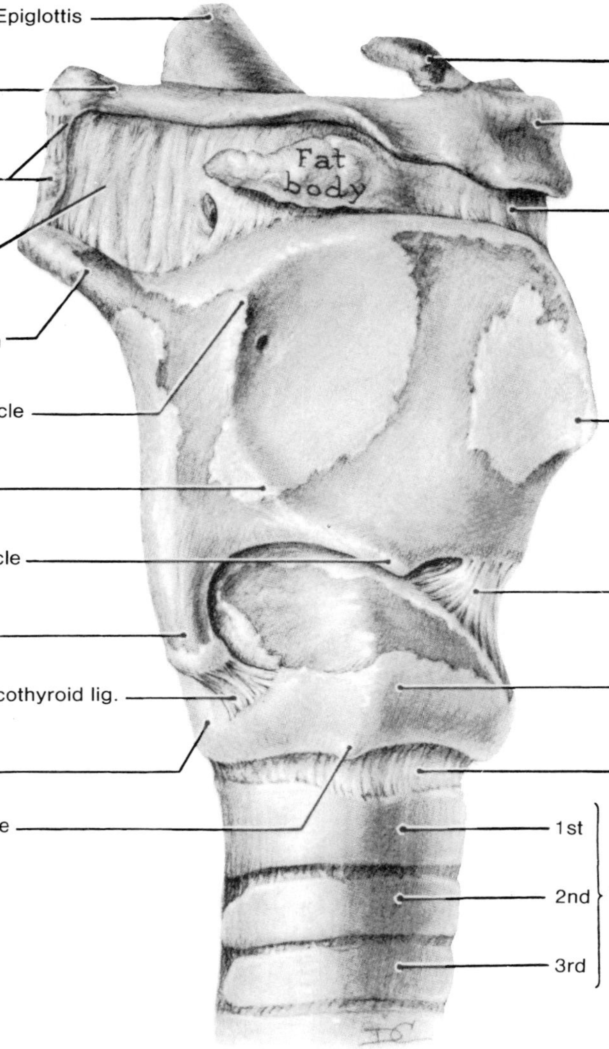

Figure 9-70. Drawing of a lateral view of the skeleton of the larynx. Note that the larynx extends vertically from the tip of the epiglottis to the lower border of the cricoid cartilage. *Understand that the hyoid bone is not a part of the larynx.* Observe the right lamina of the thyroid cartilage projecting anteriorly above the point of union with its fellow to form the laryngeal prominence (also see Fig. 9-1). Note that its posterior border is prolonged into a superior and an inferior horn. Note that the inferior horn articulates with the cricoid cartilage. Observe the thyrohyoid membrane (1) attaching the whole length of the upper border of the thyroid lamina to the upper inner border of the body and greater horn of the hyoid bone; (2) thickened anteriorly to form the median thyrohyoid ligament; (3) thickened posteriorly to form the lateral thyrohyoid ligament which contains a nodule of cartilage; (4) pierced by the internal laryngeal branch of the superior laryngeal nerve (Fig. 9-55) and its companion vessels; and (5) evaginated by a fat body. Examine the median cricothyroid ligament uniting the median parts of the adjacent border of the cricoid and thyroid cartilages.

become lodged in the pocket-like piriform recess; if sharp, they may pierce the mucous membrane and injure the **internal laryngeal nerve** (Fig. 9-69). This may result in anesthesia of the laryngeal mucous membrane as far inferiorly as the vocal folds (true vocal cords). Similarly, the nerve may be injured if the instrument used to remove the foreign body pierces the mucous membrane.

Deglutition (Swallowing). Deglutition is the complex process whereby food is transferred from the mouth through the pharynx and esophagus into the stomach. The term **bolus** is used to describe the mass of food or a quantity of liquid that is swallowed at one time. The food is mixed with saliva to form a bolus during chewing.

Stages of Deglutition. There are three stages in the act of swallowing. The **first stage is voluntary**, during which the bolus is pushed into the pharynx, mainly by movements of the tongue. The tongue is raised and pressed against the hard palate by the intrinsic muscles of the tongue. The **second stage is involuntary** and is usually rapid; it involves contraction of the walls of the pharynx. Breathing and chewing stop and successive contractions of the three pharyngeal constrictor muscles move the food through the oral and laryngeal parts of the pharynx into the esophagus. The bolus is prevented from entering the nasopharynx by the elevation of the soft palate. The tensor veli palati and the levator veli palatini muscles (Fig. 7-149) elevate the soft palate against the posterior wall of the pharynx. This closes the **pharyngeal isthmus**, thereby preventing food from entering the nasopharynx. Should a person happen to laugh during this stage, the muscles of the soft palate relax, allowing food to enter the nasopharynx. In these cases the food, especially if liquid, is expelled through the nose.

As the bolus passes through the oropharynx, the walls of the pharynx are raised. The contraction of the salpingopharyngeus muscles draws the lateral pharyngeal walls upward and inward. The hyoid and larynx are also elevated. Watch someone swallow, particularly a man, and observe that the **laryngeal prominence** (Fig. 9-1*A*) rises. Verify that upward movement of the thyroid cartilage is considerable. The palatopharyngeus and the stylopharyngeus muscles elevate the larynx and pharynx in swallowing. Palpate your hyoid bone with your thumb and forefinger as you swallow and verify that it also rises. The hyoid bone is raised and fixed in swallowing by contraction of the geniohyoid, mylohyoid, digastric, and stylohyoid muscles. Verify that elevation and forward movement of the hyoid bone precedes elevation of the larynx.

During deglutition the vestibule of the larynx (Fig. 9-79) is closed, the epiglottis is bent backward over the inlet, and the **aryepiglottic folds** are approximated (Fig. 9-68). These folds provide lateral food channels that guide the bolus from the sides of the epiglottis through the piriform recesses into the esophagus. This usually prevents food from entering the larynx.

The **third and final stage of swallowing** squeezes or "milks" the bolus from the laryngopharynx into the esophagus. This is effected by the inferior constrictor muscle (Fig. 9-55).

CLINICALLY ORIENTED COMMENTS

If the recurrent laryngeal nerves are injured (*e.g.*, during a **thyroidectomy**), paralysis of the muscles in the aryepiglottic fold occurs. As a result the inlet of the larynx does not close during swallowing, the aryepiglottic folds fall medially, and fluids tend to overflow into the larynx.

Choking on food is a common cause of **laryngeal obstruction**, particularly in persons who have consumed excessive amounts of alcohol (Case 9-4) or who have **bulbar palsy** (degeneration of motor neurons in the brain stem which supply the muscles of deglutition). Difficulty in swallowing is called **dysphagia**. Diagnostic study of swallowing is done by **cinefluoroscopy** (x-ray motion pictures of the passage of contrast material through the pharynx and esophagus).

Children swallow a variety of objects, most of which reach the stomach and pass through the gastrointestinal tract without difficulty. In some cases the foreign body stops at the inferior end of the pharynx, its narrowest part (Fig. 9-58), or in the esophagus just below the cricopharyngeus muscle, (part of the inferior constrictor, Fig. 9-69). *Foreign bodies in the esophagus* are removed under direct vision through an **esophagoscope** (an instrument for examining the interior of the esophagus).

Radiographic examinations will also reveal the presence of a *radiopaque foreign body* in the pharynx or the esophagus. When it is posterior to the soft tissues of the larynx (Fig. 9-51), the foreign body is in the laryngopharynx or the superior part of the cervical esophagus.

THE LARYNX

The larynx is a highly specialized organ between the laryngopharynx and the trachea (Fig. 9-51). Although it is an essential part of the air passages and acts as a valve for preventing swallowed food and foreign bodies from entering the lower respiratory passages, it is specifically designed for voice production (**phonation**).

The larynx is the phonating mechanism (G. *phōnē*, voice). Phonation is defined as the utterance of sounds with the aid of the **vocal folds**. Through movements of its cartilages, the larynx varies the opening between the vocal folds, thereby varying the pitch of sounds produced by the passage of air through them. These sounds are translated into intelligible speech by articulatory and resonating structures (*e.g.*, the tongue and mouth).

The larynx is located in the anterior portion of the neck. In adult males it is about 5 cm in length and is related posteriorly to the bodies of the third to sixth cervical vertebrae. The larynx is shorter in women and children and is situated slightly higher in the neck. This sex difference in the larynx normally develops at puberty in males; at this time all its cartilages enlarge.

The Skeleton of the Larynx (Fig. 9-70). The laryngeal skeleton is formed by *nine cartilages* that are joined by various ligaments and membranes. Three of the cartilages are single (thyroid, cricoid, and epiglottis) and three are paired (arytenoid, corniculate, and cuneiform).

The Thyroid Cartilage (Figs. 9-70 to 9-73). The thyroid, the largest of the laryngeal cartilages, is composed of two quadrilateral **laminae**. The inferior two-thirds of these laminae are fused anteriorly in the midline to form a subcutaneous projection called the **laryngeal prominence**. The larynx is more prominent in postpubertal males (Fig. 9-1) because the angle at which the laminae meet is smaller in males (Fig. 9-2) and the anteroposterior diameter of the laminae is greater. Immediately superior to the laryngeal prominence, the thyroid laminae diverge to form a V-shaped **thyroid notch** (Fig. 9-72). The posterior border of each lamina projects upward as the superior horn and downward as the inferior horn (Fig. 9-70). The **thyrohyoid membrane** and the lateral thyrohyoid ligaments are the posterior thickened portions of this membrane. In between the median and lateral ligaments, the superior border of the thyroid cartilage is attached to the hyoid bone by the **thyrohyoid membrane**. The **inferior horns** articulate with the cricoid cartilage at special facets that allow the thyroid cartilage to tilt or glide forward or backward in a visor-like manner (Fig. 9-71).

The lateral surface of each lamina is marked by an oblique line which provides attachment for the inferior constrictor muscle of the pharynx and the sternothyroid and thyrohyoid muscles (Fig. 9-70).

The Cricoid Cartilage (Figs. 9-70 to 9-73). The cricoid (G. ring) is *shaped like a signet ring* with its band in front. The posterior (signet) part of the cricoid is called the **lamina** and the anterior (band) part is termed the **arch**. Although much smaller than the thyroid cartilage, the cricoid is thicker and stronger. Being the most inferior of the thyroid cartilages, the cricoid forms the inferior parts of the anterior and lateral walls and most of the posterior wall of the larynx. The cricoid cartilage is attached to the inferior margin of the thyroid cartilage by the **cricothyroid ligament** and to the first tracheal ring by the **cricotracheal ligament**.

The Arytenoid Cartilages (Figs. 9-71, 9-73, and 9-74). These paired cartilages,

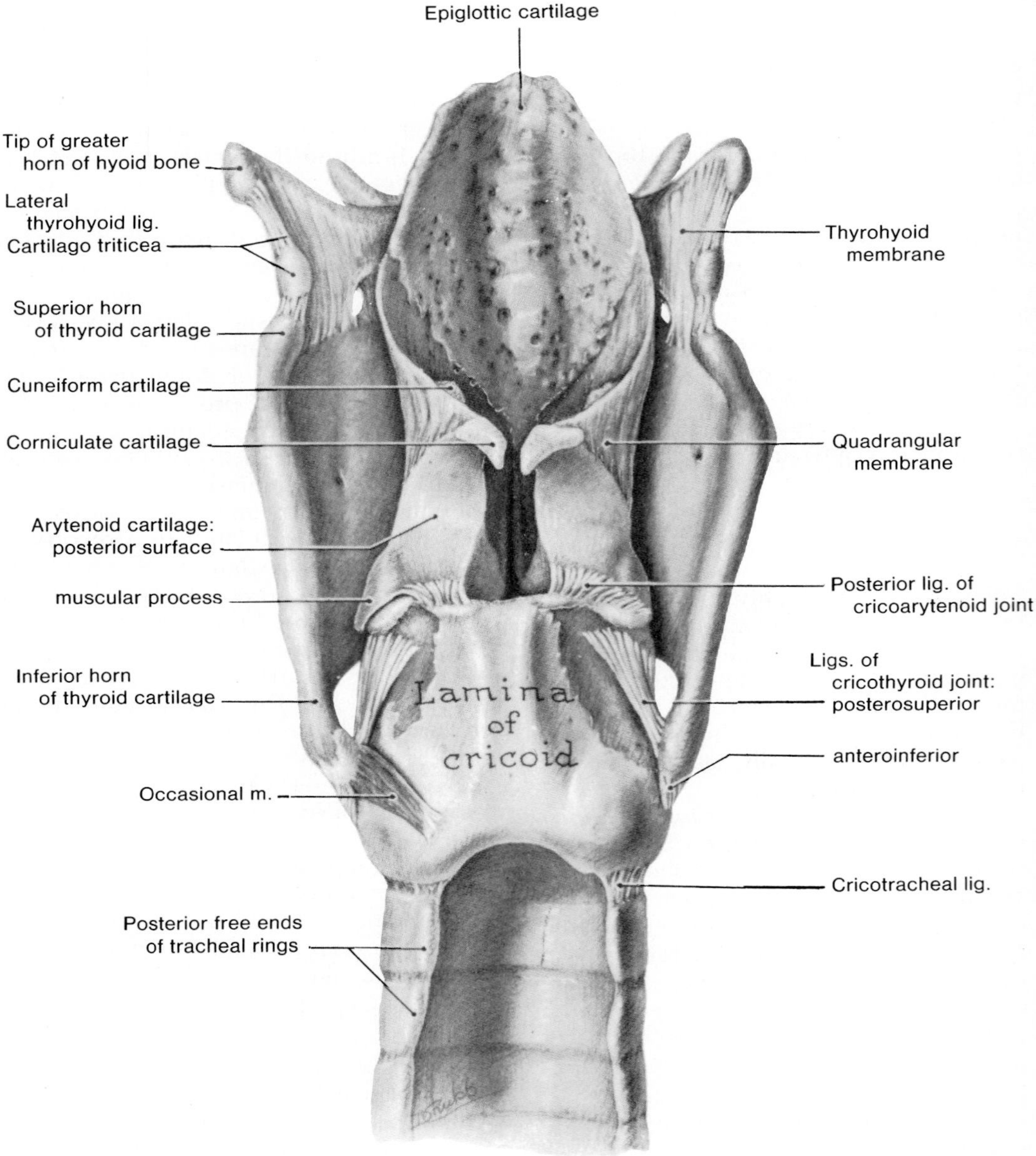

Figure 9-71. Drawing of a posterior view of the skeleton of the larynx. Observe that the thyroid cartilage shields the smaller cartilages of the larynx (epiglottic, arytenoid, corniculate, and cuneiform). The hyoid bone, although not a part of the larynx, also shields the upper part of the epiglottic cartilage. Note that the rounded posterior border of the thyroid cartilage is prolonged into superior and inferior horns. The inferior horn articulates with the cricoid cartilage at a synovial joint (cricothyroid joint). Examine the quadrangular membrane connecting the border of the epiglottic cartilage to the arytenoid and corniculate cartilages.

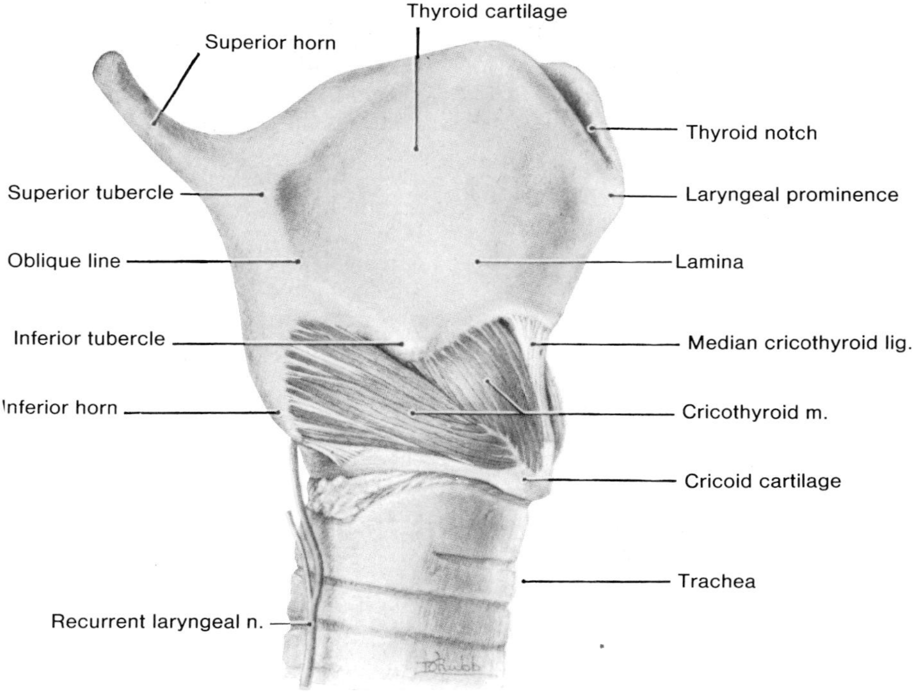

Figure 9-72. Drawing of a lateral view of the thyroid cartilage, the cricoid cartilage, and the proximal part of the trachea. Observe that the cricothyroid muscle arises from the outer surface of the arch of the cricoid cartilage and that it has a straight part inserted into the lower border of the lamina of the thyroid cartilage and an oblique part inserted into the anterior border of the inferior horn. *Observe the course of the recurrent laryngeal nerve*, which supplies all intrinsic muscles of the larynx, except the one shown here (cricothyroid).

shaped like three-sided pyramids, articulate with the lateral parts of the superior border of the lamina of the cricoid cartilage. Each has an **apex** superiorly, a **vocal process** anteriorly, and a **muscular process** laterally. The apex is attached to the aryepiglottic fold (Figs. 9-64 and 9-69), the vocal process to the **vocal ligament**, and the muscular process to the posterior and lateral **cricoarytenoid muscles**.

The Corniculate and Cuneiform Cartilages (Figs. 9-71, 9-73, and 9-74). These small cartilaginous nodules are in the posterior part of the aryepiglottic folds. The corniculate cartilages are attached to the apices of the arytenoid cartilages and serve to prolong them. The cuneiform (L. wedge-shaped) cartilages lie in the aryepiglottic folds and are approximated to the tubercle of the epiglottis when the inlet of the larynx is closed during swallowing.

The Epiglottic Cartilage (Figs. 9-69 to 9-72 and 9-74). This thin cartilage, shaped like a leaf or bicycle saddle, gives flexibility to the epiglottis. Situated posterior to the root of the tongue and the hyoid bone and anterior to the inlet of the larynx, the epiglottic cartilage forms the superior part of the anterior wall and the superior margin of the laryngeal orifice. Its broad superior end is free and its tapered inferior end is attached to the **thyroepiglottic ligament**, located in the angle formed by the thyroid laminae (Fig. 9-74). The anterior surface of the epiglottic cartilage is attached to the hyoid bone by the **hyoepiglottic ligament** (Fig. 9-75). The mucous membrane covering the epiglottis is united to the posterior part of the tongue by a median and two lateral **glossoepiglottic folds** (Fig. 9-58). Between the median and lateral folds are depressions called **epiglottic valleculae**

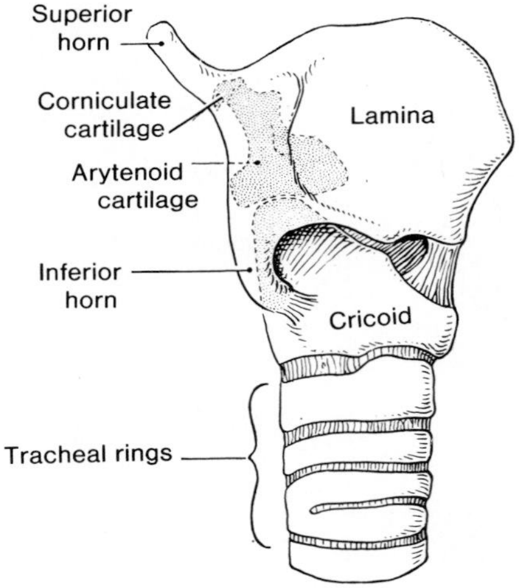

Figure 9-73. Drawing of the laryngeal skeleton illustrating how the thyroid cartilage shields the arytenoid cartilage and the superior part of the cricoid cartilage on which the arytenoid cartilage rests.

(Fig. 9-18). *Vallecula* is a Latin word meaning a little ditch, which is an appropriate term because saliva collects in them from the surface of the tongue.

The lower part of the posterior surface of the epiglottic cartilage that projects posteriorly is called the **epiglottic tubercle** (Fig. 9-78). The mucous membrane covering this tubercle bulges into the larynx and comes into contact with the cuneiform cartilages during swallowing.

CLINICALLY ORIENTED COMMENTS

The thyroid, cricoid, and most parts of the arytenoid cartilages often calcify with age. **Fractures of the laryngeal skeleton** may result from blows received during boxing, karate, or from compression by a shoulder strap during an automobile accident. These fractures produce submucous hemorrhage and edema, respiratory obstruction, hoarseness, and sometimes an inability to speak.

Joints of the Larynx. Some of the laryngeal cartilages articulate freely, thereby allowing them to move during voice production. There are two pairs of synovial joints in the larynx.

The Cricothyroid Joints (Fig. 9-71). These articulations are between the facets on the lateral surfaces of the cricoid cartilage and the inferior horns of the thyroid cartilage. Each joint has a fibrous capsule which is lined by a synovial membrane. The main movements at this joint are rotation and gliding of the thyroid cartilage at the inferior cricothyroid joints, which result in changes in the length of the vocal folds. These movements also slacken or tighten the **vocal ligaments** which pass between the arytenoid cartilages and the thyroid cartilage (Fig. 9-74).

The Cricoarytenoid Joint (Fig. 9-71). These articulations are between the bases of the arytenoid cartilages and the upper sloping surface of the lamina of the cricoid cartilage. The cricoarytenoid joints permit various movements of the arytenoid cartilages: (1) sliding toward or away from one another; (2) tilting forward and back; and (3) rotary motion. These movements are important in approximating, tensing, and relaxing the vocal folds.

The Ligaments and Membranes of the Larynx. The various laryngeal cartilages are united by several ligaments and membranes.

The Thyrohyoid Membrane (Figs. 9-70 and 9-71). This extrinsic ligament connects the thyroid cartilage and the hyoid bone, thereby suspending the larynx. It is separated from the posterior surface of the body of the hyoid by a bursa. Its thicker median part is called the **median thyrohyoid ligament** and its thickened lateral parts are called the lateral thyrohyoid ligaments. The **lateral thyrohyoid ligaments** connect the tips of the superior horns of the thyroid cartilage to the tips of the greater horns of the hyoid bone. They each contain a *triticeal* (G. kernel-like) *cartilage* which helps to close the inlet of the larynx during swallowing. These small *cartilaginous nodules* are in addition to the nine cartilages that form the skeleton of the larynx (Fig. 9-70).

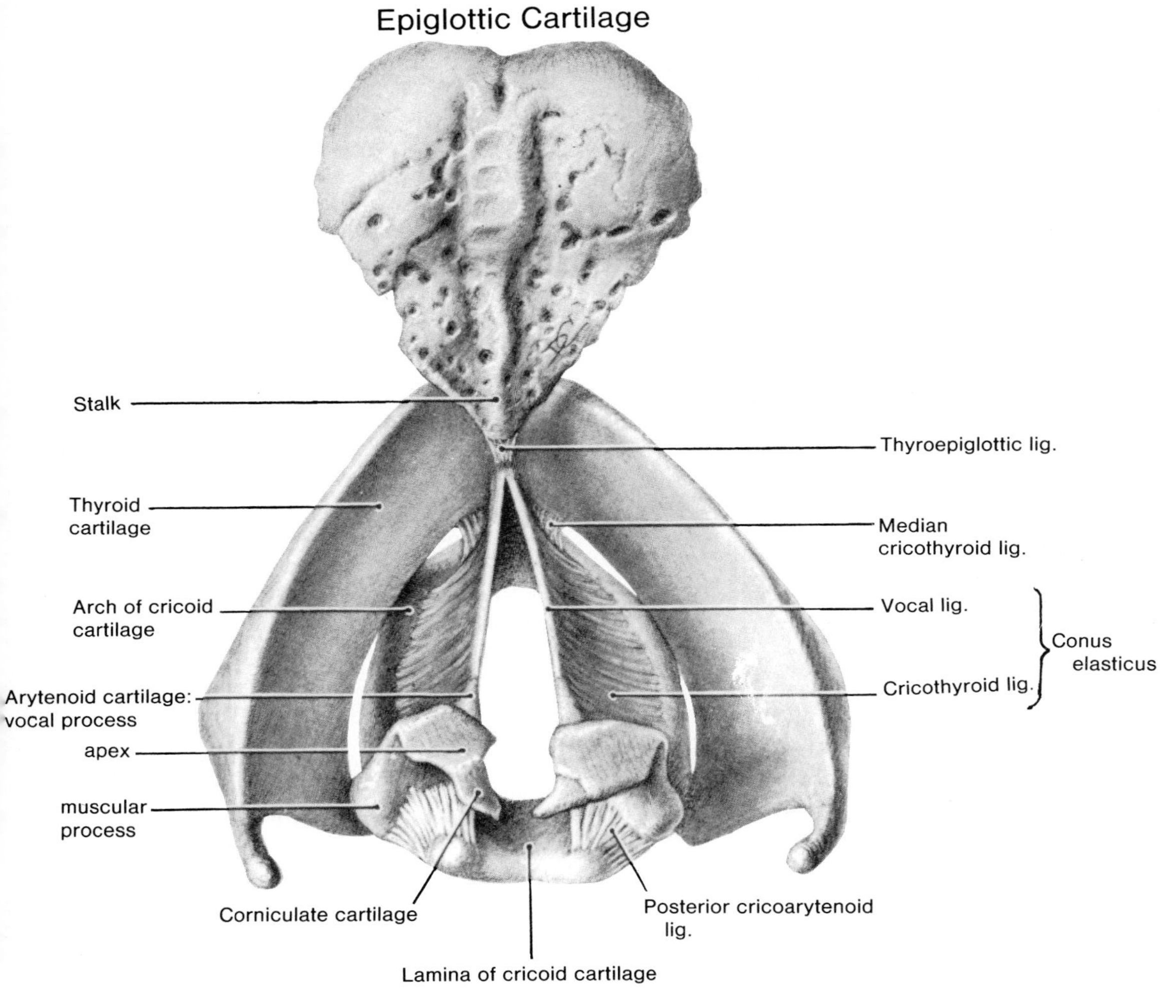

Figure 9-74. Drawing of the skeleton of the larynx from above. Note the epiglottic cartilage, shaped like a bicycle seat and showing pits for mucous glands. Observe that it is attached at its apex by ligamentous fibers to the angle of the thyroid cartilage above the vocal ligaments. Observe the paired arytenoid cartilages, which have a blunt apex prolonged as the corniculate cartilage; a rounded, lateral, basal angle called the muscular process; and a sharp, anterior basal angle called the vocal process, for the attachment of the vocal ligament. Note the strong posterior cricoarytenoid ligament which prevents the arytenoid cartilage from falling into the larynx. Observe the vocal ligament, which forms the skeleton of the vocal fold, extending from the vocal process to the "angle" of the thyroid cartilage and there joining its fellow below the thyroepiglottic ligament. Note that the cricothyroid ligament blends in front with the median cricothyroid ligament and sweeps upward from the upper border of the arch of the cricoid cartilage to the vocal ligament. Hence, when the vocal ligaments are in apposition, the membranes of opposite sides form a roof for the infraglottic section of the larynx below them.

The Cricothyroid and Cricotracheal Ligaments (Figs. 9-70 and 9-74). These ligaments connect the cricoid cartilage with the arch of the thyroid cartilage and the first tracheal ring, respectively.

CLINICALLY ORIENTED COMMENTS

If some food (*e.g.*, a piece of steak) or some other foreign object enters the larynx, the laryngeal muscles go into spasm, causing tensing of the vocal folds. As a result the **rima glottidis** (Fig. 9-77) closes and no air can enter the trachea, bronchi, and lungs; obviously the person is in danger of **asphyxiation** (called "choking to death" by laymen, Case 9-4).

If the foreign object cannot be dislodged, emergency therapy must be given to open the airway. The procedure used depends on the condition of the patient, the facilities available, and the experience of the person giving first aid. Often a large bore needle is inserted through the cricothyroid ligament to permit fast entry of air. Later a **cricothyrotomy (inferior laryngotomy)** is performed, during which an incision is made through the skin and cricothyroid ligament for more adequate relief of respiratory obstruction. Often this procedure is followed by a **tracheotomy** (Fig. 6-42) and insertion of a short curved metal tube (**tracheotomy tube**) into the trachea.

The Vocal Ligament, the Vocal Fold, and the Conus Elasticus (Figs. 9-74, 9-76, and 9-78). The elastic vocal ligament on each side extends from the junction of the laminae of the thyroid cartilage anteriorly to the vocal process of the arytenoid cartilage posteriorly. The **vocal ligament** is the fibrous core of the **vocal fold** and is the free edge of the **conus elasticus**. This elastic membrane extends upward from the cricoid cartilage to the vocal ligament.

The Quadrangular Membrane and the Vestibular Ligament (Figs. 9-71 and 9-76). This membrane is a thin submucosal sheet of connective tissue that extends from the arytenoid cartilage to the cartilage of the epiglottis. The free lower margin of this membrane constitutes the **vestibular ligament**. It is covered loosely by a **vestibular fold** of mucous membrane. This fold, lying above the vocal fold, extends from the thyroid cartilage to the arytenoid cartilage. As it may be mistaken for the vocal fold, the vestibular fold is sometimes referred to as the false vocal cord.

The cricothyroid ligament and the quadrangular membrane (Fig. 9-76), although separated by the interval between the vocal and vestibular ligaments, are referred to as the **fibroelastic membrane of the larynx**.

The Ligaments of the Epiglottis (Figs. 9-74, 9-75, and 9-78). The epiglottis has several attachments that are described with the epiglottic cartilage (p. 1179). Briefly, the epiglottis is attached to the hyoid bone by the **hyoepiglottic ligament**, to the posterior part of the tongue by the **median glossoepiglottic fold**, to the sides of the pharynx by the **lateral glossepiglottic fold**, and to the thyroid cartilage by the **thyroepiglottic ligament**.

The Interior of the Larynx (Figs. 9-76 to 9-79). The cavity of the larynx extends from the **inlet of the larynx**, through which it communicates with the laryngopharynx, to the level of the lower border of the cricoid cartilage, where it is continuous with the cavity of the trachea. The inlet lies in an almost vertical plane.

The larynx is divided into three parts by upper and lower projecting folds of mucous membrane on each side. Above the upper or **vestibular folds**, the cavity of the larynx is called the **vestibule**. Between the vestibular folds above the vocal folds is the **ventricle** of the larynx. This is the smallest of the three cavities of the larynx. It extends laterally between the two folds as the **sinus of the larynx**. From each sinus a **saccule of the larynx** passes upward between the vestibular fold and the thyroid lamina. The lower cavity of the larynx extends from the vocal folds to the lower border of the cricoid cartilage, where it is continuous with the cavity of trachea.

The Vocal Folds (Figs. 9-76 and 9-79). These folds are concerned with the produc-

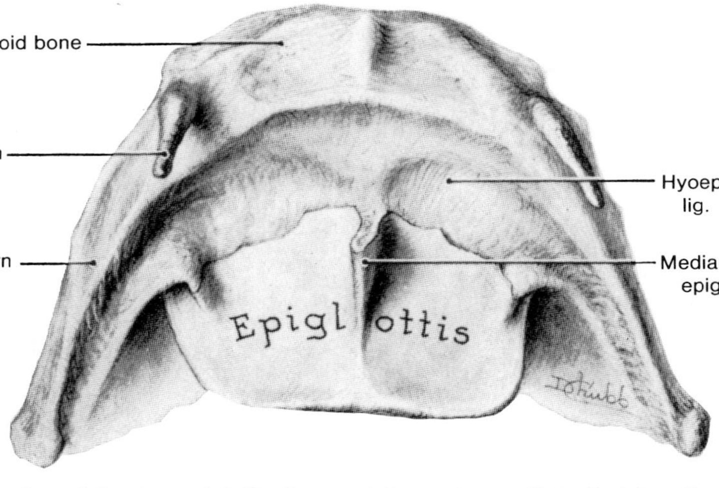

Figure 9-75. Drawing of the hyoepiglottic ligament from above. Note that it unites the epiglottic cartilage to the hyoid bone. On the *left side* observe the three parts of the hyoid bone. Also note the asymmetry of the greater and lesser horns of opposite sides.

tion of sound (phonation). The apex of each wedge-shaped vocal fold projects medially into the laryngeal cavity, and its base lies against the lamina of the thyroid cartilage. Each vocal fold consists of the vocal ligament, the conus elasticus, muscle fibers, and a covering of mucous membrane. The **rima glottidis** is the aperture between the vocal folds, whereas the term **glottis** refers to the vocal folds, the rima glottidis, and the narrow part of the larynx at the level of the vocal folds. It is the part of the larynx most directly concerned with voice production (*i.e.*, it is the **vocal apparatus**).

The shape of the rima glottidis varies according to the position of the vocal folds. During ordinary breathing, the rima glottidis is narrow and wedge-shaped; it is wide during forced respiration. The vocal folds are closely approximated during speaking so that the rima glottidis appears as a linear slit. Variation in the tension and length of the vocal folds, in the width of the rima glottidis, and in the intensity of the expiratory effort produces changes in the **pitch** of the voice. The lower range of pitch in the male voice results from the greater length of his vocal folds.

The Vestibular Folds (Figs. 9-76 to 9-79). These folds, extending between the thyroid and the arytenoid cartilages, play little or no part in voice production. They consist of two thick, pink *folds of mucous membrane* enclosing the **vestibular ligaments.** As they may be confused with the vocal folds, they used to be called the *false vocal cords.* The space between them is called the **rima vestibuli**. The vestibular folds are part of the protective mechanism by which the larynx is closed during swallowing to prevent the entry of food and foreign particles into it.

The Muscles of the Larynx (Figs. 9-20, 9-22, 9-47, 9-72, and 9-80 to 9-82). The muscles of the larynx are divided into extrinsic and intrinsic groups for descriptive purposes.

The extrinsic muscles move the larynx as a whole. The omohyoid, sternohyoid, and sternothyroid (infrahyoid muscles) are *depressors of the larynx*, whereas the stylohyoid, diagastric, mylohyoid, geniohyoid (suprahyoid muscles) and the stylopharyngeus are *elevators of the larynx.* The thyrohyoid muscle draws the hyoid bone and the thyroid cartilage together.

The intrinsic muscles are concerned with movements of the laryngeal parts, making alterations in the length and tension of the vocal folds, and in the size and

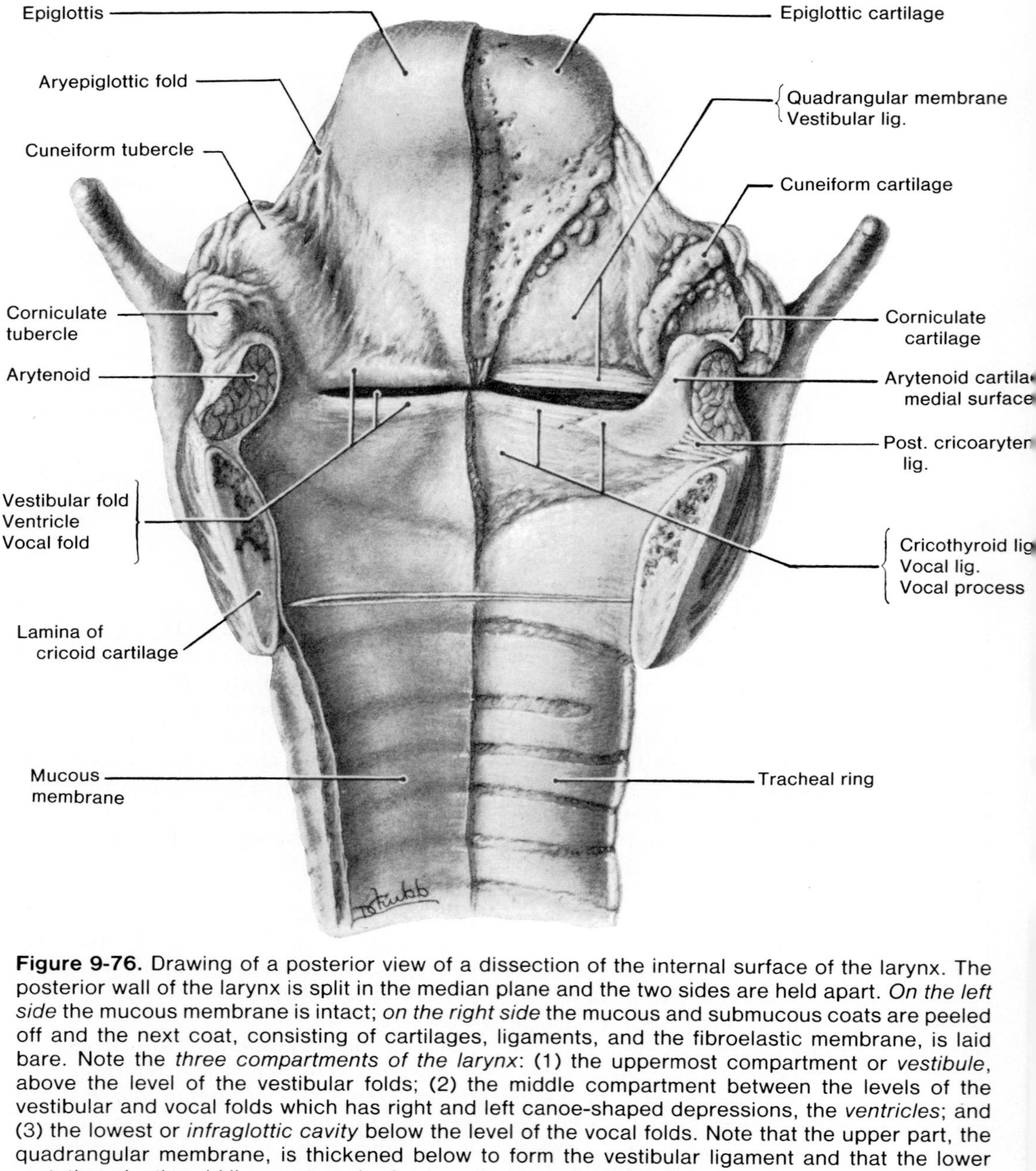

Figure 9-76. Drawing of a posterior view of a dissection of the internal surface of the larynx. The posterior wall of the larynx is split in the median plane and the two sides are held apart. *On the left side* the mucous membrane is intact; *on the right side* the mucous and submucous coats are peeled off and the next coat, consisting of cartilages, ligaments, and the fibroelastic membrane, is laid bare. Note the *three compartments of the larynx*: (1) the uppermost compartment or *vestibule*, above the level of the vestibular folds; (2) the middle compartment between the levels of the vestibular and vocal folds which has right and left canoe-shaped depressions, the *ventricles*; and (3) the lowest or *infraglottic cavity* below the level of the vocal folds. Note that the upper part, the quadrangular membrane, is thickened below to form the vestibular ligament and that the lower part, the cricothyroid ligament, ends above as the vocal ligament. Between the vocal and vestibular ligaments, the membrane lined with mucous membrane is evaginated to form the wall of the laryngeal ventricle.

shape of the rima glottidis in voice production. **All intrinsic muscles of the larynx are supplied by the recurrent laryngeal nerve**, a branch of CN X, except the cricothyroid muscle which is supplied by the **external laryngeal nerve** (Fig. 9-84). The muscles of the larynx can best be understood if they are considered as functional groups.

Muscles of the Laryngeal Inlet (Fig. 9-

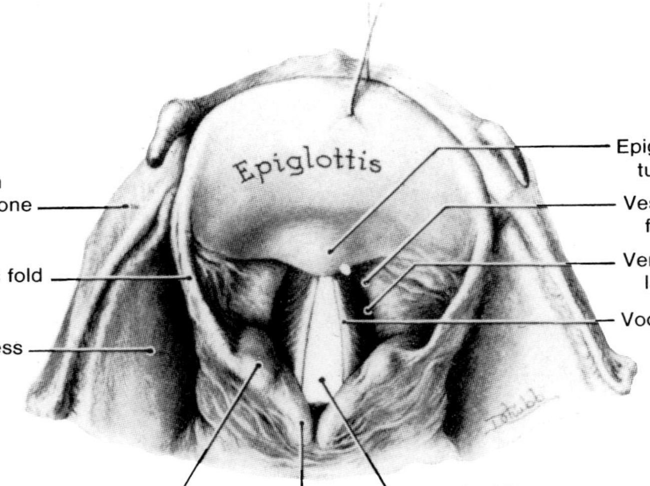

Figure 9-77. Drawing of the larynx from above. Observe the inlet of the larynx (laryngeal aditus) bounded (1) in front by the free curved edge of the epiglottis; (2) behind by the arytenoid cartilages, the corniculate cartilages which cap them, and the interarytenoid fold which unites them; and (3) on each side, by the aryepiglottic fold which contains the upper end of the cuneiform cartilage. Note that the vocal folds are closer together than the vestibular folds and, therefore, are visible below them. Observe the sharpness of the vocal folds and the fullness of the vestibular folds.

69). These muscles have a sphincteric action and *close the inlet to the larynx* as a protective mechanism in swallowing. Contraction of the transverse and oblique **arytenoid muscles** and the **aryepiglottic muscles** (prolongations of the oblique arytenoids) brings the aryepiglottic folds together and pulls the arytenoid cartilages toward the epiglottis. These movements help close the inlet.

The **transverse arytenoid muscle** (Fig. 9-69), the only unpaired muscle of the larynx, covers the arytenoid cartilages posteriorly. It extends from the posterior aspect of one arytenoid cartilage to the same region of the opposite arytenoid.

The **oblique arytenoid muscle** (Fig. 9-69), superficial to the transverse arytenoid, consists of two fasciculi which cross each other in an X-like fashion. Some oblique fibers continue as the **aryepiglottic muscle** (Fig. 9-80). The continuity of these muscles ensures that the arytenoid cartilages are brought together at the same time as the epiglottis is pulled down toward these cartilages. Hence, the inlet of the larynx is closed in two ways during swallowing, thereby preventing food from entering the larynx.

The **thyroepiglottic muscles** (Fig. 9-80) arise from the anteromedial surface of the laminae of the thyroid cartilage and insert on the lateral margin of the epiglottic cartilage. *They widen the inlet of the larynx.*

Muscles of the Vocal Folds (Figs. 9-69, 9-74, 9-78, 9-80, and 9-81). These muscles *open and close the rima glottidis.*

1. *Adductors of the Vocal Folds.* The **lateral cricoarytenoid muscles** arise from the lateral portions of the **cricoid cartilage** and insert into the **muscular processes** of the arytenoid cartilages.

Actions. **Pull muscular processes anteriorly**, **rotating arytenoids** so that their vocal processes swing medially. This adducts the vocal folds and closes the rima glottidis. This action is reinforced by the transverse arytenoid muscle, which pulls the arytenoid cartilages together.

2. *Abductors of the Vocal Folds.* The principal abductors of the vocal folds are the **posterior crioarytenoid muscles**. These muscles arise on each side from the

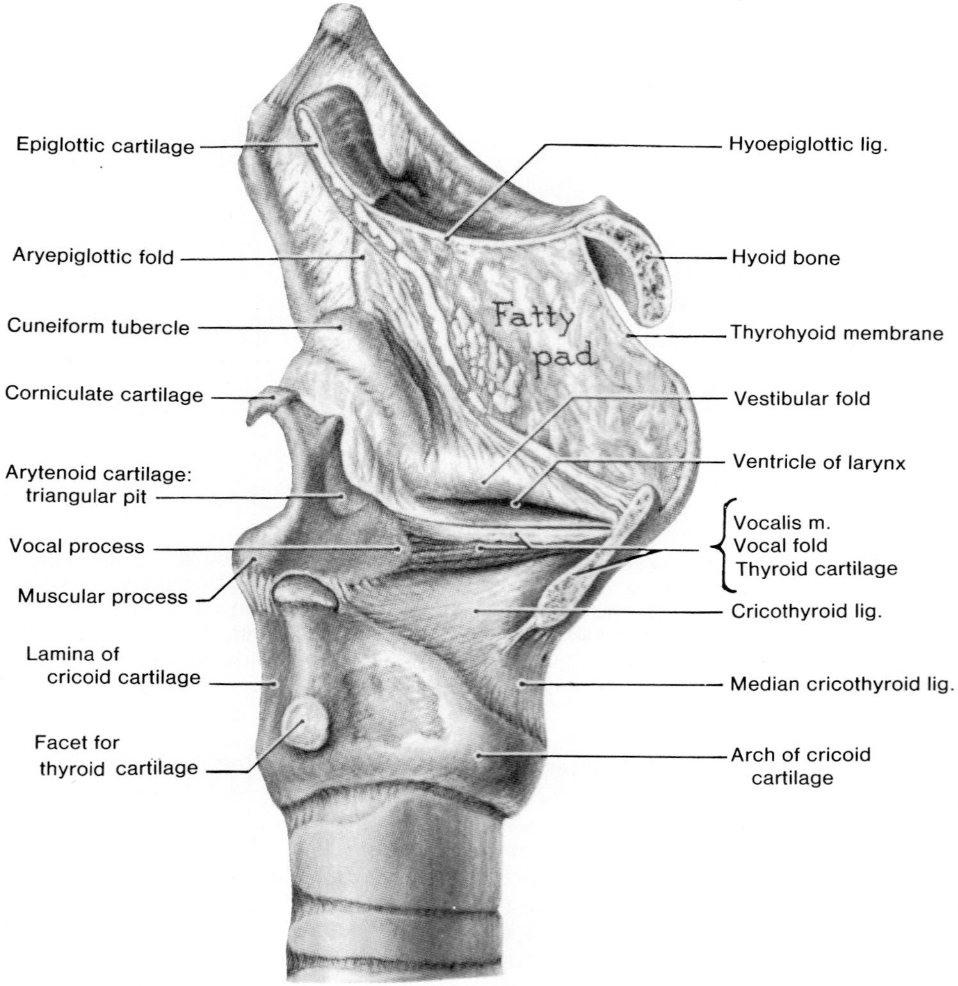

Figure 9-78. Drawing of a lateral view of the larynx. Above the vocal folds, the larynx is sectioned near the median plane and the interior of its left side is seen. Below this level, the right side of the larynx is dissected. Observe the hyoepiglottic ligament and the thyrohyoid membrane, both attached to the superior part of the body of the hyoid bone. Note the lateral aspect of the cricoid cartilage and the raised circular facet for the inferior horn of the thyroid cartilage, separating the lamina from the arch. Above this, observe the sloping facet for the arytenoid cartilage. Examine the triangular membrane, called the cricothyroid ligament, which has the vocal ligament for its upper border and blends with the median cricothyroid ligament anteroinferiorly.

posterior surface of the lamina of the **cricoid cartilage** and pass laterally and upward to insert into the **muscular processes** of the arytenoid cartilages.

Action. **Rotate arytenoid cartilages**, thereby deviating them laterally and widening the rima glottidis.

3. *Tensors of the Vocal Folds.* The main tensors of these folds are the **cricothyroid muscles**. They are located on the external surface of the larynx between the cricoid and thyroid cartilages. The muscle on each side arises from the anterolateral part of the **cricoid cartilage** and inserts into the inferior margin and anterior aspect of the inferior horn of the **thyroid cartilage**.

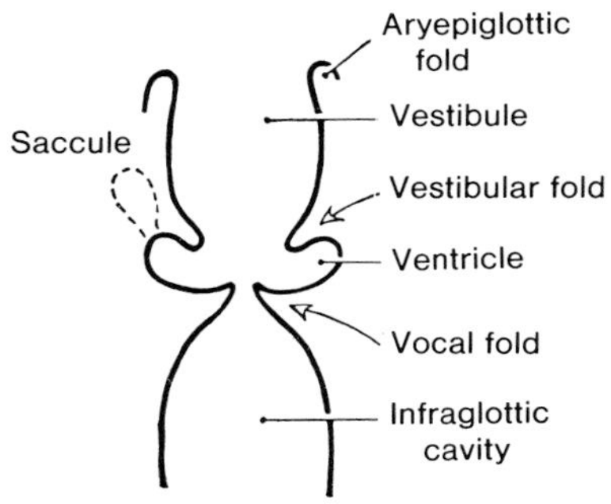

Figure 9-79. Sketch of a coronal section of the larynx showing its compartments: (1) a vestibule, (2) a middle compartment having right and left ventricles, and (3) an infraglottic cavity.

Actions. **Tilt** or **pull forward thyroid cartilage** on cricoid cartilage, increasing the distance between the thyroid and arytenoid cartilages; as a result, the vocal ligaments are elongated and tightened and the pitch of the voice is raised.

4. *Relaxors of the Vocal Folds.* The principal relaxors are the **thyroarytenoid muscles**, which arise from the posterior surface of the **thyroid cartilage** near the midline and insert into the anterolateral surfaces of the **arytenoid cartilages**. One band of fibers of each muscle, called the **vocalis** (Fig. 9-78), arises from the vocal ligament and passes to the vocal process of the arytenoid cartilage.

Actions. **Pull arytenoid cartilages anteriorly**, thereby slackening the vocal ligaments. *The vocalis produces minute adjustments of the vocal ligaments* (*e.g.*, as required in whispering).

Arterial Supply of the Larynx (Figs. 9-30 and 9-83). The superior and inferior laryngeal arteries supply the larynx. They are branches of the superior and inferior thyroid arteries, respectively.

The **superior laryngeal artery** runs with the internal branch of the superior laryngeal nerve through the thyrohyoid membrane and then ramifies to supply the internal surface of the larynx.

The **inferior laryngeal artery** runs with the inferior laryngeal nerve and supplies the mucous membrane and muscles of the inferior aspect of the larynx.

Nerves of the Larynx. The nerves are derived from (1) the internal and external branches of the **superior laryngeal nerve**, (2) the **inferior laryngeal nerve** (continuation of recurrent laryngeal), and (3) the sympathetic.

The Superior Laryngeal Nerve (Figs. 9-46 and 9-84). This branch of the vagus (CN X) arises from the middle of the inferior ganglion of the vagus at the superior end of the carotid triangle (Fig. 9-15). It divides within the carotid sheath into two terminal branches, the internal laryngeal nerve (sensory and autonomic) and the external laryngeal nerve (motor).

The **internal laryngeal nerve** (Figs. 9-30, 9-47, 9-49, and 9-84) pierces the thyrohyoid membrane with the superior laryngeal artery and supplies sensory fibers to the *laryngeal mucous membrane above the vocal folds*, including the superior surface of these folds.

The **external laryngeal nerve** (Figs. 9-30, 9-41, 9-49, 9-53, 9-55, and 9-84) is the smaller of the two terminal branches of the *superior laryngeal nerve*. It descends posterior to the sternothyroid muscle in company with the superior thyroid artery. At first it lies on the inferior constrictor muscle of the pharynx and then pierces it to supply this muscle and the cricothyroid. Recall that the cricothyroid is the only intrinsic laryngeal muscle that is not supplied by the recurrent laryngeal nerve.

The Recurrent Laryngeal Nerve (Figs. 9-49, 9-72, 9-80, and 9-84). This very important nerve ascends in the groove between the trachea and the esophagus, where it is intimately related to the medial surface of the thyroid gland (Fig. 9-41). It is vulnerable to injury during *thyroidectomy* (p. 1152), *carotid endarterectomy* (p. 1126), and other operations in the anterior cervical triangle. It enters the larynx by passing posterior to the inferior horn of the thyroid cartilage. It gives *branches to all muscles of the larynx, except the cricothyroid,* and supplies sensory fibers to the mucous membrane of the larynx below the vocal folds, including the inferior surface of these folds. The terminal part of the recurrent laryngeal is known as the **inferior laryngeal nerve**. It enters the larynx by passing deep to the inferior border of the inferior constrictor muscle of the pharynx (Figs. 9-55

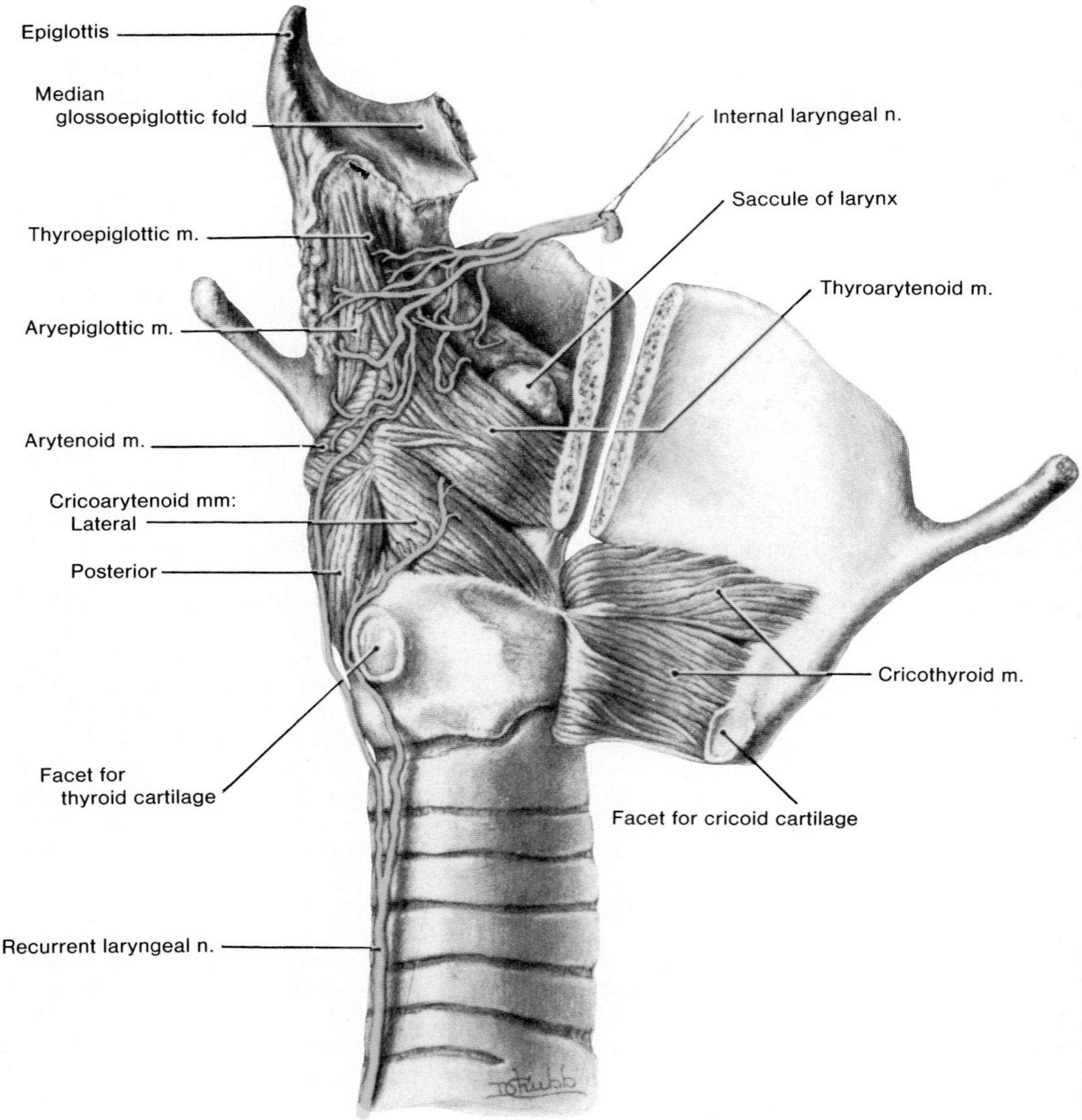

Figure 9-80. Drawing of a dissection of the muscles and nerves of the larynx. The thyroid cartilage is sawn through on the right of the median plane; the cricothyroid joint is laid open; and the right lamina of the thyroid cartilage is turned forward, stripping the cricothyroid muscles off the arch of the cricoid cartilage. Observe the lateral cricoarytenoid arising from the upper border of the arch of the cricoid cartilage and inserting with the posterior cricoarytenoid into the muscular process of the arytenoid cartilage. Note that the thyroarytenoid is inserted with the arytenoid into the lateral border of the arytenoid cartilage and that its uppermost fibers continue to the epiglottis as the thyroepiglottic muscle.

and 9-69) and divides into anterior and posterior branches. In Figure 9-49 observe that these branches accompany the inferior laryngeal artery into the larynx.

Lymphatics of the Larynx (Figs. 9-49 and 9-66). The lymph vessels *above the vocal folds* accompany the superior laryngeal artery through the thyrohyoid mem-

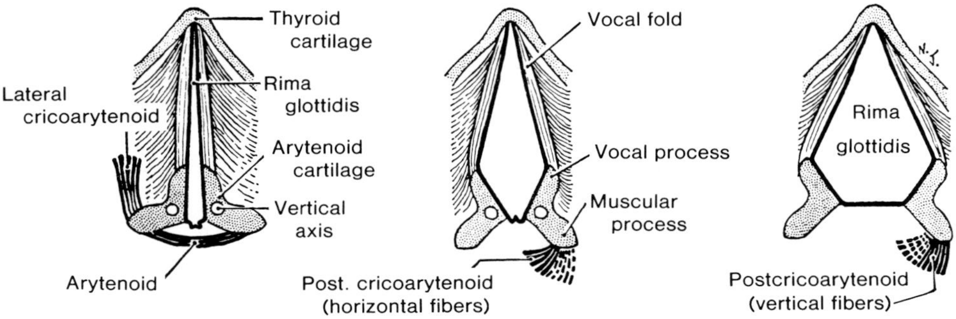

Figure 9-81. Drawings illustrating the scheme of the glottis from above and the actions of the lateral and posterior cricoarytenoid muscles.

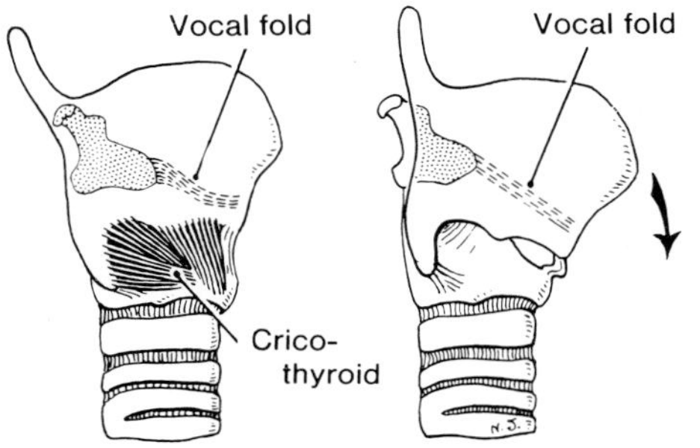

Figure 9-82. Diagrams illustrating the action of cricothyroid muscles. They act on the cricothyroid joints, tightening the vocal folds and raising the pitch of the voice.

brane and drain into the **infrahyoid** and **superior deep cervical lymph nodes**. The lymph vessels *below the vocal folds* drain into the **inferior deep cervical lymph nodes** (supraclavicular nodes) via the prelaryngeal, pretracheal, and paratracheal lymph nodes. The lymphatics of the larynx from the vocal folds do not communicate across the midline, but vessels in the posterior wall of the larynx anastomose submucously.

CLINICALLY ORIENTED COMMENTS

The larynx may be examined by **indirect laryngoscopy** (using a laryngoscopic mirrow) or by **direct laryngoscopy** (using a tubular instrument called a **laryngoscope**). The vestibular folds normally appear pink, whereas the vocal folds are pearly white in color. The size of the larynx varies somewhat from person to person and is not dependent on stature. This largely explains the difference in pitch of the voice in different persons. The larynx is larger in adult males than in adult females and the vocal ligaments are longer; however, the angle at which the laminae of the thyroid cartilage meet is greater in the female (Fig. 9-2). Because of this, the larynx is not so prominent in females as in males (Fig. 9-1*A*). In most men the vocal folds are longer than in women and children; as a result the voice of most men is deeper than most women.

Hoarseness is the most common symptom of disorders of the larynx (*e.g.*, cancer of the vocal folds). In severe cases requiring total *laryngectomy* (removal of the larynx), **esophageal speech** (regurgitation of ingested air) and other rehabilitative speech techniques can be learned.

Inhalation of foreign bodies into the larynx rapidly produces symptoms (*e.g.*, choking as in Case 9-4). If the inhaled object is sharp (*e.g.*, a chicken bone), there is usually sharp pain and progressive obstruction to breathing owing to **inflammation of the larynx**. This may cause swelling (edema) of the tissues above the glottis; however, because of the close attachment of the mucous membrane at that level, the edema does not extend below the vocal folds. The mucosa of the larynx above the

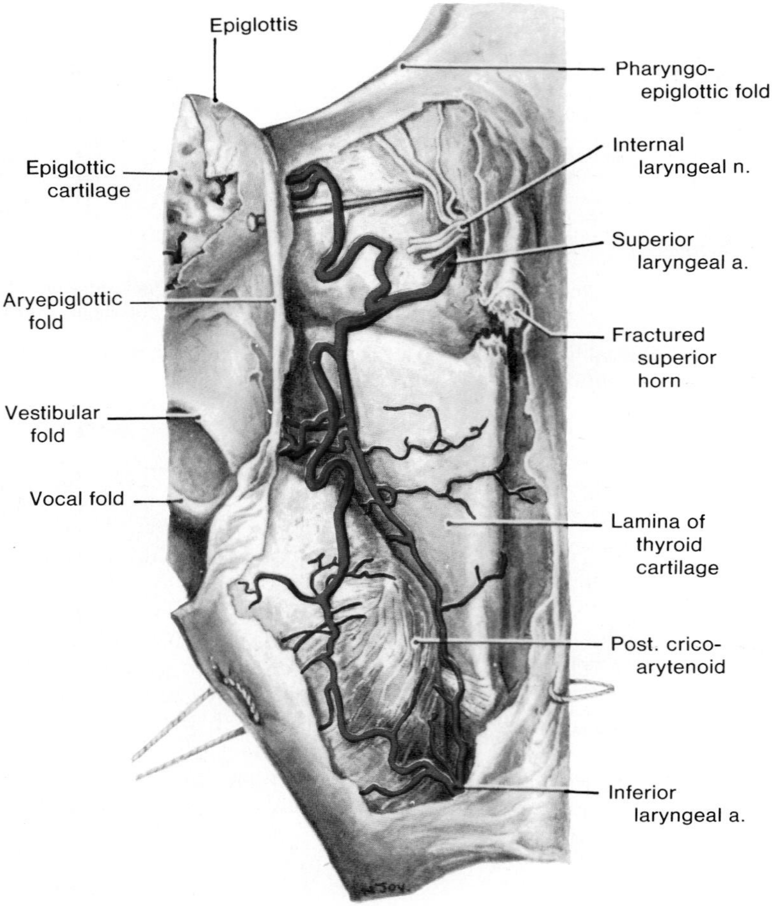

Figure 9-83. Drawing illustrating the blood supply of the larynx. Observe the anastomoses between the superior and inferior laryngeal arteries (branches of superior and inferior thyroid arteries, respectively). Arterial twigs pierce the epiglottic cartilage at the sites of the pits for the glands (Fig. 9-74).

vocal folds is extremely sensitive and contact with a foreign body immediately induces explosive coughing.

Age Changes in Larynx. The larynx grows until about the 3rd year, after which little growth occurs until about the 12th year; prior to this, there are no major laryngeal sex differences. At **puberty**, particularly in males (13 to 16 years), the walls of the larynx become strengthened, the laryngeal cavity enlarges, the vocal folds lengthen and thicken, and the laryngeal prominence becomes conspicuous in most males (Fig. 9-1*A*).

The length of the vocal folds increases gradually in both sexes up to puberty; during this period the *increase in the male is abrupt*. The pitch of the voice lowers by an octave in boys. The change in the length of the vocal folds is largely responsible for the **voice changes** occurring in boys that are familiar to everyone.

The pitch of the voice of **eunuchs** [persons in whom testes have not developed (*agonadal males*) or whose testes have been removed (*castrated males*) during childhood] does not become lower unless male hormones are administered. Similarly, these laryngeal changes do not occur in males with **seminiferous tubule degen-**

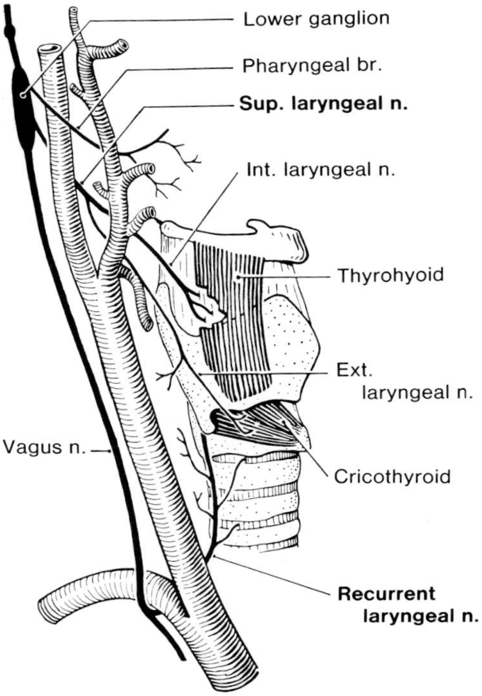

Figure 9-84. Drawing illustrating the laryngeal branches of the right vagus nerve. Note that the nerves of the larynx are the internal and external branches of the superior laryngeal nerve and the terminal branches of the recurrent laryngeal nerve. Laryngeal nerves are also derived from the sympathetic trunk (Figs. 9-41 and 9-52).

eration (47, XXY males with the **Klinefelter syndrome**) who have an inadequate production of androgens (male hormones).

PATIENT ORIENTED PROBLEMS

Case 9-1. The parents of an 8-year-old boy consulted their doctor when the child's grandmother remarked that he always *held his head tilted slightly to the right* side (Fig. 9-10).

On examination the doctor observed that one neck muscle on the right was shorter and more prominent than its partner on the left. During palpation he noted that this muscle had a fibrous consistency and that there was a firm, spindle-shaped mass in the midportion of it. When the boy was asked to straighten his head, he was unable to do so. While attempting this, the doctor noted that the origin of the muscle became prominent on the right side. During questioning the mother recalled that the child had been delivered by **breech presentation** (buttocks first) and that it had been a long and difficult birth.

Problems. What muscle was probably shortened? Describe the actions of this muscle and discuss the probable cause of its shortening. Explain anatomically the tilting of the boy's head. What would be the long term effects of shortening of this muscle if the condition was not corrected? Thinking anatomically, how do you believe the child's neck might be straightened? *These problems are discussed on page 1194.*

Case 9-2. A 22-year-old woman consulted her physician about a *swelling in the anterior midline of her neck* (Fig. 9-85). Although painless, she was concerned because it seemed to be slowly getting larger.

Physical examination revealed that the swelling was located just inferior to the hyoid bone and that it was cystic and freely movable. The doctor grasped the swelling between his forefinger and thumb and requested the patient to open her mouth and

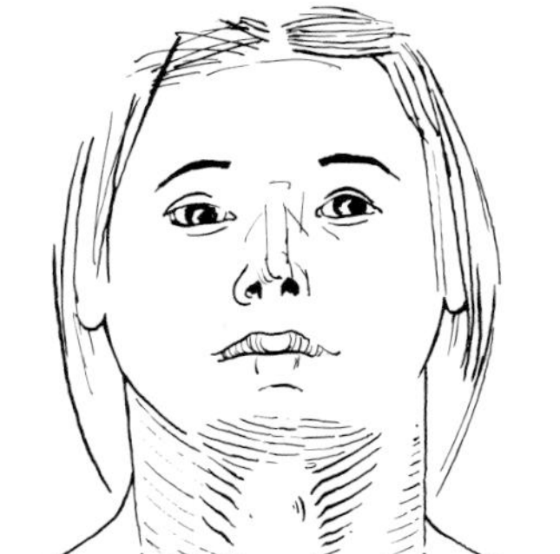

Figure 9-85. Drawing showing the infrahyoid swelling in the midline of the woman's neck.

stick out her tongue. Feeling some movement of the mass, the doctor requested the patient to stick her tongue out as far as possible and then to retract it. The doctor noted a definite upward tug on the mass as the patient's tongue protruded and that it *moved upward during swallowing.*

Fluid was aspirated from the swelling for laboratory investigation. Subsequently a diagnosis of **thyroglossal duct cyst** was made.

Problems. Explain the embryological basis of this cyst. Where are these cysts likely to be found? What is the anatomical basis for movement of the cyst upward when the patient protrudes her tongue and swallows? What would this condition be called if there had also been a midline cervical opening into the cyst? *These problems are discussed on page 1195.*

Case 9-3. A 21-year-old 2nd year dental student consulted her clinical instructor about a painless, pear-shaped *swelling inferior to the angle of her right mandible* (Fig. 9-86). As her lower third molar ("wisdom") teeth had not erupted, she thought the swelling might be caused by a dental abscess in the submandibular space or by **pericoronitis** (inflammation around the crown of a tooth). She also feared that the firm swelling might be caused by a tumor

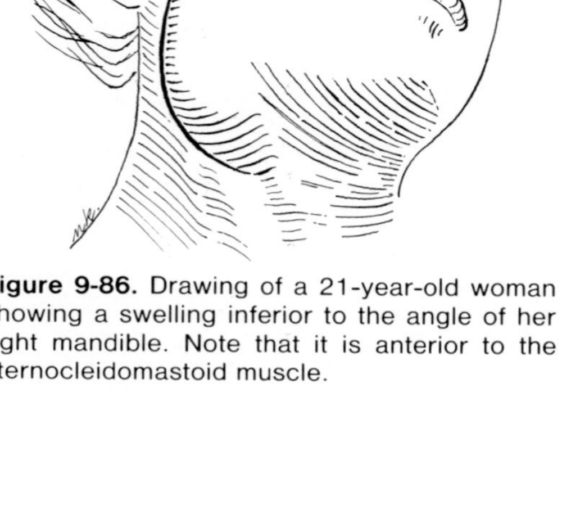

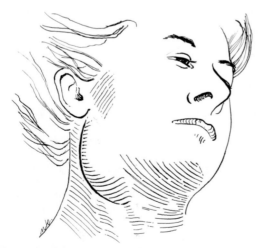

Figure 9-86. Drawing of a 21-year-old woman showing a swelling inferior to the angle of her right mandible. Note that it is anterior to the sternocleidomastoid muscle.

of the submandibular gland or of a lymph node.

Radiographs of her mandible showed the crowns of her third molars to be in contact with the posterior surfaces of her second molar teeth. The instructor recommended that her impacted teeth be surgically removed after consulting her doctor about the swelling in her submandibular region.

On examination the doctor found that the swelling was caused by a *painless fluctuant cyst* anterior to the upper one-third of her sternocleidomastoid muscle. Further investigation resulted in a diagnosis of **branchial cyst** (branchiogenic cyst). During excision of the cyst, it was discovered that a sinus tract passed superiorly from it.

Problems. Explain the embryological basis of the branchial cyst. Where does the sinus tract probably terminate? What nerve might be damaged during excision of this cyst? What signs would be present if this nerve were damaged? If the sinus tract had passed inferiorly, where would it probably open? *These problems are discussed on page 1195.*

Case 9-4. After completing your first anatomy exam, your father decided to celebrate with you and take you out for a steak dinner. Even though he had obviously had a few drinks before meeting you, he still had three drinks before dinner. You noted that his speech was slurred and that he was eating his steak very rapidly.

While telling you an off-color story and laughing loudly, you noticed your father's face change suddenly. He had a terrified look and then collapsed on the floor. At first you suspected that he had passed out from too much drinking, but as you examined him more closely you thought perhaps that he was having a stroke, a heart attack, or some other seizure. His pulse was strong and then his face began to turn blue (**cyanosis**). You now realized that he was suffering from **asphyxia** (suffocation or inability of air to reach the alveoli of the lungs in order to oxygenate the blood).

You then opened his mouth widely and observed that a large piece of steak was caught in the back of his throat. First you reached into his mouth with your finger and tried to pull it out. On being unsuccessful you rolled him into the prone position and, with your hands interlocked against his epigastrium, you gave him a forceful bear-hug, exerting pressure on his abdomen below the rib cage. This increased his intra-abdominal pressure and moved his diaphragm upward, forcing the air out of his lungs and expelling the piece of steak. He soon recovered and when he resumed eating, you cautioned him to cut his steak into small pieces and to stop drinking.

Problems. Where was the piece of steak most likely lodged? If the *"Heimlich"* maneuver had not been successful and a doctor at another table had come to help you, what life-saving measures do you think he might have taken? Discuss so-called *"restaurant deaths." These problems are discussed on page 1196.*

Case 9-5. A 30-year-old woman complained to her doctor about a *midline lump in her neck, nervousness,* and *loss of weight*. She stated that her family complains that she is irritable, excitable, and cries easily.

On examination a smooth swelling was apparent on each side of the midline of her neck, inferior to the larynx (Fig. 9-87). During palpation of the patient's neck from behind, the doctor felt an *enlarged thyroid gland* and noted that it moved up and down during deglutition (swallowing). The following signs were also detected: protrusion of the eyes (Fig. 9-87), rapid pulse, tremor of the fingers, moist palms, and loss of weight.

A diagnosis of **hyperthyroidism** (exophthalmic goiter, **Graves' disease**) was made. When the patient did not respond to medical treatment, a **subtotal thyroidectomy** was performed. After the operation the patient complained of hoarseness.

Problems. What is the anatomical basis for the swelling moving up and down during deglutition? As the patient's thyroid gland was enlarged, what nerves might have been compressed or displaced? If a **total thyroidectomy** had been done, what other endocrine glands might inadvertently have been removed along with the thyroid? What would result from this error? What was the probable cause of the patient's hoarseness? *These problems are discussed on page 1196.*

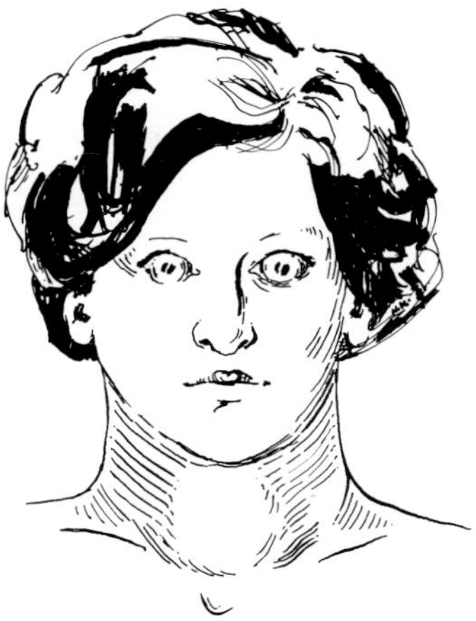

Figure 9-87. Drawing of a 30-year-old woman exhibiting the characteristic clinical features of hyperthyroidism. Note the slight protrusion of her eyes (exophthalmos) and that a rim of white (the sclera) shows above and below her iris, giving her an alarmed staring expression.

Case 9-6. A 6-year-old boy was taken to a hospital emergency department following an *abrupt onset of high fever,* difficulty in swallowing (**dysphagia**), hyperextension of the neck, and labored respirations.

The mother related a history of **nasopharyngitis** (inflammation of the nasopharynx) that had been treated with antibiotics. The doctor had given her a prescription for a 5-day supply, but she said that she had stopped giving the boy the medicine after 2 days when his temperature became normal. Later he suddenly developed a high fever and had difficulty swallowing.

On examination there appeared to be a slight *bulge in the posterior wall of the oropharynx.* A lateral radiograph of the neck showed a considerable increase in width of the retropharyngeal soft tissues, confirming the clinical suspicion of a **retropharyngeal abscess** (collection of pus in the retropharyngeal space).

Problems. Describe the retropharyngeal space. What is the function of the loose connective tissue in this space? What lymphatic structures are located in the lateral

Figure 9-88. Drawing illustrating a breech delivery during which tearing of the sternocleidomastoid muscle may occur.

extremities of the space near the base of the skull? How did the pyogenic (pus-forming) organisms probably reach the retropharyngeal space to form an abscess? To which regions would the pus spread in untreated cases? What other structures might become infected? *These problems are discussed on page 1197.*

Case 9-7. A 14-year-old girl complained to her doctor about a rounded *midline mass under her chin.* On examination the doctor noted that the mass, located just below the hyoid bone, was smooth in outline, firm in consistency, not tender, and unattached to skin. He also observed that the mass *moved up and down in swallowing.*

During careful questioning the girl said that the mass had always been in her neck, but that it seemed to enlarge monthly after she began to menstruate. When the doctor was unable to palpate her thyroid gland, he ordered a radioisotope **thyroid scan**.

The **scintigrams** showed that the cervical mass contained functioning thyroid tissue and that there was no thyroid gland in the usual location. A diagnosis of undescended or **ectopic thyroid gland** was made.

Problems. Explain embryologically this abnormal position of the thyroid gland. Where else might it have been located? What other abnormality related to descent of the thyroid gland could produce a midline swelling below the hyoid bone? What is the embryological basis of this kind of a mass? What condition would have developed if the mass had been diagnosed as a cyst or tumor and removed surgically? *These problems are discussed on page 1198.*

Case 9-8. A 10-year-old boy was admitted to hospital with a *sore throat and an earache.* He had a high fever (temperature 40.5°C or 105°F) and rapid pulse and respirations. Examination of his throat revealed diffuse redness and swelling of the pharynx, especially of the palatine tonsils. His left tympanic membrane (eardrum) was bulging.

The history revealed that the boy had had chronic symptoms of inflammation of the nasal mucous membrane (**rhinitis**), including the pharyngeal tonsil (**tonsillitis**), resulting in persistent mouth breathing. On one occasion he had had a peritonsillar abscess or **quinsy** (spread of infection beyond the tonsillar capsule with pus collection around the tonsil, usually above and behind it).

Following antibiotic treatment, the boy's infection cleared up. In view of his history, it was decided to re-admit him 3 or 4 months later for a **T&A** (tonsillectomy and adenoidectomy).

Problems. What is meant by the term tonsils? Explain the anatomical basis of the boy's earache. What lymph node in particular might be swollen and tender in this case? What is the probable source of hemorrhage in tonsillectomy? Compression of what vessel would control **severe arterial bleeding** in the tonsillar bed? *These problems are discussed on page 1199.*

DISCUSSION OF PATIENT ORIENTED PROBLEMS

Case 9-1. The child's grandmother observed a clinical condition known as **congenital torticollis** (wryneck). Considering the difficult birth of the child, the condition very likely resulted from injury to the **sternocleidomastoid** muscle during delivery. Tearing of some muscle fibers probably occurred owing to excessive stretching of the muscle during birth, because breech presentations are often difficult.

The fibrous consistency and the firm

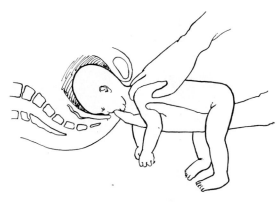

mass in the muscle probably developed gradually over several weeks after birth, during which time the necrotic (dead) part of the muscle and the blood in other parts of it were being replaced by fibrous tissue (scar tissue). As the condition originated at birth, it is designated as **congenital** (L. born with) torticollis, even though it actually started to develop after birth.

The tilting of the head and the twisting of the neck are easy to explain anatomically. *Contracture and fibrosis of the sternocleidomastoid* make it more prominent than usual in the neck. As the muscle inserts into the lateral surface of the mastoid process of the temporal bone and by a thin aponeurosis into the lateral half of the superior nuchal line of the occipital bone, it tilts the head toward the shoulder on the same side and rotates the head, turning the face to the opposite side (Fig. 9-10). Because *the contracted muscle does not grow normally in length,* it becomes relatively shorter as the cervical region of the vertebral column grows. This causes increased tilting and rotation of the head and progressive facial asymmetry during the growing years.

Obviously the muscle must be lengthened to reduce its pull on the head. Usually this is achieved by daily muscle stretching exercises during infancy. As the condition was not detected until childhood in the present case, lengthening of the muscle was achieved by sectioning its clavicular and sternal attachments.

Case 9-2. A thyroglossal duct cyst is derived from the embryonic thyroglossal duct that connects the thyroid with the base of the tongue (Fig. 9-48). Normally the thyroglossal duct atrophies and degenerates as the thyroid gland reaches its final site in the neck. Remnants of this duct may persist anywhere along the midline of the neck between the foramen cecum of the tongue and the thyroid gland (Fig. 9-45). These remnants may give rise to cysts in the tongue or in the midline of the neck, *usually just below the hyoid bone.* Often the cyst is in intimate contact with the anterior part of this bone. It may be connected superiorly by a duct with the foramen cecum of the tongue and/or inferiorly with the pyramidal lobe or the isthmus of the thyroid gland (Fig. 9-44). These connections explain why thyroglossal duct cysts move up and down during **deglutition** and when the tongue is protruded.

Sometimes a thyroglossal duct cyst develops an opening onto the surface of the skin (**thyroglossal fistula**). This results from erosion of cervical tissues following infection and rupture of the cyst (Fig. 9-48*A*).

On physical examination it may be difficult to differentiate a thyroglossal duct cyst from an abnormally positioned thyroid gland (Case 9-7 and Fig. 9-89). The location and external appearance of the mass may be similar. The aspiration of fluid from the cyst in the present case indicated that thyroid tissue was probably not present.

As the thyroid gland develops from a thickening in the floor of the primitive pharynx, where the tongue forms and normally descends into the neck, an aberrant thyroid or thyroglossal duct may be found anywhere along its usual path of descent (Fig. 9-89).

Case 9-3. All the conditions that came to the dental student's mind could have caused the swelling in the side of her neck.

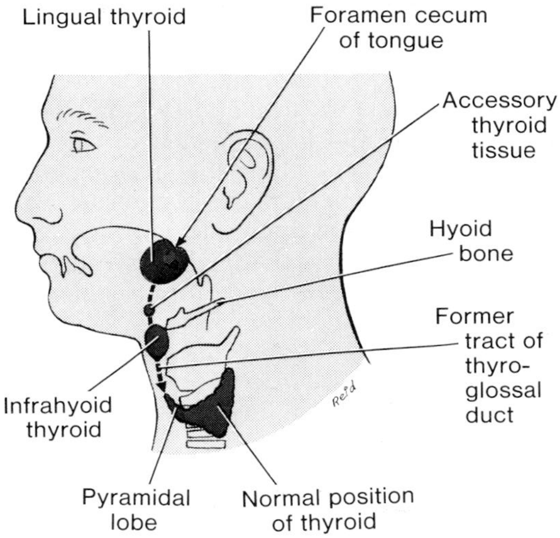

Figure 9-89. Diagrammatic sketch of the head showing the usual sites of ectopic thyroid tissue. ---- indicates the path followed by the thyroid gland during its descent and the former tract of the thyroglossal duct. Normally it reaches its usual site by the 7th week of embryonic development.

Branchial (lateral cervical) cysts may be derived from remnants of parts of the **cervical sinus**, the second branchial groove, or the second pharyngeal pouch. Although they may be associated with branchial sinuses, as in the present case, and drain through them, these cysts often lie free in the neck just below the angle of the mandible. However, they may develop at any level in the neck *along the anterior border of the sternocleidomastoid muscle*. The cyst usually extends under this muscle to deeper structures.

In the present case the cyst was probably derived from a **remnant of the second pharyngeal pouch**. The sinus tract running superiorly from it probably passed between the internal and external carotid arteries, just superior to the hypoglossal nerve and the bifurcation of the common carotid artery (Fig. 9-27). Probably it terminated in the **intratonsillar cleft** (Fig. 9-63), the adult derivative of the cavity of the second pharyngeal pouch.

During excision of these cysts the hypoglossal nerve can be injured, causing unilateral **lingual paralysis**. This would be indicated by hemiatrophy of the tongue and by deviation of the tongue to the paralyzed side when it was protruded. This results from the unopposed action of the tongue muscles on the other side (Fig. 8-24).

If the sinus tract had passed inferiorly, it probably would have opened in the lower third of the neck along the anterior border of the sternocleidomastoid muscle. Branchial sinuses that open externally are sometimes called **branchial cleft sinuses** because they are derived from remnants of the second branchial cleft.

Case 9-4. Probably *the piece of steak was lodged in the inlet of the larynx*. Choking on food is a common cause of laryngeal obstruction, particularly in children, in persons who have consumed too much alcohol, and in persons with neurological impairment.

Many "restaurant deaths," thought to be caused by heart attacks, have been shown to result from choking. Persons with dentures and/or who are drunk are less able to chew their food properly and to detect a bite that is too large.

The mucous membrane of the upper part of the larynx is very sensitive and contact by a foreign body (*e.g.*, a piece of steak) causes immediate explosive coughing to expel it. However, if there is neurological impairment or the person is drunk, this response may be reduced or absent. In rare cases, the foreign body passes through the larynx and becomes lodged in the trachea or a main bronchus. Usually, as in the present case, the piece of steak is only partly in the larynx, but entry of air into the trachea and lungs is largely prevented. The patient would likely have died within minutes, almost certainly before there was time to get him to hospital, if the piece of steak had not been dislodged enabling adequate respiration to be re-established.

Had the emergency procedure not been successful, the doctor would likely have first tried to get the piece of steak out of the patient's larynx with his finger, a long spoon, or a fork. If these procedures had failed, he would likely have done a life-saving, emergency **inferior laryngotomy**. If he had a large bore needle with him, he would have inserted it through the **cricothyroid ligament**. If not, he probably would have used a penknife or a steak knife to make an incision through the midline of the neck into the cricothyroid ligament (**cricothyrotomy**). In emergency situations, it is probably safer to incise the cricothyroid ligament than the trachea (**tracheotomy**) because the isthmus of the thyroid gland and many blood vessels cover the anterior surface of the trachea. Probably the doctor would have inserted a large plastic straw or a tube of some sort (*e.g.*, an empty ballpoint pen) to enable the patient to breathe while he was being taken to the hospital for removal of the piece of steak from his larynx and repair of the cervical wound.

Case 9-5. The tongue, hyoid, and larynx rise and fall during swallowing. As the thyroid gland is attached to the larynx by pretracheal fascia, it also moves up and down during swallowing.

Physiological enlargement of the thyroid gland is commonly seen at puberty and during pregnancy; otherwise, any enlargement of the thyroid is called a **goiter** (L.

guttur, throat). In the present case the patient's goiter resulted from hyperthyroidism. The association of hyperthyroidism with protrusion of the eyes (**exophthalmos**) was first described by an Irish physician, Dr. R.J. Graves. *The cause of exophthalmos is not precisely known;* however, a considerable increase in the size of the orbital muscles is certainly a factor.

In the surgical treatment of hyperthyroidism (Graves' disease), part of each lobe of the thyroid is removed (**subtotal thyroidectomy**), thereby leaving less glandular tissue to secrete hormones. As the four small **parathyroid glands** typically lie on the posterior surface of the thyroid gland (Fig. 9-90), posterior parts of the lobes are left so that these glands will not be inadvertently removed. At least one of them is essential for secretion of the parathyroid hormones which maintain the normal level of calcium in the blood and body fluids.

If the parathyroid glands are removed during surgery, the patient soon develops a convulsive disorder known as **tetany**. The signs are nervousness, twitching, and spasms in the facial and limb muscles.

When the thyroid gland is being removed, there is danger that important laryngeal nerves may be injured. Near the lower pole of the thyroid gland, the recurrent laryngeal nerves are intimately related to the **inferior thyroid arteries** (Fig. 9-90). The nerves may cross anterior or posterior to this artery or between its branches before ascending in or near the groove between the trachea and the esophagus.

Because of the close relationship between the recurrent laryngeal nerves and the inferior thyroid arteries, the risk of injuring them during surgery is ever present. These nerves supply all muscles of the larynx except the cricothyroids. If one of the nerves is damaged or cut, there is likely to be a serious effect on speech (*e.g.*, hoarseness as in the present case) or a change in the quality of the voice (*e.g.*, a brassy sound). Some patients also have difficulty clearing their throats. Temporary paralysis of nerves may also result from postoperative edema affecting them. It must be remembered also that a common cause of temporary hoarseness after surgery is **trauma to the mucous membrane of the larynx** by the endotracheal tube inserted by the anesthetist as an airway.

The recurrent laryngeal nerve is also vulnerable to injury during operations in the carotid triangle of the neck, *e.g.*, **carotid endarterectomy** (Case 8-1).

If both nerves are completely destroyed, breathing will be severely impaired and speech will be difficult because the vocal folds remain partly abducted (the position of complete paralysis of the intrinsic muscles); thus, the **rima glottidis** is not fully open. If the nerves are compressed as a result of inflammation or the accumulation of fluid, the breathing and speech defects will normally disappear following healing and drainage of the operative site.

Case 9-6. The **retropharyngeal space** is the most important potential space (interfascial interval) in the neck. It consists of loose *areolar connective tissue between the buccopharyngeal fascia anteriorly and the prevertebral fascia posteriorly* (Figs. 9-46, 9-50, and 9-51). It is closed laterally by the carotid sheaths. The retropharyngeal space, lying posterior to the pharynx, extends superiorly to the base of the skull and inferiorly to the posterior part of the superior mediastinum.

The loose areolar tissue in the potential retropharyngeal space permits movements of the pharynx and associated structures in swallowing. The **retropharyngeal lymph nodes**, located in the lateral regions of the retropharyngeal space (Fig. 9-46), drain the posterior nasal cavity, the nasopharynx, and the auditory tube. Efferent lymph vessels from these nodes pass to the **deep cervical lymph nodes** (Fig. 9-40*A*).

In the present case the purulent (L. festering) infection in the nasopharynx appears to have spread to the **retropharyngeal lymph nodes** via the lympatics. The pyogenic organisms then spread outside the lymphatic vessels and lymph nodes. The **inflammatory exudate** of serum and cells (*i.e.*, pus) soon collected, forming an abcess. If left untreated, the abscess might have ruptured into the pharynx, resulting in aspiration (passage into the airways) of pus.

The pus may pass (dissect) laterally and present as a mass in the anterior triangle,

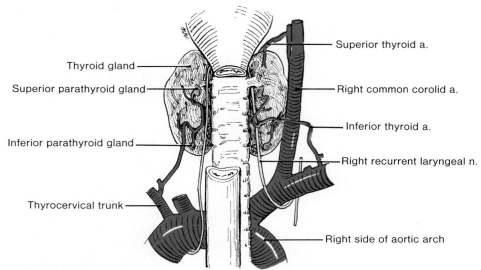

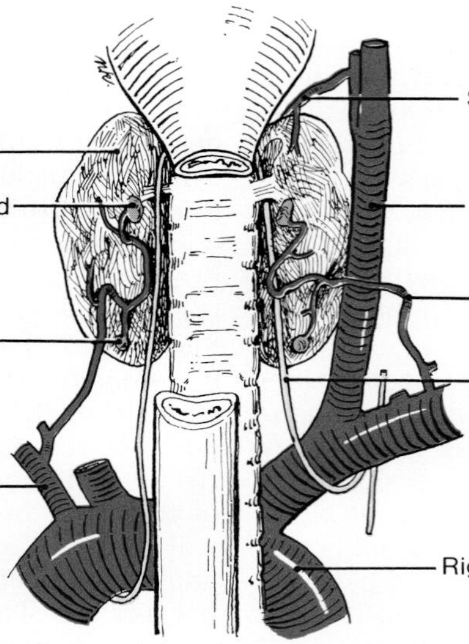

Figure 9-90. Drawing of a posterior view of the thyroid and parathyroid glands showing their relations. A thorough knowledge of the appearance, location, and blood supply of the parathyroids is essential for their preservation during operations on the thyroid gland. The superior thyroid artery is a branch of the external carotid and the inferior thyroid artery is a branch of the thyrocervical trunk. The superior parathyroids are the more constant in position and are therefore usually easy to find. The inferior parathyroids are often close to the inferior surface of the lobes of the thyroid gland (as here), but they may lie some distance below them (see Figs. 9-49 and 9-52).

but more commonly the pus dissects inferiorly into the posterior mediastinum or laterally into the posterior triangle. For this reason, the retropharyngeal space is sometimes referred to as the "danger space." The pus can pass to about the T4 level, where it is limited by the attachment of the anterior layer of the prevertebral fascia to the esophagus.

In severe cases left untreated, the infection may erode blood vessels supplying the pharynx and result in **retropharyngeal hemorrhage**. The infection may also involve the prevertebral fascia and the bodies of the cervical vertebrae, resulting in **osteomyelitis** (inflammation of bone).

Case 9-7. It is very unusual for the thyroid gland not to descend to its normal position at the level of C5 to T1 vertebrae (Fig. 9-51). *The thyroid develops from a thickening in the floor of the primitive pharynx* in the region where the tongue later develops. It normally descends through the neck until its *isthmus overlies the second and third tracheal rings* in most people (Fig. 9-43). Rarely all or part of the thyroid gland fails to descend. It may remain within the tongue (**lingual thyroid**) or descend only part way down the neck. Usually an **ectopic thyroid** gland is near the hyoid bone (*e.g.*, **infrahyoid thyroid**, Fig. 9-89).

Sometimes the thyroid gland descends to its normal position, but a part of it remains in the tongue or near the hyoid bone or the thyroid cartilage (Fig. 9-47). If an adequate amount of thyroid tissue is present in the normal position, an ectopic thyroid mass is usually removed if it is objectionable cosmetically.

The thyroglossal duct that extends from the foramen cecum of the tongue to the thyroid gland during early development (Fig. 9-45) normally disappears, but part of it may persist as a thyroglossal duct cyst (Fig. 9-48*B*), as a **pyramidal lobe of the thyroid** (Fig. 9-44), or as a fibrous cord joining the isthmus to the hyoid bone. Often these cysts are close to the hyoid bone (Fig. 9-85) and produce a swelling similar to that formed by an ectopic thyroid gland (Fig. 9-89). *Thyroglossal duct cysts transil-*

luminate ("light up" when a small light source is pressed against them), whereas an ectopic thyroid transilluminates poorly. At operation an *ectopic thyroid gland has a fleshy consistency with arteries entering it,* whereas a cyst is smooth and is not supplied by vessels.

Excision of an ectopic thyroid gland may remove all the thyroid tissue the patient has, as in the present case. If this tissue is removed, daily administration of thyroid hormone would be necessary to correct symptoms of **hypothyroidism**. The situation becomes more serious when all four parathyroid glands are intimately attached to the ectopic thyroid gland and are removed with the thyroid mass. This results in tetany and could result in early postoperative death unless the condition is recognized and treated.

Case 9-8. The term tonsil usually refers to the palatine tonsil (Fig. 9-61). The other tonsils are the lingual, the pharyngeal, and the tubal tonsils. All these tonsils form the irregular **tonsillar ring** around the faucial isthmus leading from the oral cavity into the nasopharynx. Although it is often stated that this ring acts as a barrier to infection, its function is not clearly understood; however, it is certain that this lymphatic tissue is *important in the immune reaction to infection.*

The infection in this case had spread up the auditory tube into the middle ear, producing **otitis media** and bulging of the eardrum. This would be the *chief cause of the boy's earache.* The tonsils are supplied by twigs from the glossopharyngeal nerve (CN IX) and, as the tympanic branch of this nerve supplies the mucous membrane of the tympanic cavity, some pain related to the tonsillitis may have also been referred to the ear. When the opening of the auditory tube is closed, as it probably was in the present case, pressure changes in the middle ear can also cause earache.

The numerous lymphatic vessels of the tonsil penetrate the pharyngeal wall and terminate principally in the **jugulodigastric node** of the deep cervical chain of lymph nodes (Fig. 9-66). This node lies on the internal jugular vein at the level of the greater horn of the hyoid bone, *i.e.*, just below the posterior belly of the digastric muscle (Figs. 9-17 and 9-21). Because its enlargement is commonly associated with tonsillitis, it is often called the **tonsillar node**.

The **external palatine vein** is usually the *chief source of hemorrhage* following tonsillectomy. This important and sometimes large vein descends from the soft palate and is immediately related to the lateral surface of the tonsil before it pierces the superior constrictor muscle of the pharynx (Figs. 9-58 and 9-65).

In cases of severe and uncontrolled bleeding (*e.g.*, from the tonsillar branch of the facial artery), hemorrhage may be controlled by compressing or clamping the external carotid artery at its origin because this vessel supplies blood to the tonsillar arteries (Fig. 9-29). Recall that the chief artery supplying the tonsil is the tonsillar branch of the facial artery which enters the inferior part of its lateral surface (Fig. 9-64).

SUGGESTIONS FOR ADDITIONAL READING

1. Basmajian, J. B. *Grant's Method of Anatomy*, Ed. 3, The Williams & Wilkins Co., Baltimore, 1975.

   A concise account of the neck that is well illustrated with simple, easily reproducible line drawings. Direct applications of anatomy to problems in medicine and surgery are described.

2. Fletcher, G., and Jing, B. *The Head and Neck. An Atlas of Tumor Radiology*, Year Book Medical Publishers Inc., Chicago, 1968.

   Perusal of this book will indicate how important the anatomy of the neck is to the radiologist. The discussions of diagnostic radiographic studies of the pharynx, larynx, trachea, and esophagus are fascinating, particularly those used for demonstrating tumors of the vocal folds.

3. Healey, J. E. Jr. *A Synopsis of Clinical Anatomy*, W. B. Saunders Co., Philadelphia, 1969.

   A good presentation of the regional descriptive anatomy of the neck emphasizing clinical applications of gross anatomy. This account indicates structures of prime interest to surgeons operating on the neck, *e.g.*, how to do cervical nerve blocks and a thyroidectomy.

4. Hung, W. The growth and development of the thyroid. In *Scientific Foundations of Paediatrics*, edited by J. A. Davis and J. Dobbing, W. B. Saunders Co., Philadelphia, 1974.

   This section (pp. 514–525) includes a discussion of the growth and development of the thyroid gland in the fetus, newborn infant, child, and adolescent.

5. Moore, K. L. *The Developing Human. Clinically*

Oriented Embryology, Ed. 2, W. B. Saunders Co., Philadelphia, 1977.

Most congenital malformations of the neck develop during transformation of the branchial apparatus into adult derivatives (*e.g.*, cervical cysts, ectopic thyroid, and branchial sinuses). The developmental abnormalities of the neck and many others are fully described by the author of the present text.

6. Woodburne, R. T. *Essentials of Human Anatomy*, Ed. 6, Oxford University Press, New York, 1978.

This book is known for its conciseness, accuracy, and practical organization. If you have difficulty understanding any part of the neck, you are urged to read the descriptions in this book by an outstanding anatomist.

INDEX

Main page and figure references are printed in **bold type.** In most cases items are listed under nouns rather than under descriptive adjectives; e.g., the deltoid muscle will not be found under deltoid but under the general heading **MUSCLES.** Similarly all nerves, veins, and arteries are listed under NERVES, VEINS, and ARTERIES, respectively. Widely used *eponyms* are also listed so that students can determine the meaning of terms they may hear clinicians use, e.g., the pouch of Douglas for the rectouterine pouch. Commonly used old terms are also given so that clinicians can learn the new terminology; e.g., the internal mammary artery is now called the internal thoracic artery.